Philadelphia University
Paul J. Gutman Library
Schoolhouse Lane & Henry Ave
Philadelphia, PA 19144-5497

W9-BNQ-944

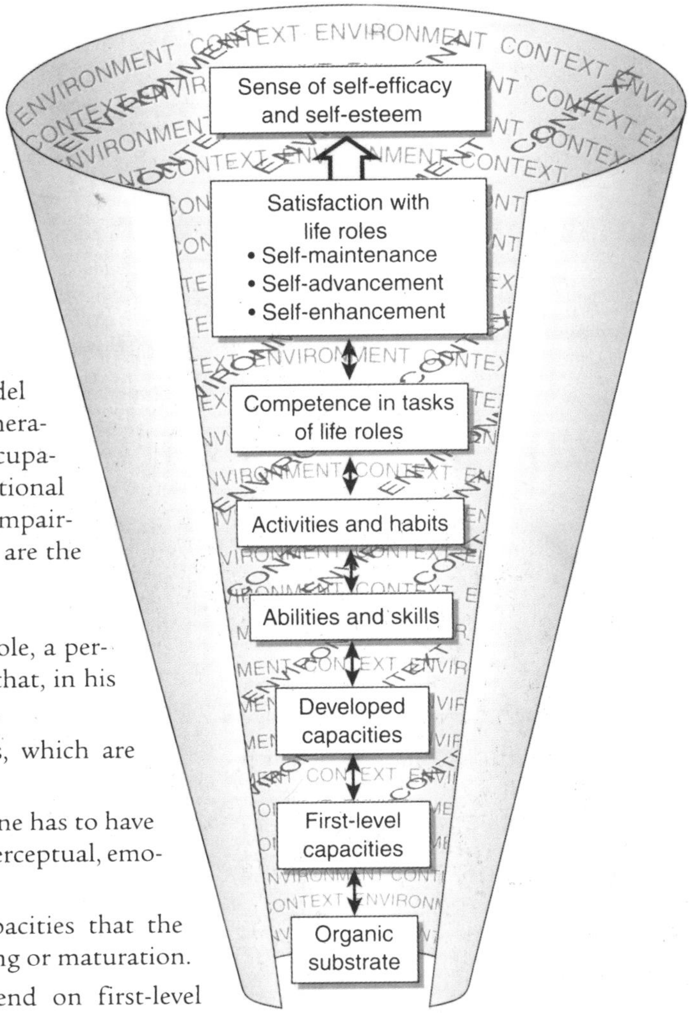

The Occupational Functioning Model (OFM) is one way that occupational therapists conceptualize the process of occupational therapy for persons with occupational dysfunction secondary to physical impairments. The propositions of the model are the following:

1. To engage satisfactorily in a life role, a person must be able to do the tasks that, in his or her opinion, make up that role.
2. Tasks are composed of activities, which are smaller units of behavior.
3. To be able to do a given activity, one has to have certain sensorimotor, cognitive, perceptual, emotional, and social abilities.
4. Abilities are developed from capacities that the person has gained through learning or maturation.
5. These developed capacities depend on first-level capacities that derive from a person's genetic endowment or spared organic substrate.
6. Personal, social, cultural, and physical contexts and environments surround and influence the life and occupational functioning of an individual.

The OFM has been chosen to provide the organization to the information in this textbook. To assist the reader in knowing where chapters fit into the OFM, a schematic algorithm of the model appears on the first page of most chapters. The particular section being emphasized in the chapter is shown in green. For example, the algorithm shown in the chapters of Sections III and IV has green arrows; the therapeutic mechanisms and therapeutic technologies that are described in those chapters move the person along from functioning at lower levels of performance to higher levels of occupational functioning. The chapters that deal with context and environment have the cone part of the algorithm emphasized (shown in green). Please refer to chapter 1 for a detailed description of the Occupational Functioning Model.

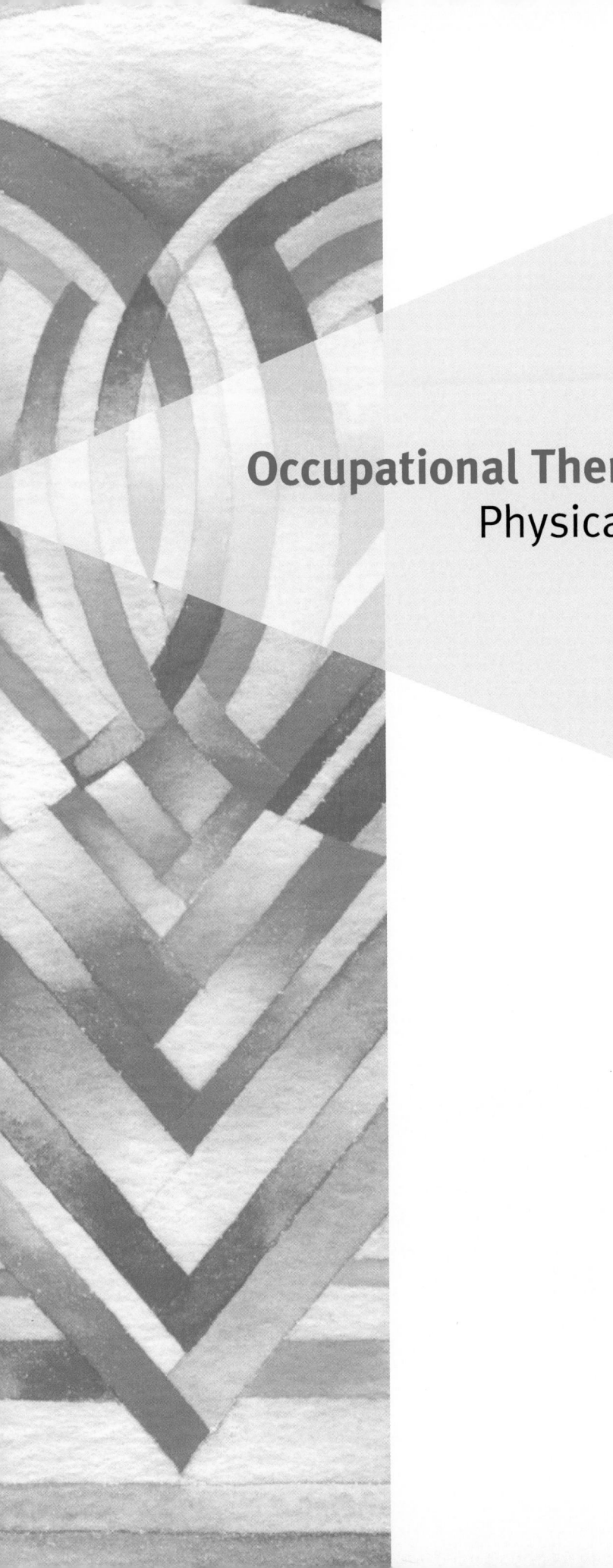

Occupational Therapy *for* Physical Dysfunction

Sixth Edition

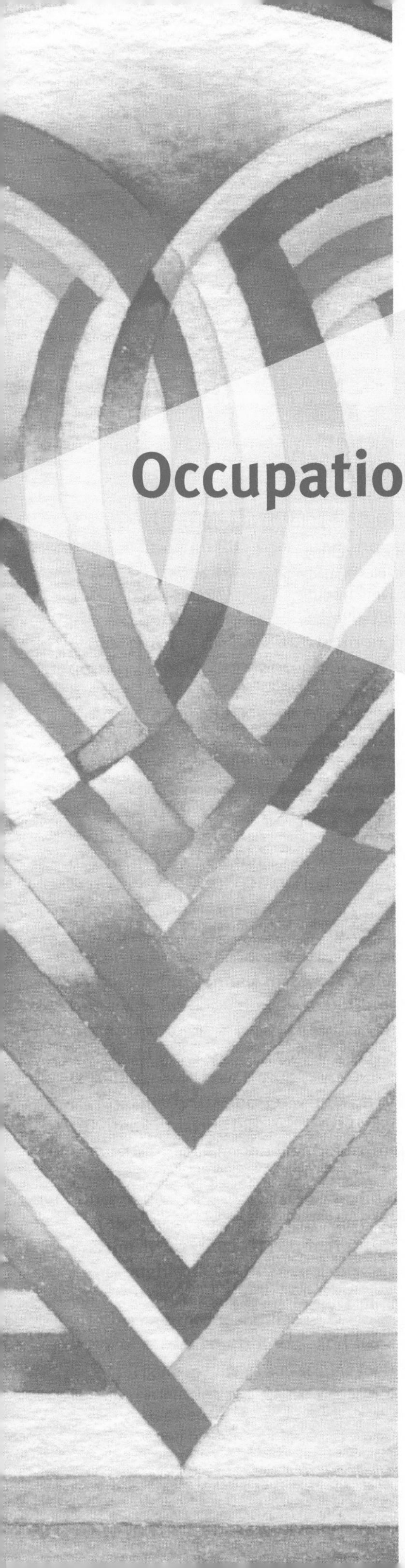

Occupational Therapy *for* Physical Dysfunction

Sixth Edition

EDITORS

Mary Vining Radomski, M. A., OTR/ L, FAOTA
Coordinator of Outcomes, Quality, and Clinical Research
Occupational therapist
Sister Kenny Rehabilitation Institute
Minneapolis, Minnesota

Catherine A. Trombly Latham, ScD, OTR/L, FAOTA
Professor Emerita
Program in Occupational Therapy
Department of Rehabilitation Science
Sargent College of Health and Rehabilitation Sciences
Boston University
Boston, Massachusetts

Wolters Kluwer Health | Lippincott Williams & Wilkins

Philadelphia • Baltimore • New York • London
Buenos Aires • Hong Kong • Sydney • Tokyo

Acquisitions Editor: Emily Lupash
Managing Editor: Andrea Klingler
Marketing Manager: Christen Murphy
Production Editor: Eve Malakoff-Klein
Designer: Risa J. Clow
Compositor: Maryland Composition, Inc.
Printer: RR Donnelley

Copyright © 2008 Lippincott Williams & Wilkins, a Wolters Kluwer business

351 West Camden Street
Baltimore, MD 21201

530 Walnut Street
Philadelphia, PA 19106

All rights reserved. This book is protected by copyright. No part of this book may be reproduced in any form or by any means, including photocopying, or utilized by any information storage and retrieval system without written permission from the copyright owner.

The publisher is not responsible (as a matter of product liability, negligence, or otherwise) for any injury resulting from any material contained herein. This publication contains information relating to general principles of medical care that should not be construed as specific instructions for individual patients. Manufacturers' product information and package inserts should be reviewed for current information, including contraindications, dosages, and precautions.

Printed in China

Fifth Edition, 2002

Library of Congress Cataloging-in-Publication Data

Occupational therapy for physical dysfunction / editors, Mary Vining Radomski, Catherine A. Trombly Latham. --6th ed.
p. ; cm.
Catherine A. Trombly Latham's name appears first in earlier ed.
Includes bibliographical references and index.
ISBN-13: 978-0-7817-6312-7
ISBN-10: 0-7817-6312-6
1. Occupational therapy. 2. People with disabilities--Rehabilitation. I. Radomski, Mary Vining. II. Latham, Catherina A. Trombly
[DNLM: 1. Occupational Therapy. 2. Disabled Persons--rehabilitation. WB 555 0143 2008]
RM735 .O33 2008
615.8'515--dc22

2006101666

The publishers have made every effort to trace the copyright holders for borrowed material. If they have inadvertently overlooked any, they will be pleased to make the necessary arrangements at the first opportunity.

To purchase additional copies of this book, call our customer service department at **(800) 638-3030** or fax orders to **(301) 223-2320**. International customers should call **(301) 223-2300**.

Visit Lippincott Williams & Wilkins on the Internet: http://www.LWW.com. Lippincott Williams & Wilkins customer service representatives are available from 8:30 am to 6:00 pm, EST.

10 11 12
5 6 7 8 9 10

RRS1001

To Kristen Trombly, OTS, and all future and practicing occupational therapists who creatively strive to restore to the highest level of occupational functioning all people who come into their care.

Catherine A. Trombly Latham

To the occupational therapists of Sister Kenny Rehabilitation Institute.

Mary Vining Radomski

Preface

Imagine:

> An occupational therapist enters a hospital room to meet Mrs. B., who sustained a stroke in the past week. The therapist sits down and knows the right questions to ask so that after their brief conversation, the therapist leaves with a general sense of Mrs. B.'s background and priorities and Mrs. B. is assured that someone on her rehabilitation team knows her beyond her current impairments. The occupational therapy evaluation continues later that day with the therapist explaining the occupational therapy assessment process to Mrs. B. and her daughter and ultimately reviewing and interpreting the results based on an appreciation of the strengths and weaknesses of tests themselves and the contextual factors that may have affected Mrs. B.'s performance. The next day, Mrs. B. and her daughter sit down with the occupational therapist to formalize the intervention plan—to discuss Mrs. B.'s priorities in light of evaluation results (from both an occupational therapy perspective as well as the perspective of other rehabilitation disciplines) and intervention options. The occupational therapist reviews what she knows about the efficacy or effectiveness of various interventions. Together, Mrs. B., her daughter, and the therapist establish short-term therapy goals with an eye toward longer-term therapy needs down the road.

This is a glimpse of occupational therapy practice to which we hope this sixth edition of *Occupational Therapy for Physical Dysfunction* contributes: practice composed of occupational therapy services provided within the context of a compassionate therapeutic relationship, informed by expert clinical reasoning that considers "why." Why use this assessment method over another? Why use this intervention approach over another? Why am I observing these results?

This edition of *Occupational Therapy for Physical Dysfunction* is designed to help occupational therapy students and practitioners acquire the skills necessary to provide occupational therapy services as well as to develop the mindset necessary to do so as a reflective practitioner.

ORGANIZATION

Similar to the previous edition, the sixth edition is composed of six sections with 50 chapters.

Section I describes the historical and social influences on the current practice of occupational therapy for those with physical impairment. This section also lays the foundation for the rest of the textbook and the theoretical foundation for practice by introducing the Model of Occupational Functioning.

Section II presents the areas of assessment for which an occupational therapist working with adults with occupational dysfunction secondary to physical impairment would be responsible. The chapters in this section begin with assessment of the person's occupational roles and competence of performance in those roles, followed by assessment of the person's abilities and capacities that support role performance, and assessment of the environmental and contextual constraints and enablers of performance.

Section III presents three mechanisms of therapeutic change: occupation and occupation as therapy, learning, and therapeutic rapport.

Section IV presents therapeutic technologies that enable and support occupational functioning: splinting, wheelchairs, adapted or assistive devices, and physical agent modalities.

Section V elucidates treatment principles and practices of therapy for persons with physical dysfunction. As in earlier editions, this section does not provide recipes for the treatment of people with particular diagnoses, but rather descriptions of best practice. The professional occupational therapist can choose from these for a particular patient who has his or her own particular goals and manifestation of a diagnosis.

Section VI includes discussions of the practice of occupational therapy for particular, major diagnostic categories, each written by a specialist in that area. These experts alert therapists who are beginning to practice with one of these populations to various commonly encountered impairments that affect occupational functioning and to the specialized assessments and treatments that have been developed for persons carrying the diagnosis. Two new chapters, "Human Immunodeficiency Virus" (Chapter 49) and "Oncology" (Chapter 50), have been added to this section since the prior edition.

NEW FEATURES

This edition also has a number of new features that emphasize the scientific and reflective foundations of clinical practice.

Chapters in Section II (Assessment of Occupational Function) include **Assessment Tables** that summarize the psychometric properties, strengths, and weaknesses of the assessment methods described in the chapter.

Evidence Tables (where evidence exists) are included in chapters in Section IV (Therapeutic Mechanisms), Section V (Treatment of Occupational Function), and Section VI (Treatment to Promote Occupational Function for Selected Diagnostic Categories). These tables summarize research studies that address the interventions mentioned in the chapters and/or Case Examples. They are not an exhaustive compendium of all research, but represent the current best evidence for the effectiveness of the interventions. Readers will find information pertaining to these tables and other features in this volume's **User's Guide**.

Finally, the **Case Examples** in this edition have been reformatted to highlight the "whys" of the assessment and intervention process. In general, Case Examples are designed to help students appreciate how various topics described in the chapter relate to and inform occupational therapy practice. Readers will find that the Case Example format in this edition describes the actions of therapy ("Occupational Therapy Process") along with the therapist's internal dialogue to explain why he or she approached occupational therapy assessment and/or intervention as he or she did ("Clinical Reasoning Process").

As in the previous edition, a **Glossary** and boxes highlighting **Clinical Reasoning** (opportunities to develop clinical reasoning skills that go beyond the material that can be looked up in the chapter), **Procedures for Practice** (how to do a particular assessment or treatment), **Definitions, Research Notes** (examples of application of research, including that from other disciplines, to practice), **Safety Notes** (precautions to be observed), and **Resources** (where to find information and equipment) are included throughout the chapters to showcase and emphasize key concepts.

ANCILLARIES

A website is available at http:www.thepoint.lww.com/trombly6e. Students can go to the site to see how an expert would answer the questions posed in Clinical Reasoning Boxes throughout the text. Instructors' Resources are also available, including Powerpoint slides that provide lecture outlines for each chapter, and an image bank containing all images and tables from the book. Also included online are the **Summary Review Questions** and **References** for each chapter.

A DVD is also included with each copy of this text, to facilitate student learning of core techniques through demonstration. It includes short video clips that help learners visualize and review key aspects of practice, including the measurement of upper extremity range of motion and hand strength, as well as how to fabricate a splint and assist clients as they transfer into and out of a wheelchair.

TERMINOLOGY

Throughout this book, readers will note an amalgam of occupational therapy terminology, derived from the *Occupational Therapy Practice Framework* (AOTA, 2002); International Classification of Functioning (WHO, 2001); *Occupational Functioning Model*; and generic "OT-speak." We are unapologetic about our aim to help develop multilingual practitioners. If you find yourself needing to think twice to do some translation, get used to it. In practice we must be proficient at adapting our language in appreciation of our audience, understanding that most of us spend our day communicating with people who have never heard of occupational therapy, much less our professional vocabulary.

Also note that we have tried to be intentional about identifying the recipients of services as patients or clients. In acute medical and inpatient rehabilitation settings, the term "patient" reflects a more passive role of the person receiving care; it is also the term used by other professionals on the health care team. The term "client" is used in reference to a person living in the community who is receiving outpatient, home-based, or community-based services. It reflects the assumption that the person receiving services is ready to assume a more directive role in organizing his or her care.

Sixty outstanding clinical and academic occupational therapists and experienced lay persons contributed to this edition. They each did so with the desire to contribute to the profession of occupational therapy by sharing their knowledge and skills with occupational therapists preparing to enter the field.

Mary Vining Radomski
Catherine A. Trombly Latham

References

American Occupational Therapy Association. (2002). Occupational therapy practice framework: Domain and process. *American Journal of Occupational Therapy, 56,* 609–639.

World Health Organization. (2001). *International Classification of Functioning, Disability and Health–Short version.* Geneva: Author.

Acknowledgements

This sixth edition is published 30 years after the first edition and 35 years after the project first began. The first edition was written in longhand on legal pads—this new edition was electronically processed. During that 35 years, it has taken dozens of people to bring the project to fruition, including contributors, photographers, videographers, models who posed for the photographs, vendors who loaned equipment and/or professional photographs of rehabilitation products, designers, artists, acquisition editors, managing editors, copy editors, art editors, production managers and their crews, typists, and reviewers (formal and informal). I owe great thanks to all of these participants.

Three people in particular contributed to the success of this project and must be acknowledged: Anna Deane Scott, M.Ed., OTR, my first co-editor; Christopher Trombly, my son; and Mary Vining Radomski, Ph.D.(cand.), OTR/L, FAOTA, my current co-editor. Anna Deane first had the idea for this textbook. We co-taught and needed to compile material for our students because there was no comprehensive book devoted to occupational therapy for those with physical dysfunction. She suggested we create that missing textbook, and Williams & Wilkins bought it.

My son Christopher grew up with this project and contributed by playing independently when I needed to work, posing for photographs at various times in his life, eating pizza, and helping out with chores. I am sure he sometimes wished life was different, as did I.

I now leave this project in Mary's capable hands. She graciously accepted co-editorship two editions ago and has brought not only her considerable knowledge about the treatment of cognitively impaired individuals, but also her high work standards, her creative ideas, her network of expert contributors, and her superb administrative skills. I have no doubt that under her leadership this textbook will continue to be an important influence on the practice of occupational therapy.

Lastly, I look forward to developing new occupational roles with my husband, John.

Catherine Trombly Latham

In addition to Jim, Lauren, and Allie Radomski, I gratefully acknowledge the contribution of my Sister Kenny family to the sixth edition of *Occupational Therapy for Physical Dysfunction*. Besides helping with photography, these remarkable therapists, social workers, doctors, and nurses tolerated the inconveniences of the video shoot, shared their expertise and resources, and continually stepped up when I came knocking with "opportunities." I also appreciate the permission to use "Warm Heart" on the cover, painted by Brom Wikstrom, which is part of the Sister Kenny permanent collection (see p. xii). A special word of thanks to occupational therapists Erin Mack, Marilyn Sicheneder (both of TRIA Orthopaedic Center), and Jennifer Theis (Sister Kenny), as well as Cheryl Smith and Rob and Marilyn Beyerl for their help with the DVD. I am grateful to Jennifer Theis for creating the Powerpoint slides that accompany the book. The rehabilitation practitioners and friends of Sister Kenny live out the kind of compassionate excellence that makes me so glad to be an occupational therapist.

I am also grateful to Catherine Trombly Latham for her confidence in me and for her example in all matters of gracious conduct (which include writing and editing). I have yet to figure out how she can be simultaneously visionary, exacting, patient, and empowering, but will give it my best to follow in her footsteps.

Mary Vining Radomski

ABOUT THE COVER ARTIST

Cover and Interior Art: Warm Heart
Artist: Brom Wilkstrom

The cover image for this volume, "Warm Heart," was painted by Brom Wilkstrom and is part of the Sister Kenny permanent collection. Brom Wilkstrom and his wife, Anne, live in Seattle, Washington. Brom studied art at Seattle Community College and was working as a sign painter in New Orleans, Louisiana, when he broke his neck swimming and became paralyzed. He now paints with his mouth and teaches in area schools. Brom exhibits his work through the International Association of Mouth and Foot Painting Artists, who also reproduce his work on greeting cards and calendars. Working at the University of Washington's Burke Museum of Natural History and Culture as an information specialist, Brom is active in many cultural organizations. He has won many awards and his work is included in many prestigious collections.

Contributors

Anne Armstrong, MA, OTR/L
Occupational Therapist
Out-Patient Service
Rehabilitation Institute of Chicago
Chicago, Illinois

Michal S. Atkins, MA, OTR/L
Clinical Specialist
Occupational Therapy Department
Rancho Los Amigos National Rehabilitation Center and Los Amigos Research and Education Institute, Inc.
Downey, California

Wendy Avery, MS, OTR/L
Occupational Therapist
Coastal Carolina Medical Center
Hardeeville, South Carolina

Julie Bass-Haugen, PhD, OTR/L, FAOTA
Professor
Department of Occupational Science and Occupational Therapy
The College of St. Catherine
St. Paul, Minnesota

Jane Bear-Lehman, PhD, OTR, FAOTA
Associate Professor
Department of Occupational Therapy
The Steinhardt School of Education
New York University
New York, New York

Karen Bentzel, MS, OTR/L
Occupational Therapist
Lancaster General Hospital
Lancaster, Pennsylvania
Heartland Home Care
York, Pennsylvania

Bette R. Bonder, Ph.D., OTR/L
Associate Dean
College of Science
Cleveland State University
Cleveland, Ohio

Alfred G. Bracciano, EdD, OTR, FAOTA
Associate Professor
School of Pharmacy and Health Professions
Creighton University
Omaha, Nebraska
Associate Clinical Professor
School of Health Technology and Management
Stony Brook University
Stony Brook, New York

Mary Ellen Buning, PhD, OTR, ATP
Assistant Professor
Health Sciences Center
University of Colorado at Denver
Denver, Colorado

Nancy Callinan, MA, OTR/L, CHT
Manager, Hand Therapy
TRIA Orthopaedic Center
Minneapolis, Minnesota

Cynthia Cooper, MFA, MA, OTR/L, CHT
Director of Hand Therapy
VibrantCare Rehabilitation
Phoenix, Arizona

Lois Copperman, PhD, OTR (L)
Clinical Associate Professor
Department of Neurology
Oregon Health and Science University
Portland, Oregon

Elin Schold Davis, OTR/L, CDRS
Occupational Therapist
Sister Kenny Rehabilitation Institute
Minneapolis, Minnesota

Jean C. Deitz, Ph.D., OTR, FAOTA
Professor
Department of Rehabilitation Medicine
University of Washington
Seattle, Washington

Lisa Deshaies, OTR/L, CHT
Clinical Specialist
Occupational Therapy Department
Rancho Los Amigos National Rehabilitation Center
Downey, CA

Brian J. Dudgeon, Ph.D., OTR, FAOTA
Assistant Professor
Department of Rehabilitation Medicine
University of Washington
Seattle, Washington

Susan E. Fasoli, ScD, OTR/L
Occupational Therapy Manager
Newton Wellesley Hospital
Newton, Massachusetts

Nancy A. Flinn, PhD, OTR/L
Associate Professor
Department of Occupational Science and Occupational Therapy
The College of St. Catherine
St. Paul, Minnesota

Susan Forwell, PhD, OT(C), FCAOT
Division of Occupational Therapy
School of Rehabilitation Sciences
University of British Columbia
Vancouver, British Columbia, Canada

Glenn Goodman, Ph.D., OTR/L
Associate Professor, Director
Master of Occupational Therapy Program
Cleveland State University
Cleveland, Ohio

Julie McLaughlin Gray, PhD (cand.), OTR/L
Instructor of Clinical Occupational Therapy
Department of Occupational Science and Occupational Therapy
University of Southern California
Los Angeles, California

Carolyn Schmidt Hanson, PhD, OTR/L
Research Coordinator
Brain Rehabilitation Research Center
North Florida/South Georgia Veterans Administration Healthcare System
Gainesville, Florida

Lucinda Hugos, MS, PT
Clinical Assistant Professor and Physical Therapist
Outpatient Therapy Center
Oregon Health and Sciences University
Portland, Oregon

Nancy Huntley, OTR/L, CES
Cardiac Rehabilitation Therapist
Fairview Southdale Hospital
Edina, Minnesota

Jeanne Jackson, PhD, OTR
Associate Professor
Department of Occupational Science and Occupational Therapy
University of Southern California
Los Angeles, California

Anne Birge James, PhD, OTR/L
Assistant Professor
Department of Occupational Therapy
Mercy College
Dobbs Ferry, New York

Sharon Kurfuerst, EdD, OTR/L
Senior Director, Clinical Services
Genesis Rehabilitation Services
Kennett Square, Pennsylvania

Catherine A. Trombly Latham, ScD, OTR/L, FAOTA
Professor Emerita
Program in Occupational Therapy
Department of Rehabilitation Science
Sargent College of Health and Rehabilitation Sciences
Boston University
Boston, Massachusetts

Lori Letts, PhD, OT Reg (Ont)
Associate Professor
School of Rehabilitation Science
McMaster University
Hamilton, Ontario, Canada

Kathryn Levit, PhD, OTR/L
Adjunct Faculty
Department of Psychology
George Mason University
Fairfax, Virginia

Joanna Bertness Lipoma, MOT, OTR
Clinical Instructor
Texas Woman's University
Dallas, Texas

Jaclyn Faglie Low, PhD, OTR, FAOTA
Retired
Houston, Texas

Mandy Lowe, MSc, OT Reg (Ont)
Clinical Educator, Occupational Therapy
Toronto Rehabilitation Institute
Toronto, Ontario, Canada

Stephen Luster, MS, OTR, CHT
Instructor/Fieldwork Coordinator
Occupational Therapy Specialty Course
US Army Academy of Health Sciences
Fort Sam Houston, Texas

Colleen Maher, MS, OTR/L, CHT, MLD
Assistant Professor
Department of Occupational Therapy
Mercy College
Dobbs Ferry, NY

Virgil Mathiowetz, PhD, OTR/L, FAOTA
Associate Professor and Assistant Director
Program in Occupational Therapy
University of Minnesota
Minneapolis, Minnesota

E. Stuart Oertli, M.S., OTR
Supervisor, Occupational Therapy
The University of Texas—M. D. Anderson Cancer Center
Houston, Texas

Karin J. Opacich, PhD, MHPE, OTR/L, FAOTA
Project EXPORT Director and Assistant Director
National Center for Rural Health Professions
University of Illinois—Rockford
Rockford, Illinois

Amy C. Orroth, OTR, CHT
Senior Burn Therapist
Massachusetts General Hospital
Boston, Massachusetts

Monica A. Pessina, Ph.D., MEd., OTR
Department of Anatomy and Neurobiology
Boston University School of Medicine
Boston, Massachusetts

Susan Lanier Pierce, OTR/L, CDRS, SCDCM
President
Adaptive Mobility Services, Inc.
Orlando, Florida

Carolyn Robinson Podolski, MA, OTR, SCDCM
Instructor
Department of Occupational Therapy
The University of Alabama at Birmingham
Birmingham, Alabama

Lee Ann Quintana, MS, OTR/L
Occupational Therapist
Total Community Care
Albuquerque, New Mexico

Mary Vining Radomski, MA, OTR/L, FAOTA
Coordinator—Outcomes, Quality, Research
Occupational therapist
Sister Kenny Rehabilitation Institute
Minneapolis, Minnesota

Valerie J. Rice, PhD, CPE, OTR/L, FAOTA
Chief, Army Research Laboratory
US Army Medical Department Center and School
Human Research and Engineering Directorate
Army Medical Department Field Element
US Army Medical Department Center and School
Fort Sam Houston, Texas

Patricia Rigby, MHSc, OT Reg (Ont)
Assistant Professor and Graduate Coordinator
Department of Occupational Science and Occupational Therapy
Faculty of Medicine
University of Toronto
Toronto, Ontario, Canada

Pamela Roberts, MSHA, OTR/L, CPHQ, FAOTA
Manager, Rehabilitation and Neurology
Cedars-Sinai Medical Center
Los Angeles, California

Kathy Longenecker Rust, MS, OT
Research Coordinator
Rehabilitation Research Design and Disability Center
University of Wisconsin—Milwaukee
Milwaukee, Wisconsin

Dory Sabata, OTD, OTR/L
Research Scientist
Georgia Institute of Technology
Center for Assistive Technology and Environmental Access
Atlanta, Georgia

Joyce Shapero Sabari, Ph.D., OTR, FAOTA
Associate Professor and Chair
Occupational Therapy Program
State University of New York
Downstate Medical Center
Brooklyn, New York

Shoshana Shamberg, OTR/L, MS
Accessibility Consultant and President
Abilities OT Services Inc.
Baltimore, Maryland

Margarette L. Shelton, Ph.D., OTR
Assistant Professor
The University of Texas—Pan American
Edinburg, Texas

Jo M. Solet, EdM, PhD, OTR/L
Clinical Instructor in Psychology
Harvard Medical School and Cambridge Health Alliance
Department of Psychiatry
Cambridge, Massachusetts

Debra Stewart, MSc, OT Reg (Ont)
Assistant Dean
Occupational Therapy Program
School of Rehabilitation Science
McMaster University
Hamilton, Ontario, Canada

Kathy Stubblefield, OTR/L
Research Occupational Therapist
Neural Engineering Center for Artificial Limbs
Rehabilitation Institute of Chicago
Chicago, Illinois

Linda Tickle-Degnen, Ph. D., OTR, FAOTA
Associate Professor
Boston School of Occupational Therapy
Tufts University
Medford, Massachusetts

Michael Williams, PhD
Research Scientist II
Georgia Institute of Technology
Center for Assistive Technology and Environmental Access
Atlanta, Georgia

Anne M. Woodson, OTR
Occupational Therapist III
Department of Occupational Therapy
University of Texas Medical Branch
Galveston, Texas

Y. Lynn Yasuda, MSEd, OTR, FAOTA
Consultant, Occupational Therapy Department
Research Occupational Therapist, Rehabilitation Engineering Center
Rancho Los Amigos National Rehabilitation Center
Downey, California

Ruth Zemke, PhD, OTR, FAOTA
Professor Emeritus
Department of Occupational Science and Occupational Therapy
University of Southern California
Los Angeles, California

User's Guide

This User's Guide introduces you to the many features of ***Occupational Therapy for Physical Dysfunction***, Sixth Edition. Taking full advantage of the text and these features, you also develop a theoretical foundation to guide your decisions.

Each chapter is loaded with features that help you focus on the key points, deepen your knowledge, and help you select the right assessment and intervention tools.

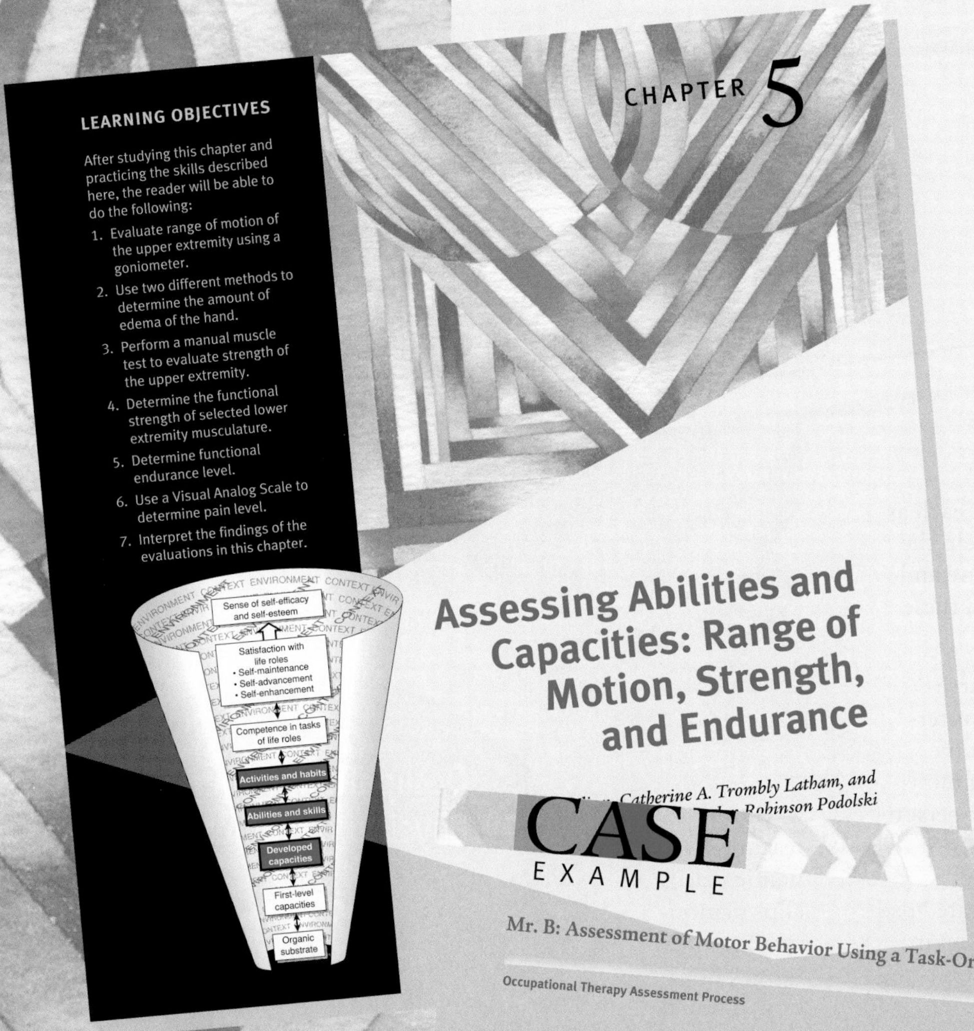

LEARNING OBJECTIVES
After studying this chapter and practicing the skills described here, the reader will be able to do the following:
1. Evaluate range of motion of the upper extremity using a goniometer.
2. Use two different methods to determine the amount of edema of the hand.
3. Perform a manual muscle test to evaluate strength of the upper extremity.
4. Determine the functional strength of selected lower extremity musculature.
5. Determine functional endurance level.
6. Use a Visual Analog Scale to determine pain level.
7. Interpret the findings of the evaluations in this chapter.
Sense of self-efficacy and self-esteem
Satisfaction with life roles
• Self-maintenance
• Self-advancement
• Self-enhancement
Competence in tasks of life roles
Activities and habits
Abilities and skills
Developed capacities
First-level capacities
Organic substrate
CHAPTER 5
Assessing Abilities and Capacities: Range of Motion, Strength, and Endurance
Catherine A. Trombly Latham, and
Robinson Podolski

LEARNING OBJECTIVES AND DIAGRAMS set forth each chapter's learning goals and how they fit within the Occupational Functioning Model.

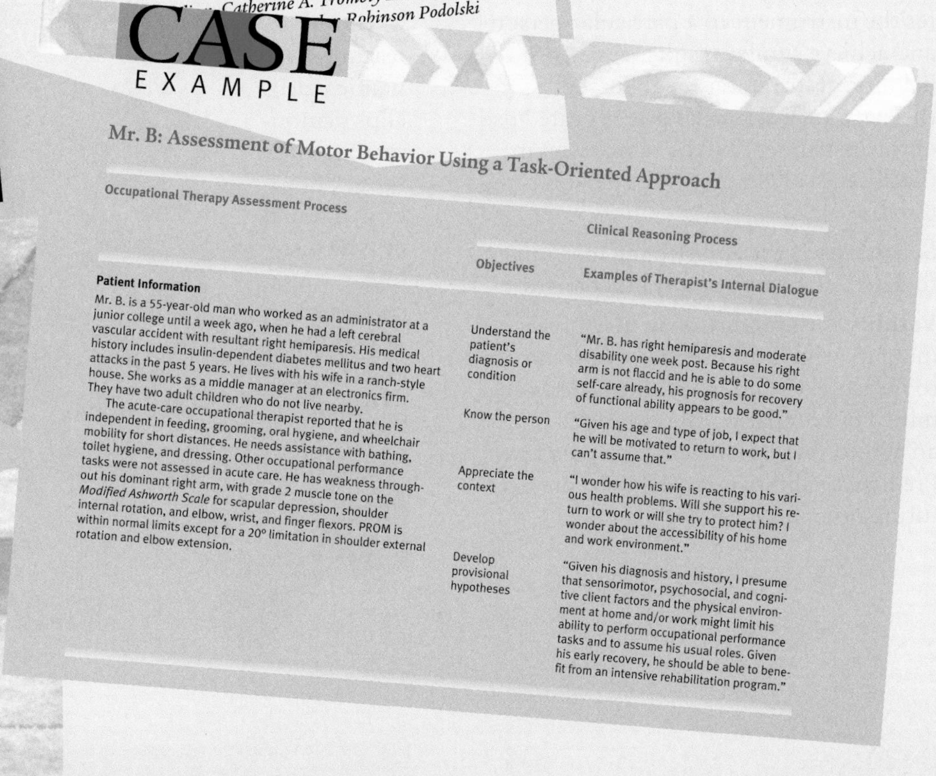

CASE EXAMPLES stress the underlying rationales of assessments and interventions and help students apply what they learn in practice.

NEW FEATURES TO HELP YOU BE A SUCCESSFUL OCCUPATIONAL THERAPIST

Occupational therapists who practice competently and ethically do so from a background of evidence that assessments are valid and reliable and treatments are efficacious. The two new table features of *Occupational Therapy for Physical Dysfunction* support evidence-based practice.

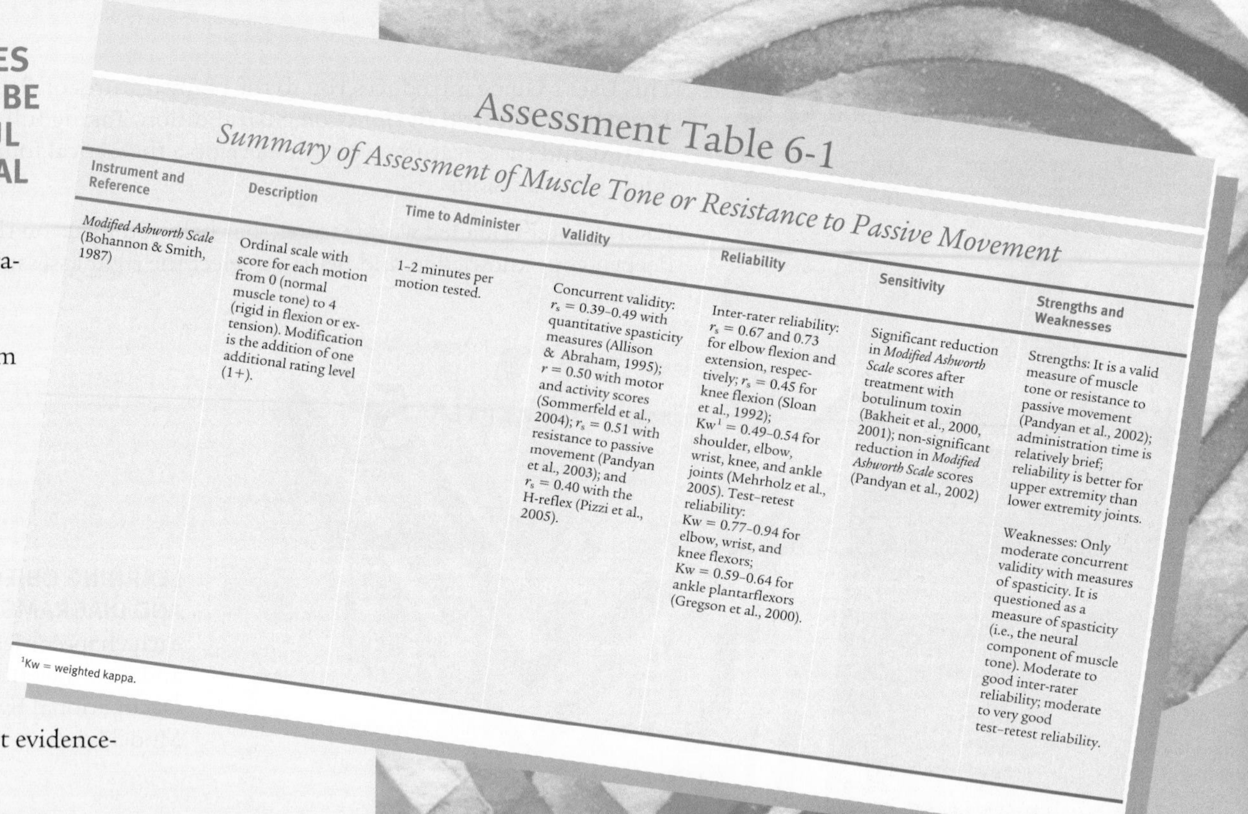

Assessment Table 6-1

Summary of Assessment of Muscle Tone or Resistance to Passive Movement

Instrument and Reference	Description	Time to Administer	Validity	Reliability	Sensitivity	Strengths and Weaknesses
Modified Ashworth Scale (Bohannon & Smith, 1987)	Ordinal scale with score for each motion from 0 (normal muscle tone) to 4 (rigid in flexion or extension). Modification is the addition of one additional rating level (1+).	1–2 minutes per motion tested.	Concurrent validity: $r_s = 0.39$–0.49 with quantitative spasticity measures (Allison & Abraham, 1995); $r = 0.50$ with motor and activity scores (Sommerfeld et al., 2004); $r_s = 0.51$ with resistance to passive movement (Pandyan et al., 2003); and $r_s = 0.40$ with the H-reflex (Pizzi et al., 2005).	Inter-rater reliability: $r_s = 0.67$ and 0.73 for elbow flexion and extension, respectively; $r_s = 0.45$ for knee flexion (Sloan et al., 1992); Kw[1] = 0.49–0.54 for shoulder, elbow, wrist, knee, and ankle joints (Mehrholz et al., 2005). Test–retest reliability: Kw = 0.77–0.94 for elbow, wrist, and knee flexors; Kw = 0.59–0.64 for ankle plantarflexors (Gregson et al., 2000).	Significant reduction in *Modified Ashworth Scale* scores after treatment with botulinum toxin (Bakheit et al., 2000, 2001); non-significant reduction in *Modified Ashworth Scale* scores (Pandyan et al., 2002)	Strengths: It is a valid measure of muscle tone or resistance to passive movement (Pandyan et al., 2002); administration time is relatively brief; reliability is better for upper extremity than lower extremity joints. Weaknesses: Only moderate concurrent validity with measures of spasticity. It is questioned as a measure of spasticity (i.e., the neural component of muscle tone). Moderate to good inter-rater reliability; moderate to very good test–retest reliability.

[1]Kw = weighted kappa.

ASSESSMENT TABLES At the end of each assessment chapter there is a table to help the therapist select an appropriate measure and to interpret the results. Terms used in these tables include:

- **Reliability** is a measure of an instrument's stability. Interobserver or inter-rater reliability refers to the outcome when two different individuals administer the instrument to a particular person and achieve similar results. Test-retest reliability, or intrarater reliability, refers to the constancy of results over repeated use of the instrument by the same tester in the absence of change in the person being tested.
- **Sensitivity** is the ability of an instrument to detect clinically important changes.
- **Validity** is the ability of an instrument to measure what it is intended or presumed to measure. Criterion validity is determined by comparing the examined test to an agreed-on *gold standard* (accepted test). Predictive validity is its ability to predict future outcomes.

STUDENT DVD features dynamic video clips demonstrating range of motion, manual muscle testing, construction of hand splints and transferring patients.

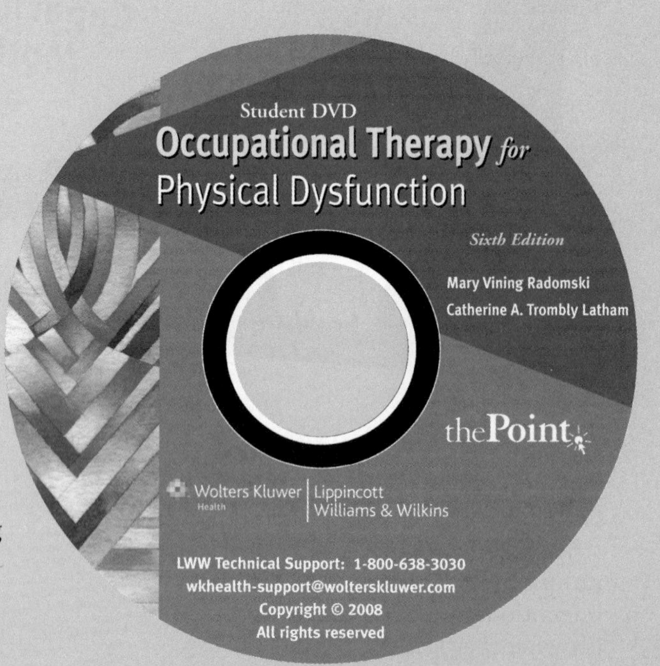

EVIDENCE TABLES

At the end of each chapter devoted to treatment or a diagnosis is a table listing some of the best evidence concerning the treatments mentioned in the chapter. Terms used in the evidence tables include:

Evidence Table 24-1
Best Evidence for Occupational Therapy Practice Regarding NDT/Bobath

Intervention	Description of Intervention Tested	Participants	Dosage	Type of Best Evidence and Level of Evidence	Benefit	Statistical Probability and Effect Size of Outcome	Reference
NDT for stroke survivors	Effectiveness of NDT in 3 areas: general treatment, upper limb recovery, and lower limb and gait.	726 acute stroke survivors; age range, 15–95 years; mean age cannot be calculated.	Ranged from 2–15 weeks.	Systematic review of 15 trials: 6 randomized controlled trials, 6 non-randomized controlled trials, and 3 case studies.	Of general effectiveness studies (n = 6), 1 found more improvement in NDT group, and 5 found no difference or more gains in alternate group; 1 of 3 studies of upper extremity effectiveness found greater benefit with NDT.	$p<0.001$ set as statistical significance level for all studies included. Effect sizes were not reported.	Paci, 2003
NDT for upper limb post stroke	Effectiveness of NDT in improving impairment (tone, strength, pain), activity limitation, and participation.	374 stroke survivors 6 weeks to 2 years post cerebrovascular accident; age range, 35–95 years; mean age cannot be calculated.	Ranged from 1 session to 20 weeks of daily 45-minute sessions.	Systematic review of 8 studies: 5 randomized controlled trials, 1 single-group crossover design trial, and 2 single case studies.	NDT more effective than proprioceptive neuromuscular facilitation but not more than general rehab at reducing muscle tone. No significant effects of NDT on motor control, upper extremity function, or participation.	Improvement in upper extremity tone using RIPs, d = 0.46.	Luke, 2004

- **Effect size** is a unit-less indication of the strength of the relationship between the treatment and the outcome (Rosenthal, 1984). There are several representations of effect size, including r, Hedges' g, Cohen's d, and h2 (eta squared). Effect size, "r," is interpreted like a correlation coefficient: 1.0 equals a perfect, strong, relationship and 0 equals no relationship (Rosenthal, 1984). An effect size of r = .10 is considered small ; of .30, medium; and of .50 large (Cohen, 1988) (h2 , eta squared, is interpreted similarly to "r").
- **Level of evidence** rating scale used in this textbook is the American Occupational Therapy Association's Evidence Based Project Scale (Trombly & Ma, 2002): Level I [highest] to Level IV [lowest]. The higher the level, the better the evidence that the intervention was the cause of the change reported. The Scale also presents grades relating to sample size, internal validity (how well the study controlled for alternate explanations of outcome), and external validity (how well the study generalizes to persons other than the study participants or to settings other than the study setting). For example, a IC2c rating means that the study was a randomized controlled trial (I), with 20 or fewer participants in each group (C), that had no strong alternative explanation for outcome, but had one or two threats to validity (2), and that the participants do not necessarily represent the population of patients of that diagnosis AND the treatment does not represent current practice OR it was carried out in an unnatural (laboratory) setting (c).
- **Statistical probability** indicates the likelihood that the outcome was due to chance. A probability level of .05 indicates that there are only 5 chances out of a hundred that the outcome occurred by chance (Rosenthal & Rosnow, 1991).

References

Cohen, J. (1988). *Statistical power analysis for the behavioral sciences* (2nd ed.). Hillsdale, NJ: Erlbaum.

Rosenthal, R. (1984). *Meta-analytic procedures for social research.* Beverly Hills; Sage Publications.

Rosenthal, R., & Rosnow, R. L. (1991). *Essentials of behavioral research: Methods and data analysis* (2nd ed.). New York: McGraw-Hill, Inc.

Trombly, C. A., & Ma, H-I. (2002). A synthesis of effects of occupational therapy for persons with stroke. Part I: restoration of roles, tasks, and activities. *American Journal of Occupational Therapy,* 56, 250-259.

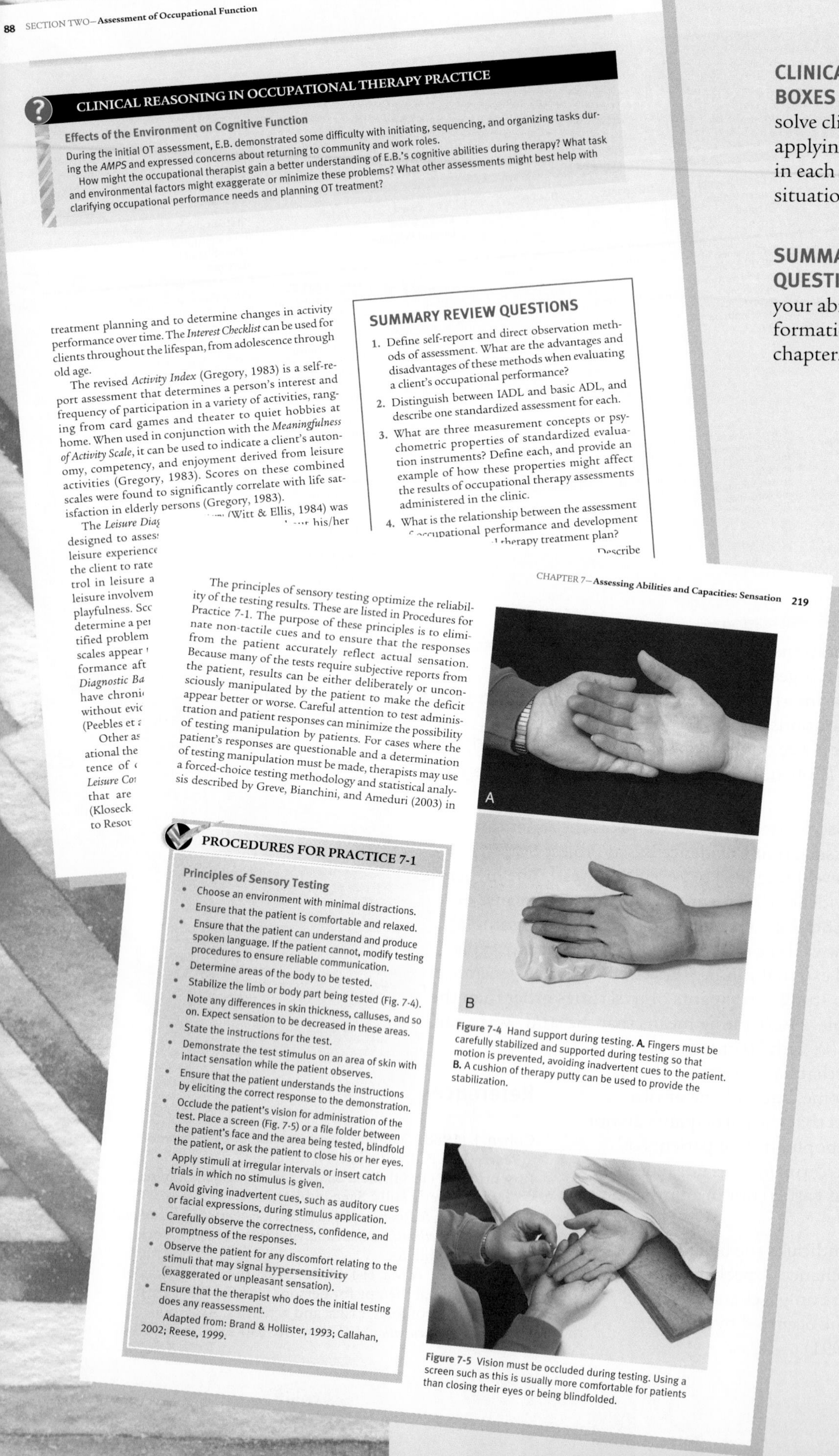

88 SECTION TWO—Assessment of Occupational Function

CLINICAL REASONING IN OCCUPATIONAL THERAPY PRACTICE

Effects of the Environment on Cognitive Function

During the initial OT assessment, E.B. demonstrated some difficulty with initiating, sequencing, and organizing tasks during the *AMPS* and expressed concerns about returning to community and work roles.

How might the occupational therapist gain a better understanding of E.B.'s cognitive abilities during therapy? What task and environmental factors might exaggerate or minimize these problems? What other assessments might best help with clarifying occupational performance needs and planning OT treatment?

treatment planning and to determine changes in activity performance over time. The *Interest Checklist* can be used for clients throughout the lifespan, from adolescence through old age.

The revised *Activity Index* (Gregory, 1983) is a self-report assessment that determines a person's interest and frequency of participation in a variety of activities, ranging from card games and theater to quiet hobbies at home. When used in conjunction with the *Meaningfulness of Activity Scale*, it can be used to indicate a client's autonomy, competency, and enjoyment derived from leisure activities (Gregory, 1983). Scores on these combined scales were found to significantly correlate with life satisfaction in elderly persons (Gregory, 1983).

The *Leisure Diag*... (Witt & Ellis, 1984) was designed to asses... his/her leisure experience... the client to rate... trol in leisure a... leisure involvem... playfulness. Sc... determine a pe... tified problem... scales appear... formance aft... *Diagnostic Ba*... have chroni... without evi... (Peebles et a... Other as... ational the... tence of... *Leisure Co*... that are... (Kloseck... to Resou...

SUMMARY REVIEW QUESTIONS

1. Define self-report and direct observation methods of assessment. What are the advantages and disadvantages of these methods when evaluating a client's occupational performance?
2. Distinguish between IADL and basic ADL, and describe one standardized assessment for each.
3. What are three measurement concepts or psychometric properties of standardized evaluation instruments? Define each, and provide an example of how these properties might affect the results of occupational therapy assessments administered in the clinic.
4. What is the relationship between the assessment of occupational performance and development ... therapy treatment plan? ... Describe

CHAPTER 7—Assessing Abilities and Capacities: Sensation 219

The principles of sensory testing optimize the reliability of the testing results. These are listed in Procedures for Practice 7-1. The purpose of these principles is to eliminate non-tactile cues and to ensure that the responses from the patient accurately reflect actual sensation. Because many of the tests require subjective reports from the patient, results can be either deliberately or unconsciously manipulated by the patient to make the deficit appear better or worse. Careful attention to test administration and patient responses can minimize the possibility of testing manipulation by patients. For cases where the patient's responses are questionable and a determination of testing manipulation must be made, therapists may use a forced-choice testing methodology and statistical analysis described by Greve, Bianchini, and Ameduri (2003) in

PROCEDURES FOR PRACTICE 7-1

Principles of Sensory Testing

- Choose an environment with minimal distractions.
- Ensure that the patient is comfortable and relaxed.
- Ensure that the patient can understand and produce spoken language. If the patient cannot, modify testing procedures to ensure reliable communication.
- Determine areas of the body to be tested.
- Stabilize the limb or body part being tested (Fig. 7-4).
- Note any differences in skin thickness, calluses, and so on. Expect sensation to be decreased in these areas.
- State the instructions for the test.
- Demonstrate the test stimulus on an area of skin with intact sensation while the patient observes.
- Ensure that the patient understands the instructions by eliciting the correct response to the demonstration.
- Occlude the patient's vision for administration of the test. Place a screen (Fig. 7-5) or a file folder between the patient's face and the area being tested, blindfold the patient, or ask the patient to close his or her eyes.
- Apply stimuli at irregular intervals or insert catch trials in which no stimulus is given.
- Avoid giving inadvertent cues, such as auditory cues or facial expressions, during stimulus application.
- Carefully observe the correctness, confidence, and promptness of the responses.
- Observe the patient for any discomfort relating to the stimuli that may signal **hypersensitivity** (exaggerated or unpleasant sensation).
- Ensure that the therapist who does the initial testing does any reassessment.

Adapted from: Brand & Hollister, 1993; Callahan, 2002; Reese, 1999.

A

B

Figure 7-4 Hand support during testing. **A.** Fingers must be carefully stabilized and supported during testing so that motion is prevented, avoiding inadvertent cues to the patient. **B.** A cushion of therapy putty can be used to provide the stabilization.

Figure 7-5 Vision must be occluded during testing. Using a screen such as this is usually more comfortable for patients than closing their eyes or being blindfolded.

CLINICAL REASONING BOXES give opportunities to solve clinical problems by applying knowledge gained in each chapter to real-life situations.

SUMMARY REVIEW QUESTIONS let you assess your ability to apply the information presented in each chapter.

PROCEDURES FOR PRACTICE BOXES provide step-by-step directions for applying concepts to practice.

Contents

SECTION VI
Treatment to Promote Occupational Function for Selected Diagnostic Categories

SECTION I: Occupational Function: Definition, Process, and History

CHAPTER 1

Conceptual Foundations for Practice

Catherine A. Trombly Latham

LEARNING OBJECTIVES

After studying this chapter, the reader will be able to do the following:

1. Describe the Occupational Functioning Model.
2. Use the language of the Occupational Functioning Model, the American Occupational Therapy Association's Occupational Therapy Practice Framework (OTPF), and the World Health Organization's International Classification of Functioning (ICF) interchangeably.
3. Organize assessment and treatment planning according to the Occupational Functioning Model.

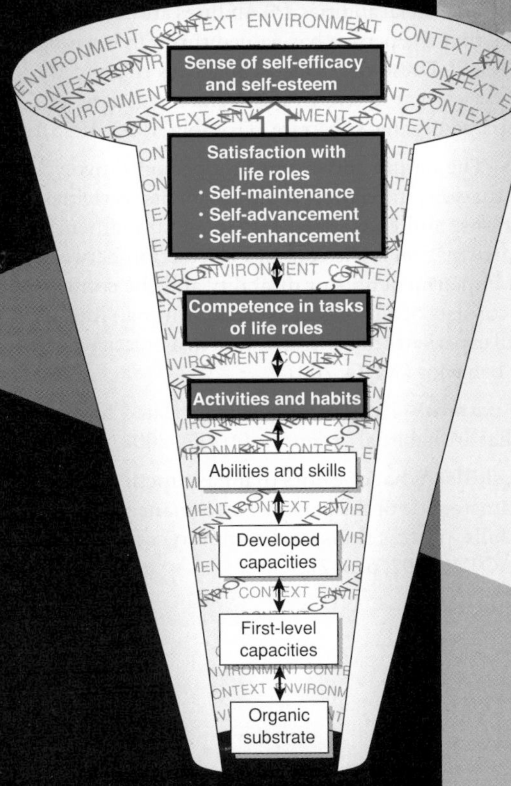

Glossary

Ability—Having sufficient power, skill, or resources to accomplish an object (Mish, 2004). A general trait an individual brings to learning a new task (Fleishman, 1972).

Activity, activities—In the Occupational Functioning Model (OFM), activities are considered small units of goal-directed behavior that make up tasks. The Occupational Therapy Practice Framework (OTPF) (AOTA, 2002) defines activity as a class of human actions that are goal directed. In the International Classification of Functioning (ICM), activity is defined as the "execution of a task or action by an individual" and includes everything a person does at any level of complexity from basic physical and mental functions of the person as a whole (e.g., acquisition of knowledge or grasp) to complex skills and behavior (e.g., driving a car or interacting with persons in formal settings) (WHO, 2001).

Activity analysis—A process used to identify the properties inherent in a given occupation, task, or activity, as well as the skills, abilities, and capacities required to complete it. Activity analysis is used to analyze and assess performance, to select occupations to remediate deficient capacities and abilities, or, knowing the person's skills, abilities, and capacities, to select and modify activity to ensure successful completion of the activity.

Adaptive therapy—Therapy that promotes a balance among a person's goals, capabilities, and environmental demands by use of assistive technology, adaptation of the environment or methods of accomplishing an activity, and/or redefinition of goals.

Augmented maturation—Therapeutic techniques that use controlled sensory stimulation and activities that promote responses in developmental postures or patterns to develop first-level capacities or developed capacities.

Capacities—Potential attributes that, once developed into abilities and skills, will contribute to occupational functioning. Capacities are the basis of performance.

Context—The circumstances surrounding an act or event (Mish, 2004). In health care, context refers to the whole situation, background, or environment that is relevant to a particular event or personality. In this sense, context has personal, social, cultural, physical, and temporal dimensions.

Environment—Surroundings; the aggregate of physical, social, and cultural conditions that influence the life of an individual (Mish, 2004).

Functioning—An umbrella term encompassing all body functions, activities, and participation (WHO, 2001).

Impairment—Any significant deviation or loss of body structure or physiological or psychological function (WHO, 2001).

Occupation—Everyday life activity (AOTA, 2002, p. 610).

Occupation-as-end—Occupation is the functional goal (activity, task) to be learned or accomplished. Its therapeutic impact comes from its characteristics of purpose and meaning (Trombly, 1995). Through repeated carrying out of an occupation, the patient will relearn the activity, or through adaptation, the activity will be possible for the person, given his current capacities and abilities. Example: Using a stocking aid, the person with a total hip replacement can don his or her stockings.

Occupation-as-means—Occupation that is used as the therapeutic change agent to remediate impaired abilities or capacities. Its therapeutic effect derives from characteristics of purpose and meaning (Trombly, 1995). It is also termed therapeutic occupation (Fisher, 1998). An example is peeling carrots to develop gross grasp by a person who likes to cook.

Occupational dysfunction—Inability to maintain one's self (i.e., care for self, dependents, and home); to advance oneself through work, learning, and financial management; or to enhance the self by engaging in self-actualizing activities that add enjoyment to life.

Occupational Functioning Model—A conceptual model that guides occupational therapy evaluation and treatment of persons with physical dysfunction. The propositions of the model are as follows: (1) To engage satisfactorily in a life role, a person must be able to do the tasks that, in his opinion, make up that role. (2) Tasks are composed of activities, which are small units of behavior. (3) To be able to do a given activity, one must have certain sensorimotor, cognitive, perceptual, emotional, and social abilities. (4) Abilities are developed from capacities that the person has gained through learning or maturation. (5) These developed capacities depend on first-level capacities that derive from a person's genetic endowment or spared organic substrate (Trombly, 1993, 1995).

Participation—The nature and extent of a person's involvement in life situations in relation to impairments, activities, health conditions, and contextual factors. A fundamental property of participation is the complex interaction between a person with impairment and/or disability and the context. Participation consists of all areas or aspects of human life, including the full experience of being involved in a practice, custom, or social behavior (WHO, 2001).

Performance patterns—Patterns of behavior related to daily life activities that are habitual or routine (AOTA, 2002, p. 632).

Performance skills—What one does that has functional purpose, not a characteristic of the person. Performance skills include motor skills, process skills, and communication/interaction skills (AOTA, 2002, p. 632).

How do occupational therapists know what to do when a person with **occupational dysfunction** secondary to a disease or injury that results in physical **impairment** is referred to them? First, they have *specific knowledge* about what the diagnosis means in terms of limitations of bodily structure or function and subsequent probable limitation of occupational performance, and they know the outcome of research on the effectiveness of interventions available—the evidence base of practice. Second, they have *specific skills* for assessing and treating persons with occupational dysfunction secondary to physical impairment. Third, they know *how therapy is organized*—the conceptual foundation for practice. The organization or process of occupational therapy is found in various conceptual models of practice. An occupational therapy model of practice is a way of conceptualizing the interrelatedness of the person, and his or her **environments**, occupations, and quality of life, to guide assessment and intervention. In this chapter, one model, the **Occupational Functioning Model (OFM)**, is described as well as how this model relates to the American Occupational Therapy Association's (AOTA) Occupational Therapy Practice Framework (OTPF) (AOTA, 2002), and the World Health Organization's (WHO) International Classification of **Functioning** (ICF) (WHO, 2001).

THE OCCUPATIONAL FUNCTIONING MODEL

The Occupational Functioning Model (OFM) guides evaluation and treatment of persons with physical dysfunction leading to competence in occupational performance. The OFM was derived from clinical practice. The primary belief is that people who are competent in their life roles experience a sense of self-efficacy, self-esteem, and life satisfaction. Research partially supports the idea that competency is related to satisfaction (Robinson-Smith, Johnston, & Allen, 2000). For example, actual performance has been found to strengthen efficacy beliefs in older adults (Resnik, 1998). Competence in occupational performance contributes to development of a person's identity (Christiansen, 1999; Toal-Sullivan & Henderson, 2004). The goal of treatment, following the OFM, is to enable satisfactory engagement in valued roles whether by restored self-performance or by directing others.

Another assumption of the OFM is that the ability to carry out one's roles and activities of life depends on basic abilities and **capacities** (e.g., strength, perception, ability to sequence information). This hierarchical organization assumes that lower-level capacities and abilities, such as strength and endurance, are related to a higher-level performance of everyday tasks and activities. This organization has been preliminarily supported by research (Dijkers, 1997, 1999; Geertzen et al., 1998; Sveen et al., 1999). Only part of the variance associated with function, however, is accounted for by any one ability. For example, Lynch and Bridle (1989) found a moderately strong ($r = -0.65$; $p < 0.01$) negative relationship between the scores of the *Jebsen-Taylor Hand Function Test* (Jebsen et al., 1969) and the scores of the *Klein-Bell ADL* (Activities of Daily Living) *Scale* (Klein & Bell, 1982). The correlation is negative because better performance on the *Jebsen-Taylor* is indicated by less time (lower score), whereas better performance on the *Klein-Bell* is indicated by a higher score. Filiatrault et al. (1991) found a similar relationship ($r = 0.6$) between the *Fugl-Meyer Motor Function Test* (upper extremity subtest) (Fugl-Meyer et al., 1975) and the *Barthel Index* (ADL) (Mahoney & Barthel, 1965). These outcomes do indicate that sensorimotor control of the upper extremities is related to self-care. But because the r^2 (0.65^2 or 0.60^2) value is only approximately 40%, other unidentified variables must account for the remaining approximately 60% variance associated with ADL. This makes sense because, in addition to upper extremity function, ADL independence requires such skills as sitting and standing balance, perception of positions of objects in space, ability to sequence steps of a procedure, environmental support, and so forth.

It appears that the relationship between two adjacent levels of performance (e.g., capacities and abilities) is stronger than between two nonadjacent levels (e.g., capacities and roles) (Dijkers, 1999). The relationship between levels is strong both at the low end of the model (Pendlebury et al., 1999) and at the high end (Dijkers, 1997, 1999). Pendlebury et al. (1999) found a strong ($r = 0.90$) relationship between deficits in organic substrate and deficits of motor capacities and abilities. In a large sample of persons with spinal cord injury, Dijkers (1999) found a moderately strong relationship ($r = 0.24$–0.42) between life satisfaction and roles related to social integration and occupation (work) but not between impairments and life satisfaction ($r = 0.04$–0.07). He concluded that "these relationships suggest a causal chain [i.e., one link leading to the next]. . . . the impact of impairment on quality of life is almost entirely through its impact on disability, and the effect of disability is largely through its impact on handicap" (Dijkers, 1999, p. 874). This suggests that the relationship between low-level capacities and abilities and higher-level tasks and roles is not direct. That is, having a particular ability such as strength does not ensure that a person can accomplish a given activity or task (Dagfinrud et al., 2005). Likewise, the ability to accomplish a single activity does not account for role performance. Many capacities contribute to the development of one ability, and many abilities are needed to engage successfully in an activity. When one capacity or ability is impaired, occupational dysfunction does not automatically occur (Rogers & Holm, 1994; Rondinelli et al., 1997). A person may adaptively use other capacities and abilities to allow accomplishment of the activity.

Research is needed to clarify the multivariate relationships among lower-level abilities and capacities and higher-level activities, tasks, and roles (Trombly, 1993, 1995). Researchers also must verify whether remediation of impaired capacities and abilities results in more complete and more versatile participation in the activities and tasks of importance to people's lives than would learning specific routines of activities in an adapted way (task-specific training). This is a key question for the practice of occupational therapy with persons having physical dysfunction.

Another assumption of the OFM is that satisfactory occupational functioning occurs only within enabling environments and **contexts** particular to the individual. True occupational functioning does not occur in a vacuum or in a controlled situation such as the clinic; occupational functioning is the successful interaction of the person with the objects, situations, and surroundings of his or her home, family, and community. Although the contexts of particular actions and occupations to regain lost abilities and capacities may be controlled at first, therapy is not complete until generalization to the person's particular environment has occurred.

Achievement of occupational functioning after injury or disease is accomplished through occupation as well as adjunctive therapies described in this textbook. In the OFM model, occupation has two natures: **occupation-as-end** and **occupation-as-means** (Trombly, 1995). Occupation-as-end equates to the higher levels of the OFM, at which the person tries to accomplish a functional goal (an activity or task) by using whatever skills, abilities, habits, and capacities he or she has. Occupation-as-means, on the other hand, is *the therapy* used to bring about changes in impaired client factors and performance skills. Occupation-as-means is based on the assumption that occupation holds within itself healing properties that will change organic or behavioral impairments. Both occupation-as-end and occupation-as-means derive their therapeutic impact from the qualities of purposefulness and meaningfulness (see Chapters 12 and 13 for discussion of these concepts).

The constructs of the occupational functioning model shown in Figure 1-1 are described next.

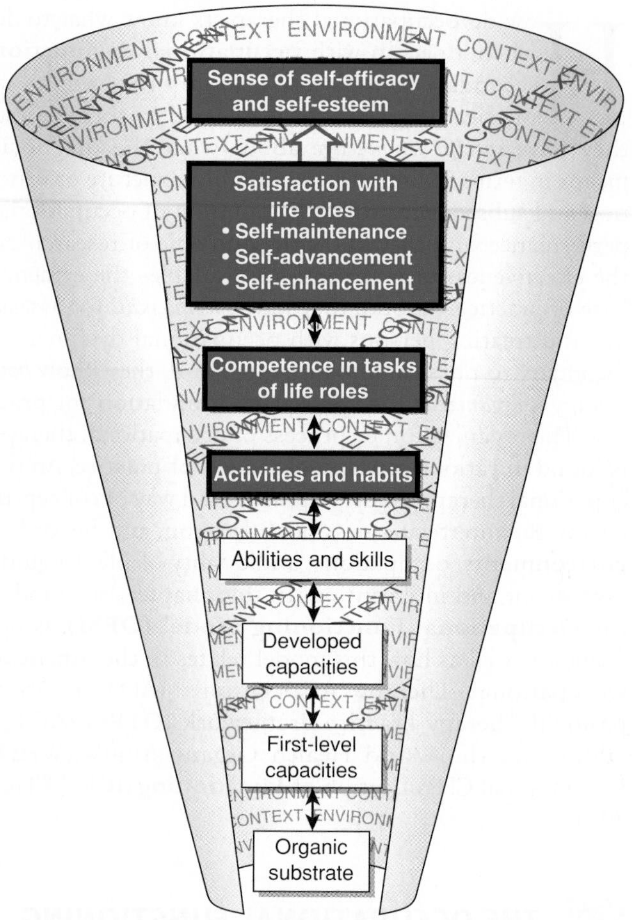

Figure 1-1 Paradigm of occupational functioning model.

Sense of Self-Efficacy and Self-Esteem

The goal of occupational therapy is the development of competence in activities and tasks of one's cherished roles, which promotes a sense of self-efficacy and self-esteem. Competence refers to effective interaction with the physical and social environments (Fig. 1-2). To be competent means to have the skills that are sufficient or adequate to meet the demands of a situation or task (White, 1959). It does not equate to excellence, normality, or the ability to do everything, and it recognizes that there are degrees of sufficiency and adequacy in people (Mocellin, 1992; White, 1971). Competence reflects people's belief in their own control rather than being controlled by the social or physical environments (Trombly, 1993). Competence develops by enabling a person to engage in graduated, goal-directed activity that is accomplishable by that person and produces a feeling of satisfaction (White, 1959). Occupational therapists help people achieve competence through graded engagement in occupation, vicarious engagement in occupation (watching others), developmental and instrumental learning with immediate and precise feedback, and therapeutic interaction with the therapist (Bandura, 1997; Radomski, 2000; Robinson-Smith, Johnston, & Allen, 2002).

When people feel competent, they are likely to esteem themselves. Self-esteem is that aspect of self-concept that attributes a negative or positive value to the self. Self-esteem is created by individuals' analyses of their competency in socially relevant areas (Gage & Polatajko, 1994). People's levels of self-esteem depend on their confidence,

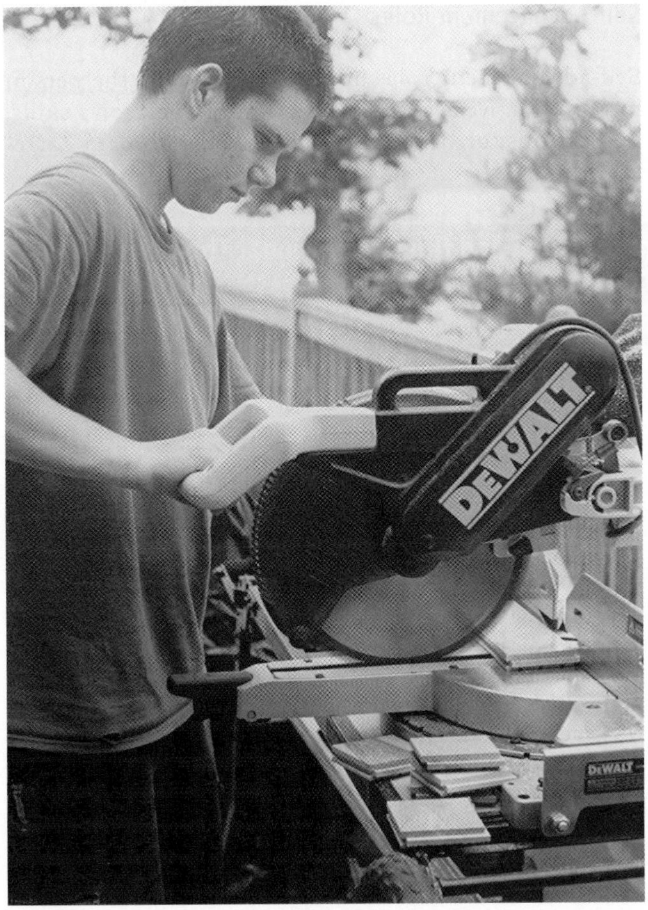

Figure 1-2 Competency in self-advancement role of contractor's helper.

based on experience, that they can make desired things happen and that others will appreciatively recognize this competence (White, 1971).

Efficacy, as it is used in the OFM, refers both to Bandura's (1977, 1997) concepts of perceived self-efficacy and outcome expectancy and Rogers' (1983) concept of response efficacy. Perceived self-efficacy refers to people's beliefs in their performance capabilities with respect to a specific task (Bandura, 1977, 1997; Gage et al., 1994; Resnik, 1998, 1999). It is concerned not with the skills one possesses but with the judgments of what one can do with those skills. Perceived self-efficacy is influenced through an ongoing evaluation of success and failure with each task people participate in over the course of their lives (Gage & Polatajko, 1994). Response efficacy and outcome expectancy refer to a judgment of the consequences that certain behavior will produce (Resnik, 1998). It is the individual's judgment of how effective his or her response to a given problem will be (Rogers, 1983). The most powerful source of efficacy expectations is past accomplishments in similar situations (Fig. 1-3).

Satisfaction with Life Roles

Being in control of one's life means being able to engage satisfyingly in one's life roles or to voluntarily reassign a role to another. Role performance is a vital component of productive independent living (Hallett et al., 1994). Various thinkers have proposed taxonomies of roles. For example, Reilly (1962) categorized occupational roles according to gender and age, identifying four: preschooler, student, housewife or paid worker, and retiree. She saw play and work roles on a continuum. The OTPF uses the phrase "areas of **occupation**" rather than roles and categorizes these areas as activities of daily living (ADL), instrumental activities of daily living (IADL), education, work, play, leisure, and social participation. The OFM sorts roles into three domains related to aspects of self-definition: self-maintenance, self-advancement, and self-enhancement (Trombly, 1993, 1995), but recognizes that the assignment of roles to a particular category is not absolute. Some roles may be classified in one domain by one person but in another domain by another person, depending on the motivation. For example, volunteering may be classified by one person as a self-advancement role because volunteering promotes skills that will be useful in a worker role. Another person may classify volunteering as self-enhancement because it promotes a sense of satisfaction without expectation of gain. The individuality of motivation underscores the importance of assessing each person from his or her own point of view, letting each define his or her roles and their meaning.

Self-Maintenance Roles

Self-maintenance roles are associated with maintenance of the self and care of the family and home. This domain

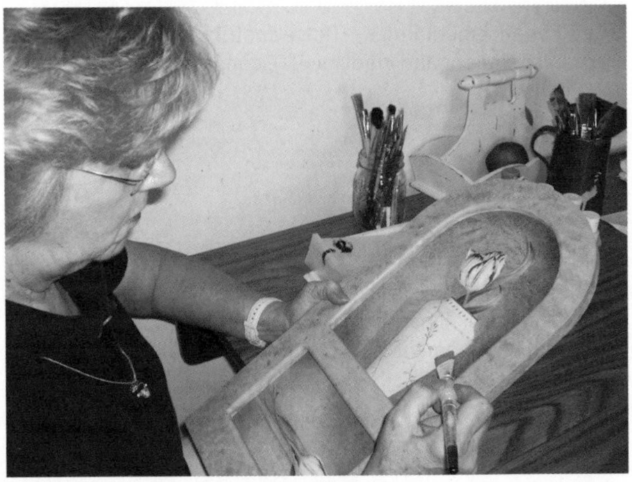

Figure 1-3 For this accomplished artist, painting a picture is a task of one of her self-advancement roles (worker). For another person for whom painting is a hobby, it would be classified as a task of a self-enhancement role (hobbyist).

equates to the OTPF areas of occupation of ADL and IADL (Table 1-1). Examples of roles in this domain are independent person, grandparent, parent, son, daughter, homemaker (Fig. 1-4), home maintainer (Fig. 1-5), exerciser, and caregiver.

Self-Advancement Roles

Self-advancement roles are those that draw the person into productive activities that add to the person's skills, possessions, or other betterment. This domain corre-

Table 1-1. The Domains of the Occupational Functioning Model and the Occupational Therapy Practice Framework

Occupational Functioning Model	Occupational Therapy Practice Framework
Competence and Satisfaction with Life Roles and Competence in the Performance of Tasks of Life Roles	***Areas of Occupation***
Self-Maintenance Roles—To maintain self, family, and home All basic activities of daily living (BADLs) and instrumental activities of daily living (IADLs) associated with self-care All IADLs associated with care of family All IADLs associated with care of home	ADL All personal care IADL Care of others Child rearing Care of pets Communication device use Community mobility Health management and maintenance Home establishment and management Meal preparation and cleanup Safety procedures and emergency responses Shopping Financial management
Self-Advancement Roles—These add to the person's skills, possessions, or other betterment. Examples are: Carpenter Tennis player Volunteer Student Shopper	Education Exploration of formal or informal educational needs and interests Participation in formal or informal education Work Employment interests and pursuits Employment seeking and acquisition Job performance Retirement preparation and adjustment Volunteer exploration and participation
Self-Enhancement Roles—These contribute to personal accomplishment and enjoyment. Examples are: Pianist Shopper Fisherman Tennis player	Play Play exploration and participation Leisure Leisure exploration and participation Social participation Family Peers, friends Community
Abilities and Skills	***Performance Skills***
Abilities and skills basic to interaction with objects and the physical environment Motor Sensory Cardiorespiratory	Motor skills—skills in moving and interacting with task objects and environment Posture: stabilizes, aligns, positions Mobility: walks, reaches, bends Coordination: coordinates, manipulates, flows

Table 1-1. *(continued)*

Abilities and skills basic to interaction with the physical, temporal, and cultural environments; to organizing life tasks; and to solving occupational problems Cognitive Perceptual Abilities and skills basic to interaction with the social and cultural environments Socioemotional	Strength and effort: moves, transports, lifts, calibrates, grips Energy: endures, paces Process skills—skills used in managing and modifying actions en route to the completion of daily life tasks Energy: paces, attends Knowledge: chooses, uses, handles, heeds, inquires Temporal organization: initiates, continues, sequences, terminates Organizing space and objects: searches/locates, gathers, organizes, restores, navigates Adaptation: notices/responds, accommodates, adjusts, benefits Communication/interaction skills—skills that convey intentions and coordinate social behavior with others Physicality: contacts, gazes, gestures, maneuvers, orients, postures Information exchange: articulates, asserts, asks, engages, expresses, modulates, shares, speaks, sustains Relations: collaborates, conforms, focuses, relates, respects
Competence in the Performance of Activities and Habits of the Tasks of Life Roles	***Performance Patterns***
Activities—occupations that are smaller units of tasks Habits—behavior patterns acquired by frequent repetition Sustain adaptive habits Release nonadaptive habits Develop new habits	Habits Useful habits Impoverished habits Dominating habits Routines—occupations with established sequences Roles—behaviors that serve a socially agreed upon function and have a code of accepted norms
The OFM has no comparable concept. Activity analysis is a basic process in therapy using the OFM (see Chapter 13).	***Activity Demands***
	Objects and their properties: tools, materials, equipment Space demands (physical): size, arrangement, temperature, etc. Sequence and timing: rules, sequences Required actions: motor, process, communicative skills Required body functions: see client factors Required body structures: organs, limbs
Developed Capacities	***Client Factors (body functions)***
Motor Sensory Cognitive Perceptual Socioemotional ***First-Level Capacities*** Sensorimotor Cognitive perceptual Socioemotional	Mental functions Global mental functions: consciousness, orientation, sleep, temperament and personality, energy and drive Specific mental functions: attention, memory, perception, thought, higher level cognition, mental functions of language and calculation, mental functions, psychomotor functions, emotional functions, experience of self and time Sensory functions and pain Seeing and related functions Hearing and vestibular functions

continued

Table 1-1. *(continued)*

Organic Substrate Central nervous system organization Integrity of skeleton, muscles, peripheral nerves, heart, lungs, skin	Other sensory function such as taste, smell, touch, and proprioception Pain Neuromusculoskeletal and movement-related functions Functions of joints and bones: mobility, stability Muscle power, tone, endurance Movement functions: motor reflexes, control of voluntary and involuntary movement, gait pattern Cardiovascular, hematological, immunological, and respiratory functions Voice and speech functions Digestive, metabolic, and endocrine functions Genitourinary and reproductive functions Skin and related structure functions
Organic Substrate—as above	***Body Structure: categories respond to body function categories (above)***
Environment and Context	***Context or Contexts***
Natural and built physical environment Requirements that tools and utensils pose for use Social relationships within family, peer group, community, therapeutic interaction Cultural and religious traditions Temporal demands of role tasks, activities and habits; balance of activity and rest	Cultural: ethnicity, family attitude, beliefs, values Physical: objects, built and natural environment Social: relationships with individuals, groups, organizations, systems Personal: age, gender, socioeconomic status Spiritual: essence of the person, higher purpose Temporal: stage of life, time of year, time of day, duration Virtual: communication occurs via air waves or computers with an absence of physical contact

sponds to the OTPF areas of occupation of work and education (Table 1-1) but extends to include the instrumental roles that enable work. Self-advancement roles correspond to the **participation** category of the ICF (Table 1-2). Examples of roles in the self-advancement role domain include worker (Figs. 1-2 and 1-6), student, intern, commuter, shopper, investor, manager, and voter.

Self-Enhancement Roles

Self-enhancement roles contribute to the person's sense of accomplishment and enjoyment (Figs. 1-3 and 1-7). This domain loosely corresponds to the OTPF areas of occupation of play, leisure, and social participation (Table 1-1) and fits within the ICF category of participation (Table 1-2). The OFM would classify activities listed by the OTPF in the education and work categories, namely informal education for personal interest and preparation for retirement, as self-enhancement activities. Examples of roles in this domain include hobbyist, friend, club member, religious participant, vacationer, golfer, moviegoer, and violinist.

Competency in Tasks of Life Roles

Roles consist of constellations of tasks. For example, the role of homemaker may include the tasks of food preparation (Fig. 1-4) and service, housecleaning, laundry, and decorating (Fig. 1-5). The tasks identified for the same role by different people may be different (Nelson & Payton, 1991; Trombly, 1993, 1995; Yerxa & Locker, 1990). The value ascribed to tasks varies among people of similar situations and may vary from what therapists consider important for patients. Because people have different values, each person must define his or her role by identifying the tasks that he or she believes are crucial to satisfactory engagement in that particular role. The therapist cannot

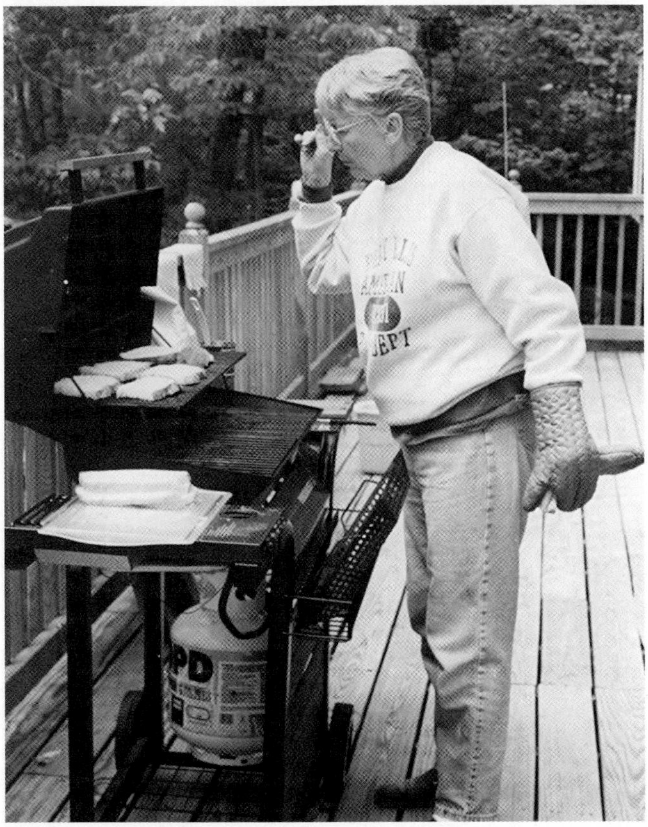

Figure 1-4 Self-maintenance role: homemaker; task: meal preparation; activity: grilling fish.

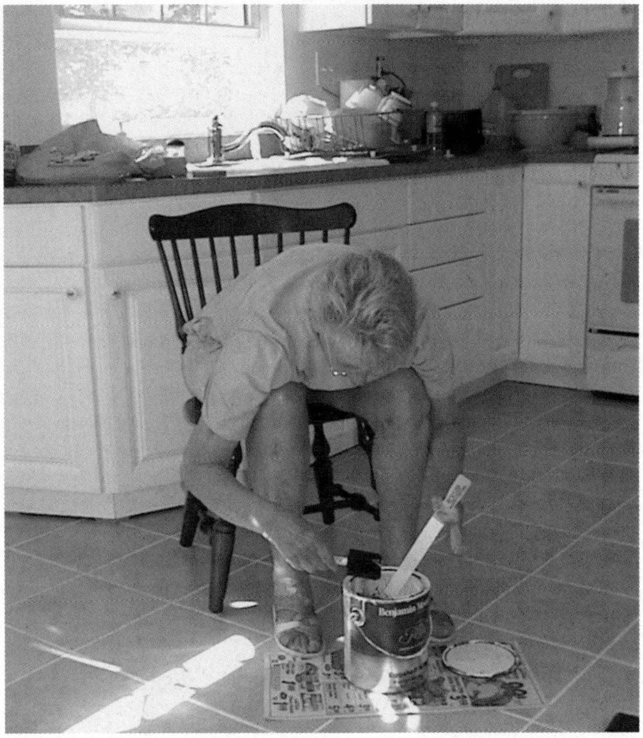

Figure 1-5 Self-maintenance role: home maintainer; task: painting the walls; activity: preparing the paint.

Table 1-2. Occupational Functioning Model Related to the World Health Organization (WHO) International Classification of Functioning (ICF) (WHO, 2001)

Occupational Functioning Model	WHO ICF Classification
Self-efficacy and self-esteem	**No corresponding concept**
Satisfaction with life roles • **Self-maintenance** • **Self-advancement** • **Self-enhancement**	**Participation:** involvement in a life situation; the nature and extent of a person's societal functioning; the interaction between the person having a disability and/or impairment with contextual factors
Competence **in tasks of life roles** Mastery of **activities and habits** Having **abilities and skills** that underlie mastery and competence	**Activity:** the execution of a task or action by an individual; the nature and extent of functioning at the level of the individual; all that a person does at any level of complexity
Developed capacities **First-level capacities** **Organic substrate**	**Bodily structure and psychological and physiological function**
Environment and context: the milieu in which occupation occurs, including natural and built physical environments, tools and utensils, social relationships, cultural situations, and time	**Contextual factors:** the complete background to a person's life and living, including both external environmental factors[a] and internal personal factors[b]. Environmental factors include all aspects of the physical, social, and attitudinal world

[a] Natural environment (weather or terrain), human-made environment (tools, furnishings, the built environment), social attitudes, customs, rules, practices and institutions, and other individuals.

[b] Age, race, gender, educational background, experiences, personality and character style, aptitudes, fitness, lifestyle, habits, upbringing, coping styles, social background, profession, and experience.

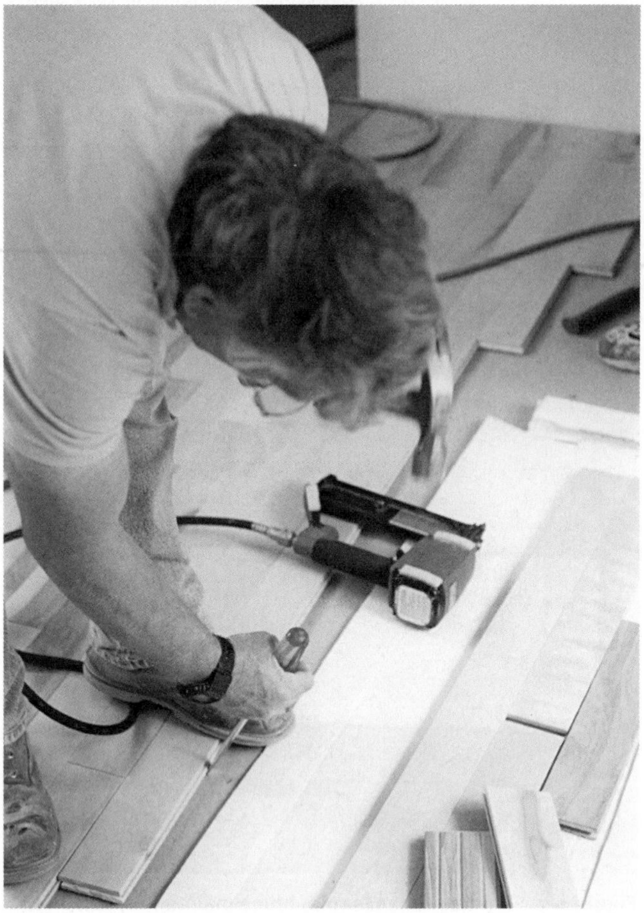

Figure 1-6 Self-advancement role: contractor; task: installing floor; activity: moving the wood into place.

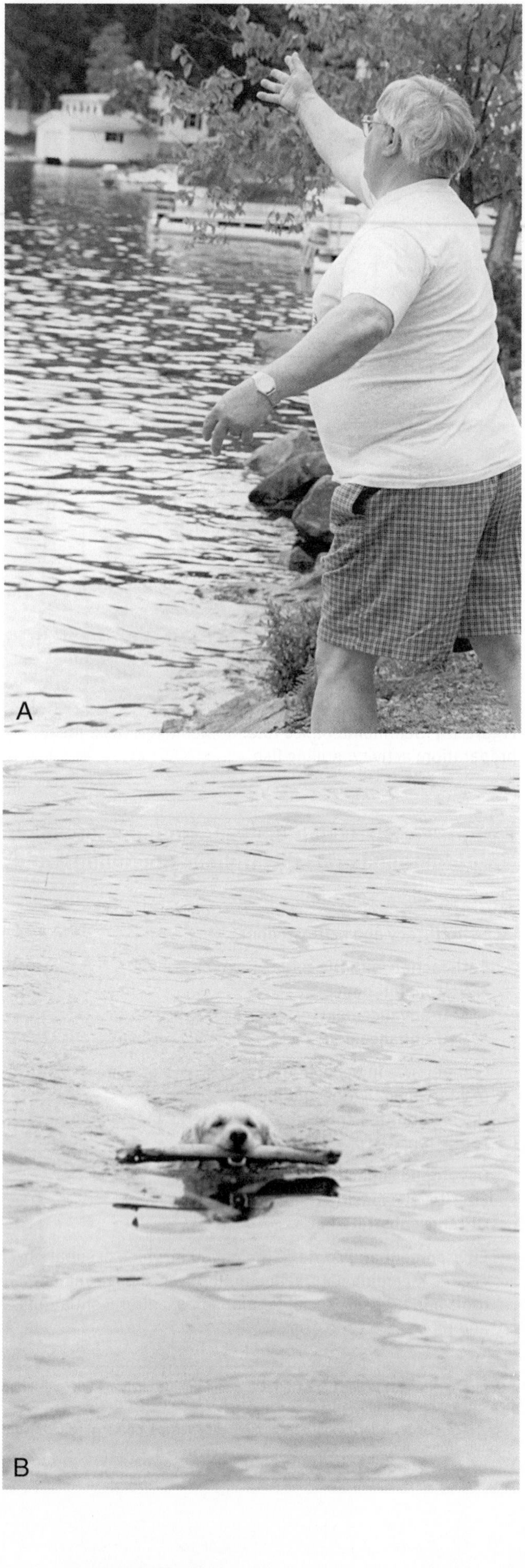

Figure 1-7 **A.** Self-enhancement role: pet owner; task: exercise dog; activity: throw the stick. **B.** Molly with stick.

assume that particular tasks are or are not important to a person's interpretation of a role.

Tasks consist of constellations of related activities and are therapeutically developed using occupation-as-end, that is, practicing the activities constituting the task in normal temporal order and environmental demand, with or without assistive technology as required.

Activities and Habits

Activities, in this model, are smaller units of goal-directed behavior that comprise tasks (Figs. 1-2 to 1-7). Activities bring together abilities and skills within a functional context. For example, one task of the gardener is pest control. Activities that make up this task include hanging lures, spreading granular insect killer, mixing and spraying liquids, and picking insects off plants. Furthermore, each of these activities consists of even smaller units of behavior, such as opening the package and pouring granular insect killer into a garden spreader. Some activities, such as picking insects off plants, require full attention. Others, called habits, do not. Habits are chains of action sequences that are so well learned that the person does not have to pay attention to do them under ordinary circumstances and in familiar contexts. Physical dysfunction disrupts habits, requiring attention to be paid to the simplest of activities of daily living. This adds to the fatigue experienced by many persons (Wallenbert & Jonsson, 2005). Occupational therapy seeks to help the person sustain or relearn adaptive habits, let go of habits that are no longer adaptive, and develop new habits, given the person's changed abilities and capacities. The OTPF term equivalent to habits is ***performance patterns***.

Activities and habits are learned using occupation-as-end, that is, "task-specific training." In task-specific training, functional and meaningful activities are practiced over and over using assistive technology, adaptive methods, or adapted environment to enable performance, if necessary. See Chapter 13 for a more complete discussion of the therapeutic use of occupation-as-end.

Abilities and Skills

Activities depend on more basic abilities (Clark, Czaja, & Weber, 1990; Fleishman, 1972; Fleishman & Quaintance, 1984; Kielhofner, 1997). A person with a great number of highly developed abilities can become proficient at a greater variety of activities. An **ability** is a general trait, such as muscle strength or memory, that individuals bring with them to a new task (Fleishman, 1972). The OFM identifies six categories of abilities and skills: motor, sensory, cognitive, perceptual, socioemotional, and cardiorespiratory. For example, remembering, solving problems, and paying attention are some of the cognitive abilities that underlie successful activity accomplishment. Actions such as reaching, stooping, grasping, pinching, manipulating, pulling, and pushing are motor abilities that underlie many activities. The OTPF terms these **performance skills** and specifies three spheres: motor, process, and communication/interaction.

In the OFM, abilities are seen as a combination of endowed talents and acquired skills. A skill is the ability to achieve a goal under a wide variety of conditions with a degree of consistency and economy (Higgins, 1991). To accomplish the activity of hanging lures in the previous example of the gardener, the person needs certain abilities, such as coordination, dexterity, and ability to follow directions. The person also needs to be able to translate these endowed talents into the skilled actions required to hang the lures. Carefully analyzed occupation-as-means is used to develop deficient abilities and skills. In the process of repeatedly accomplishing occupations that demand greater levels of the deficient ability or skill, in varying contexts, the patient gains greater levels of that ability or skill. By varying the context, the therapist encourages more robust learning. See Chapter 13 for a more complete discussion of the therapeutic use of occupation-as-means.

? CLINICAL REASONING IN OCCUPATIONAL THERAPY PRACTICE

Occupational Self-Analysis

Occupational therapists evaluate a patient's occupational profile. Practice this skill by analyzing your own occupational profile. The following directions are one way to determine the profile.

1. Make an occupational diary by listing awake hours along the left side of a piece of 11×8.5 inch paper and listing the days of the week across the top.
2. Fill in activities or tasks you do hour by hour in a typical week.
3. Classify these into role categories: self-maintenance, self-advancement, or self-enhancement.
4. Calculate what percentage of time you engaged in these role categories (hours spent in one role category/total awake hours $\times$ 100%).
5. Make another chart. Choose a favorite role. What tasks make up this role for you? Are the tasks the same as those of your classmates who chose the same role?
6. Choose the key task from your answer to Question 5. What activities comprise this task?
7. Choose one activity from your answer to Question 6. What abilities are needed to do this activity?
8. What type of impairments would prevent you from doing the activity as you usually do it?
9. What type of environmental or contextual barriers would prevent or hamper you from doing the activity?

Developed Capacities

Developed capacities reflect the organization of first-level capacities into more mature, less reflexive, and more voluntary responses. For example, to support dexterity, an ability, a person needs independent use of fingers, graded release, and pinch, which are developed capacities that derive from reflexive grasp and automatic release (first-level capacities). This organization is normally acquired through maturation. In therapy, occupation-as-means is used to develop these capacities. Therapeutic demands for gradually more mature and varied responses are made through repeated opportunities to engage in selected occupations. The equivalent OTPF term is client factors, although these appear to include not only the developed capacities of the OFM, but also the first-level capacities and organic substrate of the OFM.

First-Level Capacities

First-level capacities are the functional foundation for movement, cognition, perception, and emotional life based on the integrity of the organic substrate. In the motor domain, first-level capacities are reflex-based motor responses that reflect the organization of primary visual, sensory, and motor systems. Examples include reflexive grasp, reflexive release, primitive reaching, kicking, and stepping. They are the subroutines that Bruner (1973) described as underlying development of all voluntary movement. The ability to recognize a connection between an instrumental, nonreflexive response given consistently within a particular perceptual situation is a first-level capacity of cognition and perception. The fascination of babies with human faces is a first-level capacity of the socioemotional domain.

Organic Substrate

Organic substrate is the structural and physiological foundation for movement, cognition, perception, and emotions, including the primordial central nervous system (CNS) organization in the neonate; the CNS organization that is spared or recovers spontaneously after injury or illness; and the integrity of the skeleton, muscles, sensory and motor nerves, heart, lungs, and skin. If the organic substrate is not present, therapy cannot generate it. If it exists at all, therapy attempts to develop it into first-level capacities through techniques classified as **augmented maturation** (see Chapter 26).

Environment and Context

The words *environment* and *context* are often used interchangeably. In current health care literature, the term *context* is used to encompass all that surrounds and influences any aspect of human functioning, including the physical environment as well as social, personal, and cultural contexts. *Environment* is defined as the complex of external factors, circumstances, objects, and social and cultural beliefs and practices that influence the life of an individual. Context in the OTPF refers to cultural, physical, social, personal, spiritual, temporal, and virtual aspects of living.

Similar to the OTPF, the OFM model assumes that context and environment surround and permeate all levels of the occupational functioning hierarchy. But the OFM distinguishes between the greater influence of context and environment at the higher levels of the hierarchy and the lesser influence at the lower levels. At the lower levels, the immediate physical and personal contexts influence the actions. For example, organization of a reaching movement was shown to differ when actual, natural objects and utensils were used versus when simulated objects were used (Ma, Trombly, & Robinson-Podolski, 1999; Wu et al., 1998). Cultural and social contexts pertain less to this level. At the higher levels of activities, tasks, and roles, however, all aspects of context—personal, social, cultural, temporal, and physical—interact with the person's abilities to yield occupational functioning for the particular person. Figure 1-1 depicts these ideas within the limitations of two-dimensional representation. Chapters 10 and 35 discuss the influence of personal, social, and cultural contexts on occupational functioning, and Chapters 11 and 36 discuss the influence of physical context.

When the challenges of the environment exceed the capabilities of a person, that person is said to be disabled (Institute of Medicine, 1997). A person with impaired abilities and capacities, however, may be able to accomplish activities and tasks of his or her roles if the environment is adapted to enable that. Therefore, occupational therapy treatment may focus on changing the environment or context rather than on remediating the person's impaired abilities or capacities.

THE PROCESS OF OCCUPATIONAL THERAPY FOR PERSONS WITH PHYSICAL DYSFUNCTION

The process of occupational therapy follows the universal plan for problem solving: identify the problem, intervene, and evaluate the result. The occupational therapist, however, focuses only on problems related to the person's occupational life. What a person needs to do, wants to do, and can do are identified. Discrepancy between what the person needs or wants to do and what he or she can do identifies the problem. The occupational therapist then uses various occupational, adaptive, and adjunctive therapies to intervene. The processes of the OFM and the OTPF are similar (Table 1-3). A more thorough discussion of the OFM process follows.

Table 1-3. The Process of Occupational Therapy

Process	OFM	OTPF (AOTA, 2002)
Goal of Therapy	Satisfactorily engage in self-identified, important life roles through which the person gains a sense of self-efficacy and self-esteem	Engagement in occupation to support participation
Evaluation to Identify the Problem(s)	Top down assessment Identify roles, tasks, and activities the person wants to do or needs to do Observe and analyze the person's performance within usual context; identify inadequate performance Identify impaired abilities or capacities that contribute to inadequate performance and assess level of impairment Identify environmental or contextual enablers or hindrances	Do an occupational profile to understand the client's occupational history, patterns of daily living, interests, values, needs, problems with performance, and priorities Do an analysis of occupational performance by observation within context to specifically identify client's assets and problems Identify targeted outcomes
Plan Intervention	Plan in collaboration with the person or family to determine whether the person wants to engage in either: Remediation of impaired abilities or capacities to enhance overall performance, or Restoration of occupational performance through relearning and/or adaptation of method or environment Establish short-term goals that directly relate to the long-term goal of successful role functioning identified by the patient Select interventions that have evidence for effectiveness for the immediate goal	Develop plan with the client to guide action Base therapy on theories, frames of reference, and evidence
Implement the Intervention	Utilize therapeutic mechanisms Occupation Occupation-as-end to restore occupational functioning Occupation-as-means to optimize abilities or capacities Therapeutic rapport Learning/relearning Utilize adjunctive therapies to facilitate performance Modify contexts and environments to facilitate performance	Act to influence and support improved client performance of targeted outcomes Monitor and document client's response Review the progress toward targeted outcomes and the intervention plan
Evaluate the Result	Determine whether the targeted outcomes were achieved Determine whether the person was satisfied with his or her achievement Plan for future therapy or referral	Determine success in achieving targeted outcomes Plan future action with client Evaluate the program

Assessment

The hierarchical organization of the OFM indicates that higher level occupational functioning is established on a foundation of abilities and capacities. Assessment *always* follows a top-down approach. That is, the therapist determines what roles and tasks the person was responsible for in life before the accident or disease and what the person is expected to be and wants to be responsible for in post-rehabilitation life, including the context in which the person typically engaged in these valued roles and tasks (Coster, 1998; Mathiowetz, 1993; Mayer, Keating, & Rapp, 1986; Trombly, 1993, 1995). The *Role Checklist* (Barris, Oakley, & Kielhofner, 1988; Oakley et al., 1986), the *Canadian Occupational Performance Measure* (*COPM*) (Carswell et al., 2004; Law et al., 1998), and the *Client-Oriented Role Evaluation* (*CORE*) (Toal-Sullivan & Henderson, 2004) are assessments the therapist may use to gather this information. The therapist may also measure the patient's sense of self-efficacy concerning ability to do the tasks required to fulfill particular roles by having the patient assign a number on a visual analog scale that ranges from 0 (not at all confident) to 10 (absolutely certain) for each major task that defines a specific role (Gill et al., 1994). For example, "on this scale from 0 to 10, how confident are you that you can prepare your own lunch without help?" One such assessment is the *Self-Efficacy for Functional Activities* (*SEFA*) *Scale* (Resnick, 1999).

When evaluating a patient's competence to accomplish the roles he or she identified as important, the therapist observes the patient attempting to do the tasks and activities of those roles in the most familiar context. The *Assessment of Motor and Process Skills* (*AMPS*) (Fisher, 2003), the *Klein-Bell ADL Scale* (Klein & Bell, 1982), and the *Barthel Index* (Mahoney & Barthel, 1965; Tennant, Geddes, & Chamberlain, 1996) are examples of observational assessments of tasks and activities. Using an assessment that structures observation of performance and having knowledge of the probabilities established by the diagnosis and age of the person, the therapist detects which of the myriad abilities and capacities assumed to be related to accomplishment of these activities are impaired (the process of **activity analysis** applied to assessment; see Chapter 13) and assesses these abilities and capacities more directly. For example, if the patient's goal is to shave with an electric razor but he appears to lack the grasp strength and endurance to do so, strength and endurance are assessed according to the procedures described in Chapter 5. A person whose abilities and capacities are found deficient may be treated to optimize them, allowing not only shaving but other occupations.

Also to be considered as part of the assessment is whether the environment enables or hinders occupational functioning. Assessments of the home environment have been developed (e.g., *Safety Assessment of Function and the Environment for Rehabilitation* [*SAFER*] [Chui et al., 2002] and *Home Occupational-Environmental Assessment* [*HOEA*] [Baum & Edwards, 1998]), but assessments of other environments have not yet been developed (Letts, Baum, & Perlmutter, 2003). To assess the effects of other physical and social environments typical for the patient on occupational performance, the occupational therapist needs to observe performance under those conditions.

Treatment

Treatment may focus on changing the environment, changing the impaired skills and abilities of the person, or teaching compensatory ways to accomplish activities and tasks. Treatment to improve occupational functioning, then, may start toward the bottom of the OFM hierarchy, focusing on optimizing abilities and capacities; or it may start higher, at the activity level of the hierarchy, focusing on restoring competence in doing the activities and tasks of valued roles that the patient has identified as concerns; or it may start peripheral to the person, focusing on modifying the context or environment. The starting point should acknowledge the problem that the patient has identified as an immediate concern, although treatment may not actually start there. For example, if the patient identified resuming fishing as the goal, the therapist may choose to teach adaptive methods to enable that. If, however, in the experience of the therapist it would be more effective to start treatment by regaining finger dexterity to enable various activities related to fishing (e.g., baiting the hook and removing the fish from the line), the therapist must help the patient understand how treatment of this lower-level ability addresses the stated concern at the task level. In addition, the therapist must ensure carryover of any gained dexterity to the fishing task. Optimizing impaired abilities and capacities is accomplished through remedial therapy in which a change in physiological structure, function, or organization is sought through using occupation-as-means. If remediation of deficit abilities or capacities does not restore occupational functioning, or if economic constraints prevent such thorough treatment, or if the patient is not committed to the extensive work required to recover abilities and capacities, a degree of competence can be restored using **adaptive therapy**. Adaptive therapy seeks to find and promote a balance among the person's goals and environmental demands and his or her current capacities and abilities (Thoren-Jonsson, Moller, & Grimby, 1999). In this type of therapy, the method of doing an activity may be modified, assistive technology may be used to enable completion of the activity, and/or the physical or social environments may be modified. The person may be counseled to reassess the need to accomplish a particularly difficult activity alone and opt to employ another to do it.

Optimizing Abilities and Capacities

It is believed that remediating impaired sensorimotor, cognitive, perceptual, and emotional capacities and abilities to as high a level as a person's organic substrate allows will enable versatile performance of activities. Versatile performance allows the person to adjust to changes in the social and physical environments, whereas if a person learns only one compensatory response, adaptation to new situations is less likely. As in the typical development of these capacities and abilities, therapy engages the patient in circumscribed encounters with the environment using occupation-as-means. Using the example of the man who wanted to shave, the therapist might start treatment by providing a cuff to hold the razor to eliminate the need for grasp (adaptive therapy) and let the patient shave as much as he could. Then the occupational therapist would finish the activity. Day by day, the patient's endurance for shaving would increase, and he would do more of the task on his own (occupation used as a means of remediation). Concurrently, the therapist would engage the patient in other activities that require grasp strength until the patient was able to hold the razor.

Occupation-as-means, that is, activities that provide stretch of soft tissues, active or passive movement to preserve and restore full range of motion, resistance and other stress to strengthen weak muscles, or graduated, increasing levels of aerobic exercise to improve endurance, is used to optimize motor abilities and capacities. The evaluation and intervention techniques for optimizing abilities and capacities are described in Chapters 5, 13, and 21; adjunctive therapies that support this approach are discussed in Chapters 16 and 20; and the application of the approach, in combination with complementary approaches, is illustrated in Chapters 41 to 47. When impairment of the CNS results in the inability to move voluntarily to effect a desired change in the environment, a therapist may use sensory input and developmental postures (augmented maturation) to facilitate change in sensorimotor organization. Or the therapist may use motor learning principles to bring about change in voluntary movement behavior and thereby improve the overall functioning of the client. Two approaches apply motor learning principles and methods to treatment of persons with CNS impairment. These are the Carr and Shepherd *Motor Relearning Programme for Stroke* (1983, 1987) (see Chapter 23) and the task-oriented approach described by Horak (1991) and Bass Haugen, Mathiowetz, and Flinn (see Chapter 22). Both approaches emphasize motor performance using functional tasks, include remediation of performance components and modification of the environment to improve task performance, and stress practice that fits the nature of the task. Both approaches heed the research findings on the effect of context on the organization of movement, which indicate that practicing a skill under simplified, non-context-specific conditions is different from practicing with an actual object in a context-specific situation (Mathiowetz & Wade, 1995; Trombly & Wu, 1999; Wu et al., 1998). Other approaches use techniques such as controlled sensory input to affect motor output and ontogenetic or recovery-based developmental postures or patterns for both assessment and treatment. The approaches share the idea of the importance of the need for repetition. They emphasize the development of basic movements and postures and assume that when movement is "normalized," skilled movement and occupational performance will occur. The approaches of Bobath, Brunnstrom, Rood, and PNF (proprioceptive neuromuscular facilitation) are described in Chapters 24, 25, and 26.

Restoring Competence

Restoration of occupational functioning depends on developing competence in the valued tasks and activities of the patient's life roles. Competence in tasks and activities is synthesized through successful engagement with the environment. Occupational therapists are skilled in developing graduated encounters with objects and the surrounding physical and social environments to promote successful performance. They are also expert in teaching compensatory methods to accomplish activities. Some therapists use this approach exclusively (Mayer, Keating, & Rapp, 1986). Others believe that first optimizing the impaired abilities and capacities requires less compensation and produces more versatility of performance. There is no research to support one point of view over the other.

When activity, task, and role levels of the OFM are dysfunctional, treatment may aim at making people as independent as possible in spite of any residual impairment. If people must live with an impairment that decreases independent functioning, the occupational therapist will concentrate on helping them find ways to compensate by reorganizing activity patterns or adapting techniques, equipment, or the environment. The goal is independence. People are considered independent when they perform tasks for themselves using assistive equipment, alternative methods, or adapted environments, as required, or when they appropriately oversee completion of activities by others on their own behalf (Moyers, 1999).

Interventions to restore competence in tasks and activities are compensatory. They focus on environmental or contextual modification and on teaching physical, cognitive, and emotional adaptation. The therapist teaches the patient to recognize and use remaining abilities in adapted ways and teaches the principles and concepts of adapted methods so that the person can become an independent problem solver. Therapeutic mechanisms of change include occupation-as-end, teaching-learning, and therapeutic rapport. The assessment and treatment procedures for restoring role performance are described in Chapters 4, 10–15, 18, 19, and 30–37.

CASE EXAMPLE

Application of the OFM to a Patient with Spinal Cord Injury

Occupational Therapy Process	Mr. J is a patient with spinal cord injury (see Chapter 43 for a description of this condition, including special circumstances such as tenodesis grasp).	Clinical Reasoning—Examples of Therapist's Internal Dialogue
Obtain Information About the Patient	Diagnosis: fracture/dislocation of C 6–7 of his spine in a diving accident. Status post cervical fusion and laminectomy; medically stable. He exhibits C6 functional level.	He can become independent in self-care and other tasks and activities important to him if he's willing to work hard.
	Interview: Mr. J is 24 years old, a college graduate, who lives with his parents in a second-floor apartment in a small city. He has four older siblings who are all married. He has many friends.	He will have to relocate to a first-floor apartment or to a building with an elevator. This needs to be discussed soon and a referral made to Social Services. His sociability should make developing rapport with him easy.
Evaluation to Identify the Problem(s)	Interview: In addition to his role as independent person, Mr. J identified self-advancement and self-enhancement roles of worker and sportsman.	Mr. J values his roles as independent person, worker, friend, and sportsman. He appears ready to work to regain those roles.
	Mr. J's worker role was that of computer programmer. The company is holding his job for him. Keyboarding is the major physical task of this role.	Although he cannot do keyboarding now because of paralysis of his fingers, he should be able to resume his job with adaptations and reasonable accommodations. But he also needs to regain ADL independence and commuter activities and skills to do so.
	Swimmer, basketball player, camper, and friend are his major self-enhancement roles. The family is supportive, but they expect Mr. J. to be independent in self-care, with the prospect of resuming work, at discharge.	Because of the paralysis, he will need to learn adaptive methods of resuming his sports interests.
	Assessment: The therapist observed Mr. J's attempts to accomplish the tasks and activities associated with the independent person role and found him dependent in all basic self-care. The therapist noted that he was unable to move his lower limbs, that his upper extremities were weak, and that he was unable to grasp.	There is no need to evaluate any other activities until he can do basic self-care activities. It will only be frustrating for him. I am going to introduce him to Mr. L who has a similar disability and who is nearing discharge after gaining many skills and resuming several of his roles. It will let Mr. J see the possibilities for recovery of his own roles.

Evaluation to Identify the Problems (cont'd)	She measured Mr. J's strength and found that the proximal upper extremity musculature rated 4 to 5, with the exception of the triceps, which graded 2 (see Table 5-1, which describes muscle strength grading). Wrist extensors graded 3+ on the left and 4− on the right; wrist flexors and finger and thumb muscles graded 0 bilaterally.	He will need to learn adaptive ischial pressure relief methods and how to use tenodesis grasp.
Implement Intervention	During occupational therapy, Mr. J engaged in • occupation-as-means to remediate the weakness of his upper arms and wrists; • occupation-as-end and adaptive therapy to learn adaptive ways to accomplish important tasks and activities and to overcome environmental barriers; • group therapy for social, emotional, and practical problem solving; members are other persons with similar activity limitations.	I am going to use camping activities and simulated basketball shooting among other activities in his program to strengthen his upper extremities, especially his wrist extensors. I need to determine his openness to using adaptive devices. Relearning basic ADL may be embarrassing for him and may precipitate a depression. I need to pay attention to his emotional responses and discuss this with him. He will benefit from others' problem-solving techniques and stories of adjustment challenges and achievements. His stories will help others.
Evaluate the Result	Because of paralysis of his trunk and lower extremities, Mr. J is required to use a wheelchair, which was adapted to allow propulsion without grasp.	Mr. J was successfully rehabilitated.
	Mr. J uses gravity, momentum, and leverage to move his body in the wheelchair and on the bed.	
	The proximal upper extremity musculature recovered to normal strength.	
	Because the triceps remained at less than functional strength, he could not elevate himself off the wheelchair cushion. He learned an adaptive method of relieving ischial pressure to maintain skin integrity.	This is so important. I am glad I sent a picture sheet on adapted pressure-relief methods home with him as a reminder.
	Mr. J's wrist strength improved to 4+ bilaterally, which allowed a functional tenodesis grasp.	
	Mr. J showers using a bath bench and handheld shower head, which he holds using tenodesis grasp.	
	Has learned to manage his bowel and bladder programs.	
	Is able to dress independently using adaptive methods and devices.	His time to do this will improve with practice.

Evaluate the Result (cont'd)	He keyboards using universal cuffs with typing sticks tipped with rubber ends. His computer is adapted to allow one-key depression for all operations.	His speed will increase with practice.
	He plans on resuming work part time (noon to 4 pm).	This schedule will allow enough time for morning care.
	He plans on joining the local wheelchair basketball team	Go, Mr. J!

CLINICAL REASONING IN OCCUPATIONAL THERAPY PRACTICE

Treatment Planning for Mr. J

Mr. J has extensive impairments that prevent him from engaging in the activities and tasks of his valued roles. The occupational therapist, in conjunction with Mr. J, must decide what approach to take in treatment. What are the pros and cons of concentrating therapeutic intervention on restoration of activities, tasks, and roles versus remediation of capacities and abilities? From this deliberation, state a goal your treatment might be directed toward. Which treatments would you use to achieve that goal?

SUMMARY REVIEW QUESTIONS

1. Describe the Occupational Functioning Model (OFM).
2. In what ways are the OFM and the Occupational Therapy Practice Framework (OTPF) similar?
3. What is the overall goal of occupational therapy for persons with occupational dysfunction due to physical impairments according to the OFM? According to the OTPF?
4. Using the OFM as your model of practice, what would you assess first in a patient with stroke: level of spasticity of the upper extremity, ADL, or role history and expectations?
5. Define *ability* and *developed capacity*. Give an example of each. To what levels of the OTPF and the ICF do these correspond?
6. Define *task* and *activity*. Give an example of each. To what levels of the OTPF and the ICF do these correspond?
7. What distinguishes occupation-as-means from occupation-as-end?

ACKNOWLEDGEMENT

I am indebted to my co-editor, Mary Vining Radomski, for her contributions to this chapter, and to my family and friends for posing for the photographs.

References

American Occupational Therapy Association [AOTA]. (2002). Occupational therapy practice framework: Domain and process. *American Journal of Occupational Therapy, 56,* 609–639.

Bandura, A. (1977). Self-efficacy: Toward a unifying theory of behavior change. *Psychological Review, 84,* 191–215.

Bandura, A. (1997). *Self-efficacy*. New York: W. H. Freeman.

Barris, R., Oakley, F., & Kielhofner, G. (1988). The Role Checklist. In B. J. Hemphill (Ed.), *Mental health assessment in occupational therapy* (pp. 73–91). Thorofare, NJ: Slack.

Baum, C. M., & Edwards, D. F. (1998). *Guide for the Home Occupational-Environmental Assessment*. St. Louis, MO: Washington University Program in Occupational Therapy.

Bruner, J. (1973). Organization of early skilled action. *Child Development, 44,* 1–11.

Carr, J. H., & Shepherd, R. B. (1983). *Motor relearning programme for stroke*. Rockville, MD: Aspen.

Carr, J. H., & Shepherd, R. B. (1987). *Motor relearning programme for stroke* (2nd ed.). Rockville, MD: Aspen.

Carswell, A., McColl, M. A., Baptiste, S., Law, M., Polatajko, H., & Pollock, N. (2004). The Canadian Occupational Performance Measure: A research and clinical literature review. *Canadian Journal of Occupational Therapy, 71,* 210–222.

Christiansen, C. H. (1999). The 1999 Eleanor Clarke Slagle Lecture: Defining lives: Occupation as identity: An essay on competence, coherence, and the creation of meaning. *American Journal of Occupational Therapy, 53,* 547–558.

Chui, T., Oliver, R., Marshall, L., & Letts, L. (2002). *Safety Assessment of Function and the Environment for Rehabilitation Tool Manual*. Toronto, Ontario, Canada: COTA Comprehensive Rehabilitation and Mental health Services.

Clark, M. C., Czaja, S. J., & Weber, R. A. (1990). Older adults and daily living task profiles. *Human Factors, 32,* 537–549.

Coster, W. (1998). Occupation-centered assessment of children. *American Journal of Occupational Therapy, 52,* 337–344.

Dagfinrud, H., Kjeken, I., Mowinckel, P., Hagen, K. B., & Kvien, T. K. (2005). Impact of functional impairment in ankylosing spondylitis:

Impairment, activity limitation, and participation restrictions. *Journal of Rheumatology, 32,* 516–523.

Dijkers, M. (1997). Quality of life after spinal cord injury: A meta-analysis of the effects of disablement components. *Spinal Cord, 35,* 829–840.

Dijkers, M. P. J. M. (1999). Correlates of life satisfaction among persons with spinal cord injury. *Archives of Physical Medicine and Rehabilitation, 80,* 867–876.

Filiatrault, J., Arsenault, A. B., Dutil, E. M., & Bourbonnais, D. (1991). Motor function and activities of daily living assessments: A study of three tests for persons with hemiplegia. *American Journal of Occupational Therapy, 45,* 806–810.

Fisher, A. G. (1998). Uniting practice and theory in an occupational framework. *American Journal of Occupational Therapy, 52,* 509–521.

Fisher, A. G. (2003). *Assessment of Motor and Process Skills: Development, Standardization, and Administration Manual* (5th ed.). Fort Collins, CO: Three Star Press.

Fleishman, E. A. (1972). On the relation between ability, learning, and human performance. *American Psychologist, 27,* 1017–1032.

Fleishman, E. A., & Quaintance, M. K. (1984). *Taxonomies of human performance.* New York: Academic Press.

Fugl-Meyer, A. R., Jaasko, L., Leyman, I., Olsson, S., & Steglind, S. (1975). The post stroke hemiplegic patient: 1. A method for evaluation of physical performance. *Scandinavian Journal of Rehabilitation Medicine, 7,* 13–31.

Gage, M., Noh, S., Polatajko, H. J., & Kaspar, V. (1994). Measuring perceived self-efficacy in occupational therapy. *American Journal of Occupational Therapy, 48,* 783–790.

Gage, M., & Polatajko, H. (1994). Enhancing occupational performance through an understanding of perceived self-efficacy. *American Journal of Occupational Therapy, 48,* 452–461.

Geertzen, J. H. B., Dijkstra, P. U., van Sonderen, E. L. P., Groothoff, J. W., ten Duis, H. J., & Eisma, W. H. (1998). Relationship between impairments, disability and handicap in reflex sympathetic dystrophy patients: A long-term follow-up study. *Clinical Rehabilitation, 12,* 402–412.

Gill, D. L., Kelley, B. C., Williams, K., & Martin, J. J. (1994). The relationship of self-efficacy and perceived well-being to physical activity and stair climbing in older adults. *Research Quarterly for Exercise and Sport, 65,* 367–371.

Hallett, J. D., Zasler, N. D., Maurer, P., & Cash, S. (1994). Role change after traumatic brain injury in adults. *American Journal of Occupational Therapy, 48,* 241–246.

Higgins, S. (1991). Motor skill acquisition. *Physical Therapy, 71,* 123–139.

Horak, F. B. (1991). Assumptions underlying motor control for neurologic rehabilitation. In M. Lister (Ed.), *Contemporary management of motor control problems. Proceedings of the II STEP Conference* (pp. 11–27). Alexandria, VA: The Foundation for Physical Therapy.

Institute of Medicine. (1997). *Enabling America: Assessing the role of rehabilitation science and engineering.* Washington, DC: National Academy Press.

Jebsen, R. H., Taylor, N., Trieschmann, R., Trotter, M., & Howard, L. (1969). An objective and standardized test of hand function. *Archives of Physical Medicine & Rehabilitation, 50,* 311–319.

Kielhofner, G. (1997). *Conceptual foundations of occupational therapy* (2nd ed.). Philadelphia: F. A. Davis.

Klein, R. M., & Bell, B. (1982). Self-care skills: Behavioral measurement with Klein-Bell ADL Scale. *Archives of Physical Medicine & Rehabilitation, 63,* 335–338.

Law, M., Baptiste, S., Carswell, A., McColl, M., Polatajko, H., & Pollack, N. (1998). *Canadian Occupational Performance Measure* (3rd ed.). Ottawa, Ontario, Canada: CAOT.

Letts, L., Baum, C., & Perlmutter, M. (2003). Person-environment-occupation assessment with older adults. *OT Practice, 8,* 27–34.

Lynch, K. B., & Bridle, M. J. (1989). Validity of the Jebsen-Taylor Hand Function Test in predicting activities of daily living. *Occupational Therapy Journal of Research, 9,* 316–318.

Ma, H.-I., Trombly, C. A., & Robinson-Podolski, C. (1999). The effect of context on skill acquisition and transfer. *American Journal of Occupational Therapy, 53,* 138–144.

Mahoney, F. I., & Barthel, D. W. (1965). Functional evaluation: The Barthel Index. *Maryland State Medical Journal, 14,* 61–65.

Mathiowetz, V. (1993). Role of physical performance component evaluations in occupational therapy functional assessment. *American Journal of Occupational Therapy, 47,* 225–230.

Mathiowetz, V., & Wade, M. G. (1995). Task constraints and functional motor performance of individuals with and without multiple sclerosis. *Ecological Psychology, 7,* 99–123.

Mayer, N. H., Keating, D. J., & Rapp, D. (1986). Skills, routines, and activity patterns of daily living: A functional nested approach. In B. Uzzell & Y. Gross (Eds.), *Clinical neuropsychology of intervention* (pp. 205–222). Boston: Martinus Nijhoff.

Mish, F. C. (Ed.). (2004). *The Merriam-Webster dictionary.* Springfield, MA: Merriam-Webster.

Mocellin, G. (1992). An overview of occupational therapy in the context of the American influence on the profession: Part 2. *British Journal of Occupational Therapy, 55,* 55–60.

Moyers, P. (1999). The guide to occupational therapy practice. *American Journal of Occupational Therapy, 53,* 247–322.

Nelson, C. E., & Payton, O. D. (1991). The issue is: A system for involving patients in program planning. *American Journal of Occupational Therapy, 45,* 753–755.

Oakley, F., Kielhofner, G., Barris, R., & Reichler, R. (1986). The Role Checklist: Development and empirical assessment of reliability. *Occupational Therapy Journal of Research, 6,* 157–170.

Pendlebury, S. T., Blamire, A. M., Lee, M. A., Styles, P., & Matthews, P. M. (1999). Axonal injury in the internal capsule correlates with motor impairment after stroke. *Stroke, 30,* 956–962.

Radomski, M. V. (2000). Self-efficacy: Improving occupational therapy outcomes by helping patients say "I can." [American Occupational Therapy Association] *Physical Disabilities Special Interest Section Quarterly, 23,* 1–3.

Reilly, M. (1962). Occupational therapy can be one of the great ideas of 20th century medicine. *American Journal of Occupational Therapy, 16,* 1–9.

Resnik, B. (1998). Efficacy beliefs in geriatric rehabilitation. *Journal of Gerontological Nursing, 24,* 34–44.

Resnick, B. (1999). Reliability and validity testing of the Self-Efficacy for Functional Activities Scale. *Journal of Nursing Measurement, 7,* 5–20.

Robinson-Smith, G., Johnston, M. V., & Allen, J. (2000). Self-care self-efficacy, quality of life, and depression. *Archives of Physical Medicine and Rehabilitation, 81,* 460–464.

Rogers, R. W. (1983). Cognitive and psychological processes in fear appeals and attitude change: A revised theory of protection motivation. In J. T. Cacioppo, R. E. Petty, & D. Shapiro (Eds.), *Social psychophysiology* (pp. 153–176). New York: Guilford.

Rogers, J. C., & Holm, M. B. (1994). Accepting the challenge of outcome research: Examining the effectiveness of occupational therapy practice. *American Journal of Occupational Therapy, 48,* 871–876.

Rondinelli, R. D., Dunn, W., Hassanein, K. M., Keesling, C. A., Meredith, S. C., Schulz, T. L., & Lawrence, N. J. (1997). A simulation of hand impairments: Effects on upper extremity function and implications toward medical impairment rating and disability determination. *Archives of Physical Medicine and Rehabilitation, 78,* 1358–1363.

Sveen, U., Bautz-Holter, E., Sødring, K. M., Wyller, T. B., & Laake, K. (1999). Association between impairments, self-care ability and social activities 1 year after stroke. *Disability and Rehabilitation, 21,* 372–377.

Tennant, A., Geddes, J. M. L., & Chamberlain, M. A. (1996). The Barthel Index: An ordinal or interval measure? *Clinical Rehabilitation, 10,* 301–308.

Thoren-Jonsson, A.-L., Moller, A., & Grimby, G. (1999). Managing occupations in everyday life to achieve adaptation. *American Journal of Occupational Therapy, 53,* 353–362.

Toal-Sullivan, D., & Henderson, P. R. (2004). Client-Oriented Role Evaluation (CORE): The development of a clinical rehabilitation instrument to assess role change associated with disability. *American Journal of Occupational Therapy, 58,* 211–220.

Trombly, C. (1993). Anticipating the future: Assessment of occupational function. *American Journal of Occupational Therapy, 47,* 253–257.

Trombly, C. A. (1995). Occupation: Purposefulness and meaningfulness as therapeutic mechanisms. *American Journal of Occupational Therapy, 49,* 960–972.

Trombly, C. A., & Wu, C.-Y. (1999). Effect of rehabilitation tasks on organization of movement after stroke. *American Journal of Occupational Therapy, 53,* 333–344.

Wallenbert, I., & Jonsson, H. (2005). Waiting to get better: A dilemma regarding habits in daily occupations after stroke. *American Journal of Occupational Therapy, 59,* 218–224.

White, R. W. (1959). Motivation reconsidered: The concept of competence. *Psychological Reviews, 66,* 297–333.

White, R. W. (1971). The urge towards competence. *American Journal of Occupational Therapy, 25,* 271–274.

World Health Organization [WHO]. (2001). *International classification of functioning, disability and health (ICF).* Geneva, Switzerland: WHO.

Wu, C.-Y., Trombly, C., Lin, K.-C., & Tickle-Degnen, L. (1998). Effects of object affordances on reaching performance in person with and without cerebrovascular accident. *American Journal of Occupational Therapy, 52,* 447–456.

Yerxa, E. J., & Locker, S. B. (1990). Quality of time use by adults with spinal cord injuries. *American Journal of Occupational Therapy, 44,* 318–326.

Supplemental References

Bilbao, A., Kennedy, C., Chatterji, S., Üstün, B., Vasquez Barquero, J. L., & Barth, J. T. (2003). The ICF: Applications of the WHO model of functioning, disability and health to brain injury rehabilitation. *NeuroRehabilitation, 18,* 239–250.

Cardol, M., de Haan, R. J., van den Bos, G. A. M., de Jong, B. A., & de Groot, I. J. M. (1999). The development of a handicap assessment questionnaire: The Impact on Participation and Autonomy (IPA). *Clinical Rehabilitation, 13,* 411–419.

Daimant, R. B. (2004). Integration of the Occupational Therapy Practice Framework and international classifications of functioning concepts: Application of role performance in client-centered practice. *WFOT [World Federation of Occupational Therapists] Bulletin, 50,* 24–32.

Delany, J. V., & Squires, E. (2004). From UT-III to the Framework: Making language work. *OT Practice, 9,* 20–28.

Dumont, C., Bertrand, R., Fougeyrollas, P., & Gervais, M. (2003). Rasch modeling and measurement of social participation [the LIFE-H Scale]. *Journal of Applied Measurement, 4,* 309–325.

CHAPTER 2

Historical and Social Foundations for Practice

Pamela Roberts, Sharon Kurfuerst, and Jaclyn Faglie Low

LEARNING OBJECTIVES

After studying this chapter, the reader will be able to do the following:

1. Recall the origin of the profession of occupational therapy.
2. Identify historical and social factors that affected the development of occupational therapy for physical dysfunction.
3. Describe the historical roots of various tools of occupational therapy practice for physical dysfunction.
4. Identify economic factors that affect occupational therapy service delivery to patients with physical dysfunction.

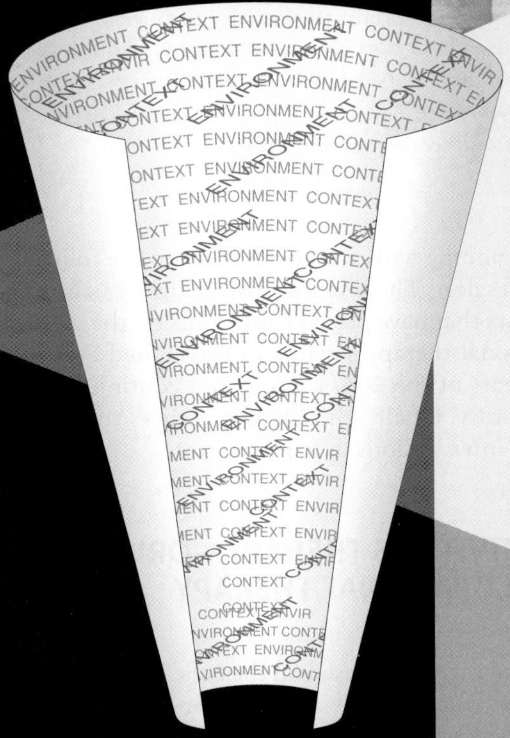

Glossary

Adaptive equipment—Equipment designed to help persons with disabilities compensate for functional limitations; equipment ranges from simple, such as a long-handled reacher for those unable to bend over, to complex, such as computerized environmental control systems.

Battle fatigue—See *War neurosis.*

Critical review—a synthesis of published outcome studies concerning a particular topic or intervention in which the strength of the evidence is critiqued and a summary judgment is made concerning whether the evidence supports or negates the use of the intervention under study.

Habit training—A regimen wherein patients hospitalized with mental illness were expected to follow a rigid daily schedule that included responsibility for personal hygiene, making one's bed, and attending treatment sessions at prescribed times; regimens were designed to help patients develop good habits as an aid to restoration of good mental health and for the therapeutic value of work and routine.

Homeopathy—Medical practice based on treating disorders with minuscule doses of substances that produce the same symptoms as the illness.

Hydrotherapy—Use of water as a therapeutic agent; hydrotherapy incorporated both the prescription of drinking water and the use of bathing to treat illness.

Meta-analysis—A statistical synthesis of published outcome studies concerning a particular research question or intervention. Meta-analysis is a set of statistical procedures for comparing and combining results from different studies (Rosenthal & Rosnow, 1991). The outcome of the meta-analysis expresses the effect of the intervention being studied in statistical terms and may also allow an estimate of the degree of relationship between the treatment and the outcome.

Moral treatment—Treatment approach for mental illness that focused on work as a therapeutic agent rather than restraint and isolation.

Neurorehabilitation—Treatment approach for persons with central nervous system dysfunction; uses specific sensory input to influence motor responses.

Orthotics—External devices fitted to specific body parts to support the body part, immobilize the body part, or facilitate movement of the body part.

Physical agent modalities—Those modalities that produce a biophysiological response through the use of light, water, temperature, sound, electricity, or mechanical devices (AOTA, 2003). Physical agent modalities are preparatory or adjunctive methods to enable a person to engage in activities and tasks of valued roles.

Prospective Payment System (PPS)—A system to pay for Medicare services based on criteria set by the government.

Purposeful activity—Activity used as treatment that is goal directed and that the patient perceives as meaningful or purposeful.

Rehabilitation—An approach to treatment for the person who has a permanent disability; focuses on training in the use of special equipment or techniques to facilitate independence rather than on remediation or correction of underlying deficits.

Third-party payer—A public or private organization that pays for or underwrites coverage for health care expenses. The client and the health care practitioner are considered the first and second parties.

War neurosis, battle fatigue—Physical and emotional responses to combat experiences.

Work hardening—Treatment program aimed at returning the injured worker to productive activity through a structured, interdisciplinary program of increasing endurance, work tolerance, and improved body mechanics.

Work therapy—Work activity with primary purpose of therapeutic benefit rather than productivity.

Occupational therapists today are concerned with their patients' abilities to resume life roles upon discharge from abbreviated hospital stays. Occupational therapists in earlier times questioned whether patients would assume vocational and other responsibilities after prolonged hospitalizations. Although the specific details of the questions have changed over time, the fundamental character of questions about the practice of occupational therapy is the same. How can we best prepare our patients to return to appropriate life roles after a life-changing illness or injury? What are the appropriate tools of practice? How do economic and social constraints affect our practice?

The roots of contemporary concerns are discernible in the experiences of our forebears. This chapter explores the social and historical foundations of physical disability practice, beginning with an introduction to the founders of the profession. The chapter also addresses the economic factors that have placed constraints on the delivery of occupational therapy services in the United States in the latter years of the 20th century and continuing into the 21st century. Finally, this chapter reviews the origins of common interventions used in practice.

ACTIVITY AS THERAPY—ORIGINS OF OCCUPATIONAL THERAPY

Occupational therapy is based on the belief that **purposeful activity** (occupation) prevents or mediates dysfunction of physical or psychological origin. Writings attributed to Hippocrates, Galen, and Aesculapius proclaimed exercise, activity treatment, and employment as important therapeutic agents. Centuries later, physicians in European asylums for the insane instituted **work therapy** for inmates. They noted that lower-class patients who were required to perform work tasks while incarcerated recovered more quickly than did idle upper-class patients. The value of physical activity and productive work was central to the **moral treatment** advanced by the French physician Phillipe Pinel in the 18th century and the Tuke family in 18th- and 19th-century England. Moral treatment is the philosophical root of occupational therapy (Bockhoven, 1971; Weinstock-Zlotnick & Hinojosa, 2004).

Ideas about the healthful value of activity were transported to colonial America. Fitness was considered necessary for optimal functioning in occupational roles determined by age, gender, and socioeconomic class. The first hospital chartered in Great Britain's North American colonies included as part of its equipment and supplies spinning wheels, wool, and flax for use by patients. Dr. Benjamin Rush, a signer of the Declaration of Independence, wrote to the managers of the Pennsylvania Hospital in 1797 and again in 1813 in support of the therapeutic value of work for patients (Dunton, 1917).

Attitudes in the United States changed as immigrants with different values and habits swelled the population of the asylums. Mental illness was seen as a permanent condition for which little could be done except to lock the sufferer away. Thus, the use of activity as therapy in institutions for the mentally ill lay dormant for decades. Dunton (1917) surmised that the decline in work as therapy from 1860 to 1890 was related to the demands of post-Civil War conditions.

Hospitals for the physically ill required work of their patients, with jobs done in the service of the institution rather than for their therapeutic benefit. As their recovery progressed, female patients were given the task of caring for sicker patients. In New York City's Bellevue and Charity hospitals, jobs for women required sewing; those for men called for maintenance skills such as carpentry, cleaning, and even rowing a boat to ferry passengers on a twice-daily schedule (Rosenberg, 1978).

Although 19th-century Americans valued work and activity, especially outdoor activity, as vital to good health, the formal idea of occupation as therapy did not emerge until the late 19th and early 20th centuries. Until the introduction of the germ theory of disease and asepsis, traditional medical care was frequently more harmful than helpful. Emphasis on curing disease through bleeding, blistering, and purging to restore the balance of the body's humors was challenged by sectarian or nontraditional approaches to health care. Health reformers advocated education, regular exercise, dress reform, and dietary restrictions in addition to specific curative practices such as **hydrotherapy** and **homeopathy**.

The Growth of the Profession of Occupational Therapy

Professions are made up of practitioners with special skills, knowledge, attitudes, and shared beliefs. Professions are not created instantaneously but evolve over time and within social, cultural, and economic contexts. Identifiable factors influenced the development of occupational therapy as a profession. These include the personalities and experiences of the individuals who recognized the idea of occupation as therapy and the world in which they lived. The late 19th and early 20th centuries were characterized by changes in the effectiveness and ways of provision of health care and influenced by burgeoning emphasis on the relation between chronological age and appropriate roles in life. These factors helped create the conditions in which the ideas and ideals of the founders could flourish.

The Founders and the Near-Founders

In the first decades of the 20th century, individuals in various fields of endeavor began almost simultaneously to practice and promote the use of occupation as therapy. George Barton, an architect with numerous health problems, was convinced that he could help others with similar problems. He opened Consolation House in Clifton Springs, New York, where he provided education, vocational assistance, and workshop activities for convalescents.

Barton assembled five like-minded individuals (Fig. 2-1) to meet with him in 1917 to establish the National Society for the Promotion of Occupational Therapy, which in 1923, was renamed the American Occupational Therapy Association (AOTA). Joining Barton was psychiatrist William Rush Dunton, Jr., a descendent and namesake of Benjamin Rush. Dunton directed the occupations program at the Sheppard and Pratt Institute in Maryland and wrote a number of books and articles on occupation as therapy

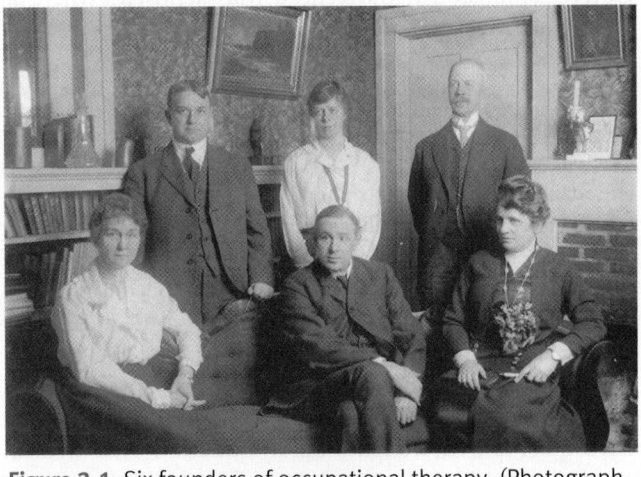

Figure 2-1 Six founders of occupational therapy. (Photograph courtesy of the Archives of the American Occupational Therapy Association, Bethesda, MD.)

and on training nurses to provide occupation. His major works included *Occupational Therapy* (1915), *Reconstruction Therapy* (1919), and *Prescribing Occupational Therapy* (1928). He also co-wrote, with Dr. Sidney Licht, *Occupational Therapy: Principles and Practice* (1950, 1957).

Also present was Eleanor Clarke Slagle. She worked with Dunton at Johns Hopkins in Baltimore, where she developed a program called **habit training** for chronically schizophrenic patients. Slagle later went to Chicago, where she directed the Henry P. Favill School of Occupations until it closed in 1920 (History, 1940). Other founding members were Susan Cox Johnson and Thomas Kidner. Johnson, director of occupations for the New York State Department of Public Charities, wrote a textbook on textiles and spent 2 years as a teacher of arts and crafts in the Philippines (Licht, 1967; Johnson, 1917). Kidner, a London-born architect, was the vocational secretary of the Canadian Military Hospitals Commission and a special adviser to the United States government on problems of rehabilitation (Licht, 1967). Isabel Newton, Barton's secretary, was also present. She later married Barton and worked with him as a teacher of occupations to invalids.

Susan Tracy, born in 1864, graduated from nurse training at the Massachusetts Homeopathic Hospital in 1889. She studied manual arts at Teachers College at Columbia University while working as a private-duty nurse. Tracy taught courses in invalid occupations for nursing students. She incorporated her course material into her textbook, *Studies in Invalid Occupations* (1910). In 1916, she introduced an occupational therapy program for general medicine patients at Michael Reese Hospital in Chicago (Occupational therapy in the general hospital, 1917, p. 425).

Although she did not attend the organizational meeting, Tracy was one of the five directors of the society listed on the certificate of incorporation. Peloquin (1991) referred to Tracy and Herbert J. Hall as near-founders because of their influence on the profession. Hall was the director of Devereux Mansion in Marblehead, Massachusetts, where he established an experimental workshop.

Rationales for Occupation as Therapy

The early practitioners of occupational therapy validated the idea of occupation as therapy in various ways. Barton emphasized the scientific aspects of occupational therapy in a speech presented at the First Consolation House Conference (March 15–17, 1917). The speech, entitled "Inoculation of the Bacillus of Work," used numerous medical metaphors, including preparation of the patient, the occupational diagnosis, occupational "applications," "hypodermics," and "lumbar punctures" (Barton, 1917). Barton compared occupational dysfunction with medical conditions and interventions. He referred to certain occupations as hypodermics, to be used, in his words, "where superficial stimulation is not sufficient, cases in which one has to get inside into the blood, or into the muscle itself" (p. 400). For even more severe problems, he termed the appropriate curative occupations "lumbar punctures" (p. 400).

Dunton acknowledged the lack of a scientific basis for occupation as therapy (Serrett, 1985) and proposed principles of occupational therapy to imbue the work with greater precision. His principles emphasized that the work be interesting, focused on cure, tailored to the patient's needs, and culminating in a useful product.

Elizabeth Upham, director of the art department at Milwaukee-Downer College, referred to "the modern science of therapeutic occupations for the handicapped" (Upham, 1917, p. 409). Other authors added their views to the debate. An unsigned history of occupational therapy credited Tracy's book *Studies in Invalid Occupation* as "the first attempt to place occupational therapy on a scientific basis" (History, 1940, p. 31). Hall defined occupational therapy as "the science of organized work for invalids" (Definitions of occupational therapy, 1940, p. 37). At an organizational level, the National Society for the Promotion of Occupational Therapy emphasized the scientific aspects of practice by selecting engineer and efficiency expert Frank Gilbreth as an honorary member in 1917 (AOTA, 1967).

Adolph Meyer, a Swiss physician, immigrated to the United States in 1892 and worked as a pathologist at the Eastern Illinois Hospital for the Insane. Later, Meyer became professor of psychiatry at Johns Hopkins University in 1921. From his early work, he was concerned with meaningful activity as the core of treatment. Hopkins (1983) indicates that Meyer described "rhythms of life that must be kept in balance even under difficulty. These were work and play, rest and sleep" (p. 6). He had extensive experiences with leaders in the occupational therapy movement including William Rush Dunton, Jr., Eleanor Clarke Slagle, and Henrietta Price. In 1921, Meyer brought together the fundamental concepts of psychobiology and wrote the paper, "The Philosophy of Occupational Therapy." In this paper, he emphasized occupation, time, and the productive use of energy with psychobiology interwoven (Meyer, 1977), contributing significantly to the identification of the core tenets of occupational therapy practice.

The Professional Literature

The directors of the National Society for the Promotion of Occupational Therapy selected the *Maryland Psychiatric Quarterly* as its official periodical. *The Modern Hospital* also carried information on occupational therapy. Articles focused equally on physical rehabilitation and mental illness, with authors emphasizing returning people to productive lives. In 1915, *The Modern Hospital* began featuring a monthly column, "Occupational Therapy, Vocational Re-Education and Industrial Rehabilitation."

A new journal, *Archives of Occupational Therapy*, appeared in 1922. Dunton owned and edited it as well as the *Maryland Psychiatric Quarterly*. *Archives of Occupational Therapy* was renamed *Occupational Therapy in Rehabilitation*. When he retired in 1947, Dunton attempted to transfer ownership of *Occupational Therapy in Rehabilitation* to the American Occupational Therapy Association, but the publisher, Williams & Wilkins, owned the copyright to the journal name and its contents (Bone, 1971). The American Occupational Therapy Association began publication of the *American Journal of Occupational Therapy* in 1947.

The founders and the near-founders contributed to the developing body of knowledge by writing books, many of which became required textbooks. Among them were *Studies in Invalid Occupation: A Manual for Nurses and Attendants* and *Rake Knitting, and Its Special Adaptation to Invalid Workers* by Susan E. Tracy, Dunton's *Occupational Therapy: A Manual for Nurses*, and Barton's *Occupational Nursing: How the Installation of Invalid Occupation Work in Institutions Will Affect the Nursing Profession, and a Practical Example of Its Therapeutic Value* and *A View of Invalid Occupation: An Explanation of the New Idea of Providing Convalescents with Occupation* (Textbooks required, 1920). Additionally, Willard and Spackman's *Occupational Therapy*, first published in 1947, serves as a core text for occupational therapy students and provides a comprehensive overview of the profession from historical perspectives to the value of research.

The first edition of this textbook, *Occupational Therapy for Physical Dysfunction*, written by Catherine Trombly and Anna Deane Scott (1977), was the first textbook specifically written to address specialty practice of occupational therapy for persons with physical disabilities. Since then, numerous textbooks have been written for all aspects of occupational therapy practice.

HISTORICAL AND SOCIAL INFLUENCES ON THE DEVELOPMENT OF THE PRACTICE OF OCCUPATIONAL THERAPY FOR PHYSICAL DYSFUNCTION

Social changes and historical events in the late 19th and early 20th centuries created an environment that fostered the development of occupational therapy for physical dysfunction. Among the social changes were changes in the organizational structure and role of the hospital, the study of human development, the increasing effectiveness of traditional medical care, the professionalization of health care providers, and the independent living movement. The First and Second World Wars provided impetus to train women to provide occupational therapy to the wounded soldiers.

The Development of Hospitals

For centuries, hospitals existed only as institutions of refuge for those without family members to care for them during illness. Little emphasis was placed on curing because there was often little that could be cured. From 1870 to 1910, two factors operated to change the role of the hospital. First, people moved to the cities in response to industrialization and thus were cut off from family support systems. Second, the introduction of aseptic techniques and anesthesia made surgery not only effective but survivable. According to Starr (1982), "The reconstitution of the hospital involved its redefinition as an institution of medical science rather than of social welfare, its reorganization on the lines of a business rather than a charity, and its reorientation to professionals and their patients rather than to patrons and the poor" (pp. 147–148).

Within the hospital, divisions of labor developed to increase efficiency. Hospitals "projected ideals of specialization and technical competence" (Starr, 1982, p. 146). Patients no longer provided their own care. Nursing as a profession emerged within the hospital setting. The population of hospitalized patients shifted from the poor to the middle class.

During the late 19th century, hospitals offered training programs for nursing students. Students did the ward work. Most nurses left the institution for private-duty work after graduation. Middle- and upper-class patients convalesced at home under the care of the hospital-trained professional nurse. By the end of the 1930s, however, the cost of private-duty nursing was prohibitive for most middle-class families (Melosh, 1984). These patients moved to hospitals for care.

Patients in hospitals of the late 19th and early 20th centuries had to work to keep the hospital functioning, so there was no place or time for occupation as therapy. Professional nurses who provided convalescent care in the home may have offered, as did Susan Tracy, invalid occupations to clients, but that was a matter of individual circumstance. It was not until hospitals became curative centers for middle-class patients that there was a place for occupational therapy.

In the mid-20th century, occupational therapists working in general hospitals dealt with a variety of diagnostic categories. Fay and March (1947) discussed grading downward for patients with neurosyphilis, a degenerative disorder, grading from large to fine movements to increase coordination for persons with hemiplegia and paraplegia, adapting activities for persons with Parkinson's disease, and focusing on muscle reeducation and avoidance of fatigue for persons with poliomyelitis. Their description of recommended management of patients with burns will be familiar to contemporary therapists: "the first object . . . is to help overcome the secondary stiffness resulting from immobilization" (p. 135). Therapists were advised to stretch contractures gently and gradually, "since the scar tissue and the new skin are sensitive and must not be torn or irritated" (p. 135). Rumsey's (1946) description of the occupational therapy principles for the treatment of peripheral nerve injuries mandated that the involved joint be kept flexible, that involved muscles be contracted and relaxed, and that the treatment plan incorporate both permanent and temporary compensatory techniques and equipment.

Emphasis on Human Development

Another influence on the development of occupational therapy practice was the introduction of concepts about the timeliness of life events. Kern (1983) identified the introduction of standard time, which occurred at the end of the 19th century, as the event that set the stage for emphasis on the temporal aspects of human development. Spokespersons in popular and professional journals began to delineate the ideal sequencing of a wide variety of experiences (Chudacoff, 1989). Emphasis on accuracy in the measurement of time created a framework in which all activities were categorized as being on time, ahead of time, or behind time. This set the stage for theories outlining appropriate times for important life events. Neugarten, Moore, & Lowe (1968) characterized the powerful influence of ideas about age- and stage-related behaviors thus: "There exists what might be called a prescriptive time-table for the ordering of major life events: a time in the life span when men and women are expected to marry, a time to raise children, a time to retire" (p. 22).

Although the study of stage theories of human development was not a part of the preparation of the founders or the early occupational therapists, implicit in the belief systems of the founders of occupational therapy was the idea that role and activity have age and stage specificity. From the beginning, occupational therapists formulated goals that focused on occupational function and selected treatment activities based on "the relation of the age, sex, interests, physical and mental limitations of the patient to the occupation selected" (Occupations for Invalids, 1916).

Historical Events that Influenced the Profession of Occupational Therapy and the Professionalization of Health Care Providers

Just as humans must adapt to various environments and challenges as they pass through the stages of life, so must professions adapt. Several significant periods in the history of occupational therapy practice influenced the profession and practitioners in significant ways. Among them are the two world wars and the period between them.

The rapid growth of occupational therapy was credited in part to World War I (Gutman, 1995). The reconstruction aides were civilian women appointed to help in therapeutic efforts for servicemen suffering from **battle fatigue**, **war neurosis**, or war-related injuries. The occupational therapy reconstruction aides used craft activities that were carefully selected to meet each patient's physical and psychological needs (Fig. 2-2). The work of one reconstruction aide, Ora Ruggles, is recounted in *The Healing Heart* (Carlova & Ruggles, 1946). The first reconstruction aides sent to France during World War I were stationed near the front lines and were charged with returning to duty as quickly as possible men suffering from war neurosis (Low, 1992). In the postwar years, the concern was for return to productive employment.

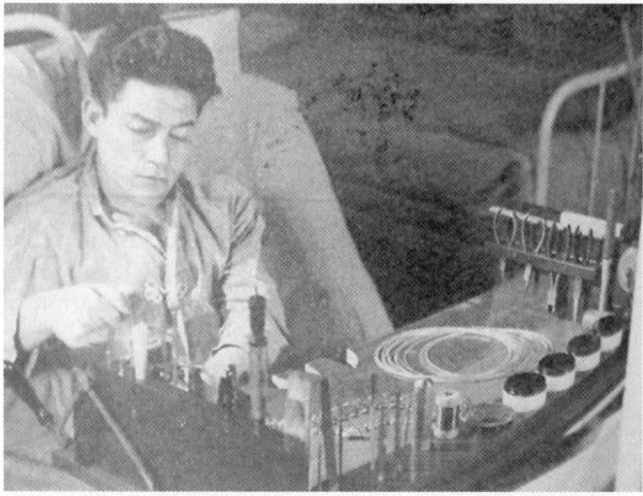

Figure 2-2 Craft activities were used in the treatment of military casualties. (Department of the Army. [1951]. *Occupational therapy*. Department of the Army Technical Manual TM 8-291, p. 8. Washington, DC: U.S. Government Printing Office.)

Women were selected for training and service as reconstruction aides on the basis of proficiency in a variety of crafts. Although training courses included psychology, specific handicapping conditions, the history of occupational therapy, and hospital etiquette, the use of crafts remained the focus (Emergency Course of Instruction for Reconstruction Aides, n.d.). An Army medical department circular dated March 27, 1918, described the job and the qualifications for appointment: "trained women to furnish forms of occupation to convalescents in long illness . . . to give to patients the therapeutic benefit of activity. . . . She shall have a High School Education, or its equivalent." In addition to the educational requirement, applicants were required to be accomplished in at least three crafts, including basketry, weaving, wood carving, block printing, and needlework.

The seriousness of purpose of occupational therapy was subject to question because the providers of occupational therapy were women and their primary tools were craft activities and their own personalities. Colonel Frank Billings (1918) of the Office of the Surgeon General characterized the work of the reconstruction aides "as diversional in character, in the form of knitting, in the form of basket weaving, etc." (p. 1925). He contrasted it with "more purposeful" activities that would serve "training of the soldier for employment after his discharge from the Army" (p. 1925).

This differentiation between women's work and men's work culminated in a distinction between bedside activities and vocational activities. Prolonged engagement in bedside activities provided by women reconstruction aides was criticized as promoting dependence and invalidism (Sexton, 1918). Vocational activities conducted by male vocational teachers prepared the men to return to economic productivity.

Following the armistice, many of the short training courses for reconstruction aides that had sprung up in response to the war emergency effort closed. Most of the reconstruction aides returned to civilian life and their former occupations of teacher, artist, or artisan. Some remained as occupational therapists employed in Veterans Bureau hospitals or public health service facilities. Although the reconstruction aides did not have military status during their service time, they were allowed to apply for credit for service time toward civil service appointments (Low, 1992).

Opportunities for occupational therapists working with the civilian population grew with the passage of the 1923 Federal Industrial Rehabilitation Act, which mandated that hospitals providing care to persons with industrial injuries or illness include occupational therapy as "an integral part of its treatment" (AOTA, 1967, p. 10). This did not immediately result in a greater number of occupational therapists working with patients with physical disabilities. In 1937, nearly 80% of occupational therapists worked in mental health settings (Reed & Sanderson, 1983).

The outbreak of World War II increased the demand for occupational therapists to care for wounded servicemen. Occupational therapy literature is replete with descriptions of programs in military hospitals. The activities and equipment described confirm emphasis on remediation of specific physical problems. Vetting (1945) described the equipment and activities of the occupational therapy clinic at the U.S. Naval Hospital at Bethesda: "A large carpentry shop . . . primarily for activities . . . to increase joint motion and muscle strength [Fig. 2-3] . . . will include workbenches designed specifically for patients who must work at shoulder height, adjustable workbenches to be used by patients who need to improve their posture . . . a height comfortable for the wheelchair patients" (p. 134). Other activities described were "Clay modeling . . . for increasing joint motions of the hands . . . floor looms adapted for shoulder and back exercise [Fig. 2-4]" (Vetting, 1945, p. 135). A report on the Naval Hospital at Jacksonville, Florida, described the use of bicycle saws (Fig. 2-5, A & B), bicycle lathes, and foot treadle looms to strengthen lower extremities (Egan, 1945).

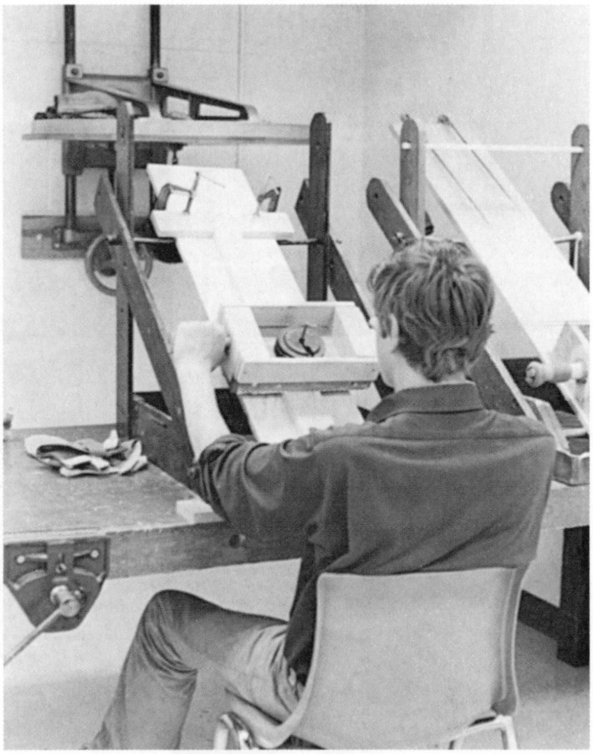

Figure 2-3 So-called purposeful activities, such as this sanding activity, were used to restore range of motion and strength of the upper extremities because they lent themselves to adaptations to achieve graded exercise. In truth, they were not meaningful to the patient, and therefore, today, would be considered poor therapy.

As its history evolved, the profession of occupational therapy developed and identified professional models to guide both service provision and research. In the late 1960s, Reilly (1969) challenged the field to distinguish occupational therapy and its purposes from medicine and to build a knowledge base that would support therapeutic

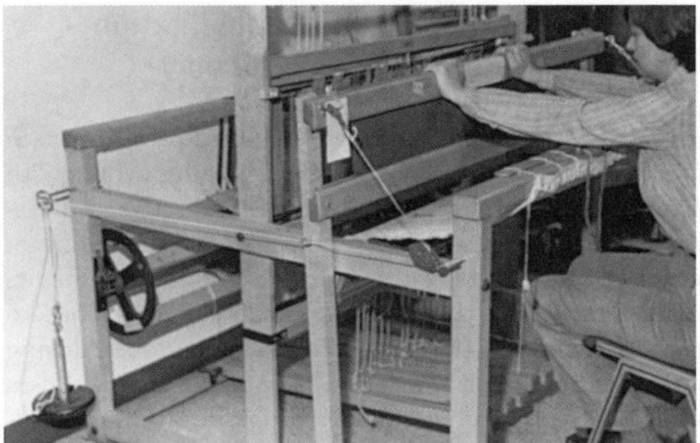

Figure 2-4 Floor loom adapted with weights and pulleys to resist elbow extension. The adaptations could be changed to resist back muscles or arm flexor muscles.

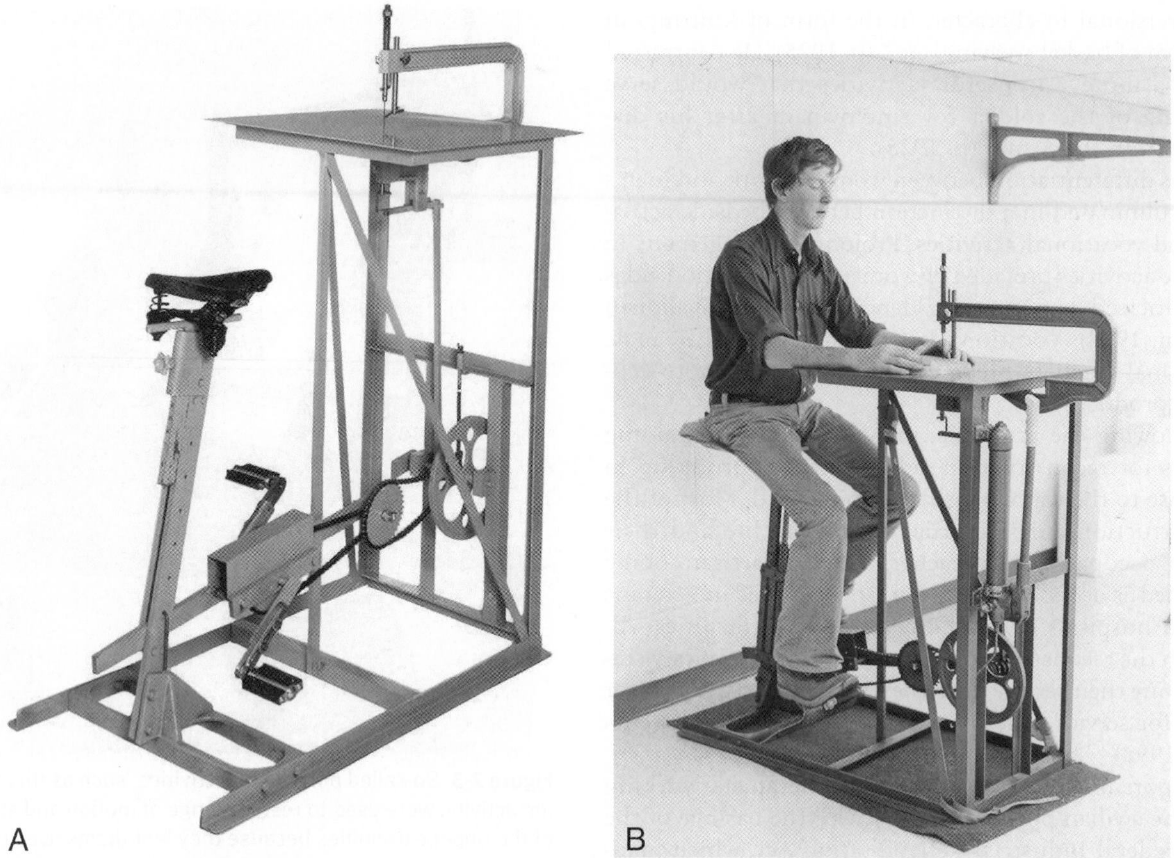

Figure 2-5 **A.** A bicycle jigsaw. (Photograph courtesy of the Archives of the American Occupational Therapy Association, Bethesda, MD.) **B.** Man using bicycle jigsaw to strengthen leg muscles while doing an interesting activity.

use of occupation. A number of professional models have evolved following this challenge. These models address assessment practices and intervention, reflect on interactions between therapists and clients, and consider these issues in the broader contexts in which the individual, family, and important occupations exist and evolve over time.

Occupational Therapy and Rehabilitation—Challenge to Professional Autonomy

Rehabilitation became a recognized medical specialty in World War II. Although the idea of helping people with handicapping conditions to become productive and useful citizens was evidenced earlier by establishment of curative workshops, histories of rehabilitation link its development not to treatment through activity but to physical medicine. The latter approach developed during the years between the world wars and encompassed uses of "physical and other effective properties of light, heat, cold, water, electricity, massage, manipulation, exercise, and mechanical devices for physical and occupational therapy in the diagnosis or treatment of disease" (Berkowitz, 1981, p. 531).

The first department of physical medicine in an American medical school was established during the 1920s at Northwestern University (Berkowitz, 1981). In 1936, the establishment of a certifying board in physical medicine was proposed before the Advisory Board of Medical Specialties. It was not approved until 1947. By 1949, 234 physicians identified themselves as specialists in this area (Stevens, 1971). Although the two specialties were not identical, the overlapping domains of physical medicine and rehabilitation resulted in the creation in 1948 of a new medical specialty board, the American Board of Physical Medicine and Rehabilitation (Stevens, 1971).

As an Army Air Force physician, Howard Rusk "received orders to minimize his patients' hospital stays and to return as many people to combat as possible" (Berkowitz, 1981, p. 532), which is reminiscent of the orders under which the reconstruction aides acted. Rusk aimed to establish convalescent centers where the wounded would be sent when their conditions stabilized sufficiently for them to leave acute care and engage in programs of reconditioning and vocational guidance. Rusk and his colleagues envisioned rehabilitation centers serving the special needs of military and civilian patients: "Unlike a general hospital, a rehabilitation clinic could contain the special facilities needed to train a paraplegic to go up and down a curb or to manipulate a wheelchair" (Berkowitz, 1981, p. 536). Occupational therapists were seen as "an important adjunct in the treatment and early recovery in injury and disease; and [occupational therapy] has an extremely important role in the modern concept of total rehabilitation" (Samberg, 1947, p. 290).

Poor relationships and communication between the physiatrists and vocational rehabilitation agencies slowed the initial growth of rehabilitation centers. In addition, territorial disputes with orthopedic surgeons caused problems. To solidify their place in the health care arena, the physiatrists attempted to assume control of both the registration of occupational therapists and the standards and structure of occupational therapy education. From 1943 through the early 1950s, the board of managers of the American Occupational Therapy Association resisted their efforts. Although successful in retaining professional autonomy, the board of managers and others in leadership positions within the association chose to avoid publicizing the actions of the physiatrists and their responses. They feared many of the rank and file occupational therapists might support the physiatrists' position because of positive interactions with physical medicine and rehabilitation doctors in military health care (Colman, 1992).

Friedland (1998) proposed that occupational therapists did in fact align themselves with rehabilitation medicine and abandoned commitment to the value of occupation in favor of reductionistic goals of increasing joint range of motion and muscle strength. This emphasis, however, along with concern for returning persons to economic productivity, was evidenced much earlier in writings that included descriptions of equipment to accomplish such goals when crafts were not sufficient (Hickinson, 1934; Taylor, 1929).

In the Rehabilitation Act of 1973, Section 504 prohibited discrimination on the basis of handicap in programs and activities of the federal government or by recipients of federal financial assistance, including work rehabilitation programs. Persons with disabilities were empowered to engage in valued leisure and work roles. As a result, occupational therapists found a greater need for their services in a variety of settings, most notably those services provided in schools and other educational settings. Around this time, the independent living movement was founded and flourished. Shapiro (1993) considered the independent living movement to be "a new civil rights movement." The need for occupational therapy again flourished because those with disabilities were in need of the skills necessary for community-based living. This movement and the disability studies movement prompted therapists to think innovatively about their work with persons with disabilities (Frieden, 1976). Emphasis again moved away from treatment of deficit conditions to enabling engagement in valued occupational roles. In 1978, Gail and Jay Fidler discussed the role of purposeful activity in self-actualization: "Doing is viewed as enabling the development and integration of the sensory, motor, cognitive, and psychological systems; serving as a socializing agent, and verifying one's efficacy as a competent contributing member of one's society" (Fidler & Fidler, 1978, p. 305).

In 1986, the National Council on the Handicapped published an assessment of federal laws and programs affecting persons with disabilities that included legislative recommendations. In 1990, the Americans with Disabilities Act (ADA) was signed into law (Smart, 2001). The ADA has five sections including employment, transportation, public accommodations and services, telecommunications, and a miscellaneous section addressing issues such as access to wilderness areas.

TOOLS OF PRACTICE

The evolution of a profession requires practitioners to be open to new tools and approaches, although transitions are rarely smooth. Professional identity may be threatened by methods perceived as radical departures from the early ideals. Incorporation of new techniques or technologies may generate territorial disputes with other professionals.

Work Programs

Work programs were part of the early history of occupational therapy. For many years, sanatoria for the treatment of tuberculosis were major employers of occupational therapists. Patients moved through a graduated regimen from bed rest to light activity to vocational training, a program easily recognizable as **work hardening**.

Work programs for other injuries simulated actual job conditions as much as possible. Goodman (1922) described a work program for industrial injuries: "[the clients] would be in the atmosphere of work all the time" (p. 200). The director of occupational therapy at a curative workshop for orthopedic conditions and industrial injuries reported on the program of physical and occupational therapy: "Our patients report for treatment at 8:00 in the morning, so that they will continue the habit of starting out early, thus making it easier for readjustment to work later on" (Taylor, 1929, p. 337). Concerns about malingering by injured patients are longstanding. Spackman (1947) noted complications arising from industrial compensation programs: "The trouble occurs in instances when it is not financially profitable for the patient to return to work" (p. 227).

More recently, the profession has returned to "work hardening" (Hanson & Walker, 1992) and has incorporated ergonomics into practice (Jacobs, 1999). Many of the clients seen today in work-hardening programs are laborers or unskilled workers; back injury is the most common reason for referral (Hanson & Walker, 1992). In addition to addressing the reconditioning needed for return to work, occupational therapists are widely engaged in injury prevention programs, using ergonomic and task analysis.

Use of Crafts and Exercise

Although expertise in activity analysis and selecting activities specific to treatment goals has been a hallmark of occupational therapy from the beginning, occupational therapists in many settings were concerned about the adequacy of handicrafts to prepare patients for occupational function. According to an editorial in a 1918 issue of *Maryland Psychiatric Quarterly*, activities used in therapy "may appear trivial" (Occupational aides, 1918, p. 27). Hall (1917), who served several times as the president of the National Society for the Promotion of Occupational Therapy, commented, "The occupations that are employed therapeutically range all the way from work in the service of the institution to virtual play in the construction of rather useless articles of the so-called arts and crafts order" (p. 383).

Practicing therapists recognized the limitations of their traditional approaches. Decrying the scarcity of crafts that required finger extension, Taylor (1929) reported, "Mechanical means are often necessary because of the limitations in occupations" (p. 337). She was equally concerned about activities for lower extremity function: "The problem ahead of us in the use of occupational therapy for functional restoration is to readapt and make jig saws, looms, etc., so that all physical exercises may be obtained through occupations" (p. 337). After describing adaptations of the loom, bicycle saw, and treadle saw for lower extremity strengthening, one director of occupational therapy noted, "As ankle flexion is usually limited, I am going to mention two ways of getting it by mechanical appliances" (Hickinson, 1934, p. 34). The first way was a cot with a pulley at one end. The patient lay on his or her side, and "a band around the patient's foot is fastened to the cord over the pulley, and a weight attached. Flexion of the foot uses the flexor muscles to pull up the weight, which may be gradually increased" (Hickinson, 1934, p. 34). The second way was described thus: "The foot may be strapped in the ankle circumductor, and the circumductor turned entirely by pulling the foot away from the pedal. [The term circumductor suggests a device that moves the ankle through full circumduction.] The handle is not used except to start. This makes a heavy exercise" (Hickinson, 1934, p. 34). Subsequent attempts at developing equipment for specific muscle patterns included such inventions as the Extensorcisor, which was described as "an apparatus to provide progressive resistive exercises for the finger extensor muscles" (Heather, Smith, & Walsh, 1962, p. 10).

Mosey (1970) noted that following World War II, "Occupational therapists were uncomfortable with their operating principle that it was good for disabled people to keep active and busy doing the things they enjoyed" (p. 235). Emphasis on crafts gave way to exercise, and practice became specialized. One of the specialized areas was the treatment of patients with poliomyelitis. Treatment, which was based on the work of Sister Elizabeth Kenny, was directed toward maintaining or improving muscle strength and joint range of motion. Exercises and activities aimed at restoring or increasing motion at specific joints required that occupational therapists be proficient in joint measurement. The first volume of the *American Journal of Occupational Therapy* included articles on joint measurement (Hurt, 1947a, 1947b, 1947c) and a printed paper goniometer with directions for cutting it out and assembling it (Goniometer, 1947). Over time, information on specific exercise techniques and equipment appeared in the professional literature.

Gradually, thinking within the profession has shifted from the earlier focus on component level therapy to functional performance, to the nature and experience of occupation within a person's life (Hasselkus, 2004). This rediscovery of our roots and rethinking of occupation has allowed occupational therapy to view practice beyond the rehabilitation clinic to the home and the community, and to serve clients beyond those with identified deficits to those who may experience occupational dysfunction because of life circumstances (e.g., aging, retirement, locating to a new community) or to groups or communities (AOTA, 2004).

Other professions have begun to see the value of meaningful occupation and are incorporating it into their practices (Basler, 2005), including the process of activity and task analysis, which occupational therapists have claimed with pride as unique to our profession. This trend will influence the profession's commitment to research and education of the public concerning the profession's expertise and contributions concerning meaningful activity as a therapeutic agent.

Adjunctive Treatment of Vision and Visual Perceptual Deficits

Historically, several people were instrumental in including remediation of visual perceptual deficits into the practice of occupational therapy. Goldstein (1942) discussed visual spatial problems with brain-injured adults following World War I. Bender, Held, Reitan, Teuber, Werner, and others improved evaluation tools to assess visual spatial organization. Hebb studied the effects of sensory deprivation on normal adults, which showed the problems with thinking and reasoning and visual perceptual difficulties (Heron

& Hebb, 1961). These studies were important for recognizing that organization of sensorimotor processing was necessary for the development of higher cortical functions. During the 1960s and 1970s, Frostig and Horne's visual perceptual programs (1965) were popular in occupational therapy practice for learning disabled children. Kephart's perceptual motor program was also widely used in the education setting (Kephart, 1960). In 1961, Ayres stressed the development of body scheme with emphasis on cognitive, visual training, and tactile and proprioceptive procedures. Ayres also recognized the importance of the vestibular system and its influence on the organization of sensory input, especially the visual system. Occupational therapists today focus not only on visual perceptual deficits but also on the role of vision and how it relates to function in daily activities. Gianutsos (1997) reported that nearly half of persons admitted to rehabilitation after brain injury had visual system deficits. Vision deficits often result in a decreased ability to function in daily activities, which leads to greater reliance on family, friends, and other social systems. Occupational therapists have incorporated the screening and treatment of visual disorders into practice preparatory to restoration of occupational functioning (Aloisio, 1998; Gianutsos, 1997).

Physical Agent Modalities

By the late 1970s and early 1980s, occupational therapists working with patients with physical disabilities began to incorporate other less traditional modalities into their treatments. To facilitate joint and muscle function, they used paraffin baths, hot and cold packs, ultrasound, and electrical stimulation. These approaches and others selected to produce changes in soft tissue were known collectively as **physical agent modalities**.

In 2003, the American Occupational Therapy Association (AOTA) reissued a position paper on the use of physical agent modalities. The techniques in question were labeled as adjunctive modalities (AOTA, 2003, p. 650) to convey that use of these techniques was considered adjunctive or supplemental to purposeful activity in meeting patients' objectives. The position paper mandated that use be restricted to "a practitioner who has documented evidence of possessing the theoretical background and technical skills for safe and competent integration of the modality into an occupational therapy intervention plan" (AOTA, 2003, p. 650).

Because, as late as 1997, a survey of occupational therapists revealed that most users of physical agent modalities had no formal training in either theoretical basis for use or technique (Cornish-Painter, Peterson, & Lindstrom-Hazel, 1997), occupational therapy education programs now incorporate specific instruction in physical agent modalities into their curricula and continuing education opportunities for clinicians are available.

Adaptive Equipment

Adaptive equipment for performing occupation-as-means and tasks and activities of daily living was first described for a patient at Michael Reese Hospital in Chicago. The patient was paralyzed by a gunshot wound. Susan Tracy strapped a polishing pad to the man's right hand and taught him to polish articles placed in front of him by moving his arm. The benefit of this was realized when, as the author reported, "This man had not been able to put anything into his own mouth for 4 months, but, with the aid of a second leather palm [Fig. 2-6] which holds a fork or spoon, he can now feed himself" (Occupational therapy in the general hospital, 1917, p. 426).

Some 30 years later, Haas provided directions for making a knife-and-fork combination (Haas, 1946). Haas published a booklet, *Equipment Aids for Those Having One Hand* (Haas, 1947, p. 1). He recommended the use of clamps, vacuum cups, and clips for stabilizing projects and proposed attaching fine sandpaper to tools to increase friction and prevent slipping (Haas, 1947).

In the years following World War II, much adapted equipment addressed the needs of disabled veterans. An unsigned article in a 1945 *Occupational Therapy and Rehabilitation* issue was illustrated with photographs of aids designed to permit war veterans with amputations to drive. The adaptations were designed by the war engineering board of the Society of Automotive Engineers, and the information was provided to occupational therapists so they could advise their patients (Simple devices enable veterans to drive motor vehicles safely, 1945).

Patients with poliomyelitis had long convalescent periods in which activities were limited by poor endurance and disability. Occupational therapists developed activity programs to provide mental stimulation without overtaxing damaged neuromuscular systems. McFarland and Lukins (1946), respectively a physician and an occupational

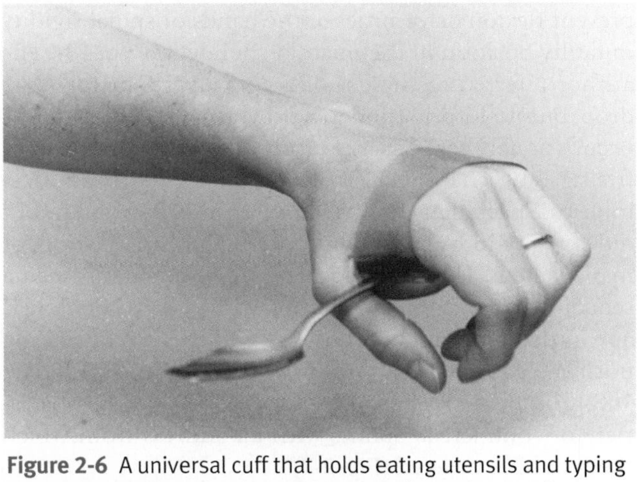

Figure 2-6 A universal cuff that holds eating utensils and typing or phone dialing sticks to enable more independent performance of some occupational tasks. This adaptation is still in use.

therapist, described a mouth-stick page turner for patients in respirators and included instructions for fabrication. MacLean (1949) described the development and adaptation of arm slings, lapboards, adjustable tables, and built-up armrests to improve functional abilities. For the next several years, adaptations to meet the needs of patients who had had poliomyelitis were frequently featured in occupational therapy literature.

New products were regularly introduced to occupational therapists in the *American Journal of Occupational Therapy*. A 1952 column of products and techniques included a collapsible reacher for the bed or wheelchair patient (Have you tried?, 1952). In 1969, Lowman and Klinger compiled and classified the extant adapted equipment into one publication that improved the selection and prescription of adapted equipment, although many of the specific devices were still made by occupational therapists. Contemporary occupational therapists have access to extensive, commercially available collections of adaptive equipment for almost every disabling condition. Today's challenges are found in selecting equipment that will achieve the goal and that is reliable, affordable, and acceptable to the patient, both functionally and cosmetically.

Orthotics

Orthotics for upper extremities were an extension of occupational therapists' design and manufacture of adaptive equipment. An article by Slagle (1938) was illustrated with a photograph of a patient identified as having a brachial plexus injury wearing an airplane splint "to rest shoulder muscles" (p. 378). The patient is engaged in an activity identified as Egyptian card weaving with the stated purpose of providing "motion of grasp, wrist and elbow flexion" (p. 378). No indication is provided that the splint is itself part of the occupational therapy program.

Writing on the management of patients with arthritis, Sammons (1945) reported, "Splints are frequently used to prevent flexion deformities of the hands or spinal rigidity in faulty position in rheumatoid spondylitis" (p. 18). The author referred to the use of a cock-up splint for wrist drop, but no information was provided as to whether the occupational therapist was involved in the fabrication or fitting. In a chapter on treating persons with physical injuries, Spackman (1947) referred to a cock-up splint but did not give information on construction, application, or management. Hand surgeon Sterling Bunnell outlined a sequence of care for hand injuries, with occupational therapy initiated once the wound had healed and continuing until the patient was "ready for work" (Bunnell, 1950, p. 148). His article was illustrated with photographs of a variety of commercial splints with an address from which they could be ordered (Fig. 2-7).

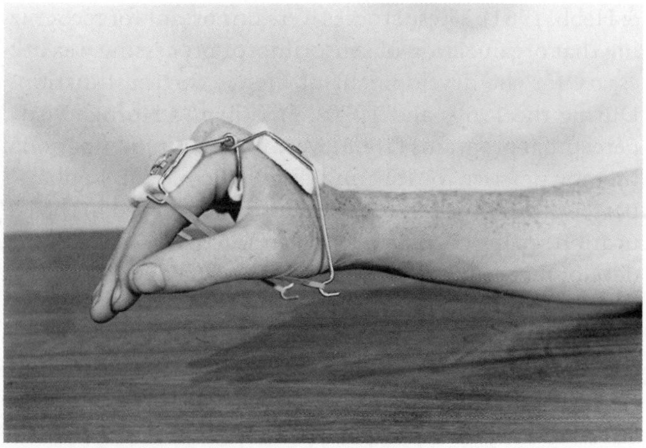

Figure 2-7 One of Bunnell's splints; this one was called a "knuckle bender."

Fabrication of orthoses was addressed in 1952. The chief of occupational therapy at the Veterans Administration Hospital in Portland, Oregon, reported on the use of plastic to fabricate splints for patients with poliomyelitis. She included principles of a well-designed splint and directions for making several splints, including an opponens cuff and a foot-drop splint (Boyce, 1952). Silverstein (1953) described clinic-made adaptations of several of Bunnell's hand splints. She noted, "It became possible . . . to adapt these splints to fit hands of unusual sizes or peculiar deformities . . . to supply these new splints quickly and at a much lower cost than previously . . . . Familiarity with the mechanics of the devices allowed alteration of the splints as the patient's condition improved" (Silverstein, 1953, p. 213).

Neurorehabilitation Techniques

As patients with head injury and stroke achieved higher rates of survival, interest in treating the sequelae of neurological insults developed. In 1948, Berta Bobath's article "The Importance of the Reduction of Muscle Tone and the Control of Mass Reflex Action in the Treatment of Spasticity" was published in *Occupational Therapy and Rehabilitation*. Subsequent writings on the management of adult hemiplegia by the Bobaths appeared in physical therapy journals.

Herbert Kabat, a physician, was among the first to introduce ideas about neuromuscular mechanisms into treatment techniques. In 1950, Kabat and occupational therapist Dorothy Rosenberg described a program aimed at "accelerating the development of voluntary motion in severely paralyzed muscles . . . [by] using reinforcement techniques for guided resistive exercise utilizing primitive mass movement patterns, certain reflexes, synergistic motions, symmetrical bilateral motions, etc." (Kabat & Rosenberg, 1950, p. 6). Patients with a variety of neurological disorders were admitted to the Kabat-Kaiser Institute for medical care, physical therapy, occupational therapy, and vocational counseling. Physical therapists helped patients establish individual motions before occupational therapists began working on movement combinations necessary for self-care. Carroll studied the efficacy of Kabat's reinforcement techniques in the treatment of hemiplegia. The techniques she used were "(1) the tonic neck reflexes, (2) the stimulation of synergists, (3) the use of resistance, and (4) rhythmic stabilization" (Carroll, 1950, p. 212). Relating inconclusive results to a limited treatment time and interruptions because of medical complications, Carroll recommended that occupational therapists "devise a variety of techniques which are based on these principles and which may lead to better results in the total rehabilitation of the hemiplegic patient" (p. 213).

In the third of a three-part series, "Proprioceptive Facilitation Elicited Through the Upper Extremities," Ayres described the selection and adaptation of "simple, normal, life-like activities" (Ayres, 1955, p. 121) using proprioceptive facilitatory mechanisms. Margaret Rood, trained as both physical therapist and occupational therapist, based her work on use of sensory input to influence motor output. Although she was not a prolific writer, her work influenced occupational therapy education (Cohen & Reed, 1996). Signe Brunnstrom, also a physical therapist, presented her theory and techniques to occupational therapists in a 1961 article, "Motor Behavior of Adult Hemiplegic Patients: Hints for Training" (Brunnstrom, 1961). Subsequent publications by occupational therapists and professionals from other disciplines provided readers further explanations of neuromuscular mechanisms and applications of theoretical information to clinical practice. Street (1963) discussed the theories of Rood, Sherrington, and others and the clinical implications of techniques for inhibiting or facilitating antagonists. In the abstract of her 1968 article, "A New Look at the Nervous System in Relation to Rehabilitation Techniques," Moore said, "More recent concepts concerning learning, plasticity and facilitatory and inhibitory systems in the nervous system are covered" (Moore, 1968, p. 489).

Contemporary research indicates that neurological functions occur concurrently at many levels of the nervous system rather than in the rigidly hierarchical model of earlier theorists. Although new information is increasing its influence on practice, occupational therapists have not discarded the works of these earlier theorists and practitioners. Techniques introduced by Kabat, the Bobaths, Brunnstrom, and Rood are still in evidence in many clinical settings and are included in this textbook.

ECONOMIC FACTORS AFFECTING HEALTH CARE SERVICE DELIVERY

Three interrelated factors affect the delivery of health care service, including occupational therapy for patients with physical dysfunction. These are governmental policies and laws concerning health care financing, third-party payer reimbursement policies and practices, and the requirement of accountability for effectiveness of service.

Governmental Policies and Laws

Access to occupational therapy services is affected by regulation and reimbursement. According to the Centers for Medicare and Medicaid Services (formerly the Health Care Financing Administration), private insurance funds approximately one third of total health care services, of which 15% is for older Americans (Federal Interagency Forum on Aging-Related Statistics, 2004). Public funds, including Medicare, contribute approximately 54%; Medicaid covers 10% of health care; out-of-pocket costs account for approximately 19%, with another 4% from other funds such as foundations (Healthcare Financing Administration, 1998; Federal Interagency Forum on Aging-Related Statistics, 2004). Managed care organizations or private insurance primarily cover children and adults under the age of 65 years who are not disabled. Depending on state law, those who are injured on the job are frequently covered under workers' compensation. Those who are uninsured may be eligible to apply for state assistance under the Medicaid system or may need to pay privately for health care services. People who are under the age of 65 and are disabled may be able to apply for state or federal assistance. Health care from the Veterans Administration is available for veterans of the United States military service. In 1966, Medicare was enacted as a means of providing health coverage for the elderly (age 65 and older) and the disabled. Older adults who meet eligibility criteria may subscribe to Medicare for their health care benefits or they may receive coverage from a managed care organization or may use a combination of benefits.

In 1983, Congress implemented the Medicare Prospective Payment System (PPS) for acute care hospitals in an effort to contain costs and standardize care. Acute care hospital PPS is based on 490+ diagnostic related groups (DRGs). Since the enactment of the DRGs, temporary exemption has been in effect for rehabilitation hospitals and units, children's hospitals and units, alcohol and drug programs, long-term care, cancer specialty hospitals, and psychiatric hospitals and units. The impact of the DRGs was significant. Hospital lengths of stay became shorter and discharges to all types of post-acute care providers rose. Current Medicare program post-acute care policy is focused on providing care based on types of providers, with the key post-acute care institutional providers being inpatient rehabilitation facilities, skilled nursing facilities, and long-term care hospitals. Each of these sites provides post-acute care to Medicare beneficiaries. The Balanced Budget Act (BBA) enacted (Balanced Budget Act of 1997, section 4421, Public Law 105-33) and mandated PPS for nursing facilities, rehabilitation hospitals and units, and home health agencies. Skilled nursing was included in the PPS in 1998 that based payment on a per diem allowance. Home health was included in 2000, and payment for that was based per episode of care. Inpatient rehabilitation was included in 2002, and payment was based on per discharge. Psychiatric hospitals and units were included in 2005.

For current occupational therapy practice, regulatory and reimbursement requirements are the basis for service delivery in institutional settings. Services are provided throughout the continuum of care, which may include emergency room, intensive care unit, acute care hospital, transitional care, inpatient rehabilitation, skilled nursing, home health, outpatient rehabilitation, assisted living, day care, inpatient psychiatric care, and long-term residential care. Standards reflect current practices and are administered through regulatory agencies such as the Joint Commission on Accreditation of Healthcare Organizations (JCAHO), the U.S. Department of Health and Human Services (DHHS), fiscal intermediaries, and the Commission on Accreditation for Rehabilitation Facilities (CARF). Occupational therapy provided in institutional settings is required to adhere to the regulations that serve as guidelines for safety and quality of care. These regulations have specific requirements to which the occupational therapist and occupational therapy assistant must adhere to ensure regulatory compliance and optimize reimbursement. For example, services must be prescribed by a physician and provided under a physician-approved plan of care; services must be performed by a qualified occupational therapist or occupational therapy assistant under the supervision of an occupational therapist; and services provided must be reasonable and necessary for the individual's illness or injury. In addition to these requirements, regulations can also place limits on the amount of therapy intervention, including the amount of time services are provided and the overall length of service provision, requiring the therapist to outline and provide a plan of care within these guidelines.

It is important for occupational therapy professionals to be aware of legislative or regulatory activities that may impact the practice of occupational therapy. For example, yearly in the *Federal Register*, revisions to payment policies under the Physician Fee Schedule are published. These revisions impact reimbursement for health care services including the delivery of occupational therapy.

Influence of the Policies of Third-Party Payers

Third-party payers have had significant influences on the delivery of occupational therapy services. Howard (1991) indicates that "reimbursement policies reflect societal influences and are shaping occupational therapy in several ways. Control has shifted to third-party payers, allowing them to define occupational therapy; use of the medical model is being rewarded by reimbursement; the language used to discuss the profession has changed to accommodate the insurance and other industries; and values that dominate society are being reinforced" (p. 875). These influences have been most notable in the past 10 years, during which an influx of new health plan products and insurers has been noted (Institute for the Future, 2003).

One of the largest payers of occupational therapy services is Medicare, a federally administered health insurance program for people age 65 and older, those of all ages with end-stage renal disease (ESRD), and those under age 65 with certain qualifying disabilities. Divided into two parts, Medicare A and Medicare B, this program helps to cover inpatient care in hospitals and skilled nursing centers, as well as some aspects of hospice and home health care, and outpatient services, including physician visits and those medically necessary services provided by occupational therapy practitioners (Centers for Medicare and Medicaid Services, 2005b). In 1997, the Balanced Budget Act (BBA) resulted in the most dramatic changes in payment for Medicare services delivered in post-acute care settings ever achieved by a single piece of legislation (Cotterill & Gage, 2002).

As a result of the BBA, there was momentum in health care to shift services to post-acute care settings, including skilled nursing facilities, inpatient rehabilitation units, and home health. These settings saw the implementation of the Prospective Payment System (PPS), a system of payment affecting services delivered to Medicare A beneficiaries. Under the PPS, post-acute health care providers are paid a daily rate, which includes all services provided to the client, including occupational therapy services. No longer can the cost of occupational therapy services be billed to the client separately.

This shift in payment structure to a prospective payment method means that a health care provider must anticipate the services that a client will need for a defined period of time and then request payment at the corresponding rate. Monitoring of the amount of time and the overall intensity of therapy delivered to Medicare A clients has become more stringent to effectively manage the overall cost of care delivery. As a result, the health care workforce, including occupational therapists and occupational therapy assistants, has been dramatically impacted. For example, in early 1998, several long-term care companies embarked on large workforce reductions as a reaction to the reimbursement changes and flooded the market with occupational therapy practitioners (Brachtesende, 2005). In response to the increased availability of therapists already in the market, academic programs experienced dips in enrollment in occupational therapy and occupational therapy assistant programs (Brachtesende, 2005). Today, post-acute care providers have learned to effectively and efficiently manage service delivery under the new reimbursement system, and the demand for occupational therapy services and occupational therapy service providers for Medicare A beneficiaries has undergone a noticeable upswing.

For Medicare B beneficiaries, including those who receive traditional outpatient services from either an independent outpatient provider or a hospital-based outpatient department, those who receive home health services, and those who are permanent residents of long-term care facilities, there have also been notable changes since the implementation of the BBA. Rehabilitation services are limited by the beneficiary cap placed on outpatient rehabilitation services, including occupational therapy. Medicare B covers 80% of the costs of therapy up to the financial limitation, or cap, and then the beneficiary must either use another insurance payer or pay privately for additional occupational therapy services (Centers for Medicare and Medicaid Services, 2005b). These financial limits have impacted the delivery of occupational therapy services by forcing some therapists and their patients to focus primarily on the most essential components of therapy, including only working on basic skills such as simple ADL activities and functional mobility (Mattson, 1999). Those clients who are most severely disabled and those with chronic conditions have also been negatively impacted as a result of the Medicare B caps and have been forced to either privately pay for additional occupational therapy services or find alternative interventions.

Another government-administered health insurance program is Medicaid. Medicaid is designed to assist low-income individuals and families who fit into specific eligibility groups that are established by federal and state law (Centers for Medicare and Medicaid Services, 2005a). Although funded by the federal government, Medicaid is administered individually by states. Each state is permitted to establish its own guidelines for both Medicaid eligibility and the coverage of services (Centers for Medicare and Medicaid Services, 2005a). Requirements can vary significantly from state to state for both recipients and service providers. Occupational therapy services may or may not be covered under Medicaid. When services are covered, the conditions warranting care are specifically identified, and there may be requirements regarding the frequency and duration of occupational therapy services for which Medicaid will pay.

In the last two decades of the 20th century, the number of Americans covered by managed care plans increased dramatically. By the mid-1990s, three quarters of those with health insurance coverage were enrolled in some form of a managed care insurance plan (Glied & Zivin, 2002). Much of the growth of these plans has been the result of increased demand for health care cost containment, a drive toward improving access to health care for all who need it, and closer scrutiny regarding the quality of care that is delivered and paid for (Frakes, 1997).

Managed care is a broad term for a variety of health care coverage arrangements where the goal is to manage and control the cost of medical care and related health care services (Krieg, 1997). It has a strong focus on prevention and wellness and uses a primary physician to help direct or "manage" the health care resources that are utilized by the client. Health Maintenance Organizations (HMOs) and Preferred Provider Organizations (PPOs) are the two primary types of managed care plans. From the inception of managed care in the 1920s, managed care has been primarily provided by private insurance companies (Krieg, 1997). More recently, government-funded health care programs, such as Medicare and Medicaid, have seen a dramatic rise in their costs and have developed their own managed care systems to help control costs and more appropriately direct the care received by beneficiaries (Krieg, 1997).

The shift in the health care climate to one of greater cost control, more efficient service delivery, and better overall management of health care resources has resulted in a plethora of changes in third-party reimbursement, which have impacted the delivery of occupational therapy services. Occupational therapy providers have seen an increase in paperwork to demonstrate compliance with payer requirements. Service intensity and duration are often dictated by the payer. Recipients of occupational therapy services may need to pay privately for additional services beyond what their insurer covers, thus requiring occupational therapy practitioners to use time with their clients effectively to insure desired clinical outcomes are achieved in the most efficient manner. Regardless of practice domain, occupational therapists and occupational therapy assistants must pay careful attention to the specifications of their client's payer source to ensure that services rendered are reimbursed timely and appropriately. The case examples in the chapters of this textbook provide practical examples of how occupational therapists plan treatment while keeping these reimbursement limitations in mind.

Accountability for Effectiveness

Requiring accountability for effectiveness has led to an emphasis on evidence-based practice throughout the medical establishment. As with other factors that have influenced occupational therapy, accountability is not a new concept in occupational therapy. In 1929, Marjorie Taylor, director of the department of occupational therapy at Milwaukee-Downer College and advisory director of the Junior League Curative Workshop in Milwaukee, exhorted: "The therapists must bend all their energies to rapidity of functional gain with every patient. In no other field is the pressure of time felt so keenly, or the loss of money through inexact or unintelligent treatment so great" (Taylor, 1929, p. 335). Although the fees charged for her program were $2.50 per day for combined treatments in occupational therapy and physical therapy, her message is both familiar and vital to occupational therapists today.

Today, the costs of therapy must be carefully assessed. Neither the government, through Medicare and Medicaid, nor the private insurance companies are willing to pay for unlimited or ineffective treatment. Whereas formerly therapists had the freedom to keep a patient under treatment until that person had obtained all benefit from therapy, now therapists are told by the insurance companies how many treatments they will be reimbursed for. Therapists are also required to demonstrate to the payers how the treatment improved the patient's functional status. Therapists must select interventions that are most likely to make a significant difference in the patient's occupational functioning. The government and the insurance carriers expect that evidence exists concerning the effectiveness of interventions. As Hasselkus said in 2002, we have entered a new therapy world called the world of evidence-based practice.

Evidence-based practice is the conscientious, explicit, and judicious use of current best evidence to make decisions about the care of individual patients (Sackett et al., 1997; Sudsawad, 2005). Although therapists did not use interventions that lacked evidence previously, the evidence was not scientific (Hasselkus, 2002). "Evidence" consisted of authority statements, a single small study, a published manual, or our own or our colleagues' experiences (Hasselkus, 2002). Now, scientific evidence is required.

Evidence-based practice involves the searching for and gathering of evidence pertinent to the therapeutic problem, the evaluation of the validity of the evidence to establish a causal relationship between the treatment studied and the outcome, the determination of best evidence available pertinent to the particular patient and intervention, and finally, the application of the evidence to the patient. Clinical experience guides that application. Clinical experience is not supplanted by scientific evidence; it makes the judgment of when and for whom the evidence applies.

Evidence-based practice requires the generation of outcome studies. As part of the effort to organize and increase outcomes research in occupational therapy, the American Occupational Therapy Association (AOTA) and the American Occupational Therapy Foundation (AOTF) funded the Center for Outcomes Research and Education (CORE) at the University of Illinois at Chicago in 1999 (Kielhofner et al., 2004). Evidence-based practice is facilitated by organized syntheses of extant evidence. In 2004, AOTA and AOTF, joined by the Agency for Healthcare Research and Quality of the United States Department of Health and Human Services, sponsored an International Conference on Evidence-Based Occupational Therapy. Therapists from 13 countries convened for 3 days to develop an international plan for the identification, review, and synthesis of scientific information and methods of making this information available to practicing therapists and students. The OTseeker database (www.otseeker.com), which was developed in Australia, was chosen as the database to become the repository of the occupational therapy evidence.

The authoritarian support for interventions, considered adequate for the first half of the 20th century, was supplanted by a growing, but still small, body of scientific evidence in the latter half of the 20th century. In the 21st century, single studies and authoritarian support are no longer adequate. Now, several studies synthesized into a **critical review** or **meta-analysis** are sought to support the effectiveness of a given intervention or class of interventions. Evidence-based occupational therapy is a worldwide effort. Individual occupational therapists as well as national organizations are contributing to the effort to generate, organize, and synthesize evidence. Examples of evidence to support assessments and interventions used in occupational therapy for physical dysfunction are included in each chapter of this textbook.

PAST, PRESENT, AND FUTURE: WILL THE QUESTIONS BE THE SAME?

Occupational therapists have met many challenges throughout the course of the profession. Today's occupational therapists are discovering that challenges once met reappear, sometimes in familiar form and sometimes in different guise. Treatment planning for short hospital stays and limited reimbursable visits are formidable tasks for occupational therapists trained in more traditional fee-for-service practices and are as daunting as the challenges our predecessors faced in preparing patients to return to productive lives after long hospitalizations. The types of diagnoses that occupational therapists see have changed with advances in health care. New technologies and treatment techniques are incorporated into practice. The value of occupation has been reinforced by research on the recovery of brain function after injury (Liepert et al., 2000), the demonstrated effects to prevent dysfunction among elders (Clark et al., 2001), the emphasis of the health care community on activity and participation (World Health Organization, 2001), the adoption by other professions of activity as therapy (Basler, 2005; Kowalske et al., 2000; Walker, 2002), and other evidence that supports occupational therapy's basic premise. Building the evidence base for the effectiveness of interventions used by occupational therapists for persons with physical dysfunction is the current focus of the profession.

SUMMARY REVIEW QUESTIONS

1. What is the basic premise of occupational therapy?
2. What social movement and historical events promoted the use of occupation as therapy?
3. How do practices of the 19th-century health reformers relate to occupational therapy in the 20th century?
4. What economic factors have affected occupational therapy practice?
5. How did adjunctive interventions, such as adaptive equipment and orthoses, enter the practice of occupational therapy for physical dysfunction?
6. Were work programs new to the practice of occupational therapy in the last decade of the 20th century? If not, what was their origin?
7. Why did early therapists have concerns about crafts as an effective modality to remediate specific physical deficits? What did they do? Is that still a concern?
8. What are physical agent modalities and when and by whom are they used?
9. What is evidence-based occupational therapy? Why is it important to practice from a base of evidence?
10. What are the economic factors affecting health care service delivery today?
11. What influence does government and third-party reimbursement have on occupational therapy practice?

ACKNOWLEDGEMENT

The authors recognize the contributions of Jean Spencer, Ph.D., OTR, FAOTA, and Catherine Trombly, Sc.D., OTR/L, FAOTA, to this chapter.

References

Aloisio, L. (1998). Visual dysfunction. In G. Gillen & A. Burkhardt (Eds.), *Stroke rehabilitation* (pp. 267–284). St. Louis, MO: Mosby-Year Book.

American Occupational Therapy Association [AOTA]. (1967). *Then–and now!* Bethesda, MD: AOTA.

American Occupational Therapy Association [AOTA]. (2003). Physical agent modalities: A position paper. *American Journal of Occupational Therapy, 57,* 650–651.

American Occupational Therapy Association [AOTA]. (2004). Scope of practice (2004). *American Journal of Occupational Therapy, 58,* 673–677.

Ayers, A. J. (1955). Proprioceptive facilitation elicited through the upper extremities. Part III: Specific application to occupational therapy. *American Journal of Occupational Therapy, 9,* 126–143.

Ayres, A. J. (1961). Development of the body scheme in children. *American Journal of Occupational Therapy, 1,* 99–128.

Balanced Budget Act of 1997. (1997). Section 4421. Public Law 105-33.

Barton, G. E. (1917). Inoculation of the bacillus of work. *The Modern Hospital, 8,* 399–402.

Basler, B. (2005). Lost & found: Promising therapy for Alzheimer's draws out the person inside. *AARP Bulletin, 46,* 10–11,17.

Berkowitz, E. D. (1981). The federal government and the emergence of rehabilitation medicine. *The Historian, 43,* 530–545.

Billings, F. (1918). Chairman's address. The national program for the reconstruction and rehabilitation of disabled soldiers. *Journal of the American Medical Association, 70,* 1924–1925.

Bobath, B. (1948). The importance of the reduction of muscle tone and the control of mass reflex action in the treatment of spasticity. *Occupational Therapy and Rehabilitation, 27,* 371–373.

Bockhoven, J. S. (1971). Legacy of moral treatment-1800s to 1910. *American Journal of Occupational Therapy, 25,* 223–225.

Bone, C. D. (1971). Origin of the *American Journal of Occupational Therapy. American Journal of Occupational Therapy, 25,* 48–52.

Boyce, M. H. (1952). Plastic splints. *American Journal of Occupational Therapy, 6,* 203–207.

Brachtesende, A. (2005). The turnaround is here! *OT Practice, 23,* 13–19.

Brunnstrom, S. (1961). Motor behavior of adult hemiplegic patients. *American Journal of Occupational Therapy, 15,* 6–12,47.

Bunnell, S. (1950). Occupational therapy of hands. *American Journal of Occupational Therapy, 4,* 145–153,177.

Carlova, J., & Ruggles, O. (1946). *The healing heart.* New York: Messner.

Carroll, J. (1950). The utilization of reinforcement techniques in the program for the hemiplegic. *American Journal of Occupational Therapy, 4,* 211–213,239.

Centers for Medicare and Medicaid Services. (2005a). Medicaid program: General information. Retrieved December 22, 2005 from www.cms.hhs.gov/MedicaidGenInfo.

Centers for Medicare and Medicaid Services. (2005b). Medicare program: General information. Retrieved December 20, 2005 from www.cms.hhs.gov/MedicareGenInfo.

Chudacoff, H. P. (1989). *How old are you? Age consciousness in American culture.* Princeton, NJ: Princeton University.

Clark, F., Azen, S. P., Carlson, M., Mandel, D., LaBree, L., Hay, J., Zemke, R., Jackson, J., & Lipson, L. (2001). Embedding health-promoting changes into the daily lives of independent-living older adults: Long-term follow-up of occupational therapy intervention. *Journal of Gerontology B: Psychological Science and Social Science, 56,* 60–63.

Cohen, H., & Reed, K. L. (1996). The historical development of neuroscience in physical rehabilitation. *American Journal of Occupational Therapy, 50,* 561–568.

Colman, W. (1992). Maintaining autonomy: The struggle between occupational therapy and physical medicine. *American Journal of Occupational Therapy, 46,* 63–70.

Cornish-Painter, C., Peterson, C. Q., & Lindstrom-Hazel, D. K. (1997). Skill acquisition and competency testing for physical agent modality use. *American Journal of Occupational Therapy, 51,* 681–685.

Cotterill, P. G., & Gage, B. J. (2002). Overview: Medicare post-acute care since the Balanced Budget Act of 1997. *Health Care Financing Review, 24,* 1–6.

Definitions of occupational therapy. (1940). *Occupational Therapy and Rehabilitation, 19,* 35–38.

Dunton, W. R. (1915). *Occupational therapy.* Philadelphia: Saunders.

Dunton, W. R. (1917). History of occupational therapy. *The Modern Hospital, 8,* 380–382.

Dunton, W. R. (1919). *Reconstruction therapy.* Philadelphia: Saunders.

Dunton, W. R. (1928). *Prescribing occupational therapy.* Baltimore: Thomas.

Dunton, W. R., & Licht, S. (1950). *Occupational therapy, principles and practices.* Springfield, IL: Charles C. Thomas.

Dunton, W. R., & Licht, S. (1957). *Occupational therapy, principles and practices* (2nd ed.). Springfield, IL: Charles C. Thomas.

Egan, H. (1945). U.S. Naval Hospital, Jacksonville, Florida. *Occupational Therapy and Rehabilitation, 25,* 143–145.

Emergency Course of Instruction for Reconstruction Aides. (n.d). American Occupational Therapy Association Archives, Series 1, Box 01, Folder 06. Rockville, MD: American Occupational Therapy Association.

Fay, E. V., & March, I. (1947). Occupational therapy in general and special hospitals. In H. S. Willard & C. S. Spackman (Eds.), *Principles of occupational therapy* (pp. 1118–1140). Philadelphia: Lippincott.

Federal Interagency Forum on Aging-Related Statistics. (2004). *Key indicators of well-being.* Federal Interagency Forum on Aging-Related Statistics. Washington, DC: U.S. Government Printing Office.

Fidler, G. S., & Fidler, J. W. (1978). Doing and becoming: Purposeful action and self-actualization. *American Journal of Occupational Therapy, 32,* 305–310.

Frakes, J. T. (1997). Managed care: Evolution and distinguishing features. *Gastroenterology Clinics of North America, 26,* 703–714.

Freiden, L. (1976). IL: Movement and programs. *American Rehabilitation, 3,* 6–9.

Friedland, J. (1998). Occupational therapy and rehabilitation: An awkward alliance. *American Journal of Occupational Therapy, 52,* 373–380.

Frostig, M., & Horne, D. (1965). An approach to the treatment of children with learning disorders. In J. Hellmuth (Ed.), *Learning disorders* (pp. 293–305). Seattle: Special Child.

Gianutsos, R. (1997). Vision rehabilitation following acquired brain injury. In M. Gentile (Ed.), *Functional visual behavior: A therapist's guide to evaluation and treatment options* (pp. 267–294). Bethesda, MD: American Occupational Therapy Association.

Glied, S., & Zivin, J. G. (2002). How do doctors behave when some (but not all) of their patients are in managed care? *Journal of Health Economics, 21,* 337–353.

Goldstein, K. (1942). *Aftereffects of brain-injuries in war.* New York: Grune and Stratton.

Goniometer. (1947). *American Journal of Occupational Therapy, 1,* 268.

Goodman, H. B. (1922). The industrial case from the accident back to the job. *Archives of Occupational Therapy, 1,* 193–204.

Gutman, S. (1995). Influence of the U.S. military and occupational therapy reconstruction aides in World War I on the development of occupational therapy. *American Journal of Occupational Therapy, 49,* 256–262.

Haas, L. J. (1946). Eating with one hand. *Occupational Therapy and Rehabilitation, 25,* 233–234.

Haas, L. J. (1947). Equipment aids for the aging person. *Occupational Therapy and Rehabilitation, 25,* 1–4.

Hall, H. J. (1917). Remunerative occupations for the handicapped. *The Modern Hospital, 8,* 383–386.

Hanson, C. S., & Walker, K. W. (1992). The history of work in physical dysfunction. *American Journal of Occupational Therapy, 46,* 56–62.

Hasselkus, B. R. (2002). Therapists awake! The challenge of evidence-based occupational therapy. *American Journal of Occupational Therapy, 56,* 247–249.

Hasselkus, B. R. (2004). Deeper into the heart of the matter. *American Journal of Occupational Therapy, 58,* 476–479.

Have you tried? (1952). *American Journal of Occupational Therapy, 6,* 281.

Healthcare Financing Administration, Office of the Actuary: National Health Statistics Group. (1998). The nation's healthcare dollar: 1998, where the healthcare dollar went. Retrieved in July, 2001, from www.hcfa.gov/stats/ nhe-oact/tables/chart.htm.

Heather, A. J., Smith, T. A., & Walsh, D. (1962). Extensorcisor. *American Journal of Occupational Therapy, 16,* 10–12.

Heron, W., & Hebb, D. O. (1961). Cognitive and physiological effects of perceptual isolation. In P. Solomon, P. E. Kubzansky, P. H. Leiderman, J. H. Mendelson, R. Trumbull, & D. Wexler (Eds.), *Sensory deprivation* (pp. 1–238). Cambridge, MA: Harvard University Press.

Hickinson, L. M. (1934). Anatomical considerations and technique in using occupations as exercise for orthopedic disabilities. *Occupational Therapy and Rehabilitation, 13,* 30–34.

History. (1940). *Occupational Therapy and Rehabilitation, 19,* 27–34.

Hopkins, H. L. (1983). An historical perspective on occupational therapy. In H. L. Hopkins & H. D. Smith (Eds.), *Willard & Spackman's occupational therapy* (pp. 3–23). Philadelphia: Lippincott.

Howard, B. S. (1991). How high do we jump? The effect of reimbursement on occupational therapy. *American Journal of Occupational Therapy, 45,* 875–881.

Hurt, S. (1947a). Considerations in muscle function and their application to disability evaluation and treatment. *American Journal of Occupational Therapy, 1,* 69–73.

Hurt, S. (1947b). Joint measurement. *American Journal of Occupational Therapy, 1,* 209–214.

Hurt, S. (1947c). Joint measurement: Part II. *American Journal of Occupational Therapy, 1,* 218–285.

Institute for the Future. (2003). *Health and health care 2010* (2nd ed.). Princeton, NJ: Jossey-Bass.

Jacobs, K. (1999). *Ergonomics for therapists* (2nd ed.). Boston: Butterworth Heinemann.

Johnson, S. (1917). Occupational therapy in New York City institutions. *The Modern Hospital, 8,* 414–415.

Kabat, H., & Rosenberg, D. (1950). Concepts and techniques of occupational therapy for neuromuscular disorders. *American Journal of Occupational Therapy, 4,* 6–11.

Kephart, N. C. (1960). *The slow learner in the classroom.* Columbus, OH: Charles E. Merrill Books, Inc.

Kern, S. (1983). *The culture of time and space.* Cambridge, MA: Harvard University.

Kielhofner, G., Hammel, J., Finlayson, M., Helfrich, C., & Taylor, R. R. (2004). Documenting outcomes of occupational therapy: The Center for Outcomes Research and Education. *American Journal of Occupational Therapy, 58,* 15–23.

Kowalske, K., Plenger, P. M., Lusby, B., & Hayden, M. E. (2000). Vocational reentry following TBI: An enablement model. *Journal of Head Trauma Rehabilitation, 15,* 989–999.

Krieg, F. J. (1997). Managed care: A brief introduction. Retrieved December 20, 2005 from www.nasponline.org/publications/cq261mancare.html.

Licht, S. (1967). The founding and founders of the American Occupational Therapy Association. *American Journal of Occupational Therapy, 21,* 269–277.

Liepert, J., Bauder, H., Miltner, W. H. R., Taub, E., & Weiller, C. (2000). Treatment-induced cortical reorganization after stroke in humans. *Stroke, 31,* 1210–1216.

Low, J. F. (1992). The reconstruction aides. *American Journal of Occupational Therapy, 46,* 45–48.

Lowman, E., & Klinger, J. (1969). *Aids to independent living.* New York: McGraw-Hill Book Co.

MacLean, F. M. (1949). Occupational therapy in the management of poliomyelitis. *American Journal of Occupational Therapy, 3,* 20–27.

Mattson, B. (1999). Caps on payment alter therapy: Medicare recipients ration their rehab to maximize treatment. Retrieved August 3, 2006 from http://www.bizjournals.com/twincities/stories/1999/06/28/focus3.html.

McFarland, J. W., & Lukins, N. M. (1946). A page turning device for respiratory patients. *Occupational Therapy and Rehabilitation, 25,* 42–44.

Melosh, B. (1984). More than "the physician's hand": Skill and authority in twentieth-century nursing. In J. W. Leavitt (Ed.), *Women and health in America* (pp. 482–496). Madison, WI: University of Wisconsin.

Meyer, A. (1977). The philosophy of occupational therapy. *American Journal of Occupational Therapy, 31,* 639–642.

Moore, J. C. (1968). A new look at the nervous system in relation to rehabilitation techniques. *American Journal of Occupational Therapy, 22,* 489–501.

Mosey, A. C. (1970). *Three frames of reference for mental health.* Thorofare, NJ: Charles B. Slack.

National Council on the Handicapped. (1986). *Toward independence: An assessment of federal laws and programs affecting persons with disabilities–with legislative recommendations.* Washington, DC: U.S. Government Printing Office.

Neugarten, B., Moore, J., & Lowe, J. (1968). Age norms, age constraints, and adult socialization. In B. L. Neugarten (Ed.), *Middle age and aging: A reader in social psychology.* Chicago: University of Chicago.

Occupational aides. (1918). *Maryland Psychiatric Quarterly, 8,* 27.

Occupational therapy in the general hospital. (1917). *The Modern Hospital, 8,* 425–427.

Occupations for invalids. (1916). School of Practical Arts, Teachers College, Columbia University. American Occupational Therapy Association Archives, Series 12, Box 101, File 733, Bethesda, MD.

Peloquin, S. M. (1991). Occupational therapy service: Individual and collective understandings of the founders, part 1. *American Journal of Occupational Therapy, 45,* 352–360.

Reed, K. L., & Sanderson, S. R. (1983). *Concepts of occupational therapy* (2nd ed). Baltimore: Williams & Wilkins.

Reilly, M. (1969). The educational process. *American Journal of Occupational Therapy, 23,* 299–307.

Rosenberg, C. E. (1978). The practice of medicine in New York a century ago. In J. W. Leavitt & R. L. Numbers (Eds.), *Sickness and health in America* (pp. 55–74). Madison, WI: University of Wisconsin.

Rosenthal, R., & Rosnow, R. L. (1991). *Essentials of behavioral research: Methods and data analysis.* New York: McGraw-Hill, Inc.

Rumsey, R. (1946). Occupational therapy in the treatment of peripheral nerve injuries. *Occupational Therapy and Rehabilitation, 25,* 180–183.

Sackett, D. L., Richardson, W. S., Rosenberg, W., & Haynes, R. B. (1997). *Evidence-based medicine: How to practice and teach EBM.* New York: Churchill Livingstone.

Samberg, H. H. (1947). Occupational therapy in a general hospital. *American Journal of Occupational Therapy, 1,* 285–290.

Sammons, D. D. (1945). Arthritis (I). *Occupational Therapy and Rehabilitation, 24,* 13–22.

Serrett, K. D. (1985). Another look at occupational therapy's history: Paradigm or pair-of-hands? *Occupational Therapy in Mental Health, 3,* 1–31.

Sexton, F. H. (1918). Vocational rehabilitation of soldiers suffering from nervous diseases. *Mental Hygiene, 2,* 265–276.

Shapiro, J. (1993). *No pity: People with disabilities forging a new civil rights movement.* New York: Random House.

Silverstein, F. (1953). Occupational therapy and the hand splint. *American Journal of Occupational Therapy, 7,* 213–216,222.

Simple devices enable veterans to drive motor vehicles safely. (1945). *Occupational Therapy and Rehabilitation, 45,* 263.

Slagle, E. C. (1938). Occupational therapy. *Trained Nurse and Hospital Review, 100,* 375–382.

Smart, J. (2001). *Disability, society, and the individual.* Gaithersburg, MD: Aspen Publishers Inc.

Spackman, C. S. (1947). Occupational therapy for patients with physical injuries. In H. S. Willard & C. S. Spackman (Eds.), *Principles of occupational therapy* (pp. 175–273). Philadelphia: Lippincott.

Starr, P. (1982). *The social transformation of American medicine.* New York: Basic Books.

Stevens, R. (1971). *American medicine and the public interest.* New Haven, CT: Yale University.

Street, D. R. (1963). Antagonistic activity in voluntary motion. *American Journal of Occupational Therapy, 17,* 10–15.

Sudsawad, P. (2005). A conceptual framework to increase usability of outcome research for evidence-based practice. *American Journal of Occupational Therapy, 59,* 351–355.

Taylor, M. (1929). Occupational therapy in industrial injuries. *Occupational Therapy and Rehabilitation, 8,* 335–338.

Textbooks required for the January 1920 term at the School of Diversional Occupation in Colorado Springs, Colorado. (1920). American Occupational Therapy Association Archives, Series 12, Box 101, File 731. Rockville, MD: American Occupational Therapy Association.

Tracy, S. (1910). *Studies in invalid occupations: A manual for nurses and attendants.* Boston: Whitcomb & Barrows.

Trombly, C. A., & Scott, A. D. (1977). *Occupational therapy for physical dysfunction.* Baltimore: Williams & Wilkins.

Upham, E. G. (1917). Some principles of occupational therapy. *The Modern Hospital, 8,* 409–413.

Vetting, M. L. (1945). U.S. Naval Hospital, N.N.M.C., Bethesda, Maryland. *Occupational Therapy and Rehabilitation, 25,* 131–135.

Walker, J. P. (2002). Case study: Functional outcome: A case for mild traumatic brain injury. *Brain Injury, 16,* 611–625.

Weinstock-Zlotnick, G., & Hinojosa, J. (2004). Bottom-up or top-down evaluation: Is one better than the other? *American Journal of Occupational Therapy, 58,* 594–599.

Willard, H. S., & Spackman, C. S. (Eds.) (1947). *Principles of occupational therapy.* Philadelphia: Lippincott.

World Health Organization [WHO]. (2001). *International classification of functioning, disability and health (ICF).* Geneva, Switzerland: WHO.

CHAPTER 3

Planning, Guiding, and Documenting Practice

Mary Vining Radomski

LEARNING OBJECTIVES

After studying this chapter, the reader will begin to be able to do the following:

1. Describe four lines of clinical reasoning that shape provision of occupational therapy services.
2. Effectively document occupational therapy services.
3. Differentiate between anticipated therapy outcomes and long- and short-term goals.
4. Consider a variety of treatment approaches in planning therapy.
5. Make a commitment to maintaining his or her professional competence.

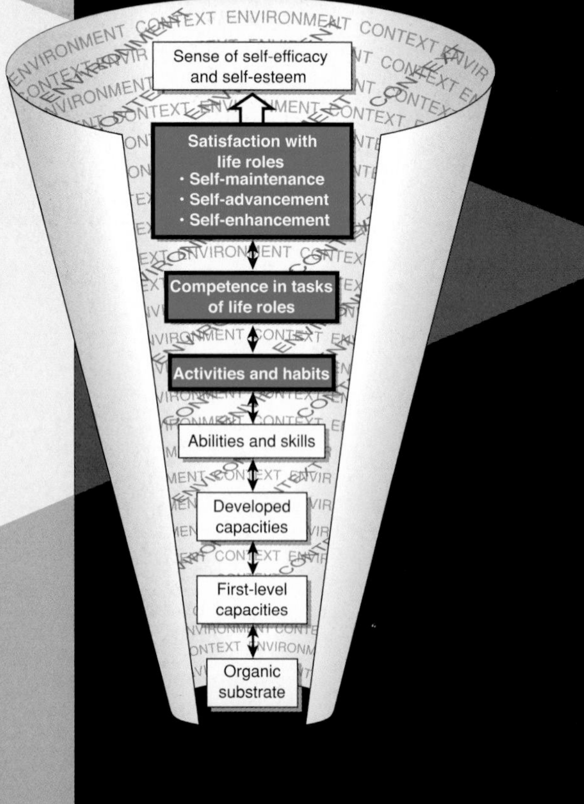

Glossary

Accreditation—A determination by an accrediting body that an eligible health care organization complies with established standards (JCAHO, 1999).

Commission on Accreditation of Rehabilitation Facilities (CARF)—Founded in 1966, CARF is a national organization whose mission is to promote the quality, value, and outcome of rehabilitation services through a consultative accreditation process that centers on enhancing the lives of persons served (CARF, 2004).

Comorbidities—Medical problems typically unrelated to the treatment diagnosis that affect the anticipated outcome and/or the treatment approach.

Continuum of care—A system of services of varying intensity that address the ongoing or intermittent needs of persons with disabilities, ranging from acute medical intervention to rehabilitation to subacute rehabilitation to home health services to outpatient treatment to community wellness opportunities (CARF, 2004).

Episode of care—A discrete interval of service provision related to the achievement of specific therapeutic goals. Patients typically participate in many episodes of care during the recovery and rehabilitation process.

Evidence-based practice—Methods and mindset that integrate research study evidence into the clinical reasoning process (Tickle-Degnen, 2000).

Goal—Narrowly defined end result of therapy to be achieved in a specified time (Bryant, 1995). Goals are usually designated as long or short term.

Joint Commission on Accreditation of Healthcare Organizations (JCAHO)—Founded in 1951, JCAHO is an independent, not-for-profit organization dedicated to improving quality of care in various health settings (JCAHO, 1999).

Length of stay—Total number of days between the date the patient is admitted to the hospital and the date he or she is discharged.

Outcome—Anticipated end result of therapy, given the client's characteristics, expected length of stay or therapy duration, and resources (funding, social support).

Plan of care—A document prepared by all members of the rehabilitation team (including the patient) that describes the interdisciplinary treatment goals, interventions, and time frames for a specific episode of care.

The caliber of the clinician's thinking about each step in the occupational therapy process will set the stage for either inspired intervention or treatment that is rote, uninteresting, and ineffective. One might argue that the ongoing behind-the-scenes thinking about assessment and intervention (known as clinical reasoning) is at least as important as what happens between the client and therapist in a typical 30-minute session.

Clinical documentation chronicles clinical reasoning about occupational therapy diagnosis (Rogers & Holm, 1991), intervention plans, actions, and results. For many clinicians (often including this author), documentation is the price paid for otherwise interesting work. Documentation, however, can be the vehicle through which clinicians think out loud: a map for planning treatment and a compass for monitoring results and shifting course.

This chapter is structured around three interrelated dimensions of occupational therapy practice: thinking, doing, and documenting. Note that Table 3-1 summarizes the ways in which clinical reasoning informs these three aspects of providing occupational therapy services and introduces the case example format used throughout the textbook. The chapter concludes with a discussion of the ways therapists use the processes of thinking, doing, and documenting to improve their clinical competence.

CLINICAL REASONING

Clinical reasoning is the thinking process by which therapists collect and use information to make decisions about care of an individual client (Rogers, 1983). Clinical reasoning is ongoing. It begins as the therapist first reads a patient's referral; extends through assessment, intervention, and discharge; and continues as the clinician reflects on the process and results of intervention with this patient as he or she plans therapy for another patient. Clinical reasoning in practice typically does not occur as a tidy progression of thoughts; it may appear cyclic or even chaotic as therapists dance back and forth between hypothesis testing and storytelling throughout their involvement in patients' care (Hagedorn, 1996). Note how the same internal questions and self-reflections in Table 3-1 are repeated at various junctures in the delivery of services.

As therapists make decisions and plans for assessment and treatment, they simultaneously employ at least four lines of clinical reasoning.

- *Scientific reasoning* refers to the logical thinking about the nature of the client's problems and optimal course of action in treatment (Mattingly, 1991; Rogers, 1983). Therapists employ scientific reasoning when they consider the reliability and validity of assessment tools and

Table 3-1. Clinical Reasoning Underlying the Process of Delivering Occupational Therapy Services

Service Delivery	Clinical Reasoning Objectives	What the Therapist. . . . *Does*	*Thinks (examples of internal questions and self-reflections)*	*Documents*
Screening	Understand the patient's diagnosis or condition	Obtain and review background information	• What do I know about the patient's medical diagnosis? • What impairments, activity limitations, and participation restrictions are typical for individuals with this diagnosis or condition? • Do the patient's records and information from referral sources suggest that occupational therapy services would be appropriate for this patient at this time?	Informal notetaking and record keeping
Assessing occupational functioning	Know the person	Interview, listen, write	• What do I need to know about this patient's current and past occupational functioning? • What does the patient's past tell me about his or her priorities, strategies, and resources under the present circumstances? • Which of the patient's current concerns relate to his or her occupational functioning? • What seem to be the patient's main priorities regarding his or her occupational functioning?	Daily contact notes
	Appreciate the context		• Are there social, cultural, and personal contextual factors that may affect the evaluation or intervention process? • Who should I talk with to better understand the patient's situation, occupational functioning, and/or needs? • Where is the patient in his or her recovery relative to onset of the condition? • What is the projected duration of this episode of care? • What sorts of resources are available to support the occupational therapy process? • What other medical, rehabilitation, and therapy services have been or are involved in the patient's care? • What have been the outcomes of past or current services?	
	Reflect on competence	Consult others (as needed)	• Do I have adequate experience, education, and training to provide occupational therapy services to this patient? • If not, should I share responsibility with someone who can provide coaching or assistance? • Should this patient be referred elsewhere for services?	
	Develop provisional hypotheses		• What physical, cognitive, and contextual barriers may be interfering with the patient's occupational function?	
	Consider the evaluation approach	Select evaluation tools and methods	• Do I want to observe function to make inferences about impairment? • Do I want to assess specific impairments to make inferences about function? • How can I use existing information from other disciplines to inform questions about barriers to occupational functioning?	Evaluation Note
	Consider the evaluation tools		• Are there standardized assessments that will help specify the nature of the barriers to occupational functioning? • What forms of evaluation or specific tools will put the patient most at ease, given what I know about his or her background?	

continued

Table 3-1. ***(continued)***

Service Delivery	Clinical Reasoning Objectives	What the Therapist. . . . *Does*	*Thinks (examples of internal questions and self-reflections)*	*Documents*
	Interpret observations	Administer evaluation; observe; take notes on performance	• How closely am I adhering to administration instructions for standardized assessments? • Does the patient seem to understand the instructions? • What physical, cognitive, and sensory processing capacities are challenged by this assessment? • What strategies or approaches does the patient use to perform the assessment?	
	Synthesize results	Write up evaluation findings	• How does the patient's performance compare to that of others? • To what extent could the patient's performance have been affected by unrelated factors (fatigue, medication, pain, distraction, etc.)? • Do patterns emerge in the patient's performance across task or assessment?	
Planning intervention	Develop intervention hypotheses		• What seem to be the most salient barriers (physical, cognitive, emotional, contextual) to the patient's occupational functioning?	Intervention plan
	Select an intervention approach or model		• What intervention approach or model has the strongest evidence of effectiveness in the rehabilitation research literature for patients similar to my current patient?	
	Reflect on competence	Consult others (as needed)	• Do I have adequate experience, education, and training to provide occupational therapy services to this patient? • If not, should I share responsibility with someone who can provide coaching or assistance? • Should this patient be referred elsewhere for services?	
	Consider the patient's appraisal of performance	Discuss evaluation impressions and findings with patient and possible course of intervention	• To what extent does the patient understand and/or agree with my hypotheses regarding barriers to his or her occupational functioning? • Given what I suspect are underlying barriers to occupational functioning, what does the patient seem to want to achieve in therapy at this time? • Are there any constraints on the length of time that I am able to provide services to this patient?	
	Consider what will occur in therapy, how often, and for how long	Specify treatment activities, time frame, and intensity	• What specific techniques or activities should be used in therapy, given the approach I've selected and what I know about the person? • What does the literature suggest about the optimal time frame, intensity, and duration of therapy needed to achieve results? • If there is no scientific evidence in this area, what do experienced clinicians recommend about time frame, intensity, and duration?	
	Ascertain patient's endorsement of interven-tion plan	Discuss with patient and modify as necessary	• What are the indicators that this patient understands the intervention plan that I've proposed? • What are the indicators that this patient (and/or significant others) endorse the plan as proposed?	

continued

Table 3-1. *(continued)*

Service Delivery	Clinical Reasoning Objectives	What the Therapist. . . . *Does*	*Thinks (examples of internal questions and self-reflections)*	*Documents*
Delivering treatment and monitoring progress	Assess the patient's comprehension	Provide instructions for therapy, exercises, tasks, and activities	• Does the patient seem to understand what I am saying? • Am I using language or expressions that likely make sense to this person?	Daily contact notes
	Understand what the patient is doing	Observe patient's performance	• What specific actions is the patient taking? • What do the actions infer about how the patient is thinking or processing? • Why does the patient appear to be performing in this manner?	Weekly and/or monthly progress notes
	Compare actual performance to expected performance	Discuss with patient; modify the treatment plan as needed	• To what extent does this patient's performance support my hypotheses regarding the nature of his or her barriers to occupational functioning? • Is the patient's performance improving at the rate I anticipated? If not, why? • To what extent is the patient complying with home recommendations, exercises, and activities?	Home programs
	Know the person		• What does the patient's performance tell me about who this patient is? • How should these insights further shape the intervention plan?	
	Appreciate the context		• Are there other possible factors that are interfering with the patient's occupational functioning? If so, what might they be? • Does the patient seem to understand what I am saying? • Am I using language or expressions that likely make sense to this person?	
	Consider alternatives to current services		• Is the patient making enough progress toward his or her occupational therapy goals to warrant continuation? Are the goals still appropriate? • Would services from other providers be beneficial?	
Discontinuing occupational therapy services	Anticipate present and future patient concerns	Write and discuss recommendations	• Given what I know about the diagnosis or condition, who he or she is, and his or her progress to date, what should this patient continue to do (or discontinue) to optimize his or her occupational functioning?	Home programs
	Analyze the patient's comprehension		• Does the patient seem to understand what I am saying? • Am I using language or expressions that likely make sense to this person? • What other people in the patient's life also need to understand this information?	Referral
	Decide if or when the patient should return for therapy	Plan for follow-up	• Do I expect the patient's occupational functioning to change at some point in such a way that therapy should then be resumed? If so, when would it make sense to reevaluate the patient's need for occupational therapy services?	Discharge summary

continued

Table 3-1. *(continued)*

Service Delivery	Clinical Reasoning Objectives	Does	What the Therapist. . . . *Thinks (examples of internal questions and self-reflections)*	*Documents*
			• Are there resources to pay for follow-up occupational therapy services? • Does the patient seem to understand under what circumstances to contact me again, or should we schedule a time at which he or she will return? • Are there other services in the community that this patient should be accessing at this point?	

when they use the patient's medical and occupational diagnoses and research evidence to shape the intervention plan (Rogers & Masagatani, 1982; Rogers & Holm, 1991).

- *Narrative reasoning* refers to thinking in story form to place the client's functioning in the context of his or her background and broader experience (Schell & Cervero, 1993). Therapists employ narrative reasoning when they try to understand the meaning of disability in the patient's life in order to link his or her goals and values to the therapy process (Mattingly, 1991).
- *Pragmatic reasoning* refers to thinking about logistics and practical aspects of delivering services to clients within a given setting or organization (Schell & Cervero, 1993). Therapists employ pragmatic reasoning when they consider norms of the department or expectations related to **accreditation**, personnel, or reimbursement factors as they provide occupational therapy services (Schell & Cervero, 1993).
- Ethical reasoning refers to idealistic thinking about what should be done on behalf of a specific individual (Rogers, 1983). A therapist employs ethical reasoning when he or she synthesizes research evidence, an appraisal of his or her competence, practical aspects of service delivery, and the patient's goals and values to answer the following question: "What, among the many things that could be done for the patient, ought to be done?" (Rogers, 1983, p. 602).

Clinical reasoning is a dynamic process, simultaneously influenced by client and therapist characteristics, experience, and background (Rogers & Holm, 1991; Roberts, 1996; Sviden & Hallin, 1999; Unsworth, 2001). For example, a middle-aged therapist with elderly parents and an equally experienced therapist with young children may arrive at different assessment conclusions and develop different treatment plans for an 80-year-old patient recovering from a pelvic fracture because of their different life experiences. Similarly, the characteristics of settings in which occupational therapists work shape clinical reasoning (Rogers & Holm, 1991). Physical, financial, and personnel resources influence assessment tools and methods, and multidisciplinary teams establish informal rules about the boundaries of each discipline's contribution (Rogers & Holm, 1991). Clearly, clinical decisions are shaped by many factors, including the clinician's professional expertise, the client's background and preferences, and research evidence (Rappolt, 2003). **Evidence-based practice** minimizes the influence of personal and environmental biases in the clinical reasoning process.

Evidence-Based Practice

Evidence-based practice (EBP) is "the conscientious, explicit, and judicious use of current best evidence in making decisions about the care of individual patients. [It integrates] individual clinical expertise with the best available external clinical evidence from systematic research" (Sackett et al., 1997, p. 2). Evidence-based practice includes both method and mindset. The method is made up of seven steps: (1) write an answerable clinical question; (2) gather best evidence to answer the question, including clinical assessment findings, systematic reviews from the literature, and primary studies; (3) evaluate the validity and clinical usefulness of the gathered evidence; (4) synthesize the findings; (5) communicate with various stakeholders, including client and family, about evidence as it relates to assessment or treatment; (6) apply findings to practice; and (7) monitor, evaluate, and document the results (Sackett et al., 1997; Tickle-Degnen, 2000). Many resources are available to clinicians, including systematic research reviews and tools for implementing EBP methods (see Resources 3-1).

Beyond the methodology, evidence-based practice reflects habits of thinking and doing that pervade the way the clinician delivers services (Cusick & McCluskey, 2000; Holm, 2000). Although evidence-based practice

RESOURCE 3-1

Evidence-Based Practice

The AGREE Collaboration (Appraisal of Guidelines Research and Evaluation)
– instrument for assessing the quality of clinical practice guidelines.
www.agreecollaboration.org

AOTA's Evidence Brief Series
– site available to members of AOTA that includes summaries of research related to occupational intervention related to various diagnostic groups.
www.aota.org

Centre for Evidence Based Medicine (EBM)
– site at University of Toronto that offers resources for understanding the steps for using evidence in practice and teaching others about this process.
www.cebm.utoronto.ca/

Cochrane Collaboration
– the site of the international organization that produces and disseminates hundreds of systematic reviews of health care interventions.
www.cochrane.org

Occupational Therapy Critically Appraised Topics (CATS)
– site containing critically appraised topics (short summaries of evidence on a topic of interest focused around a clinical question) usually developed from several critically appraised papers (CAPS) (summaries of single studies).
www.otcats.com

Occupational Therapy Evidence-Based Practice Research Group
– site created by McMaster Occupational Therapy Evidence-Based Practice Group with results of systematic reviews of research evidence in interventions used by occupational therapists and forms and guidelines to critically review qualitative and quantitative research articles.
www-fhs.mcmaster.ca/rehab/ebp/

OTseeker (Occupational Therapy Systematic Evaluation of Evidence)
– site created by a team of occupational therapists at the Universities of Queensland and Western Sydney with abstracts of systematic reviews and quality ratings of randomized controlled trials relevant to occupational therapy.
www.otseeker.com

is increasingly emphasized in the literature, it may not yet have fully infiltrated day-to-day occupational therapy practice. Many treatments do not lend themselves to controlled clinical trials, and subjects in well-designed studies tend to be unrealistically homogeneous and do not have the confounding problems or severity of impairments typical of many rehabilitation patients (Whyte, 1998). Clinicians cite insufficient time (Philibert et al., 2003; Rappolt, 2003) and difficulties understanding research (Gervais et al., 2002) as barriers to using evidence to inform practice. Many therapists put more emphasis on knowledge gained from clinical experience and consultation with others than on research literature (Dubouloz et al., 1999). They rely on previous experience and patients' input to guide decisions, using research primarily to confirm the effectiveness of practice to non-clients (Dubouloz et al., 1999).

Leaders in our profession have unambiguously charged occupational therapists to "wake up to the world of health care research and to use findings from this world of research in addition to more familiar sources of evidence to guide treatment planning" (Ottenbacher, Tickle-Degnen, & Hasselkus, 2002, p. 247). This requires individual clinicians to adhere to the ethical standards of our profession (American Occupational Therapy Association [AOTA], 2000) and take personal responsibility to know and then fully inform clients of the nature, risks, and potential outcomes of any intervention (Holm, 2000). As they adopt an evidence-oriented mindset, occupational therapists will be able to describe why they are using particular assessments and recommending particular interventions (Cusick & McCluskey, 2000) and enable clients, families, and payers to make informed decisions about occupational therapy services.

CLINICAL DOCUMENTATION

Clinical documentation in occupational therapy provides a chronological record of the patient's status and condition related to occupational functioning and details the course of therapeutic intervention (AOTA, 2004a). It reflects the clinician's reasoning and serves as the basis for judging the appropriateness, effectiveness, and necessity of intervention (AOTA, 2004a).

Occupational therapists contribute information to medical records in a number of formats: source-oriented medical records, which are organized in sections according to the department providing care; integrated medical records in chronological order; and problem-oriented medical records, which are organized according to four components, namely database, complete list of problems, plans for each problem, and progress notes (Robertson, 1997). SOAP notes are typically used to report progress in problem-oriented medical records (Robertson, 1997). (SOAP is an acronym for the four parts of a progress notes: subjective, objective, assessment, and plan.) Obviously, occupational therapists contribute documentation that complies with the structure of the medical records established for their specific work settings.

In the course of their daily work, occupational therapists produce a number of reports, including daily contact notes, evaluation summaries, weekly or monthly progress notes, and discharge summaries (Table 3-2).

Table 3-2. Overview: Types of Occupational Therapy Documentation

Documentation	Purpose	Typical Formats	Contents	When to Document
Contact, treatment, or visit note	Brief account of an individual session	Short narrative note, checklist, or flow sheet	• Amount of time spent evaluating or treating the client • Brief characterization of intervention (e.g., ADL instruction, strengthening, compensatory strategy training) • Description of client response relative to short-term goals	After each evaluation or treatment session
Evaluation report	Detailing of assessment findings, interpretation of results, estimated outcomes of intervention, goals, time frame, and treatment plan	• Therapist's observations and findings recorded on a fill-in-the-blank form • Handwritten or dictated and typed report	• Background information on the client (age, sex, diagnosis); summary of medical history, secondary problems, and **comorbidities**; precautions and contraindications • Referral source, services requested, date of referral • Date(s) of evaluation sessions and amount of time • Pre-morbid or prior level of functioning in occupational function; self-report of problems and priorities (Occupational Profile [AOTA 2002, 2004]) • Assessment results: scores, observations, summary, and analysis of assessment findings (Analysis of Occupational Performance [AOTA, 2004]) • Intervention plan: projected outcomes of therapy, goals, and time frame; statement of client participation in goal setting for therapy; general description of treatment plan (including treatment approach and recommended frequency of treatment sessions)	After completing the assessment, synthesizing the results, and collaborating with client about therapy goals
Progress report	Summary of progress toward functional goals, interventions employed, updated goals, and treatment plan	• Fill-in-the-blank form or checklist with section for handwritten comments • Flow sheet (as used with clinical pathways) • Handwritten or dictated and typed report	• Dates of service and dates of progress period • Number of treatment sessions during progress period • Overview of activities, techniques, modalities used • Summary of instruction provided to client or family • Description of adaptive equipment issued or recommended • Client's response to intervention specific to therapy goals • Recommendations regarding continuation of therapy • Revised goals and time frame for achievement • Revised treatment plan (treatment approach, recommended frequency of sessions) • Statement of client participation in goal setting for therapy	Daily, weekly, or monthly, depending on setting
Discharge report	Review of occupational therapy assessment, intervention, and outcome	• Fill-in-the-blank form or checklist with section for handwritten comments • Flow sheet (as used with critical pathways) • Handwritten or dictated and typed report	• Dates of referral, service initiation, and discontinuation • Total number of evaluation and treatment sessions • Summary of client's progress toward each therapy goal • Overview of interventions employed specific to each goal • Description of maintenance program and discharge instructions • Recommendations for follow-up, maintenance programs, referrals to other services or agencies	After the last session in an episode of care

Sources: Allen, C. A. (1997). Clinical reasoning for documentation. In J. D. Acquaviva (Ed.), *Effective documentation for occupational therapy* (2nd ed., pp. 53–62). Bethesda, MD: American Occupational Therapy Association.
American Occupational Therapy Association [AOTA]. (2002). Occupational therapy practice framework: Domain and process. *American Journal of Occupational Therapy, 56,* 609–639.
American Occupational Therapy Association [AOTA]. (2004). Guidelines for documentation of occupational therapy. In *The reference manual of the official documents of the American Occupational Therapy Association, Inc.* (10th ed., pp. 153–158). Bethesda, MD: American Occupational Therapy Association.
Wilson, D. (1997). Clinical reasoning for documentation. In J. D. Acquaviva (Ed.), *Effective documentation for occupational therapy* (2nd ed., pp. 1–3). Bethesda, MD: American Occupational Therapy Association.

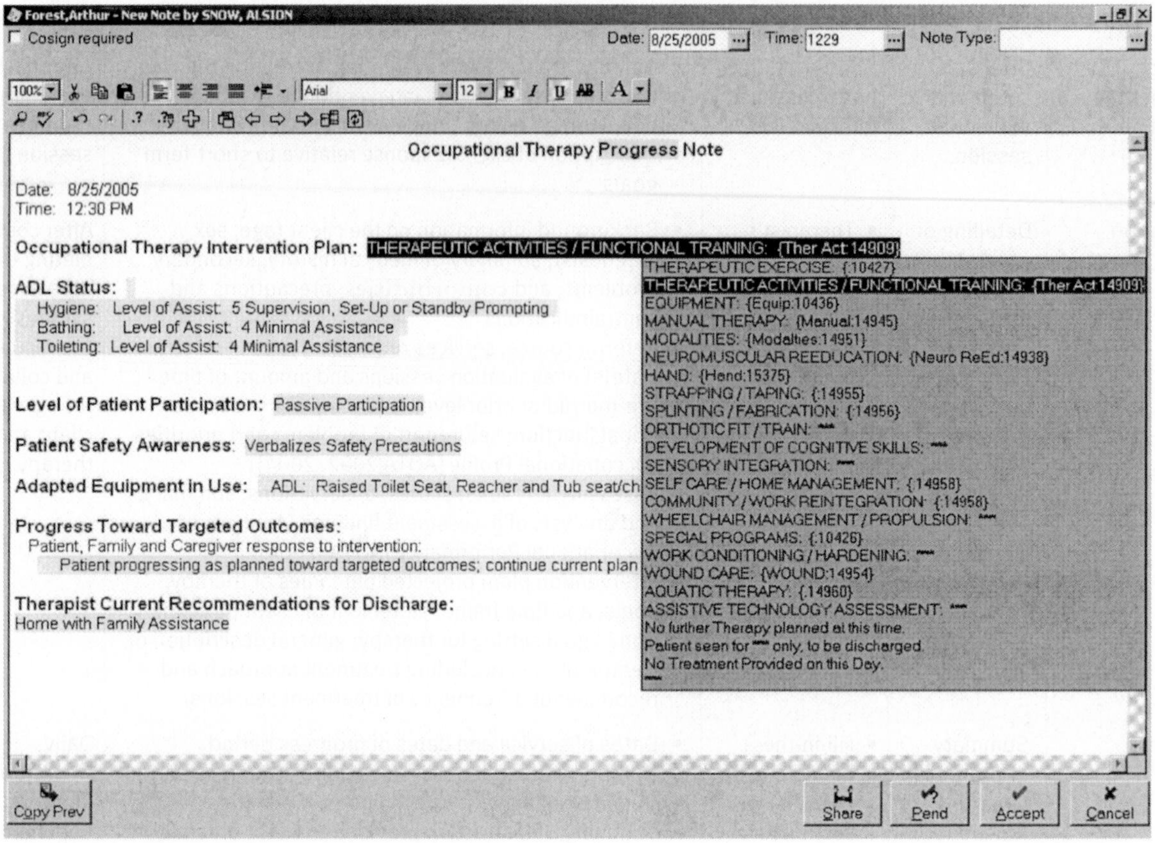

Figure 3-1 This screen shot of occupational therapy documentation in a electronic medical record depicts how clinicians use drop-down boxes to select descriptors of intervention and patient performance. (Epic Systems Corporation © 1999–2005. Reprinted with permission.)

Documentation formats include computerized records, checklists, forms, and narrative notes. (See Fig. 3-1 for an example of an occupational therapy daily progress note from a computerized medical record.) Regardless of format, to communicate in these documents, therapists must be clear about their target audience (McGuire, 1997; Robertson, 1997). That is, who will read this note and what do they need or want to know about the occupational therapy work with this patient? Clinicians aim to provide succinct descriptions of functional status, anticipated outcome, and progress to date, so that a single document meets a number of stakeholders' information needs. The reading audience may include members of the treatment team, who want to know how best to collaborate; the third-party payer, who wants to decide whether to pay for services; the accrediting agency, such as the **Joint Commission on Accreditation for Healthcare Organizations (JCAHO)** or the **Commission on Accreditation of Rehabilitation Facilities (CARF)**, which want to determine whether quality services are provided at your institution; the legal system, which wants evidence in malpractice litigation; and the patient and significant others, who want to understand the care (Robertson, 1997).

McGuire (1997) outlined six principles that reflect excellent standards for occupational therapy documentation. She suggested that clinical documentation addressing these principles meets the information requirements of a variety of stakeholders, including Medicare, the largest third-party payer in the United States. After stating each principle, I briefly summarize McGuire's recommendations for clinical documentation (Fig. 3-2).

1. Focus on function. Clinicians describe the patient's previous or premorbid level of function in key areas, review his or her current status, and/or provide estimates of potential improvements or outcomes as a result of therapy.

2. Focus on underlying causes. Clinicians combine their understanding of the patient's medical condition with results of their assessments to identify specific impairments that restrict or limit occupational performance (McGuire, 1997).

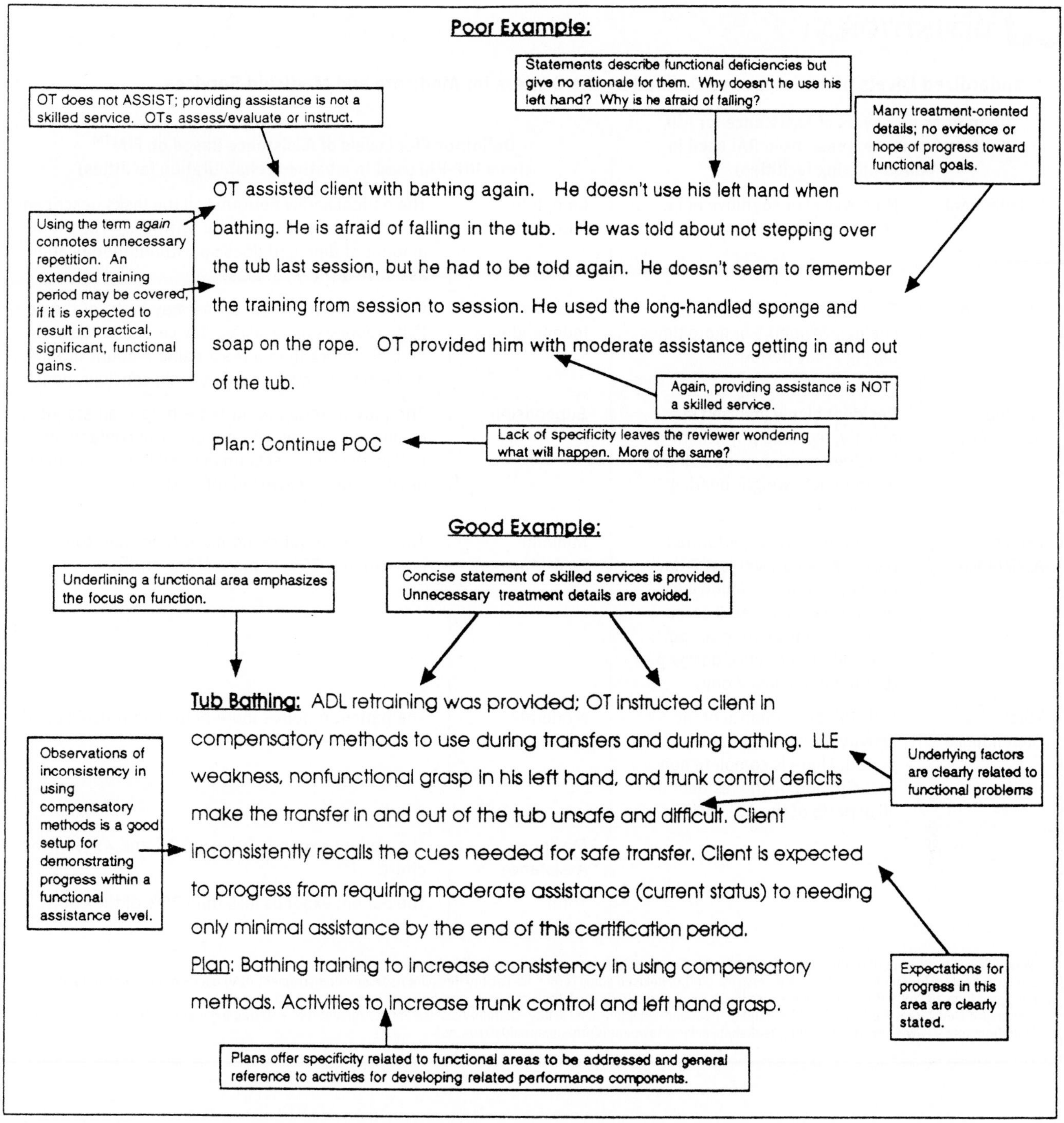

Poor Example:
OT does not ASSIST; providing assistance is not a skilled service. OTs assess/evaluate or instruct.
Statements describe functional deficiencies but give no rationale for them. Why doesn't he use his left hand? Why is he afraid of falling?
Many treatment-oriented details; no evidence or hope of progress toward functional goals.
Using the term again connotes unnecessary repetition. An extended training period may be covered, if it is expected to result in practical, significant, functional gains.
OT assisted client with bathing again. He doesn't use his left hand when bathing. He is afraid of falling in the tub. He was told about not stepping over the tub last session, but he had to be told again. He doesn't seem to remember the training from session to session. He used the long-handled sponge and soap on the rope. OT provided him with moderate assistance getting in and out of the tub.
Again, providing assistance is NOT a skilled service.
Plan: Continue POC
Lack of specificity leaves the reviewer wondering what will happen. More of the same?
Good Example:
Underlining a functional area emphasizes the focus on function.
Concise statement of skilled services is provided. Unnecessary treatment details are avoided.
Tub Bathing: ADL retraining was provided; OT instructed client in compensatory methods to use during transfers and during bathing. LLE weakness, nonfunctional grasp in his left hand, and trunk control deficits make the transfer in and out of the tub unsafe and difficult. Client inconsistently recalls the cues needed for safe transfer. Client is expected to progress from requiring moderate assistance (current status) to needing only minimal assistance by the end of this certification period.
Plan: Bathing training to increase consistency in using compensatory methods. Activities to increase trunk control and left hand grasp.
Observations of inconsistency in using compensatory methods is a good setup for demonstrating progress within a functional assistance level.
Underlying factors are clearly related to functional problems
Expectations for progress in this area are clearly stated.
Plans offer specificity related to functional areas to be addressed and general reference to activities for developing related performance components.

Figure 3-2 Features of effective progress notes. (From: McGuire, M. J. [1997]. Documenting progress in home care. *American Journal of Occupational Therapy, 51,* 444. Copyright 1997 by The American Occupational Therapy Association, Inc. Reprinted with permission.)

3. Focus on progress. Clinicians describe patients' progress toward goals according to objective measures, details of careful observation, and/or standardized levels of independence. (Definition 3-1 describes standardized definitions for levels of assistance used by the Centers for Medicare and Medicaid Services.)
4. Focus on safety. Many stakeholders look to the occupational therapist to provide information about the patient's safety and competence in self-

DEFINITION 3-1

Standardized Levels of Assistance as Defined by the Centers for Medicare and Medicaid Services

Definitions for Levels of Assistance for ADL Self-Performance Items (from RAI used in skilled nursing facilities)		Definitions for Levels of Assistance Based on FIM™ (from IRF-PAI used in inpatient rehabilitation facilities)	
Independent	No physical or cognitive help, set up, or supervision	Complete Independence	The patient safely performs all the tasks described as making up the activity within a reasonable amount of time and does so without modification, assistive devices, or aids.
Supervision	Oversight, encouragement, or cueing provided 3 or more times during 7-day period	Modified Independence	One or more of the following may be true: the activity requires an assistive device or aid, the activity takes more than a reasonable amount of time, or the activity involves safety (risk) considerations.
Limited Assistance	Resident highly involved in activity, received physical help in guided maneuvering of limbs or other non–weight-bearing assistance	Supervision	The patient requires no more help than standby, cueing, or coaxing, without physical contact; alternately, the helper sets up needed items or applies orthoses or assistive/adaptive devices.
Extensive Assistance	Although resident performed part of activity, over last 7-day period, help of the following type(s) was provided 3 or more times: weight-bearing support; full staff performance during part (but not all) of last 7 days	Minimal Assistance	The patient requires no more help than touching and expends 75% or more of the effort.
Total Dependence	Full staff performance of the activity during entire 7-day period. There is complete nonparticipation by the resident in all aspects of the ADL task.	Moderate Assistance	The patient requires more help than touching and expends 50–74% of the effort.
		Maximum Assistance	The patient expends between 25 and 49% of the effort.
		Total Assistance	The patient expends less than 25% of the effort.

Note: FIM is a trademark of Uniform Data System for Medical Rehabilitation, a division of UB Foundation Activities, Inc.
Sources: Centers for Medicare & Medicaid Services. (2002). Revised Long-Term Care Facility Resident Assessment Instrument (RAI) user's manual version 2.0. Retrieved June 28, 2005 from http://www.cms.hhs.gov/medicaid/mds20/default.asp www.cms.hhs.gov/medicaid/mds20/default.asp.
Centers for Medicare & Medicaid Services. (2004). Inpatient Rehabilitation Facility – Patient Assessment Instrument (IRF-PAI) training manual. Retrieved August 3, 2006 from http://www.cms.hhs.gov/InpatienRehabFacPPS/downloads/irfpaimanual040104.pdf

management, self-advancement, and self-enhancement roles.

5. State expectations for progress or explain slow progress or lack of progress. Occupational therapists must "document a continued expectation that the patient's condition will continue to improve significantly in a reasonable and generally predictable amount of time" (McGuire, 1997, p. 441). Therapists need to document setbacks that delay progress, such as medication changes, medical complications, and social disruptions.
6. Summarize needed skilled services. Occupational therapists avoid detailing the specific therapeutic interventions used during a given treatment session or period but emphasize the provision of skilled services. Skilled services include evaluations; direct intervention, such as training in techniques or strategies; task modification; selection or construction of equipment or orthotics;

and instructions to the patient or caregiver about maintenance programs.

PROVIDING OCCUPATIONAL THERAPY SERVICES

Clinical reasoning and documentation shape and reflect each aspect of providing occupational therapy services, including screening, assessing, planning, intervening, monitoring, and discontinuing treatment.

Screening

People are referred for occupational therapy if they have impairments, activity limitations, or participation restrictions; are at risk in these areas; or need help promoting health (Moyers, 1999). A physician's order or referral is a prerequisite to beginning services covered by third-party payers.

Screening is defined as reviewing information relevant to a prospective patient to determine the need for further evaluation and intervention (Moyers, 1999). Therapists gather this information through chart review and a brief interview.

Chart Review and Brief Interview

Occupational therapists review relevant documents in the patient's medical record before beginning assessment or treatment. Other team members' assessments (e.g., the physician's history and physical, social service or psychology intake notes, nursing assessments) help the therapist create a preliminary clinical image related to disease, severity of illness or disorder, comorbidities, age, sex, and personal and social background (Rogers & Holm, 1991). After the chart review, the occupational therapist typically introduces himself or herself to the patient and/or significant other, informs them of the referral, and briefly describes the nature of occupational therapy and the anticipated services. The purpose of this conversation is to ensure the appropriateness of the referral and obtain preliminary agreement to participate. The conversation may take place during the first few minutes of the initial assessment session, as with outpatients or patients receiving home care, or be a brief encounter in the patient's hospital room, with the assessment scheduled to take place later.

Documentation Requirements: Referral to Occupational Therapy Services

A physician's order should include the following information: the patient's diagnosis (underlying disorder, disease, or injury that contributes to occupational dysfunction); the treatment diagnosis (the likely impairment contributing to occupational dysfunction); the actual or estimated date of recent change in the level of function; a request for evaluation or treatment; the date; and the physician's signature (Allen et al., 1997).

If the screening suggests that the referral to occupational therapy is inappropriate or the patient or family defers participation, the clinician records that orders were received and a screen was performed and explains why further assessment and treatment appear unwarranted.

Assessing Occupational Function: The Four Elements

Various aspects of occupational therapy assessment have been detailed elsewhere in this text (see Chapters 4 to 11). The discussion that follows sets the four elements of assessment (interview, observation of function, evaluation, and synthesis of results) in the broader schema of providing occupational therapy services, emphasizing the clinical reasoning dimensions rather than specific tools or methods.

Interview

Using a structured interview, the clinician identifies the client's needs and goals in the context of his or her life (Fisher, 1998). Fisher extolled the value of this aspect of the assessment process: "This step is critical, and it must occur, even under the pressures of cost containment, reduced duration of care, staff cuts, and increased accountability. In fact, there is some evidence that taking more time, initially, to establish client-centered performance will result in overall outcomes being enhanced and overall costs reduced" (Fisher, 1998, pp. 515–516).

Observe Function

The occupational therapist observes the patient performing one of the activities described as important and problematic to generate hypotheses regarding underlying impairments or inefficiencies that interfere with function. For example, while observing a patient with stroke get dressed, the clinician looks for cues that point to underlying causes of performance problems (hypothesizing, for example, that difficulty locating socks, shirt, and shoes is due to left neglect).

Evaluate with Selected Tools and Methods

Based on observations of functional performance and resultant hypotheses regarding underlying causes, therapists use selected evaluation tools and methods to verify and quantify the existence of impairments or inefficiencies. In fact, clinicians evaluate only those client factors (AOTA, 2002), impairments, or inefficiencies suspected of impeding occupational function, rather than casting a wide net to identify all possible deficits.

Synthesize Results

Occupational therapists study assessment findings to draw conclusions about the patient's competence and quality of occupational function. The patient's strengths and weaknesses, likely underlying causes or explanations for performance problems, and potential barriers and enablers to improved functioning become the basis of the hypothesis for treatment (Opacich, 1991). The hypothesis for treatment reflects the therapist's understanding of the patient's problems. Although it may change as treatment gets under way, the hypothesis for treatment guides the selection of the treatment approach (Opacich, 1991).

Documentation Requirements: Record Keeping and Notes

Occupational therapists typically take notes regarding patient performance during the assessment. Sometimes these forms or protocols ultimately go directly into the medical record. Worksheets are also used for data collection (with the typed or handwritten summary produced for the medical record upon completion of the assessment). Some occupational therapy assessments and intervention plans are completed after just one evaluation session, in which case the therapist generates the documentation described in the next section. When the assessment spans multiple sessions, daily contact notes are recorded in the medical record.

Planning Intervention

After formulating a hypothesis for treatment, the occupational therapist plans intervention. Clinical reasoning is involved in estimating outcomes, setting goals, and selecting treatment approaches and methods.

Estimate Outcomes and Set Collaborative Goals

An **outcome** of therapy is an anticipated end result, given a specific set of parameters (Bryant, 1995). Outcomes are chosen in part according to expected **length of stay** or anticipated number of outpatient or home-based sessions and the type of funding available. The contemporary rehabilitation environment often requires clinicians to identify key expected outcomes for and with persons served, measure these outcomes, and determine how outcomes can be achieved in a resource-wise or cost-effective manner (Cope & Sundance, 1995). Interdisciplinary rehabilitation teams typically establish a **plan of care** for a given **episode of care** that delineates the overall patient-specific outcomes, with each discipline setting goals that contribute to these core outcomes.

The Occupational Therapy Practice Framework (AOTA, 2002) suggests that the overarching outcome of occupational therapy intervention is to enable recipients of our services to engage in occupations that allow them to participate in valued roles within their home, school, work, and/or communities (AOTA, 2002). This may be achieved through improvements related to: (1) function (remediation of impairments); (2) occupational performance (independence in activities of daily living [ADL], work, and play); (3) health and well-being (symptom status improvement and prevention of disability); and (4) quality of life (purposeful participation in community life, emotional well-being, balance of activity and rest, and life satisfaction) (Moyers, 1999). Global outcomes of occupational therapy intervention can also be identified according to resumption of self-maintenance, self-advancement, and self-enhancement roles (Trombly, 1993, 1995). In selecting and projecting outcomes of treatment, occupational therapists are urged to look beyond functional independence or relearning of physical skills as the superordinate aims of occupational therapy (Radomski, 1995) and help patients attain wholeness, autonomy, meaning, and purpose in their daily lives (Crabtree, 2000).

Predicting outcomes of therapy forces clinicians to answer two key questions in intervention planning: (1) In what broad ways will this client's life, health, and functioning improve as a result of therapy at this point in the recovery or adaptation process? (2) How long will it take to realize these benefits? The answers require an appreciation for the **continuum of care** and a realization that not every dysfunction, impairment, or inefficiency can or should be addressed within a given episode of care. For example, resumption of self-maintenance roles may be an appropriate occupational therapy outcome for a stroke patient with good family support who is expected to receive inpatient rehabilitation for 2 to 3 weeks. On the other hand, resumption of self-advancement roles would probably not be an appropriate outcome of inpatient rehabilitation. Occupational therapy services to promote work readiness can likely be provided more cost effectively when the individual is an outpatient. Furthermore, resumption of work roles typically occurs after the patient achieves medical stability, approaches maximal restoration of function, and begins the adjustment process, none of which is likely to occur within a month of a stroke. Treatment planning based on anticipated outcomes of therapy not only reflects good stewardship, but it is also required by accreditation bodies, such as CARF (2004).

Table 3-3. Example of Establishing Short-term Goals

Long-Term Goal: Independence in Lower Extremity Dressing	
Examples of Short-Term Goals Based on Impairments	***Examples of Short-Term Goals Based on Task Analysis***
• Trunk flexion and BUE forward reach adequate for LE dressing	• Client will be able to properly place trousers over feet for donning.
• Cognitive-perceptual skills adequate for positioning clothing during LE dressing	• Client will be able to spontaneously dress LLE before RLE.
• Endurance adequate for safety and independence during LE dressing	• Client will be able to pull up trousers from a standing position.
• Demonstrate compensatory methods and appropriate use of adaptive equipment for safe, independent LE dressing	• Client will be able to demonstrate proper and long handled shoe horn and complete LE use of sock donner dressing in 5 minutes without SOB.

BUE, both upper extremities; LE, lower extremity; LLE, left lower extremity; RLE, right lower extremity; SOB, shortness of breath.
From McGuire, M. J. (1997). Documenting progress in home care. *American Journal of Occupational Therapy, 51,* 483. Copyright 1997 by The American Occupational Therapy Association, Inc. Reprinted with permission.

Long- and Short-Term Goals

Once the occupational therapist and patient/family member conceptualize global outcomes of therapy, they work backward to establish a sequence of long- and short-term goals to get there (Cope & Sundance, 1995). A **goal** is a measurable, narrowly defined end result of therapy to be achieved in a specified time (Bryant, 1995). Long-term goals reflect what will be achieved by the time the patient is discharged from treatment or discharged to the next level of care on the continuum (Moorhead & Kannenberg, 1997). In occupational therapy, long-term goals always relate to expectations of the patient's functional skills and/or resumption of roles. Short-term goals are the small steps that cumulatively result in long-term goal achievement. Short-term goals are based either on expected improvements specific to client factors (AOTA, 2002) or impairments that ultimately contribute to improved function or on the patient's improved ability to perform portions of the functional task (McGuire, 1997). Table 3-3 compares these two types of short-term goals. A patient's occupational therapy goals are always linked to a predicted outcome and typically complement the work of other rehabilitation disciplines. Procedures for Practice 3-1 illustrates how long- and short-term goals support realization of outcomes. Definition 3-2 describes how to use goal attainment scaling to measure progress.

Collaborating with Clients to Set Goals

Collaborative goal setting between clients and therapists, an accreditation requirement of CARF (2004) and JCAHO (1999), presents benefits and challenges to both patients and therapists. Ponte-Allan and Giles (1999) suggested that the nature of goal setting may be linked with actual outcomes of therapy. They compared patients whose goals were functional, independence-oriented statements with patients whose goals were general, less functional statements or who made no goal statements at all. Although there were no differences in age, sex, side of lesion, or levels of disability at admission, patients who had functional goals had higher discharge scores on the Functional Independence Measure™ for grooming,

PROCEDURES FOR PRACTICE 3-1

Linking Long- and Short-Term Goals to Anticipated Rehabilitation Outcomes

P.B. is a 20-year-old man with C8 tetraplegia beginning multidisciplinary inpatient rehabilitation. The following examples of outcome and long- and short-term goals are not meant to be exhaustive lists of intervention plans but rather to illustrate the linkage between global outcome projections and therapy plans.

- Projected outcome of rehabilitation stay: In 8 weeks, P.B. will resume self-maintenance roles, requiring no more than occasional physical assistance from family members to manage in the home environment.
- Examples of long-term occupational therapy goals (to be achieved in 8 weeks):
  1) P.B. will perform upper body dressing independently and require no more than moderate assistance for lower body dressing.
  2) P.B. will use adaptive equipment to feed himself independently.
- Examples of short-term occupational therapy goals (to be achieved in 2 weeks):
  1) P.B. will don a pullover shirt with no more than general verbal cues.
  2) P.B. will participate in the evaluation of various types of adaptive equipment for self-feeding and use selected aids to feed himself independently after set up by therapist.

DEFINITION 3-2

Goal Attainment Scaling

Goal attainment scaling is a method for evaluating the effectiveness of therapy that produces a quantitative index of patient progress over time and a means by which one patient's progress can be compared with other patients in the same program (Ottenbacher & Cusick, 1990). Goal attainment scaling was developed for use in the mental health field (Kiresuk & Sherman, 1968) and has been used to measure change as a result of cognitive rehabilitation (Rockwood, Joyce, & Stolee, 1997) and brain injury rehabilitation (Joyce, Rockwood, & Mate-Kole, 1994; Trombly, Radomski, & Davis, 1998; Trombly et al., 2002).

For each goal, a 5-point behaviorally defined scale is constructed as exemplified below. Ottenbacher and Cusick (1990) provided an excellent summary regarding how quantitative outcome data can then be calculated and interpreted.

Problem area: Patient relies on other people to make transportation arrangements for her.

Predicted Attainment	Score	Goals
Most favorable outcome	+2	Patient accurately makes her own transportation arrangements without supervision or assistance.
Greater than expected outcome	+1	Patient accurately makes her own transportation arrangements with occasional cueing.
Expected outcome	0	Patient accurately makes her own transportation arrangements with ongoing supervision.
Current status	−1	Patient is provided with information about transportation arrangements made for her.
Least favorable outcome	−2	Patient is unable to successfully use transportation information provided for her.

upper and lower extremity dressing, and toilet and tub transfers. Despite the potential benefits, collaborative goal setting is challenging for newly disabled patients. Patients typically have relatively passive roles during the acute medical management of their disabling condition or illness but, upon transfer to the rehabilitation unit, are expected to actively participate in planning a process about which they are utterly unfamiliar. Patients understandably have difficulty identifying and articulating goals because to do so requires that they anticipate future functioning, tasks, and skills not needed in their current setting (Struhkamp, 2004). Patients' expectations of therapy depend on their previous experience in similar situations, background, experiences of friends and relatives (Wade, 1999), state of health and mind, and long-held priorities and values.

Collaborating with patients in goal setting is a critical counterbalance to therapist-biased expectations and priorities in treatment planning (Procedures for Practice 3-2); it reflects a philosophy of care rather than simply a periodic conversation between therapist and patient (Cott, 2004). This practice philosophy requires that therapists tolerate the stress that can occur during goal setting (Foye et al., 2002) and remain attentive and flexible as patients' goals change throughout the recovery and adaptation process (Donnelly et al., 2004). Therapists appreciate that most patients must be taught how to participate in goal setting (Nelson & Payton, 1997), probing for concerns, goals, and ideas. Asking a patient, "What are your occupational therapy goals?" is likely to be met with a perplexed look and a vague response. As one patient put it, "Asking one question about goals on an initial evaluation is probably not adequate" (Nelson & Payton, 1997, p. 582). Clearly, the time and energy invested in collaborative goal setting not only benefits patients but contributes to the empathic partnership that holds so much reward and satisfaction for therapists (Gahnstrom-Strandqvist et al., 2000).

Select Treatment Approaches and Methods

In Chapter 1, Trombly describes two broad therapy approaches that aim to improve clients' effectiveness and satisfaction with occupational roles: remedial therapy and adaptive therapy. Before proceeding with intervention, occupational therapists consider the patient's strengths and weaknesses based on assessment findings to select a treatment approach that will achieve expected outcomes and meet collaborative goals for therapy. In so doing, clinicians consider the extent to which a given treatment approach places demands on the patient's metaprocessing abilities (self-awareness, self-monitoring, and motivation), therapy time needed to improve occupational function, and potential for generalization of results.

PROCEDURES FOR PRACTICE 3-2

Suggestions for Collaborating with Clients to Set Meaningful Occupational Therapy Goals

- Incorporate life history information into the assessment process so that you are able to get a glimpse of what the patient has found meaningful and important during the course of his or her life events (Spencer, Davidson, & White, 1997). Awareness of the patient's personal context enables the clinician to discuss, frame, or propose possible therapy outcomes and goals in ways that the patient will understand.
- Appreciate that patients' ability to identify and advance their goals for therapy will be influenced by where they are in recovery and adaptation process. Individuals who are acutely ill or whose hospitalization has insulated them from the real-world impact of newly acquired disabilities will often be unable to anticipate the challenges that await them in the community. Outpatients or home-based clients are typically more able to articulate needs and hopes for therapy because of their experiences with performance gaps.
- Consider the broad continuum of care (inpatient to home health to outpatient to work reentry) as you aim to match the "right" goals with the "right" time frame by asking, "what does the person both value and need from occupational therapy at this point in his or her recovery?"
- Appreciate that most patients are unfamiliar with occupational therapy services and what we have to offer them and, therefore, are unable to independently generate goals for therapy. The therapist sometimes facilitates collaborative goal setting by proposing a menu of possible goals to address in therapy and modifying that list with the patient.
- Acknowledge the influence of cognitive function on a person's capacity to set meaningful goals. For a person to establish a meaningful goal, he or she must first accurately appraise his or her current status and compare it to past or premorbid performance. The individual must be able to imagine what is both possible and likely (given present condition and status) and how much time and effort is required to attain what is envisioned. Solicit input from family if the patient seems unable to independently determine or communicate his or her goals for therapy.
- If you are unable to arrive at consensus of broad therapy outcomes, try to agree on short-term goals. For example, a patient who is 3 months post brain injury wants only to work toward resuming his career as an air-traffic controller, a broad outcome the clinician views as unrealistic. Instead of haggling over what the future may or may not hold for this individual (which dampens energy, hope, and motivation), the patient and therapist agree that, to return to work, he needs to be able to independently get ready each morning, and begin their work there.

Remedial Therapy

Remedial therapy aims to restore an impaired capacity or ability with the expectation that this improvement will bring about general change in the patient's activities, tasks, and roles. For example, a therapist may base the treatment plan for a patient with an incomplete C8 spinal cord injury on the premise that, if upper extremity strength is optimally restored, the patient will not only become independent in grooming but also be more efficient with meal preparation and work tasks. Remedial approaches typically address body structures and functions (World Health Organization, 2001), which comprise client factors in the Occupational Therapy Practice Framework (AOTA, 2002). In general, remedial therapy places low demands on metaprocessing, but because it aims to fix underlying impairments, it may be somewhat slow to affect occupational function. A remedial approach is often emphasized when patients are in the early stages of recovery and rehabilitation.

Adaptive Therapy

Adaptive therapy is used when (1) a remedial approach does not result in full restoration of a patient's premorbid capacities and abilities or (2) the patient wants to optimize his or her level of independence while continuing to work toward restoration of fundamental capacities and abilities. For example, an inpatient with hemiplegia receives remedial therapy to improve upper extremity strength and function after a stroke but also learns one-handed dressing techniques (adaptive therapy) to facilitate independent discharge to home. Adaptive therapy entails three possible therapy actions: changing the context, reestablishing habits and routines, and acquiring compensatory skills and strategies.

Changing the Context

Context changes focus on changing factors that are external to the patient to improve occupational function (e.g., changing the demands of the task or environment, changing the tools used, changing the social supports or expectations). For example, using a range timer, which automatically turns off the stove at a predetermined time, may allow a person with memory impairment to cook without an undue safety risk. Installing grab bars in a patient's bathroom may dramatically increase the patient's ability to carry out self-maintenance tasks. Negotiating changed work responsibilities with an employer may enable a newly injured worker to keep his or her job.

Changing the context generally places low metaprocessing demands on the patient and can result in rapid improvements in occupational function, especially changes to physical aspects of context. The effects of intervention, however, are often task specific and do not necessarily generalize to other activities, tasks, and roles.

Reestablishing Habits and Routines

With enough repetition and consistency, people perform many daily occupations efficiently and accurately with little or no conscious attention (that is, automatically). For example, most people have a consistent procedure for morning hygiene and dressing that rarely changes from one day to the next. These routines or habits let people expeditiously carry out frequently performed activities with minimal attentional load. After a disabling injury or illness, many patients need assistance either to reestablish existing routines or to create new ones that better match changed capacities and abilities. (Chapter 29 has a detailed discussion of how habits and routines are reestablished or created.)

Patients need to be motivated or at least compliant enough to carry out a consistent series of steps necessary to reestablish habits and routines, but they do not necessarily need insight into their deficits and an understanding of the rationale of this approach. Because there is virtually no expectation of generalization (e.g., reestablishing a morning self-care routine will have no effect on the efficiency with which one does the laundry), patients should work on reestablishing habits and routines in the environment in which those routines will be used.

Acquiring Compensatory Skills and Strategies

Occupational therapists teach patients new skills and strategies that allow them to compensate for permanent or temporary impairments. For example, a person with lower extremity weakness or paralysis acquires new skills for moving from the wheelchair to bed. An individual with multiple sclerosis learns energy conservation strategies that allow her to optimize her productivity; a person with brain injury learns techniques that help him get to appointments on time despite ongoing memory impairment. (Chapter 14 discusses how people learn new skills and strategies.)

Learning new skills and strategies generally takes longer to affect occupational function than, for example, changing elements of the physical context. Acquiring the skills to transfer in and out of a wheelchair, however, may have benefits that generalize to a variety of activities and tasks, thus enabling performance of a number of occupational roles. To benefit from this approach, patients must appreciate the importance of the new skills and strategies, be motivated to participate in training, and be capable of recognizing opportunities in which the new skills and strategies can be used.

Determining the Optimal Treatment Approaches

Occupational therapists use diverse sources of evidence in identifying the most appropriate intervention plan for a specific client, including client perspectives and research evidence (Lee & Miller, 2003). Clinicians evaluate the available research evidence to determine the extent to which a specific research study and/or evidence review are relevant to the patient and clinical circumstances. They judge its quality based on classes of the evidence, such as randomized controlled studies, case-control research, case series, and expert opinion (Whyte, 1998). Furthermore, they evaluate the validity of a study's results by asking the following questions (Sackett et al., 1997): (1) Were patients randomly assigned to experimental and control conditions, and was the randomization concealed? (2) Were all patients who started the study accounted for at its conclusion? (3) Were patients' outcomes analyzed in the groups to which they were randomized? (4) Were the patients and clinicians blind to the experimental and control conditions? (5) Did all treatment groups receive comparable treatment except for the treatment under study? (6) Is my patient similar to those enrolled in the study?

The rehabilitation literature does not always conclusively point to a single treatment approach for a given set of problems. In such cases, Radomski and Davis (1999) suggest that clinicians weight the amount of treatment time and effort devoted to various intervention approaches based on the best available evidence and the patient's capacities, abilities, goals, and resources. They proposed the concept of a treatment fraction—the deliberate distribution of treatment efforts across appropriate treatment approaches to achieve goals. For example, with a woman acutely recovering from Guillain-Barré syndrome, the treatment fraction might look something like this: 40% of therapy efforts directed at remedial therapy (intervention focusing on improving strength and endurance); 35% directed at acquiring skills and strategies, such as learning modified self-care methods and energy conservation strategies; and 25% directed at changing the context (helping the patient make her home more accessible). When she returns to therapy as an outpatient, the treatment fraction changes: 20% of the therapy time is devoted to remedial therapy; 20% is devoted to changing the context (helping the patient's family shift roles and responsibilities around the patient's changing abilities); 25% is devoted to acquisition of skills and strategies; and 35% is devoted to reestablishing habits and routines. The distribution is dramatically different for a client with Alzheimer's disease; the therapist may choose to devote 80% of therapy time to changing the context (adapting the home environment and coaching significant others regarding how to respond when their loved one is confused) and 20% to establishing behavioral routines. Although no hard and fast rules exist for the correct weighting of therapy time and efforts, the treatment fraction illustrates the importance of deciding how to spend therapy resources in pursuit of the patient's goals rather than exclusively subscribing to one approach or mindlessly shifting focus session by session.

Required Documentation: Evaluation Note

An occupational therapy evaluation note is added to the medical record when assessment and treatment planning are complete. Table 3-2 shows the purpose of this document and what must be included.

Implementing Intervention

Once therapists collaboratively determine therapy outcomes, goals, and approaches, treatment begins. Clinicians continue to make decisions regarding how the treatment is best delivered (one-on-one or group treatment) and by whom. The exception is when a clinical pathway dictates a predetermined therapy course that dovetails with intervention of other team members (see Definition 3-3).

How Treatment Is Delivered: Individual or Group Sessions

Occupational therapy occurs during one-on-one sessions with the patient or in dyads or small groups. Although clinicians must be sensitive to costs associated with providing services, they base scheduling decisions on each patient's unique needs and goals rather than solely on the clinician's convenience or efficiency.

Individual Treatment

Clinicians typically schedule individual sessions for assessment and reassessment. Individual sessions are also appropriate when patient privacy must be protected, such as during dressing training or when the patient seems particularly vulnerable or in need of emotional support. Patients who are easily distracted, such as those in early phases of recovery from brain injury, are also best treated individually.

Group Treatment

Groups typically consist of patients engaged in parallel activities, such as performing individualized exercise regimens at the same time and place, or in collaborative activity, such as preparing a meal together. Patients tend to be grouped according to similar goals, treatment, or education needs or similar diagnoses, conditions, or limitations. Beyond its value from an economic standpoint, group treatment offers many benefits to patients. Group therapy can facilitate the exchange of social support and encouragement among patients as they derive hope for their own futures from observing others master similar challenges.

Who Delivers Treatment

Economic trends in health care require that the most appropriate person perform therapy tasks to optimize efficiency (Russell & Kanny, 1998). Occupational therapists make decisions about who will carry out the treatment plan (occupational therapist, occupational therapy assistant, and/or occupational therapy aide). Occupational therapists orchestrate the treatment plan and are ultimately responsible for service delivery (AOTA, 2004b). They typically spend their time conducting evaluations, identifying problems, planning solutions, and supervising implementation (Dunn & Cada, 1998; Glantz & Richman, 1997). Occupational therapy assistants spend most of their time delivering direct service and documenting results (Dunn & Cada, 1998; Glantz & Richman, 1997).

Required Documentation: Daily Contact Notes

Each time the patient is seen for assessment and treatment, the clinician documents the contact (Table 3-2).

Monitoring Progress

Clinicians constantly monitor clients' response to intervention and their progress toward goals. At regular intervals, typically weekly for inpatients and at least monthly for outpatients, clinicians formally reassess status relative to goals, analyze barriers and enablers to progress, evaluate effectiveness of the treatment approach, and make decisions about continuing, modifying, or discontinuing treatment. If short-term goals are met but long-term goals are not, the short-term goals are upgraded (Moyers, 1999). If short-term goals are not met or performance has leveled off, the therapist examines and possibly modifies the treatment approach, reflects on the caliber of his or her skills with the treatment methods, looks for transient explanatory factors, consults with experts, and/or considers discontinuing therapy.

Required Documentation: Weekly and/or Monthly Progress Notes

Progress notes document the formal examination of the patient's progress toward treatment goals (Allen, 1997). For outpatients with Medicare, therapists also must complete monthly recertification forms detailing the patient's progress toward goals, which must be signed by the patient's physician every 30 days.

DEFINITION 3-3

de·fin·i·tion

Critical Pathways

Critical pathways, also known as care maps, define an optimal schedule of key interventions from various disciplines for a specific diagnosis or procedure to achieve desired patient outcomes in a defined period of time (Dykes, 1997). A critical pathway represents a multidisciplinary plan in that it outlines all the tests, procedures, treatments, and teaching that the patient is expected to need during his or her hospitalization (Dykes, 1997). The treatment team documents the patient's status as compared to the plan directly on the critical pathway, with deviations recorded as a variance.

A basic assumption underlying the critical pathway is the eighty/twenty rule, which states that 80% of patients follow a predictable path 100% of the time and 20% do not (Dykes, 1997). Critical pathways provide consistency of care for most but not all patients. They are not meant to be followed blindly and can always be modified to meet the needs of individual patients (Dykes, 1997). Figure 3-3 is a portion of a critical pathway used after total knee replacement surgery.

PLACE BAR CODE HERE

PATIENT NAME:

ORTHO PAIN MANAGEMENT/ANALGESICS ROUTINE PROTOCOL:
(If patient is on Ortho Pain Protocol)

1. Assess and document pain q̄ 2h while awake. If pain is mild for 24 hours, assess q̄ 4h.
3. For unsatisfactory pain control **increase** each **scheduled** dose of morphine or hydromorphone by half (50%) of the total PRN milligrams given since the last **scheduled** dose.
4. For excessive side effects or mild pain (e.g., pain ≤ 3/10 for 12 hours), decrease **scheduled** dose by half (50%).
5. Discontinue scheduled morphine or hydromorphone when pain has been mild for 12 hours and patient tolerating other analgesics.
7. Oral "step down" analgesic(s). To begin when IV or PCA opioid is being tapered.
8. When pain is mild and patient using ≤ 3 tablets PRN during the previous 24 hours, discontinue scheduled opioid doses and give 1 to 2 tablets every 3 to 4h PRN.

LOS GUIDELINES: ***(does NOT include DOS)***
If patient DC plan is to go home with or without home care, plan on a **4 day LOS.**
If patient DC plan is to go to an extended care facility, plan on transfer after a **4 day LOS.**
Referral/DC instruction forms initiated **DAY BEFORE DISCHARGE.**

I&O / IV PROTOCOL:
Continue I&O for 48 hr. p̄ IV d/c'd.
Convert to SL when tolerates PO adequately.
Discontinue SL if:
- Antibiotics completed
- No transfusion necessary
- Pt. tolerating diet

ACTIVITY PROTOCOL

KEY:	DOS	POD #1	POD #2	POD #3	Remainder of Stay
☑ completed intervention, move to next intervention (IN PEN) △ change Ⓐ assist Ⓘ independent c̄ with s̄ without q̄ every **AEB** as evidenced by **B/4** before **BR** bedrest/bathroom **d/c** discontinue **DC** discharge **LOS** length of stay **OOB** out of bed **pt.** patient **PT** physical therapy **RT** related to **SBA** stand by assist **SR** siderail **SS** social service **W/A** when awake	**ACTIVITY PLAN:** Dangle or up to commode x1 with assist of 2 HOB up as tol Turn as tol **NO PILLOW UNDER KNEE** CPM/immobilizer as ordered	**ACTIVITY PLAN:** Transfer with assist of 1-2 for meals and therapy as ordered Use walker/transfer belt Elevate/support operated leg while sitting **NO PILLOW UNDER KNEE** If immobilizer ordered: use as directed If CPM ordered: increase 5-10 degrees/day, use 1-2 hour 2-3 x/d Quad sets and SLRs QID **PT:** BID **HYGIENE:** Pt. able to assist with upper body hygiene, full assist with lower body, back cares Remove TEDs for cares BID	**ACTIVITY PLAN:** Transfer with walker and assist of 1-2 for meals and therapy Ambulate in room x2 Use walker/transfer belt Up in chair/commode Elevate/support operated leg while sitting Sit for short intervals with feet on floor QID **NO PILLOW UNDER KNEE** If immobilizer ordered: use as directed, wear at HS only, if pt. can SLR If CPM ordered: Increase 5-10 degrees/day, Use QID for 1 hour intervals Quad sets and SLR's QID Accomplish bed mobility without use of SR/trapeze **PT:** BID **OT:** Referral prn **HYGIENE:** Pt. indep with upper body, assist with lower body Remove TEDs for cares BID	**ACTIVITY PLAN:** Transfer with walker/crutches and standby or assist of 1 Ambulate to BR No use of commode in room Up in chair for all activities, keep feet on floor Ambulate outside of room **NO PILLOW UNDER KNEE** If immobilizer ordered: wear at HS only, if pt. can SLR If CPM ordered: Increase 5-10 degrees/day, Use QID for 1 hour intervals Quad sets and SLRs QID Independent bed mobility **PT:** BID **OT:** ADL eval prn **HYGIENE:** Assist with lower extremities prn Remove TEDs for cares BID	**ACTIVITY PLAN:** Progress towards independence in bed mobility, transfers, ambulation, with walker/crutches **NO PILLOW UNDER KNEE** If CPM ordered: increase CPM 5-10 degrees/day to 90 degrees Use 3-4 times/day for minimum 1 hour intervals Progress to independent exercise program **PT:** Based on pt. need **OT:** Based on pt. need **HYGIENE:** Progress towards independence and shower before D/C

Figure 3-3 The activity protocol from a critical pathway used after total knee replacement surgery. (Reprinted with permission from Abbott-Northwestern Hospital, Minneapolis, MN.)

Discontinuing Therapy

Therapy is discontinued when goals have been met, the patient's performance has leveled off or deteriorated in such a way that he or she is not benefiting from services, or the individual chooses to stop. Ideally, the patient and family participate in discharge planning, which entails setting up a maintenance program, referring to other services, and/or planning for follow-up.

- Set up the maintenance program. Patients and families receive instructions that allow them to extend the benefits of treatment after discharge. Therapists typically provide written and oral information regarding continued exercise, recommended equipment, and strategies or techniques that optimize function.
- Refer to other services. Many patients who discontinue occupational therapy at one site continue treatment at another level of care. For example, often persons receiving inpatient rehabilitation receive additional occupational therapy in long-term care facilities, through home health agencies, or as outpatients. To continue intervention seamlessly, therapists pass information along to the next tier of intervention. Therapists may also identify areas of need that are outside their scope of practice or competence and refer patients to appropriate disciplines or specialists.
- Plan for follow-up. Implicit in intervention plans geared to addressing the right issues at the right time in a patient's recovery and adaptation is the expectation that the therapist will not treat all possible problems during a given episode of care. A scheduled occupational therapy follow-up session is a mechanism by which the clinician can screen for the need for more services. A follow-up session is necessary when the patient improves, regresses, or anticipates changed needs or goals or when the social or environmental context changes (Moyers, 1999). Some clients are ambivalent about discontinuing occupational therapy, recognizing lack of progress but fearing abandonment and stalled recovery or deterioration. Planned follow-up assures patients that occupational therapy services will be available to them if needed in the future.

Required Documentation: Home Program, Referrals, and Discharge Summary

Not only are written home programs and referrals provided to the patient and referral source, these reports are also added to the medical record. The discharge summary provides an overview of services provided, outcomes, and recommendations. Allen (1997) suggested that creating this document can be a reflective process for the clinician, who considers goals met or not and factors contributing to or interfering with progress.

USING PRACTICE EXPERIENCE TO IMPROVE COMPETENCE

You, as an occupational therapy professional, are ultimately responsible for assessing, improving, maintaining, and documenting your own competence to practice (AOTA, 1999; Youngstrom, 1998). As Holm (2000) reminded us, high standards of competence are inextricably linked to high ethical standards. Competence has many dimensions, including knowledge, critical reasoning, interpersonal abilities, performance skills, and ethical reasoning (AOTA, 1999). Like occupational therapy services, continuing competence entails assessment, goal-directed action, and documentation.

Self-Assessment: Reflecting on Practice

The cornerstone of continuing competence is reflection on yourself and your practice. Therapists deliberately and regularly take stock of their status and determine their growth edges. Clinicians interested in growth ask for feedback from peers and formally review their own performance. Schell (1992) recommended that clinicians annually outline their strengths, areas needing improvement, accomplishments of the past year, and goals for the coming year (see Procedures for Practice 3-3 for suggestions).

Goal-Directed Action

Having assessed your professional strengths and weaknesses, you have many ways to improve your competence, including the following:

- Participate in your professional national and state occupational therapy associations. During volunteer service, you will encounter other occupational therapists who are committed to their profession and their own growth.
- Become a research-sensitive practitioner (Cusick & McCluskey, 2000). Make research evidence a vital part of the way that you provide services.
- Because even the most dedicated therapists make them (Schierton, Mu, & Lohman, 2003), commit to learning from your mistakes. Reflect on your errors or inefficiencies and consider what you would do should you face similar circumstances in the future. Be willing to discuss what you learn in this process with others.
- Establish a mentoring relationship. Mentors benefit from the relationship as they expand into new areas of practice, and proteges benefit from coaching and intellectual stimulation (Smith, 1992).

PROCEDURES FOR PRACTICE 3-3

Analyzing Your Competence

Clinicians use the answers to the following questions (based on AOTA Standards of Competence [1999] and Code of Ethics [2000]) to guide their responses to unfamiliar diagnoses, conditions, or problems. They determine whether they are competent to provide independent assessment and treatment or supervised assessment and treatment or if they should refer the patient to someone with more expertise.

1. Knowledge
   - Do I have adequate and up-to-date theoretical knowledge about this diagnosis, condition, or problem?
   - Do I have knowledge regarding any legislative, legal, or regulatory issues specific to this client's diagnosis, condition, or problem?
   - Do I have knowledge of any contraindications or precautions associated with treating this diagnosis, condition, or problem?
2. Critical Reasoning
   - Will I be able to recognize the appropriate response to treatment?
   - Will I be able to recognize potentially harmful primary or secondary effects of treatment?
   - Will I be able to decide how to respond to untoward responses to treatment?
3. Interpersonal Abilities
   - Am I competent to discuss the pros and cons of various methods to assess and treat this diagnosis, condition, or problem with the client?
   - Am I competently able to collaborate with other professionals specific to this diagnosis, condition, or problem?
4. Performance Skills
   - Is specialized training or certification required or recommended for treating this diagnosis, condition, or problem?
   - Am I skilled at using modalities, devices, or technology related to treating this diagnosis, condition, or problem?
   - Is the patient at risk of harm associated with inappropriate treatment of this diagnosis, condition, or problem?
5. Ethical Reasoning
   - Is my motivation to assess or treat this patient influenced by potential personal gain or profit?
   - Is there any conflict of interest related to my decision to treat or assess this patient?

- Keep a journal to document information and questions; to reflect on ideas, concerns, and beliefs; and ultimately to identify learning needs (Tryssenaar, 1995).
- Start a journal club at work in which clinicians regularly read and discuss research articles relevant to occupational therapy practice.
- Volunteer for medical record reviews and audits. By reviewing the documentation of others and submitting your documentation to the same scrutiny, you will learn how you can make your documentation clearer and more useful.

Documentation

Crist, Wilcox, and McCarron (1998) recommended that occupational therapists use "transitional portfolios" (p. 729) to plan and document their professional competence. More than a resume or a curriculum vitae, the transitional portfolio houses artifacts of completed and exemplary work (e.g., certificates of attendance, awards, articles), in-process projects and plans for professional development, and a reflective journal with ideas, goals, feelings about one's reading, research, and work experiences. Clinicians may avail themselves of resources such as the Professional Development Tool (which includes self-assessments, professional development plans, and portfolio template) developed for members of AOTA (AOTA, 2003). By systematically collecting and organizing information and artifacts specific to accomplishments, progress, and goals, occupational therapists take responsibility for their present and future professional competence.

In summary, occupational therapists feel competent when clients achieve results that translate into meaningful improvements in their daily lives (Gahnstrom-Strandqvist et al., 2000). Such results can be achieved as clinicians combine their knowledge of evidence with their insights regarding patients' values and goals to plan and implement intervention that is not only effective but rewarding for patient and therapist alike.

CASE EXAMPLE

Clinical Reasoning and Clinical Competence

Occupational Therapy Intervention Process	Clinical Reasoning Process: Objectives	Clinical Reasoning Process: Examples of Therapist's Internal Dialogue
Patient Information N.T. is a 71-year-old man who is 15 months post onset of right cerebral vascular accident and flaccid left hemiplegia. Shortly after his stroke, N.T. received intensive inpatient rehabilitation services and, upon discharge to his home, participated in outpatient occupational therapy 3 times per week for 2 months. He was discharged from outpatient occupational therapy having achieved independence in self-care and homemaking activities. N.T. and his wife left Minnesota shortly thereafter for their winter home in Phoenix but have since returned. He was referred back to outpatient occupational therapy because of concerns about left shoulder pain and subluxation. He presented with a 2-fingerwidth left shoulder subluxation, decreased shoulder passive range of motion (−20° external rotation, −25° shoulder flexion and abduction), and pain at extremes. He reportedly was not routinely wearing a sling while walking but indicated that he tried to keep his left upper extremity supported when sitting. He also reported that he tried to perform the self range-of-motion exercises that he learned after his stroke, but pain often interfered. He described his typical level of shoulder pain as varying between 6 and 8 on a 1–10 scale. N.T. and his therapist decided to use a conservative approach to address his current shoulder problems. The therapist ordered a hemi-sling, taught him to don and doff it, and recommended N.T. wear it when walking. The therapist referred N.T. to physical therapy for ultrasound treatments, which were immediately followed by passive range-of-motion exercises in occupational therapy. N.T.'s wife attended 2 sessions and learned how to perform passive range of motion on her husband's shoulder. The therapist also helped N.T. implement strategies positioning the left upper extremity at bedtime and taught him ADL techniques that minimized the strain on his shoulder. Now after 6 sessions and 3 weeks of outpatient occupational therapy, N.T. has gained 5° in shoulder range of motion, but pain continues to interfere with daily activities as well as sleep. There has been no change in shoulder subluxation.	Appreciate the context	"It is unfortunate that N.T. has developed shoulder problems, but I know that that's a fairly common problem after stroke. I thought that his pain might lessen if he simply got in the habit of wearing a sling again and if we could improve his shoulder range of motion. His wife seemed to quickly pick up on my instructions regarding how to handle the upper extremity and how to perform pain-free passive range-of-motion exercises. But I am concerned that N.T. is still having significant shoulder pain."
	Develop intervention hypotheses	"I've been treating patients with stroke for over 3 years now, and based on my experience with other patients, I would've expected some improvement in N.T.'s shoulder pain by this point. I think that we should change the intervention plan."

Select an intervention approach	"The lead occupational therapist on my team suggested I consider trying neuromuscular electrical stimulation (NMES) on N.T.'s shoulder. I found a handful of outcome studies on PubMed and read the abstract of a systematic evidence review from the Cochrane Database. Although the 3 studies had methodologic problems (not one involved a randomized control group or standardized treatment protocol), my reading suggests that, at best, NMES might improve subluxation and decrease pain and, at worst, do no harm. It's frustrating that I can't find unequivocal direction from the literature, but between my reading and my conversations with the lead therapist, I would like to propose this course of action to N.T."
Reflect on competence	"N.T. is interested in trying NMES but I need to think through whether or not I'm the right person to provide this intervention. • I understand the rationale and research evidence for using this modality and it seems like an appropriate method of intervention, given N.T.'s pain and shoulder subluxation. (Scientific Reasoning) • N.T. appears to understand what NMES involves and seems committed to attend sessions over the next month. I'm assuming he can continue to arrange transportation to his therapy. (Narrative Reasoning) • I read the procedures, watched other therapists, and practiced applying electrodes. I am confident I can do this. However, my supervisor reminded me to check licensure requirements, and it is clear that I do not have the formal training required by the State of Minnesota to use physical agent modalities like NMES. (Pragmatic Reasoning) • Even though I think I have the knowledge and technical skills to provide this intervention, I will need to make arrangements for another therapist to do so because of the state licensure requirements. I am going to continue to explore what I need to do to get the necessary credentials for the future." (Ethical Reasoning)

CLINICAL REASONING IN OCCUPATIONAL THERAPY PRACTICE

Using Types of Clinical Reasoning as a Self-Check of Competence

Consider the case example with just one change of circumstances. Let us assume that the therapist has recently just met the state licensure requirements for using physical agent modalities but has yet to use NMES on a patient. Describe at least one competency concern in the areas of Scientific, Narrative, and Pragmatic Reasoning as well as how you recommend that the therapist address that concern.

SUMMARY REVIEW QUESTIONS

1. Describe specific aspects of occupational therapy documentation that you think are critical information for the following target audiences: referring physician, physical therapist on the interdisciplinary team, payer, and family member.
2. Summarize ways a clinician's bias may affect clinical reasoning during each phase of providing occupational therapy services.
3. Draft two long-term and two short-term occupational therapy goals for a hypothetical client with multiple sclerosis whose anticipated outcome of therapy is to return to clerical work.
4. Write a brief statement (fewer than 25 words) that you could use to describe occupational therapy to a new client as a prelude to collaborative goal setting. Compare descriptions with classmates and then share with family and friends who know little about occupational therapy.
5. Compare and contrast the treatment fractions of two patients receiving occupational therapy services: a patient with a progressive condition like amyotrophic lateral sclerosis and a patient with an acute traumatic brain injury.
6. Describe what competence looks like in action specific to knowledge, critical reasoning, interpersonal abilities, performance skills, and ethical reasoning. Describe what incompetence looks like for each area.

References

Allen, C. (1997). Clinical reasoning for documentation. In J. D. Acquaviva (Ed.), *Effective documentation for occupational therapy* (2nd ed., pp. 53–62). Bethesda, MD: American Occupational Therapy Association.

Allen, C., Foto, M., Moon, T., Wilson, D., & Thomas, V. J. (1997). Understanding the medical review process. In J. D. Acquaviva (Ed.), *Effective documentation for occupational therapy* (2nd ed., pp. 63–73). Bethesda, MD: American Occupational Therapy Association.

American Occupational Therapy Association [AOTA]. (1999). Standards of continuing competence. *American Journal of Occupational Therapy, 53,* 599–600.

American Occupational Therapy Association [AOTA]. (2000). Occupational therapy code of ethics. *American Journal of Occupational Therapy, 54,* 614–616.

American Occupational Therapy Association [AOTA]. (2002). Occupational therapy practice framework: Domain and process. *American Journal of Occupational Therapy, 56,* 609–639.

American Occupational Therapy Association [AOTA]. (2003). AOTA Professional Development Tool. Bethesda, MD: AOTA. Retrieved May 31, 2005 from www.aota.org/pdt.

American Occupational Therapy Association [AOTA]. (2004a). Guidelines for documentation of occupational therapy. In *The reference manual of the official documents of the American Occupational Therapy Association, Inc.* (10th ed., pp. 153–158). Bethesda, MD: AOTA.

American Occupational Therapy Association [AOTA]. (2004b). Guidelines for supervision, roles, and responsibilities during the delivery of occupational therapy services. *American Journal of Occupational Therapy, 58,* 663–667.

Bryant, E. T. (1995). Acute rehabilitation in an outcome-oriented model. In P. K. Landrum, N. D. Schmidt, & A. McLean (Eds.), *Outcome-oriented rehabilitation* (pp. 69–93). Gaithersburg, MD: Aspen.

Commission on Accreditation of Rehabilitation Facilities [CARF]. (2004). *2004 medical rehabilitation standards manual.* Tucson, AZ: Commission on Accreditation of Rehabilitation Facilities.

Cope, D. N., & Sundance, P. (1995). Conceptualizing clinical outcomes. In P. K. Landrum, N. D. Schmidt, & A. McLean (Eds.), *Outcome-oriented rehabilitation* (pp. 43–56). Gaithersburg, MD: Aspen.

Cott, C. A. (2004). Client-centered rehabilitation: Client perspectives. *Disability & Rehabilitation, 26,* 1411–1422.

Crabtree, J. (2000). What is a worthy goal of occupational therapy? *Occupational Therapy in Health Care, 12,* 111–126.

Crist, P., Wilcox, B. L., & McCarron, K. (1998). Transitional portfolios: Orchestrating our professional competence. *American Journal of Occupational Therapy, 52,* 729–736.

Cusick, A., & McCluskey, A. (2000). Becoming an evidence-based practitioner through professional development. *Australian Occupational Therapy Journal, 47,* 159–170.

Donnelly, C., Eng, J. J., Hall, J., Alford, L., Giachino, R., Norton, K., & Kerr, D. S. (2004). Client-centred assessment and the identification of meaningful treatment goals for individuals with spinal cord injury. *Spinal Cord, 42,* 302–307.

Dubouloz, C., Egan, M., Vallerand, J., von Zweck, C. (1999). Occupational therapists' perceptions of evidence-based practice. *American Journal of Occupational Therapy, 53,* 445–458.

Dunn, W., & Cada, E. (1998). The national occupational therapy practice analysis: Findings and implications for competence. *American Journal of Occupational Therapy, 52,* 721–728.

Dykes, P. C. (1997). Designing and implementing critical pathways: An overview. In P. C. Dykes & K. Wheeler (Eds.), *Planning, implementing, and evaluating critical pathways* (pp. 8–25). New York: Springer.

Fisher, A. G. (1998). Uniting practice and theory in an occupational framework. *American Journal of Occupational Therapy, 52,* 509–521.

Foye, S. J., Kirschner, K. L., Brady Wagner, L. C., Stocking, C., & Siegler, M. (2002). Ethical issues in rehabilitation: A qualitative analysis of dilemmas identified by occupational therapists. *Topics in Stroke Rehabilitation, 9,* 89–101.

Gahnstrom-Strandqvist, K., Tham, K., Josephsson, S., & Borell, L. (2000). Actions of competence in occupational therapy practice. *Scandinavian Journal of Occupational Therapy, 7,* 15–25.

Glantz, C. H., & Richman, N. (1997). OTR-COTA collaboration in home health: Roles and supervisory issues. *American Journal of Occupational Therapy, 51,* 446–452.

Hagedorn, R. (1996). Clinical decision making in familiar cases: A model of the process and implications for practice. *British Journal of Occupational Therapy, 59,* 217–222.

Holm, M. B. (2000). Our mandate for the new millennium: Evidence-based practice. *American Journal of Occupational Therapy, 54,* 575–585.

Joint Commission on Accreditation of Healthcare Organizations [JCAHO]. (1999). *Comprehensive accreditation manual for hospitals.* Oakbrook Terrace, IL: Joint Commission on Accreditation of Healthcare Organizations.

Joyce, B. M., Rockwood, K. J., & Mate-Kole, C. C. (1994). Use of goal attainment scaling in brain injury in a rehabilitation hospital. *American Journal of Physical Medicine and Rehabilitation, 73,* 10–14.

Kiresuk, T. J., & Sherman, R. E. (1968). Goal attainment scaling: A general method for evaluating comprehensive community mental health programs. *Community Mental Health Journal, 4,* 443–453.

Lee, C. J., & Miller, L. T. (2003). The process of evidence-based clinical decision-making in occupational therapy. *American Journal of Occupational Therapy, 57,* 473–477.

Mattingly, C. (1991). What is clinical reasoning? *American Journal of Occupational Therapy, 45,* 979–986.

McGuire, M. J. (1997). Documenting progress in home care. *American Journal of Occupational Therapy, 51,* 436–445.

Moorhead, P., & Kannenberg, K. (1997). Writing functional goals. In J. D. Acquaviva (Ed.), *Effective documentation for occupational therapy* (2nd ed., pp. 75–82). Bethesda, MD: American Occupational Therapy Association.

Moyers, P. A. (1999). The guide to occupational therapy practice. *American Journal of Occupational Therapy, 53,* 247–322.

Nelson, C. E., & Payton, O. D. (1997). The planning process in occupational therapy: Perceptions of adult rehabilitation patients. *American Journal of Occupational Therapy, 51,* 576–583.

Opacich, K. J. (1991). Assessment and informed decision-making. In C. Christiansen & C. Baum (Eds.), *Occupational therapy: Overcoming human performance deficits* (pp. 356–372). Thorofare, NJ: Slack.

Ottenbacher, K. J., & Cusick, A. (1990). Goal attainment scaling as a method of clinical service evaluation. *American Journal of Occupational Therapy, 44,* 519–525.

Ottenbacher, K. J., Tickle-Degnen, L., & Hasselkus, B. R. (2002). Therapists awake! The challenge of evidence-based occupational therapy. *American Journal of Occupational Therapy, 56,* 247–249.

Philibert, D. B., Snyder, P., Judd, D., & Windsor, M. M. (2003). Practitioners' reading patterns, attitudes, and use of research reported in occupational therapy journals. *American Journal of Occupational Therapy, 57,* 450–458.

Ponte-Allan, M., & Giles, G. M. (1999). Goal setting and functional outcomes in rehabilitation. *American Journal of Occupational Therapy, 53,* 646–649.

Radomski, M. V. (1995). There is more to life than putting on your pants. *American Journal of Occupational Therapy, 49,* 487–490.

Radomski, M. V., & Davis, E. S. (1999). *Cognitive compensatory strategies: From treatment to function.* Minneapolis, MN: Workshop presented for the Minnesota Occupational Therapy Association.

Rappolt, S. (2003). The role of professional expertise in evidence-based occupational therapy. *American Journal of Occupational Therapy, 57,* 589–593.

Roberts, A. E. (1996). Clinical reasoning in occupational therapy: Idiosyncrasies in content and process. *British Journal of Occupational Therapy, 59,* 372–376.

Robertson, S. C. (1997). Why we document. In J. D. Acquaviva (Ed.), *Effective documentation for occupational therapy* (2nd ed., pp. 29–38). Bethesda, MD: American Occupational Therapy Association.

Rockwood, K., Joyce, B., & Stolee, P. (1997). Use of goal attainment scaling in measuring clinically important change in cognitive rehabilitation patients. *Journal of Clinical Epidemiology, 50,* 581–588.

Rogers, J. (1983). Eleanor Clarke Slagle Lectureship–1983; Clinical reasoning: The ethics, science, and art. *American Journal of Occupational Therapy, 37,* 601–616.

Rogers, J. C., & Holm, M. B. (1991). Occupational therapy diagnostic reasoning: A component of clinical reasoning. *American Journal of Occupational Therapy, 45,* 1045–1053.

Rogers, J. C., & Masagatani, G. (1982). Clinical reasoning of occupational therapists during the initial assessment of physically disabled patients. *Occupational Therapy Journal of Research, 2,* 195–219.

Russell, K. V., & Kanny, E. M. (1998). Use of aides in occupational therapy practice. *American Journal of Occupational Therapy, 52,* 118–124.

Sackett, D. L., Richardson, W. S., Rosenberg, W., & Haynes, R. B. (1997). *Evidence-based medicine.* New York: Churchill Livingstone.

Scheirton, L., Mu, K., & Lohman, H. (2003). Occupational therapists' responses to practice errors in physical rehabilitation settings. *American Journal of Occupational Therapy, 57,* 307–314.

Schell, B. B. (1992). Setting realistic career goals. *Occupational Therapy Practice, 3,* 11–20.

Schell, B. A., & Cervero, R. M. (1993). Clinical reasoning in occupational therapy: An integrative review. *American Occupational Therapy Association, 47,* 605–610.

Smith, B. C. (1992). Mentoring: The key to professional growth. *Occupational Therapy Practice, 3,* 21–28.

Spencer, J., Davidson, H., & White, V. (1997). Helping clients develop hopes for the future. *American Journal of Occupational Therapy, 51,* 191–198.

Struhkamp, R. (2004). Goals in their setting: A normative analysis of goal setting in physical rehabilitation. *Health Care Analysis, 12,* 131–155.

Sviden, G., & Hallin, M. (1999). Difference in clinical reasoning between occupational therapists working in rheumatology and neurology. *Scandinavian Journal of Occupational Therapy, 6,* 63–69.

Tickle-Degnen, L. (2000). Communicating with clients, family members, and colleagues about research evidence. *American Journal of Occupational Therapy, 54,* 341–343.

Trombly, C. A. (1993). Anticipating the future: Assessment of occupational function. *American Journal of Occupational Therapy, 47,* 253–257.

Trombly, C. A. (1995). Occupation: Purposefulness and meaningfulness as therapeutic mechanisms. *American Journal of Occupational Therapy, 49,* 960–972.

Trombly, C. A., Radomski, M. V., & Davis, E. S. (1998). Achievement of self-identified goals by adults with traumatic brain injury: Phase I. *American Journal of Occupational Therapy, 52,* 810–818.

Trombly, C. A., Radomski, M. V., Trexel, C., & Burnett-Smith, S. E. (2002). Occupational therapy and achievement of self-identified goals by adults with acquired brain injury: Phase II. *American Journal of Occupational Therapy, 56,* 489–498.

Tryssenaar, J. (1995). Interactive journals: An educational strategy to promote reflection. *American Journal of Occupational Therapy, 49,* 695–702.

Unsworth, C. A. (2001). The clinical reasoning of novice and expert occupational therapists. *Scandinavian Journal of Occupational Therapy, 8,* 163–173.

Wade, D. T. (1999). Goal planning in stroke rehabilitation: How? *Topics in Stroke Rehabilitation, 6,* 16–36.

Whyte, J. (1998). *Evidence-based rehabilitation: Why not cloud the issue with facts!* Paper presented at the meeting of the American Congress of Rehabilitation Medicine, Seattle, WA.

World Health Organization. (2001). International Classification of Functioning, Disability, Health—Short version. Geneva, Switzerland: World Health Organization.

Youngstrom, M. J. (1998). Evolving competence in the practitioner role. *American Journal of Occupational Therapy, 52,* 716–720.

SECTION II: Assessment of Occupational Function

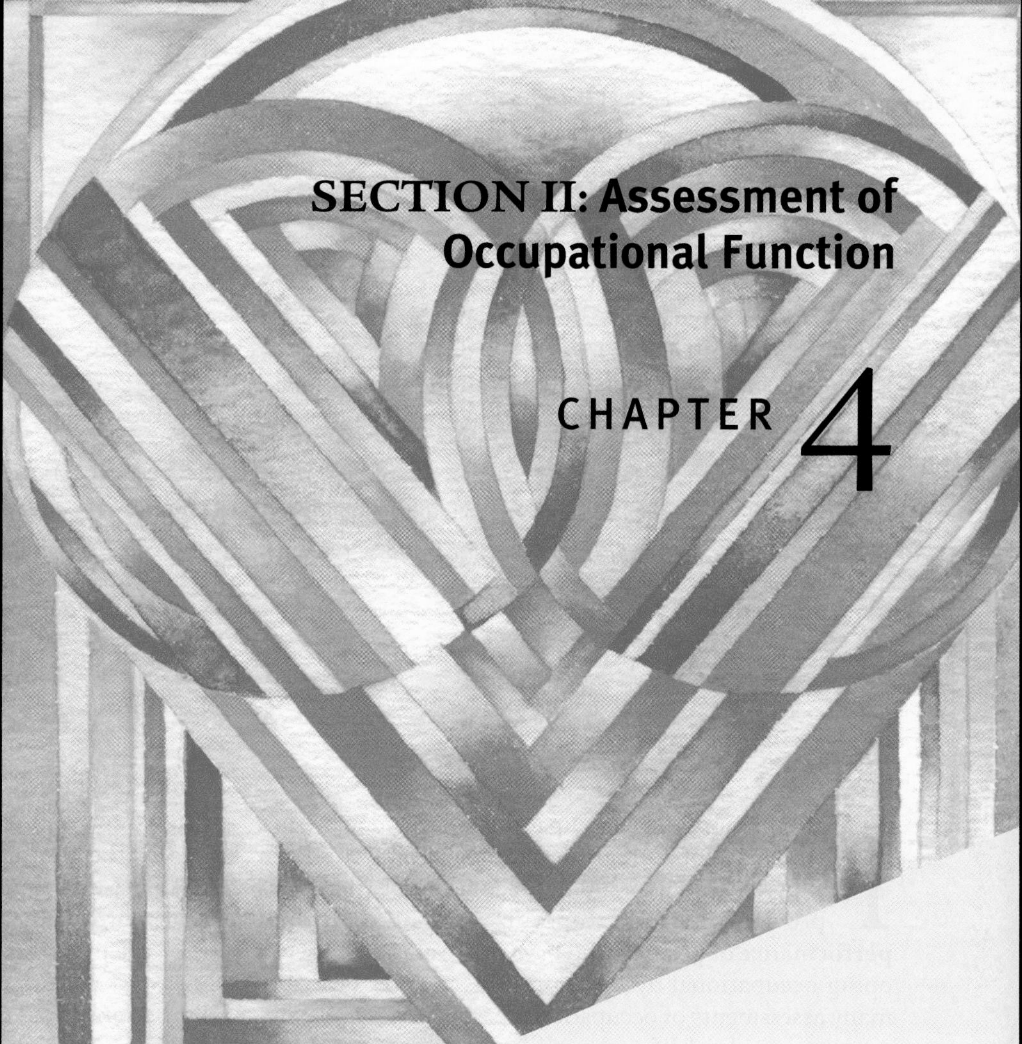

CHAPTER 4

Assessing Roles and Competence

Susan E. Fasoli

LEARNING OBJECTIVES

After studying this chapter, the reader will be able to do the following:

1. Understand the nature and importance of assessment in occupational therapy.
2. Evaluate roles, competence, and occupational functioning, beginning with clients' perception of their occupational performance issues.
3. Understand the measurement criteria necessary for reliable and valid assessments for use in occupational therapy practice.
4. Describe and select appropriate validated assessments of competence in occupational performance (roles, tasks, and activities).

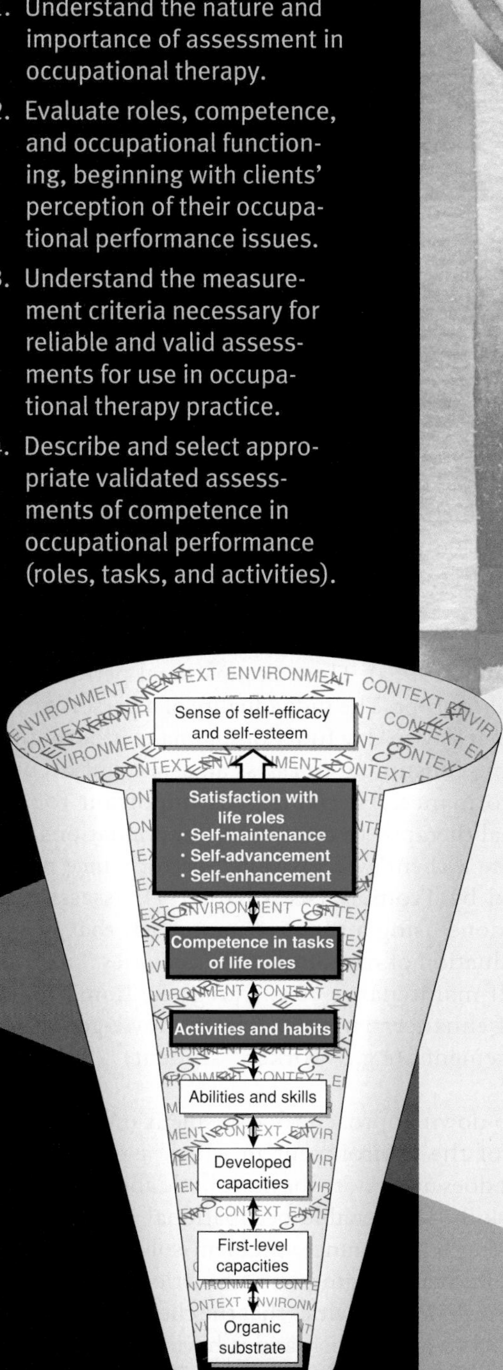

Glossary

Activities of daily living (ADL)—Activities or tasks that a person does every day to maintain personal care. Also referred to as basic activities of daily living (BADL).

Instrumental activities of daily living (IADL)—Complex activities or tasks that a person does to maintain independence in the home and community.

Leisure—Activities or tasks that are not obligatory, are intrinsically motivating, and are done for enjoyment.

Life roles—Areas of occupation associated with self-maintenance (e.g., ADL, IADL), self-advancement (e.g., work, education), and self-enhancement (e.g., leisure) that involve specific tasks and activities (see Chapter 1).

Occupational performance—Ability of individuals to satisfactorily perform purposeful daily activities (occupations). This involves the dynamic transaction among the client, the context or environment, and the activity.

Reliability—The ability of an assessment to consistently measure performance and to differentiate among clients under various conditions (Finch et al., 2002).

Validity—The extent to which an instrument measures what it is intended to measure (Finch et al., 2002).

Work—An area of occupation that includes activities needed for engaging in remunerative employment or volunteer pursuits (AOTA, 2002).

Participation in the occupations of everyday life is a vital part of human development and the lived experience (Law, 2002). Occupational therapists provide services to optimize the **occupational performance** of persons who have or are at risk for developing occupational dysfunction. This chapter describes many assessments of occupational performance and competence in valued life roles, tasks, and activities. Later chapters discuss assessment of the abilities and capacities (components of occupational function) required to carry out the tasks and activities involved in various life roles.

The goal of occupational therapy is to enable individuals to achieve competency and satisfaction in their chosen life roles and in the activities that support function and participation in these roles. Such competency and satisfaction can be achieved through personal independence or by directing others, such as an attendant. Occupational performance is the ability to carry out basic **activities of daily living (ADL or BADL)**, **instrumental activities of daily living (IADL)**, education, **work**, play or **leisure**, and social participation (American Occupational Therapy Association [AOTA], 2002). Whenever a person has a health disorder, injury, or disease that results in a physical impairment, independence in these areas of occupation may be jeopardized. The evaluation of occupational performance often begins with a semi-structured interview to assess the client's needs, problems, and concerns regarding role participation and competence in daily living tasks and activities (AOTA, 2002). During this interview, the therapist gathers valuable information from the client and family members about the tasks and roles that are most important to them and about activities that the client can and cannot do. After identifying the client's areas of difficulty in occupational performance, the therapist completes further assessments (either impairment based or disease specific) to clarify the factors that limit performance. If the limiting factors can be improved or eliminated by direct intervention, the therapist chooses an intervention approach that is appropriate for the problem. If, however, the limiting factors are not amenable to change, the therapist teaches the individual to compensate for these limitations by adapting the task or by changing the environment in which it is performed.

It is important to recognize that occupational performance, or the ability to carry out activities during daily life, depends on the individual's culture, gender, roles that he or she wishes to undertake, and environment (Law, 1991; Trombly, 1995a). Thus, occupational performance is a personal concept. The individuality of a person's roles and his or her day-to-day functioning make it both difficult and time consuming to assess all aspects of occupational performance. Therefore, it is important for the occupational therapist to carefully select evaluations that best measure a client's occupational performance needs. As outlined by Trombly (see Chapter 1), assessments should be done using a top-down approach that begins with an evaluation of roles, tasks, and activities. Life roles include self-maintenance (e.g., caregiver, home maintainer), self-enhancement (e.g., friend, movie-goer), and self-advancement (e.g., worker, student) (Trombly, 1995b).

This top-down approach to assessment includes consideration of the environment in which a person lives. Assessment does not ignore the more basic abilities, or performance skills, that enable occupational performance, such as strength, endurance, problem solving, or depth perception. Rather, it begins with a function-based assessment of the tasks and activities that the client needs, wants, or is expected to accomplish and is having difficulty performing (Law et al., 1998). Looking at this process from the perspective of the World Health Organization's International Classification of Functioning, Disability and Health (ICF) (WHO, 2001), occupational therapists first assess activities and participation, evaluating impairments in body functions (i.e., performance skills) as needed to explain difficulties in performance. By beginning with a focus on the clients' needs and considering their roles and the environment in which they live, therapists acknowledge the values and goals that these individuals bring to occupational therapy. This approach reflects a change in philosophy to a client-centered approach, recognizing that it is the person who is engaged in therapy who should articulate the goals of therapy and drive the rehabilitation process (Law, 1998).

MEASUREMENT CONCEPTS

Several important measurement concepts must be considered when choosing evaluations to assess roles and competence in occupational therapy. These concepts include whether the assessment is a standardized measure with established **reliability** and **validity**, its responsiveness to change, its level of measurement and clinical utility, and whether it involves direct observation or self-report.

A standardized measure is a published assessment tool that provides detailed instructions on test administration and scoring and has published results of reliability and validity (Finch et al., 2002). A reliable assessment is one that consistently measures the attribute under study, no matter who is scoring (inter-rater reliability) or when the assessment occurs (test-retest reliability). A valid assessment is one that measures what it purports to measure. Most evaluations of occupational performance have content validity, meaning that the test items comprehensively represent the area being tested. Some items of a valid assessment, however, may be more important than others. For example, when assessing homemaker competence during meal preparation, "can use the stove safely" is more critical in many ways than "can stir batter."

Use of the non-standardized checklists commonly found in the clinic is not recommended because of their inherent lack of reliability and validity. Because the tasks listed in non-standardized checklists are rarely operationally defined, the same methods are not necessarily used to evaluate task performance across clients and therapists. This is critical to establishing reliable and valid outcome measures. In today's demanding health care environment, it is essential that occupational therapists choose assessment tools that have strong evidence of reliably and validly evaluating changes in client performance.

An assessment that includes a wide range of test items will be more responsive to detecting impairments in occupational performance. The responsiveness of an assessment refers to its ability to detect the minimal clinically important difference (MCID) or change in performance over the course of therapy. For a therapist working on a day-to-day basis with a client to improve her ability to dress, the assessment should be sensitive enough to allow progress to be noted when different areas of the body can be dressed or different articles of clothing applied. Responsiveness is directly related to the number of items on an assessment and to the number of categories on the scoring scale. An assessment with 50 items is likely to be more responsive than one with 10 items. The level of measurement also contributes to the test's responsiveness or sensitivity in detecting clinical change. For most evaluations of roles, tasks, and activities, the level of measurement is ordinal, that is, the scores are rank-ordered to indicate the client's performance. For example, scores might range from 1 (dependent, is unable) to 7 (independent, is able). The range of ordinal scores varies depending on the assessment scale. A scoring system that uses a 1–7 Likert-type scale is likely to be more responsive to changes in performance than one using a 1–3 scale.

Periodic reevaluations are performed to monitor the client's response to therapy. At a minimum, it is important to record the level of performance at admission and discharge because these records may be used for program evaluation, to justify service to third-party payers, in legal actions, or when determining whether a patient will be discharged home or to an extended-care facility. Discharge evaluations can also aid transitions from one level of care to the next (e.g., rehabilitation hospital to home-based therapy) by providing valuable information about the client's abilities and occupational performance needs.

The clinical utility of an assessment tool is another important consideration. Clinical utility refers to all of the practical factors of an instrument, such as its cost, the training required, availability of a manual with clear instructions, and the ease of administration and interpretation. In most occupational therapy settings, managers prefer to use assessments that are time efficient and provide information useful for planning and evaluating treatment.

Assessment of roles and competence by occupational therapists can take place in many different environments, such as a hospital, rehabilitation center, workplace, school, or community setting. It is important to note that the setting in which an assessment is performed can affect a client's performance. Research indicates that the results of an assessment performed at one location (e.g., rehabilitation center) do not necessarily predict performance in another location (e.g., home) (Brown et al., 1996; Rogers et al., 2003). For example, Park, Fisher, and Velozo (1994) reported that process skills were better when older adults completed IADL tasks in the familiar environment of their homes rather than the occupational therapy clinic, while motor skills remained stable across settings. This research supports evaluation of a client's performance in the environment in which tasks ordinarily occur, whenever possible.

Standardized assessments gather information about occupational performance from either direct observation or self-report by the client or family members. Observation of activities that the client identifies as important is the most direct method of assessing competence in occupational performance. This method is preferred for accuracy, detection of inefficient or unsafe methods, and determining the underlying reason(s) that a particular task cannot be performed. Direct observation of the wide range of occupational performance areas, however, can be time consuming and costly (Law & Letts, 1989). Self-report of one's competence in occupational tasks and roles through interview is often the easiest, fastest, and least expensive method of assessing functional abilities.

There is a concern, however, that self-reports and interviews may not accurately reflect what the person can do. Studies that compared self-report ratings with direct observation of functional performance have yielded conflicting results. Some researchers reported high agreement between these two methods, especially for daily self-care tasks (Collin et al., 1988; Harris et al., 1986); others found that clients consistently overrated their abilities (Edwards, 1990; Sagar et al., 1992). If a client reports questionable data and does not permit direct observation, the therapist should verify the report with others who have knowledge of his/her actual performance. False information is not necessarily the result of a conscious intent to deceive but may reflect the fact that the client is in a health care facility and does not have an accurate sense of his or her abilities. In these cases, proxy reports and interviews with family members or caregivers can provide additional information about client performance from the family's perspective. Although self-report and direct observation in the environment where the task ordinarily occurs are preferred, the assessment methods chosen for a particular client ultimately will depend upon the nature of the disability, the supportiveness of the client's environment, and the time constraints encountered during rehabilitation.

Competence in occupational performance areas (e.g., ADL, IADL, leisure, work) is evaluated over time, based on the client's identified needs and interests. Assessments of self-care and personal mobility are usually done early because they form the basis for planning restorative therapy and/or adaptation to optimize ADL. As recovery continues and discharge plans are considered, further evaluations are used to assess a client's ability to manage home and childcare responsibilities, gain access to home and community, engage in leisure activities and family recreation, or return to valued education or work pursuits.

The assessments discussed in this chapter are generic measures that can be used to evaluate occupational performance in clients with a variety of diagnoses and levels of disablement. Refer to the chapters that follow for specific measures that assess the effects of a particular disease or condition (e.g., orthopedic injuries, COPD) on occupational performance.

ASSESSMENT METHODS AND TOOLS

A comprehensive top-down assessment of occupational performance begins with an overview and identification of a client's occupational needs, is followed by evaluation of one's engagement and competence in life roles and tasks, and continues with an assessment of the abilities or performance skills (e.g., coordination, strength, organization, etc.) needed to accomplish valued activities. See Assessment Table 4-1 for descriptions, reliability and validity data, and strengths/weaknesses of the evaluations discussed in this chapter. Resources 4-1 has contact information regarding purchase of these assessments.

Identification of Occupational Performance Needs

A client-centered occupational therapy assessment recognizes that engagement in life roles and occupations of one's choice is a personal issue and that the client's perception is an important force that drives the occupational therapy process (Law et al., 1994). Information about a person's occupational roles and tasks, developmental stage, and the environment in which he or she lives is best obtained through interview. This can be done through informal narrative interviews or through more structured interview-based assessments. Specific information about occupational performance can be further obtained via evaluations that involve direct observation.

Neistadt (1994) discussed the weaknesses of basing occupational therapy goals on informal client interviews. Her research indicated that this unstructured process often leads to goals that are vague and not specifically related to occupation. The occupational therapist is advised to select a range of standardized assessments that incorporate semi-structured interviews to identify occupational need areas, as well as direct measures of abilities and skills during observation of task performance.

Semi-Structured Interview Assessments

A semi-structured interview assessment that is widely used to evaluate a client's perception of his/her occupational performance is the *Canadian Occupational Performance Measure* (*COPM*) (Law et al., 1998). The *COPM* helps clients to identify concerns with occupational performance, assists in goal setting, and measures changes in client

RESOURCE 4-1

Assessments discussed in this chapter may be obtained either from the resources listed below or from published articles on instrument development and psychometric properties that are included in the reference list.

Assessment of Motor and Process Skills (AMPS) (5th ed., 2005)
AMPS Project International
Phone: (603) 778-2965
Fax: (603) 778-0095
E-mail: info@AMPSintl.com
www.ampsintl.com/

Canadian Occupational Performance Measure (COPM) (4th ed.)
Canadian Association of Occupational Therapists
CTTC Building, Suite 3400
1125 Colonel By Drive
Ottawa ON K1S 5R1
Canada
Phone: (613) 523-CAOT (2268)
Toll-free in Canada and the continental USA: (800) 434-CAOT (2268)
www.caot.ca

Craig Handicap Assessment and Reporting Technique (CHART)
David Mellick, MA
Craig Hospital
3425 South Clarkson
Englewood, CO 80110
Phone: (303) 789-8202
E-mail: dmellick@craighospital.org

Feasibility Evaluation Checklist and Functional Capacity Evaluations
Employment Potential Improvement Corporation
P.O. Box 3897
Ballwin, MO 63022
Phone: (636) 724-4556
Fax: (636) 898-0954
www.epicrehab.com

Functional Independence Measure (FIM)
Uniform Data System for Medical Rehabilitation
70 Northpointe Parkway, Suite 300
Amherst, NY 14228-1897
Phone: (716) 817-7800
Fax: (716) 568-0037
www.udsmr.org

Interest Checklist
MOHO Clearinghouse
Department of Occupational Therapy
College of Applied Health Sciences
University of Illinois at Chicago
See: MOHO Related Resources
www.moho.uic.edu

Kohlman Evaluation of Living Skills (3rd ed.)
AOTA
4720 Montgomery Lane
P.O. Box 31220
Bethesda, MD 20824-1220
Phone: (301) 652-2682
Fax: (301) 652-7711
www.aota.org

Leisure Competence Measure
Published by Marchard, Inc.
Idyll Arbor
39129 264th Avenue SE
Enumclaw, WA 98022
Phone: (360) 825-7797
Fax: (360) 825-5670
www.idyllarbor.com

Leisure Diagnostic Battery Users Manual
Authors: Peter Witt, Texas A&M University, and Gary Ellis, University of Utah
Venture Publishing, Inc.
1999 Cato Avenue
State College, PA 16801
Phone: (814) 234-4561
Fax: (814) 234-1651
E-mail: vpublish@venture-publish.com

Occupational Performance History Interview-II (OPHI-II) (Version 2.1, 2004)
Authors: Gary Kielhofner, Trudy Mallinson, Carrie Crawford, Meika Nowak, Matt Rigby, Alexis Henry, and Deborah Walens
MOHO Clearinghouse
Department of Occupational Therapy
College of Applied Health Sciences
University of Illinois at Chicago
www.moho.uic.edu/assessments.html

Office of Disability Employment Policy (ODEP)
U.S. Department of Labor provides a wide range of job accommodation recommendations and resources.
www.dol.gov/odep
Job Accommodation Network has suggestions for persons with various diagnoses
www.jan.wvu.edu

Role Checklist
Frances Oakley, MS, OTR, FAOTA
National Institutes of Health
Building 10, CRC, Room 1-1469
10 Center Drive MSC 1604
Bethesda, MD 20892-1604
E-mail: foakley@nih.gov

Safety Assessment of Function and the Environment for Rehabilitation (SAFER)
Community Occupational Therapy Associates (COTA)
700 Lawrence Avenue West, Suite 362
Toronto, Ontario M6A 3B4
Phone: (416) 785-9230 or 1 (888) 785-2779 (outside Toronto local calling area)
Fax: (416) 785-9358
www.cotahealth.ca

Valpar Component Work Samples
Valpar International Corporation
P.O. Box 5767
Tucson, AZ 85703
Sales Office Phone: (800) 633-3321
Fax: (262) 797-8488
E-mail: sales@valparint.com

Worker Role Interview (WRI) (Version 10.0, 2005)
Authors: Brent Braveman, Mick Robson, Craig Velozo, Gary Kielhofner, Gail Fisher, Kirsty Forsyth, and Jennifer Kerschbaum
MOHO Clearinghouse
Department of Occupational Therapy
College of Applied Health Sciences
University of Illinois at Chicago
www.moho.uic.edu/assessments.html

Assessment Table 4-1

Summary of Assessments

Instrument and Reference	Description	Time to Administer	Validity	Reliability	Sensitivity	Strengths and Weaknesses
Occupational Performance						
Canadian Occupational Performance Measure (COPM) (Law et al., 1998)	Semi-structured interview with ordinal scale to measure changes in client self-perception of performance in self-care, productivity, and leisure occupations.	20–40 minutes.	Numerous studies support *COPM* as a valid measure of occupational performance. Combined *COPM* and *FIM* scores were 65% accurate in predicting discharge status (Simmons, Crepeau, &White, 2000).	Test–retest intraclass correlation coefficients in rehabilitation setting: 0.80 for performance scores; 0.89 for satisfaction scores (Bosch, 1995).	Carswell et al. (2004) report *COPM* is more sensitive to perceived changes in client status than other disability measures, including *SF-36* and *FIM*.	Strengths: Psychometrics studied in wide range of diagnoses (Carswell et al., 2004); translated into 20 languages and used in more than 35 countries around the world.
Occupational Performance History Interview-II (OPHI-II) (Kielhofner et al., 1998)	Semi-structured interview intended to give a broad and detailed appreciation of a person's life history, the impact of disability, and the direction in which the person would like to take his or her life. Specific criteria are provided to rate performance on 3 scales: occupational competence, identity, and behavior.	45–60 minutes.	Validity for all 3 scales is excellent. More than 90% of subjects tested (with varied ages, nationalities, and diagnoses) were validly measured, and over 90% of raters used scales validly, with approximately same degree of severity or leniency (Kielhofner et al., 2001).	Refer to test manual.	Adequate. Person separation statistic showed that the scale can distinguish meaningful differences among persons of approximately 3 different levels of competence, identity, and environmental support (Kielhofner et al., 2001).	Strengths: Specific criteria assist with rating. Rasch analysis has been used to calibrate and convert ordinal scores to interval data. Weakness: Evidence of rater reliability not well reported in research literature.
Roles and Community Integration						
Role Checklist (Oakley et al., 1986)	Written inventory/checklist that provides data on client perceptions of role participation and values throughout the lifespan.	15 minutes.	Content validity of role taxonomy is based on literature review and expert opinion (AOTA, 1996)	Test–retest reliability median is $r = 0.82$ within a 2-week period.	Not established.	Strengths: Appropriate across age groups. Translated into 10 languages. Can be adapted for verbal administration by therapist.

Craig Handicap Assessment and Reporting Technique (*CHART*) (Whiteneck et al., 1992)	Interview administered in person or by phone to assess WHO dimensions of handicap. Each dimension (orientation, physical independence, mobility, occupation, social integration, and economic self-sufficiency) is scored on 100-point scale. These dimensions indicate level of participation in life situations. *CHART-SF* (short form) closely approximates scores on original *CHART* in less time.	Long form can take 45 minutes to administer and score.	*CHART* scores correlate significantly with therapist ratings of level of handicap. Rasch analysis supports construct validity of the *CHART*.	Inter-rater reliability is 0.69–0.84 between patient and family member ratings. Test–retest reliability is 0.80–0.95.	Not established.	Strengths: Allows level of handicap comparisons among and between diagnostic groups. Weaknesses: Structure doesn't allow client to specify which test items are most valued and in need of intervention. Dimension scores can only be calculated if all questions are answered.
Reintegration to Normal Living Index (*RNL*) (Wood-Dauphinee et al., 1988)	Eleven declarative statements re: how well clients return to normal living after a disabling event (e.g., "I am comfortable with how my self-care needs are met.") are rated by either a visual analog scale (VAS) or 3–4 point categorical scale. Index can be therapist administered, by self-report, or proxy. VAS scores are converted to 100-point scale for easy interpretation.	Less than 10 minutes.	Construct validity reported by significant correlations with *Quality of Life Index* and *Affect Balance Scale* (Law, Baum, & Dunn, 2001).	Test–retest reliability: $r = 0.83$ for community-dwelling elderly. Internal consistency determined by Cronbach's alpha for client, proxy, and health professional scores ranged between 0.90 and 0.95.	Not established.	Strengths: Emphasis placed on client's perceptions of autonomy in life situations. Weaknesses: Problems in *RNL* domains were more likely reported by proxy than client scores. These differed significantly at discharge and follow-up, reinforcing importance of self-report.

continued

Assessment Table 4-1

Summary of Assessments (continued)

Instrument and Reference	Description	Time to Administer	Validity	Reliability	Sensitivity	Strengths and Weaknesses
Community Integration Measure (*CIM*) (McColl et al., 2001) Primary author M. A. McColl may be contacted at: mccollm@post.queensu.ca	10-item, qualitative measure based on client-centered model of community integration. Client agreement with test statements is measured by 5-point scale. Sample items include: "I feel like part of this community, like I belong here" and "I know the rules in this community and I can fit with them."	Approximately 5 minutes.	Criterion validity supported by comparisons with *Community Integration Questionnaire* and *Satisfaction with Life Scale* (Reistetter et al., 2005). Discriminant validity supported by the ability of *CIM* to differentiate persons with brain injury from neurologically intact controls.	Cronbach's alpha for internal consistency reliability is 0.87.	Not established.	Strengths: Quick and easy to administer and score and readily understood by clients and families. Weaknesses: Psychometrics to date have only been examined with clients diagnosed with TBI, potentially limiting generalizability of this tool to other disability groups. Specific instructions to help OT relate test results with treatment planning are not provided.
Activities of Daily Living (ADL)						
Barthel Index (Mahoney & Barthel, 1965) Information available online at www.strokecenter.org/trials/scales/barthel.pdf	Self-report and direct observation used to evaluate 10 activities: feeding, bathing, grooming, dressing, bowel and bladder control, toilet use, transfers between chair and bed, mobility, and stair climbing. The total score ranges from 0 (total dependence) to 100 (total independence).	5–10 minutes if self-report; 20–60 minutes for direct observation.	Adequately classified stroke survivors as dependent or independent. Kappa = 0.77 compared to *Katz Index*. Spearman rho = 0.73 (K = 0.42) compared to *Kenny Self Care Evaluation*. (Granger, Albrecht, & Hamilton, 1979; Gresham, Phillips, & Labi, 1980).	Studies indicate excellent reliability (Fricke & Unsworth, 1996). Inter-rater reliability $r = 0.99$ with mixed diagnoses (Loewen & Anderson, 1988). Test–retest reliability Kappa = 0.98 in clients with stroke (Wolfe et al., 1991).	Lacks sensitivity to amount of assistance needed. Initially high-functioning clients can reach "ceiling" score and show no further improvement (Shah, Vanclay, & Cooper, 1989).	Strengths: Excellent reliability and validity. Widely used. Time to administer. Weaknesses: "Ceiling" effect for higher-level clients. Only fair sensitivity to change.

Functional Independence Measure (FIM) (Granger et al., 1993; Keith et al., 1987)	18 items (13 motor, 5 cognition) in the areas of self-care, sphincter control, transfers, locomotion, communication, and social cognition. A 7-point ordinal scale rates level of independence in ADL (independent without equipment = 7). Scores are based on clinical observation. Follow-up data can be gathered from phone interviews.	Approximately 45 minutes, depending on client abilities.	Excellent validity reported. Motor *FIM* able to predict level of assistance required in 83% of TBI clients tested; cognitive *FIM* predicted 77% of patients requiring supervision (Corrigan, Smith-Knapp, & Granger, 1997).	Numerous studies have reported excellent reliability in wide range of diagnostic groups. Chau et al. (1994) reported inter-rater ICC at 0.94, test–retest ICC at 0.93.	Greater sensitivity to change reported in motor than cognitive scales in persons with stroke (van der Putten et al., 1999) and multiple sclerosis (Sharrack et al., 1999).	Strengths: Extensive validation; widely recognized and used. Excellent reliability and validity in measuring disability. Weakness: *FIM* scores do not provide information re: factors (e.g., body functions, environmental support) that influence occupational performance.
Katz Index of Independence in Activities of Daily Living (Katz, 1963)	Six ADL functions are assessed through interview and observation. Test items include: bathing, dressing, toileting, transferring, continence, and feeding. Performance is rated on dichotomous scale (independent, dependent).	5–10 minutes; longer if performance is observed.	Face, construct, and concurrent validity have been reported. Predictive validity demonstrates 0.50 correlation with mobility and 0.38 with house confinement (AOTA, 1996).	Inter-rater reliability is reported to be low (Brorsson & Asberg, 1984). No report of test–retest reliability.	Although sensitive to changes in declining health status, its responsiveness to small increments of change during rehabilitation is limited.	Strength: Quick and easy to administer. Weakness: Results are too general to be useful in treatment planning.
Klein-Bell Activities of Daily Living Scale (Klein & Bell, 1982)	Behavior rating scale consists of 170 specific items to rate performance in 6 ADL areas: dressing, elimination, mobility, bathing/hygiene, eating, and emergency phone communication. Performance is observed and scored as either able or unable; scores are also weighted from 1–3 points based on item difficulty.	30 minutes depending on client's level of ability and fatigue.	Validity was established on 14 patients by comparing the total score at discharge against the hours of assistance required. A correlation of -0.86 ($p < 0.01$) was obtained, indicating that the amount of assistance decreases as the *Klein-Bell* score increases.	Inter-rater agreement = 0.92 even without extensive training (Klein & Bell, 1982).	Specificity of test items makes this test highly responsive to changes in client status.	Strengths: Highly responsive. Excellent reliability and validity. Appropriate for clinical purposes and research. Weakness: Higher level subjects may reach test "ceiling."

continued

Assessment Table 4-1

Summary of Assessments (continued)

Instrument and Reference	Instrument and Reference	Time to Administer	Validity	Reliability	Sensitivity	Strengths and Weaknesses
Instrumental Activities of Daily Living (IADL)						
The Assessment of Motor and Process Skills (*AMPS*) (Fisher, 1993, 1995)	The *AMPS* is an observational assessment that evaluates motor and process skills that directly impact occupational performance. Client chooses 2–3 IADL tasks for assessment from a list of more than 50. Computerized scoring and Rasch methods are used to generate adjusted IADL ability measures. These take into account the severity of the rater who scored performance and the relative challenge of tasks performed.	30–60 minutes for administration and scoring.	Many published studies have demonstrated the validity of the *AMPS*. Validity as a cross-cultural measure has been reported.	Intra-rater reliability is excellent ($r = 0.93$). Test–retest reliability reported to be $r = 0.88$ for motor skills and $r = 0.86$ for process skills (Fisher, 1995).	Excellent responsiveness to client change has been reported.	Strengths: Excellent reliability and validity. Evaluation tasks are chosen by client and are meaningful and relevant to his daily life situation. Appropriate for use across ages (3 years to adult) and diagnostic groups. Weaknesses: Training requirements are extensive, and this has limited its clinical utility.
The Kohlman Evaluation of Living Skills (*KELS*) (Kohlman Thomson, 1993)	Self-report and observation assessment of 17 IADL tasks in 5 areas: self-care, safety and health, money management, transportation and telephone, and work and leisure. Items such as "use of money to purchase items" or "use of phone book and telephone" are scored as 0 (independent) or 1 (needs assistance). A score of 5½ or less indicates that client is able to live independently.	30–45 minutes.	Concurrent validity studies that compared *KELS* with *Global Assessment Scale* (0.78–0.89) and *BaFPE* (−0.84) indicate high agreement.	Inter-rater reliability in multiple studies is reported to be high ($r = 0.84–1.00$) (Kohlman Thomson, 1993).	Not established.	Strengths: Easy to administer. Few materials are required. Can be used in many settings and with many diagnostic groups. Weaknesses: Tasks provide good screening of basic abilities, but higher level clients may reach test "ceiling."

Safety Assessment of Function and the Environment for Rehabilitation (*SAFER*) (Oliver et al., 1993)	The *SAFER* tool consists of an easy-to-use checklist of 97 items grouped into 14 areas of concern: living situation, mobility, kitchen, fire hazards, eating, household, dressing, grooming, bathroom, medication, communication, wandering, memory aids, and general issues. A combination of observation, interview, and task performance is used to rate each item.	Approximately 1–1.5 hours, depending on administration method, client's functioning level, and home environment.	Excellent content validity based on OT judgments and statistical methods. Construct validity has been supported in relation to cognitive impairment, but further research is needed.	Internal consistency is excellent with Kuder-Richardson coefficient of 0.83. Inter-rater and test–retest reliability demonstrated via kappa (w) or % agreement was acceptable to excellent.	Poor. The *SAFER* tool was not designed to measure changes post intervention. A revised 93-item scale, the *SAFER-HOME* v.2, is being developed (Chiu & Oliver, unpublished manuscript).	Strengths: Clear assessment guidelines and recommendations. Weaknesses: The original *SAFER* tool was a binary scale that only noted the presence or absence of a safety problem. This has been expanded into a 4-point scale on the *SAFER-HOME* v.2 to increase its sensitivity to detect change. Reliability testing of the revised scale is ongoing.
The Kitchen Task Assessment (*KTA*) (Baum & Edwards, 1993)	The *KTA* assesses 5 cognitive abilities during the task of making cooked pudding from a package: initiation, organization, inclusion of all steps, safety and judgment, and task completion. The level of support provided by the therapist is scored from 0 (independent) to 3 (not capable). Unlike the *AMPS*, this measure does not evaluate motor skills during task performance. The *KTA* was developed for persons with dementia and Alzheimer's disease.	Less than 30 minutes.	Construct validity was supported by highly significant correlations between *KTA* scores and other cognitive measures, including the *Token Test*, *Clinical Dementia Rating*, and *Blessed Dementia Scale.*	Internal consistency of the *KTA* ranges from 0.87–0.96, and inter-rater reliability for the total score is 0.85.	*KTA* scores significantly differentiated cognitive performance across all stages of dementia (Baum & Edwards, 1993). Sensitivity to client change over time has not been established.	Strengths: Good reliability and validity in lower functioning adults with dementia. Quick and easy to administer. Weaknesses: Little data to support *KTA* use with other rehabilitation populations (Duncombe, 2004). Higher functioning clients will easily reach test "ceiling."

continued

Assessment Table 4-1

Summary of Assessments (continued)

Instrument and Reference	Description	Time to Administer	Validity	Reliability	Sensitivity	Strengths and Weaknesses
Rabideau Kitchen Evaluation Revised (Neistadt, 1992, 1994)	Direct observation of meal preparation tasks, such as preparing a hot beverage and cold sandwich. Each task is broken down into component steps that are rated on a 0 (no assistance needed) to 3 scale (unable and requires direct intervention) (Neistadt, 1994). Six levels of task difficulty help guide the grading of tasks, based on client abilities (highest level involves preparation of fruit salad or baking frozen pastries).	20–30 minutes depending on tasks performed.	Criterion validity reported with the *WAIS-R* block design test ($r = -0.60$, $p = 0.0002$), suggesting that both tests measure common skills. The correlation was negative because good performance is indicated by low scores on the Rabideau and high scores on WAIS-R.	Inter-rater reliability is $r = 0.86$. Test–retest reliability on a small sample yielded $r = 0.80$ (Neistadt, 1992).	Not established.	Strengths: Reliable kitchen assessment based on information-processing theory. Dynamic assessment approach indicates amount of cognitive support needed for task completion. Weaknesses: Primarily validated with persons with TBI, limiting generalizability to other diagnostic groups. Choice of tasks is limited by test design.
Work						
VALPAR Component Work Samples (Valpar Corp.)	Direct observation of work tasks selected to evaluate client's specific job requirements and needs. Work samples are keyed to worker traits, as listed in the *Dictionary of Occupational Titles* (DOT). Each work sample consists of a scoring manual and standardized equipment ranging from common items to large equipment. Examples of the dexterity module include small parts assembly, tool manipulation, and bimanual coordination.	Dependent on number of work samples tested. Samples range in time from 20–90 minutes.	The work samples have been criterion-referenced according to the Department of Labor's DOT, yielding good face and content validity (AOTA, 1996).	Test–retest reliability for work samples 1–16 of the original series ranged from 0.70–0.99 for work rate and accuracy scores over a 1-week interval (AOTA,1996).	Measures are highly sensitive to detecting changes in client performance over time.	Strengths: High face validity and reliability. Normative tables provide error and time percentiles for each exercise. Weaknesses: High cost. Work samples emphasize physical components of work tasks and should be supplemented with assessments of worker interests, goals, and psychosocial/contextual factors influencing performance.

Worker Role Interview (Velozo, Kielhofner, & Fisher, 1998; Biernacki, 1993)	A semi-structured interview that assesses psychosocial/environmental factors of concern to the injured worker or client with a long-term disability and poor/limited work history. Complements observations made during other physical or behavioral work assessments; designed to identify specific variables influencing client's ability to return to work.	30–60 minutes and 15 minutes for scoring.	Content areas were based on a theoretical model, the *Model of Human Occupation* (*MOHO*), and extensive literature review of factors that influence return to work.	Test–retest reliability for total score with a 6- to 12-day interval was 0.95. Inter-rater reliability was 0.81 with 3 raters (Biernacki, 1993).	Not established.	Strength: Test items reflect occupational therapists' interest in the meaning of work. Weakness: Time to administer can be lengthy.
Leisure						
Interest Checklist (Matsutsuyu, 1969; Rogers, Weinstein, & Figone, 1978)	Self-report questionnaire and 80-item interview checklist. Gathers data about a client's interest patterns over time (past, present, and future). Activities range from gardening and yard work, to bowling, watching television, and driving. Modified version with 68 items is recommended for use with *Model of Human Occupation* (*MOHO*). The checklist can be used by adolescents or adults.	10–15 minutes.	Evident face validity. Rogers (1988) reports that *Interest Checklist* discriminates among diagnostic groups and normal control subjects.	Good test–retest reliability (0.92) within 3-week interval (Rogers, Weinstein, & Figone, 1978).	Not established.	Strengths: Quick to administer. Participation in wide range of activities can be assessed over time. Provides activity ideas for treatment planning (Klyczek, Bauer-Yox, & Fiedler, 1997). Weaknesses: Lack of strong validity and sensitivity data. Clients may misinterpret some items (e.g., level of participation is unclear: do clients perform vs. watch activities such as auto-racing, concerts?). Limited testing with clients who have physical vs. psychosocial disabilities.

continued

Assessment Table 4-1

Summary of Assessments (continued)

Instrument and Reference	Description	Time to Administer	Validity	Reliability	Sensitivity	Strengths and Weaknesses
Activity Index and Meaningfulness of Activity Scales (Gregory, 1983)	*Activity Index* is a self-report, ordinal measure of a client's interest and frequency of participation in a variety of leisure activities. *Meaningfulness of Activity Scale* provides additional information re: a client's autonomy, competency, and leisure enjoyment. Clients can rate up to 3 additional activities not included in the *Activity Index* list. Higher scores are moderately but significantly related to greater life satisfaction scores.	15–20 minutes.	Not established.	Test–retest reliability for the *Activity Index* was 0.70; for the *Meaningfulness of Activity Scales,* it was 0.87 (Gregory, 1983).	Not established.	Strengths: Acknowledges importance of leisure/occupational performance in retired persons. Test items are particularly relevant to elderly clients. Weaknesses: No published evidence of validity. Psychometrics only for older adults.

Leisure Diagnostic Battery (Witt & Ellis, 1984)	Self-report/interview to assess a client's perceptions about his/her leisure experiences. The first 5 subscales are used to rate perceived competence and control in leisure activities, identify needs and depth of leisure involvement, and consider self-perceptions about playfulness. Test items are scored on a 1 (strongly agree) to 5 (strongly disagree) scale. Average scores from these subscales are summed to determine a perceived freedom in leisure score and identify problems for treatment planning.	30–40 minutes.	Content validity reported through factor analysis.	Cronbach's alpha was 0.96 for the total score, indicating excellent internal consistency (Peebles et al., 1999). Test–retest reliability: intraclass correlation coefficient of 0.72.	These scales appear to be responsive to changes in leisure performance after a recreation intervention.	Strength: Well-developed measure to assess client's perception of leisure involvement. Weakness: Further testing of validity is needed.

perceptions of occupational performance over the course of therapy. The *COPM* is a generic measure that can be used with clients across all developmental stages who have a variety of disabilities. It is client centered and addresses roles, role expectations, and activity performance within the client's own environment.

The *COPM* is administered in a four-step process that includes problem definition, priority setting, scoring, and reassessment. During the initial *COPM* interview, clients or caregivers identify areas of ADL, work, and leisure that are important to them and are in need of occupational therapy intervention. For each occupational performance area, the therapist gives examples of typical activities, and the client indicates which of these he needs to, wants to, or is expected to perform. When a client identifies an activity he must do, current performance is explored. If the client is unable to perform the activity or is not satisfied with the way he completes it, that activity is listed as a problem for intervention. If a client does not report problems with activities in a given performance area, the next occupational performance area is explored. After all of the occupational performance problems are identified, clients score them in terms of importance, their perception of current performance, and satisfaction with that performance. It is important to recognize that a client with a new illness may not recognize or be ready to identify these issues. The therapist and the client may begin treatment by working on identified concerns and can return to this semi-structured interview process later to see if other issues emerge. Reassessment is completed at discharge or when the client and the therapist consider it necessary for further treatment planning (Fig. 4-1).

Another semi-structured interview assessment that is used to identify occupational performance needs is the *Occupational Performance History Interview-II* (*OPHI-II*) (Kielhofner et al., 1998). *OPHI-II* is an assessment of occupational life history in work, leisure, and daily activities that was developed using the Model of Human Occupation. The *OPHI-II* contains three valid scales that provide insight into the nature of occupational performance and adaptation. These scales measure occupational competence, occupational identity, and the settings or environments in which behaviors occur (Kielhofner et al., 2001). For example, test items explore a client's ability to organize time for responsibilities; identify interests, goals, and role expectations; recognize personal responsibilities and values; and participate in varied environments (e.g., leisure, home, and work settings). An accompanying Life History Narrative Form is used to document qualitative information from the interview. *OPHI-II* can be used with occupational therapy clients who are adolescents or older and who are seen in psychiatry, physical disability, or gerontology practices (Kielhofner et al., 1991).

Through an interview, clients identify occupational performance activities that are important to them and which they are having difficulties performing satisfactorily. These are scored on a 1–10 scale.

Activity Problems:	Importance	Performance	Satisfaction
Doing up fasteners	9	3	1
Washing face and hands	10	1	1
Preparing sandwich	5	1	4
Holding a book	7	3	5
Visiting friends	9	2	4

Figure 4-1 Example of the scores for the *Canadian Occupational Performance Measure.*

Assessing Roles and Community Integration

Trombly (1995b) sorts life roles into three domains that correspond well to the Occupational Therapy Practice Framework (OTPF) (AOTA, 2002): self-maintenance, self-advancement, and self-enhancement (see Chapter 1). The most widely used role assessments in occupational therapy include the *OPHI-II*, which was already reviewed in this chapter, and the *Role Checklist* (Oakley et al., 1986). The *Role Checklist* is a two-part self-report assessment. Part I assesses participation in 10 major life roles: student, worker, volunteer, caregiver, home maintainer, friend, family member, religious participant, hobbyist/amateur, participant in organizations, and other. Test items address past, present, and future performance of these roles. Part II measures how valuable or important each role is to the client. This assessment has been used to evaluate the client's perceptions of role participation in persons with mental illness, mothers with young children, persons with physical disabilities, and adolescents.

Community integration refers to the ability of a person to live, work, and enjoy his or her free time within the community setting. A client's competence and ability to engage in community tasks and roles after a disabling event or illness is related to intrinsic abilities or performance skills as well as characteristics of the environment in which he/she lives. Although most of the following assessments emphasize the client's perception of his/her competence in community or societal integration, others, such as the *Craig Hospital Inventory of Environmental Factors* (*CHIEF*) (Whiteneck et al., 2004), focus on environmental factors that limit community integration. Knowledge of the content and focus of these assessments will help the occupational therapist choose tools that best measure and identify occupational performance areas and skills in need of intervention.

The *Craig Handicap Assessment and Reporting Technique* (*CHART*) (Whiteneck et al., 1992) was initially developed to evaluate the World Health Organization's (WHO) dimensions of handicap. Handicap, a term that reflects one's level of participation in life situations after a disabling event (WHO, 2001), describes the total effects of social, economic, cultural, and environmental consequences of disability at the societal level (Whiteneck et al., 1992). The *CHART* assesses a client's performance according to the six dimensions of handicap, or participation, outlined by the WHO: physical independence, cognitive independence, mobility, occupation, social integration, and economic self-sufficiency. Although the *CHART* was initially developed for persons with spinal cord injuries, long and short forms of this assessment have also been validated for persons with various diagnoses, including traumatic brain injury, stroke, burn, amputation, and multiple sclerosis.

The *Reintegration to Normal Living* (*RNL*) *Index* (Wood-Dauphinee et al., 1988) is an easy-to-use 11-item assessment of how well individuals return to normal living patterns following incapacitating disease or injury. Client perceptions of reintegration are measured along the following domains: indoor, community, and distance mobility; self-care; daily activity (e.g., paid and unpaid work, school); recreational and social activities; general coping skills; family roles; personal relationships; and presentation of self to others. A visual analog scale is used by the client to rate performance (Fig. 4-2). This assessment has been tested with a wide variety of diagnostic groups including patients with arthritis, fractures, amputations, stroke, spinal cord injury, traumatic brain injury, and hip fracture.

The *Community Integration Measure* (*CIM*) (McColl et al., 2001) uses 10 items to gather qualitative information about a person's experience of community integration and participation. It is based on a theoretical model that is client centered and differs from other community assessments because it makes no assumptions about the relative importance of particular activities or relationships (McColl et al., 2001). For example, the *CIM* does not assume that independent participation is a better measure of community integration than supported or mutual participation with others. The client uses a 5-point Likert-type scale to rate his/her agreement with statements such as "I feel that I am accepted in this community" and "I know my way around this community." Although this easy-to-use measure was developed for and tested primarily with persons diagnosed with traumatic brain injury, it has been used in practice with clients who have a wide range of disabilities (McColl et al., 2001). The *CIM* is able to differentiate persons with and without disabilities and correlates significantly with other measures of community integration and life satisfaction.

Many assessments of health-related quality of life have been developed for use with persons with chronic illness. Examples of these assessments that have excellent reliability and validity include the *Sickness Impact Profile* (*SIP*) (Bergner et al., 1981) and the *Medical Outcomes Study* (*MOS*) *Short Form 36* (*SF-36*) (Jenkinson, Wright, & Coulter, 1994).

I move around my living quarters as I feel necessary. (Wheelchairs, other equipment or resources may be used.)

I am comfortable with how my self-care needs (dressing, feeding, toileting, bathing) are met. (Adaptive equipment, supervision, and/or assistance may be used.)

I spend most of my days occupied in a work activity that is necessary or important to me. (Work activity could be paid employment, housework, volunteer work, school, etc. Adaptive equipment, supervision, and/or assistance may be used.)

In general, I am comfortable with my personal relationships.

I feel that I can deal with life events as they happen.

Each item is scored with a 10-cm visual analogue, with 10 as "fully describes my situation" and 1 as "does not describe my situation."

Figure 4-2 Example of items on the *Reintegration to Normal Living Index.* (Reprinted with permission from Wood-Dauphinee, S., Opzoomer, A., Williams, J. I., Marchand, B., & Spitzer, W. O. [1988]. Assessment of global function: The Reintegration to Normal Living Index. *Archives of Physical Medicine and Rehabilitation, 69,* 583–590.)

Assessing Tasks and Activities

Occupational therapists use a variety of assessment tools to measure baseline and discharge performance in tasks and activities of importance to the client, including ADL, instrumental ADL, work, and leisure.

Activities of Daily Living (ADL)

ADL generally include mobility at home, feeding, dressing, bathing, grooming, toileting, basic communication, and personal hygiene (Trombly, 1995a). Direct observation of problem activities identified by the client should be done at the time of day when they are normally performed and, if possible, in the place where they usually occur. Remember that many people may have strong feelings of modesty regarding personal care, and those feelings should be respected. The client's endurance and safety should be closely monitored, and ADL performance can be evaluated over several therapy sessions if slow performance or fatigue occurs. Items that would be unsafe or obviously unsuccessful (such as tub transfers) are postponed until the patient's physical status improves. When the patient is not independent in a required task at the time of discharge, plans are developed to ensure that others can assist with this task and that additional therapy is received if warranted.

Most standardized ADL evaluations were designed for program evaluation to document the level of independence achieved by patients as the result of a particular program. Frequently cited ADL assessments used by occupational therapists are briefly described in the following paragraphs.

The *Barthel Index* (Mahoney & Barthel, 1965) evaluates 10 activities: feeding, bathing, grooming, dressing, bowel and bladder control, toilet use, transfers between chair and bed, mobility, and stair climbing. The total score for these 10 activities can range from 0 to 100 (total independence), and the score for each activity is weighted according to its importance for independent functioning (Gresham, Phillips, & Labi, 1980; Mahoney & Barthel, 1965). A score of 60 seems to be the transition point from dependency to assisted independence. A modified version of the *Barthel Index* has been found to be reliable and valid when administered during a telephone interview (Korner-Bitensky & Wood-Dauphinee, 1995).

The *Functional Independence Measure* (*FIM*) (Granger & Hamilton, 1992) uses a 7-point ordinal scale to evaluate occupational performance for 18 items (13 motor and five cognition items) in the areas of self-care, sphincter control, transfers, locomotion, communication, and social cognition (Granger et al., 1993; Keith et al., 1987). The *FIM* is a basic measure of the severity of disability, not impairment. The scale rates a client's performance by taking into account his/her need for assistance from another person or a device. The *FIM* instrument is intended to measure what the person with disability actually does, whatever the diagnosis or impairment, and is scored according to information gathered by members of the rehabilitation team during client observation. The *FIM* can be used during rehabilitation to track changes in activities of daily living and provide data for program evaluation. It has been shown to predict functional status at discharge and length of rehabilitation stay (Heinemann et al., 1994). The *FIM* is part of a uniform data system that collects information about rehabilitation outcomes and effectiveness and is an integral part of the *Inpatient Rehabilitation Facility–Patient Assessment Instrument* (*IRF-PAI*) (Fig. 4-3) (UB Foundation Activities, Inc., 2004).

The *Katz Index* (Katz et al., 1963) evaluates six activities of daily living: bathing, dressing, toileting, transferring, continence, and feeding. Scoring is based on ontogenetic development of self-care skills (Gresham, Phillips, & Labi, 1980; Katz et al., 1963), and a 3-point scale is used to rate performance (independent, requires assistance, dependent). The *Katz Index* has been found to predict length of hospital stay, living situation 1 year after discharge, and mortality (Brorsson & Asberg, 1984; Asberg & Nydevik, 1991). Although the *Katz Index* is sensitive to changes in declining health status, it is limited in its responsiveness to small increments of change during rehabilitation. The *Katz Index* is quick to use, but its clinical utility is somewhat limited because it does not provide detailed information for treatment planning.

The Klein-Bell Activities of Daily Living Scale (Klein & Bell, 1982) documents a client's ability to perform in six basic ADL: dressing, elimination, mobility, bathing and hygiene, eating, and emergency telephone communications. These ADL are broken down into 170 simple behavioral items, each of which is scored separately (Fig. 4-4). The large number of items makes the *Klein-Bell* one of the most responsive ADL assessments. Each item is scored as achieved (no physical or verbal assistance) or unable (assistance needed), and raw scores are converted to percentage scores to make the communication of results easier to understand. If the person can perform the test item with adapted equipment during the discharge evaluation, he or she is given credit for accomplishing that activity.

Instrumental Activities of Daily Living (IADL)

Although many IADL assessments include a few self-care items, their focus is primarily home management tasks such as meal planning, preparation, service, and cleanup; laundry; shopping for food and clothing; and routine and seasonal care of the home. Yard work and other maintenance tasks also might have been the responsibility of the patient prior to therapy and may require assessment and intervention. Frequently cited standardized IADL assessments used by occupational therapists are described in the following paragraphs.

The Assessment of Motor and Process Skills (*AMPS*) (Fisher, 1993, 1995) is an innovative observational assessment that was developed to reveal the relationship between an individual's performance of IADL tasks and the underlying process and motor skills that contribute to that performance. During the *AMPS* evaluation, motor and process skills are assessed concurrently with observation of functional performance. The client chooses to perform two or three familiar tasks from more than 50 possibilities described in the *AMPS* manual. Tasks offered to clients present a challenge to them, are not overlearned, and are appropriate to the client's environment, age, and culture (Fisher, 1993).

The *AMPS* uses a 4-point scale to assess performance of each IADL task by rating 16 motor and 20 process skill items. The motor skills (e.g., stabilizes, reaches, transports, etc.) are the actions observed during task performance that are thought to be related to underlying abilities in postural control, mobility, coordination, or strength. Process skills (e.g., sequences, initiates, adjusts) are used to organize and adapt actions during actual performance and represent the underlying attentional, conceptual, organizational, and adaptive capacities of the client (Park, Fisher, & Velozo, 1994). It is important to note that the *AMPS* is a test of skill in occupational performance and is not designed to evaluate the presence of neuromuscular, biomechanical, or cognitive impairments (e.g., strength, range of motion, memory) or underlying capacities. Unlike impairments and underlying capacities that often are evaluated sepa-

INPATIENT REHABILITATION FACILITY - PATIENT ASSESSMENT INSTRUMENT

Page 2

Function Modifiers*

Complete the following specific functional items prior to scoring the FIM™ Instrument:

	ADMISSION	DISCHARGE
29. Bladder Level of Assistance (Score using FIM Levels 1 - 7)	☐	☐
30. Bladder Frequency of Accidents (Score as below)	☐	☐

7 - No accidents
6 - No accidents; uses device such as a catheter
5 - One accident in the past 7 days
4 - Two accidents in the past 7 days
3 - Three accidents in the past 7 days
2 - Four accidents in the past 7 days
1 - Five or more accidents in the past 7 days

Enter in Item 39G (Bladder) the lower (more dependent) score from Items 29 and 30 above.

	ADMISSION	DISCHARGE
31. Bowel Level of Assistance (Score using FIM Levels 1 - 7)	☐	☐
32. Bowel Frequency of Accidents (Score as below)	☐	☐

7 - No accidents
6 - No accidents; uses device such as an ostomy
5 - One accident in the past 7 days
4 - Two accidents in the past 7 days
3 - Three accidents in the past 7 days
2 - Four accidents in the past 7 days
1 - Five or more accidents in the past 7 days

Enter in Item 39H (Bowel) the lower (more dependent) score of Items 31 and 32 above.

	ADMISSION	DISCHARGE
33. Tub Transfer	☐	☐
34. Shower Transfer	☐	☐

(Score Items 33 and 34 using FIM Levels 1 - 7; use 0 if activity does not occur) *See training manual for scoring of Item 39K (Tub/Shower Transfer)*

	ADMISSION	DISCHARGE
35. Distance Walked	☐	☐
36. Distance Traveled in Wheelchair	☐	☐

(Code items 35 and 36 using: 3 - 150 feet; 2 - 50 to 149 feet; 1 - Less than 50 feet; 0 – activity does not occur)

	ADMISSION	DISCHARGE
37. Walk	☐	☐
38. Wheelchair	☐	☐

(Score Items 37 and 38 using FIM Levels 1 - 7; 0 if activity does not occur) See training manual for scoring of Item 39L (Walk/Wheelchair)

39. FIM™ Instrument*

	ADMISSION	DISCHARGE	GOAL
SELF-CARE			
A. Eating	☐	☐	☐
B. Grooming	☐	☐	☐
C. Bathing	☐	☐	☐
D. Dressing - Upper	☐	☐	☐
E. Dressing - Lower	☐	☐	☐
F. Toileting	☐	☐	☐
SPHINCTER CONTROL			
G. Bladder	☐	☐	☐
H. Bowel	☐	☐	☐
TRANSFERS			
I. Bed, Chair, Whlchair	☐	☐	☐
J. Toilet	☐	☐	☐
K. Tub, Shower	☐	☐	☐
LOCOMOTION (W - Walk, C - wheelChair, B - Both)			
L. Walk/Wheelchair	☐ ☐	☐ ☐	☐
M. Stairs	☐	☐	☐
COMMUNICATION (A - Auditory, V - Visual, B - Both)			
N. Comprehension	☐ ☐	☐ ☐	☐
O. Expression (V - Vocal, N - Nonvocal, B - Both)	☐ ☐	☐ ☐	☐
SOCIAL COGNITION			
P. Social Interaction	☐	☐	☐
Q. Problem Solving	☐	☐	☐
R. Memory	☐	☐	☐

FIM LEVELS

No Helper
7 Complete Independence (Timely, Safely)
6 Modified Independence (Device)

Helper - Modified Dependence
5 Supervision (Subject = 100%)
4 Minimal Assistance (Subject = 75% or more)
3 Moderate Assistance (Subject = 50% or more)

Helper - Complete Dependence
2 Maximal Assistance (Subject = 25% or more)
1 Total Assistance (Subject less than 25%)

0 Activity does not occur; Use this code only at admission

*The FIM data set, measurement scale and impairment codes incorporated or referenced herein are the property of U B Foundation Activities, Inc. ©1993, 2001 U B Foundation Activities, Inc. The FIM mark is owned by UBFA, Inc.

OMB-0938-0842 (expires: 12-31-2005)

Figure 4-3 Items and scoring for the *Functional Independence Measure* (*FIM*) from the *Inpatient Rehabilitation Facilities Patient Assessment Instrument*. The *FIM* data set, measurement scale, and impairment codes incorporated herein are the property of UB Foundation Activities, Inc. (UBFA). © 1993, 2001 UBFA, Inc. The *FIM* mark is owned by UBFA, Inc.

Socks

8. Grasp sock	(1)
9. Reach sock to R foot	(2)
10. Reach sock to L foot	(2)
11. Pull sock over R toes	(2)
12. Pull sock over L toes	(2)
13. Pull sock over R foot with heel to heel	(2)
14. Pull sock over L foot with heel to heel	(2)
15. Pull sock up to full extension on R leg	(2)
16. Pull sock up to full extension on L leg	(2)

Mobility through doors

114. Operate doorknob	(1)
115. Open door toward self	(2)
116. Open door away from self	(2)
117. Close door toward self	(2)
118. Close door away from self	(1)

Scoring - Points in parentheses next to each item (either 1 or 2) are given if person is able to complete the activity. Use of equipment is allowed. Total score equals the addition of points for each item. Item is marked N/A if clearly not applicable.

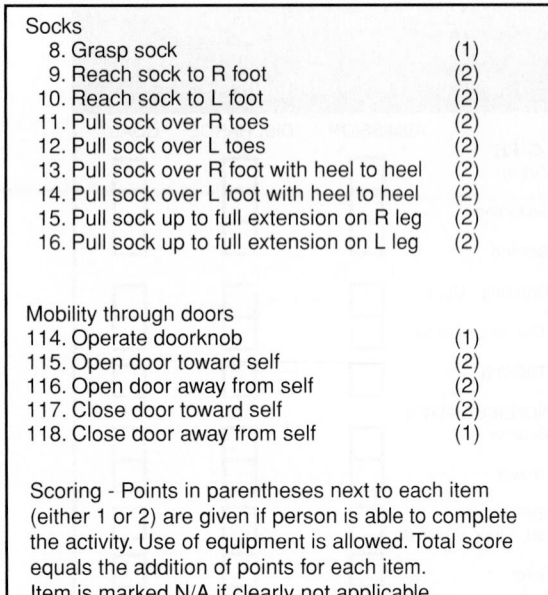

Figure 4-4 Example of items and scoring information for the *Klein-Bell ADL Scale*. (Used with permission from the University of Washington, Health Sciences for Educational Resources.)

rately from task performance, the motor and process skills of the *AMPS* are goal-directed actions that occur in the context of occupation. As a result, the *AMPS* is used to assess activities and participation, not body function or contextual factors (WHO, 2001).

Occupational therapists must attend a training workshop and become calibrated as a reliable rater before using the *AMPS*. Once trained, scoring of the *AMPS* is done by computer. The *AMPS* has been shown to discriminate well between people without disabilities and those with cognitive or physical disabilities. A significant advantage of *AMPS* is its flexibility in allowing the client to choose which tasks are used for assessment.

The Kohlman Evaluation of Living Skills (*KELS*) assesses daily activities in self-care, safety and health, money management, transportation and telephone use, and work and leisure (Kohlman Thomson, 1993). The *KELS* is a short living skills assessment that is administered through interview and direct observation. Individual items are scored as independent, needs assistance, or not applicable. Although originally created for use in short-term psychiatric units, it is also a good measure of IADL performance in elderly clients. When combined with other assessments and client input, the *KELS* data can help determine the environment that will allow a person to live as independently as possible.

The *Safety Assessment of Function and the Environment for Rehabilitation* (*SAFER*) tool was developed to provide occupational therapists with a comprehensive, consistent measure to simultaneously assess safety and occupational performance in the home (Oliver et al., 1993). The *SAFER* tool assesses safety in 15 categories, including living situation, mobility, kitchen, household management, self-care, and recreation. Items in each category assess both the environmental situation and functional ability of the client. For example, the living situation category addresses whether stairs are in good condition, the presence of scatter rugs and electric cords, and environmental clutter that might impact home safety. The instruction manual includes a list of recommendations to help the occupational therapist identify solutions to difficult problem areas.

Kitchen Tasks

Two assessments of performance during kitchen tasks have been developed for use in occupational therapy. *The Kitchen Task Assessment* (*KTA*) (Baum & Edwards, 1993) uses the task of making pudding to assess the cognitive support required by persons with Alzheimer's disease to complete a basic cooking task. Thus, the *KTA* provides information about performance as well as components of occupation, such as initiation, sequencing, organization, and problem solving. There is a significant relationship between scores on the *KTA* and other neuropsychological assessments but limited evidence of its use with clients who have physical versus psychosocial and cognitive disabilities.

The *Rabideau Kitchen Evaluation Revised* (*RKE-R*) (Neistadt, 1992, 1994) is an assessment of meal preparation that was primarily developed for adults with brain injury. It tests the ability to prepare a sandwich and a hot beverage. All task components are scored according to the number of verbal cues or amount of physical assistance required for safe completion. This quick assessment can help with discharge planning by providing information about a client's safety and independence during basic kitchen tasks.

Child Care

Childcare and parenting activities include but are not limited to the physical care and supervision of children and the use of age-appropriate activities, communication, and behaviors to facilitate child development (AOTA, 2002). Because no standard evaluations exist, the occupational therapist must work with the client to identify and assess performance needs during required and valued childcare tasks, while taking into account the ages and personalities of the children involved. The *Canadian Occupational Performance Measure* (*COPM*) can be used to assess childcare concerns and to determine what interventions and adaptations may be needed to enhance a client's competence and satisfaction in this area.

Work

Work assessments are used to determine whether an individual has the ability to perform necessary job skills and is otherwise prepared for employment in terms of work habits, work quality, ability to learn or acquire new skills, and ability to work with others as a team member, supervisor, or supervisee. Velozo (1993) described two categories of work evaluations: (1) standardized commercial evaluations such as those used in vocational rehabilitation, and (2) highly technical evaluations of physical and work capacity. He questioned whether these work evaluations truly reflect occupational therapists' interest in the meaning of work and emphasized our unique role in linking work evaluations to the psychosocial and environmental factors that contribute to client performance.

Standardized vocational evaluation systems use job analysis or work samples to determine an individual's ability to perform tasks similar to those encountered at work. In the United States, the *Dictionary of Occupational Titles* (United States Department of Labor, 1991) provides a taxonomy for measurement of work performance that lists specific job requirements, including skills and equipment. One standardized work assessment system that is often used is the *VALPAR Component Work Samples* (see Resources 4-1). The *VALPAR* system consists of a wide range of work samples that evaluate specific occupational performance skills (e.g., range of motion, problem solving, physical capacities, and mobility) during simulated job tasks. Although evidence of the reliability and validity for this standardized evaluation system is extensive, a potential disadvantage of the *VALPAR Component Work Samples* is its expense.

Because a large proportion of work evaluations are administered to clients who have musculoskeletal or soft-tissue injuries, their primary focus is on the physical capacities required for work tasks. Standardized Functional Assessments (FA) and Functional Capacity Evaluations (FCE) measure physical capacity (e.g., strength, endurance, and freedom from pain) during work-related tasks, such as lifting, sitting, and standing. In addition to evaluating a client's physical performance, however, a comprehensive work assessment must also include contextual information regarding the client's work environment, his medical condition and contraindications, and the whole person context in which he lives (e.g., information about non-work occupational activities such as homemaker, caregiver, or recreational roles) (Strong et al., 2004). Semi-structured interviews, such as the *Worker Role Interview* (Velozo, Kielhofner, & Fisher, 1998), can complement Functional Capacity Evaluations by providing important information regarding the psychosocial and environmental factors that influence return to work. This well-established tool can be used to assess other behaviors considered important for work, such as punctuality, communication ability, ability to work with others, and grooming. The *Feasibility Evaluation Checklist* (Matheson et al., 1985) assesses the feasibility of a client's return to competitive employment and his potential for improvement in 21 work behaviors, including attendance, timeliness, workplace safety, and ability to accept supervision. Although the feasibility of competitive employment is an integral component of Functional Capacity Evaluations, reliability and validity data for the *Feasibility Evaluation Checklist* is not readily available in the research literature. See Resources 4-1 for contact information.

Recently developed online services from the Office of Disability Employment Policy (ODEP) of the United States Department of Labor are good resources for clients and occupational therapists. A wide range of information is provided, including links to a Job Accommodation Network that gives specific accommodation suggestions for persons with various diagnoses (see Resources 4-1).

Leisure

Leisure involves engaging in self-chosen, motivating, and goal-directed activities for amusement, relaxation, spontaneous enjoyment, and/or self-expression. Hersch (1990) pointed out that "the concept of leisure encompasses a multitude of meanings: the leisure event itself, the amount and frequency of the activity, its meaningfulness to the participant, and the social context" in which it is performed (p. 55). In fact, Hersch (1990) and Bundy (1993) have suggested that leisure, or the playfulness of an activity, depends on the characteristics of the activity rather than the classification of an activity as leisure. Leisure serves many purposes in one's life by fulfilling physical, social, and intellectual needs, particularly for the older adult (Hersch, 1990). Participation in valued leisure pursuits has been closely related to life satisfaction. The purpose of some assessments is to identify leisure interests (Matsutsuyu, 1969; Rogers, Weinstein, & Figone, 1978; Witt & Ellis, 1984); others evaluate performance and satisfaction with leisure activities (Gregory, 1983; Kloseck, Crilly, & Hutchinson-Troyer, 2001).

The *Interest Checklist* (Matsutsuyu, 1969; Rogers, Weinstein, & Figone, 1978) gathers information about a client's level of interest and participation in 80 different activities. Activities, such as dancing, playing checkers/chess, or sewing/needlework, are rated on a 3-point scale ranging from no interest to strong interest. Interests identified by the client can be used by the occupational therapist in

CASE EXAMPLE

Optimizing Functional Recovery After Stroke

Occupational Therapy Assessment Process	Clinical Reasoning Process: Objectives	Clinical Reasoning Process: Examples of Therapist's Internal Dialogue
Patient Information E.B. is a 53-year-old married woman who experienced a left ischemic cerebrovascular accident 1 month ago while at work. She received tPA, a thrombolytic medication, within the first 3 hours of her stroke and is reported to have made excellent progress during 3 weeks of inpatient rehabilitation. She has recently been discharged home and is now being referred to outpatient rehabilitation for continued occupational, physical, and speech therapy. The OT discharge summary reports continued limitations in IADL tasks, with mild to moderate right-sided paresis and mild aphasia.	Understand the patient's diagnosis or condition	"E.B. had a pretty significant stroke and would likely have had greater limitations in motor abilities and language if she hadn't received such good care from emergency services. She is probably having difficulty using her dominant hand for daily tasks, and I wonder how she's getting around and managing at home when her husband is at work."
	Know the person	"It must have been terrible for her to have a stroke while she was at work; at least it happened during lunch and not while she was in the classroom with her students. It sounds like she was pretty busy managing multiple roles as mother, teacher, coach, and volunteer, in addition to taking care of home responsibilities. I wonder how she's dealing with this sudden change in routine."
E.B. lives with her husband and 15-year-old daughter; her 19-year-old son is a college freshman who lives 4 hours from home. E.B. is an elementary school teacher who also coaches her daughter's skating team and volunteers at the town library. Her husband has a demanding full-time job and travels 1–2 weeks per month. The occupational therapist focuses the initial occupational assessment on E.B.'s ability to resume self-maintenance roles and to engage in valued life roles and tasks now that she is home.	Appreciate the context	"It must be difficult for her husband and daughter to take on more home management tasks while she's recovering from her stroke. I wonder if they have friends or other family members who can help with shopping, driving, etc."
	Develop provisional hypotheses	"Given her diagnosis and good rate of recovery, I think she'll do well in therapy. I expect that her motor impairments will be the biggest barrier to regaining independence in home and leisure tasks. Her mild aphasia will likely limit her return to teaching, at least in the short term."
Assessment Process The therapist selected the following evaluation tools: *Canadian Occupational Performance Measure (COPM)* to obtain information about the client's perceived problems and priorities and the *Assessment of Motor and Process Skills (AMPS)* to assess IADL motor and process skills.	Consider evaluation approach and methods	"Because of her mild aphasia, it might be difficult and a bit frustrating for her to verbally describe her priorities for therapy on the *COPM*. I'll talk with the speech therapist to see if she might benefit from using a written list of activities to report concerns during this evaluation. It might also be helpful to have her husband present during the *COPM* to help clarify issues, as needed. The *AMPS* will give me the chance to observe how her right-sided paresis affects IADL performance and whether other cognitive and process-related impairments are a concern."

Assessment Results

During an interview using the *COPM*, E.B. reported that it was very important for her to resume responsibilities in managing household tasks and fulfilling her roles as wife and mother. Planning and preparing meals and grocery shopping were very important to her. She expressed frustration with the clumsiness in her dominant right hand and with her low endurance and fatigue when walking a distance with a cane. She was very concerned about returning to her job as a teacher because of her mild aphasia and expressed a strong desire to help prepare her daughter's skating team for the state finals in 2 months.

The *AMPS* revealed that process skills were mildly impaired in the sequencing and organizing of chosen tasks. Although she required additional cues/support to initiate tasks, she showed good pacing once engaged and was able to adjust and adapt her approach to tasks when difficulties arose. Motor skills were mildly to moderately impaired, as she had difficulty reaching for items at or above shoulder height, lifting a medium sized sauce pan from the stove to sink, and manipulating items with her right hand. However, she was able to use her paretic right hand to stabilize and transport items during bilateral tasks. Extra time was required for task completion because she needed frequent rest breaks when performing IADL from an ambulatory level.

Interpret observations

"E.B. seems to have good awareness of her impairments and needs for therapy and is generally able to make her needs known despite her mild aphasia and word finding problems."

"I wonder whether the problems E.B. had with sequencing and organizing tasks during the *AMPS* are related to the fact that she performed these in the rehab clinic and not at home. As she begins to take on more challenging tasks, it will be important to see how she performs in familiar versus unfamiliar settings."

"It seems like E.B.'s mild hemiparesis is having the greatest impact on her performance of IADL, and she shows great determination and desire to improve the functional use of her right arm and hand. I'll administer a couple of stroke-specific assessments to get a better handle on her motor strengths and weaknesses so we can decide on a therapy program to best address these concerns. She's a great candidate for outpatient therapy."

Occupational Therapy Problem List

1. Decreased participation and independence in IADL.
2. Impaired endurance and functional mobility, contributing to decreased productivity during IADL.
3. Reduced organizing and sequencing skills during IADL in an unfamiliar environment.
4. Mild to moderate hemiparesis RUE, impeding functional use of the limb during occupational tasks.

Synthesize results

"E.B. has experienced significant changes in her daily routine and ability to engage in important life roles and tasks since her stroke. I'll talk more with her family to see how they think she's coping with these changes. Although fatigue is common during early recovery from stroke, depression might also be affecting her initiation and reports of fatigue during IADL."

"It will be important to get a better handle on E.B.'s ability to return to her coaching and teaching roles, but this will be a longer term process. First, I'll use the Interest Checklist to help identify meaningful activities to use in therapy so we can begin to work on problem areas and help her to feel more productive as she continues to recover from her stroke."

CLINICAL REASONING IN OCCUPATIONAL THERAPY PRACTICE

Effects of the Environment on Cognitive Function

During the initial OT assessment, E.B. demonstrated some difficulty with initiating, sequencing, and organizing tasks during the *AMPS* and expressed concerns about returning to community and work roles.

How might the occupational therapist gain a better understanding of E.B.'s cognitive abilities during therapy? What task and environmental factors might exaggerate or minimize these problems? What other assessments might best help with clarifying occupational performance needs and planning OT treatment?

treatment planning and to determine changes in activity performance over time. The *Interest Checklist* can be used for clients throughout the lifespan, from adolescence through old age.

The revised *Activity Index* (Gregory, 1983) is a self-report assessment that determines a person's interest and frequency of participation in a variety of activities, ranging from card games and theater to quiet hobbies at home. When used in conjunction with the *Meaningfulness of Activity Scale*, it can be used to indicate a client's autonomy, competency, and enjoyment derived from leisure activities (Gregory, 1983). Scores on these combined scales were found to significantly correlate with life satisfaction in elderly persons (Gregory, 1983).

The *Leisure Diagnostic Battery* (Witt & Ellis, 1984) was designed to assess a client's perceptions about his/her leisure experiences. The first five subscales are used by the client to rate his/her perceived competence and control in leisure activities, identify needs and depth of leisure involvement, and consider self-perceptions about playfulness. Scores from these subscales are summed to determine a perceived freedom in leisure score, and identified problems are used for treatment planning. These scales appear to be responsive to changes in leisure performance after a recreation intervention. The *Leisure Diagnostic Battery* effectively discriminates adults who have chronic pain and physical injuries from persons without evidence of neurologic or physical dysfunction (Peebles et al., 1999).

Other assessment batteries are used primarily by recreational therapists to evaluate leisure interests and competence of clients receiving rehabilitation services. The *Leisure Competence Measure* is one example of assessments that are gaining evidence of reliability and validity (Kloseck, Crilly, & Hutchinson-Troyer, 2001). Please refer to Resources 4-1 for more information.

SUMMARY REVIEW QUESTIONS

1. Define self-report and direct observation methods of assessment. What are the advantages and disadvantages of these methods when evaluating a client's occupational performance?
2. Distinguish between IADL and basic ADL, and describe one standardized assessment for each.
3. What are three measurement concepts or psychometric properties of standardized evaluation instruments? Define each, and provide an example of how these properties might affect the results of occupational therapy assessments administered in the clinic.
4. What is the relationship between the assessment of occupational performance and development of the occupational therapy treatment plan?
5. Compare two different IADL measures. Describe the assessment and its psychometric properties, strengths, and weaknesses. Based on this information, which measure would you choose to evaluate a client recently admitted for outpatient rehabilitation services? Why?
6. A client-centered approach has been emphasized when assessing occupational roles and competence. List three ways in which this approach might influence occupational therapy intervention.

ACKNOWLEDGMENT

I thank Mary Law for her thoughtful work in developing and writing the previous edition of this chapter.

References

American Occupational Therapy Association [AOTA]. (1996). *Occupational therapy assessment tools: An annotated index* (2nd ed.). Bethesda, MD: AOTA.

American Occupational Therapy Association [AOTA]. (2002). Occupational therapy practice framework: Domain and process. *American Journal of Occupational Therapy, 56,* 609–639.

Asberg, K. H., & Nydevik, I. (1991). Early prognosis of stroke outcome by means of Katz Index of activities of daily living. *Scandinavian Journal of Rehabilitation Medicine, 23,* 187–191.

Baum, C., & Edwards, D. F. (1993). Cognitive performance in senile dementia of the Alzheimer's type: The Kitchen Task Assessment. *American Journal of Occupational Therapy, 47,* 431–436.

Bergner, M., Bobbit, R. A., Carter, W. B., & Gilson, B. S. (1981). The Sickness Impact Profile: Development and final revision of health status measure. *Medical Care, 19,* 787–805.

Biernacki, S. (1993). Reliability of the worker role interview. *American Journal of Occupational Therapy, 47,* 797–803.

Bosch, J. (1995). The reliability and validity of the Canadian Occupational Performance Measure [thesis]. Hamilton, Ontario, Canada: McMaster University.

Brorsson, B., & Asberg, K. (1984). Katz Index of independence in ADL: Reliability and validity in short term care. *Scandinavian Journal of Rehabilitation Medicine, 16,* 125–132.

Brown, C., Moore, W. P., Hemman, D., & Yunek, A. (1996). Influence of instrumental activities of daily living assessment method on judgments of independence. *American Journal of Occupational Therapy, 50,* 202–206.

Bundy, A. C. (1993). Assessment of play and leisure: Delineation of the problem. *American Journal of Occupational Therapy, 47,* 217–222.

Carswell, A., McColl, M. A., Baptiste, S., Law, M., Polatajko, H., & Pollock, N. (2004). The Canadian Occupational Performance Measure: A research and clinical literature review. *Canadian Journal of Occupational Therapy, 71,* 210–222.

Chau, N., Daler, S., Andre, J. M., and Patris, A. (1994). Inter-rater agreement of two functional independence scales: The Functional Independence Measure (FIM) and a subjective uniform continuous scale. *Disability and Rehabilitation, 16,* 63–71.

Chiu, T., & Oliver, R. (2005). Factor analysis and construct validity of the SAFER-HOME. Unpublished manuscript.

Collin, C., Wade, D. T., Davies, S., & Horne, V. (1988). The Barthel ADL index: A reliability study. *International Disabilities Studies, 10,* 61–63.

Corrigan, J. D., Smith-Knapp, K., & Granger, C. V. (1997). Validity of the functional independence measure for persons with traumatic brain injury. *Archives of Physical Medicine and Rehabilitation, 78,* 828–834.

Duncombe, L. W. (2004). Comparing learning of cooking in home and clinic for people with schizophrenia. *American Journal of Occupational Therapy, 58,* 272–278.

Edwards, M. M. (1990). The reliability and validity of self-report activities of daily living scales. *Canadian Journal of Occupational Therapy, 57,* 273–278.

Finch, E., Brooks, D., Stratford, P. W., & Mayo, N. E. (2002). *Physical rehabilitation outcome measures: A guide to enhanced clinical decision making* (2nd ed.). Hamilton, Ontario, Canada: B.C. Decker.

Fisher, A. G. (1993). The assessment of IADL motor skills: An application of many-faceted Rasch analysis. *American Journal of Occupational Therapy, 47,* 319–329.

Fisher, A. G. (1995). *Assessment of motor and process skills.* Fort Collins, CO: Three Star.

Fricke, J., & Unsworth, C. A. (1996). Inter-rater reliability of the original and modified Barthel Index and a comparison with the Functional Independence Measure. *Australian Occupational Therapy Journal, 43,* 22–29.

Granger, C. V., Albrecht, G. L., & Hamilton, B. B. (1979). Outcome of comprehensive medical rehabilitation: Measurement by PULSES Profile and the Barthel Index. *Archives of Physical Medicine and Rehabilitation, 60,* 145–153.

Granger, C. V., & Hamilton, B. B. (1992). The Uniform Data System for medical rehabilitation report of first admissions for 1990. *American Journal of Physical Medicine and Rehabilitation, 71,* 108–113.

Granger, C. V., Hamilton, B. B., Linacre, J. M., Heinemann, A. W., & Wright, B. D. (1993). Performance profiles of the Functional Independence Measure. *American Journal of Physical Medicine and Rehabilitation, 72,* 84–89.

Gregory, M. D. (1983). Occupational behavior and life satisfaction among retirees. *American Journal of Occupational Therapy, 137,* 548–553.

Gresham, G. E., Phillips, T. F., & Labi, M. L. C. (1980). ADL status in stroke: Relative merits of three standard indexes. *Archives of Physical Medicine and Rehabilitation, 61,* 355–358.

Harris, B. A., et al. (1986). Validity of self-report measures of functional disability. *Topics in Geriatric Rehabilitation, 1,* 31–41.

Heinemann, A. W., Linacre, J. M., Wright, B. D., Hamilton, B. B., & Granger, C. V. (1994). Prediction of rehabilitation outcomes with disability measures. *Archives of Physical Medicine and Rehabilitation, 75,* 133–143.

Hersch, G. (1990). Leisure and aging. *Physical and Occupational Therapy in Geriatrics, 9,* 55–78.

Jenkinson, C., Wright, L., & Coulter, A. (1994). Criterion validity and reliability of the SF-36 in a population sample. *Quality of Life Research, 3,* 7–12.

Katz, S., Ford, A. B., Moskowitz, R. W., Jackson, B. A., & Jaffe, M. W. (1963). Studies of illness in the aged: The index of ADL: A standardized measure of biological and psychosocial function. *Journal of American Medical Association, 185,* 94–99.

Keith, R. A., Granger, C. V., Hamilton, B. B., Sherwin, F. S. (1987). The functional independence measure: A new tool for rehabilitation. In M. G. Eisenberg & R. C. Grzesiak (Eds.), *Advances in clinical rehabilitation* (pp. 6–18). New York: Springer Publishing.

Kielhofner, G., Henry, A. D., Walens, D., & Rogers, E. S. (1991). A generalizability study of the Occupational Performance History Interview. *Occupational Therapy Journal of Research, 11,* 292–306.

Kielhofner, G., Mallinson, T., Crawford, D., Nowak, M., Rigby, M., & Henry, A. (1998). *User's manual for the OPHI-II.* Chicago: Model of Human Occupation Clearinghouse, University of Illinois at Chicago, Department of Occupational Therapy.

Kielhofner, G., Mallinson, T., Forsyth, K., & Lai, J.-S. (2001). Psychometric properties of the second version of the Occupational Performance History Interview (OPHI-II). *American Journal of Occupational Therapy, 55,* 260–267.

Klein, R. M., & Bell, B. (1982). Self-care skills: Behavioral measurement with Klein-Bell ADL Scale. *Archives of Physical Medicine and Rehabilitation, 63,* 335–338.

Kloseck, M., Crilly, R. G., & Hutchinson-Troyer, L. (2001). Measuring therapeutic recreation outcomes in rehabilitation: Further testing of the leisure competence measure. *Therapeutic Recreation Journal* [online]. Available at www.nrpa.org.

Klyczek, J. P., Bauer-Yox, N., & Fiedler, R. C. (1997). The interest checklist: A factor analysis. *American Journal of Occupational Therapy, 51,* 815–823.

Kohlman Thomson, L. (1993). *The Kohlman Evaluation of Living Skills* (3rd ed.). Rockville, MD: AOTA.

Korner-Bitensky, N., & Wood-Dauphinee, S. (1995). Barthel Index information elicited over the telephone: Is it reliable? *American Journal of Physical Medicine and Rehabilitation, 74,* 9–18.

Law, M. (1991). The environment: A focus for occupational therapy. *Canadian Journal of Occupational Therapy, 58,* 171–179.

Law, M., Ed. (1998). *Client-centered occupational therapy.* Thorofare, NJ: Slack.

Law, M. (2002). Participation in the occupations of everyday life. *American Journal of Occupational Therapy, 56,* 640–649.

Law, M., Baptiste, S., Carswell, A., McColl, M., Polatajko, H., & Pollock, N. (1994). *Canadian Occupational Performance Measure* (2nd ed.). Toronto, Ontario, Canada: CAOT.

Law, M., Baptiste, S., Carswell, A., McColl, M., Polatajko, H., & Pollock, N. (1998). *Canadian Occupational Performance Measure* (3rd ed.). Ottawa, Ontario, Canada: CAOT.

Law, M., Baum, C., & Dunn, W. (2001). Measuring occupational performance: Supporting best practice in occupational therapy. Thorofare, NJ: Slack.

Law, M., & Letts, L. (1989). A critical review of scales of activities of daily living. *American Journal of Occupational Therapy, 43,* 522–528.

Letts, L., Scott, S., Burtney, J., Marshall, L., & McKean, M. (1998). The reliability and validity of the Safety Assessment of Function and the Environment for Rehabilitation (SAFER). *British Journal of Occupational Therapy, 61,* 127–132.

Loewen, S. C., & Anderson, B. A. (1988). Reliability of the modified motor assessment scale and the Barthel Index. *Physical Therapy, 68,* 1077–1081.

Mahoney, F. I., & Barthel, D. W. (1965). Functional evaluation: The Barthel Index. *Maryland State Medical Journal, 14,* 61–65.

Matheson, L., Ogden, L., Violette, K., & Schultz, K. (1985). Work hardening: Occupational therapy in industrial rehabilitation. *American Journal of Occupational Therapy, 39,* 314–321.

Matsutsuyu, J. S. (1969). Interest checklist. *American Journal of Occupational Therapy, 23,* 323–328.

McColl, M., Davies, D., Carlson, P., Johnston, J., & Minnes, P. (2001). The community integration measure: Development and preliminary validation. *Archives of Physical Medicine and Rehabilitation, 82,* 429–434.

Neistadt, M. E. (1992). The Rabideau Kitchen Evaluation Revised: An assessment of meal preparation skill. *Occupational Therapy Journal of Research, 12,* 242–255.

Neistadt, M. E. (1994). A meal preparation treatment protocol for adults with brain injury. *American Journal of Occupational Therapy, 48,* 431–438.

Oakley, F., Kielhofner, G., Barris, R., & Reichler, R. K. (1986). The Role Checklist: Development and empirical assessment of reliability. *Occupational Therapy Journal of Research, 6,* 157–170.

Oliver, R., Blathwayt, J., Brockley, C., & Tamaki, T. (1993). Development of the Safety Assessment of Function and the Environment for Rehabilitation (SAFER) tool. *Canadian Journal of Occupational Therapy, 60,* 78–82.

Park, S., Fisher, A. G., & Velozo, C. A. (1994). Using the assessment of motor and process skills to compare occupational performance between clinic and home settings. *American Journal of Occupational Therapy, 48,* 697–709.

Peebles, J., McWilliams, L., Norris, L. H., & Park, K. (1999). Population specific norms and reliability of the leisure diagnostic battery in a sample of patients with chronic pain. *Therapeutic Recreation Journal* [online]. Available at www.nrpa.org.

Reistetter, T. A., Spencer, J. C., Trujillo, L., & Abreau, B. C. (2005). Examining the Community Integration Measure (CIM): A replication study with life satisfaction. *Neurorehabilitation, 20,* 139–148.

Rogers, J. C. (1988). The NPI interest checklist. In B. Hemphill (Ed.), *Mental health assessments in occupational therapy* (pp. 93–114). Thorofare, NJ: Slack.

Rogers, J. C., Holm, M. B., Beach, S., Schulz, R., Cipriani, J., Fox, A., & Starz, T. W. (2003). Concordance of four methods of disability assessment using performance in the home as the criterion method. *Arthritis and Rheumatism, 49,* 640–647.

Rogers, J. C., Weinstein, J. M., & Figone, J. J. (1978). The interest checklist: An empirical assessment. *American Journal of Occupational Therapy, 32,* 628–630.

Sagar, M. A., Dunham, N. C., Schwartes, A., Mecum, L., Halverson, K., & Harlowe, D. (1992). Measurement of activities of daily living in hospitalized elderly: A comparison of self-report and performance-based methods. *Journal of American Geriatric Society, 40,* 457–462.

Shah, S., Vanclay, F., & Cooper, B. (1989). Improving the sensitivity of the Barthel Index for stroke rehabilitation. *Journal of Clinical Epidemiology, 42,* 703–709.

Sharrack, B., Hughes, R. A. C., Soudain, S., & Dunn, G. (1999). The psychometric properties of clinical rating scales used in multiple sclerosis. *Brain, 122,* 141–159.

Simmons, D. C., Crepeau, E. B., & White, B. P. (2000). The predictive power of narrative data in occupational therapy evaluation. *American Journal of Occupational Therapy, 54,* 471–476.

Strong, S., Baptiste, S., Cole, D., Clarke, J., Costa, M., Shannon, H., Reardon, R., & Sinclair, S. (2004). Functional assessment of injured workers: A profile of assessor practices. *Canadian Journal of Occupational Therapy, 71,* 13–23.

Trombly, C. A. (1995a). Retraining basic and instrumental activities of daily living. In C. A. Trombly (Ed.), *Occupational therapy for physical dysfunction* (4th ed.). Baltimore: Williams & Wilkins.

Trombly, C. A. (1995b). Occupation: purposefulness and meaningfulness as therapeutic mechanisms. 1995 Eleanor Clarke Slagle Lecture. *American Journal of Occupational Therapy, 49,* 960–972.

UB Foundation Activities, Inc. [UBFA, Inc.]. (2004). *The Inpatient Rehabilitation Facility–Patient Assessment Instrument (IRF-PAI) training manual: Effective 4/01/04.* Buffalo, NY: U.B. Foundation Activities, Inc.

United States Department of Labor. (1991). *Dictionary of occupational titles.* (4th ed., vol. I & II). Washington, DC: United States Department of Labor.

van der Putten, J. J., Hobart, J. C., Freeman, J. A., & Thompson, A. J. (1999). Measuring change in disability after inpatient rehabilitation: Comparison of the responsiveness of the Barthel Index and the Functional Independence Measure. *Journal of Neurology, Neurosurgery, and Psychiatry, 66,* 480–484.

Velozo, C. A. (1993). Work evaluations: Critique of the states of the art of functional assessment of work. *American Journal of Occupational Therapy, 47,* 203–209.

Velozo, C., Kielhofner, G., & Fisher, G. (1998). *Worker Role Interview (WRI).* Chicago: Model of Human Occupation Clearinghouse.

Whiteneck, G., Charlifue, S., Gerhart, K., Overholser, D., & Richardson, G. (1992). Quantifying handicap: A new measure of long-term rehabilitation outcomes. *Archives of Physical Medicine and Rehabilitation, 73,* 519–526.

Whiteneck, G. G., Harrison-Felix, C. L., Mellick, D. C., Brooks, C. A., Charlifue, S. B., & Gerhart, K. A. (2004). Quantifying environmental factors: A measure of physical, attitudinal, service, productivity, and policy barriers. *Archives of Physical Medicine and Rehabilitation, 85,* 1324–1335.

Witt, P. A., & Ellis, G. D. (1984). The *Leisure Diagnostic Battery*: Measuring perceived freedom in leisure. *Society and Leisure, 7,* 109–124.

Wolfe, C. D., Taub, N. A., Woodrow, E. J., & Burney, P. G. (1991). Assessment of scales of disability and handicap for stroke patients. *Stroke, 22,* 1242–1244.

Wood-Dauphinee, S., Opzoomer, A., Williams, J. I., Marchand, B., & Spitzer, W. O. (1988). Assessment of global function: The Reintegration to Normal Living Index. *Archives of Physical Medicine and Rehabilitation, 69,* 583–590.

World Health Organization [WHO]. (2001). *International Classification of Functioning, Disability and Health (ICF).* Geneva: WHO.

CHAPTER 5

Assessing Abilities and Capacities: Range of Motion, Strength, and Endurance

Nancy A. Flinn, Catherine A. Trombly Latham, and Carolyn Robinson Podolski

LEARNING OBJECTIVES

After studying this chapter and practicing the skills described here, the reader will be able to do the following:

1. Evaluate range of motion of the upper extremity using a goniometer.
2. Use two different methods to determine the amount of edema of the hand.
3. Perform a manual muscle test to evaluate strength of the upper extremity.
4. Determine the functional strength of selected lower extremity musculature.
5. Determine functional endurance level.
6. Use a Visual Analog Scale to determine pain level.
7. Interpret the findings of the evaluations in this chapter.

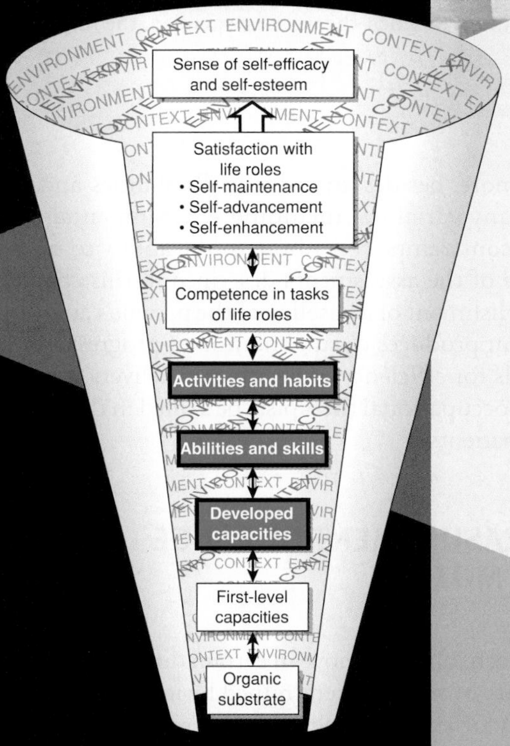

Glossary

Active range of motion (AROM)—The amount of movement possible at a joint when the patient voluntarily moves the limb by muscle contraction.

Anatomical position—Standing straight with feet together and flat on the floor, with arms by the sides and hands facing forward. The zero position for ROM measurement.

Calibrate—To set an instrument at a known value according to a standard.

Contracture—Inability to move a body part because of soft tissue shortening or bony ankylosis.

Limits of motion—The beginning and ending positions of movement at a joint.

Maximum heart rate reserve (MHRR)—The difference between resting and peak exercise heart rates; measured in beats per minute (Whaley et al., 1997).

Maximum voluntary contraction—The greatest amount of tension a muscle can generate and hold only for a moment, such as in muscle testing.

Mechanical advantage—The position in which the muscle is able to generate greatest tension, that is, when it is longer than the resting length of the muscle. In this position, the passive tension generated by the viscoelastic properties of the muscle and its tendon combine with the active tension generated by the contraction of the muscle fibers to produce a maximum voluntary contraction. When the muscle is fully lengthened or shortened, the viscoelastic, or passive, tension is reduced.

Passive range of motion (PROM)—The amount of movement possible at a joint when an outside force moves the limb.

Reliability—Characteristic of a measuring instrument, indicating the stability of the instrument's findings over time between testers when properly administered under similar circumstances (Portney & Watkins, 2000). Reliability is usually defined by a correlation coefficient (r) or an interclass correlation coefficient (ICC). An r or ICC of 1 indicates a perfect linear relationship between one variable (e.g., rater A's scores) and another variable (e.g., rater B's scores). An r of 0.85 or ICC of 0.75 is considered acceptable for measuring instruments. Reliability can be increased by controlling all variables that affect the scores other than the one being measured (e.g., change in ROM). Control is gained by keeping everything the same or by deleting some variables.

Standard deviation (SD)—A measure of dispersion indicating the variability within a set of scores. Low variability within the scores of a set of therapists indicates that the therapists are following the same protocol and the phenomenon being measured is unchanging; high variability indicates that the phenomenon being measured is unstable or that the therapists should control their test administration better.

To interpret a score, the therapist often compares it with norms (averages and SDs). The SD tells you where your patient's score falls in relation to the norm because you can relate it to the normal curve. In the bell-shaped normal curve, 1 SD is equal to approximately 68% of the area under the curve (34% on each side of the mean); 2 SD is equal to approximately 95% of the area under the curve; and 3 SD is equal to approximately 99% of the area under the curve. A score of 2 to 3 SD below the mean normative score indicates a limitation in need of treatment.

Tenodesis—The mechanical effect caused by the length of extrinsic finger flexors and extensors. When the wrist is flexed, the fingers tend to extend because the extensors are too short to allow full finger flexion and wrist flexion at the same time. Similarly, when the wrist is extended, the fingers tend to flex.

The assessments presented in this chapter are appropriate for patients who are unable to do or are restricted in doing the occupational tasks and activities important to them because of impairments in range of joint motion, strength, or endurance. Being able to move (mobility, or range of motion) and use extremities against resistance (strength) for an extended period (endurance) is essential for the completion of most occupational tasks. For example, a person who cannot fully flex the elbow, is too weak to lift a spoon to the mouth, or is too fatigued to lift the utensil repeatedly cannot eat a meal independently. Since deficits in abilities and capacities may lead to impaired occupational functioning, it is within the realm of occupational therapy to assess them. Keep in mind that occupational therapy assessments of mobility, strength, endurance, and pain focus on occupational functioning, and not on these abilities and capacities per se.

Furthermore, besides an individual's abilities and capacities, many variables, including environmental and contextual constraints, contribute to the ability to do an activity. Use of the assessments described in this chapter allows establishment of a baseline of the patient's abilities. Reassessment produces documentation of progress. With the demands for efficiency in health care delivery, it is essential that occupational therapists be skilled in their evaluations of patients.

MEASUREMENT OF RANGE OF MOTION

Normally, each joint can move in certain directions and to certain **limits of motion** determined by its structure and the integrity of surrounding tissues. Trauma or disease that affects joint structures or the surrounding tissues can decrease the amount of motion at the joint and limit occupational functioning.

Measurement of joint range may be done actively or passively. **Passive range of motion** (PROM) is the amount of motion at a given joint when the joint is moved by an outside force. **Active range of motion** (AROM) is the amount of motion at a given joint achieved by the patient using his or her own strength. If AROM is less than PROM, there is a problem of muscle weakness (or tendon integrity in hands). AROM measurement, which is used as a supplement to the measurement of the strength of muscles graded poor minus (2–) or fair minus (3–), indicates small gains that would otherwise not be noted by the muscle test.

Evaluation of ROM should start with a quick functional AROM scan (Procedures for Practice 5-1). If no limitations in ROM that would interfere with occupational functioning are found during the functional AROM scan, record the range as within normal limits; no further testing is required.

If limitations are observed, the therapist attempts to move the joint through its full ROM. If the joint is free to move to the end range, the problem is with active motion. The limited active range is measured and recorded. If the end range cannot be attained when the therapist moves the limb, the problem is with passive motion, and the limitation is measured and recorded.

A goniometer is used for measuring joint motion. Every goniometer has a protractor, an axis, and two arms. The stationary arm extends from the protractor, on which the degrees are marked. The movable arm has a center line or pointer to indicate angle measurement. The axis is the point at which these two arms are riveted together. A full-circle goniometer, which measures 0–180° in each direction, permits measurement of motion in both directions, such as flexion and extension, without repositioning the tool. When using a half-circle goniometer, it is necessary to position the protractor opposite to the direction of motion so that the indicator remains on the face of the protractor. A finger goniometer is designed with a shorter movable arm and flat surfaces to fit comfortably over the finger joints. Figure 5-1 shows each of these types of goniometers.

The therapist must place the axis and arms appropriately to ensure accuracy and **reliability** (Procedures for Practice 5-2). The specific placement of the goniometer for each joint is described and demonstrated in this chapter.

PROCEDURES FOR PRACTICE 5-1

Functional Active Range of Motion Scan

- The patient should be seated if possible.
- The patient should perform the motions bilaterally if possible. If not, the more normal side should move first to set a baseline for normal for this person.
- Observe for complete movements, symmetry of movements, and timing of movements.
- Demonstrate the movements if the patient has a language barrier or cognitive deficits.
- To estimate the amount of active movement in the following motions, give instructions such as these to the patient:

Motion	Examples of Instruction
Shoulder flexion (sagittal plane)	Lift your arms straight up in front and reach toward the ceiling.
Shoulder abduction (frontal plane)	Move your arms out to the side. Now reach over your head.
Shoulder horizontal abduction and adduction (horizontal plane)	Raise your arms forward to shoulder height. Move each arm out to the side, then back again.
External rotation	Touch the back of your head with your hand.
Internal rotation	Touch the small of your back with your hand.
Elbow flexion and extension	Start with your arms straight down by your sides. Now bend your elbows so your hands touch your shoulders.
Forearm supination and pronation	With your arms at your side and your elbows flexed to 90°, rotate your forearms so the palms of your hands face the floor and then the ceiling.
Wrist flexion and extension	Move one of your wrists up and down. Now, move the other one.
Finger flexion and extension	Make a fist, then spread your fingers out.
Finger opposition	Touch your thumb to the tip of each finger one at a time.

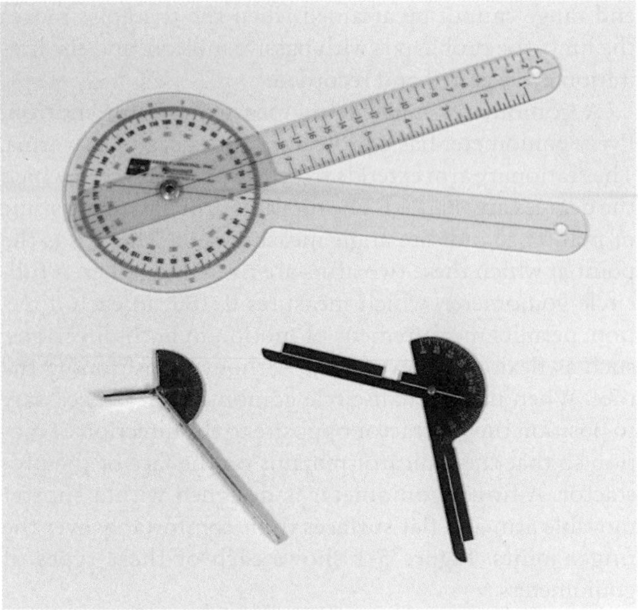

Figure 5-1 Three types of goniometers. The large full-circle goniometer (*top*) is used to measure large joints. The small finger goniometer (*bottom left*) has flat arms that fit over the fingers. The small half-circle goniometer (*bottom right*) is used to measure small joints, such as the wrist.

In addition to goniometer placement, multiple patient-related and environmental factors can affect accuracy and reliability of ROM measurements. Patient-related factors include pain, fear of pain, fatigue, and feelings of stress or tension. For the most accurate and reliable results, every effort should be made to make the patient physically and emotionally comfortable, including talking to the patient and describing the procedure that is to follow. Environmental factors include time of day, temperature of the room, type of goniometer used, and training and experience of the tester. For the most reliable pre-test–post-test information, the same tester should use the same goniometer at the same time of day.

PROCEDURES FOR PRACTICE 5-2

Principles of Goniometer Placement

- Place the axis of the goniometer over the axis of motion. The axis of motion for some joints coincides with bony landmarks, but for others, it must be found by observing movement and finding the point around which the movement occurs. In that case, the axis of motion can change position during movement, so it is acceptable for the goniometer to be repositioned at the end of range. When the two arms of the goniometer are placed correctly, they intersect at the axis of motion (Triffitt, Wildon, & Hajioff, 1999), so it is more important to have the arms line up correctly. The axis placement then automatically falls in line.
- Position the stationary arm parallel to the longitudinal axis of the body segment proximal to the joint being measured, although there are some exceptions.
- Position the movable arm parallel to the longitudinal axis of the body segment distal to the joint being measured, with some exceptions.

Reliability

Intra-rater reliability is consistently higher than inter-rater reliability for ROM testing using a universal goniometer. In one study of internal and external rotation measured in the supine position, intra-rater reliability was good (r = 0.58–0.71), and inter-rater reliability was fair to good (r = 0.41–0.66) (Awan, Smith, & Boon, 2002). In a second study, it was found that combined finger flexion measured with a ruler was a reliable measure when taken by different therapists but that goniometric measures of the finger joints were more reliable when a single therapist was involved (Ellis & Bruton, 2002).

Active motion measurements are more reliable than passive ones. In one study by Sabari et al. (1998), 30 adults were measured for both active and passive ROM for shoulder flexion and abduction in two positions, sitting and supine. The AROM measurements were more reliable than the PROM measurements for both positions (Sabari et al., 1998). Furthermore, the researchers found only a moderate range of agreement (r = 0.64–0.81) between goniometric measurements of shoulder movements with the patient sitting and supine. The authors concluded that the position of the patient can affect the ROM. Therefore, therapists should record the testing position, and the same position should be used each time the patient is retested. This chapter demonstrates measurement of shoulder ROM in a sitting patient because it measures shoulder mobility in the position more frequently used for functional task performance.

A multicenter study looked at the reliability of three goniometric techniques for measuring passive wrist flexion and extension: radial, ulnar, and volar-dorsal approaches. The study found the volar-dorsal approach to be slightly more reliable. The interclass correlation coefficient (ICC) was 0.93 for flexion and 0.84 for extension with the volar-dorsal approach, whereas the corresponding values were 0.88 and 0.80 for the radial approach and 0.89 and 0.80 for the ulnar approach (LaStayo & Wheeler, 1994). All three approaches are reliable, but they are not interchangeable. The therapist must be sure to document which approach is being used and use the same approach consistently to document progress.

It is commonly believed that experience plays a major role in the reliability of ROM measurements. A study of experience of the therapist and how it influences reliability of goniometric measurements found no dramatic difference in reliability between experienced and inexperienced therapists who were measuring foot position. All of the inexperienced therapists were uniformly trained on specific testing procedures (Somers et al., 1997). It may be inferred from this study that inter-rater reliability may be more dependent on training than experience.

Recording Range of Motion

Each measurement is accurately recorded on a ROM form, which the therapist signs and dates because a medical record is a legal document. Notation is made whether scores represent AROM or PROM. A sample form is provided in Figure 5-2. Any form should allow for recording the starting and ending positions (limits of motion) for each movement. When reading the goniometer, always state your results as a range using two numbers. The first number is the starting position of the extremity, and the second number is the limit of motion at end range. Two columns can be used for recording of initial and retest information. Both columns should be dated to allow for tracking and easy analysis of the patient's progress.

The most common method of determining ROM is the Neutral Zero Method recommended by the Committee on Joint Motion of the American Academy of Orthopaedic Surgeons (Greene & Heckman, 1994). In this method, the **anatomical position** is considered to be 0, or if a given starting position is different from anatomical position, it is defined as 0. Measurement is taken from the stated starting position to the stated end position. If the patient cannot achieve the stated starting and end positions, the actual starting and end positions are recorded to indicate limitations in movement. An example of this, using elbow flexion, is as follows:

0 to 150°: No limitation

20 to 150°: A limitation in extension (problem with the start position)

0 to 120°: A limitation in flexion (problem with end position)

20 to 120°: Limitations in flexion and extension (problems with start and end positions)

To record hyperextension of a joint, which may be occasionally seen in metacarpophalangeal or elbow joints, the American Academy of Orthopaedic Surgeons recommends a separate measurement to describe the available ROM without confusion. For example, if 20° of elbow hyperextension (an unnatural movement) is noted, it should be recorded as follows:

0 to 150° of flexion

150 to 0° of extension

0 to 20° of hyperextension

If a joint is fused, the starting and end positions are the same, with no ROM. This is recorded as fused at X°. If a joint that normally moves in two directions cannot move in one direction, the ROM-limited motion is recorded as none. For example, if wrist flexion is 15–80° with a 15° flexion **contracture**, the wrist cannot be positioned at 0 or be moved into extension; therefore, wrist extension is recorded as none.

Because there are various systems of notations, each having its own meaning, it is important to clarify the intended meaning to ensure consistency among therapists and physicians within the same facility.

MEASUREMENT OF RANGE OF MOTION OF THE UPPER EXTREMITY

This chapter addresses ROM of the upper extremity, as most functional activities require upper extremity use and manipulation skills. Lower extremity ROM is typically measured by physical therapists who are interested in the ability to walk. References listed at the end of the chapter are good sources of information concerning measurement of lower extremity ROM.

For the measurements given here, unless otherwise noted, the patient is seated with trunk erect against the back of an armless straight chair, although the measurements can be taken with the patient standing or supine, if necessary. This procedure can be done actively or passively. For active movement, take special care to ensure that there are no substitutions of movement. For PROM, the tester supports both the body part and the goniometer proximal and distal to the joint, leaving the joint free to move. Practice is required for comfortable handling of the goniometer together with the movable body segment.

On the pages that follow, the reader will find narrative and pictorial descriptions to help in understanding and practicing measurement of range of motion of the upper extremity.

Patient's Name ______________________________

Type of motion: AROM _______

PROM _______

LEFT | RIGHT

Date	Date	Joint To Be Measured		Date	Date
		Shoulder			
		Flexion	0–180		
		Extension	0–60		
		Abduction	0–180		
		Horizontal abduction	0–90		
		Horizontal adduction	0–45		
		Internal rotation	0–70		
		External rotation	0–90		
		Internal rotation (alt)	0–80		
		External rotation (alt)	0–60		
		Elbow and Forearm			
		Flexion–extension	0–150		
		Supination	0–80		
		Pronation	0–80		
		Wrist			
		Flexion	0–80		
		Extension	0–70		
		Ulnar deviation	0–30		
		Radial deviation	0–20		
		Thumb			
		CM flexion	0–15		
		CM extension	0–20		
		MP flexion–extension	0–50		
		IP flexion–extension	0–80		
		Abduction cm.			
		Opposition cm.			
		Index Finger			
		MP flexion	0–90		
		PIP flexion–extension	0–100		
		DIP flexion–extension	0–90		
		Abduction	no norm		
		Adduction	no norm		
		Middle Finger			
		MP flexion	0–90		
		PIP flexion–extension	0–100		
		DIP flexion–extension	0–90		
		Abduction	no norm		
		Adduction	no norm		
		Ring Finger			
		MP flexion	0–90		
		PIP flexion–extension	0–100		
		DIP flexion–extension	0–90		
		Abduction	no norm		
		Adduction	no norm		
		Little Finger			
		MP flexion	0–90		
		PIP flexion–extension	0–100		
		DIP flexion–extension	0–90		
		Abduction	no norm		
		Adduction	no norm		

Therapist's signature: ______________________________

Figure 5-2 Sample range of motion recording form.

Shoulder Flexion

Movement of the humerus anteriorly in the sagittal plane (0–180°, which represents both glenohumeral and axioscapular motion) (Figs. 5-3 and 5-4).

Goniometer Placement

Axis

A point around which motion occurs through the lateral aspect of the glenohumeral joint; at the start of motion, it lies approximately 1 inch below the acromion process. At the end position, the axis has moved, and the goniometer must be repositioned.

Stationary Arm

Parallel to the lateral midline of the trunk.

Movable Arm

Parallel to the longitudinal axis of the humerus on the lateral aspect.

Possible Substitutions

Trunk extension, shoulder abduction.

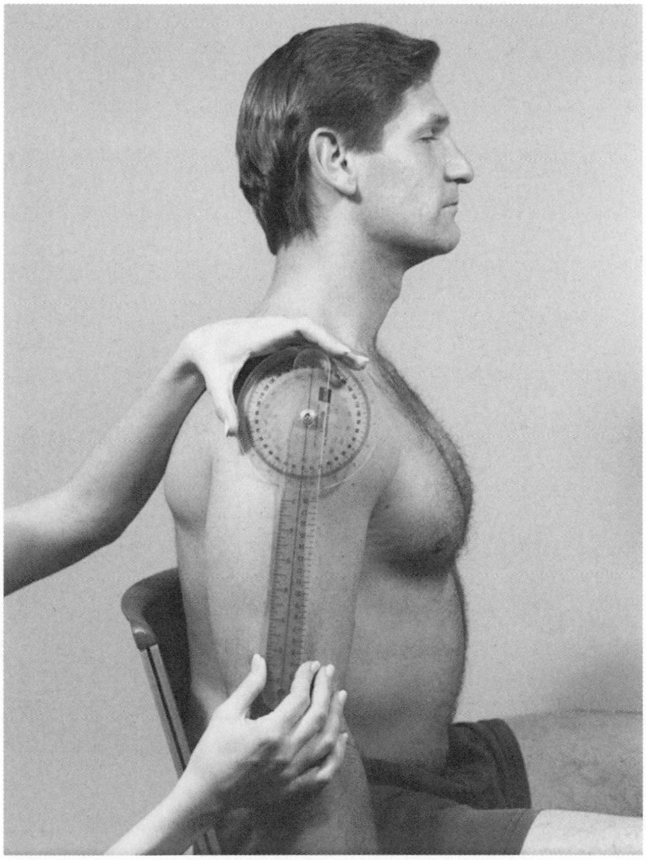

Figure 5-3 Shoulder flexion, start position.

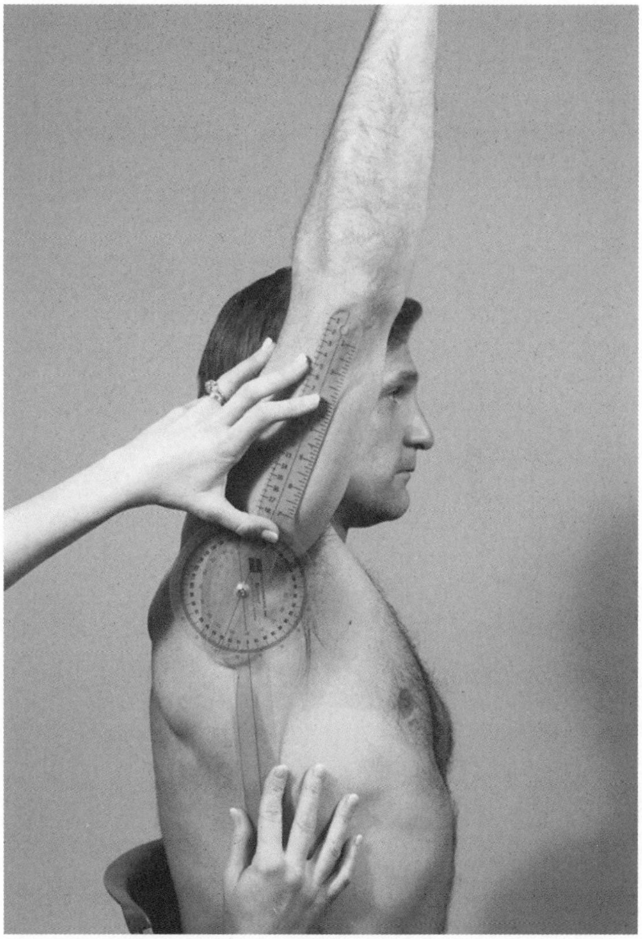

Figure 5-4 Shoulder flexion, end position.

Shoulder Extension

Movement of the humerus posteriorly in a sagittal plane (0–60°) (Figs. 5-5 and 5-6).

Goniometer Placement

Axis

A point around which motion occurs; it lies approximately 1 inch below the acromion process through the lateral aspect of the glenohumeral joint.

Stationary Arm

Parallel to the lateral midline of the trunk.

Movable Arm

Parallel to the longitudinal axis of the humerus on the lateral aspect.

Possible Substitutions

Trunk flexion, scapular elevation, and downward rotation, shoulder abduction.

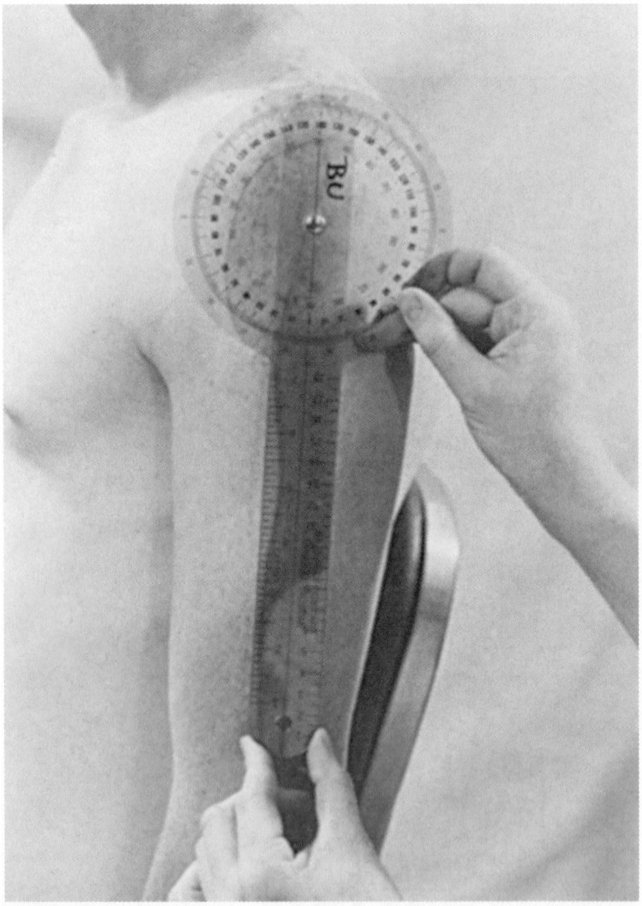

Figure 5-5 Shoulder extension, start position.

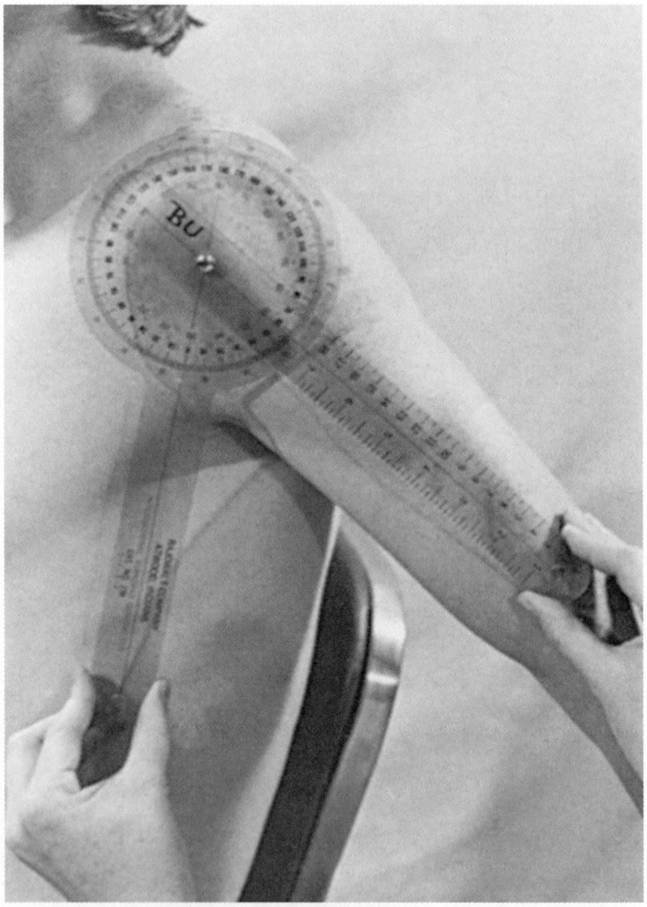

Figure 5-6 Shoulder extension, end position.

Shoulder Abduction

Movement of the humerus laterally in a frontal plane (0–180°, which represents both glenohumeral and axioscapular motion) (Figs. 5-7 and 5-8).

Goniometer Placement

Axis

A point through the anterior or posterior aspect of the glenohumeral joint. Some people consider measurement from the anterior aspect safer because the patient's back can be supported against the chair, but it is preferable to measure women from the posterior aspect.

Stationary Arm

Laterally along the trunk, parallel to the spine.

Movable Arm

Parallel to the longitudinal axis of the humerus.

Possible Substitutions

Lateral flexion of trunk, scapular elevation, shoulder flexion or extension.

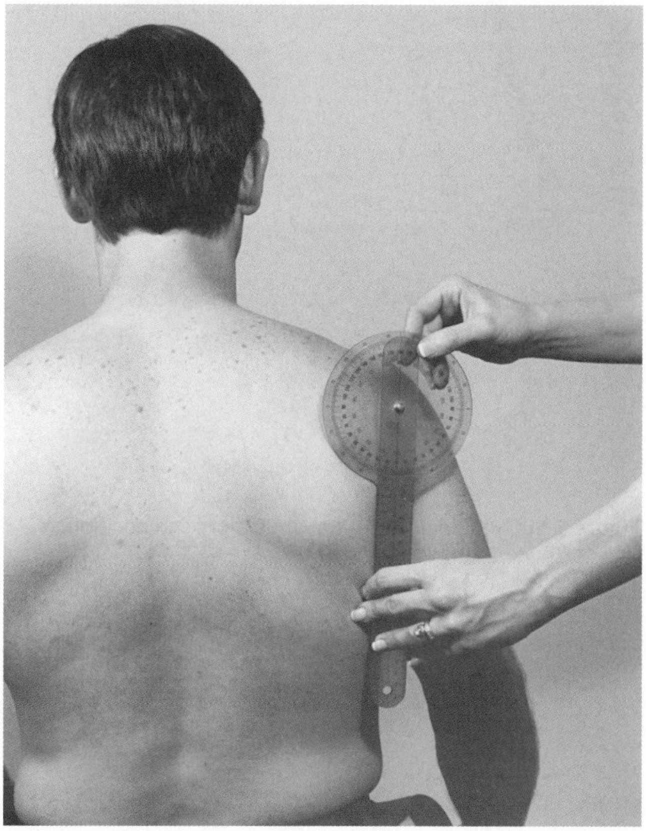

Figure 5-7 Shoulder abduction, start position.

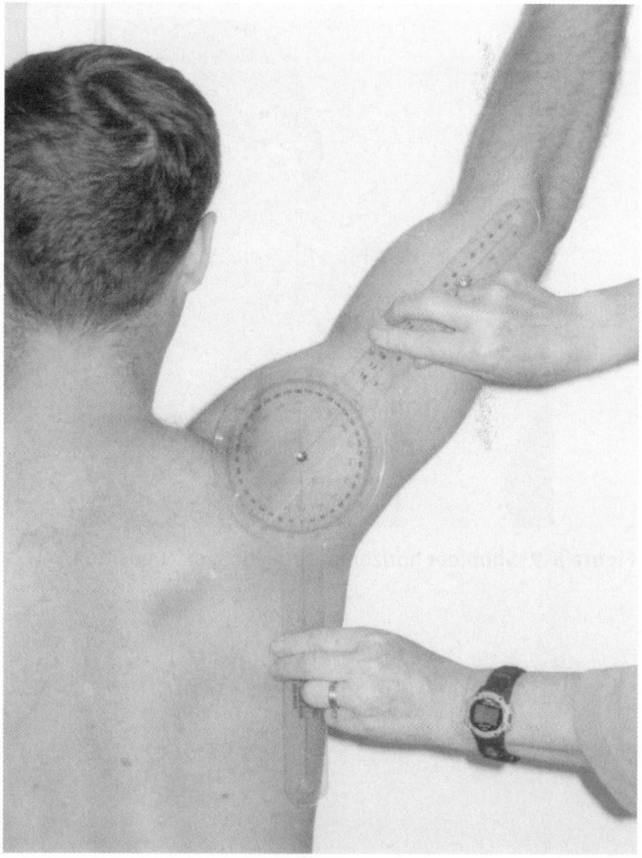

Figure 5-8 Shoulder abduction, end position.

Horizontal Abduction

Movement of the humerus on a horizontal plane from 90° of shoulder flexion to 90° of shoulder abduction and beyond to the limit of motion (0–90°) (Figs. 5-9 and 5-10).

Goniometer Placement

Axis

On top of the acromion process.

Stationary Arm

To start, the arm is parallel to the longitudinal axis of the humerus on the superior aspect and remains in that position, perpendicular to the body, although the humerus moves away. An alternative position of the stationary arm is across the shoulder, anterior to the neck and in line with the opposite acromion process. In this alternative position, the goniometer reads 90° at the start, and this must be considered when recording.

Movable Arm

Parallel to the longitudinal axis of the humerus on the superior aspect.

Possible Substitutions

Trunk rotation or trunk flexion.

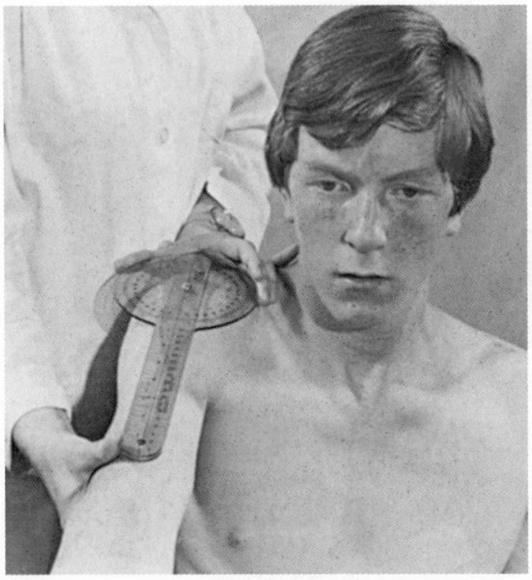

Figure 5-9 Shoulder horizontal abduction, start position.

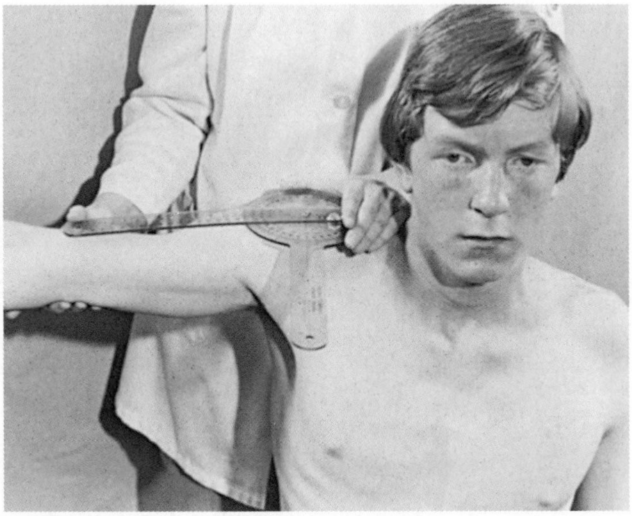

Figure 5-10 Shoulder horizontal abduction, end position.

Horizontal Adduction

Movement of the humerus on a horizontal plane from 90° of shoulder abduction through 90° of shoulder flexion, across the trunk to the limit of motion. The 90° of return motion from horizontal abduction is not measured. The motion is measured from 90° shoulder flexion across the trunk (0–45°) (Figs. 5-11 and 5-12).

Goniometer Placement

Axis

On top of the acromion process.

Stationary Arm

Parallel to the longitudinal axis on the superior aspect of the humerus in the starting position, it remains perpendicular to the body, although the humerus moves away. The alternative placement given for horizontal abduction also applies in this case.

Movable Arm

Parallel to the longitudinal axis of the humerus on the superior aspect.

Possible Substitution

Trunk rotation.

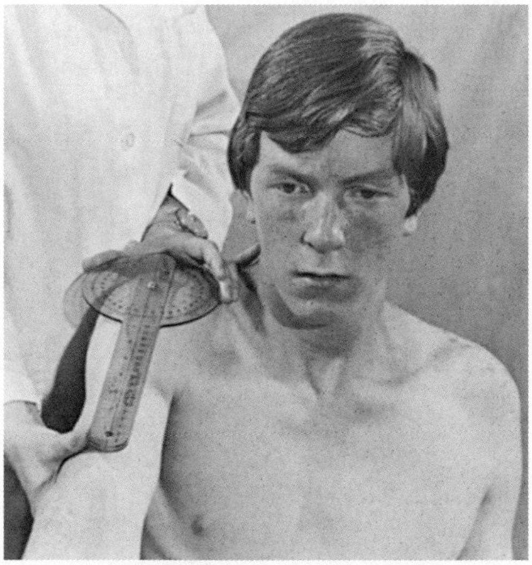

Figure 5-11 Shoulder horizontal adduction, start position.

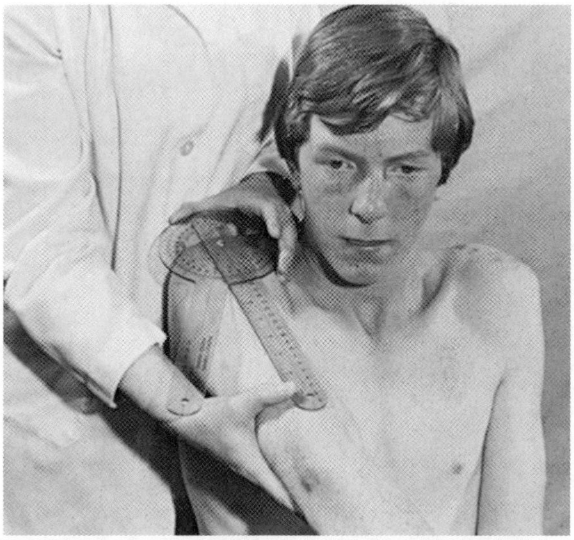

Figure 5-12 Shoulder horizontal adduction, end position.

Internal Rotation

Movement of the humerus medially around the longitudinal axis of the humerus (0–70°) (Figs. 5-13 and 5-14).

Goniometer Placement

Axis

Olecranon process of the ulna.

Stationary Arm

Perpendicular to the floor, which will be parallel to the lateral trunk if the patient is sitting up straight with hips at 90°. The goniometer reads 90° at the start, and this score must be deducted from the final score when recording ROM. *NOTE*: If the patient is supine with the shoulder abducted to 90° and the elbow flexed to 90°, the stationary arm is perpendicular to the floor, with the movable arm along the ulna. The goniometer reads 0° at the start (Boone & Smith, 2000).

Movable Arm

Parallel to the longitudinal axis of the ulna.

Possible Substitutions

Scapular elevation and downward rotation, trunk flexion, elbow extension.

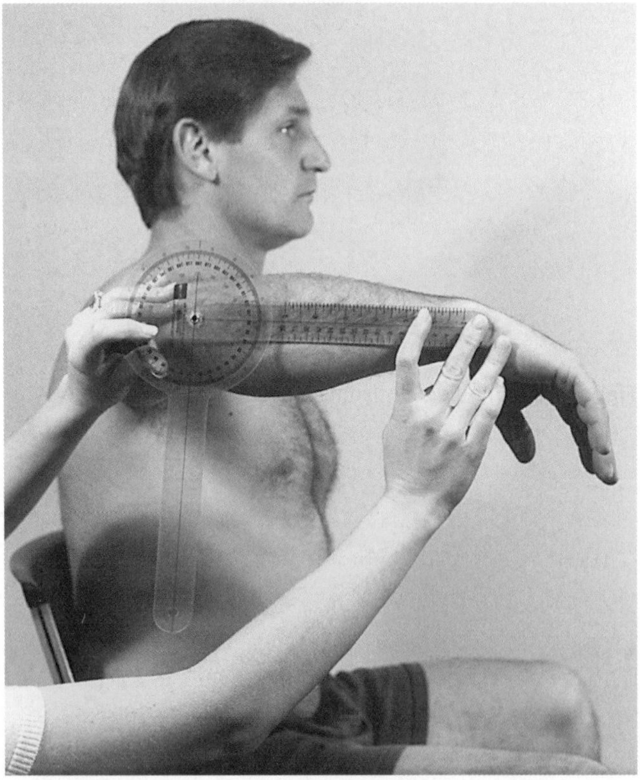

Figure 5-13 Shoulder internal rotation, start position.

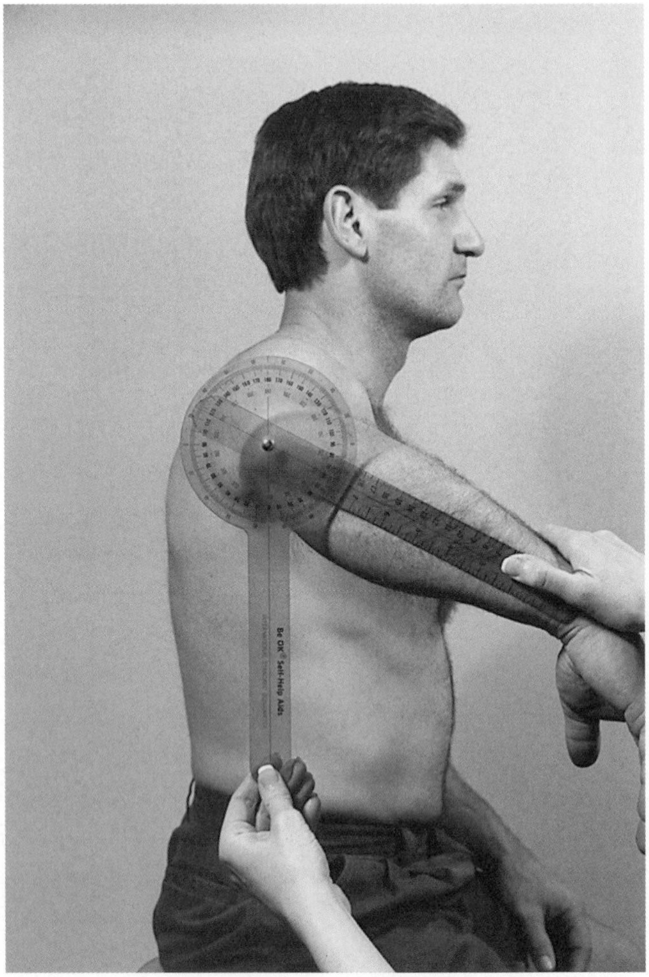

Figure 5-14 Shoulder internal rotation, end position.

External Rotation

Movement of the humerus laterally around the longitudinal axis of the humerus (0–90°) (Figs. 5-15 and 5-16).

Goniometer Placement

Axis

Olecranon process of the ulna.

Stationary Arm

Perpendicular to the floor. The goniometer will read 90° at the start, and this must be considered when recording the ROM score.

Movable Arm

Parallel to the longitudinal axis of the ulna.

Possible Substitutions

Scapular depression and upward rotation, trunk extension, elbow extension.

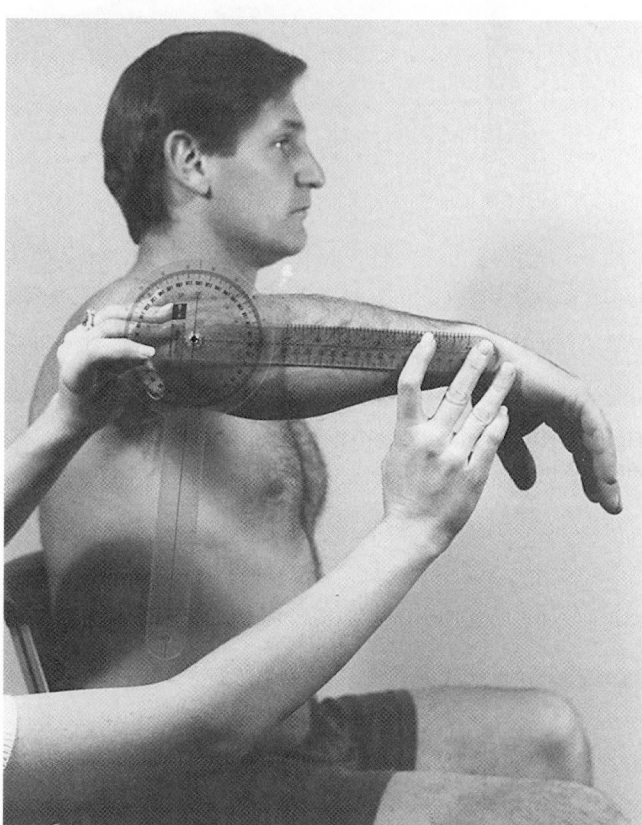

Figure 5-15 Shoulder external rotation, start position.

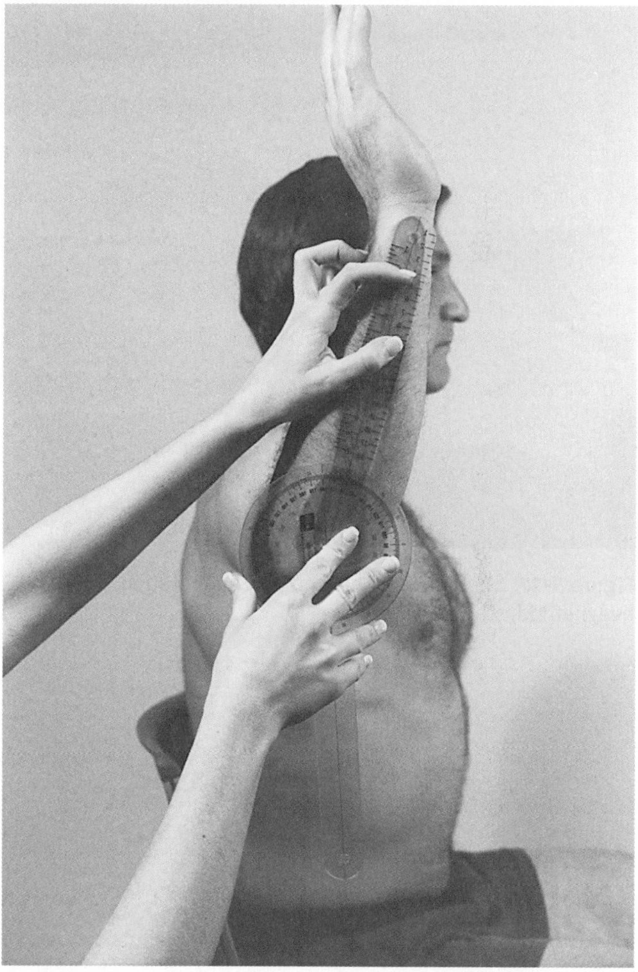

Figure 5-16 Shoulder external rotation, end position.

Internal and External Rotation: Alternative Method

If shoulder limitation prevents positioning for the previously described method, the patient may be seated with humerus adducted to the side and elbow flexed to 90° (Figs. 5-17 and 5-18). This method is inaccurate in internal rotation if the patient has a large abdomen. (Internal rotation, 0–80°; external rotation, 0–60°.)

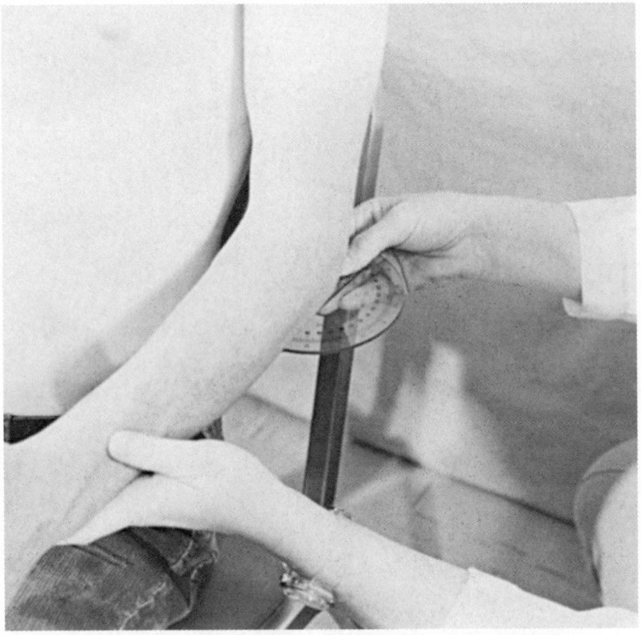

Figure 5-17 Shoulder internal and external rotation, alternative method, start position.

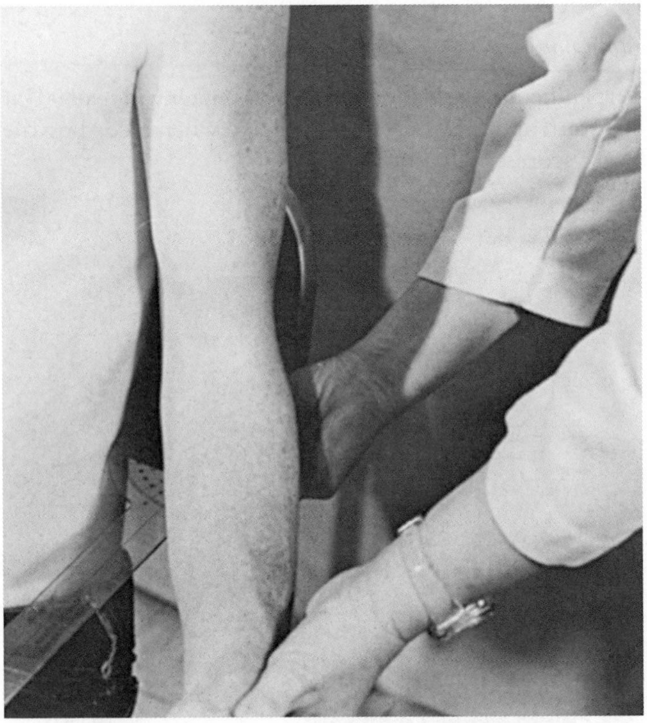

Figure 5-18 Shoulder external rotation, alternative method, end position.

Elbow Flexion–Extension

Movement of the supinated forearm anteriorly in the sagittal plane (0–150°) (Figs. 5-19 and 5-20).

Goniometer Placement

Axis

Lateral epicondyle of the humerus.

Stationary Arm

Parallel to the longitudinal axis of the humerus on the lateral aspect.

Movable Arm

Parallel to the longitudinal axis of the radius.

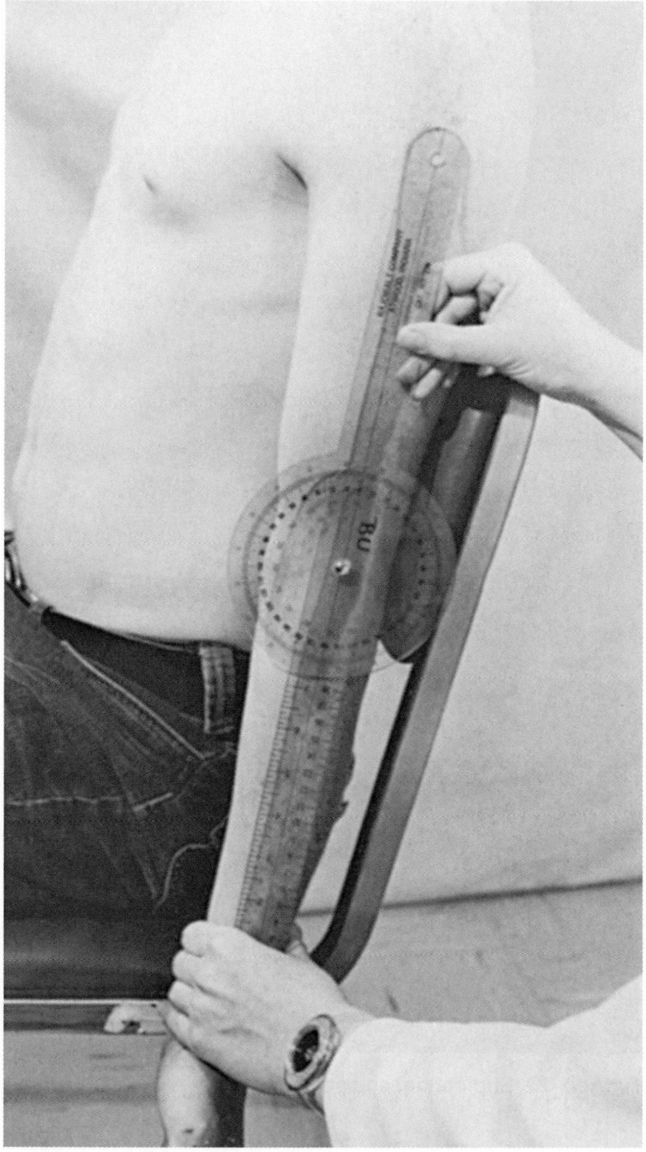

Figure 5-19 Elbow flexion, start position (elbow extension).

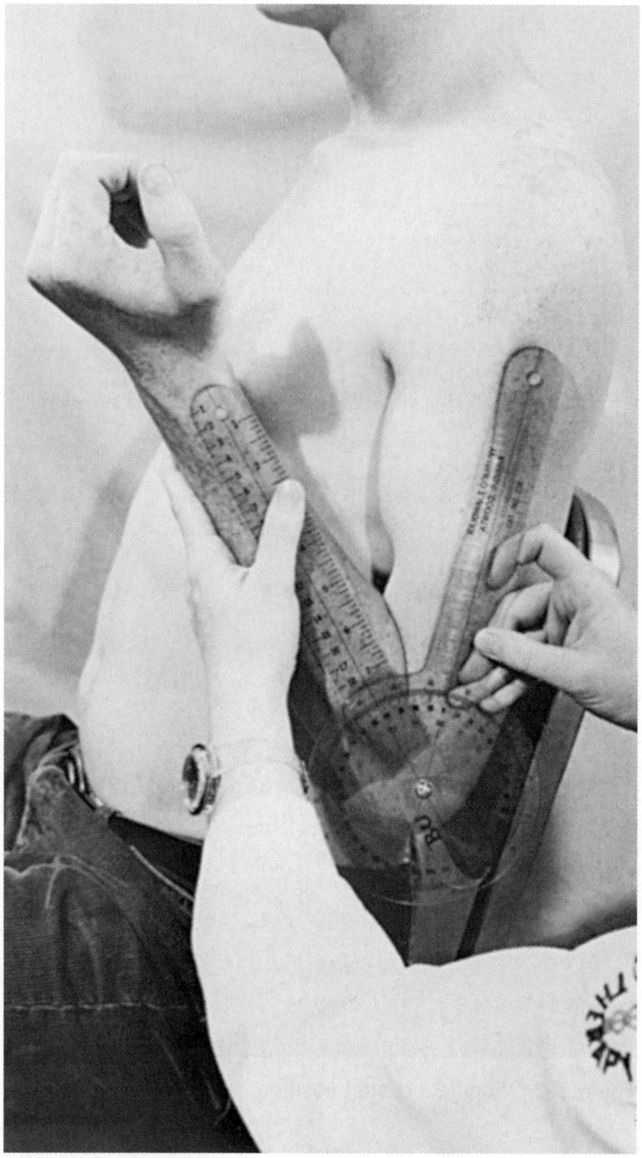

Figure 5-20 Elbow flexion, end position.

Forearm Supination

Rotation of the forearm laterally around its longitudinal axis from midposition so that the palm of the hand faces up (0–80°) (Figs. 5-21 and 5-22).

Goniometer Placement

Axis

Longitudinal axis of the forearm displaced toward the ulnar side.

Stationary Arm

Perpendicular to the floor.

Movable Arm

Across the distal radius and ulna on the volar surface.

Possible Substitutions

Adduction and external rotation of the shoulder.

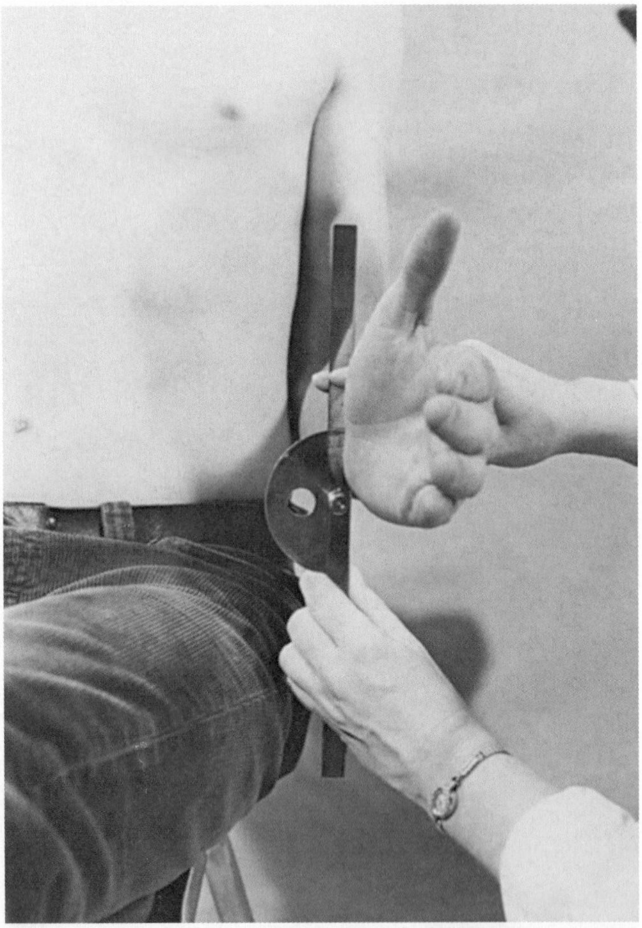

Figure 5-21 Supination, start position.

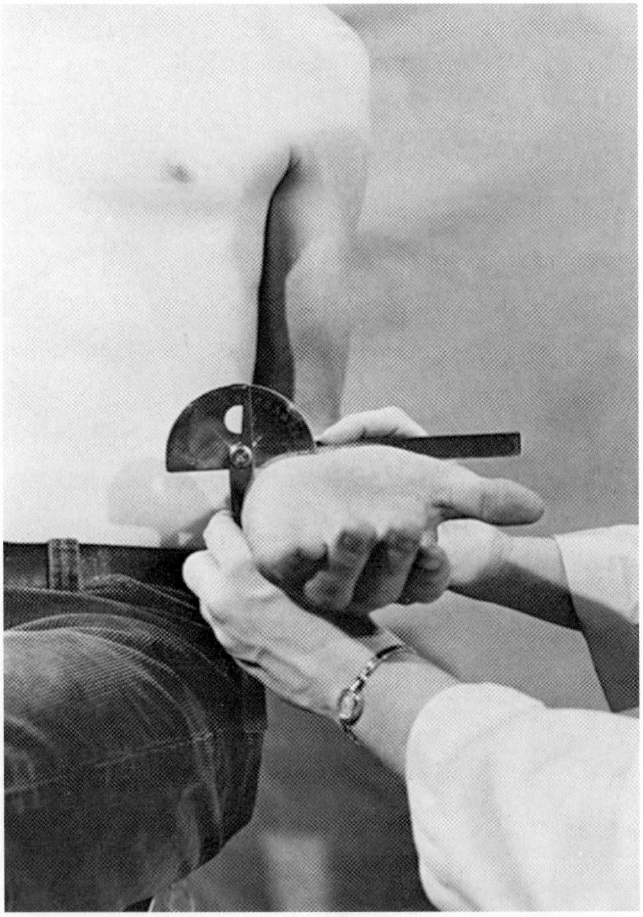

Figure 5-22 Supination, end position.

Forearm Pronation

Rotation of the forearm medially around its longitudinal axis from midposition so that the palm of the hand faces down (0–80°) (Figs. 5-23 and 5-24).

Goniometer Placement

Axis

Longitudinal axis of forearm displaced toward the ulnar side.

Stationary Arm

Perpendicular to the floor.

Movable Arm

Across the distal radius and ulna on the dorsal surface.

Possible Substitutions

Abduction and internal rotation of the shoulder.

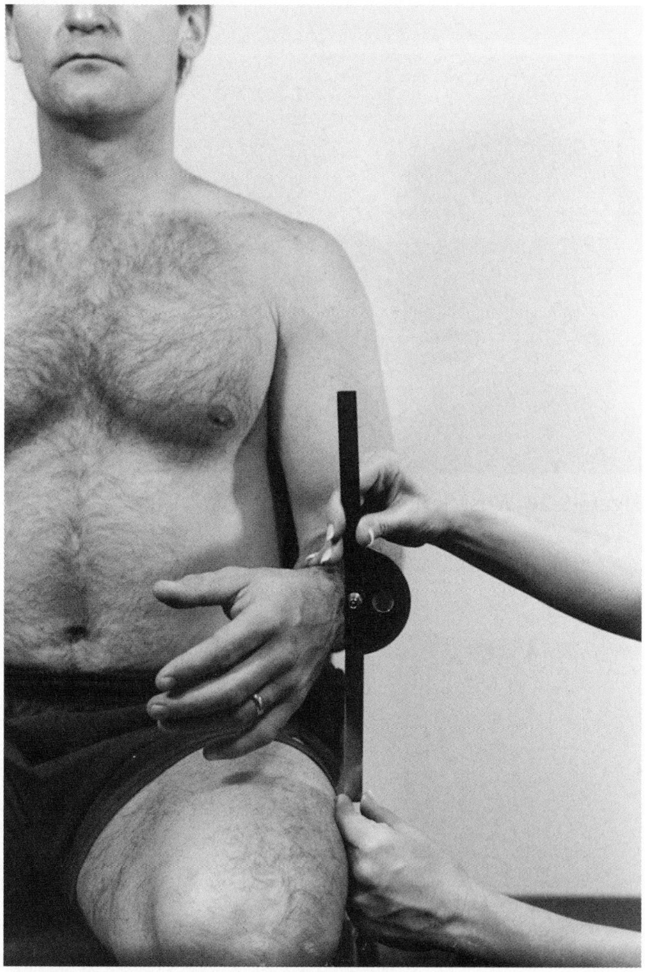

Figure 5-23 Pronation, start position.

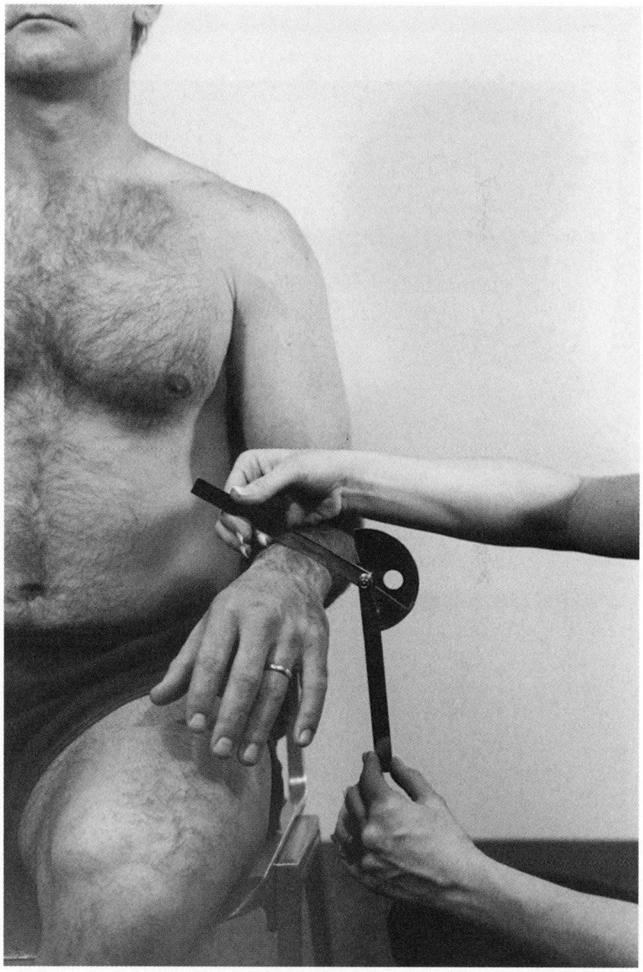

Figure 5-24 Pronation, end position.

Wrist Flexion (Volar Flexion)

Movement of the hand volarly in the sagittal plane (0–80°) (Figs. 5-25 and 5-26).

Goniometer Placement

Axis

On the dorsal aspect of the wrist joint in line with the base of the third metacarpal.

Stationary Arm

Along the midline of the dorsal surface of the forearm.

Movable Arm

Parallel to the longitudinal axis of the third metacarpal.

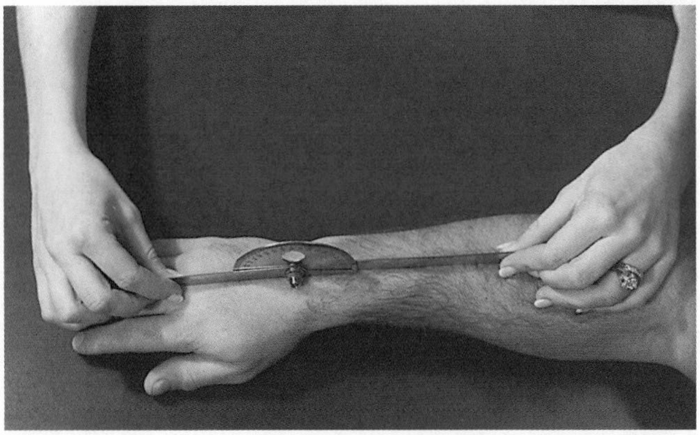

Figure 5-25 Wrist flexion, start position.

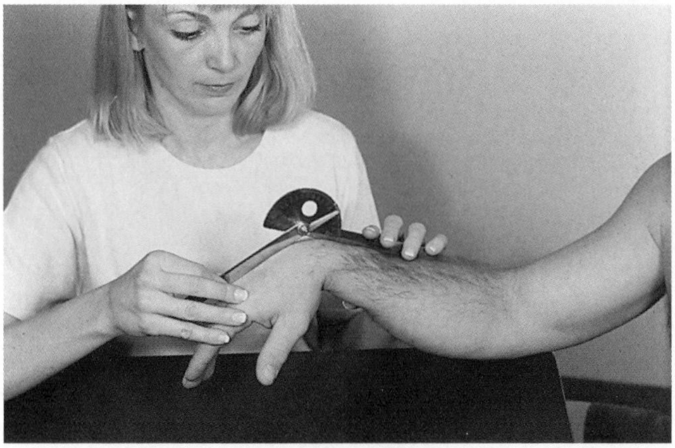

Figure 5-26 Wrist flexion, end position.

Wrist Extension (Dorsiflexion)

Movement of the hand dorsally in the sagittal plane (0–70°) (Figs. 5-27 and 5-28).

Goniometer Placement

Axis

On the volar surface of the wrist in line with the insertion of the tendon of the palmaris longus.

Stationary Arm

Along the midline of the volar surface of the forearm.

Movable Arm

Parallel to the longitudinal axis of the third metacarpal.

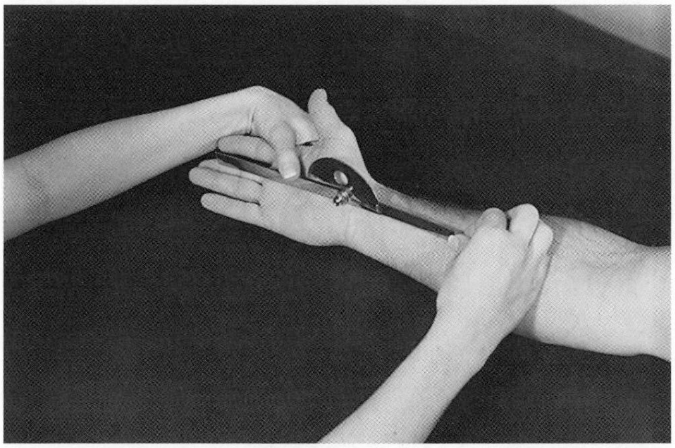

Figure 5-27 Wrist extension, start position.

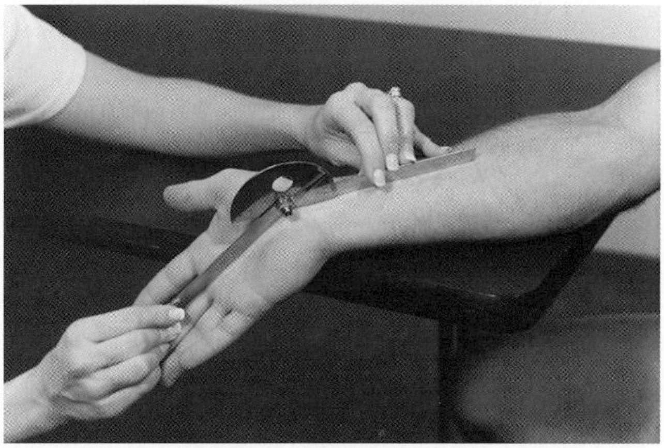

Figure 5-28 Wrist extension, end position.

Wrist Ulnar Deviation

Movement of the hand toward the ulnar side in a frontal plane (0–30°) (Figs. 5-29 and 5-30).

Goniometer Placement

Axis

On the dorsal aspect of the wrist joint in line with the base of the third metacarpal.

One Arm

Along the midline of the forearm on the dorsal surface.

Other Arm

Along the midline of the third metacarpal.

Possible Substitutions

Wrist extension, wrist flexion.

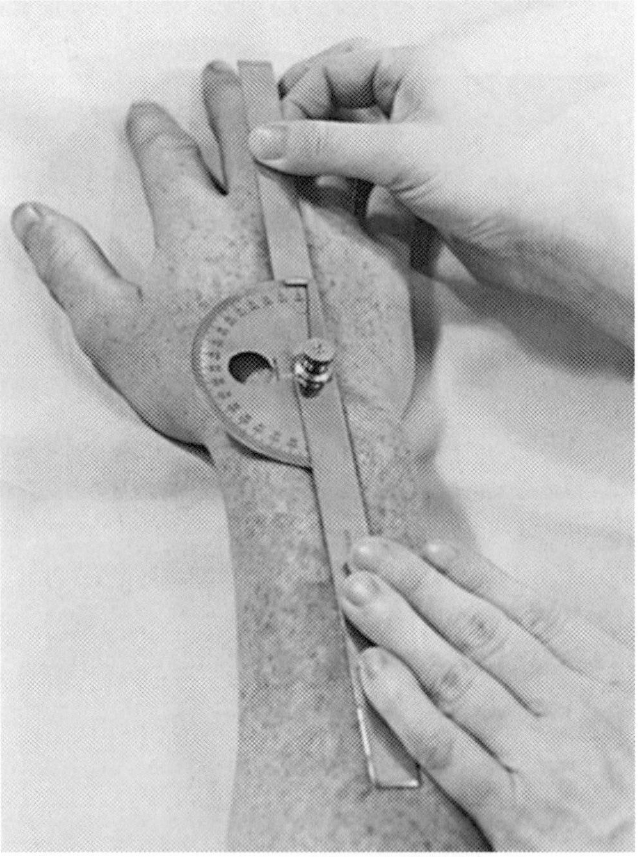

Figure 5-29 Wrist ulnar deviation, start position.

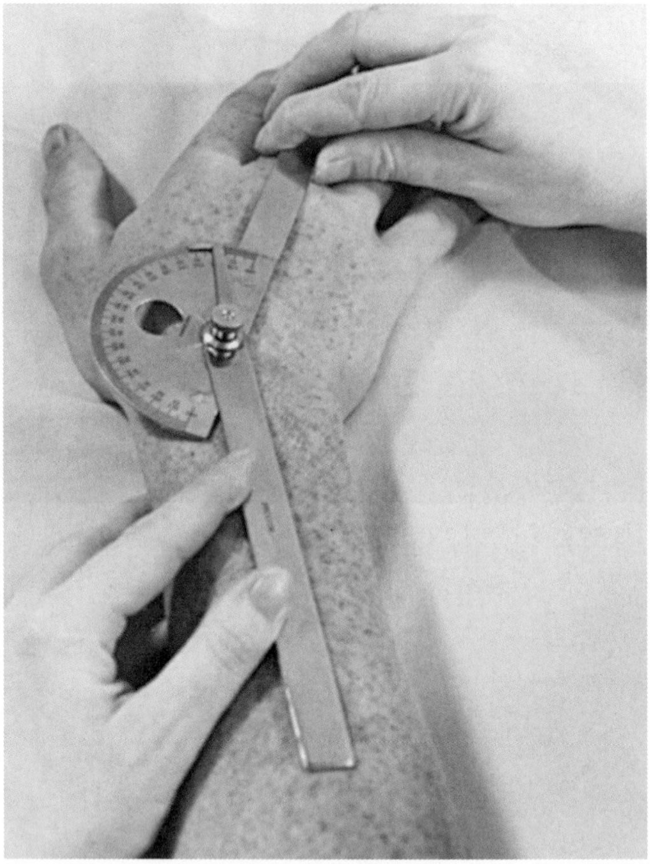

Figure 5-30 Wrist ulnar deviation, end position.

Wrist Radial Deviation

Movement of the hand toward the radial side in a frontal plane (0–20°) (Figs. 5-31 and 5-32).

Goniometer Placement

Axis

On the dorsal aspect of the wrist joint in line with the base of the third metacarpal.

Stationary Arm

Along the midline of the forearm on the dorsal surface.

Movable Arm

Along the midline of the third metacarpal.

Possible Substitution

Wrist extension.

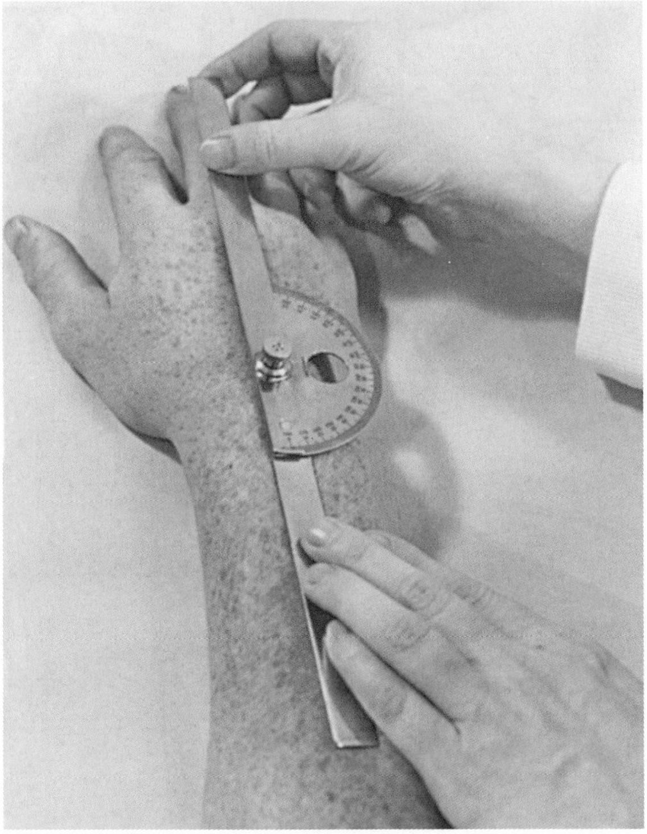

Figure 5-31 Wrist radial deviation, start position.

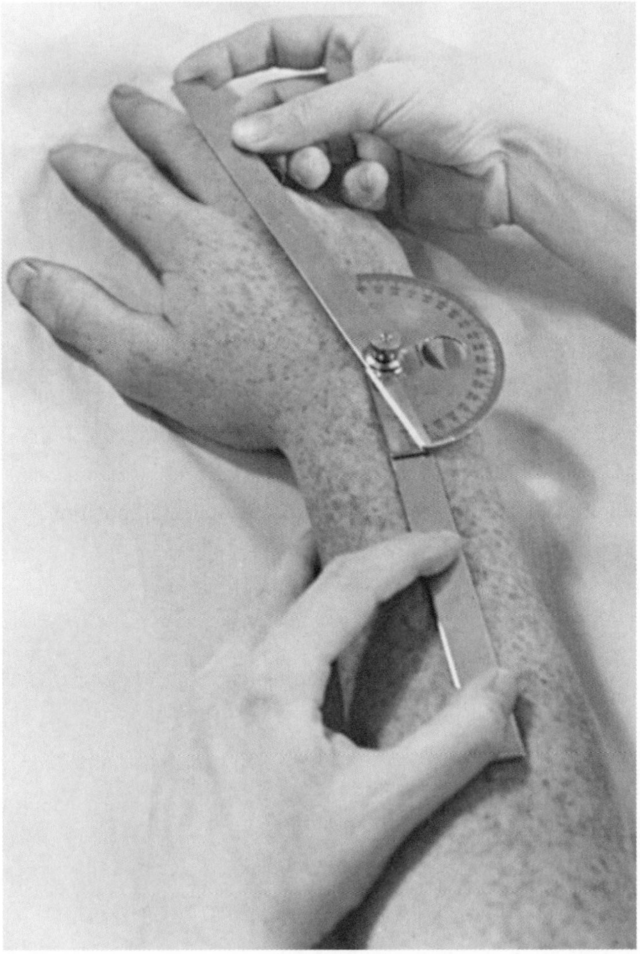

Figure 5-32 Wrist radial deviation, end position.

Thumb Carpometacarpal Flexion

Movement of the thumb across the palm in the frontal plane (0–15°) (Figs. 5-33 and 5-34).

Goniometer Placement

Axis

On the radial side of the wrist at the junction of the base of the first metacarpal and the trapezium.

Stationary Arm

Parallel to the longitudinal axis of the radius.

Movable Arm

Parallel to the longitudinal axis of the first metacarpal. For accuracy, the arms of the goniometer must remain in full contact with skin surface over the bones, but ***excessive pressure with the edge of a half-circle goniometer must be avoided.*** These statements apply to all flexion–extension measurements of the thumb and fingers.

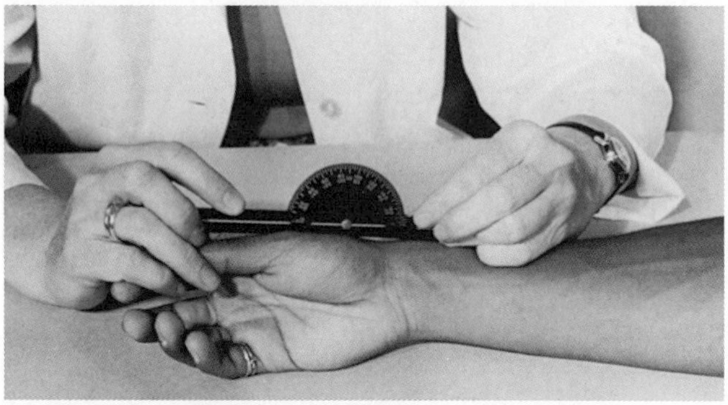

Figure 5-33 Thumb carpometacarpal flexion, start position.

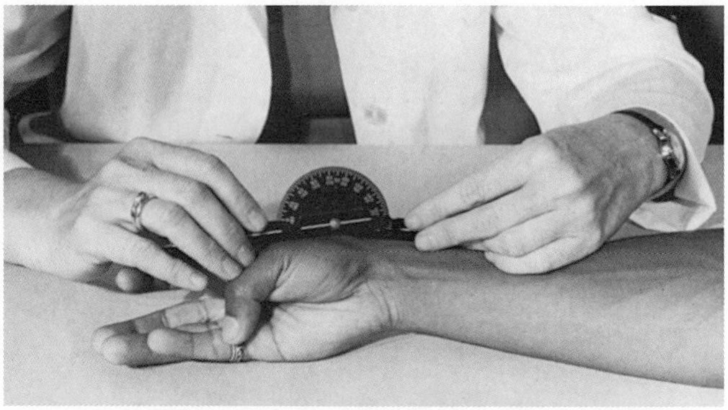

Figure 5-34 Thumb carpometacarpal flexion, end position.

Thumb Carpometacarpal Extension

Movement of the thumb away from the palm in the frontal plane (0–20°) (Figs. 5-35 and 5-36).

Goniometer Placement

Axis

On the volar side of the wrist at the junction of the base of the first metacarpal and the trapezium.

One Arm

Parallel to the longitudinal axis of the radius.

Other Arm

Parallel to the longitudinal axis of the first metacarpal.

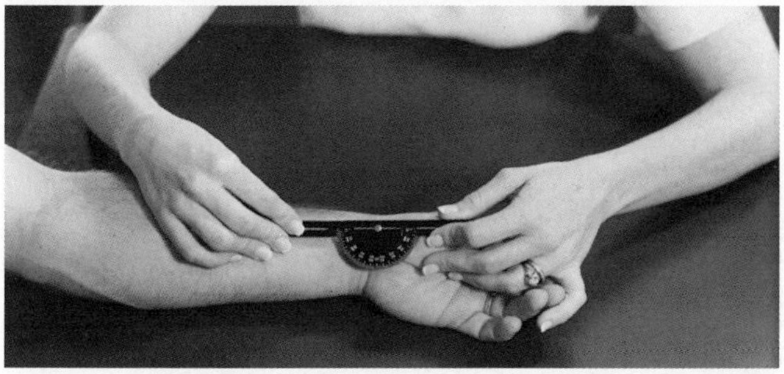

Figure 5-35 Thumb carpometacarpal extension, start position.

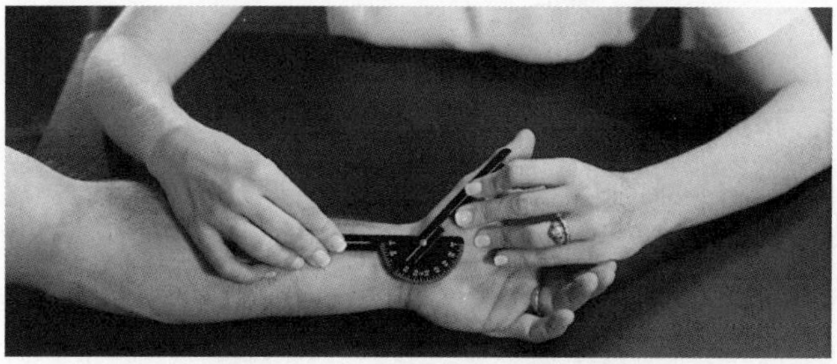

Figure 5-36 Thumb carpometacarpal extension, end position.

Thumb Metacarpophalangeal (MP) Flexion–Extension

Movement of the thumb across the palm in the frontal plane (0–50°) (Figs. 5-37 and 5-38).

Goniometer Placement

Axis

On the dorsal aspect of the MP joint.

Stationary Arm

On the dorsal surface along the midline of the first metacarpal.

Movable Arm

On the dorsal surface along the midline of the proximal phalanx of the thumb.

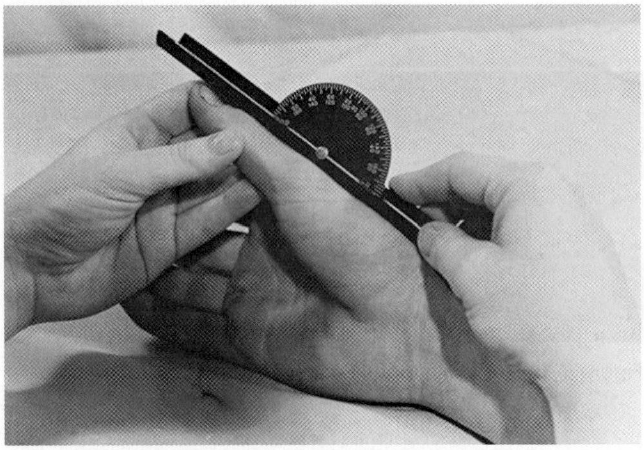

Figure 5-37 Thumb metacarpophalangeal flexion and extension start position.

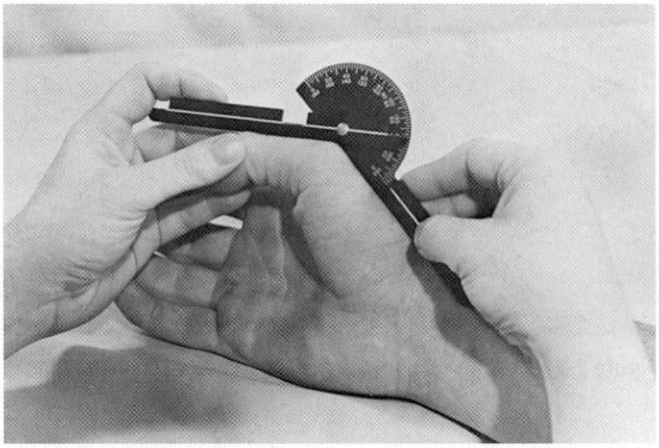

Figure 5-38 Thumb metacarpophalangeal flexion and extension, end position.

Thumb Interphalangeal (IP) Flexion–Extension

Movement of the distal phalanx of the thumb toward the volar surface of the proximal phalanx of the thumb (0–80°) (Figs. 5-39 and 5-40).

Goniometer Placement

Axis

On the dorsal aspect of the IP joint.

Stationary Arm

On the dorsal surface along the proximal phalanx.

Movable Arm

On the dorsal surface along the distal phalanx. *NOTE*: If the thumbnail prevents full goniometer contact, shift the movable arm laterally to increase accuracy. Also, thumb MP and IP flexion and extension can be measured on the lateral aspect of the thumb using lateral aspects of the same landmarks.

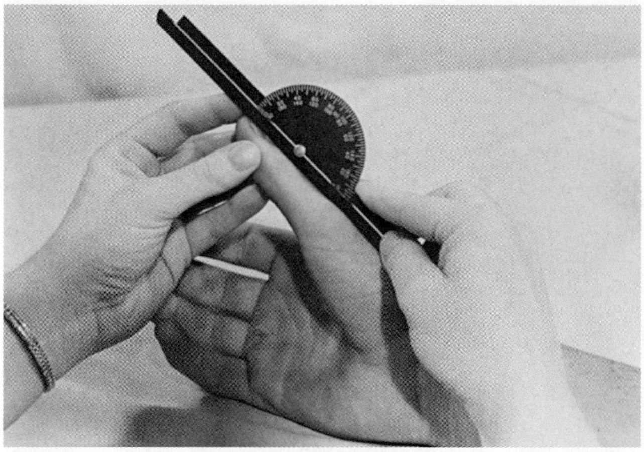

Figure 5-39 Thumb interphalangeal flexion, start position (extension).

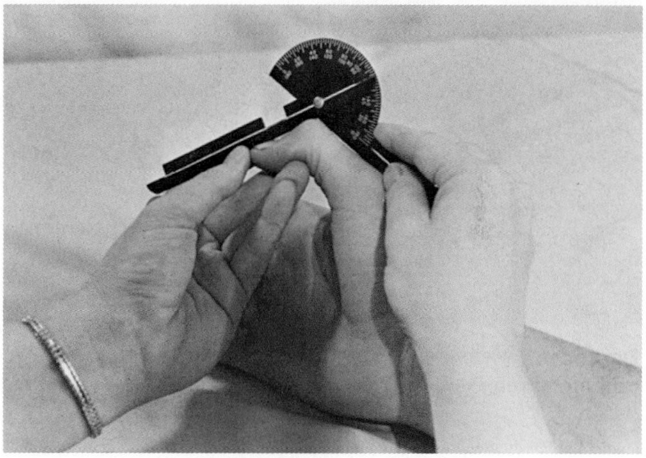

Figure 5-40 Thumb interphalangeal flexion, end position.

Thumb Abduction and Opposition: Ruler Measurements

Abduction

Take the measurement from the midpoint of the head of the first metacarpal to the midpoint of the head of the second metacarpal while the thumb is in full abduction (Fig. 5-41).

Opposition

The pad of the thumb rotates to meet the pad of each finger. The little finger rotates to better meet the pad of the thumb. As a summary measure of opposition, record the distance from the tip of the thumb (not the thumbnail) to the tip end of the little finger (Fig. 5-42).

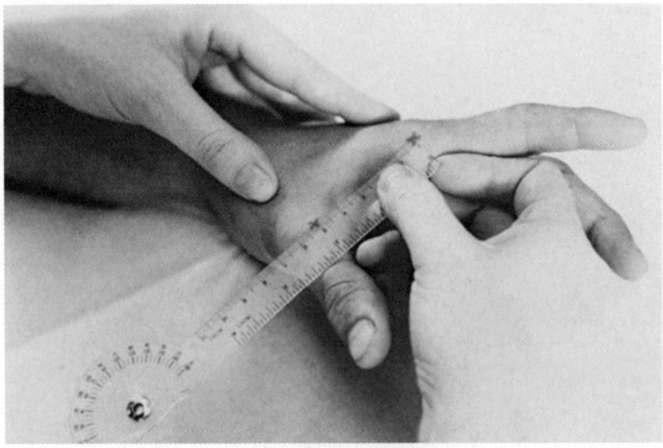

Figure 5-41 Measurement of thumb abduction using a centimeter ruler.

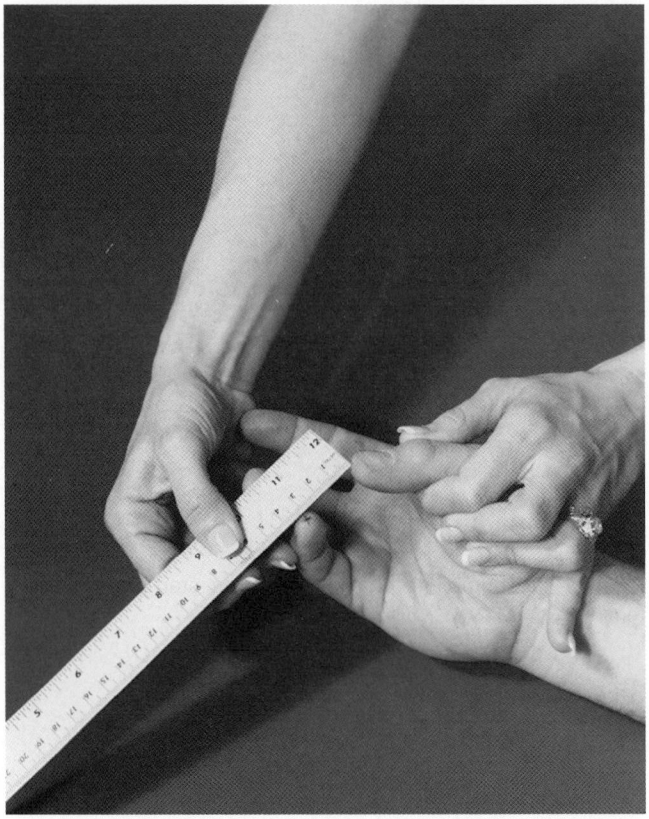

Figure 5-42 Measurement of opposition to the little finger using a centimeter ruler.

Finger Metacarpophalangeal Flexion–Extension

Movement of the finger at the MP joint in a sagittal plane (0–90°) (Figs. 5-43 and 5-44).

Goniometer Placement

Axis

On the dorsal aspect of the MP joint of the finger being measured.

Stationary Arm

On the dorsal surface along the midline of the metacarpal of the finger being measured.

Movable Arm

On the dorsal surface along the midline of the proximal phalanx of the finger being measured.

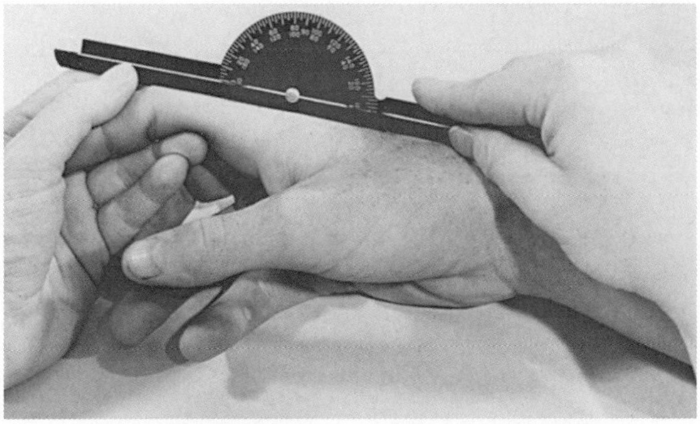

Figure 5-43 Finger metacarpophalangeal flexion, start position (extension).

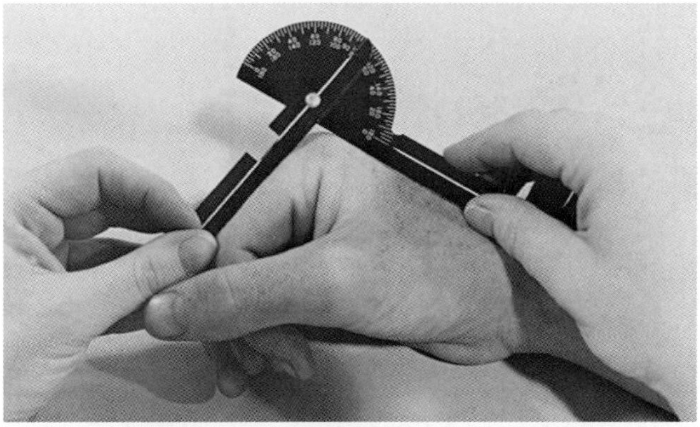

Figure 5-44 Finger metacarpophalangeal flexion, end position.

Finger Proximal Interphalangeal (PIP) Flexion–Extension

Movement of the middle phalanx toward the volar surface of the proximal phalanx in the sagittal plane (0–100°) (Figs. 5-45 and 5-46).

Goniometer Placement

Axis

On the dorsal aspect of the PIP joint of the finger being measured.

Stationary Arm

On the dorsal surface along the midline of the proximal phalanx of the finger being measured.

Movable Arm

On the dorsal surface along the midline of the middle phalanx of the finger being measured.

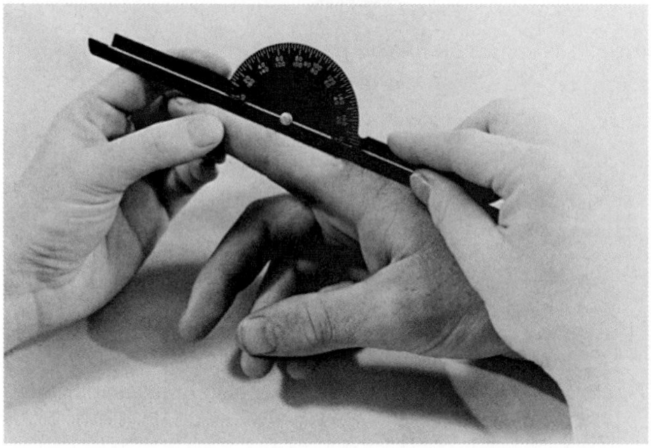

Figure 5-45 Proximal interphalangeal flexion, start position (extension).

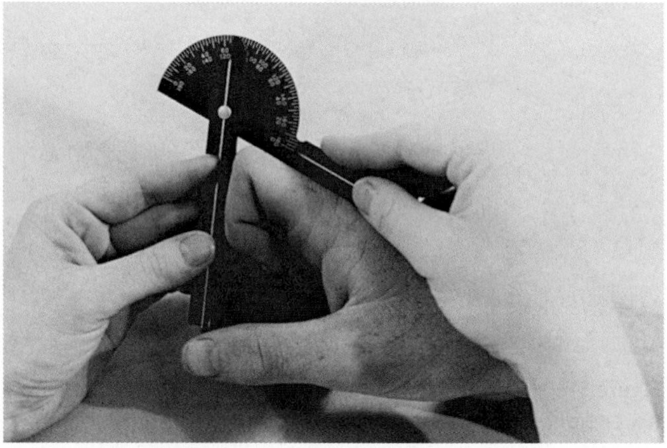

Figure 5-46 Proximal interphalangeal flexion, end position.

Finger Distal Interphalangeal (DIP) Flexion–Extension

Movement of the distal phalanx toward the volar surface of the middle phalanx in a sagittal plane (0–90°) (Figs. 5-47 and 5-48).

Goniometer Placement

Axis

On the dorsal aspect of the DIP joint of the finger being measured.

Stationary Arm

On the dorsal surface along the midline of the middle phalanx of the finger being measured.

Movable Arm

On the dorsal surface along the midline of the distal phalanx of the finger being measured. *NOTE*: If the fingernail prevents full goniometer contact, shift the movable arm laterally to increase accuracy. Also, finger PIP and DIP flexion and extension can be measured from the lateral aspect of each finger using the lateral aspect of the same landmarks. This method may be more accurate when joints are enlarged.

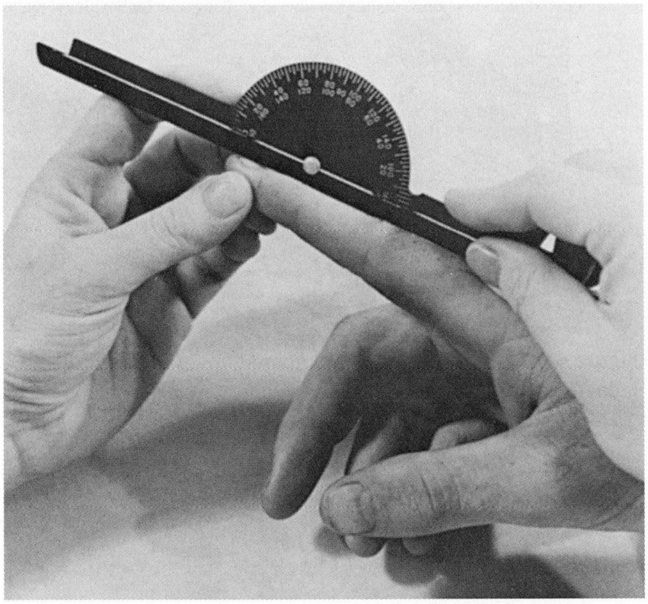

Figure 5-47 Distal interphalangeal flexion, start position (extension).

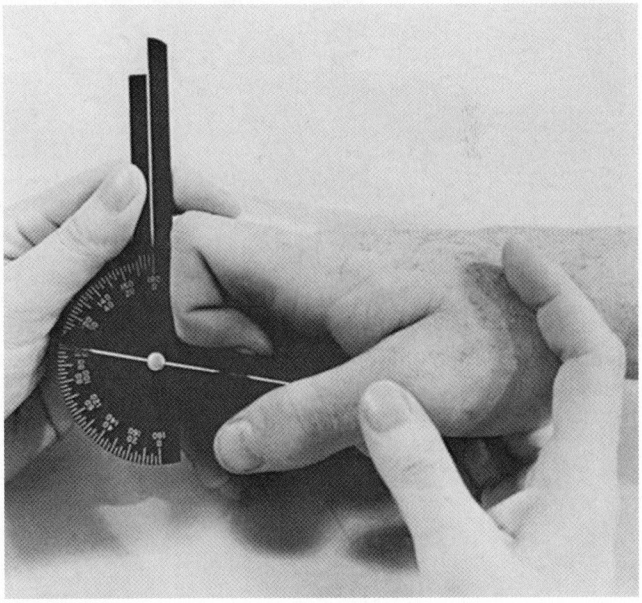

Figure 5-48 Distal interphalangeal flexion, end position.

Composite Measurement and Recording of Total Finger Flexion

A method of recording composite digital motion used by hand therapists is to sum the values for the degrees of flexion motion of the MP, PIP, and DIP joints, taking into consideration extension deficits (Ellis & Bruton, 2002). Total active motion (TAM) or total passive motion (TPM) can then be expressed by a single number. The formula for calculating these values is as follows: (MP + PIP + DIP flexion) − (MP + PIP + DIP extension deficits) = TAM or TPM.

Another method for measuring combined flexion of the PIP and DIP joints (Fig. 5-49) or combined flexion of the MP, PIP, and DIP joints (Fig. 5-50), using a centimeter ruler, is illustrated in the figures.

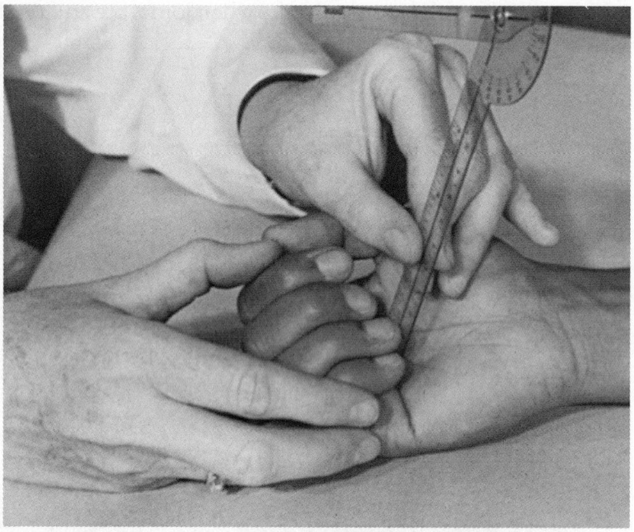

Figure 5-49 PIP and DIP combined finger flexion; ruler measurement.

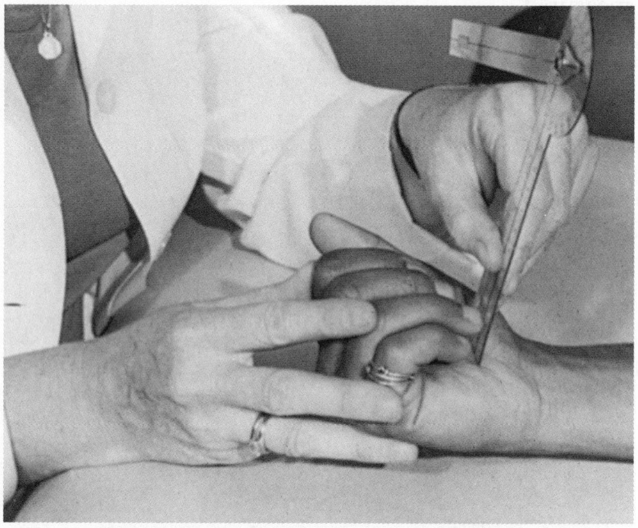

Figure 5-50 MP, PIP, and DIP combined finger flexion; ruler measurement.

Finger Abduction

Movement of the index, ring, and little fingers away from the midline of the hand in a frontal plane. The middle finger, which is the midline of the hand, abducts in both radial and ulnar directions (Figs. 5-51 and 5-52).

Goniometer Placement

Axis

On the dorsal aspect of the MP joint of the finger being measured.

Stationary Arm

Along the dorsal surface of the metacarpal of the finger being measured.

Movable Arm

Along the dorsal surface of the proximal phalanx of the finger being measured.

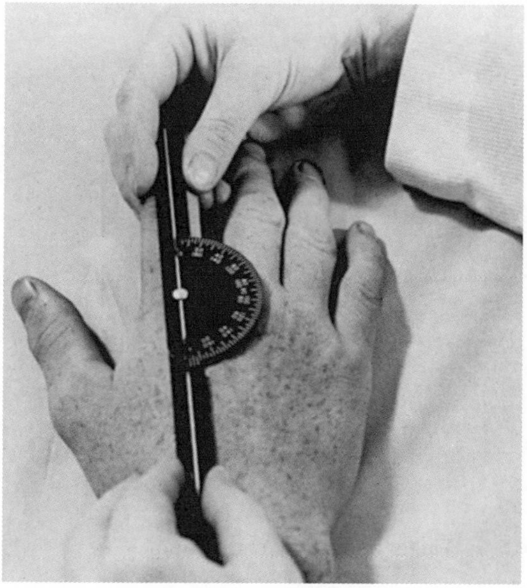

Figure 5-51 Finger abduction, start position.

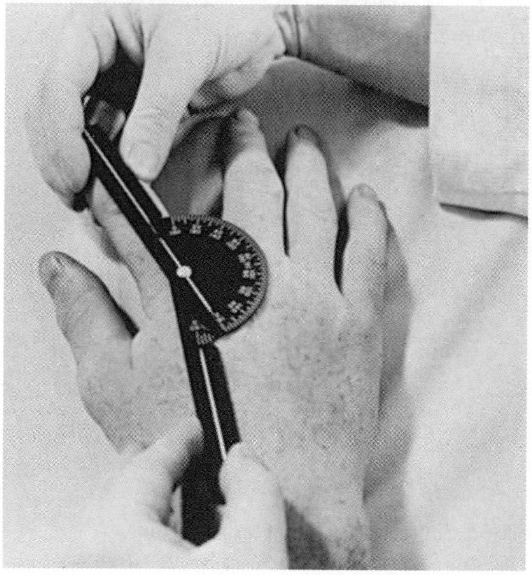

Figure 5-52 Finger abduction, end position.

Finger Adduction

Movement of the index, ring, and little fingers toward the midline of the hand in a frontal plane (Figs. 5-53 and 5-54).

Goniometer Placement

Axis

On the dorsal aspect of the MP joint of the finger being measured.

One Arm

Along the dorsal surface of the metacarpal of the finger being measured. The middle finger is not measured.

Other Arm

Along the dorsal surface of the proximal phalanx of the finger being measured.

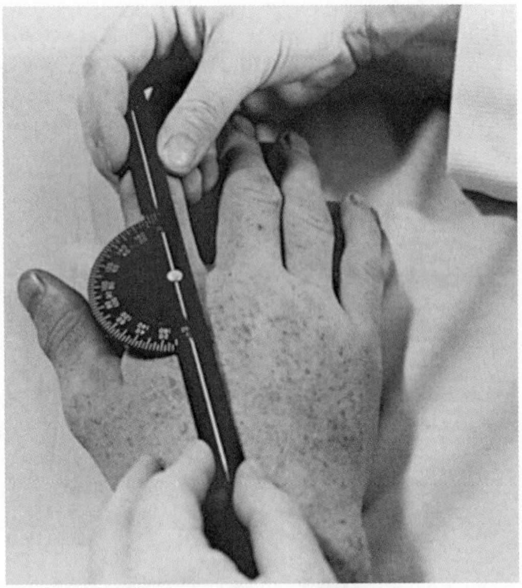

Figure 5-53 Finger adduction, start position.

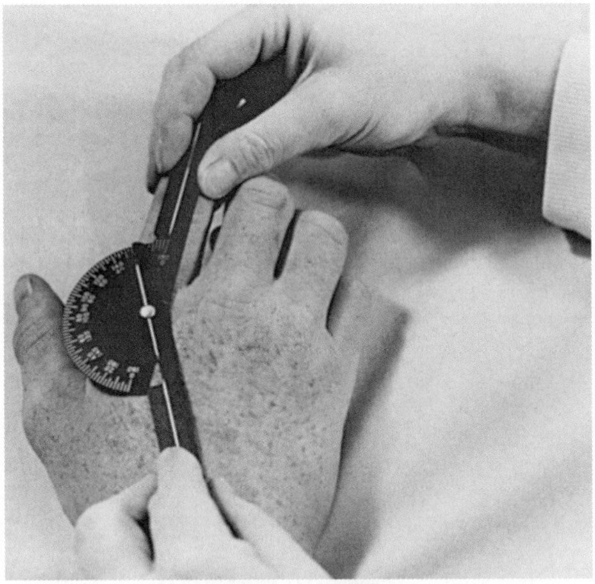

Figure 5-54 Finger adduction, end position.

MP Deviation Correction Measurement

When there is ulnar deviation deformity of the metacarpophalangeal joints, often seen in rheumatoid arthritis, this additional measurement is taken (Figs. 5-55 and 5-56).

The active range is compared with the passive range to determine whether muscle weakness is present. PROM is compared with the norm of 0° deviation to determine whether a fixed deformity exists.

Goniometer Placement

Axis

Over the MP joint of the finger being measured.

One Arm

Placed along the dorsal midline of the metacarpal.

Other Arm

Placed along the dorsal midline of the proximal phalanx.

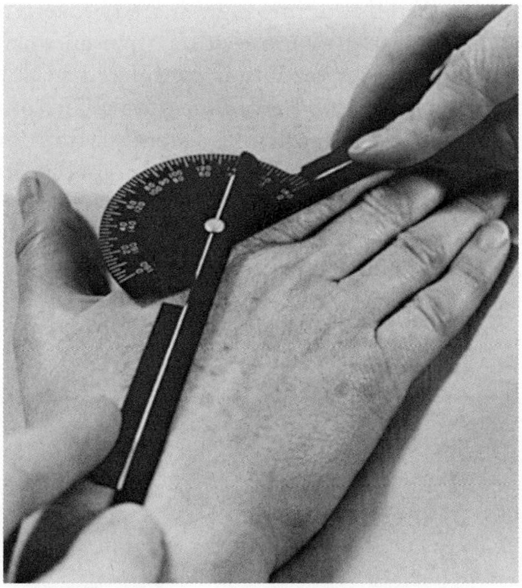

Figure 5-55 Metacarpophalangeal deviation correction, start position.

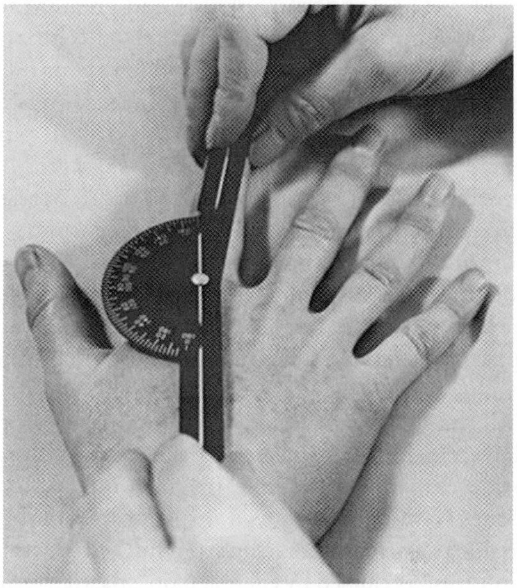

Figure 5-56 Metacarpophalangeal deviation correction, end position.

Interpreting the Results

The initial evaluation is interpreted by reviewing the recording form to identify which joints have significant limitation. A significant limitation is one that decreases occupational functioning or may lead to deformity. The therapist notes whether the limitation is the result of tissue changes (PROM < norms) or muscle weakness (AROM < PROM).

Limits of motion scores can be used in several ways. First, the therapist can compare the scores of the involved to the uninvolved extremity. A study of more than 1000 healthy male subjects, however, found a significant difference in ROM between the dominant and nondominant sides. The nondominant side had greater range in many of the upper extremity joints tested (Gunal et al., 1996). This information should be kept in mind when comparing the two sides. The patient's scores can be compared with the average limits (norms) expected for each motion. The average limits stated by the Committee on Joint Motion of the American Academy of Orthopaedic Surgeons (Greene & Heckman, 1994) are commonly used and are included here. However, patients may be functional with less ROM than is noted in the norms for particular joints. The emphasis in occupational therapy is to enable occupational functioning.

With the significant limitations and probable cause in mind, treatment goals that reflect the identified problem can be developed. For example, if skin, joint, and/or muscle tissues have shortened as a result of immobilization, the goal is to increase range by stretching these tissues. If the limitation is caused by edema, pain, spasticity, or muscle weakness, the primary goal is to reduce or correct the underlying problem, and the secondary goal is to prevent loss of ROM caused by the immobility imposed by the primary condition. If the cause is bony ankylosis or longstanding contracture, the goal is to teach the patient methods of compensation, as these conditions do not respond to nonsurgical treatment.

It is important to compare initial evaluation scores to mid- and post-treatment scores to assess the outcome and redirect treatment if necessary. Interpretation of a reevaluation that shows improvement following treatment must be tempered, however, with the realization that changes may occur simply as a result of remeasurement. For measurements of ROM to be considered to reflect actual change, the amount of change must exceed measurement error, which was found to be 5° for both the upper and lower extremities (Aalto et al., 2005; Groth et al., 2001). For example, if in a reevaluation the patient has shown an increase of 10° in shoulder flexion, it is considered a minimal improvement, as 5° may be accounted for by measurement error.

EDEMA

Edema, one cause of limited ROM, is quantified using circumferential or volumetric measurements. A millimeter tape is used to measure the circumference of a body part not easily submerged. It is essential to measure at exactly the same place from test to test.

Volumetric measures document changes in the mass of a body part by use of water displacement. It is most often used to measure hand edema. A water vessel that is large enough to allow submersion of the whole hand is used (Fig. 5-57). It has a spillover spout near the top of the water level. When the hand is placed in the vessel, water is displaced and spills out into a graduated beaker. An edematous hand displaces more water than an unswollen hand, so that a lower reading is considered an improvement. Dodds et al. (2004) examined the ability of therapists to orient the extremity consistently within the volumeter and to measure the displaced water accurately. In this protocol, the measurement was done with the participant standing; trunk support was provided by a therapist to maintain a stable position; and a micropipette was used to measure the water. There was high reliability over

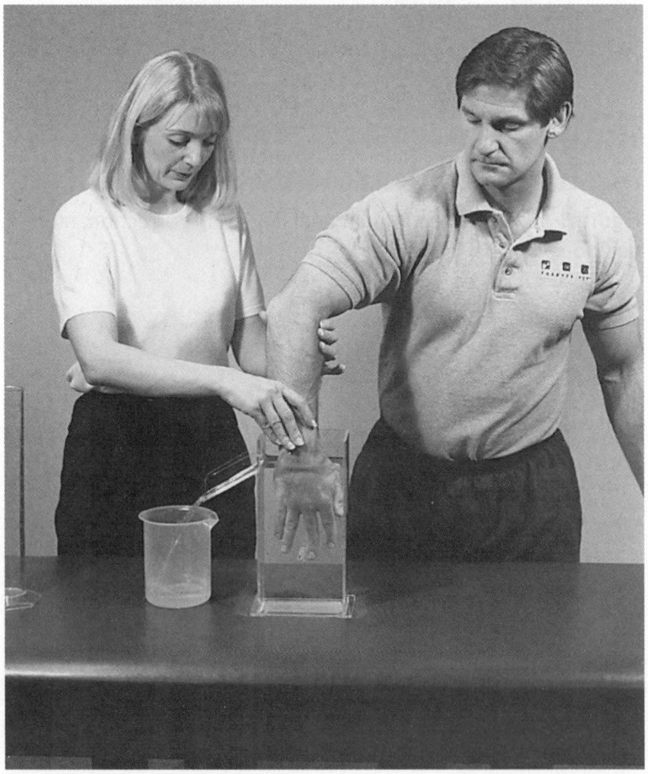

Figure 5-57 Measuring edema of the hand using a volumeter. Note the water being displaced into the graduated beaker as the hand is submerged.

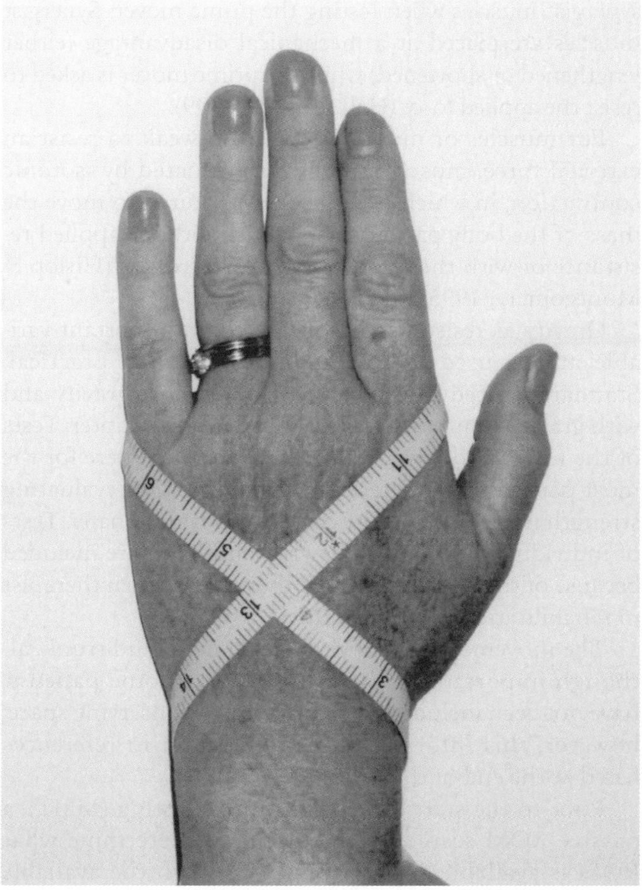

Figure 5-58 Measuring edema of the hand using a tape measure.

two repeated tests on 50 hands, showing a inter-rater reliability of 0.99 (Dodds et al., 2004). To interpret findings, compare the measurement of the affected part with that of its contralateral counterpart. If edema is present, the short-term goal of treatment may be, for example, to decrease edema more than 10 mL, which is slightly more than the identified within-patient variance of 3 mL (Dodds et al., 2004), or to reduce measurement by X mL.

A second method of measuring edema of the whole hand is the figure-of-eight technique (Pellecchia, 2004). Using a ¼-inch wide fiberglass tape measure and the wrist in neutral and fingers adducted, the tape is started at the medial aspect of the wrist just distal to the ulnar styloid. The tape is then run across the ventral surface of the wrist to the most distal point of the radial styloid, then run diagonally across the dorsum of the hand to the fifth metacarpophalangeal joint. The tape is then run across the heads of the metacarpals to the second metacarpophalangeal joint, and then back across the dorsum of the hand to the starting point. The measurement recorded is the distance measured by the tape (Fig. 5-58). The inter-tester and the intra-tester reliabilities for this method were high (r = 0.98–0.99) (Pellecchia, 2004; Leard et al., 2004). When the figure-of-eight measurement was compared to the submersion method, the two methods were highly correlated (r = 0.94–0.95) (Maihafer et al., 2004). The figure-of-eight measurement technique may be especially appropriate in cases of open wounds or skin conditions but would not be appropriate if the edema was localized to a single finger.

PAIN

Pain is another possible cause of ROM limitations. Pain or fear of pain may affect a person's willingness to move. The International Association for the Study of Pain (IASP) defines pain as "an unpleasant sensory and emotional experience associated with actual or potential tissue damage" (Merskey & Bogduk, 1994). Because pain is subjective, self-report measures provide the most valid measure of the experience (Katz & Melzack, 1999). The several self-report measures include the *Visual Analog Scale* (*VAS*), *Faces Test, Color Scale*, and the *Adjective Test* (Gordon et al., 1998). The most frequently used method to measure the intensity of pain is the *VAS* (Gordon et al., 1998; Katz & Melzack, 1999). It is quick and simple to use. It consists of a 10-cm line, with 0 and 10 noted at each end of the line. The zero end is designated as "no pain at all"; the other end is designated as "the worst pain I ever felt" (Fig. 5-59). The patient marks on the line the point that represents the intensity of the pain he or she feels. The score is obtained by measuring the line from the zero point to the patient's mark in cm. For example, if the mark is made at 4.6 cm on the 10-cm line, the score could be 4 or the more exact 4.6, depending on the practice at the facility. There are no norms for this scale, and it cannot be used to compare different patients, but it is useful in monitoring the progress of the same patient over time (Wittink & Michel, 1997).

MUSCLE STRENGTH

The Quick Reference Dictionary for Occupational Therapy defines strength as "demonstrating a degree of muscle power when movement is resisted, as with objects or gravity" (Jacobs & Jacobs, 2004, p. 225). Weakness is a lack or reduction of the power of a muscle or muscle group. When weakness limits or impairs the individual's occupational

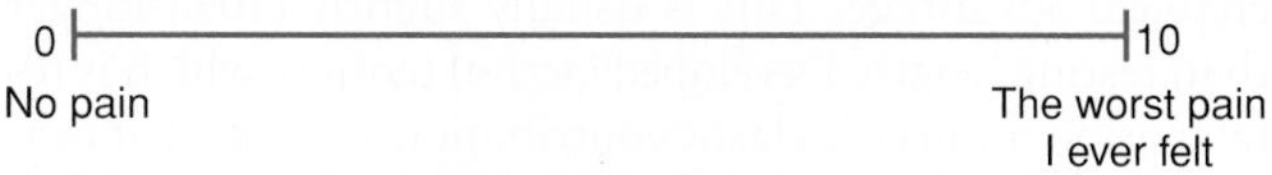

Figure 5-59 A Visual Analog Scale used to quantify the phenomenological experience of pain.

functioning, it is necessary to determine the degree and distribution of weakness to establish an appropriate intervention plan. Treatment can be focused on remediating the weakness, or it can focus on alternative ways of accomplishing the task. Weakness can be manifested in several forms. It can be general, such as with Guillain-Barré syndrome, or it can be local, such as with a peripheral nerve lesion. In the former case, muscles throughout the body are assessed; in the latter case, just the muscles innervated by the involved nerve are tested. In both cases, the muscles to be tested are the ones contributing to the functional limitations on which treatment will focus.

A **maximum voluntary contraction** (MVC), the maximum amount of tension that can be produced under voluntary control, is commonly used to measure strength (Wilmore & Costill, 1999). Because muscle testing is a measurement of voluntary contraction of an isolated muscle or muscle group, strength testing is inappropriate for patients who lack the ability to contract a single muscle or a muscle group in isolation, such as patients who exhibit patterned movement.

In this chapter, a technique called the break test is used. In the break test, the muscle to be tested is positioned at its greatest **mechanical advantage**. Once the extremity is positioned, the patient is asked to hold the position as the tester imparts an external force to overcome the contractile force of the muscle or muscle group using his or her hand. In other words, the therapist tries to break the patient's isometric contraction (Bohannon, 1988).

Another method of strength measurement is the make test, and it is the preferred method when using a hand-held dynamometer (Andrews, Thomas, & Bohannon, 1996). The joint is placed in a gravity-eliminated position, and the hand-held dynamometer is placed perpendicular to the limb segment. The patient is asked to build a maximum contraction against the dynamometer for a 1- to 2-second period and then to hold that contraction against the dynamometer for 4–5 seconds. The recorded measure is the maximum isometric value that was achieved by the patient. This type of measurement is particularly helpful for quantifying antigravity strength (grades 3+ to 5) (Hayes et al., 2002).

The term mechanical advantage refers to the length-tension relationship of a muscle. Total tension of a muscle is the sum of the passive tension exerted by the elastic components in the lengthened muscle and surrounding tissue and the active tension generated by the contractile elements of the contracting muscle (Hall & Brody, 1999). A muscle is able to generate its greatest total tension or sustain the heaviest load when positioned at a length that gives it optimal mechanical advantage. This is usually slightly (10%) longer than resting length. Developed (active) tension, which is total tension minus the elastic contribution, is greatest at resting length but decreases as the muscle shortens or lengthens. The length-tension principle is used to elicit the best response from prime movers during muscle testing. Furthermore, this principle is used to reduce the contribution of synergist muscles when testing the prime mover. Synergist muscles are placed at a mechanical disadvantage (either lengthened or shortened) while the prime mover is asked to resist the applied force (Hall & Brody, 1999).

For muscles or muscle groups too weak to resist an external force, muscle strength is evaluated by isotonic contraction, in which the muscle is required to move the mass of the body part against gravity without applied resistance or with the effect of gravity decreased (Hislop & Montgomery, 1995; Kendall et al., 2005).

Gravity as resistance is considered an important variable and is used to test all motions when practical. Standard procedures for evaluation against gravity and with gravity eliminated are described in this chapter. Tests of the upper and lower extremities described here for the most part are motion tests for the purpose of evaluating strength in terms of ability to perform functionally. Tests of individual muscles in the wrist and hand are included because of the responsibility of the occupational therapist in rehabilitation of hand injuries.

The movements of the face, head, neck, and trunk, although important in the assessment of some patients, have not been included in the interest of conserving space; however, this information can be found in references listed at the end of this chapter.

Prior to the start of manual muscle testing (MMT), a passive ROM scan should be done to determine what ROM is available at each joint. Although the available range is considered to be full ROM for the purposes of muscle testing, a notation should be made of any limitation. The muscle or muscle group is assigned a grade, according to the amount of resistance it can take. Two grading systems are presented here; Table 5-1 equates the Medical Research Council (1976) Oxford system to the descriptive grading system (Clarkson, 2000).

Procedures for Practice 5-3 shows the sequence of steps for testing every muscle or muscle group to ensure reliability and accuracy. There are additional considerations when performing a manual muscle test. First, although fatigue differs for each person and each muscle, a rest of 2 minutes between maximum effort of the same muscle is considered adequate (Milner-Brown, Mellenthin, & Miller, 1986). Second, for the comfort and convenience of the patient, all testing in one position is done before the patient changes to another position. Also, position of head, neck, and proximal parts are usually kept the same from test to test, although preliminary study results indicated that this does not affect tension development (Anderson & Bohannon, 1991; Bohannon, Warren, & Cogman, 1991).

Reliability

Reliability is essential for meaningful evaluation. Most important to the reliability of the scores of repeated tests is strict adherence to the exact procedures of testing. In

Table 5-1. Muscle Testing Grading System

Grade	Definition	Description
5	Normal	The part moves through full ROM against gravity and takes maximal resistance.
4	Good	The part moves through full ROM against gravity and takes moderate resistance.
4−	Good minus	The part moves through full ROM against gravity and takes less than moderate resistance.
3+	Fair plus	The part moves through full ROM against gravity and takes minimal resistance before it breaks.
3	Fair	The part moves through full ROM against gravity and is unable to take any added resistance.
3−	Fair minus	The part moves less than full range of motion against gravity.
2+	Poor plus	The part moves through full ROM in a gravity-eliminated plane and takes minimal resistance, then breaks.
2	Poor	The part moves through full ROM in a gravity-eliminated plane with no added resistance.
2−	Poor minus	The part moves less than full ROM in a gravity-eliminated plane.
1	Trace	Tension is palpated in the muscle or tendon, but no motion occurs at the joint.
0	Zero	No tension is palpated in the muscle or tendon.

PROCEDURES FOR PRACTICE 5-3

Muscle Testing Procedures

1. Explain the procedure and demonstrate the desired movement.
2. Position the patient so the direction of movement will be against gravity.
3. Stabilize proximal to the joint that will move to prevent substitutions.
4. Instruct the patient to move actively to the end position. If the patient cannot move actively against gravity, place the patient in a gravity-eliminated position and ask the patient to move actively in this position.
5. If the patient can move actively against gravity, tell the patient to hold the contraction at the end position.
6. Apply resistance:
   - to the distal end of the segment into which the muscle inserts
   - in the direction the movement came from
   - by starting with light resistance and increase to maximal resistance over a 2- to 3-second period
7. Palpate over the prime mover to determine whether the muscle is contracting or whether gravity and/or synergistic muscles are substituting.
8. Record the appropriate grade according to the resistance tolerated before the muscle broke or by the amount of movement achieved without resistance in an against-gravity or gravity-eliminated position.

addition, reliability of muscle testing scores is affected by the interest and cooperation of the patient and by the experience and tone of voice of the tester (Johannson, Kent, & Shepard, 1983). The most suitable environment is free of distractions, is at a comfortable temperature, and has proper lighting. Other factors known to affect outcome are posture, fatigue, the patient's ability to understand directions, the therapist's operational definitions of various grades, and test positions (Kendall et al., 2005). For reliability, these variables must be controlled from test to test and among therapists at the same facility. It is necessary for the inexperienced therapist to develop a kinesthetic sense of minimal, moderate, and maximal resistances by working with experienced therapists, each testing the same patient and discussing the grade to be assigned.

Manual muscle testing (MMT) is a valid and reliable procedure to measure muscle strength (Herbison et al., 1996; Marx, Bombardier, & Wright, 1999; Schwartz et al., 1992). A study of reliability for testing intrinsic hand muscles found the correlation for intra-rater reliability to range from .71 to .96, and from .72 to .93 for inter-rater reliability (Brandsma et al., 1995). Florence et al. (1992) performed MMT on patients with Duchenne's muscular dystrophy. Using a standard method of testing and the modified Medical Research Council grading scale (Table 5-1), reliability for muscle grades 0 to 5 ranged from .80 to .99. The most reliable graders were 3 and below, with the least reliable grades being 3+ (.80), 4- (.83), and 5- (.83), those that involve a developed kinesthetic sense of minimal, moderate, and maximal resistance.

CLINICAL REASONING IN OCCUPATIONAL THERAPY PRACTICE

Planning a Muscle Testing Strategy

Testing of shoulder, elbow, and lower extremity musculature may require the patient to lie prone or supine or to sit up, depending on whether you are testing in an antigravity or gravity-eliminated position. It would be too tiring for the patient to keep switching postures between lying and sitting during a muscle test as presented in this chapter. Devise a practical strategy you will use in muscle testing that will be least fatiguing for a patient. The strategy will list the order of muscles to be tested and for what grade, according to position.

Recording Muscle Strength Scores

The grade is accurately recorded in the appropriate place on a form that has columns to record grades for both the right and left sides of the body. The therapist must sign and date each test; if a test continues over several days, the form should reflect that. A sample form is presented in Figure 5-60. On that form, the peripheral nerve and spinal segmental levels are listed beside each muscle to assist the therapist in interpreting the results of the muscle test.

On the pages that follow, the reader will find narrative and pictorial descriptions to help in understanding and practicing measurement of upper extremity strength.

Patient's Name: ______________________ Age: ________

LEFT | RIGHT

Date	Date		Date	Date
		Scapula		
		ELEVATION		
		Upper trapezius (accessory) CN XI, C3-4		
		Levator scapulae (dorsal scapular) C5, C3-4		
		DEPRESSION		
		Lower trapezius (accessory) CN XI, C3-4		
		Latissimus dorsi (thoracodorsal) C6-8		
		ADDUCTION		
		Middle trapezius (accessory) CN XI, C3-4		
		Rhomboids (dorsal scapular) C5		
		ABDUCTION		
		Serratus anterior (long thoracic) C5-7		
		Shoulder		
		FLEXION		
		Anterior deltoid (axillary) C5-6		
		Coracobrachialis (musculocutaneous) C5-6		
		Pectoralis major-clavicular (pectoral) C5-6		
		Biceps (musculocutaneous) C5-6		
		EXTENSION		
		Latissimus dorsi (thoracodorsal) C6-8		
		Teres major (lower subscapular) C5-6		
		Posterior deltoid (axillary) C5-6		
		Triceps-long head (radial) C7-8		
		ABDUCTION		
		Supraspinatus (suprascapular) C5-6		
		Middle deltoid (axillary) C5-6		
		ADDUCTION		
		Latissimus dorsi (thoracodorsal) C6-8		
		Teres major (lower subscapular) C5-6		
		Pectoralis major (pectoral) C5-T1		
		HORIZONTAL ABDUCTION		
		Posterior deltoid (axillary) C5-6		

Figure 5-60 Sample form for recording manual muscle strength.

Patient's Name: ______________________ Age: __________

LEFT Date	LEFT Date		RIGHT Date	RIGHT Date
		HORIZONTAL ADDUCTION		
		Pectoralis major (pectoral) C5-T1		
		Anterior deltoid (axillary) C5-6		
		EXTERNAL ROTATION		
		Infraspinatus (suprascapular) C5-6		
		Teres minor (axillary) C5-6		
		Posterior deltoid (axillary) C5-6		
		INTERNAL ROTATION		
		Subscapularis (upper, lower subscapular) C5-7		
		Teres major (lower subscapular) C6-7		
		Latissimus dorsi (thoracodorsal) C6-8		
		Pectoralis major (pectoral) C5-T1		
		Anterior deltoid (axillary) C5-6		
		Elbow		
		FLEXION		
		Biceps (musculocutaneous) C5-6		
		Brachioradialis (radial) C5-7		
		Brachialis (musculocutaneous) C5-6 (radial) C7-8		
		EXTENSION		
		Triceps (radial) C6-8		
		Forearm		
		PRONATION		
		Pronator teres (median) C6-7		
		Pronator quadratus (median) C8-T1		
		SUPINATION		
		Supinator (radial) C5-6		
		Biceps (musculocutaneous) C5-6		
		Wrist		
		EXTENSION		
		Ext. carpi radialis longus (radial) C6-7		
		Ext. carpi radialis brevis (radial) C7-8		
		Ext. carpi ulnaris (radial) C7-8		
		FLEXION		
		Flexor carpi radialis (median) C6-7		
		Palmaris longus (median) C7-8		
		Flexor carpi ulnaris (ulnar) C8-T1		
		Fingers		
		DIP FLEXION		
		1st flexor profundus (median) C8-T1		
		2nd flexor profundus (median) C8-T1		
		3rd flexor profundus (ulnar) C8-T1		
		4th flexor profundus (ulnar) C8-T1		
		5TH MP FLEXION		
		Flexor digiti minimi (ulnar) C8-T1		
		PIP FLEXION		
		1st flexor superficialis (median) C7-T1		
		2nd flexor superficialis (median) C7-T1		
		3rd flexor superficialis (median) C7-T1		
		4th flexor superficialis (median) C7-T1		
		ABDUCTION		
		1st palmar interosseus (ulnar) C8-T1		
		2nd palmar interosseus (ulnar) C8-T1		
		3rd palmar interosseus (ulnar) C8-T1		

Figure 5-60 *(continued)*

Patient's Name: ______________________ Age: ________

LEFT | RIGHT

Date	Date		Date	Date
		ABDUCTION		
		1st dorsal interosseus (ulnar) C8-T1		
		2nd dorsal interosseus (ulnar) C8-T1		
		3rd dorsal interosseus (ulnar) C8-T1		
		4th dorsal interosseus (ulnar) C8-T1		
		MP EXTENSION		
		1st extensor digitorum (radial) C7-8		
		2nd extensor digitorum (radial) C7-8		
		3rd extensor digitorum (radial) C7-8		
		4th extensor digitorum (radial) C7-8		
		Extensor digiti minimi (radial) C7-8		
		IP EXTENSION		
		1st lumbrical (median) C8-T1		
		2nd lumbrical (median) C8-T1		
		3rd lumbrical (ulnar) C8-T1		
		4th lumbrical (ulnar) C8-T1		
		Thumb		
		EXTENSION		
		Extensor pollicis longus (radial) C7-8		
		Extensor pollicis brevis (radial) C7-8		
		FLEXION		
		Flexor pollicis longus (median) C8-T1		
		Flexor pollicis brevis (median) C8-T1		
		ABDUCTION		
		Abductor pollicis longus (radial) C7-8		
		Abductor pollicis brevis (median) C8-T1		
		ADDUCTOR		
		Adductor pollicis (ulnar) C8-T1		
		OPPOSITION		
		Opponens pollicis (median) C8-T1		
		Opponens digiti minimi (ulnar) C8-T1		
		Hip		
		FLEXION		
		Iliopsoas (femoral) L2-3		
		EXTENSION		
		Gluteus maximus (inf. gluteal) L5-S2		
		Knee		
		FLEXION		
		Hamstrings (tibial) L5-S2		
		EXTENSION		
		Quadriceps (femoral) L2-4		
		Ankle		
		DORSIFLEXION		
		Tibialis anterior (deep peroneal) L4-S1		
		Extensor digitorum longus (deep peroneal) L4-S1		
		Extensor hallucis longus (deep peroneal) L4-S1		
		PLANTARFLEXION		
		Gastrocnemius (tibial) S1-2		
		Soleus (tibial) S1-2		

Therapist's signature: ______________________ Date: ____________

Reprinted with permission from Pansky, B. (1996). *Review of Gross Anatomy* (6th ed.) New York: McGraw-Hill.

Figure 5-60 *(continued)*

MEASUREMENT OF THE PROXIMAL UPPER EXTREMITY

Scapular Elevation

Prime Movers

Upper trapezius

Levator scapulae

Against-Gravity Position (Fig. 5-61)

Start Position

Patient sitting erect with arms at side.

Stabilize

Trunk is stabilized against the plinth or chair back.

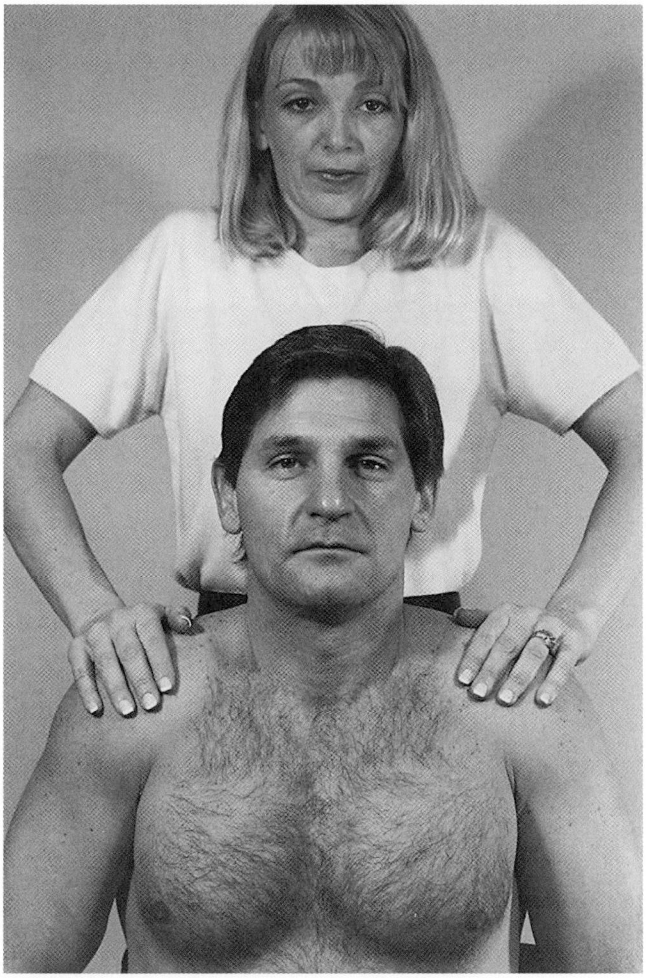

Figure 5-61 Scapular elevation against gravity.

Instruction

"Lift your shoulders toward your ears. Don't let me push them down."

Resistance

The therapist places his or her hands over each acromion and pushes down toward scapular depression. A normal trapezius of an adult cannot be broken.

Substitution

A substitution is the use of an alternate muscle or position a patient may use to complete a motion. In this case, it could appear that the patient's shoulders elevated if he or she pushed on the knees with his or her hands.

Gravity-Eliminated Position (Fig. 5-62)

Start Position

Prone with arms at side and therapist supporting under the shoulder.

Stabilize

The trunk is stabilized against the mat.

Instruction

"Lift your shoulder toward your ear."

Palpation

The upper trapezius is palpated on the shoulder at the curve of the neck. The levator scapulae is palpated posterior to the sternocleidomastoideus on the lateral side of the neck.

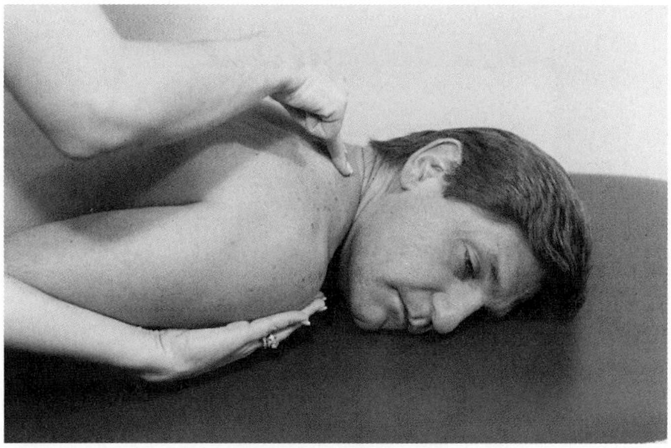

Figure 5-62 Scapular elevation, gravity eliminated.

Scapular Depression

Prime Movers

Lower trapezius

Latissimus dorsi

Resistance Test (Fig. 5-63)

Start Position

This movement is tested in a gravity-eliminated position as the patient cannot be positioned to move against gravity. The patient lies prone with arms by the sides.

Stabilize

The trunk is stabilized by the mat.

Instruction

"Reach your hand down toward your feet."

Resistance

The therapist's hand cups the inferior angle of the scapula; the therapist pushes up toward scapular elevation. When the inferior angle is not easily accessible because of tissue bulk, apply resistance at the distal humerus if the shoulder joint is stable and pain free.

Palpation

Palpate the lower trapezius lateral to the vertebral column as it passes diagonally from the lower thoracic vertebrae to the spine of the scapula. Palpate the latissimus dorsi along the posterior rib cage or in the posterior axilla as it attaches to the humerus.

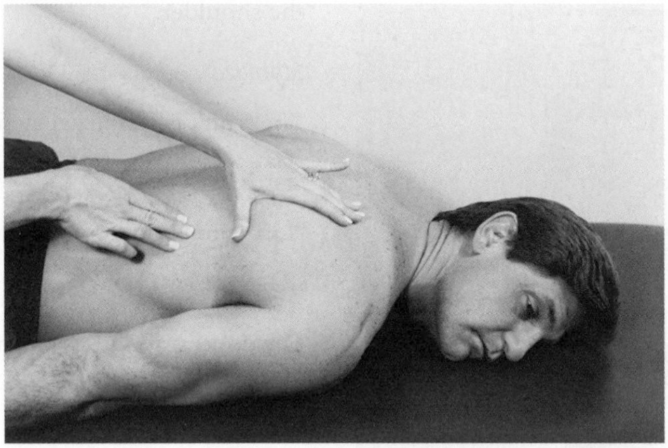

Figure 5-63 Scapular depression.

Scapular Adduction: Retraction

Prime Movers

Middle trapezius

Rhomboids

Against-Gravity Position for the Middle Trapezius (Fig. 5-64)

Start Position

Prone on a mat with the shoulder abducted to 90° and the elbow flexed to 90°.

Stabilize

The trunk is stabilized against the mat. Additional stabilization over the contralateral scapula provides counterpressure during action and resistance.

Instruction

"Raise your elbow toward the ceiling. Don't let me push it down."

Resistance

Apply resistance laterally at the vertebral border of the scapula or, if the shoulder is stable and pain free, downward at the distal humerus.

Palpation

With your hand over the vertebral border of the scapula, feel to see whether the scapula stays adducted during resistance. Palpate the middle trapezius between the vertebral column and vertebral border of the scapula at the level of the spine of the scapula.

Against-Gravity Position for the Rhomboids (Fig. 5-65)

Start Position

Prone on the mat with the shoulder internally rotated and with the back of the hand resting on the lumbar region.

Stabilize

The trunk is stabilized against the mat. Additional stabilization over the contralateral scapula will provide counterpressure during action and resistance.

Instruction

"Lift your hand off of your back. Don't let me push it down."

Resistance

Apply downward resistance against the distal humerus or, if the shoulder is unstable or painful, against the vertebral border of the scapula in the direction of scapular abduction.

Palpation

Palpate the rhomboids along the vertebral border of the scapula near the inferior angle.

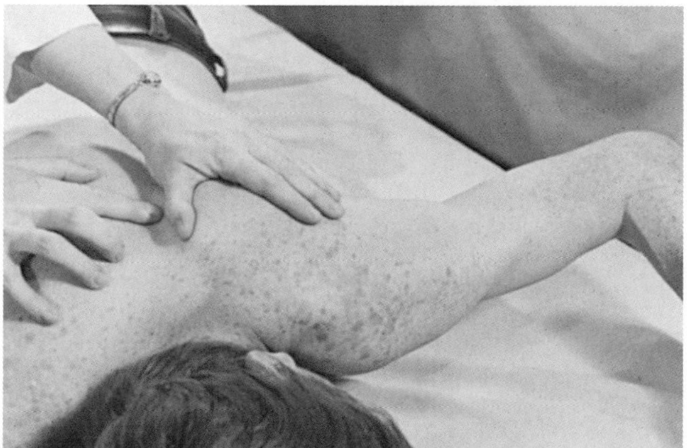

Figure 5-64 Scapular adduction, test for middle trapezius.

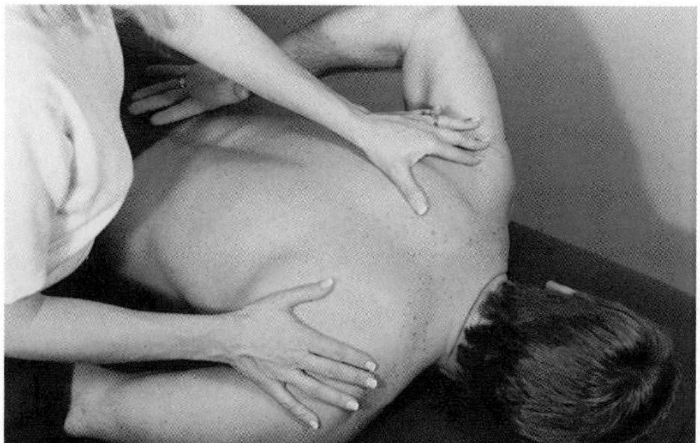

Figure 5-65 Scapular adduction, test for rhomboids.

Gravity-Eliminated Position for the Middle Trapezius and Rhomboids (Fig. 5-66)

Start Position

Sitting erect with the humerus abducted to 90° and supported.

Stabilize

The trunk is stabilized by the chair.

Instruction

"Try to move your arm backward."

Grading

If the scapula moves toward the spine, give a grade of 2. If no movement is noted, palpate the scapular adductors.

Palpation

Same as previously described.

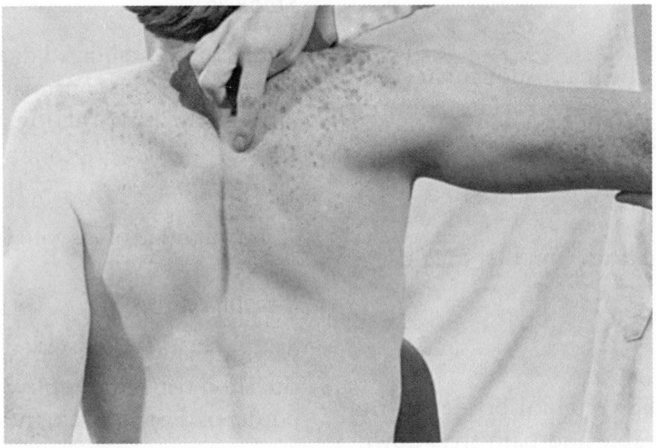

Figure 5-66 Scapular adduction, gravity eliminated. The therapist is pointing to the middle trapezius.

Scapular Abduction: Protraction

Prime Mover

Serratus anterior

Against-Gravity Position (Fig. 5-67)

Start Position

Supine with the humerus flexed to 90°. The elbow may be flexed or extended.

Stabilize

The trunk is stabilized on the mat.

Instruction

"Reach your arm toward the ceiling."

Resistance

According to the rule, resistance should be applied along the axillary border of the scapula. Because it is difficult to apply resistance there, therapists often resist this motion either by grasping the distal humerus or by cupping the hand over the patient's elbow and pushing down or back toward scapular adduction. ***Of course, this method is not used if the glenohumeral joint is unstable or painful.***

Gravity-Eliminated Position (Fig. 5-68)

Start Position

Sitting erect with the humerus flexed to 90° and supported.

Stabilize

The trunk is stabilized against the chair.

Instruction

"Try to reach your arm forward."

Grading

Movement of the scapula into abduction receives a grade of 2. If no movement occurs, palpate the serratus anterior.

Palpation

Palpate the serratus anterior on the lateral ribs just lateral to the inferior angle of the scapula.

Substitution

In the gravity-eliminated position, this motion can be achieved by inching the arm forward on a supportive surface using the finger flexors.

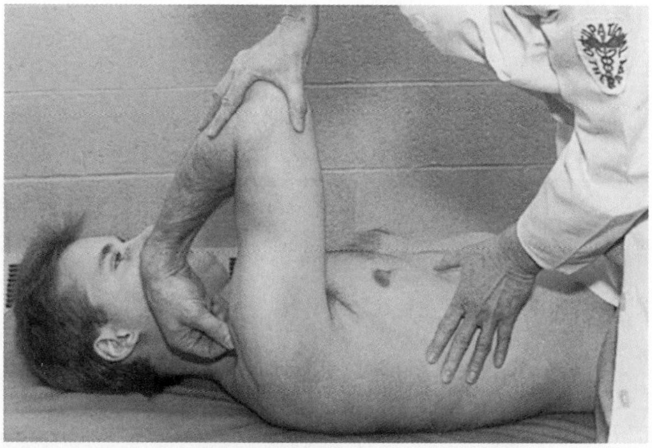

Figure 5-67 Scapular abduction against gravity.

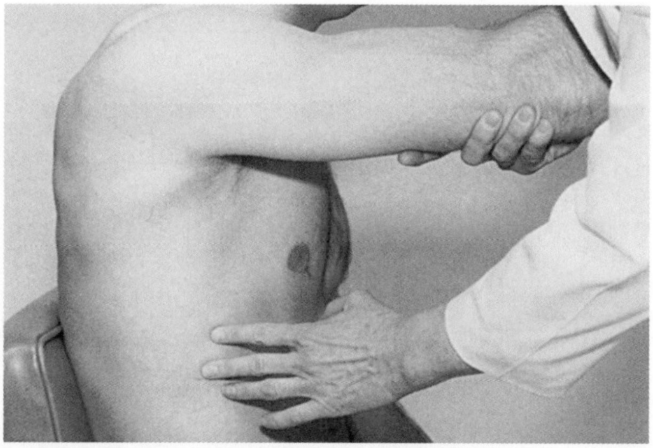

Figure 5-68 Scapular abduction, gravity eliminated.

Shoulder Flexion

Prime Movers

Anterior deltoid
Coracobrachialis
Pectoralis major, clavicular head
Biceps, both heads

Against-Gravity Position (Fig. 5-69)

Start Position

Sitting in a chair with the arm down at the side in midposition.

Stabilize

Over the clavicle and the scapula.

Instruction

"Lift your arm in front of you to shoulder height. Don't let me push it down."

Resistance

The therapist's hand, placed over the distal end of the humerus, pushes down toward extension. Movement above 90° involves scapular rotation; these motions are separated for muscle testing, although they are not separated for ROM measurement.

Substitutions

Shoulder abductors, scapular elevation, or trunk extension.

Gravity-Eliminated Position (Fig. 5-70)

Start Position

Side-lying with the arm along the side of the body in midposition; therapist supports the arm under the elbow.

Instruction

"Try to move your arm so your hand is at the level of your shoulder."

Palpation

Palpate the anterior deltoid immediately anterior to the glenohumeral joint. Coracobrachialis may be palpated medially to the tendon of the long head of the biceps, which is palpated on the anterior aspect of the humerus. The clavicular head of the pectoralis major may be palpated below the clavicle on its way to insert on the humerus below the anterior deltoid.

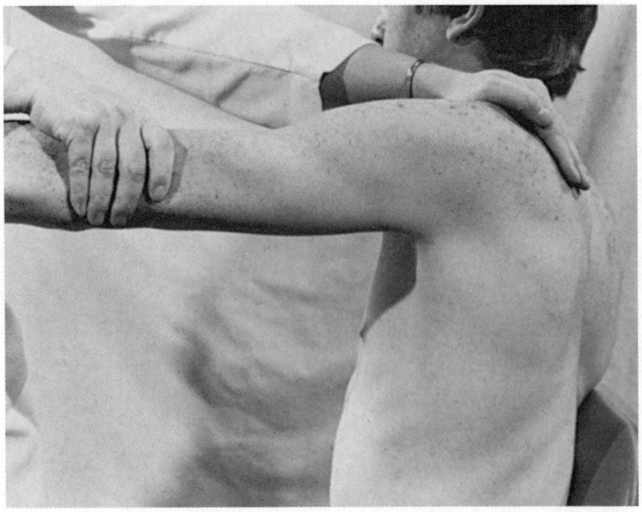

Figure 5-69 Shoulder flexion against gravity.

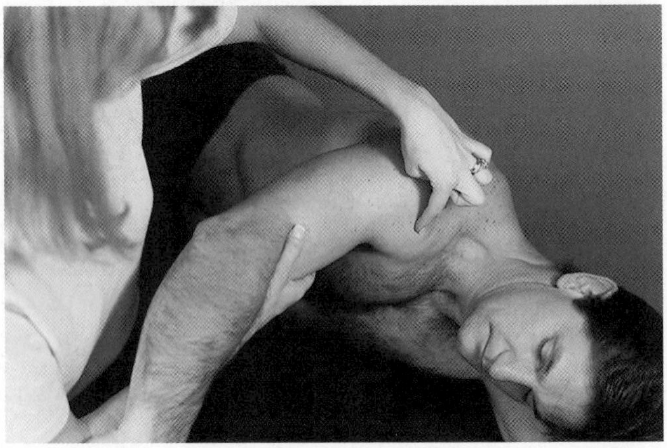

Figure 5-70 Shoulder flexion, gravity eliminated.

Shoulder Extension

Prime Movers

Latissimus dorsi

Teres major

Posterior deltoid

Triceps, long head

Against-Gravity Position (Fig. 5-71)

Start Position

Sitting with the arm by the side and the humerus internally rotated.

Stabilize

Over the clavicle and scapula; make sure the patient remains upright.

Instruction

"Move your arm straight back as far as it will go. Keep your palm facing the back wall."

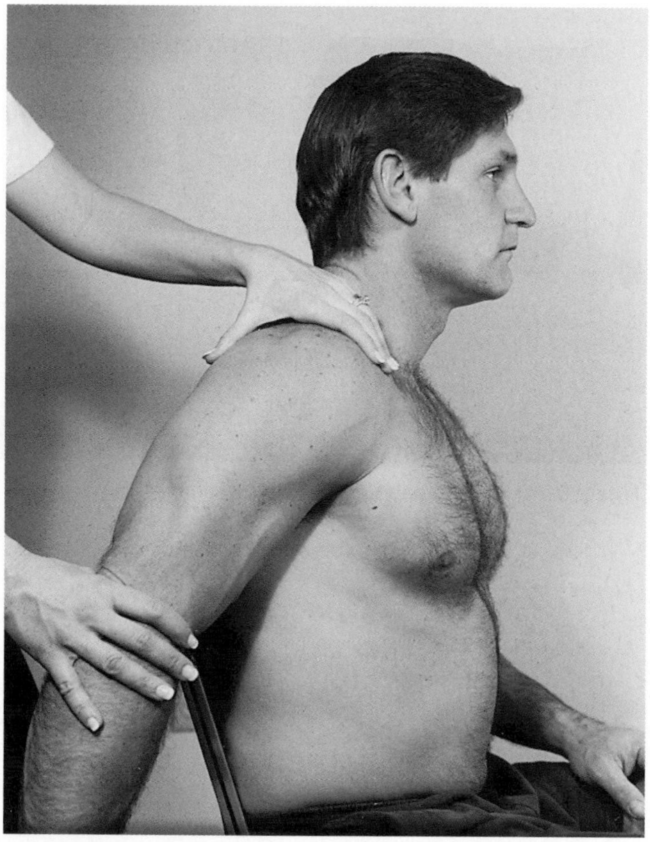

Figure 5-71 Shoulder extension against gravity.

Resistance

The therapist's hand, placed over the distal end of the humerus, pushes forward toward flexion.

Substitutions

Shoulder abductors, tipping the shoulder forward, bending the trunk forward.

Gravity-Eliminated Position (Fig. 5-72)

Start Position

Side-lying with the arm along the side of the body and in internal rotation. Therapist supports the elbow during the motion.

Instruction

"Try to move your arm backward."

Palpation

The latissimus dorsi and teres major form the posterior border of the axilla. The latissimus dorsi is inferior to the teres major. The posterior deltoid is immediately posterior to the glenohumeral joint. The triceps are palpated on the posterior aspect of the humerus.

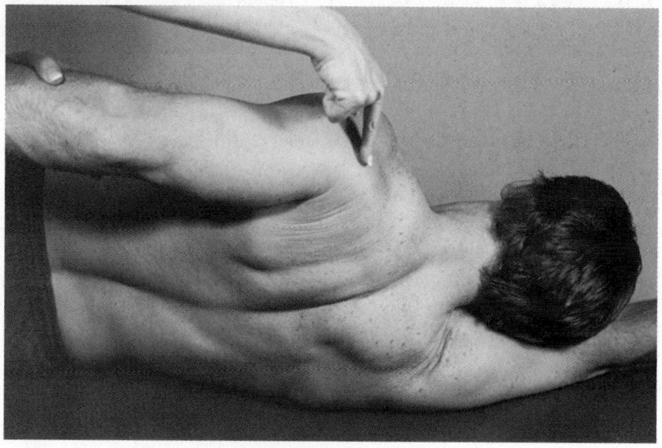

Figure 5-72 Shoulder extension, gravity eliminated.

Shoulder Abduction

Prime Movers

Supraspinatus
Middle deltoid

Against-Gravity Position (Fig. 5-73)

Start Position

Sitting erect with the arm down at the side and in midposition.

Stabilize

Over the clavicle and the scapula.

Instruction

"Raise your arm out to the side to shoulder level. Don't let me push it down."

Resistance

The therapist's hand, placed over the distal end of the humerus, pushes the humerus down toward the body. Movement above 90° involves scapular rotation and is not measured.

Substitutions

The long head of the biceps can substitute if the humerus is allowed to move into external rotation; trunk lateral flexion.

Gravity-Eliminated Position (Fig. 5-74)

Start Position

Supine with the arm supported at the side in midposition. The therapist supports the elbow during the motion.

Instruction

"Try to move your arm out to the side."

Palpation

The supraspinatus lies too deep for easy palpation. Palpate the middle deltoid below the acromion and lateral to the glenohumeral joint.

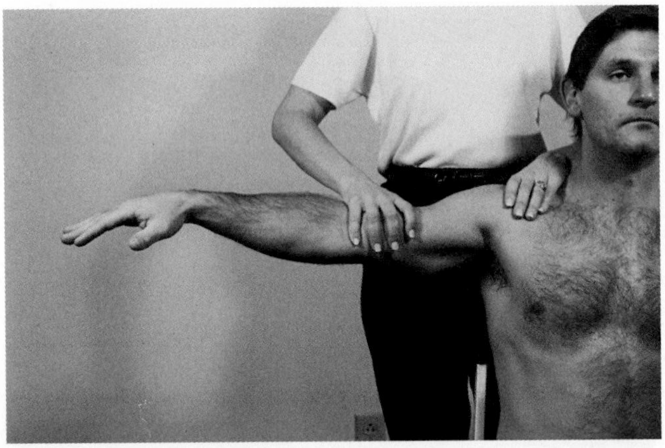

Figure 5-73 Shoulder abduction against gravity.

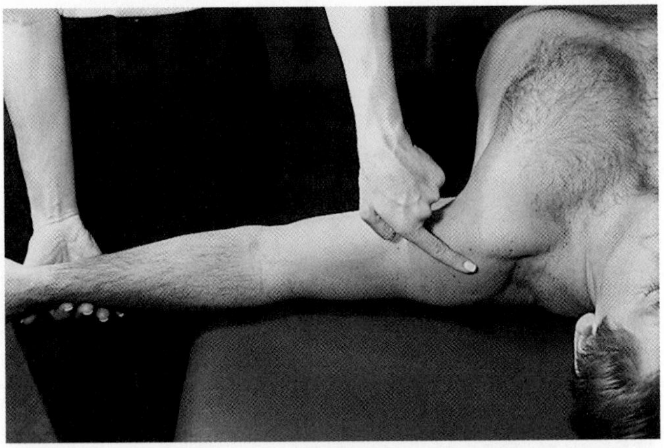

Figure 5-74 Shoulder abduction, gravity eliminated.

Shoulder Adduction

Prime Movers

Pectoralis major

Teres major

Latissimus dorsi

Gravity-Eliminated Position (Fig. 5-75)

The patient cannot be positioned for this motion against gravity.

Start Position

Supine with the humerus abducted to 90° and the forearm in midposition.

Stabilize

The trunk is stabilized by the mat.

Instruction

"Bring your arm down to your side, and don't let me pull it away."

Resistance

The therapist's hand, placed on the medial side of the distal end of the humerus, attempts to pull the humerus away from the patient's body.

Palpation

The pectoralis major forms the anterior border of the axilla, where it may be easily palpated. Palpation of the teres major and the latissimus dorsi is described earlier in the chapter.

Grading

Antigravity grades can only be estimated; a question mark should be entered beside the grade on the form. With experience, the therapist develops the skill to estimate reliably.

Substitutions

On a supporting surface, the arm can be inched down using the finger flexors.

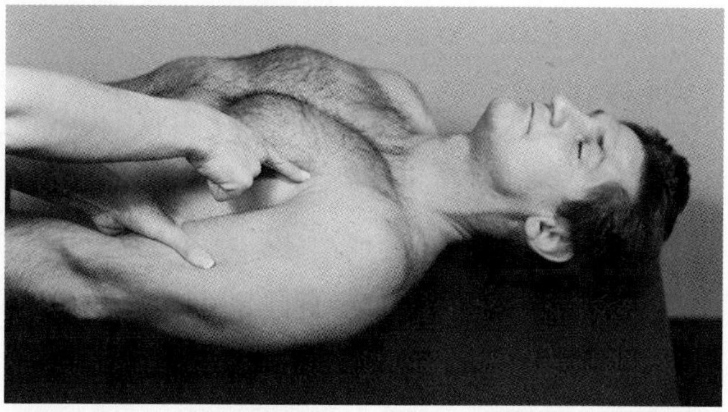

Figure 5-75 Shoulder adduction.

Shoulder Horizontal Abduction

Prime Mover

Posterior deltoid

Against-Gravity Position (Fig. 5-76)

Start Position

Prone with the arm over the edge of the plinth. The shoulder is abducted to 90°, and the elbow is flexed to 90°.

Stabilize

The scapula and trunk are stabilized by the mat. Counterpressure over the contralateral scapula is helpful during action and resistance.

Instruction

"Raise your elbow toward the ceiling."

Resistance

The therapist's hand, placed on the posterior surface of the distal end of the humerus, pushes the arm down toward horizontal adduction.

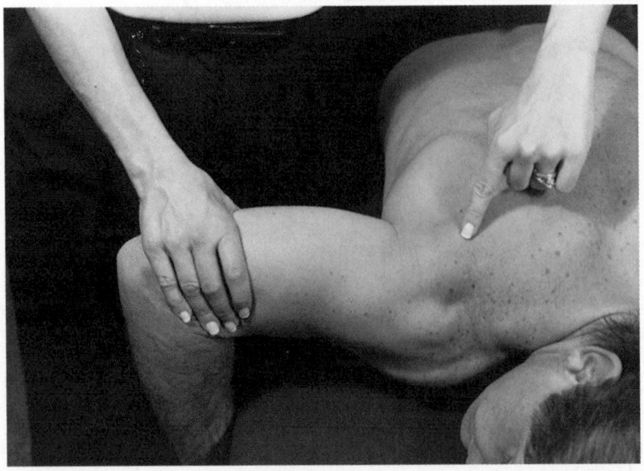

Figure 5-76 Shoulder horizontal abduction against gravity.

Gravity-Eliminated Position (Fig. 5-77)

Start Position

Sitting in a chair with the humerus supported in 90° of flexion and the elbow straight. The therapist supports the elbow.

Stabilize

The trunk is stabilized against the back of the chair.

Instruction

"Try to move your arm out to the side."

Palpation

Palpate the posterior deltoid immediately posterior to the glenohumeral joint.

Substitution

Trunk rotation.

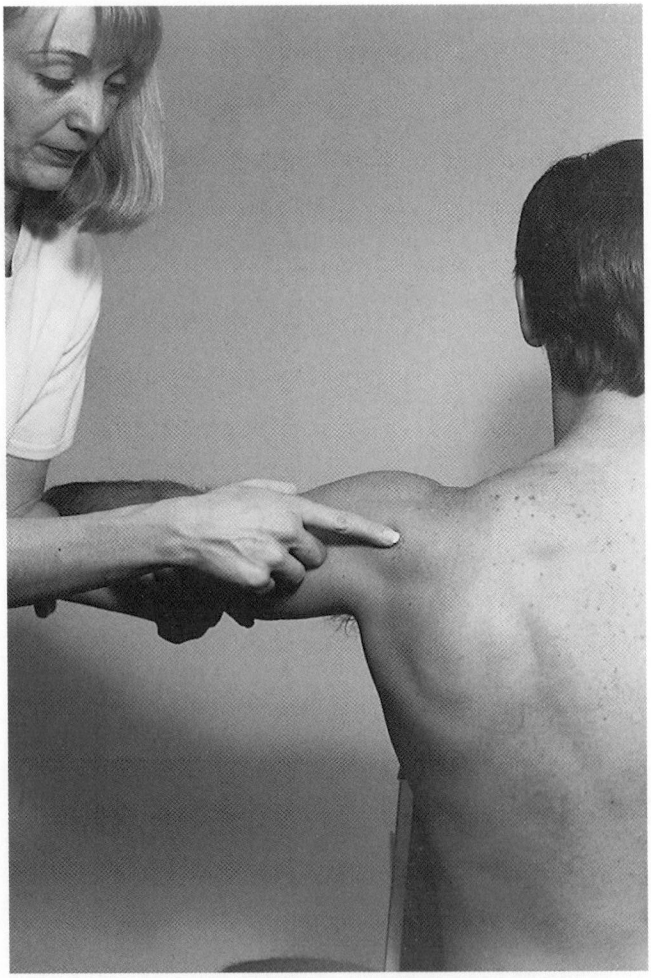

Figure 5-77 Shoulder horizontal abduction, gravity eliminated.

Shoulder Horizontal Adduction

Prime Movers

Pectoralis major
Anterior deltoid

Against-Gravity Position (Fig. 5-78)

Start Position

Supine with the humerus abducted to 90° in neutral rotation and the elbow extended.

Stabilize

The table stabilizes the scapula and trunk. If the elbow extensors are weak, be sure to support the distal end of the forearm so the hand doesn't fall into the patient's face during horizontal adduction.

Instruction

"Move your arm in front of you and across your chest."

Resistance

The therapist's hand, placed on the anterior surface of the distal end of the humerus, pulls the arm out toward horizontal abduction.

Gravity-Eliminated Position (Fig. 5-79)

Start Position

Sitting in a chair with the arm abducted to 90°.

Stabilize

The trunk is stabilized against the back of the chair. The therapist supports the arm under the elbow.

Instruction

"Try to bring your arm across your chest."

Palpation

Palpate the pectoralis major along the anterior border of the axilla. The anterior deltoid is immediately anterior to the glenohumeral joint below the acromion process and superior to the pectoralis major.

Substitutions

Trunk rotation can substitute. The arm can be inched across a supporting surface using the finger flexors.

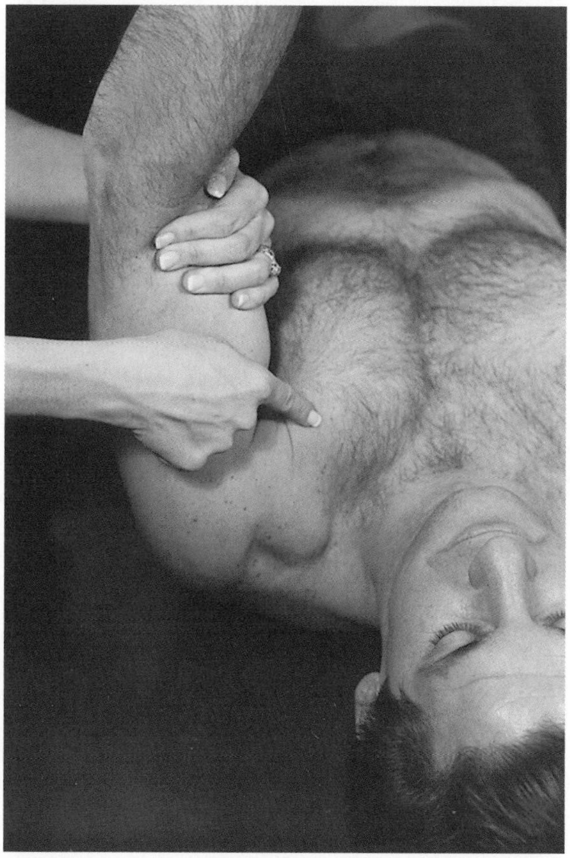

Figure 5-78 Shoulder horizontal adduction against gravity.

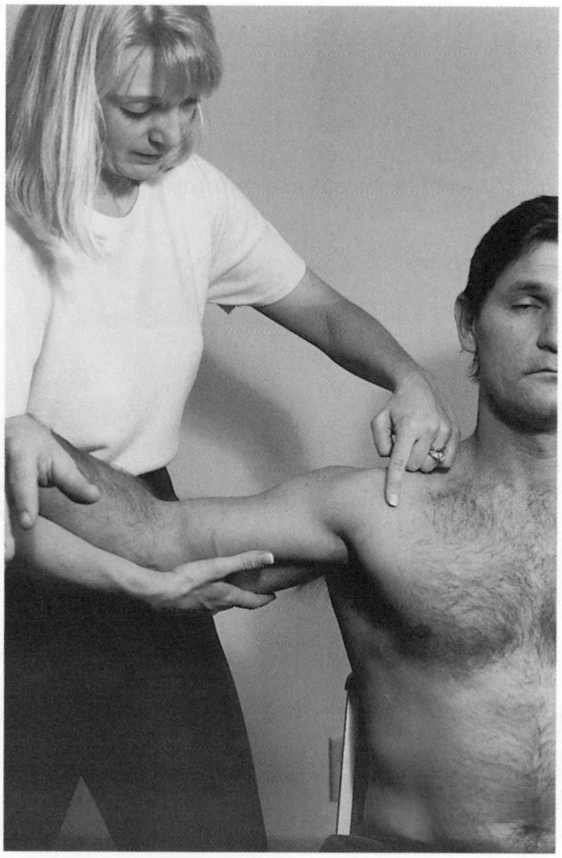

Figure 5-79 Shoulder horizontal adduction, gravity eliminated.

Shoulder External Rotation

Prime Movers

Infraspinatus

Teres minor

Posterior deltoid

Against-Gravity Position (Fig. 5-80)

Start Position

Prone with the humerus abducted to 90° and supported by the mat. The elbow is flexed to 90° and is hanging over the edge of the table.

Stabilize

The humerus is held just proximal to the elbow to allow only rotation.

Instruction

"Lift the back of your hand toward the ceiling."

Resistance

The therapist's hand, placed on the dorsal surface of the distal end of the forearm, pushes toward the floor. The therapist's other hand keeps the patient's elbow supported and flexed to 90° to prevent supination.

Substitutions

Scapula adduction combined with downward rotation can substitute. The triceps may substitute when resistance is applied.

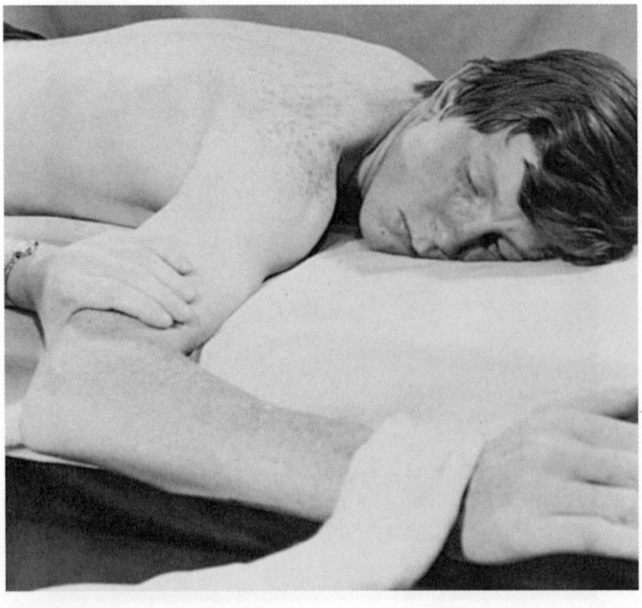

Figure 5-80 Shoulder external rotation against gravity.

Gravity-Eliminated Position (Fig. 5-81)

Start Position

Prone with the entire arm hanging over the edge of the mat. The arm is in internal rotation.

Stabilize

The trunk and scapula are stabilized on the plinth.

Instruction

"Try to turn your palm outward."

Palpation

Palpate the infraspinatus inferior to the spine of the scapula. Palpate the teres minor between the posterior deltoid and the axillary border of the scapula; it is superior to the teres major. Palpation of the posterior deltoid was described earlier.

Substitution

Supination may be mistaken for external rotation in a gravity-eliminated position.

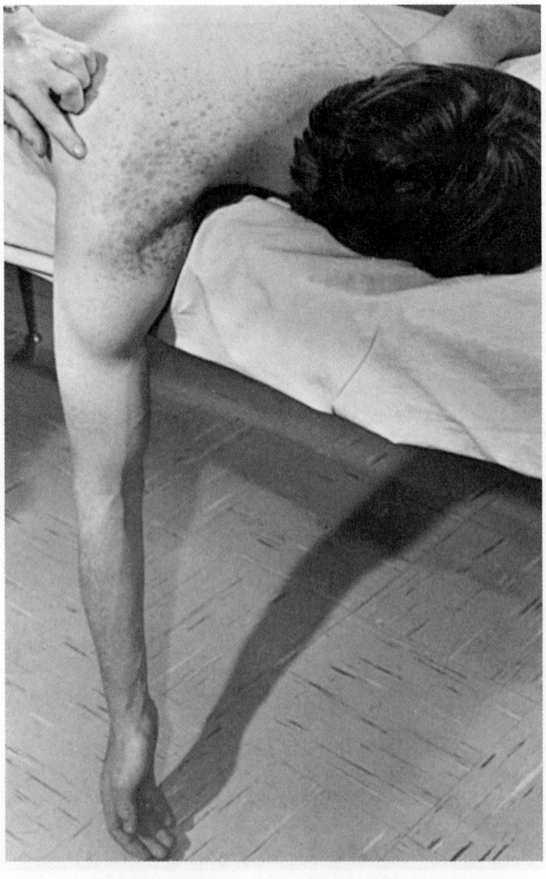

Figure 5-81 Shoulder external rotation, gravity eliminated.

Alternative Gravity-Eliminated Position (Fig. 5-82)

Start Position

Sitting in a chair with the humerus adducted to the side and the elbow flexed to 90°.

Stabilize

The distal end of the humerus is held against the body to allow only rotation.

Instruction

"Try to move the back of your hand out to the side."

Palpation

Same as previously described.

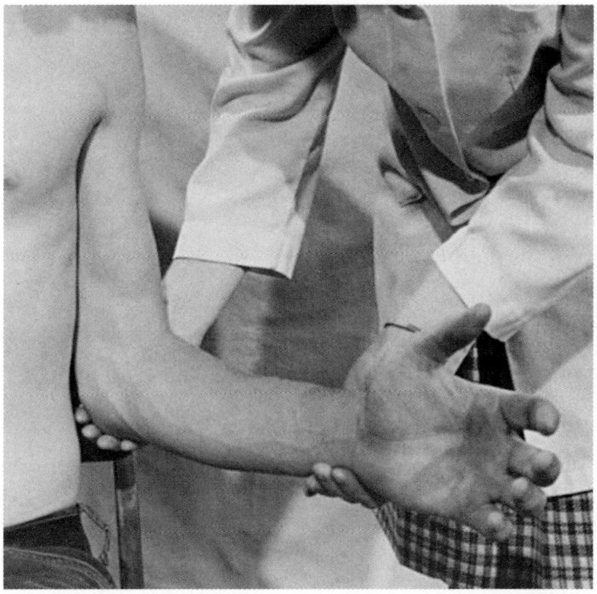

Figure 5-82 Shoulder external rotation, alternative position with gravity eliminated.

Shoulder Internal Rotation

Prime Movers

Subscapularis

Teres major

Latissimus dorsi

Pectoralis major

Anterior deltoid

Against-Gravity Position (Fig. 5-83)

Start Position

Prone with the humerus abducted to 90° and supported by the mat. The elbow is flexed to 90° and hangs over the edge of the mat.

Stabilize

The humerus is held just proximal to the elbow to allow only rotation.

Instruction

"Lift the palm of your hand toward the ceiling."

Resistance

The therapist's hand, placed on the volar surface of the distal end of the forearm, pushes toward the floor. The therapist's other hand keeps the patient's elbow supported and flexed to 90° to prevent supination.

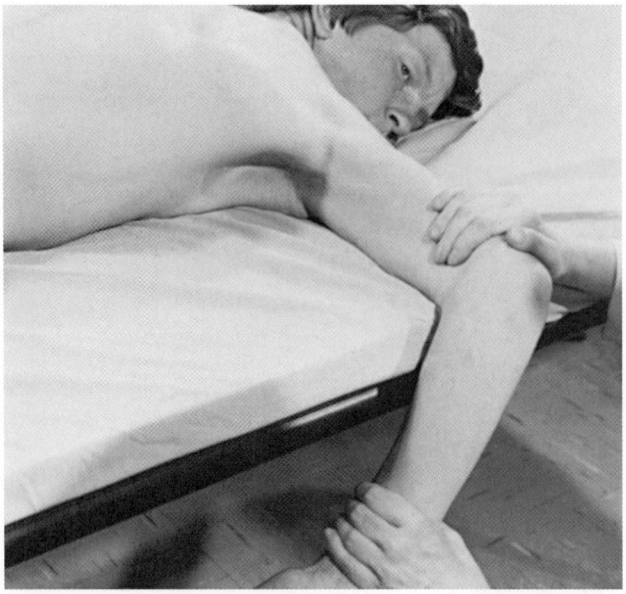

Figure 5-83 Shoulder internal rotation against gravity.

Substitutions

Scapular abduction combined with upward rotation can substitute. The triceps can substitute as in external rotation.

Gravity-Eliminated Position (Fig. 5-84)

Start Position

Prone with the entire arm hanging over the edge of the mat. The arm is in external rotation.

Stabilize

The trunk and scapula are stabilized by the mat.

Instruction

"Try to turn your palm inward."

Palpation

The subscapularis is not easily palpated but may be found in the posterior axilla. Palpate the teres major, latissimus dorsi, pectoralis major, and anterior deltoid as previously described.

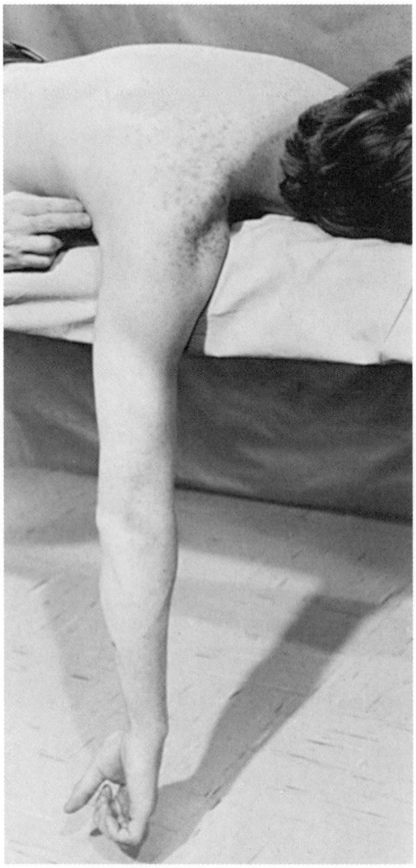

Figure 5-84 Shoulder internal rotation, gravity eliminated.

Substitutions

Scapular abduction combined with upward rotation can substitute. Pronation may be mistaken for internal rotation in a gravity-eliminated position.

Alternative Gravity-Eliminated Position (Fig. 5-85)

Start Position

Sitting in a chair with the humerus adducted to the side and the elbow flexed to 90°.

Stabilize

The distal end of the humerus is held against the body to allow only rotation.

Instruction

"Try to move the palm of your hand in toward your stomach."

Palpation

Same as previously described.

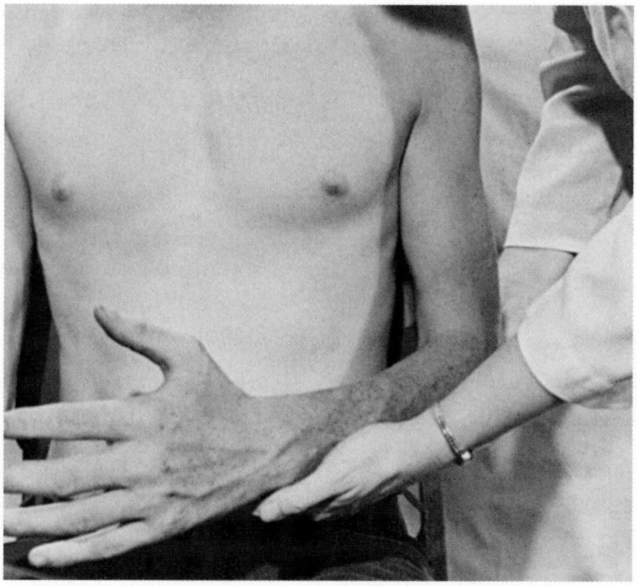

Figure 5-85 Shoulder internal rotation, alternative position with gravity eliminated.

Elbow Flexion

Prime Movers

Biceps
Brachialis
Brachioradialis

Against-Gravity Position (Fig. 5-86)

Start Position

Sitting in a chair with the arm at the side. The position of the forearm determines which muscle is working primarily: forearm in supination, biceps brachii; forearm in pronation, brachialis; forearm in midposition, brachioradialis.

Stabilize

Stabilize the distal end of the humerus during the action. While applying resistance, provide counterpressure at the front of the shoulder.

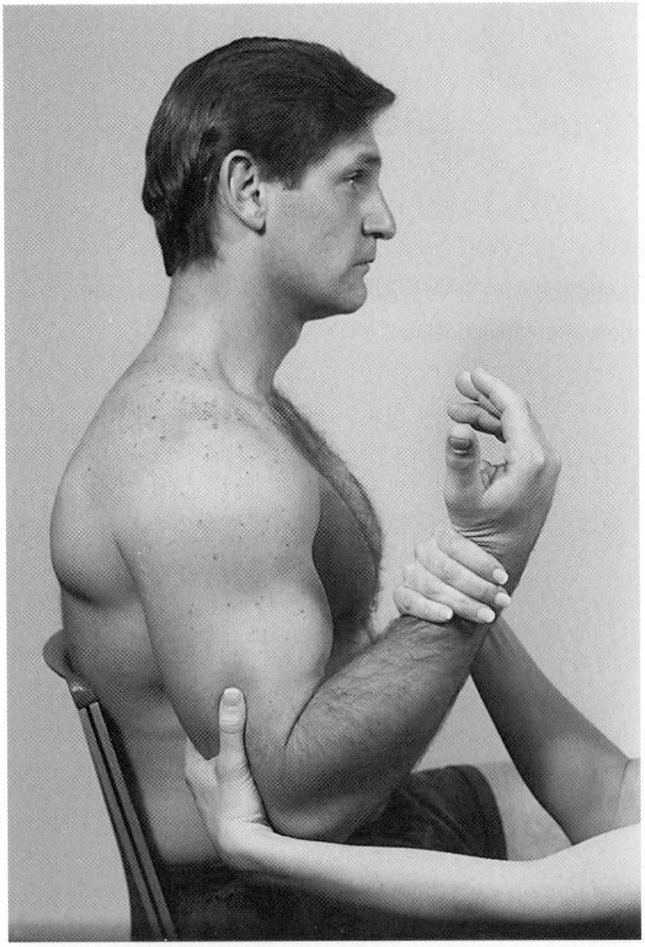

Figure 5-86 Elbow flexion against gravity.

Instruction

While the patient is in each of the three forearm positions, say, "Bend your elbow to touch your shoulder and don't let me pull it back down."

Resistance

For each of the three positions, the therapist's hand is placed on the distal end of the forearm and pulls out toward extension.

Gravity-Eliminated Position (Fig. 5-87)

Start Position

Sitting with the arm supported by the therapist in 90° of abduction and elbow extension. The position of the forearm determines which muscle is working, as described earlier.

Stabilize

Distal humerus.

Instruction

"Try to move your hand toward your shoulder."

Palpation

The biceps is easily palpated on the anterior surface of the humerus. With the biceps relaxed and the forearm pronated, palpate the brachialis just medial to the distal biceps tendon. With the forearm in midposition, palpate the brachioradialis along the radial side of the proximal forearm.

Substitution

In a gravity-eliminated plane, the wrist flexors may substitute.

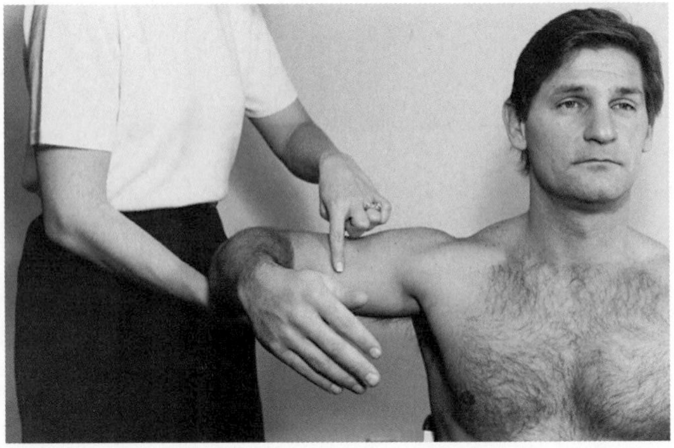

Figure 5-87 Elbow flexion, gravity eliminated.

Elbow Extension

Prime Mover

Triceps

Against-Gravity Position (Fig. 5-88)

Start Position

Prone with humerus abducted to 90° and supported on the table. The elbow is flexed, and the forearm is hanging over the edge of the table.

Stabilize

Support the arm under the anterior surface of the distal humerus.

Instruction

"Straighten your arm, and don't let me push it back down."

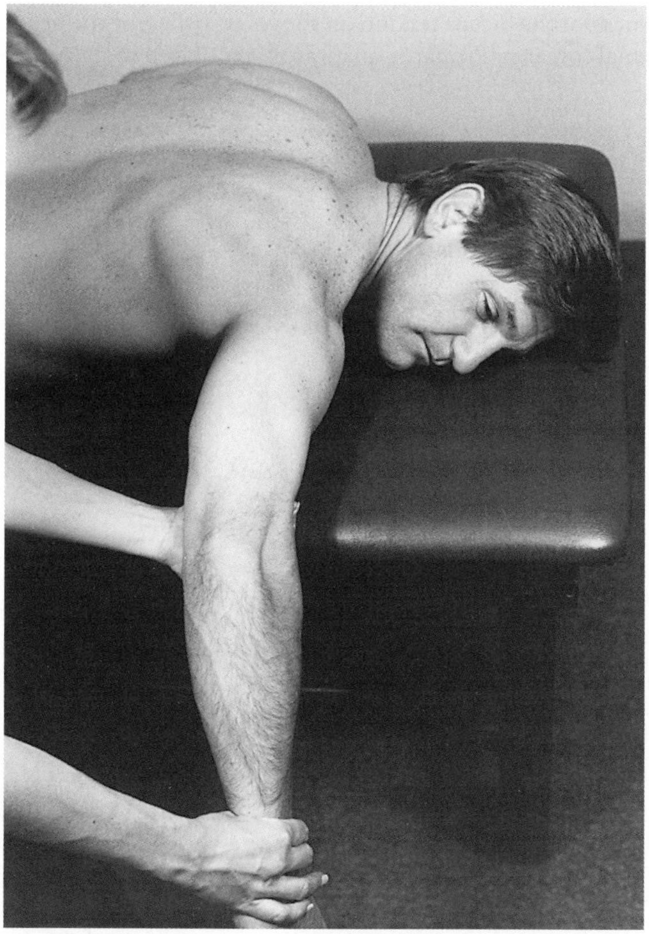

Figure 5-88 Elbow extension against gravity.

Resistance

Apply resistance with the elbow at 10–15° less than full extension so that the elbow does not lock into position, which may indicate greater strength than the patient actually has. The therapist's hand, placed on the dorsal surface of the patient's forearm, pushes toward flexion.

Gravity-Eliminated Position (Fig. 5-89)

Start Position

Sitting, with the humerus supported by the therapist in 90°of abduction. The elbow is fully flexed.

Stabilize

The humerus is supported and stabilized.

Instruction

"Try to straighten your elbow."

Palpation

The triceps are easily palpated on the posterior surface of the humerus.

Substitutions

In the gravity-eliminated position, no external rotation of the shoulder is permitted, so as to avoid letting the assistance of gravity produce extension. On a supporting surface, finger flexion may be used to inch the forearm across the surface.

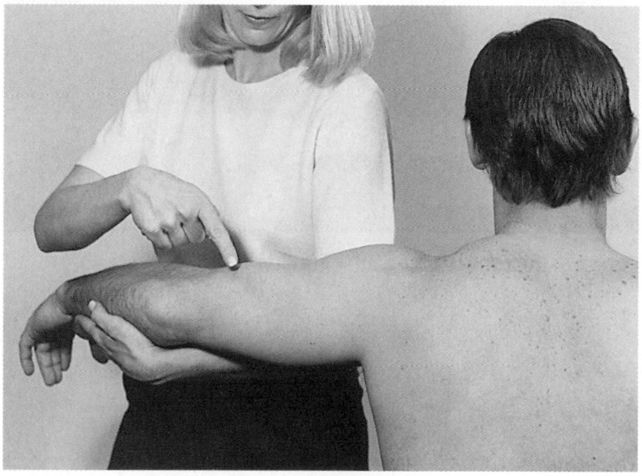

Figure 5-89 Elbow extension, gravity eliminated.

Pronation

Prime Movers

Pronator teres
Pronator quadratus

Against-Gravity Position (Fig. 5-90)

Start Position

Sitting with the humerus adducted, elbow flexed to 90°, and forearm supinated. The wrist and fingers are relaxed.

Stabilize

The distal humerus is stabilized to keep it adducted to the body.

Instruction

"Turn your palm to the floor, and don't let me turn it back over."

Resistance

The therapist's hand encircles the patient's volar wrist with the therapist's index finger extended along the forearm. The therapist applies resistance in the direction of supination.

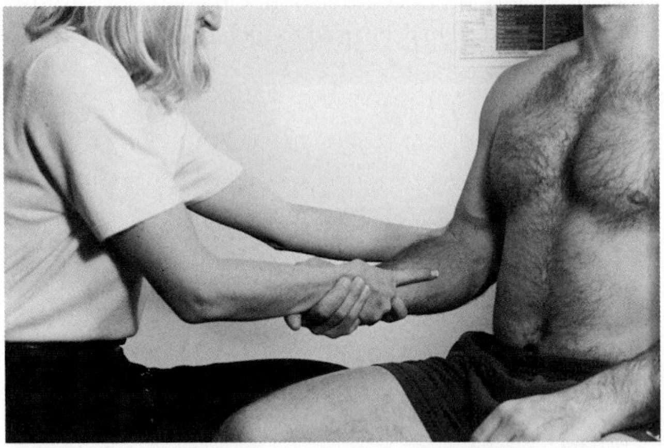

Figure 5-90 Pronation against gravity.

Substitutions

Shoulder abduction or wrist and finger flexion may substitute.

Gravity-Eliminated Position (Fig. 5-91)

Start Position

Sitting with the humerus flexed to 90° and supported. The elbow is flexed to 90° and the forearm is in full supination. The wrist and fingers are relaxed.

Stabilize

The humerus is stabilized.

Instruction

"Try to turn your palm away from your face."

Palpation

The pronator teres is palpated medial to the distal attachment of the biceps tendon on the volar surface of the proximal forearm. Pronator quadratus is too deep to palpate.

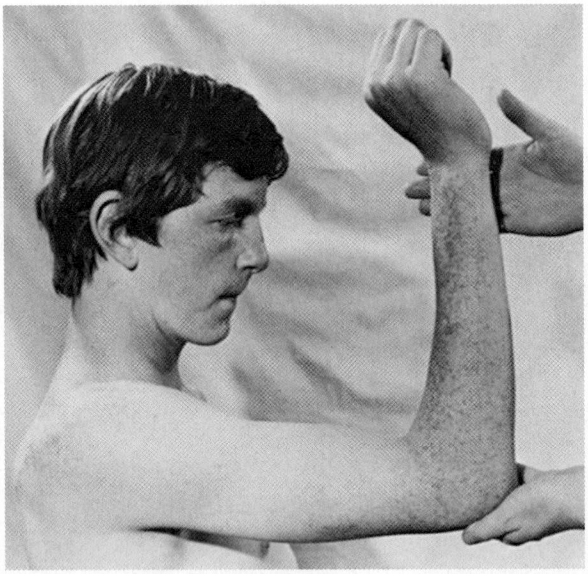

Figure 5-91 Pronation, gravity eliminated.

Supination

Prime Movers

Supinator
Biceps

Against-Gravity Position (Fig. 5-92)

Start Position

Sitting, with the humerus adducted, elbow flexed to 90°, and forearm pronated. The wrist and fingers are relaxed. To differentiate the supinator from the supination function of the biceps, isolate the supinator by extending the elbow. The biceps does not supinate the extended arm unless resisted (Kendall et al., 2005).

Stabilize

The distal humerus is stabilized.

Instruction

"Turn your palm up toward the ceiling, and don't let me turn it back over."

Resistance

Same as for pronation except that resistance is in the direction of pronation.

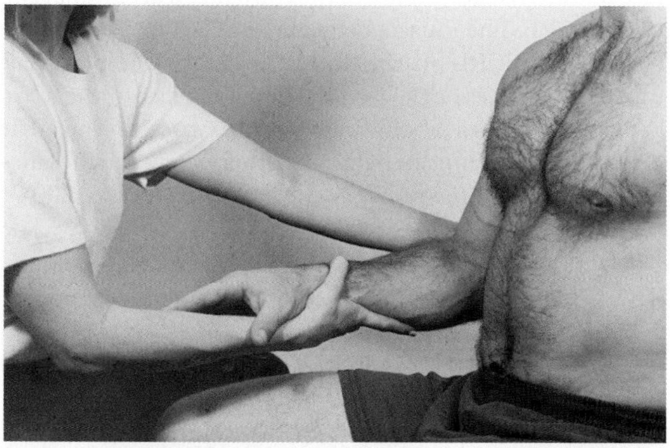

Figure 5-92 Supination against gravity.

Substitutions

The wrist and finger extensors may substitute.

Gravity-Eliminated Position (Fig. 5-93)

Start Position

Sitting with the humerus flexed to 90° and supported. The elbow is flexed to 90°, and the forearm is in full pronation. The wrist and fingers are relaxed.

Stabilize

The humerus is stabilized and supported.

Instruction

"Try to turn your palm toward your face."

Palpation

The supinator is palpated on the dorsal surface of the proximal forearm just distal to the head of the radius. Palpation of the biceps was described earlier.

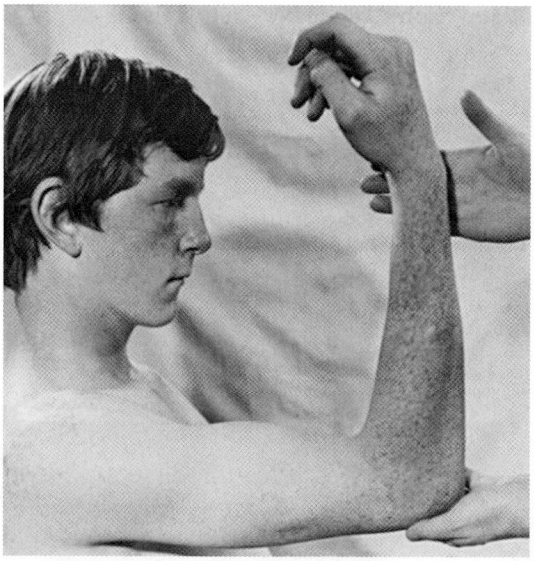

Figure 5-93 Supination, gravity eliminated.

MEASUREMENT OF THE WRIST AND HAND

Many tendons of the wrist and hand cross more than one joint. For this reason, test positions for individual muscles must include ways to minimize the effect of other muscles crossing the joint. As a general rule, to minimize the effect of a muscle, place it opposite the prime action. For example, to minimize the effect of the extensor pollicis longus on extension of the proximal joint of the thumb, flex the distal joint.

Wrist Extension

Prime Movers

Extensor carpi radialis longus (ECRL)
Extensor carpi radialis brevis (ECRB)
Extensor carpi ulnaris (ECU)

Against-Gravity Position (Figs. 5-94 and 5-95)

Start Position

The forearm is supported on a table in full pronation with fingers and thumb relaxed or slightly flexed.

Stabilize

The forearm is stabilized on the table.

Instruction

"Lift your wrist as far as you can, and don't let me push it down."

Resistance

To test the ECRL, which extends and radially deviates, apply resistance to the dorsum of the hand on the radial side in the direction of flexion and ulnar deviation (Fig. 5-94). To test the ECRB, apply resistance on the dorsum of the hand and push into flexion. To test the ECU, which extends and ulnarly deviates, apply resistance to the dorsum of the hand on the ulnar side and push in the direction of flexion and radial deviation (Fig. 5-95).

Substitutions

Extensor pollicis longus, extensor digitorum.

Gravity-Eliminated Position

Start Position

The forearm is supported on the table in midposition with the wrist in a slightly flexed position.

Instruction

"Try to bend your wrist backward."

Palpation

Palpate the tendon of the ECRL on the dorsal surface of the wrist at the base of the second metacarpal. The muscle belly is on the dorsal proximal forearm adjacent to the brachioradialis. Palpate the tendon of the ECRB on the dorsal surface of the wrist at the base of the third metacarpal adjacent to the ECRL. The muscle belly of the ECRB is distal to the belly of the ECRL on the dorsal surface of the proximal forearm. Palpate the ECU on the dorsal surface of the wrist between the head of the ulna and the base of the fifth metacarpal. The muscle belly is approximately 2 inches distal to the lateral epicondyle of the humerus (Rybski, 2004).

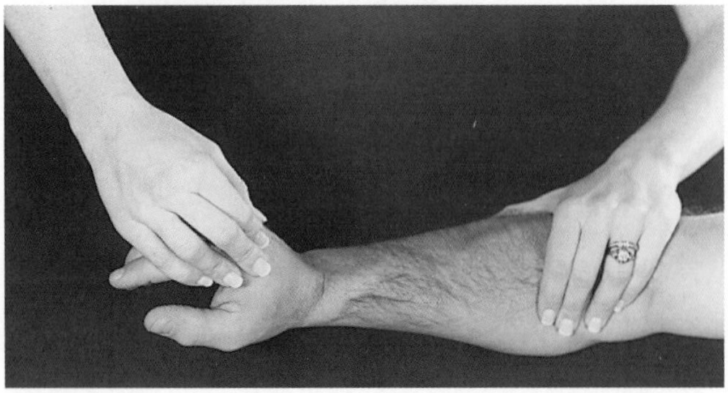

Figure 5-94 Wrist extension. Resistance is being given to the extensor carpi radialis.

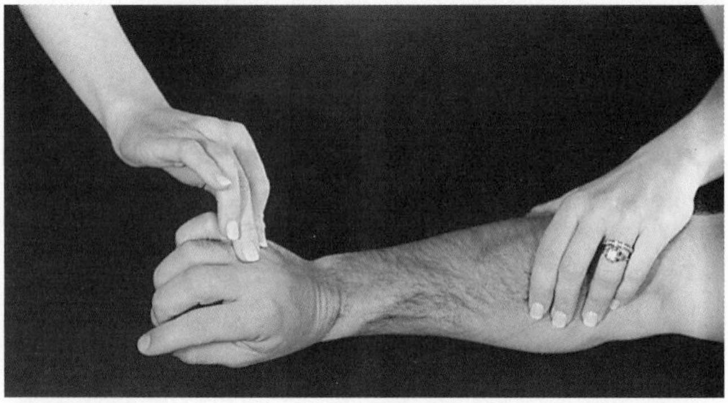

Figure 5-95 Wrist extension. Resistance is being given to the ECU.

Wrist Flexion

Prime Movers

Flexor carpi radialis (FCR)
Palmaris longus
Flexor carpi ulnaris (FCU)

Against-Gravity Position (Figs. 5-96 and 5-97)

Start Position

The forearm is supinated, the wrist is extended, and fingers and thumb are relaxed.

Stabilize

The forearm is stabilized on the table with the back of the hand raised off the table to allow the wrist to go into slight extension.

Instruction

"Bend your wrist all the way forward, and don't let me push it back."

Resistance

To test the FCR and palmaris longus, the therapist applies resistance over the heads of the metacarpals on the volar surface of the hand toward extension. To test for the FCU, the therapist applies resistance over the head of the fifth metacarpal on the volar surface of the hand toward wrist extension and radial deviation.

Substitutions

Abductor pollicis longus, flexor pollicis longus, flexor digitorum superficialis, and flexor digitorum profundus.

Gravity-Eliminated Position

Start Position

Forearm in midposition, wrist extended, and fingers and thumb relaxed.

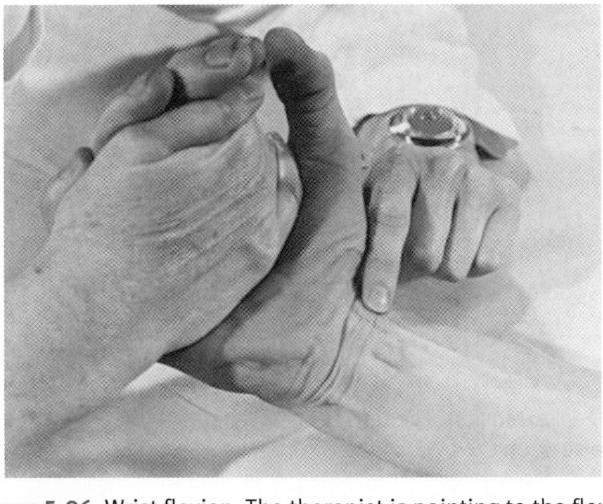

Figure 5-96 Wrist flexion. The therapist is pointing to the flexor carpi radialis longus tendon as she gives resistance.

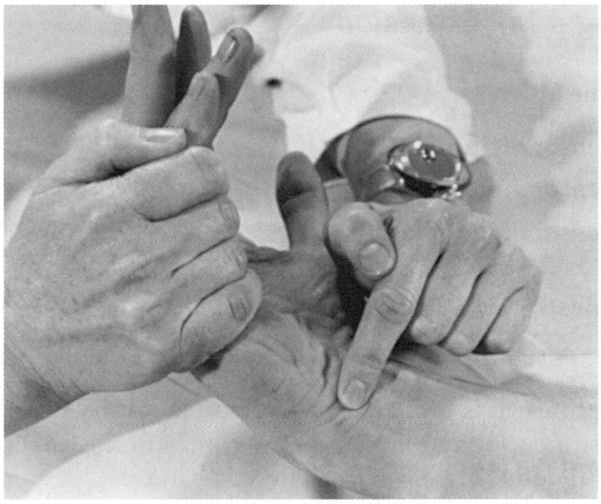

Figure 5-97 Wrist flexion. The therapist is pointing to the FCU tendon as she gives resistance.

Stabilize

The forearm rests on the table.

Instruction

"Try to bend your wrist forward."

Palpation

Palpate the FCR on the volar surface of the wrist in line with the second metacarpal and radial to the palmaris longus (if present) (Fig. 5-96). Palpate the FCU on the volar surface of the wrist just proximal to the pisiform bone (Fig. 5-97). The palmaris longus is a weak wrist flexor. The tendon crosses the center of the volar surface of the wrist (Fig. 5-98). It is not tested for strength and may not even be present; if it is present, it will stand out prominently in the middle of the wrist when wrist flexion is resisted or the palm is cupped.

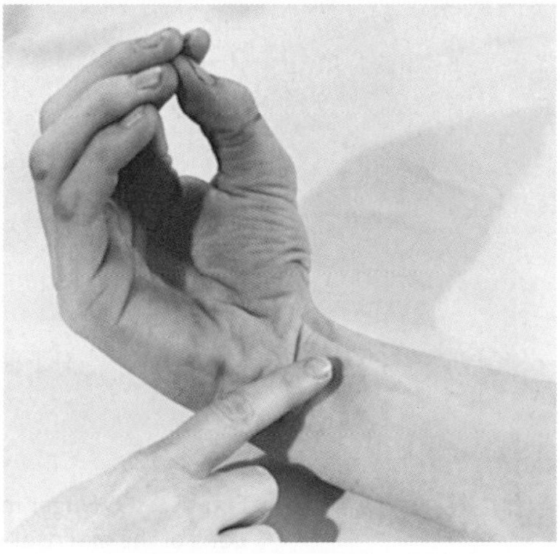

Figure 5-98 The therapist is pointing to the tendon of the palmaris longus as the patient cups his hand in an effort to make his tendon stand out.

Finger MP Extension

Prime Movers

Extensor digitorum (ED)
Extensor indicis proprius
Extensor digiti minimi

Against-Gravity Position (Fig. 5-99)

Start Position

The forearm is pronated and supported on the table. The wrist is supported in neutral position, and the finger MP and IP joints are in a relaxed flexed posture.

Stabilize

Wrist and metacarpals.

Instruction

"Lift this knuckle straight as far as it will go [touch the finger that is to be tested]. Keep the rest of your fingers bent. Don't let me push your knuckle down." (Be sure to demonstrate this action.)

Resistance

Using one finger, the therapist pushes the head of each proximal phalanx toward flexion, one at a time.

Substitution

Apparent extension of the fingers can result from the rebound effect of relaxation following finger flexion. Flexion of the wrist can cause finger extension through **tenodesis** action.

Gravity-Eliminated Position

Start Position

Forearm supported in midposition, wrist in neutral position, and fingers flexed.

Stabilize

Wrist and metacarpals.

Instruction

"Try to move your knuckles back as far as they will go, one at a time. Keep the rest of your fingers bent."

Palpation

Palpate the muscle belly of the ED on the dorsal–ulnar surface of the proximal forearm. Often the separate muscle bellies can be discerned. The tendons of this muscle are readily seen and palpated on the dorsum of the hand. The extensor indicis proprius tendon is ulnar to the extensor digitorum tendon. Palpate the belly of this muscle on the mid to distal dorsal forearm between the radius and ulna. Palpate the extensor digiti minimi tendon ulnar to the ED. Actually, it is the tendon that looks as if it were the ED tendon to the little finger because the ED to the little finger is only a slip from the ED tendon to the ring finger.

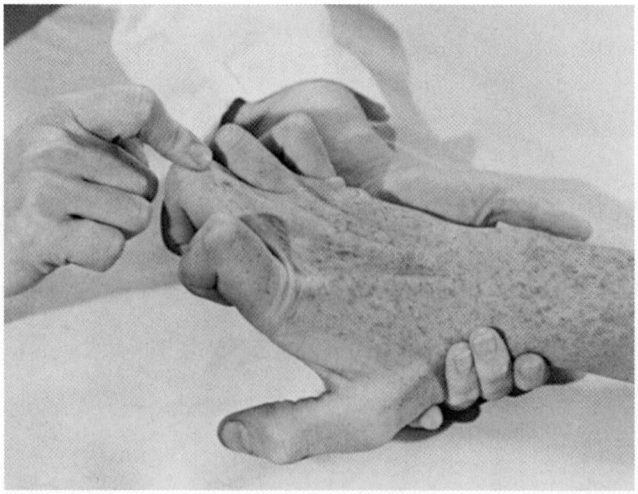

Figure 5-99 Finger metacarpophalangeal extension. The tendons of the extensor digitorum can be seen on the back of the patient's hand.

Finger Interphalangeal Extension

Prime Movers

Lumbricales

Interossei

Extensor digitorum

Extensor indicis proprius

Extensor digiti minimi

According to electromyographic evidence, the intrinsics, especially the lumbricales, are the primary extensors of the interphalangeal joints (Long, 1968; Long & Brown, 1962). Except for the lumbricales and interossei, the other muscles have been discussed. The interossei are discussed under their alternative action of finger abduction and adduction. The lumbricales, arising as they do from the flexor profundus and inserting on the extensor digitorum, have a unique action in regard to finger extension. Contracting against the noncontracting flexor profundus, the lumbricales pull the tendons of the profundus toward the fingertips. This slackens the profundus tendons distal to the insertion of the lumbricales, allowing the extensor digitorum to extend the interphalangeal joints fully, regardless of the position of the MP joints (Landsmeer & Long, 1965; Long, 1968). The interossei flex the MP joints while extending the interphalangeal joints and, in fact, operate to extend only when the MP joints are flexed or flexing (Long, 1968).

Against-Gravity Position for the Lumbricales

There is no reliably good test for lumbrical function. Test 1 is traditional. Test 2 is suggested in accordance with electromyographic evidence.

Start Position

The forearm is supinated and supported. The wrist is in neutral position. Test 1: MPs are extended with the IPs flexed. Test 2: MPs are flexed with the IPs extended.

Stabilize

Metacarpals and wrist.

Instruction

Test 1: "Bend your knuckles and straighten your fingers at the same time." (Be sure to demonstrate this movement.) Test 2: "Straighten your knuckles and keep your fingers straight at the same time."

Resistance

Test 1: The therapist holds the tip of the finger being tested and pushes it toward the starting position. Test 2: The therapist places one finger on the patient's fingernail and pushes toward flexion (Fig. 5-100).

Substitution

Nothing substitutes for DIP extension in the event of the loss of lumbrical function when the MP joint is extended. Other muscles of the dorsal expansion can substitute for DIP extension when the MP joint is flexed.

Palpation

Lumbricales lie too deep to be palpated.

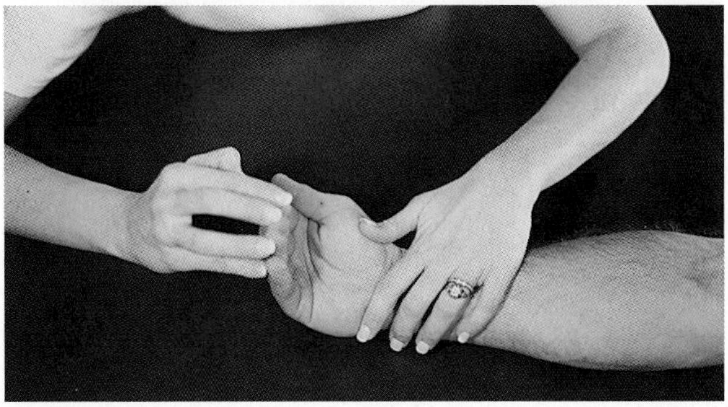

Figure 5-100 Finger interphalangeal extension. Resistance is given to the lumbricales as described for test 2.

Finger DIP Flexion

Prime Mover

Flexor digitorum profundus (FDP)

Against-Gravity Position (Fig. 5-101)

Start Position

Forearm supinated and supported on a table; wrist and interphalangeal joints relaxed.

Stabilize

Firmly support the middle phalanx of each finger as it is tested to prevent flexion of the proximal interphalangeal joint; wrist should remain in neutral position.

Instruction

"Bend the last joint on your finger as far as you can."

Resistance

The therapist places one finger on the pad of the patient's finger and applies resistance toward extension.

Substitutions

Rebound effect of apparent flexion following contraction of extensors. Wrist extension causes tenodesis action.

Gravity-Eliminated Position

Start Position

The forearm is in midposition, resting on the ulnar border on a table. The wrist and interphalangeal joints are relaxed in neutral position.

Stabilize

Same as previously described.

Instruction

Same as previously described.

Palpation

Palpate the belly of the FDP just volar to the ulna in the proximal third of the forearm. The tendons are sometimes palpable on the volar surface of the middle phalanges.

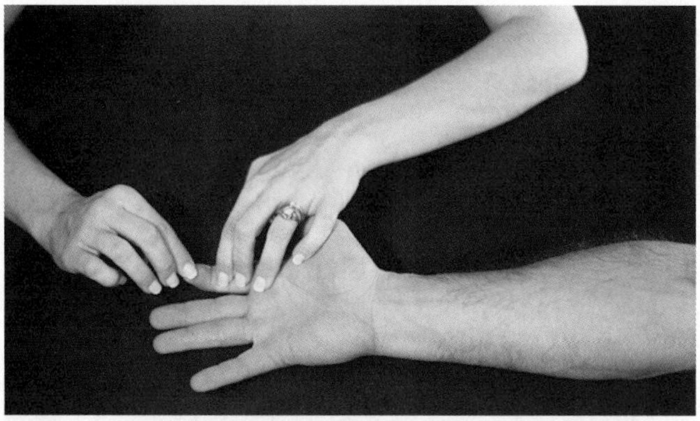

Figure 5-101 Finger distal interphalangeal flexion. The other joints of the finger are prevented from flexing.

Finger PIP Flexion

Prime Movers

Flexor digitorum superficialis (FDS)

Flexor digitorum profundus

Against-Gravity Position for the Flexor Digitorum Superficialis (Fig. 5-102)

Start Position

Forearm supinated and supported on the table; wrist and metacarpophalangeal joints relaxed and in zero position. To rule out the influence of the profundus when testing the superficialis, hold all interphalangeal joints of the fingers not being tested in full extension. Because the profundus is essentially one muscle with four tendons, preventing its action in three of the four fingers prevents it from working in the tested finger. In fact, the patient cannot flex the distal joint of the tested finger at all. In some people, the profundus slip to the index finger is such that this method cannot rule out its influence on the PIP joint of the index finger. This should be noted on the test form.

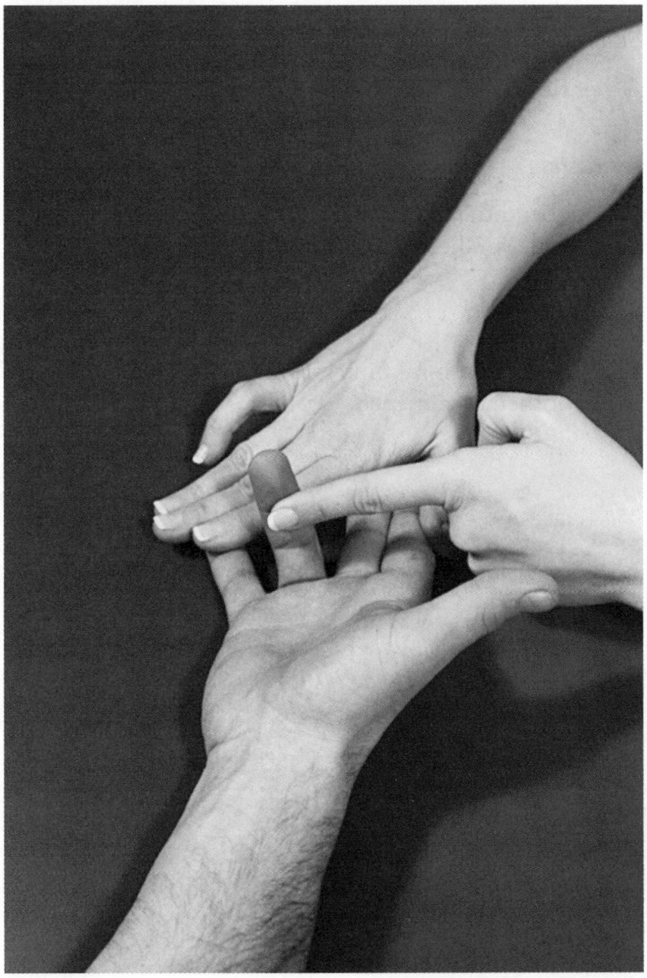

Figure 5-102 Finger proximal interphalangeal flexion. The flexor profundus is prevented from substituting because the therapist is holding in extension all fingers not being tested.

Stabilize

All IP joints of the other digits of the hand.

Instruction

Point to the PIP joint and say, "Bend just this joint."

Resistance

Using one finger, the therapist applies resistance to the head of the middle phalanx toward extension.

Substitutions

Flexor digitorum profundus. Wrist extension causes tenodesis action.

Gravity-Eliminated Position

Start Position

Forearm supported in midposition, with the wrist and MP joints relaxed in neutral position. Again, rule out the influence of the FDP by holding all the joints of the untested fingers in extension.

Stabilize

Proximal phalanx of the finger being tested as well as all IP joints of the other digits of the hand.

Instruction

Point to the PIP joint and say, "Try to bend just this joint."

Palpation

Palpate the superficialis on the volar surface of the proximal forearm toward the ulnar side. Palpate the tendons at the wrist between the palmaris longus and the flexor carpi ulnaris.

Finger MP Flexion

Prime Movers

Flexor digitorum profundus

Flexor digitorum superficialis

Dorsal interossei

Volar (palmar) interossei

Flexor digiti minimi

The tests for the first four muscles are discussed under their alternative actions. The flexor of the little finger has no other action and is described here.

Against-Gravity Position for the Flexor Digiti Minimi (Fig. 5-103)

Start Position

Forearm supported in supination.

Stabilize

Other fingers in extension.

Instruction

"Bend the knuckle of your little finger toward your palm while you keep the rest of the finger straight."

Resistance

Using one finger, the therapist pushes the head of the proximal phalanx toward extension. The therapist must be sure the interphalangeal joints remain extended.

Substitutions

The flexor digitorum profundus, flexor digitorum superficialis, or third volar interosseus may substitute.

Gravity-Eliminated Position

Start Position

Forearm supported in midposition.

Stabilize

Other fingers in extension.

Instruction

"Try to bend the knuckle of your little finger toward your palm while you keep the rest of the finger straight."

Palpation

The flexor digiti minimi is found on the volar surface of the hypothenar eminence.

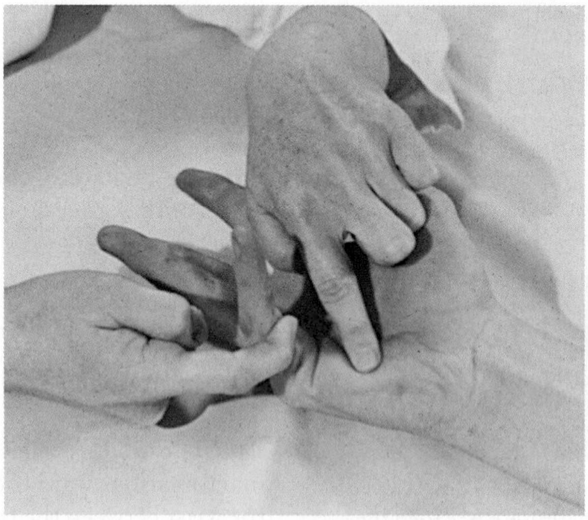

Figure 5-103 Flexor digiti minimi. The therapist is pointing to the muscle belly.

Finger Abduction

Prime Movers

Dorsal interossei (4)

Abductor digiti minimi

Gravity-Eliminated Position (Fig. 5-104)

Start Position

The pronated forearm is supported with the wrist neutral. The fingers are extended and adducted. Be sure the MP joints are in neutral or slight flexion.

Stabilize

The wrist and metacarpals are gently supported.

Instruction

"Spread your fingers apart, and don't let me push them back together."

Action

Because the midline of the hand is the third finger and abduction is movement away from midline, the action of each finger is different. It is important to know which dorsal interossei (DAB) you are testing. The first dorsal interosseus (DAB 1) abducts the index finger toward the thumb. The DAB 2 abducts the middle finger toward the thumb. The DAB 3 abducts the middle finger toward the little finger. The DAB 4 abducts the ring finger toward the little finger. The abductor digiti minimi abducts the little finger ulnarly.

Resistance

Using the thumb and index finger to form a pincer, the therapist applies resistance at the radial or ulnar side of the head of the proximal phalanx in an attempt to push the finger toward midline. Applying resistance to the radial side of the heads of the index and middle fingers tests DABs 1 and 2. Applying resistance to the ulnar side of the middle, ring, and little fingers tests DABs 3 and 4 and the abductor digiti minimi.

Substitutions

Extensor digitorum.

Grading

Normal finger abductors do not tolerate much resistance. If the fingers give way to resistance but spring back when the resistance is removed, the grade is 5. The grade is 4 if the muscle takes some resistance. The grade is 3 when there is full AROM. The grade is 2 if there is partial AROM. The grade is 1 when contraction is felt with palpation. The grade is 0 when no contractile activity is palpable.

Palpation

DAB 1 fills the dorsal web space and is easy to palpate there. Palpate the abductor digiti minimi on the ulnar border of the fifth metacarpal. The other interossei lie between the metacarpals on the dorsal aspect of the hand, where they may be palpated; on some people, the tendons can be palpated as they enter the dorsal expansion near the heads of the metacarpals. When the DABs are atrophied, the spaces between the metacarpals on the dorsal surface appear sunken.

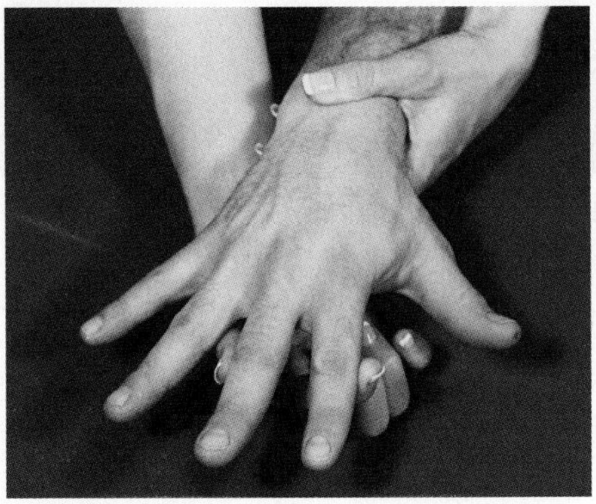

Figure 5-104 Finger abduction.

Finger Adduction

Prime Movers

Volar (palmar) interossei (3)

Gravity-Eliminated Position (Fig. 5-105)

Start Position

The forearm is pronated, and the MPs are abducted and in extension.

Stabilize

Both of the therapist's hands are needed for resistance. The forearm and wrist can be supported on a table.

Instruction

"Bring your fingers together and hold them. Don't let me pull them apart."

Action

Because the midline of the hand is the third finger and adduction is movement toward midline, the action of each finger is different. Palmar interosseus (PAD) 1 adducts the index finger toward the middle finger. PAD 2 adducts the ring finger toward the middle finger. PAD 3 adducts the little finger toward the middle finger.

Resistance

The therapist holds the heads of the proximal phalanx of two adjoining fingers and applies resistance in the direction of abduction to pull the fingers apart. For the index and middle finger pair, PAD 1 is tested. For the middle and ring finger pair, PAD 2 is tested. For the ring and little finger pair, PAD 3 is tested.

Substitutions

Extrinsic finger flexors.

Grading

Same as with the finger abductors.

Palpation

The palmar interossei are usually too deep to palpate with certainty. When these muscles are atrophied, the areas between the metacarpals on the volar surface appear sunken.

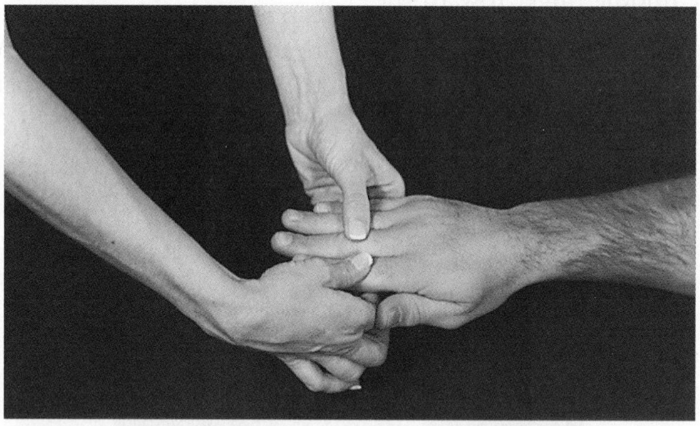

Figure 5-105 Finger adduction.

Thumb IP Extension

Prime Mover

Extensor pollicis longus (EPL)

Against-Gravity Position (Fig. 5-106)

Start Position

Forearm supported in midposition, wrist flexion of 10–20°, and thumb MP and IP flexion.

Instruction

"Straighten the end of your thumb."

Stabilize

Proximal phalanx into MP flexion.

Resistance

The therapist places one finger over the dorsum of the distal phalanx (thumbnail) and pushes only the DIP toward flexion.

Substitutions

Relaxation of the flexor pollicis longus produces apparent extensor movement as a result of rebound effect. Because the abductor pollicis brevis, adductor pollicis, and flexor pollicis brevis insert into the lateral aspects of the dorsal expansion, they may produce thumb IP extension when the extensor pollicis longus is paralyzed. To prevent this, the position of maximal flexion of the carpometacarpal and MP joints, wrist flexion of 10–20°, and full forearm supination are used to put these synergists in a shortened, disadvantaged position while testing the EPL (Howell et al., 1989).

Gravity-Eliminated Position

Start Position

Forearm supinated, thumb flexed.

Instruction

"Try to straighten the end of your thumb."

Palpation

The tendon of the EPL may be palpated on the ulnar border of the anatomical snuffbox and on the dorsal surface of the proximal phalanx of the thumb.

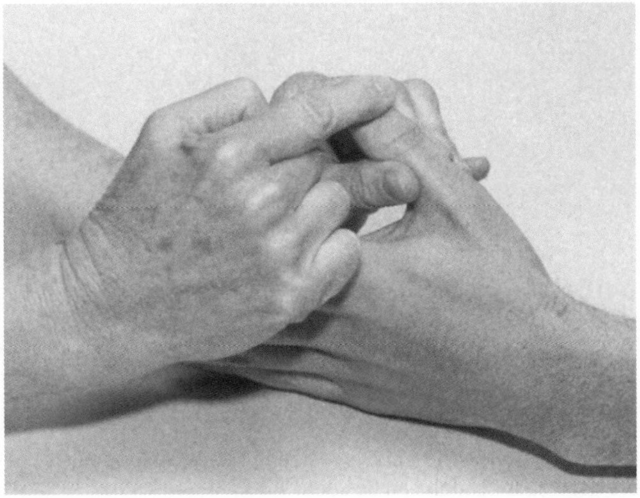

Figure 5-106 The therapist is resisting the extensor pollicis longus, whose tendon is prominent.

Thumb MP Extension

Prime Movers

Extensor pollicis brevis (EPB)
Extensor pollicis longus

Against-Gravity Position for the Extensor Pollicis Brevis (Fig. 5-107)

Start Position

Forearm supported in midposition, MP and IP joints flexed.

Stabilize

Firmly support the first metacarpal in abduction.

Instruction

"Straighten the knuckle of your thumb while keeping the end joint bent." You may have to move the thumb passively a few times for the patient to get the kinesthetic input regarding the movement.

Resistance

The therapist's index finger, placed on the dorsal surface of the head of the proximal phalanx, pushes toward flexion.

Substitution

Extensor pollicis longus.

Gravity-Eliminated Position

Start Position

Forearm supinated, MP and IP joints flexed.

Stabilize

First metacarpal in abduction.

Instruction

"Try to straighten the knuckle of your thumb while keeping the end joint bent."

Palpation

Palpate the tendon of the EPB on the radial border of the anatomical snuffbox medial to the tendon of the abductor pollicis longus. The EPB may not be present.

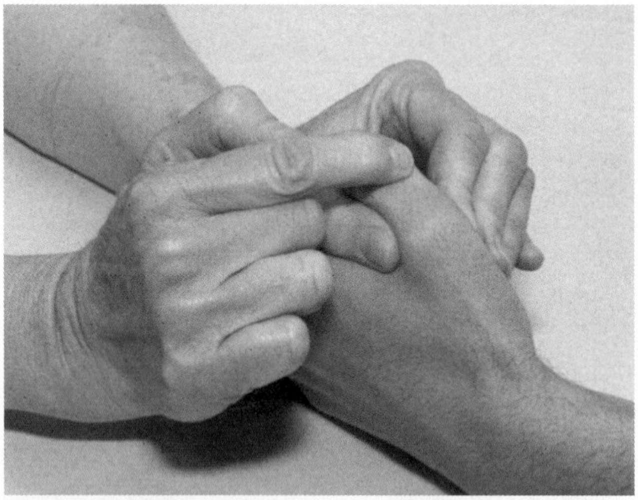

Figure 5-107 The therapist is resisting the extensor pollicis brevis, whose tendon can be seen.

Thumb Abduction

Prime Movers

Abductor pollicis longus

Abductor pollicis brevis

Against-Gravity Position for the Abductor Pollicis Longus (Fig. 5-108)

Start Position

Forearm supinated, wrist in neutral position, thumb adducted.

Stabilize

Support the wrist on the ulnar side and hold it in neutral position.

Instruction

"Bring your thumb away from your palm. Don't let me push it back in."

Action

Patient abducts the thumb halfway between thumb extension and palmar abduction. The therapist may have to demonstrate this action while giving the instructions.

Resistance

The therapist's finger presses the head of the first metacarpal toward adduction.

Substitutions

Abductor pollicis brevis, extensor pollicis brevis.

Gravity-Eliminated Position

Start Position

Forearm in midposition, wrist in neutral position, thumb adducted.

Stabilize

Support the wrist on the ulnar side and hold it in neutral position.

Instruction

"Try to bring your thumb away from your palm."

Palpation

Palpate the tendon of the abductor pollicis longus at the wrist joint just distal to the radial styloid and lateral to the EPB.

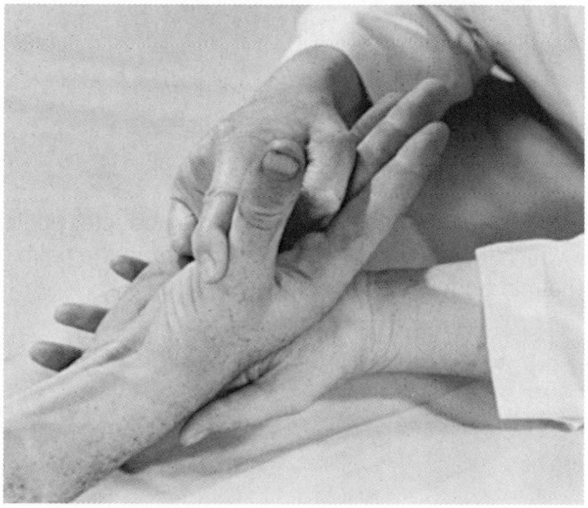

Figure 5-108 The therapist is resisting the abductor pollicis longus, which moves the thumb away from the palm halfway between extension and palmar abduction.

Against-Gravity Position for the Abductor Pollicis Brevis (Fig. 5-109)

Start Position

Forearm is supported in supination, wrist in neutral position, and thumb adducted.

Stabilize

Support the wrist in neutral position by holding it on the dorsal and ulnar side.

Instruction

"Lift your thumb directly out of the palm of the hand. Don't let me push it back in."

Resistance

The therapist's finger presses the head of the first metacarpal toward adduction.

Substitution

Abductor pollicis longus.

Gravity-Eliminated Position

Start Position

Forearm is supported in midposition, wrist in neutral position, thumb adducted.

Stabilize

Support the wrist in neutral position by holding it on the dorsal and ulnar side.

Instruction

"Try to move your thumb away from the palm of your hand."

Palpation

Palpate the abductor pollicis brevis over the center of the thenar eminence.

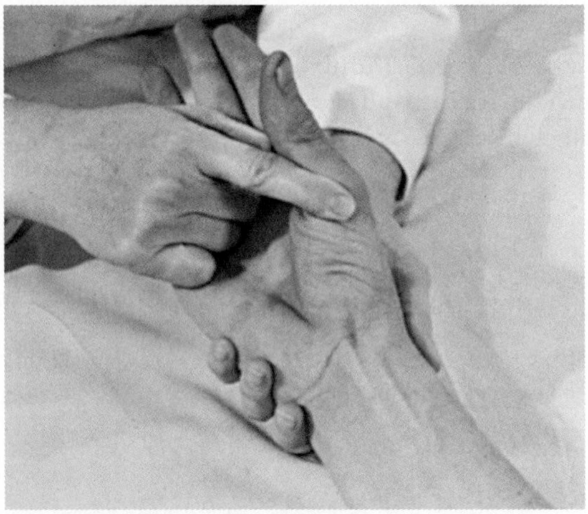

Figure 5-109 The therapist is resisting the abductor pollicis brevis, which moves the thumb directly up from the palm of the hand (palmar abduction).

Thumb IP Flexion

Prime Mover

Flexor pollicis longus

Against-Gravity Position (Fig. 5-110)

Start Position

Elbow flexed and supported on a table. Forearm supinated so that the palmar surface of the thumb faces the ceiling; thumb extended at the MP and IP joints.

Stabilize

Proximal phalanx, holding MP joint in extension.

Instruction

"Bend the tip of your thumb as far as you can, and don't let me straighten it."

Resistance

The therapist's finger pushes the head of the distal phalanx toward extension.

Substitution

Relaxation of the extensor pollicis longus causes apparent rebound movement.

Gravity-Eliminated Position

Start Position

Forearm supinated to 90° so that the thumb can flex across the palm.

Stabilize

Proximal phalanx, holding MP joint in extension.

Instruction

"Try to bend the tip of your thumb as far as you can."

Palpation

Palpate the flexor pollicis longus on the palmar surface of the proximal phalanx.

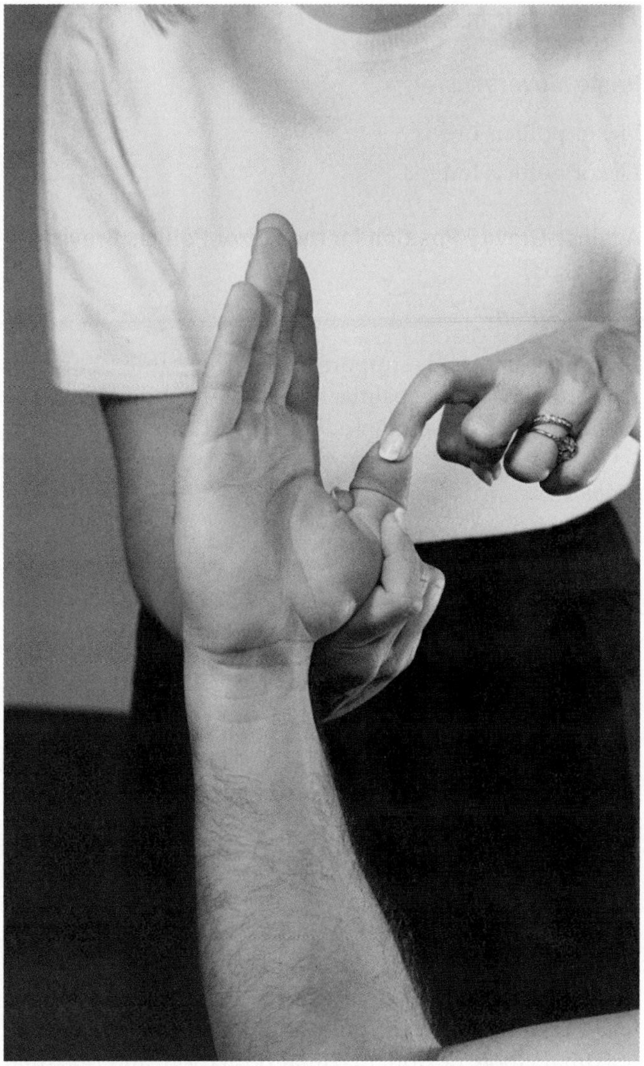

Figure 5-110 The therapist is resisting the flexor pollicis longus.

Thumb MP Flexion

Prime Movers

Flexor pollicis brevis
Flexor pollicis longus

Against-Gravity Position for the Flexor Pollicis Brevis (Fig. 5-111)

Start Position

Elbow flexed and supported on the table. Forearm supinated so that the palmar surface of the thumb faces the ceiling; thumb is extended at both the MP and IP joints.

Stabilize

Firmly support the first metacarpal.

Instruction

"Bend your thumb across your palm, keeping the end joint of your thumb straight. Don't let me pull it back out."

Resistance

The therapist's finger pushes the head of the proximal phalanx toward extension.

Substitution

Flexor pollicis longus; the abductor pollicis brevis and the adductor pollicis through insertion into the extensor hood. To rule out the effect of the flexor pollicis longus when testing the flexor pollicis brevis, a test position of maximal elbow flexion, maximal pronation, and maximal wrist flexion has been recommended (Howell et al., 1989).

Gravity-Eliminated Position

Start Position

Forearm supinated to 90° so that the thumb can flex across the palm.

Stabilize

First metacarpal.

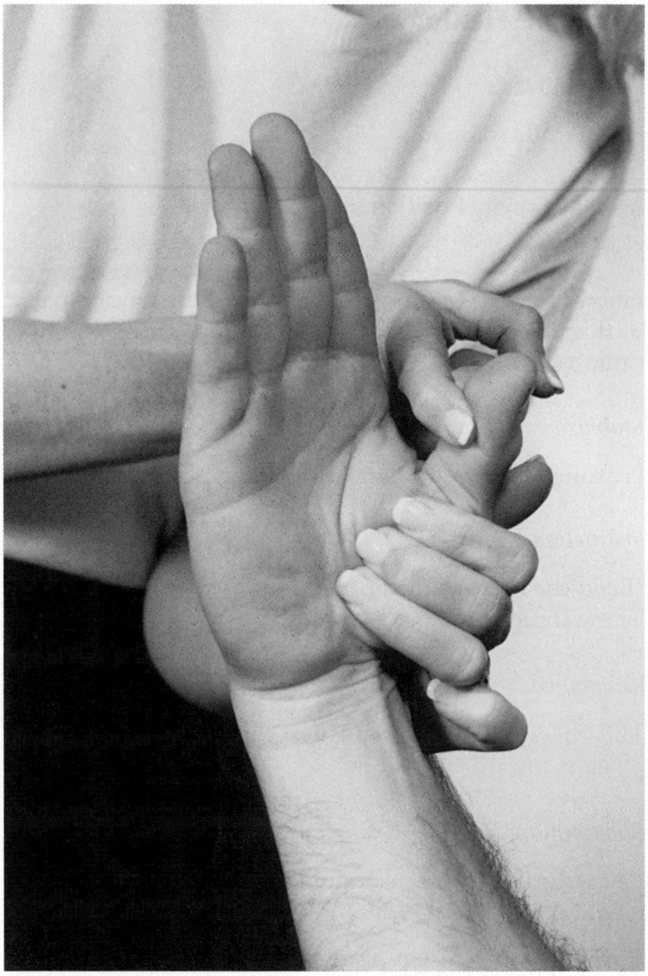

Figure 5-111 The therapist is resisting the flexor pollicis brevis.

Instruction

"Try to bend your thumb into your palm, keeping the end joint of your thumb straight."

Palpation

Palpate the flexor pollicis brevis on the thenar eminence just proximal to the MP joint and medial to the abductor pollicis brevis.

Thumb Adduction

Prime Mover

Adductor pollicis

Against-Gravity Position (Fig. 5-112)

Start Position

Forearm pronated, wrist and fingers in neutral position, thumb abducted, and MP and IP joints of the thumb in extension.

Stabilize

Metacarpals of fingers, keeping the MP joints in neutral.

Instruction

"Lift your thumb into the palm of your hand, and don't let me pull it out."

Resistance

The therapist grasps the head of the proximal phalanx and tries to pull it away from the palm toward abduction.

Substitutions

The extensor pollicis longus, flexor pollicis longus, or flexor pollicis brevis may substitute.

Gravity-Eliminated Position

Start Position

Same except forearm is in midposition.

Stabilize

Metacarpals of fingers, keeping the MP joints in neutral.

Instruction

"Try to bring your thumb into the palm of your hand."

Palpation

Palpate the adductor pollicis on the palmar surface of the thumb web space.

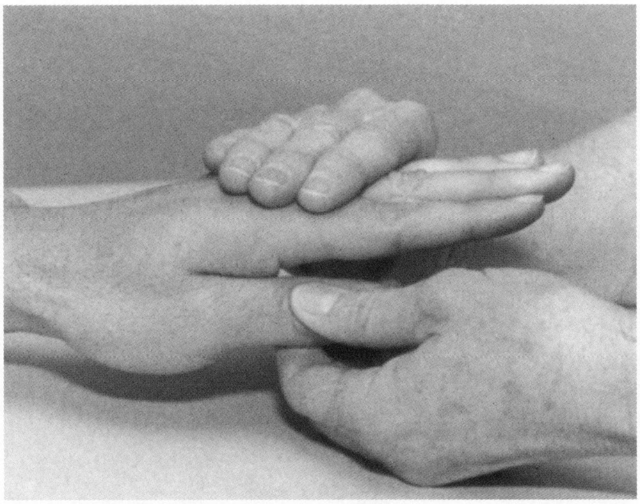

Figure 5-112 The therapist is resisting the adductor pollicis.

Opposition

Prime Movers

Opponens pollicis
Opponens digiti minimi

Against-Gravity Position (Fig. 5-113)

Start Position

Forearm supinated and supported, wrist in neutral position, thumb adducted and extended.

Stabilize

Hold the wrist in a neutral position.

Instruction

"Touch the pad of your thumb to the pad of your little finger. Don't let me pull them apart."

Resistance

The therapist holds along the first metacarpal and derotates the thumb or holds along the fifth metacarpal and derotates the little finger. These can be resisted simultaneously using both hands.

Substitutions

The abductor pollicis brevis, flexor pollicis brevis, or flexor pollicis longus may substitute.

Gravity-Eliminated Position

Start Position

Elbow resting on the table with forearm perpendicular to the table, wrist in neutral position, thumb adducted and extended.

Stabilize

Hold the wrist in a neutral position.

Instruction

"Try to touch the pad of your thumb to the pad of your little finger."

Palpation

Place fingertips along the lateral side of the shaft of the first metacarpal where the opponens pollicis may be palpated before it becomes deep to the abductor pollicis brevis. The opponens digiti minimi can be palpated volarly along the shaft of the fifth metacarpal.

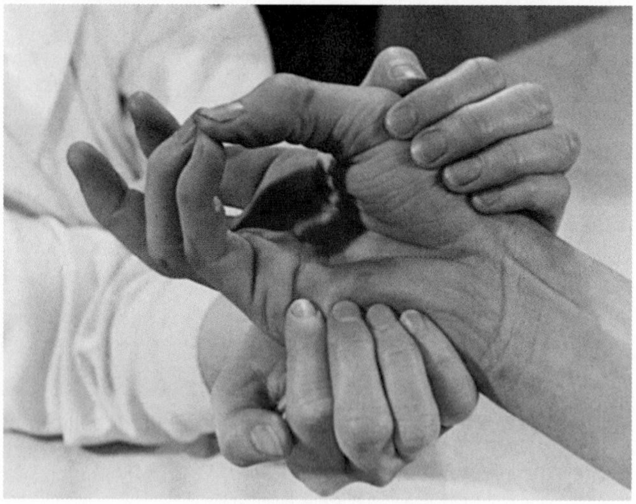

Figure 5-113 The therapist is resisting both the opponens pollicis and the opponens digiti minimi.

MEASUREMENT OF SELECTED LOWER EXTREMITY MUSCLE GROUPS

Muscle testing of the flexors and extensors of the three major joints of the lower extremity is described here because of their importance to functions required for completion of certain activities of daily living, such as climbing stairs and curbs, dressing, bathing, sitting, standing, and transferring. Only against-gravity testing is described. Muscles weaker than 3 (fair) are too weak for functional activities in occupational therapy, and in these cases, adaptive methods of doing activities of daily living are the most efficient therapeutic intervention.

Hip Flexion

Prime Movers

Iliopsoas

Iliacus

Psoas major

Against-Gravity Start Position

Sitting on the plinth with lower leg hanging down.

Stabilize

The pelvis is stabilized on the plinth.

Instruction

"Lift your knee toward the ceiling, keeping your knee bent. Don't let me push your leg back down."

Resistance

The therapist presses the distal anterior thigh down toward extension (Fig. 5-114).

Palpation

The iliacus is too deep to be palpated. With the patient sitting, the psoas major can be palpated if the patient bends forward and relaxes the abdominal muscles. The therapist's fingers lie at the waist between the ribs and the iliac crest, and the therapist applies pressure posteriorly to feel the contraction of the psoas major as the hip flexes (Smith, Weiss, & Lehmkuhl, 1996).

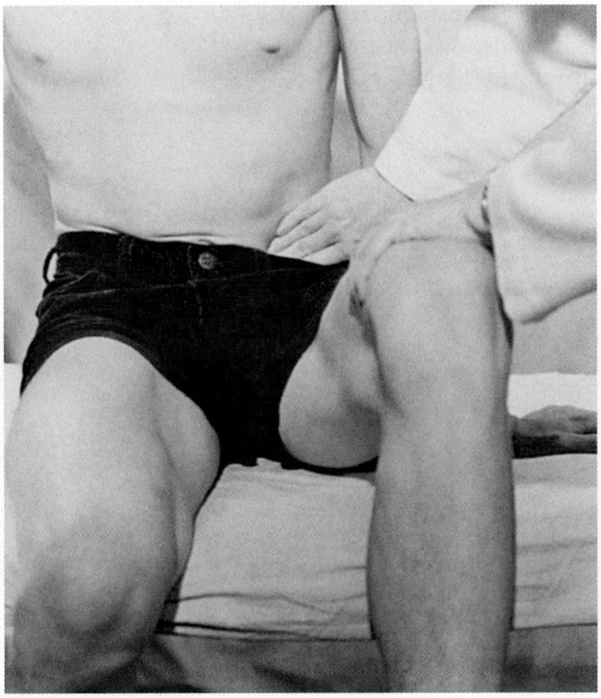

Figure 5-114 The therapist is attempting to palpate the psoas major while resisting hip flexion.

Hip Extension

Prime Movers

Gluteus maximus

Biceps femoris

Against-Gravity Start Position for the Gluteus Maximus

The patient lies prone with the knee flexed to 90° or more (Kendall et al., 2005).

Stabilize

The pelvis and lumbar spine are stabilized on the plinth.

Instruction

"Lift your leg off the table as high as you can. Keep your knee bent."

Resistance

The therapist presses the distal posterior thigh down toward flexion (Fig. 5-115).

Palpation

The gluteus maximus, the large muscle of the buttocks, can be easily palpated.

Substitutions

Extension of the lumbar spine. The other hamstrings, the semimembranosus and the semitendinosus, assist resisted hip extension if the hip is internally rotated (Kendall et al., 2005).

Start Position for Combined Gluteus Maximus and Biceps Femoris Action

The patient lies supine with the leg to be tested in full extension and holds the other leg in flexion at the hip and knee (Diekmeyer, 1978).

Stabilize

The pelvis and lumbar spine are stabilized by the plinth.

Instruction

"Do not let me lift your leg off the plinth."

Resistance

The therapist holds the thigh just above the knee and attempts to raise the leg off the plinth (Fig. 5-116).

Grading

Hip extension is graded as 5 (normal) if the trunk rather than the leg comes up off the plinth and as 3 (fair) if the hip gives as the trunk begins to come up off the table.

Palpation

Palpate the biceps femoris on the posterior aspect of the thigh; its tendon bounds the popliteal fossa laterally (Kendall et al., 2005).

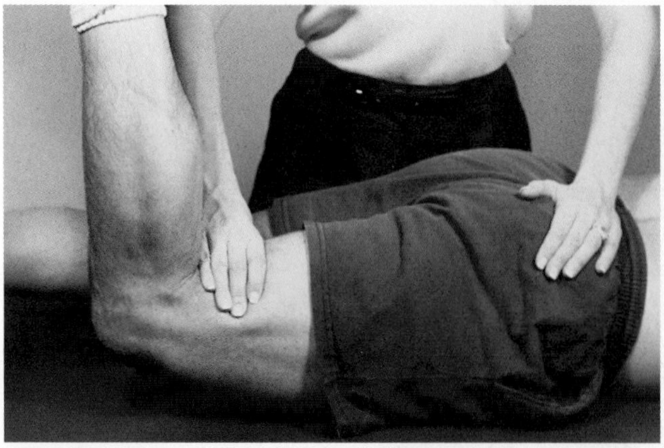

Figure 5-115 The therapist is resisting hip extension with the knee flexed to test the gluteus maximus.

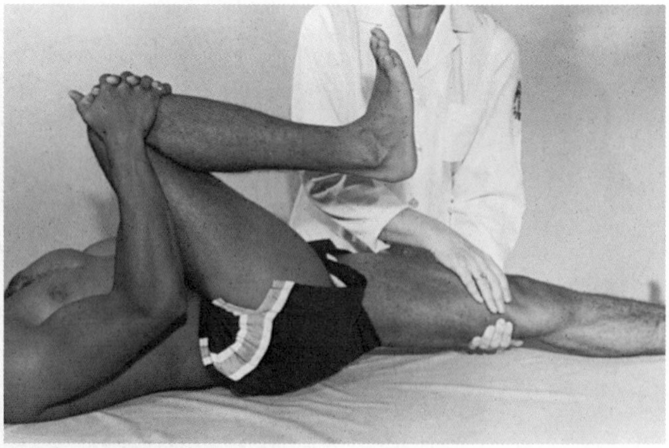

Figure 5-116 During testing of the gluteus maximus and the biceps femoris together, the patient lies supine and holds the hip and knee of the untested leg flexed. The therapist tries to lift the extended leg off of the plinth.

Knee Flexion

Prime Movers

Hamstrings

Semimembranosus

Semitendinosus

Biceps femoris

Against-Gravity Start Position

The patient lies prone, with both hips and knees extended.

Stabilize

The thigh is stabilized against the plinth.

Instruction

"Bend your knee. Hold it. Don't let me push it back to the plinth."

Resistance

The therapist's hand, placed on the distal end of the posterior surface of the tibia, pushes toward extension. If resistance is applied to one side, medially or laterally, either the lateral or medial hamstrings will contract more strongly (Fig. 5-117).

Grading

In deciding between a 3− and 3 grade, the therapist must make an educated guess unless the patient can stand up and demonstrate knee flexion to 120°, that is, full flexion, against gravity.

Palpation

Palpate these three muscles on the posterior surface of the thigh. Palpate the tendon of the biceps femoris on the lateral side of the popliteal space and the tendon of the semitendinosus on the medial side of the popliteal space. Both tendons become prominent when resistance is applied. Isolate the biceps femoris from the other muscles by rotating the lower leg externally with respect to the femur. The semitendinosus contracts more prominently if the lower leg is rotated internally with respect to the femur. The semimembranosus lies deep to the semitendinosus, but its lower portion is palpable on both sides of the semitendinosus (Kendall et al., 2005).

Substitutions

When the patient is prone, gravity assists flexion beyond 90°. When the patient is sitting, gravity can flex the knee.

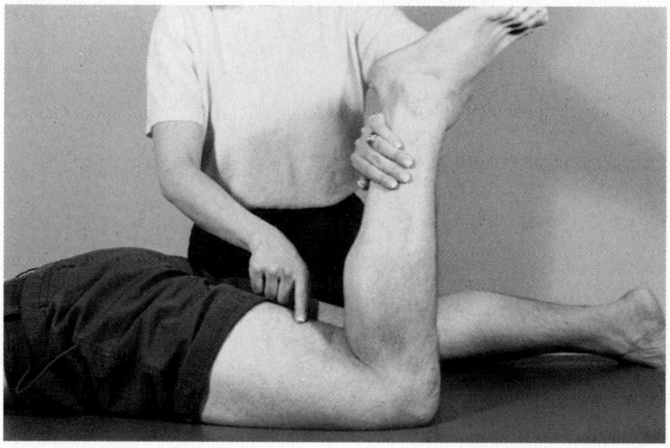

Figure 5-117 Knee flexion against gravity.

Knee Extension

Prime Movers

Quadriceps

Rectus femoris
Vastus medialis
Vastus intermedius
Vastus lateralis

Against-Gravity Start Position

The patient sits on the plinth with the knee flexed and lower leg hanging down.

Stabilize

The thigh is stabilized on the plinth.

Instruction

"Straighten your knee. Don't let me bend it."

Resistance

After the patient achieves full extension, the knee is flexed approximately 10–15° before resistance is applied. The therapist's hand is placed at the distal end of the anterior surface of the tibia (Fig. 5-118). Resistance is applied slowly to build up to the patient's maximum to avoid injury to the knee. ***Applying sudden or excessive resistance can injure the knee.*** It is almost impossible to break a normal quadriceps (Hines, 1965).

Palpation

Palpate the tendon of the quadriceps as it approaches the patella. Except for the vastus intermedius, the muscle bellies can be palpated on the anterior surface of the thigh. The rectus femoris is in the center and lies over the vastus intermedius. Palpate the other vasti medially and laterally to the rectus femoris.

Substitutions

None.

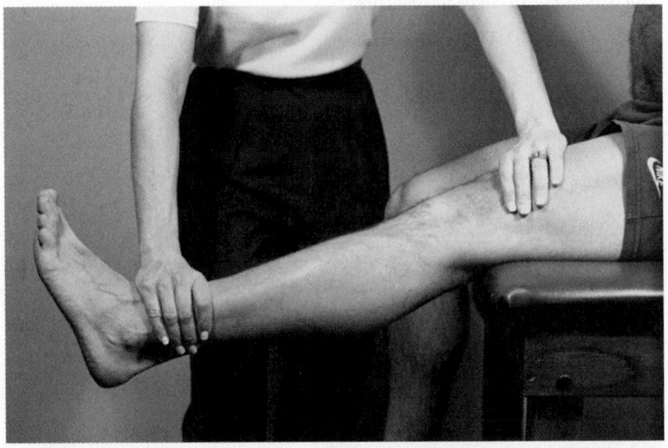

Figure 5-118 Knee extension against gravity.

Ankle Dorsiflexion

Prime Movers

Tibialis anterior

Extensor hallucis longus

Extensor digitorum longus

Against-Gravity Start Position

The patient sits on the plinth with the lower leg hanging down. The foot is perpendicular to the lower leg.

Stabilize

Lower leg just proximal to the ankle.

Instruction

"Lift your foot up so your toes point to the ceiling."

Resistance

The therapist's hand lies on the forefoot and pushes toward plantar flexion without allowing the foot to invert or evert (Fig. 5-119).

Palpation

Palpate the belly of the tibialis anterior immediately lateral to the shaft of the tibia. Palpate its large tendon on the anterior surface of the ankle, medial to the tendon of the extensor hallucis longus. Palpate the latter in the middle of the anterior surface of the ankle. The extensor digitorum longus tendon is prominent on the lateral side of the anterior aspect of the ankle. The tendons of the extensor hallucis longus and extensor digitorum longus can be traced to their insertions on the toes.

Substitutions

None.

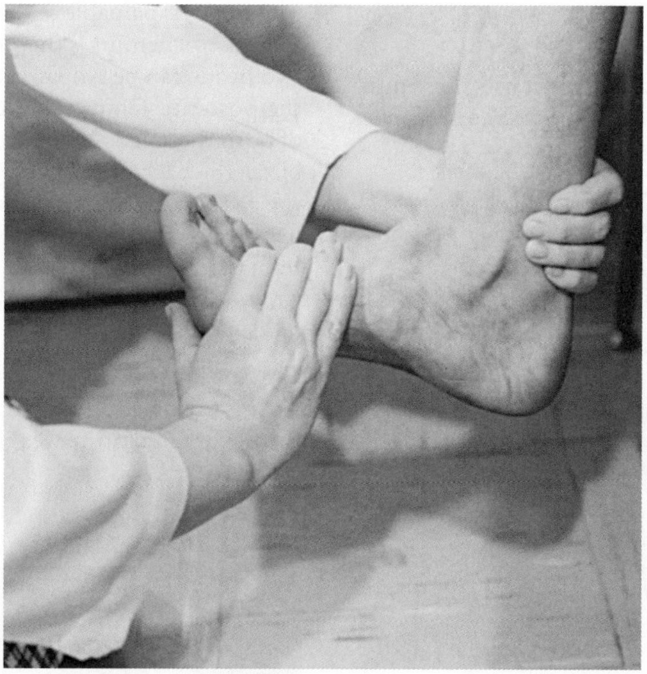

Figure 5-119 Ankle dorsiflexion against gravity.

Ankle Plantar Flexion

Prime Movers

Gastrocnemius

Soleus

Against-Gravity Start Position

There are two ways to test plantar flexion: (1) The patient stands. (2) The patient who cannot stand lies prone on the plinth with the foot off the end of the plinth.

Stabilize

In the standing test, the patient may have to hold onto something for balance. In the prone test, stabilize the lower leg just above the ankle.

Instruction

(1) "Stand on your tiptoes. Do it 20 times." (2) "Press down with your foot as if you were pressing on the gas pedal of a car. Don't let me push it back."

Resistance

In the standing test, the full body weight resists these muscles (Fig. 5-120). In the prone test, the therapist applies manual resistance against the distal portion of the foot and pushes the foot toward dorsiflexion (Fig. 5-121).

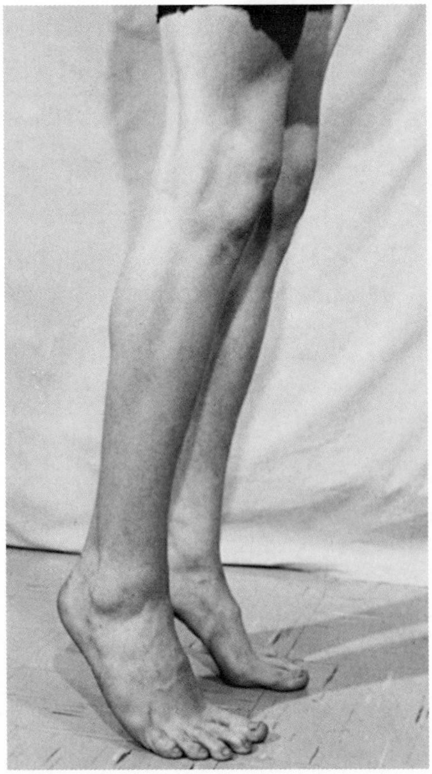

Figure 5-120 Ability to stand on tiptoe indicated grade 5 ankle plantar flexion.

Grading

According to Hislop and Montgomery (1995), the grade is 5 (normal) if the patient completes 20 heel raises through full ROM without rest or fatigue. Other therapists grade 5 if the person can go up on tiptoes and maintain the position longer than momentarily. Hislop and Montgomery give a grade of 4 (good) if the patient completes 10 to 19 heel raises through full ROM without rest or fatigue. The grade is 3 (fair) if 1 to 9 heel raises are completed correctly without rest or fatigue. If the patient is unable to complete full ROM in any one repetition, the grade drops automatically to the next lower level. If the patient cannot complete one heel raise, the grade must be less than 3, and the patient is tested prone. In the prone test, the grade is 2+ (poor plus) if the patient can complete full range and hold against maximal resistance. If the patient completes full range but cannot take any resistance, the grade is 2 (poor).

Palpation

The soleus is palpable at the distal portion of the lower leg. The gastrocnemius is the superficial muscle of the calf; the two heads can be palpated at their origin on either side of the posterior femur. The Achilles tendon is the insertion of both the soleus and gastrocnemius and is readily palpable at the back of the ankle. To minimize the influence of the gastrocnemius when testing for the soleus, the patient lies prone with the knee flexed. Slight resistance is applied to plantar flexion (Kendall et al., 2005).

Substitutions

Gravity substitutes when the person is lying supine or is sitting with feet off the supporting surface. The extrinsic toe flexors substitute weakly.

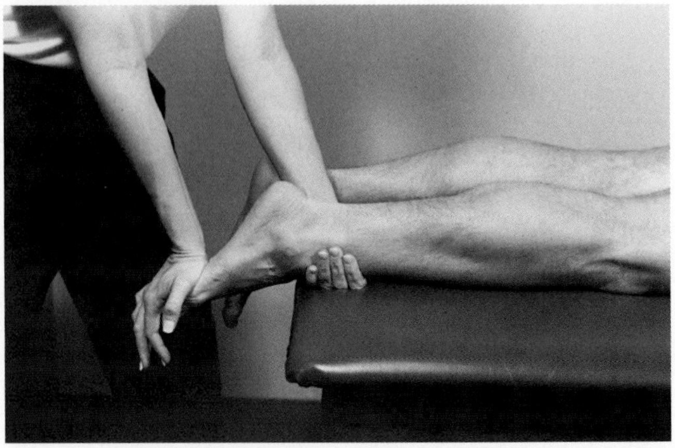

Figure 5-121 Ankle plantarflexion against gravity.

Interpreting the Muscle Test

After recording all muscle test scores, the therapist reviews the scores and looks for the weak muscles and the distribution and significance of the weakness. Any muscle that grades good minus (4−) or below is considered weak. Good plus (4+) muscles are functional and usually require no therapy. Good (4) muscles may or may not be functionally adequate for the patient, depending on his or her occupational task requirements. The pattern of muscle weakness is important. The pattern may indicate general weakness caused by disuse secondary to immobilization, or it may reflect the level of spinal innervation in a patient after spinal cord injury or the distribution of a peripheral nerve in the case of peripheral nerve injury. A pattern of imbalance of forces in agonist and antagonist muscles may be deforming; therefore, counterpositioning or splinting should be considered along with strengthening of the weak muscles.

The pattern of significant strengths is also important. For example, a muscle test of a patient with injured spinal cord that indicates some strength in a muscle innervated by a segment below the diagnosed level of injury is hopeful for more recovery. Or, because muscles are reinnervated proximally to distally after peripheral nerve injury, findings showing beginning return of strength in particular muscles help to track the progress of nerve regeneration.

Short-term goals move the patient from the level of strength determined by testing to the next higher level; for example, if a muscle grades 3, the short-term goal is to improve strength to 3+; if it grades 3+, the goal is to increase strength to 4−, and so on. The required strength for occupational functioning must always be kept in mind when establishing goals.

If the muscle test is a reevaluation, the scores are compared with those of the previous test. The frequency of reevaluation depends on the nature of expected recovery. Expected rapid recovery requires frequent reevaluation. If the repeated muscle test shows that the patient is making gains, the program is considered beneficial and its demands are upgraded. If repeated muscle tests show no gains despite program adaptations, the patient is considered to have reached a plateau and to no longer benefit from remedial therapy. In that case, the focus of treatment shifts to teaching the patient compensatory strategies to enable participation in desired tasks and activities.

Patients with degenerative diseases are expected to get weaker; therefore, therapy is aimed at maintaining their strength and function for as long as possible. Repeated muscle tests confirm that effect of therapy. A plateau for these patients is desirable; it indicates that the therapy is effective for maintaining strength and should be continued.

MEASUREMENT OF GRASP AND PINCH STRENGTH

Therapists supplement manual strength testing with dynamometric evaluations of grip and pinch strength that are valid and reliable (Bellace et al., 2000; Peolsson, Hedlund, & Öberg, 2001) and for which norms have been established (Mathiowetz et al., 1985). Abbreviated versions of the norms are listed in Tables 5-2 and 5-3. Although these norms were originally established using a specific version of the Jamar dynamometer, it has now been established that the Jamar (Blair, 1989), Rolyan (Mathiowetz, 2002), Dexter (Bellace et al., 2000), BTE-Primus (Schechtman et al., 2003), or Baseline (Mathiowetz, Vizenor, & Melander, 2000) models can be used with these grip strength norms. Because variations in measurement between models have been reported (Schechtman, Gestewitz, & Kimble, 2005), therapists are cautioned to use the same dynamometer consistently with any specific patient. The pinch norms can be used with the B & L, JTech, and NK pinch meters because they have been

Table 5-2. Dynamometer Norms in Pounds: Mean of Three Trials

Norms at Age:		20	25	30	35	40	45	50	55	60	65	70	75+
Men	Right	121	121	122	120	117	110	114	101	90	91	75	66
	SD	21	23	22	24	21	23	18	27	20	21	21	21
	Left	104	110	110	113	113	101	102	83	77	77	65	55
	SD	22	16	22	22	19	23	17	23	20	20	18	17
Women	Right	70	74	79	74	70	62	66	57	55	50	50	43
	SD	14	14	19	11	13	15	12	12	10	10	12	11
	Left	61	63	68	66	62	56	57	47	46	41	41	38
	SD	13	12	18	12	14	13	11	12	10	8	10	9

N = 628; age range = 20–94 years.
Reprinted with permission from Mathiowetz, V., Kashman, N., Volland, G., Weber, K., Dowe, M., & Rogers, S. (1985). Grip and pinch strength: Normative data for adults. *Archives of Physical Medicine and Rehabilitation, 66,* 69–74.

Table 5-3. Pinch Meter Norms in Pounds: Mean of Three Trials

		Norms at Age:	20	30	40	50	60	70	75+
Tip	Men	Right	18	18	18	18	16	14	14
		Left	17	18	18	18	15	13	14
	Women	Right	11	13	11	12	10	10	10
		Left	10	12	11	11	10	10	9
Lateral	Men	Right	26	26	26	27	23	19	20
		Left	25	26	25	26	22	19	19
	Women	Right	18	19	17	17	15	14	13
		Left	16	18	16	16	14	14	11
Palmar	Men	Right	27	25	24	24	22	18	19
		Left	26	25	25	24	21	19	18
	Women	Right	17	19	17	17	15	14	12
		Left	16	18	17	16	14	14	12

Tip pinch average standard deviation (SD): men, 4.0; women, 2.5. Lateral pinch average SD: men, 4.6; women, 3.0. Palmar pinch average SD: men, 5.1; women, 3.7. N = 628; age range = 20–94.
Reprinted with permission from Mathiowetz, V., Kashman, N., Volland, G., Weber, K., Dowe, M., & Rogers, S. (1985). Grip and pinch strength: Normative data for adults. *Archives of Physical Medicine and Rehabilitation, 66*, 69–74.

found to be interchangeably reliable: for symptomatic subjects ($r < 0.90$) and for non-symptomatic subjects ($r > 0.80$) (MacDermid, Evenhuis, & Louzon, 2001).

As with any tool of measurement, the instrument must be **calibrated** and set at 0 to start. Dynamometers and pinch meters can be calibrated by placing known weights on or suspending them from the compression part of the meter (Fess, 1987). With this procedure, the Jamar dynamometer was found to be accurate to within ±7% (Schechtman, Gestewitz, & Kimble, 2005), and the B & L pinch meter was found to accurate to within ±1% (Mathiowetz, Vizenor, & Melander, 2000).

The standard method of measurement used in the study from which the norms were established reflects the recommendations of the American Society of Hand Therapists (Fess, 1992). Test-retest (1 week) reliability of this method using the Jamar hydraulic dynamometer was found to be 0.88; inter-rater reliability (two raters, same time) was 0.99. Inter-rater (two raters, same time) reliability of averaged B & L pinch meter scores was 0.98, and test-retest (1 week) reliability was 0.81 (Mathiowetz et al., 1984).

A vigorimeter is an acceptable alternative hand strength-measuring device for patients whose diagnoses contraindicate stress on joints and/or skin. It requires the patient to squeeze a rubber bulb rather than a steel handle. The vigorimeter is a commercially available instrument for which norms have been published (Fike & Rousseau, 1982).

Another adapted sphygmomanometer for measuring grip strength of patients with rheumatoid arthritis was found to have a strong linear relationship ($r = 0.83$ for the right hand; $r = 0.84$ for the left hand) to the Jamar when tested on 88 patients. Agnew and Maas (1991) used linear regression equations to develop conversion tables to relate scores of the Jamar to the sphygmomanometer.

Position can be a factor in the results of a grip strength test. Su et al (1994) examined the effects of different positions of the elbow and shoulder on grip strength using the Jamar dynamometer. The researchers found significant differences in the highest mean grip strength recorded in various positions. This study demonstrates the importance of consistency in the position used for grip testing. If the shoulder or elbow is positioned differently from test to test, the scores will not be reliable, and if the patient is not positioned as in the study that established the norms, the norms are unusable.

Lamoreaux and Hoffer (1995) looked at wrist deviation and its effects on grip and pinch strength. They found no statistical difference in pinch strength when the wrist was deviated, but wrist radial and ulnar deviation significantly decreased grip strength. This research is clinically relevant because certain patients in occupational therapy practice, such as those with Colles' fractures and rheumatoid arthritis, are prone to develop wrist deviations.

A study by Nitschke et al. (1999) addressed how much change in a grip score is necessary to result in a functional change. The study consisted of 42 female participants; 32 were healthy, and 10 had nonspecific regional pain. The authors concluded that at least a 13-pound change in grip strength was necessary to be sure the improvement was not a chance occurrence.

With occupational therapy practice moving into the community and home, the need for valid tools that are quick, portable, and easy to use is increasing. Bohannon (1998) examined the validity of using the Jamar dynamometer to assess upper extremity strength as compared to manual muscle testing in adult home care patients. There were significant correlations between grip dynamometry and manual muscle testing, with the highest correlation between the dynamometer and manual tests of grip for the left hand ($r = 0.80$) and for the right hand ($r = 0.78$). Therefore, the handgrip dynamometer was found to be a good predictor of overall strength.

Grasp (Fig. 5-122; Table 5-2)

The patient should be seated with his or her shoulder adducted and neutrally rotated, the elbow flexed at 90°, and the forearm and wrist in neutral position. Grip strength varies with elbow position, so a standardized position is necessary (Su et al., 1994). The handle of the dynamometer is set at the second position (Mathiowetz et al., 1984, 1985). The task is demonstrated to the patient. After the dynamometer is positioned in the patient's hand, the therapist says, "Ready? Squeeze as hard as you can," and urges the patient on throughout the attempt. The patient squeezes the dynamometer with as much force as he or she can three times, with a 2- to 3-minute rest between trials. The score is the average of the three trials.

Pinch

Three types of pinch are typically evaluated because they are involved in accomplishing occupational tasks and activities efficiently.

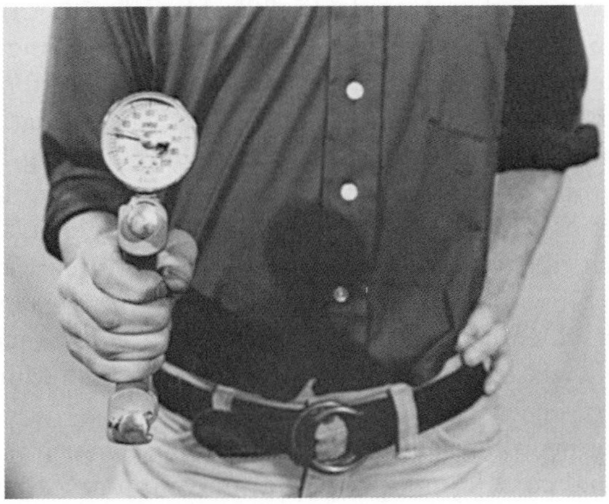

Figure 5-122 Measuring grasp using a dynamometer. The patient's upper arm is close to his body, and the elbow is flexed to 90°.

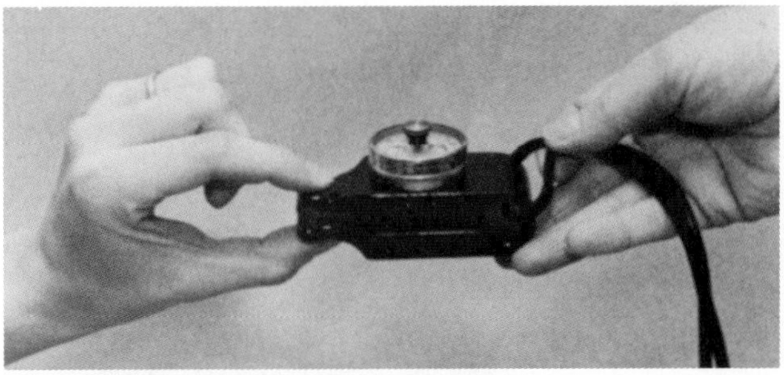

Figure 5-123 Measuring tip pinch with a pinch meter.

Tip Pinch (Fig. 5-123; Table 5-3)

The patient pinches the ends of the pinch meter between the tips of the thumb and index finger (Mathiowetz et al., 1985) or between the thumb and the index and middle fingers (MacDermid, Evenhuis, & Louzon, 2001). The test is administered by first giving the patient instructions and a demonstration. Then the therapist says, "Ready? Pinch as hard as you can." The patient is urged on as he or she attempts to pinch. Three trials, with a rest between each trial, are completed. The average of three trials is recorded.

Lateral Pinch (Fig. 5-124; Table 5-3)

The patient pinches the meter between the pad of the thumb and the lateral surface of the index finger. The instructions and procedure are the same as for tip pinch.

Palmar Pinch: Three-Jaw Chuck (Fig. 5-125; Table 5-3)

The patient pinches the meter between the pad of the thumb and the pads of the index and middle fingers. The instructions and procedure are the same as for tip pinch.

Interpretation of Grasp and Pinch Scores

Scores are compared with those of the other hand or to norms to ascertain whether the patient has a significant

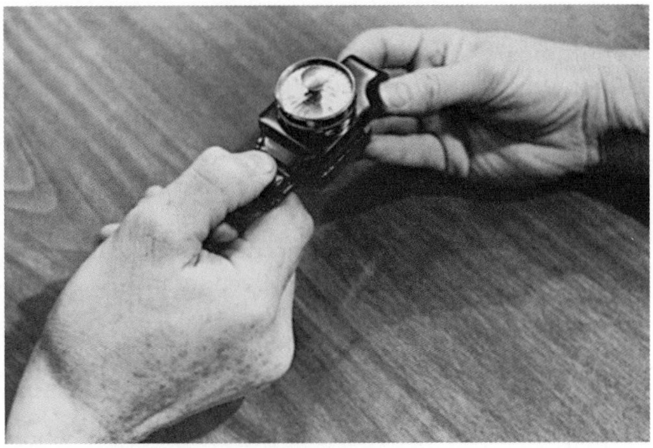

Figure 5-124 Measuring lateral pinch.

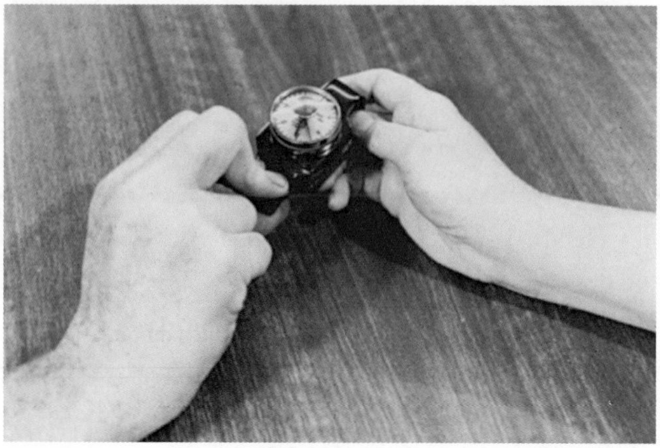

Figure 5-125 Measuring palmar pinch or three-jaw chuck pinch.

limitation. The accuracy of the Jamar dynamometer was found to be ±7%, which means that, if the patient scored 50 pounds, the actual strength may range from 46.5 to 53.5 pounds (Schechtman, Gestewitz, & Kimble, 2005). Grasp and pinch scores are considered abnormal if they are associated with a functional limitation and/or if they are ±3 **standard deviations** (SD) from the mean. For example, suppose a 40-year-old man had a grasp score of 50 pounds when you averaged the three trials for his dominant right hand. Table 5-2 shows that the average score for his age group is 117 pounds, so the patient's grasp score was 67 pounds less than the mean normal score on the table. When you divide the difference in his score (62) by the SD given in the table (21), you find that he is 3.2 SD below the mean. This is more than 3 SD below the mean, so he has a significant limitation. Grasp and pinch measurements can be quickly and easily reevaluated over time to monitor the progress of the patient and the effectiveness of the treatment plan.

MEASUREMENT OF ENDURANCE

Endurance is the ability to sustain effort and to resist fatigue (Wilmore & Costill, 1999). It is related to cardiopulmonary and muscular function. The better cardiopulmonary and muscular function a person has, the better the endurance. Many of the patients seen in occupational therapy have endurance limitations. A variety of conditions, including cardiac or pulmonary impairments, a major trauma or illness requiring bed rest, loss of significant muscle function, or the need to use prostheses or adapted equipment, can affect one's endurance.

Cardiopulmonary Aspects of Endurance

Cardiopulmonary endurance is the ability of the whole body to sustain prolonged rhythmical activity (Wilmore & Costill, 1999). Muscular work creates a demand for oxygen. As an immediate effect of activity, the heart rate and stroke volume increase. Heart rate increases to deliver the required amount of oxygenated blood to the active muscles. Stroke volume, or amount of blood pumped per heartbeat, increases because of increased venous flow into the heart during diastole (the period of relaxation when the chambers fill) (American College of Sports Medicine, 2000). As the intensity of muscular work increases, more oxygen is required. There is, however, a maximal amount of oxygen that a person can take in and dispense to muscles during exercise. Termed maximal oxygen uptake, it is abbreviated $\dot{V}O_{2max}$. $\dot{V}O_{2max}$ is a standard measure of cardiovascular fitness (American College of Sports Medicine, 2001). It increases with physical training and decreases with bed rest and age. With physical training, the heart rate becomes lower for the same level of work, which is referred to as the training effect. The training effect indicates improvement in efficiency of the circulatory system (American College of Sports Medicine, 2000).

There is a linear relationship between oxygen uptake and heart rate for various intensities of light to moderately heavy exercise. Therefore, heart rate can be used to estimate $\dot{V}O_2$. However, the heart rate of those who are physically unfit increases faster for a given level of oxygen uptake; therefore, the relationship is individual (American College of Sports Medicine, 2001).

Muscular Aspects of Endurance

Endurance of a muscle or muscle group is its ability to sustain intensive activity (Wilmore & Costill, 1999); endurance may be decreased because of local trauma or reduction of innervation. In normal muscle contraction against low resistance, only a few of the available motor units are needed at any one time. The active and resting units take turns. Fatigue rarely occurs in conditions required for activities of daily life. If the person sustains a contraction that exceeds 15–20% MVC for the muscle group involved, however, blood flow to the working muscle decreases, causing a shift to anaerobic metabolism, which limits duration of contraction. The limitation is signaled by symptoms of muscle fatigue (cramping, burning, and tremor, which are secondary to the accumulation of lactic acid) and slowed nerve conduction velocity to the muscle fibers, which reduce tension and eventually result in inability to hold the contraction (American College of Sports Medicine, 2001). Strength and endurance are closely related. As a muscle gains strength, its endurance for a given level of work also increases.

For neurologically disadvantaged muscle, such as after a spinal cord injury, peripheral nerve injury, or stroke, fewer motor units or muscle fibers may be available than are required for daily activity. Such muscles work at as much as 50–75% MVC to do otherwise low-intensity work (Trombly & Quintana, 1985).

The Evaluation

Endurance can be measured dynamically or statically. Dynamic assessments include the number of repetitions per unit of time or the percentage of maximal heart rate generated by an aerobic activity or exercise or metabolic equivalent (MET) level. Static assessment is the amount of time a contraction can be held (American College of Sports Medicine, 2000; Fletcher et al., 2001).

Intensity, duration, and frequency of the activity are considerations in evaluation of endurance. Intensity is related to both resistance and speed. The heavier the resistance or the faster the pace is, the higher the intensity. The intensity of the test activity must be kept constant from test to test to gauge improvement.

Intensity of an activity is estimated in terms of light, moderate, or heavy work or number of METs. One MET equals basal metabolic rate (American College of Sports Medicine, 2001). Basal metabolic rate is the amount of oxygen consumption necessary to maintain the metabolic processes (e.g., respiration, circulation, peristalsis, temperature regulation, glandular function) of the body at rest and is quantified as 3.5 mL of oxygen per kilogram of body weight per minute. The energy cost of activities or exercise can be rated using multiples of METs. An exercise that is rated 4 METs requires 4 times the amount of oxygen per kilogram of body weight per minute than the basal rate. The oxygen consumption of daily living, recreational, and vocational tasks has been measured for normal subjects, and the METs required for each task have been calculated (Table 5-4). These costs are estimates that vary with environmental conditions, such as humidity and temperature, and personal conditions, such as anger.

Heart rate is a simple means to quantify the physiological demand of a dynamic activity for a particular person (Hall & Brody, 1999). Because heart rate relates linearly to $\dot{V}O_{2max}$ except at the upper limits (80–90%) of maximal capacity, if a person's heart rate is 70% of maximal heart rate (HR_{max}), he or she is using approximately 70% of $\dot{V}O_{2max}$. HR_{max} is estimated by subtracting the person's age from 220. The pulse taken immediately after aerobic large-muscle exercise is then related to the person's HR_{max} as percent-

Table 5-4. Metabolic Equivalents

Energy Level	Activities of Daily Living	Occupational Activities	Recreational Activities
1–2 MET	Eating Dressing and undressing Washing hands and face Sweeping the floor	Desk and phone work Keyboard operation Riding in a car Watch repair	Standing Walking (strolling 1 mile/hr) Playing cards and board games Painting
2.5–3.5 MET	Showering Food preparation Making beds Ironing Cleaning windows	Welding Small-parts assembly Bricklaying and plastering Playing a musical instrument	Walking (2 miles/hr) Cycling (5.5 miles/hr) Horseback riding (walk) Billiards Bowling Golf (pulling bag cart)
4–5 MET	Raking leaves Hoeing Walking downstairs Beating carpets	Heavy assembly work Painting Light carpentry Paperhanging	Walking (3 miles/hr) Cycling (9 miles/hr) Golf (carrying clubs) Ballroom dancing Table tennis
5.5–6.5 MET	Walking with braces and crutches Mowing lawn by hand mower	Carpentry Chopping wood	Walking (4 miles/hr) Tennis Horseback riding (trot) Folk dancing Ice or roller skating
7–8 MET		Shoveling (22 pounds for 10 minutes) Digging	Jogging (5 miles/hr) Skiing (vigorous) Horseback riding (gallop)
8.5–9.5 MET		Shoveling (31 pounds for 10 minutes)	Running (7.5 miles/hr) Squash Fencing Football Basketball

MET, metabolic equivalents.
Adapted with permission from Wilmore, J. H., & Costill, D. L. (1999). *Physiology of sport and exercise* (2nd ed.). Champaign IL: Human Kinetics.

age of maximum. A constant heart rate obtained during exercise indicates a steady state, that is, a balance of oxygen intake and consumption (Fletcher et al., 2001). Heart rate is measured by placing the index and middle fingers lightly but firmly over the radial artery at the wrist (lateral to the flexor carpi radialis) and counting the number of beats per minute (bpm). It is most accurate to count for a full minute, but an exercise heart rate can be counted for only 10 to 15 seconds, as the return to resting rate occurs quickly after stopping exercise. In that case, the obtained value is multiplied by 6 for 10 seconds or 4 for 15 seconds to arrive at the bpm (American College of Sports Medicine, 2001).

The relation between heart rate and oxygen uptake does not hold for patients with chronic obstructive pulmonary disease, who, because of reduced expiration and expulsion of carbon dioxide waste, have greater ventilatory requirements. These patients have limited exercise capacity (American College of Sports Medicine, 2001).

Whether to measure dynamically or statically depends on the functional goal of the patient and his or her cardiopulmonary status. If the patient's self-advancement and self-enhancement roles require mostly isotonic activity, endurance should be evaluated dynamically. To measure endurance in terms of number of repetitions, use a light repetitive activity such as the *Box and Block Test*, which is described in Chapter 42. It can be adapted to measure upper extremity endurance for light work by counting the number of blocks the patient can transfer before becoming fatigued.

If the patient expects to return to a job or hobby that requires maintained grasp or holding loads (isometric contractions), static endurance should be tested. To measure statically, the amount of time a person can hold an object or position requiring a certain level MVC is noted. Normally, a person can hold 25% MVC for 5 to 6 minutes, 50% MVC for 1 to 2 minutes, and 100% MVC only momentarily (Dehn & Mullins, 1977).

Isometric holding increases blood pressure and stresses the cardiopulmonary system (Pollock et al., 2000) (Safety Tip 5-1). This is true especially if the person holds his or her breath (Valsalva maneuver) while holding the contraction. Therefore, persons being tested should talk (e.g., count or sing) while doing an isometric contraction to preclude breath holding. Isometric testing can produce arrhythmias and, therefore, electrocardiogram and blood pressure should be monitored during isometric testing of patients with heart disease or abnormalities. The results of isometric testing cannot be extrapolated to gauge isotonic aerobic exercise capacity (Pollock et al., 2000).

Another way to assess dynamic endurance is to ascertain the individual's perception of how hard he or she is working. Scales of ratings of perceived exertion (RPE), such as the *Rating of Perceived Exertion* (Borg, 1985), are based on psychophysics or the relating of a physical property to a subjective property via scaling procedures (Russell, 1997). The *Borg* (15-point) *Scale of Perceived Exertion* ranges from 6 (no exertion at all) to 20 (maximal exertion) (Wilmore & Costill, 1999). This scale allows the person to assign one of a consecutive set of numbers with a corresponding descriptor of amount of exertion to the ongoing activity (e.g., 11, fairly light; or 17, very hard). The American Heart Association (2001) and the American College of Sports Medicine (2000) suggest that an RPE of 12–16 on the 15-point *Borg Scale* is associated with a physiological training effect (Whaley et al., 1997). Therapists should be aware, however, that perceived exertion for a given level of oxygen uptake is higher for arm work than leg work (Russell, 1997). For dynamic activities, the *Borg Scale* has been found over the years to correlate validly with heart rate and oxygen uptake (Finucane, Fiddler, & Lindfield, 2005). Lamb, Eston, and Corns (1999) looked at test–retest reliability and found it to differ by as much as 3 RPE when level of agreement between trials was examined and the scores of the two trials were not merely correlated. Whaley et al. (1997) tested the validity of the oxygen consumption associated with each score on the 15-point *Borg Scale*. They found interindividual differences that ranged from a rating of 6 to 20 for 60% **maximum heart rate reserve** (MHRR) and from 8 to 20 for 80% MHRR in both normal healthy adults and cardiac patients. Nevertheless, these scales provide a good estimate when used repeatedly for the same patient and, therefore, may be used clinically during ongoing continuous activity, such as walking, bicycling, scrubbing floors, painting a wall, mowing the lawn, raking leaves, and calisthenic exercises. These scales do not apply to activities composed of sporadic variable movements.

The therapist should orient the person to the scale using standardized instructions published by Borg (1985) prior to the start of the activity. The scale should be enlarged and posted so that it can be seen easily from where the person is exercising. At 1- or 2-minute intervals, the therapist prompts the patient to rate exertion at that moment. The decision to continue depends on the goal and precautions for the particular patient.

SAFETY NOTE 5-1

Precautions for Isometric Testing

- If the patient exhibits dyspnea, weakness, changes in sensorium, angina, decreased heart rate (HR) for increased workload, increased ventricular arrhythmias, pallor, or cyanosis, his or her cardiopulmonary capacity has been exceeded (American College of Sports Medicine, 2001).
- Endurance testing in occupational therapy should not reach this level, but if any of these symptoms are observed or reported by the patient, the intensity of work should be immediately reduced to a comfortable level.

Assessment Table 5-1

Summary of Assessment of Abilities and Capacities

Instrument & Reference	Description	Time to Administer	Validity[a]	Reliability[b]	Sensitivity[c]	Strengths & Weaknesses
Measurement of Range of Motion	Interval scale, ranges vary with joint being measured.	Full evaluation of all joints in the upper extremity, 45 minutes to an hour.	Gold standard.	Intra-rater reliability for shoulder external rotation, ICC = 0.58–0.67, internal rotation ICC = 0.63–0.71. Inter-rater reliability for external rotation = 0.41–0.66, internal rotation ICC = 0.41–0.66 (Awan, Smith, & Boon, 2002).	In the upper and lower extremities, measurement error is estimated at 5° (Aalto et al., 2005; Groth et al., 2001).	Strengths: Relatively fast and inexpensive measure. Measurements are consistently more accurate when done by a single therapist, with the patient in the same position from test to test. Weaknesses: Inter-rater reliability is consistently lower than intra-rater reliability. Accuracy of measurement is dependent on the consistent placement of the goniometer.
Hand Volumetry (Dodds et al., 2004)	Interval scale because it is a direct measure of the volume of water displaced.	15–20 minutes.	Direct measurement of hand volume.	Test–retest reliability, $r = 0.99$ (Dodds et al., 2004).	Variation of measurement, 3–5 mL (Dodds et al., 2004).	Strength: Gold standard for edema measurement. Weaknesses: Hand must be immersed in water, so cannot be used with open wounds, skin conditions, etc. Takes considerable time.

continued

Assessment Table 5-1

Summary of Assessment of Abilities and Capacities (continued)

Instrument & Reference	Description	Time to Administer	Validity[a]	Reliability[b]	Sensitivity[c]	Strengths & Weaknesses
Figure-of-Eight Technique to Measure Hand Edema (Pellecchia, 2004)	Interval scale.	3–4 minutes.	Correlation coefficient between figure-of-eight technique and hand volumetry, ICC = 0.94–0.95 (Maihafer et al., 2004).	Intra-tester ICC for figure-of-eight ICC = 0.98–0.99; inter-tester reliability ICC = 0.99 (Leard et al., 2004).	Not established.	Strengths: Fast measurement; can be used with individuals with open wounds or skin conditions. Weakness: Sensitivity not established.
Visual Analog Scale for Pain Measurement	Interval scale with scores from 1–10.	1 minute.	Gold standard.	Not established.	Not established.	Strengths: Fast measurement and can be used to monitor changes in pain in a single patient. Weakness: Cannot be used to compare pain levels between patients.
Manual Muscle Testing	Ordinal scale from 0–5.	Depending on the number of muscles being tested, up to 1 hour.	Gold standard.	In a reliability test for intrinsic hand muscles, intra-rater r = 0.71–0.96 and inter-rater r = 0.72–0.93 (Brandsma et al., 1995). In an evaluation of reliability for the deltoid muscles, Pollard et al. (2005) found that two testers agreed exactly 82% of the time ($\kappa = 0.62$).	Not established.	Strength: No equipment needed. Weakness: Dependent on training and experience of the tester.

continued

Hand-Held Dynamometry	Interval scale, measurement is in kilograms.	Depending on the number of muscles being tested, up to 1 hour.	Direct measure of strength.	Inter-rater reliability ICC = 0.79–0.96; intra-rater reliability ICC = 0.87–0.98 (Ottenbacher, et al., 2002).	Norms established (Bohannon, 1998).	Strength: Reliable testing device. Weaknesses: Validity and sensitivity not established; expense of device.
Grip Strength Test	Interval scale, measures resistance in pounds or kilograms.	5 minutes.	Recommended by American Society of Hand Therapy as a valid measure of hand strength (Fess, 1992).	Test–retest reliability of Jamar dynamometer = 0.88; inter-rater reliability = 0.99 (Mathiowetz et al., 1984).	Norms established (Mathiowetz et al., 1985).	Strengths: Quick and easy measure; norms available. Weakness: Dynamometers need to be calibrated regularly to be accurate.
Pinch Test	Interval scale, measures resistance in pounds or kilograms	5 minutes.	Recommended by American Society of Hand Therapy as a valid measure of pinch strength (Fess, 1992).	Inter-rater reliability = 0.98; test–retest reliability = 0.81 (Mathiowetz et al., 1984).	Norms established (Mathiowetz, et al., 1985).	Strengths: Quick and easy measure; norms available. Weaknesses: Pinchmeters need to be calibrated regularly to be accurate.
Borg Rating of Perceived Exertion Scale	Ordinal scale, from 6–20.	1 minute.	Valid measure of exercise intensity (Chen, Fan, & Moe, 2002).	Not established.	Not established.	Strength: Good measure for individuals. Weakness: Not consistent between individuals.

[a] Validity is the ability of an instrument to measure what it is intended and presumed to measure. Criterion validity is determined by comparing its results to an agreed-on g*old standard* (accepted test). Predictive validity is its ability to predict future outcomes.
[b] Reliability is a measure of an instrument's stability. Inter-observer or inter-rater reliability refers to the ability of two different individuals to administer the instrument to a particular person and achieve similar results. Test–retest reliability refers to the constancy of results over repeated use of the instrument in the absence of change in the patient.
[c] Sensitivity to change is the ability of an instrument to detect clinically important change.

CASE EXAMPLE

Occupational Therapy Assessment Process	Clinical Reasoning Process: Objectives	Clinical Reasoning Process: Examples of Therapist's Internal Dialogue
Patient Information Mrs. B. is a 58-year-old right-handed woman with a 5-year history of primary degenerative joint disease (DJD), or osteoarthritis. She complains of upper extremity weakness, stiffness, and Heberden's nodes over several DIP joints. She also complains of pain and fatigue that are increasingly limiting her self-maintenance, self advancement, and self-enhancement roles.	Understand the patient's diagnosis or condition	"Mrs. B is very active, and the increasing problems she is having because of the progression of her DJD are probably very frustrating to her. I wonder how much she knows about DJD?"
	Know the person	"Mrs. B. lives alone and is used to taking care of herself. I wonder if she stops activities due to pain and fatigue, or works through it?"
She is a divorced fifth-grade teacher who lives alone in a one-story house. She has two grown children and enjoys gardening, reading, and shopping for antiques. She has a referral for occupational therapy services because of the occupational dysfunction and has been approved for four outpatient visits.	Appreciate the context	"I bet teaching in a fifth grade classroom is a challenging environment, and I think it might be difficult to adapt the classroom to her limitations, for example, her need for rest, or stopping when she has pain. I wonder if she has any help with the heavy work around the house-heavy cleaning, lawn-mowing, snow shoveling, etc."
	Develop provisional hypotheses	"She has had this diagnosis for 5 years, and it sounds like she is having increasing problems. I wonder if she is limiting her activities due to pain and fatigue, and therefore losing more strength and endurance?"
Assessment Process To determine Mrs. B.'s perception of her occupational dysfunction and her priorities, the therapist administered the Canadian Occupational Performance Measure (COPM). To determine to what extent strength and endurance problems affected Mrs. B.'s occupational functioning, a manual muscle test on selected muscle groups, grip and pinch strength assessment, visual analogue pain rating scale, and the Borg Perceived Exertion Scale for endurance during activities were administered.	Consider evaluation approach and methods	"I need to get a picture of what occupations are important to her. I also need to know exactly how her arms are functioning in terms of strength in her shoulders, elbows, and wrists, as well as her grip and pinch strength. I'd like to know how much pain she is having at rest and during activity, and what her endurance is for important activities."
Assessment Results The results of the COPM are as follows: Difficulty writing on the chalk board, which she does 2 to 3 hours a day (performance 4, satisfaction 3) Difficulty with morning activities of daily living, including showering and dressing. She has problems reaching overhead, manipulating bottle caps, doing buttons and zippers, and putting on jewelry (performance 6, satisfaction 5)	Interpret observations	"Mrs. B. is involved in lots of gross and fine motor activities during the day, and seems to be having problems with all of them."

Difficulty decorating her classroom bulletin boards and doing arts and crafts at school because of the cutting and stapling (performance 5, satisfaction 5)

Inability to do many meal preparation activities, including manipulating kitchen appliances, cutting vegetables, and carrying dishes (performance 4, satisfaction 4)
Unable to garden as desired, specifically planting, digging with a trowel, and weeding (performance 3, satisfaction 2)

The results of Mrs. B.'s manual muscle test are displayed below. Grip strength using a Jamar dynamometer was 18 pounds on the right and 45 pounds on the left. Tip pinch strength was 3 pounds on the right, 9 pounds on the left. Lateral pinch was 5 pounds on the right, 12 pounds on the left. Palmar pinch was 4 pounds on the right, 13 pounds on the left.

Manual muscle strength	Right	Left
Shoulder flexion	3-	4-
Shoulder abduction	3-	4-
Shoulder external rotation	3-	4
Elbow flexion	4	4+
Elbow extension	3+	4
Forearm supination	3+	4+
Forearm pronation	4	4+
Wrist flexion	3+	4
Wrist extension	3+	4

Mrs. B. reported a 2 on the visual analog scale (VAS) for pain at rest but stated that pain in her hands and shoulders increases to 4 during morning activities of daily living, 5 during meal preparation, and 6 when she uses scissors or gardening tools.

Using the Borg Scale, Mrs. B. rated bathing and dressing this morning a 13; teaching an hour math lesson using the blackboard, a 14; and gardening for a half an hour, a 17.

"Mrs. B. is weak in all of the muscle groups of the right arm and proximally in her left arm. The weakness of her right shoulder would interfere with writing on the blackboard, and with washing and brushing her hair. The dynamometer test showed a significant decrease in grip strength for her right hand, which is her dominant hand, but was within normal limits for her left hand. Her right hand pinches were also significantly limited compared to the left or to the norms, while all three pinches of her left hand were within normal limits. The weakness in her right hand also contributes to her difficulty in many occupational tasks, such as using scissors or a stapler, opening jars, and manipulating garden tools."

"Mrs. B.'s scores on the VAS indicate increased pain in her hands and shoulders during many functional activities, with decreased pain at rest. The results of the Borg Scale indicate low endurance, which contributes to her fatigue and decreased ability to perform a number of tasks, including standing while bathing, teaching, and gardening. The fact that she has pain during most of these activities would also increase her fatigue."

Occupational Therapy Problem List

Decreased ability to perform morning activities of daily living, including bathing and dressing, because of shoulder weakness and low endurance.

Decreased ability to perform meal preparation tasks because of weak grasp and pinch.

Decreased ability to perform work-related tasks, including writing on the blackboard, decorating bulletin boards, and arts and crafts, because of weak shoulders bilaterally, poor endurance, and pain.

Decreased ability to garden because of weakness and pain.

Synthesize results

"Mrs. B. has problems with weakness, pain, and fatigue, which are all interrelated, and are all interfering with the activities she wants to be able to do. I will need to find out if she would be willing to make some adaptations to some of these occupations to reduce her pain and fatigue. I'm concerned that if I just add a home program to address her problems with strength, it will just compound her problems with endurance and fatigue."

"I need to find out how flexible her work environment is, and whether she has any control of her daily schedule or activities when she is in the classroom. Maybe the students could help out with writing on the board or demonstrating the arts and crafts?"

"I wonder if there are any things that she is doing that are going well—any occupations with which she isn't have trouble? If not, I'm concerned about her emotional well-being."

SUMMARY REVIEW QUESTIONS

1. Describe in general the correct placement of a goniometer.
2. What does it mean if AROM is less than PROM?
3. ROM limitations can be caused by a number of underlying conditions. State the short-term goal for treatment of elbow flexion contracture after removal of a cast used to immobilize a fractured humerus.
4. How is a break test used to determine strength?
5. Of what importance is the length-tension relationship of a muscle in manual muscle testing?
6. Describe the standardized procedures for testing muscle strength.
7. For what muscle test grades is treatment to increase strength an appropriate goal?
8. How is dynamic endurance measured?
9. How is static endurance measured?
10. What is your maximum heart rate? What percentage of $\dot{V}O_{2max}$ do you use to vacuum a room? Take a shower? Wash the dishes?

ACKNOWLEDGMENTS

Over the many editions of this textbook, several photographers have contributed to this chapter. They are Anne Fisher, ScD, OTR; Lucia Grochowska-Littlefield; Judith La Drew; and Keith Weaver. The models for the photographs are Brian Despres, OTR; Mark Erikson; Sam Fitzpatrick; Jim Morando; James Polga; and Christopher Trombly. To all of these people, without whom we could not have produced this chapter, we give our deepest thanks.

References

Aalto, T. J., Airaksinen, O., Härkönen, T. M., & Arokoski, J. P. (2005). Effect of passive stretch on reproducibility of hip range of motion measurements. *Archives of Physical Medicine and Rehabilitation, 86,* 549–557.

Agnew, P. J., & Maas, F. (1991). Jamar dynamometer and adapted sphygmomanometer for measuring grip strength in patients with rheumatoid arthritis. *Occupational Therapy Journal of Research, 11,* 259–270.

American College of Sports Medicine. (2000). *Guidelines for Exercise Testing and Prescription* (6th ed.). Baltimore: Lippincott, Williams & Wilkins.

American College of Sports Medicine. (2001). *ACSM's Resource Manual for Guidelines for Exercise Testing and Prescription* (4th ed.). Philadelphia: Lippincott, Williams & Wilkins.

American Heart Association. (2001). Exercise standards testing and training: A statement for health care professionals from the American Heart Association. *Circulation, 104,* 1694–1740.

Anderson, L. R. III, & Bohannon, R. W. (1991). Head and neck position does not influence maximum static elbow extension force measured in healthy individuals tested while prone. *Occupational Therapy Journal of Research, 11,* 121–126.

Andrews, A. W., Thomas, M. W., & Bohannon, R. W. (1996). Normative values for isometric muscle force measurements obtained with hand-held dynamometers. *Physical Therapy, 76,* 248–259.

Awan, R., Smith, J., & Boon, A. J. (2002). Measuring shoulder internal rotation range of motion: A comparison of 3 techniques. *Archives of Physical Medicine and Rehabilitation, 83,* 1229–1234.

Bellace, J. V., Healy, D., Byron, T., & Hohman, L. (2000). Validity of the Dexter evaluation system's Jamar dynamometer attachment for assessment of handgrip strength in a normal population. *Journal of Hand Therapy, 13,* 46–51.

Blair, S. M. (1989). Comparison of Jamar dynamometers: Inter-instrument reliability [unpublished Master's thesis]. Richmond, VA: Virginia Commonwealth University.

Bohannon, R. W. (1988). Make tests and break tests of elbow flexor muscle strength. *Physical Therapy, 68,* 193–194.

Bohannon, R. W. (1998). Hand-grip dynamometry provides a valid indication of upper extremity strength impairment in home care patients. *Journal of Hand Therapy, 11,* 258–260.

Bohannon, R. W., Warren, M., & Cogman, K. (1991). Influence of shoulder position on maximum voluntary elbow flexion force in stroke patients. *Occupational Therapy Journal of Research, 11,* 73–79.

Boone, A. J., & Smith, J. (2000). Manual scapular stabilization: Its effect on shoulder rotational range of motion. *Archives of Physical Medicine and Rehabilitation, 81,* 978–983.

Borg, G. A. V. (1985). *An introduction to Borg's RPE-Scale.* New York: Mouvement.

Brandsma, J. W., Schreuders, T. R., Birke, J. A., Piefer, A., & Oostendorp, P. (1995). Manual muscle strength testing: Intraobserver and interobserver reliabilities for the intrinsic muscles of the hand. *Journal of Hand Therapy, 8,* 185–190.

Chen, M. J., Fan, I., & Moe, S. T. (2002). Criterion-related validity of the Borg ratings of perceived exertion scale in healthy individuals: A meta-analysis. *Journal of Sports Sciences, 20,* 873–899.

Clarkson, H. M. (2000). *Musculoskeletal assessment: Joint range of motion and manual muscle strength* (2nd ed.). Philadelphia: Lippincott, Williams & Wilkins

Dehn, M. M., & Mullins, C. B. (1977). Physiologic effects and importance of exercise in patients with coronary artery disease. *Cardiovascular Medicine, 2,* 365–371, 377–387.

Diekmeyer, G. (1978). Altered test position for hip extensor muscles. *Physical Therapy, 58,* 1379.

Dodds, R. L., Nielsen, K. A., Shirley, A. G., Stefaniak, H., Falconio, M. J., & Moyers, P. A. (2004). Test-retest reliability of the commercial volumeter. *Work, 22,* 107–110.

Ellis, B., & Bruton, A. (2002). A study to compare the reliability of composite finger flexion with goniometry for measurement of range of motion in the hand. *Clinical Rehabilitation, 16,* 562–570.

Fess, E. E. (1987). A method of checking Jamar dynamometer calibration. *Journal of Hand Therapy, 1,* 28–32.

Fess, E. E. (1992). Grip strength. In J. S. Casanova (Ed.), *Clinical assessment recommendations* (2nd ed., pp. 41–45). Chicago: American Society of Hand Therapists.

Fike, M. L., & Rousseau, E. (1982). Measurement of adult hand strength: A comparison of two instruments. *Occupational Therapy Journal of Research, 2,* 43–49.

Finucane, L., Fiddler, H., & Lindfield, H. (2005). Assessment of the RPE as a measure of cardiovascular fitness in patients with low back pain. *International Journal of Therapy and Rehabilitation, 12,* 106–111.

Fletcher, G. F., Balady, G. J., Amsterdam, E. A., Chaitman, B., Eckel, R., Fleg, J., Froelicher, V. F., Leon, A. S., Piña I. L., Rodney, R., Simons-Morton, D. G., Williams, M. A., & Bazzarre, T. (2001). AHA Scientific Statement: Exercise standards for testing and training: A statement for healthcare professionals from the American Heart Association. *Circulation, 104,* 1694–1740.

Gordon, M., Greenfield, E., Marvin, J., Hester C., & Lauterbach, S. (1998). Use of pain assessment tools: Is there a preference? *Journal of Burn Care Rehabilitation, 19,* 451–454.

Greene, W. B., & Heckman, J. D. (Eds.). (1994). *The clinical measurement of joint motion.* Rosemont, IL: American Academy of Orthopaedic Surgeons.

Groth, G. N., VanDeven, K. M., Phillips, E. C., & Ehretsman, R. L. (2001). Goniometry of the proximal and distal interphalangeal joints: Part III. Placement preferences, interrater reliability and concurrent validity. *Journal of Hand Therapy, 14,* 23–29.

Gunal, I., Kose, N., Erdogan, O., Gokturk, E., & Seber, S. (1996). Normal range of motion of the joints of the upper extremity in male subjects, with special reference to side. *Journal of Bone and Joint Surgery, 78-A,* 1401–1404.

Hall, C. M., & Brody, L. T. (1999). *Therapeutic exercise: Moving toward function*. Philadelphia: Lippincott, Williams & Wilkins.

Hayes, K., Walton, J. R., Szomor Z. L., & Murrell, G. A. C. (2002). Reliability of 3 methods for assessing shoulder strength. *Journal of Shoulder and Elbow Surgery, 11,* 33–39.

Herbison, G. J., Issac, Z., Cohne, M. E., & Ditunno, J. F. (1996). Strength post-spinal cord injury: Myometer versus manual muscle test. *Spinal Cord, 34,* 543–548.

Hines, T. (1965). Manual muscle examination. In S. Licht (Ed.), *Therapeutic exercise* (2nd ed., pp. 163–256). Baltimore: Waverly.

Hislop, H., & Montgomery, J. (Eds.). (1995). *Daniel's and Worthingham's muscle testing* (6th ed.). Philadelphia: W. B. Saunders Co.

Howell, J. W., Rothstein, J. M., Lamb, R. L., & Merritt, W. H. (1989). An experimental investigation of the validity of the manual muscle test positions for the extensor pollicis longus and flexor pollicis brevis muscles. *Journal of Hand Therapy, 3,* 20–28.

Jacobs, K., & Jacobs L. (Eds.). (2004). *Quick reference dictionary for occupational therapy* (4th ed.). Thorofare, NJ: Slack.

Johannson, C. A., Kent, B. E., & Shepard, K. F. (1983). Relationship between verbal command volume and magnitude of muscle contraction. *Physical Therapy, 63,* 1260–1265.

Katz, J., & Melzack, R. (1999). Measurement of pain. *Surgical Clinics of North America, 79,* 231–252.

Kendall, F. P., McCreary, E. K., Provance, P. G., Rodgers, M. M., & Romani, W. A. (2005). *Muscles: Testing and function with posture and pain* (5th ed.). Baltimore: Lippincott, Williams & Wilkins.

Lamb, K. L., Eston, R. G., & Corns, D. (1999). Reliability of ratings of perceived exertion during progressive treadmill exercise. *British Journal of Sports Medicine, 33,* 336–339.

Lamoreaux, L., & Hoffer, M. M. (1995). The effect of wrist deviation on grip and pinch strength. *Clinical Orthopaedics and Related Research, 314,* 152–155.

Landsmeer, J. M. F., & Long, C. (1965). The mechanism of finger control based on electromyograms and location analysis. *Acta Anatomica (Basel), 60,* 330–347.

LaStayo, P. C., & Wheeler, D. L. (1994). Reliability of passive wrist flexion and extension goniometric measurements: A multicenter study. *Physical Therapy, 74,* 162–176.

Leard, J. S., Breglio, L., Fraga, L., Ellrod, N., Nadler, L., Yasso, M., Fay, E., Ryan, K., & Pellecchia, G. L. (2004). Reliability and concurrent validity of the figure-of-eight method of measuring hand size in patients with hand pathology. *Journal of Orthopaedic and Sports Physical Therapy, 34,* 335–340.

Long, C. (1968). Intrinsic-extrinsic muscle control of the fingers. *Journal of Bone and Joint Surgery, 50A,* 973–984.

Long, C., & Brown, M. E. (1962). EMG kinesiology of the hand: Part III. Lumbricales and flexor digitorum profundus to the long finger. *Archives of Physical Medicine and Rehabilitation, 43,* 450–460.

MacDermid, J. C., Evenhuis, W., & Louzon, M. (2001). Inter-instrument reliability of pinch strength scores. *Journal of Hand Therapy, 14,* 36–42.

Maihafer, G. C., Llewellyn, M. A., Pillar, W. J., Scott, K. L., Marina, D. M., & Bond, R. M. (2004). A comparison of the figure-of eight method and water volumetry in measurement of hand and wrist size. *Journal of Hand Therapy, 16,* 305–310.

Marx, R. G., Bombardier, C., & Wright, J. G. (1999). What do we know about the reliability and validity of physical examination tests used to examine the upper extremity? *Journal of Hand Surgery, 24-A,* 185–193.

Mathiowetz, V. (2002). Comparison of Rolyan and Jamar dynamometers for measuring grip strength. *Occupational Therapy International, 9,* 201–209.

Mathiowetz, V., Kashman, N., Volland, G., Weber, K., Dowe, M., & Rogers, S. (1985). Grip and pinch strength: Normative data for adults. *Archives of Physical Medicine and Rehabilitation, 66,* 69–74.

Mathiowetz, V., Vizenor, L., & Melander, D. (2000). Comparison of baseline instruments to Jamar dynamometer and the B & L Engineering pinch gauge. *Occupational Therapy Journal of Research, 20,* 147–162.

Mathiowetz, V., Weber, K., Volland, G., & Kashman, N. (1984). Reliability and validity of grip and pinch strength evaluations. *Journal of Hand Surgery, 9A,* 222–226.

Medical Research Council. (1976). *Aids to the examination of the peripheral nervous system*. London: Her Majesty's Stationary Office.

Merskey, H., & Bogduk, N. (1994). *Classification of chronic pain* (2nd ed.). Seattle, WA: International Association for the Study of Pain.

Milner-Brown, H. S., Mellenthin, M., & Miller, R. G. (1986). Quantifying human muscle strength, endurance and fatigue. *Archives of Physical Medicine and Rehabilitation, 67,* 530–535.

Nitschke, J. E., McMeeken, J. M., Burry, H. C., & Matyas, T. A. (1999). When is a change a genuine change? A clinically meaningful interpretation of grip strength measurements in healthy and disabled women. *Journal of Hand Therapy, 12,* 25–30.

Ottenbocher, K. J., Branch, L. G., Ray, L., Gonzales, V. A., Peek, M. K., & Hinman, M. R. (2002). The reliability of upper- and lower-extremity strength testing in a community survey of older adults. *Archives of Physical Medicine and Rehabilitation, 83,* 1423–1427.

Pellecchia, G. L. (2004). Figure-of-eight method of measuring hand size: Reliability and concurrent validity. *Journal of Hand Therapy, 16,* 300–304.

Peolsson, A., Hedlund, R., & Öberg, B. (2001). Intra- and inter-tester reliability and reference values for hand strength. *Journal of Rehabilitation Medicine, 33,* 36–41.

Pollard, H., Lakay, B., Tucker, F., Wilson, B., & Bablis, P. (2005). Interexaminer reliability of the deltoid and psoas muscle test. *Journal of Manipulative and Physiological Therapy, 25,* 52–56.

Pollock, M. L., Franklin, B. A., Balady, G. J., Chaitman, B. L., Fleg, J. L., Fletcher, B., Limacher, M., Piña, I. L., Stein, R. A., Williams, M., & Bazzarre, T. (2000). Resistance exercise in individuals with and without cardiovascular disease: Benefits, rationale, safety, and prescription. *Circulation, 101,* 828–833.

Portney, L. G., & Watkins, M. P. (2000). *Foundations of clinical research: Applications to practice* (2nd ed.). Upper Saddle River, NJ: Prentice Hall.

Russell, W. D. (1997). On the current status of rated perceived exertion. *Perceptual and Motor Skills, 84,* 799–808.

Rybski, M. (2004). *Kinesiology for occupational therapy*. Thorofare, NJ: SLACK.

Sabari, J. S., Maltzev, I., Lubarsky, D., Liszkay, E., & Homel, P. (1998). Goniometric assessment of shoulder range of motion: Comparison of testing in supine and sitting positions. *Archives of Physical Medicine and Rehabilitation, 79,* 647–651.

Schechtman, O., Davenport, R., Malcolm, M., & Nabavi, D. (2003). Reliability and validity of the BTE-Primus grip tool. *Journal of Hand Therapy, 16,* 36–42.

Schechtman, O., Gestewitz, L., & Kimble, C. (2005). Reliability and validity of the DynEx dynamometer. *Journal of Hand Therapy, 18,* 339–347.

Schwartz, S., Cohen, M. E., Herbison, G. J., & Shah, A. (1992). Relationship between two measures of upper extremity strength: Manual muscle testing compared to hand held myometry. *Archives of Physical Medicine and Rehabilitation, 73,* 1063–1068.

Smith, L. K., Weiss, E. L., & Lehmkuhl, L. D. (1996). *Brunnstrom's clinical kinesiology* (5th ed.). Philadelphia: F. A. Davis Company.

Somers, D. L., Hanson, J. A., Kedzierski, C. M., Nestor, K. L., & Quinlivan, K. Y. (1997). The influence of experience on the reliability of goniometric and visual measurement of forefoot position. *Journal of Orthopedic Sports Physical Therapy, 25,* 192–202.

Su, C. Y., Lin, J. H., Chien, T. H., Cheng, K. F., & Sung, Y. T. (1994). Grip strength in different positions of elbow and shoulder. *Archives of Physical Medicine and Rehabilitation, 75,* 812–815.

Triffitt, P. D., Wildin, C., & Hajioff, D. (1999). The reproducibility of measurement of shoulder movement. *Acta Orthopaedica Scandinavica, 70,* 322–324.

Trombly, C. A., & Quintana, L. A. (1985). Differences in response to exercise by post-CVA and normal subjects. *Occupational Therapy Journal of Research, 5,* 39–58.

Whaley, M. H., Brubaker, P. H., Kaminsky, L. A., & Miller, C. R. (1997). Validity of rating of perceived exertion during graded exercise testing in apparently healthy adults and cardiac patients. *Journal of Cardiopulmonary Rehabilitation, 17,* 261–267.

Wilmore, J. H., & Costill, D. L. (1999). *Physiology of sport and exercise* (2nd ed.). Champaign, IL: Human Kinetics.

Wittink, H., & Michel, T. (1997). *Chronic pain management for physical therapists*. Boston: Butterworth-Heinemann.

CHAPTER 6

Assessing Abilities and Capacities: Motor Behavior

Virgil Mathiowetz and Julie Bass-Haugen

LEARNING OBJECTIVES

After studying this chapter, the reader will be able to do the following:

1. Contrast the reflex-hierarchical and systems models of motor control.
2. Describe various types of motor dysfunction seen in persons with central nervous system lesions.
3. Compare the neuromaturational and systems theories of motor development.
4. Contrast the assumptions of the neurophysiological and task-related approaches to treatment.
5. Describe the different evaluation strategies that are used by the neurophysiological and task-related approaches.
6. Describe some additional evaluation strategies that are not associated directly with either approach.

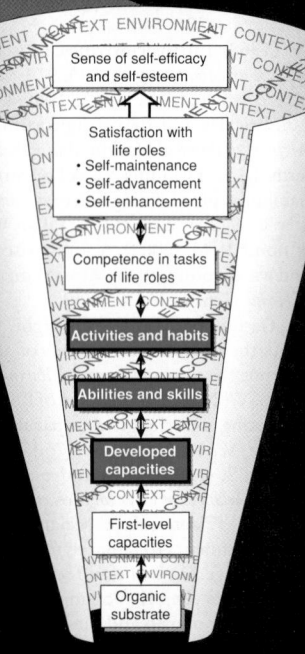

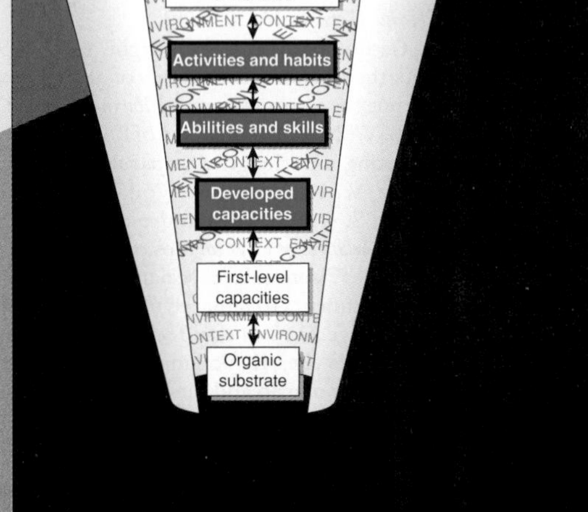

Glossary

Closed-loop system—A control system that utilizes feedback to correct movement errors and achieve the planned movement (Schmidt, 1991).

Control parameter—A variable that changes behavior from one pattern of behavior to another. It does not control the change but acts as an agent for the shift in behavior (Heriza, 1991).

Coordinative structures—Groups of muscles, usually spanning several joints, that are constrained to act as a single functional unit (Magill, 2004; Turvey, 1977).

Degrees of freedom—Elements of a control system that are free to vary.

Heterarchical system or model—A system in which control is distributed among many systems; control emerges from the interaction of various subsystems; there is no strict order of command; subsystems in charge vary with task requirements.

Hierarchical system or model—A system with several levels of control, with each level subordinate to the one above it.

Knowledge of results (KR)—Awareness of the outcome of movement in relation to the goal.

Muscle tone—Resistance of a muscle to passive elongation or stretching.

Open-loop system—A control system that utilizes preprogrammed instructions (i.e., anticipatory, or feed-forward, control) to an effector; does not use feedback or error-detection processes (Schmidt, 1991).

Phase shift—Change, which is often nonlinear, from one preferred coordinated pattern to another (Heriza, 1991).

Self-organization—The idea that a system composed of a number of subsystems can organize itself through the dynamic interaction of the subsystems (i.e., no higher level control or motor program is required) (Heriza, 1991).

Splinter skill—The ability to do a specific task that does not generalize to other tasks.

Our understanding of motor behavior—motor control, motor development, motor learning, and motor skill—continues to evolve (VanSant, 1991a). Sophisticated technology has led to an explosion of information about the control, development, and acquisition of movement (Lister, 1991). Human movement scientists, neurophysiologists, neuropsychologists, and others contribute to this effort. In an attempt to impose order on the many pieces of information, they deduce models and theories of motor behavior. As these models and theories change, therapeutic approaches also must change.

As a result of changes in the motor behavior literature, some (e.g., Gordon, 1987; Shumway-Cook & Woollacott, 2001) have questioned the assumptions underlying the neurophysiological approaches, which include Rood's (1954) sensorimotor approach, Knott & Voss' (1968) proprioceptive neuromuscular facilitation, Brunnstrom's (1970) movement therapy, and Bobath's (1978, 1990) neurodevelopmental treatment. Two task-related approaches, a task-oriented approach (Horak, 1991; Mathiowetz & Bass-Haugen, 1994) (see Chapter 22) and Carr and Shepherd's (1987, 1998, 2003) approach (see Chapter 23), are proposed as alternatives to the neurophysiological approaches. The assumptions of these new approaches are derived from a systems model of motor control, systems theories of motor development, and recent motor learning theories.

Definition 6-1 provides an overview of this chapter, which contrasts the assumptions of the neurophysiological and task-related approaches, the models and theories of motor behavior that they are based on, and the evaluation strategies associated with each approach. We believe the evaluation strategies used by the neurophysiological approaches still continue to influence clinical practice. Task-related evaluation strategies, however, have an increasing influence on current practice.

NEUROPHYSIOLOGICAL APPROACHES

Assumptions of the Neurophysiological Approaches

Definition 6-1 includes the assumptions of the four neurophysiological approaches as described by their original proponents. It is recognized that these approaches have evolved over time. For example, the neurodevelopmental treatment approach recently rejected most of the assumptions of the neurophysiological approaches and adopted most of the assumptions of the occupational therapy (OT) task-oriented approach (Howle, 2002). As a result, the theoretical differences between these approaches are much smaller today than they were 10 years ago. Unfortunately, clinical practice tends to lag behind changes in theory. Therefore, it is important to understand the differences between the neurophysiological approaches of the past and the current OT task-oriented approach. To understand the neurophysiological approaches, one must understand the reflex-**hierarchical model** of motor control and neuromaturational theories of motor development

DEFINITION 6-1

Comparison of the Neurophysiological and OT Task-Oriented Approaches

Neurophysiological Approaches	OT Task-Oriented Approach
Models of Motor Control	
Reflex-Hierarchical • Movements are elicited by sensory input or controlled by central programs. • Open-loop and closed-loop control is used. • Feedback and feed-forward influence movements. • Central nervous system (CNS) is hierarchically organized, with higher centers controlling lower centers. • Reciprocal innervation is essential for coordinated movement.	**Systems** • Personal and environmental systems interact to achieve functional goals. • Movement emerges from the interaction of many systems. • Systems are dynamical, self-organizing, and heterarchical. • Movement used for a task is the preferred means for achieving a functional goal. • Changes in one or more systems can alter behavior.
Theories of Motor Development	
Neuromaturational • Changes are due to CNS maturation. • Development follows a predictable sequence (e.g., cephalocaudal, proximal-distal). • CNS damage leads to regression to lower levels and more stereotypical behaviors.	**Systems** • Changes are due to interaction of multiple systems. • Progression varies because person and environmental contexts are unique. • CNS damage leads to attempts to use remaining resources to achieve functional goals.
Assumptions of Therapeutic Approaches	
• CNS is hierarchically organized. • Sensory stimuli inhibit spasticity and abnormal movement and facilitate normal movement and postural responses. • Repetition of movement results in positive permanent changes in CNS. • Recovery from CNS damage follows a predictable sequence. • Behavioral changes after CNS damage have a neurophysiological basis.	• Personal and environmental systems, including the CNS, are heterarchically organized. • Functional tasks help organize behavior. • Occupational performance emerges from the interaction of persons and their environment. • Experimentation with various strategies leads to optimal solutions to motor problems. • Recovery is variable because personal characteristics and environmental contexts are unique. • Behavioral changes reflect attempts to compensate and to achieve task performance.
Evaluation	
Primary focus on performance components • Abnormal muscle tone. • Abnormal reflexes and stereotypical movement patterns lead to incoordination. • Postural control. • Sensation and perception. • Memory and judgment. • Stage of recovery or developmental level.	**Primary focus on role and occupational performance using a client-centered view** • Task analysis to determine performance components and contexts that limit function and to identify preferred movement patterns for specific tasks in varied contexts. • Variables that cause transitions to new patterns.
Secondary focus on occupational performance	**Secondary focus on selected occupational performance components and contexts that limit function**

from which these treatment approaches originated. A discussion of the motor learning theories that influenced the neurophysiological and task-related approaches is covered in Chapter 14.

Reflex-Hierarchical Model of Motor Control

Figure 6-1 illustrates a reflex-hierarchical model (Trombly, 1989), which synthesizes the basic science literature of the 1970s and 1980s. This model evolved from earlier separate reflex and hierarchical models, which were unsuccessful in explaining the variety of movements available to human beings. This combined model assumes that the central nervous system (CNS) is hierarchically organized and movement is controlled by central programs or elicited by sensory input. The model utilizes both **closed-loop** and **open-loop systems** to explain how slow and fast movements are controlled. Each step of the reflex-hierarchical model is discussed conceptually, using the example of a person reaching for a bottle of water. See the references listed at the end of this chapter for greater detail.

Motivation to Move Is Generated

Purposeful movement does not occur in the absence of a need to move, which is generated from within the person or as a response to external stimuli (Marsden, 1982). Thus, a person who is thirsty (internal stimulus) or sees a cold bottle of water (external stimulus) becomes motivated to reach for the bottle.

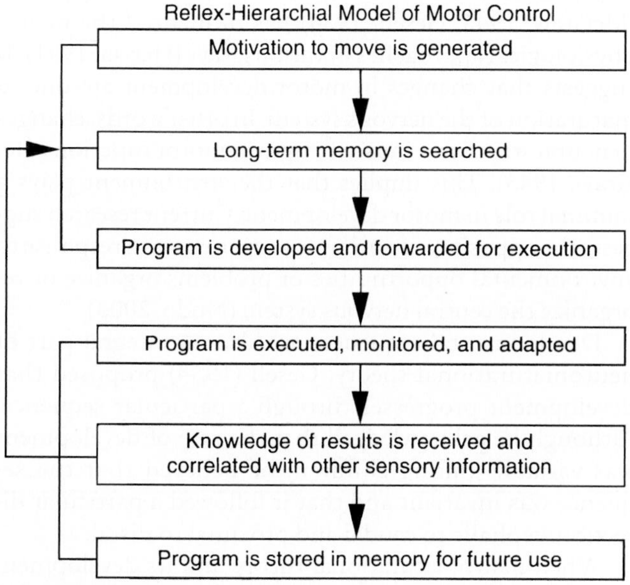
Reflex-Hierarchial Model of Motor Control
Motivation to move is generated
Long-term memory is searched
Program is developed and forwarded for execution
Program is executed, monitored, and adapted
Knowledge of results is received and correlated with other sensory information
Program is stored in memory for future use

Figure 6-1 Reflex-hierarchical model of motor control, adapted from Trombly (1989), includes both open-loop and closed-loop control.

Long-Term Memory Is Searched

Once the person is motivated, the executive or programming center searches long-term memory (LTM) for a pattern of movement that would enable reaching for the bottle. All previous efforts to reach a bottle were stored in a generalized motor program that contains an abstract representation about the order, relative timing, and relative force of the reaching movement (Schmidt, 1988). It also includes the postural adjustments that will be needed, so that the person does not overbalance while reaching for the bottle.

A Program Is Developed and Forwarded for Execution

Using the selected generalized motor program, the reaching movement is organized and planned (Marsden, 1982). The program is adapted to take into account environmental factors and to designate the specific muscles needed, the force of the contractions, and the overall duration of the movement. In this way, the generalized motor program is modified to meet the requirements of this specific action (reaching for a bottle of water on a table in front of the person).

Postural muscles are activated automatically as part of the program to provide a stable base from which movement may occur. In addition, the γ-motor neurons are programmed so that spindle sensitivity is set and accurate information concerning the length and speed of length change can be continually monitored (Fredericks & Saladin, 1996). Different types of movements and environmental factors require different control strategies (Brooks, 1986). Strategies also differ among people and between trials by the same person.

Program Is Executed, Monitored, and Adapted

As the program for reaching a bottle of water is executed, the movements are monitored via cutaneous input, visual and auditory cues, and ongoing proprioceptive input (Brooks, 1986). If the movement appears to be progressing successfully (the bottle of water is reached and picked up), the program is continued as planned. If the movement is sensed to be wrong (e.g., the hand misses the target) or an unexpected event occurs (e.g., the bottle is empty instead of full), an adjustment is made while the movement is still in progress. In the latter case, it is the α-γ coactivation that keeps the muscle spindle sensitive to the unexpected event. The agonist lifter muscles were programmed to lift a full bottle. The antagonist muscles were programmed to relax enough to allow the movement and then to contract to brake the movement as the bottle reached the mouth. Because the bottle was lighter than expected, the person lifted faster initially than was programmed. As a result, the muscle spindles of the agonist muscles went slack because the agonists shortened faster than expected, while the muscle spindles of the antagonist muscles stretched because they lengthened faster than was programmed. This information was returned to various levels of the CNS, which made adjustments for this unexpected event.

It is important to understand how the CNS adjusts for unexpected events because it is the basis of some therapeutic procedures and because it illustrates why active rather than passive movement is used for therapy. When the motor program is executed, the α- and γ-motor neurons are coactivated and excite the extrafusal and intrafusal muscle fibers according to the plan. When active movement is stopped by an unexpectedly full bottle of water or a therapist's hand (i.e., external stretch), the extrafusal muscle fibers are mechanically prevented from shortening as programmed. Meanwhile, the intrafusal fibers keep contracting as programmed. Soon the discrepancy between their length and the length of the extrafusal fibers is signaled to higher centers. Because the muscle spindle is held in place by connective tissue attached to the extrafusal muscle fibers, the spindle is mechanically prevented from shortening despite the intrafusal muscle contractions (i.e., internal stretch). As a result, external and internal stretch of the midportions of the spindle fibers add together, and stretch reflexes are activated (Brooks, 1986). Therapists use this technique to increase the strength of muscle contraction.

Knowledge of Results Is Received and Correlated with Other Sensory Information

Knowledge of results (KR) is awareness of the outcome of movement in relation to the goal. Open-loop movements are learned first as closed-loop movements in which attention is focused on the sensory feedback during the movement. Then the feedback is correlated to the outcome of the movement—KR—and the plan is modified for future movements. An open-loop movement can be executed exactly as programmed and yet be inaccurate for accomplishing the goal (Schmidt, 1988). For example, the person reaching for the bottle of water may miss the target, which illustrates the importance of KR and sensory feedback for improving motor learning.

The Program Is Stored in Memory for Future Use

Movements are generated from past experiences if success has been recognized (Brooks, 1986). Memories of successful movement are stored in long-term memory (LTM). "Successful" indicates that the sensory feedback generated by the movement matched the sensory outflow at the time the program was generated and accomplished the goal (Gentile, 1972). If attention is directed to the movement so that information concerning it remains in short-term memory (STM) for a time, the memory becomes stored in LTM for future use. If the information is lost from STM, however, it does not become part of LTM, and learning does not take place (Schmidt, 1988). The learned motor skill must be practiced to be retained at the same level of expertise (Brooks, 1986). Expertise is improved by practice with intention to improve.

Reflex-hierarchical models of motor control have been challenged by three inter-related questions. (1) How can the CNS control the many **degrees of freedom** of each movement (i.e., the large number of joints, planes of motion within each joint, muscles that control each joint, and single motor units within each muscle) without specifying the details of the muscle activation pattern (Bernstein, 1967)? If the CNS does specify the details, each motor program would be extremely complex. (2) How many motor programs would be needed to perform the numerous tasks that humans perform in everyday life? It is likely that an extremely large number would be necessary, which creates a storage problem for the brain. (3) How many motor programs would be needed to perform a given task in varied contexts? Studies (Marteniuk, MacKenzie, & Jeannerod, 1987; Mathiowetz & Wade, 1995) have demonstrated that small changes in environmental context can result in unique movement patterns during simple reaching tasks. Thus, the environment has a larger role in motor control than the reflex-hierarchical model would suggest, and it seems that an incomprehensible number of motor programs would be necessary to respond to various contexts (Newell, 2003). Does the brain have unlimited storage capacity to accommodate all of the motor programs, even generalized motor programs? The answer is probably not; an alternative explanation of motor behavior is explored after the neurophysiological approach is fully presented.

Neuromaturational Theory of Motor Development

The neuromaturational theory of motor development (McGraw, 1945; Gesell, 1954) has influenced the neurophysiological approaches in various ways (Heriza, 1991). It suggests that changes in motor development are due to maturation of the nervous system. In other words, changes in neural structures cause changes in motor function (McGraw, 1945). This implies that the environment plays a minimal role in motor development. Current research suggests the opposite; sensorimotor experiences in response to environmental opportunities or problems organize or reorganize the central nervous system (Nudo, 2003).

Developmental sequences are also an integral part of neuromaturational theory. Gesell (1954) proposed that development progresses through a particular sequence. Although he acknowledged that the rate of development was variable among children, he believed that the sequence was invariant and that it followed a particular direction: cephalic to caudal and proximal to distal.

When neuromaturational theory and its developmental sequences are used as a guide in therapy, it is assumed that treatment must start at the patient's current developmental level. Developmental and reflex testing serve as primary assessment tools (Bobath, 1978; Fiorentino, 1973). For treatment, it is assumed a patient must master the current developmental level before progressing to the next level (Rood, 1954). If patients master the developmental sequence, these motor skills are assumed to generalize to task performance. It is thought that working on specific functional tasks will result in **splinter skills**, which will not generalize and may in fact interfere with a child's progression through the developmental sequence. As a result, the development of movement skills is emphasized at the expense of functional performance.

Neuromaturational theories have also been used to explain motor problems seen in adults with CNS damage. It is believed that CNS damage frees lower centers from higher level control, resulting in a release of primitive reflexes and abnormal muscle tone (Bobath, 1990). Neurophysiological approaches focus on a progression through the developmental sequence, inhibition of primitive reflexes and spasticity, and facilitation of higher level control. Some of these concepts still influence practice; others have been modified or discarded.

Motor Dysfunction Caused by CNS Lesions

The view of the neurophysiological approaches is that motor dysfunctions that follow CNS damage (Definition 6-2) are understood best by knowing the site and extent of the lesions (Cheney, 1985). It is assumed that specific areas of the brain serve specific functions. Therefore, if a given area of the brain is damaged, its associated function is expected to be impaired.

Cortical Lesions

Local cortical lesions, such as occur as a result of cerebrovascular accident or penetrating injury, result in deficits in motor planning or execution of voluntary goal-directed movement, depending on the particular cortical area damaged. Although patients may be unable to move a segment of a limb in isolation, they are often able to move the whole limb in a stereotyped way because lower levels of the CNS that control this function are spared. Even in patients who seem to have similar lesions, however, dysfunction varies because of the complexity of the control options available to the CNS and the way each individual uses them (Scholz & Campbell, 1980). Diffuse lesions, such as those seen after closed head injury, can result in extensive damage to cortical areas and deeper structures of the brain. The motor dysfunction includes deficits described earlier plus any deficits associated with the lower level areas involved.

The motor deficits of cortical damage can be described as both positive and negative (Burke, 1988). The positive features are phenomena that are released from the inhibitory control of the cortex: exaggerated reflexes, spasticity, and the hemiplegic posture. The negative features are weakness and abnormal coordination. The neurophysiological approaches assume that the positive symptoms have the most devastating effect on the motor function of cortically damaged patients. They also assume that, until the positive symptoms are corrected, the negative deficits cannot be improved (Bobath, 1978). There is growing evidence to doubt these assumptions (Bourbonnais & Vanden Noven, 1989; Shumway-Cook & Woollacott, 2001). In fact, Burke (1988) suggested that the negative features affect function more than the positive features.

Motor behavior is abnormal not only because of the motor deficits but also because of deficits in sensation, cognition, and perception. Patients with sensory loss due to a cortical lesion cannot use the affected limb spontaneously, but can compensate for the loss using intact sensory systems when directed to do so (Jeannerod, Michel, & Prablanc, 1984). The sensory loss seriously affects the ability to sustain a constant level of force needed to hold an object or to maintain a posture. In the case of impaired sensation, movement is affected by the distortion, and the patient needs to relearn the meaning of the new sensations through active movement. No relearning occurs during passive movement, even if the patient watches the movement (Gentile, 1972). Sensory problems are covered in more detail in Chapters 7 and 27.

Deficits in cognitive and perceptual processing can affect motor behavior as well. Perceptual processing entails accurate interpretation of sensory stimuli from the internal and external environment. A patient with poor depth perception has problems in reaching for objects. Cognitive processing involves orientation, attention span, memory, and problem solving. Patients with impaired memory have problems learning new tasks because they can't remember how they were instructed to perform them or the task itself. Cognition and perception are covered in more detail in Chapters 8, 9, 28, and 29.

Cerebellar Lesions

Symptoms of cerebellar lesions (Definition 6-2) reflect timing abnormalities and problems with the rate, range, and force of a movement. The basis for these deficits is a combination of delayed initiation of preprogrammed patterns and delayed termination of agonistic muscular activity, which results in delayed or missing initiation of the antagonist (Brooks, 1986). These patients are able to carry out voluntary programmed movement of a limb but lack the fine adjustments needed for end-point accuracy.

Basal Ganglia Lesions

The basal ganglia control automatic rhythmical patterned movements and the initiation of automatic (learned) movements. Lesions of the basal ganglia (e.g., Parkinson's disease) result in problems of voluntary movement, such

DEFINITION 6-2

Motor Dysfunction Due to CNS Lesions

Cortical Lesions

- *Hemiplegic posture or pattern of spasticity* includes retraction and depression of the scapula; internal rotation of the shoulder; flexion of the elbow, wrist, and fingers; pronation of the forearm; lateral flexion of the trunk toward the involved side; elevation and retraction of the pelvis; internal rotation of the hip; extension of the hip and knee; supination of the foot; and plantar flexion of the ankle and toes (Bobath, 1990).
- *Hypotonia* (decreased muscle tone or flaccidity) is less than normal resistance to passive elongation; the affected limb feels limp and heavy.
- *Hypertonia* (increased muscle tone) is more than normal resistance of a muscle to passive elongation. Both neural (spasticity) and mechanical (soft tissue stiffness) factors cause it.
- *Spasticity*, the neural component of hypertonus, is characterized by a velocity-dependent increase in tonic stretch reflexes and exaggerated tendon reflexes (Katz & Rymer, 1989). It is commonly accompanied by muscle clonus and the clasp knife reflex.
- *Clonus* is the oscillating contraction and relaxation of a limb segment due to the alternating pattern of stretch reflex and inverse stretch reflex of a spastic muscle.
- *Clasp knife phenomenon or reflex* is resistance to passive stretch of a spastic muscle that suddenly gives way, like the blade of a jackknife.
- *Weakness* is the inability to generate the necessary force for effective motor action.
- *Loss of fractionation* is the inability to move a single joint without producing unnecessary movements in other joints, resulting in stereotyped movement patterns instead of selective, flexible movement patterns.
- *Apraxia* is the inability to perform goal-directed motor activity in the absence of paresis, ataxia, sensory loss, or abnormal muscle tone. Apraxia is characterized by omissions, disturbed order of submovements within a sequence, clumsiness, perseveration, and inability to gesture or use common tools or utensils.
- *Lead pipe rigidity* is characterized by hypertonus in both agonist and antagonist muscles, with resistance to movement that is not velocity dependent and that is felt throughout the range of motion.

Cerebellar Lesions

- *Intention tremor* is the rhythmic oscillating movement that develops during precise intentional movements due to involuntary alternating contractions of opposing muscles.
- *Dysmetria* is the inability to judge distances accurately; it results in overshooting or undershooting a specific target.
- *Decomposition of movement*, or *dyssynergia*, is characterized by movements that are broken up into a series of successive simple movements rather than one smooth movement involving multiple joints.
- *Dysdiadochokinesia* is impairment in the ability to perform repeated alternating movements, such as pronation and supination, rapidly and smoothly.
- *Adiadochokinesia* is the loss of ability to perform rapid alternating movements.
- *Ataxia* is unsteadiness, incoordination, or clumsiness of movement.
- *Ataxic gait* is a wide-based, unsteady, staggering gait with a tendency to veer from side to side.

Lesions of the Basal Ganglia

- *Tremors at rest* or *non-intention tremors* stop at the initiation of voluntary movement but resume during the holding phase of a motor task when attention wanes or is diverted to another task. Tremors at rest are fatiguing.
- *Cogwheel rigidity* is characterized by rhythmic interrupted resistance of the muscles being stretched when the wrist or elbow is flexed quickly.
- *Hypokinesia* is slowness or poverty of movement. It includes *akinesia*, difficulty initiating voluntary movements, and *bradykinesia*, slowness in carrying out movements. These symptoms are reflected in lack of facial expression, monotone speech, reduced eye movements, diminished arm swing during walking, and decreased balance and equilibrium responses seen in Parkinson's disease.
- *Festinating gait* is characterized by small, fast, shuffling steps that propel the body forward at an increasing rate and by difficulty stopping or changing directions.
- *Athetosis* is characterized by slow, writhing involuntary movements, particularly in the neck, face, and extremities. Athetosis ceases during sleep. Muscle tone may be increased or decreased.
- *Dystonia* is characterized by powerful, sustained contractions of muscles that cause twisting and writhing of a limb or of the whole body, often resulting in distorted postures of the trunk and proximal extremities.
- *Chorea* is characterized by sudden involuntary, purposeless, rapid, jerky movements and/or grimacing, primarily in the distal extremities and face (e.g., Huntington's chorea).
- *Hemiballismus* is unilateral chorea in which there are violent, forceful, flinging movements of the extremities on one side of the body, particularly involving the proximal musculature.

Primary source: Fredericks & Saladin, 1996.

as akinesia and bradykinesia, and of involuntary movements, such as tremor at rest and rigidity (Phillips & Stelmach, 1996).

For the most part, diseases of the cerebellum or basal ganglia are degenerative, and recovery arising from neural changes is not expected. Therefore, treatment focuses on compensation for the deficits. In contrast, some recovery is expected after traumatic injury to the cerebellum and basal ganglia.

View of Recovery after CNS Lesions

The view of the neurophysiological approaches is that recovery after CNS lesions is due to changes in the CNS. Recovery from cortical lesions is believed to follow a developmental sequence from reflex to voluntary control, from mass to discrete movements, and from proximal to distal control. Recovery can stop at any level along the continua, and this is not totally predictable. The speed of early spontaneous recovery offers a clue to the ultimate level of function to be gained (Twitchell, 1951). This view of recovery is not supported by current neuroscience research (Nudo, 2003).

Evaluations Used by Neurophysiological Approaches

Given the assumptions of the neurophysiological approaches (Definition 6-1), the evaluations of patients focus primarily on abilities and capacities impaired by CNS damage. These include muscle tone, abnormal reflexes and movement patterns, postural control, sensation (see Chapter 7), perception (see Chapter 8), and cognition (see Chapter 9). In addition, it is important to determine the patient's stage of recovery or developmental level. Finally, areas of occupation (see Chapter 4) are evaluated secondarily on the assumption that any deficits in these areas are due to impaired performance skills. This bottom-up evaluation framework is not consistent with the model of occupational functioning (see Chapter 1).

Muscle Tone Evaluations

Muscle Tone and Associated Factors

Muscle tone is defined as the resistance of a muscle to passive elongation or stretching (Shumway-Cook & Woollacott, 2001). Slight resistance in response to passive movement characterizes normal muscle tone. When the therapist moves the arm, it feels relatively light, and if the therapist lets go of it, it is able to maintain the position. Hypotonia is less than normal resistance to passive elongation. When the therapist moves the arm, it feels floppy and heavy. If the therapist lets go of it, it cannot maintain the position or resist the effects of gravity. Hypertonia, which is more than normal resistance of a muscle to passive elongation, is due to neural and mechanical factors. The neural factor (i.e., spasticity) is due to hyperactive stretch reflexes frequently seen after CNS damage. In a spastic muscle, there is a range of free movement, then a strong contraction of the muscle in response to stretch (i.e., stretch reflex), and free movement again when the muscle suddenly relaxes (i.e., clasp knife phenomenon or reflex) (Fredericks & Saladin, 1996). Spasticity is not synonymous with hypertonus or muscle tone (Burridge et al., 2005). The mechanical factors of hypertonus are the elastic properties of connective tissue and the viscoelastic properties of muscle. The mechanical factors change if a muscle is immobilized in a shortened or lengthened position (i.e., there is increased or decreased resistance to passive stretching). The neural changes after CNS damage—spasticity—contribute to abnormal positioning of limbs, which causes secondary changes in the mechanical factors. Together the neural and mechanical factors account for increased resistance to passive elongation—hypertonus—that is seen after CNS damage (Burridge et al., 2005).

Muscle tone is measured clinically by observing the response of a muscle to passive stretch. A problem in measuring hypertonus, especially the neural factor, is the high variation in spasticity from day to day in the same subject. The reliability of a test is affected by the speed of the passive test movement because the tonic stretch reflexes are velocity dependent (Katz & Rymer, 1989). Reliability is also affected by effort, emotional stress, temperature, fatigue, changes in concurrent sensory stimulation, urinary tract infections, and head position (Sloan et al., 1992). Rigid standardization of the test procedure must be the rule; otherwise, the findings may be misleading (Burridge et al., 2005). Poor evaluation techniques that allow high test-retest variability may obscure therapeutic effectiveness. Although there are many assessments of muscle tone and spasticity described in the literature, most are not practical for clinical use and the *Modified Ashworth Scale* is the most widely used (van Wijck et al., 2001).

Modified Ashworth Scale

Ashworth (1964) proposed a qualitative scale for assessing the degree of spasticity as part of a drug study. The resistance encountered to passive movement through the full available range was rated on a 5-point scale (0–4). Although it was developed and described as a measure of spasticity, the scale is a measure of muscle tone or the resistance to passive movement (Burridge et al., 2005; Pandyan et al., 2002). Bohannon and Smith (1987) modified the Ashworth scale (Procedures for Practice 6-1) by adding an additional level (1+), by incorporating the angle at which resistance first appeared, and by controlling the speed of the passive movement with a 1-second count. The examiner performs five to eight repetitions of the movement before assigning the rating. Assessment Table 6-1 describes the psychometric properties of the *Modified*

PROCEDURES FOR PRACTICE 6-1

Modified Ashworth Scale for Grading Spasticity

Grade	Description
0	No increase in muscle tone
1	Slight increase in muscle tone manifested by a catch and release or by minimal resistance at the end of the range of motion when the affected part or parts are moved in flexion or extension
1+	Slight increase in muscle tone manifested by a catch, followed by minimal resistance throughout the remainder (less than half) of the ROM
2	Marked increase in muscle tone through most of the ROM, but affected parts are easily moved
3	Considerable increase in muscle tone; passive movement difficult
4	Affected part or parts rigid in flexion or extension

Reprinted with permission from Bohannon, R. W., & Smith, M. B. (1987). Interrater reliability of a Modified Ashworth Scale of muscle spasticity. *Physical Therapy*, 67, 207. Copyright 1987 by American Physical Therapy Association.

Ashworth Scale, which has modest evidence of concurrent validity. Despite its limitations, the *Modified Ashworth Scale* is the best available measure of muscle tone and the most widely cited in the literature (Sloan et al., 1992).

Evaluation of Motor Function

Fugl-Meyer Assessment

The *Fugl-Meyer Assessment* (*FMA*) was developed to evaluate motor function, balance, some aspects of sensation, and joint function in persons after stroke (Fugl-Meyer et al., 1975). The items were based on earlier studies on the sequential stages of motor recovery after stroke (e.g., Brunnstrom, 1970; Twitchell, 1951). The maximum points are 66 for the upper extremity, 34 for the lower extremity, 14 for balance, 24 for sensation, 24 for position sense, 44 for range of motion, and 44 for joint pain (total possible score, 250). Each section can be scored separately. See Fugl-Meyer et al. (1975) for test procedures and scoring criteria. The procedures for the upper extremity subtest are described in Chapter 25. Assessment Table 6-2 describes the psychometric properties of the *FMA*. The *FMA* is the second most frequently used assessment of motor deficits of persons with central nervous system impairments (van Wijck et al., 2001), is widely used in outcome studies, and is a recommended assessment of motor function in the Agency for Health Care Policy and Research clinical practice guidelines for post-stroke rehabilitation (Gresham et al., 1995).

TASK-RELATED APPROACHES

Assumptions of the Task-Related Approaches

The assumptions of the occupational therapy (OT) task-oriented approach are listed in Definition 6-1. They originate from a systems model of motor behavior, a systems view of motor development, and recent motor learning theories. Carr and Shepherd's (1987) *Motor Relearning Programme for Stroke* (see Chapter 23) is also based on this research. The assumptions of their program are (p. 5):

- Regaining the ability to perform motor tasks, such as walking, reaching, and standing up, is a learning process, and the disabled have the same learning needs as those who are not disabled; that is, they need to practice, get feedback, understand goals, and so on.
- Motor control is exercised in both anticipatory and ongoing modes, and postural adjustments and focal limb movements are inter-related.
- Control of a specific motor task can best be regained by practice of that specific motor task, and such tasks should be practiced in their various environmental contexts.
- Sensory input related to the motor task helps modulate action.

To understand the evaluation framework of the task-related approaches, it is important to understand the origins of the assumptions of these approaches.

Systems Model of Motor Control

Over the past 30 years, a new model of motor control has evolved from the ecological approach to perception and action (Gibson, 1979; Turvey, 1977) and from the study of complex dynamical systems in mathematics and the sciences (Gleick, 1987). The new model emphasizes the interaction between persons and environments and suggests that motor behavior emerges from people's multiple systems interacting with unique task and environmental contexts (Newell, 1986). Thus, the systems model of motor control is more interactive or **heterarchical** and emphasizes the role of the environment more than the reflex-hierarchical model.

In the systems model, the nervous system is only one system among many that influence motor behavior. The nervous system itself is organized heterarchically so that higher centers interact with the lower centers but do not

Assessment Table 6-1

Summary of Assessment of Muscle Tone or Resistance to Passive Movement

Instrument and Reference	Description	Time to Administer	Validity	Reliability	Sensitivity	Strengths and Weaknesses
Modified Ashworth Scale (Bohannon & Smith, 1987)	Ordinal scale with score for each motion from 0 (normal muscle tone) to 4 (rigid in flexion or extension). Modification is the addition of one additional rating level (1+).	1–2 minutes per motion tested.	Concurrent validity: $r_s = 0.39–0.49$ with quantitative spasticity measures (Allison & Abraham, 1995); $r = 0.50$ with motor and activity scores (Sommerfeld et al., 2004); $r_s = 0.51$ with resistance to passive movement (Pandyan et al., 2003); and $r_s = 0.40$ with the H-reflex (Pizzi et al., 2005).	Inter-rater reliability: $r_s = 0.67$ and 0.73 for elbow flexion and extension, respectively; $r_s = 0.45$ for knee flexion (Sloan et al., 1992); Kw[1] = 0.49–0.54 for shoulder, elbow, wrist, knee, and ankle joints (Mehrholz et al., 2005). Test–retest reliability: Kw = 0.77–0.94 for elbow, wrist, and knee flexors; Kw = 0.59–0.64 for ankle plantarflexors (Gregson et al., 2000).	Significant reduction in *Modified Ashworth Scale* scores after treatment with botulinum toxin (Bakheit et al., 2000, 2001); non-significant reduction in *Modified Ashworth Scale* scores (Pandyan et al., 2002)	Strengths: It is a valid measure of muscle tone or resistance to passive movement (Pandyan et al., 2002); administration time is relatively brief; reliability is better for upper extremity than lower extremity joints. Weaknesses: Only moderate concurrent validity with measures of spasticity. It is questioned as a measure of spasticity (i.e., the neural component of muscle tone). Moderate to good inter-rater reliability; moderate to very good test–retest reliability.

[1]Kw = weighted kappa.

Assessment Table 6-2

Summary of Assessments of Motor Function

Instrument and Reference	Description	Time to Administer	Validity	Reliability	Sensitivity	Strengths and Weaknesses
Arm Motor Ability Test (*AMAT*) (Kopp et al., 1997)	13 unilateral and bilateral functional tasks scored on performance time, functional ability, and quality of movement (latter two on a 6-point scale).	30–45 minutes.	Concurrent validity: $r_s = 0.92–0.94$ with FMA[1] (Chae, Labatia, & Yang, 2003); $r_s = 0.45–0.61$ with Motricity Index: Arm score (Kopp et al., 1997).	Inter-rater reliability: $r_s = 0.97–0.99$; K = 0.68–0.77. Test–retest reliability: $r = 0.93–0.99$. Internal consistency: K = 0.94–0.99 (Kopp et al., 1997).	Significant improvement in scores after 1 or 2 weeks of intensive therapy (Kopp et al., 1997); significant improvement in scores after constraint-induced movement therapy (Kunkel et al., 1999).	Strengths: Use of functional tasks; excellent reliability; evidence of validity. Weaknesses: Ceiling and floor effects for performance time (Chae, Labatia, & Yang, 2003); less sensitive to change than the *WMFT*[2] (Morris et al., 2001).
Fugl-Meyer Motor Assessment (*FMA*) (Fugl-Meyer et al., 1975)	Most items are scored on a 3-point ordinal scale (0, cannot be performed; 1, performed partly; 2, performed faultlessly).	34–110 minutes for total *FMA*; 30–45 minutes for the upper and lower extremity sections; 8–12 minutes for the upper extremity alone.	Actual motor recovery post stroke parallels the test items (Fugl-Meyer et al., 1975). Concurrent validity: $r_s = 0.88$ with total *MAS* (Poole & Whitney, 1988) and $r = 0.68–0.85$ with the Barthel Index (Wood-Dauphinee, Williams, & Shapiro, 1990).	Inter-rater reliability: $r = 0.79–0.99$ for the upper and lower extremity subtests; intra-rater reliability: $r = 0.86–0.99$ across three test times and non-significant differences among the three means (Duncan, Probst, & Nelson, 1983).	Significantly greater improvement in experimental vs. control group at 6- and 12-month follow-ups (Feys et al., 1998).	Strengths: Administration time for upper extremity is acceptable; evidence supports its reliability, validity, and sensitivity. Weaknesses: Administration time for total *FMA* is lengthy; items have little relevance to everyday activities; validity of balance subscale was questioned (Malouin et al., 1994).

Motor Assessment Scale (MAS) (Carr et al., 1985)	8 areas of motor function are rated on a 7-point hierarchical scale: 0 = easiest task and 6 = hardest task.	15–30 minutes for total *MAS* (Carr et al., 1985); 18–60 minutes for total *MAS* (Malouin et al., 1994).	Concurrent validity: $r_s = 0.88$ with the total *FMA*[3]; $r_s = 0.91$ for total upper extremity; $r_s = 0.28$ for balanced sitting (Poole & Whitney, 1988); $r_s = 0.96$ with the total *FMA* (Malouin et al., 1994). Predictive validity: arm function at 1 week ($r_s = 0.84$) and at 1 month ($r_s = 0.91$) are good predictors of arm function at discharge (Loewen & Anderson, 1990).	Inter-rater reliability: $r = 0.95$ and average of 87% agreement between raters (Carr et al., 1985); $r_s = 0.99$ between raters (Poole & Whitney, 1988). Test–retest reliability: ($r = 0.98$) on clients post stroke (Carr et al., 1985).	Significant improvements for clients post stroke on all subtests as a result of clinical interventions (Ada & Westwood, 1992; Dean & Mackey, 1992).	Strengths: Items are functionally relevant; administration time is shorter. Evidence supports its reliability, validity, and sensitivity. Weakness: Sequence of the scoring hierarchy of the hand function and advanced hand activities scales was questioned (Dean & Mackey, 1992; Sabari et al., 2005).
Wolf Motor Function Test (WMFT) (Wolf et al., 2001)	6 timed upper extremity movements and 9 timed functional tasks (Wolf et al., 2001). Modification includes adding functional ability scale (Morris et al., 2001).	30–45 minutes.	Discriminant validity: between normal subjects and persons post stroke (Wolf et al., 2001).	Inter-rater reliability: $r = 0.95–0.99$ (Wolf et al., 2001); ICC ≥ 0.93; test–retest reliability: $r = 0.90–0.95$; internal consistency: Chronbach's $\alpha = 0.86–0.92$ (Morris et al., 2001).	Significant improvement in scores after constraint-induced movement therapy (Kunkel et al., 1999; Taub et al., 1993).	Strengths: Combination of simple and complex movements; excellent reliability; more sensitive to change than the *AMAT* (Morris et al., 2001). Weaknesses: 9 individual items had less than adequate inter-rater reliability (Morris et al., 2001); several modifications of the test have been reported.

[1] FMA = Fugl-Meyer Motor Assessment
[2] WFMT = Wolf Motor Function Test
[3] FMA = Fugl-Meyer Motor Assessment

control them. Closed-loop and open-loop systems work cooperatively, and both feedback and feed-forward control are used to achieve task goals. The CNS interacts with multiple personal and environmental systems as a person attempts to achieve a goal.

Ecological Approach to Perception and Action

The ecological approach to perception and action emphasizes the study of interaction between the person and the environment during everyday functional tasks and the close linkage between perception and action (i.e., purposeful movement). Gibson recognized the role of functional goals and the environment in the relationship between perception and action. He stated that direct perception entails the active search for *affordances* (Gibson, 1977), which is defined as the functional utility of objects for persons and their unique characteristics (Warren, 1984). Thus, Gibson's concept of affordances explains the close relationship between perception and action in terms of what the information in the environment means to a specific person.

Bernstein (1967) recognized the importance of the environment and personal characteristics other than the CNS in motor behavior. He suggested that the role a particular muscle plays in a movement depends on the context or circumstances. Bernstein identified three possible sources of variability in muscle function. A first source is anatomical factors. For example, from kinesiology you know that the pectoralis major muscle will either flex or extend the shoulder, depending on the initial position of the arm. Another example relates to adducting the shoulder. If you want to adduct the shoulder quickly or against resistance, the latissimus dorsi contracts. In contrast, if you adduct the shoulder slowly against no resistance, the deltoid muscles contract eccentrically, and the latissimus dorsi does not contract. In both cases, the role of the muscle depends on the context in which it is used. A second source of variability is mechanical factors. Many non-muscular forces, such as gravity and inertia, determine the degree to which a muscle must contract. For example, a muscle must exert much more force to contract against gravity than in a gravity-eliminated plane. Likewise, because of the effects of inertia, the contraction of the elbow flexor muscles is different if the shoulder is flexing or extending at the same time. Again, the effect of a muscle contraction depends on the context. A third source of variability is physiological factors. When higher centers send down a command for a muscle to contract, middle and lower centers have the opportunity to modify the command. Lower and middle centers receive peripheral sensory feedback. Thus, the effect of the command on the muscle varies depending on the context and degree of influence of the middle and lower centers. As a result, the relationship between higher center or executive commands and muscle action is not one-to-one. Trombly and Wu (1999) demonstrated the influence of context on movement. They reported that goal-directed, object-present activity elicited different and more efficient movement patterns than non–goal-directed exercise.

Thus, postures and movements are not triggered by external stimulation or central commands, as suggested by the reflex-hierarchical model, but instead, they are **coordinative structures** that are capable of adapting to changing circumstances. When learning a new task, a person tends to constrain or stiffen many joints to reduce the degrees of freedom to be controlled. This use of a coordinative structure enables the person to focus on controlling a limited number of joints. Natural tenodesis grasp and release is an example of a coordinative structure. The long flexor and extensor muscles of the forearm are constrained to work together for functional grasp and release. Fitch, Tuller, and Turvey (1982) suggested that perceptual information could modulate or tune the coordinative structures without intervention from the executive or higher centers. Reed (1982) suggested that postures and movements are modulated as needed by updated perceptual information to achieve the functional goal. Thus, the study of motor behavior or action evolved into "the study of how organisms use available information to modulate their actions" (Reed, 1982, p. 110).

Dynamical Systems Theory

The study of dynamical systems originated in mathematics, physics, biology, chemistry, psychology, and kinesiology, and it has been applied to occupational therapy, physical therapy, nursing, adapted physical education, and some areas of medicine (Burton & Davis, 1992; Lister, 1991). It has influenced the systems model of motor control as well. Dynamical systems theory proposes that behaviors emerge from the interaction of many systems. Because the behavior is not specified but emergent, it is considered to be self-organizing (Kamm, Thelen, & Jensen, 1990). This concept of **self-organization** is not compatible with the assumptions of the reflex-hierarchical model, which suggests that higher centers or motor programs prescribe movements. Evidence of self-organization is seen in the relatively stable patterns of motor behavior seen in many tasks in spite of the many degrees of freedom available to a person (Thelen & Ulrich, 1991). When we eat or write, we have many choices of ways to perform these tasks, yet we tend to use preferred patterns.

Behavior can change from stable to less stable as a result of aging or CNS damage. In fact, throughout life, behaviors shift between periods of stability and instability. It is during unstable periods, characterized by a high variability of performance, that new types of behaviors may emerge, either gradually or abruptly. These transitions in behavior, called **phase shifts**, are changes from one preferred pattern of coordinated behavior to another. An example of a gradual phase shift is when an infant decreases automatic stepping between 2 and 4 months of age. An example of an abrupt phase shift is when a person in a hurry walks faster and faster and suddenly changes to a running pattern. How can these changes in behavior be explained?

In the dynamical systems view, **control parameters** are variables that shift behavior from one form to another. They do not control the change but act as agents for reorganization of the behavior to a new form (Heriza, 1991). Control parameters are gradable in some way. In the case of the infant, Thelen and Fisher (1982) demonstrated that the decrease in automatic stepping was due in part to the rapid weight gain during this time. Because infants' muscles are not strong enough to move the heavier body, automatic stepping decreases. This control parameter, the increase in body weight, shifts the behavior from automatic stepping to no stepping. In the other example, increasing the speed of locomotion elicits the change from a walking to a running pattern. Consequently, speed is considered a control parameter as well.

Explanations of changes in motor behavior in the systems model of motor control are quite different from earlier models. Thelen (1989) stated that an important characteristic of a system perspective is that the shift from one preferred movement pattern to another is marked by discrete, discontinuous transitions. These transitions in motor behavior are the result of changes in only one or a few personal or environmental systems (i.e., control parameters) (Davis & Burton, 1991). Thus, two important points are: (1) systems themselves are subject to change, and (2) there is no inherent ordering of systems in terms of their influence on motor behavior.

Systems View of Motor Development

A systems view of motor development suggests that changes over time are caused by multiple factors or systems such as maturation of the nervous system, biomechanical constraints and resources, and the influences of the physical and social environment (Heriza, 1991). A systems view also suggests that normal development does not follow a rigid intertask sequence, as the motor milestones suggest (VanSant, 1991b). In fact, children follow variable developmental sequences arising from their unique personal characteristics and environmental contexts. If the traditional inter-task developmental sequences are no longer sufficient as a guide for working with children, then they are certainly not appropriate as a guide for working with adults with CNS dysfunction (VanSant, 1991b). In contrast, intra-task sequences—developmental sequences within a single skill, such as rising without assistance or reaching to grasp an object—do provide guides for age-appropriate movement patterns (VanSant, 1991b).

Systems Model of Motor Behavior

Figure 6-2 depicts the theoretical basis of the OT task-oriented approach. It illustrates the interaction between the systems of the *Person* (cognitive, psychosocial, and sensorimotor) and the systems of the *Environment* (physical, socioeconomic, and cultural). *Occupational Performance Tasks* (i.e., activities of daily living, work, and play/leisure) and *Role Performance* emerge from the interaction between the person and the environment. Changes in any one of these systems can affect occupational performance tasks and ultimately role performance. In some cases, only one primary factor may determine occupational performance. In most cases, occupational performance tasks emerge from the interaction of many systems. The ongoing interactions among all components of the model reflect its heterarchical nature.

In addition, any occupational performance task affects the environment in which it occurs and the person acting. For example, a client with hemiplegia who has just become independent in making his own lunch may free his spouse from coming home from work during her lunch hour. It also may mean that certain objects in the kitchen must be kept in accessible places, and the kitchen may not be as orderly as the spouse is used to. Thus, the task of making lunch affects people and objects in the environment. It also affects the person and the associated performance skills and patterns. The ability to be less dependent on his spouse may improve the client's self-esteem (i.e., psychosocial subsystem). The process of making lunch provides the client the opportunity to solve problems and to discover optimal strategies for performing tasks. This influences a client's cognitive and sensorimotor subsystems and the ability to perform other functional tasks.

The various parts of the systems model of motor behavior can be related to the Occupational Therapy Practice Framework (OTPF) (American Occupational Therapy Association [AOTA], 2002) and the Occupational Functioning Model (OFM) (see Chapter 1). OTPF terminology has been added to the model in parentheses (Fig. 6-2). Thus, the *person* system includes client factors, performance skills, and performance patterns. The *sensorimotor* system includes components such as strength, endurance, range of motion, coordination, sensory awareness, postural control, and perceptual skills. The *psychosocial* system includes a person's values, interests, self-concept, social interactions, and self-management skills that can affect occupational performance tasks. The *cognitive* system includes orientation, attention span, memory, problem-solving skills, and learning ability. The *person* system in this model includes the four lowest levels of the OFM: organic substrate, first-level capacities, developed capacities, and abilities and skills. The *environment* system includes physical, socioeconomic, and cultural contexts and the related personal, spiritual, temporal, and virtual contexts that influence client performance. The *physical*

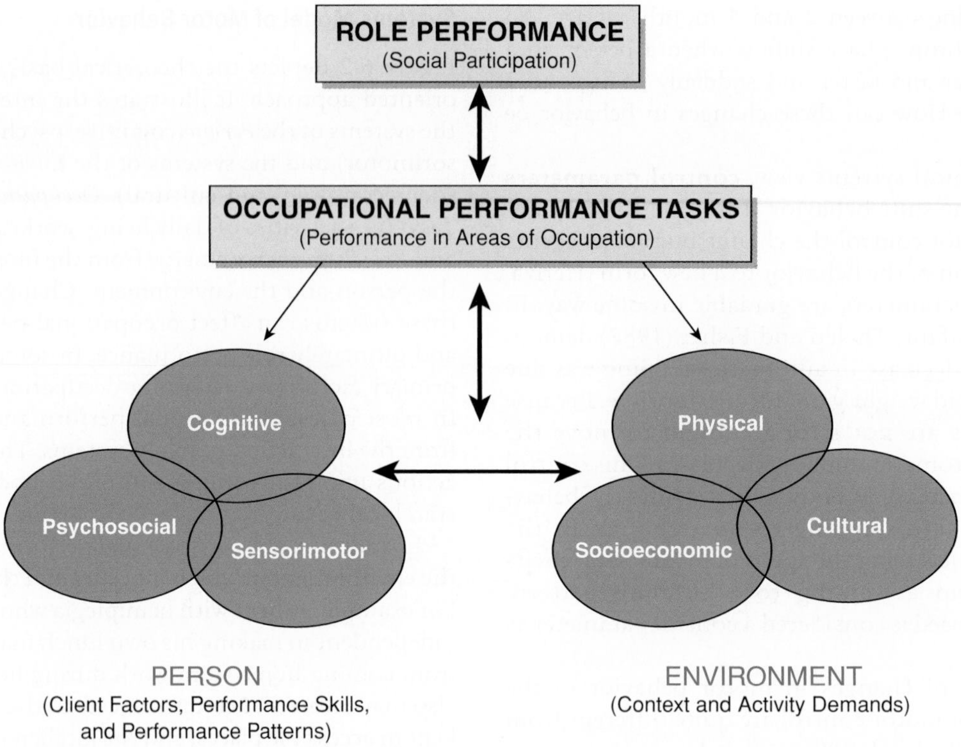

Figure 6-2 Systems model of motor behavior, which supports the OT task-oriented approach, emphasizes that occupational performance tasks and role performance emerge from an interaction of the person and the environment. In addition, occupational performance tasks impact the person and environment as well. There is a continuous interaction between role performance and occupational performance tasks. These interactions are ongoing across time. Adapted with permission from Mathiowetz and Bass-Haugen (2002).

environment system includes objects, tools, and the natural and built environment, which may limit or enhance task performance. The *cultural* environment system includes ethnicity, family, attitudes, beliefs, values, customs, and societal expectations, which also could affect occupational performance tasks. Finally, the *socioeconomic* system includes social supports provided by the family, friends, caregivers, social groups, and community and financial resources, which may influence choice in activities. The *environment* system is consistent with the OFM: environment and context.

The *Occupational Performance Tasks* are consistent with OTPF areas of occupation (activities of daily living, instrumental activities of daily living, education, work, play, and leisure), except for social participation, which we include under *Role Performance*. The *Occupational Performance Tasks* include the OFM activities and habits needed to perform the tasks required to fulfill self-maintenance, self-advancement, and self-enhancement roles. *Role Performance* includes the highest levels of the OFM: sense of self-efficacy and satisfaction with life roles.

The inclusion of *Role Performance* in this model (Fig. 6-2) reflects an occupational therapy perspective and does not originate from the motor behavior literature. Occupational therapists believe the roles that persons want and need to fulfill determine the occupational performance tasks and activities that they need to do. Conversely, the tasks and activities persons are able to do determine what roles they are able to fulfill. Although this model may have applications to all areas of occupational therapy practice and to occupational therapy theory development, the focus of this chapter is its application to individuals with CNS dysfunction.

View of Recovery after CNS Dysfunction

A client with a damaged CNS attempts to compensate for the lesion to achieve functional goals. Recovery from brain damage is a process of discovering what abilities and capacities remain to enable performance of activities and tasks. CNS damage affects each system differently relative to occupational performance. Therapists must consider all systems as potential variables to explain behavior of each client at a specific time. For example, the flexor pattern of spasticity commonly seen after a stroke is caused by various factors in addition to spasticity, such as inability to recruit appropriate muscles, weakness, soft tissue tightness, and perceptual deficits (Bourbonnais & Vanden Noven, 1989; Shumway-Cook & Woollacott, 2001). This pattern may become obligatory because of abnormal positioning and decreased use in functional contexts. Because each client is a unique person and functions in a unique environment, therapists should expect recovery for each client to vary even if the CNS damage is similar.

There is increasing evidence that neural reorganization after a brain lesion reflects the functional demands on the CNS. For example, forced use of the involved limb has improved functional performance in persons more than a year post stroke (Liepert et al., 2000; Taub et al., 1993). These changes can hardly be attributed to spontaneous recovery. Thus, providing appropriately challenging tasks and environments for those with CNS dysfunction, both in the hospital and at home, appears critical to the maximal rehabilitation of our clients (Bach-y-Rita, 1993; Nudo, 2003).

Evaluations

Evaluation Using the OT Task-Oriented Approach

Evaluation is conducted using a top-down approach consistent with the model of occupational functioning (see Chapter 1). A framework for evaluation is described in Procedures for Practice 6-2. Evaluation efforts focus initially on role and occupational performance because they are the goals of motor behavior. A thorough understanding of the roles that a client wants, needs, or is expected to perform and of the tasks needed to fulfill those roles enables therapists to plan meaningful and motivating treatment programs. After a client has identified the most important role and occupational performance limitations, therapists use task analysis to identify which person and/or environmental factors are limiting functional performance. This process may indicate the need for evaluation of selected person and/or environmental factors (Fisher & Short-DeGraff, 1993). The emphasis on role and occupational performance in the OT task-oriented approach suggests that evaluation in occupational therapy should be primarily at the participation and activities levels rather than the body functions and structures (impairment) level, using the World Health Organization (2001) terminology. The evaluation process necessitates use of both qualitative and quantitative measures (VanSant, 1990). Therefore, therapists use interviews, skilled observations, and standardized assessments to evaluate their clients. Although the client is the primary source of information, other sources, including the client's records, caregivers, family members, and the client's environment, contribute as well. Next, each step of the evaluation framework is described in more detail.

The first step in evaluation is the assessment of role performance. Trombly (1993) states that satisfactory fulfillment of roles is necessary for clients to achieve a sense of efficacy (i.e., competence and self-esteem). These roles may serve a variety of purposes, including development and maintenance of self (self-care), advancement of self or pro-

PROCEDURES FOR PRACTICE 6-2

Evaluation Framework for the OT Task-Oriented Approach Based on a Systems Model of Motor Behavior

1. Role Performance
   - Identify past roles and whether they can be maintained or must be changed.
   - Determine how future roles will be balanced: worker, student, volunteer, home maintainer, hobbyist, amateur, participant in organizations, friend, family member, caregiver, religious participant, other.
2. Occupational Performance Tasks: Areas of Occupation
   - ADL: feeding, grooming, functional mobility, dressing, oral and toilet hygiene, bowel and bladder management, and bathing/showering.
   - Instrumental activities of daily living: care of others and/or pets, communication device use, community mobility, home management, meal preparation and clean-up, safety procedures, and shopping.
   - Work: employment seeking and acquisition, job performance, volunteer exploration and participation, and retirement preparation and adjustment.
   - Play/leisure: exploration and participation.
3. Task Selection and Analysis
   - What performance components and/or performance contexts limit or enhance occupational performance?
4. Person: Performance Components
   - Cognitive: orientation, attention span, memory, problem solving, learning, and generalization.
   - Psychosocial: values, interests, self-concept, interpersonal skills, self-expression, coping skills, time management, and self-control.
   - Sensorimotor: strength, endurance, range of motion, sensory awareness and processing, perceptual processing, and postural control.
5. Environment: Performance Context
   - Physical: objects, tools, devices, animals, and built and natural environment.
   - Socioeconomic: social supports, including family, friends, caregivers, social groups, and community, and financial resources.
   - Cultural: ethnicity, family, attitudes, beliefs, values, customs, and societal expectations.

ductivity (work), and enhancement of self (leisure). Therapists must determine which roles clients had prior to the onset of disability and which roles they can and cannot do at this time. A discussion of which roles clients want or need to perform in the future helps therapists to determine which roles are most important to their clients. In addition, therapists must explore how any role changes have affected or will affect their client and their families, especially the primary caregivers. Jongbloed, Stanton, and Fousek (1993, p. 76) suggested that therapists ask questions such as the following: "How have roles changed since the disability? How have family members reacted to these changes? Is there role flexibility when needed? How competently do family members perform roles?" These questions may have to be adapted to the respondent's level of understanding.

Although role performance can be assessed using a non-standardized, semi-structured interview, a standardized assessment tool, such as the *Role Checklist* (Barris, Oakley, & Kielhofner, 1988), is recommended. The *Role Checklist* is a written inventory designed for adolescents and adults with physical dysfunction. In part 1, clients indicate which of 10 roles (Procedures for Practice 6-2) they have performed in the past, are performing in the present, and plan to perform in the future. In part 2, clients indicate the value of each role to them. Other role assessment tools may be appropriate depending on the type of client and the setting. For example, if a client is undergoing major role changes and there is sufficient time for a comprehensive assessment, the *Role Change Assessment* for older adults (Rogers & Holm, 1999) or *Client-Oriented Role Evaluation* (*CORE*) (Toal-Sullivan & Henderson, 2004) are recommended. Detailed information on the assessment of role performance and other role assessment tools is presented in Chapter 4. After clients have identified the roles that they want or need to perform, it is easier for them to identify the tasks and activities needed to fulfill each role.

The second step in the evaluation process is the assessment of occupational performance tasks: activities of daily living (ADL), instrumental activities of daily living (IADL), work, and play/leisure (Procedures for Practice 6-2). Because roles, tasks, activities, and their contexts are unique to each person, a client-centered assessment tool, such as the *Canadian Occupational Performance Measure* (*COPM*) (Law et al., 1998) is recommended. It was designed to measure a client's perception of his or her occupational performance over time. A semi-structured interview is used to administer the *COPM*. First, clients are asked to identify problem areas in self-care, productivity, and leisure. Second, the importance of each problem area is rated. Third, clients rate their own performance and their satisfaction with the performance. The importance ratings assist therapists in setting treatment priorities. The performance and satisfaction ratings can be used as outcome measures to assess change across time. When therapists are concerned that a client may not provide accurate information because of a cognitive impairment, a caregiver may be interviewed or direct observation of selected activities can be used to validate the information. The information elicited by the *COPM* is unique to each client and his or her environmental context, which is critical to the OT task-oriented approach.

The *Assessment of Motor and Process Skills* (*AMPS*) is another recommended measure of occupational performance, specifically personal and instrumental ADL (Bray, Fisher, & Duran, 2001; Fisher, 2003). It is a client-centered assessment because the person chooses two or three ADL tasks to be performed, which ensures familiarity and relevance to the person being evaluated. The purpose of the *AMPS* is to determine whether or not a person has the necessary motor and process skills to effortlessly, efficiently, safely, and independently perform the ADL tasks needed for community living (Fisher, 2003). Because the *AMPS* has been standardized internationally and cross-culturally, it is appropriate for persons from diverse backgrounds and with diverse needs and interests. A unique feature of the *AMPS* is that it can adjust, through Rasch analysis, for the difficulty of tasks performed and the severity of the rater who scores the client's performance. In addition, it allows a therapist to compare the performance of clients who performed one set of tasks on initial evaluation with the results of a reevaluation on a different set of tasks. A limitation of the *AMPS* is that it requires a 5-day training and calibration workshop to learn how to administer the assessment reliably and validly. Computer software, which is required to score the *AMPS*, is provided with the workshop. Because the *AMPS* requires observation of clients performing occupational performance tasks, it also assists the third step in the evaluation process.

While evaluating occupational performance tasks, therapists must observe both the outcome and the process (i.e., the preferred movement patterns, their stability or instability, the flexibility to use other patterns, efficiency of the patterns, and ability to learn new strategies) to understand the motor behaviors used to compensate and to achieve functional goals. It is important to determine the stability of the motor behavior because it will help determine the feasibility of achieving behavioral change in treatment. Behaviors that are very stable require a great amount of time and effort to change. Behaviors that are unstable are in transition, which is the optimal time for eliciting behavioral change. Thus, a compensatory approach may be most appropriate when behaviors are stable, and a remediation approach may be more appropriate when behaviors are unstable. Evaluation of the process of task performance is likely to require use of both quantitative and qualitative measures.

The third step is task selection and analysis. The tasks selected for observation should be ones that clients have identified as important but difficult. In most cases, observation of performance will happen as part of the second step. Therapists use task or activity analysis (see Chapter 13) to determine whether there is a match between task requirements and personal characteristics that enables task performance within a relevant environment. If not, therapists attempt to determine which personal and/or environmental factors are interfering with occupational performance tasks. In dynamical systems theory, these are considered the critical control parameters or the variables that have the potential to shift behavior to a new level of task performance. Each person with CNS dysfunction has unique strengths, limitations, and environmental context. As a result, the critical control parameters that limit or support occupational performance tasks are also unique. As persons and their environments change over time, the critical control parameters also change.

The identification of critical control parameters is the most challenging part of the evaluation. Evidence in the research literature suggests that some performance components and/or environmental variables may be critical control parameters for persons with CNS dysfunction. Gresham et al. (1979) reported that psychosocial and environmental factors were significant determinants of functional deficits long after stroke. In a review, Gresham et al. (1995) reported that 11–68% of individuals post stroke have depression, with 10–27% meeting the criteria for major depression. In the cognitive area, Rao et al. (1991) reported that 43% of patients with multiple sclerosis had cognitive impairments of recent memory and sustained attention. In the sensorimotor area, weakness (Olsen, 1990), fatigue (Ingles, Eskes, & Phillips, 1999), impaired motor function (Bernspang et al., 1987), and visuospatial deficits (Titus et al., 1991) are associated with poorer functional outcomes. For example, Bernspang et al. (1987) reported that motor function measured with the *FMA* was moderately correlated ($r = 0.64$) with self-care ability.

One caution is that most of these studies were correlational, indicating relationships between these variables and functional performance, but they do not establish a causal link. Also, most correlations were moderate or low, which indicates that any one variable explains a relatively small percentage of the variance associated with functional performance. Reding and Potes (1988), however, provided evidence that, as the number of performance component impairments increased, functional outcomes decreased. Thus, multiple variables contribute to functional performance for most individuals with CNS dysfunction. The challenge is to identify the variables that are most important to your clients. Case studies by Flinn (1995) and Gillen (2000, 2002) illustrate the search for critical control parameters.

Bobath (1990) suggested that spasticity is the primary cause of motor deficits in individuals with CNS dysfunction and that weakness and decreased range of motion are due to spastic antagonists. However, there is increasing evidence that spasticity is not a critical control parameter (Bourbonnais & Vanden Noven, 1989). For example, Sahrmann and Norton (1977) reported EMG findings indicating that movements were limited not by antagonist stretch reflexes (spasticity) but by delayed initiation and cessation of agonist contraction. Similarly, Fellows, Kaus, and Thilmann (1994) found no relation between movement impairments and passive muscle hypertonia in the antagonist muscles. O'Dwyer, Ada, and Neilson (1996) found no relation between spasticity and either weakness or loss of dexterity. Thus, research evidence challenges the assumption that spasticity causes the weakness and decreased range of motion often seen in individuals with CNS dysfunction.

After identifying the variables that support or constrain occupational performance, the therapist must assess the interactions of these systems. Consider two clients who have small limitations in shoulder flexion. The role and tasks of client as worker may or may not be affected. If the worker is a carpenter, the interaction of this personal limitation with the demands of the work environment is likely to make nailing overhead, installing cabinets, and hanging doors difficult or impossible. A worker who does word processing, however, probably can do most tasks adequately because the interaction of personal characteristics and the performance context does not interfere with task performance. This part of the evaluation requires a qualitative assessment and clinical reasoning by the therapist using the information gathered.

The fourth step in the evaluation process is to perform specific assessments of the personal and/or environmental factors that are thought to be critical control parameters. The critical control variables are the only ones that must be evaluated. The evaluation of selected variables according to the OT task-oriented approach contrasts with bottom-up approaches that evaluate all component variables. This selective approach eliminates the need to evaluate variables that have little functional implication and saves therapists' time, which is critical for cost containment.

It is likely that occupational therapists will use a variety of measures in their evaluation of the client factors and/or environmental contexts that constrain or support occupational performance tasks or functioning. Some assessments are designed to examine one or more components within the context of occupational performance. The *Fatigue Impact Scale* (Fisk et al., 1994) was developed to evaluate the perceived effect of fatigue on the everyday lives of those with multiple sclerosis. Assessment of cognitive function through a functional task is the focus of the *Allen Cognitive Level Scale* (Allen, 1985; Allen, Kehrberg, & Burns, 1992). The *A-One Evaluation* (Arnadattoir, 1990) facilitates evaluation of perceptual and cognitive systems within the context of ADL. From a task-oriented perspective, these are preferred assessment tools because they closely link client factors to occupational performance. In contrast, most assessments of client factors are conducted independent of occupational performance (see Chapters 5 and 7–9 for specific assessments).

Evaluation of a client's environment is an important part of the fourth step of the evaluation. The inclusion of physical, social, cultural, personal, spiritual, temporal, and virtual environments in AOTA (2002) clinical practice guidelines acknowledges their important influence on occupational performance. Dunn (1993) and Spencer, Krefting, and Mattingly (1993) emphasized the importance of assessing environmental context as part of the overall evaluation process. Chapters 10 and 11 review assessments for these variables.

Evaluation Using Carr and Shepherd's Approach

Carr and Shepherd (1987, 1998, 2003) developed their approach in response to disillusionment with the neurophysiological approaches and attempts to apply recent motor behavior research to clinical practice. Although Carr and Shepherd are physical therapists, their approach to optimizing motor performance is relevant to occupational therapy because it emphasizes the relearning of daily activities and provides a task-related strategy for improving motor control (Sabari, 2002). Carr and Shepherd (1998) described in detail how they approach evaluation. Their most important contribution to evaluation is their *Motor Assessment Scale* (*MAS*), a recommended test of motor function in the Agency for Health Care Policy and Research (AHCPR) clinical practice guidelines for post-stroke rehabilitation (Gresham et al., 1995). In addition, they deserve credit for their strong emphasis on task analysis as part of the evaluation (see Chapter 23).

Motor Assessment Scale (Assessment Table 6-2)

Carr et al. (1985) developed the *MAS* as an easily administered and relatively brief (15–30 minutes) assessment relevant to everyday motor activities (Procedures for Practice 6-3). The original version of the *MAS* included a ninth subtest, muscle tone, which has been deleted because it had poor reliability and questionable validity (Carr & Shepherd, 1998). The psychometric properties of *MAS* are described in Assessment Table 6-2. Because reliability and validity data for individual subtests of the *MAS* are available, one or more subtests can be used with each client, but the *MAS* total score across the subtests should not be used because it is an ordinal scale (Carr & Shepherd, 1998).

Assessments of Motor Function (Assessment Table 6-2)

The *Arm Motor Ability Test* (*AMAT*) was developed as an assessment of functional ability and quality of movement as a result of constraint-induced movement therapy (Kopp et al., 1997). Some of the 13 functional tasks are simulated (e.g., Cut Meat uses Play-Doh) and thus are not as natural as most functional assessments.

The *Wolf Motor Function Test* (*WMFT*) "quantifies upper extremity movement ability through timed single- or multiple-joint motions and functional tasks" (Wolf et al., 2001, p. 1635). It was also developed to assess the effects of constraint-induced movement therapy.

PROCEDURES FOR PRACTICE 6-3

Scoring Sheet for the Motor Assessment Scale

Each subtest is scored on a 7-point scale according to specific criteria.

Subtests	0	1	2	3	4	5	6
Supine to side-lying onto intact side							
Supine to sitting on side of bed							
Balanced sitting							
Sitting to standing							
Walking							
Upper arm function							
Hand movements							
Advanced hand activities							

Reprinted with permission from Carr, J. H., Shepherd, R. B., Nordholm, L., & Lynne, D. (1985). Investigation of a new Motor Assessment Scale for stroke patients. *Physical Therapy*, 65, 175–180. Copyright 1985 by American Physical Therapy Association.

Assessments of Balance (Assessment Table 6-3)

The *Balance Scale* (Berg et al., 1992) is not associated with a particular neurophysiological or task-related approach. It is compatible with the task-related approaches because it evaluates clients' performance on 14 items common in everyday life. The items include "the subject's ability to maintain positions of increasing difficulty by diminishing the base of support from sitting, to comfortable stance, to standing with feet together, and finally tandem standing (i.e., one foot in front of the other) and single leg stance, the two most difficult items. Other items assess how well the subject is able to change positions from sitting to standing, transfer from chair to chair, turn, pick up an object from the floor, and sit down" (Berg et al., 1992, p. 1074). The *Balance Scale* is a recommended assessment of balance in the AHCPR clinical practice guidelines for post-stroke rehabilitation (Gresham et al., 1995).

The *Functional Reach Test* (Duncan et al., 1990) was developed as a quick, clinical measure of dynamic balance that uses a continuous scoring system to assess the risk of falls in the elderly. It was intended to be an alternative to sophisticated laboratory-based assessments of falls, which are not feasible for clinical use. For a broader review of balance assessments, see Whitney, Pool, and Cass (1998).

Assessment Table 6-3

Summary of Assessments of Balance

Instrument and Reference	Description	Time to Administer	Validity	Reliability	Sensitivity	Strengths and Weaknesses
Balance Scale (Berg et al., 1992)	14 items common in everyday life are "graded on a five-point scale, 0 to 4. Points are based on the time the position can be maintained, the distance the arm is able to reach forward, or the time to complete the task" (Berg et al., 1992, p. 1075).	About 15 minutes to administer and requires only a stopwatch and ruler.	Concurrent validity: $r = 0.91$ with the *Tinetti Balance Subscale* (Tinetti, 1986); $r = .67$ with *Barthel Mobility*; $r = 0.76$ with *Timed Up-and-Go Test* (Podsiadlo & Richardson, 1991); and $r = 0.55$ average with 8 of 10 laboratory tests of balance. Discriminant validity: among persons using various types of walking aids (Berg et al., 1992).	Inter-rater reliability: ICC[1] = 0.98 for total scale; ICC = 0.71–0.99 for individual items. Test–retest reliability: ICC = 0.99 for total scale. Internal consistency: Cronbach's $K^2 = 0.96$ (Berg et al., 1989).	Significant changes in scores at 6 and 12 weeks post stroke (Wood-Dauphinee et al., 1997).	Strengths: Measures many aspects of balance; excellent reliability; evidence of validity. Weakness: Longest administration time.
Functional Reach Test (Duncan et al., 1990)	"The maximal distance one can reach forward beyond arm's length while maintaining a fixed base of support in the standing position" (Duncan et al., 1990, p. M192).	1–2 minutes to administer and requires a 48-inch leveled ruler mounted on the wall at shoulder height (Weiner et al., 1993).	Concurrent validity: $r = 0.71$ with center of pressure excursion (Duncan et al., 1990); discriminant validity: significant difference between persons with high and low risk of falls; predictive validity: score ≤6 inches predictive of falls in elderly (Duncan et al., 1992).	Inter-rater reliability: $r = 0.98$; test–retest reliability: ICC = 0.92 (Duncan et al., 1990).	Marginal significant change ($p = 0.07$) after physical rehabilitation; responsiveness index = 0.97 (Weiner et al., 1993).	Strengths: Brief, functional test; excellent reliability; evidence of validity. Weakness: Sensitivity is borderline.

[1] ICC = intraclass correlation coefficient, a reliability index that depicts consistency of agreement

[2] K = kappa

CASE EXAMPLE

Mr. B: Assessment of Motor Behavior Using a Task-Oriented Approach

Occupational Therapy Assessment Process	Clinical Reasoning Process: Objectives	Clinical Reasoning Process: Examples of Therapist's Internal Dialogue
Patient Information		
Mr. B. is a 55-year-old man who worked as an administrator at a junior college until a week ago, when he had a left cerebral vascular accident with resultant right hemiparesis. His medical history includes insulin-dependent diabetes mellitus and two heart attacks in the past 5 years. He lives with his wife in a ranch-style house. She works as a middle manager at an electronics firm. They have two adult children who do not live nearby. The acute-care occupational therapist reported that he is independent in feeding, grooming, oral hygiene, and wheelchair mobility for short distances. He needs assistance with bathing, toilet hygiene, and dressing. Other occupational performance tasks were not assessed in acute care. He has weakness throughout his dominant right arm, with grade 2 muscle tone on the *Modified Ashworth Scale* for scapular depression, shoulder internal rotation, and elbow, wrist, and finger flexors. PROM is within normal limits except for a 20° limitation in shoulder external rotation and elbow extension.	Understand the patient's diagnosis or condition	"Mr. B. has right hemiparesis and moderate disability one week post. Because his right arm is not flaccid and he is able to do some self-care already, his prognosis for recovery of functional ability appears to be good."
	Know the person	"Given his age and type of job, I expect that he will be motivated to return to work, but I can't assume that."
	Appreciate the context	"I wonder how his wife is reacting to his various health problems. Will she support his return to work or will she try to protect him? I wonder about the accessibility of his home and work environment."
	Develop provisional hypotheses	"Given his diagnosis and history, I presume that sensorimotor, psychosocial, and cognitive client factors and the physical environment at home and/or work might limit his ability to perform occupational performance tasks and to assume his usual roles. Given his early recovery, he should be able to benefit from an intensive rehabilitation program."
Assessment Process		
The *Role Checklist* was used to identify which roles were most important to him and to identify the tasks and activities that are associated with those roles. The *COPM* was used to determine the occupational performance tasks he wanted or needed to do and to determine his perception of his ability. Task analysis was used with specific tasks he perceived as difficult or impossible. The therapist observed him for client factors that might be limiting function and explored environmental factors that could support or limit his performance.	Consider evaluation approach and methods	"The primary aim of the assessment in the rehabilitation unit was to determine which roles and occupational performance tasks were most important to Mr. B. and to determine his ability on those tasks. The secondary aim was to determine if specific client or environmental factors were supporting or limiting his functional performance."
Assessment Results		
It was clear from the *Role Checklist* that Mr. B.'s work role was important to him. His concerns about returning to work included problems with writing, word processing, and removing heavy manuals from shelves above his desk. His wife, however, was pushing him to consider early retirement because of his increasing health problems. He and his wife enjoyed entertaining friends at home, at which times	Interpret observations	"It is clear that work and cooking tasks are priorities for this client, followed by self-care tasks. It is not yet clear whether he will be able to return to work. Decreased strength and impaired sensation are limiting the function of the right hand. Decreased PROM

he was the primary chef. This was an important activity for both of them. Although he was responsible for many home and yard maintenance tasks, these were not important to him. He thought friends would help them or they could hire help. On the *COPM,* return to work was ranked as most important, followed by cooking, toilet hygiene, dressing, and driving. He rated his performance and satisfaction for all of these tasks as very low.

His performance on several work-related, cooking, and self-care tasks were observed. He had difficulty holding a regular pen. A trial with an enlarged pen with a rubber grip, however, enabled him to hold a pen for about 3 minutes and write with very poor legibility. He was unable to use his right hand for keyboarding because he could not isolate individual fingers. He became frustrated while performing a simple cooking task (i.e., making pudding) because he could not walk and had difficulty using his right hand for bilateral tasks. He was able to toilet himself with verbal cueing and standby assistance. During dressing, he had difficulty raising his right arm, reaching down to put on his socks (concerned appropriately about balance), and difficulty performing bilateral tasks (e.g., tying his shoelaces). He complained about the time and energy needed to complete functional tasks. He used his right hand in half of the bilateral tasks he attempted. Thus, it appeared that sensorimotor client factors might be the cause of the difficulty performing occupational performance tasks, so these were evaluated further.

There was no evidence of unilateral visual neglect on a line bisection test. Sensory testing indicated loss of protective sensation and diminished light touch in the right hand (Semmes-Weinstein monofilaments) and impaired proprioception in the wrist and fingers only. Selective muscle testing indicated grade 3+ in scapular elevation, elbow flexion, and extension; 3− in shoulder flexion, abduction, and external rotation; and wrist flexion and extension. Grip strength in the right hand was 5 pounds, and in the left hand, it was 80 pounds; key pinch on the right was 3 pounds, and on the left, it was 19 pounds. He was able to reach forward nine inches on the *Functional Reach Test.*

of the shoulder external rotation is a concern because it is often associated with development of a painful shoulder. There is no evidence of cognitive or perceptual deficits. He has a mild deficit in balance. I chose the *Functional Reach Test* instead of the *Berg Balance Scale* to assess balance because it was specific to the balance problems observed and administration time is brief. Selected subscales of the *MAS* were considered because they are more functional than the other motor function assessments, but the two subscales—Hand Movements and Advanced Hand Activities—that would have provided the most useful information on Mr. B. have questionable validity. Therefore, I chose not to use the *MAS* with this client."

Occupational Therapy Problem List

1. Decreased ability to perform work, cooking, and self-care tasks because of sensorimotor impairments
2. Decreased strength, PROM, sensibility, and dexterity in his right upper extremity; decreased endurance for activity; mild impairment of sitting balance
3. Insufficient information on home environments to prepare adequately for discharge

Synthesize results — "Although I have sufficient information to begin treatment with Mr. B., I will need additional information from him and his employer about job requirements and work environment. In addition, more details about the home environment, home management roles and responsibilities, and other leisure interests are necessary."

CLINICAL REASONING IN OCCUPATIONAL THERAPY PRACTICE

Impact of Theoretical Assumptions on Clinical Assessments

Post-acute care assessments for Mr. B. were approached using the assumptions of the OT task-oriented approach. How would the assumptions and assessment differ if you used a neurophysiological approach with Mr. B.? What would be the primary and secondary focus of assessments? Would those assessments make a difference in the problems you identified?

CLINICAL REASONING IN OCCUPATIONAL THERAPY PRACTICE

Choice of Motor Function Assessment

Post-acute care assessments for Mr. B. were approached using the assumptions of the OT task-oriented approach. Which assessments of motor function, if any, would you choose for Mr. B.? Why?

SUMMARY REVIEW QUESTIONS

1. How do the reflex-hierarchical and systems models of motor control differ?
2. How do the neuromaturational and systems theories of motor development differ?
3. What types of motor dysfunction are associated with cortical, cerebellar, and basal ganglia lesions of the CNS?
4. What might account for the recovery seen after CNS damage?
5. What are at least four assumptions of the neurophysiological approaches?
6. How would you evaluate abnormal muscle tone and movement patterns?
7. What are at least four assumptions of the OT task-oriented approach?
8. How do evaluations used by the neurophysiological and task-related approaches differ?

ACKNOWLEDGMENT

We thank Nancy Flinn, PhD, OTR/L, who uses the OT task-oriented approach in her clinical practice and has provided us with constructive feedback.

References

Ada, L., & Westwood, P. (1992). A kinematic analysis of recovery of the ability to stand up following stroke. *Australian Physiotherapy, 38,* 135–142.

Allen, C. (1985). *Occupational therapy for psychiatric diseases: Measurement and management of cognitive disabilities.* Boston: Little, Brown.

Allen, C., Kehrberg, K., & Burns, T. (1992). Evaluation instruments. In K. A. Allen, C. A. Earhart, & T. Blue (Eds.), *Occupational therapy treatment goals for the physically and cognitively disabled.* Rockville, MD: American Occupational Therapy Association.

Allison, S. C., & Abraham, L. D. (1995). Correlation of quantitative measures with the Modified Ashworth Scale in the assessment of plantar flexor spasticity in patients with traumatic brain injury. *Journal of Neurology, 242,* 699–706.

American Occupational Therapy Association [AOTA]. (2002). Occupational therapy practice framework: Domain and process. *American Journal of Occupational Therapy, 56,* 609–639.

Arnadattoir, G. (1990). *The brain and behavior: Assessing cortical dysfunction through activities of daily living.* St. Louis: Mosby.

Ashworth, B. (1964). Preliminary trial of carisoprodol in multiple sclerosis. *Practitioner, 192,* 540–542.

Bach-y-Rita, P. (1993). Recovery from brain damage. *Journal of Neurological Rehabilitation, 6,* 191–199.

Bakheit, A. M., Thilmann, A. F., Ward, A. B., Poewe, W., Wissel, J., Muller, J., Benecke, R., Collin, C., Muller, F., Ward, C.D., & Neumann, C. (2000). A randomized, double-blind, placebo-controlled, dose ranging study to compare the efficacy and safety of three doses of botulinum toxin type A (Dysport) with placebo in upper limb spasticity after stroke. *Stroke, 31,* 2402–2406.

Bakheit, A. M., Pittock, S., Moore, A. P., Wurker, M., Otto, S., Erbguth, F., & Coxon, L. (2001). A randomized, double-blind, placebo-controlled study of the efficacy and safety of botulinum toxin type A in upper limb spasticity in patients with stroke. *European Journal of Neurology,* 8, 559–565.

Barris, R., Oakley, F., & Kielhofner, G. (1988). The Role Checklist. In B. J. Hemphill (Ed.), *Mental health assessment in occupational therapy* (pp. 73–91). Thorofare, NJ: Slack.

Berg, K., Maki, B., Williams, J. I., Holliday, P. J., & Wood-Dauphinee, S. (1992). Clinical and laboratory measures of postural balance in an elderly population. *Archives of Physical Medicine and Rehabilitation, 73,* 1073–1080.

Berg, K., Wood-Dauphinee, S., Williams, J. I., & Gayton, D. (1989). Measuring balance in the elderly: Preliminary development of an instrument. *Physiotherapy Canada, 41,* 301–311.

Bernspang, B., Asplund, K., Eriksson, S., & Fugl-Meyer, A. R. (1987). Motor and perceptual impairments in acute stroke patients: Effects on self-care ability. *Stroke, 18,* 1081–1086.

Bernstein, N. (1967). *The coordination and regulation of movements.* Elmsford, NY: Pergamon.

Bobath, B. (1978). *Adult hemiplegia: Evaluation and treatment* (2nd ed.). London: Heinemann Medical.

Bobath, B. (1990). *Adult hemiplegia: Evaluation and treatment* (3rd ed.). Oxford: Butterworth Heinemann.

Bohannon, R. W., & Smith, M. B. (1987). Interrater reliability of a modified Ashworth scale of muscle spasticity. *Physical Therapy, 67,* 206–207.

Bourbonnais, D., & Vanden Noven, S. (1989). Weakness in patients with hemiparesis. *American Journal of Occupational Therapy, 43,* 313–319.

Bray, K., Fisher, A. G., & Duran, L. (2001). The validity of adding new tasks to the Assessment of Motor and Process Skills. *American Journal of Occupational Therapy, 55,* 409–415.

Brooks, V. B. (1986). *The neural basis of motor control.* New York: Oxford University.

Brunnstrom, S. (1970). *Movement therapy in hemiplegia.* New York: Harper & Row.

Burke, D. (1988). Spasticity as an adaptation to pyramidal tract injury. In S. G. Waxman (Ed.), *Advances in neurology. Vol. 47: Functional recovery in neurological disease* (pp. 401–423). New York: Raven.

Burridge, J. H., Wood, D. E., Hermens, H. J., Voerman, G. E., Johnson, G. R., van Wijck, F., Platz, T., Gregoric, M., Hitchcock, R., & Pandyan, A. (2005). Theoretical and methodological considerations in the measurement of spasticity. *Disability and Rehabilitation, 27,* 69–80.

Burton, A. W., & Davis, W. E. (1992). Optimizing the involvement and performance of children with physical impairments in movement activities. *Pediatric Exercise Science, 4,* 236–248.

Carr, J. H., & Shepherd, R. B. (1987). *A motor relearning programme for stroke* (2nd ed.). Rockville, MD: Aspen.

Carr, J. H., & Shepherd, R. B. (1998). *Neurological rehabilitation: Optimizing motor performance.* Oxford: Butterworth Heinemann.

Carr, J. H., & Shepherd, R. B. (2003). *Stroke rehabilitation: Guidelines for exercise and training to optimize motor skill.* Oxford: Butterworth Heinemann.

Carr, J. H., Shepherd, R. B., Nordholm, L., & Lynne, D. (1985). Investigation of a new Motor Assessment Scale for stroke patients. *Physical Therapy, 65,* 175–180.

Chae, J., Labatia, I., & Yang, G. (2003). Upper limb motor function in hemiparesis. *American Journal of Physical Medicine and Rehabilitation, 82,* 1–8.

Cheney, P. D. (1985). Role of cerebral cortex in voluntary movements: A review. *Physical Therapy, 65,* 624–635.

Davis, W. E., & Burton, A. W. (1991). Ecological task analysis: Translating movement behavior theory into practice. *Adapted Physical Activity Quarterly, 8,* 154–177.

Dean, D., & Mackey, F. (1992). Motor Assessment Scale scores as a measure of rehabilitation outcome following stroke. *Australian Journal of Physiotherapy, 38,* 31–35.

Duncan, P. W., Propst, M., & Nelson, S. G. (1983). Reliability of the Fugl-Meyer Assessment of the sensorimotor recovery following cerebrovascular accident. *Physical Therapy, 63,* 1606–1610.

Duncan, P. W., Studenski, S., Chandler, J., & Prescott, B. (1992). Functional Reach: Predictive validity in a sample of elderly male veterans. *Journal of Gerontology: MEDICAL SCIENCES, 47,* M93–M98.

Duncan, P. W., Weiner, D. K., Chandler, J., & Studenski, S. (1990). Functional Reach: A new clinical measure of balance. *Journal of Gerontology: MEDICAL SCIENCES, 45,* M192–M195.

Dunn, W. (1993). Measurement of function: Actions for the future. *American Journal of Occupational Therapy, 47,* 357–359.

Fellows, S. J., Kaus, C., & Thilmann, A. (1994). Voluntary movement at the elbow in spastic hemiparesis. *Annals of Neurology, 36,* 397–407.

Feys, H. M., De Weerdt, W. J., Selz, B. E., Steck, G., Spichiger, R., Vereeck, L. E., Putman, K. D., & Van Hoydonck, G. A. (1998). Effect of a therapeutic intervention for the hemiplegic upper limb in the acute phase after stroke. *Stroke, 29,* 785–792.

Fiorentino, M. R. (1973). *Reflex testing methods for evaluating CNS development* (2nd ed.). Springfield, IL: Charles C. Thomas.

Fisher, A. G. (2003). *Assessment of Motor and Process Skills: Development, standardization, and administration manual* (5th ed.). Fort Collins, CO: Three Star Press.

Fisher, A. G., & Short-DeGraff, M. (1993). Improving functional assessment in occupational therapy: Recommendations and philosophy for change. *American Journal of Occupational Therapy, 47,* 199–201.

Fisk, J. D., Pontefract, A., Ritvo, P., Archibald, C., & Murray, T. (1994). The impact of fatigue on patients with multiple sclerosis. *Canadian Journal of Neurological Science, 21,* 9–14.

Fitch, H. L., Tuller, B., & Turvey, M. T. (1982). The Bernstein perspective: III. Tuning of coordinative structures with special reference to perception. In J. A. S. Kelso (Ed.), *Human motor behavior: An introduction* (pp. 271–281). Hillsdale, NJ: Erlbaum.

Flinn, N. (1995). A task-oriented approach to the treatment of a client with hemiplegia. *American Journal of Occupational Therapy,* 49, 560–569.

Fredericks, C. M., & Saladin, L. K. (Eds.). (1996). *Pathophysiology of the motor systems: Principles and clinical presentations.* Philadelphia: Davis.

Fugl-Meyer, A. R., Jaasko, L., Leyman, I., Olsson, S., & Steglind, S. (1975). The post-stroke hemiplegic patient: A method for evaluation of physical performance. *Scandinavian Journal of Rehabilitation Medicine, 7,* 13–31.

Gentile, A. M. (1972). A working model of skill acquisition with application to teaching. *Quest, 17,* 3-23.

Gesell, A. (1954). The ontogenesis of infant behavior. In L. Carmichael (Ed.), *Manual of Child Psychology* (2nd ed., pp. 335-373). New York: Wiley.

Gibson, J. J. (1977). The theory of affordances. In R. Shaw & J. Bransford (Eds.), *Perceiving, acting, and knowing* (pp. 67–82). Hillsdale, NJ: Erlbaum.

Gibson, J. J. (1979). *The ecological approach to visual perception.* Boston: Houghton Mifflin.

Gillen, G. (2000). Improving activities of daily living performance in an adult with ataxia. *American Journal of Occupational Therapy, 54,* 89–96.

Gillen, G. (2002). Improving mobility and community access in an adult with ataxia. *American Journal of Occupational Therapy, 56,* 462–466.

Gleick, J. (1987). *Chaos: Making a new science.* New York: Penguin.

Gordon, J. (1987). Assumptions underlying physical therapy interventions: Theoretical and historical perspectives. In J. H. Carr, R. B. Shepherd, J. Gordon, A. M. Gentile, & J. M. Held (Eds.), *Movement science: Foundations for physical therapy in rehabilitation* (pp. 1–30). Rockville, MD: Aspen.

Gregson, J. M., Leathley, M. J., Moore, A. P., Smith, T. L., Sharma, A. K., & Watkins, C. L. (2000). Reliability of measurements of muscle tone and muscle power in stroke patients. *Age and Ageing, 29,* 223–228.

Gresham, G. E., Duncan, P. W., Stason, W. B., et al. (1995). *Post-stroke rehabilitation: Clinical practice guidelines no. 16.* Rockville, MD: U.S. Department of Health and Human Services. AHCPR Publication 95-0662.

Gresham, G. E., Phillips, T., Wolf, P., McNamara, P., Kannel, W., & Dawber, T. (1979). Epidemiologic profile of long-term stroke disability: The Framingham study. *Archives of Physical Medicine and Rehabilitation, 60,* 487–491.

Heriza, C. (1991). Motor development: Traditional and contemporary theories. In M. J. Lister (Ed.), *Contemporary management of motor control problems: Proceedings of the II STEP Conference* (pp. 99–126). Alexandria, VA: Foundation for Physical Therapy.

Horak, F. B. (1991). Assumptions underlying motor control for neurologic rehabilitation. In M. J. Lister (Ed.), *Contemporary management of motor control problems: Proceedings of the II Step Conference* (pp. 11–27). Alexandria, VA: Foundation for Physical Therapy.

Howle, J. (2002). Neurodevelopmental treatment approach: Theoretical foundations and principles of clinical practice. Laguna Beach, CA: Neurodevelopmental Treatment Association.

Ingles, J. L., Eskes, G. A., & Phillips, S. J. (1999). Fatigue after stroke. *Archives of Physical Medicine and Rehabilitation, 80,* 173–178.

Jeannerod, M., Michel, F., & Prablanc, C. (1984). The control of hand movements in a case of hemianesthesia following a parietal lesion. *Brain, 107,* 899–920.

Jongbloed, L., Stanton, S., & Fousek, B. (1993). Family adaptation to altered roles following stroke. *Canadian Journal of Occupational Therapy, 60,* 70–77.

Kamm, K., Thelen, E., & Jensen, J. L. (1990). A dynamical systems approach to motor development. *Physical Therapy, 70,* 763–775.

Katz, R. T., & Rymer, W. Z. (1989). Spastic hypertonia: Mechanism and measurement. *Archives of Physical Medicine and Rehabilitation, 70,* 144–155.

Knott, M., & Voss, D. E. (1968). *Proprioceptive neuromuscular facilitation* (2nd ed.). New York: Harper & Row.

Kopp, B., Kunkel, A., Flor, H., Platz, T., Rose, U., Mauritz, K.-H., Gresser, K., McCulloch, K. L., & Taub, E. (1997). The Arm Motor Ability Test: Reliability, validity, and sensitivity to change of an instrument for assessing disabilities in activities of daily living. *Archives of Physical Medicine and Rehabilitation, 78,* 615–620.

Kunkel, A., Kopp, B., Muller, G., Villringer, K., Villringer, A., Taub, E., & Flor, H. (1999). Constraint-induced movement therapy for motor recovery in chronic stroke patients. *Archives of Physical Medicine & Rehabilitation, 80,* 624–628.

Law, M., Baptiste, S., Carswell, A., McColl, M., Polatajko, H., & Pollock, N. (1998). *Canadian Occupational Performance Measure* (3rd ed.). Ottawa, Ontario, Canada: CAOT.

Liepert, J., Bauder, H., Wolfgang, H., Miltner, W., Taub, E., & Weiller, C. (2000). Treatment-induced cortical reorganization after stroke in humans. *Stroke, 31,* 1210–1216.

Lister, M. J. (Ed.). (1991). *Contemporary management of motor control problems: Proceedings of the II STEP Conference.* Alexandria, VA: Foundation for Physical Therapy.

Loewen, S. C., & Anderson, B. A. (1990). Predictors of stroke outcome using objective measurement scales. *Stroke, 21,* 78–81.

Magill, R. A. (2004). *Motor learning and control: Concepts and applications* (7th ed.). Boston: McGraw-Hill.

Malouin, F., Pickard, L., Bonneau, C., Durand, A., & Corriveau, D. (1994). Evaluating motor recovery early after stroke: Comparison of the Fugl-Meyer Assessment and the Motor Assessment Scale. *Archives of Physical Medicine and Rehabilitation, 75,* 1206–1212.

Marsden, C. D. (1982). The mysterious motor function of the basal ganglia: The Robert Wartenberg lecture. *Neurology, 32,* 514–539.

Marteniuk, R. G., MacKenzie, C. L., & Jeannerod, M. (1987). Constraints on human arm trajectories. *Canadian Journal of Psychology, 41,* 365–368.

Mathiowetz, V., & Bass-Haugen, J. (1994). Motor behavior research: Implications for therapeutic approaches to CNS dysfunction. *American Journal of Occupational Therapy, 48,* 733–745.

Mathiowetz, V., & Bass-Haugen, J. (2002). Assessing abilities and capacities: Motor behavior. In C. A. Trombly & M. V. Radomski (Eds.), *Occupational therapy for physical dysfunction* (5th ed., pp. 137–158). Baltimore: Lippincott Williams & Wilkins.

Mathiowetz, V. G., & Wade, M. (1995). Task constraints and functional motor performance of individuals with and without multiple sclerosis. *Ecological Psychology, 7,* 99–123.

McGraw, M. B. (1945). *The neuromuscular maturation of the human infant.* New York: Hafner.

Mehrholz, J., Major, Y., Meissner, D., Sandi-Gahun, S., Koch, R., & Pohl, M. (2005). The influence of contractures and variation in measurement stretching velocity on the reliability of the Modified Ashworth Scale in patients with severe brain injury. *Clinical Rehabilitation, 19,* 63–72.

Morris, D. M., Uswatte, G., Crago, J. E., Cook, E. W., & Taub, E. (2001). The reliability of the Wolf Motor Function Test for assessing upper extremity function after stroke. *Archives of Physical Medicine and Rehabilitation, 82,* 750–755.

Newell, K. M. (1986). Constraints on the development of coordination. In M. G. Wade & H. T. A. Whiting (Eds.), *Motor development in children: Aspects of coordination and control* (pp. 341–360). Dordrecht, the Netherlands: Martinus Nijhoff.

Newell, K. M. (2003). Schema theory (1975): Retrospectives and prospectives. *Research Quarterly of Exercise and Sport, 74,* 383–389.

Nudo, R. J. (2003). Adaptive plasticity in motor cortex: Implications for rehabilitation after brain injury. *Journal of Rehabilitation Medicine, 41 (Suppl.),* 7–10.

O'Dwyer, N. J., Ada, L., & Neilson, P. D. (1996). Spasticity and muscle contracture following stroke. *Brain, 119,* 1737–1749.

Olsen, T. S. (1990). Arm and leg paresis as outcome predictors in stroke rehabilitation. *Stroke, 21,* 247–251.

Pandyan, A. D., Price, C. I. M., Barnes, M. P., & Johnson, G. R. (2003). A biomechanical investigation into the validity of the Modified Ashworth Scale as a measure of elbow spasticity. *Clinical Rehabilitation, 17,* 290–294.

Pandyan, A. D., Vuadens, P., van Wijck, F., Stark, S., Johnson, G. R., & Barnes, M. P. (2002). Are we underestimating the clinical efficacy of botulinum toxin (type A)? Quantifying changes in spasticity, strength and upper limb function after injections of Botox to the elbow flexors in a unilateral stroke population. *Clinical Rehabilitation, 16,* 654–660.

Phillips, J. G., & Stelmach, G. E. (1996). Parkinson's disease and other involuntary movement disorders of the basal ganglia. In C. M. Fredericks & L. K. Saladin (Eds.), *Pathophysiology of the motor systems: Principles and clinical presentations* (pp. 203–216). Philadelphia: Davis.

Pizzi, A., Carlucci, G., Falsini, C., Verdesca, S., & Grippo, A. (2005). Evaluation of the upper-limb spasticity after stroke: A clinical and neurophysiologic study. *Archives of Physical Medicine and Rehabilitation, 86,* 410–415.

Podsiadlo, D., & Richardson, S. (1991). The timed "up and go": A test of basic mobility for frail elderly persons. *Journal of the American Geriatrics Society, 39,* 142–148.

Poole, J. L., & Whitney, S. L. (1988). Motor Assessment Scale for stroke patients: Concurrent validity and interrater reliability. *Archives of Physical Medicine and Rehabilitation, 69,* 195–197.

Rao, S. M., Leo, G., Bernardin, L., & Unverzagt, F. (1991). Cognitive dysfunction in multiple sclerosis: I. Frequency, patterns, and prediction. *Neurology, 41,* 685–691.

Reding, M. J., & Potes, E. (1988). Rehabilitation outcomes following initial unilateral hemispheric stroke: Life table analysis approach. *Stroke, 19,* 1354–1358.

Reed, E. S. (1982). An outline of a theory of action systems. *Journal of Motor Behavior, 14,* 98–134.

Rogers, J. C., & Holm, M. B. (1999). Role Change Assessment: An interview tool for older adults. In B. J. Hemphill-Pearson (Ed.), *Assessments in occupational therapy mental health: An integrated approach* (pp. 73–82). Thorofare, NJ: Slack.

Rood, M. S. (1954). Neurophysiological reactions as a basis for physical therapy. *Physical Therapy Review, 34,* 444–449.

Sabari, J. S. (2002). Optimizing motor control using the Carr and Shepherd approach. In C. Trombly & M. V. Radomski (Eds.), *Occupational therapy for physical dysfunction* (5th ed., pp. 501–519). Baltimore: Lippincott Williams & Wilkins.

Sabari, J. S., Lim, A. L., Velozo, C. A., Lehman, L., Kieran, O., & Lai, J. (2005). Assessing arm and hand function after stroke: A validity test of the hierarchical scoring system used in the Motor Assessment Scale for stroke. *Archives of Physical Medicine and Rehabilitation, 86,* 1609–1615.

Sahrmann, S. A., & Norton, B. J. (1977). The relationship of voluntary movement to spasticity in the upper motor neuron syndrome. *Annals of Neurology, 2,* 460–465.

Schmidt, R. A. (1988). *Motor control and learning: A behavioral emphasis* (2nd ed.). Champaign, IL: Human Kinetics.

Schmidt, R. A. (1991). *Motor learning and performance: From principles to practice.* Champaign, IL: Human Kinetics.

Scholz, J. P., & Campbell, S. K. (1980). Muscle spindles and the regulation of movement. *Physical Therapy, 60,* 1416–1424.

Shumway-Cook, A., & Woollacott, M. (2001). *Motor control: Theory and practical application* (2nd ed.). Baltimore: Lippincott Williams & Wilkins.

Sloan, R. L., Sinclair, E., Thompson, J., Taylor, S., & Pentland, B. (1992). Inter-rater reliability of the Modified Ashworth Scale for spasticity in hemiplegic patients. *International Journal of Rehabilitation Research, 15,* 158–161.

Sommerfeld, D. K., Eek, E., Svensson, A., Holmqvist, L. W., & von Arbin, M. H. (2004). Spasticity after stroke: Its occurrence and association with motor impairments and activity limitations. *Stroke, 35,* 134–140.

Spencer, J., Krefting, L., & Mattingly, C. (1993). Incorporation of ethnographic methods in occupational therapy assessment. *American Journal of Occupational Therapy, 47,* 303–309.

Taub, E., Miller, N. E., Novack, T. A., Cook, E. W., Fleming, W., Nepomuceno, C., Connell, J., & Crago, J. (1993). Technique to improve chronic motor deficit after stroke. *Archives of Physical Medicine and Rehabilitation, 74,* 347–354.

Thelen, E. (1989). Self-organization in developmental processes: Can systems approaches work? In M. R. Gunnar & E. Thelen (Eds.), *Systems and development* (pp. 77–117). Hillsdale, NJ: Erlbaum.

Thelen, E., & Fisher, D. M. (1982). Newborn stepping: An explanation for a "disappearing reflex." *Developmental Psychology, 18,* 760–775.

Thelen, E., & Ulrich, B. D. (1991). Hidden skills. *Monograph of the Society for Research in Child Development, 56* (Serial 223). Chicago: University of Chicago.

Tinetti, M. E. (1986). Performance-oriented assessment of mobility problems in elderly patients. *Journal of American Geriatrics Society, 34,* 119–126.

Titus, M. N., Gall, N. G., Yerxa, E. J., Roberson, T. A., & Mack, W. (1991). Correlation of perceptual performance and activities of daily living in stroke patients. *American Journal of Occupational Therapy, 45,* 410–418.

Toal-Sullivan, D., & Henderson, P. R. (2004). Client-Oriented Role Evaluation (CORE): The development of a clinical rehabilitation instrument to assess role change associated with disability. *American Journal of Occupational Therapy, 58,* 211–220.

Trombly, C. A. (1989). Motor control therapy. In C. Trombly (Ed.), *Occupational therapy for physical dysfunction* (3rd ed., pp. 72–95). Baltimore: Williams & Wilkins.

Trombly, C. A. (1993). The issue is anticipating the future: Assessment of occupational function. *American Journal of Occupational Therapy, 47,* 253–257.

Trombly, C. A., & Wu, C. (1999). Effect of rehabilitation tasks on organization of movement after stroke. *American Journal of Occupational Therapy, 53,* 333–344.

Turvey, M. T. (1977). Preliminaries to a theory of action with reference to vision. In R. Shaw & J. Bransford (Eds.), *Perceiving, acting, and knowing* (pp. 211–265). Hillsdale, NJ: Erlbaum.

Twitchell, T. E. (1951). The restoration of motor function following hemiplegia in man. *Brain, 74,* 443–480.

VanSant, A. (1990). Life-span development in functional tasks. *Physical Therapy, 70,* 788–798.

VanSant, A. (1991a). Motor control, motor learning, and motor development. In P. C. Montgomery & B. H. Connolly (Eds.), *Motor control and physical therapy: Theoretical framework and practical applications* (pp. 13–28). Hixson, TN: Chattanooga Group.

VanSant, A. (1991b). Should the normal motor developmental sequence be used as a theoretical model to progress adult patients? In M. J. Lister (Ed.), *Contemporary management of motor control problems: Proceedings of the II STEP Conference* (pp. 95–97). Alexandria, VA: Foundation for Physical Therapy.

van Wijck, F. M. J., Pandyan, A. D., Johnson, G. R., & Barnes, M. P. (2001). Assessing motor deficits in neurological rehabilitation: Patterns of instrument usage. *Neurorehabilitation and Neural Repair, 15,* 23–30.

Warren, W. H. (1984). Perceiving affordances: Visual guidance of stair climbing. *Journal of Experimental Psychology: Human Perception and Performance, 10,* 683–703.

Weiner, D. K., Bongiorni, D. R., Studenski, S., Duncan, P. W., & Kochersberger, G. G. (1993). Does functional reach improve with rehabilitation? *Archives of Physical Medicine and Rehabilitation, 74,* 796–800.

Whitney, S. L., Poole, J. L., & Cass, S. P. (1998). A review of balance instruments for older adults. *American Journal of Occupational Therapy, 52,* 666–671.

Wolf, S. L., Catlin, P. A., Ellis, M., Archer, A. L., Morgan, B., & Piacentino, A. (2001). Assessing Wolf Motor Function Test as outcome measure for research in patients after stroke. *Stroke, 32,* 1635–1639.

Wood-Dauphinee, S., Berg, K., Bravo, G., & Williams, I. (1997). The Balance Scale: Responsiveness to clinically meaningful changes. *Canadian Journal of Rehabilitation, 10,* 35–50.

Wood-Dauphinee, S. L., Williams, J. I., & Shapiro, S. H. (1990). Examining outcome measures in a clinical study of stroke. *Stroke, 21,* 731–739.

World Health Organization. (2001). *International classification of functioning, disability and health (ICF).* Geneva: World Health Organization.

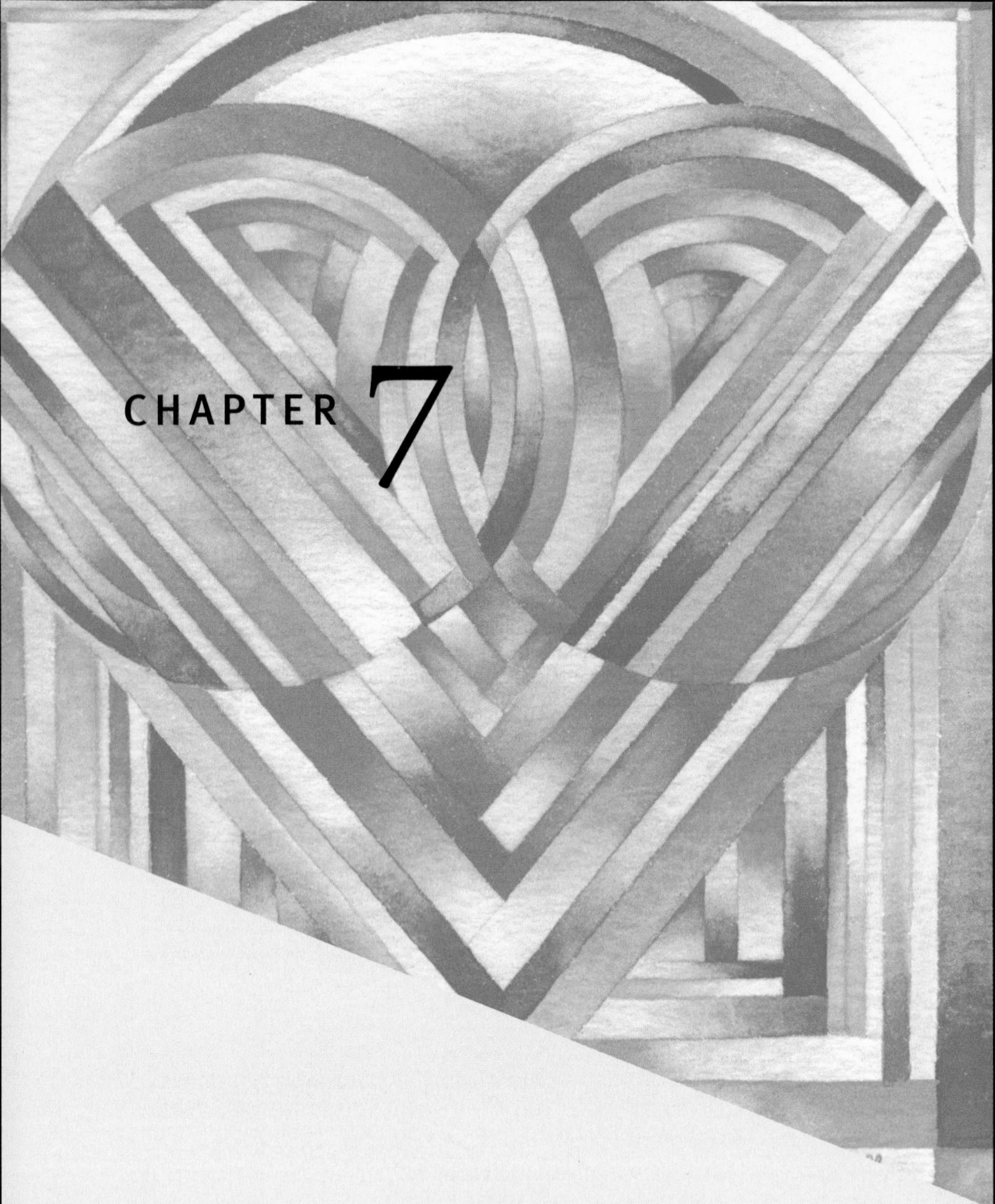

CHAPTER 7

LEARNING OBJECTIVES

After studying this chapter, the reader will be able to do the following:

1. Describe the effects of sensory loss on occupational function.
2. Predict the pattern of sensory loss based on diagnosis or described lesion in the somatosensory system.
3. Demonstrate appropriate sensory testing techniques for tactile sensation when provided with appropriate tools or equipment.
4. Differentiate standardized and nonstandardized tactile tests.
5. Choose appropriate sensory testing techniques for a given patient or situation.
6. Correctly interpret the results of sensory testing for treatment planning.

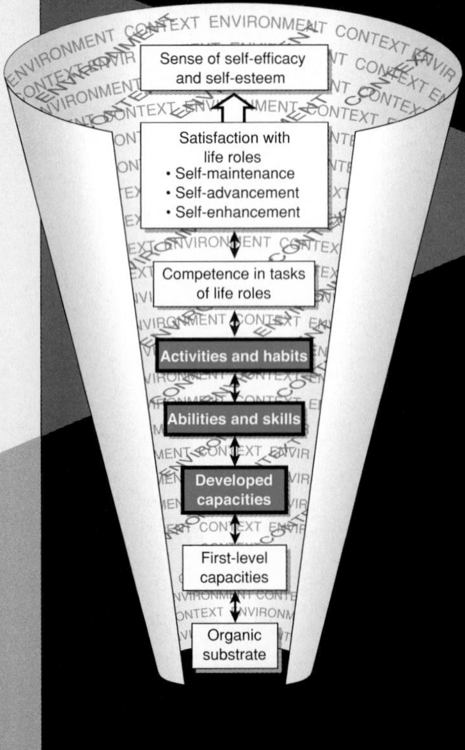

Assessing Abilities and Capacities: Sensation

Karen Bentzel

Glossary

Aesthesiometer—Instrument designed for sensory testing. The term usually indicates a tool consisting of a ruler type of scale and two prongs that can be moved progressively closer or farther apart that is used for assessing two-point discrimination (Fig. 7-7). Monofilaments are occasionally called pressure aesthesiometers in the literature.

Hypersensitivity, hyperesthesia—A condition in which an exaggerated or unpleasant sensation is experienced in response to ordinary stimuli.

Kinesthesia—The ability to identify "the excursion and direction of joint movement" (AOTA, 1994, p. 1053).

Monofilament—Thin nylon strand resembling fishing line, of graded thicknesses, attached to a handle and used in testing the threshold of light touch sensation.

Paresthesia—An abnormal sensation such as a feeling of pins and needles, tingling, or tickling in the absence of tactile stimulation or in response to tactile stimuli that ordinarily do not evoke tingling or tickling.

Proprioception—Interpreting stimuli originating in muscles, joints, and other internal tissues that give information about the position of one body part in relation to another (AOTA, 1994, p. 1052).

Stereognosis—The ability to identify objects through proprioception, cognition, and the sense of touch (AOTA, 1994). Astereognosis is the term used to describe the absence of this ability.

Vibrometer—Instrument designed to test the threshold of vibration sensation. It consists of a vibrating head that is applied to the patient's skin and a control unit that allows for gradual changes in the amplitude and frequency of vibration.

The American Occupational Therapy Association [AOTA] (1994, p. 1052) defines tactile sensory processing as "interpreting light touch, pressure, temperature, pain, and vibration through skin contact/receptors." The tactile sense is necessary throughout the body for occupational functioning but is especially important in the hands. Moberg described hands without sensation as being like eyes without vision (Dellon, 1988).

Immediately after birth, an infant is bombarded with tactile sensations that are different from those in utero. Within a few months, the infant learns to interpret a multitude of tactile stimuli, such as soothing touch from a parent that brings comfort and contentment. This developed capacity supports further development of abilities and skills, as the infant uses touch to grasp an object, bring two hands together at midline, and reach out to stroke a parent's face. These abilities are necessary for self-maintenance, self-enhancement, and self-advancement roles in childhood and throughout adulthood.

ROLE OF SENSATION IN OCCUPATIONAL FUNCTIONING

The role of sensation in occupational functioning is dramatically described in Cole's (1991) account of Ian Waterman, who at 19 years of age acquired a rare neurological illness that resulted in the loss of all sensation of touch in his body from the neck down. He had no awareness of the positions of his arms, legs, or body. Although his muscles were not affected, any attempt at movement was wildly uncontrolled. Ian's initial attempt at standing up resulted in him falling "in a heap . . . like a pile of wet clothes" (Cole, 1991, p. 11). He was unable to feed himself, get dressed, or do any functional activity requiring control of movement. Over several years, Waterman learned how to complete functional activities by substituting vision for his lost sensation. Every movement had to be carefully watched and consciously controlled. The high level of concentration required and the energy expended to complete daily self-care and work activities led Cole to name the account of Waterman's life, *Pride and a Daily Marathon*.

Although a loss of sensation like Waterman's without any motor loss is unusual, it exemplifies the close connection between the motor and sensory systems. With sensory loss in the hand, fine motor coordination is impaired, and manipulative ability is decreased (Chapman, Tremblay, & Ageranioti-Belanger, 1996; Jones, 1996). The amount of force needed to maintain grasp on an object also depends on sensory feedback. Usually, we use force that is just sufficient to overcome the pull of gravity, taking into account the amount of friction afforded by the surface texture. Without adequate tactile sensation, the force used to grip an object is either lower or higher than the force needed, resulting in objects slipping from grasp, delicate objects (such as a plastic foam cup) being crushed by excessive grip force, or muscles developing fatigue from overactivity (Johansson, 1996).

Some activities require sensory feedback because they are totally dependent on the sense of touch, such as determining the temperature of a bowl taken from the microwave. Tactile sensations let us know whether the food is warm and whether the bowl is too hot to carry to the table. Finding coins or other objects in a pocket and fastening a necklace or closing a back zipper are examples of activities for which vision is not used; therefore, we rely entirely upon sensory feedback. It is the tactile sense that tells us when our new shoes are a bit too tight and we had better remove them or we will get a blister. Impairment in the somatosensory system not only hinders movement but also increases the risk of injury.

PURPOSES OF SENSORY EVALUATION

The purposes of sensory testing, as defined by Cooke (1991), are as follows:

- Assess the type and extent of sensory loss.
- Evaluate and document sensory recovery.
- Assist in diagnosis.
- Determine impairment and functional limitation.
- Provide direction for occupational therapy intervention.
  - Determine time to begin sensory reeducation.
  - Determine need for education to prevent injury during occupational functioning.
  - Determine need for desensitization.

Before considering sensory evaluation, therapists need a good understanding of the neural structures responsible for tactile sensation.

NEUROPHYSIOLOGICAL FOUNDATIONS OF TACTILE SENSATION

Receptors for tactile sensation are present within skin, muscles, and joints. Each tactile receptor is usually specialized for a single type of sensory stimulation such as touch, temperature, or pain (Fredericks, 1996a). The types of sensation, specific kinds of receptors, and corresponding neurons that connect the sensory receptors with the spinal cord and ultimately with the cerebral cortex appear in Table 7-1. Neural impulses follow the described pathways to the brain, where the sensations are perceived and interpreted.

Each sensory neuron and its distal and proximal terminations can be considered a sensory unit. Each sensory unit has an area of skin that encompasses its defined receptive field. A stimulus anywhere in the field may evoke a response, but stimuli applied to the center of the receptive field produce sensations more easily. In other words, the center of a receptive field has a lower threshold than the periphery. Adjacent receptive fields overlap; therefore, a single stimulus evokes a profile of responses from overlapping sensory units.

The variation in the number of sensory units in a given area of skin is called innervation density. The face, hand, and fingers have high innervation densities. Areas with high innervation density are highly sensitive and have a proportionately large representation area within the somatosensory area of the cortex, the postcentral gyrus of the parietal lobe (Fredericks, 1996a). Figure 7-1 shows the organization within the cortex of sensory receptors from various regions of the body.

Table 7-1 and the description of sensory pathways simplify a complex process. For example, tactile stimuli of sufficient strength elicit responses from both constant and moving touch receptors and perhaps also from the pain receptors (Fredericks, 1996a). Extremes of hot and cold stimuli activate the pain receptors rather than the temperature receptors (Lindblom, 1994). Perception of joint motion (**kinesthesia**) and joint position (**proprioception**) appear to be a result of information from multiple kinds of receptors. Researchers disagree about the relative contributions of joint, muscle, and skin receptors to proprioception and kinesthesia (Fredericks, 1996a; Jones, 1996).

RESOURCE 7-1

Sensory Evaluation Instrument Suppliers

AliMed (monofilaments)
297 High Street
Dedham, MA 02026
Phone: (800) 225-2610
www.alimed.com

Biomedical Instrument Co. (Biothesiometer **vibrometer**)
15764 Munn Road
Newbury, OH 44065
Phone: (216) 543-9443

Lafayette Instrument Company (Disk-Criminator, **aesthesiometer**, picking-up test)
P.O. Box 5729
Lafayette, IN 47903
Phone: (800) 428-7545
Fax: (765) 423-4111
www.lafayetteinstrument.com

NK Biotechnical Corporation (pressure-specified sensory device)
10850 Old County Road 15
Minneapolis MN 55441
Phone: (800) 462-3751
Fax: (763) 541-0868
www.nkb.com

North Coast Medical (monofilaments, Disk-Criminator, aesthesiometer, testing shield)
18305 Sutter Boulevard
Morgan Hill, CA 95037-2845
Phone (800) 821-9319
Fax: (877) 213-9300
www.ncmedical.com

Sammons Preston Rolyan (monofilaments, Disk-Criminator, aesthesiometer, tuning forks, picking-up test, hot and cold probes, testing shield)
270 Remington Blvd, Suite C
Bolingbrook, IL 60440-3593
Phone: (800) 323-5547
Fax: (800) 547-4333
www.sammonspreston.com

Sensortek, Inc. (Vibratorn II)
2528 Vassar Place
Costa Mesa, CA 92626
Phone: (714) 444-2276
Fax: (714) 444-2278
www.easitek.com

WR Medical Electronics Co. (Case IV System)
123 North Second Street
Stillwater, MN 55082
Phone: (651) 430-1200
Fax: (651) 439-9733
www.wrmed.com

Ztech, L.C. (Automated Tactile Tester)
P.O. Box 581215
Salt Lake City, UT 84148
Phone: (801) 581-5928

Table 7-1. Neural Pathways of Sensory Stimuli

Type of Sensation	Sensory Receptor	Type of Afferent Neuron	Pathway	Termination of Pathway
Constant touch or pressure Moving touch or vibration	Merkel's cell Ruffini's end organ Meissner's corpuscles Pacinian corpuscles Hair follicles	Type A-beta slowly adapting I and II myelinated neurons Type A-beta rapidly adapting I and II myelinated neurons	Ascend in dorsal column and medial lemniscus of spinal cord in posterior pyramidal tract, cross to opposite side in medulla	Thalamus and somatosensory cortex
Proprioception and kinesthesia	Same as both moving and constant touch or vibration plus touch receptors found in skin and joint structures Muscle spindles Golgi tendon organs	Same as for moving touch or vibration plus A-alpha myelinated neurons	Same as for moving touch or vibration plus spinocerebellar tract	Same as for moving touch or vibration plus cerebellum
Pain (pinprick) Pain (chronic) Temperature	Free nerve endings Free nerve endings Free nerve endings Warm receptors Cold receptors	Type A-delta myelinated neurons Type C unmyelinated fibers Type A-delta myelinated neurons and type C unmyelinated fibers	Immediately cross to opposite side and pass upward in anterior spinothalamic tracts of spinal cord	Brainstem, thalamus, and somatosensory cortex

Based on information in Dellon, A. L. (1997). *Somatosensory testing and rehabilitation.* Bethesda, MD: American Occupational Therapy Association; Chapman, C. E., Tremblay, F., & Ageranioti-Bélanger, A. (1996). Role of primary somatosensory cortex in active and passive touch. In A. M. Wing, P. Haggard, & J. R. Flanagan (Eds.), *Hand and brain: The neurophysiology of hand movements* (pp. 329–347). San Diego: Academic; Fredericks, C. M. (1996). Basic sensory mechanisms and the somatosensory system. In C. M. Fredericks & L. K. Saladin (Eds.), *Pathophysiology of the motor systems: Principles and clinical presentations* (pp. 78–106). Philadelphia: Davis; and Fredericks, C. M. (1996). Disorders of the spinal cord. In C. M. Fredericks & L. K. Saladin (Eds.), *Pathophysiology of the motor systems: Principles and clinical presentations* (pp. 394–423). Philadelphia: Davis.

Therapists use a solid understanding of the neurophysiology of the tactile system to choose evaluation and treatment techniques for sensory deficits. They combine this understanding with knowledge of typical patterns of impairment from injury and illness prior to implementing assessment of sensation.

SOMATOSENSORY DEFICIT PATTERNS

Any interruption along the ascending sensory pathway or in the sensory areas of the cortex can lead to a decrease or loss of sensation. The extent and severity of the sensory deficit can generally be predicted in accordance with the mechanism and location of the lesion or injury. Patterns of sensory impairment are directly related to the involved neuroanatomical structures, which could be anywhere in the central or peripheral nervous system.

Cortical Injury

Patients with brain lesions caused by cerebrovascular accident (CVA) or head trauma demonstrate sensory losses related to loss of functioning of specific neurons within the central nervous system. Approximately 60% of patients with stroke in the carotid artery system, which includes the anterior and middle cerebral arteries, have sensory deficits (Garrison et al., 1988). Effects of CVA on sensation depend on specific disruption of blood supply. For instance, occlusion of the middle cerebral artery (the most common site of CVA) is often associated with contralateral impairment of all sensory modalities on the face, arm, and leg. Occlusion of the anterior cerebral artery tends to cause more loss of sensation in the contralateral leg than in the arm because of this artery's supply to the medial aspect of the cerebral cortex (Fig. 7-1) (Saladin, 1996a). Patterns of sensory loss following head trauma are less predictable because of the more diffuse areas of brain damage associated with this condition (Saladin, 1996b). For patients with either CVA or head injury, perception of fine touch and proprioception are most affected, temperature sensation is affected less, and pain sensibility is affected least (Fredericks, 1996a).

Sterzi et al. (1993) compared patients with left and right CVA and found that loss of proprioception and pain perception were more common following right CVA than left CVA. Left neglect, an inability to recognize and use perceptions from the left side of the body and environment, was proposed as a factor underlying this difference. The study of Beschin et al. (1996) provides evidence to support the existence of tactile neglect; patients with right

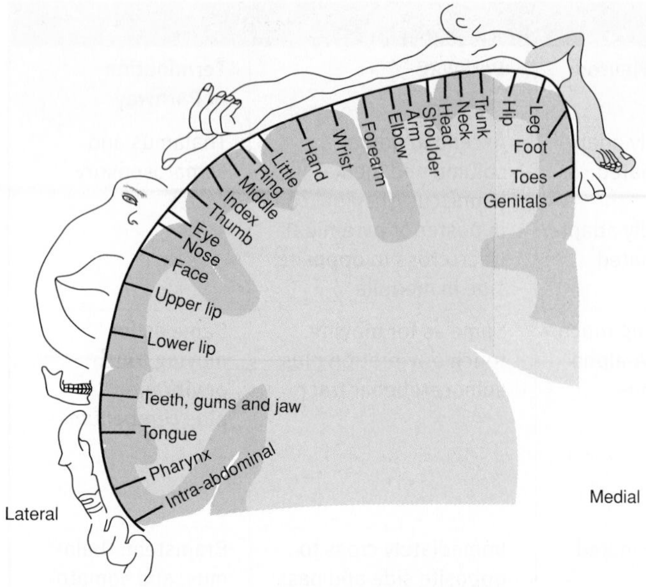

Figure 7-1 The areas responsible for sensation of body parts within the postcentral gyrus of the cerebral cortex. (Reprinted with permission from Kingsley, R. E. [1996]. *Concise text of neuroscience* [p. 185]. Baltimore: Williams & Wilkins.)

brain damage tend to ignore left space during active tactile exploration.

Partial recovery of sensation following cortical injury is attributed to decreased edema, improved vascular flow, cortical plasticity (adaptability of neurons to assume new functions), and relearning (Carr & Shepherd, 1998). Recovery of pain and temperature perception usually precedes recovery of proprioception and light touch (Fredericks, 1996a).

Use the following guidelines in planning assessments for patients with cortical injury:

- Quickly screen those areas of the body where sensation is likely to be intact, followed by a more thorough evaluation only if a deficit is found during screening.
- Assess more thoroughly those areas most likely to be affected, usually the side contralateral to the injury.
- If fine touch and proprioception are intact, assessment of temperature and pain is not necessary, as these protective sensations will also be intact. For patients with mild cortical impairment, begin the sensory assessment with light touch and/or proprioception.
- If pain and temperature are absent, assessment of light touch and proprioception is not necessary as these will also be absent. For patients with severe cortical impairment, begin with assessment of pain and temperature for greatest efficiency.
- Use the recovery sequence of pain and temperature before light touch and proprioception during reassessment to document recovery.

Spinal Cord Injury

Patients with complete lesions of the spinal cord demonstrate a total absence of sensation in the dermatomes (Fig. 7-2) below the level of the lesion. The level of the lesion determines the extent of the sensory loss, with the greatest loss occurring in patients with the lesions in the highest cervical regions of the spinal cord. **Paresthesia** (tingling or pins and needles sensation) may occur in the dermatome associated with the level of the lesion (Fredericks, 1996c).

Incomplete spinal cord lesions result in sensory losses that are related to damage within specific spinal tracts. For instance, damage to the anterior part of the spinal cord usually results in loss of pain and temperature sensation below the level of the lesion, whereas touch, vibration, and proprioception remain intact. Conversely, patients who have damaged the posterior portion of the spinal cord cannot feel light touch and vibration but can feel differences in temperature and painful stimuli. Patients with damage to one side of the spinal cord (Brown Sequard syndrome) display loss of touch, vibration, and proprioception on the side of the lesion and loss of temperature and pain sensation on the side opposite the lesion. This occurs because of the differences in the pathways of the ascending sensory fibers; neurons carrying temperature and pain sensations cross to the opposite side of the spinal cord immediately after entering it, whereas neurons carrying touch sensations ascend to the medulla before crossing to the opposite side (Fredericks, 1996c). Damage to the central spinal cord often results in bilateral loss of pain and temperature sensation below the level of the lesion because the neurons cross to the opposite side through the central portion of the cord. Mild to moderate compression of the spinal cord may result in decreased or absent sensation in the single dermatome at the level of the compression or could also involve dermatomes below the compressed area (Fredericks, 1996c).

Any sensory recovery following traumatic spinal cord injury usually occurs within the first year, with the greatest recovery in the first 6 months (Waters et al., 1993). Recovery of sensation is thought to occur because of resolution of ischemia and edema within the spinal cord.

Use the following guidelines in planning assessments for patients with spinal cord injury:

- Use a test with a strong stimulus (pinprick, cotton ball) to determine level of injury.
- The American Spinal Injury Association recommends key sensory points within each dermatome to utilize when assessing injury level. See Chapter 43 for further details.
- Bilateral testing is necessary following spinal cord injury because results may differ from side to side.
- For patients with known complete lesions, there is no need to test multiple sensory modalities.

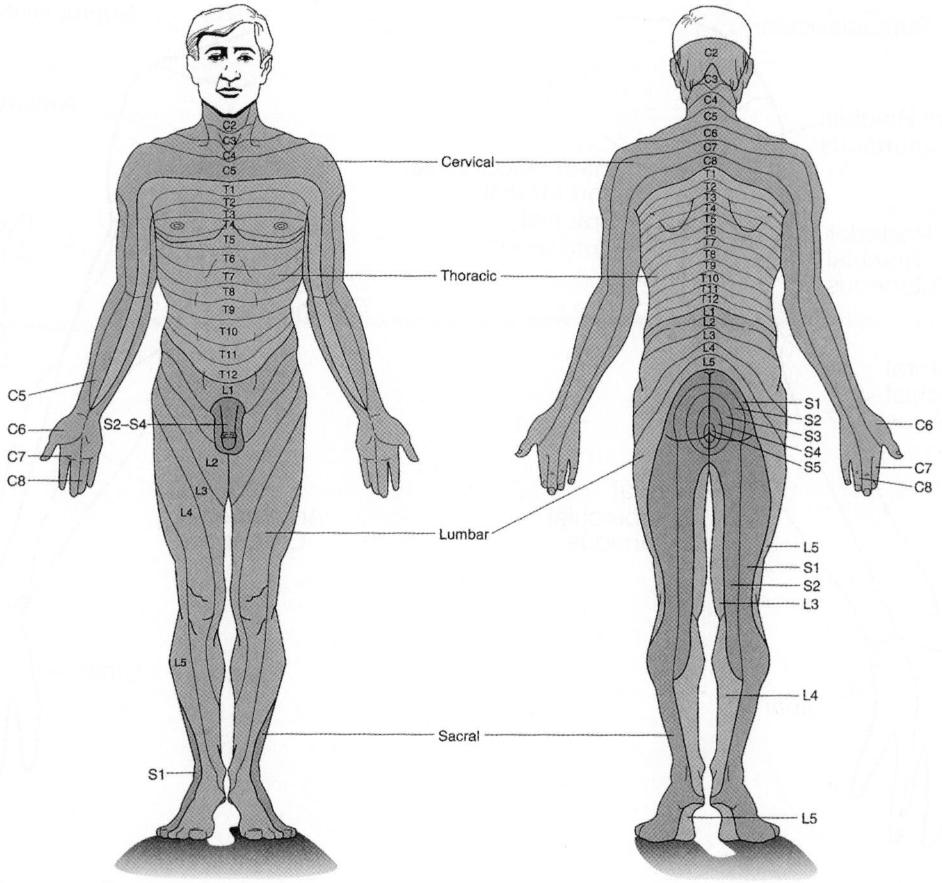

Figure 7-2 Typical dermatome distribution. (Reprinted with permission from Bear, M. F., Connors, B. W., & Paradiso, M. A. [1996]. *Neuroscience: Exploring the brain* [p. 322]. Baltimore: Williams & Wilkins.)

- For patients with incomplete or unknown lesions, test for multiple sensory modalities, including at least one pain or temperature assessment and at least one measure of touch, vibration, or proprioception.

Peripheral Nerve Injury

Patterns of sensory loss following peripheral nerve injury vary with the nerve or nerves involved. Damage to a single nerve root as it exits the spinal cord affects sensation on one side of the body within a single dermatome (Fig. 7-2). Damage to a peripheral nerve distal to the brachial plexus affects sensation within the appropriate peripheral nerve distribution (Fig. 7-3) (Adams, Victor, & Ropper, 1997). For instance, in carpal tunnel syndrome, compression of the median nerve at the wrist produces sensory symptoms in the thumb, index, middle, and half of the ring finger on the affected side. For information about the typical patterns of sensory loss related to lesions of the trunks and cords of the brachial plexus, Callahan's chapter in *Rehabilitation of the Hand and Upper Extremity* (2002) is an excellent reference.

The severity of the sensory loss can vary widely. A complete transection of a peripheral nerve results in a total loss of tactile sensation within the region. A mild nerve compression, such as in early stages of carpal tunnel syndrome, produces a slightly elevated threshold for sensing light touch or vibration. As the compression persists or increases in severity, further loss of sensation will occur, the threshold of light touch sensation will be higher, and the patient will begin to report symptoms such as frequently dropping items from the hand. Eventually, if the compression is not relieved, numbness and loss of protective sensation will develop.

Recovery of sensation following release of a nerve from compression is very likely if the compression was brief and mild. Significant recovery following prolonged compression is common, but sensory perception does not always reach normal levels. Recovery of sensation following total transection of a nerve is possible only with surgical intervention and adequate regrowth of neurons (Smith, 1995). Sensation of temperature and pain generally (but not always) recovers first, followed by touch sensation, because regrowth of pain fibers averages 1.08 mm per day, and regrowth of touch fibers averages 0.78 mm per day (Waylett-Rendall, 1988). Moving touch recovers before light touch. Accurate touch localization recovers last (Callahan, 2002).

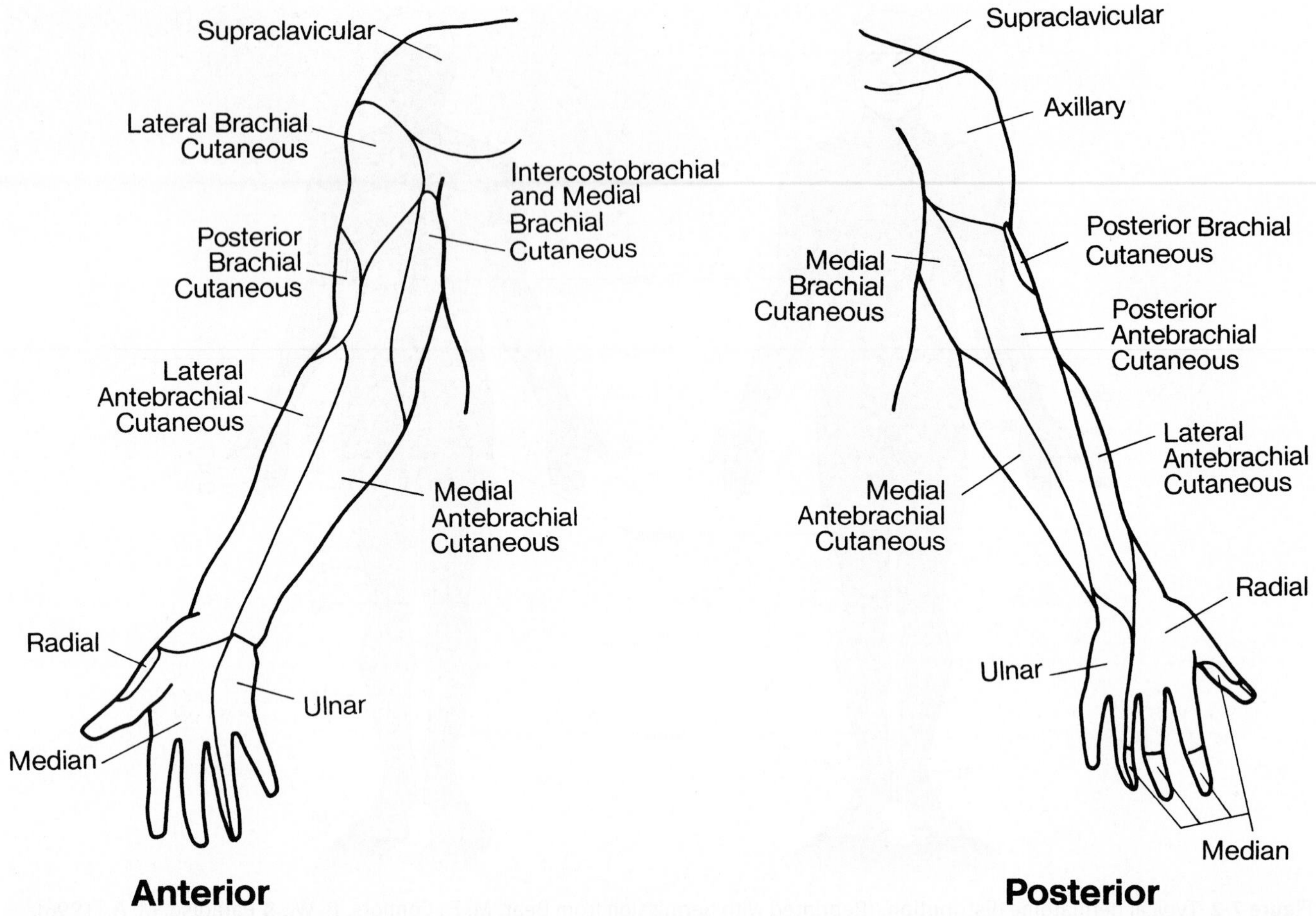

Figure 7-3 Typical sensory distribution of peripheral nerves within the upper extremity. (Reprinted with permission from Sieg, K. W., & Adams, S. R. [1996]. *Illustrated essentials of musculoskeletal anatomy* [3rd ed., p. 79.]. Gainesville, FL: Megabooks.)

The pattern of sensory loss occurring as a result of peripheral polyneuropathies, which are associated with chronic conditions such as diabetes mellitus and alcoholism, is typically bilateral and symmetrical, usually beginning in the feet and hands (glove-and-stocking distribution) and spreading proximally. Paresthesia and pain may accompany peripheral neuropathy. Because of the chronic conditions associated with peripheral neuropathy, recovery of sensation is generally not expected (Fredericks, 1996b).

Use the following guidelines in planning assessments for patients with peripheral nerve injury:

- The purpose of evaluation in clients with peripheral polyneuropathy is to establish the impact of disease on protective sensation, so choose an assessment of protective sensation.
- The desired outcome of sensory evaluation in clients with involvement of a single peripheral nerve is an accurate map of both the body area and severity of sensory loss.
- Evaluation of nerve compression and subsequent recovery requires measures that are highly sensitive to show small changes in sensory function.
- Because functional tests of sensation requiring object or texture identification are completed with the thumb, index, and middle fingers, these assessments provide information about the functioning of the C6, C7, and C8 nerve roots and the median nerve.
- In documenting recovery of peripheral nerve function, keep in mind the recovery sequence of pain → moving touch → light touch → touch localization.

EVALUATION TECHNIQUES

There are numerous methods of testing sensation. Some are intended to evaluate a specific type of sensory receptor, such as the test for vibration awareness using a tuning fork that is believed to be specific to the Meissner's and Pacinian corpuscles (Dellon, 1997). Some are intended to evaluate the use of sensation in skills that support occupational functioning, such as the use of the hand to identify objects by touch in the test of **stereognosis**. Some are designed to detect very small changes in sensory perception, such as the touch threshold test using **monofilaments** (fine nylon strands).

The principles of sensory testing optimize the reliability of the testing results. These are listed in Procedures for Practice 7-1. The purpose of these principles is to eliminate non-tactile cues and to ensure that the responses from the patient accurately reflect actual sensation. Because many of the tests require subjective reports from the patient, results can be either deliberately or unconsciously manipulated by the patient to make the deficit appear better or worse. Careful attention to test administration and patient responses can minimize the possibility of testing manipulation by patients. For cases where the patient's responses are questionable and a determination of testing manipulation must be made, therapists may use a forced-choice testing methodology and statistical analysis described by Greve, Bianchini, and Ameduri (2003) in

PROCEDURES FOR PRACTICE 7-1

Principles of Sensory Testing

- Choose an environment with minimal distractions.
- Ensure that the patient is comfortable and relaxed.
- Ensure that the patient can understand and produce spoken language. If the patient cannot, modify testing procedures to ensure reliable communication.
- Determine areas of the body to be tested.
- Stabilize the limb or body part being tested (Fig. 7-4).
- Note any differences in skin thickness, calluses, and so on. Expect sensation to be decreased in these areas.
- State the instructions for the test.
- Demonstrate the test stimulus on an area of skin with intact sensation while the patient observes.
- Ensure that the patient understands the instructions by eliciting the correct response to the demonstration.
- Occlude the patient's vision for administration of the test. Place a screen (Fig. 7-5) or a file folder between the patient's face and the area being tested, blindfold the patient, or ask the patient to close his or her eyes.
- Apply stimuli at irregular intervals or insert catch trials in which no stimulus is given.
- Avoid giving inadvertent cues, such as auditory cues or facial expressions, during stimulus application.
- Carefully observe the correctness, confidence, and promptness of the responses.
- Observe the patient for any discomfort relating to the stimuli that may signal **hypersensitivity** (exaggerated or unpleasant sensation).
- Ensure that the therapist who does the initial testing does any reassessment.

Adapted from: Brand & Hollister, 1993; Callahan, 2002; Reese, 1999.

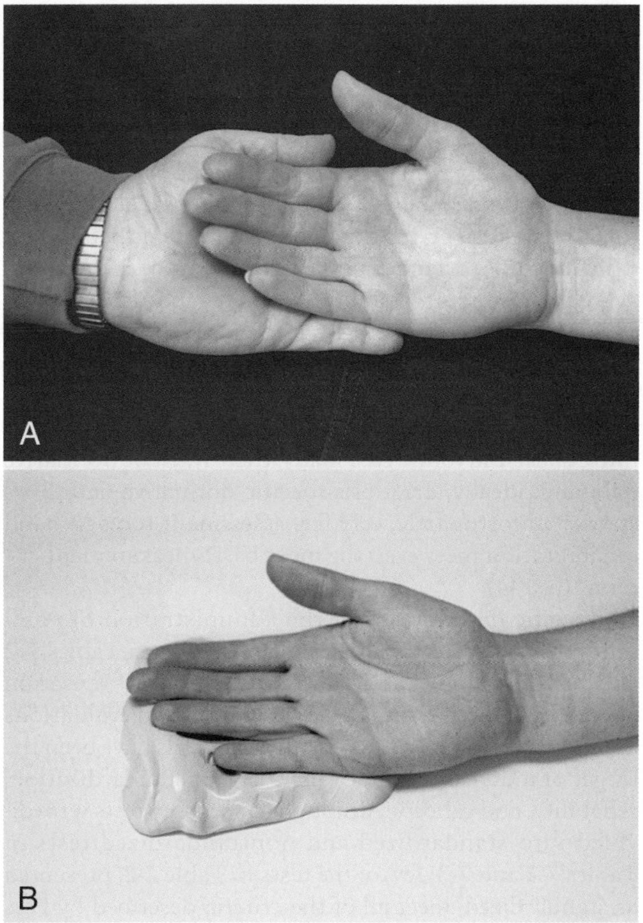

Figure 7-4 Hand support during testing. **A.** Fingers must be carefully stabilized and supported during testing so that motion is prevented, avoiding inadvertent cues to the patient. **B.** A cushion of therapy putty can be used to provide the stabilization.

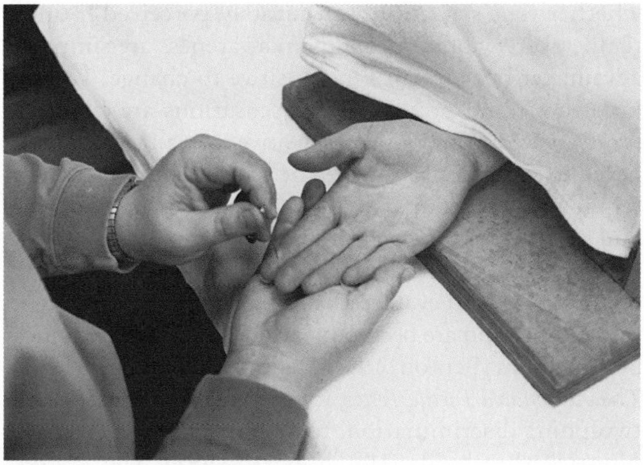

Figure 7-5 Vision must be occluded during testing. Using a screen such as this is usually more comfortable for patients than closing their eyes or being blindfolded.

which patients are required to identify whether they are touched with one finger or two. A statistically low percentage correct suggests an invalid response, since someone without sensation who merely guessed would be likely to get approximately 50% correct.

Fess (1995), in her article "Guidelines for Evaluating Assessment Instruments," describes four essential criteria for all assessment instruments. The first is reliability, which includes accuracy of the instrument measurements as well as test–retest stability and inter-rater repeatability. Second, she describes validity as the tool's ability to measure the sensory modality for which it was designed. Third, standards for the manufacture, administration, and scoring of the assessment and interpretation of the results must be set and followed. Finally, there must be normative data and, ideally, diagnosis-specific normative data. Fess states, "unfortunately, very few assessment tools in hand rehabilitation meet even the most basic measurement criteria" (p. 144).

Specific descriptions of the administration of commonly used sensory evaluations are shown in Tables 7-2 and 7-3. The more standardized evaluations of sensation appear in Table 7-2, and the less standardized evaluations are shown in Table 7-3. Sensory testing tools have been the target of much criticism for their lack of standardization, reliability, and validity. Although the sensory tests were divided into standardized and nonstandardized tests in Tables 7-2 and 7-3, few of the tests in Table 7-2, presented as standardized, meet all of the criteria described by Fess (1995).

Therapists must consider various qualities of the types of sensory tests as they choose and administer them. Threshold tests determine the smallest stimuli that can be noticed by the patient. They are the most sensitive and have numeric results that can easily be compared over time. Two-point discrimination measures innervation density in the fingers and is quite sensitive to change. Touch localization evaluates not only sensation but also whether that sensation is accurately perceived. Touch, temperature, vibration, and pain awareness are simple to administer but are not very sensitive to change. Tests of kinesthetic and proprioceptive sensations are less commonly used and are not very sensitive to change but are believed to be related to the specific type of sensory feedback required for coordinated movement. The picking-up test and stereognosis test are more functional but require combined motor and sensory function in the hand.

Computerized evaluations of sensation are often used for research and are becoming available in a limited number of clinics (Benton, 1994; Dellon, 1997; Riggle, 1999). The *Automated Tactile Tester*, for instance, measures touch, two-point discrimination, temperature, vibration, and pinprick thresholds (Horch et al., 1992). The *Pressure Specified Sensory Device* measures pressure threshold for one-point and two-point discrimination (Dellon, 1997).

Although sensory tests are usually administered with the patient rested and in a comfortable, supported position, exceptions to this principle occur in the case of patients with peripheral nerve compression. Provocative testing, which determines whether increases in symptoms occur as a result of additional stress or compression on the peripheral nerve, is completed. Increased sensory loss in the median nerve distribution with the wrist in flexion implicates compression of that nerve in the carpal tunnel area. Elbow flexion is the stress position for suspected cubital tunnel syndrome, which is compression of the ulnar nerve in the elbow area. Manual pressure over the nerve can be combined with the provocative position to further increase stress on the nerve (Callahan, 2002; Novak & Mackinnnon, 2005; Szabo et al., 1999).

Recording Assessment Results

Documentation should include the type of test, the skin area tested, and the response. One easy way to document touch threshold testing with monofilaments is to use a color code on a drawing of the body part (Fig. 7-9). Standard colors used to document results for the Semmes Weinstein Monofilaments and Weinstein Enhanced Sensory Test (WEST) are indicated in Table 7-4. A series of sensory maps can easily and quickly demonstrate sensory recovery.

For standardized tests, results can be compared with norms; however, age should be taken into account because studies show a decline in sensation with age (Desrosiers et al., 1996). Normative monofilament expectations for adults over age 60 are shown in Table 7-5. For both standardized and nonstandardized tests, results from the affected area of the patient can be compared with results from an unaffected area.

Sensory evaluation findings are often summarized as absent, intact, or impaired. *Absent* describes a total loss of sensation or inability to detect a specific sensory modality. *Intact* describes normal sensation. Sensation is *impaired* when the patient is able to detect some but not all of the stimuli or when the perception of the stimulus is different from that of an area of skin that has intact sensation.

Interpretation of Evaluation Findings and Treatment Planning

In analyzing sensory evaluation findings, compare the results with those expected based upon the patient's diagnosis. If the results differ from what was expected, further testing might be recommended. Individual sensory distributions sometimes vary from the illustrations of typical sensory distributions included in this and other texts. Furthermore, although there are clear lines of demarcation on the illustrations, humans generally have some overlapping

Table 7-2. Standardized Sensory Testing Techniques

Sensory Test	Test Instrument	Stimulus (S) and Response (R)	Scoring and Expected Results
Touch Threshold Measures threshold of light touch sensation (Bell-Krotoski, 1995; Tomancik, 1987; Weinstein, Drozdenko, & Weinstein, 1997)	Semmes-Weinstein monofilaments OR Weinstein Enhanced Sensory Test (WEST)	Semmes-Weinstein S: Begin testing with filament marked 2.83; hold filament perpendicular to skin, apply to skin until filament bends (Fig. 7-6). Apply in 1.5 seconds, hold 1.5 seconds, and remove in 1.5 seconds. Repeat three times at each testing site, using thicker filaments if the patient does not perceive thin ones (except for filaments marked >4.08, which are applied one time to each site). R: Patient says yes upon feeling the stimulus. WEST S: Patient is prompted to stimulus, then filament is slowly applied perpendicular to skin and held for 1 second, then slowly lifted. Catch trials consisting of prompt without filament application are randomly inserted within test sequence. R: Patient responds with yes or no to indicate whether stimulus was felt.	Semmes-Weinstein Score is either the marking number or the actual force of the thinnest filament detected at least once in three trials; results are usually recorded according to a standard color code using colored pencils or markers and a diagram of the hand (Table 7-5 and Fig. 7-9). Normal touch threshold for adults is perception of the filament marked 2.83 (force 0.08 g) except for the sole of the foot, where the normal threshold is the filament marked 3.61 (force 0.21 g). WEST Results are recorded according to the color of the filament. Normal touch threshold is perception of the thinnest monofilament. There are two WEST devices, one for the hand and another for the foot.
Static Two-Point Discrimination Measures innervation density of slowly adapting fibers of the hand (Callahan, 2002; Dellon, 1997)	Disk-Criminator OR aesthesiometer (Fig. 7-7)	Static Two-Point Discrimination S: Begin with a 5-mm separation of points. Lightly (just to the point of blanching) apply one or two points (randomly sequenced) in a transverse or longitudinal orientation on the hand; hold for at least 3 seconds or until patient responds. Gradually adjust distance of separation to find least distance that patient can correctly perceive. R: Patient responds by saying 1, 2, or I can't tell.	Score is smallest distance at which perception of one or two points is better than chance. When the patient's responses become hesitant or inaccurate, require 2 of 3, 4 of 7, or 7 of 10 correct responses. Static Two-Point Discrimination Norms 3–5 mm in fingertips ages 18–70 (Bell-Krotoski, 1997) 5–6 mm in fingertips ages 70 and above (Desrosiers et al., 1996) 5–9 mm for middle and proximal phalanges in adults ages 18–60; 0–12 mm for middle and proximal phalanges in adults ages 60 and above (Shimokata & Kuzuya, 1995)

continued

Table 7-2. Standardized Sensory Testing Techniques *(continued)*

Sensory Test	Test Instrument	Stimulus (S) and Response (R)	Scoring and Expected Results
Moving Two-Point Discrimination Measures innervation density of quickly adapting fibers of fingertips (Callahan, 2002; Dellon, 1988, 1997)		Moving Two-Point Discrimination S: Beginning with a 5–8 mm distance, move one or two points randomly from proximal to distal on the distal phalanx with points side by side and parallel to the long axis of the finger; use just enough pressure for the patient to appreciate the stimulus. Gradually adjust distance of separation to find least distance that patient can correctly perceive. R: Patient responds by saying 1, 2, or I can't tell.	Moving Two-Point Discrimination Norms 2–4 mm for ages 4–60 (Dellon, 1997; Hermann, Novak, & Mackinnon, 1995) 4–6 mm for ages 60 and above (Dellon, 1997; Desrosiers et al., 1996)
Touch Localization Measures spatial representation of touch receptors in the cortex (Nakada, 1993)	Semmes-Weinstein Monofilament number 4.17 or pen, pencil eraser	S: Apply touch to patient's skin. R: Patient remembers location of stimulus. With vision no longer occluded, patient uses index finger or marking pen to point to spot just touched.	Score is the measured distance in millimeters between location of stimulus and location of response. Normal response is approximately 3–4 mm in digit tips, 7–10 mm in palm of hand, and 15–18 mm in forearm (Schady, 1994; Sieg & Williams, 1986).
Vibration Threshold Measures threshold of rapidly adapting fibers (Callahan, 2002; Dellon, 1997; Horch et al., 1992)	Vibrometer, Biothesiometer, Vibratron II, Automated Tactile Tester, Case IV System	Protocols vary with instrument. S: Generally, vibrating head is applied to area to be tested. Stimulus intensity is gradually increased or decreased. R: Patient indicates when vibration is first felt or no longer felt.	Scoring varies with instrument; norms usually provided by manufacturer.
Modified Picking Up Test (Dellon) Dellon's modification of Moberg's picking-up test measures the interpretation of sensation in the distribution of the median nerve (Dellon, 1988)	A small box and 12 standard metal objects: wing nut, screw, key, nail, large nut, nickel, dime, washer, safety pin, paper clip, small hex nut, and small square nut	Part 1 S: Tape small and ring digits to palm to prevent use. With patient using vision, have him or her pick up and place objects in a box as quickly as possible; time performance on two trials. R: Patient picks up each object and deposits it in the box as quickly as possible. Part 2 S: With patient's vision occluded, place one object at a time between three-point pinch in random order and measure speed of response. R: Patient manipulates object and names it as rapidly as possible.	Part 1 Score is total time to pick up and place all 12 objects in the box for each of 2 trials. Normal response: Trial 1, 10–19 seconds Trial 2, 9–16 seconds Part 2 Score is time to recognize each object on each of two trials (up to a maximum of 30 seconds). Normal response: 2 seconds per object

Table 7-3. Nonstandardized Sensory Testing Techniques

Sensory Test	Test Instruments	Stimulus (S) and Response (R)	Scoring and Expected Results
Touch Awareness General awareness of touch input (Adams, Victor, & Ropper, 1997)	Cotton ball or swab, fingertip, pencil eraser	S: Light touch to a small area of the patient's skin. R: Patient says yes or makes agreed-upon nonverbal signal each time stimulus is felt.	Score is number of correct responses in relation to number of applied stimuli. Expected score is 100%.
Pinprick or Pain Awareness Measures discrimination of sharp and dull stimuli, which indicates protective sensation (Brand & Hollister, 1993; Reese, 1999)	New or sterilized safety pin	S: Randomly apply sharp and blunt ends of safety pin, perpendicular to skin, at pressure necessary to elicit correct response on uninvolved side of body. R: Patient says "sharp" or "dull" after each stimulus.	Score is number of correct responses divided by number of stimuli. Expected score is 100%. Correct responses to sharp stimuli indicate intact protective sensation; incorrect responses to sharp stimuli indicate some awareness of pressure but absent protective sensation.
Temperature Awareness (Fig. 7-8) Measures discrimination of warm and cool stimuli (Waylett-Rendall, 1988)	Hot and Cold Discrimination Kit or glass test tubes filled with warm and cool water	S: Apply cold (40°F) or warm (115–120°F) stimulus to patient's skin. R: Patient indicates hot or cold after each stimulus.	Score is number of correct responses divided by number of stimuli. Normal response is 100%.
Vibration Awareness Measures awareness of input to rapidly adapting A-beta fibers (Dellon, 1988)	Tuning forks: 30 cycles per second 256 cycles per second	S: Strike tuning fork with force to cause vibration; place prong tangentially to fingertip of injured and then uninjured hand; ask patient, "Does this feel the same or different?" R: Patient responds same or different and describes difference in perception.	Scoring is normal if stimuli to both hands feel the same or altered if stimuli feel different. The 30-cps tuning fork is used to test the Meissner afferents, and the 256-cps tuning fork is used to test the Pacinian afferents.
Stereognosis Measures the ability to identify objects, which requires interpretation of sensory input. Motor function is prerequisite. (Eggers, 1984)	A number of small objects known to the patient	S: Place a small object in the hand to be tested. R: Patient may manipulate object within the hand; patient names object.	Scoring is number of correct responses divided by total number of objects presented or time to identify each object. Normal response is correct identification of almost all objects within 2–3 seconds (Lederman & Klatzky, 1996).
Moberg's Picking-Up Test Measures the function of slowly adapting A-beta fibers in medial nerve injury (Callahan, 2002; Dellon, 1988)	An assortment of small objects and a small box	S: Instruct patient to pick up objects as rapidly as possible and place them in the box, using right and left hands, with and without vision. R: Patient quickly picks up objects and places them in box.	Scoring is total time to pick up objects. Compare scores of left and right hands and those with and without vision. Mean times for 12 standard objects were found by Ng, Ho, and Chow (1999) to be 10–12 seconds with vision and 20–23 seconds without vision.

continued

Table 7-3. Nonstandardized Sensory Testing Techniques *(continued)*

Sensory Test	Test Instruments	Stimulus (S) and Response (R)	Scoring and Expected Results
Proprioception Measures sense of joint position, which relies upon input from an unknown combination of muscle, joint, and skin receptors (Adams, Victor, & Ropper, 1997)	None	S: Hold body segment being tested on the lateral surfaces; move the part into different positions and hold. R: Patient duplicates position with opposite extremity.	Graded as intact, impaired, or absent. Usually, reproduction of position can be accomplished within a few degrees. One study of the knee joint found, on average, 4 degrees of error in subjects under age 30 and 7 degrees of error in subjects over age 60 (Kaplan et al., 1985).
Kinesthesia Measures sense of joint motion, which relies on input from an unknown combination of muscle, joint, and skin receptors (Adams, Victor, & Ropper, 1997)	None	S: Hold body segment being tested on the lateral surfaces; move the part through angles of varying degrees. R: Patient indicates whether part is moved up or down.	Graded as intact, impaired, or absent. Nearly 100% correct identification is expected.

areas of innervation along the borders of sensory receptive areas (Adams, Victor, & Ropper, 1997).

Consider whether the actual and expected results are different enough to suggest that there might be neural issues other than the diagnosis. If a peripheral nerve is compressed at one site, it is more sensitive to compression at other sites. Double and multiple neural compression sites can produce unexpected patterns of sensory impairment (Novak & Mackinnon, 2005).

Touch threshold testing with monofilaments can be interpreted based upon categories of sensory loss as indicated in Table 7-4. With decreased light touch, patients often do not realize that they have a loss of sensation. There is no effect on the motor use of the hand, and patients can identify temperatures, textures, and objects by touch. Diminished protective sensation results in decreased motor coordination, as evidenced by slower manipulation and dropping objects from grasp. Identification of temperatures and painful stimuli is intact. Loss of protective sensation causes an inability to use the hand when it is not in view. Patients will feel pinpricks and deep pressure but will be less able or unable to determine temperatures. Those patients who cannot feel the thickest monofilament may or may not be able to feel a pinprick but have no other feeling and require visual guidance for all hand function (Bell-Krotoski, 2002).

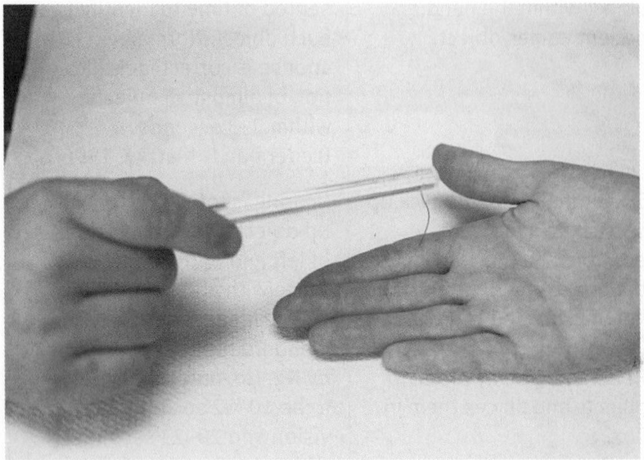

Figure 7-6 Testing of the median nerve distribution using Semmes-Weinstein monofilaments.

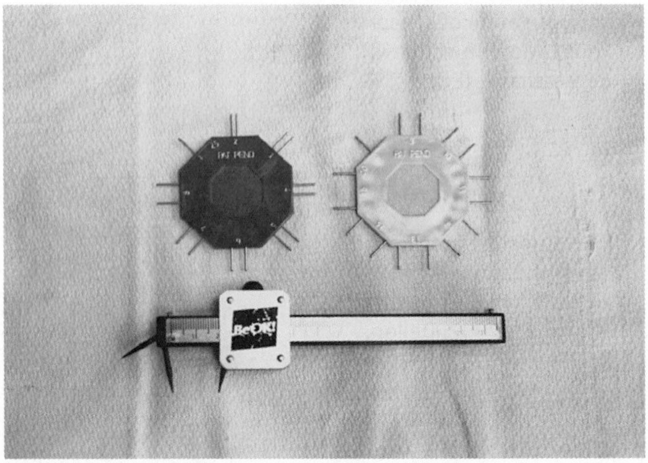

Figure 7-7 Tools used in two-point discrimination tests: a Disk-Criminator (*top*) and an aesthesiometer (*bottom*).

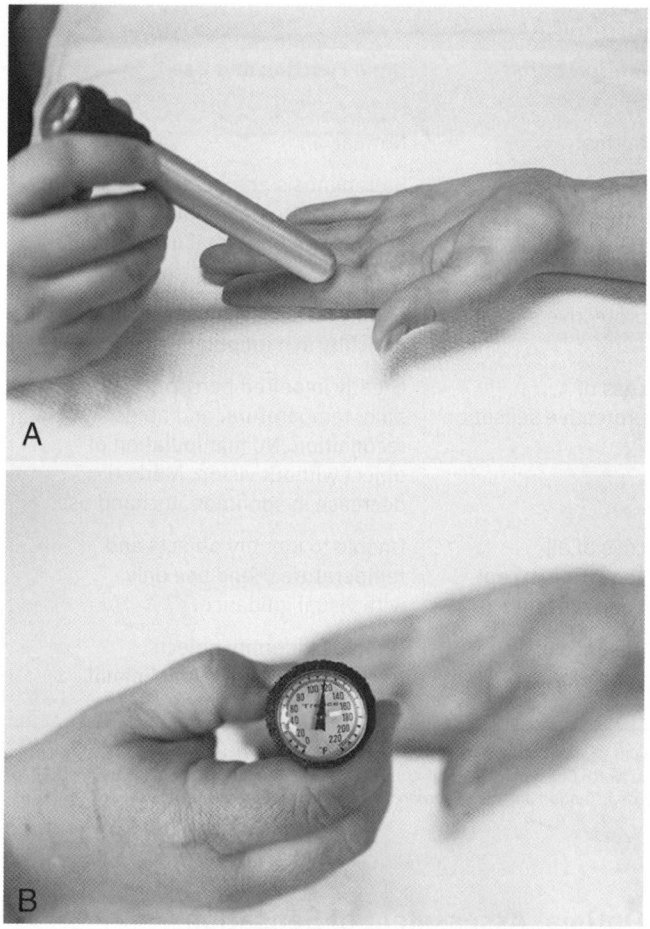

Figure 7-8 Temperature awareness testing. **A.** Metal probe is heated or cooled in water. **B.** The thermometer at the top helps to maintain consistency in testing.

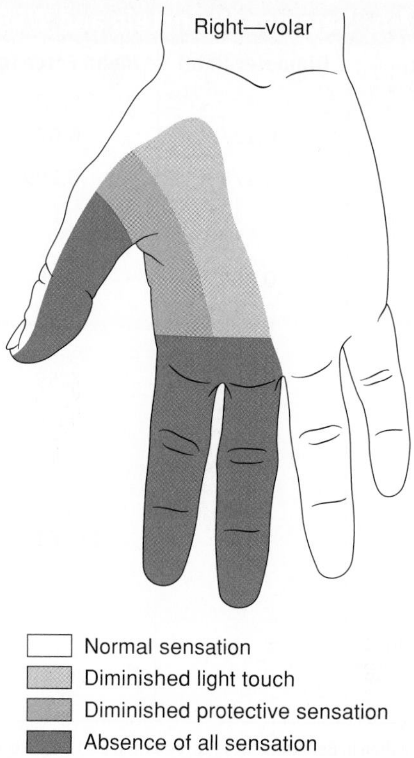

Figure 7-9 Results of monofilament testing for Mr. T. (see Case Example) 6 weeks following median nerve laceration and surgery.

In planning treatment, diminished or lost protective sensation or absence of sensation indicates that the patient is at risk for injury of the affected body part or parts. The patient must be taught to use vision and an adapted environment to compensate for lost sensation and avoid injury. Results that indicate impaired sensation need further investigation to determine the appropriate course of intervention. If there is hypersensitivity of the body part, a program of desensitization is indicated. If there is a decrease but not total loss of sensation within an area, the patient may be a candidate for sensory retraining, as long as the diagnostic prognosis indicates that there is a potential for improvement. Chapter 27 describes each of these interventions in detail.

CHOOSING EVALUATION METHODS

Therapists use clinical reasoning to select appropriate sensory evaluation techniques for each patient. Diagnostic and procedural reasoning suggest that certain tests are best at answering certain kinds of clinical questions. Ethical reasoning suggests that the tests should be the best available for each patient and that the practitioner has developed competence in test administration and interpretation. Pragmatic reasoning suggests that tests should be readily available and quickly administered (Schell, 1998).

Before choosing an evaluation method, decide why the test is necessary and what information is needed. Consider the diagnosis and the patient's description of the problem. For instance, for a patient with spinal cord injury, it is important to know whether sensation is present or absent in each region of skin. A touch awareness or pinprick test is common, with the results recorded on a drawing of the body (Waters et al., 1993).

If the purpose is to assist in the diagnosis of a nerve compression, such as carpal tunnel syndrome, it is necessary to use a highly sensitive test, such as a monofilament test. Sensation can be evaluated in positions that are likely to provoke more symptoms, for example with the wrist flexed (Szabo et al., 1999). A self-report of sensory loss has also been found useful in the diagnosis of carpal tunnel syndrome (Katz & Stirrat, 1990).

During observation of dressing or grooming by a patient with a diagnosis of CVA, a suspicion may arise that the observed errors are related to a loss of proprioception. An evaluation of proprioception can confirm or refute this hypothesis. For this same patient, it is important to know

Table 7-4. Semmes-Weinstein and WEST Hand Monofilaments

Filament Number	Diameter (mm)	Mean Force (g)	Color Code	Interpretation	Hand Function and Use
2.83	0.127	0.076	Green	Normal	Normal
3.61	0.178	0.209	Blue	Diminished light touch	Stereognosis and perception of temperature and pain are good, close to normal use of hand.
4.31	0.305	2.35	Purple	Diminished protective sensation	Decreased recognition of objects and painful stimuli, difficulty in manipulating objects.
4.56	0.356	4.55	Red	Loss of protective sensation	Greatly impaired perception of pain, temperature, and object recognition. No manipulation of object without vision. Marked decrease in spontaneous hand use.
6.65	1.143	235.61	Red-orange	Loss of all sensation except deep pressure	Unable to identify objects and temperature. Hand use only with visual guidance.
No response to 6.65	—	—	Red lines	Absence of all sensation	Unable to identify objects, temperature, and pain. Minimal hand use.

Based on information in Bell-Krotoski, J., & Tomancik, E. (1987). Repeatability of testing with Semmes-Weinstein monofilaments. *Journal of Hand Surgery, 12A,* 155–161; Tomancik, L. (1987). *Directions for using Semmes-Weinstein monofilaments.* San Jose, CA: North Coast Medical; Bell-Krotoski, J. A. (1997). Correlating sensory morphology and tests of sensibility with function. In J. M. Hunter, L. H. Schneider, & E. J. Mackin (Eds.), *Tendon and nerve surgery in the hand: A third decade* (pp. 49–62). St. Louis; Mosby.

whether there is risk of injury because of a loss of pain and temperature sensation (protective sensation). Either a pinprick and temperature test or monofilament test can provide this information. The monofilament test is more standardized and therefore a better choice, although it usually takes more time.

A test of stereognosis is most appropriate to predict, for example, whether a patient with a hand injury who is a mechanic can feel for and locate unseen automobile parts. The result of a two-point discrimination test or a monofilament test correlates with but does not totally predict the ability to identify objects (Bell-Krotoski, 1997; Van Heest, House, & Putnam, 1993).

Table 7-5. Semmes-Weinstein Results for Subjects Over 60: Median Monofiliament Marking Number by Gender and Age

Age	Women	Men
60–69	3.22	3.61
70–79	3.61	3.61
80+	3.61	3.84

Based on information from Desrosiers, J., Hébert, R., Bravo, G., & Dutil, É. (1996). Hand sensibility of healthy older people. *Journal of the American Geriatrics Society, 44,* 974–978.

Optimal Assessment of Sensation

Ideally, patients are thoroughly assessed using standardized, reliable assessments that are easy to perform and that provide a complete understanding of sensation. A battery of tests is recommended if it is desirable to get a complete understanding of tactile sensation because no one test can assess this complex sense (Callahan, 2002; Lundborg & Rosen, 1994; Rosen, 1996). In clinical practice, however, therapists must sometimes balance the ideal with practical constraints. Schell (1998) described pragmatic constraints that affect assessment and treatment, including sensory testing, in occupational therapy. These include the availability of equipment and supplies, the availability of treatment time, team roles and responsibilities, reimbursement, trends within the profession, culture of the health care organization, and the therapist's clinical competencies or preferences.

Brand and Hollister (1993) charge that much time is wasted in sensory testing and the results are open to question. Therapists should carefully assess their practices periodically to ensure that they are providing intervention that is as close to the ideal as possible despite pragmatic constraints. Great improvements can and should be made in tests of sensation so that they are meaningful, quantitative, and meet the criteria for good test instruments (Peripheral Neuropathy Association, 1993).

Assessment Table 7-1

Summary of Assessments of Sensation

Instrument and Reference	Description	Time to Administer	Validity	Reliability	Sensitivity	Strengths and Weaknesses
Monofilaments Available from AliMed, North Coast Medical, or Sammons Preston Rolyan	Measures low threshold of touch perception on an ordinal scale. Results can be documented with a color-coded drawing or with numbers. 2.83 represents normal sensation and >6.65 represents absent sensation.	5–30 minutes or more, depending on area tested.	Using Semmes-Weinstein monofilaments, diminished light touch associated with longer response time for object identification (King, 1997). WEST Monofilament testing compared to Distal Motor Latency using Electoneurometer revealed r = 0.659–0.886 for individual fingers (Schulz, Bohannon, & Morgan, 1998).	Repeatability of the force of application was demonstrated by Bell-Krotoski and Buford (1997). Test–retest reliability reported by Novak et al. (1993), r = 0.78–0.89, and inter-rater reliability, intra-class correlation (ICC) = 0.965.	72% sensitive in diagnosis of carpal tunnel syndrome (MacDermid & Wessel, 2004).	Strengths: Excellent reliability and validity; widely used. Weaknesses: Relies on subjective responses from patient. Filaments are easily damaged.
Disk-Criminator and Aesthesiometer Available from Lafayette Medical Instruments, North Coast Medical, or Sammons Preston Rolyan	Measures two-point discrimination in millimeters, a ratio scale.	5–10 minutes.	Not established.	Test–retest reliability for two-point discrimination using the Disk-Criminator was reported as: r = 0.961 for static and 0.922 for moving by Dellon, Mackinnon, and Crosby (1987); inter-rater reliability ICC = 0.989 for static and 0.991 for moving (Novak, et al., 1993); test–retest reliability of aesthesiometer in children, ICC = 0.54 (Menier, Forget, & Lambert, 1996).	Study by MacDermid & Wessel (2004) reported static testing has 24% sensitivity and 62% specificity in diagnosis of carpal tunnel syndrome.	Strengths: Excellent reliability; widely used; inexpensive, durable; useful in documenting nerve regeneration; most useful on fingertips. Weakness: Variation in force of application has been shown by Bell-Krotoski & Buford (1997), which may affect results.

continued

Assessment Table 7-1

Summary of Assessments of Sensation (continued)

Instrument and Reference	Description	Time to Administer	Validity	Reliability	Sensitivity	Strengths and Weaknesses
Tuning Forks Available from Sammons Preston Rolyan	Indicates whether or not vibration is perceived, a nominal scale.	5 minutes.	Not established.	Not established.	Sensitivity for diagnosis of carpal tunnel syndrome is reported at 55% and specificity at 81% (MacDermid & Wessel, 2004).	Strength: Low frequency useful to document regeneration of nerve. Weaknesses: Relies on subjective responses from patient; unknown validity and reliability; application techniques are not standardized.
Hot and Cold Temperature Probes Available from Sammons Preston Rolyan	Indicates whether or not temperature is perceived, a nominal scale.	5 minutes.	Not established.	Not established.	Not established.	Strengths: Assesses functional sensation; useful to identify loss of protective sensation. Weaknesses: Relies on subjective responses from patient. Tool does not test fine gradations of temperature discrimination and, therefore, may not be sensitive to change.

Vibrometer Biomedical Instrument Company, Sensortek, Inc., or WR Medical Electronics	Determines lowest intensity of vibration that can be perceived, an interval scale.	20 minutes.	Not established.	Inter-rater reliability using Vibratron II, ICC = 0.982 (Novak et al., 1993).	In diagnosis of carpal tunnel syndrome, sensitivity is 50%, and specificity is 73% (MacDermid & Wessel, 2004).	Strengths: Multiple kinds; manufacturers provide protocols for testing; small gradations of scale. Weaknesses: Limited availability in OT clinics; expense.
Automated Tactile Testing Device Ztech, LC	Multiple modalities are tested, including temperature, pain, touch, vibration, and two-point discrimination.	15–30 minutes or more, depending on areas tested.	r = 0.470–0.529 when compared with monofilament and discriminator (Horch et al., 1992).	Test–retest reliability of Ztech using specific protocol, ICC = 0.86–0.89 (Hubbard et al., 2004). Intra-subject r = 0.659 (Horch et al., 1992).	In patients with carpal tunnel syndrome, 71% had abnormal results on the Automated Tactile Tester (Hardy et al., 1992).	Strengths: Computerized; quantifiable; tests multiple sensory modalities. Weaknesses: Limited availability in OT clinics; expense.
Pressure-Specified Sensory Device Neurotherapy DX	Measures pressure threshold and ability to feel and distinguish the distance between two points, with results graphically generated by a computer and quantified on an interval scale score with a range of 0.1–100 g/mm2 for touch threshold.	10–20 minutes.	Results correlate well with timed object identification, r = 0.691. (Dellon, 1997).	Inter-test reliability is r = 0.93 for moving two-point discrimination, r = 0.97 for single-point static touch threshold test. Inter-rater reliability is r = 0.61 (Dellon, 1997).	In diagnosis of nerve entrapment, sensitivity is 100% (Tassler & Dellon, 1995).	Strengths: Computerized; quantifiable; measures both threshold and innervation density; excellent sensitivity. Weaknesses: Limited availability in OT clinics; expense.
Moberg Picking-Up Test (Dellon, 1988; Ng, Ho, & Chow, 1999) Available from Lafayette Instrument Company or Sammons Preston Rolyan	Picking up and identifying objects are timed, which results in an interval scale score.	10 minutes.	Not established.	Inter-rater reliability, r = 0.67 with eyes open and r = 0.80 with eyes closed (Ng, Ho, & Chow, 1999).	Not established.	Strengths: Simple, quick to administer; functional; easy to replicate; inexpensive; useful to assess function of median nerve. Weaknesses: Useful for limited diagnostic category; lack of standardized protocol.

CASE EXAMPLE

Mr. T. : Sensory Problems Following Median Nerve Laceration

Occupational Therapy Assessment Process	Clinical Reasoning Process: Objectives	Clinical Reasoning Process: Examples of Therapist's Internal Dialogue
Patient Information Mr. T. is a 25-year-old married man with a son aged 2. Mr. T.'s right wrist was injured by a broken window, resulting in a complete laceration of the median nerve and the flexor digitorum superficialis tendons to the middle and ring fingers. Both the nerve and tendons were repaired surgically the day after the injury.	Understand the patient's diagnosis or condition	"This was a really serious hand injury. Since the splinting was discontinued, the tendon and nerve repairs must have healed well."
Immediately after the injury, movement was restricted throughout the hand due to tendon healing precautions and protective splinting. Sensation was absent in the median nerve distribution of the palm and fingers, and there was loss of innervation to the thenar muscles. Mr. T. had a 7-cm incision scar on his volar wrist and palm area.	Know the person	"Mr. T. seems like a hard-working man. His work is physically demanding. I wonder how he is dealing with being off from work for so long."
Mr. T. graduated from vocational-technical school with training in major appliance repair. At the time of his injury, he was working for a local company doing in-home repairs of refrigerators, washers, and dryers. His wife works in a secretarial position. He is right-handed, but he reported that since the injury, he has been using his left hand successfully in basic activities of daily living, such as feeding, dressing, and hygiene. He has not attempted using his right hand for any work, home management, or child care.	Appreciate the context	"I wonder how this hand injury affects the relationship Mr. T. has with his wife and son?"
At 6 weeks after injury, protective splinting is discontinued, and Mr. T. is allowed to begin to use his right hand in functional activities with light resistance. The occupational therapist is now performing a comprehensive reassessment to determine the level of motor and sensory recovery of the median nerve, the sensibility and sensitivity around the area of the scar, and Mr. T.'s ability to use his right hand in functional activities.	Develop provisional hypotheses	"Given the history, I would expect that there has been about 1 1/2 inches of neural regrowth beyond the laceration. This should mean there will be some sensation in the palm but not yet in the fingers."
Assessment Process The occupational therapist selected the following sensory evaluation tools: Touch threshold test using Semmes-Weinstein monofilaments Static and moving two-point discrimination Touch localization Dellon's modification of the Moberg picking-up test	Consider evaluation approach and methods	"This is a good time to do a thorough sensory assessment because it will indicate how the neurons are regrowing and whether there are areas that still lack protective sensation. The monofilaments will give reliable information about all areas of the hand and indicate whether protective sensation is present or reduced. Because perception of moving touch recovers first, two-point discrimination testing might show recovery. The touch localization test will show how the brain is interpreting tactile sensations. The picking-up test relates sensation to functional hand use. These four tests will give good information for treatment planning and will demonstrate sensory recovery over time."

Assessment Results The results of the Semmes-Weinstein monofilament test for the right palm and fingers are shown in Figure 7-9. Touch pressure threshold testing over the area of the scar revealed that Mr. T. disliked touch directly on the scar. The area was rubbed with textured items, and Mr. T. reported a marked preference for soft textures and no tolerance for rough textures, such as burlap and Velcro. Mr. T. was unable to feel the Disk-Criminator anywhere on the fingertips in the moving test and did not feel anything on the fingers or thumb in the static test. Touch localization in the radial portion of the right palm measured 18–25 mm. Mr. T.'s scores on Dellon's modification of the picking-up test were as follows: Part 1: Left/Right Trial 1: 17 seconds/55 seconds Trial 2: 15 seconds/60 seconds Part 2: No objects could be identified without vision	Interpret observations	"Sensation is returning pretty much as I expected it would. Return of some protective sensation in the palm is a positive sign that neuron regrowth is occurring. I expected absent sensation in the fingertips, because I remember the rate of regrowth is about 1 mm per day, or an inch per month. Mr. T. can use visual guidance to pick up small objects despite the sensory loss, but his movements are awkward. That incoordination could be due to either motor or sensory deficits. Because of lack of sensation in the fingertips, object identification is not possible now, but hopefully, Mr. T. will regain this ability because I suspect he will need to use his hand in places where he cannot see in his work as an appliance repairman."
Occupational Therapy Problem List 1. Absent and decreased protective sensation in the thumb, index, and middle fingers and radial palm 2. Mislocalization of touch sensations in the radial portion of the palm 3. Hypersensitivity in the area of the scar 4. Decreased ability to pick up and manipulate objects 5. Decreased use of the right hand in functional activities	Synthesize results	"Mr. T. is probably at some risk for injury to the fingertips because he can now start using his hand in more functional tasks but lacks any protective sensation in the digit tips, which is a likely place for thermal injuries or lacerations. The presence of some protective sensation in the palm and the mislocalization of touch stimuli suggest that retraining of sensation in this area can now be started. He might have a tendency to avoid using his right hand due to his hypersensitivity and decreased coordination. I'll need to provide functional activities to encourage bilateral functional use. Perhaps some work simulation activities will be motivating for Mr. T."

CLINICAL REASONING IN OCCUPATIONAL THERAPY PRACTICE

Interpretation and Treatment Planning for Peripheral Sensory Problem

Mr. T.'s touch threshold test performed 6 weeks post injury is shown in Figure 7-9. How will the mapping likely change when Mr. T. is reassessed after 6 more weeks? What kind of sensation (pain or touch) will he be able to feel first in his fingertips? Compare his current functional hand use with his expected hand use when his fingertips regain touch sensation.

SUMMARY REVIEW QUESTIONS

1. What pattern of sensory loss would be expected in a patient with a T10 complete spinal cord injury?
2. What pattern of sensory loss would be expected in a patient with peripheral polyneuropathy?
3. Which patient will have a better prognosis for recovery of sensation, one with a peripheral nerve compression or one with a middle cerebral artery stroke?
4. Name and describe the purposes of at least three standardized and three nonstandardized sensory tests.
5. Describe or demonstrate the administration and scoring of a touch threshold test, a pain awareness test, and a touch localization test.
6. Which sensory test or tests would you select for a patient with peripheral polyneuropathy? Justify your response.
7. What type of intervention is needed for a patient with absent protective sensation?

ACKNOWLEDGMENT

I extend my appreciation to Paul Petersen and Melanie Seltzer for their assistance with the photography for this chapter.

References

Adams, R. D., Victor, M., & Ropper, A. H. (1997). *Principles of neurology* (6th ed.). New York: McGraw-Hill.

American Occupational Therapy Association [AOTA]. (1994). Uniform terminology for occupational therapy (3rd ed.). *American Journal of Occupational Therapy, 48,* 1047–1054.

Bell-Krotoski, J. A. (1995). Sensibility testing: Current concepts. In J. M. Hunter, E. J. Mackin, & A. D. Callahan (Eds.), *Rehabilitation of the hand: Surgery and therapy* (4th ed., pp. 109–128). St. Louis: Mosby.

Bell-Krotoski, J. A. (1997). Correlating sensory morphology and tests of sensibility with function. In J. M. Hunter, L. H. Schneider, & E. J. Mackin (Eds.), *Tendon and Nerve surgery in the hand: A third decade* (pp. 49–62). St. Louis: Mosby.

Bell-Krotoski, J. A. (2002). Sensibility testing with the Semmes-Weinstein Monofilaments. In E. J. Mackin, A. D. Callahan, T. M. Skirven, L. H. Schneider, A. L. Osterman, & J. M. Hunter (Eds.), *Rehabilitation of the hand and upper extremity* (5th ed., pp. 194–213). St. Louis: Mosby.

Bell-Krotoski, J. A., & Buford, W. L. (1997). The force/time relationship of clinically used sensory testing instruments. *Journal of Hand Therapy, 10,* 297–309.

Bell-Krotoski, J., & Tomancik, E. (1987). Repeatability of testing with Semmes-Weinstein monofilaments. *Journal of Hand Surgery, 12A,* 155–161.

Benton, S. (1994). Computerized assessment holds promise. *Rehab Management, 7,* 37.

Beschin, N., Cazzani, M., Cubelli, R., Sala, S. D., & Spinazzola, L. (1996). Ignoring left and far: An investigation of tactile neglect. *Neuropsychologia, 34,* 41–49.

Brand, P. W., & Hollister, A. (1993). *Clinical mechanics of the hand* (2nd ed.). St. Louis: Mosby.

Callahan, A. D. (2002). Sensibility assessment for nerve lesions-in-continuity and nerve lacerations. In E. J. Mackin, A. D. Callahan, T. M. Skirven, L. H. Schneider, A. L. Osterman, & J. M. Hunter (Eds.), *Rehabilitation of the hand and upper extremity* (5th ed., pp. 214–239). St. Louis: Mosby.

Carr, J., & Shepherd, R. (1998). *Neurological rehabilitation: Optimizing motor performance.* Oxford: Butterworth-Heinemann.

Chapman, C. E., Tremblay, F., & Ageranioti-Belanger, A. (1996). Role of primary somatosensory cortex in active and passive touch. In A. M. Wing, P. Haggard, & J. R. Flanagan (Eds.), *Hand and brain: The neurophysiology of hand movements* (pp. 329–347). San Diego: Academic.

Cole, J. (1991). *Pride and a daily marathon.* Cambridge, MA: MIT.

Cooke, D. (1991). Sensibility evaluation battery for the peripheral nerve injured hand. *Australian Occupational Therapy Journal, 38,* 241–245.

Dellon, A. (1988). *Evaluation of sensibility and re-education of sensation in the hand.* Baltimore: Lucas.

Dellon, A. L. (1997). *Somatosensory testing and rehabilitation.* Bethesda, MD: American Occupational Therapy Association.

Dellon, A. L., Mackinnon, S. E., & Crosby, P. M. (1987). Reliability of two-point discrimination measurements. *Journal of Hand Surgery, 12A,* 693–698.

Desrosiers, J., Hebert, R., Bravo, G., & Dutil, A. A. E. (1996). Hand sensibility of healthy older people. *Journal of the American Geriatrics Society, 44,* 974–978.

Eggers, O. (1984). *Occupational therapy in the treatment of adult hemiplegia.* Rockville, CO: Aspen Systems.

Fess, E. E. (1995). Guidelines for evaluating assessment instruments. *Journal of Hand Therapy, 8,* 144–148.

Fredericks, C. M. (1996a). Basic sensory mechanisms and the somatosensory system. In C. M. Fredericks & L. K. Saladin (Eds.), *Pathophysiology of the motor systems: Principles and clinical presentations* (pp. 78–106). Philadelphia: Davis.

Fredericks, C. M. (1996b). Disorders of the peripheral nervous system: The peripheral neuropathies. In C. M. Fredericks & L. K. Saladin (Eds.), *Pathophysiology of the motor systems: Principles and clinical presentations* (pp. 346–372). Philadelphia: Davis.

Fredericks, C. M. (1996c). Disorders of the spinal cord. In C. M. Fredericks & L. K. Saladin (Eds.), *Pathophysiology of the motor systems: Principles and clinical presentations* (pp. 394–423). Philadelphia: Davis.

Garrison, S. J., Rolak, L. A., Dodaro, R. R., & O'Callaghan, A. J. (1988). Rehabilitation of the stroke patient. In J. A. DeLisa, D. M. Currie, B. M. Gans, P. F. Gatens, J. A. Leonard, & M. C. McPhee (Eds.), *Rehabilitation medicine: Principles and practice* (pp. 565–584). Philadelphia: Lippincott.

Greve, K. W., Bianchini, K. J., & Ameduri, C. J. (2003). Use of a forced-choice test of tactile discrimination in the evaluation of functional sensory loss: A report of 3 cases. *Archives of Physical Medicine and Rehabilitation, 84,* 1233–1236.

Hardy, M., Jiminez, S., Jabaley, M., & Horch, K. (1992). Evaluation of nerve compression with the Automated Tactile Tester. *Journal of Hand Surgery, 17A,* 838–842.

Hermann, R. P., Novak, C. B., & Mackinnon, S. E. (1995). Establishing normal values for moving two-point discrimination in children and adolescents. *Southern Medical Journal, 88,* S97 (Abstr).

Horch, K., Hardy, M., Jiminez, S., & Jabaley, M. (1992). An Automated Tactile Tester for evaluation of cutaneous sensibility. *Journal of Hand Surgery, 17A,* 829–837.

Hubbard, M. C., MacDermid, J. C., Kramer, J. F., & Birmingham, T. B. (2004). Quantitative vibration threshold testing in carpal tunnel syndrome: Analysis strategies for optimizing reliability. *Journal of Hand Therapy, 17,* 24–30.

Johansson, R. S. (1996). Sensory control of dexterous manipulation in humans. In A. M. Wing, P. Haggard, & J. R. Flanagan (Eds.), *Hand and brain: The neurophysiology of hand movements* (pp. 381–414). San Diego: Academic.

Jones, L. (1996). Proprioception and its contribution to manual dexterity. In A. M. Wing, P. Haggard, & J. R. Flanagan (Eds.), *Hand and brain: The neurophysiology of hand movements* (pp. 349–362). San Diego: Academic.

Kaplan, F. S., Nixon, J. E., Reitz, M., Rindfleish, L., & Tucker, J. (1985). Age-related changes in proprioception and sensation of joint position. *Acta Orthopaedica Scandinavia, 56,* 72–74.

Katz, J. N., & Stirrat, C. R. (1990). A self-administered hand diagram for the diagnosis of carpal tunnel syndrome. *Journal of Hand Surgery, 15A,* 360–363.

King, P. (1997). Sensory function assessment: A pilot comparison study of touch pressure threshold with texture and tactile discrimination. *Journal of Hand Therapy, 10,* 24–28.

Lederman, S. J., & Klatzky, R. L. (1996). Action for perception: Manual exploratory movements for haptically processing objects and their features. In A. M. Wing, P. Haggard, & J. R. Flanagan (Eds.), *Hand and brain: The neurophysiology of hand movements* (pp. 431–446). San Diego: Academic.

Lindblom, U. (1994). Analysis of abnormal touch, pain, and temperature sensation in patients. In J. Boivie, P. Hansson, & U. Lindblom (Eds.), *Touch, temperature, and pain in health and disease: Mechanisms and assessment* (pp. 63–84). Seattle: IASP.

Lundborg, G., & Rosen, B. (1994). Rationale for quantitative sensory tests in hand surgery. In J. Boivie, P. Hansson, & U. Lindblom (Eds.), *Touch, temperature, and pain in health and disease: Mechanisms and assessment* (pp. 151–162). Seattle: IASP.

MacDermid, J. C., & Wessel, J. (2004). Clinical diagnosis of carpal tunnel syndrome: A systematic review. *Journal of Hand Therapy, 17,* 309–319.

Menier, C., Forget, R., & Lambert, J. (1996). Evaluation of two-point discrimination in children: Reliability effects of passive displacement and voluntary movement. *Developmental Medicine and Child Neurology, 38,* 523–537.

Nakada, M. (1993). Localization of a constant-touch and moving-touch stimulus in the hand: A preliminary study. *Journal of Hand Therapy, 6,* 23–28.

Ng, C. L., Ho, D. D., & Chow, S. P. (1999). The Moberg Pickup Test: Results of testing with a standard protocol. *Journal of Hand Therapy, 12,* 309–312.

Novak, C. B., & Mackinnon, S. E. (2005). Evaluation of nerve injury and nerve compression in the upper quadrant. *Journal of Hand Therapy, 18,* 230–240.

Novak, C. B., Mackinnon, S. E., Williams, J. I., & Kelly, L. (1993). Establishment of reliability in the evaluation of hand sensibility. *Plastic and Reconstructive Surgery, 92,* 311–322.

Peripheral Neuropathy Association. (1993). Quantitative sensory testing: A consensus report from the Peripheral Neuropathy Association. *Neurology, 43,* 1050–1052.

Reese, N. B. (1999). *Muscle and sensory testing.* Philadelphia: Saunders.

Riggle, M. (1999). Review of the book *Somatosensory Testing and Rehabilitation. American Journal of Occupational Therapy, 53,* 412.

Rosen, B. (1996). Recovery of sensory and motor function after nerve repair: A rationale for evaluation. *Journal of Hand Therapy, 9,* 315–327.

Saladin, L. K. (1996a). Cerebrovascular disease: Stroke. In C. M. Fredericks & L. K. Saladin (Eds.), *Pathophysiology of the motor systems: Principles and clinical presentations* (pp. 486–512). Philadelphia: Davis.

Saladin, L. K. (1996b). Traumatic brain injury. In C. M. Fredericks & L. K. Saladin (Eds.), *Pathophysiology of the motor systems: Principles and clinical presentations* (pp. 467–485). Philadelphia: Davis.

Schady, W. (1994). Locognosia: Normal precision and changes after peripheral nerve injury. In J. Boivie, P. Hansson, & U. Lindblom (Eds.), *Touch, temperature, and pain in health and disease: Mechanisms and assessment* (pp. 143–150). Seattle: IASP.

Schell, B. B. (1998). Clinical reasoning: The basis of practice. In M. E. Neistadt & E. B. Crepeau (Eds.), *Willard & Spackman's occupational therapy* (9th ed., pp. 90–100). Philadelphia: Lippincott.

Schulz, L. A., Bohannon, R. W., & Morgan, W. J. (1998). Normal digit tip values for the Weinstein Enhanced Sensory Test. *Journal of Hand Therapy, 11,* 200–205.

Shimokata, H., & Kuzuya, F. (1995). Two-point discrimination test of the skin as an index of sensory aging. *Gerontology, 41,* 267–272.

Sieg, K., & Williams, W. (1986). Preliminary report of a methodology for determining tactile location in adults. *Occupational Therapy Journal of Research, 6,* 195–206.

Smith, K. L. (1995). Nerve response to injury and repair. In J. M. Hunter, E. J. Mackin, & A. D. Callahan (Eds.), *Rehabilitation of the hand: Surgery and therapy* (4th ed., pp. 609–626). St. Louis: Mosby.

Sterzi, R., Bottini, G., Celani, M. G., Righetti, E., Lamassa, M., Ricci, S., & Vallar, G. (1993). Hemianopia, hemianesthesia, and hemiplegia after right and left hemisphere damage: A hemispheric difference. *Journal of Neurology, Neurosurgery, and Psychiatry, 56,* 308–310.

Szabo, R. M., Slater, R. R., Farver, T. B., Stanton, D. B., & Sharman, W. K. (1999). The value of diagnostic testing in carpal tunnel syndrome. *Journal of Hand Surgery, 24A,* 704–714.

Tassler, P. L., & Dellon, A. L. (1995). Correlation of measurements of pressure perception using the pressure-specified sensory device with electrodiagnostic testing. *Journal of Occupational and Environmental Medicine, 37,* 862–866.

Tomancik, L. (1987). *Directions for using Semmes-Weinstein monofilaments.* San Jose, CA: North Coast Medical.

Van Heest, A., House, J., & Putnam, M. (1993). Sensibility deficiencies in the hands of children with spastic hemiplegia. *Journal of Hand Surgery, 18A,* 278–281.

Waters, R., Adkins, R., Yakura, J., & Sie, I. (1993). Motor and sensory recovery following complete tetraplegia. *Archives of Physical Medicine and Rehabilitation, 74,* 242–247.

Waylett-Rendall, J. (1988). Sensibility evaluation and rehabilitation. *Orthopedic Clinics of North America, 19,* 43–56.

Weinstein, S., Drozdenko, R., & Weinstein, C. (1997). Evaluation of sensory measures in neuropathy. In J. M. Hunter, L. H. Schneider, & E. J. Mackin (Eds.), *Tendon and nerve surgery in the hand: A third decade* (pp. 63–76). St. Louis: Mosby.

CHAPTER 8

Assessing Abilities and Capacities: Vision, Visual Perception, and Praxis

Lee Ann Quintana

LEARNING OBJECTIVES

After studying this chapter, the reader will be able to do the following:

1. Understand the importance of evaluating the visual foundation skills prior to higher level visual cognitive skills.
2. Identify and describe evaluation techniques for visual acuity, visual fields, and ocular motor control.
3. Describe and evaluate the two subtypes of unilateral neglect: sensory and motor.
4. Describe and evaluate apraxia.

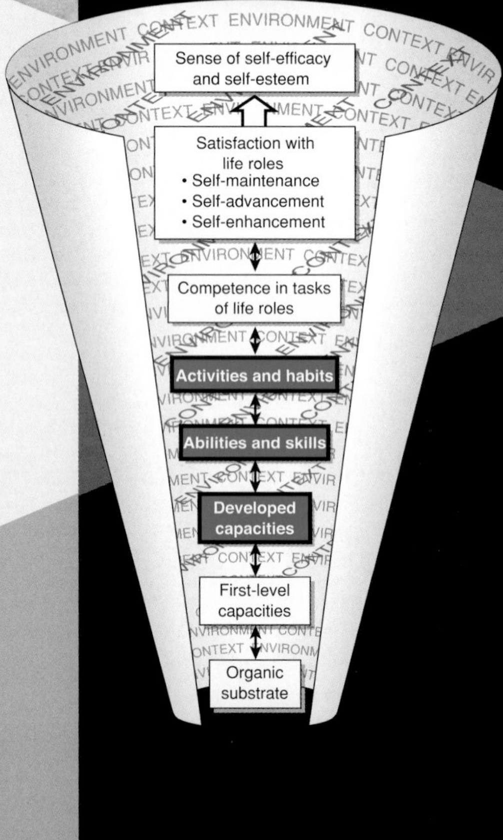

Glossary

Accommodation—ability to adjust focus of vision at different distances; age related, and decreases with age.

Apraxia—the inability to carry out skilled movement in the presence of intact sensation, movement, and coordination.

Binocular vision—ability to resolve two images (one from each eye) into one.

Contrast sensitivity—ability to see with differing amounts of contrast.

Oculomotor control—ability of the eyes to move smoothly and in a coordinated manner through full range of motion.

Unilateral neglect—a constellation of symptoms that is manifested by a failure to respond or orient to stimuli presented contralateral to a brain lesion.

Visual acuity—ability of the eyes to make what is seen sharp and clear.

Visual fields—the scope of vision in each eye; central visual field: central 20° of vision; peripheral: area seen other than central vision.

Visual foundation skills—primary visual skills of visual acuity, visual fields, and oculomotor control upon which higher-level visual perception is built.

Vision is a critical channel by which we gather information from the environment. We depend heavily on vision for learning, decision making, social interactions, motor control, and postural control because of its critical role in attention, information processing, and movement detection (Titcomb, Okoye, & Schiff, 1997; Warren, 1999). It is the means by which we register information and decide what will happen next (e.g., move out of the way of a moving car, comfort a friend who is crying, pick up a tool lying on the table). Because of vision's importance to almost all activities of daily living, occupational therapists must know the basic status of the visual system of their clients.

The purpose of this chapter is to review evaluation of the visual system with more emphasis on **visual foundation skills** and less on the higher level visual cognitive skills. In addition, the chapter discusses assessment of praxis (motor planning).

VISUAL PERCEPTUAL HIERARCHY

Warren (1993a) developed a hierarchy of visual perception (Fig. 8-1), with each level built on and dependent on the one below it. Visual cognition, the highest level, is "the ability to mentally manipulate visual information and integrate it with other sensory information to solve problems, formulate plans, and make decisions" (Warren, 1993a, p. 43). Visual memory is below visual cognition in the hierarchy. If the car doesn't start and you look under the hood to check the battery, you need a picture in your memory of what a battery looks like, or you would fumble around for quite a while trying to find what was wrong. Likewise, pattern recognition subserves memory. You must be able to identify the features of an object before storing it in memory. To identify the features of an object, you must be able to scan it thoroughly. To scan thoroughly, you must be alert and attentive. All of these higher skills depend upon the visual foundation skills: (1) **visual acuity**, which assures the accuracy of information sent to the brain; (2) **visual fields** (VF), which let the brain know what's going on in the environment; and (3) **oculomotor control**, which ensures efficient eye movements (Warren, 1993a).

Visual impairment changes the quality and amount of visual input to the brain and therefore decreases our ability to use vision to adapt (Warren, 1999) (Definition 8-1). If a person has poor **contrast sensitivity**, he or she may no longer want to go out in the evening because of the difficulty of maneuvering in poor light. Patients generally have

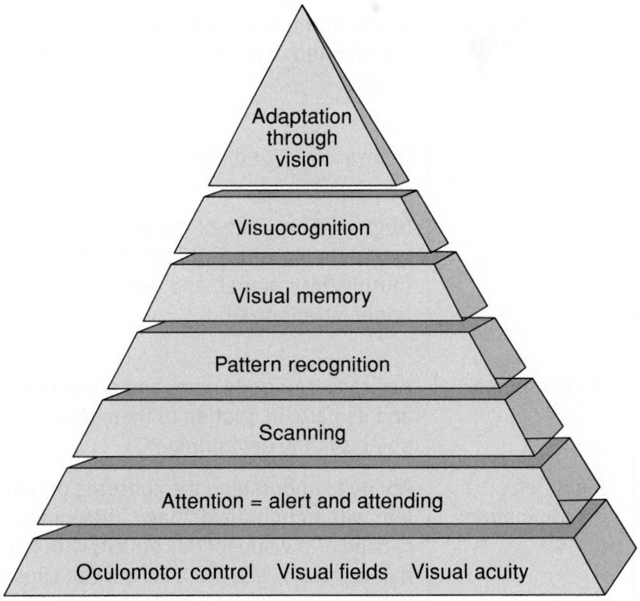

Figure 8-1 Hierarchy of visual perception. (From Warren, M. [1993a]. A hierarchical model for evaluation and treatment of visual perceptual dysfunction in adult acquired brain injury, Part 1. *American Journal of Occupational Therapy, 47,* 43. Copyright 1993 by the American Occupational Therapy Association, Inc. Reprinted with permission.)

DEFINITION 8-1

de·fin·i·tion

Definitions and Descriptions of Vision, Visual Perception, and Praxis Deficits

Area of Deficit	Definition	Functional Description of Deficit
Visual acuity	Ability of the eyes to make what is seen sharp and clear.	Client complaints: blurred vision (near or far); print too small, too faint; headaches, squinting. Effect on function: holds objects too close to the face; ↓ facial recognition; fear of new environments; lack of interest in environment; difficulty localizing objects; ↓ interest in reading; vision fluctuates throughout the day; bumps into low-contrast objects.
Visual fields	Area that one sees when looking out into the environment. Central visual field (VF): central 20° where vision is clear and focused; peripheral VF: area seen other than central where vision is not as clear but used for motion detection and orientation in space.	Client complaints: bumps into objects; can't find things; difficulty reading. Effect on function: difficulty moving in crowded or busy environments; anxiety; startle response; difficulty with self-care; unsafe.
Binocular vision	Ability to resolve two images (one from each eye) into one. Motor component: muscles and nerves that align the eyes with the object. Sensory component: activity within the cortex that allows perception of one image.	Client complaints: double vision; difficulty sustaining visual work effort; eye fatigue with sustained work, eyes look crossed; blurred vision; headaches. Effect on function: poor eye contact; inability to concentrate; avoidance of activities at near distance; loss of vision; difficulty with activities requiring depth perception.
Accommodation	Ability to adjust focus of vision at different distances.	Client complaints: headaches; eye strain; difficulty with sustained activity at near distance; print moves while reading. Effect on function: under- and over-reaching; frustration when maneuvering in visually stimulating environments; road fatigue.
Ocular motility	Ability of the eyes to move smoothly and in a coordinated manner through full range of motion.	Client complaints: headaches; difficulty keeping eyes focused; dizziness; balance problems. Effect on function: excessive head movements; frequent loss of place and skipping lines when reading.
Anosognosia	Unawareness or denial of deficits.	Functional activities are unsafe; unable to learn compensatory techniques.
Unilateral neglect	Neglect of one side of the body or extrapersonal space. Types: motor (output/intentional) and perceptual (input/attentional).	Shaves only one side of face, dresses only one side of the body; eats food from only half of the plate; reads only a half of a page or half of a word; transfers and functional mobility are unsafe; bumps into objects on one side.
Body scheme	Awareness of body parts and position of body and its parts in relation to themselves and objects in the environment.	May result in dressing apraxia; may not recognize body parts or relationship between them; transfers may be unsafe.
Right/left discrimination	Ability to understand the concepts of right and left; with right brain damage (RBD), may be caused by a visuospatial deficit; with left brain damage (LBD) and aphasia, may be caused by language deficitsor by general mental impairment.	May have difficulty dressing and understanding concepts of right and left.
Body part identification	Ability to identify parts on self and/or others.	May respond incorrectly when told to move a specific body part.

continued

DEFINITION 8-1 (continued)

Definitions and Descriptions of Vision, Visual Perception, and Praxis Deficits

Area of Deficit	Definition	Functional Description of Deficit
Position in space	Ability to understand the concepts of over and under, above and below, etc.	Difficulty moving through a crowded area; difficulty with dressing; difficulty following directions using these terms.
Spatial relations	Ability to perceive self in relation to other objects.	As above; transfers unsafe.
Topographical orientation	Ability to find one's way from one place to another.	Difficulty finding the way to a room, to therapy, or from one room to another.
Figure-ground perception	Ability to distinguish foreground from background.	Unable to find object in cluttered drawer, white washcloth on white sheet, brakes on wheelchair, food in refrigerator, etc.
Limb apraxia	Inability to carry out purposeful movement in the presence of intact sensation, movement, and coordination.	May experience difficulty with functional tasks involving objects, as client does not know how to use objects or attempts to use the incorrect object (e.g., uses knife to eat soup); difficulty with production and understanding gestures; may be clumsy and have trouble with writing, knitting, etc.
Constructional apraxia	Deficit in constructional activities: graphic and assembly; RBD: drawings are complex but exhibit disorganized spatial relations and poor orientation in space; LBD: drawings are simplified with few details.	May result in dressing apraxia; difficulty setting a table, making a dress, wrapping a gift, arranging numerical figures for mathematical processing, making a sandwich, assembling a craft project from a kit, etc.
Dressing apraxia	Inability to dress oneself.	Attempts to put clothes on inside out, backwards, or in the wrong order; dresses only one half of the body.

the most difficulty in dynamic environments. At home, we are best able to control and compensate for the deficits; community activities, such as shopping and driving, present more of a problem.

In the past, therapists often evaluated higher level visual perceptual skills without a good understanding of the optical system and how it provides the foundation for these skills (Warren, 1999). A deficit in one of the higher level visual perceptual skills, such as figure-ground or spatial relations, may be the result of a problem in one of the foundation skills. For example, clients who do poorly on a figure-ground test may have decreased visual acuity and be unable to get a clear picture of what they see or have poor convergence and therefore difficulty with any close work.

ASSESSING VISION AND VISUAL PERCEPTION

If higher level visual cognitive skills are the result of the integration of the skills that subserve them in the visual hierarchy, it seems that the therapist's limited time is best spent evaluating the foundation skills, rather than higher level visual cognitive skills (Warren, 1993b). Evaluation includes the following:

- A basic eye history, including premorbid visual conditions (e.g., congenital strabismus, ocular trauma)
- Interviews with the client and/or family as to complaints or symptoms (e.g., difficulty concentrating, double vision, eyestrain, bumping into objects on one side)
- Observation of the client during functional activities
- Screening of the foundation skills

The therapist bases plans for further evaluation and intervention on the results and the client's goals and lifestyle. For example, if the client is 35 years old, has had a stroke, and works as a mechanic, the therapist may evaluate his constructional abilities in depth. If the client is 75 years old and retired and spends his time reading and watching television, detailed evaluation of constructional abilities may not be indicated. This idea is carried over into treatment as well. The 35-year-old mechanic will need a higher level of constructional skills than the 75-year-old retiree. In addition, the therapist may find that the client performs adequately on a test but exhibits difficulty in a functional situation. This also indicates the need for further evaluation.

All neurologically impaired clients should have their visual foundation skills screened. Screening is also considered for older clients whose vision may have been affected by age. How in depth of a screening may depend on the team members who care for the patient. If working in a rehabilitation facility with the services of an eye care professional, the occupational therapist may only refer the patient to the eye care professional and collaborate on the findings and development of a treatment plan. On the other hand, the occupational therapist may be the only one on the team to specifically look at vision and its effects on functional activities. In this case, the occupational therapist may choose to screen all clients and, at any sign of difficulty, refer the client to an eye care professional.

Eye Care Professionals

The eye care professionals include the ophthalmologist and optometrist. The ophthalmologist is a medical doctor whose major concern is eye health (e.g., cataracts, macular degeneration, infections). Generally, "ophthalmologists are rarely trained, experienced or interested in visual system rehabilitation or function" (Gianutsos, 1997, p. 273). Optometrists receive 4 years of postgraduate training on diagnosis and treatment of eye disease, but the focus is on function and how vision affects performance and quality of life (Scheiman, 1999). Even with this focus, most optometrists specialize in refraction and contact lenses, and only a small percentage of optometrists do vision therapy (Scheiman, 1999). To find eye care professionals with a similar frame of reference, ask them questions such as these (Scheiman, 2002, p. 88):

- Do you have experience working with patients with acquired brain injury?
- Do you test accommodative amplitude and facility?
- Do you evaluate fusional vergence and facility?
- Do you evaluate visual information processing skills?
- Do you offer vision therapy as a service in your practice?

Once the decision has been made to refer the client to an eye care professional, therapists ideally go to the appointment with the client or send information such as this:

- Practical information: diagnosis, method of communication and reliability of responses, ability to transfer, and medications
- Description of functional behaviors that may indicate a problem with vision
- Visual history

If the therapist is able to attend the appointment, he or she can take notes, act as an interpreter between the client and family and the eye doctor, and interact with the doctor to discuss treatment plans (Gianutsos, 1997). The therapist provides input on function and follows through with recommendations. If unable to attend the appointment, the therapist might send a form with the client for the doctor to complete, requesting information such as the following (Warren, 1999):

- Visual acuity
- Ocular motility
- Visual fields
- Pertinent ocular diagnoses
- Recommendations for follow-up and treatment

Visual Foundation Skills

The visual foundation skills include visual acuity, visual fields, and oculomotor control. Although deficits in these areas can affect function, clients may not complain of any problems, or they may make complaints that appear unrelated to vision and/or appear to be due to something else (Definition 8-1). Therefore, it is important that these areas are screened even if the client denies difficulty seeing things.

Visual Acuity

Visual acuity is the ability of the eyes to make what is seen sharp and clear. Most of us are familiar with the concept of 20/20 vision. The numerator denotes the distance at which the client recognizes the stimulus, and the denominator is the distance at which it would be recognized by someone with normal vision. For instance, a person with 20/200 vision is able to recognize a stimulus at 20 feet that a person with normal vision could recognize at 200 feet. Deficits in visual acuity may be the result of refractive errors, poor eye health with inability to process the image (e.g., cataract, macular degeneration, diabetic retinopathy), or poor transmission of the image by the optic nerve (Warren, 1999).

Visual acuity is most often screened using conventional letter charts (e.g., Snellen Chart). Test cards are available that use symbols rather than letters for use with aphasic, non-English-speaking, and severely impaired clients (e.g., Lea Symbol Test). Visual acuity should be examined in each eye for both near (16 inches or less) and far (20 feet or more) vision. Near acuity is important for any table top activity, and far vision is especially important for activities such as driving. Testing of visual acuity should be carried out with the best correction available; clients should wear their glasses. If the glasses are not available, have the client look through a pinhole in a piece of paper, as this helps the focusing power of the eye (Simon, Aminoff, & Greenberg, 1999).

Since conventional letter charts measure acuity by determining the smallest high-contrast detail a person can perceive at a given distance and most settings do not provide such high contrast, contrast sensitivity should

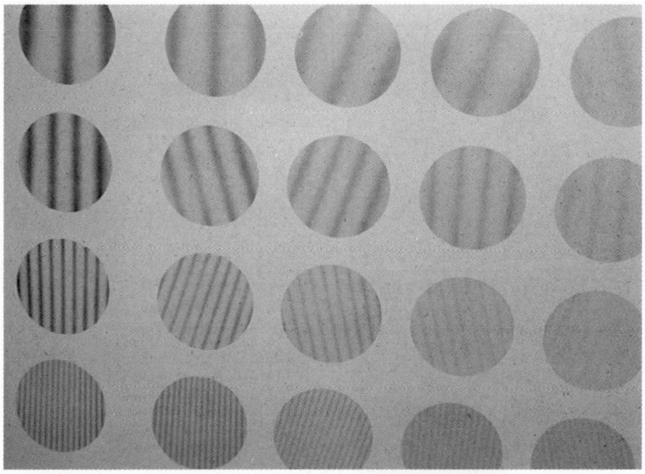

Figure 8-2 Contrast sensitivity test. (Reprinted with permission from Vistech Consultants, Inc., Dayton, OH.)

be evaluated as well. It indicates the person's ability to see objects in various levels of contrast and how he or she will perform functionally. The tester presents a series of sine wave gratings that vary in orientation, contrast, and frequency. The client must indicate the orientation of the grating; the poorer the acuity, the more contrast required to detect the orientation of the grating (Fig. 8-2). In addition, Warren (1996), in *Brain Injury Visual Assessment Battery for Adults* (biVABA), presents some clinical tasks and observations that can indicate a person's level of contrast sensitivity .

Visual Fields

Confrontation testing is typically used to screen for visual field deficits (Fig. 8-3). Visual fields are measured one eye at a time, and the client's visual fields are compared to the examiner's supposedly normal visual fields (Procedures for Practice 8-1). The normal limits of visual field are 60° superior, 75° inferior, 60° nasal, and 100° temporal (Simon, Aminoff, & Greenberg, 1999). Confrontation testing has been found to be relatively unreliable (Trobe et al., 1981) and should therefore be used in conjunction with functional observations. Scheiman (2002) has suggested a method of confrontation testing with two examiners when possible. Warren (1999) suggests observation of the client during a dynamic functional activity, such as walking through a crowded area with moving objects, as a means of screening for visual field deficit. Warren also presents some other methods of confrontation testing as part of the biVABA (1996).

Automated perimetry provides a more accurate description and printout of the client's visual field deficit. Figure 8-4 shows the results of a client with visual field

PROCEDURES FOR PRACTICE 8-1

Screening Visual Field Deficits: Confrontation Testing

Equipment

- Eye patch or patches.
- Interesting target mounted on a wand.

Set-Up

- Patient seated directly opposite examiner, approximately 20′′ eye to eye.
- Background behind examiner should be dark and distraction free.

Procedure

- Patch the patient's left eye, and close or patch your own right eye.
- Instruct patient to look at your left eye, and tell him or her you will be moving a target in from the side and the patient is to indicate when the target is first seen.
- Move target in from all angles (e.g., begin at 12 o'clock, then 2, 4, 6, 8, 10).
- Compare the patient's response with yours.
- Position hands at 3 and 9 o'clock so that you can just see your fingers. Ask the patient how many fingers you are holding up.
- Patch the patient's right eye, and close or patch your own left eye. Repeat the previous 4 steps.
- A problem is indicated if the patient cannot see the target when you do or if the patient does not see both fingers simultaneously.

Adapted from Scheiman, 2002.

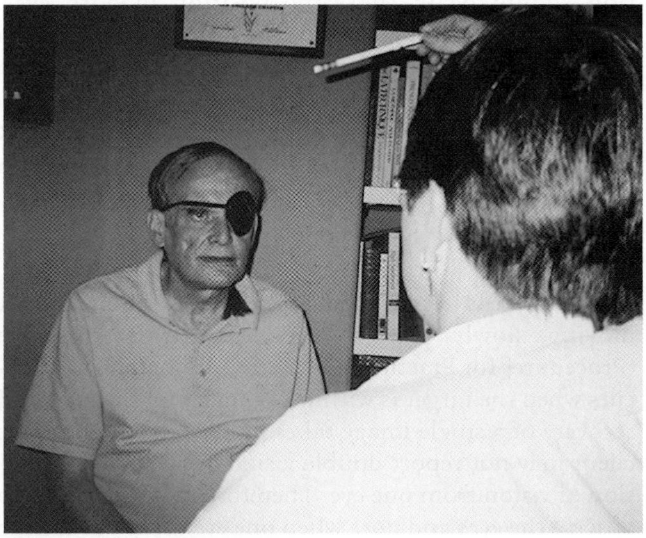

Figure 8-3 Confrontation test.

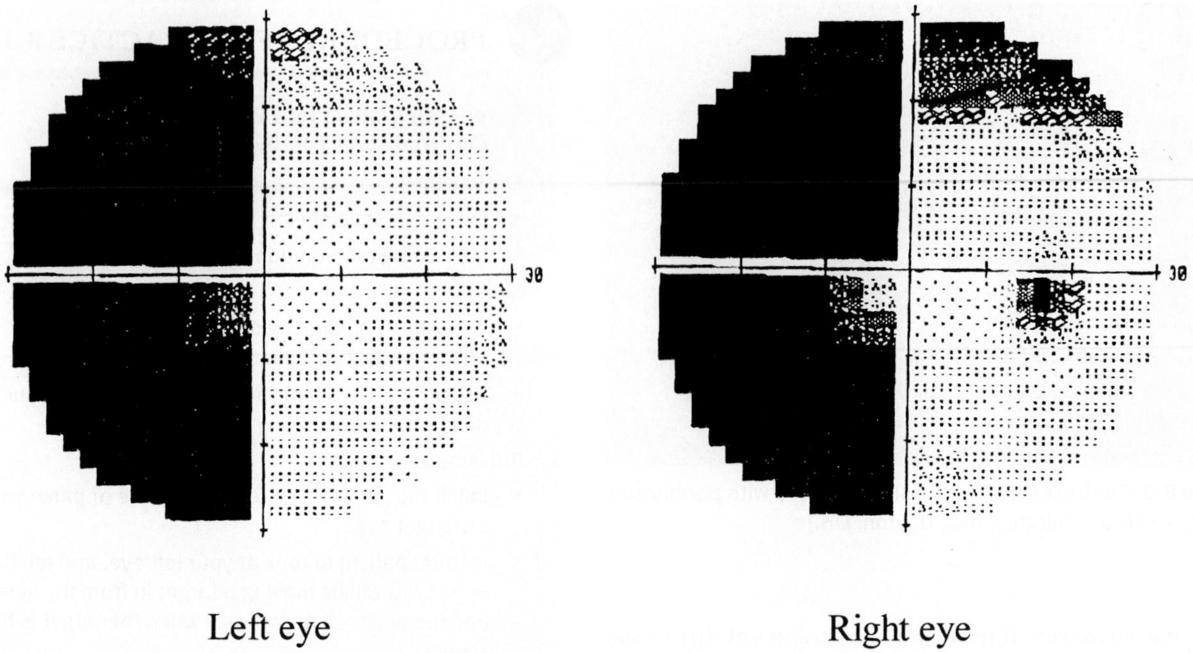

Figure 8-4 Automated perimetry results of a patient with RBD. The patient is unable to see anything in darkened areas (almost entire left visual field). There is some macular sparing on the left and a loss in the superior visual field in the right eye.

deficit. The results of the test are effectively used to teach the family and client regarding visual field losses. There are several limitations:

1. The test can require up to 20 minutes of sustained concentration if there are significant deficits, and therefore, clients unable to maintain that level of concentration cannot be accurately tested.
2. The test requires a motor response to push a button within 1–3 seconds of the presentation, which could exclude evaluation of clients with significantly delayed motor responses or motor planning deficits.
3. The equipment is expensive.

The client is generally referred to an eye care professional for perimetry testing. If the automated perimetry results are not available, the therapist can use the confrontation test along with close observation of the client during daily activities.

Oculomotor Control

Control of eye movements depends upon a complex interaction at cortical and subcortical levels. The role of the occupational therapist in screening oculomotor function is "not to diagnose the deficit, but to describe its functional effect and formulate the critical questions for the ophthalmologist or optometrist" (Warren, 1993b, p. 68). **Binocular vision** allows us to resolve two images, one from each eye, into one. It depends on good eye alignment and the ability of the eyes to converge and adjust focus at different distances. The therapist screens binocular vision, including eye alignment and convergence, and **accommodation**, smooth pursuits, and saccades.

Eye Alignment

Eye alignment is generally measured by observation of the reflection of light on the cornea. Seated in front of the client, the therapist asks him to gaze at a penlight held in different quadrants of the visual field. The therapist observes the light reflection in each eye; the reflection should be in the same position in both eyes. Directions that the eye or eyes turn are noted (Definition 8-2). Scheiman (2002) describes a method of evaluation of alignment using phoria cards (near and far), penlight, and a red Maddox Rod. Using this method, the therapist should be able to determine the amount of strabismus present.

Convergence

Convergence is tested by having the client follow a target moving slowly toward and away from the face (Procedures for Practice 8-2). Double vision normally occurs when the target is within 2–4 inches of the face, and recovery of a single image takes place at 4–6 inches. The client may not report double vision because of suppression of vision from one eye. Therefore, it is important to observe the eyes and note when one eye drifts out during convergence and pulls back in with fusion.

DEFINITION 8-2

Eye Movement

- Accommodation: ability of the eye to adjust focus at different distances.
  - Accommodative facility: speed of response and ability to maintain response over time.
  - Accommodative amplitude: amount of accommodation available (decreases with age).
- Convergence: ability to maintain focus as an object moves toward you.
  - Convergence insufficiency: unable to focus on a "near" object due to an exophoria at near distance.
- Diplopia: double vision.
- Phoria: tendency for the eyes to turn that is controlled with muscular effort.
  - Esophoria: tendency for the eye to turn inward.
  - Exophoria: tendency for the eye to turn outward.
  - Hyperphoria: tendency for the eye to turn upward.
  - Hypophoria: tendency for the eye to turn downward.
- Presbyopia: age-related loss of accommodation.
- Saccades: quick eye movements that change the fixation from one point to another and allow us to redirect our line of sight.
- Smooth pursuits: those eye movements that maintain continued fixation on a moving target.
- Stereopsis: depth perception; visual perception of three-dimensional space.
- Strabismus: misalignment of the eyes.
- Suppression: visual information from one eye is ignored (usually when there is a discrepancy between the two eyes).
- Tropia: synonym for strabismus.
  - Esotropia: strabismus in which the eye turns inward.
  - Exotropia: strabismus in which the eye turns outward.
  - Hypertropia: strabismus in which the eye turns upward.
  - Hypotropia: strabismus in which the eye turns downward.

Accommodation

Accommodation is the ability to adjust the focus of vision at a range of distances, such as the automatic focusing of the eyes when you look up from the speedometer to the road while driving. It decreases with age. Presbyopia, a condition of decreased near vision secondary to decreased accommodative ability, sets in at around 40–45 years of age. Information regarding the client's

PROCEDURES FOR PRACTICE 8-2

Screening: Convergence

Equipment

- Penlight or target.
- Ruler

Set-Up

- Patient seated directly opposite the therapist.
- Patient's head should be vertically erect.

Procedure

- Slowly move the penlight or target toward patient at eye level (do not shine light directly into the patient's eyes; direct it at the brow slightly above eye level).
- Ask patient to keep eyes on the light and to report when two lights are seen. Note the distance at which diplopia occurs.
- Once two lights are seen, move the target in another inch or so and begin to move it away from the patient.
- Ask patient to let you know when he or she can see one light again. Note the distance at which the patient reports single vision.

Adapted from Scheiman, 2002.

accommodative ability is typically picked up by observing and listening to the client's complaints. If the client is over 40–45 years old, expect accommodation to be decreased. With younger clients, Scheiman (2002) presents a method for the occupational therapist to determine their accommodation.

Visual Tracking

Visual tracking (smooth pursuits) are eye movements that maintain continued fixation on a moving target. Smooth pursuits, which are influenced by age, attention, and motivation, play a significant role in activities entailing movement of either the person or the object of regard (e.g., driving, playing sports). If smooth pursuits are impaired, acuity is impaired when motion is involved (Haarmeier & Thier, 1999). Smooth pursuits are usually evaluated by asking the client to track a moving object (Procedures for Practice 8-3). Warren (1999) suggests using a penlight in a slightly darkened room. Scheiman (2002) presents a method of scoring in which performance is scored on: (1) ability to complete two rotations in both directions; (2) accuracy (number of refixations required); and (3) head and body movement during the test.

PROCEDURES FOR PRACTICE 8-3

Screening: Smooth Pursuits and Visual Tracking

Equipment

- Small, interesting target.

Set-Up

- Patient seated directly in front of the examiner.
- Hold target approximately 16 inches from the patient's face.

Procedure

- Give no instructions regarding head movement.
- Tell patient, "Watch the target and don't take your eyes off it."
- Move target clockwise for two rotations and counter-clockwise for two rotations.
- Observe:

  Number of rotations the patient is able to complete.

  Ability to maintain fixation, that is, the number of times the patient has to refixate.

  Movement of the head or body.

Adapted from Scheiman, 2002.

PROCEDURES FOR PRACTICE 8-4

Screening: Saccades

Equipment

- Two interesting targets (e.g., two tongue depressors, one with a green circle on the end and the other with a red circle on the end).

Set-Up

- Patient seated directly in front of the examiner.

Procedure

- Hold wands approximately 16 inches from the face, separated by approximately 8 inches.
- Give no instructions regarding head movement.
- Tell patient, "Look at the red dot when I say red. Look at the green dot when I say green, and remember to wait until I say to look."
- Tell patient to look from one target to the other for a total of 10 fixations, 5 round trips.
- Observe:

  Ability to complete 5 round trips.

  Accuracy of eye movements (overshooting or undershooting target).

  Movement of the head or body.

Adapted from Scheiman, 2002.

Saccades

Saccades are quick eye movements that change fixation from one point to another and allow us to redirect our line of sight. These eye movements are more closely related to reading and close work and may appear more problematic following brain injury (Gianutsos, 1997). Saccades are tested by holding up two targets and asking the client to keep looking from one target to another (Procedures for Practice 8-4). Performance of saccades is scored on: (1) ability to complete five round trips; (2) accuracy (amount of over- and undershooting); and (3) head and body movement during the test (Scheiman, 2002).

Considerations for the Minimally Responsive Patient

Because visual testing requires attention and cooperation, it is often put off until clients have recovered and their neurological systems have settled down. It is imperative that we begin to look at the visual system as early as possible. How much better may clients do in therapy if corrective action is taken early in their stay? Whyte and DiPasquale (1995) present a method of assessing vision in minimally responsive clients (Procedures for Practice 8-5). The evaluation takes only a short time to administer and can be given frequently by various team members to provide a pattern of responses that are "more interpretable than clinician's unstructured observations" (Whyte and DiPasquale, 1995, p. 810). The relationship between side, stimulus, and frequency of eye movements is analyzed: (1) total number of eye movements in each direction (unequal distribution of eye movements suggests gaze preference, asymmetric visual fields, or visual attention deficit); (2) frequency of eye movement to stimulus side (contingent orienting); (3) difference in orienting to photos versus cards (as evidence of visual perception); and (4) comparison of bilateral to unilateral presentations. The authors found that they were able to identify hemifield deficits, extinction, and monocular pathology with this method (Whyte & DiPasquale, 1995).

Unilateral Neglect

Visual attention allows us to determine the what (object identification) and where (orientation in space) of things in our environment (Warren, 1999). Visual attention is influenced by general alertness, both nonspatial and spatial. It is evaluated through scanning tasks because a change in

PROCEDURES FOR PRACTICE 8-5

Assessment of Vision in Minimally Responsive Patients

Equipment

- Six brightly colored snapshots from patient's family.
- Plain white card, same size as photos.
- Eye patch as needed.

Set-Up

- Examiner stands 6 feet in front of patient, at patient's visual midline.
- Use eye patch for patients with dysconjugate gaze.

Procedure

- Pictures are presented at ear level, 30–40° lateral to midline.
- May give alerting stimulation prior to presentation as needed.
- Pictures are present in 6 combinations (order can be varied from session to session):

Left Field	Right Field
Photo	—
—	Photo
Card	—
—	Card
Photo	Card
Card	Photo

- Record the direction of the first lateral eye movement for each presentation. Record "no response" if there is no movement in 5 seconds.

Adapted from Whyte & DiPasquale, 1995.

visual attention is manifested as a change in visual search (Warren, 1999). Visual attention can be influenced by the perceptual load, whether it be visual, tactile, or auditory (Mattingley et al., 1997; Robertson et al., 1997).

Unilateral neglect, a constellation of symptoms affecting both perceptual and exploratory behavior, has variously been called unilateral neglect, hemispatial neglect, and hemi-inattention. It is a heterogeneous condition that includes both behavioral components and related disorders (Table 8-1). Unilateral neglect manifests as a failure to respond or orient to stimuli presented contralateral to a brain lesion (Heilman, Watson, & Valenstein, 1993). It is observed functionally in the client who eats the food on only half of the plate, shaves only one side of his face, and so on. It is most commonly caused by a lesion in the right hemisphere; it does occur following left brain damage (LBD), although the deficit is usually not as severe as for right brain damage (RBD) (Heilman, Watson, & Valenstein, 1997; Mennemeier et al., 1997; Stone, Halligan, & Greenwood, 1993).

The incidence of neglect varies widely in the literature. This is most likely because of a lack of a common definition, differences among tests used to evaluate neglect, and/or laterality of motor response (Mercier, Hebert, & Gauthier, 1995; Maeshima et al., 2001).

Although it is generally agreed that neglect is related to a deficit in attention, just how this happens is still under discussion. Kinsbourne (1993) proposes a model in which attention to right and left space is controlled by the contralateral hemisphere. When one hemisphere is damaged, the other becomes disinhibited and biases attention toward the contralateral side. Another view focuses on the hyporesponsiveness of the damaged hemisphere (Heilman & Watson, 1977). Posner and Rafal (1987) suggest that the problem is an inability to disengage attention from objects in ipsilateral space.

Visual field deficits and unilateral neglect frequently occur together and are difficult to separate. Warren (1999) suggests that it is possible to differentiate the two by observing how clients organize their search patterns during a scanning task (Table 8-2). A client who exhibits the behaviors listed for visual field deficit probably has no more than mild neglect, whereas if he or she demonstrates the neglect behaviors, you cannot assume that there are no field cuts.

Table 8-1. Unilateral Neglect Syndrome

Main Behavioral Components:

- Hemi-inattention: inability to orient to or respond to stimuli from one side of the environment, irrespective of the modality.
- Hemispatial visual neglect: inability to orient to relevant contralateral visual stimuli.
- Extinction: failure to report a contralesional stimulus when it occurs simultaneously with a more ipsilateral stimulus, even though able to do so if either is presented alone.
- Allesthesia: consistently attributing sensory stimuli on one side of the body to the other side, or moving limbs on one side when requested to move the limb on the other side.
- Hemiakinesia: motor neglect.

Related Disorders:

- Anosognosia: lack of awareness or denial of hemiparesis.
- Gaze paresis.
- Visual field deficit.

Adapted from Stone, Halligan, & Greenwood, 1993; Stone et al., 1998.

Table 8-2. Scanning: Visual Field Deficit Versus Unilateral Neglect

Visual Field Deficit	Unilateral Neglect
Abbreviated scanning pattern	Disorganized, random scanning pattern
Scanning pattern is organized	Asymmetrical search pattern in hemispace
Re-scanning is observed	Scanning pattern is carried out with reduced effort and little or no re-scanning
Length of time/effort are appropriate for the task	Task is completed swiftly, or if patient is aware of deficit, will take an inordinate amount of time in an attempt to compensate

Adapted from Warren, 1999.

Sensory Neglect

Two major subtypes of unilateral neglect have been described: sensory (input or attentional) and motor (output or intentional) (Bisiach et al., 1990; Coslett et al., 1990; Tegner & Levander, 1991). Sensory neglect can include awareness of all stimuli on one side of the space (spatial neglect) or be confined to one side of the body (personal neglect) (Heilman, Watson, & Valenstein, 1997). It may be evident in any of the modalities, including auditory, tactile, and visual. Historically, neglect has generally been referred to in the horizontal (right–left) dimension, although some research has been done on neglect in the vertical and radial (near and far space) dimensions (Cowey, Small, & Ellis, 1994; Kageyama et al., 1994; Ladavas, Carletti, & Gori, 1994). Neglect of visual imagery (e.g., mental images of familiar places, spelling, drawing from memory) has been termed representational neglect (Beschin et al., 1997).

Evaluating neglect can be confusing because the client can exhibit neglect in one situation but not in another (Halligan & Marshall, 1998; Riddoch & Humphreys, 1994). Neglect can vary as follows:

- Locus of lesion: The inferior and posterior parietal cortex are critical for monitoring and directing attention in the visual environment; anterior and frontal lesions result in difficulty executing movement in or toward the side contralateral to the lesion.
- Task: For example, verbal tasks versus spatial tasks; complexity and perceptual load of the task (e.g., one object vs. several objects).
- Mode of response: Verbal versus contralateral extremity versus ipsilateral extremity.
- Modality: Visual, auditory, tactile.

Unilateral neglect has traditionally been evaluated in a variety of ways, largely with paper and pencil tasks, including drawing tasks, cancellation tasks, line bisection, and reading (Chatterjee & Mennemeier, 1997).

Drawing and Copying Tasks

Drawing and copying tasks, although easy to give, are subjective in their scoring. In all such tasks, the therapist looks for omissions and errors concentrated to one side (Fig. 8-5). The therapist also observes how the client approaches the task, variations between copying and free drawing, and missing elements on one side of the picture or on one side of objects within the picture. These tasks can alert you to a moderate or severe neglect but should be used in conjunction with other tests of neglect and functional activities to provide a clear picture of mild neglect.

Cancellation Tasks

Another common evaluation method is cancellation tasks. These tests are easy to administer and score and are sensitive to neglect (Sea, Henderson, & Cermak, 1993; Stam & Bakker, 1990; Ferber & Karnath, 2001; Maeshima

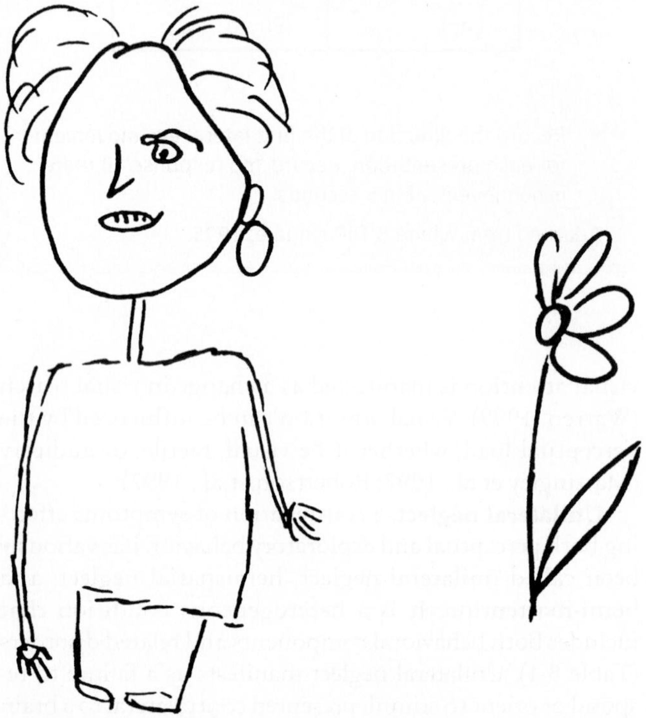

Figure 8-5 Drawings by patients with RBD and unilateral neglect.

et al., 2001). The client is presented with a sheet of paper with several lines of letters or shapes and is asked to mark a specific stimulus letter or shape that is scattered randomly throughout the page. Cancellation tasks can be varied in many ways, including overall density, whether the display is organized or random, density of stimuli in ipsilateral space, complexity of stimuli in ipsilateral space, and amount of similarity between the target and distracters (Dawson & Tanner-Cohen, 1997; Heilman, Watson, & Valenstein, 1997; Kartsounis & Findley, 1994). The score is usually based on the number of omissions (targets not marked) and commissions (cancellations of items other than the target) as well as where on the page the errors are made. Because of these many variations, it is important that various tasks, as part of a neglect battery, should be used to fully detect neglect (Maeshima et al., 2001).

DEFINITION 8-3

Motor Neglect

- Limb akinesia—failure to move limb.
- Hypokinesia—limb moves but only after a long delay and much encouragement.
- Hypometria—movements are of decreased amplitude.
- Impersistence—inability to maintain a movement or posture.
- Motor perseveration—inability to disengage from a motor activity.
- Motor extinction—delay or failure to move the contralesional limb when also required to move the ipsilateral limb.

Adapted from Heilman, Watson, & Valenstein, 1997.

Line Bisection

Line bisection, another traditional test, requires the client to divide a line or lines in the center (Schenkenberg, Bradford, & Ajax, 1980). The therapist will note the direction and amount of deviation from center. The following factors can increase the percentage of error on line bisection tests: longer line, line placement in contralesional space, and cues placed on the ipsilateral end of the line (Heilman, Watson, & Valenstein, 1997). Ferber and Karnath (2001) compared line bisection tests with cancellation tests and found that cancellation tests were better able to detect spatial neglect than line bisection. They felt that line bisection could be influenced by such things as presence of a visual field deficit or what hand was used.

Functional Tests

Appelros et al. (2003) stress the "importance of not relying completely on test instruments when diagnosing unilateral neglect" (p. 478). As a result, there has been an emphasis on evaluation of unilateral neglect during functional activities (Assessment Table 8-1). The occupational therapist is in a position to observe the client in a variety of daily activities that can provide vital information for the team. A client is likely to perform differently in a quiet test room than in an everyday situation, such as dressing or preparing a simple meal.

Motor neglect

Motor neglect presents as impaired initiation or execution of movement into contralateral hemispace by either limb (Bisiach et al., 1990; Tegner & Levander, 1991). Heilman, Watson, and Valenstein (1997) describe several types of motor neglect (Definition 8-3). It is often difficult to differentiate between sensory and motor neglect because tests of motor neglect entail some form of sensory input. Consequently, the therapists wonder whether clients fail to respond to a stimulus on the involved side because they don't see it or because they cannot initiate movement toward it. If motor neglect is suspected, one way to distinguish between the two entails contrasting a task that requires a hand response with one that has minimal motor response (e.g., naming letters on the involved side as opposed to pointing to the same letters). In other words, the stimulus (letters on the involved side) stays the same, and the motor response is varied (Riddoch & Humphreys, 1994).

Although there are no standardized tests of motor neglect (Appelros et al., 2003), observations of clients and how they use the extremity can provide insight into the presence of motor neglect. One may note reluctance to move the arm and movement only after a delay (hypokinesia) or movement only with strong encouragement (akinesia), a tendency to undershoot a target when asked to move along a given line (hypometria), or inability to sustain a posture (impersistence) (Heilman, Watson, & Valenstein, 1997). Different limbs can be observed, as can the direction of the movement required (ipsilateral vs. contralateral) and the hemispace in which the movement is to occur (ipsilateral vs. contralateral).

ASSESSING PRAXIS

People rapidly conceive of and plan motor acts in response to the environment (Crepeau, 1998). This innate capacity is referred to as praxis. **Apraxia** is the inability to carry out skilled movement in the presence of intact sensation, movement, and coordination (Heilman & Rothi, 1993). Apraxia is generally seen in patients with LBD (Goodglass & Kaplan, 1972; Haaland, Harrington, & Yeo, 1987; Poeck,

Assessment Table 8-1

Summary of Functional Assessments for Unilateral Neglect

Instrument and Reference	Description	Time to Administer	Validity	Reliability	Sensitivity	Strengths and Weaknesses
Catherine Bergego Scale (*CBS*) (Azouvi et al., 1996; Azouvi et al., 2002; Azouvi et al., 2003)	10 items from everyday life situations (e.g., grooming left side of face, collisions with people or objects on the left). Unilateral neglect scored on 4-point scale: 0 = no neglect observed; 3 = severe neglect; client only able to access right hemispace.	Unknown, but would be observed during the occupational therapist's evaluation of ADLs.	Internal consistency: Rho ranged from 0.58–0.88. *CBS* score correlated significantly with performance on 5 paper and pencil tests (Rho = 0.50–0.74). Significant correlation between *CBS* and *Barthel Index* (Rho = −0.63)	Inter-rater reliability: K ranged from 0.59–0.99 (Rho = 0.96).	Authors found it more sensitive than conventional paper and pencil tests.	Strengths: It is a direct observation of a client's function during everyday activities and provides the client with insight into their deficits. Weaknesses: Training recommended for inexperienced therapists unfamiliar with unilateral neglect. Difficulty differentiating sensory and motor neglect.
Wheelchair Collision Test (*WCT*) (Qiang et al., 2005)	Patient propels a wheelchair around 4 chairs arranged in 2 rows placed at 2 different distances apart (120 cm and 140 cm). Patient collisions with chairs are considered abnormal.	10 minutes.	Relationship between number of collisions and *CBS* total score: $r = 0.72$ at 120 cm and $r = 0.75$ at 140 cm.	Test–retest reliability = 0.68–0.97.	Not established.	Strengths: Easy to set-up and score in clinic setting; short time to complete. Weaknesses: Small number of subjects (19); no scoring range given; possible learning effect; only looked at one aspect of neglect; did not address RBD.

Baking Tray Task (Tham & Tegner, 1996)	Patient is asked to spread out 16 'buns' on a 'baking tray.' The number of cubes in each half field are counted. Distribution of cubes skewed greater than 7 on one side and 9 on the other is considered abnormal.	Task is not timed.	Did not significantly correlate with conventional neglect tests (e.g., line cancellation, line bisection, drawing).	Not established.	Relative sensitivity for visual spatial neglect is 66.7% (Bailey, Riddoch, & Crome, 2000).	Strengths: Short and easy to present and evaluate. Weaknesses: Addresses one area of neglect only; doesn't correlate with other tests of neglect; task is somewhat gender specific.
Comb & Razor/ Compact Test (Beschin & Robertson, 1997)	Patient is asked to comb the hair and shave (males) or use a compact (females) for 30 seconds. The number of strokes and where they occurred (right, left, and ambiguous) are counted. Score is determined by dividing the number of strokes on the left by the total of all strokes. A score of <0.35 indicates neglect.	30 seconds for each of 2 tasks plus set-up and explanation.	Significant difference between 4 groups of experimental subjects (F = 18.0; d.f. = 3,57; $p < 0.0001$).	Test–retest: $r = 0.94$.	Not established.	Strength: Short, simple test of personal neglect. Weakness: Must be combined with tests of extrapersonal neglect for clear picture of neglect.
Behavioral Inattention Test (BIT) (Wilson, Cockburn, & Halligan, 1987)	15-item standardized test battery: 6 pen and paper tests and 9 behavioral tasks. Cut-off scores are used to indicate neglect.	Approximately 30 minutes.	Correlation between *BIT* and *Barthel Index*: $r = 0.642$ (Cassidy et al., 1999); correlation between *BIT* behavior subtests and items on an ADL checklist: $r = 0.77$ (Hartman-Maeir & Katz, 1995).	Test–retest: $r = 0.99$; inter-rater reliability: $r = 0.99$.	Behavioral subtests were found to differ between groups: neglect and no neglect (Hartman-Maeir & Katz, 1995).	Strength: Includes functional as well as conventional tests. Weaknesses: Two subtests (map navigation and picture scanning) were found to not correlate with a functional ADL activity (Hartman- Maeir & Katz, 1995); measures neglect in peripersonal space only and cannot distinguish between sensory and motor neglect.

1985). These patients generally can spontaneously use the extremity in such everyday tasks as eating, shaving, or opening a door, but if they are asked to pantomime an activity or carry out a series of steps, their performance is not correctly or smoothly executed.

Research has shown that LBD patients are clumsy, with more dexterity errors than normal controls (Sunderland et al., 1999). When meal-time eating behavior of apraxic patients was compared to that of normal subjects, the patients were found to be less efficient, be less well organized when sequencing activities, and produce more action errors (Foundas et al., 1995). These findings suggest that limb apraxia can affect activities of daily living. How it impacts a particular client depends upon his or her goals and lifestyle. For instance, if the client is aphasic as well, understanding and production of gestures is an important part of communication with others, and apraxia may need to be considered more closely.

There are five types of apraxia: verbal, buccofacial, limb, constructional, and dressing. The first two, which are usually evaluated by a speech and language pathologist, are not discussed in this chapter.

Limb Apraxia

Limb apraxia is usually associated with LBD in right-handed patients and RBD in left-handed patients (Heilman, Rothi, & Watson, 1997), although variations have been described (Marchetti & Della Sala, 1997). According to Heilman, Rothi, & Watson (1997), there are six types of limb apraxia: limb kinetic, ideomotor,

Table 8-3. Types of Limb Apraxia

Type of Apraxia	Error Type	How Elicited	Functional Example
Ideomotor	Production errors	Most errors are made on pantomiming transitive tasks; improves with imitation and usually does best with the actual object.	Movements will be awkward but will bear a resemblance to the intended movement. Able to use tools to complete tasks but may appear clumsy or awkward.
Conceptual	Content errors: • Tool-action knowledge • Tool-association knowledge • Mechanical knowledge • Tool fabrication	Use of tools; actions associated with specific tools, association between tool and object.	Patient has obvious difficulty with tool use: may use a tube of toothpaste to brush teeth, comb hair with fork, etc.
Disassociation	Thought to be a disconnection between hemispheres; therefore, there is no recognizable movement on command.	Pantomime to command is impaired; imitation and use of object will be much better.	Unable to pantomime movements, but since able to imitate and use tools, minimal effect on functional activities.
Conduction	Difficulty decoding and understanding gestures.	Impaired imitation of gestures; does better when asked to pantomime.	A client with aphasia might have difficulty understanding and using gestures.
Ideational	Difficulty with a series of tasks.	Tasks requiring a series of activities (e.g., clean pipe, put in tobacco, and light pipe).	Task may be completed more skillfully than with ideomotor apraxia, but client will have difficulty sequencing steps in the correct order (e.g., client might try to light the empty pipe, then put the tobacco in, then clean it).

Adapted from Heilman, Watson, & Rothi, 1997.

ideational, dissociation, conduction, and conceptual (Table 8-3). Limb kinetic apraxia is characterized by a loss of ability to make finely graded precise finger movements and is thought to be a motor problem rather than a true apraxia (Heilman, Watson, & Rothi, 1997).

Testing has traditionally consisted of gesture production. The client is asked to pantomime a task on command (e.g., "Show me how you comb your hair"), to imitate the tester, or to use an object. These assessments require various types of gestures, including transitive gestures that entail object use (e.g., "Show me how a man shaves"), intransitive gestures that are meant to express ideas or feelings (e.g., "Show me how you wave goodbye"), meaningless or nonsymbolic gestures (e.g., "Put your hand under your chin"), proximal gestures (e.g., "Show me how you bounce a ball"), and distal gestures (e.g., "Show me how you would use a telegraph key"). Transitive gestures are especially sensitive to apraxia (Haaland, 1993). Generally, clients with apraxia would have least difficulty with proximal intransitive gestures away from the body (e.g., waving goodbye) and most difficulty with distal transitive gestures on the body (e.g., putting on makeup) (Haaland, 1993; Helm-Estabrooks & Albert, 1991). In the last decade, gesture comprehension and discrimination have been added to the list of apraxia testing methods (Heilman & Rothi, 1993; York & Cermak, 1995; Joseph, 1996; Heilman, Watson, & Rothi, 1997) (Table 8-4).

Apraxia often occurs in conjunction with aphasia, and it is sometimes difficult to distinguish between the two. Therefore, it is important when evaluating a client with aphasia to include (besides the regular commands, e.g., "show me how you would . . . ") questions that can be answered by yes/no responses and by pointing at the correct answers (Heilman & Rothi, 1993). If the client performs poorly but can answer yes/no questions, he or she may be apraxic. Similarly, if the client is unable to respond to yes/no questions, failure to make the appropriate movement to command may be due to a language problem rather than apraxia. If the client has only a mild language deficit but uses a body part as object or makes a

Table 8-4. Apraxia Testing Methods

Method	Example
Gesture to command: Should include both transitive movements (tool use) and intransitive movements (nonverbal communication).	Transitive: "Show me how you would open the door with a key, use a hammer." Intransitive: "Show me how you hitchhike, salute, wave good-bye."
Gesture to imitation	Examiner produces a gesture and asks the client to "do it the same way I do it; don't name the gesture and don't start until I'm finished"; can be familiar gestures or nonsense gestures (e.g., hand to the forehead).
Gesture in response to tool	Visual: Examiner shows the tool and says, "Show me how you use this." Tactile: With eyes closed or covered, client examines the tool by hand and examiner says, "Show me how you use this."
Gesture in response to seeing object on which the tool acts: tool selection task	Examiner presents client with object representing an incomplete action (e.g., if the target is sawing, client is shown a partially cut piece of wood); client must choose the correct tool from a choice of three, one of which is the saw.
Actual tool use	Patient is given a tool (e.g., hammer) and asked, "Show me how you use this."
Gesture decision: discrimination between correctly and incorrectly pantomimed movements	Examiner makes a gesture and asks the client, "Is this the correct way to. . ." (e.g., use a pair of scissors).
Gesture comprehension	Examiner makes a gesture and asks the client, "Tell me what I am doing." "What tool am I using?" "Am I using a hammer or a saw?"
Serial acts	Examiner tells client, "Fold letter, put it in an envelope, seal envelope, and place stamp on it."

Adapted from Heilman & Rothi, 1993; Rothi, Raymer, & Heilman, 1997.

Table 8-5. Sample Items from the *Florida Apraxia Screening Test–Revised*

Show me:
How you salute.
How to use a saw to cut a piece of wood out in front of you.
How you hitchhike.
Stop.
How to use a salt shaker to salt food on a table out in front of you.
How to use a spoon to stir coffee on a table out in front of you.

Rothi, Raymer, & Heilman, 1997.

clumsy but recognizable response, it is probably due to apraxia rather than language. When assessing people with severe aphasia, provide a model for the client to imitate or place the object out of reach and ask the client to pantomime its use. Use the tactile modality in testing by having the client handle the object while blindfolded and then show how it is used.

There are few standardized tests available for limb apraxia. Rothi and her colleagues have developed the *Florida Apraxia Screening Test–Revised* (*FAST-R*) for use in the research of neurologically impaired patients (Rothi, Raymer, & Heilman, 1997). This test consists of 30 items that are presented verbally (Table 8-5). The patient uses the dominant arm if possible. Prior to testing, patients practice pantomiming such that they pretend they hold the imagined tool and act on the imagined object. This rehearsal is important to discourage use of a body part as the imagined tool itself. Normal subjects may use a body part as tool, but with instruction, they correct their performance, whereas apraxic patients continue to do so even with the instruction (Raymer et al., 1997). Scoring for the *FAST-R* includes multiple error types based on content of the pantomime, timing and sequencing of the response, and spatial features (Table 8-6).

Tests of apraxia described in the literature all rely on observer judgment of errors made during movement performance (Assessment Table 8-2). Some researchers suggest more than one observer or even videotaping the response during testing. Butler (2002) advises to not rely on one test of apraxia, but rather to consider functional indices in ADL tasks as more clinically relevant. van Heugten et al. (1999b) developed an assessment of disability in stroke patients with apraxia that looks at an independence measure and three aspects (initiation, execution, and control) of four activities (personal hygiene, dressing, preparing food, and another activity that is chosen by the therapist). This allows the therapist to determine in what area the person is having difficulty and better focus treatment.

Constructional Apraxia

Constructional apraxia is a specific deficit in spatial-organizational performance (Benton & Tranel, 1993). Patients with constructional apraxia have difficulty with copying, drawing, and constructing designs in two and three dimensions. Constructional apraxia has been found to correlate with deficits of activities of daily living (Baum & Hall, 1981; Neistadt, 1993; Warren, 1981). It can be seen functionally as difficulty with such activities as setting a table, making a sandwich, and making a dress and with any mechanical activity in which parts are to be combined into a whole.

Constructional apraxia can be found in both RBD and LBD patients. Because of qualitative differences noted in the performance of RBD and LBD patients (Definition 8-1), constructional apraxia in RBD is believed to be the result of visuospatial deficits, while that in LBD is thought to be caused by an executive or conceptual disorder (Benton, 1967; Piercy, Hecaen, & Ajuriaguerra, 1960). Constructional apraxia has often been found to be more frequent and more severe in RBD patients (Arrigoni & DeRenzi, 1964; Benton & Fogel, 1962; Piercy, Hecaen, & Ajuriaguerra, 1960; Warrington, James, & Kinsbourne, 1966).

There are two types of constructional activities used in assessment: graphic tasks (e.g., copying line drawings and drawing to command) and assembly tasks (e.g., block and stick designs). Both types are included in an evaluation of constructional apraxia. The most common example of a graphic task is copying geometric shapes (from simple to complex) and drawing without a model (e.g., house, clock, flower). It is best to use a simple task (e.g., simple geometric figures, three-dimensional block design) because a more complex task involves a greater number of skills and becomes less specific (DeRenzi, 1997).

Goodglass and Kaplan (1972) describe the test of drawing to command. This test includes having the client draw a clock, daisy, elephant, cross, cube, and house; scoring criteria are given in Table 8-7.

Assembly tasks include such activities as stick arrangement and three-dimensional block designs. Common errors on stick arrangement include selecting sticks of incorrect length; failing to reproduce parts of

Table 8-6. Apraxia Error Types

Error Type	Description
Content Errors	
Perseveration	Patient's response includes all or part of a previously produced pantomime.
Related	Pantomime is correctly produced but only related to the action requested (e.g., playing the trombone instead of playing a bugle).
Nonrelated	Pantomime is accurately produced but unrelated to request (e.g., playing the trombone for shaving).
Hand	Performs the action without use of a real or imagined tool (e.g., turning a screw with the fingers rather than an imaginary screwdriver).
Temporal	
Sequencing	Addition, deletion, or transposition of the movement elements of a sequence.
Timing	Any alteration in the timing or speed of a pantomime: abnormally increased, decreased, or irregular rate of production.
Occurrence	Any multiplication of characteristically single-cycle movements (e.g., unlocking a door) or reduction of a characteristically repetitive cycle (e.g., screwing in a screw) to a single event.
Spatial	
Amplitude	Any increase, decrease, or irregularity of the characteristic movement.
Internal Configuration	Any abnormality of the required finger/hand posture and its relationship to the target tool (e.g., when pretending to brush the teeth, the hand may be closed tightly into a fist with no space allowed for the imagined toothbrush handle).
Body Part as Tool	Patient uses finger, hand, or arm as the imagined tool, even when requested to pretend he or she is holding the object (e.g., uses the finger to brush the teeth).
External Configuration	Difficulties orienting the fingers/hand/arm to the object or in placing the object in space (e.g, brushing teeth with the hand so close to the mouth as to not allow room for the imagined toothbrush).
Movement	Any disturbance of the characteristic movement used when acting on an object (e.g., movement at incorrect joint; when pantomiming a screwdriver and rotation occurs at the shoulder rather than at the forearm).
Other	
Concretization	Patient performs pantomime not on an imagined object but, instead, on a real object not normally used in the task (e.g., instead of pretending to saw wood, they pantomime sawing on their leg).
No Response	
Unrecognizable	Response shares no temporal or spatial features of the target; it is unrecognizable.

Adapted from Rothi, Raymer, & Heilman, 1997.

the model, especially lateral; making lines more oblique than the model indicates; tending to remove part of the model to make the copy; and crowding in (the client's copy rests on top of or touches the model) (Critchley, 1966). Assembly tasks can be varied in numerous ways. For example, constructing from memory may be more difficult than copying from a model (representational or actual). Patients may be asked to choose the correct pieces from a large number of blocks and sticks versus providing them with the correct number and type of blocks and sticks, which would structure the task and make it simpler.

In general, these tasks are not standardized and rely on subjective judgment of the results. It is important to note the client's method of completing the task; the client's comments; any emotional display, hesitancy, indecision, and change of mind; and the type of errors made.

The *Lowenstein Occupational Therapy Cognitive Assessment* (*LOTCA*) battery was standardized on brain-injured adults and contains a section on visuomotor organization (Katz et al., 1989). This section contains block design, copying, drawing, and pegboard design (see Assessment Table 9.1 in Chapter 9).

Assessment Table 8-2

Summary of Assessments for Apraxia

Instrument and Reference	Description	Time to Administer	Validity	Reliability	Sensitivity	Strengths and Weaknesses
Florida Apraxia Screening Test–Revised (FAST-R) (Rothi, Raymer, & Heilman, 1997)	30-item, gesture to verbal command test: 20 transitive and 10 intransitive pantomime items; scored on multiple error types. Normal cut-off score is 15 out of 30 correct.	Unknown; includes time to train and practice pantomime and then to complete a 30-item test.	Not established.	Not established. Recommend that the responses are videotaped for later scoring.	Not established.	Strength: Can be completed with one hand only. Weaknesses: Coexisting aphasia can be a problem due to verbal presentation. Relates to limb apraxia only. Scoring can be difficult and requires too much time for clinic use. No psychometric characteristics established.
Screening for Apraxia (Almeida, Black, & Roy, 2002)	5 gestures (3 transitive, 2 intransitive); 5 dimensions for each task are scored on a 3-point scale (see Roy et al., 1998 for scoring).	Authors feel that this can be used to detect apraxia and then decision can be made to follow-up with a more comprehensive assessment battery.	Not established.	Not established on screen; kappa coefficient for inter-rater reliability ranged from 0.71–0.78 on the full battery (Roy et al., 1998).	Not established.	Strength: Short 5-item screening test. Weakness: Scoring is unclear and requires knowledge and practice on the part of the examiner.

Assessment of Apraxia (van Heugten et al., 1999a)	2 subtests: demonstration of object use (3 sets of objects presented under 3 different conditions) and imitation of gestures (6 gestures to be imitated). Each is scored from 0 (movement not recognizable) to 3 (performance is correct and appropriate). Maximum subscore is 54 for object use and 36 for imitation of gestures, with a total score of 90. Total score below 86 is considered to identify apraxia.	Unknown.	Not established.	Internal consistency good (Cronbach's alpha = 0.96; Mokken coefficient of reliability, Rho = 0.96); interrater reliability kappa > 0.60 on all but 3 items (Zwinkels et al., 2004).	At cut-off score of 86 (mean score − one standard deviation), sensitivity was 91%.	Strength: Uses common gestures and objects. Weakness: Includes items for ideational and ideomotor apraxia only.
Assessment of Disabilities in Stroke Patients with Apraxia (van Heugten et al., 1999b)	Set of standard ADL observations for assessment of disabilities due to apraxia: personal hygiene, dressing, preparing food, and another of the therapist's choice. Scoring: 4 measures (independence, initiation, execution, and control) scored from 0 (no observable problems) to 3 (therapist has to take over). Then these scores can be added together to get a total score.	Unknown, but could easily be observed during the occupational therapist's evaluation of ADL.	Not established.	Coefficient of reliability, Rho = 0.94. Interrater reliability: kappa value highest for independence scores (0.81–0.97), increased variability on aspect (initiation, execution, control) scores.	Not established.	Strengths: Can be easily incorporated into the therapist's ADL evaluation; task specifically related to the client can be addressed; allows therapist to determine where the breakdown is occurring (initiation, execution, or control) to develop treatment program. Weakness: Training is recommended to improve reliability.

Table 8-7. Scoring for Drawing to Command

Shape	Instruction	Scoring
Clock	"Draw the face of a clock showing the numbers and the two hands."	0 to 3: one point each for approximately circular face, symmetry of number placement, and correctness of numbers
Daisy	"Draw a daisy."	0 to 2: one point each for general shape (center with petals around it) and symmetry of petal arrangement
Elephant	"Draw an elephant."	0 to 2: one point each for general shape (legs, trunk, head, body) and relative proportions correct
Cross	"You know what the Red Cross looks like? Draw an outline of it without taking your pencil off the paper."	0 to 2: one point each for basic configuration and ability to form all corners adequately with a continuous line
Cube	"Draw a cube-shaped block in perspective, as it would look if you could see the top and two sides."	0 to 2: one point each for grossly correct attempt and correctness of perspective
House	"Draw a house in perspective, so you can see the roof and two sides."	0 to 2: one point each for grossly correct features of house and accuracy of perspective

Dressing Apraxia

Dressing apraxia refers to an inability to dress oneself. It is usually due to RBD and secondary visuospatial disorganization. It is evaluated functionally by watching clients dress themselves. The underlying problem needs to be determined (e.g., visual deficits, unilateral neglect, apraxia, constructional apraxia), rather than evaluating dressing apraxia per se.

CASE EXAMPLE

Assessing Vison After Stroke

Occupational Therapy Assessment Process	Clinical Reasoning Process: Objectives	Clinical Reasoning Process: Examples of Therapist's Internal Dialogue
Patient Information S.D. is a 21-year-old male who suffered a right CVA as a result of an arterial malformation 15 months ago. He was in a coma for 4 months. After the coma, he was in acute rehabilitation for 2 months and subsequently in outpatient therapy. Prior to the CVA, S.D. attended college where he was a math major and a basketball player. He is currently living with his family, taking one class at college, and is beginning	Understand the patient's diagnosis or condition	"S.D. had a stroke involving the right side of his brain. From the history, he has been left with severe physical impairments that require a PCA. What visual skills might be affecting his ability to read, participate in school, and carry out self-care tasks? What type of neglect does he demonstrate and how does it affect personal independence and ability to interact in the community? Is he aware of the neglect and/or visual

to assist in coaching sports at a local school. He has a personal care attendant (PCA) 2–4 hours a day who assists with self-care activities.		deficits and does he become very frustrated? Or is he unaware and does he put himself in dangerous situations?"
He presents with left hemiplegia, moderate tone throughout the left side, with little controlled movement in either extremity. He is unable to walk and uses the wheelchair for all mobility. He has a left neglect and mild cognitive deficits, especially in short-term memory.	Know the person	"It must be difficult for someone who was a sports player to be in a wheelchair and sit on the sidelines coaching others. There is no mention of any behavior problems. I wonder what roles he plays now and how he is dealing with the changes."
He was referred to occupational therapy by his physiatrist because S.D.'s vision and left neglect were limiting him in school and with mobility.	Appreciate the context	"Given health care today, I wonder how long S.D. will have the services of a PCA? Is his family willing and/or able to provide personal care?"
	Develop provisional hypotheses	"S.D.'s visual skills/deficits, level of neglect, and level of awareness of his deficits appear to be his biggest barriers to school and mobility."

Assessment Process The occupational therapist wanted to determine the status of S.D.'s visual system and how it impacts on his daily functioning. The therapist used a symptom questionnaire to determine the patient's symptoms and complaints, as well as interview to determine his level of daily functioning. She then evaluated the visual foundation skills, including: acuity (near and far), visual fields, binocular vision, convergence, scanning, saccades, and pursuits. Because reading was a particular concern, she also included the *Pepper Test*, which is a standardized reading test used to determine accuracy and reading rate with unfamiliar text. Observations of where errors occur, how and where he uses his right upper extremity, and when and if he becomes frustrated will be made during the assessment.	Consider evaluation approach and methods	"Because he is having difficulty in school and with mobility, the visual foundation skills need to be assessed first to determine their effect on his ability to read and complete self-care tasks. If he does well on these but continues to have difficulty with self-care tasks and reading, then I would look at neglect in more depth."

Assessment Results Based on the interview, S.D. indicated that he had difficulty with eating (secondary to not always seeing the entire plate), mobility, reading, doing his homework, and being able to track the kids he was coaching. The symptom questionnaire appeared to indicate problems with accommodation, ocular motility, and visual fields.	Interpret observations	"His difficulty with convergence and poor ocular motor skills indicate that he would have a problem reading." "His accommodation deficits impact his ability to copy work from blackboard to table top, and it is not surprising that he has difficulty in the classroom."
Acuity: Within normal limits with the glasses that he wears at all times for distance.		"Visual field deficit or neglect? It's difficult to know at this time; he does demonstrate neglect, which can impact how well he does on confrontation testing."
Visual fields: On confrontation testing, he exhibits moderate difficulty with stimuli on the left, especially in the lower left quadrant.		"His inefficient scanning and left neglect impacts on his mobility and ability to successfully track the kids he is coaching."
Binocular vision: No diplopia or suppression present, but he appears somewhat impaired on test of stereopsis/depth perception. Convergence: Tested with 5 trials. Right eye broke at 8″, 3″, and 3 times at 6″, which indicates convergence insufficiency.		"Although S.D. appeared to be aware that he had difficulty with functional tasks such as eating, reading, and coaching, he was unable to compensate fully for the visual deficits or the neglect. I feel that he is a good candidate for outpatient therapy at this time."

Scanning: During all scanning tasks, he exhibited an inefficient scanning pattern; during table top activities, he missed 75% of items on the left side of the page; and when scanning the room for specific numbers sequentially, although he located all numbers, he required maximum cues and increased time.

Pursuits: He demonstrated a lag and occasionally lost the item, especially in lower left quadrant. He has great difficulty following with his eyes and usually will turn his head.

Saccades: He was unable to shift vision between two pens without head movement.

Reading test: 60 WPM with 80% accuracy.

Throughout testing, he was cooperative and motivated. He demonstrates awareness of his neglect but still requires maximum cues and increased time to compensate

Occupational Therapy Problem List

1. Decreased ocular motor skills
2. Decreased convergence
3. Inefficient scanning skills
4. Decreased accommodation
5. Unilateral neglect

Synthesize results

"Overall, S.D. demonstrates convergence insufficiency, poor ocular motor skills, decreased accommodation, inefficient scanning and left neglect. I think that he would benefit from an evaluation by an optometrist who specializes in vision therapy and who can work with S.D. and me to provide what S.D. needs to manage school and sports."

"Because of the neglect and decreased awareness at 15 months post injury, I am afraid that he will not be able to overcome the neglect and will require compensation from within, in which case activities will take a long time to complete, or he will require ongoing compensation from without, provided by others such as family or PCA. It will be important to determine which activities are most important to him."

CLINICAL REASONING IN OCCUPATIONAL THERAPY PRACTICE

Effects of Functional Roles on Assessment of Vision, Visual Perception, and Praxis

S.D. was 21 years old, a math major in college, and involved in playing basketball at the time of his CVA. How might the evaluation have differed if he had been 71 years old, retired, and enjoyed watching TV? Or 45 years old with an active dental practice?

SUMMARY REVIEW QUESTIONS

1. What are the visual foundation skills and why should they be evaluated before higher-level visual perceptual skills?
2. Your head-injured client does poorly on a test of figure-ground. List at least four possible reasons this might happen.
3. Why is it important to assess contrast sensitivity?
4. Under what circumstances might you evaluate visual foundation skills in a neurologically intact person?
5. Who are the eye care professionals and in what ways would you interact with them? What information might you request, and what information might you be able to give them?
6. How might you try to differentiate between a visual field deficit and unilateral neglect?
7. Why is it important to screen vision as early as possible?
8. What are the two major types of unilateral neglect, and how is each evaluated?
9. Your client has LBD with resultant right hemiparesis and non-fluent aphasia. Why and how would you evaluate for the presence of apraxia?
10. When should you include evaluation of apraxia in a client?

ACKNOWLEDGMENT

Thanks to Stephanie Singleton, OTR, for her assistance with research.

References

Almeida, Q. J., Black, S. E., & Roy, E. A. (2002). Screening for apraxia: A short assessment for stroke patients. *Brain and Cognition, 48,* 253–631.

Appelros, P., Nydevik, I., Karlsson, G. M., Thorwalls, A., & Seiger, A. (2003). Assessing unilateral neglect: Shortcomings of standard test methods. *Disability and Rehabilitation, 25,* 473–479.

Arrigoni, G., & DeRenzi, E. (1964). Constructional apraxia and hemispheric locus of lesions. *Cortex, 1,* 170–197.

Azouvi, P., Marchal, F., Samuel, C., Morin, L., Renard, C., Louis-Dreyfus, A., Jokie, C., Wiart, L., Pradat-Diehl, P., Deloche, G., & Bergego, C. (1996). Functional consequences and awareness of unilateral neglect: Study of an evaluation scale. *Neuropsychological Rehabilitation, 6,* 133–150.

Azouvi, P., Olivier, S., de Montety, G., Samuel, C., Louis-Dreyfus, A., & Tesio, L. (2003). Behavioral assessment of unilateral neglect: Study of the psychometric properties of the Catherine Bergego Scale. *Archives of Physical Medicine and Rehabilitation, 84,* 51–57.

Azouvi, P., Samuel, C., Louis-Dreyfus, A., Bernati, T., Bartolomeo, P., Beis, J.-M., Chokron, S., Leclercq, M., Marchal, F., Martin, Y., de Montety, G., Olivier, S., Perennou, D., Pradat-Diehl, L., Prairial, C., Rode, G., Sieroff, E., Wiart, L., & Rousseaux, M. (2002). Sensitivity of clinical and behavioral tests of spatial neglect after right hemisphere stroke. *Journal of Neurology, Neurosurgery and Psychiatry, 73,* 160–166.

Bailey, M. J., Riddoch, M. J., & Crome, P. (2000). Evaluation of a test battery for hemineglect in elderly stroke patients for use by therapists in clinical practice. *NeuroRehabilitation, 14,* 139–150.

Baum, B., & Hall, K. M. (1981). Relationship between constructional praxis and dressing in the head-injured adult. *American Journal of Occupational Therapy, 35,* 438–442.

Benton, A. L. (1967). Constructional apraxia and the minor hemisphere. *Confinia Neurologica, 29,* 1–16.

Benton, A. L., & Fogel, M. L. (1962). Three-dimensional constructional praxis. *Archives of Neurology, 7,* 347–354.

Benton, A., & Tranel, D. (1993). In K. M. Heilman & E. Valenstein (Eds.), *Clinical neuropsychology* (3rd ed., pp. 165–213). New York: Oxford University Press.

Beschin, N., Cocchini, G., Sala, S. D., & Logie, R. H. (1997). What the eye perceives, the brain ignores: A case of pure unilateral representational neglect. *Cortex, 33,* 3–26.

Beschin, N., & Robertson, I. H. (1997). Personal versus extrapersonal neglect: A group study of their dissociation using a reliable clinical test. *Cortex, 33,* 379–384.

Bisiach, E., Geminiani, G., Berti, A., & Rusconi, M. L. (1990). Perceptual and premotor factors of unilateral neglect. *Neurology, 40,* 1278–1281.

Butler, J. A. (2002). How comparable are tests of apraxia? *Clinical Rehabilitation, 16,* 389–398.

Chatterjee, A., & Mennemeier, M. (1997). Diagnosis and treatment of spatial neglect. In T. E. Fineberg & M. J. Farah (Eds.), *Behavioral neurology and neuropsychology* (pp. 597–612). New York: McGraw-Hill.

Coslett, H. B., Bowers, D., Fitzpatrick, E., Haws, B., & Heilman, K. M. (1990). Directional hypokinesia and hemispatial inattention in neglect. *Brain, 113,* 475–486.

Cowey, A., Small, M., & Ellis, S. (1994). Left visuo-spatial neglect can be worse in far than in near space. *Neuropsychologia, 32,* 1059–1066.

Crepeau, E. B. (1998). Activity analysis: A way of thinking about occupational performance. In M. E. Neistadt & E. B. Crepeau (Eds.), *Willard & Spackman's occupational therapy* (pp. 135–147). Philadelphia: Lippincott.

Critchley, M. (1966). *The parietal lobes.* New York: Hafner.

Dawson, D. R., & Tanner-Cohen, C. (1997). Visual scanning patterns in an adult Chinese population: Preliminary normative data. *Occupational Therapy Journal of Research, 17,* 264–279.

DeRenzi, E. (1997). Visuospatial and constructional disorders. In T. E. Feinberg & M. J. Farah (Eds.), *Behavioral neurology and neuropsychology* (pp. 297–307). New York: McGraw Hill.

Ferber, S., & Karnath, H.-O. (2001). How to assess spatial neglect: Line bisection or cancellation tasks? *Journal of Clinical and Experimental Neuropsychology, 23,* 599–607.

Foundas, A. L., Macauley, B. L., Raymer, A. M., Maher, L. M., Heilman, K. M., & Rothi, L. J. G. (1995). Ecological implications of limb apraxia: Evidence from mealtime behavior. *Journal of the International Neuropsychology Society, 1,* 62–66.

Gianutsos, R. (1997). Vision rehabilitation following acquired brain injury. In M. Gentile (Ed.), *Functional visual behavior* (pp. 267–294). Bethesda, MD: American Occupational Therapy Association, Inc.

Goodglass, H., & Kaplan, E. (1972). *The assessment of aphasia and related disorders.* Philadelphia: Lea & Febiger.

Haaland, K. (1993). Typology and assessment of individuals with limb apraxia. Paper presented at the AOTA Neuroscience Institute conference: Treating Adults with Apraxia, Baltimore.

Haaland, K. Y., Harrington, D. L., & Yeo, R. (1987). The effects of task complexity on motor performance in left and right CVA patients. *Neuropsychologia, 25,* 783–794.

Haarmeier, T., & Thier, P. (1999). Impaired analysis of moving objects due to deficient smooth pursuit eye movements. *Brain, 122,* 1490–1505.

Halligan, P. W., & Marshall, J. C. (1998). Visuospatial neglect: The ultimate deconstruction? *Brain and Cognition, 37,* 419–438.

Hartman-Maeir, A., & Katz, N. (1995). Validity of the Behavioral Inattention Test (BIT): Relationships with functional tasks. *American Journal of Occupational Therapy, 49,* 507–516.

Heilman, K. M., & Rothi, L. J. G. (1993). Apraxia. In K. M. Heilman & E. Valenstein (Eds.), *Clinical neuropsychology* (3rd ed., pp. 141–163). New York: Oxford University Press.

Heilman, K. M., Rothi, L. J. G., & Watson, R. T. (1997). Apraxia. In S. C. Schachter & O. Devinsky (Eds.), *Behavioral neurology and the legacy of Norman Geschwind* (pp. 171–182). Philadelphia: Lippincott-Raven.

Heilman, K. M., & Watson, R. T. (1977). The neglect syndrome: A unilateral defect of the orienting response. In S. Hardned, R. W. Doty, L. Goldstein, J. Janynes, & G. Kean Thamer (Eds.), *Lateralization in the nervous system*. New York: Academic Press.

Heilman, K. M., Watson, R. T., & Rothi, L. G. (1997). Disorders of skilled movements: Limb apraxia. In T. E. Fineberg & M. J. Farah (Eds.), *Behavioral neurology and neuropsychology* (pp. 227–235). New York: McGraw-Hill.

Heilman, K. M., Watson, R. T., & Valenstein, E. (1993). Neglect and related disorders. In K. M. Heilman & E. Valenstein (Eds.), *Clinical neuropsychology* (3rd ed., pp. 297–336). New York: Oxford University Press.

Heilman, K. M., Watson, R. T., & Valenstein, E. (1997). Neglect: Clinical and anatomic aspects. In T. E. Fineberg & M. J. Farah (Eds.), *Behavioral neurology and neuropsychology* (pp. 309–317). New York: McGraw-Hill.

Helm-Estabrooks, N., & Albert, M. L. (1991). *Manual of aphasia therapy*. Austin, TX: Pro-ed.

Joseph, R. (1996). *Neuropsychiatry, neuropsychology, and clinical neuroscience* (2nd ed.). Baltimore: Williams & Wilkins.

Kageyama, S., Imagase, M., Okubo, M., Takayama, Y. (1994). Neglect in three dimensions. *American Journal of Occupational Therapy, 48,* 206–210.

Kartsounis, L. D., & Findley, L. V. (1994). Task specific visuospatial neglect related to density and salience of stimuli. *Cortex, 30,* 647–659.

Katz, N., Itzkovich, M., Averbach, S., & Elazar, B. (1989). Lowenstein Occupational Therapy Cognitive Assessment (LOTCA) battery for brain injured patients: Reliability and validity. *American Journal of Occupational Therapy, 43,* 184–192.

Kinsbourne, M. (1993). Orientation bias model of unilateral neglect: Evidence from attentional gradients within hemispace. In I. H. Robertson & J. C. Marshall (Eds.), *Unilateral neglect: Clinical and experimental studies* (pp. 63–86). Hove, UK: Lawrence Erlbaum Associates, Publishers.

Ladavas, E., Carletti, M., & Gori, G. (1994). Automatic and voluntary orientating of attention in patients with visual neglect: Horizontal and vertical dimensions. *Neuropsychologia, 32,* 1195–1208.

Maeshima, S., Truman, G., Smith, D. S., Dohi, N., Shigeno, K., Itakura, T., & Komai, N. (2001). Factor analysis of the components of 12 standard test batteries, for unilateral spatial neglect, reveals that they contain a number of discrete and important clinical variables. *Brain Injury, 15,* 125–137.

Marchetti, C., & Della Sala, S. (1997). On crossed apraxia: A description of a right-handed apraxic patient with right supplementary motor area damage. *Cortex, 33,* 341–354.

Mattingley, J. B., Driver, J., Beschin, N., & Robertson, I. H. (1997). Attentional competition between modalities: Extinction between touch and vision after right hemisphere damage. *Neuropsychologia, 35,* 867–880.

Mennemeier, M., Vezey, E., Chatterjee, A., Rapcsak, S. Z., & Heilman, K. M. (1997). Contributions of the left and right cerebral hemispheres to line bisection. *Neuropsychologia, 35,* 703–715.

Mercier, L., Hebert, R., & Gauthier, L. (1995). Motor free visual perception test: Impact of vertical answer cards position on performance of adults with hemispatial visual neglect. *Occupational Therapy Journal of Research, 15,* 223–237.

Neistadt, M. E. (1993). The relationship between constructional and meal preparation skills. *Archives of Physical Medicine & Rehabilitation, 74,* 144–148.

Piercy, M., Hecaen, H., & Ajuriaguerra, J. (1960). Constructional apraxia associated with unilateral cerebral lesions: Left and right sided cases compared. *Brain, 83,* 225–242.

Poeck, K. (1985). Clues to the nature of disruptions to limb praxis. In E. A. Roy (Ed.), *Neuropsychological studies of apraxia and related disorders* (pp. 99–109). Amsterdam: Elsevier.

Posner, M. I., & Rafal, R. D. (1987). Cognitive theories of attention and the rehabilitation of attentional deficits. In M. J. Meier, A. L. Benton, & L. Diller (Eds.), *Neuropsychological rehabilitation* (pp. 182–201). New York: Churchill Livingston.

Qiang, W., Sonoda, S., Suzuki, M., Okamoto, S., & Saitoh, E. (2005). Reliability and validity of a wheelchair collision test for screening behavioral assessment of unilateral neglect after stroke. *American Journal of Physical Medicine & Rehabilitation, 84,* 161–166.

Raymer, A. M., Maher, L. M., Foundas, A. L., Heilman, K. M., & Rothi, L. J. (1997). The significance of body part as tool errors in limb apraxia. *Brain and Cognition, 34,* 287–292.

Riddoch, M. J., & Humphreys, G. W. (1994). Towards an understanding of neglect. In M. J. Riddoch & G. W. Humphreys (Eds.), *Cognitive neuropsychology and cognitive rehabilitation* (pp. 125–147). Hove, UK: Laurence Erlbaum Associates.

Robertson, I. H., Manly, T., Beschin, N., Daini, R., Haeski-Deivick, H., Homberg, V., Jehkonen, M., Pizzamiglio, G., Shiel, A., & Weber, E. (1997). Auditory sustained attention is a marker of unilateral spatial neglect. *Neuropsychologia, 35,* 1527–1532.

Rothi, L. J. G., Raymer, A. M., & Heilman, K. M. (1997). Limb praxis assessment. In L. J. G Rothi & K. M. Heilman (Eds.), *Apraxia: The neuropsychology of action* (pp. 61–73). East Sussex, UK: Psychology Press Publishers.

Roy, E. A., Black, S. E., Blair, N., & Dimeck, P. (1998). Analyses of deficits in gestural pantomime. *Journal of Clinical and Experimental Neuropsychology, 20,* 628–643.

Scheiman, M. (1999). Understanding and managing visual deficits: Theory, screening, procedures, intervention techniques. Jacksonville, FL: Conference of Vision Education Seminars.

Scheiman, M. (2002). *Understanding and managing vision deficits: A guide for occupational therapists* (2nd ed.). Thorofare, NJ: Slack, Inc.

Schenkenberg, T., Bradford, D. C., & Ajax, E. T. (1980). Line bisection and unilateral visual neglect in patients with neurologic impairment. *Neurology, 30,* 509–517.

Sea, M.-J. C., Henderson, A., & Cermak, S. A. (1993). Patterns of visual spatial inattention and their functional significance in stroke patients. *Archives of Physical Medicine & Rehabilitation, 74,* 355–360.

Simon, R. P., Aminoff, M. J., & Greenberg, D. A. (1999). *Clinical neurology* (4th ed.). Stamford, CT: Appleton & Lange.

Stam, C. J., & Bakker, M. (1990). The prevalence of neglect: Superiority of neuropsychological over clinical methods of examination. *Clinical Neurology and Neurosurgery, 92,* 229–235.

Stone, S. P., Halligan, P. W., & Greenwood, R. J. (1993). The incidence of neglect phenomena and related disorders in patients with an acute right or left hemisphere stroke. *Age and Aging, 22,* 46–52.

Stone, S. P., Halligan, P. W., Marshall, J. C., & Greenwood, R. J. (1998). Unilateral neglect: A common but heterogeneous syndrome. *Neurology, 50,* 1902–1905.

Sunderland, A., Bowers, M. P., Sluman, S. M., Wilcock, D. J., & Ardron, M. E. (1999). Impaired dexterity of the ipsilateral hand after stroke and the relationship to cognitive deficit. *Stroke, 30,* 949–955.

Tegner, R., & Levander, M. (1991). Through a looking glass: A new technique to demonstrate directional hypokinesia in unilateral neglect. *Brain, 114,* 1943–1951.

Tham, K., & Tegner, R. (1996). The baking tray task: A test of spatial neglect. *Neuropsychological Rehabilitation, 6,* 19–25.

Titcomb, R. E., Okoye, R., & Schiff, S. (1997). Introduction to the dynamic process of vision. In M. Gentile (Ed.), *Functional visual behavior* (pp. 3–39). Bethesda MD: American Occupational Therapy Association, Inc.

Trobe, J. D., Acosta, P. C., Krischer, J. P., & Trick, G. L. (1981). Confrontation visual field techniques in the detection of anterior visual pathway lesions. *Annals of Neurology, 10,* 28–34.

van Heugten, C. M., Dekker, J., Deelman, B. G., Stehmann-Saris, J. C., & Kinebanian, A. (1999a). A diagnostic test for apraxia in stroke patients: Internal consistency and diagnostic value. *The Clinical Neuropsychologist, 13,* 182–192.

van Heugten, C. M., Dekker, J., Deelman, B. G., Stehmann-Saris, J. C., & Kinebanian, A. (1999b). Assessment of disabilities in stroke patients with apraxia: Internal consistency and inter-observer reliability. *Occupational Therapy Journal of Research, 19,* 55–73.

Warren, M. (1981). Relationship of constructional apraxia and body scheme disorders to dressing performance in adult CVA. *American Journal Occupational Therapy, 35,* 431–437.

Warren, M. (1993a). A hierarchical model for evaluation and treatment of visual perceptual dysfunction in adult acquired brain injury, Part 1. *American Journal of Occupational Therapy, 47,* 42–54.

Warren, M. (1993b). A hierarchical model for evaluation and treatment of visual perceptual dysfunction in adult acquired brain injury, Part 2. *American Journal of Occupational Therapy, 47,* 55–66.

Warren, M. (1996). *Brain injury visual assessment battery for adults.* Lenexa, KS: visABILITIES Rehab Services.

Warren, M. (1999). Evaluation and treatment of visual perceptual dysfunction in adult brain injury, Part 1. Nashville, TN: Conference of visABILITIES Rehab Services, Inc.

Warrington, E. K., James, M., & Kinsbourne, M. (1966). Drawing disability in relation to laterality of cerebral lesion. *Brain, 89,* 53–82.

Whyte, J., & DiPasquale, M. C. (1995). Assessment of vision and visual attention in minimally responsive brain injured patients. *Archives of Physical Medicine and Rehabilitation, 76,* 804–810.

Wilson, B., Cockburn, J., & Halligan, P. (1987). Development of a behavioral test of visuospatial neglect. *Archives of Physical Medicine & Rehabilitation, 68,* 98–102.

York, C. D., & Cermak, S. A. (1995). Visual perception and praxis in adults after stroke. *American Journal of Occupational Therapy, 49,* 543–550.

Zwinkels, A., Geusgens, C., van de Sande, P., & van Heugten, C. (2004). Assessment of apraxia: Inter-rater reliability of a new apraxia test, association between apraxia and other cognitive deficits and prevalence of apraxia in a rehabilitation setting. *Clinical Rehabilitation, 18,* 819–827.

CHAPTER 9

Assessing Abilities and Capacities: Cognition

Mary Vining Radomski

LEARNING OBJECTIVES

After studying this chapter, the reader will be able to do the following:

1. Describe specific cognitive capacities and abilities and analyze their influence on occupational function.
2. Select cognitive assessment methods and tools based on individual clients' characteristics and requirements.
3. Anticipate and describe factors that may confound performance during cognitive assessment.
4. Distinguish occupational therapy's contribution to multidisciplinary cognitive assessment from that of other rehabilitation disciplines.

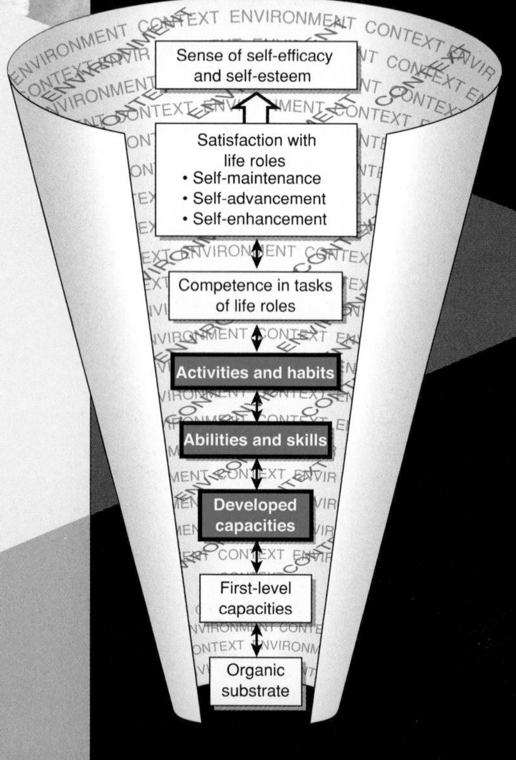

Glossary

Attention—The ability to deploy limited mental resources for purposes of concentration. Human activities have various attentional demands, including sustained attention (length of time), selective attention (competing stimuli), divided attention (multiple simultaneous stimuli), and alternating attention (shifts back and forth to various stimuli).

Cognition—The general term that reflects the mental enterprises related to absorbing information, thinking, and goal-directed action.

Concept formation—The ability to analyze relationships between objects and their properties (Sohlberg & Mateer, 1989).

Executive function—Metaprocess that enables a person to initiate, plan, self-monitor, and correct his or her approach to goal-directed tasks. Executive disorders often result from frontal lobe damage and are evidenced by problems with self-control, self-direction, and organization (Lezak, 1995).

Higher order thinking abilities—Complex mental operations that include problem solving, reasoning, and concept formation. Thinking generally entails the manipulation of remembered information (Mayer, 1992) and depends on intact primary cognitive capacities (orientation, attention, and memory) (Sohlberg & Mateer, 1989).

Memory—The result of interactive cognitive systems that receive, code, store, and retrieve information.

Neuropsychological evaluation—A long battery of standardized tests for purposes of diagnosis, patient care and planning, rehabilitation evaluation, and research (Lezak, 1995). Typically, the examiner is a doctor of psychology with specialized training in cognitive processes and brain-behavior relationships.

Orientation—The awareness of self in relation to one's physical and temporal environment that depends upon reliable integration of attention, memory, and perception (Lezak, 1995). Impaired orientation is strongly suggestive of cerebral dysfunction (Lezak, 1995).

Problem solving—The multistage process consisting of identifying a problem, generating possible solutions, implementing a preferred solution, and evaluating the results. Everyday problem solving, however, does not always follow this logical sequence of steps.

Reasoning—The ability to draw inferences or conclusions from known or assumed facts.

Self-awareness—The capacity to objectively perceive the self (Prigatano & Schacter, 1991) and (with a reasonable degree of accuracy) to compare that conception to a pre-morbid standard.

Cognition refers to the integrated functions of the human mind that together result in thought and goal-directed action. Simply put by Diller (1993), "Cognition involves the acquisition, processing, and application of information in daily life" (p. 9). Cognition is at the core of an individual's essence or personhood. In fact, Schacter (1996) suggested that without the capacity to remember the past, humans lose a sense of self. Cognition not only influences what a person chooses to do (Bandura, 1986), but it also dictates how an experience is remembered and interpreted.

Cognition clearly influences the selection, performance, analysis, and learning of everyday activities. In addition to its central role in occupational functioning, a person's cognitive function influences the acquisition of new activities of daily living (ADL) skills after the onset of disability (Walker, Walker, & Sunderland, 2003) and a person's capacity to perform IADL with progressive conditions such as dementia (Nygard et al., 1998) and human immunodeficiency virus (HIV) (Heaton et al., 2004). Cognition also predicts rehabilitation outcome after injury and illness. MacNeill and Lichtenberg (1997) found that, for geriatric inpatients, levels of cognitive function predicted ability to return home alone at discharge from rehabilitation. Sandstrom and Mokler (1999) also described cognitive function as a key outcome variable for persons with severe motor stroke, and Hanks et al. (1999) found that cognition predicted functional abilities and social integration 6 months after discharge from acute rehabilitation. To identify and remove barriers that interfere with occupational functioning and to anticipate rehabilitation outcomes, occupational therapists examine patients' cognitive function as part of a comprehensive occupational therapy assessment.

This chapter begins with descriptions of specific cognitive capacities and abilities and follows with a discussion of various influences on cognitive function. I review clinical reasoning considerations pertinent to cognitive assessment and describe specific methods and tools based on two complementary approaches to cognitive assessment.

DEFINING COGNITIVE CAPACITIES AND ABILITIES

Cognition consists of an interactive hierarchy (Ben-Yishay cited in Goldstein & Levin, 1987) that includes primary cognitive capacities (orientation, attention, and memory), higher level thinking abilities (reasoning, concept formation, and problem solving), and metaprocesses (executive functions and self-awareness).

Primary Cognitive Capacities

The primary cognitive capacities of orientation, attention, and memory largely reflect the neuroanatomical and physiological integrity of the brain (Radomski, 1998). They are thought to be prerequisite to higher level thinking abilities and to influence metaprocessing.

Changes in primary cognitive capacities are seen in many recipients of occupational therapy services. After a severe traumatic brain injury (TBI), many patients enter a confusional stage of recovery in which they are disoriented (Levin, O'Donnell, & Grossman, 1979). Stroke and TBI often result in problems with attention, memory, and language (Capruso & Levin, 1992; Claesson et al., 2005; Hochstenbach et al., 1998). Persons with chronic conditions, such as multiple sclerosis (Benedict et al., 2005), epilepsy (Helmstaedter et al., 2003), systemic lupus erythematosus (McLaurin et al., 2005), and HIV/acquired immunodeficiency syndrome (AIDS) (Heaton et al., 2004; Poutiainen et al., 1996), may also experience deterioration in attention and memory.

Orientation

Orientation refers to the awareness of self in relation to person, place, time, and circumstance (Sohlberg & Mateer, 1989). Orientation deficits are typically symptoms of brain dysfunction, with disorientation to time and place being most common (Lezak, 1995).

Attention

Attention is the deployment of mental resources for concentration. Each person is thought to have a limited capacity for consciously attending to information—a hard-wired upper limit that dictates how many inputs can be simultaneously processed (Lezak, 1995). Let us examine four levels of attention in the context of preparing a meal.

1. *Sustained attention* is the capacity to maintain attentional performance over time (Sohlberg & Mateer, 2001). To prepare a meal with several dishes, an individual must stay focused for the duration of the task.
2. *Selective attention* occurs when an individual concentrates on one set of stimuli while ignoring competing stimuli (Sohlberg & Mateer, 2001), as when the cook ignores the noise from the television while measuring or counting ingredients.
3. *Divided attention* allows a person to respond to more than one task at a time and is a more complex mental skill than sustained and selective attention (Sohlberg & Mateer, 2001). The cook browns the meat while talking with a family member.
4. *Alternating attention* is necessary as one flexibly shifts attention between multiple operations (Sohlberg & Mateer, 2001). The cook interrupts meal preparation to answer the telephone and then quickly resumes setting the table while monitoring the status of food simmering on the stove.

Memory

Memory broadly refers to information storage and retrieval (Lezak, 1995). There are many conceptions of the way this process occurs (Baddeley, 1990; Lezak, 1995). Atkinson and Shiffrin's (1971) Information-Processing Model of memory highlights stages of acquiring and employing new knowledge and skills (Fig. 9-1). Definition 9-1 outlines terms commonly used in the discussion of memory.

Sensory Registers

Information from the environment is briefly (milliseconds) held in registers (or stores) specific to the human senses (Lezak, 1995). This registration stage has been called the intake valve for determining what data from the

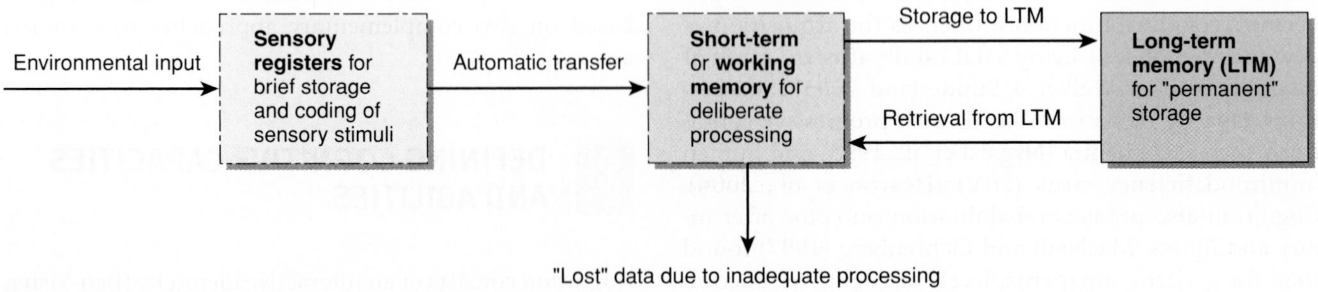

Figure 9-1 Human information-processing diagram.

DEFINITION 9-1

Memory Terms

Term	Definition
Memory	
Recent	Usually corresponds to long-term memory; includes memory hours to months post stimulus presentation
Remote	Very long-term memory, as from childhood
Episodic	Memory of one's personal history (e.g., what you had for breakfast this morning)
Semantic	Personal knowledge of the world (e.g., that horses are big and ants are small)
Amnesia	
Retrograde (RA)	Loss of ability to recall events that occurred before the trauma
Anterograde	Decreased memory of events occurring after trauma
Post-traumatic (PTA)	Period following trauma during which the patient is confused and disoriented and seems to lack the ability to store and retrieve new information

environment are ultimately stored. This phase is influenced by acuity of the senses (such as hearing and vision), affective set, and perception.

Short-Term Memory

The short-term phase of information processing has many labels: immediate memory, short-term memory, and working memory. The term *working memory* connotes the effortful deployment of cognitive resources during this stage. In short, for input from sensory registers to proceed to storage in long-term memory, it must be the subject of deliberate concentration in working memory for approximately 30 seconds (Lezak, 1995). Without this focused attention, the memory trace decays, and the memory is not retained (Lezak, 1995). Unlike long-term memory, which is thought to have an infinite capacity, working memory has a restricted holding capacity of seven plus or minus two chunks of information (Miller, 1956). In addition to its role in information processing, working memory is the seat of conscious thought used in concentration and problem solving (Baddeley, 1990). Based on electrochemical activity in the brain, working memory reflects the contribution of attention to the memory process (Lezak, 1995).

Long-Term Memory

Whereas data in working memory has a short shelf life, information in long-term memory can be stored for a lifetime (Lezak, 1995). When we remember information (an event that occurred an hour ago or a year ago), we have located and retrieved data from long-term memory and are holding it for conscious attention and thought in limited-capacity working memory. Storage in long-term memory is based on relatively permanent changes in brain cell structure (Glover, Ronning, & Bruning, 1990), although there does not appear to be a single local storage site for stored memories (Lezak, 1995). Long-term memory is thought to consist of two subsystems, declarative memory and procedural memory. Declarative memory holds factual information, which is subdivided into episodic memory (knowledge of personal information and events) and semantic memory (knowledge of facts about the world) (Eysenck & Keane, 1990). Procedural memory holds information related to knowing how to do things; it allows us to learn and perform skilled motor actions (Eysenck & Keane, 1990).

Higher Level Thinking Abilities

Higher level thinking abilities are the result of complex and dynamic interactions between a number of brain structures united in functional systems (Hochstenbach et al., 1998); they depend on intact primary cognitive capacities (Sohlberg & Mateer, 1989). After brain injury, people may have difficulty with reasoning and abstraction (Scherzer et al., 1993) and with sequencing and categorization (Adamovich, Henderson, & Auerbach, 1985), all of which interfere with higher level thought. Sohlberg and Mateer (1989) described three inter-related categories of higher level thinking abilities: problem solving, reasoning, and concept formation.

Problem Solving

Most people use problem-solving skills hundreds of times a day. Problem solving occurs whenever the situation is different from a desired situation or goal and the person does not immediately know what series of actions to take (Bransford & Stein, 1984). In fact, at a basic level, all human responses that are not routine or habitual can be construed as problem solving (Radomski, 1998). Problem solving is usually conceptualized as the following multistage process:

- Identify the problem
- Define the problem
- Generate possible solutions and select one
- Implement the preferred solution
- Evaluate the outcome against the desired goal

Everyday problem solving, however, does not always follow this logical sequence. In his discussion of managerial problem solving, Wagner (1991) reported that high-level managers most often employ nonlinear problem solving in which they rely on tacit knowledge and base their actions and decisions on intuition rather than deliberation. Therefore, occupational therapists use the aforementioned sequence to organize their observations during assessment of problem solving rather than as a singular "right" sequence against which to judge effectiveness.

Reasoning

Reasoning entails drawing inferences or conclusions from known or assumed facts. It can make use of sequencing, categorization, and deduction (Sohlberg & Mateer, 1989). Sequencing is ordering information properly (Sohlberg & Mateer, 1989), whereas categorization involves grouping objects or ideas according to characteristics (Goverover, 2004). During deductive reasoning, a thinker uses evidence to make inferences, that is, uses available information to generate and test hypotheses (Goverover, 2004). For example, a client who is doing a task observes the therapist signaling that a high degree of accuracy is required. The client deduces from general feedback that she should slow down and periodically check the work.

Concept Formation

Closely linked to reasoning, concept formation is the ability to analyze relationships between objects and their properties (Sohlberg & Mateer, 1989). Sohlberg and Mateer (1989) suggested that "forming a concept requires that an individual identify critical features of instances of that concept and also determine how those features interrelate" (p. 267). A person forms a concept when sorting a box of assorted kitchen tools, for example, determining whether to organize them by function, size, or color. Thinking can be further qualified on a continuum of concrete to abstract (Mosey, 1993). Concrete thinking is characterized by the tendency to be bound to obvious stimulus properties and the inability to remove oneself from the immediate task (Sohlberg & Mateer, 1989); it is the most common sign of impaired conceptual thinking (Lezak et al., 2004). On the other end of the continuum, abstract thinking involves the ability to transcend the immediate situation, appreciate various aspects of the problem, and think symbolically (Sohlberg & Mateer, 1989). In the sorting example, a concrete thinker might choose to organize the kitchen tools by color, whereas the more abstract thinker might organize by common function.

Metaprocessing Abilities

Executive functions and self-awareness are metaprocesses that contribute initiation, planning, monitoring, reflection, and self-evaluation to cognitive function (Sternberg, 1990). Bewick et al. (1995) depicted these abilities as cognitive directors because they facilitate the interplay of primary cognitive capacities and higher level thinking in the execution of complex tasks.

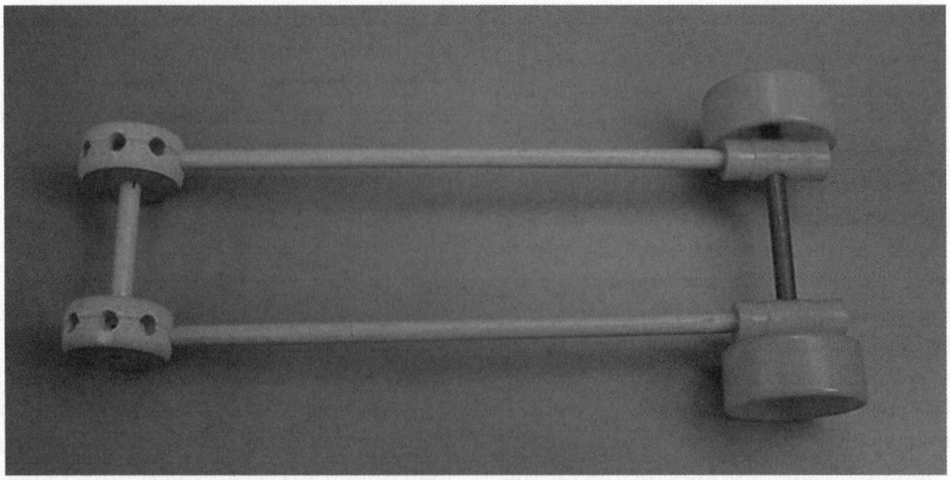

Figure 9-2 Tinker toy test.

The importance of executive functions and self-awareness to satisfying and productive role performance cannot be overstated. Impairments in executive functions are major factors associated with loss of everyday competence (Goverover, 2004), social autonomy, and inability to return to work long after TBI (Mazaux et al., 1997). Decreased self-awareness after TBI prevents the survivor from recognizing the deficits that limit performance and diminishes motivation to participate in rehabilitation therapies. Interestingly, some family members view unawareness as a blessing in persons with dementia (Fleming, Strong, & Ashton, 1996), whereas for other caregivers, it is associated with higher levels of subjective distress (Prigatano et al., 2005).

Executive Functions

Intact executive functions are necessary for the successful performance of unstructured multistep tasks (such as the Tinkertoy test in Fig. 9-2) and an array of everyday occupations. Lezak et al. (2004) described four components of executive functions: volition, planning, purposive action, and effective performance.

1. Volitional behavior is dictated by determining what one needs or wants and then formulating a goal or an intention to act (Lezak et al., 2004). It is influenced by self-awareness because needs, wants, and goals are often moderated by people's understanding of their circumstances and the ability to realize an objective (Lezak et al., 2004).
2. Planning is identifying and sequencing steps to move toward the goal or end point (Lezak et al., 2004).
3. Purposive action is "the translation of an intention or plan into productive, self-serving activity [requiring] the actor to initiate, maintain, switch, and stop sequences of complex behavior in an orderly and integrated manner" (Lezak, 1995, p. 658).
4. Effective performance requires that an individual monitor and self-correct while regulating the intensity, speed, and strategies used during the task (Lezak, 1995).

Self-Awareness

Prigatano and Schacter (1991) suggested that self-awareness is the highest of all integrated activities of the brain. It is the ability to process information about the self and compare it to a longstanding self-evaluation (Dougherty & Radomski, 1993). Self-awareness has two primary dimensions: (1) appreciation of personal attributes, such as physical and cognitive strengths and weaknesses; and (2) initiation of compensatory strategies in response to known personal attributes. In general, persons with TBI tend to be more aware of physical deficits than cognitive or emotional changes (Anderson & Tranel, 1989), and typically, the more severe the brain injury, the more problems the individual has with self-awareness (Sherer et al., 2005).

Crosson et al. (1989) proposed a three-level self-awareness hierarchy consisting of intellectual awareness, emergent awareness, and anticipatory awareness:

1. Intellectual awareness is a person's ability to understand at some level that a particular function is impaired. Severe deficits in memory impede intellectual awareness because such awareness requires recall of the past.
2. Emergent awareness is the ability of a person to recognize a problem when it is actually happening.
3. Anticipatory awareness, which depends on the existence of intellectual and emergent awareness, is the ability to anticipate a challenge or problem resulting from physical or cognitive impairments.

Metacognition, knowledge and regulation of one's own cognitive capacities and strategies (Ownsworth & Fleming, 2005; Katz, 2005), is closely linked to anticipatory awareness. For a person to begin taking notes in response to novel instructions (a metacognitive strategy), he or she must appreciate vulnerability from memory deficits and anticipate the challenge the activity represents (intellectual and anticipatory awareness).

Executive functions reciprocally influence self-awareness. Self-knowledge informs the selection of reasonable goals for a given undertaking and drives selection of strategies that best facilitate performance. Ongoing monitoring of task performance with adjustment of strategies and incorporation of feedback can in turn affect self-awareness, altering percepts of personal strengths and weaknesses.

MULTIPLE-DETERMINANT MODEL OF COGNITIVE FUNCTION

The dissection of specific cognitive capacities and abilities for purposes of description belies the complexity of their inter-relationships and redundancies. In actuality, an individual's cognitive state is dynamic, determined by many interacting variables, including neurobiological, affective, experiential, social, and cultural influences, all of which are mediated by the task and environment. Changes in any of these domains improve or detract from a person's cognitive state and thereby his or her occupational functioning. To assess cognition and interpret findings, occupational therapists must appreciate how variables can affect performance during cognitive assessment. What follows is a brief summary of each influence, supported with specific examples from the literature.

Neurobiological Influence on Cognition

The neurobiological influence on cognition is best understood as foundational cognitive capacities resulting from dynamic neural networks (Hochstenbach et al., 1998). This influence is most apparent following changes to the anatomy and physiology of the brain, as with injury and aging. Persons with stroke have local damage to brain tissue that often results in predictable and specific cognitive deficits, such as frontal lobe damage leading to executive dysfunction and temporal lobe damage affecting memory. Neurobiological changes that accompany aging also seem to affect thinking abilities and memory. Crystallized intelligence (well-practiced, overlearned skills and knowledge) is reportedly maintained or strengthened into the eighth decade of life, whereas fluid intelligence, which entails reasoning and problem solving for unfamiliar challenges, begins a slow decline in the sixth decade of life (Lezak, 1995). Small et al. (1999) found that healthy adults aged 70 and older demonstrated a decline in specific aspects of memory performance when compared with subjects 60–69 years old. They suggest that this profile of age-related memory decline is related to changes in the hippocampal formation (Small et al., 1999).

Changes or deterioration of other functions of the human body have secondary neurobiological influences on cognition. For example, visual-perceptual impairments alter the inputs into the memory process, limiting what a person can accurately remember. Medications can also have a neurobiological influence on cognition. Researchers suggest a link between adjuvant chemotherapy for operative primary breast cancer and cognition (Schilling et al., 2005).

Affective Influences on Cognition

Although it is clear that emotions affect cognition, the underlying mechanism is not known. Anxious people differ from others in several aspects of attentional functioning. Anxious people are more likely to attend to threat-related stimuli and use limited-capacity working memory for worry, self-concern, and other task-irrelevant distractions (Eysenck & Keane, 1990). Persons with depression also frequently complain about poor memory but often do not demonstrate memory deficits on neuropsychological testing (Lezak, 1995). Depressed individuals are thought to show passive disengagement with the environment in that their attentional focus is on internal concerns rather than environmental events (Eysenck & Keane, 1990). Depressed people also demonstrate a negative recall bias (a tendency to recall more negative information about themselves than others do) (Baddeley, 1990; Eysenck & Keane, 1990). Memory problems associated with depression seem to have a secondary effect on executive processes. Channon and Green (1999) found that otherwise healthy but depressed individuals performed worse than controls who were not depressed on three measures of executive function. They explained this difference as possibly related to alterations in neurotransmitter activities and/or distractions by dysfunctional negative thoughts that occupy limited-capacity working memory during problem solving and task performance.

Similarly, transient mental distractions can impair cognition. Pain and fatigue are thought to be irrelevant inputs that diminish the function of limited-capacity working memory by occupying attention that is therefore unavailable to incoming data (Denburg, Carbotte, & Denburg, 1997). Therefore, clients who are exhausted or in physical or emotional pain are unlikely to be able to demonstrate their cognitive capabilities during assessment, with or without neurobiological impairments (Bryant, Chiaravalloti, & DeLuca, 2004; Heyer et al., 2000).

Experiential, Social, and Cultural Influence on Cognition

Feuerstein (1980) hypothesized that experience and sociocultural background play superordinate roles in the development of cognitive capacities and habits. An Israeli psychologist–educator, Feuerstein became convinced that the large number of "retarded" adolescent immigrants after World War II lacked cognitive skills primarily because of poverty and socially deprived surroundings. Participants in his 2-year intervention program, which focused on acquisition of cognitive habits and strategies, demonstrated improvements in general intellectual aptitude, interpersonal conduct, self-sufficiency, and adaptation (Perkins, 1995).

Experts also suggest that basic processes of perception and cognition are influenced by culture. Nisbett and Masuda (2003) summarized a series of studies that illustrate information-processing differences in East Asian and Western cultures. They suggested that Americans tended to focus their attention on objects and object attributes, but Japanese subjects tended to focus on the field, background, relationship, or context of the objects. Consider the impact that culture also has on self-awareness. Prigatano, Ogano, and Amakusa (1997) suggested that, because incompetence in personal care is a sign of disgrace in Japan, Japanese patients with TBI tended to overestimate their abilities in this realm. On the other hand, because Japanese generally view high estimations of social and interpersonal skills as impolite, Japanese patients with TBI tended to underestimate their abilities in this realm.

Task and Environment as Contextual Mediators of Cognition

People bring their neurobiological, emotional, experiential, social, and cultural predispositions to all information processing, but performance at a given moment is mediated by characteristics of the task and environmental contexts. In her Dynamic Interactional Model of Cognition, Toglia (2005) suggested that, in addition to a person's neurological capacity, personal context, self-awareness, and processing strategies, his or her cognitive functioning is also influenced by the activity and environment. Task variables that influence cognition include complexity, arrangement, and movement demands (Toglia, 1998). Here is an example of task-cognition interplay. When a task is familiar, the thinker requires relatively little attention to recognize a problem type and determine a hypothesis and plan of action (Mayer, 1992). A familiar task or problem prompts the individual to retrieve a large number of interconnected units of knowledge, both related facts and previous solutions (Mayer, 1992). Tasks that optimally challenge an individual's cognitive capacities and abilities and engage his or her interest elicit an individual's peak cognitive performance (Csikszentmihalyi, 1990).

The environment similarly affects cognition. Contextual cues in the environment enhance recall of similar tasks or previously effective techniques or solutions. The stimulus-arousal properties of the environment also influence cognitive function. Lighting and noise can focus attention or, as is often the case for persons with brain injury, provide distractions that derail thinking.

In summary, cognition consists of specific but interrelated capacities and abilities that are influenced by neurobiological, affective, experiential-sociocultural variables and task and environmental contexts. This discussion, although not exhaustive, highlights the complexity, if not the mystery, of cognitive function, which is an appreciation necessary for assessing cognitive capacities and abilities in occupational therapy. In judging the cognitive status of another person, teasing out performance confounders is as important as selecting and correctly administering the assessment tool. Whereas assigning and summing scores on standardized instruments requires the attentiveness of a trained technician, observing and interpreting performance during assessment requires the insight of a professional.

THE PROCESS OF COGNITIVE ASSESSMENT

Occupational therapists in clinical practice assess cognition for three primary reasons:

1. To establish a baseline against which to measure change
2. To inform intervention and discharge planning
3. To identify those who would benefit from more detailed neuropsychological evaluation

As previously discussed, many persons requiring the attention of medical and rehabilitation professionals have cognitive deficits that interfere with function. Cognitive changes can be temporary, relatively static, or progressive. Occupational therapists use a combination of static and dynamic assessments to get a comprehensive picture of the client. Static assessments are standardized evaluations that provide a snapshot of the client's functioning at a specific period of time (Kolakowsky, 1998). Dynamic assessments focus on client performance at two or more points in time (Kolakowsky, 1998) and examine learning potential and the client's ability to transfer or generalize new skills (Toglia, 2005). Rather than adhering to a strict standardized administration, dynamic assessments allow clinicians to manipulate person, environment, and activity variables to ascertain how those variables might be modified to optimize the client's level of functioning (Polatajko, Mandich, & Martini, 2000; Toglia, 2005). Static assessments typically result in a numeric score that enables the clinician to characterize the nature and extent of cognitive impairment before, during, and after intervention. Dynamic assessments help occupational therapists determine what problems to address and to select specific intervention strategies.

Occupational therapists exchange information about their findings with the family and other rehabilitation professionals so that the rehabilitation team together can create a comprehensive picture of the client's function. For example, language is inextricably linked to almost every aspect of cognitive function. Occupational therapists review the results of speech and language assessment to understand the language capacities and abilities of a given patient and the influence of any impairment on cognitive assessment. Neuropsychology is informed by occupational therapists' observations of cognitive function in the context of daily life tasks and life roles. Neuropsychologists use a variety of standardized tests to diagnose localized deficits and differentiate between neurological and psychiatric symptoms. A full neuropsychological evaluation, which typically entails 2–8 hours of tests, guides decision making prior to major rehabilitation transitions (return to work or moving from supervised to independent living or vice versa) and establishes the permanence of cognitive impairments for legal purposes. Because neuropsychological evaluation is so expensive, occupational therapists often assess cognition on behalf of the team during acute rehabilitation, when cognitive capacities and abilities are in a period of rapid change.

Clinicians select the most appropriate cognitive assessment methods and tools based on the objectives of assessment and specific needs and characteristics of the client.

Occupational therapists use two complementary approaches to assessing cognition: (1) assessing function to make inferences about cognitive capacities and abilities and (2) assessing cognitive capacities and abilities to make inferences about function.

Methods and Tools for Assessing Function to Make Inferences about Cognition

Occupational therapists begin any new assessment by identifying the client's goals and priorities as well as his or her roles and performance in occupations (American Occupational Therapy Association, 2002). Assessment of cognition is part of that process. Informal and formal functional assessments provide opportunities to make hypotheses about cognitive strengths and weaknesses, allowing the clinician to identify domains warranting further evaluation. For example, during an activities of daily living (ADL) or homemaking evaluation, occupational therapists observe attention to task by counting episodes of distractions, memory for instructions, and evidence of organization and planning. Of course, informal functional assessments of cognition are highly subjective and easily influenced by the clinician's definition of "normal" and his or her acumen in using the observable (behavior) to make inferences about internal cognitive processes. This method of cognitive assessment, however, is preferable for patients who cannot understand verbal or written instructions, as with communication deficits or speaking another language.

Three standardized functional assessments help clinicians simultaneously examine function and cognition: the *Arnadottir OT-ADL Neurobehavioral Evaluation* (*A-ONE*) (Arnadottir, 1990), the *Rabideau Kitchen Evaluation–Revised* (Neistadt, 1992), and the *Kitchen Task Assessment* (Baum & Edwards, 1993).

Arnadottir OT-ADL Neurobehavioral Evaluation

The *A-ONE* evaluates performance of ADL and examines the effect of neurobehavioral dysfunction on task performance. There are two parts of the instrument; part 2 is considered optional. During part 1, the occupational therapist observes the patient performing dressing, hygiene, transfer and mobility, feeding, and communication tasks and completes the *Functional Independence Scale* by assigning a numerical score (0–4) for each aspect of the various tasks. For example, a score is assigned to each of the activities of dressing (donning shirt, pants, socks, and shoes; fastening clothing). While observing the patient's performance of each component, the therapist also rates the patient in terms of presence of neurobehavioral impairments, again using a 0–4 scale. For example, the patient is scored on each of the following possible neurobehavioral impairments specified for the task of dressing: motor apraxia, ideational apraxia, unilateral body neglect, somatoagnosia, spatial relations, unilateral spatial neglect, abnormal tone, perseveration, and organization and sequencing. The scores on the *Functional Independence* and *Neurobehavioral* scales are not additive but used to establish patterns of performance and impairment. Occupational therapists may use the results of part 1 to localize cerebral dysfunction based on functional performance (part 2). Part 1 of the *A-ONE*, which takes approximately 25 minutes to administer, was standardized on patients with cortical central nervous system dysfunction. Its author recommends that therapists attend a training seminar before using the tool (Arnadottir, 1990).

Rabideau Kitchen Evaluation–Revised

The *Rabideau Kitchen Evaluation–Revised* (*RKE-R*) requires that persons with brain injury synthesize an array of cognitive capacities and abilities in the context of preparing a simple meal, a cold sandwich with two fillings and a hot beverage. Each of the 40 component activities is rated on a 0–3 scale indicating level of assistance or cueing required, and the total time for completion is recorded. Neistadt (1994) recommended that therapists use scores on the *RKE-R* to determine where to begin with a treatment protocol designed to improve meal preparation skills but suggested that this test may not be sensitive enough to use with persons who have subtle cognitive or perceptual deficits (Neistadt, 1992).

Kitchen Task Assessment

The *Kitchen Task Assessment* (*KTA*) measures the cognitive support necessary for the patient to prepare cooked pudding. Specific neurobehavioral components, such as initiation, organization, and safety, are scored on a 0–3 scale, reflecting the degree of cueing or physical assistance required for that aspect of the task. This test was standardized on patients with Alzheimer's disease.

Work Simulations

Work simulations are another method for assessing cognition through functional activity. Nadeau and Buckheit (1995) recommended a three-phase *Work Simulation Model* for outpatients with TBI as a means to observe executive functions. In the set-up phase, after patients are provided with a workspace and scheduled work time, they make a list of supplies they need for the job. Before beginning the simulation phase, patients predict their performance on projects that are somewhat similar to work tasks they would have done before the injury. In the post-simulation phase, patients rate actual performance and compare self-ratings to that of the therapist. Dougherty and Radomski

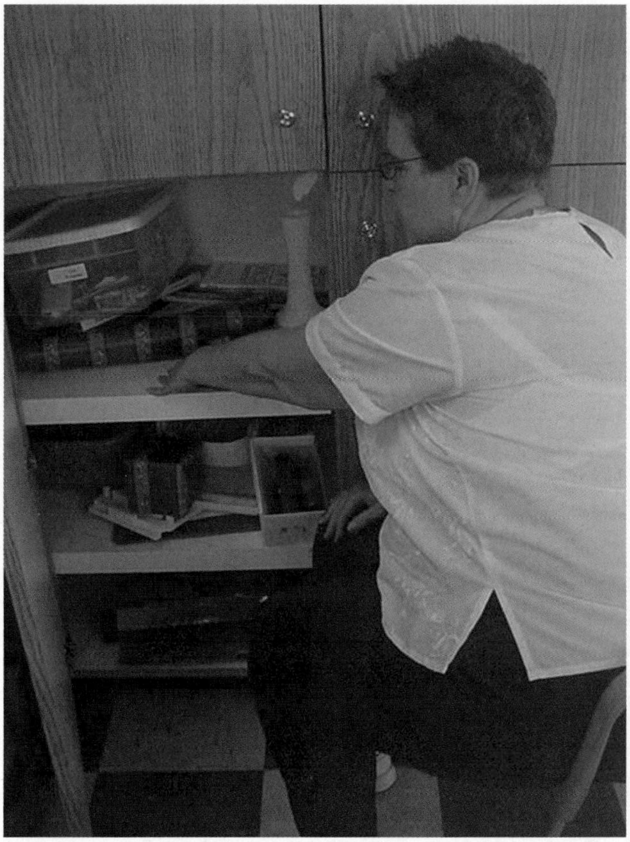

Figure 9-3 Messy cupboard.

(1993) described a similar assessment of work behaviors in which following directions, accuracy, and vigilance are rated in the context of four tasks: balancing a checkbook and using a calculator, the Yellow Pages, and transportation schedules.

Dynamic Investigative Approach

Finally, therapists can convert any task (such as organizing the messy cupboard in Fig. 9-3) to an opportunity for cognitive assessment by using a dynamic investigative approach (Toglia, 1989). Therapists deliberately manipulate performance variables related to task, environment, strategies, and cueing to determine in what conditions the patient performs at his or her best (Dougherty & Radomski, 1993). *Dynamic Interactional Assessment* (*DIA*) (Toglia, 1998) is a formal example of a dynamic investigative approach. *DIA* consists of awareness questioning, cueing and task grading, and strategy investigation (Toglia, 1998). During awareness questioning, patients answer increasingly specific questions that tap their intellectual awareness of potential problems. They also predict their performance before beginning the assessment task. Graded verbal cues are offered as needed once the patient begins work, and parameters of the task are changed, if necessary, to buoy the patient's performance. During task performance, the therapist seeks to understand what strategies or approaches the patient uses by asking strategy questions. Toglia incorporates *DIA* into a number of the standardized assessment tools she developed, including the *Contextual Memory Test* (Toglia, 1993) and the *Toglia Category Assessment* (Toglia, 1994).

When using methods and tools for assessing function to make inferences about cognition, occupational therapists generally seek to determine what the patient can do given various supports and conditions. These less structured approaches to evaluation allow for observation of metaprocesses and qualitative aspects of performance that are not easily captured using more structured methods. Because of their foundation in function, such methods capitalize on the unique expertise of occupational therapists. Hajek, Gagnon, and Ruderman (1997), however, suggested that functional assessments may not be sufficient for identifying cognitive disability and that rehabilitation outcome would be better predicted if the results of functional assessment were coupled with a detailed assessment of specific cognitive capacities and abilities.

Methods and Tools for Assessing Cognitive Capacities and Abilities to Make Inferences about Function

Based on the results of assessing performance of tasks and activities, clinicians generate hypotheses as to what specific barriers or impairments interfere with a patient's optimal occupational function. Tools and methods that assess specific cognitive capacities and abilities are then used to verify these hypotheses and establish a baseline against which to measure improvement. Many instruments have demonstrated reliability and validity, and standardized scoring criteria greatly reduce therapist bias. Assessments of specific cognitive capacities and abilities, however, may be predicated on a serious theoretical fallacy—the notion that these constructs can be separated from one another. Based on the inter-relatedness of various aspects of human cognition, one questions whether, for example, memory can be assessed apart from attention. Assessment Table 9-1 provides examples of various measures of specific cognitive capacities and abilities, including a cognitive screen and three microbatteries. A cognitive screen takes less than 15 minutes to administer and provides the clinician with a general sense of a patient's cognitive status but little information about what specific areas may be impaired. A microbattery may take up to 45 minutes to administer and consists of a number of subtests, typically associated with an array of cognitive capacities and abilities.

Assessment Table 9-1

Summary of Assessments of Cognition

Instrument and Reference	Description	Time to Administer	Validity	Reliability	Sensitivity	Strengths and Weaknesses
Selected Tools for Assessing Cognitive Capacities and Abilities to Make Inferences about Function						
Galveston Orientation and Amnesia Test (*GOAT*) (Levin, O'Donnell, & Grossman, 1979)	A widely used measure of orientation to person, place, time, and memory for events preceding and following injury. 10 questions with weighted error points deducted from a total of 100 points.	10–15 minutes.	Performance on the *GOAT* strongly related to aspects of the *Glasgow Coma Scale* (for eye opening, $\chi^2 = 21.09$, $p < 0.00001$; for verbal responding, $\chi^2 = 19.53$, $p < 0.000001$).	Good inter-rater reliability (Kendall τ coefficient = 0.99, $p < 0.001$).	Well suited to track fluctuations in confusional period after traumatic brain injury (TBI).	Strength: Brief test that evaluates PTA and RA (see Definition 9-1). Weakness: Designed for use after TBI and may be difficult to use with other populations of rehabilitation patients.
Orientation Log (*O-Log*) (Jackson, Novack, & Dowler, 1998)	10-item scale that is designed for repeated administration that evaluates orientation to place, time, and situation in terms of cueing needed for correct responses. Range of scores = 0–30.	~5 minutes.	Significant correlation with the *GOAT* ($r = 0.901$, $p < 0.001$) (Novack et al., 2000).	Good inter-rater reliability for total *O-Log* score (Spearman Rho = 0.993).	No psychometric data available regarding the test's sensitivity. As the patient receives points for responding to cues, however, the test may be sensitive to progress.	Strength: Applicable to a wide range of rehabilitation patients. Weakness: Less well known than *GOAT*.

Test of Everyday Attention (*TEA*) (Robertson et al., 1996)	Test of sustained, selective, and divided attention based on 8 ecologically plausible subtests such as Map and Telephone Search (selective attention), Elevator Counting and Lottery (sustained attention), and Telephone Dual Task (divided attention).	45–60 minutes.	Concurrent validity: moderate to moderately strong correlation between *TEA* subtests and other measures of attention ($r = 0.42$–0.63). Discriminant validity: Statistically significant differences between older healthy controls and older stroke patients on all subtests ($p < 0.001$) and on 5 of 8 subtests with younger paired subjects.	Test–retest reliability (across parallel forms of the test) is strong across subtests of the parallel versions ($r = 0.66$–0.90).	There are 3 parallel forms of the *TEA* to prevent patients from learning the test with repeated administration.	Strengths: Development of *TEA* was based on investigations for functional-neuroanatomical specialization of attention. Subtests have ecological validity for clients. Weaknesses: Not appropriate for patients with significant visual problems; rather lengthy assessment of one dimension of cognitive function.
Rivermead Behavioral Memory Test (*RBMT*) (Wilson, Cockburn, & Baddeley, 1985)	Assesses memory skills necessary for everyday life including remembering names, faces, routes, and appointments.	30–45 minutes.	Wilson et al. (1989) found statistically significant differences between persons with brain injury and healthy controls on all *RBMT* subtests ($p < 0.001$).	Inter-rater reliability: 100% agreement when 40 subjects with brain injury were scored separately but simultaneously by 2 raters (Wilson et al., 1989).	There are 4 parallel forms of the *RBMT* to prevent patients from learning the test with repeated administration.	Strengths: Subtests are similar to everyday tasks; useful in the characterization of memory disorders for a wide range of diagnostic groups (Lezak et al., 2004). Weakness: Requires intact visual and verbal skills.
Contextual Memory Test (Toglia, 1993)	Dynamic assessment of recall, awareness of memory capacity, and memory strategy use in which client tries to remember 20 objects related to 1 of 2 themes (ADL routine or restaurant).	30–40 minutes.	Concurrent validity: strongly correlated with the *RBMT* ($r = 0.80$–0.84).	Reliability for parallel forms of test ($r = 0.73$–0.81). Test–retest reliability for persons with brain injury ($r = 0.85$–0.94).	Not established.	Strength: One assessment that provides information about memory and information about meta-memory. Weakness: Potential for cultural bias-associated pictures (Josman & Hartman-Maeir, 2000).

continued

Assessment Table 9-1

Summary of Assessments of Cognition (continued)

Instrument and Reference	Description	Time to Administer	Validity	Reliability	Sensitivity	Strengths and Weaknesses
Selected Tools for Assessing Cognitive Capacities and Abilities to Make Inferences about Function						
Toglia's Category Assessment (*TCA*) (Toglia, 1994)	Dynamic assessment related to concept formation and ability to switch conceptual sets. 18 plastic utensils in 3 colors are sorted according to size, color, and type.	10–25 minutes to administer *TCA* and *DR* together.	Concurrent validity: positive significant correlation with the *Risk Object Classification* test, a static measure of categorization ($r = 0.51, p < 0.01$). Failed to detect significant differences between persons with schizophrenia and brain injury (Josman, 1998).	Inter-rater reliability of 0.87 (Josman, 1998).	Not established.	Strength: Involves use of familiar, functional objects to assess abstract concept. Weakness: Less predictive of IADL performance than *DR* test for persons with brain injury (Goverover & Hinojosa, 2002).
Toglia's Deductive Reasoning Test (DR) (Toglia, 1994)	*TCA* subtest designed to assess deductive reasoning. The client is asked to determine which utensil the examiner is thinking about by asking the fewest possible yes or no questions. Scores range from 1 (cannot obtain the right answer with maximum cues and task modification) to 7 (correct answer with 5 questions) for each of 3 trials.	10–25 minutes to administer *TCA* and *DR* together.	Adequate discriminant validity: significant differences in scores for persons with brain injury as compared to healthy controls ($F [1, 91] = 52.68, p < .001$) (Goverover & Hinojosa, 2004).	Interclass correlation coefficient computed to determine inter-rater reliability was statistically significant based on interclass correlation coefficient reliability test ($F [30] = 352.28, p < .001$) (Goverover & Hinojosa, 2004).	No information.	Strength: Score on *DR* test was found to be predictive of IADL performance in persons with brain injury (Goverover & Hinojosa, 2002). Weakness: Focuses on only one dimension of cognitive function.

Tinkertoy Test (*TTT*) (Lezak, 1982; Lezak et al., 2004)	Unstructured assessment of executive functions in which the patient is provided with 50 specific Tinkertoy pieces and given 2 instructions: "Make whatever you want with these" and "You will have at least 5 minutes and as much more time as you wish to make something." The patient's approach is observed, and the final construction is assigned a numerical score based on its complexity and sophistication, including mobility and symmetry (0–12 points).	At least 5 minutes.	Mixed findings. Bayless, Varney, and Roberts (1989) found statistically different *TTT* scores between 2 groups: healthy controls and employed persons 2 years post TBI versus unemployed persons who were 2 years post TBI. Spikman, Deelman, and van Zomeren (2000), however, found that *TTT* scores were not statistically different when comparing the scores of persons with TBI and healthy controls.	Moderately strong to strong inter-rater reliability on 3 of 7 subscores (three-dimensional ICC = 0.95, $p = 0.00$; name ICC = 0.71, $p = 0.00$; moving parts ICC = 0.78, $p = 0.00$) (Koss et al., 1998). (Note: inter-rater agreement was not evaluated on the other 4 subscores.)	No information.	Strength: Unstructured nature allows for observations related to executive functioning. Weakness: Adult patients may perceive constructional task involving Tinkertoys as childish or insulting.
Patient Competency Rating Scale (*PCRS*) (Prigatano et al., 1986)	The patient is asked to answer 30 questions related to everyday tasks, rating how easy or difficult each is (can't do, very difficult, some difficulty, fairly easy, can do with ease). A person familiar with the patient's abilities (family or staff) also rates the patient's proficiency with the 30 tasks. The magnitude of differences between self-ratings and those of the relative or staff quantifies the patient's awareness of deficits. Average perceived behavioral competency is calculated by computing the mean rating of competency across all 30 items.	15–20 minutes.	Moderate correlation between scores on the *PCRS* and the *Awareness Questionnaire* for patients (Spearman correlation coefficient = 0.50, $p < 0.01$) and informant (Spearman correlation coefficient = 0.62, $p < 0.01$) (Sherer, Hart, & Nick, 2003).	Strong inter-rater reliability (average $r = 0.92$) (Fordyce & Roueche, 1986). Strong 1-week test–retest reliability for total scores (ICC = 0.85 for persons 3 months post TBI; ICC = 0.95 for staff) (Fleming & Strong, 1999).	The original instrument has been modified for use with patients on an acute rehab unit (Borgaro & Prigatano, 2003).	Strengths: Formal methods of ascertaining discrepancies between patient, staff, and family perceptions of competence; could be used as a vehicle for discussion of incongruencies. Weakness: It is necessary to be familiar with the patient to judge the accuracy of his or her self-ratings.

continued

Assessment Table 9-1

Summary of Assessments of Cognition (continued)

Instrument and Reference	Description	Time to Administer	Validity	Reliability	Sensitivity	Strengths and Weaknesses
Selected Tools for Assessing Cognitive Capacities and Abilities to Make Inferences about Function						
Self-Awareness of Deficits Interview (*SADI*) (Fleming, Strong, & Ashton, 1996)	Tool designed to obtain both qualitative and quantitative data on status of self-awareness. The patient is asked about self-awareness of deficits, self-awareness of functional limitations because of deficits, and ability to set realistic goals. A therapist familiar with the patient's level of functioning assigns a score in each realm (0–3, with 0 representing full awareness).	10 minutes.	*SADI* moderately correlated with the *Dysexecutive Questionnaire* (*DEX*) ($r = 0.40$, $p < 0.05$). Regression analyses indicated that *SADI* scores were significantly predicted by a set of executive functioning measures ($p < 0.01$, $R^2 = 0.31$) (Bogod, Mateer, & MacDonald, 2003).	Strong inter-rater reliability (ICC = 0.82). Strong test–retest reliability (ICC = 0.94) (Simmond & Fleming, 2003).	No information.	Strength: Brief semi-structured interview with questions that are relevant to treatment planning. Weakness: Potential for bias because clinician judges the extent to which patient responses reflect level of self-awareness disorder.
Mini-Mental State Examination (*MMSE*) (Folstein, Folstein, McHugh, 1975).	Screening tool involving a therapist-administered interview comprised of 11 questions related to orientation, attention, learning, calculation, abstraction, information, construction, and delayed recall. Scores of 0–30 with scores of 24 or below suggestive of possible cognitive disorder (Tombaugh & McIntyre, 1992).	5–10 minutes.	Concurrent validity: *MMSE* score is highly correlated with *Weschler Adult Intelligence Scale* (for Verbal IQ, Pearson $r = 0.776$, $p < 0.0001$; for Performance IQ, Pearson $r = 0.660$, $p < 0.001$).	24-hour test–retest reliability, Pearson $r = 0.887$. Inter-rater reliability, Pearson $r = 0.827$.	Concerns about sensitivity of *MMSE* with scores < 24 (Kukull et al., 1994). Improved sensitivity with the *MMSE* (Teng & Chui, 1987) and in combination with draw a clock (Suhr & Grace, 1999; Watson, Arfken, & Birge, 1993).	Strengths: Widely used and understood by many rehabilitation and medical disciplines; brief screen that is helpful in determining need for more in-depth cognitive assessment (Zwecker et al., 2002). Weaknesses: Bias toward verbal items and, therefore, insensitive to damage in right hemisphere; poor sensitivity to mild cognitive deficits.

Loewenstein Occupational Therapy Cognitive Assessment (*LOTCA*) (Katz et al., 1989)	Microbattery consisting of 20 subtests in four areas: orientation, perception, visuomotor operations, and thinking operations.	30–45 minutes.	All subtests, except identification of objects, differentiated between patients with craniocerebral injury (CCI) and healthy controls and stroke patients and healthy controls using Wilcoxon two-sample tests ($p < 0.0001$).	Strong inter-rater reliability (Spearman's rank correlation coefficient ranged from 0.82–0.97 for various subtests).	Katz et al. (1989) observed improved test scores between test scores at admission and after 2 months for TBI and stroke patients.	Strength: Provides a snapshot of a number of cognitive capacities in a relatively short amount of time. Weaknesses: Does not pick up subtle cognitive deficiencies on persons with mild injuries; does not include measure of memory.
Cognitive Assessment of Minnesota (*CAM*) (Rustad et al., 1993)	Microbattery consisting of 17 subtests including attention, memory, orientation, neglect, following directions, money and math skills, planning and abstract reasoning, and problem solving.	45 minutes.	Concurrent validity: moderate correlation of *CAM* total score with the *Porteus Maze Test Quotient* ($r = 0.5016, p = 0.048$) and *MMSE* ($r = 0.4355$, $p = 0.046$).	A paired t-test comparing total *CAM* scores given by 2 raters indicated no statistically significant differences (suggesting adequate inter-rater reliability).	Discriminant analysis: results of the discriminant model indicate that 95.48% were correctly classified as having or not having cognitive impairment.	Strengths: Provides an overview of cognitive functioning; performance is reported in a profile format indicating presence or extent of impairment. Weakness: Possible ceiling effect for mild or subtle cognitive deficits; little literature on its use in rehabilitation.
Cognistat (*Neurobehavioral Cognitive Status Examination*) (Kiernan et al., 1987)	Microbattery that comprises 10 subtests in the areas of orientation*, attention, comprehension*, repetition*, naming*, construction, memory, calculation, similarities, and judgment.	20–25 minutes.	Discriminant analysis: Wilcoxon analysis suggested that 4 of the subtests (see*) discriminated between elderly persons with stroke and healthy independent elderly (Katz, Elazar, & Itzkovich, 1996); statistically significant mean scores for healthy controls, persons with Alzheimer's type dementia, and neurosurgical patients on 9 of 10 subtests (Katz et al., 1997).	No information.	Found to be more sensitive than *MMSE* with neurosurgical patients (Schwamm et al., 1987).	Strengths: Scores are presented in a profile of performance in each domain (average, mild, moderate, and severe impairment); normative data available for healthy elderly persons (Eisenstein et al., 2002). Weaknesses: Some test items (construction subtest) may be too difficult for both stroke patients and healthy elderly persons (Osman et al., 1992); not appropriate for geriatric or psychiatric patients (Engelhart, Eisenstein, & Meininger, 1994).

continued

Assessment Table 9-1

Summary of Assessments of Cognition (continued)

Instrument and Reference	Description	Time to Administer	Validity	Reliability	Sensitivity	Strengths and Weaknesses
Selected Tools for Assessing Function to Make Inferences about Cognition						
Arnadottir OT-ADL Neurobehavioral Evaluation (A-ONE) (Arnadottir, 1990)	Two parts to the instrument. Part 1 involves observing ADL performance and completing the (1) *Functional Independence Scale* and (2) *Neurobehavioral Specific Impairment Subscale*. Part 2 is optional, enabling the clinician to cross link the neurobehavioral impairment to the most likely lesion site.	25 minutes.	Content validity established through expert input. Concurrent validity: compared scores of 50 persons with stroke and 79 healthy controls. Significant Mann-Whitney *U* test suggests *A-ONE* discriminates between groups for all items of the *Functional Independence Scale* and all but 6 items of the *Neurobehavioral Subscale*.	Inter-rater reliability: *Functional Independence Scale*, kappa = 0.83); *Neurobehavioral Specific Impairment Subscale* (kappa = 0.86). Test–retest reliability within 1 week (r_s = 0.85).	No information.	Strength: Standardized methods for combining assessment of ADL with assessment of some areas of cognition so that therapists can assess both areas at the same time. Weakness: Neurobehavioral subscale does not include assessment in key cognitive capacities such as memory and attention.
Rabideau Kitchen Evaluation–Revised (RKE-R) (Neistadt, 1992)	Observational tool designed to assess the functional sequencing of adults with TBI in the context of preparing a sandwich and hot beverage (score range of 0–120).	30–45 minutes.	Criterion-related validity demonstrated by statistically significant association between scores on the *RKE-R* and the Block Design subtest of the *Weschler Adult Intelligence Scale–Revised* ($r = -0.60$, $p = 0.0002$).	Inter-rater agreement of 86% for the total score, with agreement on individual component steps ranging from 46–100%.	Not established.	Strength: Standardized tool for determining where to begin a meal preparation intervention protocol. Weakness: May not be sensitive enough to use with persons with subtle cognitive deficits.

Executive Function Route-Finding Task (EFRT) (Boyd & Sautter, 1993)	Patient is asked to find an unfamiliar location within the rehabilitation or health care setting as efficiently as possible. The therapist accompanies and observes the patient but may not answer questions about how to get there. Performance is rated in a number of domains including task understanding, information seeking, retaining directions, and error detection and correction, on-task behavior.	5–20 minutes (depending upon distance of unfamiliar location and patient's proficiency with route finding).	In a study involving persons with TBI, *EFRT* score was moderately correlated with Perceptual Organization ($r = 0.50, p < 0.05$) and Verbal Comprehension ($r = 0.44, p < 0.05$) subtest scores of the *Weschler Adult Intelligence Scale–Revised.* Spikman, Deelman, and van Zomeren (2000) found that scores on the *ERFT* were statistically different in two domains when comparing the scores of persons with TBI and healthy controls (Judgment of Route, $p < 0.01$; Frequency of Cues, $p < 0.005$).	Good inter-rater reliability (Pearson $r = 0.94, p < 0.001$).	No information.	Strengths: Unstructured nature allows for observations related to executive functioning; ecologically valid assessment task. Weakness: No information about sensitivity or predictiveness relative to ADL and IADL functioning.
Kitchen Task Assessment (KTA) (Baum & Edwards, 1993)	Measures cognitive support necessary for patient to prepare cooked pudding (neurobehavioral components are scored on a 0–3 scale, with total scores ranging from 0–18).	30–45 minutes.	Moderate to moderately strong correlation between *KTA* and 5 neuropsychological tests and 2 dementia rating scales (−0.46 to −0.68, $p < 0.001$).	Strong inter-rater reliability (0.853); strong internal consistency (correlation coefficients among subtests ranged from 0.72–0.84).	*KTA* scores are sensitive to stages of senile dementia of the Alzheimer's type ($p < 0.0001$).	Strength: Involves familiar, multistep functional task. Weakness: *KTA* was standardized on persons with dementia, and its appropriateness for other populations has not been established

continued

Assessment Table 9-1

Summary of Assessments of Cognition (continued)

Instrument and Reference	Description	Time to Administer	Validity	Reliability	Sensitivity	Strengths and Weaknesses
Observed Tasks of Daily Living–Revised (*OTDL-R*) (Diehl et al., 2005)	An assessment of everyday problem solving in which the patient performs 9 tasks related to medication use, telephone use, and financial management.	25–30 minutes.	*OTDL-R* scores were associated with measure of executive functioning (moderate correlation with the *Toglia Category Assessment*, $r = 0.506$, and moderately strong correlation with the *Deductive Reasoning Test*, $r = 0.796$) (Goverover & Hinojosa, 2002). *OTDL-R* scores were significantly different among 4 groups (community dwelling older adults, older adults living in nursing homes, individuals with schizophrenia, and individuals with brain injury) ($p < 0.001$) (Goverover & Josman, 2004).	Internal consistency for the total measure (Chronbach's $\alpha = 0.82$).	Not established.	Strength: Measure of everyday cognition that can be administered at bedside. Weakness: Does not provide a comprehensive picture of cognitive function, especially related to unstructured situations.

CASE EXAMPLE

Assessing Cognitive Function

Occupational Therapy Assessment Process	Clinical Reasoning Process	
	Objectives	**Examples of Therapist's Internal Dialogue**
Patient Information D.B. is a 26-year-old single male who sustained a TBI as a result of a pedestrian–auto accident. Upon admission to the emergency room, he had a Glasgow Coma Scale score of 6, and records indicate that he was in a coma for approximately 10 days. In addition to the brain injury, D.B. sustained fractures in both legs, a tibia-fibula fracture on the right and fracture of the femur on the left. D.B. participated in inpatient rehabilitation for 3 weeks.	Understand the patient's diagnosis or condition	"D.B. had a severe brain injury and will likely have significant, long-term cognitive impairments. He sounds like someone who is used to being active and mobility restrictions may be confusing and frustrating. I wonder how he is getting around now that he is 3 months post injury."
D.B. graduated from college with a degree in law enforcement and worked in a rural community as a police officer at the time of his injury. His former girlfriend broke off the relationship approximately 1 month ago.	Know the person	"I know that I have certain stereotyped expectations of cops. I expect him to be sort of rigid and reluctant to take instructions from women. I know that I may be wrong about that. I wonder if D.B.'s girlfriend couldn't handle the changes related to the TBI or if there were longstanding issues that led to the recent breakup. Either way, D.B. must feel sad and isolated."
Unable to return to his own apartment because of concerns about safety, D.B. was discharged from the inpatient rehabilitation unit to his brother's home. At approximately 3 months post TBI, D.B. was referred to outpatient occupational therapy to assess readiness for independent living. The occupational therapist focuses the assessment on D.B.'s ability to assume self-maintenance roles and identification of cognitive deficits interfering with role and task performance.	Appreciate the context	"I wonder what transpired during the past 2 months at the brother's home. How much of a role is the brother willing to play in this transition?"
	Develop provisional hypotheses	"Given his diagnosis and history, I presume that D.B.'s cognitive impairments are the biggest barriers to potential for independent living."
Assessment Process The therapist selected the following evaluation tools: *Canadian Occupational Performance Measure (COPM)* to obtain information about the client's perceived problems and priorities; *Kohlman Evaluation of Living Skills (KELS)*; *Cognitive Assessment of Minnesota (CAM)* to obtain a general picture of cognitive capabilities; and systematic observation of the client's response to the presentation of homework.	Consider evaluation approach and methods	"Because he hasn't been assessed in occupational therapy for over 2 months, I want to get a full picture of his occupational functioning. The *COPM* will tell me about his priorities and give me a snapshot of his awareness of deficits. The *KELS* will give me a chance to observe him in a number of IADL-related tasks. *CAM* will give me a sense of his cognitive strengths and weaknesses and be useful in benchmarking cognitive change. His response to homework will help me observe his use of compensatory cognitive strategies."

Assessment Results Based on an interview using the COPM, D.B. indicated that his ability to function independently was limited because of lower extremity fractures. He was dissatisfied with his inability to drive; the slowness with which he donned lower extremity clothing; his low stamina when walking outside the home; and lack of avocational outlets because of mobility limitations. When queried about known dependence on family members to take medications and his lack of initiation of self-maintenance tasks, D.B. quickly dismissed these reports as awkwardness associated with being a guest in their home. D.B. needed assistance to perform two activities in the Money Management component of the *KELS* (use of banking forms, payment of bills). He seemed capable to carrying out basic arithmetic operations but made transcription errors that he did not detect or correct on his own. In areas of Self-Care and Safety and Health, he demonstrated adequate awareness of and responses to personal and household hazards. On the *CAM,* D.B.'s scores in the areas of recall/recognition, problem solving, and abstract thinking ranked in the moderate to severe categories of impairment. Performance ranked within normal limits for such domains as orientation, following directions, immediate memory, temporal awareness, auditory memory and sequencing, and simple math and money skills. During each of his two outpatient evaluation sessions, the therapist gave D.B. oral instructions specific to three homework assignments to complete at home, all of which he agreed to do but did not make note of. He completed none of them. He seemed motivated throughout the assessment and did not appear distracted by pain or emotional distress during his sessions.	Interpret observations	"D.B. seems to be quite aware about concrete changes in his mobility but less aware of possible cognitive changes related to initiation and memory of medications. I wonder how much family members are helping to prevent any errors in daily life that might otherwise give him feedback about his cognitive changes." "Simply because D.B. 'passed' the Self-Care and Health and Safety components of the *KELS* doesn't mean I should set aside any concerns. This is a fairly structured test, and he might perform quite differently in a situation that required initiation and problem solving. I'll want to look at this further over time." "D.B.'s performance on the CAM doesn't surprise me all that much given the severity of his TBI. He seems to have a number of cognitive strengths that I think will really help him participate in the therapy process." "I'm guessing that D.B. has not had to take responsibility for keeping track of information in recent months; no doubt his brother has done that for him. I bet he hasn't had much experience with his memory changes and doesn't appreciate that he needs to compensate for these changes. He seems to be a really good candidate for outpatient rehabilitation at this point."
Occupational Therapy Problem List 1. Decreased initiation of ADL and IADL 2. Decreased productivity due to poor stamina and limited repertoire of appropriate avocational outlets 3. Memory inefficiency and inadequate repertoire of memory compensation strategies 4. Decreased awareness of cognitive deficits interfering with compensatory strategy use	Synthesize results	"Overall, D.B. seems to have rather superficial awareness of his limitations; he acknowledges physical but not cognitive changes. His brother's report of D.B.'s need for supervision with medications and prompts for ADL and IADL seem consistent with what I saw on his performance of the CAM. I don't really feel like I have a good handle on his problem-solving capabilities because most of the evaluations were very structured in nature. I'll want to incorporate opportunities for dynamic assessment into the treatment plan. I need to talk a little more with D.B.'s brother about the role he'd like to play in the therapy program. Maybe he needs a break and wants the team to take a more dominant role for a while."

CLINICAL REASONING IN OCCUPATIONAL THERAPY PRACTICE

Effects of Environment on Cognitive Function

During his inpatient rehabilitation, D.B. was observed to have decreased attentional capacities, especially with complex tasks. How might this problem be evident during the occupational therapy homemaking assessment? What factors in the environment might exaggerate these problems? What factors might minimize them?

SUMMARY REVIEW QUESTIONS

1. Analyze bill paying and grocery shopping in terms of the specific cognitive capacities and abilities required.
2. Compare the advantages and disadvantages of the two approaches to cognitive assessment described in this chapter.
3. Describe each variable that influences a person's ability to think. How would you expect these variables to affect cognitive assessment of an elderly illiterate client? How would you expect these variables to affect cognitive assessment of a college student?
4. Explain the occupational therapist's contribution to the rehabilitation team in the realm of cognitive assessment. Specifically, outline the ways in which occupational therapy complements the assessments of other professionals and the unique elements of occupational therapy.

References

Adamovich, B. B., Henderson, J. A., & Auerbach, S. (1985). *Cognitive rehabilitation of closed head injured patients*. San Diego: College-Hill.

American Occupational Therapy Association (2002). Occupational Therapy Practice Framework. *American Journal of Occupational Therapy, 56,* 609–639.

Anderson, S. W., & Tranel, D. (1989). Awareness of disease states following cerebral infarction, dementia, head trauma: A standardized assessment. *Clinical Neuropsychologist, 3,* 327–339.

Arnadottir, A. (1990). *The brain and behavior: Assessing cortical dysfunction through activities of daily living*. St. Louis: Mosby.

Atkinson, R. C., & Shiffrin, R. M. (1971). The control of short-term memory. *Scientific American, 225,* 82–90.

Baddeley, A. (1990). *Human memory: Theory and practice*. Boston: Allyn & Bacon.

Bandura, A. (1986). *Social foundations of thought and action: A social cognitive theory*. Englewood Cliffs, NJ: Prentice-Hall.

Baum, C., & Edwards, D. F. (1993). Cognitive performance in senile dementia of the Alzheimer's type: The Kitchen Task Assessment. *American Journal of Occupational Therapy, 47,* 431–436.

Bayless, J. D., Varney, N. R., & Roberts, R. J. (1989). Tinker toy test and performance and vocational outcome in patients with closed head injuries. *Journal of Clinical and Experimental Neuropsychology, 11,* 913–917.

Benedict, R. H., Wahlig, E., Bakshi, R., Fishman, I., Munschauer, F., Zivadinov, R., & Weinstock-Guttman, B. (2005). Predicting quality of life in multiple sclerosis: Accounting for physical disability, fatigue, cognition, mood-disorder, personality, and behavior change. *Journal of the Neurological Sciences, 231,* 29–34.

Bewick, K. C., Raymond, M. J., Malia, K. B., & Bennett, T. L. (1995). Metacognition as the ultimate executive: Techniques and tasks to facilitate executive functions. *NeuroRehabilitation, 5,* 367–375.

Bogod, N. M., Mateer, C. A., & MacDonald, S. W. S. (2003). Self-awareness after traumatic brain injury: A comparison of measures and their relationship to executive functions. *Journal of the International Neuropsychological Society, 9,* 450–458.

Borgaro, S. R., & Prigatano, G. P. (2003). Modification of the Patient Competency Rating Scale for use on an acute neurorehabilitation unit: The PCRS-NR. *Brain Injury, 17,* 847–853.

Boyd, T. M., & Sautter, S. W. (1993). Route-finding: A measure of everyday executive functioning in the head-injured adult. *Applied Cognitive Psychology, 7,* 171–181.

Bransford, J. D., & Stein, B. S. (1984). *The IDEAL problem solver: A guide for improving thinking, learning, and creativity*. New York: Freeman.

Bryant, D., Chiaravalloti, N. D., & DeLuca, J. (2004). Objective measurement of cognitive fatigue in multiple sclerosis. *Rehabilitation Psychology, 49,* 114–122.

Capruso, D. X., & Levin, H. S. (1992). Cognitive impairment following closed head injury. *Neurologic Clinics, 10,* 879–893.

Channon, S., & Green, P. S. S. (1999). Executive function in depression: The role of performance strategies in aiding depressed and non-depressed participants. *Journal of Neurology, Neurosurgery, and Psychiatry (London), 66,* 162–171.

Claesson, L., Linden, T., Skoog, I., & Blomstrand, C. (2005). Cognitive impairment after stroke: Impact on activities of daily living and costs of care for elderly people. The Goteborg 70+ Stroke Study. *Cerebrovascular Diseases, 19,* 102–109.

Crosson, B., Barco, P. P., Velozo, C. A., Bolesta, M. M., Cooper, P. V., Werts, D., & Brobeck, T. C. (1989). Awareness and compensation in postacute head injury rehabilitation. *Journal of Head Trauma Rehabilitation, 4,* 46–54.

Csikszentmihalyi, M. (1990). *Flow: The psychology of optimal experience*. New York: Harper Collins.

Denburg, S. D., Carbotte, R. M., & Denburg, J. A. (1997). Cognition and mood in systemic lupus erythematosus. *Annals of the New York Academy of Sciences, 823,* 44–59.

Diehl, M., Marsieke, M., Horgas, A. L., Rosenberg, A., Saczynski, J. S., & Willis, S. L. (2005). The Revised Observed Tasks of Daily Living: A performance-based assessment of everyday problem solving in older adults. *The Journal of Applied Gerontology, 24,* 211–230.

Diller, L. (1993). Introduction to cognitive rehabilitation. In C. Royeen (Ed.), *AOTA self-study series: Cognitive rehabilitation*. Rockville, MD: American Occupational Therapy Association.

Dougherty, P. M., & Radomski, M. V. (1993). *The cognitive rehabilitation workbook*. Gaithersburg, MD: Aspen.

Eisenstein, N., Engelhart, C. I., Johnson, V., Wolf, J., Williamsom, J., & Losonczy, M. B. (2002). Normative data for healthy elderly persons with the Neurobehavioral Cognitive Status Exam (Cognistat). *Applied Neuropsychology, 9,* 110–113.

Engelhart, C., Eisenstein, N., & Meininger, J. (1994). Psychometric properties of the Neurobehavioral Cognitive Status Exam. *The Clinical Neuropsychologist, 8,* 405–415.

Eysenck, M. W., & Keane, M. T. (1990). *Cognitive psychology: A student's handbook*. London: Lawrence Erlbaum.

Feuerstein, R. (1980). *Instrumental enrichment: An intervention program for cognitive modifiability*. Baltimore: University Park.

Fleming, J. M., Strong, J., & Ashton, R. (1996). Self-awareness of deficits in adults with traumatic brain injury: How best to measure? *Brain Injury, 10,* 1–15.

Fleming, J. M., & Strong, J. (1999). A longitudinal study of self-awareness: Functional deficits underestimated by persons with brain injury. *Occupational Therapy Journal of Research, 19,* 3–17.

Folstein, M. F., Folstein, S. E., & McHugh, P. R. (1975). "Mini-Mental State": A practical method for grading cognitive state of patients for the clinician. *Journal of Psychiatric Research, 12,* 189–198.

Fordyce, D. J., & Roueche, J. (1986). Changes in perspectives of disability among patients, staff, and relatives during rehabilitation of brain injuries. *Rehabilitation Psychology, 31,* 217–229.

Glover, J. A., Ronning, R. R., & Bruning, R. H. (1990). *Cognitive psychology for teachers*. New York: Macmillan.

Goldstein, F. C., & Levin, H. S. (1987). Disorders of reasoning and problem-solving ability. In M. J. Meier, A. L. Benton, & L. Diller (Eds.), *Neuropsychological rehabilitation* (pp. 327–354). New York: Guilford.

Goverover, Y. (2004). Categorization, deductive reasoning, and self-awareness: Association with everyday competence in persons with acute brain injury. *Journal of Clinical and Experimental Neuropsychology, 26,* 737–749.

Goverover, Y., & Hinojosa, J. (2002). Categorization and deductive reasoning: Predictors of instrumental activities of daily living performance in adults with brain injury. *American Journal of Occupational Therapy, 55,* 509–516.

Goverover, Y., & Hinojosa, J. (2004). Interrater reliability and discriminant validity of the Deductive Reasoning Test. *American Journal of Occupational Therapy, 58,* 104–108.

Goveroer, Y., & Josman, N. (2004). Everyday problem solving among four groups of individuals with cognitive impairments: Examination of the discriminant validity of the Observed Tasks of Daily Living-Revised. *Occupational Therapy Journal of Research, 24,* 103–112.

Hajek, V. E., Gagnon, S., & Ruderman, J. E. (1997). Cognitive and functional assessments of stroke patients: An analysis of their relation. *Archives of Physical Medicine and Rehabilitation, 78,* 1331–1337.

Hanks, R. A., Rapport, L. J., Millis, S. R., & Deshpande, S. A. (1999). Measures of executive functioning as predictors of functional ability and social integration in a rehabilitation sample. *Archives of Physical Medicine and Rehabilitation, 80,* 1030–1037.

Heaton, R. K., Marcotte, T. D., Mindt, M. R., Sadek, J., Moore, D. J., Bentley, H., McCutchan, J. A., Reicks, C., & Grant, I. (2004). The impact of HIV-associated neuropsychological impairment on everyday functioning. *Journal of the International Neuropsychological Society, 10,* 317–331.

Helmstaedter, C., Kurthen, M., Lux, S., Reuber, M., & Elger, C. E. (2003). Chronic epilepsy and cognition: A longitudinal study in temporal lobe epilepsy. *Annals of Neurology, 54,* 425–432.

Heyer, E., Sharma, R., Winfree, C. J., Mocco, J., McMahon, D. J., McCormick, P. A., Quest, D. Q., McMurtry, J. G., Riedel, C. J., Lazar, R. M., Stern, Y., & Connolly, E. S. (2000). Severe pain confounds neuropsychological test performance. *Journal of Clinical and Experimental Neuropsychology, 22,* 633–639.

Hochstenbach, J., Mulder, T., van Limbeek, J., Donders, R., & Schoonderwaldt, H. (1998). Cognitive decline following stroke: A comprehensive study of cognitive decline following stroke. *Journal of Clinical and Experimental Neuropsychology, 20,* 503–517.

Jackson, W. T., Novack, T. A., & Dowler, R. N. (1998). Effective serial measurement of cognitive orientation in rehabilitation: The Orientation Log. *Archives of Physical Medicine and Rehabilitation, 79,* 718–720.

Josman, N. (1998). Reliability and validity of the Toglia Category Assessment test. *Canadian Journal of Occupational Therapy, 66,* 33–42.

Josman, N. & Hartman-Maeir, A. (2000). Cross-cultural assessment of the Contextual Memory Test. *Occupational Therapy International, 7,* 246–258.

Katz, N. (2005). Higher level cognitive functions: Awareness and executive functions enabling engagement in occupation. In N. Katz (Ed.), *Cognition and occupation across the life span* (pp. 3–26). Bethesda, MD: American Occupational Therapy Association.

Katz, N., Elazar, B., & Itzkovich, M. (1996). Validity of the Neurobehavioral Cognitive Status Examination (COGNISTAT) in assessing patients post CVA and healthy elderly in Israel. *Israel Journal of Occupational Therapy, 5,* E185–E198.

Katz, N., Hartman-Maeir, A., Weiss, P., & Armon, N. (1997). Comparison of cognitive status profiles of healthy elderly persons with dementia and neurosurgical patients using the neurobehavioral cognitive status examination. *NeuroRehabilitation, 9,* 179–186.

Katz, N., Itzkovich, M., Averbuch, S., & Elazar, B. (1989). Loewenstein Occupational Therapy Cognitive Assessment (LOTCA) battery for brain-injured patients: Reliability and validity. *American Journal of Occupational Therapy, 43,* 184–192.

Kiernan, R. J., Mueller, J., Langston, J. W., & Van Dyke, C. (1987). The Neurobehavioral Cognitive Status Examination: A brief but differentiated approach to cognitive assessment. *Annals of Internal Medicine, 107,* 481–485.

Kolakowsky, S. A. (1998). Assessing learning potential in patients with brain injury: Dynamic assessment. *NeuroRehabilitation, 11,* 227–238.

Koss, E., Patterson, M. B., Mack, J. L., Smyth, K. A., & Whitehouse, P. J. (1998). Reliability and validity of the Tinkertoy Test in evaluating individuals with Alzheimer's disease. *The Clinical Neuropsychologist, 12,* 325–329.

Kukull, W. A., Larson, E. B., Teri, L., Bowen, J., McCormick, W., & Pfanschmidt, M. L. (1994). The Mini-Mental State Examination Score and the clinical diagnosis of dementia. *Journal of Clinical Epidemiology, 47,* 1061–1067.

Levin, H. S., O'Donnell, V. M., & Grossman, R. G. (1979). The Galveston Orientation and Amnesia Test. *Journal of Nervous and Mental Disease, 167,* 675–684.

Lezak, M. D. (1982). The problem of assessing executive functions. *International Journal of Psychology, 17,* 281–297.

Lezak, M. D. (1995). *Neuropsychological assessment* (3rd ed.). New York: Oxford University.

Lezak, M. D., Howieson, D. B., Loring, D. W., Hannay, H. J., & Fischer, J. S. (2004). *Neuropsychological assessment* (4th ed.). New York: Oxford University Press.

MacNeill, S. E., & Lichtenberg, P. A. (1997). Home alone: The role of cognition in return to independent living. *Archives of Physical Medicine and Rehabilitation, 78,* 755–758.

Mayer, R. E. (1992). *Thinking, problem solving, cognition.* New York: Freeman.

McLaurin, E. Y., Holliday, S. L., Williams, P., & Brey, R. L. (2005). Predictors of cognitive dysfunction in patients with systemic lupus erythematosus. *Neurology, 64,* 297–303.

Mazaux, J. M., Masson, F., Levin, H. S., Alaoui, P., Maurette, P., & Barat, M. (1997). Long-term neuropsychological outcome and loss of social autonomy after traumatic brain injury. *Archives of Physical Medicine and Rehabilitation, 78,* 1316–1320.

Miller, G. A. (1956). The magical number seven, plus or minus two: Some limits on our capacity for processing information. *Psychological Review, 63,* 81–97.

Mosey, A. C. (1993). Working taxonomies. In C. Royeen (Ed.), *AOTA self study series: Cognitive rehabilitation* (pp. 23–35). Rockville, MD: American Occupational Therapy Association.

Nadeau, B., & Buckheit, C. (1995). Work simulation as a diagnostic tool in the rehabilitation setting. *Occupational Therapy in Health Care, 9,* 37–44.

Neistadt, M. E. (1992). The Rabideau Kitchen Evaluation–Revised: An assessment of meal preparation skill. *Occupational Therapy Journal of Research, 12,* 242–253.

Neistadt, M. E. (1994). A meal preparation treatment protocol for adults with brain injury. *American Journal of Occupational Therapy, 48,* 431–438.

Nisbett, R. E., & Masuda, T. (2003). Culture and point of view. *National Academy of Sciences, 100,* 1163–1170.

Novack, T. A., Dowler, R. N., Bush, B. A., Tannahill, G., & Schneider, J. J. (2000). Validity of the Orientation Log relative to the Galveston Orientation and Amnesia Test. *Journal of Head Trauma Rehabilitation, 15,* 957–961.

Nygard, L., Amberla, K., Bernspang, B., Almkvist, O., & Winblad, B. (1998). The relationship between cognition and daily activities in cases of mild Alzheimer's disease. *Scandinavian Journal of Occupational Therapy, 5,* 160–166.

Osmon, D. C., Smet, I. C., Winegarden, B., & Gandhavadi, B. (1992). Neurobehavioral Cognitive Status Examination: Its use with unilateral stroke patients in a rehabilitation setting. *Archives of Physical Medicine and Rehabilitation, 73,* 414–418.

Ownsworth, T., & Fleming, J. (2005). The relative importance of metacognitive skills, emotional status, and executive function in psychosocial adjustment following acquired brain injury. *Journal of Head Trauma Rehabilitation, 20,* 315–332.

Perkins, D. (1995). *Outsmarting IQ.* New York: Free Press.

Polatajko, H. J., Mandich, A., & Martini, R. (2000). Dynamic performance analysis: A framework for understanding occupational performance. *American Journal of Occupational Therapy, 54,* 65–72.

Poutiainen, E., Elovaara, I., Raininko, R., Vilkki, J., Lahdevirta, J., & Iivanainen, M. (1996). Cognitive decline in patients with symptomatic HIV-1 infection: No decline in asymptomatic infection. *Acta Neurologica Scandinavica, 93,* 421–427.

Prigatano, G. P., Borgaro, S., Baker, J., & Wethe, J. (2005). Awareness and distress after traumatic brain injury: A relative's perspective. *Journal of Head Trauma Rehabilitation, 20,* 359–367.

Prigatano, G. P., Fordyce, D. J., Zeiner, H. K., Rouche, J. R., Pepping, M., & Wood, B. C. (1986). *Neuropsychological rehabilitation after brain injury.* Baltimore: John Hopkins University.

Prigatano, G. P., Ogano, M., & Amakusa, B. (1997). A cross-cultural study on impaired self-awareness in Japanese patients with brain dysfunction. *Neuropsychiatry, Neuropsychology, and Behavioral Neurology, 10,* 135–143.

Prigatano, G. P., & Schacter, D. L. (1991). *Awareness of deficit after brain injury: Clinical and theoretical issues.* New York: Oxford University.

Radomski, M. V. (1998). Problem-solving deficits: Using a multidimensional definition to select a treatment approach. *Physical Disabilities Special Interest Section Quarterly, 21,* 1–4.

Robertson, I. H., Ward, T., Ridgeway, V., & Nimmo-Smith, I. (1996). The structure of normal human attention: The Test of Everyday Attention. *Journal of the International Neuropsychological Society, 2,* 525–534.

Rustad, R. A., DeGroot, T. L., Jungkunz, M. L., Freeberg, K. S., Borowick, L. G., & Wanttie, A. M. (1993). *The cognitive assessment of Minnesota.* Tucson: Therapy Skill Builders.

Sandstrom, R., & Mokler, P. J. (1999). Cognitive function and key rehabilitation outcomes: Understanding the structure of human disability after sever motor stroke. *Journal of Rehabilitation Outcomes, 3,* 22–26.

Schacter, D. L (1996). *Searching for memory: The brain, the mind, and the past.* New York: Basic Books.

Scherzer, B. P., Charbonneau, S., Solomon, C. R., & Lepore, F. (1993). Abstract thinking following severe traumatic brain injury. *Brain Injury, 7,* 411–423.

Schilling, V., Jenkins, V., Morris, R., Deutsch, G., & Bloomfield, D. (2005). The effects of adjuvant chemotherapy on cognition in women with breast cancer: Preliminary results of an observational longitudinal study. *Breast, 14,* 142–150.

Schwamm, L. H., Van Dyke, C., Kiernan, R. J., Muerrin, E. L., & Mueller, J. (1987). The neurobehavioral cognitive status examination: Comparison with the cognitive capacity screening examination and the mini-mental status examination in a neurosurgical population. *Annals of Internal Medicine, 107,* 486–490.

Sherer, M., Hart, T., & Nick, T. G. (2003). Measurement of impaired self-awareness after traumatic brain injury: A comparison of the patient competency rating scale and the awareness questionnaire. *Brain Injury, 17,* 25–37.

Sherer, M., Hart, T., Whyte, J., Nick, T. G., & Yablon, S. A. (2005). Neuroanatomic basis of impaired self-awareness after traumatic brain injury. *Journal of Head Trauma Rehabilitation, 20,* 287–300.

Simmond, M., & Fleming, J. (2003). Reliability of the self-awareness of deficits interview for adults with traumatic brain injury. *Brain Injury, 17,* 325–337.

Small, S. A., Stern, Y., Tang, M., & Mayeux, R. (1999). Selective decline in memory function among healthy elderly. *Neurology, 52,* 1392–1396.

Sohlberg, M. M., & Mateer, C. A. (1989). *Introduction to cognitive rehabilitation theory and practice.* New York: Guilford.

Sohlberg, M. M., & Mateer, C. A. (2001). *Cognitive rehabilitation.* New York: Guilford Press.

Spikman, J. M., Deelman, B. G., & van Zomeren, A. H. (2000). Executive functioning, attention and frontal lesions in patients with chronic CHI. *Journal of Clinical and Experimental Neuropsychology, 22,* 325–338.

Sternberg, R. J. (1990). *Metaphors of mind: Conceptions of the nature of intelligence.* New York: Cambridge University.

Suhr, J. A., & Grace, J. (1999). Brief cognitive screening of right hemisphere stroke: Relation to functional outcome. *Archives of Physical Medicine and Rehabilitation, 80,* 773–776.

Teng, E. L., & Chui, H. (1987). The Modified Mini-Mental State (3MS) Examination. *Journal of Clinical Psychiatry, 48,* 314–318.

Toglia, J. P. (1989). Approaches to cognitive assessment of the brain-injured adult. *Occupational Therapy Practice, 1,* 36–55.

Toglia, J. P. (1993). *The contextual memory test.* Tucson: Therapy Skill Builders.

Toglia, J. P. (1994). *Dynamic assessment of categorization skills: The Toglia category assessment.* Pequannock, NJ: Maddak.

Toglia, J. P. (1998). A dynamic interactional model to cognitive rehabilitation. In N. Katz (Ed.), *Cognition and occupation in rehabilitation.* Bethesda, MD: American Occupational Therapy Association.

Toglia, J. P. (2005). A dynamic interactional approach to cognitive rehabilitation. In N. Katz (Ed.), *Cognition and Occupation Across the Life Span* (pp. 29–72). Bethesda, MD: American Occupational Therapy Association.

Tombaugh, T. N., & McIntyre, N. J. (1992). The Mini-Mental State Examination: A comprehensive review. *Journal of the American Geriatric Society, 40,* 922–935.

Wagner, R. K. (1991). Managerial problem solving. In R. J. Sternberg & P.A. Frensch (Eds.), *Complex problem solving: Principles and mechanisms* (pp. 159–183). Hillsdale, NJ: Lawrence Erlbaum.

Walker, C. M., Walker, M. F., & Sunderland, A. (2003). Dressing after stroke: A survey of current occupational therapy practice. *British Journal of Occupational Therapy, 66,* 263–268.

Watson, Y. I., Arfken, C. L., & Birge, S. J. (1993). Clock completion: An objective screening test for dementia. *Journal of the American Geriatric Society, 41,* 1235–1240.

Wilson, B. A., Cockburn, J., & Baddeley, A. (1985). *The Rivermead Behavioral Memory Test.* Reading, UK: Thames Valley Test; Gaylord, MI: National Rehabilitation Services.

Wilson, B. A., Cockburn, J., Baddeley, A., & Hiorns, R. (1989). The development and validation of a test battery for detecting and monitoring everyday memory problems. *Journal of Clinical and Experimental Neuropsychology, 11,* 855–870.

Zwecker, M., Levenkrohn, S., Fleisig, Y., Zeilig, G., Ohry, A., & Adunsky, A. (2002). Mini-Mental State Examination, Cognitive FIM Instrument, and the Loewenstein Occupational Therapy Cognitive Assessment: Relation to functional outcome of stroke patients. *Archive of Physical Medicine and Rehabilitation, 83,* 342–345.

CHAPTER 10

Assessing Context: Personal, Social, and Cultural

Mary Vining Radomski

LEARNING OBJECTIVES

After studying this chapter, the reader will be able to do the following:

1. Describe the components of personal, social, and cultural context that influence occupational therapy assessment and guide treatment planning.
2. Employ methods for quantifying the influence of various contextual factors on performance.
3. Recognize the role of contextual factors in the development of conditional reasoning in clinical practice.
4. Examine his or her own contextual fabric—the personal, social, and cultural factors that shape the therapist's everyday experiences.

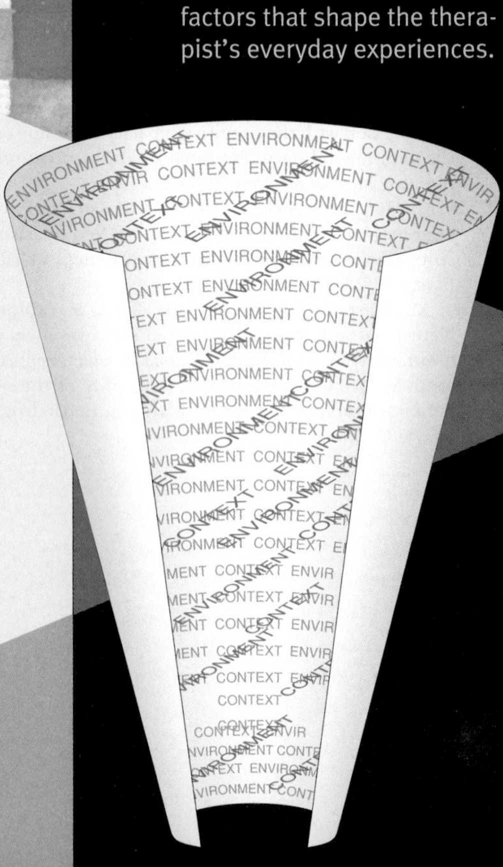

Glossary

Context—The whole situation, background, or environment that is relevant to a particular event or personality (Webster's New World Dictionary, 1994).

Culture—The norms, values, and behavior patterns that serve as guidelines for people's interactions with others and their environments (Krefting, 1991).

Cultural context—Stable and dynamic norms, values, and behaviors associated with the community or societal environments in which occupational functioning occurs.

Ethnicity—Membership by virtue solely of one's birth in a racial, religious, national, or linguistic group (McGruder, 1998). In and of itself, ethnicity does not predict cultural identity.

Personal context—A person's internal environment, derived from stable and dynamic factors such as sex, age, mood, and cultural identity.

Social context—The social environment consisting of stable and dynamic factors such as premorbid roles, social network, and support resources.

Social network—An interactive web of people who provide each other with helpfulness and protection. Social networks typically vary in terms of reciprocity, complexity, intensity, and density (Heaney & Israel, 1997).

Social support—The aid and assistance (emotional, instrumental, information, and appraisal) exchanged through a social network (Heaney & Israel, 1997).

Spirituality—Beliefs and practices that give a person transcendent meaning in life (Puchalski, 1996).

Much as a phrase, punch line, or couplet can be understood only in the larger **context** of a story, joke, or poem, a client's performance during occupational therapy assessment can be interpreted only in light of the broader context of his or her life and background. For example, lack of eye contact during an initial interview can easily be misinterpreted as lack of interest or motivation unless the therapist appreciates the contribution of cultural background—that avoiding eye contact is a way of showing respect in some **cultures**, including the Vietnamese culture (Farrales, 1996). Difficulty selecting clothing during a dressing assessment may be erroneously attributed to a patient's poor decision-making skills unless the therapist appreciates the contribution of social role experiences—that for 50 years, the patient's wife set out his clothing each morning.

The term *context* refers to the whole situation, background, or environment that is relevant to a particular event or personality; it has its roots in the Latin word *contexere*, to weave together (*Webster's New World Dictionary*, 1994). Occupational therapists appreciate that a person's function at any moment is shaped by a tapestry of contextual factors, and not solely by his or her capacities, acquired skills, and abilities. Without deliberate attention to these personal, social, cultural, and physical mediators of performance, therapists may misunderstand what they observe during assessment and risk assigning erroneous labels of dysfunction.

This chapter describes the personal, social, and cultural contextual factors that help or hinder performance during occupational therapy assessment. (Chapter 11 focuses on assessing contextual factors associated with the built or physical environment.) After summarizing the role of context in human functioning, this chapter discusses specific examples of personal, social, and cultural context in terms of their potential for influencing occupational therapy assessment and intervention. Using these examples, readers are encouraged to reflect on other contextual factors not discussed herein. The role of context in occupational function cannot be exhaustively explored in one chapter; whole texts and careers have been devoted to each of these complex constructs. This overview, however, has one superordinate aim: to inspire therapists to try to interpret clients' performance in the broader context of their background, changing circumstances, and envisioned futures.

CONTEXT AND OCCUPATIONAL FUNCTION

Occupational function is always embedded in context, with physical, cultural, social, and personal factors shaping its form (Nelson, 1988). Figure 10-1 depicts the interweaving of personal, social, cultural, and physical context that creates the parameters of a given occupational experience. Consider how minor changes in any dimension change the tapestry: a middle-aged homemaker preparing eggs and toast for her children before they leave for school versus a middle-aged homemaker preparing the same breakfast as part of an occupational therapy assessment.

The important role of context in occupational function is described by a number of models and frameworks from occupational therapy, rehabilitation, and health fields. Each of the models or frameworks summarized in Table 10-1 emphasizes the dynamic relationship between a person; his or her cultural, social, and physical contexts; and the continuum of function to disability relative to chosen roles and tasks.

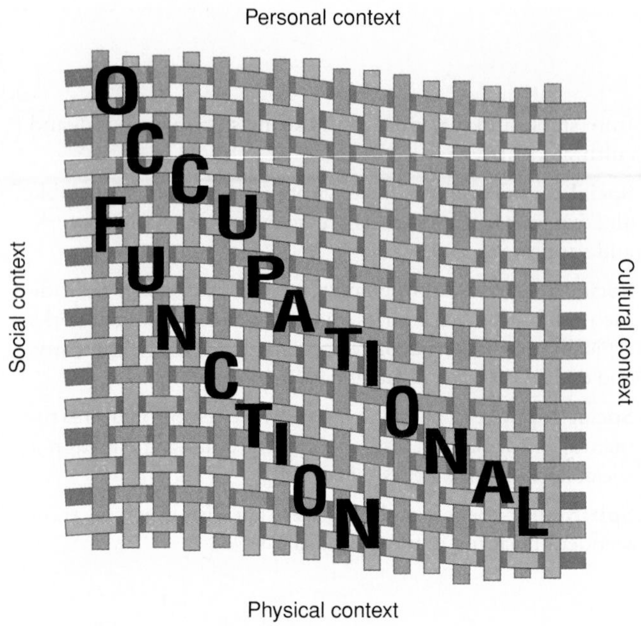

Figure 10-1 Interwoven tapestry of personal, social, cultural, and physical contextual factors.

The aforementioned models universally downplay the contribution of physical impairments and elevate the role of context in the explanation of human functioning and disablement but use slightly different terminology. In this chapter, contextual factors are presumed to be peripheral or unrelated to clients' primary diagnoses or disabling conditions (World Health Organization, 2001) but central to the broad realms within which people carry out their lives.

- **Personal context** reflects an individual's internal environment derived from his or her gender, values, beliefs, cultural background, or state of mind.
- **Social context** refers to factors in the human environment (roles, resources, and structure) that enable or deter the person's occupational function.
- **Cultural context** has to do with the norms, values, and behaviors related to the community or society in which the occupational function occurs.

The convenience of describing personal, social, and cultural contextual factors as separate and distinct entities

Table 10-1. Selected Models or Frameworks that Specifically Include Context as an Element in Human Function

Models and Frameworks	Synopsis of Role of Context in Occupation and/or Human Function
Ecology of Human Performance (Dunn, Brown, & McGuigan, 1994)	The interaction between a person and the environment affects his or her behavior and performance. Human performance can be understood only through the "lens" of context, which includes temporal (age, development, health status), physical, cultural, and social features that operate external to a person. In essence, the inter-relationship between person and context determines which tasks fall within the individual's performance range.
Person-Environment-Occupation Model of Occupational Performance (Law et al., 1996)	Occupational function is the result of the transactive relationship "between people, their occupations and roles, and the environments in which they live, work, and play" (p. 9). This model emphasizes the interdependence of person and environment (defined as those contexts and situations which occur outside the individual such as cultural, socioeconomic, institutional, and social considerations). It also recognizes the temporal or changing nature of person, environment, occupation characteristics, and their inter-relationships.
Occupational Therapy Intervention Process Model (Fisher, 1998)	Occupational performance occurs as a "transaction between the person and the environment as he or she enacts a task" (p. 514). Therapists must be aware of the client's performance context (comprised of temporal, environmental, cultural, societal, social, role, motivational, capacity, and task dimensions) to understand, evaluate, and interpret a person's occupational performance.
International Classification of Functioning, Disability, and Health (World Health Organization, 2001)	"A person's functioning and disability are conceived as a dynamic interaction between health conditions and contextual factors" (p. 10). Contextual factors include personal and environmental factors. Personal factors are internal influences of functioning that are not part of a health condition or functional state such as gender, age, social background, fitness, lifestyle, and habits. Environmental factors, external influences on functioning, include features of the physical, social, and attitudinal world.
Occupational Therapy Practice Framework (American Occupational Therapy Association, 2002)	The overarching outcome of occupational therapy is to advance clients' engagement in occupation to support life participation in the context of their unique situations. As such, "context" (cultural, physical, social, personal, spiritual, temporal, virtual) is included in the domain of occupational therapy. Context is viewed as affecting occupational performance as well as an underlying influence on the process of service delivery.

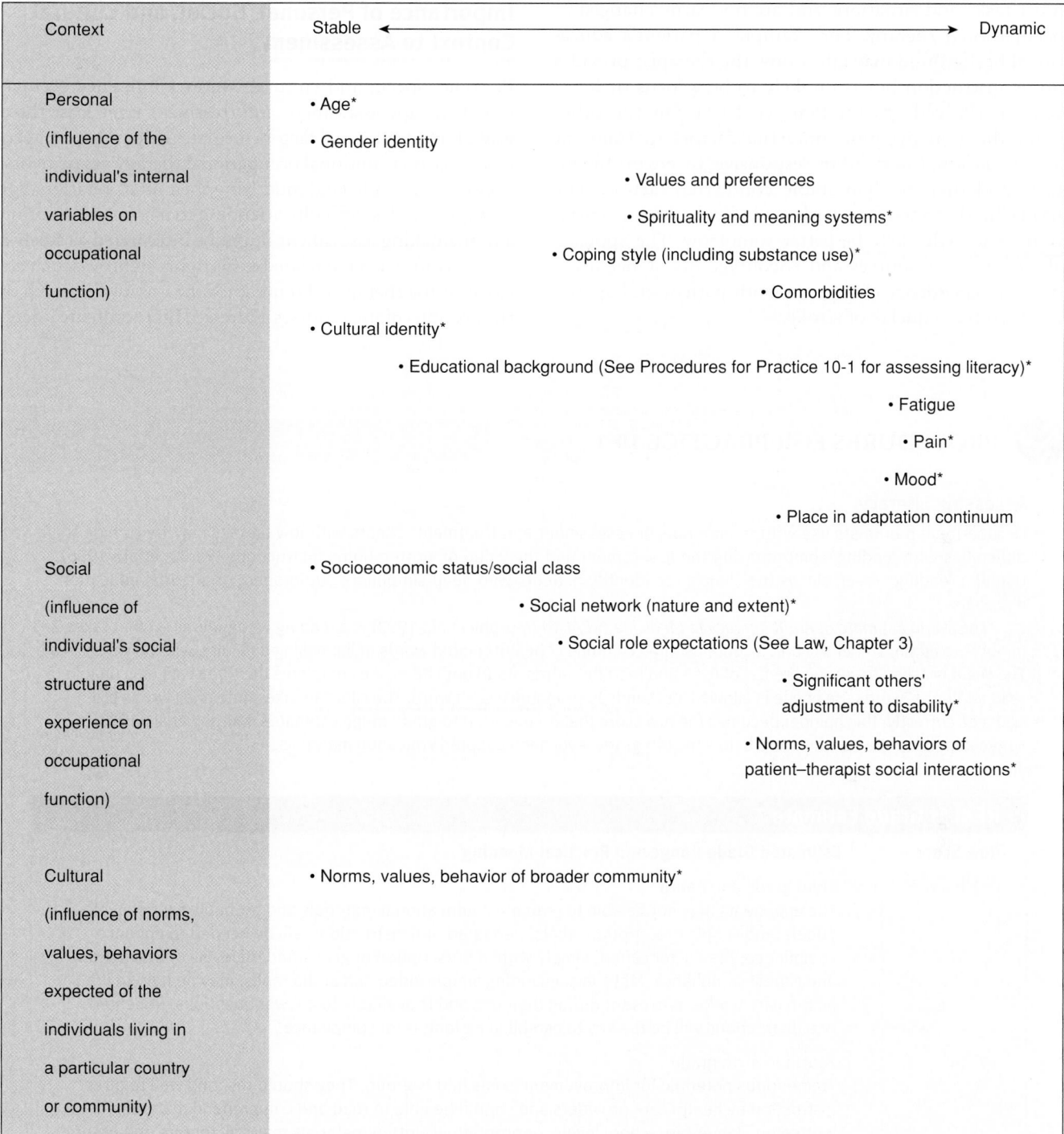

Context	Stable ⟷ Dynamic
Personal (influence of the individual's internal variables on occupational function)	• Age* • Gender identity • Values and preferences • Spirituality and meaning systems* • Coping style (including substance use)* • Comorbidities • Cultural identity* • Educational background (See Procedures for Practice 10-1 for assessing literacy)* • Fatigue • Pain* • Mood* • Place in adaptation continuum
Social (influence of individual's social structure and experience on occupational function)	• Socioeconomic status/social class • Social network (nature and extent)* • Social role expectations (See Law, Chapter 3) • Significant others' adjustment to disability* • Norms, values, behaviors of patient–therapist social interactions*
Cultural (influence of norms, values, behaviors expected of the individuals living in a particular country or community)	• Norms, values, behavior of broader community*

* These factors are discussed in this chapter.

Figure 10-2 Examples of interrelated personal, social, and cultural contextual factors.

belies their complexity, inter-relatedness, and interactive influences (Fig. 10-2). Krefting (1991) described the pervasive influence of culture on community, families (norms, values, and behaviors related to social context), and individuals (such as distinctive food preferences, humor, definition of personal space; in this chapter, considered to be a part of personal context). Likewise, personal context may influence social and cultural context. For example, a person's spiritual beliefs often shape his or her **social network**, preferred roles, and definitions of acceptable behavior.

Personal, social, and cultural contextual factors can be examined on a continuum of highly stable to highly dynamic. The relatively stable factors, such as age, gender identity, and premorbid coping style, tend to pervade most tasks and situations and are not easily changed in occupational therapy. For example, a patient's educational background may affect how the therapist provides home instruction but is unlikely to be a focus of intervention (Procedures for Practice 10-1). On the other hand, the more dynamic contextual factors are transient and situational and more responsive to environment, task, and therapy than stable contextual factors. The headache that interferes with an individual's concentration today will likely be better tomorrow. The spouse's ability to use resources and encourage his or her loved one's independence changes as both patient and spouse adapt to the sequelae of stroke.

Importance of Personal, Social, and Cultural Context to Assessment

Personal, social, and cultural contexts influence occupational therapy assessment and treatment in at least three ways. First, contextual factors mediate (help or hinder) performance on traditional occupational therapy assessments, skewing the results and muddying their interpretation. For example, Mr. J.'s difficulty attending to instructions during a homemaking assessment might be interpreted as solely a cognitive impairment related to his right cerebrovascular accident if the therapist did not know he was awake much of the previous night as nurses addressed his roommate's dete-

PROCEDURES FOR PRACTICE 10-1

Assessing Literacy

Occupational therapists use written materials in assessment and treatment. Clients with low literacy may try to hide their difficulties with reading, compromising the assessment and the value of written home instructions (Parikh et al., 1996). Use of a reading screen allows the clinician to identify patients who need simplified, audiotaped, or pictorial education materials.

The *Rapid Estimate of Adult Literacy in Medicine (REALM)* (Murphy et al., 1993) is a reading recognition test that takes 2–3 minutes to administer and score. It contains three columns of health-related words of increasing difficulty, with 66 words in all. The client is asked to start at the top of list 1 and read the words aloud until he or she completes the three lists or is unable to read additional words. He or she is allowed 5 seconds to pronounce each word. The clinician takes note of all words pronounced correctly; this number becomes the raw score that is converted to grade range estimates. Murphy et al. (1993) suggested that patients who score below the 9th-grade level need adapted education materials.

REALM Grade Estimate

Raw Score	Estimated Grade Range and Practical Meaning
0–18	Third grade and below These patients may not be able to read most educational materials and probably cannot even understand simple prescription labels. Repeated oral instructions will be needed to enhance compliance; the doctor cannot simply write a prescription or give standard levels of instruction and expect compliance. Materials, including simple video and audio tapes, may be helpful if a health care worker is present during their use and is available to answer questions. Repeated oral instructions will be the key to establishing long-term compliance.
19–44	Fourth to sixth grade Tremendous potential for improvement exists in this group. They should respond well to direct instruction by health care providers and should be able to read and comprehend materials written on elementary school levels. Appropriately written materials may still require one-on-one counseling for adequate understanding.
45–60	Seventh to eighth grade These patients will certainly benefit from appropriately written materials, but material (both oral and written) should not be too simple (e.g., first grade) or too complex. Material written for a fourth- to sixth-grade level may be appropriate.
61–66	Ninth grade and above These readers can understand much high school–level material presented to them; therefore, current educational brochures may be effective. These individuals should also be able to converse with their physicians about matters of lifestyle.

riorating medical condition. Second, contextual factors may be facilitators or barriers to function and therefore targets of occupational therapy intervention. Consider the influence of social context on occupational therapy goals. Despite adequate strength and technical skills, Mrs. S. remains dependent in lower extremity dressing after her total hip replacement because her husband, fearful that she may overexert, insists on assisting with dressing. The home health therapist, who brings his or her own biases regarding the goal of independence, ultimately collaborates with Mr. and Mrs. S. regarding their expectations of therapy. Should they choose to work toward complete independence in self-care, the therapist helps Mr. S. become comfortable with Mrs. S. dressing herself and helps Mrs. S. improve her skills. Finally, throughout the assessment, occupational therapists trawl for glimpses of what clients find meaningful—lures to hook them into therapy. Each dimension of context holds such possibilities as goals are set and intervention is planned.

Conditional Reasoning

Awareness of interwoven contextual factors is a foundation for what Mattingly and Fleming (1994) describe as conditional reasoning: viewing the client as a complex composite of premorbid characteristics and preferences, condition-specific limitations, and future potentialities.

"Therapists try to understand what is meaningful to the patients, and to their perceptions of themselves and others in the physical and social contexts in which they experience their lives. To do this, therapists need an ability to imagine the clients, both as they were before the illness, and as they could be in the future. They also need to be able to enlist the patients in imagining a possible future for themselves" (Mattingly & Fleming, 1994, p. 197).

Conditional reasoning enables the therapist to appreciate the wholeness of the client and his or her situation. Although it is more often employed by experienced therapists than novices (Mattingly & Fleming, 1994), one may presume that desire to learn may expedite the acquisition of this mindset.

Looking in the Mirror: Therapist as Contextually Influenced Being

Appreciation for the influence of personal, social, and cultural context requires that therapists acquire a complex combination of knowledge, attitudes, and skills. The goal is to shift from viewing how a client can fit into the therapist's world to examining how the therapist can understand and fit into the client's world (St. Clair & McKenry, 1999). To accomplish this shift, therapists must acknowledge and inventory the personal, social, and cultural factors that influence their own function. As I become aware of my own beliefs and biases, social background, and culturally based expectations, I will be able to appreciate their influence on collaborations with patients and coworkers (Odawara, 2005).

In summary, clinicians need not obsess about correctly labeling or pigeonholing each and every contextual factor. Rather, therapists aim to tease out various contributions to clients' performance during assessment so as to inform intervention planning by asking whether this person's present performance is influenced by the following:

- Personal, social, or cultural factors that obscure identification of strengths or weaknesses in occupational function
- Longstanding personal, social, or cultural factors that are unlikely to change as a result of therapy
- Personal, social, or cultural factors that are transient or situational; factors that may be affected by occupational therapy intervention
- The therapist's personal, social, or cultural contextual factors

PERSONAL CONTEXT

> "Life is suddenly reduced to a one dimension picture, known as physical function, and continually referred to as 'outcome.' The typical outcome process ignores . . . emotional and interpersonal needs and skills. Within those parameters lies the answer to true recovery . . . I refuse to have an 'outcome.' I do have a *life*!" (Cannon, 1994, p. 3)

Personal context refers to the intrapersonal environment that shapes an individual's experience. These factors play a role in determining the client's unique response to the onset of illness or impairment and contribute to his or her ability to adapt (National Center for Medical Rehabilitation and Research, 1993). Some aspects of a person's internal environment, such as age and longstanding beliefs, are stable; others, such as pain, mood, and adaptation to illness or injury (see Chapter 35), may be constantly in flux.

Personal Demographics: Age

A person's age influences his or her occupational functioning in three primary ways: (1) age-related changes in capacities and abilities; (2) developmental shifts in goals, values, and priorities; and (3) the individual's generation-based worldview.

Table 10-2 summarizes typical changes in capacities and abilities associated with normal aging. In tandem with physiological changes in capacities, Royeen (1995) hypothesized that people undergo "occupational shifts" (p. 11) during the life cycle that lead to major changes in patterns

Table 10-2. Age-Related Changes in Physical and Cognitive Capacities and Abilities

Age Group	Physical Development	Cognitive Development
20s	• Fully developed body shape and proportions (except weight and body mass, which fluctuate throughout a person's life) • Peak muscle strength achieved • Fully mature reproductive systems, with both sexes experiencing involuntary cyclic alterations in sex hormone production	• Peak brain cell development (although the final number of neurons and supportive cells that a person possesses is determined by the end of the first year of life) • Memory capacity peaks with the brain's greatest mass • Gradual shrinkage of brain cells at aroundage 30, but because of the vast number of unused brain cells, these changes do not impact function
30s and 40s	• Gradual slowing of body functions (dependent on diet, exercise, stress, genetic predisposition, and presence of disease) • Without regular exercise, gradual loss of muscle size and strength and bone mass and density • Decreasing elasticity in cardiorespiratory system, resulting in gradually decreasing respiratory capacity and increasing blood pressure • Beginnings of hearing loss (first limited to high pitches) • Beginnings of presbyopia (affecting near vision), which necessitates reading glasses or bifocals	• Continued gradual brain shrinkage but increasing life experiences result in high mental acumen
50s and 60s	• Physical changes of previous decades continue at a faster rate and to a greater extent • Fewer calories are required (necessitating changes in intake and/or activities to maintain weight) • Changes in amounts and patterns of hormone production affecting metabolism, energy, sexuality, and reproduction	• Continued brain shrinkage offset by reservoir of life experience, wisdom, and judgment
70s and older	• Loss of vestibular function in inner ears, resulting in decreased balance • Steady deterioration of vision and hearing • Loss of cartilage and connective tissue, leading to decreased range of motion, pain, and postural changes • Reduced appetite due to inactive taste buds and changes in digestion • Changes in metabolism, making it more difficult to adapt to changing temperatures	• Decreasing memory capacity • Decreasing abilities in areas of abstract reasoning and novel problem solving • Enriched perspectives based on lifelong learning and integrated experiences

Summarized from Freiberg, 1987.

of activity. She posited that early adulthood is characterized by establishing worker roles while realigning social roles to adjust to marriage and parenthood. In middle adulthood, people maintain work and leisure roles but may undergo sudden occupational shifts related to caregiving roles of parents, children, and grandchildren. During maturity (45 years to retirement), people continue their work and leisure roles, but occupational shifts arise from death of family members, loss of provider status, and adjustments in life goals. Persons in old age must adjust to changes in role performance commensurate with deterioration of physical and mental capacities.

Finally, a person's age location in history may influence his or her personality and beliefs (Lancaster & Stillman, 2002; Strauss & Howe, 1991). Although clinicians avoid jumping to conclusions about patients based on age, consider the ways in which generational identity may influence participation in occupational therapy for five contemporary generational groups in the United States:

- G. I. elders (born 1901–1924) strive for public harmony and cooperative social discipline and subscribe to a philosophy that optimism and hard work guarantee goal achievement.

- Silent midlifers (born 1925–1942) appreciate a variety of mindsets, virtues, and flaws and subscribe to a philosophy that promotes compromise and consensus as means to happy endings.
- Boomer adults (born 1943–1960) view their own opinions and perspectives as morally correct and subscribe to a philosophy suggesting that adherence to moral ideals leads to satisfying experience.
- Generation Xers (born 1961–1981) typically identify the need for personal determinism and subscribe to a philosophy that elevates the acquisition of money to personal survival in response to perceived uncertainties in their economic future.
- Millennials (born 1981–2000), who tend to be practical and techno-savvy, have a unique appreciation for diversity—variety in people, environments, and activities. They are accustomed to participant-oriented decision making and expect to work in collaboration with others in their endeavors (Lancaster & Stillman, 2002).

Of course, generalizations about patterns of aging may or may not apply to specific individuals, and therapists are cautioned against age-related patient biases (Rybarczyk et al., 2001). Human function over time is influenced by an array of factors, such as lifetime habits related to diet and exercise, stress, genetic predispositions, and sociocultural background (Freiberg, 1987). Catastrophic loss of function, as with illness or disability, takes place against a backdrop of other age-related changes, developmental tasks, and worldviews. For example, a person's adaptation to a spinal cord injury may occur as he or she is also adapting to a new marriage or career. An elderly patient's efforts to relearn motor skills and standing balance may be complicated by declines in capacities associated with age and beliefs that, if a person works hard enough, he or she will always achieve goals. A client who has lived and aged with a long-standing disability will likely have different health concerns and vulnerabilities than a young person with a new injury (Amsters et al., 2005).

Coping Strategies and Beliefs

Premorbid coping styles and long-term spiritual beliefs and meaning systems influence peoples' reactions to catastrophic injury and chronic illness.

Coping Style

The ways that people typically face stressful circumstances affect whether they seek health-related services and the extent to which they follow professionals' advice (Lerman & Glanz, 1997). Coping styles are relatively stable characteristics of a person and are thought to mediate the effects of stress on function (Lerman & Glanz, 1997). (Procedures for Practice 10-2 describes assessment of substance use, a maladaptive coping style.)

Lerman and Glanz (1997) summarized two aspects of coping. Consider how each of them contributes to or derails occupational therapy assessment and treatment when they are part of the client or therapist's longstanding coping style.

- Optimism is the tendency to have positive rather than negative expectations for outcomes. Optimism is associated with relatively few physical symptoms during stress, and it predicts psychological adjustment. Optimists tend to use active coping strategies, such as planning, problem solving, and acceptance rather than avoidance.
- Locus of control is a general belief about one's ability to control relevant life circumstances and events. People with an internal locus of control are likely to take

PROCEDURES FOR PRACTICE 10-2

Assessing Possible Substance Abuse

Alcohol use is a risk factor for spinal cord and brain injury (Bogner et al., 2001; Kolakowsky-Hayner et al., 1999). Kolakowsky-Hayner et al. found alarmingly high rates of pre-injury heavy drinking among patients who were treated in a Level I trauma center and subsequently in rehabilitation (57% of patients admitted with spinal cord injury, 42% of patients admitted with traumatic brain injury). Pre-injury substance abuse has been associated with worse rehabilitation outcomes (Bogner et al., 2001; Moyers & Stoffel, 1999) and predicts post-injury substance abuse (Kolakowsky-Hayner et al., 1999). Despite the implications for rehabilitation, health care providers are often reluctant to ask patients about substance use because of time constraints, lack of knowledge, and reluctance to intervene (Taj, Devera-Sales, & Vinson, 1998).

An occupational therapist who suspects that a patient is a substance abuser has an ethical obligation (Moyers & Stoffel, 1999) to perform a screening test and, if indicated, refer the patient for further assessment and intervention. Here are two screening methods.

- Ask a pointed question. Taj, Devera-Sales, and Vinson (1998) were able to identify 74% of at-risk or problem drinkers when physicians incorporated a simple question into their routine examinations ("On any single occasion during the past 3 months, have you had more than 5 drinks containing alcohol?"). They presented the alcohol screening question between two other general health questions ("In the past 3 months, have you used tobacco?" and "Do you regularly wear your seat belt when riding in the car?") (p. 329).
- Use a mnemonic when interviewing clients about suspected alcohol abuse. The CAGE *Questionnaire* (Ewing, 1984) asks 4 questions related to patients' perceptions of need to **cut** down, **annoyance** with criticism, **guilt** about drinking, and need for a drink as an **eye-opener** first thing in the morning.

responsibility for change, while those with an external locus of control tend to expect other people or factors ultimately to determine a particular outcome. The assumption that one can affect one's circumstances leads to active coping and goal-directed activity that influence outcome.

Spirituality

Spirituality refers to the beliefs and practices about the world and one's place in it that give a person transcendent meaning in life (Egan & Swedersky, 2003; Puchalski, 1996). These beliefs may be expressed as a religious faith or directed toward nature, family, or community. It reflects a person's overriding system of meaning that influences use of time, choice of actions, and perceptions of purpose. As such, spirituality is central to a person's occupational function (Christiansen, 1997). In a survey of 270 registered occupational therapists in the United States, 84% of the respondents viewed spirituality as an important dimension of health and rehabilitation, but fewer than 40% of the respondents thought their patients' spiritual needs were within their scope of practice (Engquist et al., 1997). Even therapists who believe that spirituality has a role in occupational therapy practice express concerns about their lack of experience or education in addressing clients' spiritual concerns (Collins, Paul, & West-Frasier, 2001).

Therapists who do incorporate spirituality into their practice do so by dealing with clients' religious concerns, encouraging patients' core sense of self, and addressing or confronting patients' experience of suffering (Egan & Swedersky, 2003). In a survey of 112 occupational therapists, over 63% of the respondents reported that they had occasionally or frequently discussed the fear of death and dying, meaning or purpose of illness, or faith, belief, or religion with their patients (Collins, Paul, & West-Frasier, 2001). These connections with clients become opportunities for the therapist's development as well (Egan & Swedersky, 2003).

Riley et al. (1998) suggested that knowledge of a client's spiritual beliefs informs treatment planning and intervention and "is clearly too important a variable to be neglected in the rehabilitation process" (p. 263). Procedures for Practice 10-3 suggests ways to discuss coping, spiritual belief, and meaning systems with patients.

Cultural Background and Identity

Culture is an information-based system that provides guidelines for peoples' interactions with others and their environments (Baumeister, 2005; Krefting, 1991). Although socialization teaches these guidelines for values, beliefs, and behavior patterns, culture is emergent, dynamic, and interactional (Bonder, Martin, & Miracle, 2004). Culture is not biologically inherited or determined by geography or **ethnicity** (Krefting, 1991). Ethnicity is defined as "membership, conveyed by birth, in a racial, religious, national, or linguistic group" (McGruder, 1998, p. 55). It may have implications in economic, social, and political realms, but contributes little to a therapist's appreciation of a patient's personal context. Furthermore, clinicians are cautioned about the reliability and accuracy of ethnic designations in hospital records (Stansbury et al., 2004). Because there is as much variation within ethnic groups as between them (McGruder, 1998), a person's ethnic background is not a reliable gauge of his or her cultural identity.

The influence of culture on a person's experience is hard to state precisely. Although cultural rules are learned, they are also graded, flexible, task- and environment-specific, and often self-selected. For example, the degree to which immigrants have assimilated the customs and patterns of behavior of their new country or region is determined by how recently they emigrated, the primary language spoken at home, and the amount of contact with their homeland (Krefting, 1991). People adopt the culture of specific subgroups and environments; the expectations for behavior of a clinician in an occupational therapy clinic are different from expectations for a broker working at the New York Stock Exchange. The dynamic influence of culture on human experience requires that clinicians resist attempts to characterize or stereotype clients based on ethnic or geographical background. Rather, occupational therapists attempt to recognize and then step outside of their own cultural backgrounds and biases to appreciate and accept the culturally based customs, values, and beliefs of each client (Procedures for Practice 10-4).

Many occupational therapy evaluation tools are based on norms developed for a white middle-class population (Krefting, 1991; Paul, 1995). Culturally reflective clinicians assess the cultural validity of their standardized assessment tools (Krefting, 1991) and select criterion-referenced and norm-referenced tests appropriate for the person's background (Paul, 1995). Paul described the challenges of devising culturally unbiased tests that include only items that reflect knowledge, experiences, and skills common to all cultures. He recommended the use of culture-specific evaluation tools, which include items relevant to a specific cultural group, when available. Practically speaking, it is impossible to locate culture-specific tools for all of the diverse cultural groups in North America. Therefore, therapists must make every effort to attempt to understand a client's individual cultural background before interpreting performance on the most appropriate standardized tests.

Pain

Pain, acute and chronic, interferes with occupational function and quality of life for many people receiving occupational therapy services (Ehde et al., 2003). People with spinal cord injury who use manual wheelchairs report upper

PROCEDURES FOR PRACTICE 10-3

Assessing Patients' Coping, Spiritual Beliefs, and Meaning Systems

People typically share personal information with those they trust. Therefore, to explore patients' beliefs and meaning systems, therapists invest in establishing therapeutic rapport (see Chapter 15). Without the rapport that comes with time and consistency of care providers, patients may perceive questions about their spirituality, for example, as intrusive or offensive. Therapists who are aware of their own coping strategies and belief systems will be best able to comfortably discuss these issues with their patients.

In general, discussions of these very personal and potentially sensitive matters begin at a superficial level and progress to deeper, more personal levels as dictated by the patient and therapist's comfort with each other and the subject matter. Here are examples of this progression.

- Ask the client to provide an hour-by-hour account of a typical day prior to the injury or onset of illness (Radomski, 1995). How a person is used to spending his or her time richly defines his or her valued activities and priorities.
- Take a brief life history, asking the patient to give you an overview of his or her life course, including past goals and obstacles (Kleinman, 1988). People often use stories or narratives to make connections and meaning attributions between a series of life events (Mattingly, 1991).
- Ask the patient about his or her explanatory model of the illness or disability. Kleinman (1988) suggested that faced with illness, disability, or suffering, people attempt to construct models to explain the whys of their experiences. They make attributions about causation and outcome that are more likely to be based on personal beliefs and culture than on facts or medical information. For example, patients may feel responsible for permanent impairments because they didn't try hard enough in rehabilitation to overcome them (Luborsky, 1997). If the person views onset of illness or disability as God's punishment for a past sin or mistake, he or she may not feel empowered to invest in rehabilitation efforts. Only as patients' explanatory models are acknowledged may they be negotiated with the therapist or health care team (Kleinman, 1988).
- Cox and Waller (1991, p. 86) suggested that clinicians ask patients about past experiences in which their coping skills were taxed:
  1. When you're discouraged and feeling despondent, what keeps you going?
  2. Where have you found strength in the past?
  3. What have you done in the past when you've lost someone or something important?
  4. What do you think the message in this is for you?
- Puchalski and Romer (2000) recommended an acronym for aspects of a spiritual assessment (*F*, Faith; *I*, Importance and influence; *C*, Community; and *A*, Address).
  - F. What things do you believe in that give meaning to your life?
  - I. How have your beliefs influenced your behavior during this illness? What roles do your beliefs play in regaining your health?
  - C. Are you a part of a spiritual or religious community? Is this a support to you and how?
  - A. How would you like me, your health care provider, to address these issues in your health care?

extremity pain, with the most severe pain occurring while pushing the wheelchair up an incline and during sleep (Curtis et al., 1999). Dalyan, Cardenas, and Gerard (1999) found that upper extremity pain was associated with lower employment rates and greater disability for outpatients with spinal cord injury. Finally, many stroke patients have upper extremity pain as well, typically beginning 2 weeks after the onset of stroke (Chantraine et al., 1999). In addition to its contribution to disability and to decreased quality of life, pain is linked to depression (Dalyan, Cardenas, & Gerard, 1999) and inefficiencies in information processing (Luoto et al., 1999).

Pain is a highly personal experience (Dudgeon et al., 2002); an individual's pain in the present is influenced by his or her recollections of past pain, expectations of pain, and perceptions regarding its cause (Smith, Gracely, & Safer, 1998). Many people with disabilities are used to living with pain, differentiating between usual pain and unexpected pain (Dudgeon et al., 2006). Because many recipients of occupational therapy services may be reluctant to mention their concerns about pain to therapists (Dudgeon et al., 2002), therapists take responsibility to routinely ask and/or assess.

Million et al. (1982) described two categories of pain assessment techniques: (1) those that assess the patient's subjective experience with pain and limitations in activities and (2) those that quantify physical signs, such as moving during a physical examination and biochemical

PROCEDURES FOR PRACTICE 10-4

Cultural Assessment

Experts advise against using cultural cookbooks to gain insights about culturally based habits and behaviors of various ethnic groups, as they can lead to stereotyping individual patients (Krefting, 1991; Lipson, 1996). Instead, therapists consider the unique influence of culture on each individual's experience by carefully attending to nuances of body language, word choice, and gestures and adopting an attitude of curiosity about each client's situation and background (Bonder, Martin, & Miracle, 2004).

Lipson (1996, p. 3) suggested the following questions as key elements of a cultural assessment of any patient. Occupational therapists may get the answers to these questions in the medical record or talk directly with patients or loved ones.

- Where was the person born? If an immigrant, how long has the patient lived in this country?
- What is the patient's ethnic affiliation, and how strong is the patient's ethnic identity?
- Who are the client's major support people, family members, or friends? Does he or she live in an ethnic community?
- What are the primary and secondary languages and the speaking and reading ability?
- How would you characterize the nonverbal communication style?
- What is the person's religion, its importance in daily life, and current practices?
- What are his or her food preferences and prohibitions?
- What is the person's economic situation, and is the income adequate to meet the needs of the patient and family?
- What are the health and illness beliefs and practices?
- What are the customs and beliefs around such transitions as birth, illness, and death?

changes during activity. Beyond observing function and behavior, the former methods seem most appropriate for occupational therapists. Two commonly used subjective measures of pain are described: the *McGill Pain Questionnaire–Short Form* (*MPQ-SF*) (Melzack, 1987) and the *Visual Analog Scale* (*VAS*) (Huskisson, 1974; Million et al., 1982).

McGill Pain Questionnaire–Short Form

The *MPQ-SF*, adapted from the *McGill Pain Questionnaire* (Melzack, 1975), is widely used to measure pain and response to pain interventions (Melzack, 1987). The tool has three components. First, patients are asked to rate descriptors from two categories that best describe the characteristics of their pain. These 15 descriptors are rated on a 0 to 3 intensity scale and then summed. The following are examples: throbbing, shooting, cramping, and sickening. The patients also complete two indices of the overall intensity of their pain (*Present Pain Index* and *VAS*).

Visual Analog Scale

The *VAS* is a self-administered measure of pain intensity. Patients are asked to indicate the severity of their pain by marking a point on a 10-cm line on which the end points are labeled "Pain as bad as it could be" or "No pain" (Huskisson, 1974). The rating is converted to a score by measuring the distance of the mark from the origin of the scale. Million et al. (1982) suggested that asking patients to provide one global rating of pain demands that they provide a singular estimate of their pain experience across time and situation, when in reality, pain varies with time and activity. Therefore, they developed 15 questions related to severity of pain associated with various activities, each accompanied by a *VAS*. Each question is answered as the patient marks the *VAS* based on the continuum of symptoms or limitations. The ends of each scale are described with extreme answers to the question. Here are two examples:

- Does your back pain interfere with your freedom to walk? (Complete freedom to walk—completely unable to walk)
- To what extent does your pain interfere with your work? (No interference at all—totally incapable of work) (Million et al., 1982, pp. 211-212).

Because it is brief, reliable, and valid, the *VAS* is often used to screen inpatients and outpatients for acute pain-related concerns, in compliance with hospital accreditation requirements (Joint Commission on Accreditation of Healthcare Organizations, 2005). The *VAS* will likely not provide adequate information to inform occupational therapy assessment or intervention for persons with chronic or variable pain.

Questionnaires and numerical or *VAS* scales should be the catalysts for, rather than replacements of, more in-depth conversations with clients about their experience with pain. A one-time rating of pain often does not represent the variability of pain that some clients experience (Zelman et al., 2004). Occupational therapists will be best equipped to interpret occupational assessment findings if they go beyond obtaining a snapshot of a client's static pain. Conversations to explore the extent to which pain levels are manageable or tolerable will be a prelude to problem solving about the kinds of strategies that might help (Zelman et al., 2004).

Mood

Many people who receive occupational therapy services have mood disorders, such as depression and anxiety (Arruda, Stern, & Sommerville, 1999). Almost one third of geriatric rehabilitation inpatients are thought to be depressed (Cully et al., 2005). Persons with spinal cord injury, traumatic brain injury (Kreuter et al., 1998), and Parkinson's disease (Meara, Michelmore, & Hobson, 1999) tend to be more depressed than the general population. Early identification and treatment of mood disorders is important, as depression and anxiety appear to interfere with attention and concentration during assessment (Eysenck & Keane, 1990) and negatively influence outcome of intervention (Lai et al., 2002). Although occupational therapists do not diagnose mood disorders, they have numerous opportunities to observe behavior. According to Scherer and Cushman (1997), certain patterns of behavior may indicate psychological distress and warrant referral to a psychologist or psychiatrist for further assessment and treatment.

Depression

People feeling transitory sadness and discouragement or normal grief may display signs that are similar to those of depression, but will differ in terms of persistence of symptoms and their effect on self-esteem (Gorman, Sultman, & Luna-Raines, 1989). That is, sadness and normal grief resolve with time and generally do not lead to lowered self-esteem, as suggested by the following signs of possible clinical depression (Gorman, Sultman, & Luna-Raines, 1989; Scherer & Cushman, 1997):

- Significant declines in functioning lasting 2 weeks or more
- Feelings of worthlessness, inadequacy, self-doubt
- Diminished interest in virtually all activities, even formerly enjoyable activities
- Depressed or irritable mood most of the time
- Vegetative disturbances: lethargy; insomnia or excessive sleep; change of appetite with weight change of more than 5%; periods of excessive activity or slowness almost every day
- Very poor concentration
- Withdrawal from social interaction
- Recurrent thoughts of death or suicide

Anxiety

Anxiety is defined as a "subjectively painful warning of impending danger, real or imagined, that motivates the individual to take corrective action to relieve the unpleasant feelings and is experienced both psychologically and physiologically" (Gorman, Sultman, & Luna-Raines, 1989, p. 51). Anxiety is different from fear. Anxiety is characterized by a diffuse feeling of dread, whereas fear is a reaction to a specific temporary external danger (Gorman, Sultman, & Luna-Raines, 1989). Here are some signs of possible anxiety disorder (Gorman, Sultman, & Luna-Raines, 1989; Scherer & Cushman, 1997) that may prompt referral to a psychiatrist or psychologist:

- Panic attack (choking feeling, nausea, dizziness, palpitations or chest pain, fear of dying or losing control)
- Distorted, unrealistic fears or perceptions of a situation or object
- Disruption of normal routines or daily activities associated with irrational fears

Despite their best intentions, occupational therapists often have difficulty recognizing these disorders. Therefore, occupational therapists are advised to use standardized screens to identify patients in need of psychological or psychiatric services (Ruchinskas, 2002). The *Hospital Anxiety and Depression Scale* (Zigmond & Snaith, 1983) and the *Beck Depression Index-FastScreen for Medical Patients* (Beck, Steer, & Brown, 2000) are good examples.

SOCIAL CONTEXT

> "In the acute stages of an illness, it's easy to be a good friend—exhausting but rewarding to nurse a loved one back to health. But her health never returned and chronic care takes tenacious strength when you're also battling grief. I often feel unequal to the challenge." (Osborne, 1998, p. 46)

Social context, including the person's social resources, roles, and preferences, influences occupational pursuits, satisfaction, health, and well-being (Helliwell & Putnam, 2004). For example, some people select tasks and activities that put them in contact with a social network; others select occupations that allow them to avoid social interaction, as in the case of individual preferences for hobbies or careers. Social networks may facilitate an individual's chosen occupations through emotional support, assistance, or instruction; unfortunately, some social relationships interfere with a person's optimal function. Only if occupational therapists are aware of the social context in which occupational function occurs can they orchestrate intervention that will outlive their own involvement in a client's recovery and adaptation.

Social Network and Support

The characteristics of a person's social network are relatively stable social contextual factors that influence his or her identity, opportunities, and function. Langford et al.

(1997) suggested that a social network is an interactive web of people who provide each other with help and protection; that is, they give and receive **social support**. Social networks vary in terms of the following characteristics: reciprocity (extent to which resources and support are both given and received); intensity (extent to which social relationships offer emotional closeness); complexity (extent to which social relationships serve many functions); and density (extent to which network members know and interact with each other) (Heaney & Israel, 1997).

Social support is defined as aid and assistance exchanged through social relationships and interactions (Heaney & Israel, 1997). The four types of social support are: (1) emotional (expressions of empathy, love, trust, and caring); (2) instrumental (tangible aid and service); (3) information (including advice and suggestions); and (4) appraisal (feedback and affirmation) (Heaney & Israel).

During the assessment, occupational therapists first try to identify the composition and characteristics of the client's social network (i.e., who these individuals are and the nature of their relationships). Occupational therapists must step outside of their own biases and expectations to appreciate that patients' social networks take many forms, including traditional nuclear families, same-sex partners, friendships, and acquaintances. Such biases remain prevalent, insidious, and hurtful. For example, despite our profession's stance on nondiscrimination and inclusion (American Occupational Therapy Association, 2004), Jackson (2000) described many occupational therapy clinics as noninclusive environments in which a heterosexist perspective pervades conversations, humor, and assumptions.

Second, therapists attempt to determine the types of support that individuals in the social network are willing and able to provide. For example, longstanding intimate ties typically provide emotional support and long-term assistance, while neighbors and friends most often provide short-term instrumental and informational support (Heaney & Israel, 1997). Key players in the social network assume as much or as little responsibility as they are able, and the patient–family unit becomes the primary recipient of occupational therapy services (Brown, Humphry, & Taylor, 1997). Therapists can learn a lot about patients' social networks and resources by simply talking with them. An alternative method of assessing a patient's social network and resources is the *Norbeck Social Support Questionnaire* (Norbeck, Lindsey, & Carrieri, 1981). It is a standardized, self-administered questionnaire consisting of nine items and taking about 10 minutes to complete. Patients list individuals in their personal network and specify the nature of these relationships. Patients then indicate the extent to which each person listed provides emotional, appraisal, and instrumental support.

Finally, occupational therapists appreciate that some social relationships are harmful to patients. Accredited hospitals and rehabilitation facilities are mandated to have policies in place to respond to patients considered to be vulnerable adults or potential victims of intimate partner violence (Joint Commission on Accreditation of Healthcare Organizations, 2005). Therapists must familiarize themselves with employers' policies and procedures that describe how to report, document, and respond to cases of suspected maltreatment. For example, at Mercy and Unity Hospitals in suburban Minneapolis, physical and occupational therapists are expected to screen all outpatients for family violence (Fig. 10-3) (J. L. Miller, personal communication, February 3, 2006).

Caregiver Adaptation: A Dynamic Social Factor

Longstanding intimate ties in the patient's social network (hereafter also referred to as family) are critical to patients' ability to adapt to chronic illness and disability. Families influence outcome of services because they provide a context for individual change and because they represent continuity in patients' lives (Brown, Humphry, & Taylor, 1997). The ability of significant others to provide needed support, however, is dictated in part by their own emotional and physical health and place in the adaptation process (Grant et al., 2000). Many relatives of persons with traumatic brain injury (Webster, Daisley, & King, 1999), stroke (Grant et al., 2000), and Alzheimer's disease (Pruchno & Potashnik, 1989), for example, experience significant levels of subjective burden and mood disorders as well as role changes in work, leisure, and social life (Frosch et al., 1997). To contribute to patients' long-term quality of life, occupational therapists assess family members' adaptation needs on an ongoing basis.

All of the personal, social, and cultural contextual factors described in Figure 10-2 can be applied to the significant other's occupational functioning as caregiver. That is, a spouse's ability to learn and reinforce new techniques and strategies is affected by his or her own health concerns and distractions, age and generation, sex, mood, cultural background, makeup of the social network, and culture of the community (Murray, Manktelow, & Clifford, 2000). Furthermore, caregivers' goals and perceptions of need from health providers change as they adapt to the patient's illness or injury.

Corbin and Strauss (1988) described the work of adapting to chronic disability over time as "a set of tasks performed by an individual or couple, alone or in conjunction with others, to carry out a plan of action designed to manage one or more aspects of the illness" (p. 9). This work consists of not only adjustments to self-maintenance tasks and roles but also the work involved in redefining one's identity. Corbin and Strauss used the term *illness trajectory* to refer to the sequence of physiological changes associated with an illness, injury, or disorder and the adaptive work demanded of a patient and family that accompanies each

Family Violence Screening and Response Tool

ALLINA
HEALTH SYSTEM

What to do: RADAR mnemonic *

Routinely ask. Inquiring about family violence can be an intervention. You're signaling that violence is inappropriate; you may be helping to end the isolation.
Affirm and support patients who acknowledge abuse.
Document objective findings; patient statements in quotes.
Address your patient's safety.
Refer the patient to people skilled in family violence and safety planning.

When do you screen?

- ➤ Patient must always be alone. The exception is with infants or nonverbal toddlers.
- ➤ Screen all adults—both males and females.

When do you introduce the screening?

An introductory statement will lead you into asking the screening questions. This statement gives the patient the following messages:

- ➤ Violence in the home is a major health care issue;
- ➤ I care about you;
- ➤ All patients are asked these questions; and
- ➤ This is a safe place.

STATE: *We at (name clinic/hospital) are concerned about the violence that is impacting the health of many of our patients, so we routinely ask everyone the following confidential questions.*

Screening Questions

- ➤ Have you ever been hit, kicked, pushed, or otherwise hurt or mistreated by someone important to you?
- ➤ Is someone important to you yelling at you, threatening you, or otherwise trying to control your life?

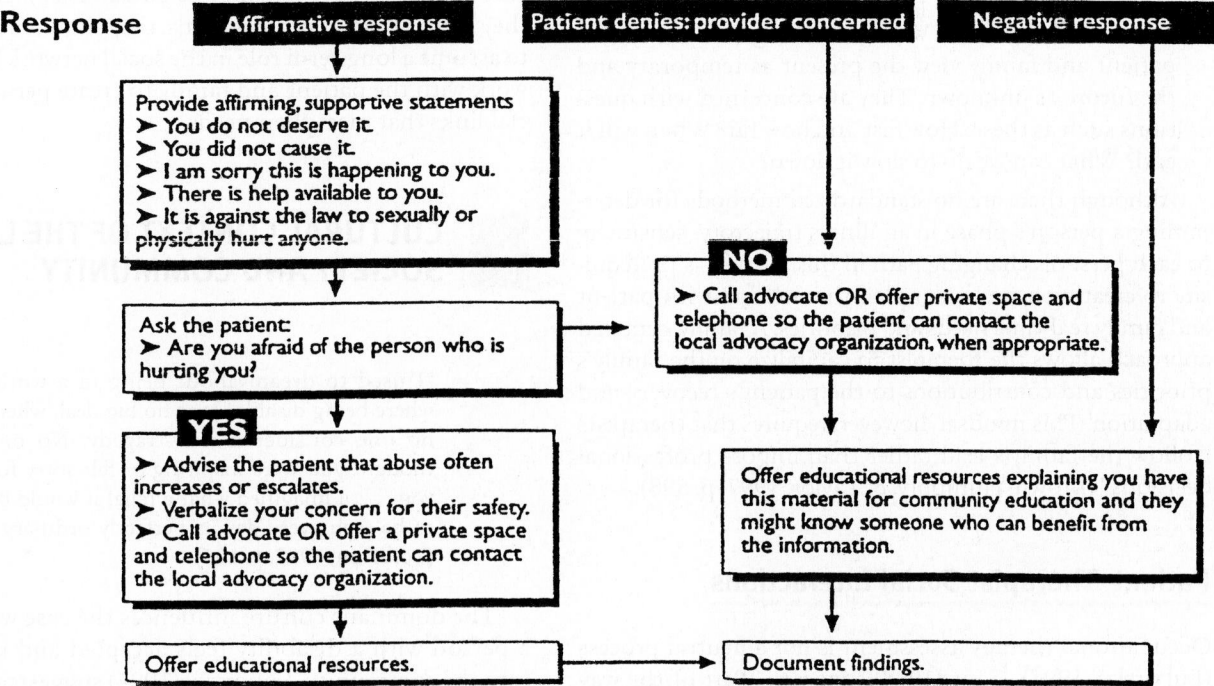

Response

Affirmative response

Provide affirming, supportive statements
- ➤ You do not deserve it.
- ➤ You did not cause it.
- ➤ I am sorry this is happening to you.
- ➤ There is help available to you.
- ➤ It is against the law to sexually or physically hurt anyone.

Ask the patient:
- ➤ Are you afraid of the person who is hurting you?

YES
- ➤ Advise the patient that abuse often increases or escalates.
- ➤ Verbalize your concern for their safety.
- ➤ Call advocate OR offer a private space and telephone so the patient can contact the local advocacy organization.

Offer educational resources. → Document findings.

Patient denies: provider concerned

NO
- ➤ Call advocate OR offer private space and telephone so the patient can contact the local advocacy organization, when appropriate.

Negative response

Offer educational resources explaining you have this material for community education and they might know someone who can benefit from the information.

Document findings.

* Alpert, E.J. (1999). *Partner Violence: A Guide for Physicians and Other Health Care Professionals (3rd Edition) – Use Your "RADAR".* Waltham, MA: Massachusetts Medical Society.

Figure 10-3 Family Violence Screening and Response Tool. (Reprinted with permission from Allina Health System, Minneapolis, MN.)

phase. They further suggested that most trajectories have five types of phases, distinctly ordered according to various diagnoses and individual courses: acute, comeback, stable, unstable, and downward.

- *Acute phase.* The patient requires immediate medical attention and focuses on physiological stabilization and recovery. Patient and family may wonder how life will change because of the illness, injury, or disorder.
- *Comeback phase.* The patient is in the midst of physical and emotional recovery and focuses on getting physically well and regaining functional abilities. Patient and family may ask questions such as these: Will I (he or she) come back? How long will it take before I (he or she) peak? "In the comeback trajectory, the present is seen as overbearing, and the future is put on hold while one awaits answers to the foregoing questions" (Corbin & Strauss, 1988, p. 46).
- *Stable phase.* The patient undergoes very few changes in course of illness or functional abilities, as in the remission phase of multiple sclerosis or permanent spinal cord injury. Patient and family focus on maintaining stable health while wondering how long the phase will last and what can be done to extend it.
- *Unstable phase.* The patient has periodic but erratic downturns in function or exacerbations of illness (as might come, for example, with bladder infection). Unstable phases hamper normal living, and people in this phase ask questions like these: How long until we get this under control? How much longer can I (or we) go on like this?
- *Downward phase.* The patient slowly or rapidly loses health and function. With increasing incapacity, the patient and family view the present as temporary and the future as unknown. They are concerned with questions such as these: How fast and how far? When will it end? What can we do to slow it down?

Although there are no standardized methods for determining a person's phase in an illness trajectory, sensitivity to each person's changing path in this journey is prerequisite to creating a treatment plan that meshes with patient and family real-time needs and priorities. A family-centered approach allows the therapist to capitalize on the family's priorities and contributions to the patient's recovery and adaptation. This mindset, however, requires that therapists "follow the family's lead rather than impose professional decisions" (Brown, Humphry, & Taylor, 1997, p. 598).

Patient–Therapist Social Interactions

Occupational therapy assessment is not a neutral process (Luborsky, 1997). Gans (1998) suggests, "Part of the way the patient behaves with you is a function of the way you are with the patient. This effect may comprise 75%, 25%, or 2% of what goes on between you and the patient, but it is there" (p. 4). Social convention and cultural norms organize the patient's self-report of problems and symptoms and the therapist's response to these concerns (Luborsky, 1997). The therapist is endowed with power to shape the interaction by selecting certain questions and omitting others (Luborsky, 1995), to judge or evaluate the responses of the patient, and even to determine whose expectations and "reality" are correct (Abberley, 1995).

Occupational therapists monitor the extent to which their own needs infiltrate social interactions with patients. Perhaps to meet self-imposed expectations around outcome, Abberley (1995) suggested that some occupational therapists unwittingly define the client as the problem and themselves as the solution, with failure of intervention always attributed to the patient and success always credited to the clinician's efforts. Gans (1998) believes that a primary source of clinician gratification should stem from "the privilege of participating intimately in another person's life" (p. 5). He further suggests that, when the work no longer feels like a privilege, one should try to figure out why (e.g., volume of caseload, private life that is distracting or burdensome, burnt out, or ethically questionable employer expectations that corrode integrity).

Clinicians also examine their expectations of their own supportive roles in patients' lives. They recognize that professional helpers are typically not able to provide support over long periods. They realize that professional–lay relationships are not characterized by reciprocity typical of social networks and often entail invisible but palpable power differentials that interfere with the provision of genuine emotional support (Heaney & Israel, 1997). In essence, they realize that, as professionals, they should not attempt to assume a long-term role in the social network but rather work with the patient and family to create permanent social links that meet their needs.

CULTURAL CONTEXT OF THE LARGER SOCIETY AND COMMUNITY

> "I used to dream about being in a world where being disabled was no big deal, where no one considered it a tragedy. No one thought you were inspiring or felt sorry for you . . . . I imagined what a relief it would be to be seen every day as perfectly ordinary." (Tollifson, 1997, p. 105)

The dominant culture influences the ease with which a person with a disability feels accepted and integrated into the community. Luborsky (1994) suggested that culturally based requirements for status of full adult person in Europe and North America, such as self-sufficiency, activity, and upright posture, are often at odds with full participation for persons with disabilities. Adapted equipment may be rejected because of its appearance and acceptability in public rather than its functional value (Luborsky, 1994, 1997). Patients and family may respond to embarrassment or guilt over disability by attempting to keep the disability private and denying help from friends or neighbors (Armstrong & Fitzgerald, 1996). Loss of social status is further compounded when insidious cultural beliefs hold persons with disabilities responsible for their impairments. "At a deep level there is a bias that either they are culpable for the cause of the impairment, or for not working harder at rehabilitation to be able to 'overcome' the odds regardless of how realistic that is" (Luborsky, 1994, p. 251). As abhorrent and illogical as such notions are, patients, families, and occupational therapists are not immune to the subtle but pervasive influences of the sociocultural context in which they live.

Occupational therapists are challenged to check many of their own assumptions about people with disabilities. For example, Kielhofner (2005) reminds us that the person-first terminology that therapists are urged to use is objectionable to some disability activists and scholars who suggest that the term "disabled person" more accurately reflects his or her true minority status. Many people resent the notion that their impairments reflect some sort of personal tragedy (Wakefield, 2005; Watson, 2002) and, instead, view their disability with pride as a part of their identity (Eddey & Robey, 2005). Even the concept of rehabilitation and remediation of impairments can be interpreted as an effort to remove a flaw or a negative characteristic, a round-about way of suggesting abnormality or imperfection (Kielhofner, 2005).

GENERAL COMMENTS ON ASSESSING PERSONAL, SOCIAL, AND CULTURAL CONTEXT

If nothing else, the discussion of assessing personal, social, and cultural context underscores that occupational therapists ought to not get too comfortable with their findings, scores, or impressions and learn to tolerate the ambiguity of "it just depends." The imposing influence of contextual variables serves to keep us humble and on guard against jumping to the wrong conclusions about assessment findings and our clients.

Occupational therapists struggle to balance their preeminent concerns for service to patients with very real demands for efficiency and productivity. Clinicians typically devote 30 minutes to 3 hours assessing each patient; the short lengths of stay in acute settings allow less time; inpatient rehabilitation settings (with possibly longer stays) allow somewhat more. How does one have time to assess the web of personal, social, and cultural contextual factors on top of all pertinent areas of occupational function (roles, tasks, activities, abilities and skills, and capacities)? Here are some general guidelines:

- Review the assessments of other professionals. Many patients who are referred to occupational therapy are also assessed by social workers, psychologists, speech-language pathologists, physical therapists, physicians, therapeutic recreation specialists, chaplains, and/or nurses. Reviewing the assessments of team members greatly adds to the occupational therapist's ability to understand a patient's personal, social, and cultural context without using limited assessment time to do so.
- Use specific tools (many discussed in this chapter) to measure contextual factors that appear to bias or confound performance during assessment or that are expected to be targets of occupational therapy intervention (to establish a baseline).
- Take advantage of informal conversations with patients. Luborsky (1997) pointed out the value of attending to patients' informal remarks made during structured assessments. He described how a patient's comments during transitions between various standardized tools provide insights not captured by the tools themselves. He further stated that patients' informal remarks "can be essential to gaining an understanding of the way subjects make sense of the assessment; to providing us with important information on the validity of the assessment tool; and to identifying important areas for clinical intervention" (p. 12).

It is advisable to use each and every moment with patients to try to understand who they are, where they come from, and how they are interpreting their experience in therapy. Gans (1998) links this investment to patient outcome: "our ongoing, relentless determination to understand the uniqueness of each patient is what the patient, to the degree he or she can, experiences as love . . . [and] patients who feel cared about and valued make the most gains in therapy" (p. 5). It is unrealistic to expect therapists to unravel the mysteries of a client's contextual fabric during an arbitrarily defined assessment period. The richness of conversations that relate to personal, social, and cultural context grows as the therapeutic relationship deepens and continues to inform the intervention process.

CASE EXAMPLE

Appreciating Context During Assessment

Occupational Therapy Assessment Process	Objectives	Clinical Reasoning Process: Examples of Therapist's Internal Dialogue
Patient Information Mrs. N., a 30-year-old wife and mother of three young children, was referred to outpatient occupational therapy for assessment and treatment approximately 6 months after a suspected brain injury. She was injured when a shelf at a convenience store broke and its contents fell on her head. After the accident, Mrs. N. frequently complained of headaches, fatigue, and dizziness accompanied by dramatic decrease in her activity level and was observed to be forgetful, even unsafe (e.g., leaving stove burners turned on, losing track of her children, forgetting to take medication). With a high school education, Mrs. N. worked full time as a teaching assistant at a day care center but was unable to return to work following her injury. As a recent immigrant from Saudi Arabia, Mrs. N. spoke very little English. (She speaks and writes in Arabic.) The consulting neuropsychologist opted not to perform a battery of standardized cognitive assessments because of concerns about communication, cultural biases of the tests themselves, and possible religious discomfort associated with spending hours of assessment time with the neuropsychologist, a man. Therefore, assessment and observations in occupational therapy were particularly important in establishing her rehabilitation needs.	Understand the patient's diagnosis or condition	"Mrs. N.'s complaints and presentation are certainly consistent with a brain injury. It appears that she did not seek medical attention immediately after the accident and that she has never received any rehabilitation services. These symptoms must be frightening for her."
	Know the person	"It is going to be challenging for me to try to get to know Mrs. N. and to provide the kind of encouragement and support that I feel is so important to my approach with patients, given our language barriers."
	Appreciate the context	"I realize that I need an assessment strategy that is different from what I am used to. It would not make much sense for me to rely on scores from standardized tests. I will also be sensitive to the fact that it's possible that some of what Mrs. N. says to me may be lost in translation."
	Develop provisional hypotheses	"My guess is that some of Mrs. N.'s problems can be attributed to brain injury but I wonder what effect anxiety and/or depression may have on her overall functioning."
Assessment Process Mrs. N. appeared to doze in the waiting room prior to her initial occupational therapy session. She was cooperative and soft spoken; she was able to respond in English to approximately 30% of the questions. She stayed awake for most of each of the three 1-hour assessment sessions. Mr. N., also a native of Saudi Arabia, served as translator but often dominated interactions with details of his own stress related to his wife's status. He appeared to be on the verge of tears on at least two occasions as he described his inability to work full time because of his wife's need for supervision, assistance, and transportation to medical appointments.	Consider evaluation approach and methods	"I think that I can learn the most about Mrs. N.'s functioning with a dynamic assessment approach—observing her response to various demands and challenges that I set up."

Patient's and Husband's Report of Abilities and Limitations

Through her husband, Mrs. N. indicated that she was primarily concerned about her memory and endurance and that her ultimate goals were to completely resume her roles as mother, homemaker, and worker. (At the time of her assessment, Mr. N. prepared all of the family meals, and their oldest daughter, age 9, did most of the household chores.) Through her husband, Mrs. N. indicated that she had very little activity or routine in her day. She woke anywhere between 8:00 AM and noon. After rising, she sat for approximately half an hour, avoiding movement so as to avoid dizziness. She did not prepare meals for herself, eating only a cookie with tea instead of breakfast or lunch. She typically spent her afternoons napping, sitting alone at the window, or watching television. She fell asleep at approximately 9:00 PM, but her husband reported that he regularly found her crying in the middle of the night. Her inactivity contrasted dramatically with reports of her premorbid status: working full time, attending language and driving classes, managing all household tasks, caring for her children, and socializing with friends. With the patient's permission, the therapist also contacted Mrs. N.'s American-born, English-speaking sister-in-law, who confirmed the dramatic decline in Mrs. N.'s activity level and abilities, Mr. N.'s understandable stress given these changes, and her own willingness to serve as a resource.

"Descriptions of Mrs. N.'s premorbid activities and her self-reports of long-term goals contradict my assumptions about Muslim women from the Middle East. Prior to meeting Mrs. N., I expected that Mrs. N.'s narrow sphere of activities would center exclusively on her home and children. Mrs. N.'s premorbid engagement in work outside of her home and language and driving lessons and her goals to return to these roles reminds me of the importance of trying to understand each patient as an individual rather than drawing conclusions based on cultural or ethnic stereotypes."

"It is helpful to get a snapshot of Mrs. N.'s functioning through her husband and her sister-in-law. I feel fairly confident that I'm following all that Mr. N. is telling me, as his sister-in-law tells me much the same thing."

Observations of Cognitive Function

Mrs. N. performed the *Contextual Memory Test* (CMT) (Toglia, 1993), a test of immediate and delayed recall of 20 pictures associated with morning hygiene. Her performance on this test suggested moderate memory deficits but adequate awareness of these limitations. Her husband translated instructions to a 10-step task to which she jotted notes. After a 25-minute delay and interference activities, she was able to use her own notes to carry out the task with 70% accuracy. She appeared to make errors because she did not carefully review her notes and approached two steps in what appeared to be a hasty and impulsive manner.

"I know that I am supposed to follow the CMT's administration protocol, but under these circumstances, I just can't. However, the picture format of this test might give me a sense of her ability to learn new information. I appreciate that the veracity of assessment findings are in question, as all responses were reported through her husband."

Observations of Performance of Functional Tasks

The therapist requested that Mrs. N. select a familiar stove-top meal to prepare in occupational therapy and asked her to bring necessary supplies and ingredients to one of her assessment sessions. Mr. N. reportedly reminded Mrs. N. to do so. As instructed by the therapist, Mrs. N. made an obvious effort to remember to turn off the stove burner once she finished preparing her dish. She sat next to the stove throughout the task, but having removed the pan from the stove to serve the food, she did not return to turn off the burner (which was left on for 5 minutes, until the therapist turned it off). She appeared well organized in her approach to the task, removing all ingredients and supplies from the cupboard ahead of time and cleaning up as she proceeded. Despite these efforts, she forgot to add one of the ingredients she had set out on the table and asked the therapist whether she had added another.

Interpret observations

"I thought it would be a good idea to have Mrs. N. prepare a familiar dish so as to remove at least one novelty variable. I am impressed that she is willing to try every activity that I propose and that says a lot to me about her motivation to use therapy to improve her functioning."

Mrs. N. frequently requested rest during occupational therapy sessions that entailed physical activity. She generally tolerated approximately 5 minutes of standing or walking before requesting to sit and rest because of fatigue and dizziness. During one of the three sessions, Mrs. N. complained of headache and intermittently rested her head on the table.

Analysis of Results

Mrs. N.'s performance of functional tasks in occupational therapy seemed consistent with the kinds of problems reported at home by Mrs. N., her husband, and her sister-in-law. Specifically, Mrs. N.'s performance on pencil-and-paper and kitchen tasks were marked by forgetfulness, absent-mindedness, and poor endurance. Furthermore, given her dramatic decline in activity, reports of frequent crying, and decreased appetite, the therapist was concerned about depression. Given his own stress, the therapist questioned whether Mr. N. would be able to maintain all of the roles he had assumed since his wife's injury.

The following recommendations were suggested as pre-requisite to commencing occupational therapy treatment:

- Referral to a woman psychologist for further evaluation and treatment of possible mood disorder.
- Referral to a neurologist specializing in balance disorders (she had never had this complaint exhaustively evaluated).
- Schedule of a family conference with Mrs. N.'s sister-in-law, brother-in-law, and attorney to make arrangements to assist Mr. N. at home, enabling him to put in more hours at work.
- Work with the hospital patient representative to provide a translator for future occupational therapy sessions.
- Schedule an occupational therapy home safety evaluation.

"I requested an interpreter from the Patient Representative but it has taken a little longer than I would like to find someone. Our policies and procedures recommend against using a family member as an interpreter and I can see that logic. Mr. N. has his own stresses and maybe his own agenda. He needs to be freed up to take care of his other responsibilities, and I think it would be beneficial for Mrs. N. to participate in occupational therapy sessions on her own."

"I am concerned that Mrs. N. may not make substantive progress towards her goals if she is depressed, and so I recommended that she see a psychologist or psychiatrist before beginning occupational therapy intervention. Similarly, her complaints about dizziness have never been medically evaluated, and we need to find out what is going on. Given what Mr. and Mrs. N. have told me and what I've seen of Mrs. N.'s performance, I am very concerned about her safety at home. I am not confident in offering any definitive suggestions until I observe her in her own environment."

Occupational Therapy Problem List

1. Decreased memory and concentration capabilities and inadequate strategies to compensate for these problems.
2. Deconditioning associated with prolonged inactivity complicated by poor nutrition.
3. Lack of structure or routine for daily activities and inability to judge independently which tasks were within her competence level.

Synthesize results

"I have addressed similar issues with other clients, and I am confident I can help Mrs. N. address these problems as well."

CLINICAL REASONING IN OCCUPATIONAL THERAPY PRACTICE

Adapting Assessment to Contextual Factors

The occupational therapist working with Mrs. N. used only one standardized assessment tool because of concerns related to language barriers and cultural biases. How might the assessment have been different if Mrs. N. had presented the same symptoms and complaints but was born in Pittsburgh and spoke English all of her life?

Assessment Table 10-1

Assessing Personal, Social, and Cultural Contexts

Instrument and Reference	Description	Time to Administer	Validity	Reliability	Sensitivity	Strengths and Weaknesses
Rapid Estimate of Adult Literacy in Medicine (*REALM*) (Murphy et al., 1993)	Reading recognition test that allows clinicians to estimate patients' reading skills.	2–3 minutes.	Concurrent validity: significant correlation ($p < 0.0001$) between *REALM* and standardized measures of reading, including the *Peabody Individual Achievement Test–Revised* ($r = 0.97$), *Wide Range Achievement Test–Revised* ($r = 0.88$), and *Slosson Oral Reading Test–Revised* ($r = 0.96$) (Davis et al., 1993).	Excellent test–retest reliability ($r = 0.99$, $p < 0.001$).	No information.	Strengths: Brief; minimal training needed Weakness: Assesses literacy in English only
CAGE Questionnaire (Ewing, 1984)	Involves asking 4 questions to persons seeking medical services to identify possible alcohol abuse.	5–10 minutes.	Convergent validity for 4 *CAGE* questions with alcohol-related items of the *Army's Health Risk Appraisal* ranged from: Φ coefficient 0.1713–0.3496 (moderately weak). Criterion validity: persons with cut-off score of 2 were at 3.5 times greater risk for military discharge due to alcoholism (Bell et al., 2003).	Good rest–retest reliability (2–30 days) for 4 questions (*r* ranged from 0.73–0.83) (Bell et al., 2003).	In a study of individuals with traumatic brain injury, specificity and sensitivity of *CAGE* were high (86% and 91%, respectively) (Ashman et al., 2004).	Strength: Appropriate for use with clinical populations Weaknesses: Poor sensitivity when modified to detect drug abuse or when used to determine pre-injury substance abuse (Ashman et al., 2004); *CAGE* was shown to be unable to discriminate between heavy drinkers and non-heavy drinkers in the general population (Bisson, Nadeau, & Demers, 1999).

continued

Assessment Table 10-1

Assessing Personal, Social, and Cultural Contexts (continued)

Instrument and Reference	Description	Time to Administer	Validity	Reliability	Sensitivity	Strengths and Weaknesses
Visual Analog Scale (*VAS*) to measure pain (Huskisson, 1974)	Presented as a 10-cm line, anchored with "no pain" on one end of the continuum and "worst imaginable pain" on the other end. Patient marks a line to indicate pain intensity, which is measured in millimeters (with zero at the "no pain" anchor).	Approximately 2 minutes.	High correlation between *VAS* and numerical rating scale for pain ($r = 0.94$; 95% CI, 0.93–0.95) (Bijur Latimer, & Gallagher, 2003).	High reliability (intraclass correlation coefficient for paired *VAS* scores = 0.97; 95% CI, 0.96–0.98) (Bijur, Silver, & Gallagher, 2001).	Statistically significant differences between changes in *VAS* scores (in mm) by verbal descriptors of pain (F = 79.4, $p < 0.001$) (Gallagher et al., 2002; Pizzi et al. 2005).	Strengths: Brief screening tool; widely used and understood by patients and professionals. Weaknesses: Limited research regarding reliability and validity with rehabilitation populations; may not be reliable measure of pain in patients with cognitive impairments (Williamson & Hoggart, 2005); not an appropriate tool for analyzing differences in pain across individuals (Kane et al., 2005).

McGill Pain Questionnaire (*MPQ-SF*) (Melzack, 1987)	Self-report tool designed to measure pain and response to intervention that has 3-part dimensions: *SF* (word identification), *Pain Intensity Index* (*PII*), and *VAS*.	2–5 minutes.	Moderately strong to strong correlation between subscales of SF and long form (Melzack, 1975) for 4 diagnostic groups ($r = 0.65$–0.88, $p < .001$). Persons with disability use many but not all of the pain descriptors included in the *MPQ-SF* when verbally describing their pain experience (Dudgeon et al., 2005).	Strong inter-rater reliability (intra-class correlation coefficient of 0.98 when *MPQ-SF* was readministered within 5 minutes by a second therapist) (Gridley & van den Dolder, 2001).	Responsive to pain-related intervention. Statistically significant differences before and after intervention with 3 diagnostic groups on 3 components of test (*SF*, $p < 0.001$, *PII*, $p < 0.001$, *VAS*, $p < 0.001$) (Melzack, 1987).	Strengths: Brief; measures quality of the pain in addition to intensity. Weaknesses: Melzack (1975) cautions that simply asking the patient to fill out the questions by him or herself may yield unreliable information and suggests that the clinician read each subset of questions/instructions to the patient. Patient must be able to read.
The Hospital Anxiety and Depression Scale (*HADS*) (Zigmond & Snaith, 1983)	Self-administered questionnaire designed to detect depression and anxiety in a medical outpatient clinic setting. Comprised of 16 questions related to psychological rather than somatic complaints.	Less than 20 minutes.	Moderate correlation between patient self-ratings on *HADS* and psychiatric interview assessment for anxiety ($r = 0.54, p < 0.05$); moderately strong for depression ($r = 0.79, p < 0.01$).	Good internal consistency (Cronbach's $\alpha = 0.83$ for anxiety subscale and 0.84 for depression subscale) (Pallant & Bailey, 2005).	Good sensitivity and specificity for separate subscales with cut-off score of ≥ 8 (*HADS*-anxiety: sensitivity, 0.89; specificity, 0.88; *HADS*-depression: sensitivity, 0.80; specificity, 0.88) (Olssøn, Mykletun, & Dahl, 2005).	Strengths: Brief screen, such that patient could complete while waiting for appointment; has been translated into Arabic, Dutch, French, German, Hebrew, Swedish, Italian, and Spanish; appropriate for wide range of medical diagnoses. Weaknesses: Patients must be able to read to complete the *HAD*; use of total score not adequately sensitive in identifying cases of psychiatric illness (Poole & Morgan, 2006).

continued

Assessment Table 10-1

Assessing Personal, Social, and Cultural Contexts (continued)

Instrument and Reference	Description	Time to Administer	Validity	Reliability	Sensitivity	Strengths and Weaknesses
Beck Depression Index (BDI) – FastScreen for Medical Patients (Beck, Steer, & Brown, 2000)	Self-report tool that screens for depression in adults and adolescents. Comprised of 7 items extracted from the 21 item *Beck Depression Inventory–II.*	Less than 5 minutes to complete.	Construct validity: moderately strong correlation between *BDI-FastScreen* and *HADS* ($r = 0.62$, $p < 0.001$).	Good internal consistency (alphas of the *BDI-FastScreen* for family practice, internal medicine, and pediatric patients were 0.85, 0.85, and 0.88, respectively) (Beck, Steer, & Brown, 2000).	*BDI-FastScreen* cut-off score of ≥ 4 had 100% sensitivity and 84% specificity rates (Scheinthal et al., 2001).	Strengths: Very brief with good psychometric properties; responses to *BDI-FastScreen* not related to sex, ethnicity, age, or total number of medical conditions (Beck, Steer, & Brown, 2000). Weaknesses: Does not specifically inform occupational therapy intervention planning; serves only to identify persons in need of referral for more in-depth psychiatric assessment.
Norbeck Social Support Questionnaire (NSSQ) (Norbeck, Lindsey, & Carrieri, 1981)	Self-administered questionnaire consisting of 9 items. Patients list individuals in their personal network and specify the nature of their relationship. Measures 3 functional types of social support (affect, affirmation, and aid).	Approximately 10 minutes.	Results of factor analysis support a 3-factor model (affect, affirmation, aid) ($\chi^2 = 8.42$, df = 6, $p = 0.208$) (Gigliotti, 2002). (Note: A significant chi-square test suggests that variables are not independent. In this study, the results were *not* significant.)	High degree of test–retest reliability (0.85–0.92). High internal consistency within 3 types of support (0.89–0.97) (Norbeck, Lindsey, & Carrieri, 1981).	No information.	Strengths: Based on conceptual definitions of social support proposed by Kahn (1979); instrument may provide useful structure for interviewing clients about the nature of their social support. Weakness: Specific subscale scores may be more relevant to research than practice.

SUMMARY REVIEW QUESTIONS

1. Consider your morning self-care routine—the activities you performed today to get ready to leave for school or work. List the personal, social, and contextual factors that influenced your performance. If someone who did not know you judged your performance, what aspects might they consider unusual? What aspects might he or she consider normal for someone of your age and background?
2. Review Figure 10-2 and write a paragraph describing the possible influences on occupational functioning of one of the contextual factors not discussed in this chapter. For example, how might social class or gender help or hinder performance?
3. Outline circumstances in which you would use standardized instruments to assess contextual factors and those in which you would use more informal methods.
4. Make a private list of your own biases. What assumptions do you have about people who are different from you in terms of age, sex, cultural and educational background, sexual orientation, and abilities (physical, cognitive, emotional)? List the steps you can take to debunk these biases and measures to minimize their effects during interactions with patients.
5. Observe the interactions of another clinician and patient during assessment. What, if any, comments made by the therapist could be attributed to his or her personal, social, and cultural context? What comments made by the patient could be attributed to his or her personal, social, and cultural context?

References

Abberley, P. (1995). Disabling ideology in health and welfare: The case of occupational therapy. *Disability and Society, 10,* 221–232.

American Occupational Therapy Association [AOTA]. (2002). Occupational Therapy Practice Framework: Domain and process. *American Journal of Occupational Therapy, 56,* 609–639.

American Occupational Therapy Association [AOTA]. (2004). Occupational therapy's commitment to nondiscrimination and inclusion. *American Journal of Occupational Therapy, 58,* 668.

Amsters, D. I., Pershouse, K. J., Price, G. L., & Kendall, M. B. (2005). Long duration spinal cord injury: Perceptions of functional change over time. *Disability and Rehabilitation, 27,* 489–497.

Armstrong, M. J., & Fitzgerald, M. H. (1996). Culture and disability studies: An anthropological perspective. *Rehabilitation Education, 10,* 247–304.

Arruda, J. E., Stern, R. A., & Sommerville, B. A. (1999). Measurement of mood states in stroke patients: Validation of the Visual Analog Mood Scale. *Archives of Physical Medicine and Rehabilitation, 80,* 676–680.

Ashman, T. A., Schwartz, M. E., Cantor, J. B., Hibbard, M. R., & Gordon, W. A. (2004). Screening for substance abuse in individuals with traumatic brain injury. *Brain Injury, 18,* 191–202.

Baumeister, R. F. (2005). *The cultural animal: Human nature, meaning, and social life.* New York: Oxford University Press.

Beck, A. T., Steer, R. A., & Brown, G. K. (2000). *BDI-Fast Screen for Medical Patients.* San Antonio, TX: The Psychological Corporation.

Bell, N. S., Williams, J. O., Senier, L., Strowman, S. R., & Amoroso, P. J. (2003). The reliability and validity of the self-reported drinking measures in the Army's Health Risk Appraisal survey. *Alcoholism: Clinical and Experimental Research, 27,* 826–834.

Bijur, P. E., Latimer, C. T., & Gallagher, J. (2003). Validation of a verbally administered numerical rating scale of acute pain for use in the emergency department. *Academic Emergency Medicine, 10,* 390–392.

Bijur, P. E., Silver, W., & Gallagher, J. (2001). Reliability of the visual analog scale for measurement of acute pain. *Academic Emergency Medicine, 8,* 1153–1157.

Bisson, J., Nadeau, L., & Demers, A., (1999). The validity of the CAGE scale to screen for heavy drinking and drinking problems in a general population survey. *Addiction, 94,* 715–722.

Bogner, J. A., Corrigan, J. D., Mysiw, J., Clinchot, D., & Fugate, L. (2001). Comparison of substance abuse and violence in the prediction of long-term rehabilitation outcomes after traumatic brain injury. *Archives of Physical Medicine and Rehabilitation, 82,* 571–577.

Bonder, B. R., Martin, L., & Miracle, A. W. (2004). Culture as emergent in occupation. *American Journal of Occupational Therapy, 58,* 159–168.

Brown, S. M., Humphry, R., & Taylor, E. (1997). A model of the nature of family-therapist relationships: Implications for education. *American Journal of Occupational Therapy, 51,* 597–603.

Cannon, P. (1994). If I live, does the injury take my life? *Viewpoints: Issues in Brain Injury Rehabilitation, 26,* 3–4.

Chantraine, A., Baribeault, A., Uebelhart, D., & Gremion, G. (1999). Shoulder pain and dysfunction in hemiplegia: Effects of functional electrical stimulation. *Archives of Physical Medicine and Rehabilitation, 80,* 328–331.

Christiansen, C. (1997). Acknowledging a spiritual dimension in occupational therapy practice. *American Journal of Occupational Therapy, 51,* 169–172.

Collins, J. S., Paul, S., & West-Frasier, J. (2001). The utilization of spirituality in occupational therapy: Beliefs, practices, and perceived barriers. *Occupational Therapy in Health Care, 14,* 73–92.

Corbin, J. M., & Strauss, A. (1988). *Unending work and care: Managing chronic illness at home.* San Francisco: Jossey-Bass.

Cox, B. J., & Waller, L. L. (1991). *Bridging the communication gap with the elderly.* Chicago: American Hospital.

Cully, J. A., Gfeller, J. D., Heise, R. A., Ross, M. J., Teal, C. R., & Kunik, M. E. (2005). Geriatric depression, medical diagnosis, and functional recovery during acute rehabilitation. *Archives of Physical Medicine and Rehabilitation, 86,* 2256–2260.

Curtis, K. A., Drysdale, G. A., Lanza, D., Kolber, M., Vitolo, R. S., & West, R. (1999). Shoulder pain in wheelchair users with tetraplegia and paraplegia. *Archives of Physical Medicine and Rehabilitation, 80,* 453–457.

Dalyan, M., Cardenas, D. D., & Gerard, B. (1999). Upper extremity pain after spinal cord injury. *Spinal Cord, 37,* 191–195.

Davis, T. C., Long, S. W., Jackson, R. H., Mayeaux, E. J., George, R. B., Murphy, P. W., & Crouch, M. A. (1993). Rapid estimate of adult literacy in medicine: A shortened screening instrument. *Family Medicine, 25,* 391–395.

Dudgeon, B. J., Ehde, D. M., Cardenas, D. D., Engel, J. M., Hoffman, A. J., & Jensen, M. P. (2005). Describing pain with physical disability: Narrative interviews and the McGill Pain Questionnaire. *Archives of Physical Medicine and Rehabilitation, 86,* 109–115.

Dudgeon, B. J., Gerrard, B. C., Jensen, M. P., Rhodes, L. A., & Tyler, E. J. (2002). Physical disability and the experience of chronic pain. *Archives of Physical Medicine and Rehabilitation, 83,* 229–235.

Dudgeon, B. J., Tyler, E. J., Rhondes, L. A., & Jensen, M. P. (2006). Managing usual and unexpected pain with physical disability: A qualitative analysis. *American Journal of Occupational Therapy, 60,* 92–103.

Dunn, W., Brown, C., & McGuigan, A. (1994). The ecology of human performance: A framework for considering the effect of context. *American Journal of Occupational Therapy, 48,* 595–607.

Eddey, G. E., & Robey, K. L. (2005). Considering the culture of disability in cultural competence education. *Academic Medicine, 80,* 706–712.

Egan, M., & Swedersky, J. (2003). Spirituality as experienced by occupational therapists in practice. *American Journal of Occupational Therapy, 57,* 525–533.

Ehde, D. M., Jensen, M. P., Engel, J. M., Turner, J. A., Hoffman, A. J., & Cardenas, D. D. (2003). Chronic pain secondary to disability: A review. *The Clinical Journal of Pain, 19,* 3–17.

Engquist, D. E., Short-DeGraff, M., Gliner, J., & Oltjenbruns, K. (1997). Occupational therapists' beliefs and practices with regard to spirituality and therapy. *American Journal of Occupational Therapy, 51,* 173–180.

Ewing, J. A. (1984). Detecting alcoholism: The CAGE questionnaire. *Journal of the American Medical Association, 252,* 1905–1907.

Eysenck, M. W., & Keane, M. T. (1990). *Cognitive psychology: A student's handbook.* London: Lawrence Erlbaum.

Farrales, S. (1996). Vietnamese. In J. G. Lipson, S. L. Dibble, & P. A. Minarik (Eds.), *Culture & nursing care: A pocket guide* (pp. 280–290). San Francisco: UCSF Nursing.

Fisher, A. G. (1998). Uniting practice and theory in an occupational framework. *American Journal of Occupational Therapy, 52,* 509–521.

Freiberg, K. L. (1987). *Human development: A life-span approach* (3rd ed.). Boston: Jones & Bartlett.

Frosch, S., Gruber, A., Jones, C., Myers, S., Noel, E., Westerlund, A., & Zavisin, T. (1997). The long term effects of traumatic brain injury on the roles of caregivers. *Brain Injury, 11,* 891–906.

Gallagher, E. J., Bijur, P. E., Latimer, C., & Silver, W. (2002). Reliability and validity of a visual analog scale for acute abdominal pain in the ED. *American Journal of Emergency Medicine, 20,* 287–290.

Gans, J. S. (1998). Enhancing the therapeutic value of talking with patients in the rehabilitation setting. *Rehabilitation Outlook, Summer,* 4–5.

Gigliotti, E. (2002). A confirmation of the factor structure of the Norbeck Social Support Questionnaire. *Nursing Research, 51,* 276–284.

Gorman, L. M., Sultman, D., & Luna-Raines, M. (1989). *Psychosocial nursing handbook for the nonpsychiatric nurse.* Baltimore: Williams & Wilkins.

Grant, J. S., Bartolucci, A. A., Elliot, T. R., & Giger, J. N. (2000). Sociodemographic, physical, and psychosocial characteristics of depressed and non-depressed family caregivers of stroke survivors. *Brain Injury, 14,* 1089–1100.

Gridley, L., & van den Dolder, P. A. (2001). The Percentage Improvement in Pain Scale as a measure of physiotherapy treatment effects. *Australian Journal of Physiotherapy, 47,* 133–136.

Heaney, C. A., & Israel, B. A. (1997). Social networks and social support. In K. Glanz, F. M. Lewis, & B. K. Rimer (Eds.), *Health behavior and health education* (pp. 179–205). San Francisco: Jossey-Bass.

Helliwell, J. F., & Putnam, R. D. (2004). The social context of well-being. *Philosophical Transactions of the Royal Society B, 359,* 1435–1446.

Huskisson, E. C. (1974). Measurement of pain. *Lancet, 2,* 1127–1131.

Jackson, J. (2000). Understanding the experience of noninclusive occupational therapy clinics: Lesbians' perspectives. *American Journal of Occupational Therapy, 54,* 26–35.

Joint Commission on Accreditation of Healthcare Organizations (2005). *Comprehensive accreditation manual for hospitals.* Oakbrook Terrace, IL: Joint Commission on Accreditation of Healthcare Organizations.

Kane, R. L., Bershadsky, B., Rockwood, T., Saleh, K., & Islam, N. C. (2005). Visual Analog Scale pain reporting was standardized. *Journal of Clinical Epidemiology, 58,* 618–623.

Kielhofner, G. (2005). Rethinking disability and what to do about it: Disability studies and its implication for occupational therapy. *American Journal of Occupational Therapy, 59,* 487–496.

Kleinman, A. (1988). *The illness narratives: Suffering, healing, and the human condition.* New York: Basic Books.

Kolakowsky-Hayner, S. A., Gourley, E. V., Kreutzer, J. S., Marwitz, J. H., Cifu, D. X., & McKinley, W. O. (1999). Pre-injury substance abuse among persons with brain injury and spinal cord injury. *Brain Injury, 13,* 571–581.

Krefting, L. (1991). The culture concept in the everyday practice of occupational and physical therapy. *Physical and Occupational Therapy in Practice, 11,* 1–16.

Kreuter, M., Sullivan, M., Dahllof, A. G., & Siosteen, A. (1998). Partner relationships, functioning, mood and global quality of life in persons with spinal cord injury and traumatic brain injury. *Spinal Cord, 36,* 252–261.

Lai, S. M., Duncan, P. W., Keighley, J., & Johnson, D. (2002). Depressive symptoms and independence in BADL and IADL. *Journal of Rehabilitation Research and Development, 39,* 589–596.

Lancaster, L. C., & Stillman, D. (2002). *When generations collide.* New York: Harper Collins Publishers, Inc.

Langford, C. P. H., Bowsher, J., Maloney, J. P., & Lillis, P. (1997). Social support: A conceptual analysis. *Journal of Advanced Nursing, 25,* 95–100.

Law, M., Cooper, B., Strong, S., Stewart, D., Rigby, P., & Letts, L. (1996). The person-environment-occupation model: A transactive approach to occupational performance. *Canadian Journal of Occupational Therapy, 63,* 9–23.

Lerman, C., & Glanz, K. (1997). Stress, coping, and health behavior. In K. Glanz, F. M. Lewis, B. K. Rimer (Eds.), *Health behavior and health education* (pp. 113–138). San Francisco: Jossey-Bass.

Lipson, J. G. (1996). Culturally competent nursing care. In J. G. Lipson, S. L. Dibble, and P. A. Minarik (Eds.), *Culture and nursing care: A pocket guide* (pp. 1–10). San Francisco: UCSF Nursing.

Luborsky, M. R. (1994). The cultural adversity of physical disability: Erosion of full adult personhood. *Journal of Aging Studies, 8,* 239–253.

Luborsky, M. R. (1995). The process of self-report of impairment in clinical research. *Social Science Medicine, 40,* 1447–1459.

Luborsky, M. (1997). Attuning assessment to the client: Recent advances in theory and methodology. *Generations, 21,* 10–15.

Luoto, S., Taimela, S., Hurri, H., & Alaranta, H. (1999). Mechanisms explaining the association between low back trouble and deficits in information processing. *Spine, 24,* 255–261.

Mattingly, C. (1991). The narrative nature of clinical reasoning. *American Journal of Occupational Therapy, 45,* 998–1005.

Mattingly, C., & Fleming, M. H. (1994). *Clinical reasoning.* Philadelphia: Davis.

McGruder, J. (1998). Culture and other forms of human diversity in occupational therapy. In M. E. Neistadt & E. B. Crepeau (Eds.), *Willard and Spackman's occupational therapy* (pp. 54–66) (9th Ed.). Philadelphia: Lippincott.

Meara, J., Michelmore, E., & Hobson, P. (1999). Use of the GDS-15 geriatric depression scale as a screening instrument for depressive symptomatology in patients with Parkinson's disease and their carers in the community. *Age and Ageing, 28,* 35–38.

Melzack, R. (1975). The McGill Pain Questionnaire: Major properties and scoring methods. *Pain, 1,* 277–299.

Melzack, R. (1987). The short-form McGill Questionnaire. *Pain, 30,* 191–197.

Million, R., Hall, W., Nilsen, K. H., Baker, R. D., & Jayson, M. I. V. (1982). Assessment of the progress of the back pain patient. *Spine, 7,* 204–212.

Moyers, P. A., & Stoffel, V. C. (1999). Alcohol dependence in a client with a work-related injury. *American Journal of Occupational Therapy, 53,* 640–645.

Murphy, P. W., Davis, T. C., Long, S. W., Jackson, R. H., & Decker, B. C. (1993). Rapid Estimates of Adult Literacy in Medicine (REALM): A quick reading test for patients. *Journal of Reading, 37,* 124–130.

Murray, S. A., Manktelow, K., & Clifford, C. (2000). The interplay between social and cultural context and perceptions of cardiovascular disease. *Journal of Advanced Nursing, 32,* 1224–1233.

National Center for Medical Rehabilitation Research. (1993). Research plan for the National Center for Medical Rehabilitation Research (NIH Publication 93-3509). Bethesda: MD: National Center for Medical Rehabilitation Research.

Nelson, D. L. (1988). Occupation: Form and performance. *American Journal of Occupational Therapy, 42,* 633–641.

Norbeck, J. S., Lindsey, A. M., & Carrieri, V. L. (1981). The development of an instrument to measure social support. *Nursing Research, 30,* 262–269.

Odawara, E. (2005). Cultural competency in occupational therapy: Beyond a cross-cultural view of practice. *American Journal of Occupational Therapy, 59,* 325–334.

Osborne, C. L. (1998). *Over my head.* Kansas City, MO: Andrews McMeel.

Olssøn, I., Mykletun, A., & Dahl, A. A. (2005). The hospital anxiety and depression rating scale: A cross-sectional study of psychometrics and case finding abilities in general practice. *BMC Psychiatry, 5,* 46.

Pallant, J. F., & Bailey, C. M. (2005). Assessment of the structure of the Hospital Anxiety and Depression Scale in musculoskeletal patients. *Health and Quality of Life Outcomes, 3,* 82.

Parikh, N. S., Parker, R. M., Nurss, J. R., Baker, D. W., & Williams, M. V. (1996). Shame and health literacy: The unspoken connection. *Patient Education and Counseling, 27,* 33–39.

Paul, S. (1995). Culture and its influence on occupational therapy evaluation. *Canadian Journal of Occupational Therapy, 62,* 154–161.

Pizzi, A., Carlucci, G., Falsini, C., Verdesca, S., & Grippo, A. (2005). Application of a volar static splint in poststroke spasticity of the upper limb. *Archives of Physical Medicine and Rehabilitation, 86,* 1855–1859.

Poole, N. A., & Morgan, J. F. (2006). Validity and reliability of the Hospital Anxiety and Depression Scale in a hypertrophic cardiomyopathy clinic: The HADS in a cardiomyopathy population. *General Hospital Psychiatry, 28,* 55–58.

Pruchno, R. A., & Potashnik, S. L. (1989). Caregiving spouses: Physical and mental health in perspective. *Journal of the American Geriatrics Society, 37,* 697–705.

Puchalski, C., & Romer, A. L. (2000). Taking a spiritual history allows clinicians to understand patients more fully. *Journal of Palliative Medicine,* 3, 129–137.

Radomski, M. V. (1995). There is more to life than putting on your pants. *American Journal of Occupational Therapy, 49,* 487–490.

Riley, B. B., Perna, R., Tate, D. G., Forchheimer, M., Anderson, C., & Luera, G. (1998). Types of spiritual well-being among persons with chronic illness: Their relation to various forms of quality of life. *Archives of Physical Medicine and Rehabilitation, 79,* 258–264.

Royeen, C. B. (1995). The human life cycle: Paradigmatic shifts in occupation. In C. B. Royeen (Ed.), *The practice of the future: Putting occupation back into therapy.* Bethesda, MD: American Occupational Therapy Association.

Ruchinskas, R. (2002). Rehabilitation therapists' recognition of cognitive and mood disorders in geriatric patients. *Archives of Physical Medicine and Rehabilitation, 83,* 609–612.

Rybarczyk, B., Haut, A., Lacey, R. F., Fogg, L. F., & Nicholas, J. J. (2001). A multifactorial study of age bias among rehabilitation professionals. *Archives of Physical Medicine and Rehabilitation, 82,* 625–632.

Scheinthal, S. M., Steer, R. A., Giffin, L., & Beck, A. T. (2001). Evaluating geriatric medical outpatients with the Beck Depression Inventory-Fastscreen for medical patients. *Aging and Mental Health, 5,* 143–148.

Scherer, M. J., & Cushman, L. A. (1997). A functional approach to psychological and psychosocial factors and their assessment in rehabilitation. In S. S. Dittmar & G. E. Gresham (Eds.), *Functional assessment and outcome measures for the rehabilitation health professional* (pp. 57–67). Gaithersburg, MD: Aspen.

Smith, W. B., Gracely, R. H., & Safer, M. A. (1998). The meaning of pain: Cancer patients' rating and recall of pain intensity and affect. *Pain, 78,* 123–129.

Stansbury, J. P., Reid, K. J., Reker, D. M., Duncan, P. W., Marshall, C. R., & Rittman, M. (2004). Why ethnic designation matters for stroke rehabilitation: Comparing VA administrative data and clinical records. *Journal of Rehabilitation Research and Development, 41,* 269–278.

St. Clair, A., & McKenry, L. (1999). Preparing culturally competent practitioners. *Journal of Nursing Education, 38,* 228–234.

Strauss, W., & Howe, N. (1991). *Generations.* New York: William Morrow.

Taj, N., Devera-Sales, A., & Vinson, D. C. (1998). Screening for problem drinking: Does a single question work? *Journal of Family Practice, 46,* 328–335.

Toglia, J. P. (1993). *The Contextual Memory Test.* Tucson, AZ: Therapy Skill Builders.

Tollifson, J. (1997). Imperfection is a beautiful thing: On disability and meditation. In K. Fries (Ed.), *Staring back: The disability experience from the inside out.* New York: Penguin Putnam.

Wakefield, D. (2005). *I remember running: The year i got everything i ever wanted–and ALS.* New York: Marlowe & Company.

Watson, N. (2002). Well, I know this is going to sound very strange to you, but I don't see myself as a disabled person: Identity and disability. *Disability and Society, 17,* 509–527.

Webster's new world dictionary of American English (3rd college ed). (1994). New York: Prentice Hall.

Webster, G., Daisley, A., & King, N. (1999). Relationship and family breakdown following acquired brain injury: The role of the rehabilitation team. *Brain Injury, 13,* 593–603.

Williamson, A., & Hoggart, B. (2005). Pain: A review of three commonly used pain rating scales. *Issues in Clinical Nursing, 14,* 798–804.

World Health Organization. (2001). *International Classification of Functioning, Disability and Health–Short version.* Geneva: World Health Organization.

Zelman, D. C., Smith, M. Y., Hoffman, D., Edwards, L., Reed, P., Levine, E., Siefeldin, R., & Dukes, E. (2004). Acceptable, manageable, and tolerable days: Patient daily goals for medication management of persistent pain. *Journal of Pain and Symptom Management, 28,* 474–487.

Zigmond, A. S., & Snaith, R. P. (1983). The Hospital Anxiety and Depression Scale. *Acta Psychiatrica Scandinavia, 67,* 361–370.

Supplemental References

Brandt, E. N., & Pope, A. M. (Eds.) (1997). *Enabling America.* Washington, DC: National Academy.

CHAPTER 11

Assessing Environment: Home, Community, and Workplace Access

Patricia Rigby, Mandy Lowe, Lori Letts, and Debra Stewart

LEARNING OBJECTIVES

After studying this chapter, the reader will be able to do the following:

1. Describe the roles and responsibilities of the occupational therapist in the evaluation of environmental access.
2. Identify factors that act as environmental barriers and supports to occupational performance.
3. Apply critical appraisal when selecting assessment instruments appropriate for use in evaluating access to home, community, and workplace.
4. Explain how legislation and building standards influence the degree of environmental access that is available for people with disabilities.

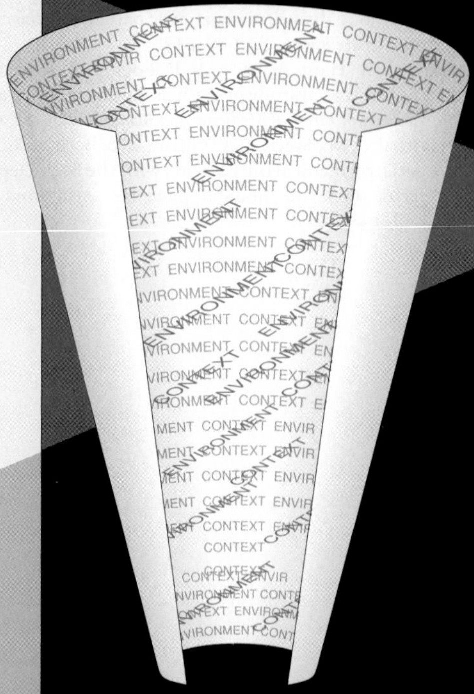

Glossary

Accessibility—The ease with which the physical environment may be reached, entered, and used by all individuals.

Accommodations (environmental)—Removal of environmental barriers and provision of environmental supports and resources to enable a person with a disability to enjoy equal opportunity.

Barrier-free design—Design features of the built environment that remove physical barriers to full and equal accessibility for all persons with disabilities.

Environmental barrier—Any component of the environment that impedes optimal occupational functioning.

Environmental support—Any component of the environment that encourages, facilitates, or provides assistance to allow a person to achieve optimal occupational functioning.

PEO fit—The goodness of fit between personal factors (e.g., functional, social, and psychological), the characteristics of the environment (e.g., barriers and supports), and the characteristics of the chosen occupation.

Physical environment—The natural or human-made features of the environment within which occupational functioning occurs.

Standardization—The process of making an assessment available in a manual with standard procedures for testing, scoring, and interpreting the results. Environmental assessments do not usually undergo a normative process because of the variability in environments, yet many are based on standards developed by the ANSI, government building codes, and interpretations of the ADA.

Transactive—Integrated, co-dependent (of a relationship).

Universal design—Design features of the built environment that enhance optimal function and convenience for all individuals, regardless of their ability.

The environment influences human behavior and provides the context within which all roles are performed. In occupational therapy, the environment is broadly defined as having physical, social, cultural, organizational, and institutional dimensions. These dimensions interact with each other and are difficult to tease apart; that is, they are said to be **transactive** (Law et al., 1996).

A number of occupational therapy theories specifically address the issue of environmental influences on occupational functioning (e.g., American Occupational Therapy Association [AOTA], 2002; Canadian Association of Occupational Therapists [CAOT], 1997; Dunn, Brown, & McGuigan, 1994; Law et al., 1996). These vary slightly in terminology and approach, but all agree on the importance of environmental considerations in the practice of occupational therapy (Rigby & Letts, 2003). Central to these theories is the notion that **environmental barriers** to occupational performance for people with disabilities can be modified or eliminated more easily than most other negative influences. Also, the theories all emphasize that **environmental supports** promote optimal occupational performance.

The examination of occupational performance involves analysis of the goodness of fit for the person-environment-occupation (PEO) relationship (Law et al., 1996). The better the **PEO fit**, the more optimal the occupational performance. Occupational therapists are frequently called upon to determine the fit between people with disabilities, their chosen occupations, and the various environments in which they live, work, and play. In this capacity, the therapist's role is as follows:

- To identify and evaluate barriers that may challenge the competency and ability of individuals to carry out their chosen occupations and roles
- To identify and evaluate resources that will support occupational performance and occupational functioning
- To develop strategies to eliminate or ameliorate barriers
- To utilize resources and supports to improve the goodness of PEO fit

This chapter focuses on the assessment of the environment for occupational performance. Specifically, it will consider the environment that is external to the client when assessing occupational functioning: the physical, social, and institutional attributes of the environment. The assessment measures selected are those that we consider the best available and that reflect the transactive nature of the relationship between people, their chosen occupations, and the environment in which these occupations are performed.

EVALUATION OF THE ENVIRONMENT

The environment provides the context for occupational functioning. Consequently, an assessment of its attributes should be augmented with information about those who will use the environment and the functions they will carry out there. In the practice of occupational therapy, it is important to begin this process with the person.

Client-Centered Approach

The client is central to all occupational therapy services, and much has been written about the need to engage and involve clients in all stages of the occupational therapy process (Law, 1998). The client-therapist interaction begins with an interview and assessment so that the therapist can gain an understanding of the client's occupational profile (AOTA, 2002). This involves determining what roles and occupations the client previously had and what the client currently wants or is expected to be able to do. Clinicians find that collaborative goal setting is an important stage in establishing client-centered occupational therapy (Wressle et al., 2002).

Once the occupational profile is established, the occupational therapist then completes an analysis of occupational performance to better understand the client's performance skills, patterns, and challenges, considering the contexts within which activities and roles will be carried out. It is at this time that environmental assessment may be deemed necessary. For example, a therapist and client could focus on community mobility and access because it is important to the client to continue participating in a volunteer role at the local public library. The therapist would consider the client's abilities by assessing his or her mobility using a wheelchair in the hospital setting, assessing the client's ability to access community transportation systems, and possibly assessing the library's accessibility to ensure that the client could negotiate the entrances, work areas, and public washrooms.

Roles

The roles carried out by clients address purposeful activities related to self-maintenance, self-enhancement, and self-advancement. Each individual ascribes different meaning to his/her roles. Specific features of the environment can support or hinder the fulfillment of valued roles within the home, community, and workplace.

Environmental Barriers and Supports

The occupational therapist must be able to identify the key environmental barriers and supports that influence the occupational functioning of clients. In clinical practice, barriers and supports are broadly defined. This chapter, however, discusses barriers and supports in the external environment; other contextual barriers and supports are described in Chapter 10.

The International Classification of Functioning, Disability and Health (ICF) classifies environmental factors as assistive products and technology; the natural and human-made environments; supports and relationships; attitudes; and services, systems, and policies (World Health Organization, 2001). The therapist is encouraged to consider these factors during assessment. For example, physical barriers in the natural environment can prevent or impede a person with a disability from participating in daily activities, while human-made resources can improve **accessibility**. Consider the challenge that stairs or rocky paths impose on a person using a wheelchair. These barriers can be removed or reduced by adding supports such as elevators or ramps to replace stairs and a ramped bridge across the rocks to allow access for a wheelchair.

Access that is discriminatory or inconvenient, such as when persons with physical disabilities must use freight elevators or ramped entrances at the back of buildings, is no longer considered a viable solution to eliminating access barriers. Improved accessibility through the use of **universal design** and **barrier-free design** is preferred. These two terms are similar but not synonymous. Universal design refers to features of the built environment that enhance optimal function and convenience for everyone, regardless of ability. Barrier-free design refers to features of the built environment that remove physical barriers to allow full and equal accessibility for all persons with disabilities. Universal design can encompasses barrier-free design, but the converse is not necessarily true. For this reason, it is preferable to promote the use of universal design (Resource 11-1).

RESOURCE 11-1

Internet Resources for Assessing Access to Home, Community, and Workplace

Adaptive Environments: Human-centered design
www.adaptenv.org
Provides access to resources on universal design and on accessibility and the ADA (e.g., book titled, *Achieving Physical and Communication Accessibility*).

Americans with Disabilities Act (ADA)
www.usdoj.gov/crt/ada/adahom1.htm
Provides information and technical assistance on the ADA and the ADA standards for accessible design.

Center for Universal Design
www.design.ncsu.edu/cud/
Includes overviews of the principles of universal design, publications, and information on fair housing and home modifications.

Fair Housing FIRST
www.fairhousingfirst.org
Provides information and resources to support implementation of the Fair Housing Act amendments, such as the Fair Housing Act Design Manual (Revised April 1998).

International Code Council
www.iccsafe.org/e/catalog.html
Provides catalogue of materials on accessibility such as the *California Disabled Accessibility Guidebook 2003*.

National Highway Traffic Safety Administration
www.nhtsa.dot.gov/

United States Department of Transportation
www.dot.gov
Phone: (202) 366-4000.

Influences on Environmental Accessibility

Various societal and cultural attitudes influence the degree to which the **physical environment** is made accessible to people with disabilities. Occupational therapy practice standards also reflect these global views. These influences manifest as national and state or provincial legislation, building standards, and professional practice requirements.

Legislation

The Americans with Disabilities Act (ADA) (1990), is a civil rights law designed to increase the integration and successful community living of people with disabilities in American society. In other countries, similar civil rights laws may prohibit discrimination toward persons with disabilities and guarantee equal rights and provisions for **accommodations** in society.

For example, the ADA mandates that a qualified person with a disability cannot be discriminated against when seeking or participating in employment. The intent of the law is to create equal opportunity and equal access to public environments, services, and transportation for persons with disabilities. The ADA is a dynamic legal document that focuses on achieving integration and independent living for people with disabilities through societal change.

The key phrase in the ADA is the obligation of society to provide reasonable accommodation to ensure that public services, facilities, transportation, employment, accommodations, and telecommunications are accessible. Reasonable accommodations ensure that no person with a disability is excluded from or denied services, segregated, or otherwise treated differently from the general population because of the absence of auxiliary aids or services.

Titles II and III of the ADA detail the steps to be taken by public and private sector services, programs, and facilities to comply with and implement the requirements of the ADA. They address the accommodations required and the availability of resources; modifications to policies, practices, and procedures; the removal of barriers; and alternative forms of services, such as accessible transit services when mainline public facilities are unavailable. Legal parameters are developed through challenge on a case-by-case basis.

These regulations were expected, over time, to eliminate barriers and improve accessibility for people with disabilities. Analysis of the impact of the ADA 10 years later is mixed. Persons with disabilities do not, as yet, perceive that the ADA has been very effective in improving accessibility (Hinton, 2003). Analysis of social policy, however, demonstrates that attitudes and practices of Americans have changed and that the ADA has improved the quality of life for persons with disabilities (Harrison, 2002). See Resources 11-1 for further information on the ADA.

Although the ADA does not mandate professional involvement in achievement of the criteria it sets forth, occupational therapists, who are skilled in occupational analysis, environmental assessment, and determining PEO fit, are well suited to assist with meeting the requirements of the ADA. When occupational therapists were surveyed, however, they demonstrated a lack of knowledge about the ADA and reported inaction in implementing ADA provisions (Redick, McClain, & Brown, 2000). Because the ADA and similar laws are critical for improving accessibility, independence, and empowerment of persons with physical disabilities, it is imperative that occupational therapists take action to better utilize such legislation.

Building Standards

In 2004, the United States Access Board released the updated ADA-ABA (Architectural Board Act) Accessibility Guidelines for new or altered buildings, which provide the accessibility requirements for public and private facilities (United States Access Board, 2004a). The specifications in these guidelines are based upon adult and child dimensions and anthropometrics and should be applied during the design and construction or alteration of buildings and facilities covered by titles II and III of the ADA. Specifications are provided for most aspects of the built environment including space required for maneuvering wheelchairs in corridors and rooms (Figs. 11-1 and 11-2), washrooms, building entrances, and parking lots.

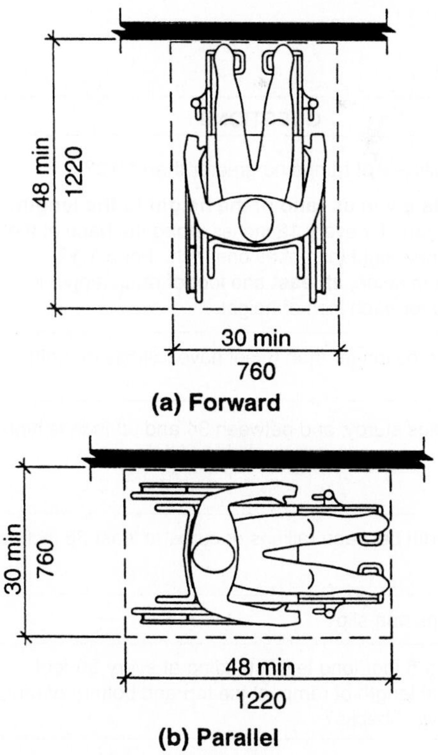

Figure 11-1 Position—clear space of a minimum of 30 × 48 inches (760 × 1220 mm) for either forward or parallel approach to an element. (Adapted from the ADA-ABA Accessibility Guidelines [United States Access Board, 2004a].)

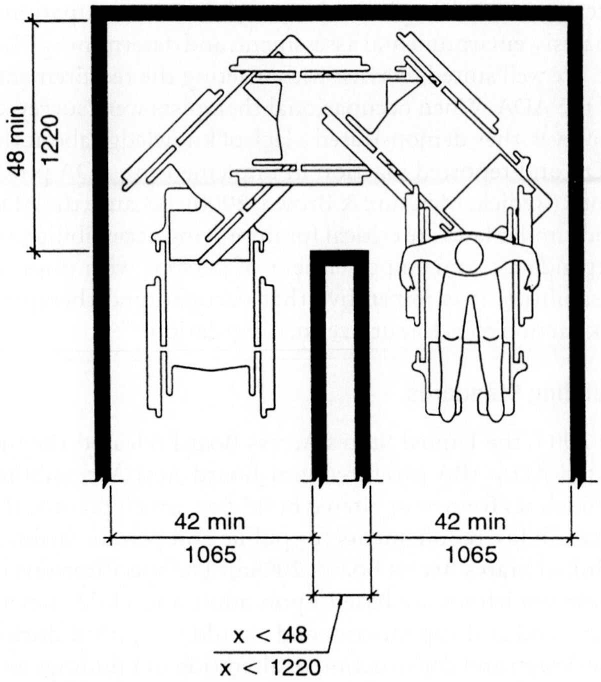

Figure 11-2 Clear width of a minimum of 42 inches (1065 mm) at approach to turn, and 48 inches (1220 mm) at turn. (Adapted from the ADA-ABA Accessibility Guidelines [United States Access Board, 2004a].)

Other standards have been developed for specific environments, such as the workplace. For example, the National Institute of Occupational Safety and Health (NIOSH) publishes criteria directed at reducing the rate of workplace injuries. Occupational therapists who work in these environments must become familiar with the standards and guidelines relevant to their area of practice.

The *Americans with Disabilities Act Checklist for Readily Achievable Barrier Removal* (Adaptive Environments, 1995) was developed for owners and managers of public buildings and businesses to identify barriers in their facilities. This survey tool is based on the older ADA Accessibility Guidelines (ADAAG) (United States Access Board, 2002) and provides easy-to-use measurement guides to identify accessibility barriers and suggestions for "readily achievable" access solutions. For example, requirements for a ramped entrance to a building are shown in the checklist in Figure 11-3. The occupational therapist can assist businesses to use this tool and set priorities for achieving accessibility. It would be important and reasonably easy to cross-reference this checklist with the new ADA-ABA Accessibility Guidelines (United States Access Board, 2004a).

RAMPS

QUESTIONS	MEASUREMENT	YES	NO	POSSIBLE SOLUTIONS
Are the slopes of ramps no greater than 1:12? **Slope is given as ratio of the height to the length.** 1:12 means for every 12 inches along the base of the ramp, the height increases one inch. For a 1:12 maximum slope, **at least** one foot of ramp length is needed for each inch of height.	slope = _____			☐ Lengthen ramp to decrease slope. ☐ Relocate ramp. ☐ If available space is limited, reconfigure ramp to include switchbacks.
Do all ramps longer than 6 feet have railings on both sides?				☐ Add railings.
Are railings sturdy, and between 34 and 38 inches high?	height = _____			☐ Adjust height of railing if not between 30 and 38 inches. ☐ Secure handrails in fixtures.
Is the width between railings or curbs at least 36 inches?	width = _____			☐ Relocate the railings. ☐ Widen the ramp.
Are ramps non-slip?				☐ Add non-slip surface material.
Is there a 5-foot-long level standing at every 30-foot horizontal length of ramp, at the top and bottom of ramps and at switchbacks?	length = _____			☐ Remodel or relocate ramp.
Does the ramp rise no more than 30 inches between landings?	rise = _____			☐ Remodel or relocate ramp.

Figure 11-3 Accessible approach ramps. (Adapted from the *Americans with Disabilities Act Checklist for Readily Achievable Barrier Removal* [Adaptive Environments Center, 1995].)

Professional Practice Requirements

The practice of occupational therapy is also guided by professional regulations. Standards of practice, core competencies, and functions expected of therapists are developed at the national and state/provincial levels and provide performance evaluation criteria. These guidelines are usually generic in nature and apply to all therapists, regardless of the area, setting, or focus of practice (AOTA, 1995; CAOT, 1996). Knowledge of and ability to perform assessments of context/environment are considered to be core competencies and functions of practice for all occupational therapists (AOTA, 1995; Association of Canadian Occupational Therapy Regulatory Organizations, 2000).

ASSESSMENTS OF ENVIRONMENT

Ideally, the occupational therapist should select instruments with **standardization** that assess PEO fit to take into consideration the goodness of fit between the personal factors and characteristics of the environment and the occupation. The PEO relationship is dynamic, complex, and interwoven and, therefore, more difficult to measure than interactions that can be understood by assessing discrete components. Few measures have been developed to assess this complex PEO relationship. Thus, we have included not only those measures in this chapter, but also an array of very useful tools that measure the person–environment relationship or specific characteristics of the environment.

In this chapter, the assessments have been categorized by setting: those suitable for assessing homes (Assessment Table 11-1), the community (Assessment Table 11-2), and the workplace (Assessment Table 11-3). Key information about each assessment, including an analysis of the tool's strengths and weaknesses, was included in the tables to assist occupational therapists in identifying the most appropriate tool(s) for their purposes. The critique of each tool was guided by using the Outcomes Measures Rating Form and Guidelines (Law, 2004). Most measures included here have established psychometric properties. We have, however, included some unique measures that have good content validity and clinical utility but for which formal studies of psychometric properties are unavailable or incomplete. Each table follows its related narrative.

Assessment of Access to Home

A home assessment completed by an occupational therapist can be an important component of the occupational therapy process. Home assessments are often completed as part of a discharge planning process from rehabilitation. It is vital to ensure that clients' home environments are able to provide them with the supports they need while they recover from or live with disabilities. The overriding purpose of a home assessment is to identify the degree of fit for the person completing his or her daily roles within the home environment and to recommend modifications to the environment to ensure optimal independence and safety. A home assessment may also provide opportunities to prevent secondary injuries resulting from home hazards or unsafe practices. Research on the effectiveness of home assessments to prevent falls in older adults demonstrated that home assessments may reduce the risk of falls, especially in people who have a history of past falls (Cumming et al., 1999). Other research has described varying patterns of home modification recommendations resulting from home assessments when comparing clients insured through public or private insurance systems, suggesting that occupational therapists tend to make recommendations that can be practically implemented considering the financial resources available to the client (Lysack & Neufeld, 2003). In a study comparing assessment results between home-based performance assessment, client and proxy report, and clinic-based performance assessment, Rogers et al. (2003) found that home-based performance assessment provides an accurate reflection of the clients' ability to manage in that setting, which cannot be replaced by self-report, caregiver proxy, or clinic-based performance assessments. See Safety Note 11-1 for considerations related to visiting a client's home.

Standardized home assessments are now available for occupational therapists to use with clients and families to identify occupational performance problems in the home. Researchers have discussed the limited use of standardized home assessments by occupational therapists (Mitchell & Unsworth, 2004) and called for the use of dynamic and criterion-referenced assessments (Rogers, Holm, & Stone, 1997). In clinical practice, where service provision needs to be justified, the use of standardized home assessments can be important to ensure that a comprehensive assessment is completed to meet the needs of the client and to justify requests for equipment and home modifications. A review of assessment tools to guide home adaptations (Rousseau et al., 2001) presented information on 16 different assessments, although 10 of these had no psychometric studies reported. While some home assessments focus almost exclusively on the physical environment (e.g., accessibility and home hazards), a number are now available that take into consideration such environmental factors as social supports provided by caregivers and the attitudes within the environment.

Home assessments typically involve the examination of PEO fit for a client within his or her home environment and recommendations related to home modifications. The *Housing Enabler* (Iwarsson & Isacsson, 1996) and *EASE3* (Christenson, 2002) are both measures that address environmental factors explicitly in relationship to clients' needs and ability. Both include separate components that

SAFETY NOTE 11-1

Therapist Safety on Home Visits

Therapists are often the only health professionals involved when conducting home visits, so safety of the therapist and client need to be considered. Although a therapist may be very confident about her/his safety with the client, other occupants of the home, building, or even the neighborhood (including animals) may put the therapist at risk. Home and community settings can present risks because they are complex and often unfamiliar to the therapist. Therefore, it is always advisable for therapists to maintain vigilance about their personal safety when conducting home visits. The following points are useful to ensure that the therapist and client are safe during home visits:

- Ensure that someone knows the location and approximate times for your home visit. It is good practice when a visit is conducted outside of normal business hours to phone that person when you have completed a visit and are on your way to let him/her know that you are safe.
- Carry a mobile phone to use in case of emergency during the travel or home visit. Keep the battery charged.
- If traveling by car, ensure that it is in good repair, prepared for emergency, and has at least a half tank of gas.
- Park as close as you safely can to the client's home.
- If taking public transportation, follow safety recommendations related to its use.
- When you arrive at the home, assess the surroundings and inside the home to identify any potential hazards.
- Throughout the visit, ensure that you are aware of exits and escape routes.
- Have the client lead you to different areas of the home, including up and down stairways.
- Try to limit the amount of material that you bring into the home or have outside of a carrying bag at any time.
- If possible, wear footwear inside the home, even if that means removing outdoor footwear at the door and donning a second pair of indoor shoes.
- If you feel unsafe or uncomfortable at any time, leave the situation immediately.
- Adhere to any policies or procedures of your employer, including conducting joint visits, and report any unusual or unsafe situations immediately.

first address the client's abilities and disabilities and then examine the home environment in relation to these factors. Both tools are administered through an interview; the *Housing Enabler* also involves observation of the physical environment. To rate items on the *Safety Assessment of Function and the Environment for Rehabilitation* (*SAFER*), *Home Fast*, and *Westmead*, clinicians integrate information about the client's abilities with observations about the environment. For example, in determining if an item such as toileting is a problem on the *SAFER* (or the extent to which it is a problem on the *SAFER-HOME*), the therapist must consider the client's ability to safely transfer on to and use the toilet while simultaneously considering the availability of physical supports (such as grab bars) and social supports (family caregiver assistance) and how willing the client is to make use of the supports available (see Fig. 11-4 for an example of this tool). Ideally, all of these assessments should be conducted in the client's home. In clinical settings where it is not possible to visit the home, the occupational therapist may choose to conduct an interview using the items of the *SAFER* or *EASE3* with the client and/or a family member or friend selected by the client who knows the client's home well. The interview, however, cannot be used as a substitute to determine whether or not a client can manage safely at home or what modifications may be needed. Rather, it can be used to highlight issues that clients and/or caregivers need to consider in the home. Other options include self-assessment guides to home adaptation, which can be used in collaboration with a client (e.g., *Maintaining Seniors' Independence through Home Adaptation: A Self-Assessment Guide* [Canadian Mortgage and Housing Corporation, 2003] and *A Consumer's Guide to Home Adaptation* [Adaptive Environments Center, 2002]). These tools provide practical suggestions for home adaptations in relation to functional problems, such as difficulty entering the bathtub, as shown in Figure 11-5. The therapist could help the client to select solutions that best fit his or her situation. See overview of home assessments in Assessment Table 11-1.

Housing options can also be reviewed with home assessments to determine the best fit for the client. Options are numerous and most communities have innovative, barrier-free housing with access to attendant care and other support services, meals, and recreation. Many seniors and persons with severe physical disabilities choose to live in these housing projects since they can more easily achieve independence within a supportive system. Transitional housing programs also assist clients to develop independent living skills and to develop knowledge of available resources. The occupational therapist can use assessment tools such as the *Housing Enabler* (Iwarsson & Isacsson, 1996) and *EASE3* (Christenson, 2002) for such purposes.

The United States Office of Fair Housing and Equal Opportunity administers the federal laws and policies that

COMPREHENSIVE REHABILITATION
COTA
AND MENTAL HEALTH SERVICES

700 Lawrence Avenue West, Suite 362,
Toronto, ON M6A 3B4, Phone: 416-785-9230
Fax: 785-9358, Email: info@cotarehab.on.ca

SAFER TOOL
☑ *Safety Assessment of Function & the Environment for Rehabilitation*

© COTA Comprehensive Rehabilitation and Mental Health Services

CLIENT'S NAME:

Mrs. P.

MMSE score: Not completed

TYPE OF HOUSING: __House x Apartment __Other

ADDRESSED - A
NOT APPLICABLE - NA
PROBLEM - P

		A	NA	P	COMMENTS
	LIVING SITUATION				**Score** 1
1.	Access/entrance/security	✔			
2.	Lives alone/with others	✔			Lives with husband. Daughter lives nearby - very supportive
3.	Support – family/friends	✔			
4.	Stairs/ramps - condition	✔			
5.	- railings	✔			
6.	Elevator	✔			
7.	Environment cluttered	✔			
8.	Scatter rugs/flooring	✔		x	Hallway rug - corners curled
9.	Wires/cords	✔			
	MOBILITY				**Score** 2
10.	Positioning	✔			
11.	Transfers	✔		x	Sometimes forgets to put brakes on during transfers.
12.	Walking/devices	✔			
13.	Wheelchair/scooter	✔			Wheelchair is used primarily
14.	Venturing outside	✔			Husband drives
15.	Public/disabled transport	✔			No disabled persons parking permit
16.	Car/driving	✔		x	License under medical suspension

Figure 11-4 Case example of home assessment using the *SAFER* tool (Chui et al., 2001). (Reprinted with permission from COTA Health, Toronto, Ontario, Canada, www.cotahealth.com.)

COTA SAFER Tool Client name:

		A	NA	P	COMMENTS
	KITCHEN				Score 2
17	Toaster/toaster oven	✔			Husband cooks
18	Microwave	✔			
19	Stove - gas/electric	✔		x	Has forgotten to turn off stove 2 times
20	- readable controls	✔		x	(and has turned on wrong element 3 times)
21	- removable dials/fuses	✔			
22	- grease & clutter	✔			
23	Evidence of burns or fires	✔			
24	Kettle – manual/electric/shut off	✔			
25	Storage – accessible/safe	✔			
26	Knives/scissors - safe storage/use	✔			
27	Food supply-fridge/cupboards	✔			
28	Garbage – storage/disposal	✔			
29	Evidence of alcohol	✔			
	FIRE HAZARDS				Score 1
30	Smoking/candles/signs of burns	✔			
31	Smoke&carbon monoxide detectors	✔		x	No batteries in smoke detector
32	Wiring/plugs	✔			No carbon monoxide detector
33	Electric blanket/pad/heater	✔			
34	Furnace/thermostat/fireplace	✔			
35	Fire exit	✔			
	EATING				Score 0
36	Liquids/food - to mouth/swallowing	✔			
37	Nutrition	✔			
	HOUSEHOLD				Score 3
38	Preparation – hot drinks	✔		x	Spilled hot tea & soup on self on 2
39	- meals	✔		x	occasions.
40	Carrying drinks/meals	✔		x	Not safe carrying drinks/meals
41	Meals On Wheels	✔	✔		
42	Shopping	✔			Daughter shops for them
43	Handling money/safekeeping	✔			Husband manages money - Mrs. P. satisfied with this arrangement.
44	Financial management/abuse	✔			
45	Bed making	✔			
46	Cleaning – light/heavy	✔			Husband/daughter doing cleaning & laundry
47	Laundry	✔			
48	Iron - manual/auto shut-off	✔			

Figure 11-4 *(Continued)*

COTA SAFER Tool Client name:

		A	NA	P	COMMENTS
	DRESSING				Score **0**
49	Dress	✔			Mr. P. provides minimal assistance for dressing - safe & comfortable with this
50	Undress	✔			
51	Appropriate selection	✔			
	GROOMING				Score **0**
52	Hair care	✔			Not currently using curling iron due to left arm paralysis
53	Nail care	✔			
54	Shaving		✔		
55	Teeth - oral hygiene	✔			
	BATHROOM				Score **4**
56	Sponge bath/shower/bath	✔			Moderate assistance provided by husband for bathing - no concerns
57	- seating/transfer aid	✔			
58	- shower extension	✔			
59	- grab bar	✔			
60	- non-skid aid	✔		x	No non-skid aid
61	Continence - bladder	✔			
62	- bowel	✔			
63	Toiletting	✔			
64	- raised toilet seat	✔		x	Difficulty getting up from toilet - no aid
65	- versaframe/grab bar	✔		x	on toilet
66	Door lock	✔		x	No emergency unlocking mechanism for door
67	Safe water temperature	✔			
68	Taps	✔			
	MEDICATION				Score **0**
69	In use as prescribed/dosette	✔			Mr. P. reminds Mrs. P. regularly to take medication.
70	Safe storage of family drugs	✔			
71	Ordering/delivery	✔			
	COMMUNICATION				Score **4**
72	Use of telephone	✔			
73	- location(s)	✔			
74	- emergency # posted/readable	✔		x	Not posted
75	- ability to dial 911/emergency #	✔			
76	Speech	✔			
77	Vision	✔		x	Complains of visual problems. Not checked in 6 years.
78	Hearing	✔			Problems reading
79	Reading	✔		x	

Figure 11-4 *(Continued)*

COTA | SAFER Tool | Client name:

		A	NA	P	COMMENTS
80	Writing	✔			
81	Alert system	✔		x	No personal emergency response system
82	TV/radio	✔			
	WANDERING				**Score** 0
83	Night/day	✔	✔		
84	Wandering person's registry	✔	✔		
85	Neighbours aware	✔	✔		
86	Medic alert/identification	✔	✔		
87	Windows/doors	✔	✔		
88	Enclosed yard	✔	✔		
89	Local traffic	✔	✔		
	MEMORY AIDS				**Score** 1
90	Clocks/can tell time	✔			Doesn't use memory aids; forgets appointments
91	Calendar/date book/notes	✔		x	
	GENERAL				**Score** 1
92	Intercom/call button	✔			No night light
93	Lighting/night light	✔		x	
94	Bulbs/fuses/snow/grass	✔			
95	Storage of dangerous substances	✔			
96	Leisure	✔			
97	Abuse	✔			

Category	SAFER Score	95th percentile	99th percentile
Living situation	1	3	5
Mobility	2	3	4
Kitchen	2	3	7
Fire Hazards	1	1	2
Eating	0	1	2
Household	3	4	7
Dressing	0	2	3
Grooming	0	2	4
Bathroom	4	4	6
Medication	0	1	3
Communication	4	4	6
Wandering	0	3	5
Memory aids	1	1	2
General	1	2	3
SAFER Total Score	**19**	**19**	**32**

Susan Smith	*Susan Smith, OT Reg (Ont.)*	12/05/05
Therapist's name (Please print)	Therapist's signature & designation	Date (dd/mm/yy)

Figure 11-4 *(Continued)*

Assessment Table 11-1

Access to Home

Assessment and Reference	Description	Time to Administer	Validity	Reliability	Sensitivity	Strengths and Weaknesses
The Housing Enabler (Slaug & Iwarsson, 2001) Ordering and pricing information are available through the Enabler web page: www.enabler.nu/index.html	Questionnaire to assess the congruence or fit between an individual with a functional impairment and his or her home environment. Measures functional limitations (15 items) and physical environmental barriers (188 items). Available in several languages. Scoring level: dichotomous ratings for Steps 1 and 2 and ordinal scale (4-point predetermined Likert scale) for Step 3. Summary scores are best calculated with the use of *Housing Enabler* Software. Range of scores: dependent on the number of functional limitations, use of mobility aids, and the number of environmental barriers.	Up to 2 hours depending on functional limitations and physical environment. In particular, Step 2 can be time consuming to administer since 188 environmental items need to be reviewed.	Content: Item selection based on literature review and expert opinion; adjusted after pilot studies. Step 1 and 2 subscores can be used independently. Convergent: Swedish accessible housing standards provide the gold standard against which the environmental assessments are measured. Construct: Established theoretical agreement for person–environment relationship and for construct of housing accessibility. References: Iwarsson & Isacsson, 1998; Iwarsson, Isacsson, & Lanke, 1998.	Inter-rater: Three studies reported in Iwarsson & Isacsson (1996) with excellent results ranging from 81–100% agreement; pilot 2 (n = 440 occupational therapists and 26 cases) overall mean kappa = 0.76 for person and 0.55 for - environment; pilot 3 (n = 430 occupational therapists and 30 cases) mean kappa = 0.82 for person, 0.68 for environment (188 items), and 0.87 for accessibility problems; ICC range = 0.92–0.98. A multi-national study in 5 countries with raters with different professional backgrounds (n = 64) resulted in moderate to good overall inter-rater reliability (Iwarsson, Nygren, & Slaug, 2005). Test–retest: ICC = 0.92–0.98 (Iwarsson & Isacsson, 1996).	Not established.	Strengths: Meticulous development and testing; up-to-date web site; widely used in Europe; Step 3 provides a predictive score of accessibility problems and measure of handicap; useful for both clinical and research purposes. Weaknesses: Rater training more difficult to arrange outside of Europe; Step 2 can be time consuming to administer.

continued

Assessment Table 11-1

Access to Home (continued)

Assessment and Reference	Description	Time to Administer	Validity	Reliability	Sensitivity	Strengths and Weaknesses
Home Falls and Accidents Screening Tool (HOME FAST) (Mackenzie, Byles, & Higginbotham, 2000). The appendix of the article includes all items of the *HOME FAST* along with definitions.	Assessment of the home hazards that may contribute to falls and, therefore, fall prevention interventions. Scoring level: Nominal (items are scored as a hazard, not a hazard, or not applicable). Scores range from 0–25 (indicating the number of items for which hazards are identified).	20–30 minutes.	Content: Based on compilation of items from the literature, field testing with 83 older adults, and review of content and field testing data by an expert panel to reduce the number of items (Mackenzie, Byles, & Higginbotham, 2000). Content was further examined through a cross-national validation (Australia, Canada, and United Kingdom) that asked occupational therapists, physiotherapists, and nurses to respond to a survey regarding the content and weighting of *HOME FAST* items (Mackenzie, Byles, & Higginbotham, 2002a). Convergent: Not established. No gold standard exists. Construct: Initial evidence suggests that the *HOME FAST* may be useful in identifying relative risk for falls associated with exposure to home hazards, based on 99% confidence intervals	Inter-rater: Evaluated (n = 40) using kappa for individual items and weighted kappa for the total number of hazards. The overall weighted kappa was 0.56 (considered fair to good agreement); kappas for individual items indicated that 4 items had excellent reliability, 20 had fair to good reliability, and one item (hazardous outside paths) had poor reliability (Mackenzie, Byles, & Higginbotham, 2002b). Test–retest: Not established.	Not established.	Strengths: Can be quickly administered as a screening assessment. Research has been conducted in various countries. Initial psychometric research is positive. Weakness: Further examination of construct and predictive validity would strengthen our understanding of the measure.

			(Mackenzie, Byles, & Higginbotham, 2000). Further research in this area is required with larger sample sizes and with longitudinal information rather than cross-sectional data.			
Life EASE 3.2 Basic and *3.2 Deluxe* www.lifease.com/lifease-home.html Author: Margaret Christenson (mchristenson@lifease.com)	Computer-based questionnaire to assess personal needs and abilities as well as potential home environment problems. Based on these data, program recommends solutions. Scoring level: Basic scoring is nominal (yes/no) rating whether or not the person can perform the functional activity; deluxe version involves a 5-point Likert scale for each item related to the person's ability to function. An individualized environmental checklist is then created based on the functional abilities of the person. Range of scores: no summary score is provided.	Varies depending on extent of activity limitations and number of rooms in the home.	Content: Excellent item selection including: comprehensive assessment of physical characteristics of home; functional actions needed for doing ADL at home; and provides a wide range of design and AT products and solutions. Constantly under review. Convergent: Not established. Construct: Not established.	Not established.	Not established.	Strengths: Practical, comprehensive, and popular. Power Point slides for occupational therapists available through company and AOTA. Weakness: Lacks psychometric testing.

continued

Assessment Table 11-1

Access to Home (continued)

Assessment and Reference	Description	Time to Administer	Validity	Reliability	Sensitivity	Strengths and Weaknesses
Safety Assessment of Function and the Environment for Rehabilitation (*SAFER* tool) and *SAFER-HOME* (Chiu et al., 2001) COTA Health, 700 Lawrence Ave. West, Suite 362, Toronto, Ontario, M6A 3B4; Telephone: 416-785-9230. E-mail: info@cotahealth.ca Order form can be downloaded from Products at www.cotahealth.ca	The *SAFER* tool is designed to identify and describe safety concerns of individuals in their own homes and to collect information to plan interventions and recommendations to improve safety (14 sections: living situation, mobility, kitchen, fire hazards, eating, household, dressing, grooming, bathroom, medication, communication, wandering, memory aids, and general). The *SAFER-HOME* is designed to measure change in safety over time (10 domains: meal preparation, awareness of safety hazards, mobility and toileting, cognitive impairment, homemaking support, emergency communication, functional communication, personal care, family assistance, and medication).	45–90 minutes.	Content: For both the *SAFER* and the *SAFER-HOME*, content validity has been established through review by experts and clinicians, as well as statistical analysis of completed measures. Criterion: Not established (as no gold standard exists). Construct: *SAFER*: Total scores have been associated with cognitive status and independent living in houses, but not directly to ADLs or IADLs (Letts & Marsall, 1995; Letts et al., 1998). *SAFER-HOME*: Total scores were compared to functional status scores using the Functional Autonomy Measurement System (SMAF) (Hebert, Carrier, & Bilodeu, 1988). The correlation was weak, which confirmed that the *SAFER-HOME* is measuring more than functional abilities (Chui & Oliver, in press).	*SAFER*: Inter-rater: kappa or % agreement: acceptable to excellent for 92 items (Letts et al., 1998). Test–retest: kappa or % agreement: acceptable to excellent for 90 items (Letts et al., 1998). *SAFER-HOME*: Internal consistency: coefficient alpha for total scores = 0.8593; subscales ranged from 0.539–0.789 (Chui & Oliver, in press).	Not established: It is hypothesized that the *SAFER-HOME* will be more sensitive to change with its 4-point rating for each item.	Strengths: Comprehensive coverage of home safety. Both tools developed and tested rigorously Weaknesses: Length of administration may be problematic in some clinical situations. Further research on responsiveness to change needed.

	Scoring level: *SAFER*: Nominal for each item (problem or not a problem); *SAFER-HOME*: Ordinal (4-point rating scale [0–3]: no problem, mild problem, moderate problem, severe problem). Ranges of scores: *SAFER*: 0–97; *SAFER-HOME*: 0–279.					
Westmead Home Safety Assessment Co-ordinates Publications, a division of Co-ordinates Therapy Services Pty Ltd, P.O. Box 59, West Brunswick, Victoria 3055; Telephone: 011 61 3 93801127; Fax: 011 61 3 93874829; www.therapybookshop.com/coordinates.html	Assessment to identify fall hazards in the home environments of older adults. Scoring level: Nominal (dichotomized relevant or not; each relevant item is rated as a hazard or not; hazards are presented by type). Ranges of scores: No summary score.	One home visit required.	Content: Established through content analysis of the literature and a rigorous expert review process (Clemson, Fitzgerald, & Heard, 1999). Criterion: Not established (as no gold standard exists). Construct: Not established.	Inter-rater: tested in a sample of 21 clients' homes; kappa values of >0.75 for 34 items; and between 0.4 and 0.75 for 31 items; kappa could not be calculated for some items (Clemson et al., 1999). Test–retest: Not established.	Not established.	Strengths: Comprehensive and systematic assessment of home hazards specific to falls in older adults. Manual is helpful and provides operational definitions for key hazards. Weaknesses: Does not address home hazards besides falls. Further evaluation of reliability, construct validity, and responsiveness to change would be helpful.

Do you have any difficulty stepping into or out of the bathtub?

☐ **No** ➢ If no, go to next question

☐ **Yes** If yes, check the adaptations below which would help you

- ☐ Install a vertical and an horizontal or angled grab bar by the tub
- ☐ Install non-slip flooring throughout the bathroom
- ☐ Install a non-slip surface in the bathtub
- ☐ Install a commercial or custom-made transfer bench so that the tub can be entered from a seated position
- ☐ Replace bathtub with a shower stall, if difficulty is severe
- ☐ Install a separate shower stall, if difficulty is severe
- ☐ Other (describe)

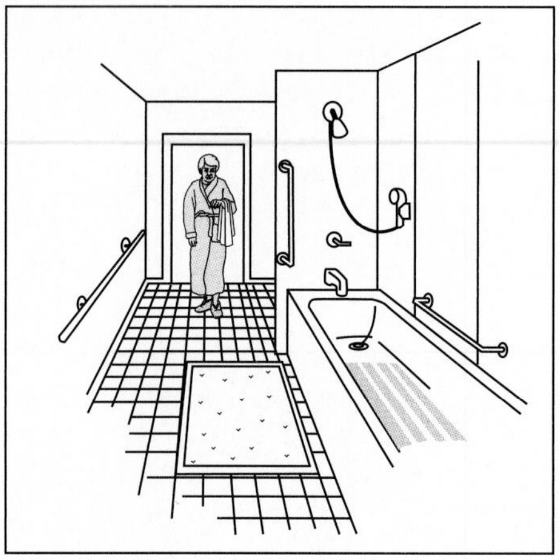

A vertical grab bar provides support when entering the tub, while an horizontal (or angled) bar helps you to complete the entrance and lower yourself onto a shower seat or to the bottom of the tub.

Figure 11-5 Using the bathroom: accessing the bathtub. (Adapted from *Maintaining Seniors' Independence through Home Adaptations: A Self-Assessment Guide*. Canadian Mortgage and Housing Corporation, 2003.)

make sure persons with a physical disability have equal access to the housing of their choice (United States Department of Housing and Urban Development [HUD], 2001). Specific accessibility requirements have been established to ensure that the design and construction of new residential buildings comply with the Fair Housing Act (e.g., buildings must have an accessible entrance on an accessible route). Occupational therapists conducting an environmental assessment of an apartment should also remember to evaluate building access, parking, halls, facilities, and fire routes to ensure that these requirements have been met. Many of the home assessments presented in this chapter offer items relevant to single family as well as multi-unit dwellings.

Assessment of Access to Community

Occupational therapists are becoming more involved in changing environments to facilitate their clients' roles within their communities. This may be particularly important toward achieving community participation and the realization of self-enhancement roles. Persons with disabilities may not be aware that community businesses and services must be made accessible to them (ADA, 1990). Occupational therapists can assume consultation or advocacy roles with groups seeking to make educational, cultural, commercial, and religious facilities accessible. The concept of universal design is also gaining increased attention in communities, and occupational therapists can play an important role in promoting this mainstreaming approach to design (Ringaert, 2003).

The transportation needs of persons with disabilities should not be overlooked in communities (Iwarsson, 2003). Useful information about standards and devices for vehicular transportation for persons with physical disabilities can be sought from the United States Department of Transportation and the National Highway Traffic Safety Administration. Commercial transportation companies, such as airlines, buses, and trains, must also comply with accessibility standards and make reasonable accommodations according to the ADA.

The occupational therapist should be familiar with the new ADA-ABA Accessibility Guidelines to ensure community structures are in line with ADA requirements (United States Access Board, 2004a, 2004b). A new instrument for assessing urban public transport accessibility, the *Travel Chain Enabler*, has been successfully piloted by occupational therapist Suzanne Iwarsson and her colleagues in Sweden (Iwarsson, Jensen, & Stahl, 2000). The therapist can also ask the client's opinions about community access and supports by using the *Craig Hospital Inventory of Environmental Factors* (*CHIEF*) (Craig Hospital Research Department, 2001) and can measure a client's perceptions of environmental facilitators and obstacles to their social participation and daily occupation using the *Measure of*

Quality of the Environment (Fougeyrollas et al., 1999). The *Multidimensional Scale of Perceived Social Support* (Zimet et al., 1988) is useful for quickly identifying clients' perceptions of social supports available from their family and friends and to lead into a discussion of social resources toward enabling greater community participation. Some of these assessment instruments and their sources are presented in Assessment Table 11-2.

Assessment of Access to Workplace

Occupational therapists play an important role in enabling clients to fulfill self-advancement roles by assisting them to seek or return to work. On-site assessment of workplace accessibility is critical, as workplace environments can differ significantly (Innes & Straker, 1998). Workplace assessment is a key step in helping the occupational therapist learn how workplace factors impact work performance (Bootes & Chapparo, 2002). See Procedures for Practice 11-1 and 11-2 for suggestions related to conducting work site assessments.

Knowledge of the ADA and the supporting guidelines is critical for guiding workplace assessment. For practical assessment purposes, the occupational therapist may wish to use the guidelines together with the *Americans with Disabilities Act Checklist for Readily Achievable Barrier Removal*, as mentioned earlier in this chapter (Adaptive Environments Center, 1995). Other tools, such as the *ADA Work-Site Assessment* (Jacobs, 1999a) or the *Job Analysis during Employer Site Visit* (Jacobs, 1999b), may also be used to help the occupational therapist focus on specific environmental factors in addition to work demands that may influence work performance. Unfortunately, these checklists have incomplete psychometric validation.

Occupational therapists recognize that a range of environmental factors can affect one's ability to work. Therefore, it is also important to assess the sociocultural environment, including social supports, staff interactions, and attitudes of co-workers and supervisors (Bootes & Chapparo, 2002). Tools such as the *Life Stressors and Social Resources Inventory*, *Work Environment Scale*, *Work Experience Survey*, and *Workplace Environment Impact Scale* (refer to Assessment Table 11-3 for details) are not limited to physical access issues because they also address areas such as social environments and resources.

Persons with disabilities may also face challenges while volunteering at or attending school. Many of the tools previously discussed to address work environments or community access may be of use in these instances. Occupational therapists may also use tools such as the *Accessibility Checklist* from the North Carolina State University, Disability Services for Students (1997). This informal checklist briefly addresses physical, policy/programmatic, information, and attitudinal environments from a post-secondary school perspective.

PROCEDURES FOR PRACTICE 11-1

Preparing for a Site Visit

The occupational therapist is asked to perform a work site assessment to determine accommodations that may be necessary for successful return to work of a client. The following background information should be gathered:

- Description of job (e.g., duties, responsibilities, sequence, temporal patterns, risks, variations in complexity of tasks, essential competencies, etc.)
- Description of workstation and work site (e.g., structure, ambiance, layout, environmental hazards, location, etc.)
- Consent of employer/business/industry representatives and client (including nature of client's wishes regarding information to be shared)—often written
- Understanding worker and employer perspectives (e.g., expectations, issues, abilities, etc.)
- Arrangements for visit (including consent and preparatory planning with appropriate personnel) should be conducted well in advance of visit
- Presence of a contact person during visit (e.g., supervisor, occupational health personnel, etc.)
- Evaluation framework, including list of questions, activities, safety concerns, and so on
- Charts/assessment forms to record findings
- Consideration of contributions from second person (e.g., physiotherapist)—dependent on nature of assessment

PROCEDURES FOR PRACTICE 11-2

Supplies and Materials Required for Site Visit

Planning with employer (including a preliminary understanding of the work site) may help to determine with greater accuracy what supplies and materials may or may not be required in advance of the visit.

- Paper, pens, pencils, and clipboard
- Measuring tape and wheeled measuring device
- Stopwatch
- Force gauge dynamometer
- Personal protective equipment as appropriate (e.g., steel-toed footwear)
- Thermometer
- Digital camera (with video recording capacity), tripod
- Photo release forms
- Laptop computer (Aja, 1996; Jacobs, 1994.)

(Aja, 1996; Jacobs, 1994.)

Assessment Table 11-2

Access to Community

Assessment	Description	Time to Administer	Validity	Reliability	Sensitivity	Strengths and Weaknesses
Craig Hospital Inventory of Environmental Factors (*CHIEF* and *CHIEF Short Form*) The Center for Outcome Measurement in Brain Injury (http://tbims.org/combi/chief) at Craig Hospital: (www.craighospital.org/Research/Disability/CHIEF%20Manual.pdf), (www.craighospital.org/Research/Disability/DISCHIEF.asp), (www.tbims.org/combi/chief/CHIEF.pdf)	Assessment of the frequency and magnitude of a broad range of environmental characteristics that act to impede accomplishment of daily activities and social roles. Self-administered or administered by interview. Full *CHIEF*: 25 items. *Short Form*: 12 items.	Self-administered, 10 minutes. Interview administered, 15 minutes. *Short Form*: 5 minutes for self-administration, 10 minutes for interview.	Content validity established by literature review and consultation with experts. Four advisory panels involved. Construct validity addressed when subscales were established: showed differences in reported frequency and magnitude of environmental barriers between groups with different impairments and activity limitations (Whiteneck, Gerhart, & Cusick, 2004; Whiteneck et al., 2004).	Internal consistency: moderate to high ratings for total score (0.93) and subscales (ranging from 0.76–0.81). Authors recommend that proxies should not be used to complete *CHIEF*. Study of test–retest reliability showed an overall ICC of 0.926 for total score, and ICCs for individual items ranged from 0.332–0.882 (Whiteneck et al., 2004).	No evidence.	Strengths: Based on *ICF*. Comprehensive inventory of environmental factors. Quick and easy to administer and score. Appropriate for both population-based or individual-focused assessment and research. Weaknesses: Further evaluation of psychometric properties needed. Scale for assessing magnitude of barriers has only 2 points (little vs. big problem).

Measure of Quality of the Environment (MQE) (Fougeyrollas et al., 1999) Available from authors: Kathy Boschen (boschen.kathy@torontorehab.on.ca); or Luc Noreau (Luc.Noreau@rea.ulaval.ca)	Measures environmental facilitators and obstacles to social participation and accomplishment of daily activities. Environment is defined broadly to include social, attitudinal, institutional, technical, and physical factors in the environment. Interview format: can be administered with client in context of home, community, or workplace.	Less than 30 minutes.	Content based conceptually on the Disability Creation Process model and input from individuals with SCI and clinicians (Fougeyrollas, Noreau, & Boschen, 2002). Construct validity has been demonstrated (Noreau, Fougeyrollas, & Boschen, 2002).	Moderate concordance scores across items. Good test–retest reliability (Boschen, Noreau, & Fougeyrollas, 1998).	No evidence.	Strengths: Tool is easy to administer. Some evidence of validity and reliability. Weaknesses: Not published and only available from authors; no method for summarizing and interpreting scores. Further examination of psychometric properties is recommended.
Multidimensional Scale of Perceived Social Support (MSPSS) (Zimet et al., 1988)	Assessment of perceptions of social support from 3 sources: family, friends, and significant other. Inventory/list of 12 statements of relationships. Each item rated on 7-point Likert-type scale.	2–5 minutes.	Content validity established through factor analysis. Multiple studies established construct validity with numerous health constructs, psychopathology, suicidal behavior, anxiety, and depression. Marginalized groups demonstrate lower perceived social support.	Internal consistency good, with Cronbach's alpha ranging from 0.81–0.91 in multiple studies. Test–retest reliability in one study with undergraduate psychology students was good for total score (0.85) and subscales (0.72, 0.85, and 0.75) (Zimet et al., 1988). Good reliability shown in study with older adults (Stanley, Beck, & Zebb, 1998).	No evidence.	Strengths: Simple to use and score in a short time. Has been used primarily with mental health populations; appears to have utility for populations with physical disability. Weaknesses: Need to be wary of socially desirable responses. Requires evaluation of sensitivity to change and utility as an outcome measure.

continued

Assessment Table 11-3

Access to Workplace

Instrument and Reference	Description	Time to Administer	Validity	Reliability	Sensitivity	Strengths and Weaknesses
Americans with Disabilities Act (ADA) *Work-Site Assessment* (Jacobs, 1999a)	Used for work-site assessments based on *ADA Checklist* and short answer format.	Information not available.	Not available.	Not available.	Not available.	Strength: Observations guided by ADA. Weakness: Lacks psychometric validation.
Job Analysis during Employer Site Visit (Jacobs, 1999b)	Checklist to analyze a range of factors during work site visit. Factors include environmental conditions, social conditions, job tasks, physical and cognitive demands, classification of work by amount of strength required, and physical barriers.	Information not available.	Not available.	Not available.	Not available.	Strength: Structures observations. Weakness: Lacks psychometric validation.
Life Stressors and Social Resources Inventory–Adult Form (*LISRES-A*) (Moos & Moos, 1998) Psychological Assessment Resources (PAR) Inc., 16204 N. Florida Ave., Lutz, FL 33549; www.parinc.com; Telephone: 1-800-331-8378 or (813) 968-3003.	Questionnaire designed to provide an overview of an individual's life context, including life stressors (9 measures) and social resources (7 measures). Self-report or therapist administered; 200 items (uses dichotomous and Likert-type scales).	30 minutes to administer; 10–15 minutes to score.	Face and content validity addressed through descriptions of domains and placing of domains in non-overlapping dimensions. Construct validity has been demonstrated (Moos, Finney, & Moos, 2000).	Internal consistency averaged 0.82 for stressors and 0.79 for resource measures (Moos & Moos, 1998).	Not established; however, commonly used to evaluate social resource/stress reduction interventions.	Strengths: Examines both stressors and social supports in one tool. Modified ICIDH format. Well standardized. Internally consistent, relatively stable tool. Weaknesses: Further research needed with broader populations. No spirituality items.

Work Environment Scale (*WES*) (Moos, 1994) CPP, Inc., 1055 Joaquin Rd., Suite 200, Mountain View, CA 94043; Telephone: (650) 969-8901; Toll Free: 1-800-624-1765; Fax: (650) 969-8608	Questionnaire to assess employees' perceptions of social environments across work settings. Self-administered questionnaire (90 items, true/false); 10 subscales (e.g., work pressure, supervisor support, and physical comfort)	15–20 minutes; 5–10 minutes to score.	Face validity established in manual; tools based on *Social Climate Scales*. Multiple studies demonstrate construct validity (e.g., Staten et al., 2003).	Cronbach's alpha coefficients for test–retest reliability (1 month) fell between 0.69 and 0.83 At 12 months, test–retest coefficients ranged from 0.51–0.63 Test–retest reliability: ICC > 0.70 (Moos, 1994).	No information found.	Strengths: Standardized; established psychometric properties; readily available, portable. Promotes discussion and identifies clients' views. Useful on an individual basis, with groups, or with organizations. Weaknesses: Scores alone should not provide direction for intervention. Need further study with populations with physical disability.
Work Experience Survey (*WES*) (Roessler & Gottcent, 1994; Roessler, 1996) Available from The National Clearinghouse of Rehabilitation Training Materials http://shopping.netsuite.com/s.nl/c.392723/sc.1/.f	Interview used to identify job accommodation needs (worksite accessibility, performance of essential functions, job mastery, and job satisfaction). Based on several tools or sources of information that have been adapted and included in the *WES* (Roessler & Gottcent, 1994).	30–60 minutes.	Has been used across groups of clients with a range of diagnoses (e.g., MS, blindness, arthritis) and frequently cited as a valid tool, although specific psychometric data could not be located.	Coefficient alphas for assessing job mastery and assessing job satisfaction reported as 0.74 and 0.78, respectively, in one study (Roessler, 1996).	Not available.	Strengths: Literature cites its use in several case studies. Facilitates identification of barriers and reasonable accommodations. Assists in empowering clients to address work barriers with employers. Has been used in individuals with a variety of disabilities Weaknesses: Need to look at utility of *WES* in follow-up interviews. Additional psychometric data required.

continued

Assessment Table 11-3

Access to Workplace (continued)

Instrument and Reference	Description	Time to Administer	Validity	Reliability	Sensitivity	Strengths and Weaknesses
Workplace Environment Impact Scale (*WEIS*) (Kielhofner et al., 1998). Model of Human Occupation Clearinghouse, University of Illinois at Chicago; www.moho.uic.edu/; www.moho.uic.edu/assess/weis.html	Semi-structured interview and rating scale. Addresses individuals' experiences and perceptions of their work environments. Designed for use with individuals with physical or psychosocial disabilities who are employed or are planning to return to work after an interruption in employment (due to injury/illness). 17 items scored on 4-point ordinal scales.	30–45 minutes to conduct interview (depending on interviewer's abilities and the client); 15 minutes to complete scoring.	Construct validity established (based on Rasch analysis in which infit MnSq = 1.6 and Zstd = 3.0) (Kielhofner et al., 1998). Found to measure a single construct (none of 17 items fit criteria for misfit) (Corner, Kielhofner, & Lin, 1997); found to be valid across 2 distinct cultures (Kielhofner et al., 1998).	Rasch analysis: Item separation statistic was 2.77 (reliability of 0.88); items were consistently separated into distinct (non-overlapping) groups (Kielhofner et al., 1998). Found to lack ability to discriminate between groups, although population was found to be homogeneous (Corner, Kielhofner, & Lin, 1997).	Not established.	Strengths: Items work well to measure the construct of work environment impact. The scale is suitably matched to the clients and effectively discriminates different levels of work environment. Both language versions of the *WEIS* are equal and free of cultural bias. Manual includes suggested questions (www.moho.vic.edu/moho_pub_respond.php). Weakness: Need to be very familiar with interview and scale to ensure appropriate use.

Through partnering with clients and employers, occupational therapists help identify environmental factors that can affect one's ability to work. A range of strategies, such as work-station modifications and assistive technologies, can be implemented to reduce performance barriers. (See Chapter 36 for discussion of specific strategies.) Additional research is required to better understand how environmental factors affect work outcomes (Shaw & Polatajko, 2002).

Looking Ahead

Many occupational therapists rely mainly on experience, observation, and interviews when called on to evaluate the environment. While these strategies are necessary

CLINICAL REASONING IN OCCUPATIONAL THERAPY RACTICE

Professional Issues to Consider When Making a Work Site Assessment

During a site visit, the occupational therapist observed department store clerks performing a full range of duties. What environmental factors should be noted and evaluated? In particular, consider transportation; access to the building, offices, and public areas; workstations and work areas; and the essential tasks of the job. What methods should be used to collect data? What additional sources of information could be sought and considered to determine the degree of PEO fit present?

CASE EXAMPLE

Assessment of the Home Environment

Occupational Therapy Assessment Process	Clinical Reasoning Process: Objectives	Clinical Reasoning Process: Example of Therapist's Internal Dialogue
Patient Information Mrs. P. is an 85-year-old woman who sustained a right-sided cerebrovascular accident (CVA) 2 months ago, resulting in left-sided hemiparesis. She was recently discharged from the rehabilitation center to an apartment that she has shared with her husband for more than 30 years. Results from the *Functional Independence Measure* (*FIM*™) (conducted at time of	Understand the patient's diagnosis or condition	"Although Mrs. P. is still early in her recovery, I would expect that her hemiparesis and any cognitive and perceptual changes will limit her basic personal care, homemaking, and community living skills and safety. Depression is possible after stroke, so I will need to be on the lookout for any mood changes as well."
discharge) are available from the referral (see Fig. 11-6). Her total *FIM*™ score improved from 70 (at time of admission) to 97 on discharge. Mr. P. and their daughter are presently doing the housekeeping and most of the meal preparation. Mr. P. would like to hire an attendant to work a few hours a day to assist with Mrs. P.'s personal care and to help with the housekeeping, but financial constraints do not allow for this. Both Mr. P. and their daughter have reported becoming increasingly frustrated and fatigued. They both say that they don't believe that they can leave Mrs. P. alone because of their concerns about her safety and inde-	Know the person	"She seems like someone for whom her abilities to care for herself and her family were extremely important to her. I wonder how she is coping now. Since she may have been the person who took care of everything and everyone at home, I wonder how well her daughter and husband are managing all of this. I haven't worked with many older people and realize that I may have some stereotyped expectations of her readiness to change; I will need to be careful as I could very well be wrong about this. However, I am a bit concerned about how willing she will be to make modifications to her home if I suggest them."
pendence. Prior to her stroke, Mrs. P. prided herself on her ability to care for her husband and her home. Mrs. P. is becoming increasingly concerned about becoming too much of a burden on her family and thinks that they are being overly protective. Mrs. P. has been referred to the community occupational therapist to address concerns about her independence and safety in her home environment.	Appreciate the context	"I want to know more about her relationships with her husband and her daughter. How have they been affected by the changes? As Mrs. P. uses a quad cane to walk in her home, I also wonder about how well she is able to get around because apartments can be quite small. I may also want to consult with the OT who worked with Mrs. P. at the rehabilitation center for more information."

FIM™ instrument

LEVELS		
	7 Complete Independence (Timely, Safely) 6 Modified Independence (Device)	**NO HELPER**
	Modified Dependence 5 Supervision (Subject = 100%+) 4 Minimal Assist (Subject = 75%+) 3 Moderate Assist (Subject = 50%+) **Complete Dependence** 2 Maximal Assist (Subject =25%+) 1 Total Assist (Subject = less than 25%)	**HELPER**

	ADMISSION	DISCHARGE	FOLLOW-UP
Self-Care			N/A
A. Eating	5	6	
B Grooming	3	4	
C. Bathing	2	3	
D. Dressing - Upper Body	3	4	
E. Dressing - Lower Body	2	4	
F. Toileting	4	5	
Sphincter Control			
G. Bladder Management	5	7	
H. Bowel Management	5	7	
Transfers			
I. Bed, Chair, Wheelchair	3	5	
J. Toilet	3	5	
K. Tub, Shower	1	4	
Locomotion	(W Walk / C Wheelchair / B Both)	(W Walk / C Wheelchair / B Both)	(W Walk / C Wheelchair / B Both)
L. Walk/Wheelchair	2 W	6 B	
M. Stairs	2	5	
Motor Subtotal Score	40	65	
Communication	(A Auditory / V Visual / B Both)	(A Auditory / V Visual / B Both)	(A Auditory / V Visual / B Both)
N. Comprehension	7 B	7 B	
	(V Vocal / N Nonvocal / B Both)	(V Vocal / N Nonvocal / B Both)	(V Vocal / N Nonvocal / B Both)
O. Expression	7 B	7 B	
Social Cognition			
P. Social Interaction	7	7	
Q. Problem Solving	4	5	
R. Memory	5	6	
Cognitive Subtotal Score	30	32	
TOTAL FIM Score	70	97	

NOTE: Leave no blanks. Enter 1 if patient not testable due to risk

FIM™ Instrument. Copyright © 1997 Uniform Data System for Medical Rehabilitation, a divison of U B Foundation Activities, Inc. Reprinted with the permission of UDSMR, University at Buffalo, 232 Parker Hall, 3435 Main Street, Buffalo, NY 14214.

Figure 11-6 Case example of Functional Independence Measure (FIM™) assessment. (Reprinted with permission from Uniform Data Systems, 1993.)

	Develop provisional hypotheses	"Given her diagnosis, I am assuming that there may be cognitive and perceptual impairments in addition to the more obvious physical problems that will impact Mrs. P.'s occupational performance. I also think that the environment will play a big role in how independent and safe she is at home."
Assessment Process The therapist decided to use the *Canadian Occupational Performance Measure (COPM)* (Law et al., 1998) to identify Mrs. P.'s perceptions and priorities for therapy. The *SAFER* tool was chosen to assess Mrs. P.'s ability to safely engage in occupations in her home.	Consider evaluation approach and methods	"I would like to get a sense of her priorities and learn more about her abilities to advocate for herself and make her ideas heard. The *COPM* will be ideal for this. The *SAFER* tool will provide me with information about her home environment and safety. It allows us to discuss her abilities and challenges and to demonstrate a variety of occupations in her home. It will help me identify areas of concern and make recommendations to enhance safety and independence."
Assessment Results Based on the *COPM,* Mrs. P. indicated that her priorities were to bathe, prepare meals, complete housekeeping, and do the laundry. The *SAFER* tool highlighted areas of safety concern that Mrs. P. had not raised previously, including issues associated with medication use, vision, and ability to remember to turn off appliances (refer to Figure 11-4, the *SAFER* tool results for this case study).	Interpret observations	"Mrs. P. seems to have limited awareness of any cognitive, visual or perceptual changes since her stroke. However, she is very aware of physical changes. Further assessment may be helpful to explore cognitive, visual, and perceptual difficulties impacting occupational performance. I was surprised that Mrs. P. was having difficulties remembering to turn off the stove, as she doesn't seem to have memory problems in more social situations. She is occasionally missing things on the left, so I am wondering whether she has any visual attention difficulties as well."
Occupational Therapy Problem List 1. Decreased independence in self-care, particularly in bathing and toileting. 2. Decreased independence in IADLs including meal preparation, laundry, and housekeeping. 3. Physical barriers to independence and safety identified in home (particularly kitchen and bathroom). 4. Limited funds available for assistive devices, home modifications, and purchase of services. 5. In addition to changes in motor function since CVA, cognitive, visual, and perceptual difficulties may also be impacting safety and independence in daily occupations.	Synthesize results	"Overall, Mrs. P. seems to benefit from occupational therapy intervention. She clearly has many areas she would like to address and is very motivated to work on these areas. The safety concerns I have identified should be addressed as soon as possible. Although Mrs. P. does not seem to be as concerned about the safety concerns, she is open to addressing them if only to help her husband and daughter feel a bit better. I will need to develop a plan to address the areas where I suspect that more assessment would be beneficial. I can also use the database provided in the EASE 3.2 software to find design modifications and AT products that can improve the accessibility of Mrs. P.'s home. I should consult with a colleague regarding options for funding. I wonder what programs Mrs. P. may qualify for that will supplement funding for equipment I may recommend. I am glad that I used the *SAFER* and the *COPM* as I can re-administer both of these tools in the future as part of my outcome evaluation."

CLINICAL REASONING IN OCCUPATIONAL THERAPY PRACTICE

Effects of the Physical Environment on Performance of Meal Preparation

Mrs. P. is an 85-year-old woman with left-sided hemiparesis who can walk short distances using a cane (see Case Example). Considering the occupational therapist's assessment findings, what would a therapist expect to observe if Mrs. P. tried to make a light meal in her apartment kitchen? What environmental factors might help or hinder her performance? How might family members help or hinder the process? What environmental modifications would you suggest to facilitate her task?

components of good practice, they cannot stand alone. The use of well-validated, standardized instruments is also necessary. Although there is limited availability of well-developed measures for assessing the environment, new instruments may soon be created to assess both barriers and resources in the environment (WHO, 2001).

SUMMARY REVIEW QUESTIONS

1. Why would an occupational therapist assess the environment?
2. List seven examples of environmental barriers that a person with mobility impairment might encounter when returning to work.
3. List seven examples of environmental supports that would allow a senior with arthritis to continue to live at home.
4. What assessments would you use to evaluate whether a client with a spinal cord injury can live independently in the community?
5. As an occupational therapist consultant to an assisted-living facility, what assistance could you offer the facility's administration regarding their plans to renovate the building?
6. What are some reasonable accommodations mandated by the ADA with which occupational therapists should be familiar?

References

Adaptive Environments Center. (1995). *Americans with Disabilities Act Checklist for Readily Achievable Barrier Removal.* Boston: Adaptive Environments Center. Retrieved May 2, 2005 from www.usdoj.gov/crt/ada/checkweb.htm or from www.adaptenv.org/index.php?option=Resource&articleid=226&topicid=30.

Adaptive Environments Center. (2002). *A consumer's guide to home adaptation.* Boston: Adaptive Environments Center. Retrieved June 15, 2005 from www.adaptenv.org/documents/aepuborder.html.

Aja, D. (1996). Finding a niche in job-site analysis. *OT Practice,* July, 36–41.

American Occupational Therapy Association [AOTA]. (1995). *Developing, maintaining, and updating competency in occupational therapy: A guide to self-appraisal.* Bethesda, MD: AOTA.

American Occupational Therapy Association [AOTA]. (2002). Occupational therapy practice framework: Domain and process. *American Journal of Occupational Therapy, 56,* 609–639.

Americans with Disabilities Act. (1990). *Public Law 101-336, 42 U.S.C. 12101.* Washington, DC: United States Department of Justice. Retrieved March 11, 2005 from www.usdoj.gov/crt/ada/adahom1.htm.

Association of Canadian Occupational Therapy Regulatory Organizations. (2000). *Essential competencies of practice for occupational therapists in Canada.* Association of Canadian Occupational Therapy Regulatory Organizations.

Bootes, K., & Chapparo, C. J. (2002). Cognitive and behavioral assessment of people with traumatic brain injury in the work place: Occupational therapists' perceptions. *Work, 19,* 255–268.

Boschen, K., Noreau, L., & Fougeyrollas, P. (1998). A new instrument to measure the quality of the environment for persons with physical disabilities. *Archives of Physical Medicine and Rehabilitation, 79,* 1331.

Canadian Association of Occupational Therapists [CAOT]. (1996). Profile of occupational therapy practice in Canada. *Canadian Journal of Occupational Therapy, 63,* 2, 79–95.

Canadian Association of Occupational Therapists [CAOT]. (1997). *Enabling occupation: An occupational therapy perspective.* Ottawa, Ontario, Canada: CAOT Publications ACE.

Canadian Mortgage and Housing Corporation. (2003). *Maintaining seniors' independence through home adaptations: A self-assessment guide.* Ottawa, Ontario, Canada: Canadian Mortgage and Housing Corporation. Retrieved June 14, 2005 from www.cmhc.ca.

Chiu, T., & Oliver, R. (in press). Factor analysis and construct validity of the SAFER-HOME. *Occupational Therapy Journal of Research.*

Chiu, T., Oliver, R., Marshall, L., & Letts, L. (2001). *Safety assessment of function and the environment for rehabilitation tool manual.* Toronto, Ontario, Canada: COTA Comprehensive Rehabilitation and Mental Health Services.

Christenson, M. (2002) EASE3.2. Retrieved March 3, 2005 from www.lifease.com/lifease-home.html.

Clemson, L., Fitzgerald, M. H., & Heard, R. (1999). Content validity of an assessment tool to identify home fall hazards: The Westmead home safety assessment. *British Journal of Occupational Therapy, 62,* 171–179.

Clemson, L., Fitzgerald, M. H., Heard, R., & Cumming, R.G. (1999). Inter-rater reliability of a home fall hazards assessment tool. *Occupational Therapy Journal of Research, 19,* 83–100.

Corner, R., Kielhofner, G., & Lin, F. L. (1997). Constuct validity of a work environment impact scale. *Work, 9,* 21–34.

Craig Hospital Research Department. (2001). *Craig Hospital Inventory of Environmental Factors (CHIEF) manual version 3.0.* Englewood, CO: Craig Hospital. Retrieved May 2, 2005 from www.tbims.org/combi/chief/.

Cumming, R. G., Thomas, M., Szonyi, G., Salkeld, G., O'Neill, E., Westbury, C., & Frampton, G. (1999). Home visits by an occupational therapist for assessment and modification of environmental hazards: A randomized trial of falls prevention. *Journal of the American Geriatrics Society, 47,* 1397–1402.

Dunn, W., Brown, C., & McGuigan, A. (1994). The ecology of human performance: A framework for considering the effect of context. *American Journal of Occupational Therapy, 48,* 595–607.

Fougeyrollas, P., Noreau, L., & Boschen, K. (2002). Interaction of environment with individual characteristics and social participation: Theoretical perspectives and applications in persons with spinal cord injury. *Topics in SCI Rehabilitation, 7,* 1–16.

Fougeyrollas, P., Noreau, L., St Michel, G., & Boschen, K. (1999). *Measure of the quality of the environment, version 2.* Author.

Harrison, T. C. (2002). Has the Americans with Disabilities Act made a difference? A policy analysis of quality of life in the post-Americans with Disabilities Act era. *Policy, Politics, & Nursing Practice, 3,* 333–347.

Hebert, R., Carrier, R., & Bilodeau, A. (1988). Functional autonomy rating scale (SMAF): Description and validation of an instrument for the measurement of handicaps. *Age and Aging, 17,* 293–302.

Hinton, C. A. (2003). The perceptions of people with disabilities as to the effectiveness of the Americans with Disabilities Act. *Journal of Disability Policy Studies, 13,* 210–220.

Innes, E., & Straker, L. (1998). A clinician's guide to work-related assessments: 2-design problems. *Work, 11,* 191–206.

Iwarrson, S. (2003). Accessible transportation: Novel occupational therapy perspectives. In L. Letts, P. Rigby, & D. Stewart (Eds.), *Using environments to enable occupational performance* (pp. 235–251). Thorofare, NJ: Slack Inc.

Iwarsson, S., & Isacsson, A. (1996). Development of a novel instrument for occupational therapy assessment of the physical environment in the home: A methodologic study on "The Enabler." *Occupational Therapy Journal of Research, 16,* 227–244.

Iwarsson, S., & Isaacsson, A. (1998). Housing standards, environmental barriers in the home, subjective general apprehension of housing situation among the rural elderly. *Scandinavian Journal of Occupational Therapy, 3,* 52-61.

Iwarsson, S., Isacsson, A., & Lanke, J. (1998). ADL dependence in the elderly: The influence of functional limitations and physical environmental demand. *Occupational Therapy International, 5,* 1173-1193.

Iwarrson, S., Jensen, G., & Stahl, A. (2000). Travel chain enabler: Development of a pilot instrument for assessment of urban public transportation accessibility. *Technology and Disability, 12,* 3-12.

Iwarsson, S., Nygren, C., & Slaug, B. (2005). Cross-national and multiprofessional inter-rater reliability of the Housing Enabler. *Scandinavian Journal of Occupational Therapy, 12,* 29-39.

Jacobs, K. (1994). Job analysis. *Rehab Management, 7,* 113-114.

Jacobs, K. (1999a). Americans with Disabilities Act work-site assessment. In K. Jacobs (Ed.), *Ergonomics for therapists* (2nd ed., pp. 345-354). Boston: Butterworth-Heinemann.

Jacobs, K. (1999b). Job analysis during employer site visit. In K. Jacobs (Ed.), *Ergonomics for therapists* (2nd ed., pp. 356-364). Boston: Butterworth-Heinemann.

Kielhofner, G., Lai, J., Olson, L., Haglund, L., Ekbadh, E., & Hedlund, M. (1998). Psychometric properties of the work environment impact scale: A cross-cultural study. *Work: A Journal of Prevention, Assessment, and Rehabilitation 12,* 71-77.

Law, M. (1998). *Client-centered occupational therapy.* Thorofare, NJ: Slack.

Law, M. (2004). *Outcome Measures rating form and guidelines.* Hamilton, Ontario, Canada: CanChild. Retrieved January 5, 2005 from http://bluewirecs.tzo.com/canchild/patches/measguid.pdf.

Law, M., Baptiste, S., Carswell, A., McColl, M., Polatajko, H., & Pollock, N. (1998). *Canadian Occupational Performance Measure* (3rd ed.). Toronto Ontario, Canada: CAOT Publications ACE.

Law, M., Cooper, B., Strong, S., Stewart, D., Rigby, P., & Letts, L. (1996). The Person-Environment-Occupation Model: A transactive approach to occupational performance. *Canadian Journal of Occupational Therapy, 63,* 9-23.

Letts, L., & Marshall, L. (1995). Evaluating the validity and consistency of the SAFER tool. *Physical and Occupational Therapy in Geriatrics, 13,* 49-66.

Letts, L., Scott, S., Burtney, J., Marshall, L., & McKean, M. (1998). The reliability and validity of the Safety Assessment of Function and the Environment for Rehabilitation (SAFER) tool. *British Journal of Occupational Therapy, 61,* 127-132.

Lysack, C. L., & Neufeld, S. (2003). Occupational therapist home evaluations: Inequalities, but doing the best we can? *American Journal of Occupational Therapy, 57,* 369-379.

Mackenzie, L., Byles, J., & Higginbotham, N. (2000). Designing the Home Falls and Accidents Screening Tool (HOME FAST): Selecting the items. *British Journal of Occupational Therapy, 63,* 260-269.

Mackenzie, L., Byles, J., & Higginbotham, N. (2002a). Professional perceptions about home safety: Cross-national validation of the Home Falls and Accidents Screening Tool (HOME FAST). *Journal of Allied Health, 31,* 22-28.

Mackenzie, L., Byles, J., & Higginbotham, N. (2002b). Reliability of the Home Falls and Accidents Screening Tool (HOME FAST) for identifying older people at increased risk of falls. *Disability and Rehabilitation, 24,* 266-274.

Mitchell, R., & Unsworth, C. A. (2004). Role perceptions and clinical reasoning of community health occupational therapists undertaking home visits. *Australian Occupational Therapy Journal, 51,* 13-24.

Moos, R. (1994). *Work Environment Scale manual* (3rd ed.). Palo Alto, CA: Consulting Psychologists Press.

Moos, R., Finney, J., & Moos, B. (2000). Inpatient substance abuse care and the outcome of subsequent community residential and outpatient care. *Addiction, 95,* 833-846.

Moos, R. H., & Moos, B. S.(1998). Life Stressors and Social Resources Inventory. In C. P. Zalaquett & R. J. Woo (Eds.), *Evaluating stress: A book of resources, volume one* (pp. 177-190). Lanham, MD: Scarecrow Press, Inc.

Noreau, L., Fougeyrollas, P., & Boschen, K. (2002). Perceived influence of the environment on social participation among individuals with spinal cord injury. *Topics in SCI Rehabilitation, 7,* 56-72.

North Carolina State University, Disability Services for Students. (1997). *Accessibility Checklist.* Retrieved April 21, 2005 from http://www.ncsu.edu/dso/accommodations/desk_ref/endtro.html#check.

Redick, A. G., McClain, L., & Brown, C. (2000). Consumer empowerment through occupational therapy: The Americans with Disabilities Act Title III. *American Journal of Occupational Therapy, 54,* 207-213.

Rigby, P., & Letts, L. (2003). Environment and occupational performance: Theoretical considerations. In L. Letts, P. Rigby, & D. Stewart (Eds.), *Using environments to enable occupational performance* (pp. 17-32). Thorofare, NJ: Slack Inc.

Ringaert, L. (2003). Universal design of the built environment to enable occupational performance. In L. Letts, P. Rigby, & D. Stewart (Eds.), *Using environments to enable occupational performance* (pp. 97-115). Thorofare, NJ: Slack Inc.

Roessler, R. T. (1996). The role of assessment in enhancing vocational success of people with multiple sclerosis. *Work, 6,* 191-201.

Roessler, R. T., & Gottcent, J. (1994). The Work Experience Survey: A reasonable accommodation/career development strategy. *Journal of Applied Rehabilitation Counseling, 25,* 16-21.

Rogers, J. C., Holm, M. B., Beach, S., Schulz, R., Cipriani, J., Fox, A., & Starz, T. W. (2003). Concordance of four methods of disability assessment using performance in the home as the criterion method. *Arthritis & Rheumatism (Arthritis Care & Research), 49,* 640-647.

Rogers, J. C., Holm, M. B., & Stone, R. G. (1997). Evaluation of daily living tasks: The home care advantage. *American Journal of Occupational Therapy, 51,* 410-422.

Rousseau, J., Potvin, L., Dutil, E., & Falta, P. (2001). A critical review of assessment tools related to home adaptation issues. *Occupational Therapy in Health Care, 14,* 93-104.

Shaw, H., & Polatajko, H. (2002). An application of the Occupation Competence Model to organizing factors associated with return to work. *The Canadian Journal of Occupational Therapy, 69,* 158-167.

Slaug, B., & Iwarsson, S. (2001). *Housing Enabler 1.0: A tool for housing accessibility analysis. Software for PC.* Staffenstorp & Navlinge: Slaug Data.

Stanley, M. A., Beck, J. G., & Zebb, B. J. (1998). Psychometric properties of the MSPSS in older adults. *Aging and Mental Health, 2,* 186-193.

Staten, D. R., Mangalindan, M. A., Saylor, C., & Stuenkel, D. L. (2003). Staff nurse perceptions of the work environment: A comparison among ethnic backgrounds. *Journal of Nursing Care Quality, 18,* 202-208.

Uniform Data Systems. (1993). *Guide for the Uniform Data Set for medical rehabilitation.* Buffalo, NY: University of Buffalo Foundation.

United States Access Board. (2002). *ADA Accessibility Guidelines for Buildings and Facilities (ADAAG).* Retrieved March 5, 2005 from www.access-board.gov/adaag/html/adaag.htm.

United States Access Board. (2004a). *ADA-ABA accessibility guidelines.* Retrieved March 5, 2005 from www.access-board.gov/ada-aba/final.pdf.

United States Access Board. (2004b). *A guide to the new ADA-ABA accessibility guidelines.* Retrieved March 5, 2005 from www.access-board.gov/ada-aba/summary.htm.

United States Department of Housing and Urban Development. (2001). Fair housing and equal opportunity: People with disabilities. Retrieved June 8, 2005 from www.hud.gov/offices/fheo/disabilities/sect504.cfm.

Whiteneck, G. G., Gerhart, K. A., & Cusick, C. P. (2004). Identifying environmental factors that influence the outcomes of people with traumatic brain injury. *Journal of Head Trauma Rehabilitation, 19,* 191-204.

Whiteneck, G. G., Harrison-Felix, C. L., Mellick, D. S., Brooks, C. A., Charlifue, S. B., & Gerhart, K. A. (2004). Quantifying environmental factors: A measure of physical, attitudinal, service, productivity and policy barriers. *Archives of Physical Medicine and Rehabilitation, 85,* 1324-1335.

World Health Organization. (2001) *International Classification of Functioning, Disability and Health.* Geneva: World Health Organization. Retrieved January 30, 2005 from www.who.int/classification/icf/.

Wressle, E., Eeg-Olofsson, A. M., Marcusson, J., & Henriksson, C. (2002). Improved client participation in the rehabilitation process: Using a client centred goal formulation structure. *Journal of Rehabilitation Medicine, 34,* 5-11.

Zimet, G. D., Dahlem, N. W., Zimet, S. G., & Farley, G. K. (1988). The Multidimensional Scale of Perceived Social Support. *Journal of Personality Assessment, 52,* 30-41.

SECTION III: Therapeutic Mechanisms

CHAPTER 12

Occupation: Philosophy and Concepts

Catherine A. Trombly Latham

LEARNING OBJECTIVES

After studying this chapter, the reader will be able to do the following:

1. Define occupation.
2. Discuss the importance of occupation in people's lives.
3. Discuss occupation as a therapeutic medium.
4. Characterize occupation-as-end and occupation-as-means.
5. Discuss the therapeutic qualities of occupation: purposefulness and meaningfulness.
6. Cite evidence that supports the use of occupation as therapy.
7. Describe how therapeutic occupation is implemented in practice.

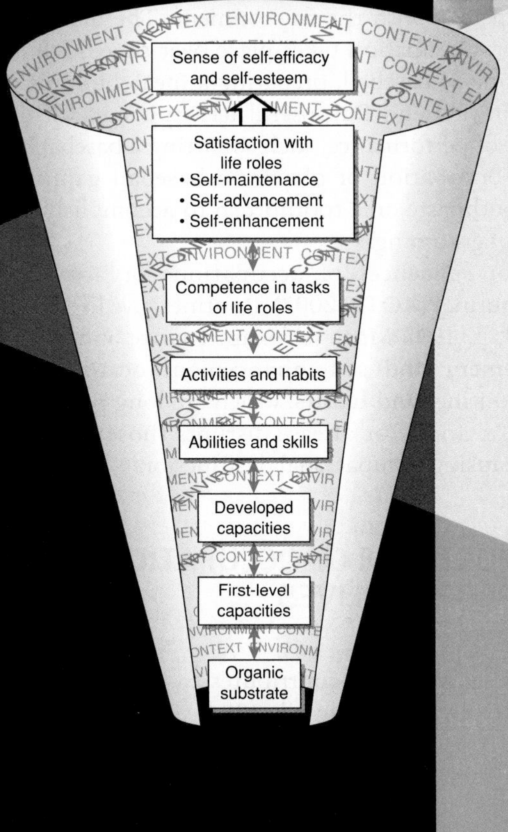

Glossary

Activity analysis—A process by which properties inherent in a given activity, task, or occupation may be gauged for their ability to elicit individual motivation and to fulfill patient's needs in occupational performance and performance components (Llorens, 1993).

Constraints—Limitations imposed on purposeful movement or the completion of occupational performance. Extrinsic constraints include the physical and sociocultural environment and task demands. Intrinsic constraints include biomechanical and neuromuscular aspects of a person's body, as well as other personal contextual factors (Newell, 1986).

Habit—A usual manner of behavior (Mish, 2004).

Phase planes—Graphs of movement, with velocity of the end point on the ordinate and displacement on the abscissa. Movements using the same motor plan produce replicable phase planes, but movements using different plans produce unique phase planes.

Purposeful activity—Purposeful activity is a general class of human actions that are goal directed. A person may participate in activities to achieve an occupational goal, but these activities, on their own, do not assume a place of central importance or meaning for the person (AOTA, 2002, p. 610).

Task demands—The context (e.g., objects, surroundings, ritual, tools, materials) that evokes certain maneuvers required to accomplish the goal of the task.

OCCUPATION DEFINED

Occupation is defined by the general public as an activity in which one engages, especially one's work (Mish, 2004). Occupational therapists define *occupation* "as activities of everyday life, named, organized and given value and meaning by individuals and a culture. Occupation is everything people do to occupy themselves, including looking after themselves, enjoying life and contributing to the social and economic fabric of their communities" (American Occupational Therapy Association [AOTA], 2002; Law et al., 1997, p. 32). Occupational therapists believe that "occupation is a source of meaning and purpose, choice and control" (Hammell, 2004, p. 299). The term *occupation* applies to the integration of the person's abilities, motivations, goals, and the environment to enable role performance. Personal identity emerges from "an harmonious balance" of the many meaningful occupations in which a person engages over time (Christiansen, 1999; Unruh, 2004, p. 294). People engaged in occupation not only define their identity but also achieve a sense of competence and report a sense of satisfaction and fulfillment (AOTA, 2002). Occupational therapists work with people who have experienced a significant crisis in occupational identity (Unruh, 2004). It is the role of the occupational therapist to help the person to grieve his or her loss and to reconstruct an acceptable occupational identity.

Although the terms *occupation* and **purposeful activity** are used interchangeably by most therapists, the American Occupational Therapy Association (2002) has distinguished between the two on the basis of meaningfulness. It defines occupation as activity having unique meaning and purpose in a person's life. Occupations are central to a person's identity and competence, and they influence how one spends time and makes decisions (AOTA, 2002, p. 610). Purposeful activity, or activity, is a general class of human actions that are goal directed. A person may participate in activities to achieve a goal, but these activities do not assume a place of central importance or meaning for the person (AOTA, 2002, p. 610). Each occupation is composed of several purposeful activities.

Purposeful activity is circumscribed; it demands particular responses within particular contexts and is used therapeutically to facilitate change in impairments and functional limitations. In this text, occupation-as-end is equated to *occupation*, and occupation-as-means is equated to *purposeful activity*.

Both occupation and purposeful activity involve interaction by a person with the environment. The temporal aspects differ. Occupation takes place over time, such as playing a game of baseball, preparing a meal, building a house, or being a friend. Purposeful activity occurs within the moment of performance, such as hitting a baseball as part of the occupation of playing a baseball game or spreading toothpaste on a toothbrush to accomplish the occupation of grooming.

Strings or sequences of occupations or activities constitute routines (AOTA, 2002). Routines give life order (Segal, 2004, p. 499). Most self-maintenance and many self-advancement and self-enhancement occupations depend on routines and **habits**, which are long practiced and automatic. Injury or disease disrupts those routines and habits, causing occupational dysfunction.

IMPORTANCE OF OCCUPATION IN PEOPLE'S LIVES

Occupational engagement contributes to the experience of a life worth living (Hammell, 2004). Engagement in positive occupations (e.g., care of self, others, and property; creative endeavors; work) that the person has the capabilities to accomplish and chooses to accomplish regulates the rhythm of personal and community life. Such occupations absorb attention and evoke creativity, promote feelings of satisfaction with achievement, and contribute to a sense of self-esteem and self-efficacy (Fig. 12-1). These occupations are potentially therapeutic.

Time-use studies indicate that people who are mentally able to envision goals fill their time with activities and tasks (Grady, 1992; McKinnon, 1992; Pentland et al., 1999; Yerxa & Baum, 1986; Yerxa & Locker, 1990). Beyond the organization and positive feelings generated by engagement in occupation, there is evidence that social and productive occupations are independently associated with survival. A study followed 2,761 men and women in one U.S. city over 13 years. The researchers controlled all other variables that could possibly explain the survival rate and found that social activities, defined as going to church, cinema, and restaurants; taking trips; playing cards and other games; and participating in social groups and productive activities (defined as gardening, preparing meals, and shopping), conferred survival advantages equivalent to those of fitness activities. They concluded that social and productive activities exert an independent protective effect not due exclusively to the associated physical activity (Glass et al., 1999). In an explorative study of older Swedish adults with functional impairments, researchers found that some persons continued to engage in meaningful occupation despite reduced capacities, although others failed to do so (Borell et al., 2001). Failure to do so was associated with a reduced sense of hope. In the absence of social and productive occupation (as occurs, for example, early in retirement or in the acute stage of motor disability, or immediately after a profound loss [Hoppes, 2005]), a person may experience a sense of disorganization, depression, and loss of a sense of self-worth.

Not all occupation or purposeful activity is beneficial. Attempts to engage in occupations beyond one's capabilities lead to frustration, anxiety, and depression (Rebeiro & Polgar, 1998). Engagement in negative occupation (e.g., crime, destruction) disrupts personal and community life.

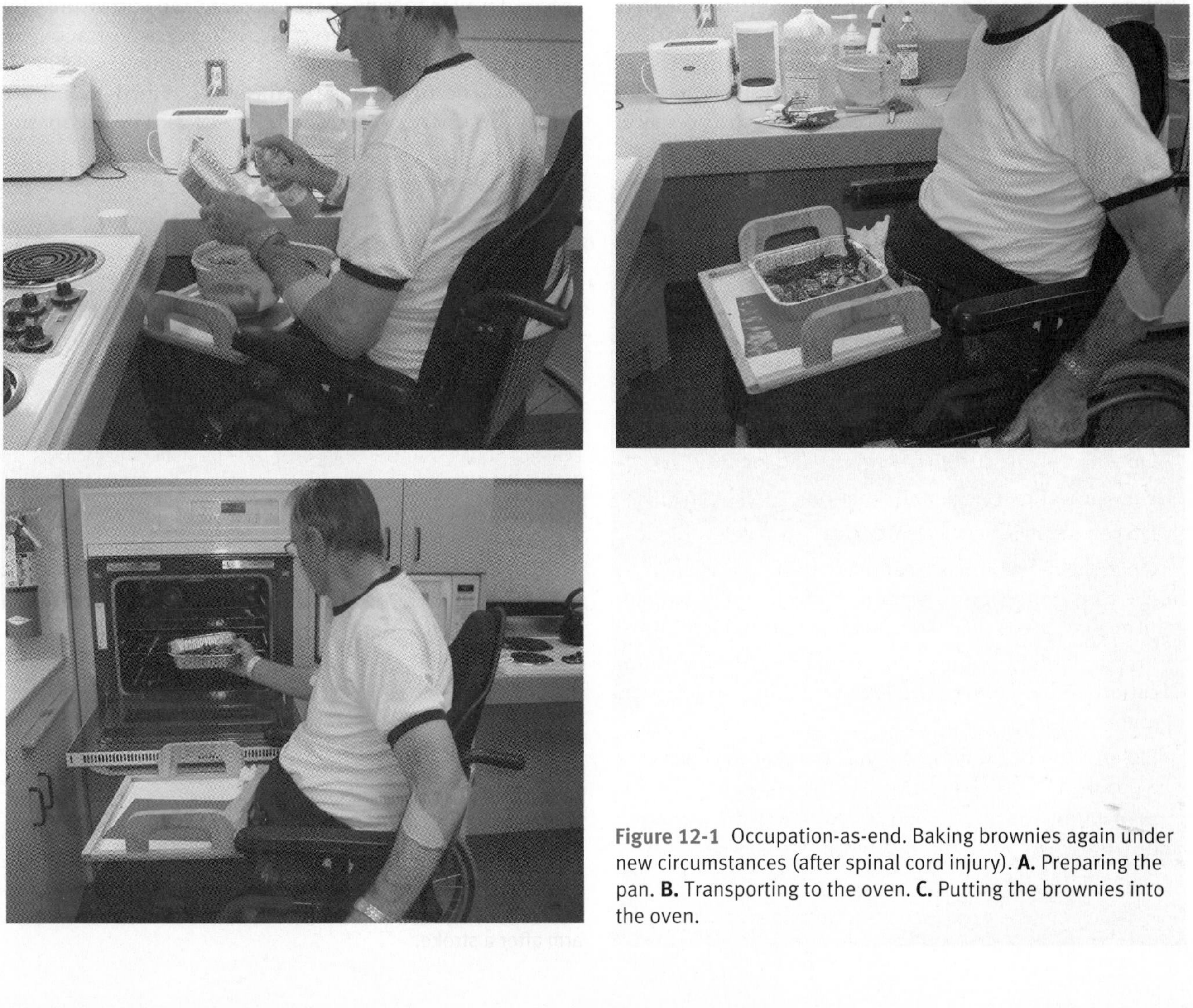

A B C

Figure 12-1 Occupation-as-end. Baking brownies again under new circumstances (after spinal cord injury). **A.** Preparing the pan. **B.** Transporting to the oven. **C.** Putting the brownies into the oven.

Doing the same activity repetitively beyond the requirements of the task, as seen in obsessive-compulsive disorder (OCD), reinforces pathology. Imposition of unsuitable, negatively meaningful activities (e.g., children's games for elderly patients) fails to build a sense of self-esteem and satisfaction. These types of occupation are not therapeutic. Therapeutic occupation, a special type of occupation, is defined as the use of positive, meaningful, and purposeful activities to improve a person's occupational functioning or to improve abilities and capacities to enable improved occupational functioning.

Occupation as Therapy

Occupation is the unique therapeutic medium of occupational therapy (National Society for the Promotion of Occupational Therapy, 1917; Reilly, 1962). Long before there was scientific evidence, occupational therapists believed that occupation maintained or restored health and gave meaning and quality to one's life (Rebeiro, 1998). Even now, the evidence is meager (Rebeiro, 1998).

What about occupation maintains or restores health? That question is still debated, but one suggestion is that occupation is therapeutic when it appeals to the patient (has meaning for the patient); when it advances therapeutic goals (makes demands on the system needing improvement); and when it is carried out in the space, time, and sociocultural conditions that it would be in real life (fulfills a purpose in the person's life) (Pierce, 1998). Another aspect of the therapeutic experience is the "just right" challenge, the optimal fit between demands of the occupation and the skills of the person (Rebeiro & Polgar, 1998). An occupation is therapeutic when it requires effort for the patient to accomplish but is possible for the patient to accomplish. By accomplishing it, the patient improves the impaired ability or capacity being challenged. By succeeding in the challenge, the patient is motivated to continue or repeat the experience (Rebeiro & Polgar, 1998). See Chapter 13 concerning selection and grading of occupation. A successful therapeutic occupation results in feelings of self-satisfaction, self-esteem, and self-efficacy.

Today, as in the past, occupational therapists help people achieve satisfying occupational lives in several ways. One way is to adapt the environment or tools and teach the person how to use these contextual adaptations or other adapted methods to accomplish activities and tasks of daily life (Clark et al., 1997; Jackson et al., 1998; Moyers, 1999). In this case, occupation is both the treatment and the end goal (occupation-as-end). The second way is to remediate impaired capacities and abilities that prevent successful performance of activities and tasks required of a patient's roles (Moyers, 1999). In this case, occupation is the means to remediate impairment (occupation-as-means) (Fig. 12-2). The occupation

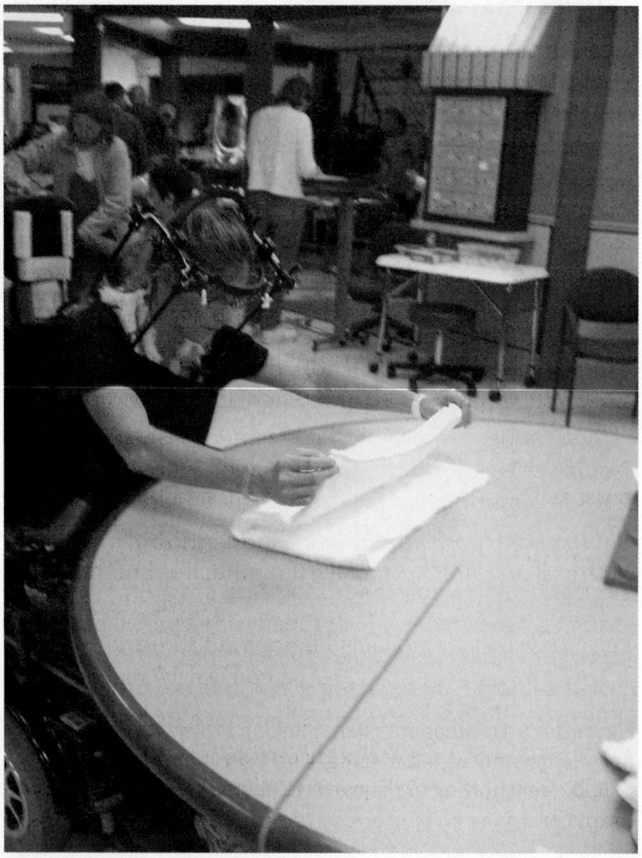

A

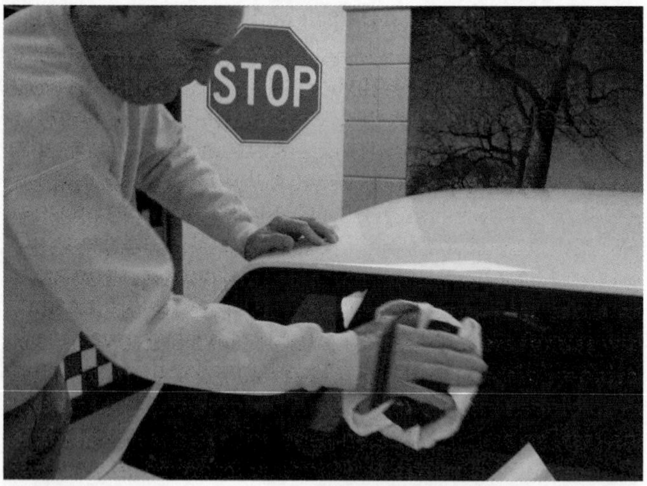

B

Figure 12-2 Occupation-as-means. **A.** Folding towels as a means to improve sitting balance for a person with spinal cord injury. **B.** Polishing the car to gain movement control of a weak arm after a stroke.

used may actually be the same, for instance, chopping apples to make a pie. If the goal is to relearn how to make an apple pie, then we consider it occupation-as-end. If the goal is to improve strength of grasp to enable multiple other life occupations, then we consider chopping apples occupation-as-means.

Occupation-As-End

Occupation-as-end is the complex activities and tasks that comprise roles (Fig. 12-3). Learning the occupation within the customary environment is the goal. Occupation-as-end is more or less equivalent to *areas of occupation* of the Occupational Therapy Practice Framework (AOTA, 2002) and *activities and participation* of the World Health Organization's International Classification of Functioning (ICF; World Health Organization, 2001) (see Chapter 1). Occupation-as-end is a person's functional goal that he or she tries to accomplish in a given environment using what abilities and capacities he or she has and any adaptations that may be necessary (Fig. 12-4).

An explorative study of Swedish adults aged 42 to 82 years old who had suffered a stroke found that patients were frustrated in their daily occupations because they were not able to carry out their former habits due to their impairments (Wallenbert & Jonsson, 2005). They resisted making adaptations or developing new habits, however, because they feared doing so would diminish gains they could make for their physical impairments. They saw development of new habits as a symbol of dependence. The possibility of this type of thinking needs to be explored with patients who resist the benefits of engaging in occupation-as-end. Occupation-as-end may remediate impairments, but this benefit is serendipitous, and the occupation is not chosen for that purpose. Occupation-as-end achieves its therapeutic effect from the qualities of purposefulness and meaningfulness (Definition 12-1). Purposefulness is hypothesized to organize behavior, and meaningfulness is hypothesized to motivate performance (Trombly, 1995).

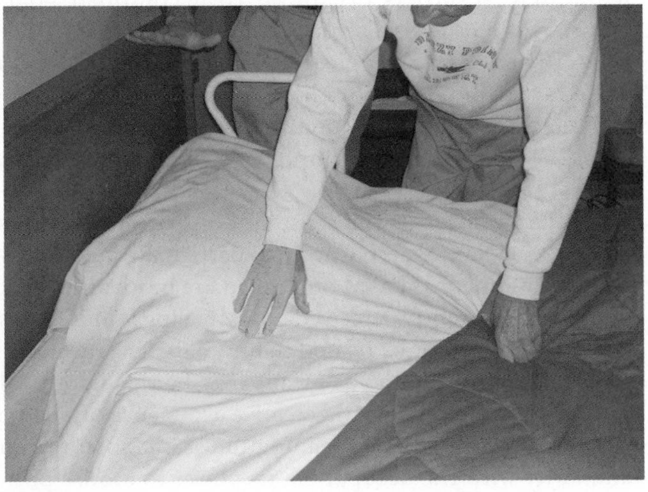

Figure 12-3 Occupation-as-end. Relearning to make the bed after stroke.

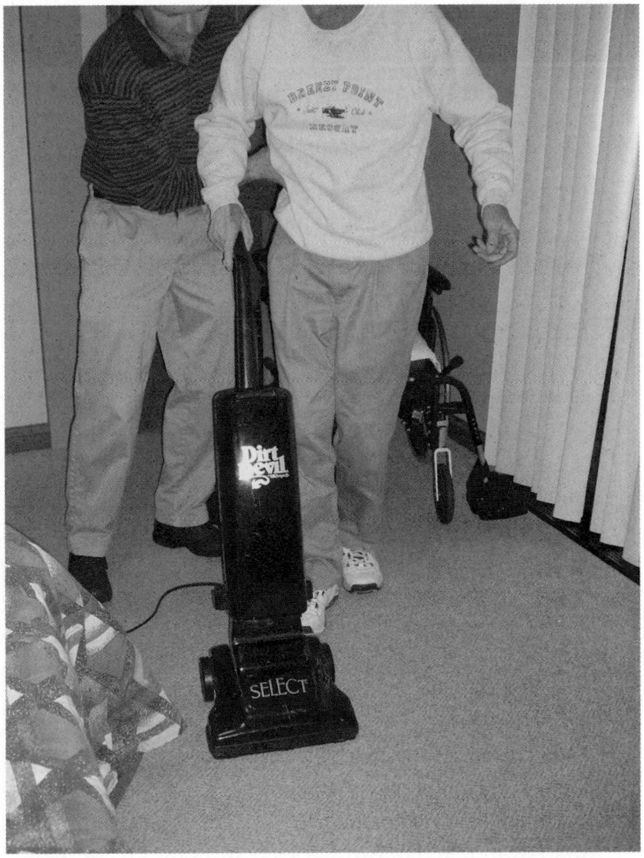

Figure 12-4 Occupation-as-end. Relearning to vacuum after stroke.

Occupation-as-end is purposeful by virtue of its focus on accomplishing activities and tasks. Purposeful occupation-as-end organizes a person's behavior, day, and life (Meyer, 1922, 1977; Slagle, 1914; Yerxa & Baum, 1986; Yerxa & Locker, 1990). Although there are no studies on how occupational therapists use occupation-as-end to organize people's lives, there is some anecdotal evidence that occupation-as-end does organize people's lives. For example, an occupational therapist and a patient reported on how the patient reorganized her own life after traumatic brain injury using a synergistic mix of occupation and narration (Price-Lackey & Cashman, 1996).

Occupation-as-end is not only purposeful but also meaningful because it is the performance of activities or tasks that a person sees as important. Only meaningful occupation remains in a person's life repertoire. Meaningfulness of occupation-as-end is based on a person's values acquired from family and cultural experiences. Meaningfulness also springs from a person's sense of the importance of participating in certain occupations or performing in a particular manner, from the person's

DEFINITION 12-1

Therapeutic Characteristics and Effects of Occupation-As-Means and Occupation-As-End

	Occupation-As-Means	Occupation-As-End
Purposefulness	Organizes abilities and capacities, e.g., movement, cognition, perception	Organizes capacities and abilities into activities, tasks, roles
Meaningfulness	Motivates engagement in therapeutic occupation	Motivates engagement in activities, tasks, life roles
Effect	Occupation, through task demand, remediates capacities and abilities	Occupation, through adaptation or education, restores activities and tasks of life roles

estimate of his or her reward in terms of success or pleasure, and possibly from a threat of bad consequences if the occupation is not engaged in. Meaning is individual (Bruner, 1990), and although the occupational therapist can guess what may be meaningful to the patient based on the person's life history, the therapist must verify with each patient that the particular occupation *is* meaningful to that person *now* and verify that the person sees value in relearning it. The therapist cannot substitute his or her own values in selecting appropriate occupational goals for the patient.

One study has determined that individualized, meaningful occupation-as-end used preventatively resulted in significant benefits across various health, function, and quality of life domains compared with no treatment or group social activity for well elderly participants (Clark et al., 1997). Meaningfulness is not only a psychological term but also a mechanism of change. It affects neurological functioning, as was seen in a positron emission tomography (PET) study by Decety et al. (1997) who discovered that brain activation differed with the meaning of an action regardless of subjects' strategies. Meaningful actions strongly engaged the frontal and temporal regions of the left hemisphere, while meaningless action activated mainly the right occipitoparietal areas.

Few studies in occupational therapy have tested the hypothesis that meaningful occupation-as-end motivates behavior. One qualitative study of the experience of occupational engagement for persons with mental illness reports that the participants experienced a sense of competency secondary to engagement in activities they believed at first to be beyond their capabilities. They were eager to attend therapy to continue working on their projects (Reberio & Cook, 1999). Related studies indicate that life satisfaction is at least partially defined in terms of competent role performance. One can extrapolate from this indication that, if a particular role is satisfying, one would be motivated to do the tasks associated with that role. For example, in the study by Yerxa and Baum (1986) of 15 subjects with spinal cord injury and their 12 nondisabled friends, a significant moderate correlation ($r = 0.44$) was found between satisfaction with performance in home management and overall life satisfaction. A slightly higher correlation ($r = 0.62$) was found between community skills and overall life satisfaction.

Occupation-As-Means

Occupation-as-means is the use of occupation as a treatment to improve a person's impaired capacities and abilities to enable eventual occupational functioning. Occupation-as-means refers to occupation acting as the therapeutic change agent. Various arts, crafts, games, sports, exercise routines (Figs. 12-5 and 12-6), and daily activities that are systematically selected and tailored to each individual are used as occupation-as-means (Cynkin & Robinson, 1990). The capacities and abilities that are required to complete the activity or task are improved when the person engages repeatedly in the activity or task.

Occupation-as-means is therapeutic when the activity has a purpose or goal that makes a challenging demand yet has a prospect for success. Because the central nervous system (CNS) is organized to accomplish goals (Granit, 1977), the goal or purpose seems to organize the most efficient response, given the **constraints** of person and context. Furthermore, if an activity has meaning and relevance to the individual who is to change, it motivates the will to learn and improve (Cynkin & Robinson, 1990).

Meaningfulness in the sense of occupation-as-means has an immediate aspect. Choice to participate in an activity at the moment is based on immediate motivation that is guided by currently perceived needs, feelings, and desires that may or may not be related to life goals. The meaningful aspect of occupation-as-means may be the emotional value that an interesting and creative experience offers the patient (Ayres, 1958). Or meaningfulness may stem from familiarity with the occupation, its power to arouse positive associations, the likelihood that completion of it will

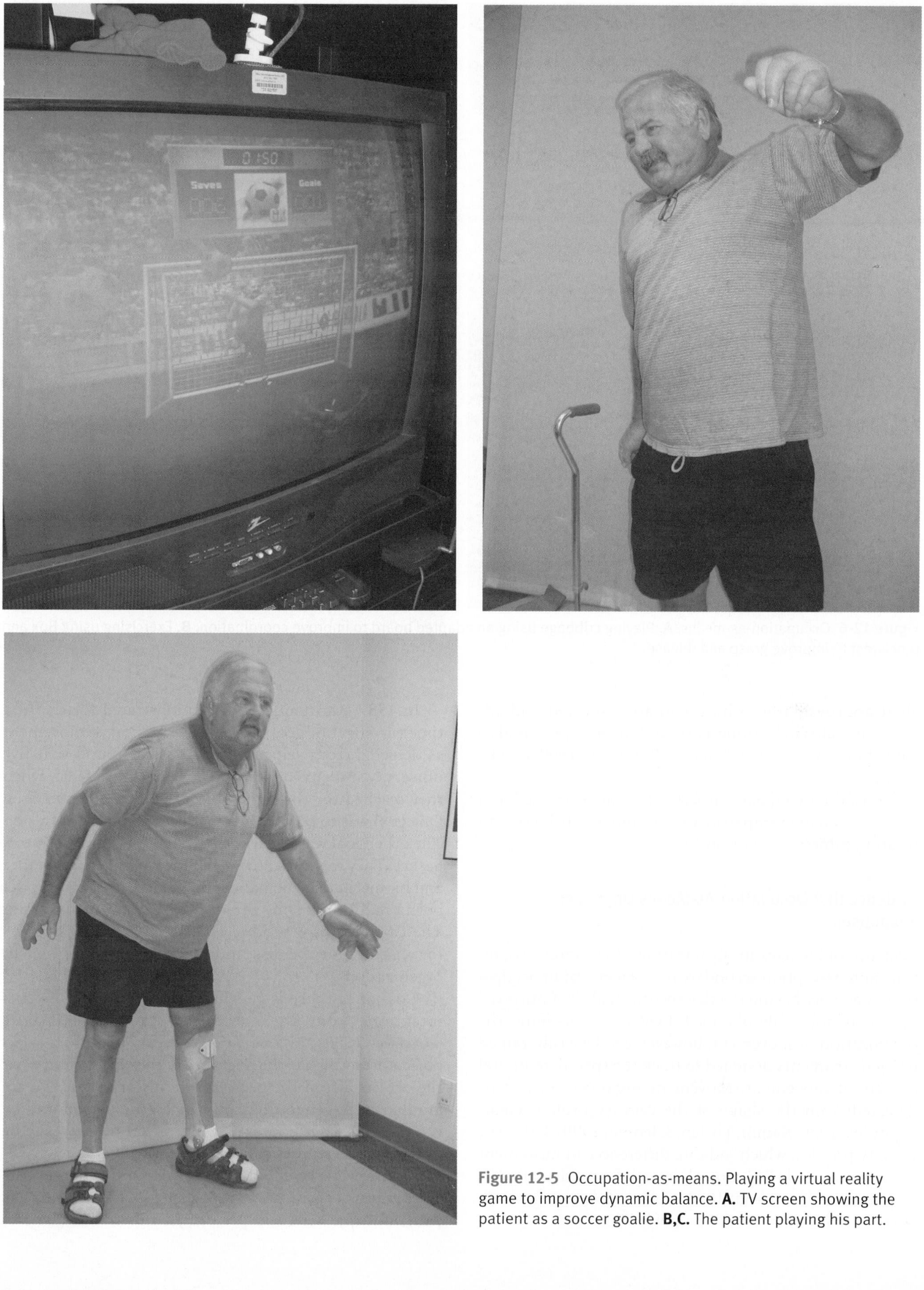

A B C

Figure 12-5 Occupation-as-means. Playing a virtual reality game to improve dynamic balance. **A.** TV screen showing the patient as a soccer goalie. **B,C.** The patient playing his part.

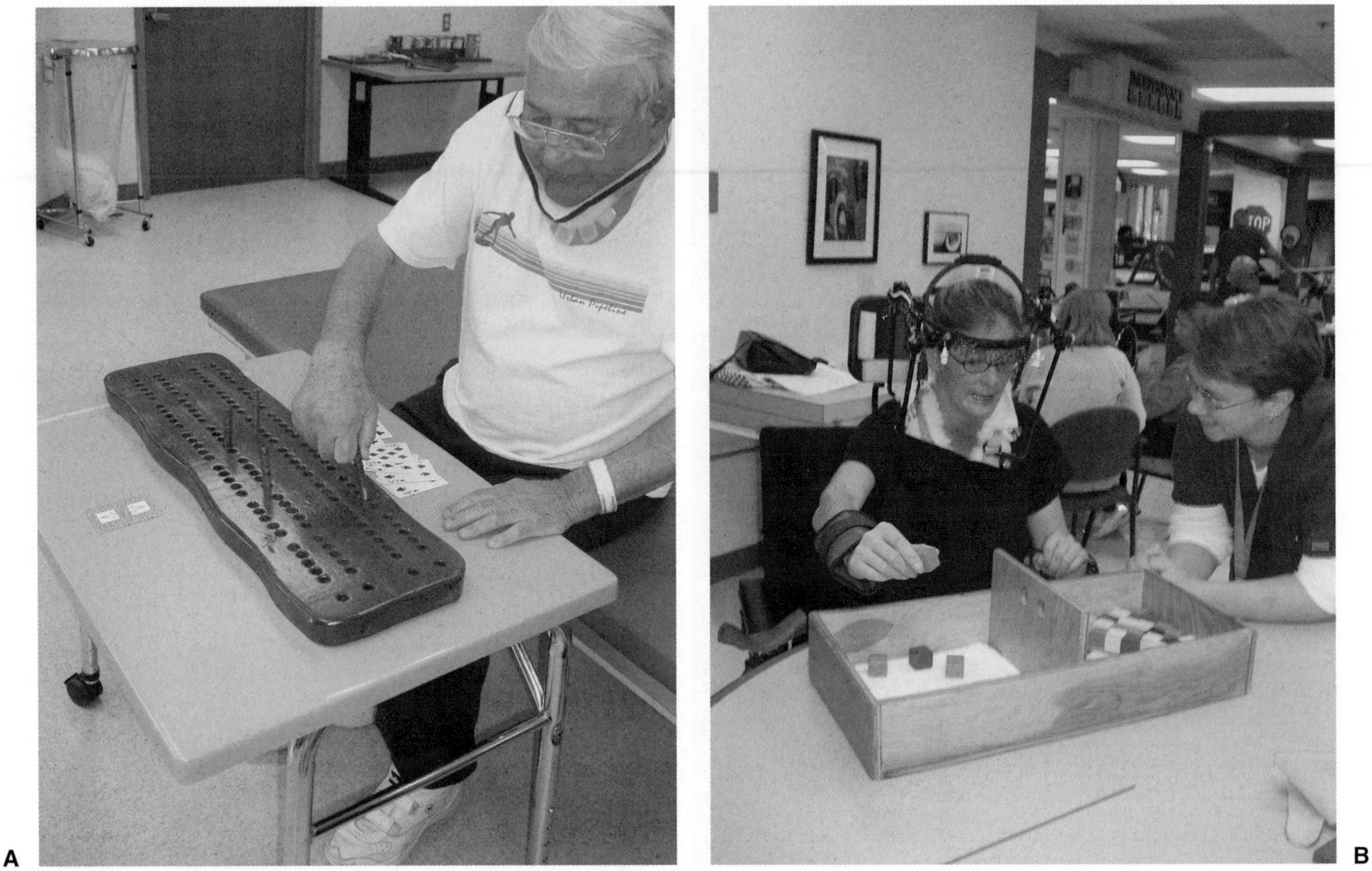

Figure 12-6 Occupation-as-means. **A.** Playing cribbage using an adapted board to improve coordination. **B.** Exercising using Box and Block test to improve grasp and release.

elicit approval from others who are respected and admired, its value in learning a prized skill, or its potential to contribute to recovery (Cynkin & Robinson, 1990; Grady, 1992).

Thus, the therapeutic aspects of occupation used as a means to change impairments are purposefulness and meaningfulness (Definition 12-1).

Evidence that Occupation-As-Means Organizes Responses

Evidence of changes in organization of emotions, cognition, and perception secondary to engagement in occupation or activity having the therapeutic quality of purposefulness is not easily obtained. Evidence concerning the organization of movement, however, can be easily gained using instruments designed to track the spatial-temporal aspects of movement. Movement organization can be detected from the shape of the velocity profile (Georgopoulos, 1986; Kamm, Thelan, & Jensen, 1990). Different velocity profiles, which indicate differences in movement organization and CNS control, emerge for particular goals or purposes (Jeannerod, 1988; Nelson, 1983) (Fig. 12-7). Some of that evidence will be reported here.

In 1987, Marteniuk et al. demonstrated for the first time the effect of goal on the organization of movement as detected from velocity profiles. They found that five university students organized movement differently when they reached for the same object for different purposes. One goal was to pick up a 4-cm disk and place it in a slot. The other goal was to pick up the disk and throw it into a basket. They measured the reach to the disk. The distance and biomechanical demands were exactly the same under both conditions. Only intent after reach was different. The two purposes produced different velocity profiles for reaching for the disk, indicating different movement organizations.

Goal or purpose is generated from the patient's own intention, from the therapist's directions (Fisk & Goodale, 1989), or from the context, including what objects are available, the relevance of the objects, and what the objects afford the person in terms of action. We are familiar with generation of goals by the person and by the therapist, but contextual indication of goal may be unfamiliar, so studies concerning this will be reviewed.

Mathiowetz and Wade (1995) tested whether the same motor organization was elicited when 20 subjects with multiple sclerosis performed functional tasks in

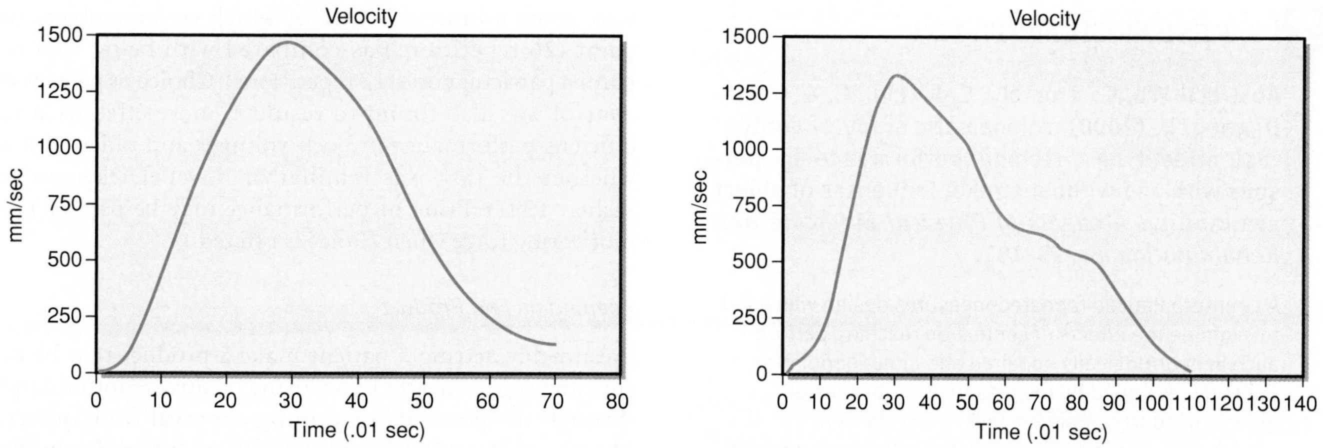

Figure 12-7 Velocity profiles. The profile on the left is symmetrical and bell-shaped, which is commonly seen in planned reach to a stationary, large target. The peak of the velocity profile (end of the acceleration phase) occurs between 33% and 50% of the reach. The profile on the right is left-shifted, which is commonly seen in guided reach to a small target. The peak velocity occurs early in the reach, and the deceleration phase is extended as the person guides the hand to the target.

natural, impoverished, partial, and simulated conditions. In the natural condition, the subjects actually ate applesauce from a dish with a spoon; in the impoverished condition, they pretended to eat applesauce, with no applesauce, spoon, or dish; in the partial condition, they pretended to eat applesauce using a dish and spoon but no applesauce; in the simulated condition, they performed the feeding subtest of the *Jebsen-Taylor Hand Function Test*, which has the subject pick up kidney beans with a spoon and transfer them to a can. The different contexts transmitted the idea of different goals to the subjects. Because subjects produced unique spatial-temporal maps (**phase planes**), which are indicative of different movement organization, in each context, the researchers concluded that subjects perceived each as a unique activity having a different goal.

Trombly and Wu (1999) examined, in two conditions, the movement organization of 14 people who had had a stroke. The conditions were goal object present and goal object absent (rote exercise). In the goal object–present condition, participants were asked to reach forward to take a piece of food off the plate and bring it to the mouth. In the goal object–absent condition, they were asked to reach forward to the same place but without the food goal. Although the two conditions were biomechanically equivalent, the reach was organized differently (smoother, faster, more forceful, and more planned) when the goal object was present compared with when it was absent. These findings have been verified in other studies (Ma, Trombly, & Robinson-Podolski, 1999; Wu et al., 1998, 2000). At least in terms of motor responses, then, purposiveness, as transmitted by context, does appear to organize behavior. Of course, much more study is required to verify this and confirm it to be true for other performance skills.

Evidence that Occupation-As-Means Motivates Participation

Although the meaningfulness of occupation to a person must be determined by interview and discussion with that person, *meaningfulness* has been operationalized in occupational therapy research in four ways: (1) provide enjoyment; (2) offer a choice; (3) offer the end product to keep; and (4) enhance the context or make the context more applicable to the person's life. The response, *motivation*, is measured as the number of repetitions or length of time engaged in the occupation or the effort expended.

Fun or Enjoyment

Fun is immediately motivating. Several studies confirm that fun or enjoyment derived from play motivates attempts to perform an action or prolongs engagement in an action. King (1993) treated 146 patients in a hand clinic using either a computer game that required the person to pinch or grasp to play the game or by using pinch or grip-strengthening devices. Both treatments lasted 3 minutes. Those who participated in the game did significantly more repetitions (237.2 grips, 240.5 pinches) than those who did the exercise without the game (170.7 grips, 203.2 pinches). Hoppes (1997) studied 10 elderly women who were unable to maintain a functional standing position. They alternatively played a game of their choice or did other chosen, non-playful activities, such as reading, conversing, or folding towels, all while standing at a raised table. Although the difference in standing tolerance was only a minute and a half, it was significantly greater for playing the game (386.5 seconds) than for the other activities (294.3 seconds).

RESEARCH NOTE 12-1

Abstract: Wu, C., Trombly, C. A., Lin, K., & Tickle-Degnen, L. (2000). A kinematic study of contextual effects on reaching performance in persons with and without stroke: Influences of object availability. *Archives of Physical Medicine and Rehabilitation, 81*, 95–101.

A counterbalanced repeated-measures design was used to examine the effects of context on reaching performance in neurologically impaired and intact populations. Context was varied by the presence or absence of objects used to complete a task. Subjects were 14 people with stroke and 25 neurologically intact persons. In a motor control laboratory in a university setting, each participant was tested under two conditions: presence of the object, in which the participant reached forward with the impaired arm or corresponding arm to scoop coins off the table into the other hand; and absence of the object, in which the participant reached forward to a place where the coins would be placed if the object were present. The dependent variables were kinematic variables of movement time, total displacement, peak velocity, percentage of reach where peak velocity occurs, and movement units derived from acceleration data for the reaching part of the activity. The condition of object present elicited significantly better ($p < 0.0055$) performance of reaching movements than the condition of object absent. Better performance was defined as faster (shorter movement time), more direct (less total displacement), more planned and less guided (greater percentage of reach where peak velocity occurs), and smoother (fewer movement units). Peak velocity (forcefulness) was not significantly different between conditions ($p = 0.2791$).

Application to Practice

- Occupation provides significant performance advantage over rote exercise.
- Tasks that use real objects elicit improved organization of movement.
- Treatment in simulated contexts using simulated objects and simulated goals may not help a patient learn occupational performance for real life.

Choice

Provision of a choice presumably creates emotional value because the person is likely to choose an activity that is interesting and creative and/or arouses positive associations from the past. Zimmerer-Branum and Nelson (1995) gave 52 elderly nursing home residents a choice between a simulated basketball game chosen to encourage shoulder flexion and rote shoulder flexion exercises. After trying both, 69% chose the game for the actual treatment session. LaMore and Nelson (1993) found a significant increase in repetitions when 22 adult subjects with mental disabilities were given a limited choice of which ceramic object to paint (26 repetitions) as compared with being told to paint a particular one (17 repetitions). Choice or perceived control was also found to result in more effective and efficient performance in both younger and older adults whether the task was familiar or novel (Dickerson & Fisher, 1997). Pride of performance may be part of the motivating force when choice is offered.

Keeping an End Product

Presumably, letting a patient make a product that he or she can keep motivates by arousing positive emotions and through the potential of gaining approval from others. Murphy et al. (1999) found that 50 college-aged subjects worked significantly longer on a craft project of their choice when they could keep the product (21.2 minutes) than when they could not (16.9 minutes). However, this was true for only two of the four activities from which the subjects could choose, and only 80% of the subjects reported being interested in keeping the end product. So it is not safe to assume that offering an opportunity to keep an end product is motivational; one must ask.

Enriched Context

Enriched or natural contexts motivate through the positive emotions associated with familiarity and arousal of positive associations with one's home, culture, or previous life. Lang, Nelson, and Bush (1992) tested the responses of 15 elderly nursing home residents under three conditions: kicking a red balloon, kicking a described imagined balloon, and exercise in which they kicked as demonstrated. A significantly greater number of repetitions was associated with really kicking the balloon (54) versus in the imagery or exercise conditions (26 and 18, respectively). This study was later replicated by DeKuiper et al. (1993) with similar results. A number of other researchers demonstrated significantly greater numbers of repetitions or duration of performance under enhanced context conditions (Bloch, Smith, & Nelson, 1989; Kircher, 1984; Miller & Nelson, 1987; Steinbeck, 1986; Thomas, Vander Wyk, & Boyer, 1999; Yoder, Nelson, & Smith, 1989).

Meaningfulness, as operationalized by fun and enjoyment, enhanced context, and possibly choice, appears to motivate continued performance, but more research is needed.

EFFECTIVENESS OF THERAPEUTIC OCCUPATION

For occupational therapists to take pride in their work, they must have confidence that the therapy they offer is effective in improving occupational functioning for their patients. Each therapist's personal experience nurtures that belief. In this age of evidence-based health practice, however, we need to offer our patients, the payers, and the public more substantial proof of that effectiveness than our anecdotal experiences.

Evidence that Occupation Restores a Sense of Self-Efficacy or Self-Esteem

The qualitative study by Rebeiro and Cook (1998), mentioned earlier, provides the best evidence we have at this time that engagement in occupation restores a sense of self-efficacy and self-esteem. The participants were eight long-time members of an outpatient Women's Group at a mental health facility who engaged in a cooperative occupational project—making a quilt. On interview after 25 weeks of participation, the participants reported that engagement in the occupation gave them a sense of self-confidence and competency because of their accomplishment, which they did not have before the introduction of occupation to the group.

Evidence that Occupation-As-End Restores Self-Maintenance, Self-Enhancement, and Self-Advancement Roles

Direct evidence of the effectiveness of occupation-as-end to restore life roles is sparse. One study reported successful resumption of role performance in 17 randomly selected chronically disabled community-living elders after receiving home-based occupational therapy (Levine & Gitlin, 1993). As a result of the program, participants engaged in a greater range of tasks, such as wine making, visiting relatives, attending church, and cleaning, than they did before the intervention. They became more engaged in life, as shown by their volunteerism and increased social activities. See Evidence Table 12-1 for examples of studies from which evidence concerning the effectiveness of occupation to restore role resumption can be gleaned.

Evidence that Occupation-As-Means Remediates Impairments

Studies of the effects of occupation-as-means on persons with physical impairments are few and scattered; two are described in Evidence Table 12-1.

IMPLEMENTATION OF THERAPEUTIC OCCUPATION IN PRACTICE

Lyons, Phipps, and Berro (2004) described ways of organizing one clinic to efficiently utilize occupation therapeutically. The treatment areas in the clinic were rearranged to resemble a homelike environment (e.g., bedroom, living room, nursery). The therapists prepared "occupation kits," which were large plastic boxes containing all the props necessary to engage in an occupation. Occupation kits were made for gardening, letter writing, pet care, fishing, scrapbooking, and car care, which were the most commonly named activities by their clients. Therapists in this clinic were encouraged to work with the patients in the various areas of the hospital campus and surrounding environment, the larger community, and the client's own community (barbershop, market, place of worship) to provide meaningful occupation-based interventions in the clients' natural contexts.

Occupation-as-end is implemented by teaching the activity or task directly, using whatever abilities the patient has, or by providing whatever adaptations are necessary to enable performance. Because occupation occurs within a person–task–environment interaction, change in any one of these variables may result in successful performance. Implementation of occupation-as-end focuses on changing the **task demands** and/or the environment, whereas occupation-as-means focuses on changing the person. Therapeutic principles for application of occupation-as-end derive from cognitive information processing and learning theories. It is the rehabilitative approach (Trombly & Scott, 1977). In this approach, occupations are analyzed to ensure that they are within the capabilities of the patient, but they are not used to bring about change in these capabilities per se. The patient learns, with the help of the therapist as teacher and adaptor of the task demands and context. In the therapeutic encounter, the therapist:

- Ensures that the task is within the person's capabilities
- Organizes the subtasks to be learned so the person will succeed
- Provides clear instructions
- Provides feedback to promote successful outcome

CLINICAL REASONING IN OCCUPATIONAL THERAPY PRACTICE

Implementing Therapeutic Occupation in Practice

One way to incorporate occupation into practice is to use "occupation kits," as suggested by Lyons, Phipps, & Berro (2004). Occupational kits are used to implement occupation-as-means. Describe the contents of occupational kits designed for these occupations:

1. Needlework
2. Home entertainment
3. Home repair

State why each object is included (the therapeutic benefit).

Evidence Table 12-1

Selected Evidence for Occupational Therapy Practice Regarding Occupation

Intervention	Description of Intervention Tested	Participants	Dosage	Type of Best Evidence and Level of Evidence	Benefit	Statistical Probability and Effect Size of Outcome	Reference
Occupation-as-end: Goal-specific training to achieve valued occupational goals	Experimental: long-term ADL goals valued by the participants and carers and considered amenable by the staff were worked toward via a series of written contracts that specified interim and short-term goals. Carried out in homes, day centers, and work place. Control: booklet that listed resources with those particular to the participant highlighted.	94 (75.5% male) persons with moderate to severe TBI aged 16–65 years, in acute to chronic stages of recovery. Randomized to group.	2–6 hours per week for a mean of 28 weeks for experimental group and 1 visit for control group.	Randomized controlled trial. IA2a	Yes. Community rehabilitation after severe TBI can yield benefits that outlive the active treatment period even if offered years after injury.	35% of the experimental participants versus 20% of the control group improved on the *Barthel Index* (Mann-Whitney $U = 831, p < 0.05$). The experimental participants scored significantly better than the control on the total *BICRO-39* score (Mann-Whitney $U = 517, p < 0.05$) and self-organization (Mann-Whitney $U = 474, p < 0.05$) and psychological well-being (Mann-Whitney $U = 469, p < 0.05$) subscales. Effect sizes could not be calculated from data provided.	Powell, Heslin, & Greenwood, 2002

Occupation-as-end: Training in leisure activities to regain hobby roles	Experimental: practice skills and use of equipment to improve participation in self-identified hobbies and interests at home. Control #1: ADL practice and perceptual drills at home. Control #2: no treatment.	65 persons with acute stroke (23 LCVA; 41 RCVA; 1 other); mean age = 65.9 years. Randomized to group.	30 minutes once a week for 12 weeks after discharge from hospital and 30 minutes every 2 weeks for the next 12 weeks.	Randomized controlled trial. IB2a	Yes. The experimental group scored significantly higher than the two control groups on the *Nottingham Health Profile*, a measure of psychological well-being.	Experimental > Control #1: $p = 0.0002$, $r = 0.39$; Experimental > Control #2: $p = 0.0011$, $r = 0.34$.	Drummond & Walker, 1996
Occupation-as-end: Training to resume adult roles of family member and worker	Three parts: (1) adaptation of computer programs, keyboard, and monitor; (2) instruction in adapted word processing and e-mailing; (3) computer-related activities designed to enhance participation in desired social roles.	1 male after traumatic brain injury, with obsessive compulsive disorder and ADHD since childhood, left hemiparesis, left hemianopsia, and speech deficits; living in a residential setting.	2-hour weekly sessions for 4 months.	Case study. VC3c	Yes. The participant was able to reestablish his roles of brother and adult son; develop and maintain an extended family of others beyond his family of origin; create a satisfying adult work role that brought greater meaning to his life.	No statistical analysis. Anecdotal evidence. No controls to allow one to accept with confidence that the treatment caused the outcome.	Gutman, 2000

continued

Evidence Table 12-1

Selected Evidence for Occupational Therapy Practice Regarding Occupation (continued)

Intervention	Description of Intervention Tested	Participants	Dosage	Type of Best Evidence and Level of Evidence	Benefit	Statistical Probability and Effect Size of Outcome	Reference
Occupation-as-means: Game to increase arm reach	Condition #1: participant reached to a point 3 in above the center of the table placed to require full forward reach. Condition #2: participant reached the same distance to play the Simon® computer-controlled game of flashing lights and sounds.	20 (17 men; 3 women) brain-injured adults with mild to moderate spasticity of the upper extremity.	10 trials of each condition in a laboratory setting.	Non-randomized, counterbalanced design. IIC2c	Yes. The use of the game elicited significantly more range of motion of the affected upper extremity than the rote exercise. The results support the use of an occupationally embedded intervention.	$t_{(19)} = 5.77$, $p < 0.001$, $r = 0.80$.	Sietsema et al., 1993
Occupation-as-means: Game to decrease pronator spasticity and to increase supination (external rotation) ROM	Experimental: bilaterally assisted supination exercise in the context of a dice game that required the subjects to supinate to dump out the dice for a score. Control: bilaterally assisted supination exercise using the same apparatus without the game.	26 women in acute stage after stroke (11 LCVA; 15 RCVA); mean age = 68.4 years. Participants were randomly assigned in a stratified balanced way to either the experimental or control condition.	Two sets of 10 trials for each condition; different days.	Randomized controlled trial. IC2c	Yes. Those who participated in the game demonstrated significantly greater handle rotation [supination] (95.3°) than the controls (81.9°).	Mean gain of 13.4° in handle rotation by the experimental group ($p = 0.016$, $r = 0.42$)	Nelson et al., 1996

ADL, activities of daily living; TBI, traumatic brain injury; LCVA, left cerebral vascular accident; RCVA, right cerebral vascular accident; ADHD, attention deficit hyperactivity disorder; ROM, range of motion.

- Structures the practice to ensure improved performance and learning
- Makes adaptations as necessary.

To implement occupation-as-means, occupations of interest are analyzed to determine that they demand particular responses from the person and that the responses demanded are slightly more challenging than what the person can easily produce. The therapist provides the opportunity to engage in the potentially therapeutic occupation (Meyer, 1922, 1977), and as the person makes the effort and succeeds, the particular impairment the occupation-as-means was chosen to remediate is reduced. In the therapeutic encounter, the therapist:

- Ascertains the patient's interests
- Selects occupations that reflect those interests
- Analyzes the occupations to determine which would be appropriate to achieve the patient's goal
- Lets the patient choose from among several offered occupations
- Instructs the patient in the correct procedure for doing the activity to derive the most therapeutic benefit
- Grades the occupation to increase the challenge as the patient improves.

See the Case Example of how occupation as therapy is implemented in practice. The processes involved in using occupation therapeutically are **activity analysis**, selection and gradation, and adaptation. Guidelines for these processes are presented in Chapter 13.

CASE EXAMPLE

Ms. C.: Using Occupation Therapeutically

Occupational Therapy Intervention Process	Clinical Reasoning Process: Objectives	Clinical Reasoning Process: Examples of Therapist's Internal Dialogue
Patient Information Ms. C. is a 55-year-old, right-handed woman who began inpatient rehabilitation after a left cerebral vascular accident (LCVA). She was originally from the Philippines, where she worked as a school teacher. For the past few years, she has been living in the U.S. with one of her daughters. Evaluation: 1. *Occupational history interview.* She described her life through a series of stories, allowing her self story to become evident. Several themes of meaning and important occupations emerged: (a) theme of being a teacher, which was evident in her communication style, her previous role as teacher, and the educational play she described with her grandchildren; (b) theme of cleanliness and efficiency, which was evident through her report that she had to finish all the housework before playing with her grandchildren; and (c) theme of spirituality when she discussed the importance of daily church attendance.	Appreciate the context	"Ms. C. is a relatively young woman who has experienced a stroke affecting her dominant side. She is depressed because she fears the loss of important roles and occupations. I chose to use a narrative approach to begin the evaluation so that I can understand Ms. C. as an occupational being and she can gain hope that someone is going to help her resume her life activities. Three themes of meaning emerged as she talked—teaching, home management, and spirituality. These will become important components of the treatment planning process."

2. *Description of a typical day* in chronological sequence revealed that her routine consisted of cooking breakfast for her granddaughters, doing housework, playing with her grandchildren, going to church in the evening, and sending text messages to her friends in the Philippines.
3. *Evaluation of impairments* revealed: (a) decreased motor control but developing volitional movement throughout her right arm; (b) decreased sensation; (c) poor muscle tone of the right side of her body, but able to stand for short periods of time; (d) impaired but improving expressive language; and (e) poor executive cognitive functioning.

Develop intervention hypotheses	"Occupation-based treatment will initiate the development of Ms. C.'s new view of herself as someone who could now continue to participate in her roles and occupations. This new vision of herself will lighten her depression and assist her in setting goals for her future. I notice that by providing Ms. C. with the opportunity to make decisions regarding her goals and preferences for treatment, she is becoming empowered and demonstrates increased motivation to participate in therapy."
Select an intervention approach	"I will use a client-centered, occupation-based approach."
Reflect on competence	"I have treated many patients of Ms. C.'s age with similar disability. My client-centered, occupation-based approach has been universally successful with them; therefore, I am competent to treat Ms. C."

Recommendations

Ms. C. will attend inpatient occupational therapy for 60- to 90-minute treatment sessions, 6 times a week for 3 weeks.

Long-term goal is to return home and resume valued roles of grandmother, homemaker, and church attendee.

Consider the patient's appraisal of performance	"I have helped Ms. C. notice that she is able to incorporate her returning motor, cognitive, and language skills directly into occupation-based treatment so that her impairments will improve as she relearns the activities and tasks of her valued roles. This pleases her."
Consider what will occur in therapy, how often, and for how long	"Intensive therapy during her brief inpatient hospitalization is warranted. Ms. C. agrees with this plan."
Ascertain the patient's endorsement of plan	

Summary of Short-Term Goals and Progress

Goal setting was accomplished using the *COPM (Canadian Occupational Performance Measure)*. Ms. C.'s goals included the following most valued occupations:

1. performing household chores
2. cooking
3. storytelling with her grandchildren
4. sending text messages to the Philippines
5. going to church
6. using public transportation

The initial occupation-based session with Ms. C. involved engaging in household management occupations. To prepare for engaging in these roles at home, she began cleaning, vacuuming, and doing laundry in a homelike setting within the clinic.

Know the person

"We are using occupation-as-means, so by performing valued activities, Ms. C. is improving motor control by incorporating her right arm into activity completion. She is also learning how to structure her day to complete the activities she wants to include in her day. She is using the household management "occupation kit" to practice opening containers of laundry products, which promotes fine motor skills as well as prepares her for an important activity. Vacuuming is challenging her dynamic balance. Ms. C. told me that she saw her new role as an assistant in home management so, through the use of occupation-as-end, Ms. C. is beginning to form a new self-identity and vision for her future."

A subsequent intervention session was held in a simulated living room environment. Her daughter brought her two children, along with some of their storybooks. During the session, Ms. C. had difficulty maintaining the attention of the children and physically calming them down. She then used her teaching skills to explain to her grandchildren her new participation level in her role as grandmother and taught them to help hold her right hand as they played together.

Appreciate the context

"In the play session with her grandchildren, Ms. C. gained insight into the process of role resumption for this activity at home. In addition, her family was able to see her potential for participating in the children's play."

One of Ms. C.'s final intervention sessions involved going on a market outing to prepare for a cooking activity. This session provided Ms. C. with opportunities to relearn how to push a grocery cart, reach for and manipulate items in the store, attend to tasks despite increased ambient noise, and practice mobility within the store.

"The shopping session allowed Ms. C. to carry over some of the skills that she had learned in the clinic into the real world. The experience supported her continual formation of herself as an occupational being, and it provided her with hope for participation in this role."

Next Steps

Again, using the COPM, these short-term goals were identified for outpatient rehabilitation:

1. clean the bottom of her bathtub
2. clean the bathroom sink
3. carry a heavy laundry basket
4. carry heavy grocery bags long distances
5. cut vegetables with her right dominant hand
6. write letters to friends in the Philippines (communication had stopped because of cost of text messaging)
7. find transportation to attend church daily
8. kneel to pray and read the Bible in church
9. volunteer in a local hospital

Anticipate present and future patient concerns

Analyze patient's comprehension

Decide if he or she should continue or discontinue therapy and/or return in the future

"At discharge from inpatient rehabilitation, Ms. C. believed she would be able to return to her chosen occupations, such as self-care, light household management, playing with her grandchildren, and preparing light meals. She was able to initiate and integrate the use of her right side, so she expected she could participate in her typical day when she returned home. Armed with strategies and ideas regarding how to more fully participate in her life roles and occupations, she felt that she had a good foundation to return home. However, Ms. C. found that the transition from the structure of the inpatient rehabilitation setting to home and community settings presented greater challenges to her participation than she had anticipated. She was tearful about diminished participation in occupations that held considerable meaning for her life. Outpatient occupational therapy was required, and I recommended that she be seen for 60- to 120-minute sessions, once a week for 4 weeks to facilitate the transition."

Adapted with permission from the American Occupational Therapy Association (publisher) and the authors. Lyons, A., Phipps, S. C., & Berro, M. (2004). Using occupation in the clinic. *OT PRACTICE*, 9, 11–15.

SUMMARY REVIEW QUESTIONS

1. Define occupation and purposeful activity.
2. State some reasons why occupation is important in a person's life.
3. Define occupation-as-end.
4. Define occupation-as-means.
5. Therapeutic occupation is both purposeful and meaningful. What effects do these qualities produce?
6. List two examples of evidence that occupation is therapeutic.

ACKNOWLEDGMENTS

I thank my former students Dr. Steven Cope, Dr. Susan Fasoli, Janice Ferguson, Yvonne Fuller, Dr. Hui-Ing Ma, Dr. Susan Murphy, Julie Pope, Natalia Ramsbey, Ellen Rosenberg, Dr. Pimjai Sudsawad, Dr. Pei-Luen Tsai, and Dr. Ching-Yi Wu for their assistance and conversations about occupation. I am also especially indebted to the occupational therapists and patients of the Sister Kenny Institute in Minneapolis, MN, for allowing me to photograph them or for facilitating the photography. Specifically, I thank Cindy Bemis, Arlan Berg, Michelle Brown, M.Ed., OTR/L, Larry Chaney, Anthony Drong, Larry Larkin, Robb Miller, OTR/L, Mary Radomski, M.A., OTR/L, Jennifer Theis, M.S., OTR/L, and Sharon E. Gowdy Wagener, OTR/L.

References

American Occupational Therapy Association [AOTA]. (2002). Occupational therapy practice framework: Domain and process. *American Journal of Occupational Therapy, 56,* 609–639.

Ayres, A. J. (1958). Basic concepts of clinical practice in physical disabilities. *American Journal of Occupational Therapy, 12,* 300–302,311.

Bloch, M. W., Smith, D. A., & Nelson, D. L. (1989). Heart rate, activity, duration, and affect in added-purpose versus single-purpose jumping activities. *American Journal of Occupational Therapy, 43,* 25–30.

Borell, L., Lilja, M., Sviden, G. A., & Sadlo, G. (2001). Occupations and signs of reduced hope: An explorative study of older adults with functional impairments. *American Journal of Occupational Therapy, 55,* 311–316.

Bruner, J. (1990). *Acts of meaning.* Cambridge, MA: Harvard University.

Christiansen, C. H. (1999). The 1999 Eleanor Clarke Slagle Lecture—Defining lives: Occupation as identity: An essay on competence, coherence, and the creation of meaning. *American Journal of Occupational Therapy, 53,* 547–558.

Clark, F., Azen, S. P., Zemke, R., Jackson, J., Carlson, M., Mandel, D., Hay, J., Josephson, K., Cherry, B., Hessel, C., Palmer, J., & Lipson, L. (1997). Occupational therapy for independent-living older adults: A randomized controlled trial. *Journal of the American Medical Association, 278,* 1321–1326.

Cynkin, S., & Robinson, A. M. (1990). *Occupational therapy and activities health: Toward health through activities.* Boston: Little, Brown.

Decety, J., Grezes, J., Costes, N., Perani, D., Jeannerod, M., Procyk, E., Grassi, F., & Fazio, F. (1997). Brain activity during observation of actions: Influence of action content and subject's strategy. *Brain, 120,* 1763–1777.

DeKuiper, W. P., Nelson, D. L., & White, B. E. (1993). Materials-based occupation versus imagery-based occupation versus rote exercise: A replication and extension. *Occupational Therapy Journal of Research, 13,* 183–197.

Dickerson, A. E., & Fisher, A. G. (1997). Effects of familiarity of task and choice on the functional performance of younger and older adults. *Psychology and Aging, 12,* 247–254.

Drummond, A., & Walker, M. (1996). Generalisation of the effects of leisure rehabilitation for stroke patients. *British Journal of Occupational Therapy, 59,* 330–334.

Fisk, J. D., & Goodale, M. A. (1989). The effects of instructions to subjects on the programming of visually directed reaching movements. *Journal of Motor Behavior, 21,* 5–19.

Georgopoulos, A. P. (1986). On reaching. *Annual Review of Neurosciences, 9,* 147–170.

Glass, T. A., Mendes de Leon, C., Marottoli, R. A., & Berkman, L. F. (1999). Population based study of social and productive activities as predictors of survival among elderly Americans. *British Journal of Medicine, 319,* 478–483.

Grady, A. P. (1992). Nationally speaking: Occupation as vision. *American Journal of Occupational Therapy, 46,* 1062–1065.

Granit, R. (1977). *The purposive brain.* Cambridge, MA: MIT.

Gutman, S. A. (2000). Using a computer as an environmental facilitator to promote post-head injury social role resumption: A case report. *Occupational Therapy in Mental Health, 15,* 71–89.

Hammell, K. W. (2004). Dimensions of meaning in the occupations of daily life. *Canadian Journal of Occupational Therapy, 71,* 296–305.

Hoppes, S. (1997). Can play increase standing tolerance? A pilot study. *Physical and Occupational Therapy in Geriatrics, 15,* 65–73.

Hoppes, S. (2005). When a child dies the world should stop spinning: An autoethnography exploring the impact of family loss on occupation. *American Journal of Occupational Therapy, 59,* 78–87.

Jackson, J., Carlson, M., Mandel, D., Zemke, R., & Clark, F. (1998). Occupation in lifestyle redesign: The well elderly study occupational therapy program. *American Journal of Occupational Therapy, 52,* 326–336.

Jeannerod, M. (1988). *The neural and behavioral organization of goal-directed movements.* Oxford, UK: Clarendon.

Kamm, K., Thelen, E., & Jensen, J. L. (1990). A dynamical systems approach to motor development. *Physical Therapy, 70,* 763–775.

King, T. I. (1993). Hand strengthening with a computer for purposeful activity. *American Journal of Occupational Therapy, 47,* 635–637.

Kircher, M. A. (1984). Motivation as a factor of perceived exertion in purposeful versus nonpurposeful activity. *American Journal of Occupational Therapy, 38,* 165–170.

LaMore, K. L., & Nelson, D. L. (1993). The effects of options on performance of an art project in adults with mental disabilities. *American Journal of Occupational Therapy, 47,* 397–401.

Lang, E. M., Nelson, D. L., & Bush, M. A. (1992). Comparison of performance in materials-based occupation, imagery-based occupation, and rote exercise in nursing home residents. *American Journal of Occupational Therapy, 46,* 607–611.

Law, M., Polatajko, H., Baptiste, W., & Townsend, E. (1997). Core concepts of occupational therapy. In E. Townsend (Ed.), *Enabling occupation: An occupational therapy perspective* (pp. 29–56). Ottawa, Ontario, Canada: Canadian Association of Occupational Therapists.

Levine, R. E., & Gitlin, L. N. (1993). A model to promote activity competence in elders. *American Journal of Occupational Therapy, 47,* 147–153.

Llorens, L. A. (1993). Activity analysis: Agreement between participants and observers on perceived factors in occupation components. *Occupational Therapy Journal of Research, 13,* 198–211.

Lyons, A., Phipps, S. C., & Berro, M. (2004). Using occupation in the clinic. [American Occupational Therapy Association]. *OT PRACTICE, 9,* 11–15.

Ma, H., Trombly, C. A., & Robinson-Podolski, C. (1999). The effect of context on skill acquisition and transfer. *American Journal of Occupational Therapy, 53,* 138–144.

Marteniuk, R. G., MacKenzie, C. L., Jeannerod, M., Athenes, S., & Dugas, C. (1987). Constraints on human arm movement trajectories. *Canadian Journal of Psychology, 41,* 365–378.

Mathiowetz, V., & Wade, M. G. (1995). Task constraints and functional motor performance of individuals with and without multiple sclerosis. *Ecological Psychology, 7,* 99–123.

McKinnon, A. L. (1992). Time use for self care, productivity, and leisure among elderly Canadians. *Canadian Journal of Occupational Therapy, 59,* 102–110.

Meyer, A. (1922, 1977). The philosophy of occupational therapy. *Archives of Occupational Therapy, 1,* 1–10; *American Journal of Occupational Therapy, 31,* 639–642.

Miller, L., & Nelson, D. L. (1987). Dual-purpose activity versus single-purpose activity in terms of duration of task, exertion level, and affect. *Occupational Therapy in Mental Health, 1,* 55–67.

Mish, F. C. (Ed.). (2004). *The Merriam-Webster dictionary*. Springfield, MA: Merriam-Webster, Incorporated.

Moyers, P. A. (1999). The guide to occupational therapy practice. *American Journal of Occupational Therapy, 53,* 247–322.

Murphy, S., Trombly, C. A., Tickle-Degnen, L., & Jacobs, K. (1999). The effect of keeping as end-product on intrinsic motivation. *American Journal of Occupational Therapy, 53,* 153–158.

National Society for the Promotion of Occupational Therapy. (1917). *Constitution of the National Society for the Promotion of Occupational Therapy*. Baltimore: Sheppard Hospital.

Nelson, W. L. (1983). Physical principles for economies of skilled movements. *Biological Cybernetics, 46,* 135–147.

Nelson, D. L., Konosky, K., Fleharty, K., Webb, R., Newer, K., Hazboun, V. P., Fontane, C., & Licht, B. C. (1996). The effects of an occupationally embedded exercise on bilaterally assisted supination in persons with hemiplegia. *American Journal of Occupational Therapy, 50,* 639–646.

Newell, K. M. (1986). Constraints on the development of coordination. In M. G. Wade & H. T. A. Whiting (Eds.), *Motor development in children: Aspects of coordination and control* (pp. 341–360). Boston: Martinus Nijhoff.

Pentland, W., Harvey, A. S., Smith, T., & Walker, J. (1999). The impact of spinal cord injury on men's time use. *Spinal Cord, 37,* 786–792.

Pierce, D. (1998). The Issue Is: What is the source of occupation's treatment power? *American Journal of Occupational Therapy, 52,* 490–491.

Powell, J., Heslin, J., & Greenwood, R. (2002). Community based rehabilitation after severe traumatic brain injury: A randomized controlled trial. *Journal of Neurology, Neurosurgery, and Psychiatry, 72,* 193–202.

Price-Lackey, P., & Cashman, J. (1996). Jenny's story: Reinventing oneself through occupation and narrative configuration. *American Journal of Occupational Therapy, 50,* 306–314.

Rebeiro, K. L. (1998). Occupation-as-means to mental health: A review of the literature, and a call for research. *Canadian Journal of Occupational Therapy, 65,* 12–19.

Rebeiro, K. L., & Cook, J. V. (1999). Opportunity, not prescription: An exploratory study of the experience of occupational engagement. *Canadian Journal of Occupational Therapy, 66,* 176–187.

Rebeiro, K. L., & Polgar, J. M. (1998). Enabling occupational performance: Optimal experiences in therapy. *Canadian Journal of Occupational Therapy, 65,* 14–22.

Reilly, M. (1962). Occupation can be one of the great ideas of 20th century medicine. *American Journal of Occupational Therapy, 16,* 1–9.

Segal, R. (2004). Family routines and rituals: A context for occupational therapy interventions. *American Journal of Occupational Therapy, 58,* 499–508.

Sietsema, J. M., Nelson, D. L., Mulder, R. M., Mervau-Scheidel, D., & White, B. E. (1993). The use of a game to promote arm reach in persons with traumatic brain injury. *American Journal of Occupational Therapy, 47,* 19–24.

Slagle, E. C. (1914). History of the development of occupation for the insane. *Maryland Psychiatric Quarterly, 4,* 14–20.

Steinbeck, T. M. (1986). Purposeful activity and performance. *American Journal of Occupational Therapy, 40,* 529–534.

Thomas, J. J., Vander Wyk, S., & Boyer, J. (1999). Contrasting occupational forms: Effects on performance and affect in patients undergoing phase II cardiac rehabilitation. *The Occupational Therapy Journal of Research, 19,* 187–202.

Trombly, C. A. (1995). Occupation: Purposefulness and meaningfulness as therapeutic mechanisms. *American Journal of Occupational Therapy, 49,* 960–972.

Trombly, C. A., & Scott, A. D. (1977). *Occupational therapy for physical dysfunction*. Baltimore: Williams & Wilkins.

Trombly, C. A., & Wu, C. (1999). Effect of rehabilitation tasks on organization of movement after stroke. *American Journal of Occupational Therapy, 53,* 333–344.

Unruh, A. M. (2004). Reflections on: "So . . . what do you do?" Occupation and the construct of identity. *Canadian Journal of Occupational Therapy, 71,* 290–295.

Wallenbert, I., & Jonsson, H. (2005). Waiting to get better: A dilemma regarding habits in daily occupations after stroke. *American Journal of Occupational Therapy, 59,* 218–224.

World Health Organization [WHO]. (2001). *International Classification of Functioning, Disability and Health (ICF)*. Geneva, Switzerland: World Health Organization.

Wu, C., Trombly, C. A., Lin, K., & Tickle-Degnen, L. (1998). Effects of object affordances on reaching performance in persons with and without cerebrovascular accident. *American Journal of Occupational Therapy, 52,* 447–456.

Wu, C., Trombly, C. A., Lin, K., & Tickle-Degnen, L. (2000). A kinematic study of contextual effects on reaching performance in persons with and without stroke: Influences of object availability. *Archives of Physical Medicine and Rehabilitation, 81,* 95–101.

Yerxa, E. J., & Baum, S. (1986). Engagement in daily occupations and life satisfaction among people with spinal cord injuries. *Occupational Therapy Journal of Research, 6,* 271–283.

Yerxa, E. J., & Locker, S. (1990). Quality of time use by adults with spinal cord injuries. *American Journal of Occupational Therapy, 44,* 318–326.

Yoder, R. M., Nelson, D. L., & Smith, D. A. (1989). Added-purpose versus rote exercise in female nursing home residents. *American Journal of Occupational Therapy, 43,* 581–586.

Zimmerer-Branum, S., & Nelson, D. L. (1995). Occupationally embedded exercise versus rote exercise: A choice between occupational forms by elderly nursing home residents. *American Journal of Occupational Therapy, 49,* 397–402.

CHAPTER 13

Occupation as Therapy: Selection, Gradation, Analysis, and Adaptation

Catherine A. Trombly Latham

LEARNING OBJECTIVES

After studying this chapter, the reader will be able to do the following:

1. Select occupation-as-means to achieve particular goals.
2. Grade occupations to challenge the person's abilities to improve performance.
3. Analyze occupations to determine their value for remediation of impaired abilities and capacities.
4. Analyze occupations to determine whether they are within the capabilities of a particular person.
5. Adapt occupations to increase their therapeutic value or to bring them within the capability of a person.

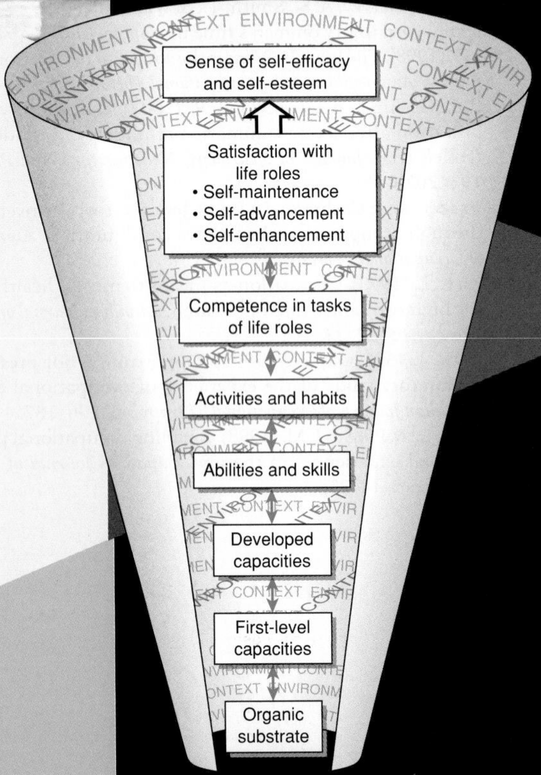

Glossary

Activity analysis—A process by which properties inherent in a given activity, task, or occupation may be gauged for their ability to elicit individual motivation and to fulfill patients' needs in occupational performance and performance components (Llorens, 1993).

Closed task—A closed task involves the least interaction with environment (Gentile, 1987). A closed task is one in which the task demands remain constant and for which habits can develop so that little conscious control is required once learned.

Constraints—Limitations imposed on purposeful movement or the completion of occupational performance. Extrinsic constraints include the physical and sociocultural environment and task demands. Intrinsic constraints include biomechanical and neuromuscular aspects of a person's body, as well as other personal contextual factors (Newell, 1986).

Electromyographic—Pertaining to recording the electrical activity produced by a contracting muscle. When a muscle is at rest, no electrical activity is recorded. As the muscle contracts, the electrical activity increases proportionately.

Kinematic—Spatial and temporal description of movement measured by optoelectric or videographic instruments that allows detection of strategies for the organization of movement (Georgopoulos, 1986; Jeannerod, 1988).

MET (metabolic equivalent)—The amount of energy expended when a person is engaged in activity. At rest in a semireclined position and with the extremities supported (basal state), that amount is 3.5 mL of oxygen per minute per kilogram of body weight (1 MET). Energy expenditure of activities is rated in terms of multiples of METs.

Occupation-as-end—Activities and tasks that constitute the roles of a given individual (Trombly, 1995).

Occupation-as-means—Activities and tasks chosen to remediate deficient abilities or capacities (Trombly, 1995).

Open task—Task with most interaction between the performer and environment (Gentile, 1987). An open task is one for which the environment and/or objects may vary during performance and between trials. Open tasks require attention and vigilance.

Task analysis—Similar to activity analysis; term used primarily in relation to work assessment (ergonomics). Analysis of the dynamic relationship among a person, a selected task or occupation, and a specific context or environment (Watson & Wilson, 2003).

Task demands—The context (e.g., objects, surroundings, ritual) that evokes certain maneuvers required to accomplish the goal of the task.

As described in the previous chapter, occupation is the therapeutic medium of occupational therapy with the goal of facilitating participation in life (American Occupational Therapy Association [AOTA], 2002). The therapist must select the appropriate occupation for the patient to remediate deficit abilities or capacities (**occupation-as-means**) or to enable independent performance of valued occupations (**occupation-as-end**). To be able to *select* an appropriate occupation, the therapist must be able to *analyze* activities. To improve subnormal abilities and capacities, the occupation must challenge those abilities and capacities and continue to do so as the patient improves. The therapist controls the challenge by *grading* the activity along particular therapeutic continua and/or by *adapting* the methodology. To enable performance of occupation-as-end, when the patient's impairments prevent usual engagement in the occupation, therapists adapt activities, tools, or context/environment. This chapter instructs on how to select, analyze, grade, and adapt occupation.

SELECTION AND GRADATION

The therapist skilled in activity analysis can match the patient's abilities with activities and tasks the patient needs or wants to do (occupation-as-end) and select the most appropriate activity for remediation from those that are available and are of interest to the patient (occupation-as-means).

Selection of Occupation-As-End

Occupations-as-end are activities and tasks that constitute the patient's life roles. The patient and therapist identify key tasks and activities that would enable the patient to engage in the role. Through activity analysis, the therapist matches the particular patient's capabilities to the demand level of each activity. The comparison between **task demands** within the usual environment and the patient's capabilities determines whether the patient will be able to do the activity independently, with adaptation, or not at all. A person feels best when engaging in activity if his or her skills match the situational challenges posed by the activity and the challenge of the activity matches the person's skills—called "flow" by Csikszentmihalyi (1990; Moneta & Csikszentmihalyi, 1996).

Selection and Gradation of Occupation-As-Means

An activity that is to be used to restore one or more abilities or capacities must challenge the patient's level of ability so that, through effort and/or practice, the patient improves

RESOURCE 13-1

Additional Sources of Information Concerning Activity Analysis

Harnish, S. (2001). Gardening for life: Adaptive techniques and tools. *OT PRACTICE, 6,* 12–15. A compilation of adapted techniques and tools to enable gardening.

Fecko, A., Errico, P., & Jacobs, K. (2004). Everyday ergonomics for therapists. *OT PRACTICE, 9,* 16–18. A detailed list of ergonomic considerations for everyday life.

Lyons, A., Phipps, S. C., & Berro, M. (2004). Using occupation in the clinic. *OT PRACTICE, 9,* 11–15. Description of one facility's readoption of a focus on occupation. Excellent case example.

Walters, L. (2001). One-hand typing: Adapt the technology or the client? *OT PRACTICE, 6,* 20–21.

Sorenson, V., Ingvaldsen, R. P., & Whiting, H. T. (2001). The application of co-ordination dynamics to the analysis of discrete movements using table-tennis as a paradigm skill. *Biological Cybernetics, 85,* 27–38.

(see Definition 13-1). Some specific characteristics for the goals commonly addressed by occupational therapists who treat persons with physical disabilities are listed here and are summarized in Procedures for Practice 13-1. The dimensions along which the activity is to be graded are also listed. When more than one dimension is listed, the therapist should be careful to grade the changes one dimension at a time so that the patient has more of a chance at success. The best activity for remediation is one that intrinsically demands the exact response that has been determined to need improvement and that allows incremental gradations starting where the patient can be successful. Contrived methods of doing an ordinary activity to make it therapeutic may diminish the value of the activity in the eyes of the patient. Contrived methods also require the patient constantly to focus directly on the process rather than the goal of the activity, undermining the therapeutic value.

CLINICAL REASONING IN OCCUPATIONAL THERAPY PRACTICE

Selecting and Adapting Occupation-As-End

Mrs. B. is experiencing increased occupational dysfunction secondary to degenerative joint disease. One of Mrs. B.'s goals is to resume gardening. Given her abilities and capacities, as described in the Case Example in Chapter 5, what key factors must pertain to gardening activities to enable participation? How could these key factors be implemented?

DEFINITION 13-1

Characteristics of Therapeutic Occupation

Generally, activities should:

- Have the necessary inherent characteristics to evoke the desired response
- Allow gradation of response to progress the patient to the next higher level of function
- Be within the patient's capabilities
- Be meaningful to the person
- Be as repetitive as required to evoke the therapeutic benefit

To Retrain Sensory Awareness and/or Discrimination

The activity must provide components that offer a variety of textures, shapes, and sizes, graded from large, distinct, common shapes to small, less common shapes with less distinct differences between them. The texture of the various objects should be graded from diverse coarse materials to similar smooth materials. The patient and the therapist must also involve themselves in a teaching–relearning interactive experience in which the characteristics of the objects are discussed and correct identification by touch is rewarded.

To Decrease Hypersensitivity

The activity should involve objects or media whose textures can be graded from those that the patient perceives to be least noxious to textures perceived to be tolerably noxious. Another plan grades textures and objects from soft to hard to rough and grades the contact with the objects from touching them to rubbing them to tapping them.

CLINICAL REASONING IN OCCUPATIONAL THERAPY PRACTICE

Selecting and Grading Occupation-as-Means

Mrs. B., who is described in Chapter 5, has gardening as one of her self-enhancement goals. Currently she is experiencing weakness of her dominant upper extremity, low endurance (fatigue), and pain that interfere with achieving this goal. Although she could engage in some gardening activities using adaptations to the tools, method, and context, she could engage in more activities with less adaptation if her impairments were improved. What key factors must the occupation-as-means offer to improve these impairments? What occupation-as-means could you offer to Mrs. B. to implement this treatment? How could this activity be graded as she improves?

PROCEDURES FOR PRACTICE 13-1

Selecting and Grading Therapeutic Occupation-As-Means

Remediation Goal	Key Factors of the Activity
To retrain sensory awareness or discrimination	Offer various textures, sizes, shapes. Grade from diverse, coarse, large to similar, smooth, small.
To decrease hypersensitivity	Offer various textures and degrees of hardness or softness. Grade from acceptable to barely tolerable.
To reacquire skilled voluntary movement	Require sought-after, goal-directed response; allow feedback. Grade from simple to complex movements.
To improve coordination and dexterity	Require ROM the patient can control. Grade from slow, gross movement involving limited number of joints to fast, precise movement involving a greater number of joints.
To increase passive ROM	Provide controlled stretch or traction. Grade from lesser to greater ROM.
To increase strength	Require movement or holding against resistance. Grade from lesser to greater resistance or from slow to fast movement.
To improve cardiopulmonary endurance	Use activities rated at the patient's current MET level. Grade by increasing duration, frequency, then intensity (METs).
To improve muscular endurance	Require movement or holding against 50% or less of maximal strength. Grade by increasing repetitions or duration.
To decrease edema	Allow use of the extremity in an elevated position and require isotonic contraction.
To improve problem solving	Require performance at the outside edge of the patient's current skill. Grade from simple (one step) to complex (multiple steps) and from concrete to abstract.

To Relearn Skilled Voluntary Movement

Organization of voluntary movement depends both on the unique problem or goal and the **constraints** operating at a given time (Jordan & Newell, 2004; Newell, 1986). The activity must have a clear goal or purpose, demand the sought-after movement or movements, and offer opportunity to self-monitor success (feedback). The contextual and task constraints should support natural responses. Grading should provide increasingly more difficult motor challenges (e.g., moving the body in various directions, moving the limbs in various directions, isolated movement of particular joints, faster movement, more accurate movement in more challenging contexts, or greater number of submovements [Ma & Trombly, 2004]).

Sensorimotor learning requires practice, so opportunities for vast amounts of varied practice should be provided. The activity may provide an opportunity for practice simply through the accomplishment of the intended goal. For example, weaving requires multiple passes of the shuttle to produce the desired product and offers good practice of bilateral horizontal abduction and adduction. For other activities, the goal may be achieved quickly, so practice is sought through repetition of the whole action, as with ironing, polishing silverware, throwing a ball, and other activities of daily living. Variable practice promotes learning. Unvaried (blocked) practice improves performance within a session but does not improve long-term learning. Blocked practice is used to begin to develop a new movement or skill (see Chapter 14).

To Increase Coordination and Dexterity

The activity should allow as much range of motion (ROM) as the patient can control and allow grading from slow, gross motions to precise, fast movements involving greater ROM or action at more joints. At first, if you are grading along the continuum of increasing speed, expect accuracy to suffer. A speed–accuracy trade-off is basic to the organization of the central nervous system (CNS) (Fitts, 1954).

To Increase Active ROM

The activity must require that the part of the body being treated move to its limit repeatedly and be graded, naturally or through adaptations, to demand greater amounts of movement as the patient's limit changes.

To Increase Passive ROM or Elongate Soft Tissue Contracture

The activity must provide controlled stretch or traction to the part being treated and be held at the end of range for several seconds. ***Stretch should be slow and gentle to avoid tearing the tissue.*** Grade from lesser to greater ROM.

To Increase Strength

Stress to muscle tissue increases strength. Stress can be graded by increasing the velocity and/or resistance needed to complete the activity or, for very weak muscles, by increasing the number of repetitions of an isotonic contraction or the amount of time an isometric contraction is held.

To Increase Cardiopulmonary Endurance

The metabolic demand of the activity (**MET** level) should match the patient's status. The demand can be graded by increasing the duration of a task, by increasing the frequency of doing the task, by changing the muscles used in the task (smaller muscles increase metabolic demand), or by increasing the intensity (METs). The metabolic intensities (METs) of 605 physical activities, including activities of daily living and sexual activity, occupation (work), transportation, volunteering, religious activities, and sports and recreational activities, have been measured and reported (Ainsworth et al., 1993, 2000). Some MET levels are listed in Chapter 5.

To Increase Muscular Endurance

The activity must be repetitious over a controlled number of times or period. Resistance should be held to 50% or less of maximal strength.

To Decrease Edema

The activity should entail repetitive isotonic contractions of the muscles in the edematous part. An activity that requires repeated movement of the extremity into an elevated position helps to drain the fluid out of the extremity.

To Improve Perceptual Impairments or Problem-Solving Strategies

The activity should involve varied practice of information processing or perceptual processing at the outside edge of the person's capability. For example, if the person has impaired figure–ground discrimination skill, practice may start with detecting one figure from a plain background and progress through finding multiple figures on a plain background or finding one figure in more complex backgrounds until the person has developed the level of functional ability he or she requires (e.g., able to find the scissors in a kitchen "junk" drawer). Gradation is along a continuum of increasing complexity (more stimuli).

If the person has impaired problem-solving skills, practice may start with concrete problems involving objects that the person can see and touch, such as the problem of getting soup out of a can, with can, manual can opener, and electrical can opener at hand. The patient figures out that he or she must open the can to get the soup, selects a can opener, and figures out through exploration how to use the can opener. Therapy may proceed to a higher level of abstraction by asking the person to figure out how many pills he or she needs for the week if he or she should take one (or two or more) pill(s) every day. The pill bottle, calendar, and weekly pill minder container are present. The patient may solve the problem in one of several ways: using arithmetic (unlikely, since the patient is in treatment for cognitive deficits); using a calendar, taking out the pill or pills for each day and lining them up on the calendar and counting them; or putting a pill in each compartment of the pill minder and then counting them.

Gradation is along a continuum of concrete to abstract and few objects or ideas to multiple objects or ideas. See Chapters 28 and 29 for suggestions for particular impairments.

ANALYSIS

Activity analysis, or **task analysis**, is a fundamental skill of occupational therapists. Occupational therapists analyze an activity because they want to know (1) whether the patient, given certain abilities, can be expected to do the activity or (2) whether the activity can challenge latent abilities or capacities and thereby improve these. Through activity analysis, one gains an appreciation of the activity's components and characteristics (Greene, 1990).

Activity analysis developed from industrial time-and-motion study methods. Military occupational therapists applied these methods to rehabilitation of injured soldiers during World War I (Creighton, 1992) at the suggestion of

CLINICAL REASONING IN OCCUPATIONAL THERAPY PRACTICE

Activity Analysis

Analyze planting tulip bulbs in a raised garden area according to the format in Procedures for Practice 13-2 and the example in Procedures for Practice 13-3.

Context: The garden measures 10 feet by 18 inches and is 2 feet above ground level. It is surrounded by a stone wall. The dirt is well cultivated. There are no other plants in the garden at this time. No squirrels live in the vicinity, so the gardener does not have to treat the bulbs or cover the garden with wire.

The gardener sits on a rolling garden stool so that, when seated, the top of the garden is equal to the gardener's mid-chest level.

Discuss your analysis with your classmates and professor. If you disagree, determine why and clarify your analysis.

Gilbreth and Gilbreth (1920), industrial engineers who observed injured soldiers in military hospitals. Gilbreth (1911) listed these steps for analyzing a task: "(1) Reduce. . .practice to writing; (2) enumerate motions used; (3) enumerate variables which affect each motion" (p. 5). Variables considered were characteristics of the worker, the surroundings, and the motion. This method has been used by occupational therapists for many years when focusing the analysis on the activity. Other methods of occupational analyses that focus on the performance of the patient are Performance Analysis (Fisher, 1998), Ecological Task Analysis (Burton & Davis, 1996; Davis & Burton, 1991), and Dynamic Performance Analysis (Polatajko, Mandich, & Martini, 2000). These analyses require extensive training and skill. Both activity and performance analyses entail unnesting the component tasks and activities that constitute the occupation and determining what abilities, skills, and capacities are needed to do the specified activity or that may improve if the person does the activity (Mayer, Keating, & Rapp, 1986; Trombly, 1995). The activity-focused analysis is presented in this chapter because it demonstrates the process to the inexperienced activity analyst, with the expectation that therapists will continue to educate themselves concerning this important therapeutic skill.

Analyzing for the abilities and capacities required to carry out the activity presupposes that activities have reliably identifiable inherent therapeutic qualities. This belief is stated in a position paper of the American Occupational Therapy Association (1995): "Whether physical or mental in nature, the behaviors necessary for completion of tasks in daily occupations can be analyzed according to specific components related to moving, perceiving, thinking, and feeling" (p. 1015). Although tasks and activities require particular performance skills, abilities, and capacities, identification of these (activity analysis) is a high-level skill that requires practice under supervision. A survey of 120 experienced therapists indicated that there was limited consensus on which performance skills, abilities, or capacities were required by particular activities (Tsai, 1994). Neistadt et al. (1993) also reported discrepancies among therapists in identifying components of common activities. Research on activity analysis and greater emphasis on activity analysis in educational programs are needed.

Activity-Focused Analysis

Using an analytical approach, the therapist examines an activity to determine its components and the level of capability demanded. The outcome can be used to select activities for remediation or to match a particular person's skills with the demands of the task.

All analyses should occur within some conceptual framework to give them direction, coherence, and meaning (Mosey, 1981). For example, planting a tulip bulb in a plant pot can be analyzed from various frames of reference. The biomechanical approach prompts the therapist to examine the physical aspects, such as grasp and ROM, whereas the cognitive-perceptual approach examines the activity according to its cognitive or perceptual demands. The Model of Human Occupation might focus the therapist's attention on how this planting activity may meet the patient's nurturing needs and values.

Whereas biomechanical analysis observes joint ROM and estimates muscle contraction used to carry out the activity based on knowledge of anatomy and kinesiology, **electromyographic** (EMG) and **kinematic** research indicates that this type of analysis may not be wholly valid because of individual differences in muscle action and differences in movement strategies secondary to learning, maturation, injury, and perception of goal (Illyes & Kiss, 2005; Jordan & Newell, 2004; Kelly et al., 2005; Trombly & Quintana, 1983) that are not detectable by an observer without instrumentation. Each person's CNS plans movement to accomplish the goal with the resources the person has. Reaching for a glass of milk on the table may or may not activate the anterior deltoid. If that muscle is weak, the patient may accomplish the goal by substituting other muscles or strategies, such as turning sidewise to the table to make use of the stronger middle deltoid to reach the glass. The substitutions listed in the muscle testing section of Chapter 5 are common ways people accomplish the movement goal when the prime mover is weak. The idea that doing a certain activity will always exercise a certain weak muscle may be naive. If it is essential that a particular muscle of a particular patient be contracting to a certain level of activity, as may be the case in tendon transfer rehabilitation, it is best to monitor the muscle directly using EMG biofeedback as the patient does the activity (Trombly & Cole, 1979; Trombly & Quintana, 1983).

On average, certain motions and muscle actions are more probable than others and, therefore, an analysis can be based on observation if the therapist realizes that actual performance of a particular patient must be verified and not assumed. As instrumentation to measure human movement is too complex to be used clinically at this time, by default, the traditional biomechanical activity analysis continues to be the method used by practicing therapists and is described here (Procedures for Practice 13-2 and 13-3).

The therapist begins the biomechanical analysis by stating the goal (purpose) and by identifying the task demands, that is, the constraints that will impinge on performance. Some constraints to be considered are the size and type of tools, placement of the selected tools and equipment in relation to the patient, the speed at which the activity is to be accomplished, the complexity of the task, and the context in which it will be carried out. Changes in any of these variables change the task demands and require a different analysis. The prerequisite abilities and capacities

PROCEDURES FOR PRACTICE 13-2

Activity-Focused Analysis

1. Name the activity goal.
2. Describe the task demands:
   - Task constraints: How are the person and materials positioned, especially in relation to one another?
   - Task constraints: What utensils/tools/materials are normally used to do this activity?
   - Environmental constraints: Where is this activity usually carried out?
   - Contextual constraints: Does this activity or the way it is carried out hold particular meaning for certain cultures or social roles? Is there a time factor involved in carrying out the activity?
3. What capacities and abilities are prerequisite to successful accomplishment of this activity?
4. List the steps of the activity.
5. Describe the biomechanical internal constraints for the most therapeutic or repetitive step.

Motions	ROM	Primary Muscles	Gravity Assists, Resists, No Effect	Minimal Strength Required	Type of Contraction

6. What must be stabilized to enable doing this activity, and how will that stabilization be provided?
7. For which ages is this activity appropriate?
8. What is the estimated MET level of this activity?
9. What precautions must be considered when using this activity in therapy?
10. For which short-term goal or goals is this activity appropriate?
11. How can this activity be graded to improve the following:
    - Strength
    - Active ROM
    - Passive ROM
    - Endurance
    - Coordination and dexterity
    - Edema
    - Perceptual abilities
    - Cognitive skills

for accomplishing the whole activity are identified. If these prerequisite abilities are lacking and the goal is to accomplish the activity (occupation-as-end), then the way the goal is to be accomplished would have to be modified (e.g., if the patient is blind). Alternatively, if the goal is to improve one or more of the required abilities (occupation-as-means), then the activity would be adapted to reduce the demands to just challenge the patient's level of performance.

The first step of an activity analysis is to identify the exact activity. For example, the steps of vacuuming the carpet while standing are listed under no. 4 in Procedures for Practice 13-3. The potential repetitions of each motion are noted. Only the fourth step, pushing the vacuum cleaner back and forth, would be analyzed further if vacuuming were going to be used as occupation-as-means because it is the repetitive, therapeutic aspect of this activity. The other steps occur too infrequently to be therapeutic. Each repetitive step is subdivided into motions. For example, pushing the vacuum back and forth involves shoulder flexion with elbow extension, shoulder extension with elbow flexion, and trunk flexion and extension, although trunk movement may be eliminated, depending on how the person moves in relation to the machine. Wrist stabilization (co-contraction) in extension and cylindrical grasp are also "motions" associated with vacuuming.

The range of each motion is estimated by observing another person or by doing the activity oneself. Each motion is further analyzed to determine which muscle or muscles are likely responsible, based on anatomical, kinesiological, and electromyographical knowledge. Examining the effect of gravity allows estimation of the minimal strength necessary to do the motion. The kind of contraction demanded for each muscle group in each motion is established by definition.

PROCEDURES FOR PRACTICE 13-3

An Example of an Activity-Focused Analysis

1. Name the goal: Vacuuming the hallway carpet using a lightweight vacuum with a 25-foot cord.
2. Describe the task demands:
   - Task constraints: How are the person and materials positioned, especially in relation to one another?
     - The vacuum cleaner is in a closet next to the area to be cleaned.
     - The electrical plug is halfway between the two ends of the hallway, 5 inches from the floor.
     - When vacuuming, the person will be directly behind the machine.
   - Task constraints: What utensils, tools, and materials are normally used to do this activity?
     - A lightweight vacuum cleaner
   - Environmental constraints: Where is this activity usually carried out?
     - The hallway is 30 feet long and 3 feet wide.
     - No furniture is in the way.
     - The carpet is a flat pile.
   - Contextual constraints: Does this activity or how it is carried out hold particular meaning for certain cultures or social roles? Is there a time factor involved in carrying out the activity?
     - The person takes pride in a clean, well-vacuumed home.
     - The person is not willing to switch to a lighter, nonmotorized carpet sweeper because of the feeling that it doesn't do a proper job.
     - There is no limiting time factor involved in the activity under normal circumstances.
3. What capacities and abilities are prerequisite to successful accomplishment of this activity?
   - Standing balance
   - Ability to bend over and straighten up
   - Ability to grasp
   - Ability to walk forward and backward on carpeting
   - Ability to move dominant arm against gravity and moderate resistance
   - Vision[1]
4. List the steps.
   1. Get the vacuum cleaner from the closet.
   2. Unwind the cord.
   3. Plug cord into wall socket and turn vacuum cleaner on.
   4. Push the vacuum cleaner back and forth.
   5. Unplug it and wind the cord.
   6. Return the vacuum cleaner to the closet.
5. Describe the biomechanical internal constraints for pushing the vacuum back and forth (step #4).

Motions	ROM (degrees), Distances	Primary Muscles	Gravity Assists, Resists, No Effect	Minimal Strength Required	Type of Contraction
Shoulder flexion	0–75	Anterior deltoid, coracobrachialis, pectoralis major	Resists	4− to 4	Concentric
Elbow extension	90–0	Triceps	Assists	4− to 4	Concentric
Scapular protraction	1.5 in	Serratus anterior	No effect	4− to 4	Concentric
Shoulder extension	0–45	Posterior deltoid	Assists	4− to 4	Concentric
		Latissimus dorsi	No effect		
		Teres major	Resists		
Elbow flexion	90–120	Biceps, brachialis	Resists	4− to 4	Concentric
Scapular retraction	1.5 in	Middle trapezius	No effect	4− to 4	Concentric
Cylindrical grasp		Finger flexors, finger extensors, interossei	No effect	4− to 4	Isometric
Wrist stabilize		All wrist muscles	No effect	4− to 4	Isometric
Trunk flexion	0–30	Back extensors	Assists	3+ to 4−	Eccentric
Trunk extension	30–0	Back extensors	Resists	4− to 4	Concentric

[1]The blind person needs to use adaptive methods for knowing which sections of the carpet have been cleaned and which have not.

PROCEDURES FOR PRACTICE 13-3 *(continued)*

6. What must be stabilized to enable doing this activity, and how will that stabilization be provided?
   - Nothing
7. For which ages is this activity appropriate?
   - 18+ years primarily
   - 10–17 years secondarily
8. What is the estimated MET level of this activity?
   - 2–3 METs
9. What precautions must be considered when using this activity in therapy?
   - If standing balance and bending over are not well developed, the patient must be guarded.
   - A patient who is apt to lose balance walking on carpet must be guarded.
   - A patient who has low back pain must be taught to do the activity without bending forward.
   - A patient with low endurance needs to rest periodically.
10. For which short-term goal or goals is this activity appropriate?
    - Strengthening of upper extremity musculature
    - Developing dynamic standing balance
    - Improving grip strength
    - Improving central and peripheral endurance
    - Learning proper back mechanics
11. How can this activity be graded to improve the following?
    - Strength
      - Heavier vacuum cleaner
      - Thicker carpet
    - Active ROM
      - At limit
    - Passive ROM
      - Not applicable
    - Endurance
      - Increase amount of carpeting vacuumed before resting
    - Coordination, dexterity
      - Place furniture in the area so patient has to change directions of the vacuum to go around the obstacles
    - Edema
      - Not applicable
    - Improve perceptual abilities (examples)
      - Change the color of the "dirt" on the carpet, e.g., spread bits to be vacuumed either in contrasting colors or closer to the color of the carpet (figure–ground)
      - Put objects in the way for the person to figure out how to move around them (spatial relations)
    - Improve cognitive skills
      - Not applicable

Activities selected to restore motor function must also take into account the person's cognitive and perceptual abilities, emotional status, cultural background, and interests. Some cognitive aspects of the activity to be considered include the number and complexity of the steps involved in doing the activity, the requirements for organizing and sequencing of the steps or stimuli, and the amount of concentration and memory required. Some perceptual factors to be considered are whether the activity requires the patient to distinguish figure from ground, determine position in space, construct a two- or three-dimensional object, or follow verbal or spatial directions. Other cognitive-perceptual considerations are found in Chapters 28 and 29. Some psychosocial aspects of an activity that may be important to patients include whether the activity must be done alone or in a group, the length of time required to complete the activity, whether fine detailed work or large expansive movements are involved, how easily errors can be corrected, the value of the activity from the person's particular cultural and social background, and the likelihood of producing a satisfying outcome.

Other methods of analysis of activities have been published. Gentile (1987) has provided a detailed taxonomy of task analysis to be used for evaluation and selection of functionally relevant activities. The taxonomy is related to the learning of motor tasks. Her taxonomy is briefly described here, although the reader should see the original material for a complete description and rationale. The taxonomy consists of 16 categories comprised of movement types and environmental regulatory constraints. The dimensions are presented separately in Definition 13-2 for the sake of clarity, but they are meant to be combined. The easiest tasks are repetitive ones done in a stationary environment with the body in a stable position, such as sitting and brushing one's hair. Tasks are graded by changing one at a time the various parameters (e.g., environmental regulatory conditions, differences in performance between trials, body orientation, manipulation demands). The

DEFINITION 13-2

Examples of Tasks Described According to the Taxonomy of Gentile

Environmental Regulatory Dimension		
Environmental Regulatory Conditions During Performance	**No Differences in Performance Between Trials**	**Differences in Performance Between Trials**
Stationary: the objects people, and/or apparatus do not move	**Closed tasks** Climbing stairs at home Brushing teeth Unlocking the front door Turning on the bedroom light	Tasks in which objects are different but stationary during performance: Walking on different surfaces Drinking from mugs, glasses, cups Putting on shirt, sweater
Motion: the objects, people, and/or apparatus move	Tasks in which objects move consistently over repeated encounters: Stepping onto an escalator Lifting luggage from the conveyer belt at the airport Moving through a revolving door	**Open Tasks** Propelling a wheelchair down a crowded hall Catching a ball Carrying a wiggling child
Movement Type Dimension		
Body Orientation	**No Manipulation**	**Manipulation**
Stability: body is positioned in one place	Body stability: Sit Stand Lean on table	Body stability plus manipulation: Hold object while standing Reach for hairbrush while sitting Keyboard sitting at computer
Transport: body is moving through space	Body transport: Walk Run Propel wheelchair	Body transport plus manipulation: Run to catch a ball Drive an automobile Dial phone while walking

Adapted with permission from Gentile, A. M., Higgins, J. R., Miller, E. A., & Rosen, B. (1975). Structure of motor tasks. In *Mouvement Actes du 7e Symposium Canadien en Appentissage Psycho-motor et Psychologie du Sport* (pp. 11–28). Quebec, Canada (out of print). Also printed in Gentile, A. (1987). Skill acquisition: Action, movement and neuromotor processes. In J. H. Carr, R. B. Shepherd, J. Gordon, A. M. Gentile, & J. M. Held (Eds.), *Movement science: Foundations for physical therapy in rehabilitation* (pp. 93–154). Rockville, MD: Aspen Systems.

most demanding tasks are those done in an environment that changes with the performance, with requirements that change between trials, and with the body in motion while manipulating an object, such as playing basketball.

Neistadt et al. (1993) published a model for analyzing activities in relation to cognitive and perceptual demands. Watson and Wilson (2003) published a task-analysis form based on the American Occupational Therapy Association's Occupational Therapy Practice Framework.

Some therapists keep files of activity analyses, which they adapt to particular patients, while others prefer to analyze specifically for a particular patient in a particular context. Some activity analyses have been published: Hi-Q game (Neistadt et al., 1993); macramé (Chandani & Hill, 1990); planting a small garden (Nelson, 1988); using a computer for skill development, education, and prevocational training (Okoye, 1993); hand activities (Trombly & Cole, 1979); donning a sock (Greene, 1990); and bilateral inclined sanding (Spaulding & Robinson, 1984).

Performance-Focused Analysis

Using an analytic approach, the therapist observes the patient's performance of role-related occupations. Figure 13-1 and Procedures for Practice 13-4 depict analysis of role performance using the Occupational Functioning Model as the basis (Trombly, 1993). The first step is to determine whether the person is accomplishing the role as he or she wants, needs, or expects to. If not, the patient identifies the tasks and activities within the role that are

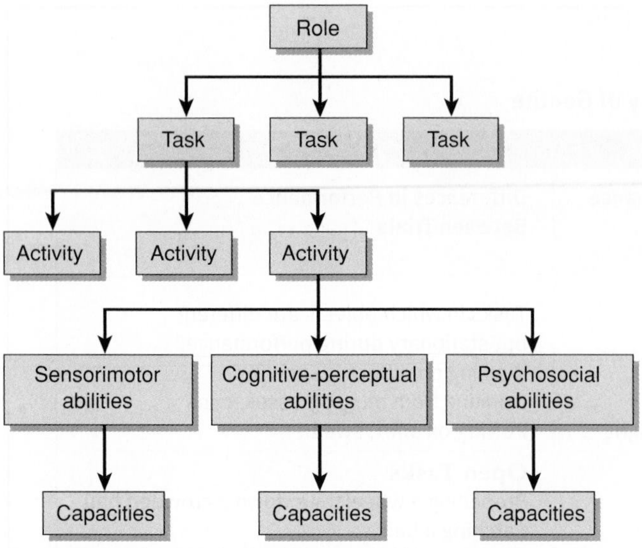

Figure 13-1 Performance-focused analysis according to the Occupational Performance Model. One role is composed of several tasks. Each task consists of several activities. Each activity depends on varying degrees of sensorimotor, cognitive-perceptual, and psychosocial abilities. Those abilities depend on supporting capacities. The performance-focused analysis examines these from the top down by observing the patient. When the patient has difficulty performing, the therapist examines the next lower levels and/or the environment as possible constraints to the performance.

not being accomplished to criterion. Observing the person's attempt gives the therapist clues about which abilities and capacities may need further evaluation and treatment. This is the assessment described in Chapter 1. It is similar to the Dynamic Performance Analysis (DPA) proposed by Polatajko, Mandich, and Martini (2000). The DPA is described as a performance-based dynamic iterative process of analysis that is carried out as the client performs an occupation. The steps are: (1) establish whole-task performer prerequisites (motivation and knowledge of the task), (2) analyze observed performance to identify where the patient demonstrates performance difficulties, and (3) establish the source of the difficulties within the relationship between client abilities and the environmental or occupational supports or demands. Analysis according to the Occupational Functioning Model is also similar to the analysis based on the Occupational Therapy Practice Framework (Watson & Wilson, 2003) but is less complicated.

The Performance Analysis proposed by Fisher (1998) involves observational evaluation of the "transaction between the client and the environment as the client performs a task that is familiar, meaningful, purposeful and relevant" (p. 517). To do this, Fisher uses a standardized performance analysis, the *Assessment of Motor and Process Skills* (*AMPS*) (Fisher, 1997; Merritt & Fisher, 2003), although it can also be done by informal observation. The quality of performance, not the person's underlying capacities, is graded, although the capacities are considered when interpreting the outcome and planning treatment.

The Ecological Task Analysis (ETA) is based on ideas of the dynamical systems theory of movement and Gibson's (1977) theory of affordances (Burton & Davis, 1996; Davis and Burton, 1991). This analysis examines the interacting constraints (limitations and enablers) of performer, environment, and task as the occupation is undertaken. The ETA is based on the premise that there are many solutions to a particular task, determined by the unique interaction of performer and environment with the goal or intent of the action. The steps are as follows. (1) The therapist selects and establishes the task goal, structures the physical and social environments, and provides verbal and other cues to allow for an understanding of the task goal by the patient. (2) The patient practices the task, with the therapist allowing the patient to choose movement solutions. (3) The therapist manipulates the performer, environment, or task variables to find the optimal performance. The therapist identifies specific contexts in which the person can always (sometimes, never) accomplish the task and discovers by perturbation (e.g, increase speed, force, or other potentially controlling variable) the importance of performer or environmental variables on the performance of the task or movement. (4) The therapist provides direct instructions of other possibilities of movement solutions. See Chapter 22 for application of this analysis and teaching process.

PROCEDURES FOR PRACTICE 13-4

Performance-Focused Analysis According to the Occupational Functioning Model

1. Name the role.
2. List the tasks the person identifies as important to this role.
3. List the activities the person identifies as part of a key task.
4. Observe the person performing one of the activities.
5. If the person is able to perform the activity, observe another of the activities. When the person is unable to do an activity, one of two directions can be taken:
   - Teach the person adapted methods to accomplish the activity
   - Remediate impaired abilities and capacities to enable performance
5. If remediation is chosen, analyze what ability limitations are interfering with performance.
7. After identifying particular ability limitations, measure those abilities to confirm the limitation.
8. If the ability is significantly limited, analyze what deficit capacities are causing that limitation.
9. Measure those capacities. Treat when verified.

ADAPTATION

Activity adaptation is the process of modifying an activity of daily living, craft, game, sport, or other occupation to enable performance, accomplish a therapeutic goal, or prevent cumulative trauma injury (Definition 13-3). Although we may like to think that occupational therapists devised this process, actually Gilbreth devised it in the early 1900s (Creighton, 1992, 1993). He proposed adapting activity to suit the anatomy of workers to make work more efficient (Gilbreth, 1911).

There are four reasons to adapt an activity in the treatment of the physically disabled. One is to modify the activity to make it therapeutic when ordinarily it would not be so. Many examples of this can be seen in occupational therapy clinics. For example, in wall checkers, the board is mounted on the wall and has pegs at each square to hold the checkers. Tic-tac-toe can be adapted similarly by drawing the grid on the wall and using Velcro-backed Xs and Os or Xs and Os drawn on sticky notes (Fig. 13-2).

The second reason for adaptation is to graduate the exercise offered by the activity along therapeutic continua to accomplish goals. Grading of activity for this purpose is an original principle of occupational therapy (Creighton, 1993). For example, to increase coordination, the activity must be graded along a continuum from gross, coarse movement to fine, accurate movement. Checkers and other board games lend themselves easily to such gradations. For example, checkerboards or cribbage boards and the pieces can be changed in size so that the aficionado can continue a favorite game while continuing to benefit therapeutically (Fig. 13-3, A & B).

The third reason for adapting activities is to enable a person with physical impairments to do an activity or task he or she would be unable to do otherwise. For example, after having a stroke that causes paresis of one upper limb, a patient can learn a new method of putting on a shirt that requires only one hand. Or the environment in which a favorite activity was accomplished can be modified to allow engagement. For example, a gardener who undergoes bilateral lower extremity amputation because of diabetes can continue to garden from a wheelchair if the beds are raised (Harnish, 2001). Figures 13-4 and 13-5 show other examples of contextual adaptation to enable performance. See Chapters 30 to 34 for ways to compensate for particular disabilities to enable role performance.

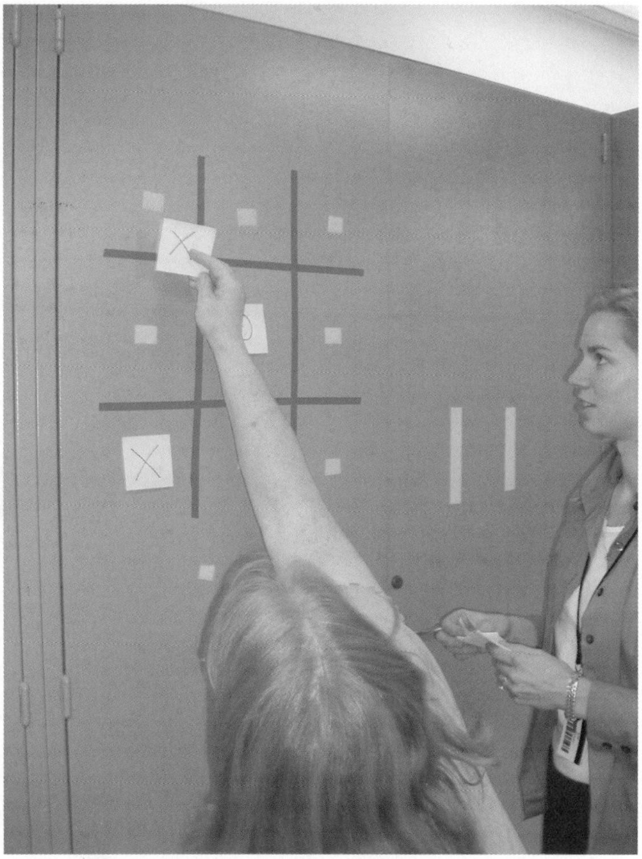

Figure 13-2 Therapist and patient playing tic-tac-toe in an adapted way that requires reaching up.

The fourth reason for adapting activities, especially work activities that are engaged in for long periods of time, is to prevent cumulative trauma injury. Examples of such adaptation are changing the table height to reduce strain on the back or upper extremities or doing the work task while seated to reduce stress on the low back.

As with all therapeutic techniques, it is vital for the patient to understand the reason why an activity is adapted (Peloquin, 1988). Ways to modify activities are described here and summarized in Procedures for Practice 13-5.

DEFINITION 13-3

Characteristics of a Good Adaptation

- Accomplishes the specific goal
- Does not encourage or require odd movements or postures
- Is not dangerous to the patient
- Intrinsically demands a certain response that the patient does not have to concentrate on
- Does not demean the patient; some contrived adaptations seem ridiculous to the patient and thus are embarrassing

Positioning the Task Relative to the Person

The position of the person relative to the work to be done dictates the movement demanded by the activity, and

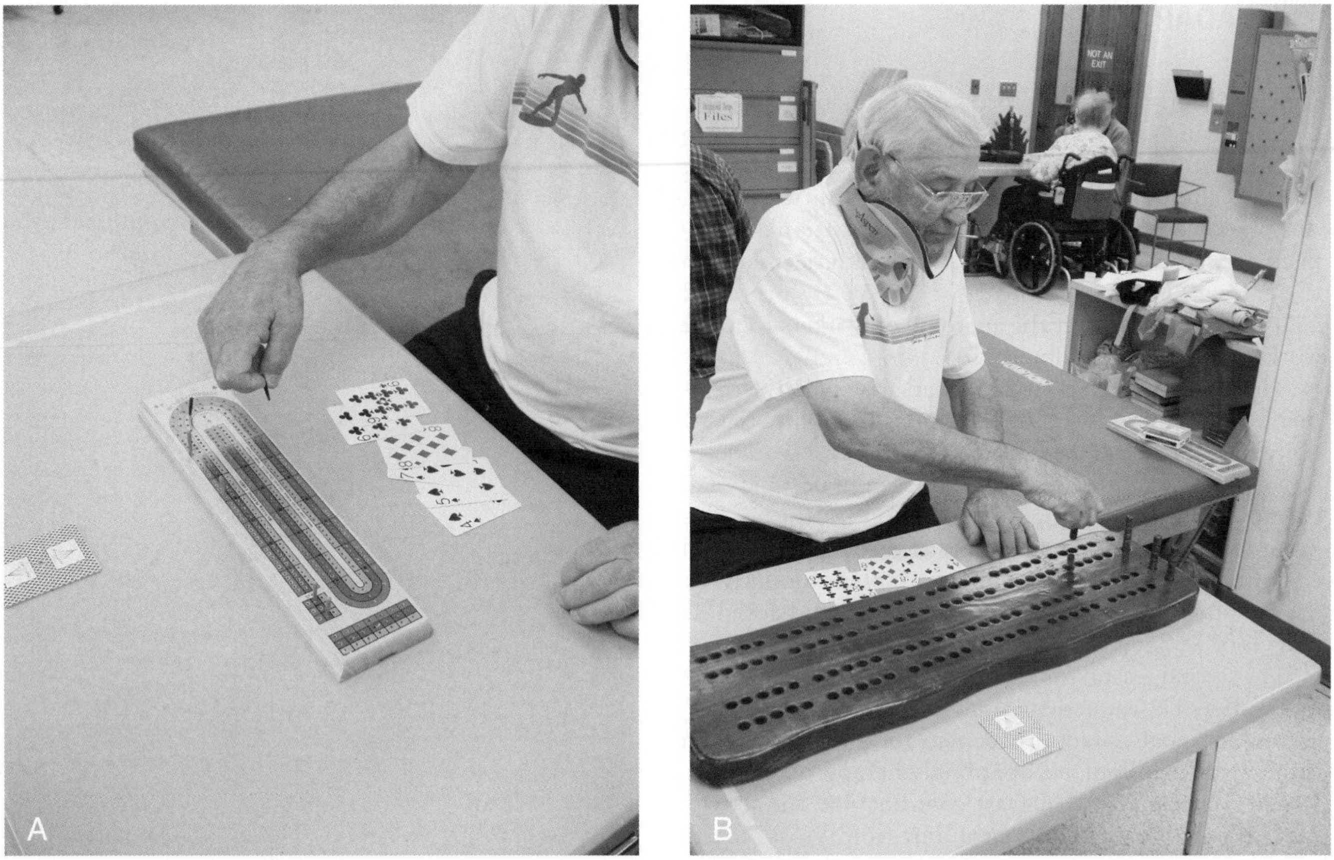

Figure 13-3 **A.** Standard-sized cribbage board demands fine coordination. **B.** Enlarged cribbage board and pegs allow a person with deficient fine coordination to play (occupation-as-end) or demand greater range of motion of reaching (occupation-as-means).

therefore, which muscle groups are likely to be used (McGrain & Hague, 1987). Poor positioning of work equipment relative to the size of the person may result in musculoskeletal discomfort or repeated stress injuries (Sung et al., 2003). Adaptation by positioning refers to changes in incline of work surface, height of work surface, location of work equipment, or placement of pieces to be added to the project.

Activities that are usually done on a flat surface, such as finger painting, board games, and sanding wood, can be made more or less resistive by changing the incline of the surface. For example, if the surface is inclined down and away from the patient, resistance is given to shoulder extension and elbow flexion. If the incline is up and toward the patient, resistance is given to shoulder flexion and elbow extension.

The standard horizontal work surface itself can be raised or lowered to make demands on certain muscle groups or to alter the effect of gravity. For example, a table raised to axilla height allows flexion and extension of the elbow on a gravity-eliminated plane and may enable a person with grade 3+ muscles to eat independently.

Placing items, such as nails, mosaic tiles, pieces of yarn, beads, darts, bean bags, and paint brushes, in various locations changes the motion required to reach them when performing the activity in an otherwise standard manner. Placement may be high enough to encourage shoulder flexion or abduction; lateral to encourage shoulder rotation, trunk rotation, or horizontal motion; or low to encourage trunk flexion or lateral trunk flexion. All of the placements would encourage improvement in dynamic balance (Fig. 13-6).

Arrangement of Objects Relative to Each Other

To grade an activity for increasing perceptual skills (e.g., figure-ground discrimination, unilateral neglect), the arrangement of objects to be used, the printing on a page, and so on can be graded from sparse to dense (i.e., fewer objects or words with space between versus many objects or words with no space between). Putting game pieces on the right side of the game board encourages use of the right hand, while placement on the left encourages use of the left hand. Placement of ingredients on a

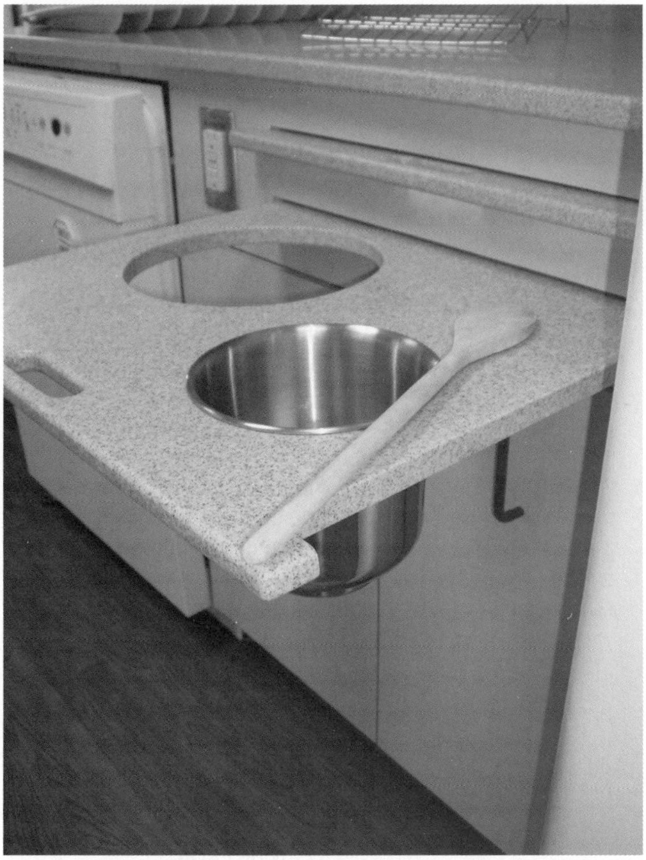

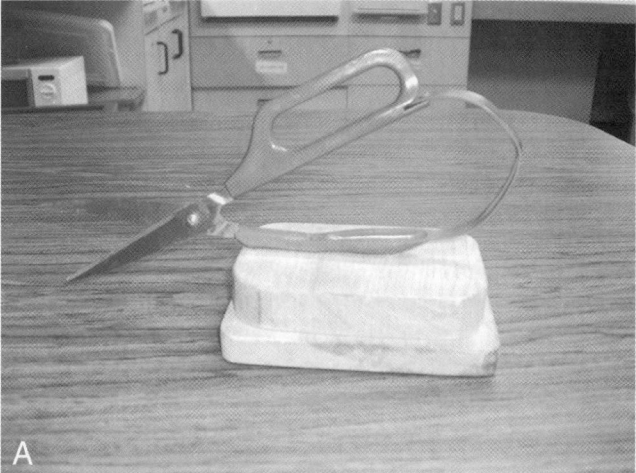

Figure 13-4 A pull-out shelf with holes that accommodate bowls or pots enables a person confined to a wheelchair to cook efficiently.

kitchen counter across the room from the mixing bowl encourages walking in the kitchen that would not occur if all were together. On the other hand, placing all objects needed for a task together reduces the energy required to do the task.

Changing Length of the Lever Arm

The amount of work a muscle or muscle group is doing depends on the resistance. Resistance is determined by the pull of gravity on the limb and the implements the patient is using, which together act as the resistance lever arm. The effect of a given amount of resistance can be altered by lengthening or shortening the resistance arm. The longer the resistance arm, the greater the force required to counterbalance it. The resistance arm can be altered by shortening or lengthening the limb; for example, flexing the knee, which shortens the limb, offers less resistance to hip extension than if the knee were extended. Another example is carrying an object close to the body, which

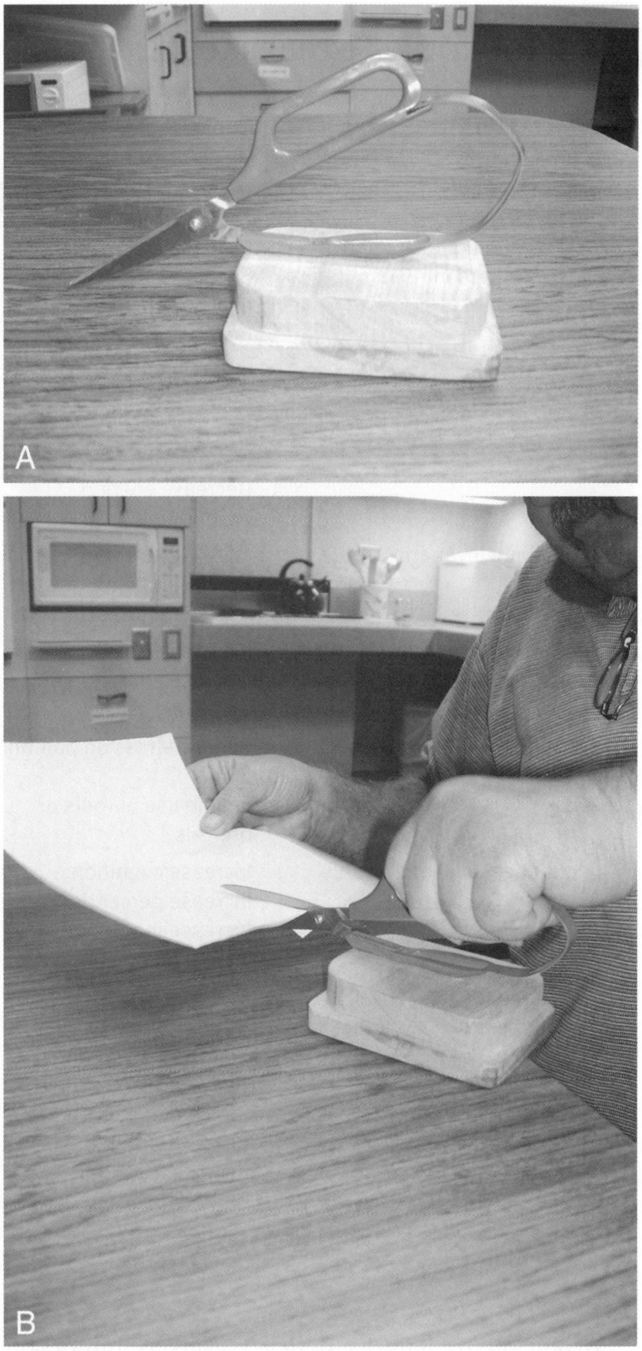

Figure 13-5 **A, B.** Scissors have been stabilized in a wooden block to enable cutting by a person who lacks finger dexterity.

requires less activity of back muscles than if the object is carried at arm's length.

On the other hand, increasing the length of the force lever arm decreases the muscle activity needed to accomplish a task. For example, in Figure 13-7, if the clothespin were adapted to have longer handles, less pinch force would be required to open it the same distance.

PROCEDURES FOR PRACTICE 13-5

Adaptations for Therapeutic Purpose

Adaptation	Therapeutic Purpose	Adaptation	Therapeutic Purpose
Position the task relative to the person	Increase ROM Specify muscles, motions Enable person to do the task	Change color contrast between objects	Improve figure–ground discrimination Enable performance by those with low vision
Arrange objects in relation to others	Improve perceptual responses Require specific movements Decrease energy expenditure	Change method of doing the activity	Enable person to do the task Increase strength Increase ROM Increase coordination, dexterity Increase cognitive-perceptual demands
Change lever arms	Increase strength Reduce strength needed Prevent injuries	Modify tool	Enable the person to do the task Prevent deformity Prevent cumulative trauma disorders
Change materials or texture of materials	Increase strength Increase coordination Challenge sensory system		
Padding handles of tools	Reduce stress on painful joints Enable use of tools or utensils	Add weights	Increase strength Reduce incoordinated movements Provide PROM
Change level of difficulty	Increase cognition Increase perception Increase motor planning Enable person to do the task	Add springs or rubber bands	Increase strength Reduce incoordinated movements Provide PROM Assist weak muscles
Change the size or shape of objects	Improve dexterity Enable activities, such as feeding, with enlarged handles on utensils Increase strength Increase ROM		

Attention to lengths of lever arms is important not only in adapting an activity to make it more therapeutic but also in adapting utensils and tools used in daily life tasks to enable weak persons to use them (Fig. 13-8). Furthermore, this idea guides workers in methods of lifting and handling on their jobs to avoid musculoskeletal injuries. See illustrations of lever arms in Chapter 21.

Change of Materials or Texture of Materials

Gradation along the strengthening continuum may be accomplished by selection of material by type and also by variations of texture or density to change resistance. Resistance can be changed, for example, by starting a cutting project with tissue paper and then progressing to heavier materials. Metal tooling can be graded for resistance by choosing materials in grades from thin aluminum to thick copper. Sandpaper is graded from extra fine to coarse, and resistance increases as the grade coarsens. Mixing can be graded from making gelatin dessert to scrambled eggs to biscuit batter and so on. If materials are graded in the opposite direction, that is, from heavy to light, the activity demands increased coordination from the patient. Weaving may begin using rug roving and be graded toward fine linen threads as the patient progresses in coordination.

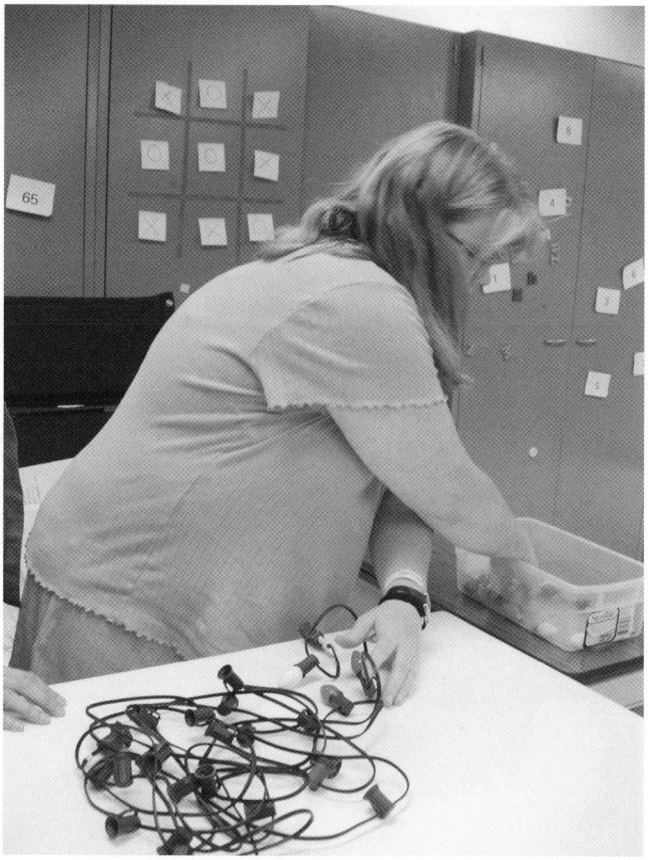

Figure 13-6 Christmas tree lights are placed to the left of a right-handed person to encourage reaching and development of dynamic standing balance.

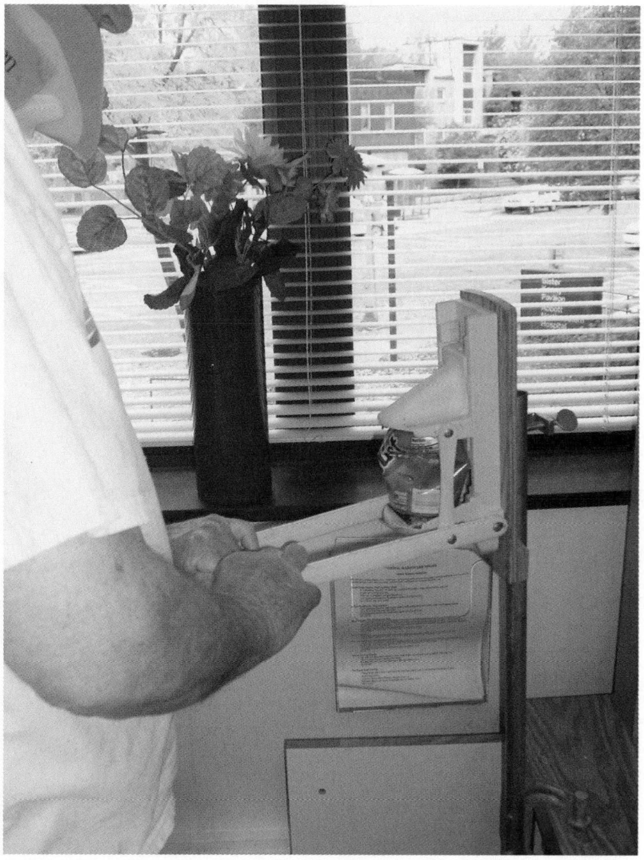

Figure 13-8 A patient who has weak upper extremities is able to crush cans for recycling because the handle (force arm) of the crusher has been elongated.

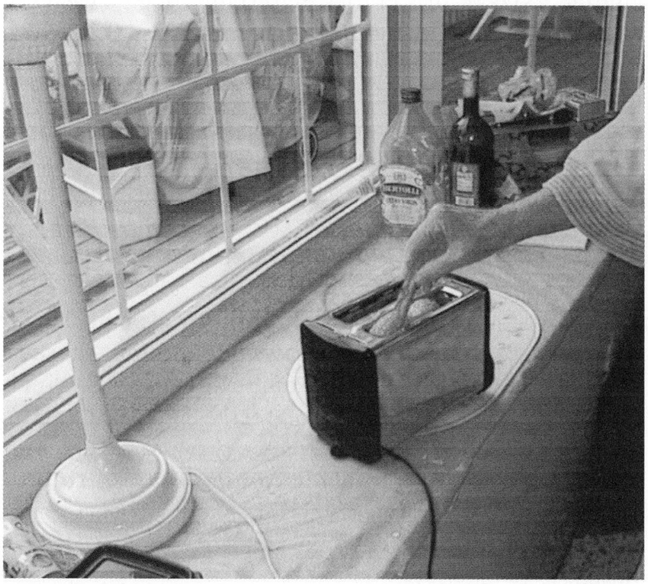

Figure 13-7 Retrieving toast with a spring clothespin.

Cutaneous stimulation changes with the amount of texture of objects or surfaces. By making balls from yarn or terry toweling, carpeting the surfaces the person works on, padding handles with textured material, and so on, the therapist adapts the activity to increase sensory stimulation.

Pad Handles of Tools or Utensils

Padding the handles of utensils or tools with high-density foam or other firm but soft material (Fig. 13-9, A & B) reduces stress on painful finger joints and/or enables persons with poor grip to use the utensil or tool.

Change in Level of Difficulty

Patterns for craft activities, game rules, extent of task (e.g., prepare instant coffee versus espresso), and level of creativity can be downgraded to enable the patient to succeed or upgraded to demand per-

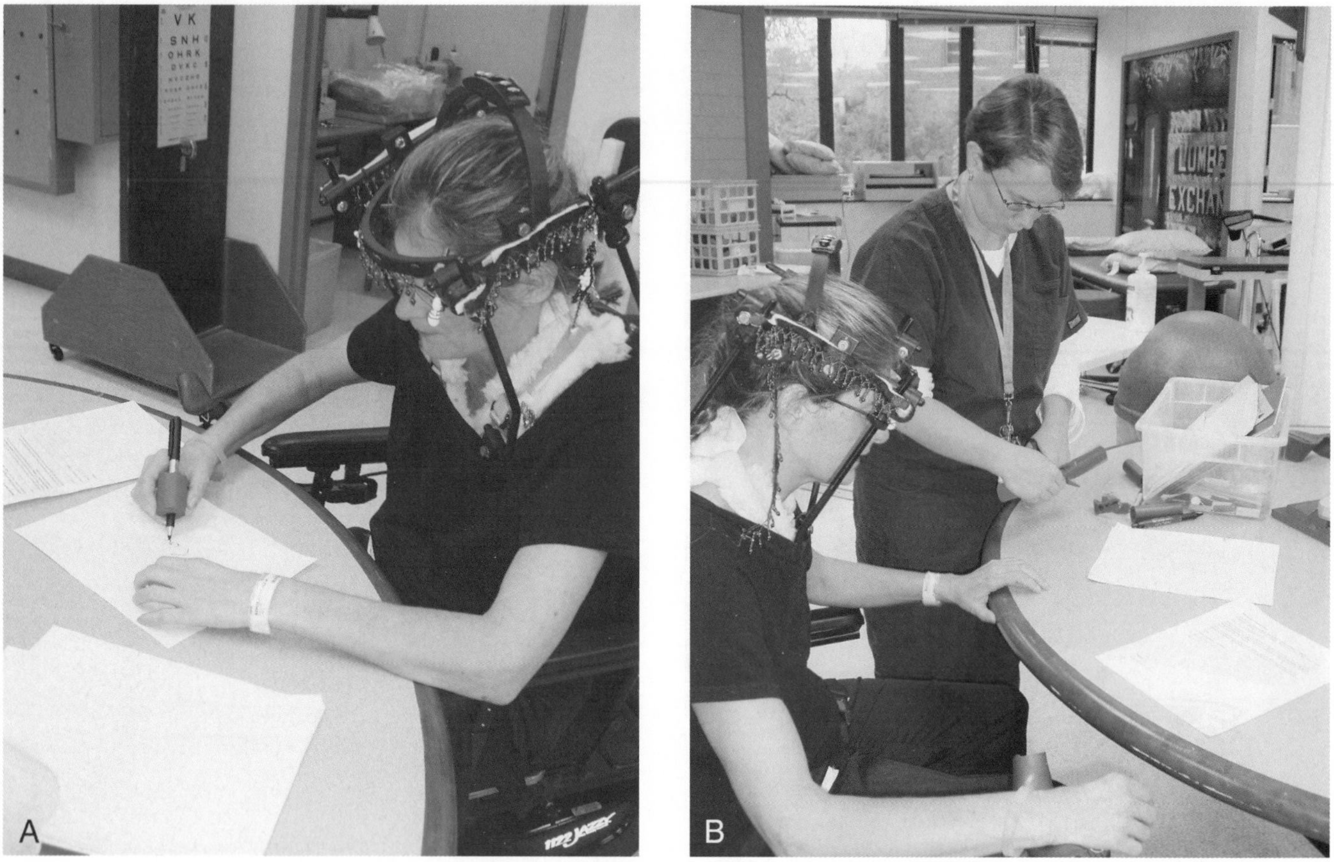

Figure 13-9 **A.** Writing using a built-up handle. **B.** Therapist adapting the pen.

formance at higher levels. Changing the difficulty entails changing the number of pieces or the ideas that must be manipulated, changing the problem-solving level from concrete reasoning to abstract reasoning, changing the directions from specific to general, and so on. For example, a patient with traumatic brain injury may be unable to pay the bills if the top of the desk is littered with bills and papers but may be able to manage if one bill is taken out at a time.

Change the Size or Shape of Objects

Playing pieces of board games can vary in size and shape and can therefore offer a therapeutic benefit that the standard objects would not. For example, checkers, which are usually flat pieces approximately 2.5 cm in diameter, can be cylinders, squares, cubes, or spheres; can range in size from tiny to as large as a person's grasp permits; or can have handles attached (Fig. 13-10, A & B).

Reducing the size or changing the shape of the pieces being worked on facilitates the goals of increased dexterity and fine coordination. Therapists creatively change sizes of craft materials (e.g., weaving thread, tiles, paint-by-number guidelines, and ceramic pieces) and recreational materials (e.g., puzzle pieces, chess pieces, and target games) to increase coordination. Tools and utensils can be adapted by changing the length, diameter, or shape of their handles or by adding handles to tools that do not normally have them.

The actual size of the tool can be chosen to offer more or less resistance. For example, saws range in size from small coping saws and hacksaws to large cross-cut and rip saws. Resistance of saws can also be graded by the number of teeth per inch on the blade; the fewer the teeth, the greater the resistance. Woodworking planes vary in size, and the amount of exposed blade can be adjusted to provide resistance. Size of scissors, screwdrivers, stirring spoons, and other tools and utensils can also be varied.

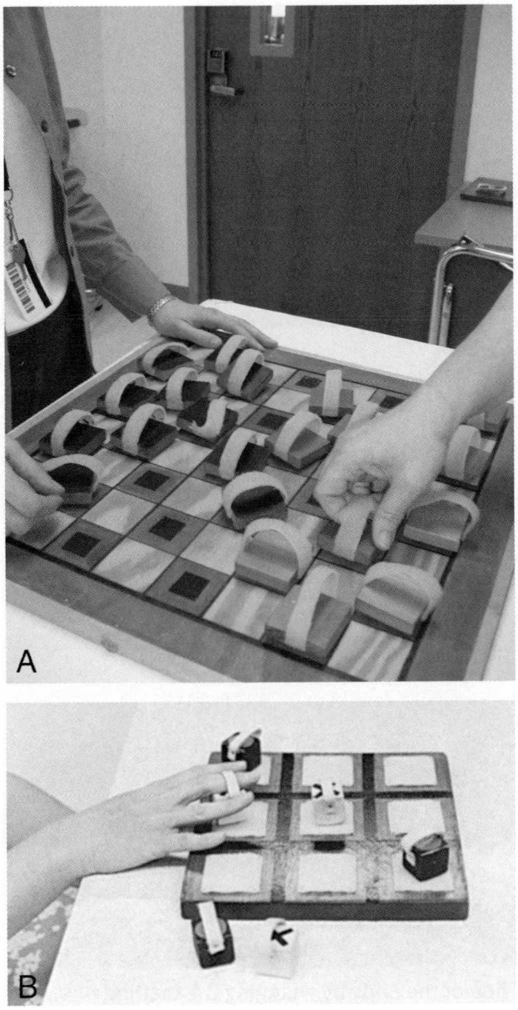

Figure 13-10 **A, B.** Checkers and tic-tac-toe pieces adapted with handles. This enables a person to play who otherwise could not (occupation-as-end) or challenges abilities not used when playing standard games (occupation-as-means).

Change of Color of Multiple Objects

Neistadt et al. (1993) suggested grading challenge to figure-ground discrimination ability by changing game objects from contrasting colors to increasingly similar colors.

Change of Method of Doing the Activity; Change Physical Context

Change of method is used both for occupation-as-means (Fig. 13-2) and for occupation-as-end (Figs. 13-3B, 13-4, 13-11, A & B, and 13-12). Such compensatory adaptation allows performance of an activity that would otherwise be impossible because of the person's disability. Bowling, basketball, and many other sports can be done seated instead of standing. Change of rules adapts some sports, such as track and field events, to certain requirements of the physically impaired. Sewing and needlework, normally bilateral activities, can be made unilateral by adaptations that hold the material steady for the working hand (Fig. 13-13). Books, notebook computers, or other tools can be transported via a rolling backpack or rolling table instead of carrying them.

By altering the physical context, individuals are able to move at the edge of their competence (Nilsen, Kaminiski, & Gordon, 2003). For example, if a person cannot flex his shoulder against gravity, by placing him in a side-lying position, the effects of gravity are minimized, allowing the movement. Movement organization in a gravity-eliminated plane, however, differs from movement in an against-gravity context.

Movement organization is also different in simulated contexts using simulated objects compared with natural contexts with actual objects (Dunn, Brown, & McGuigan, 1994; Flinn, 1999; Ma, Trombly, & Robinson-Poldolski, 1999; Mathiowetz & Wade, 1995; Trombly & Wu, 1999; Wu et al., 1998, 2000). As movement organization is sensitive to contextual changes (Nilsen, Kaminiski, & Gordon, 2003), some rehabilitation centers now have manufactured "real" environments or have renovated their clinic spaces to allow patients to practice in realistic contexts to enable best performance and to facilitate carry over to actual contexts (Fig. 13-14).

Use of Modified or Supplemental Tools and Utensils

Using tools when normally none are used or modifying tools or utensils enables a person to accomplish activities and tasks that he or she would not be able to do otherwise. For example, toast can be retrieved from a toaster by use of a wooden spring clothespin when sensory precautions are in effect (Fig. 13-7). Angling the handles on carving knives allows a person with rheumatoid arthritis to cut meat or vegetables without putting deforming forces on the wrist and fingers. Changing keyboard or mouse designs can prevent carpal tunnel syndrome. Including the tool in a specially designed splint can reduce symptoms caused by prolonged holding (Bockman, 2004). Although manufacturers are offering tools and household utensils designed to enable persons with weak grasp or arthritic pain to use them comfortably, therapists must not assume that tools labeled "ergonomic" produce better positioning or less discomfort than nonadapted tools. Patients' perceptions of comfort and ease of use need to guide the selection (Tebben & Thomas, 2004).

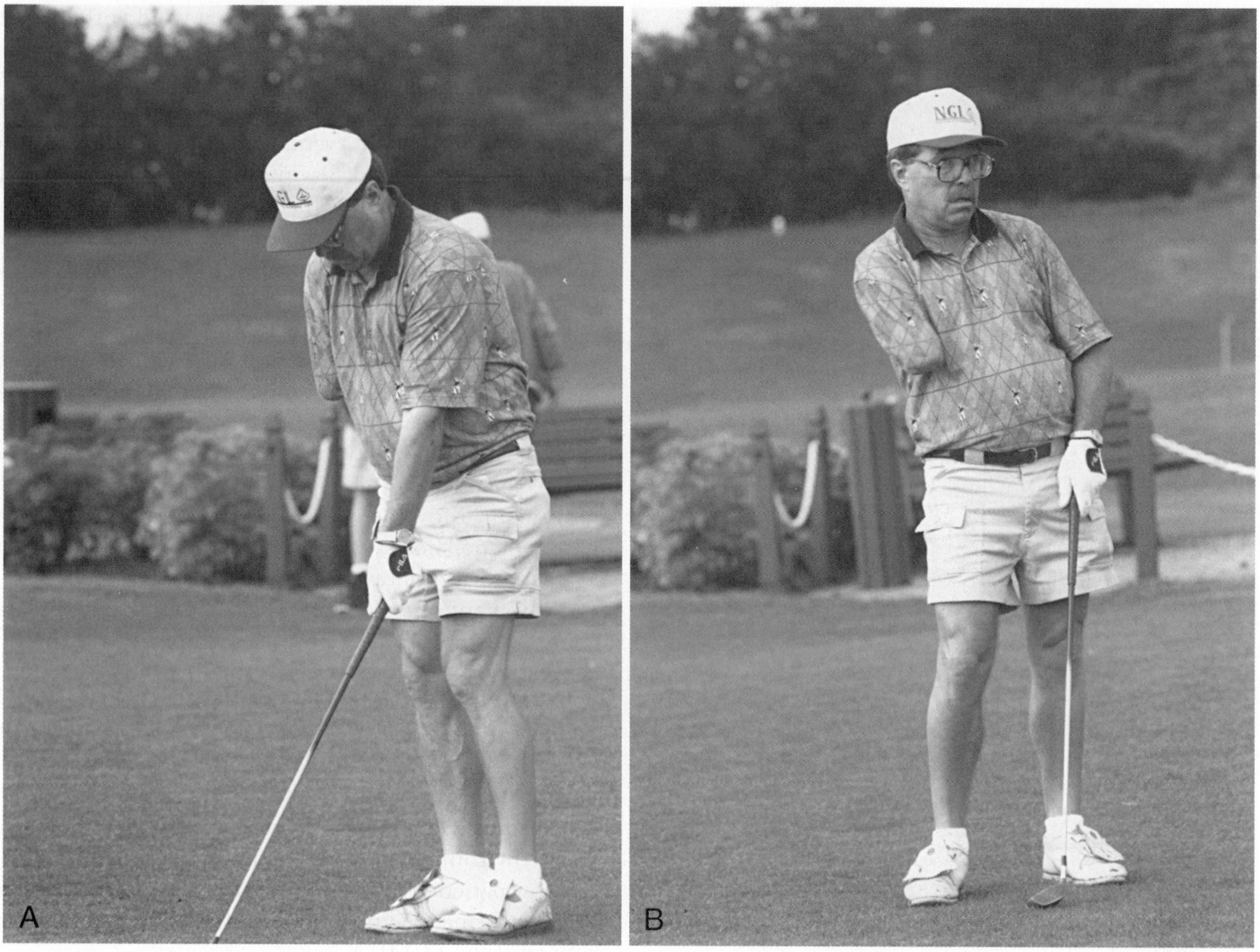

Figure 13-11 **A.** Golf is made possible for a person with the use of only one side of the body by changing the method of swinging the club. **B.** Watching the ball land. (Photographs by Jim Hanson.)

Add Weights

The addition of weights adapts an activity to meet such goals as increase of strength, promotion of co-contraction, and increase of passive ROM by stretch. Some nonresistive activities can be made resistive by adding weights to the apparatus directly or by use of pulleys; others may be made resistive by adding weights to the person, as with weighted cuffs (Fig. 13-15). Tools also are weights, and they can be selected or adjusted to offer graded resistance; for instance, hammers range from lightweight tack hammers to heavy claw hammers.

Add Springs or Rubber Bands

Springs and rubber bands are means of adapting activity to increase strength through resistance, to assist a weak muscle, or to stretch muscle and other soft tissue to increase passive ROM. When offering resistance, the spring or rubber band is positioned so that its pull is opposite to the pull of motion of the target muscle group, whereas if used for assistance, the spring or rubber band is set to pull in the same direction as the contracting muscle group. Springs and rubber bands applied for the purpose of stretching are placed so the pull is against the tissue to be stretched.

Springs of graduated tensions may be applied directly to larger pieces of equipment. Rubber bands can be added to smaller pieces of equipment and can be graded from thin with light tension to thick with heavy tension. For example, a rubber band can be wrapped around the pincer end of a spring-type clothespin to add resistance when it is used in games involving picking up small pieces.

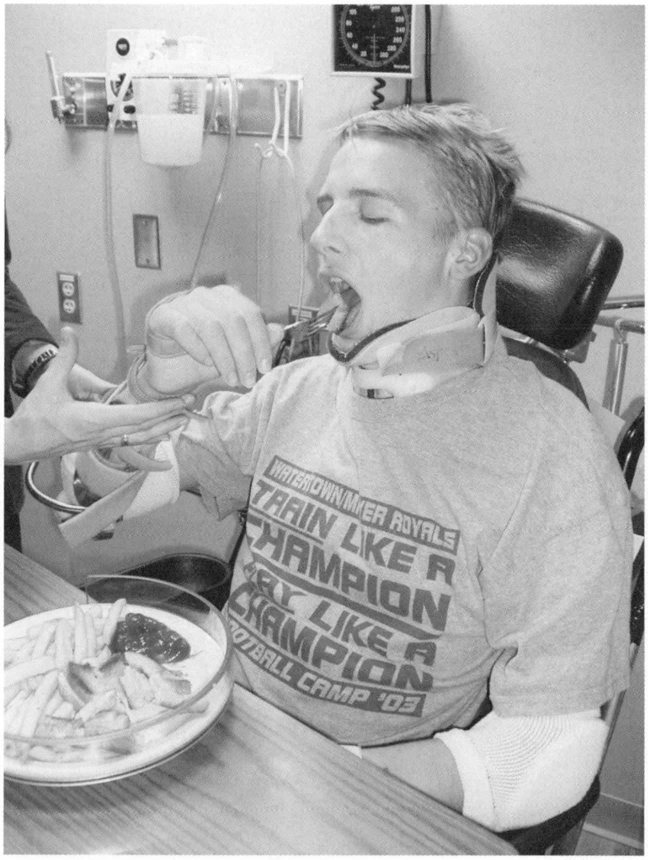

Figure 13-12 A patient with spinal cord injury is learning to feed himself in a new way. He is using a mobile arm support, a fork held in a universal cuff, and a plate guard to prevent food from being pushed off the plate.

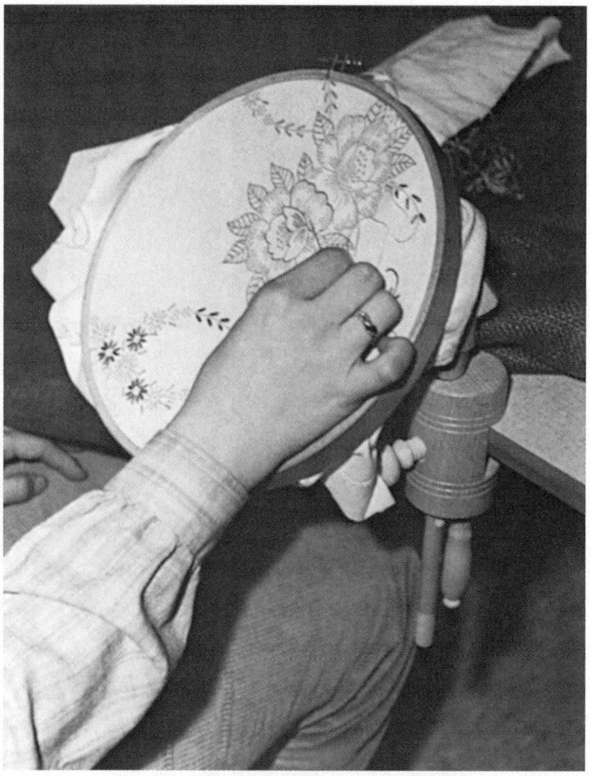

Figure 13-13 An adapted hoop that fastens to the table enables a person with the use of only one hand to embroider.

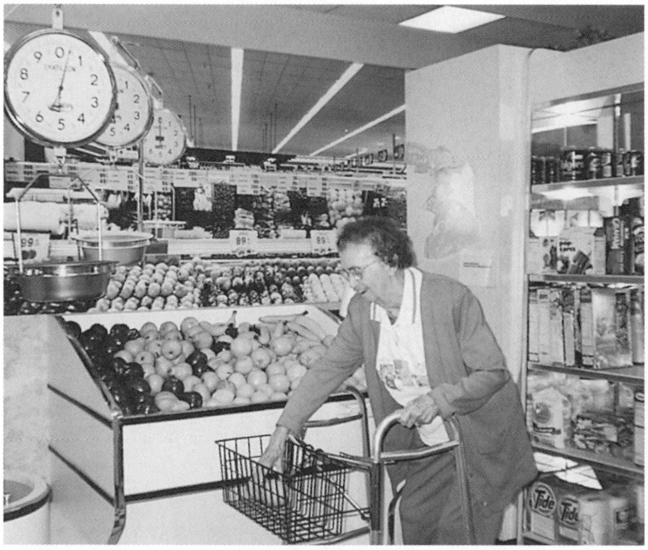

Figure 13-14 "Shopping" at Independence Square Market, a manufactured "real" environment to promote best performance in preparation to return to the community. (Photo by Mary Vining Radomski.)

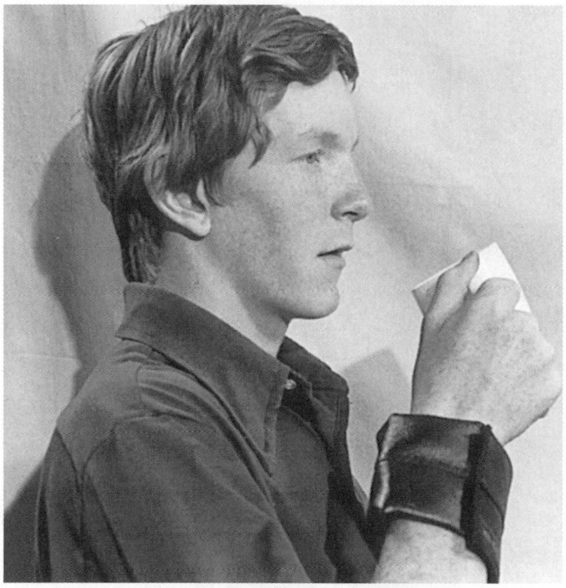

Figure 13-15 Weight cuff used to damp intention tremor or other uncoordinated movements or to add resistance to an action that is not normally resistive.

Evidence Table 13-1
Best Evidence for Occupational Therapy Practice Regarding Selection, Gradation, and Adaptation of Occupation

Intervention	Description of Intervention Tested	Participants	Dosage	Type of Best Evidence and Level of Evidence	Benefit	Statistical Probability and Effect Size of Outcome	Reference
Task constraints: #1–different sized handles; #2–different weight cups	#1: three ceramic cups 12 cm high, weighing 309.0 g, having handles of 2 cm, 4 cm, and 8 cm. #2: two cups, 12 cm high with 2-cm handles, weighing 309.0 g and 705.9 g when filled with water.	30 healthy women aged 20–45 years.	3 trials for each cup. Carried out in a laboratory.	One group, repeated-measures design, randomized to condition. 1B1b	Mixed. #1: Yes. The size of the handle significantly affected the number of fingers being placed through the handle; the larger the handle, the more fingers. #2: No. Weight did not significantly affect the number of fingers used to support the cup.	#1: $\chi^2_{(2)} = 49.8$, $p < 0.001$; effect size could not be calculated. #2: not significant.	Fuller & Trombly, 1997
Exercise apparatus adapted into a game	Experimental: Exercise using a game apparatus that required supination to dump dice out to score. Control: Exercise using the same apparatus without the game.	30 patients with acute stroke, mean age = 68.4 years.	Two sets of 10 trials for each condition; different days.	Randomized controlled trial. IC2c	Yes. The game significantly increased the degrees of handle rotation (supination) achieved. Mean of 13.4° more in experimental group compared with control group.	$p = 0.016$, $r = 0.42$.	Nelson et al., 1996

Functional activity (goal object present) vs. rote exercise (goal object absent)	Present: Reach to scoop coins off the table in the laboratory. Absent: Reach forward without functional goal in a laboratory.	14 patients with chronic stroke, mean age = 61.8 years. 24 healthy persons, mean age = 63.2 years.	10 trials within 1 day.	Randomized controlled trial. IC1c	Yes. Both groups demonstrated significantly better movement organization with goal object present. Results are reported for the stroke patients only: The force of movement did not differ significantly.	Overall effect size = 0.63. Speed, $p = 0.003$, $r = 0.70$; straightness of path, $p = 0.002$, $r = 0.72$; smoothness, $p = 0.005$, $r = 0.66$; automaticity of movement, $p = 0.001$, $r = 0.75$. Force of movement, $p = 0.28$, $r = 0.17$.	Wu et al., 2000
Grade speed of action; grade work surface	Condition: 1: rest 2: unilateral horizontal sanding at 15 cycles/min 3: same as 2 at 30 cycles/min 4: unilateral sanding with board inclined to 15° at 15 cycles/min 5: same as 4 at 30 cycles/min.	8 patients with stroke of unknown chronicity, mean age = 67.6 years.	3 minutes each of 5 conditions with rests between; all conditions within 1 day.	One group, repeated-measures design without randomization to condition. IIC2c	Mixed. When tested together, speed and angle significantly increased cardiopulmonary measures above resting. When separated, only different velocities affected the outcome.	$p < 0.01$; effect size could not be calculated. No statistical information available concerning the tests of angle and speed separately.	Muraki et al., 1990
Weighted cuff	Weighted cuff applied to forearm to decrease tremors and increase functional feeding in adults. Each person ate ½ the meal with the weighted cuff and ½ without the cuff. Weight determined individually by trial and error.	5 adults aged 30–81 years. All had tremor secondary to various diagnoses.	8 or 16 meals.	AB single-case design; conditions alternated randomly. IVC3b	Partial benefit for some participants. Time to acquire food on utensil decreased significantly for 4/5 participants. The number of spills decreased significantly for 2/5 participants. The amount of food consumed did not change significantly.	Time to acquire food on utensil: $p < 0.013$; effect size for 4, $r = 0.97$. Number of spills: $p < 0.012$; effect size for 2, $r = 0.96$.	McGruder et al., 2003

SUMMARY REVIEW QUESTIONS

1. What are the general characteristics required of an activity to be used to treat motor impairments?
2. How does analysis relate to selection of an occupation or activity?
3. What would a therapist need to know to select occupation-as-end for a particular patient?
4. What goal(s) might be accomplished by engaging a patient in occupation-as-means that requires moving at different speeds?
5. What are two reasons for adapting an occupation used as means? Occupation-as-end?
6. What are the five characteristics of good adaptations?
7. What therapeutic goals can be accomplished by the following?
   - Changing the position of the task relative to the person
   - Adding weights to tools or game pieces
   - Adding springs or rubber bands to craft equipment or tools
   - Changing the length of lever arms of tools, equipment, or the limb itself
   - Changing the material to be used in a project
   - Changing the method of doing an activity

ACKNOWLEDGMENTS

I thank my former students Dr. Steven Cope, Dr. Susan Fasoli, Janice Ferguson, Yvonne Fuller, Dr. Hui-Ing Ma, Dr. Susan Murphy, Julie Pope, Natalia Ramsbey, Ellen Rosenberg, Dr. Pimjai Sudsawad, Dr. Pei-Luen Tsai, and Dr. Ching-Yi Wu for their research assistance and conversations about occupation. I am especially indebted to the occupational therapists and patients at Sister Kenny Institute, Minneapolis, MN, for their assistance with photography for this chapter. Specifically, I thank Jake Beckstrom, Cindy Bemis, Arlan Berg, Tricia Bonavoglia, OTR/L, Michelle Brown, M.Ed., OTR/L, Krista Elfink, M.S., OTR/L, Larry Larkin, Mary Vining Radomski, M.A., OTR/L, Jennifer Theis, M.S., OTR/L, and Valerie Wheeler.

References

Ainsworth, B. E., Haskell, W. L., Leon, A. S., Jacobs, D. R., Montoye, H. J., Sallis, J. F., & Paffenbarger, R. S. (1993). Compendium of physical activities: Classification of energy costs of human physical activities. *Medicine and Science in Sports and Exercise, 25,* 71–80.

Ainsworth, B. E., Haskell, W. L., Whitt, M. C., Irwin, M. L., Swartz, A. M., Strath, S. J., O'Brien, W. L., Bassett, D. R. Jr., Schmitz, K. H., Emplaincourt, P. O., Jacobs, D. R. Jr., & Leon, A. S. (2000). Compendium of physical activities: An update of activity codes and MET intensities. *Medicine and Science in Sports and Exercise, 32 (Suppl. 9),* S498–S504.

American Occupational Therapy Association [AOTA]. (1995). Position paper: Occupation. *American Journal of Occupational Therapy, 49,* 1015–1018.

American Occupational Therapy Association [AOTA]. (2002). Occupational therapy practice framework: Domain and process. *American Journal of Occupational Therapy, 56,* 609–639.

Bockman, T. (2004). Splinting the tool to the worker. *OT PRACTICE, 9,* 22.

Burton, A. W., & Davis, W. E. (1996). Ecological task analysis: Utilizing intrinsic measures in research and practice. *Human Movement Science, 15,* 285–314.

Chandani, A., & Hill, C. (1990). What really is therapeutic activity? *British Journal of Occupational Therapy, 53,* 15–18.

Creighton, C. (1992). The origin and evolution of activity analysis. *American Journal of Occupational Therapy, 46,* 45–48.

Creighton, C. (1993). Looking back: Graded activity: Legacy of the sanatorium. *American Journal of Occupational Therapy, 47,* 745–748.

Csikszentmihalyi, M. (1990). *Flow: The psychology of optimal experience.* New York: Harper & Row.

Davis, W. E., & Burton, A. W. (1991). Ecological task analysis: Translating movement behavior theory into practice. *Adapted Physical Activity Quarterly, 8,* 154–177.

Dunn, W., Brown, C., & McGuigan, A. (1994). The ecology of human performance: A framework for considering the effect of context. *American Journal of Occupational Therapy, 48,* 595–607.

Fisher, A. G. (1997). *Assessment of motor and process skills* (2nd ed.). Fort Collins, CO: Three Star.

Fisher, A. G. (1998). Uniting practice and theory in an occupational framework. *American Journal of Occupational Therapy, 52,* 509–521.

Fitts, P. M. (1954). The information capacity of the human motor system in controlling the amplitude of movement. *Journal of Experimental Psychology, 47,* 381–391.

Flinn, N. A. (1999). Clinical interpretation of "Effect of rehabilitation tasks on organization of movement after stroke." *American Journal of Occupational Therapy, 53,* 345–347.

Fuller, Y., & Trombly, C. A. (1997). Effect of object characteristics on female grasp patterns. *American Journal of Occupational Therapy, 51,* 481–487.

Gentile, A. (1987). Skill acquisition: Action, movement and neuromotor processes. In J. H. Carr, R. B. Shepherd, J. Gordon, A. M. Gentile, & J. M. Held (Eds.), *Movement science: Foundations for physical therapy in rehabilitation* (pp. 93–154). Rockville, MD: Aspen Systems.

Gentile, A. M., Higgins, J. R., Miller, E. A., & Rosen, B. (1975). Structure of motor tasks. In *Mouvement Actes du 7e Symposium Canadien en Appentissage Psycho-motor et Psychologie du Sport* (pp. 11–28). Quebec, Canada (out of print).

Georgopoulos, A. P. (1986). On reaching. *Annual Review of Neurosciences, 9,* 147–170.

Gibson, J. J. (1977). The theory of affordances. In R. E. Shaw & J. Bransford (Eds.), *Perceiving, acting, and knowing: Toward an ecological psychology* (pp. 67–82). Hillsdale, NJ: Lawrence Erlbaum.

Gilbreth, F. B. (1911). *Motion study.* New York: Van Nostrand.

Gilbreth, F. B., & Gilbreth, L. M. (1920). *Motion study for the handicapped.* London: Routledge.

Greene, D. (1990). A clinically relevant approach to biomechanical analysis of function. *Occupational Therapy Practice, 1,* 44–52.

Harnish, S. (2001). Gardening for life: Adaptive techniques and tools. *OT PRACTICE, 6,* 12–15.

Illyes, A., & Kiss, R. M. (2005). Shoulder muscle activity during pushing, pulling, elevation and overhead throw. *Journal of Electromyography and Kinesiology, 15,* 282–289.

Jeannerod, M. (1988). *The neural and behavioral organization of goal-directed movements.* Oxford, UK: Clarendon.

Jordan, K., & Newell, K. M. (2004). Task goal and grip force dynamics. *Experimental Brain Research, 156,* 451–457.

Kelly, B. T., Williams, R. J., Cordasco, F. A., Backus, S. I., Otis, J. C., Weiland, D. E., Altchek, D. W., Craig, E. V., Wickiewicz, T. L., &

Warren, R. F. (2005). Differential patterns of muscle activation in patients with symptomatic and asymptomatic rotator cuff tears. *Journal of Shoulder and Elbow Surgery, 14,* 165–171.

Llorens, L. A. (1993). Activity analysis: Agreement between participants and observers on perceived factors in occupation components. *Occupational Therapy Journal of Research, 13,* 198–211.

Ma, H., & Trombly, C. A. (2004). Effects of task complexity on reaction time and movement kinematics in elderly people. *American Journal of Occupational Therapy, 58,* 150–158.

Ma, H., Trombly, C. A., & Robinson-Podolski, C. (1999). The effect of context on skill acquisition and transfer. *American Journal of Occupational Therapy, 53,* 138–144.

Mathiowetz, V., & Wade, M. G. (1995). Task constraints and functional motor performance of individuals with and without multiple sclerosis. *Ecological Psychology, 7,* 99–123.

Mayer, N. H., Keating, D. J., & Rapp, D. (1986). Skills, routines, and activity patterns of daily living: A functional nested approach. In B. Uzzell & Y. Gross (Eds.), *Clinical neuropsychology of intervention* (pp. 205–222). Boston: Martinus Nijhoff.

McGrain, P., & Hague, M. A. (1987). An electromyographic study of the middle deltoid and middle trapezius muscles during warping. *Occupational Therapy Journal of Research, 7,* 225–233.

McGruder, J., Cors, D., Tiernan, A. M., & Tomlin, G. (2003). Weighted wrist cuffs for tremor reduction during eating in adults with static brain lesions. *American Journal of Occupational Therapy, 57,* 507–516.

Merritt, B. K., & Fisher, A. G. (2003). Gender differences in the performance of activities of daily living. *Archives of Physical Medicine and Rehabilitation, 84,* 1872–1877.

Moneta, G. B., & Csikszentmihalyi, M. (1996). The effect of perceived challenges and skills on the quality of subjective experience. *Journal of Personality, 64,* 275–310.

Mosey, A. C. (1981). *Occupational therapy: Configuration of a profession.* New York: Raven.

Muraki, T., Kujime, K., Su., M., Kaneko, T., & Ueba, Y. (1990). Effect of one hand sanding on cardiometabolic and ventilatory functions in the hemiplegic elderly: A preliminary investigation. *Physical and Occupational Therapy in Geriatrics, 9,* 37–48.

Neistadt, M. E., McAuley, D., Zecha, D., & Shannon, R. (1993). An analysis of a board game as a treatment activity. *American Journal of Occupational Therapy, 47,* 154–160.

Nelson, D. L. (1988). Occupation: Form and performance. *American Journal of Occupational Therapy, 42,* 633–641.

Nelson, D. L., Konosky, K., Fleharty, K., Webb, R., Newer, K., Hazboun, V. P., Fontane, C., & Licht, B. C. (1996). The effects of an occupationally embedded exercise on bilaterally assisted supination in persons with hemiplegia. *American Journal of Occupational Therapy, 50,* 639–646.

Newell, K. M. (1986). Constraints on the development of coordination. In M. G. Wade & H. T. A. Whiting (Eds.), *Motor development in children: Aspects of coordination and control* (pp. 341–360). Boston: Martinus Nijhoff.

Nilsen, D. M., Kaminiski, T. R., & Gordon, A. M. (2003). The effect of body orientation on a point-to-point movement in healthy elderly persons. *American Journal of Occupational Therapy, 57,* 99–107.

Okoye, R. L. (1993). Computer applications in occupational therapy. In H. L. Hopkins & H. D. Smith (Eds.), *Willard and Spackman's occupational therapy* (8th ed., pp. 341–353). Philadelphia: Lippincott.

Peloquin, S. M. (1988). Linking purpose to procedure during interactions with patients. *American Journal of Occupational Therapy, 42,* 775–781.

Polatajko, H. J., Mandich, A., & Martini, R. (2000). Dynamic performance analysis: A framework for understanding occupational performance. *American Journal of Occupational Therapy, 54,* 65–72.

Spaulding, S. J., & Robinson, K. L. (1984). Electromyographic study of the upper extremity during bilateral sanding: Unresisted and resisted conditions. *American Journal of Occupational Therapy, 38,* 258–262.

Sung, C. Y. Y., Ho, K. K. F., Lam, R. M. W., Lee, A. H. Y., & Chan, C. C. H. (2003). Physical and psychosocial factors in display screen equipment assessment. *Hong Kong Journal of Occupational Therapy, 13,* 2–10.

Tebben, A. B., & Thomas, J. J. (2004). Trowels labeled ergonomic versus standard design: Preferences and effects on wrist range of motion during a gardening occupation. *American Journal of Occupational Therapy, 58,* 317–323.

Trombly, C. A. (1993). The issue is: Anticipating the future: Assessment of occupational function. *American Journal of Occupational Therapy, 47,* 253–257.

Trombly, C. A. (1995). Occupation: Purposefulness and meaningfulness as therapeutic mechanisms. *American Journal of Occupational Therapy, 49,* 960–972.

Trombly, C. A., & Cole, J. M. (1979). Electromyographic study of four hand muscles during selected activities. *American Journal of Occupational Therapy, 33,* 440–449.

Trombly, C. A., & Quintana, L. A. (1983). Activity analysis: Electromyographic and electrogoniometric verification. *Occupational Therapy Journal of Research, 3,* 104–120.

Trombly, C. A., & Wu, C. (1999). Effect of rehabilitation tasks on organization of movement after stroke. *American Journal of Occupational Therapy, 53,* 333–344.

Tsai, P.-L. (1994). Activity analysis and activity selection among occupational therapists: A survey. Unpublished Master's thesis. Boston: Boston University.

Watson, D. E., & Wilson, S. A. (2003). *Task analysis: An individual and population approach* (2nd ed.). Bethesda, MD: American Occupational Therapy Association.

Wu, C., Trombly, C. A., Lin, K., & Tickle-Degnen, L. (1998). Effects of object affordances on reaching performance in persons with and without cerebrovascular accident. *American Journal of Occupational Therapy, 52,* 447–456.

Wu, C., Trombly, C. A., Lin, K., & Tickle-Degnen, L. (2000). A kinematic study of contextual effects on reaching performance in persons with and without stroke: Influences of object availability. *Archives of Physical Medicine and Rehabilitation, 81,* 95–101.

CHAPTER 14

Learning

Nancy Ann Flinn and Mary Vining Radomski

LEARNING OBJECTIVES

After studying this chapter, the reader will be able to do the following:

1. Differentiate between patient[1] performance and patient learning.
2. Outline clinical considerations necessary for planning patient-specific teaching.
3. Explain the roles of context, feedback, and practice in the acquisition of both task-specific skills and general strategies.
4. List phases of teaching patients and describe the advantages and disadvantages of various teaching technologies.
5. Identify strategies for facilitating caregiver education and training.

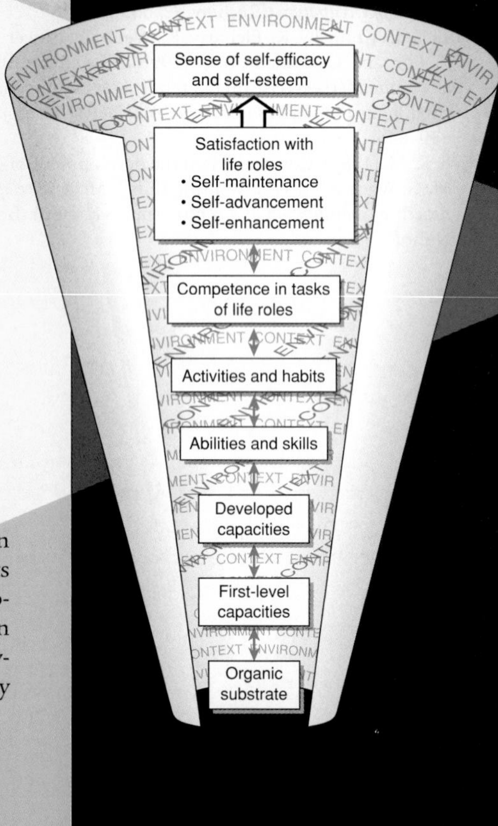

[1] Readers will note that the terms "patient" and "client" are used at various points in this chapter. In acute medical and rehabilitation settings, the term "patient" reflects a more passive role of the person receiving care; it is also the term used by other professionals on the health care team. The term "client" is used in reference to a person living in the community who is receiving outpatient, home-based, or community-based services. It reflects the assumption that the person receiving services is ready to assume a more directive role in organizing his or her care.

Glossary

Automaticity—The phase of learning resulting from numerous consistent repetitions in which a person accurately carries out a skill or task with little or no cognitive effort (Sternberg, 1986).

Contextual interference—Changes across trials in intrinsic and extrinsic factors that force learners to use multiple and variable processing strategies (Shea & Morgan, 1979).

Encoding—Processes in which stimulation of our senses is translated into codes and then stored in memory (Mann & Sabatino, 1985).

Encoding specificity—A phenomenon of information processing wherein we store a given memory along with information about the context in which the memory occurred and, as a result, elements of the context may trigger recall and recognition of that memory in the future.

Feedback—Intrinsic or extrinsic information that patients receive while learning to perform a new skill or strategy.

Generalization—The ability to apply a skill or strategy to an altogether new task in an environment that is different from the one in which the original training occurred.

Learning—The result of processes associated with practice or experience that leads to relatively permanent changes in a person's knowledge, skills, and behavior (Schmidt, 1988).

Performance—Temporary changes in response during practice.

Practice—The repetition of a to-be-learned task, a key ingredient in the learning of skills and strategies.

Retrieval—The search for and location of information stored in long-term memory that occurs when people remember (recall or recognize) something that they have learned (Eysenck & Keane, 1990).

Transfer—The ability to perform a new skill in an environment that is different from the training environment.

Learning is a primary therapeutic mechanism underlying many, if not all, occupational therapy interventions. Occupational therapists teach patients to use adaptive equipment, new ways to move, and a variety of compensatory skills and strategies. As teachers, therapists must determine whether and when learning has taken place. For example, after a 30-minute dressing session, a patient who has had total knee replacement surgery is able to don his pants, socks, and shoes. From a traditional learning perspective, the patient's performance at the end of the session reflects the extent to which he or she has learned the desired skill or strategy. However, what if a nurse later reports that the patient is unable to carry out the activities he demonstrated proficiency with the day before? One can easily deduce that while within-session performance was buoyed by cues and practice, true learning did not occur.

Schmidt's (1988) contemporary definition of motor learning allows us to differentiate learning from within-session performance. According to Schmidt (1988), "motor learning is a set of processes associated with practice or experience leading to relatively permanent changes in the capability for responding" (p. 346). Based on this definition of learning, we would expect the knee replacement patient to demonstrate similar levels of proficiency after the occupational therapy session as during. The term *performance* is used to describe what is seen during training, that is, short-term capabilities resulting from instruction, cues, or assistance. For occupational therapy to help patients resume occupational roles, therapists must understand the process of transforming performance into learning and employ teaching methods that help the patient learn the skills.

This chapter discusses the role of information processing in learning and then summarizes the array of variables that affect the patient-specific teaching plan. We detail key influences on learning and conclude with specific applications to occupational therapy practice. Regarding issues of learning, there has been a traditional division in the research between motor tasks and cognitive tasks. In clinical practice, however, it is unusual to find motor tasks that do not have a cognitive component or cognitive tasks that do not have a motor component. As this distinction does not translate well into practice and because principles in the two areas are similar, they are reviewed together in this chapter.

HUMAN INFORMATION PROCESSING MODEL OF LEARNING

Learning is inextricably linked to memory, specifically the **encoding** and **retrieval** of information. As explained in Chapter 9, people hold environmental stimuli very briefly in a series of short-term sensory stores before transferring it to limited-capacity working memory (Atkinson & Shiffrin, 1971). In working memory, also called short-term memory, people may use control processes to encode information for storage in long-term memory (Schneider & Shiffrin, 1977). These control processes include but are not limited to rehearsal, coding, and imaging (Atkinson & Shiffrin, 1971). Rehearsal is rote repetition of information, whereas coding entails linking the new information to something already meaningful. Imaging transforms verbal information to visual images that are stored in memory. Craik and Tulving (1975) found that the durability of the memory trace is a function of depth of processing. That is, deep processing, as in the time-consuming process of linking new information to personally relevant old knowledge, results in better retention than shallow processing, such as rote rehearsal. If the learner does not use some form of conscious control, the memory trace quickly fades from working memory and cannot be recovered or stored (Atkinson & Shiffrin, 1971). From the standpoint of human information processing, learning is the transfer of information from short-term or working memory to long-term memory (Shiffrin & Schneider, 1977).

Controlled Versus Automatic Information Processing

Consider the attentional resources required of you the first time you drove a car compared with the attention required for the same task now. After years of experience, the car seems to drive itself, freeing the driver to concentrate on plans for the day or talk to a passenger. This example typifies the difference between controlled and automatic processing.

Controlled Processing

A controlled process is technically a temporary activation of a series or sequence of elements in long-term memory under the control and attention of the thinker (Schneider & Shiffrin, 1977). For example, the new driver must actively recall specific rules and instructions and direct his or her attention to each motor sequence of the task. Controlled processing is limited by the capacity of working memory and, therefore, effortful but flexible in handling novel situations. When learning a new task or skill that requires effortful concentration, people employ controlled processing. Thus, patients learning new skills or behaviors can process only a limited number of inputs (instructions, cues, environmental distractions) at a time.

Automatic Processing

With enough controlled processing, a task requires less and less concentration to carry out (Shiffrin & Schneider, 1977). That is, the task becomes increasingly automatic, as in the example of the proficient driver. Automatic processing occurs when specific contextual stimuli internal or external to the person trigger the activation of a specific learned sequence in long-term memory (Schneider & Shiffrin, 1977). Given enough repetition, the individual performs the skill or task in a consistent manner with little or no attention. Sternberg (1986) suggested that development of a full level of automatization requires at least 200 trials of a task but that automatization begins in as few as 10 trials, so long as those trials involve consistency. With fully automatic skills, people cannot stop themselves from performing the overlearned sequence unless control processes are employed to override it. Definition 14-1 discusses implications related to helping patients with memory impairment to reacquire skills.

According to Giles (2005), overlearning is practice of a skill or strategy well beyond demonstration of learning or proficiency; it increases the likelihood that the skill or strategy will become automatic. These automatic skills and strategies become the easiest behaviors to initiate from an array of possible behaviors (Giles, 2005), minimizing demands on attention and decision making. Habits and routines are examples of automatic motor sequences that, according to Kielhofner, Barris, and Watts (1982), organize a person's tasks, space, and time. Characteristic of automatic skills and strategies, habits and routines are responsive to the environmental conditions under which they are learned and develop with repetition (Kielhofner, Barris, & Watts, 1982; Wood, Quinn, & Kashy, 2002). Habit learning is a form of implicit learning, which is described in Definition 14-2. Occupational therapists often help patients resume or relearn self-maintenance tasks so that they are once again automatic. See Chapter 29 for a more thorough discussion of that process.

DEFINITION 14-1

Errorless Learning

Errorless learning is a technique that involves encoding new information without error (Tailby & Haslam, 2003). Learners are helped to do it right each time the new skill is performed by introducing and then fading preemptive cues and/or assistance. Wilson and Evans (1996) propose errorless learning methods for persons with severe memory impairments. They suggest that these individuals have difficulty remembering what they learned if they made errors during the training process. Guessing and trial-and-error are avoided, and because training generally occurs in the context in which the new skills will be used, expectations of transfer are minimized.

Implications of the Information Processing Memory Model

Attention and memory play important roles in many aspects of learning. Therefore, occupational therapists assess these domains before they try to teach patients skills or strategies. Sensitivity to distractions, such as pain, fatigue, and noise, allows therapists to optimize the likelihood that patients will use limited-capacity cognitive resources to hold and ultimately store stimuli related to the new skills or strategies. Therapists also facilitate memory storage and retrieval by helping patients use effective control processes,

DEFINITION 14-2

Implicit and Explicit Learning

People learn through two key processes that are supported by separate brain structures and have very different characteristics.

Explicit learning (sometimes called declarative learning) refers to the conscious encoding and recollection of specific events, task rules, and facts (Deckersbach et al., 2002; Eldridge, Masterman, & Knowlton, 2002). It relies on the integrity of the medial temporal lobe and diencephalic structures, particularly the hippocampus (Eldridge, Masterman, & Knowlton, 2002). It can be facilitated by a therapist through direct instruction about key environmental features, task-relevant feedback, and cues (Reber & Squire, 1994). Explicit learning is more flexible than implicit learning and has been shown to generalize more easily, probably because it is not as context dependent (Squire, 1994).

Implicit learning (also called procedural learning) refers to an unconscious change in behavior resulting from repetition within a stable context. There appear to be several forms of implicit learning including skill and habit learning, some forms of conditioning, and the phenomenon of priming (Squire, Knowlton, & Musen, 1993). Much of the learning of a motor task is thought to be implicit, including the dynamics of force production in the task, which is the interaction of active and passive components of the multiple joints involved in the task. The therapist facilitates implicit learning by structuring the environment to create consistent cues and frequent opportunities for appropriate task practice (Gentile, 1998). Implicit learning is more robust than explicit learning and retains its strength even when the explicit knowledge about a task has decayed (Lee & Vakoch, 1996). The basal ganglia support implicit learning rather than the medial temporal lobe (Packard & Knowlton, 2002). This suggests that even people with impaired explicit memory systems (e.g., Alzheimer's disease) are capable of implicit learning (Eldridge, Masterman, & Knowlton, 2002).

such as linking the new information to something they already know. Finally, therapists recognize that, for many skills, the learning end point is not proficiency but **automaticity**. Therapists ultimately enable their patients to carry out these tasks with accuracy and ease if they encourage consistency in performance (consistent environment, consistent sequence of steps).

CLINICAL CONSIDERATIONS IN TEACHING CLIENTS

In advance of every teaching intervention, occupational therapists make deliberate decisions regarding appropriate teaching methods. These decisions are based on the characteristics of the learner, anticipated length of intervention, desired learning outcome (specific task vs. general strategy), and expectations for **transfer** and **generalization**.

Learner Characteristics

A client's learning potential is determined by many factors. Variables affecting cognitive status (reviewed in Chapter 9) are critical contributors to learning potential. They include neurobiological, affective, experiential, and sociocultural influences. In brief, the *neurobiological influences* on cognitive function are largely associated with the physiological and anatomical integrity of a person's brain. *Affective influences* may interfere with learning because depression and anxiety, for example, distract a person from attending to new information and storing that information in memory. Therapists consider other personal affective influences with similar effects on learning, such as motivation to improve function and pain and fatigue. (Chapter 10 discusses assessing these aspects of personal context.) Finally, each individual brings his or her *experiential sociocultural* background to the lesson. Remember, all of these considerations apply to family caregivers as well as patients (see Procedures for Practice 14-1). Literacy is one important dimension of the experiential sociocultural influence on learning, with many implications regarding teaching methods. (Again, see Chapter 10 regarding assessing literacy.) Neistadt (1995) suggested that occupational therapists attempt to answer four questions regarding patients' learning capacities during the course of their traditional evaluation. These questions include the following:

1. What modes of input (e.g., visual, auditory, tactile) can this patient process most easily?
2. What approaches to tasks (outputs or behaviors) are still available to this patient?
3. What tasks remain meaningful or are most likely to facilitate learning for this patient?
4. How well is this patient able to transfer learning, that is, apply specific skills to a variety of tasks under a variety of circumstances?

Anticipated Length of Treatment

Occupational therapists also consider how many teaching sessions are likely to be available. Typically this is dictated by expected length of stay at the hospital, rehabilitation center, or nursing facility; insurance coverage of rehabilitation services; acuteness of medical condition; and learning potential of the patient. Awareness of time constraints for teaching allows the clinician to anticipate what stage of learning the patient will attain by the completion of treatment. Discharge planning then incorporates recom-

PROCEDURES FOR PRACTICE 14-1

Caregiver Education and Training

Ever-decreasing hospital lengths of stay continue to increase the demands and responsibilities of family caregivers (Clark et al., 2004). Occupational therapists and other rehabilitation professionals can contribute to clients' quality of life by providing multidimensional education and training to their caregivers (Kalra et al., 2004; Pasacreta et al., 2000). Here are some important considerations and strategies:

- Acknowledge and validate the pivotal role that family caregivers play in the recovery and quality of life of your client. Make sure that your occupational therapy intervention plan incorporates specific goals, strategies, and timelines for caregiver training.
- Appreciate the complex demands placed on people when they assume caregiver roles. Remember that family caregivers typically have to juggle the needs of other family members and their own jobs and activities in addition to their caregiving responsibilities (Carter & Nutt, 1998; Pasacreta et al., 2000). Adjust your teaching methods in consideration of these demands and distractions on caregivers and expect that you will need to repeat information and instructions more than once.
- Try to empathize with the emotional burden often carried by family caregivers. Appreciate that they often carry an array of worries about their loved one's condition, the quality of care their loved one is receiving, and what the future holds in terms of their caregiving responsibilities (Hong, 2005). Make a point of structuring your education and training efforts to address these worries.
- Incorporate caregiver education and training into your intervention from day 1 by showing family members how to participate in providing care. Ask family members to attend therapy sessions and include them as active participants. Show them how they can extend the benefits of occupational therapy intervention by, for example, prompting and assisting with activities of daily living or reinforcing the use of adaptive equipment.
- Collaborate with other health care professionals to ensure that caregiver education and training is multifaceted and ongoing. Appreciate that current and premorbid family functioning is an important predictor of caregiver stress and adjustment (Clark et al., 2004). Refer caregivers and their family members to counselors, psychologists, and social workers when necessary.
- Take responsibility for helping family caregivers to transfer what they have learned in the hospital or clinic setting to their home and family contexts. Consider making a home visit before discontinuing your services to review information and techniques within the client's home environment.
- Set up a caregiver education plan that extends beyond the duration of occupational therapy intervention. Identify possible resources for continued caregiver education and support in the future.

mendations for continuing and extending the learning that began in treatment.

Stages of Learning

In 1967, Fitts and Posner described three sequential stages of learning, or acquisition, of motor skills: cognitive, associative, and autonomous; each of the stages requires different kinds of attention resources (Eversheim & Bock, 2001). During the cognitive stage, the patient tries to understand the requirements of the task. The patient uses conscious control to acquire the new skill or strategy: thinking through or verbalizing the steps, attending to visual and verbal **feedback** from the therapist, and determining what cues to heed.

In the associative stage, the patient has determined the most effective way of doing the task and begins to make refinements in performance. The learner relies less on vision and verbal feedback and begins to use internal feedback mechanisms. During this stage, practice takes on primary importance; this important dimension of learning is discussed in more detail later in this chapter.

During the autonomous stage, the new skill or strategy becomes increasingly automatic or habitual. The patient can accurately perform most of the skill or strategy without thinking about it and is less subject to interference from other activities or environmental distractions.

Desired Learning Outcomes: Task-Specific Skills Versus General Strategy Related to Expectations for Transfer and Generalization

Recipients of occupational therapy services have a variety of learning needs. Two categories of learning end points include acquisition of task-specific skills and acquisition of general strategies. Therapists deliberately determine the patient-specific learning end point because it dictates teaching methods, length of treatment, and expectations for transfer and generalization.

Task-Specific Skills and Transfer of Training

After a stroke, many patients receive occupational therapy services to learn task-specific skills such as how to dress themselves using only one hand. Acquired skills are expected to enhance function solely within the training tasks. For example, a client who receives home-based treatment may learn techniques specific to donning her housecoat and slippers (her usual attire) at the side of her bed, which rests on shag carpeting. Teaching in this situation (within the environment and context that the skill will be used) is task specific. The learning process is embedded in the performance environment, with surroundings and objects becoming cues. The therapist does not expect the client to apply skills learned in this sequence to a whole host of new tasks, and therefore, training time is minimized. Typically the therapist hopes that, given enough consistent repetition, the routine will be carried out automatically.

However, occupational therapy intervention, such as activities of daily living (ADLs) training, typically begins while the patient is hospitalized. Patients often learn one-handed dressing techniques from hospital beds in rooms with very different characteristics from those of their homes. For the intervention to improve the patient's level of independence after discharge, the therapist must train to transfer. That is, therapists employ teaching techniques that optimize patients' chances of being able to apply the task-specific dressing skills learned at the hospital when they get home.

Transfer of learning refers to a person's ability to carry out the same task in a different environment. According to Toglia (1991), transfer is not an all-or-none phenomenon. She described four levels of transfer—near, intermediate, far, and very far—based on the number of differences in the surface characteristics between the learning and real-life environments. In general, near transfer requires the person to apply the same skill in very similar circumstances, whereas far transfer implies greater differences in application environment (Perkins, 1995). Transfer is associated with perceptual similarities of tasks, not similarities in underlying principles (Perkins, 1995). Therefore, transfer places minimal demands on metaprocessing abilities (see Chapter 9) and requires less training time than generalization of newly learned strategies (Saloman & Perkins, 1989).

Strategies and Generalization of Learning

Whereas acquisition of task-specific skills involves learning targeted behavioral sequences, the acquisition of strategies entails learning rules or principles that can be broadly applied. For example, many therapists expect persons with stroke to learn this general strategy: dress the weak side first, and undress the weak side last. This rule or principle enables patients to don and doff sweatshirts, dress shirts, slacks, and outwear, but it presumes generalization of learning.

Generalization occurs when the person is able to apply the newly learned strategy to a new task in a new environment. For example, the patient who demonstrates the ability to get dressed one-handed in the hospital can use the same strategies to put on a raincoat at home. Generalization, as it is here defined, depends on the learner's mindful abstraction of a principle and is based on conceptual similarities between the learning task and environment and the real-world application (Perkins, 1995). Generalization of learning places greater demands on patients' metaprocessing abilities (Saloman & Perkins, 1989). In fact, the more abstract the strategy, the more difficult it is to learn (Kirby, 1984). (It is easier for a patient to learn to dress the weak extremity before the strong one than to learn to use a higher order problem-solving strategy.)

FUNDAMENTALS OF THE TEACHING-LEARNING PROCESS

Clearly, the value of occupational therapy intervention will largely be judged by the extent to which new skills and strategies are carried out in patients' real-life environments. Therapists interested in helping patients achieve transfer and generalization objectives incorporate research findings about critical constructs in teaching-learning theory. These constructs relate to the therapeutic use of context, feedback, and practice.

Therapeutic Use of Context

The term "context" broadly refers to the setting in which an event or activity occurs. Many conceptions of context as a facilitator or barrier to function can be found in the occupational therapy and rehabilitation literature (American Occupational Therapy Association [AOTA], 2002; Dunn, Brown, & McGuigan, 1994; Fisher, 1998; World Health Organization, 1997) (see Chapters 10 and 11). The Occupational Therapy Practice Framework (AOTA, 2002) suggests that context has many dimensions: cultural, physical, social, personal, spiritual, temporal, and virtual. It also defined activity demands in terms of objects and their properties, space demands, social demands, sequencing and timing, and required actions as influencing the performance of skills and patterns. We now briefly discuss the influence of environmental context and activity demands on learning.

Role of Context in Learning

Research indicates that objects used in activities, the characteristics of those objects, and the goals of the activities performed have a strong influence on motor performance and must be carefully manipulated in treatment. Wu, Trombly, & Lin (1994) demonstrated that college students elicited smoother and faster arm movements when using real objects in movement tasks. Students were asked to perform three movements: picking up a pencil and preparing to write their name (materials-based task), pretend picking up a pencil and preparing to write their name (imagery-based task), and moving the arm forward to a target (exercise task). Students performed the three tasks differently, with the material-based task eliciting the smoothest and fastest movements. In addition, other groups of students were more successful in learning to eat with chopsticks if they used real food items during practice than if they had practiced manipulating non-food items (Ma, Trombly, & Robinson-Podolski, 1999)

The finding that the use of real objects elicits different movements and learning than imagery-based tasks or rote exercise has also been demonstrated by persons with disabilities such as cerebral palsy, stroke, and multiple sclerosis (Mathiowetz & Wade, 1995; Trombly & Wu, 1999; van der Weel, van der Meer, & Lee, 1991; Wu et al., 2000). Mathiowetz & Wade (1995) demonstrated that both subjects with multiple sclerosis and those without benefited from the information provided by real objects. Subjects were asked to eat applesauce, with a spoon, bowl, and applesauce available (materials-based task); pretend to eat applesauce, with a spoon and bowl available (partial-support task); and pretend to eat applesauce without a spoon or bowl (imagery-based task). Again, the movement patterns in the three conditions were significantly different. Trombly and Wu (1999) demonstrated that subjects who had strokes benefited from having objects to reach to rather than just reaching for a point in space. These findings support occupational therapy approaches that emphasize the significance of real-life tasks in optimizing function (Mathiowetz & Haugen, 1994). (See Chapters 6 and 22 for more about this approach.)

Environmental context is equally important to cognitive learning. In a classic study by Godden and Baddeley (1975), scuba divers who learned lists of words while underwater recalled them better underwater than on dry land, while divers who learned the lists on dry land recalled them better in that setting. These and previous findings are likely explained by two important principles: **encoding specificity** and **contextual interference**.

Encoding Specificity

The principle of encoding specificity suggests that events are stored in memory in such a way as to be inseparable from their contexts (Tulving & Thompson, 1973). That is, people encode features of the learning task and environment along with the newly acquired skill or strategy. Encoding specificity limits transfer and generalization because new tasks and environments do not have the same cueing properties as those present during original learning, making retrieval from long-term memory more difficult. For example, imagine that a therapist works with a patient on the same grasp and release task every day; even the work space is consistent. Although the patient improves performance on the task, the information about control of grasp and release is stored along with the context of the practice task and environment, and he or she may not be able to elicit these skills during ADL.

Contextual Interference

One way to mitigate the influence of encoding specificity on learning is to employ high contextual interference training (Battig, 1978). Low contextual interference occurs when the context and training task are invariant, allowing the learner to perform the same task repetitively in a consistent environment, as in the previous example. On the other hand, high contextual interference occurs when the task and environment keep changing throughout the learning process. This principle asserts that task and environmental variation force people to use multiple and varied information processing strategies, which makes retrieval easier. Contextual interference forces elaborate processing strategies, and transfer is facilitated.

Put another way, high contextual interference is a barrier to rote responding because it introduces problem-solving demands with each change of the context (Lee, Swanson, & Hall, 1991). Had the therapist from the previous example provided a variety of grasp and release activities in a variety of settings, the patient would have used more complex processing strategies during the learning process. Information about many similar grasp and release movements would be stored in memory along with a variety of environments and objects. As a result, the patient would be more likely to use the newly learned skills to solve problems within the inevitable variety of the real world. Therefore, to facilitate transfer of task-specific skills and generalization of newly learned strategies, therapists deliberately vary the learning tasks and environments.

Therapeutic Use of Feedback

Feedback also can enhance or interfere with learning. Occupational therapists understand the functions of feedback and deliberately select the types and schedules of feedback in designing a patient's learning experience. Procedures for Practice 14-2 discusses videotaped feedback.

Functions of Feedback

Feedback regarding performance has several functions (Salmoni, Schmidt, & Walter, 1984). It has a temporary motivating or energizing effect and a guidance effect that

PROCEDURES FOR PRACTICE 14-2

Teaching Technologies: Videotape Feedback

Many researchers have investigated the use of videotape for feedback to improve learning (Brotherton et al., 1988; Morgan & Salzberg, 1992; Tham & Tegner, 1997). It has been applied to a broad variety of situations and a large number of patient populations. These studies have consistently demonstrated that videotape feedback can improve a patient's awareness of his or her performance. However, researchers have also found that simply showing a videotape of performance does not lead to improvements. Effective feedback must be structured by the clinician to focus the attention of the patient on pertinent actions and events. The advantage of videotape feedback is that the therapist can stop the tape at critical points, focus attention on specific features, and ask the subject to analyze and suggest appropriate changes. For example, in an investigation of the effectiveness of videotape feedback in the treatment of neglect syndrome, patients were videotaped performing a simulated cooking task that involved arranging pastries on a baking tray (Tham & Tegner, 1997). Therapists showed the subjects structured videotapes of their performance and provided feedback during the viewing. Subjects improved on follow-up on this test, but no generalization was noted.

Videotape has also been used to assist with social skills training of patients with brain injuries and severe mental retardation (Brotherton et al., 1988; Morgan & Salzberg, 1992). In both cases, the videotape feedback was used to help patients identify problematic behaviors, which was followed by rehearsal of appropriate behaviors. Again, in these cases, the therapist structured viewing of the videotape, with identification of the problems and the appropriate behaviors, as part of an ongoing dialogue. Rehearsal of appropriate responses was also part of the training program.

Finally, videotape may be especially helpful in teaching complex motor skills. Hodges, Chua, and Franks (2003) used video to facilitate learning and retention of a complex bimanual activity. Those participants who had access to the video during training performed significantly better on the post-test and were better able to able to identify errors in performance than those individuals who did not have access to video feedback during training. This was especially true for those individuals who performed worst at the pre-test. It is suggested that, by using video feedback, participants were able to formulate a model of the action they were to perform and were then able to come closer to that model during training and retention trials.

As these studies show, the use of videotaped feedback can assist in the teaching process, but it must be used in a structured and purposeful way. Showing patients specific sections of tape, pointing out relevant details, and asking patients to describe their behavior and solve problems are all effective ways to use videotape. Furthermore, if reasonable for the specific task, rehearsal of appropriate responses provides patients with a repertoire of appropriate behaviors.

informs the learner how to correct an error on the next trial. However, feedback can permanently impair motor learning if provided beyond the point that the person has a rough idea of the desired motion.

Types of Feedback

To help patients learn and sustain skills and strategies, therapists initially provide extrinsic feedback on performance but ultimately facilitate the development of intrinsic feedback.

Extrinsic Feedback: Knowledge of Results and Knowledge of Performance

Therapists typically provide feedback about performance in verbal form. Extrinsic information presented after task completion falls into two categories, knowledge of results and knowledge of performance. This feedback allows subjects to alter or adapt their responses or behaviors on subsequent trials. Knowledge of results provides information about outcome, such as "You've got your shirt on" or "You took the cap off that jar." A second type of feedback, knowledge of performance, is related to qualitative descriptions of a performance, such as "You shifted your weight too far to the left" or "You bent your elbow." This information directs patients' attention not to outcome but to components of movement that they need to change or attend to. This type of feedback duplicates information patients already have available through intrinsic feedback but on which they may not be focusing.

Other external information provided to patients during practice falls into the category of encouragement. It is important that patients and therapists do not confuse encouragement ("Keep going") with feedback ("You're doing great"), especially if the latter is not true, as incorrect feedback is highly detrimental to learning (Buekers, Magill, & Hall, 1992).

Intrinsic Feedback

Intrinsic feedback, or internal feedback, is information that patients receive through their own senses, such as seeing an egg break as it hits the floor after dropping it or feeling the pain of hitting the ground after an unsuccessful transfer. Although this information is readily available to patients, they may need cueing to focus on the most important components of a skill or strategy, such as learning to use vision when moving an anesthetic limb. Intervention that incorporates self-monitoring and self-estimation (task difficulty, completion time, accuracy score, amount of cueing, or assistance needed) enables patients to create mechanisms for self-generated feedback (Cicerone & Giacino, 1992; Toglia, 1998), lessening dependence on therapists for successful performance.

Feedback Schedules

The frequency and content of feedback are critical to the learning process and must be considered when a teaching situation is planned.

Immediate and Summary Feedback

The frequency and time at which feedback is given can profoundly influence the acquisition and learning of task-specific skills and strategies. Studies in this area evaluate learning during a "retention trial," which is done some time after teaching is completed. For example, Lavery (1962) wanted to know which schedule of feedback best facilitated learning: immediate feedback provided after each trial was completed, also referred to as constant feedback; summary feedback provided after a number of trials were completed; or both. Lavery found that subjects who received immediate or combined feedback improved their performance of the task more quickly during the acquisition phase than the group receiving only summary feedback. However, when tested for retention of the task 4, 37, and 93 days after training, the subjects who received only summary feedback did significantly better than those who received either immediate feedback or both types.

Lavery hypothesized that people who received immediate feedback came to rely on it when performing the task and those that received only summary feedback were forced to analyze their own movements. The subjects who received both immediate and summary feedback did just as poorly as those who received only immediate feedback, suggesting that the immediate feedback interfered with the processing of the summary feedback. Beyond its implications about the schedule of feedback, these findings support the idea that performance during the training phase does not reflect actual learning of the skill.

Faded Feedback

Therapists are often concerned that providing only summary feedback after a series of trials will not help their patients understand tasks that are complex or new. Winstein and Schmidt (1990) evaluated the effectiveness of feedback given on 50% and 100% of trials on the learning of a task by college students. The 50% feedback was faded, with the feedback given on every trial initially and then decreased to no feedback at the end of training, with feedback being given on an overall average of 50% of all the trials. They found a slight advantage for the 100% feedback group during acquisition of the skill, but there were significant differences during the retention phase, which is the true test of learning. The group that received faded feedback performed significantly better than the immediate feedback group on the retention trials; the trials were performed at 10 minutes and 2 days, with the effect at 2 days more noticeable. Remember that, from the standpoint of encoding specificity, subjects who were on the 50% schedule received no feedback at the end of the acquisition phase and were performing the task in exactly the same way as they did during the retention phase. Also, these findings point out an important irony: factors that degrade performance during acquisition may improve learning.

Bandwidth Feedback

With bandwidth feedback, an acceptable range of performance is defined, and the subject receives feedback only when performance is outside of that range. As the subject's performance improves, feedback is provided less frequently. Research Note 14-1 further discusses this point (Goodwin & Meeuwsen, 1995).

Therapeutic Use of Practice

In addition to planning feedback, the design of a treatment session factors in the nature of instructions and a plan for practicing the material.

Internally or Externally Focused Instructions

Recent research supports instruction that is focused on the task rather than on the patient's performance (Wulf et al., 2002). For example, Fasoli et al. (2002) found that persons who had had a stroke reached faster and more smoothly when cued to focus on an object and what they were going to do with it, rather than focusing on their arm as they did the task. This means that the instructions given to patients should focus their attention on the objects and the task, rather than on the movements that they will be using to achieve the goal.

Blocked Versus Random Practice

As discussed earlier, traditional models of learning did not distinguish between learning and performance. These models also promoted blocked forms of practice, such as drill, as the most efficient schedule for learning a task.

RESEARCH NOTE 14-1

Abstract: Goodwin, J. E., & Meeuwsen, H. J. (1995). Using bandwidth knowledge of results to alter relative frequencies during motor skills acquisition. *Research Quarterly for Exercise and Sport, 66,* 99–104.

Goodwin and Meeuwsen (1995) examined the effect of using bandwidth feedback on a golfing task. Subjects were assigned to four groups. The first group received feedback on every trial that did not hit the hole, whereas the second group received feedback on every trial in which the ball was more than 18 inches from the hole. The third group was given feedback on a shrinking bandwidth schedule, tolerating increasingly smaller errors (initially if the ball missed the hole by 27 inches, then 18 inches, 9 inches, and 0 inches). The fourth group received feedback on an expanding schedule, tolerating increasingly larger errors, starting with 0 inches and then increasing to 9 inches, 18 inches, 27 inches, and finally 36 inches. Interestingly, the groups that received the least feedback (i.e., the group that got feedback only when the ball was more than 18 inches from the hole and the expanding [fourth] group) performed the best during the retention phase. The third (shrinking) group performed similarly to the group that received feedback whenever the ball did not hit the hole. These findings led the authors to suggest that receiving high frequencies of feedback at the end of the acquisition phase increases the subject's dependence on that feedback and is as detrimental to learning as providing high frequencies of feedback throughout the acquisition phase.

Implications for Practice

- Frequent indiscriminate feedback seems detrimental to learning. Therefore, therapists must monitor the timing and frequency of comments to patients as they learn new skills and strategies.
- When it comes to feedback, it appears that less is more. Patients who receive less feedback may increasingly rely on intrinsic feedback and be more likely to retain the new skill or strategy than persons who get a lot of feedback when they make errors. Therapists should provide opportunities for patients to determine when and why they have made errors.

Using a blocked format, the same skill or strategy is practiced over a number of repetitions, after which the next skill or strategy is rehearsed. As such, blocked practice is a form of practice with low contextual interference.

Shea and Morgan (1979) studied whether increasing the contextual interference by random practice during skill acquisition leads to improved retention and transfer of motor skills. Their experiments entailed knocking over wooden barriers with a tennis ball held in the hand. In brief, they found that blocked practice provided low contextual interference, whereas random practice provided high contextual interference, requiring subjects to formulate a new movement plan for each trial. Subjects who practiced with high contextual interference demonstrated better retention and transfer than those who used blocked practice. This study demonstrated two important findings: (1) performance during acquisition of a skill does not necessarily relate to later learning; and (2) conditions that may improve performance during acquisition do not necessarily create better learning. In fact, structuring training to improve performance during practice by using blocked practice schedules is actually detrimental to learning.

The advantage of random practice over blocked practice was also demonstrated for patients with hemiplegia (Hanlon, 1996). Patients practiced a multistep functional activity that consisted of reaching for a cupboard door, opening it, picking up a coffee cup by the handle, transferring it to a counter, and releasing the handle. The subjects practiced these steps in either a blocked or a random pattern. The random pattern group performed significantly better than either the blocked or control group on both the 2-day and 7-day retention trials.

Part-Whole Practice

Therapists also decide whether patients practice the whole task or components of a task (referred to as part-whole training). Ma and Trombly (2004) evaluated the characteristics of movement under part and whole task conditions. The task involved reaching for a pen, bringing the pen to paper, and signing the name. The three segments of movement were performed separately and then as a single task for each individual. The performance of the whole task elicited greater efficiency of movement, greater force during the task, and smoother movements. Mane, Adams, & Donchin (1989) manipulated two dimensions of practice while teaching a task: whole versus part task and speed of performance. Participants learned to play a goal-directed computer game. The part-whole study examined the extent to which practicing part of the task improved performance of the whole game. In this study, subjects who practiced a critical skill extracted from the game did improve performance on the overall game. However, changing the speed of practice was met with varying success. Practice at the slowest speed fundamentally changed the demands of the task, leading to poor transfer of skills to the task at original speeds. On the other hand, slight slowing of task speed during training enhanced learning.

Winstein et al. (1989) examined the effect of part-task practice with gait training. One group of patients with hemiplegia received traditional physical therapy gait training. The second group received traditional physical therapy and specific training in standing balance symmetry (proposed as a reasonable critical component of symmetrical gait). After several weeks of training, the group that had practiced symmetry in standing showed improvement in that component of the activity, but there was no carryover to the whole task of gait. There was no significant difference in gait symmetry between the two groups.

These findings demonstrate that, although part-whole training may work in some situations, such as the computer game, it is not successful in all situations. Furthermore, therapists may not be able to identify the specific critical components that would improve overall learning. It will require much more research to identify the components that will transfer to the whole task before part-task training can be the preferred method. Winstein et al. (1989) suggested that tasks that are continuous and cannot be easily separated into component parts may not be appropriate for part training. Examples of this type of movement include walking or driving a car—tasks that require many adjustments with components that occur simultaneously and cannot be easily separated.

MAKING PERSONAL CHANGE

Employing a newly learned skill or strategy is fundamentally a personal change. Using a new skill or strategy in daily life depends not only on recall, transfer, or generalization but also on learners' beliefs about their competence and their stage in the change process.

Bandura (1977) posited that people's beliefs about their ability to handle a new situation largely determine whether they attempt the new task and their ultimate performance. Self-percepts of efficacy (self-perceptions of competence) predict success with a wide range of acquired health behaviors, including smoking cessation (Stewart, Borland, & McMurray, 1994), exercise maintenance (McAuley, 1993), medication compliance (DeGeest et al., 1994), and use of energy-conservation techniques to manage fatigue (Mathiowetz, Matuska, & Murphy, 2001). Bandura (1977) demonstrated that people make judgments about their competence (self-efficacy) by thinking about past accomplishments, vicarious experience (observing others who are similar), verbal persuasion, and emotional arousal, such as anxiety. Since self-percepts of competence seem to explain the discrepancy between what people can do and what they actually do (Bandura, 1982), occupational therapists actively create opportunities for patients to demonstrate to themselves that they are indeed competent with the new skill or strategy.

Many patients served by occupational therapists have had sudden onset of changes in physical functioning. Persons who are insulated from ramifications of these changes (perhaps those who have been hospitalized continuously since onset) may not fully appreciate the need for the skills and strategies therapists are attempting to teach them. The Stages of Change Model (Prochaska & DiClemente, 1982) helps therapists target their teaching-learning interventions to address the learning predispositions of the client and family.

This model identifies four stages of change: contemplation, determination, action, and maintenance. During the first stage, clients become aware of the problem or concern; in the determination stage, they resolve to do something about it; during the action stage, clients work to address the problem or issue; and clients must still put forth some degree of effort to sustain the desired skill or behavior during the maintenance stage. The researchers suggested that verbal intervention strategies are most appropriate during the first two stages (pointing out the problem and discussing possible approaches), whereas action-oriented behavioral interventions are most helpful during the last two stages. For example, before a client routinely employs strategies for scanning the left visual field, he or she must believe that parts of the environment are missing or that personal safety is in jeopardy. Merely elucidating the problem is not enough. Once convinced and motivated, the client is taught specifically how to handle the problem.

OCCUPATIONAL THERAPIST AS TEACHER

The extent to which occupational therapy contributes to a client's resumption of roles depends to a large extent on the effectiveness of the therapist as a teacher. Principles of teaching parallel therapy: assessment, goal setting, intervention, and evaluation (Redman, 1997). Although this process rarely follows a predictable, orderly sequence, these steps serve as a checklist to ensure that therapists consider variables affecting the outcome of their teaching efforts (Redman, 1997).

Assess Learning Needs and Readiness

Before teaching begins, therapists complete a traditional occupational therapy assessment so as to understand the client's occupational needs, priorities, capacities, skills, and competencies. Therapists attempt to identify barriers to learning, such as low literacy; distracters, such as pain and fatigue; lack of human or financial support; awareness of problem areas; and incongruous values between patient and therapist (Vanetzian, 1997). Dynamic assessment provides information about the circumstances (task, environment, strategies, and cueing) in which the patient

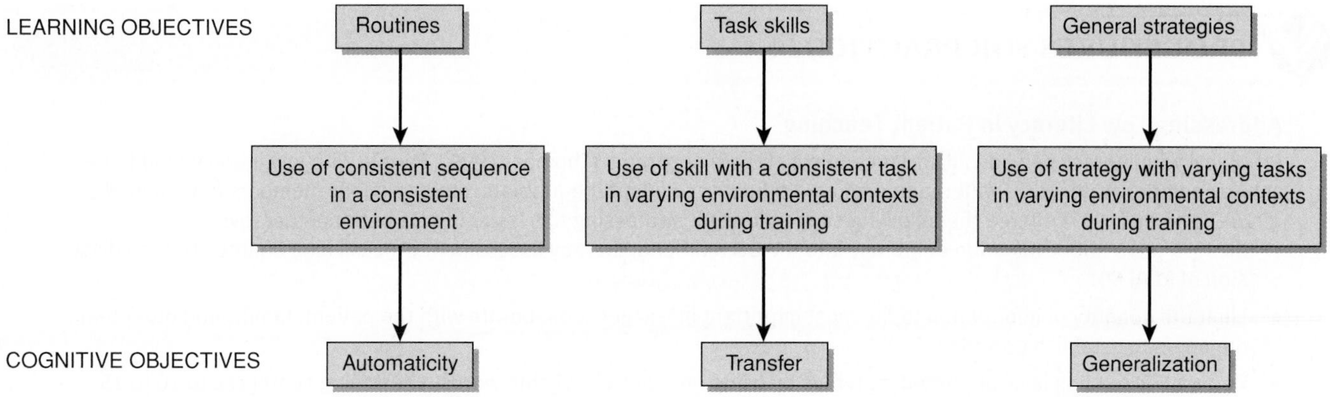

Figure 14-1 Teaching objectives in occupational therapy.

is best able to learn (Toglia, 1989) (see Chapter 9). Therefore, the therapist determines who will be the subject or subjects of the teaching—the patient, family member (if the patient seems unlikely to retain the information), or both.

Set Client-Specific Learning Goals

Therapists use the results of their assessments and estimates of the treatment time available to set learning and cognitive objectives for each patient (Fig. 14-1). Therapists plan treatment around transfer and generalization goals by identifying reinforcements in the natural environment and incorporating into the treatment stimuli common to both training and real-world environments (Sohlberg & Raskin, 1996). If the intervention ultimately is to change an existing routine, skill, or strategy, the therapist attempts to determine where in the process of change the learner is. For example, a patient with little or no awareness of a memory problem is likely to have minimal interest in learning to use compensatory memory techniques. Therefore, the therapist sets goals that move the patient toward the contemplative stage of change by allowing him or her to take the consequences of forgetting. Finally, therapists merely recommend learning goals. Goals that direct teaching-learning efforts are set in collaboration with patients and their families.

Create Learning Opportunities Throughout Intervention

Therapists deliberately use context, feedback, and practice to help patients meet learning goals (Procedures for Practice 14-3). They try to enhance motivation and recall by linking new skills or strategies with patients' specific interests, knowledge, and abilities. Effective teachers also make an effort to overcome barriers to learning. They select the optimal time of day and environment for teaching

PROCEDURES FOR PRACTICE 14-3

Therapeutic Use of Context, Feedback, and Practice to Promote Transfer and Generalization

- Vary the training environmental context to achieve transfer; vary training tasks and environments to achieve generalization of new strategies.
- Provide extrinsic feedback just until the learner understands the desired movement, skill, or strategy. Use cueing and the patient's own performance prediction and analysis to help the learner increasingly rely on intrinsic feedback.
- Provide summary feedback when possible. Tolerate a slower or longer acquisition phase of learning, appreciating the later benefits in terms of retention, transfer, and generalization.
- Fade therapist feedback and cues so that these elements of training do not get encoded with the new skill or strategy.
- Attempt to teach movement, skills, and strategies within whole tasks. Address components or subskills only when they are critical to whole-task performance.

PROCEDURES FOR PRACTICE 14-4

Addressing Low Literacy in Patient Teaching

Problems with literacy pervade all socioeconomic and ethnic groups (Thomas, 1999). People with low literacy tend to be ashamed of their difficulties with reading and are reluctant to admit the problem, even to family members (Parikh et al., 1996). Thomas (1999) offered the following suggestions for addressing this issue in occupational therapy:

- Incorporate a brief evaluation of literacy into the occupational therapy assessment process (see Chapter 10 for a discussion of REALM).
- Limit the quantity of information to the most important messages. Collaborate with the patient, family, and other team members to establish priorities.
- Reduce the reading level of printed materials by using one- or two-syllable words, shortening sentences to 10 to 15 words, and targeting materials to the fifth- or sixth-grade reading level.
- Make sure text and graphics are well organized. Davis et al. (1998) found both preference for and improved comprehension with a question-and-answer list format over a paragraph format for text.
- Use materials that are racially and culturally sensitive. As recommended by Thomas (1999), "make sure that patients can 'see themselves' in materials provided."

and change their schedules occasionally to adapt to family needs. Clinicians recognize that literacy affects comprehension and use of health-related written materials for many adults (Davis et al., 1998). Citing the results of the 2003 National Adult Literacy Survey, Schneider (2005) reported that 13% of all Americans had "Below Basic" English literacy for prose material. This means that 30 million Americans cannot do much more than sign a form or review a document to see what they are allowed to drink before a medical procedure (Schneider, 2005). Another 22% had only "Basic" literacy, meaning, at best, they can find information in a pamphlet about how jurors were selected for a jury pool (National Center for Education Statistics, 2005). Therefore, clinicians create and use written materials that are well organized and limit the demands on reading (Procedures for Practice 14-4). Finally, to achieve transfer and generalization goals, therapists use the continuum of care to reinforce long-term learning. Often this means teaching family members how to extend the learning process and providing copies of the discharge instructions to other providers, such as the home health occupational therapist, vocational specialist, and nurse case manager.

Evaluate Achievement of Learning Goals

Effective teachers routinely assess clients' progress toward learning goals, typically by changing the training task or environment and evaluating carryover. Family members perform return demonstrations of new techniques, such as transfers. Based on performance or other changes in learning status, therapists adjust learning goals throughout the intervention.

Evidence Table 14-1

Intervention	Description of Intervention Tested	Participants	Dosage	Type of Best Evidence and Level of Evidence	Benefit	Statistical Probability and Effect Size of Outcome	Reference
Videotape feedback	Experimental group received videotaped feedback after performance of a task; control group did not.	14 consecutive stroke survivors, all RCVA, 7 in experimental arm and 7 in control arm. Mean age = 67.9 years.	A single episode of video feedback, with follow-up testing 3 hours after feedback session.	Randomized controlled study. IC1b	Yes. The treatment group improved more than the control group but only on the trained task.	Baking Tray Task: $p = 0.02$, $r = 0.81$.	Tham & Tegner, 1997
Training in a task in a natural or simulated context	Participants practiced an eating task using chopsticks in a natural or simulated context.	40 right-handed college students without disabilities and without previous experience with using chopsticks. Mean age = 23.75 years.	60 training trials on 1 day, 24-hour retention measured on a transfer task.	Randomized controlled study. IB1c	Participants in natural context performed better than those in a simulated context on the transfer task.	Natural context: $p = 0.03$, $r = 0.30$ for success rate at retention trial in the transfer task.	Ma, Trombly, & Robinson-Podolski, 1999
Effect of goal-directed action	Experiment 1: Subjects reached in a goal-directed action or to a spatial location. Experiment 2: Subjects reached for phone, disconnected receiver, and a stick.	14 stroke survivors (9 LCVA, 4 RCVA, 1 bilateral CVA). Mean age = 65 years; average time since onset of stroke = 39 months.	Each participant tested under several conditions.	Randomized controlled repeated measures counterbalanced design. IC1b	Participants reaching for an object were faster, smoother, and took less time to reach peak speed than when they reached for a point in space.	Experiment 1: number of movement units, $p = 0.05$, $r = 0.55$; movement time $p = 0.02$, $r = 0.62$; percentage of reach to peak velocity, $p = 0.04$, $r = 0.57$; peak velocity, $p = 0.01$, $r = 0.66$. Experiment 2: no effect.	Trombly & Wu, 1999

continued

Evidence Table 14-1 (*continued*)

Intervention	Description of Intervention Tested	Participants	Dosage	Type of Best Evidence and Level of Evidence	Benefit	Statistical Probability and Effect Size of Outcome	Reference
Presence or absence of objects used in movements	Participants evaluated for movements with object or without object.	14 stroke survivors (9 LCVA, 5 RCVA, and 1 bilateral CVA) and 25 neurologically intact adults.	Each participant was tested under 2 conditions: reaching to scoop up coins and reaching to where the coins would have been.	Randomized controlled repeated measures counterbalanced design. IC1b	Using real objects elicited better performance of reaching, as measured by decreased movement time, decreased displacement, higher velocity, and fewer movement units.	Stroke survivor data: movement time, $p = 0.0028$, $r = 0.70$; total displacement, $p = 0.0019$, $r = 0.72$; percentage of reach where peak velocity occurs, $p = 0.0011$, $r = 0.75$; movement units, $p = 0.0055$, $r = 0.66$.	Wu et al., 2000

RCVA, right cerebral vascular accident; LCVA, left cerebral vascular accident; CVA, cerebral vascular accident.

CASE EXAMPLE

Learning as Part of Home-Based Intervention for a Client with Motor and Perceptual Deficits

Occupational Therapy Intervention Process

Client Information

Mr. O. is a 69-year-old married man seen by occupational therapy in home care 1 month post stroke. He had received therapy in both the acute hospital setting and in a rehabilitation unit. During his initial interview, Mr. O. indicated that he wanted to resume the following pre-morbid roles: working as the head of an advertising agency, golfing, driving, and being independent at home. He indicated that his goals for therapy included being safe during short periods of being left alone, being able to walk and drive independently, and being independent in self-care, light meal preparation, and going to the bathroom. He also wanted to use his involved left arm like he did before. He viewed these skills and tasks as pre-requisite to resumption of his identified roles.

Mr. O. was assessed at home with the following results:

- ADL: Mr. O. was able to dress with minimal assistance and cues but needed maximal assistance in toileting, bathing, and meal preparation.
- Upper extremity function: He did not use his left arm in any functional activities, although he did have active movement and strength of muscle grades 3 to 4 throughout. He had difficulty using the available motion in tasks requiring movement at more than one joint.
- Walking and mobility: He was able to stand with moderate assistance but was unable to propel his wheelchair in the house. He walked with moderate assistance and a wide-based quad cane.
- IADL: Driving was not evaluated. Due to his need for assistance in standing, golf was not evaluated initially.
- Patient's safety: Mr. O. fell several times in the hospital and had been labeled impulsive. However, conversation with the patient revealed that the problem was not so much impulsivity as awareness. As he put it, "I forget that my leg and arm don't work when I stand up but remember as I'm falling."
- Problems in performance were related to severe left neglect, which the patient strongly denied. He knew adapted dressing techniques but needed cues regarding neglect of his left arm. There were also environmental barriers to using the wheelchair, and adaptive equipment was needed for the bathroom.

Clinical Reasoning Process

Objectives	Examples of Therapist's Internal Dialogue
Appreciate the context	"Mr. O. struck me as someone who is used to being in charge—doing what he wants, when he wants. I could tell that he was frustrated with his dependence on his wife and by the fact that he continued to need supervision. I was not interested in arguing with him about goals that I viewed as unrealistic at this time (especially the driving) but instead helped him focus on the first steps of managing himself independently at home." "I was actually surprised by how much strength Mr. O. had in his left arm because I never observed him using it during functional activities. It was clear to me that Mr. O. could be much more self-reliant once we installed some adaptive equipment in the bathroom. It seems that Mr. O's left neglect is a real barrier to his safety, however. The neglect appears to be at the heart of his need for ongoing supervision and certainly interferes with his use of his left arm. He seems to get rather defensive at the suggestion that neglect is a problem. Again, I have no intention of arguing with Mr. O. about this but will try to teach him about the impact of his neglect if and when situations arise.
Develop intervention hypotheses	1. By providing adaptive equipment, I thought I could help Mr. O. to become more independent in a number of the ADLs that matter to him. 2. I figured that if I can help Mr. O. become more aware of his left neglect, he may learn to compensate for it and realize improved upper extremity function and safety.
Select an intervention approach	The following are intervention approaches that I used: 1. Change the physical environment/context 2. Teach compensatory skills 3. Restore left upper extremity function
Reflect on competence	"I have never treated someone whose left neglect is so profound but have worked with clients with brain injury who have similar problems with awareness, so I feel competent to provide services to Mr. O."

Recommendations

Home-based occupational therapy was recommended for four times a week for 3 weeks, then two or three times a week for 3 weeks, followed by transition to outpatient occupational therapy. Short-term goals for home care (3 weeks) were identified as (1) minimal assistance in toileting and clothing adjustment, (2) standby assistance with showering, (3) safety and independence for short periods during the day (30–60 minutes), and (4) independence in light meal preparation.

Consider the client's appraisal of performance

Consider what will occur in therapy, how often, and for how long

Ascertain the client's endorsement of plan

"Even though Mr. O. didn't initially appreciate the significance of his left neglect, he seemed very committed to his therapy program and quite clear about his goals. He'd have me come every day, if my schedule permitted."

"I recommended a fairly intense home-based therapy program to start with because we really had a lot to do. Both Mr. and Mrs. O. were frustrated with his level of assistance, especially in the bathroom, and I knew that it would take a few visits to get that in order. But since we were practicing in his own home, I felt that Mr. O. could make good progress quickly."

Summary of Short-Term Goals and Progress

The first week of therapy focused on environmental adaptations so that Mr. O. could move about the house in his wheelchair. Also, a raised tub seat, raised toilet seat, and grab bars were installed in the bathroom to increase safety and decrease his dependence on his wife. Attempts to increase his awareness of neglect were integrated into almost all contacts. He did make some improvements in compensation for the left neglect, specifically as it related to wheelchair propulsion and toileting.

During the second week of home care, the patient attempted to walk without assistance and fell. He received a large gash to his face and ear and spent the night in the emergency room. When the occupational therapist arrived the next day, he announced that this "left neglect thing" might be more of a problem than he had thought and that he was now willing to work on it. A number of functional tasks were practiced, including playing cards and doing crossword puzzles, activities he had previously enjoyed. Over the next 2 weeks, he became more aware of his left visual space, compensating spontaneously in most simple activities around the house and becoming much safer at home.

During this same 2-week period, he continued to make gains in gait and all ADL. Improvements in both strength and compensation for neglect allowed him to go to the bathroom and transfer into and out of the bathtub with minimal assistance. However, he continued to need constant cueing to incorporate his left arm into most activities. When cued to use his arm, he insisted that it had been involved with the activity or that he always did that task with only his right arm.

In summary, after 3 weeks of home-based therapy, Mr. O. met his goals related to toileting and clothing adjustment (requiring just minimal assistance) and remaining safe and independent for brief periods of time. He had made progress toward his other goals related to showering and meal preparation.

Assess the client's comprehension

Understand what he is doing

Compare actual to expected performance

Know the person

Appreciate the context

"Both Mr. and Mrs. O. were very pleased with the bathroom equipment. Mr. O.'s brother is a home-repair expert, and he came over to install the grab bars in the shower/tub area. I just don't feel comfortable installing anything into ceramic tile myself. The equipment made an immediate difference in Mr. O.'s independence."

"I was relieved that Mr. O.'s fall didn't result in a more severe injury; he was lucky, and he knew it. This incident 'put the fear in him,' and I tried to capitalize on that in therapy. He was willing to do the table top activities that I gave him as homework, which safely occupied him while Mrs. O. did the laundry in the basement."

"Even though I'm seeing progress in terms of Mr. O.'s safety and independence in self-care activities, I'm really not seeing the gains I had hoped to in terms of his arm function. Again, the left neglect is the big barrier and Mr. O. seems to be tiring of my pointing out issues that he simply can't see. He strikes me as someone who doesn't like to be prompted or cajoled; for that matter, I suppose I wouldn't like that either."

Next Steps

1. Use visual feedback to improve awareness of left neglect

   In an attempt to increase his awareness of the use of the left arm, video feedback was employed during a golfing task. The client tried putting several times, and these attempts were videotaped. The client consistently neglected his left hand but insisted that he was using it. Following the unsuccessful cues, four more putts were taped. Mr. O. was then shown the videotape as a form of summary feedback. He was surprised by his lack of use of his arm and hand and identified that as part of the cause of his poor performance. Following the viewing of the tape, he putted some more. The client consistently incorporated his left arm into the

Anticipate present and future client concerns

"I wanted to allow Mr. O. to see what I was seeing relative to his left arm use and function so that he might begin to prompt himself rather than simply endure what seemed like endless nagging from me. I specifically chose to videotape his performance during a golfing task because I knew that that activity really mattered to him. Mr. O. received important feedback in two key ways: seeing himself on tape and then observing his own improved task performance when he used both arms. He and I came up with a silly verbal prompt to task, and his performance improved. Most surprisingly, this awareness transferred to other activities, increasing his safety and efficiency in a variety of tasks, including transfers, walking, meal preparation, and emptying the dishwasher.

2. Continue with revised goals

After the first 3 weeks of treatment, new goals for therapy were set. They included: (1) independence in light meal preparation, (2) independence in toileting, (3) standby assistance for transfers in and out of shower, and (4) safety and independence for short periods (1–2 hours).

Analyze client's comprehension Decide if he or she should continue or discontinue therapy and/or return in the future	use whenever he seemed to be neglecting his arm. It is something like, 'sometimes the right hand doesn't know what the left hand is doing.' Mrs. O. uses it now too, and Mr. O. doesn't mind. Now that Mr. O. is more aware of his tendency to neglect the left side, I think he's ready to tackle more complex activities such as meal preparation and getting in and out of the shower."

CLINICAL REASONING IN OCCUPATIONAL THERAPY PRACTICE

Differentiating Between the Acquisition of Skills Versus Strategies

Mr. O.'s assessment suggested a number of learning needs related to his self-identified goals. List learning needs characterized as task-specific skills. List learning needs that are best characterized as general strategies. Compare Mr. O.'s learning processes for the task-specific skills and general strategies in terms of speed and ease of acquisition and teaching methods.

CLINICAL REASONING IN OCCUPATIONAL THERAPY PRACTICE

Training for Transfer and Generalization

Mr. O.'s treatment took place in his home in the context of his everyday activities. Describe how encoding specificity contributed to the acquisition of skills and strategies in this setting. Imagine that Mr. O. works toward similar goals while a patient in a rehabilitation unit. In what ways should his treatment program change to optimize the likelihood of transfer and generalization of skills and strategies?

SUMMARY REVIEW QUESTIONS

1. List the types of practice patterns and discuss the advantages and disadvantages of each.
2. Design two ADL training sessions, one for learning a specific task and the second for learning a general strategy.
3. Discuss the different feedback schedules and compare their advantages and disadvantages.
4. Identify Fitts and Posner's three stages of learning. Describe the characteristics of performance that you might see as patients learn to use a piece of adaptive equipment.
5. List characteristics of practice mostly likely to facilitate transfer and generalization of practice.
6. Describe the influences on the learning readiness of a family caregiver. What will you do to optimize the learning process in response to these influences?

References

American Occupational Therapy Association [AOTA]. (2002). Occupational therapy practice framework: Domain and process. *American Journal of Occupational Therapy, 56,* 609–639.

Atkinson, R. C., & Shiffrin, R. M. (1971). The control of short-term memory. *Scientific American, 225,* 82–90.

Bandura, A. (1977). Self-efficacy: Toward a unifying theory of behavior change. *Psychological Review, 84,* 191–215.

Bandura, A. (1982). Self-efficacy mechanism in human agency. *American Psychologist, 37,* 122–147.

Battig, W. F. (1978). The flexibility of the human memory. In L. S. Cermak & F. I. M. Craik (Eds.), *Levels of processing and human memory* (pp. 23–44). Hillsdale, NJ: Erlbaum.

Brotherton, F. A., Thomas, L. L., Wisotzek, I. E., & Milan, M. A. (1988). Social skills training in the rehabilitation of patients with traumatic closed head injury. *Archives of Physical Medicine and Rehabilitation, 69,* 827–832.

Buekers, M. J. A., Magill, R. A., & Hall, K. G. (1992). The effect of erroneous knowledge of results on skill acquisition when augmented information is redundant. *Quarterly Journal of Experimental Psychology, 44,* 105–117.

Carter, J. H., & Nutt, J. G. (1998). Family caregiving: A neglected and hidden part of health care delivery. *American Academy of Neurology, 51,* 1245–1246.

Cicerone, K. D., & Giacino, J. T. (1992). Remediation of executive function deficits after traumatic brain injury. *NeuroRehabilitation, 2,* 12–22.

Clark, P. C., Dunbar, S. B., Shields, C. G., Viswanathan, B., Aycock, D. M., & Wolf, S. (2004). Influence of stroke survivor characteristics and family conflict surrounding recovery on caregivers' mental and physical health. *Nursing Research, 53,* 406–413.

Craik, F. I. M., & Tulving, E. (1975). Depth of processing and retention of words in episodic memory. *Journal of Experimental Psychology: General, 104,* 268–294.

Davis, T. C., Fredrickson, D. D., Arnold, C., Murphy, P. W., Herbst, M., & Bocchini, J. A. (1998). A polio immunization pamphlet with increased appeal and simplified language does not improve comprehension to an acceptable level. *Patient Education and Counseling, 33,* 25–37.

Deckersbach, T., Savage, C. R., Curran, T., Bohne, A., Wilhelm, S., Baer, L., Jenike, M. A., & Rauch, S. L. (2002). A study of parallel implicit and explicit information processing in patients with obsessive-compulsive disorder. *American Journal of Psychiatry, 159,* 1780–1782.

DeGeest, S., Abraham, I., Gemoets, H., & Evers, G. (1994). Development of the long-term medication behavior self-efficacy scale: Qualitative study for item development. *Journal of Advanced Nursing, 19,* 233–238.

Dunn, W., Brown, C., & McGuigan, A. (1994). The ecology of human performance: A framework for considering the effect of context. *American Journal of Occupational Therapy, 48,* 595–607.

Eldridge, L. L., Masterman, D., & Knowlton, B. J. (2002). Intact implicit habit learning in Alzheimer's disease. *Behavioral Neuroscience, 116,* 722–726.

Eversheim, U., & Bock, O. (2001). Evidence for processing stages in skills acquisition: A dual-task study. *Learning and Memory, 8,* 183–189.

Eysenck, M. W., & Keane, M. R. (1990). *Cognitive psychology: A student's handbook.* East Sussex, UK: Lawrence Erlbaum.

Fasoli, S. E., Trombly, C. A., Tickle-Degnen, L., & Verfaellie, M. H. (2002). Effect of instructions on functional reach in persons with and without cerebrovascular accident. *American Journal of Occupational Therapy, 56,* 380–390.

Fisher, A. G. (1998). Uniting practice and theory in an occupational framework. *American Journal of Occupational Therapy, 52,* 509–521.

Fitts, P. M., & Posner, M. I. (1967). *Human performance.* Belmont, CA: Brooks/Cole.

Gentile, A. M. (1998). Implicit and explicit processes during acquisition of functional skills. *Scandinavian Journal of Occupational Therapy, 5,* 7–16.

Giles, G. M. (2005). A neurofunctional approach to rehabilitation following severe brain injury. In N. Katz (Ed.), *Cognition and occupation across the life span* (pp. 139–165). Bethesda, MD: American Occupational Therapy Association.

Godden, D. R., & Baddeley, A. D. (1975). Context-dependent memory in two natural environments: On land and underwater. *British Journal of Psychology, 66,* 325–331.

Goodwin, J. E., & Meeuwsen, H. J. (1995). Using bandwidth knowledge of results to alter relative frequencies during motor skills acquisition. *Research Quarterly for Exercise and Sport, 66,* 99–104.

Hanlon, R. E. (1996). Motor learning following unilateral stroke. *Archives of Physical Medicine and Rehabilitation, 77,* 811–815.

Hodges, N. J., Chua, R., & Franks, I. M. (2003). The role of video in facilitating perception and action of a novel coordination movement. *Journal of Motor Behavior, 35,* 247–260.

Hong, L. (2005). Hospitalized elders and family caregivers: A typology of family worry. *Journal of Clinical Nursing, 14,* 3–8.

Kalra, L., Evans, A., Perez, I., Melbourn, A., Patel, A., Knapp, A., & Donaldson, N. (2004). Training carers of stroke patients: Randomised controlled trial. *British Journal of Medicine, 328,* 1099.

Kielhofner, G., Barris, R., & Watts, J. H. (1982). Habits and habit dysfunction: A clinical perspective for psychosocial occupational therapy. *Occupational Therapy in Mental Health, 2,* 1–21.

Kirby, J. R. (1984). Educational roles of cognitive plans and strategies. In J. R. Kirby (Ed.), *Cognitive strategies and educational performance* (pp. 51–88). Orlando, FL: Academic.

Lavery, J. J. (1962). Retention of simple motor skills as a function of type of knowledge of results. *Canadian Journal of Psychology, 16,* 300–311.

Lee, T. D., Swanson, L. R., & Hall, A. L. (1991). What is repeated in a repetition? Effects of practice conditions on motor skill acquisition. *Physical Therapy, 71,* 150–156.

Lee, Y., & Vakoch, D. A., (1996). Transfer and retention of implicit and explicit learning. *British Journal of Psychology, 87,* 637–651.

Ma, H., Trombly, C. A., & Robinson-Podolski, C. (1999). The effect of context on skill acquisition and transfer. *American Journal of Occupational Therapy, 53,* 138–144.

Ma, H. I., & Trombly, C. A. (2004). Effects of task complexity on reaction time and movement kinematics in elderly people. *American Journal of Occupational Therapy*, 58, 150–158.

Mane, A. M., Adams, J. A., & Donchin, E. (1989). Adaptive and part-whole training in the acquisition of a complex perceptual-motor skill. *Acta Psychologica, 71,* 179–196.

Mann, L., & Sabatino, D. A. (1985). *Foundations of cognitive process in remedial and special education.* Rockville, MD: Aspen Systems Corporation.

Mathiowetz, V., & Haugen, J. B. (1994). Motor behavior research: Implications for therapeutic approaches to central nervous system dysfunction. *American Journal of Occupational Therapy, 48,* 733–745.

Mathiowetz, V., Matuska, K., & Murphy, M. E. (2001). Efficacy of an energy conservation course for persons with multiple sclerosis. *Archives of Physical Medicine and Rehabilitation, 82,* 449–456.

Mathiowetz, V., & Wade, M. G. (1995). Task constraints and functional motor performance of individuals with and without multiple sclerosis. *Ecological Psychology, 7,* 99–123.

McAuley, E. (1993). Self-efficacy and the maintenance of exercise participation in older adults. *Journal of Behavioral Medicine, 16,* 103–113.

Morgan, R. L., & Salzberg, C. L. (1992). Effects of video-assisted training on employment-related social skills of adults with severe mental retardation. *Journal of Applied Behavioral Analysis, 25,* 365–383.

National Center for Education Statistics. (2005). *National Assessment of Adult Literacy (NAAL): A first look at the literacy of America's adults in the 21st century.* Department of Education, Institute of Education Sciences Publication No. NCES 2006-470. Pittsburgh, PA: U.S. Government Printing Office.

Neistadt, M. E. (1995). Assessing learning capabilities during cognitive and perceptual evaluations for adults with traumatic brain injury. *Occupational Therapy in Health Care, 9,* 3–16.

Packard, M. G., & Knowlton, B. J. (2002). Learning and memory functions of the basal ganglia. *Annual Review of Neuroscience, 25,* 563–593.

Parikh, N. S., Parker, R. M., Nurss, J. R., Baker, D. W., & Williams, M. V. (1996). Shame and health literacy: The unspoken connection. *Patient Education and Counseling, 27,* 33–39.

Pasacreta, J. V., Barg, F., Nuamah, I., & McCorkcle, R. (2000). Participant characteristics before and 4 months after attendance at a family caregiver cancer education program. *Cancer Nursing, 23,* 295–303.

Perkins, D. (1995). *Outsmarting IQ: The emerging science of learnable intelligence.* New York: Free Press.

Prochaska, J. O., & DiClemente, C. C. (1982). Transtheoretical therapy: Toward a more integrative model of change. *Psychotherapy: Theory, Research and Practice, 19,* 276–288.

Reber P. J., & Squire, L. R. (1994). Parallel brain systems for learning with and without awareness. *Learning and Memory, 1,* 217–229.

Redman, B. K. (1997). *The practice of patient education.* St. Louis, MO: Mosby.

Salmoni, A. W., Schmidt R. A., & Walter, C. B. (1984). Knowledge of results and motor learning: A review and critical reappraisal. *Psychological Bulletin, 95,* 355–386.

Saloman, G., & Perkins, D. N. (1989). Rocky roads to transfer: Rethinking mechanisms of a neglected phenomenon. *Educational Psychologist, 24,* 113–142.

Schmidt, R. A. (1988). *Motor control and learning: A behavioral emphasis* (2nd ed.) Champaign, IL: Human Kinetics.

Schneider, M. (2005). 2003 National Assessment of Adult Literacy (NAAL) results. Accessed June 2, 2006 from http://nces.ed.gov/whatsnew/commissioner/remarks2005/12_15_2005.asp.

Schneider, W., & Shiffrin, R. M. (1977). Controlled and automatic human information processing: I. Detection, search, and attention. *Psychological Review, 84,* 1–66.

Shea, J. B., & Morgan, R. L. (1979). Contextual interference effects on the acquisition, retention and transfer of a motor skill. *Journal of Experimental Psychology: Human Learning and Memory, 5,* 179–187.

Shiffrin, R. M., & Schneider, W. (1977). Controlled and automatic human information processing: II. Perceptual learning, automatic attending, and a general theory. *Psychological Review, 84,* 127–190.

Sohlberg, M. M., & Raskin, S. A. (1996). Principles of generalization applied to attention and memory interventions. *Journal of Head Trauma Rehabilitation, 11,* 65–78.

Squire, L. R. (1994). Declarative and nondeclarative memory: Multiple brain systems support learning and memory. In D. Schacter & E. Tulving (Eds.), *Memory systems 1994* (pp. 203–231). Cambridge, MA: MIT.

Squire, L.R., Knowlton, B. J., & Musen, G. (1993). The structure and organization of memory. *Annual Review of Psychology, 44,* 453–495.

Sternberg, R. J. (1986). *Intelligence applied: Understanding and increasing your intellectual skills.* New York: Harcourt Brace Jovanovich.

Stewart, K., Borland, R., & McMurray, N. (1994). Self-efficacy, health locus of control, and smoking cessation. *Addictive Behaviors, 19,* 1–12.

Tailby, R., & Haslam, C. (2003). An investigation of errorless learning in memory-impaired patients: Improving the technique and clarifying theory. *Neuropsychologia, 41,* 1230–1240.

Tham, K., & Tegner, R. (1997). Video feedback in the rehabilitation of patients with unilateral neglect. *Archives of Physical Medicine and Rehabilitation, 78,* 410–413.

Thomas, J. J. (1999). Enhancing patient education: Addressing the issue of literacy. *Physical Disabilities Special Interest Section Quarterly, 22,* 3–4.

Toglia, J. P. (1989). Approaches to cognitive assessment of the brain-injured adult. *Occupational Therapy Practice, 1,* 36–55.

Toglia, J. P. (1991). Generalization of treatment: A multicontext approach to cognitive perceptual impairment in adults with brain injury. *American Journal of Occupational Therapy, 45,* 505–516.

Toglia, J. P. (1998). A dynamic interactional model to cognitive rehabilitation. In N. Katz (Ed.), *Cognition and occupation in rehabilitation.* Bethesda, MD: American Occupational Therapy Association.

Trombly, C. A., & Wu, C. (1999). Effect of rehabilitation tasks on organization of movement after stroke. *American Journal of Occupational Therapy, 53,* 333–344.

Tulving, E., & Thompson, D. (1973). Encoding specificity and retrieval processes in episodic memory. *Psychological Review, 80,* 352–373.

van der Weel, F. R., van der Meer, A. L. H., & Lee, D. N., (1991). Effect of task on movement control in cerebral palsy: Implications for assessment and therapy. *Developmental Medicine and Child Neurology, 33,* 419–426.

Vanetzian, E. (1997). Learning readiness for patient teaching in stroke rehabilitation. *Journal of Advanced Nursing, 26,* 589–594.

Wilson, B. A., & Evans, J. J. (1996). Error-free learning in the rehabilitation of people with memory impairments. *Journal of Head Trauma Rehabilitation, 11,* 54–64.

Winstein, C. J., Gardner, E. R., McNeal, D. R., Barto, P. S., & Nicholson, D. E. (1989). Standing balance training: Effect on balance and locomotion in hemiparetic patients. *Archives of Physical Medicine and Rehabilitation, 70,* 755–762.

Winstein, C. J., & Schmidt, R. A. (1990). Reduced frequency of knowledge of results enhances motor skill learning. *Journal of Experimental Psychology: Learning, Memory, and Cognition, 16,* 677–691.

Wood, W., Quinn, J. M., & Kashy, D. A. (2002). Habits in everyday life: Thought, emotion, and action. *Journal of Personality and Social Psychology, 83,* 1281–1297.

World Health Organization [WHO]. (1997). *ICIHD-2: International Classification of Impairments, Activities, and Participation (Beta-1 draft for field trials).* Geneva: World Health Organization.

Wu, C., Trombly, C. A., & Lin, K. (1994). The relationship between occupational form and occupational performance: A kinematic perspective. *American Journal of Occupational Therapy, 48,* 679–687.

Wu, C., Trombly, C. A., Lin, K., Tickle-Degnan, L. (2000). A kinematic study of contextual effects on reaching performance in persons with and without stroke: Influences of object availability. *Archives of Physical Medicine and Rehabilitation, 81,* 95–101.

Wulf, G., McConnel, N., Gartner, M., Schwartz, A. (2002). Enhancing the learning of sport skills through external focus feedback. *Journal of Motor Behavior, 34,* 171–182.

CHAPTER 15

Therapeutic Rapport

Linda Tickle-Degnen

LEARNING OBJECTIVES

After studying this chapter, the reader will be able to do the following:

1. Define high therapeutic rapport.
2. Describe how rapport influences intervention and the client's occupational functioning.
3. Describe how collaboration between therapist and client contributes to achieving high therapeutic rapport.
4. Select methods to enhance rapport with a client.
5. Identify therapists' and clients' attributes that can influence the development of rapport.
6. Apply knowledge of ethics of practice to the therapeutic relationship.

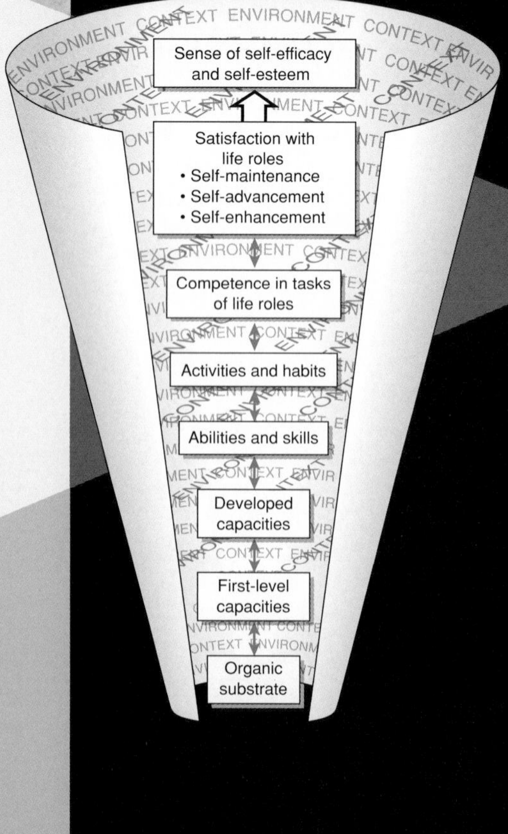

Glossary

Mutuality—Interaction between the client and therapist in which they influence one another.

Nonverbal communication—The process of interpreting another's nonverbal behavior and expressing one's own thoughts and emotions through nonverbal behavior. Nonverbal behavior includes positions and movements of the face and body and qualities of the voice, such as vocal tone, intensity, and speed.

Therapeutic rapport—The qualities of experience and behavior between client and therapist that affect the client's performance and involvement in therapy.

Verbal communication—Interpreting another's words and expressing one's own thoughts and emotions through words.

Working alliance—Working together to achieve agreed upon goals.

The origins of the term *rapport* reflect an emphasis on communication and connection between individuals (*Oxford English Dictionary,* 2005). Individuals who are finely tuned to one another's actions and ideas, such that they respond to one another "immediately, spontaneously, and sympathetically" (Park & Burgess, 1924, p. 893), are said to be in rapport with one another.

Although rapport can occur in any social situation, the type of rapport developed in therapy has its own special characteristics. Rapport is one *mechanism,* or means, by which a client achieves positive therapeutic outcomes, or in the case of occupational therapy, confident and competent occupational functioning. It involves the interpersonal influences arising between client and therapist that can support the client's desire to try occupational therapy, to maintain continued involvement in therapy despite the need for considerable effort and courage, and to participate with the therapist in constructing a new vision of life possibilities that project into the client's occupational future (Mattingly & Fleming, 1994; Peloquin, 2002).

A client who shares a high rapport with the therapist at the point of assessment may want to try therapy simply because of an initial liking for the therapist and, once in the midst of therapy, carry through with the work because of having a competent and caring ally in the achievement of mutually derived occupational goals. In addition, many, if not most, daily life occupations are conducted in a social milieu. People do occupations together and in the presence of one another, and their occupations are supported naturally by their immediate, spontaneous, and sympathetic responses to one another. The therapist can provide this natural supportive function while expertly guiding occupation-as-means to achieving therapeutic goals.

This chapter defines the behaviors and feelings associated with therapeutic rapport, describes conditions affecting its development, and discusses the ethics of a therapeutic relationship. Although this chapter focuses on therapeutic rapport with a single client, its content can be applied to developing rapport with caregivers and family members as well (Clark, Corcoran, & Gitlin, 1995).

DEFINITION OF HIGH THERAPEUTIC RAPPORT

High **therapeutic rapport** (Definition 15-1) involves the mutual experience and behavior of the client and therapist as they interact with each other as well as the outcome of the interaction for the client:

1. It is an optimal interpersonal *experience* for both the client and the therapist that involves concentration, masterful communication, and enjoyment (Csikszentmihalyi, 1990; Tickle-Degnen, 2006).
2. It occurs with *behavior* that reflects high levels of mutual attentiveness, interpersonal coordination, and mutual positivity (Tickle-Degnen & Gavett, 2003; Tickle-Degnen & Rosenthal, 1992).
3. It has a *beneficial effect* on client performance and follow-through with intervention plans (Ambady et al., 2002; Di Blasi et al., 2001; Feinberg, 1992; Hall, Harrigan, & Rosenthal, 1995; Martin, Garske, & Davis, 2000; Porszt-Miron, Florian, & Burton, 1988).

MUTUALITY AND THERAPEUTIC RAPPORT

Mutuality in the relationship between client and therapist is relatively new in the espoused philosophy of occupational therapy. In the first half of this century, occupational therapists were expected to be friendly and cheerful but not intimate with clients (Aitken, 1948; American Occupational Therapy Association, 1948). Therapists and clients were not to affect each other through the force of their personal attributes. Starting at mid-century, the "therapeutic use of self" (Frank, 1958) became the prevailing philosophical position guiding the therapeutic relationship. Therapists recognized that not only modalities but also their own selves could be agents of therapeutic change in their clients. By being role mod-

DEFINITION 15-1

High Therapeutic Rapport

Qualities of Experience	
Concentration	The client and therapist experience a deep and effortless concentration on the interaction. Distractions, worries, and self-concern disappear.
Masterful communication	They are challenged by the interaction yet feel skillful in meeting the challenge. The goals of the interaction are experienced as clear and shared by both. Each understands immediately how well these goals are being met.
Enjoyment	They experience the interaction with deep satisfaction.
Qualities of Verbal and Nonverbal Behavior	
Attentiveness	The client and therapist demonstrate verbally and nonverbally that their attention is focused on the other.
Interpersonal coordination	They demonstrate a highly tuned responsiveness to each other such that behavior and emotional expression are highly coordinated between the two.
Positivity	They demonstrate verbally and nonverbally that their feelings are positive toward one another and the interaction.
Beneficial Effects for the Patient	
Enhanced client performance	Qualities of the client–therapist interaction are beneficial if they improve client performance during evaluation and intervention.
Client follow-through with therapeutic activities	Qualities of the client–therapist interaction are beneficial if they support clients' continued involvement in activities that enable them to make progress toward their goals.

els to their clients and by behaving in certain ways, they could help clients change. Although therapists could influence clients, therapists were to remain somewhat professionally detached to ensure that they themselves were not unduly affected by clients.

Starting in the late 1960s, with the inception of the human rights, human potential, and consumer movements, and continuing into the early 2000s, occupational therapy's view of the therapeutic relationship has been undergoing a major transformation. The profound shift has been toward viewing the relationship as a mutual and collaborative exchange between equals, a perspective exemplified by Yerxa's (1973) work: "The therapist allows himself to feel real emotion as he enters into mutual relation with the client. . . . The authentic occupational therapist is involved in the process of caring and to care means to be affected just as surely as it means to affect" (p. 8).

The current philosophy of the therapeutic relationship has advanced the mutuality perspective to the image of covenanting partner or friend (Peloquin, 2002). This image is revolutionary in that it conveys that the client and therapist *together* engage in mutually satisfying occupation and interaction (e.g., Clark, 1993). Although the relationship between client and therapist can embody a mutual respect similar to that of good friends, it usually does not involve the same reciprocity of a typical social friendship; rather, it is *client centered* (Egan et al., 1998). A client and an occupational therapist usually meet and grow to know one another because the therapist is expected to provide a service to the client. This service relationship may arise when it is difficult for the client, because of suffering or impairment, to experience or communicate feelings that contribute to the development of rapport (Rosa & Hasselkus, 2005). Finally, the therapist usually is paid for the services, and is accountable to institutional and professional systems that are charged with monitoring therapy and tracking clients' response to therapy.

Despite a therapeutic focus on the client, clients and therapists mutually influence one another. Evidence suggests that, if either the client or the therapist is not attentive, responsive, or positive, or perceived as such by the other, high therapeutic rapport is difficult to achieve (Tickle-Degnen & Rosenthal, 1992).

EXPERIENTIAL AND BEHAVIORAL QUALITIES OF HIGH THERAPEUTIC RAPPORT

Health care research findings and client autobiographical accounts demonstrate that both the therapist and client contribute to the development of a relationship. The following sections discuss therapist and client rapport qualities.

Therapist Concentration and Attentiveness

A person who is paying attention to another will tend to orient his or her body and eyes toward the other to pick up information coming from the other person. In therapy, this type of behavior enables the therapist to watch the client and to pick up emotion and thought cues from the client's face and body. Therapists also show that they are paying attention to clients by taking the time to sit down and talk with them (Figs. 15-1 and 15-2). Verbal and nonverbal attentiveness has been found to be positively associated with client disclosure about the subjective experience of illness (Duggan & Parrott, 2000), participation in occupational therapy (Feinberg, 1992), client satisfaction (Hall, Roter, & Katz, 1988), and occupational performance outcomes (Ambady et al., 2002).

Paying attention to a client goes beyond conducting a standardized evaluation, and it goes beyond physical attention. It requires listening carefully to what the client has to say about his or her life, the illness, and the experience of intervention (Crepeau, 1991; Kleinman, 1988; Padilla, 2003) and remaining open to changing one's own therapeutic ideas in response to what is heard (Rosa & Hasselkus, 2005). Without this kind of attentiveness, the therapist may apply a "cookbook" intervention that is not individualized to the needs of the client, as happened to McCrum (1998) during rehabilitation following a stroke. During therapy, McCrum felt like a 3-year-old child playing with letters of the alphabet:

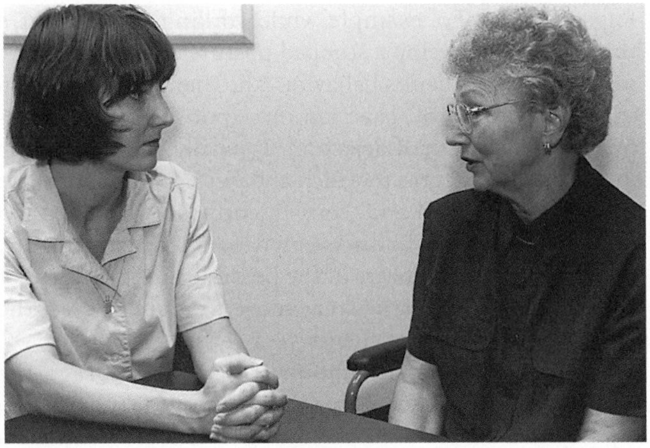

Figure 15-1 Mutual attentiveness by therapist and client forms the basis for effective communication and the development of a successful working relationship.

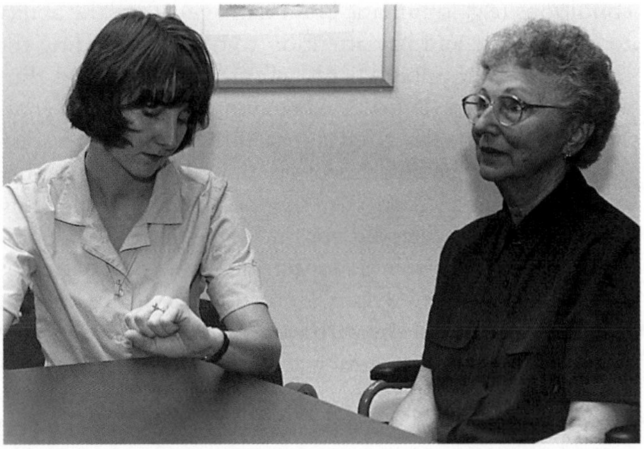

Figure 15-2 The therapist who is distracted by time pressure or other concerns loses the interpersonal connection with the client.

> "Sitting in my wheelchair with my Day-Glo letter-blocks I could not escape reflecting on the irony of the situation. If only Milan Kundera, Kazuo Ishiguro, or Mario Vargas Llosa, whose texts I had pored over with their authors, could have seen their editor at that moment!" (p. 139)

Simple tabletop activities in and of themselves are not at fault here. They can be exactly what a particular client needs although in this case, they apparently were not. Therapists usually are well intentioned, but unless their intentions are consistent with what the client perceives to be important, they may be less than beneficial. Reflecting upon her hospital experiences as a child with spina bifida, Saxton (1987) considered the saddest aspect of her experiences to be that so many practitioners were trying to help her, yet:

> "They never asked me what I wanted for myself. They never asked me if I wanted their help. . . . I just wish all disabled children would say to their helpers: 'Before you do anything else, just listen to me.'" (p. 55)

Craig (1991) described how her husband's nurse, during each home visit, listened and heard:

> "[S]he began by listening. And anything Ed wanted to tell her was relevant. She let him tell her, in his own way and in his own time, about everything that was happening to his body. And in that way, she came to know his soul." (p. 241)

Client Concentration and Attentiveness

Therapists need attention from their clients as well. A client who does not attend to the therapist cannot give or get important information from him or her. Many pathological conditions (e.g., traumatic brain damage) affect the ability to concentrate and pay attention to others, including the therapist. In addition, clients who feel anxious and thus avoid eye contact (Baker & Edelmann, 2002; Bernieri et al., 1996) may not be able to engage attentively with a therapist.

Clients may be more involved and attentive when they value their therapy than when they do not value it. McCrum (1998), quoted earlier, did not find value in the form of his therapy, particularly in juxtaposition to his occupation as an editor for brilliant writers. Unfortunately, it appears that the therapist did not engage the client collaboratively in the determination of intervention activities. Despite strong collaborative values and ethics in occupational therapy, research finds that therapists often fall short of fully and collaboratively involving clients and their families in decision making (Brown & Bowen, 1998; Hasselkus, 1991; Northern et al., 1995; Rosa & Hasselkus, 2005).

Therapist Communication and Interpersonal Coordination

It is impossible for even the most attentive therapist to apprehend and feel exactly what the client feels about his or her own illness and life. Likewise, the client cannot fully comprehend the personal experience and role obligations of the therapist. Each is a unique individual with a unique life history and perspective. Despite these differences, the therapist and client can teach each other their personal perspectives through **verbal** and **nonverbal communication** (Crepeau, 1991; Padilla, 2003).

The fundamental condition for the therapist to communicate effectively with the client is for the therapist to direct her attention toward the client. The next step is for the therapist to *interpret* accurately the client's verbal and nonverbal behavior (Tickle-Degnen & Rosenthal, 1992; Tickle-Degnen & Lyons, 2004). This interpretation process involves first the observation of how another person has behaved, and then the translation of this observation into an inference about the other's thoughts and emotions (Fig. 15-3). Svidén and Säljö (1993) found that, over 18 months, the impressions of occupational therapy students about clients became increasingly complex. For example, at a student's first viewing of a client's videotaped behavior, her impression consisted of the following seven words: "It was rather difficult for her psychologically" (p. 495). That same student's impression 18 months after beginning her training consisted of at least 71 words. It included a description of the client's gaze and vocal behavior and conjectures about the feelings the client may have had, such as hopelessness, confusion, lack of happiness, and embarrassment. By this second viewing, the student had a better articulated and more complex impression of the client and, as a result, would have been able to engage in a more effective dialogue with the client to confirm or refute elements of the impression.

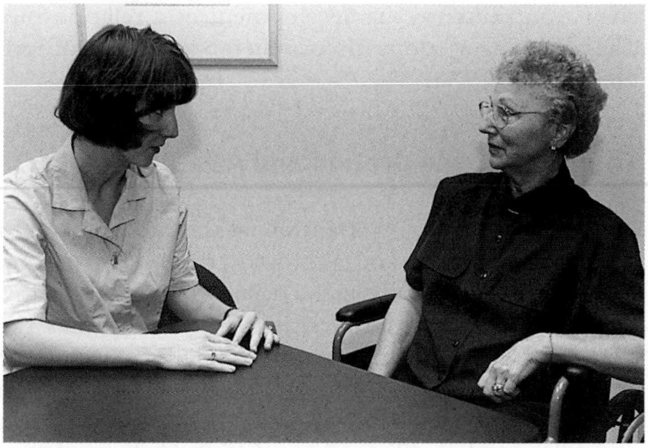

Figure 15-3 The client's backward lean may indicate that she is withdrawing from the therapist or from the information the therapist is giving her. The therapist must determine whether or not the client's behavior is a sign of withdrawal and then whether to adjust her own behavior to maintain rapport. This therapist may decide to become less confrontational, relaxing her posture and making less intense eye contact.

Therapists rapidly form impressions of a client's emotional and social attributes, and these impressions can be accurate or inaccurate (Lyons et al., 2004; Tickle-Degnen & Lyons, 2004). Accuracy can be enhanced if the client gives feedback to the therapist about the accuracy of the therapist's impressions (Marangoni et al., 1995). If the client cannot give verbal feedback to the therapist about the accuracy of the therapist's interpretations, the therapist may be able to learn what the client is feeling simply by reflecting on what the therapist's own emotions are. More than likely, what the therapist feels is very similar to what the client feels because the therapist and client unconsciously and subtly coordinate their bodily and facial movements to one another (Bernieri & Rosenthal, 1991; Dijksterhuis & Bargh, 2001) and literally feel their way into one another's emotions (Hatfield, Cacioppo, & Rapson, 1994). For example, while working with a client, a therapist may develop a stooped posture through a subtle mimicry of the client's behavior. The therapist may begin to have a feeling of dejection in response to the client's own bodily pattern of dejection. Typically, individuals are unaware of the degree to which another person's emotions influence their own and, consequently, do not reflect on their own emotions to discover what another person's are. Yet if therapists are aware of the possibility of this form of emotional influence, they may more accurately detect the unspoken emotions of clients.

After accurate interpretation of a client's message, the next step in effective communication is for the therapist to *express* her own emotions and thoughts in a manner that is clear to and beneficial for the client (Tickle-Degnen & Rosenthal, 1992; Tickle-Degnen & Gavett, 2003). When a therapist feels positive, hopeful, and engaged in treatment

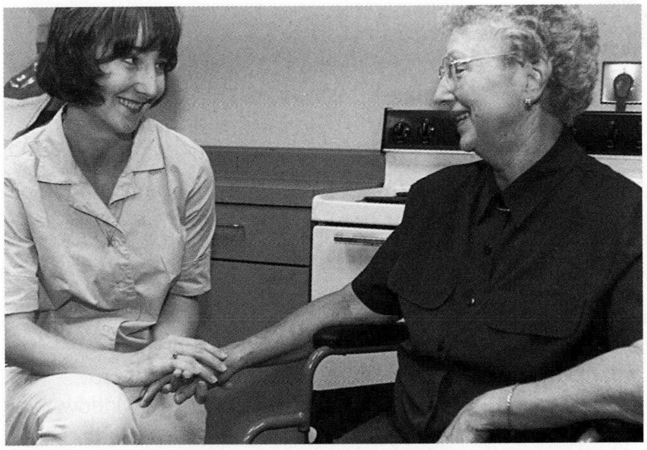

Figure 15-4 The therapist and client show mutual positivity through their facial expressions and physical contact. Social physical contact, like holding a client's hand, is appropriate if it is an expression of professional warmth and the client gains comfort from it. Not all clients like being touched in this manner.

and is expressive of these feelings in an unambiguous manner, clients tend to have similar reactions and respond favorably (Fig. 15-4) (Ambady et al., 2002; Di Blasi et al., 2001; Hall, Harrigan, & Rosenthal, 1995). Nonverbal messages are typically conveyed more rapidly than verbal ones (Ambady, Bernieri, & Richeson, 2000), and they are usually conveyed unconsciously (Lakin & Chartrand, 2003). Watt (1996), a man in severe pain, described his favorite nurse:

> "I believed she would make things better. It was never anything she said. It was something in her face." (p. 13)

The combination of verbal and nonverbal behavior that the therapist uses to express his or her feelings and attitudes toward the client can be profoundly moving for the client. Brack (Brack & Collins, 1981), a woman with multiple sclerosis, described how her physical therapist conveyed a sense of compassion and hope after a long period of hard work but little progress in therapy. As Brack was waiting for therapy in a line of wheelchairs, she could not suppress her tears of despair and shame at not being able to regain her ability to walk. Her therapist quickly pulled her chair out of the line and wheeled it down to the therapy office, where together they wept:

> "Our eyes met. 'Do you want to quit?' [the therapist] said. 'I know it's tough and you know you may never get any better. But shall we try a little longer?' Right away I knew I had to. I smiled damply and dried my eyes. What a friend!" (pp. 71–72)

The therapist in this example does not simply say, "Keep trying, I know you can do it." Because she had worked with this client for a long time, she could express her understanding of the client's feelings in a heartfelt and intimate manner, by weeping with the client. Brack continued her description by explaining how she and her therapist kept working at the parallel bars, never giving up. Eventually she was able to walk again. This example demonstrates that effective communication occurs not only through verbal and nonverbal behavior but also through the activities in which the therapist and client engage. The act of engaging in therapy, even when it seems that hope is lost, is a message to the client that hope is *not* lost.

Likewise, messages are conveyed through the tools that occupational therapists offer their clients. When an occupational therapist gives a buttonhook to a client, several messages are offered; among these messages is that the client is capable of using a buttonhook and that dressing independently is a valued goal of the client. In high-rapport and effective interactions, the client is aware of the goals of the interaction, feels control during the interaction, and feels that the therapist has an empathic understanding of the client's thoughts and feelings (Greenberg et al., 2001; Martin, Garske, & Davis, 2000; Tickle-Degnen & Gavett, 2003). Thus, the performance of activities that are clearly consistent with the client's goals communicates that the therapist understands the client's perspective, and the client may respond with renewed energy and engagement in therapy. Hanlan (1979), a man with amyotrophic lateral sclerosis, wanted to maintain his daily functioning:

> "Of increasing importance to me is the help of occupational therapists. . . . My first OT, a man with a direct and kind manner, provided me with a buttonhook, so I could button and unbutton my clothing. I had an almost childlike, happy response to discovering this little tool." (p. 40)

Client Communication and Interpersonal Coordination

Some clients cannot accurately interpret a therapist's social behavior. Individuals with brain damage, particularly in the right hemisphere, have difficulty perceiving and interpreting social nonverbal cues (Brozgold et al., 1998). Among individuals with left hemispheric damage, those with a receptive form of aphasia may be unable to understand the therapist's speech. It is difficult for clients with these types of problems to make sense of the therapist's social overtures and respond appropriately to them. For clients who have interpretation difficulties, the therapist must make frequent and multimedia attempts to communicate (Tham & Kielhofner, 2003). For example, the therapist can express information verbally, nonverbally, in writing, and in picture form.

Likewise, problems of expression could interfere with the development of rapport. Right brain damage and Parkinson's disease have been found to interfere with an individual's ability to nonverbally express interpretable emotions to others (Brozgold et al., 1998; Tickle-Degnen & Lyons, 2004). DeGroat, Lyons, and Tickle-Degnen (2006) found that people with Parkinson's disease appear to be able to express verbally their emotions and preferences quite well during an interview about meaningful activities (Research Note 15-1). Clients with an expressive aphasia, however, may have difficulty communicating verbally their thoughts and needs and may need to rely on nonverbal gestures. For clients in general, it is wise for the therapist to seek information from multiple communication channels, such as through the verbal, facial, and bodily behavior of the client.

Therapist Enjoyment and Positivity

Individuals who are genuine and openly expressive inspire cooperative effort and trust, whereas those who hold back and are indifferent inspire disengagement and distrust (Boone & Buck, 2003). In the therapeutic encounter, the expression of positive feelings and warmth is particularly important. A study of occupational therapy students found that those who tended to express negative feelings, as opposed to those who tended to express positive or neutral feelings, had less rapport with their colleagues and were rated as being less clinically skilled by fieldwork supervisors (Tickle-Degnen & Puccinelli, 1999).

Practitioners may express their warmth and liking through a variety of nonverbal behaviors, such as leaning forward and smiling (Fig. 15-4). Clients interpret these and other types of friendly verbal and nonverbal behavior as positive (Ambady et al., 2002) and respond with increased follow-through with intervention regimens (Feinberg, 1992) and with more successful occupational performance (Ambady et al., 2002) and health outcomes (Di Blasi et al., 2001).

Peloquin (1993a) has eloquently described how health professionals can act in a manner that distances rather than connects them to their clients and saps their clients' courage. Beisser (1989), a man with polio, found that his dependency on hospital attendants for physical survival had a profound effect on his day-to-day view of himself and the world:

> "Everything that affected them affected me. If I was cared for willingly and without reluctance, I felt good and the world was sunny. If my care was given grudgingly or irritably, in a callous way, powerful feelings of degradation swept over me." (p. 34)

In Beisser's experience (1989), the helpers who enjoyed their work and were nurtured by their relationships with clients were most effective. With them, Beisser felt human again, able to reciprocate their warmth and concern. The body of evidence on therapeutic rapport suggests that connecting to clients in a respectful and positive manner, per the seminal work of Carl Rogers (1957), contributes to therapeutic effectiveness. The reverse is true as well: being effective contributes to a feeling of connectedness with clients (Rosa & Hasselkus, 1996, 2005).

What may be most important in therapists' expression of positivity toward clients is the genuine feeling and

RESEARCH NOTE 15-1

Abstract: DeGroat, E., Lyons, K. D., & Tickle-Degnen, L. (2006). Verbal content during favorite activity interview as a window into the identity of people with Parkinson's disease. *Occupational Therapy Journal of Research: Occupation, Participation, and Health 26*, 56–68.

Abstract

The purpose of this study was to document the degree to which a brief segment of an occupational therapy interview about favorite activities served as a window into personal identity and experience in clients with Parkinson's disease. Two-minute segments of videotaped interviews of 12 participants with Parkinson's disease were transcribed and analyzed. The results indicated that the favorite activity interview served as a window primarily into the socio-emotional identity of the client. Client extraversion was positively correlated with the mention of social activities and activities occurring in the public domain; positive affect was positively correlated with the positive tone of the verbal content, as well as the number of positive words spoken during the interview, and negative affect was positively related to the negative tone of words.

Implications for Practice

- Client's preferences, feelings, and personality are quickly expressed during an interview about favorite activities.
- For example, a person who is extraverted and sociable, but who may not seem sociable in his or her nonverbal behavior, may talk about a favorite activity that is done with other people, while a person who is more introverted may talk about a solitary activity.
- It is important not to infer that clients are sociable or solitary, or have positive or negative feelings, based upon their interpersonal styles if they have nonverbal expressive disorders.
- When clients have nonverbal expressive disorders such as Parkinson's disease, therapists may be able to get to know the client by listening to the content of the client's words rather than focusing on the client's nonverbal behavior, such as facial expressions and bodily posturing.

communication of concern and caring (Peloquin, 2002). For example, Ambady et al. (2002) found that therapist nonverbal behavior that was more expressive and concerned, including both more smiling and frowning, predicted better outcomes for geriatric clients. Genuine feelings are not necessarily uniformly cheery and positive. Tickle-Degnen and Gavett (2003) found that moderate levels of positivity were more characteristic of speech therapy dyads with secure therapeutic alliances, whereas very high or very low levels of positivity were more characteristic of dyads with insecure alliances.

It is not easy to achieve a high level of concern and caring in today's health care system, which emphasizes cost containment and adherence to protocol and provides little recognition for caring involvement (Peloquin, 1993b; Sachs & Labovitz, 1994). A supportive system composed not only of the therapist's personal commitment to caring but also of a societal and institutional commitment to caring are needed to sustain a therapeutic level of caring.

Client Enjoyment and Positivity

Clients who are very anxious or depressed demonstrate relatively little warmth nonverbally. For example, they smile infrequently and make little eye contact. Practitioners, especially those who are inexperienced and unlikely to interpret this behavior as a normal response to illness or a sign of disease, may take personally this lack of warmth by some clients (Rosa & Hasselkus, 2005).

Misery from illness may encompass the client's life, reducing the ability to respond warmly to others. As Brack, who was suffering from multiple sclerosis, noted:

> "'Thanks' is a near-forgotten word among us clients as we wallow in our private miseries." (Brack & Collins, 1981, p. 47)

From an ethical and professional standpoint, practitioners are expected to rise above petty responses to unpleasant behavior in clients, but unfortunately, they may begin to resent those that they are supposed to help (Rosa & Hasselkus, 2005).

For example, Beisser (1989) found that his helpers on the polio ward had a powerful form of retribution for clients who were thought to be difficult:

> "You cannot get mad in hospitals. If you do, you may be in trouble. . . . Angry clients come last. So I quickly learned to smile patiently. . . . I had to be careful, for they were more in control of my body than I was." (p. 19)

Even practitioners who do not engage in this form of retribution may find it hard to work with a client who lacks warmth and happiness. Schindler, Hohenberger-Sieber, and Hahlweg (1989), for example, found that during a first therapeutic encounter, the more frequently clients gave reports of success and the less frequently they merely described their problems, the more positive the therapists felt. Rosa and Hasselkus (2005) similarly found that both novice and expert occupational therapists preferred clients who were enthusiastic and ready participants in therapy. These therapist responses may have unfortunate effects on a client who is feeling poorly. Research suggests that creating a climate in which a person must suppress negative emotions, as what Beisser (1989) experienced in the hospital, actually impairs rapport and increases the blood pressure of both interaction partners (Butler et al., 2003).

In occupational therapy, clients may have strong negative reactions to the frustrations of trying to perform what they perceive to be simple tasks (Darragh, Sample, & Krieger, 2001). Puller (1991), a Vietnam veteran with bilateral upper extremity amputations, reports:

> "There were times in OT when I felt like screaming as I tried to learn how to button clothes or to thread a needle." (p. 181)

Such frustration is bound to impinge on the client's view of therapy and the therapist, and it should not be ignored. The therapist may have to reevaluate the balance of the emotional costs and physical benefits of particular forms of activity and to confirm that these activities support the client's own goals.

Evidence suggests that practitioners must be careful not to view all expressions of frustration, sadness, or anger as confirmation of pathology (Langer & Abelson, 1974). For example, Widome (1989) described how a nurse responded to an emotional outburst that apparently was Widome's expression of anger at being in the horrible predicament of having cancer. As Widome was walking down a hospital corridor, the nurse asked him how he was feeling:

> "I let loose with a tirade of words. . . . Wouldn't she prefer no life to a thread of existence? . . . The nurse made a notation on my chart that I had made a decision to end my life, that I was considering self-destruction. I was now a marked man—suicidal." (pp. 99-100)

Expressions of frustration and anger may be indeed be signs of a pathological process that requires diagnosis, or they may be normal responses to the experience of illness and intervention.

BENEFICIAL EFFECT AND HIGH THERAPEUTIC RAPPORT

Listed next are three of the possible reasons attentive, coordinated, and positive client-therapist interactions may have a beneficial effect on the client's performance and follow-through with intervention:

1. The interaction provides the external scaffolding necessary for skill development by directing attention to important aspects of a task problem, by communicating the information necessary to solve the problem, and by giving motivational support for pursuing problem solution (Tham & Kielhofner, 2003; Tickle-Degnen, 2006; Tickle-Degnen & Coster, 1995).
2. The interaction improves physiological and emotional health, thus enabling individuals to focus energy and effort on occupation. Evidence is accruing that an individual's health is a mind-body-social dynamic (e.g., Di Blasi et al., 2001). Rapport involves bringing the therapist and client together in a close and meaningful relationship. The health effects of positive therapeutic relationships, including direct effects on immune and physiological functioning and indirect effects on adherence to health interventions, appear to be very similar to health effects of social support provided by positive familial relationships (DiMatteo, 2004).
3. The interaction creates a self-fulfilling prophecy of improved performance (Ambady et al., 2002; Harris & Rosenthal, 1985). Through verbal and nonverbal communication, a therapist conveys his or her expectations for the progress of a client, with the effect that the client's actual performance conforms to those expectations. Informative, warm, and respectful behavior may affirm to the client that he or she is a capable and valued human being, which mobilizes the client's psychological and physical resources toward fulfillment of those qualities.

DEVELOPMENT OF A HIGH THERAPEUTIC RAPPORT RELATIONSHIP

All relationships take time to develop. Yet evidence suggests that the critical development of rapport and a working alliance, that is, the experience of working collaboratively toward mutually agreed upon goals, is achieved within the first three to five sessions of therapy (Horvath & Luborsky, 1993; Tickle-Degnen & Gavett, 2003). First meetings tend to be somewhat superficial and rigidly constrained by role expectations. The therapist most likely performs an evaluation, and the client most likely tries to answer the questions or perform the activities of the evaluation. Through close adherence to cultural scripts of friendly, polite behaviors, they offer their identities to one another as valuable and likable (Clark, Pataki, & Carver, 1996).

In the first meeting, the client may convey private information to the therapist, but the depth of intimacy and mutuality continues to grow over subsequent interactions, although not in a linear fashion (Altman, 1993). A dialectical tension between the desires for intimacy and autonomy appears to manifest itself in a cyclical pattern of intimate and more distant behavior. After the first few therapeutic encounters, there appears to be a period of much fluctuation in the nature of the interpersonal interaction (Tickle-Degnen & Gavett, 2003), as if client and therapist are trying out different patterns of relating to one another. It also may be that these fluctuations are a result of shifts between therapeutic work and socializing. There is evidence that the grueling, attentive, task-focused work of therapy requires off-task periods of rest and recovery with opportunities for chit-chat. This chit-chat may serve to affirm the social connection between therapist and client (Hall, Roter, & Milburn, 1999).

Relationships that endure, whether they are personal or therapeutic, seem to have one primary attribute in common: the ability to control and manage the development of emotions, especially negative ones (Gottman, 1994). Although individuals in both successful and failing relationships have negative emotions and behavior, in successful relationships, people have interpersonal strategies for rapidly repairing the hurt or negative consequences of these emotions and preventing an escalation of negativity. In failing ones, the individuals are unable to curtail this escalation.

Therapists' and clients' characteristics and conditions in the therapy setting can facilitate or inhibit the development of high rapport. One study (Tickle-Degnen, 1998) found that occupational therapy students who were quiet and empathically concerned attained the highest supervisory ratings in physical rehabilitation settings. Different attributes appeared to be needed in other types of settings. These results suggest that therapists must adapt their interpersonal styles to different therapeutic contexts. Through self-reflection; feedback from supervisors, colleagues, and clients; and reflective clinical experience, the therapist should be able to learn how to make these adaptations.

Based on the evidence presented here, Procedures for Practice 15-1 gives guidelines for enhancing the development of rapport. It is not the client's responsibility to change to enhance the rapport; it is the therapist's. Therefore, the guidelines are directed at actions the therapist can take.

Typically, therapeutic relationships work toward a planned end to the relationship as goals are achieved or services are no longer needed. As discharge approaches, the therapist should work actively with the client to transform their relationship appropriately, so that the client does not feel abandoned (e.g., Clark, 1993; Klein,

PROCEDURES FOR PRACTICE 15-1

Therapist Guidelines for Facilitating the Development of High Therapeutic Rapport

Create Conditions that Maximize Therapist's and Client's Concentration and Attention

1. Set aside time to listen to client.
2. Reduce distractions in therapy setting.
3. Reduce potential for client's embarrassment or anxiety.
4. Position own body to see and hear client clearly.
5. Position client so that client can see and hear therapist clearly.
6. Listen for issues that are most important to client.

Create Conditions that Maximize Therapist and Client Masterful Communication and Interpersonal Coordination

1. Remain open and sensitive to verbal and nonverbal messages from the client.
2. Provide assistance as needed for the client to express emotions and thoughts.
3. Check with the client to see whether therapist's interpretation of client's messages is accurate.
4. Clearly express emotions and thoughts that are consistent with the needs and goals of the client.
5. Check with the client to see whether the client is interpreting the therapist's messages accurately.
6. Create a challenging and interesting interaction, but one in which the client can interact skillfully.
7. Involve the client collaboratively in the development of goals and the planning of intervention.

Create Conditions that Maximize Therapist and Client Enjoyment and Positivity

1. Find a satisfying, fulfilling aspect to every interaction with a client.
2. Express genuine concern and caring for the client through verbal and nonverbal behavior.
3. Resolve personal problems and fulfill personal social needs outside of the client–therapist interaction.
4. Determine whether client's sadness or anger is normal or pathological, and respond appropriately to alleviate suffering.
5. Engage client in activities and interactions that are inherently enjoyable for the client.
6. During required activities that are not enjoyable, provide periodic opportunities for rest and off-task recovery.
7. Manage negativity so that it can be expressed as needed in a constructive manner and does not escalate.

1995). The form this transformation takes depends on the setting. For example, the therapist may help the client to develop other fulfilling relationships in the community or may keep in contact with the client through the phone or occasional clinic visits.

ETHICS AND THE THERAPEUTIC RELATIONSHIP

The Occupational Therapy Code of Ethics (American Occupational Therapy Association, 2005) outlines the key ethical elements of the therapeutic relationship. The ethical principles covered here are the ones most relevant to the therapeutic relationship.

Principle 1

Occupational Therapy Personnel Shall Demonstrate a Concern for the Safety and Well-Being of the Recipients of Their Services

A key element of this principle is that therapists must provide services in an equitable manner to all individuals. A therapist may have fears or negative attitudes about a particular client population, for example, such as individuals with AIDS (Hansen, 1990). Despite these feelings, it is the ethical imperative of therapists to provide services.

Although there is no ethical imperative to feel rapport with clients, the imperative to demonstrate a concern for the well-being of the recipient of services suggests that the therapist should make every effort to create a climate of therapeutic rapport. As a therapist works to create rapport, it is important that the therapist realize that his or her own beliefs about what is important for well-being and occupation are not necessarily equivalent to the beliefs held by the client, especially clients from different cultures (Iwama, 2003).

Principle 2

Occupational Therapy Personnel Shall Take Measures to Ensure a Recipient's Safety and Avoid Imposing or Inflicting Harm

The therapist should consider changing jobs or clinical specialization if he or she is unable to overcome negative feelings with clients typically seen in a particular setting or specialization area. Negative feelings may result in negative outcomes for the client. If the therapist has made an honest but unsuccessful attempt to support high therapeutic rapport, he or she may consider referring the client to a different therapist, perhaps one that is a specialist in such cases (Rosa & Hasselkus, 2005).

Another element of this principle is that therapists must maintain relationships that do not exploit the client sexually, physically, emotionally, financially, socially, or in any other manner. Mutuality of feeling, behavior, and goals is critical to the development of a relationship of high therapeutic rapport; interdependency or the expectation of reciprocal benefits, however, is not. The therapist who becomes dependent on a client for meeting a personal need is exploitive because of his or her higher power relative to the client's position of vulnerability. Furthermore, although the therapist is ethically responsible for helping the client, the client is not expected to help the therapist in any manner.

Principle 3

Occupational Therapy Personnel Shall Respect Recipients to Assure Their Rights

One element of the third ethical principle is autonomy. Respect for the client's autonomy requires therapeutic relationships in which clients collaborate to the best of their ability in the determination of goals and priorities during intervention. For clients to be able to collaborate, they must be informed about the nature, risks, and potential outcomes of the intervention and have the opportunity to suggest, reject, or refuse services or elements of services. This standard is both ethical and consistent with the nature of therapeutic rapport and the effective working alliance. Collaborative decisions are carried out not because of external pressures but because of an active feeling of personal control and responsibility (Fig. 15-5).

Other elements of this principle are privacy and confidentiality. During a relationship of high therapeutic rapport, the client may tell the therapist about matters that are private and confidential. The therapist must protect the confidentiality of information by not discussing it in an inappropriate context (for example, in a public elevator conversation) or manner (for example, laughing at the client's capabilities) with a colleague or any other person.

Principle 4

Occupational Therapy Personnel Shall Achieve and Continually Maintain High Standards of Competence

A relationship of high therapeutic rapport is a trusting one. The client trusts that the therapist is doing the best that can be done for him or her. It is the ethical responsibility of the therapist to uphold this trust by performing services competently. Part of this competence involves being able to critically examine current emerging knowledge relevant to practice and then being able to use this knowledge to engage the client in a collaboration based upon accurate information (Tickle-Degnen, 2000).

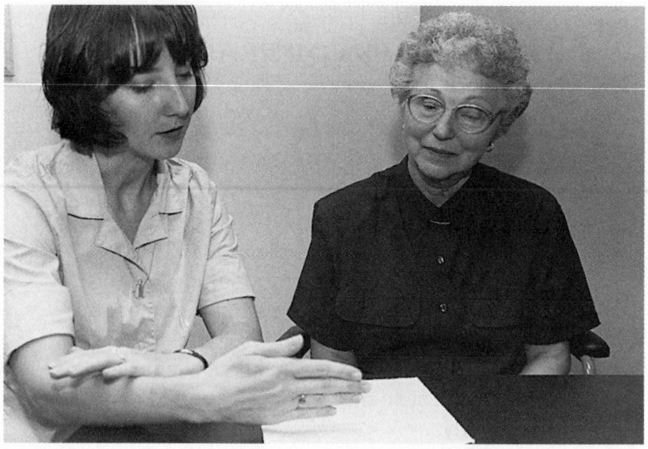

Figure 15-5 In a collaborative relationship, the therapist and client discuss the benefits and risks of participating in various occupational therapy interventions so that the client can make informed decisions about participating in these interventions.

SUMMARY

High therapeutic rapport develops as the therapist and client are mutually attentive, coordinated to one another, and mutually positive. It is one mechanism by which the client achieves confident and competent occupational functioning. It supports the client's desire to try occupational therapy, to maintain continued involvement in therapy, and to participate with the therapist in constructing a new vision of life possibilities. Although rapport is based upon a perspective of mutuality and collaboration between client and therapist, it is the therapist's responsibility to manage oneself, guide the client, and modify the environment to support attentiveness, coordination, and positivity. Through self-reflection, feedback from others, reflection about clinical practice, and careful adherence to ethical standards, the therapist can learn to facilitate therapeutic rapport with a variety of clients in a variety of practice settings.

CASE EXAMPLE

Establishing Rapport with a Reluctant Client

Occupational Therapy Intervention Process	Clinical Reasoning Process	
	Objectives	**Examples of Therapist's Internal Dialogue**
Client Information Mrs. K., a 75-year-old woman (widowed) with Parkinson's disease, was referred to the adult day program by her physician and her children who were concerned about her social isolation and reluctance to do basic grooming and self-care despite the physical and cognitive capacity to do so. The diagnosis of depression was ruled out. Mrs. K. moved slowly with a rigid, shuffling gait, had the facial mask of Parkinson's disease, and had bilateral tremor in her hands. Mrs. K. stated to the occupational therapist that she did not want to attend the program but was trying it out only because of her children's desires. Her favorite activity was to visit with her grandchildren and her best friend, Jane, yet she rarely visited them. On a health-related quality of life measure designed for people with Parkinson's disease, Mrs. K. identified that she felt stigmatized by her movement disorder and would prefer to stay home rather than let others see her, even friends and family. The assessment process identified that she had not learned compensatory strategies for handling the community and social aspects of the symptoms of Parkinson's disease.	Appreciate the context	"Since Mrs. K. did not have cognitive or emotional impairment, I expected that she would be able to reflect upon and discuss her occupational functioning. To understand her limited functioning, it was important to hear and understand her perspective. The quality of life assessment procedure was appropriate for eliciting her reflection and generating a client-centered discussion."
	Develop intervention hypotheses	"Mrs. K's social isolation and self-care issues may be related specifically to the stigmatizing aspects of the movement disorder of Parkinson's disease. I can't tell from her affect what interests her, and probably other people in her life can't either. Her eyes rarely move, there is little expression around the mouth, and her responses are slow to come, making it difficult to carry on an easy conversation with her. It seems that she doesn't like me, but that might be due to the effect of the disease on her ability to smile and be physically expressive. She appears to be engaged with me when talking about stigma and how to reduce it. Her verbal behavior tells me that she has the capacity to express interest and engagement."
	Select an intervention approach	"I find that I can engage Mrs. K's interest through my eye contact and body positioning. I'll try to keep an unconditional positive and concerned feeling toward her and be my usual expressive self. It is necessary to establish a strong therapeutic alliance as a basis for gaining her commitment to examining and working on her occupational functioning. To establish this alliance, I must collaborate with Mrs. K., establish an affective bond, and work with her toward developing mutually acceptable intervention goals and tasks."

	Reflect on competence	"I have not worked with many clients with Parkinson's disease. I see that there may be many stigmatizing aspects to this disease. Mrs. K. is teaching me new things about what it is like to live with the disease."
Recommendations Because of a high risk of Mrs. K. refusing intervention, the occupational therapist suggested to Mrs. K. that they meet once per week for 3 weeks to get to know one another better before starting the day program. The immediate goal was to establish rapport and a strong working alliance, after which the therapist and Mrs. K. could address directly her occupational functioning needs.	Consider the patient's appraisal of performance Consider what will occur in therapy, how often, and for how long Ascertain the patient's endorsement of plan	"Mrs. K. is willing to meet with me for no more than three weekly 1-hour sessions before deciding about whether or not to participate in the day program. I plan to meet with her in an area where she can see what other participants in the program are doing. I believe that if she became familiar with the day program in a non-pressured manner, she might start to see how it might be helpful for her."
Summary of Short-Term Goals and Progress 1. *Mrs. K. and the therapist will complete a task that is mutually interesting to one another.* The therapist and Mrs. K. each completed an interest checklist and then discussed their responses with one another. They noted five mutual interests, one being an interest in poetry. They each brought a favorite poem to the following session to read to the other. At the end of the task, both agreed that they found the task interesting and then selected another task to do with one another in the following week. 2. *Mrs. K. and the therapist will have decided mutually upon one goal of intervention by the end of the third session.* The therapist and Mrs. K. ended each session with discussing and writing down two possible goals of intervention. Tentatively they selected one potential goal by the end of the third session: the reduction of stigma associated with eating a meal in a restaurant. Mrs. K. did not see this goal as the one that she wanted to make a commitment to achieving as of yet. 3. *Mrs. K. and the therapist will have at least one positive experience during each session.* The therapist and Mrs. K. agreed to try to do something that made them feel good or happy at least once during each session. They would assess their achievement of this goal during each session. At each session, they identified several times during which they experienced positive feelings. Therapeutic rapport was developing in a satisfactory manner by the third session. Mrs. K. continued to be reluctant to make a commitment to attend the day program but agreed to try it out for an additional 4-week period at two half-day sessions per week.	Assess the patient's comprehension Understand what she is doing Compare actual to expected performance Know the person Appreciate the context	"Mrs. K. has come to every scheduled session. It has gotten easier to work with her as I have learned what cues indicate that she is happy, sad, angry, or frightened. Her positive attributes are easiest to see whenever we discuss or do things related to her favorite activities and interests. Mrs. K. appears to understand my role and the tasks involved in intervention. She responds positively to clear explanations and my undivided attention." "I think her reluctance to attend the program is partly because she has not recently practiced socially interacting with her peers and, as a result, has not had the experience of seeing that others accept her despite the symptoms of Parkinson's disease."

Next Steps Revised short-term goals: 1. *Mrs. K. will express interest in participating in a group activity on identifying goals for daily living.* 2. *Mrs. K. will communicate about her ideas with the group members.* 3. *Mrs. K. will have a pleasant social interaction with at least one of the other group members.*	Anticipate present and future patient concerns Analyze patient's comprehension Decide if he or she should continue or discontinue therapy and/or return in the future	"I feel that Mrs. K. and I have developed a good rapport with one another and that now she understands she may be able to participate in friendly interactions with other people. She is ready to try a group activity in the day program. I must prepare for the possibility that Mrs. K. will decide not to continue the program after 1 month. I will discuss her concerns about the day program with her family and physician to determine how best to support her involvement in goal setting and to determine what alternatives are available for helping Mrs. K. to participate fully in her life activities."

CLINICAL REASONING IN OCCUPATIONAL THERAPY PRACTICE

When to Refer to Another Therapist

The therapist suspects that one reason that Mrs. K. does not want to be involved in the day program is because the therapist is of a different ethnicity than that of Mrs. K., who seems to have a negative attitude toward the therapist's ethnic group. How should the therapist attempt to deal with this possibility? What can be done to promote rapport? At what point and under what conditions should the therapist attempt to refer the client to another therapist or program?

CLINICAL REASONING IN OCCUPATIONAL THERAPY PRACTICE

An Ethical Dilemma

Mrs. K. refuses involvement in the day program despite the therapist's, the family members', and the physician's encouragement for her to participate. What should the therapist do? What is the therapist's ethical responsibility? How will the therapist's decision affect the therapeutic relationship with Mrs. K.?

Evidence Table 15-1
Best Evidence for Occupational Therapy Practice Regarding Therapeutic Rapport

Intervention	Description of Intervention Tested	Participants	Dosage	Type of Best Evidence and Level of Evidence	Benefit	Statistical Probability and Effect Size of Outcome	Reference
Therapeutic alliance	A therapeutic relationship characterized by: (1) client–therapist collaboration; (2) affective bond; and (3) shared understanding of therapy goals and tasks to achieve the goals. Construct of therapeutic alliance grew out of client-centered approach in psychotherapy and is consistent with current client-centered occupational therapy approach.	4771 clients (66% females) primarily from psychiatric populations. One study involved a head trauma population (Prigatano et al., 1994).	Average of 22.18 sessions (SD = 18.76).	Meta-analysis of 79 studies.	Yes. Clients who have stronger alliances with their therapists have better therapy outcomes than clients who have weaker alliances.	Mean weighted effect size was $r = 0.22$, equivalent to a 22% success rate over control treatment.	Martin, Garske, & Davis, 2000

Therapeutic nonverbal behavior	Physical therapist (PT) distancing behavior (not smiling, looking away, and remaining seated) during a single therapy session with each client, an indicator of consistent therapist behavior toward each client.	28 female and 20 male inpatients who were 75 years of age and older with mobility disorders, and 8 female and 3 male PTs.	Average of 9.3 days of inpatient therapy.	Correlational design (IIB3a) in which amount of PT distancing behavior was used to predict change in patient physical and cognitive functioning from admission to discharge and from admission to 3 months post intervention. Also was used to predict psychological functioning at discharge only (no change measured). Other behaviors besides distancing were measured. Distancing had some of the most consistent findings.	Yes. The less distancing the PT behavior, the greater the positive change in activities of daily living (ADL), the greater the reduction of confusion, and the less depression at discharge. There was little association with mobility. Similar findings were seen for the admission to 3 months post intervention period. Confounding is an alternative explanation: e.g., perhaps patients with less potential for change create a difficult communication context for PT.	Admission to discharge: ADL (Physical Self-Maintenance Scale), $p < 0.001$, $r = -0.34$; confusion (blinded interviewer judgment), $p < 0.05$, $r = 0.29$; mobility (Mobility Assessment Scale), $p > 0.05$, $r = 0.02$; correlation with discharge: depression (Geriatric Depression Scale), $p < 0.05$, $r = -0.27$.	Ambady et al., 2002

SUMMARY REVIEW QUESTIONS

1. What are the elements of high therapeutic rapport?
2. How has the view of the client-therapist relationship changed over time?
3. How are the therapist's experience and behavior related to rapport?
4. How are the client's experience and behavior related to rapport?
5. What are three reasons high rapport may be beneficial for clients?
6. How can the therapist facilitate the development of high therapeutic rapport?
7. What are two ethical responsibilities that a therapist holds in a relationship with a client?

ACKNOWLEDGMENTS

The ideas in this chapter evolved during a Mary Switzer Research Fellowship supported by the National Institutes for Disability and Rehabilitation Research. A special thanks to Irene Zombek and Melissa Muns, who searched clients' autobiographies for excerpts. The photographer for this chapter was Robert Littlefield.

References

Aitken, A. N. (1948). Values of occupational therapy in the rehabilitation of the tuberculosis client. *American Journal of Occupational Therapy, 2,* 219–222.

Altman, I. (1993). Dialectics, physical environments, and personal relationships. *Communication Monographs, 60,* 26–34.

Ambady, N., Bernieri, F. J., & Richeson, J. A. (2000). Toward a histology of social behavior: Judgmental accuracy from thin slices of the behavioral stream. *Advances in Experimental Social Psychology, 32,* 201–271.

Ambady, N., Koo, J., Rosenthal, R., & Winograd, C. H. (2002). Physical therapists' nonverbal communication predicts geriatric patients' health outcomes. *Psychology and Aging, 17,* 443–452.

American Occupational Therapy Association [AOTA]. (1948). Professional attitudes. *American Journal of Occupational Therapy, 2,* 97–98.

American Occupational Therapy Association [AOTA]. (2005). Occupational therapy code of ethics. Retrieved August 7, 2006, from http://www.aota.org/general/docs/ethicscode05.pdf.

Baker, S. R., & Edelmann, R. J. (2002). Is social phobia related to lack of social skills? Duration of skill-related behaviors and ratings of behavioural adequacy. *British Journal of Clinical Psychology, 41,* 243–257.

Beisser, A. R. (1989). *Flying without wings: Personal reflections on being disabled.* New York: Doubleday.

Bernieri, F. J., Gillis, J. S., Davis, J. M., & Grahe, J. E. (1996). Dyad rapport and the accuracy of its judgments across situations: A lens model analysis. *Journal of Personality and Social Psychology, 71,* 110–129

Bernieri, F. J., & Rosenthal, R. (1991). Interpersonal coordination: Behavior matching and interactional synchrony. In R. Feldman & R. Rime (Eds.), *Fundamentals of nonverbal behavior* (pp. 401–432). Cambridge, UK: Cambridge University.

Boone, T., & Buck, R. (2003). Emotional expressivity and trustworthiness: The role of nonverbal behavior in the evolution of cooperation. *Journal of Nonverbal Behavior, 27,* 163–182.

Brack, J., & Collins, R. (1981). *One thing for tomorrow: A woman's personal struggle with MS.* Saskatoon, Saskatchewan, Canada: Western Producer Prairie.

Brown, C., & Bowen, R. E. (1998). Including the consumer and environment in occupational therapy treatment planning. *Occupational Therapy Journal of Research, 18,* 44–62.

Brozgold, A. Z., Borod, J. C., Martin, C. C., Pick, L. H., Alpert, M., & Welkowitz, J. (1998). Social functioning and facial emotional expression in neurological and psychiatric disorders. *Applied Neuropsychology, 5,* 15–23.

Butler, E. A., Egloff, B., Wilhelm, F. H., Smith, N. C., Erickson, A., & Gross, J. J. (2003). The social consequence of expression suppression. *Emotion, 3,* 48–67.

Clark, C. A., Corcoran, M., & Gitlin, L. N. (1995). An exploratory study of how occupational therapists develop therapeutic relationships with family caregivers. *American Journal of Occupational Therapy, 49,* 587–594.

Clark, F. (1993). Eleanor Clarke Slagle Lecture: Occupation embedded in real life: Interweaving occupational science and occupational therapy. *American Journal of Occupational Therapy, 47,* 1067–1078.

Clark, M. S., Pataki, S. P., & Carver, V. H. (1996). Some thoughts and findings on self-presentation of emotions in relationships. In G. J. O. Fletcher & J. Fitness (Eds.), *Knowledge structures in close relationships: A social psychological approach* (pp. 247–274). Malwah, NJ: Lawrence Erlbaum.

Craig, J. (1991). *Between hello and goodbye.* Los Angeles: Tarcher.

Crepeau, E. B. (1991). Achieving intersubjective understanding: Examples from an occupational therapy treatment session. *American Journal of Occupational Therapy, 45,* 1016–1025.

Csikszentmihalyi, M. (1990). *Flow: The psychology of optimal experience.* New York: Harper Collins.

Darragh, A. R., Sample, P. L., & Krieger, S. R. (2001). "Tears in my eyes 'cause somebody finally understood": Client perceptions of practitioners following brain injury. *American Journal of Occupational Therapy, 55,* 191–199.

DeGroat, E., Lyons, K. D., & Tickle-Degnen, L. (2006). Verbal content during favorite activity interview as a window into the identity of people with Parkinson's disease. *Occupational Therapy Journal of Research: Occupation, Participation, and Health, 26,* 56–68.

Di Blasi, Z., Harkness, E., Ernst, E., Georgious, A., & Kleijnen, J. (2001). Influence of context effects on health outcomes: A systematic review. *Lancet, 357,* 757–762.

Dijksterhuis, A., & Bargh, J. A. (2001). The perception-behavior expressway: Automatic effects of social perception on social behavior. In M. Zanna (Ed.), *Advances in experimental social psychology* (Vol. 33, pp. 1–40). San Diego, CA: Academic Press.

DiMatteo, M. R. (2004). Social support and patient adherence to medical treatment: A meta-analysis. *Health Psychology, 23,* 207–218.

Duggan A. P., & Parrott, R. L. (2000). Research note: Physician's nonverbal rapport building and patients' talk about the subjective component of illness. *Human Communication Research, 27,* 299–311.

Egan, M., Dubouloz, C.-J., von Zweck, C., & Vallerand, J. (1998). The client-centered evidence-based practice of occupational therapy. *Canadian Journal of Occupational Therapy, 55,* 191–199.

Feinberg, J. (1992). Effect of the arthritis health professional on compliance with use of resting hand splints by clients with rheumatoid arthritis. *Arthritis Care and Research, 5,* 17–23.

Frank, J. D. (1958). The therapeutic use of self. *American Journal of Occupational Therapy, 12,* 215–225.

Gottman, J. M. (1994). *What predicts divorce? The relationship between marital processes and marital outcomes* (pp. 409–440). Hillsdale, NJ: Lawrence Erlbaum.

Greenberg, L. S., Elliott, R., Watson, J. C., & Bohart, A. C. (2001). Empathy. *Psychotherapy, 38,* 380–384.

Hall, J. A., Harrigan, J. A., & Rosenthal, R. (1995). Nonverbal behavior in clinician-client interaction. *Applied and Preventive Psychology, 4,* 21–37.

Hall, J. A., Roter, D. L., & Katz, N. R. (1988). Meta-analysis of correlates of provider behavior in medical encounters. *Medical Care, 26,* 657–675.

Hall, J. A., Roter, D. L., & Milburn, M. A. (1999). Illness and satisfaction with medical care. *Current Directions in Psychological Science, 3,* 96–99.

Hanlan, A. J. (1979). *Autobiography of dying.* New York: Doubleday.

Hansen, R. A. (1990). The ethics of caring for patients with HIV or AIDS. *American Journal of Occupational Therapy, 44,* 239–242.

Harris, M. J., & Rosenthal, R. (1985). Mediation of interpersonal expectancy effects: 31 meta-analyses. *Psychological Bulletin, 97,* 363–386.

Hasselkus, B. R. (1991). Ethical dilemmas in family caregiving for the elderly: Implications for occupational therapy. *American Journal of Occupational Therapy, 45,* 206–212.

Hatfield, E., Cacioppo, J. T., & Rapson, R. L. (1994). *Emotional contagion.* Paris: Cambridge University.

Horvath, A. O., & Luborsky, L. (1993). The role of the therapeutic alliance in psychotherapy. *Journal of Counseling and Clinical Psychology, 61,* 561–573.

Iwama, M. (2003). Toward culturally relevant epistemologies in occupational therapy. *American Journal of Occupational Therapy, 57,* 582–588.

Klein, B. S. (1995). Reflections on . . . An ally as well as a partner in practice. *Canadian Journal of Occupational Therapy, 62,* 283–285.

Kleinman, A. (1988). *The illness narratives.* New York: Basic Books.

Lakin, J. L., & Chartrand, T. L. (2003). Using nonconscious behavioral mimicry to create affiliation and rapport. *American Psychological Society, 14,* 334–339.

Langer, E. J., & Abelson, R. P. (1974). A client by any other name. . .: Clinician group differences in labeling bias. *Journal of Consulting and Clinical Psychology, 42,* 4–9.

Lyons, K. D., Tickle-Degnen, L., Henry, A., & Cohn, E. (2004). Impressions of personality in Parkinson's disease: Can rehabilitation practitioners see beyond the symptoms? *Rehabilitation Psychology, 49,* 328–333.

Marangoni, C., Garcia, S., Ickes, W., & Teng, G. (1995). Empathic accuracy in a clinically relevant context. *Journal of Personality and Social Psychology, 68,* 854–869.

Martin, D. J., Garske, J. P., & Davis, M. K. (2000). Relation of the therapeutic alliance with outcome and other variables: A meta-analytic review. *Journal of Consulting and Clinical Psychology, 68,* 438–450.

Mattingly, C., & Fleming, M. H. (1994). *Clinical reasoning: Forms of inquiry in a therapeutic practice.* Philadelphia: Davis.

McCrum, R. (1998). *My year off.* New York: Norton.

Northern, J. G., Rust, D. M., Nelson, C. E., & Watts, J. H. (1995). Involvement of adult rehabilitation patients in setting occupational therapy goals. *American Journal of Occupational Therapy, 49,* 214–220.

Oxford English Dictionary. (2005). Oxford, UK: Oxford University. Retrieved May 5, 2005 from http://www.askoxford.com.

Padilla, R. (2003). Clara: A phenomenology of disability. *American Journal of Occupational Therapy, 57,* 413–423.

Park, R. E., & Burgess, E. W. (1924). *Introduction to the science of sociology.* Chicago: University of Chicago.

Peloquin, S. M. (1993a). The depersonalization of patients: A profile gleaned from narratives. *American Journal of Occupational Therapy, 47,* 830–837.

Peloquin, S. M. (1993b). The patient-therapist relationship: Beliefs that shape care. *American Journal of Occupational Therapy, 47,* 935–942.

Peloquin, S. M. (2002). Reclaiming the vision of 'Reaching for Heart as Well as Hands.' *American Journal of Occupational Therapy, 56,* 517–526.

Porszt-Miron, L., Florian, M., & Burton, J. (1988). A pilot study on the effect of rapport on the task performance of an elderly confused population. *Canadian Journal of Occupational Therapy, 55,* 255–258.

Prigatano, G. P., Klonoff, P. S., O'Brien, K. P., Altman, I. M., Amin, K., Chiapello, D., Shepherd, J., Cunningham, M., & Mora, M. (1994). Productivity after neuropsychologically oriented milieu rehabilitation. *Journal of Head Trauma Rehabilitation, 9,* 91–102.

Puller, L. B. (1991). *Fortunate son.* New York: Grove Weidenfeld.

Rogers, C. (1957). The necessary and sufficient conditions of therapeutic change. *Journal of Consulting Psychology, 21,* 95–105.

Rosa, S. A., & Hasselkus, B. R. (1996). Connecting with patients: The personal experience of professional helping. *Occupational Therapy Journal of Research, 16,* 245–260.

Rosa, S. A., & Hasselkus, B. R. (2005). Finding common ground with patients: The centrality of compatibility. *American Journal of Occupational Therapy, 59,* 198–208.

Sachs, D., & Labovitz, D. R. (1994). The caring occupational therapist: Scope of professional roles and boundaries. *American Journal of Occupational Therapy, 48,* 997–1005.

Saxton, M. (1987). The something that happened before I was born. In M. Saxton & F. Howe (Eds.), *With wings: An anthology of literature by and about women with disabilities* (pp. 51–55). New York: Feminist.

Schindler, L., Hohenberger-Sieber, E., & Hahlweg, K. (1989). Observing client-therapist interaction in behaviour therapy: Development and first application of an observational system. *British Journal of Clinical Psychology, 28,* 213–226.

Svidén, G., & Säljö, R. (1993). Perceiving clients and their nonverbal reactions. *American Journal of Occupational Therapy, 47,* 491–497.

Tham, K., & Kielhofner, G. (2003). Impact of the social environment on occupational experience and performance among persons with unilateral neglect. *American Journal of Occupational Therapy, 57,* 403–412.

Tickle-Degnen, L. (1998). Working well with others: The prediction of students' clinical performance. *American Journal of Occupational Therapy, 52,* 133–142.

Tickle-Degnen, L. (2000). Evidence-based practice forum: Communicating with clients, family members, and colleagues about research evidence. *American Journal of Occupational Therapy, 54,* 341–343.

Tickle-Degnen, L. (2006). Nonverbal behavior and its functions in the ecosystem of rapport. In M. L. Patterson & V. Manusov (Eds.), *Handbook of nonverbal communications* (pp. 381–399). Thousans Oaks, CA: Sage.

Tickle-Degnen, L., & Coster, W. (1995). Therapeutic interaction and the management of challenge during the beginning minutes of sensory integration treatment. *Occupational Therapy Journal of Research, 15,* 122–141.

Tickle-Degnen, L., & Gavett, E. (2003). Changes in nonverbal behavior during the development of therapeutic relationships. In P. Philippot, R. S. Feldman, and E. J. Coats (Eds.), *Nonverbal behavior in clinical settings* (pp. 75–110). Oxford, UK: Oxford University Press.

Tickle-Degnen, L., & Lyons, K. D. (2004). Practitioners' impressions of patients with Parkinson's disease: The social ecology of the expressive mask. *Social Science and Medicine, 58,* 603–614.

Tickle-Degnen, L., & Puccinelli, N. (1999). The nonverbal expression of negative emotions: Peer and supervisor responses to occupational therapy students' emotional attributes. *Occupational Therapy Journal of Research, 19,* 18–39.

Tickle-Degnen, L., & Rosenthal, R. (1992). Nonverbal aspects of therapeutic rapport. In R. S. Feldman (Ed.), *Applications of nonverbal behavioral theories and research* (pp. 143–164). Hillsdale, NJ: Lawrence Erlbaum.

Watt, B. (1996). *Patient.* New York: Grove.

Widome, A. (1989). *The doctor/the client.* Miami: Editech.

Yerxa, E. J. (1973). The 1966 Eleanor Clarke Slagle Lecture: Authentic occupational therapy. In American Occupational Therapy Association (Ed.), *The Eleanor Clarke Slagle Lectures: 1955–1972* (pp. 155–173). Dubuque, IA: Kendall/Hunt.

Supplemental References

Peloquin, S. M. (1990). The client-therapist relationship in occupational therapy: Understanding visions and images. *American Journal of Occupational Therapy, 44,* 13–21.

Tickle-Degnen, L. (2002). Evidence-based practice forum: Client-centered practice, therapeutic relationship, and the use of research evidence. *American Journal of Occupational Therapy, 56,* 470–474.

Tickle-Degnen, L., & Rosenthal, R. (1990). The nonverbal correlates of rapport. *Psychological Inquiry, 1,* 285–293.

SECTION IV: Therapeutic Technologies

CHAPTER 16

Upper Extremity Orthoses

Lisa D. Deshaies

LEARNING OBJECTIVES

After studying this chapter, the reader will be able to do the following:

1. Define and discuss key concepts and terms related to orthoses.
2. Identify major purposes for using orthoses.
3. Explain general precautions relative to the use of orthoses.
4. Identify key factors to consider when selecting the most appropriate orthosis.
5. Given a photograph or illustration, identify the orthosis and a clinical problem for which it may be used.
6. Select an appropriate orthosis for a given diagnosis based on a specific clinical need.

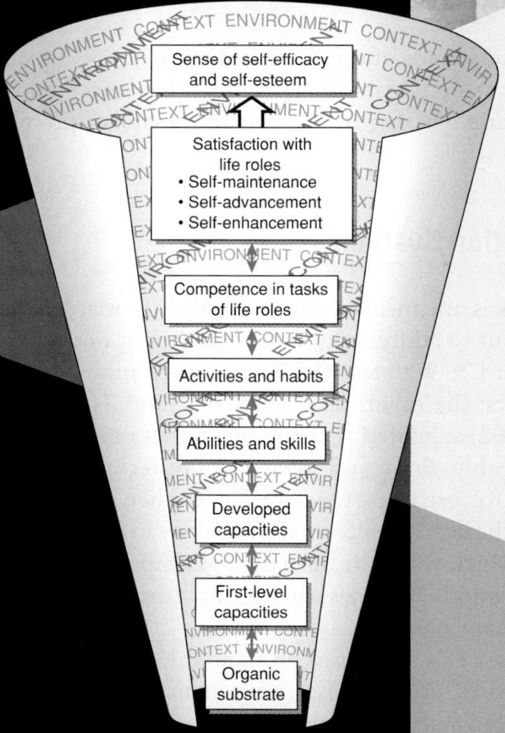

Glossary

Arm sling—An orthosis that supports the proximal upper extremity to restrict motion, reduce pain, or prevent or reduce shoulder subluxation.

Arm trough—An upper extremity positioning device attached to a wheelchair armrest.

Dynamic splint—Orthosis that has moving parts; primarily used to regain joint mobility or facilitate function.

Lapboard—A portable tabletop that is applied to a wheelchair to provide a working surface or support an upper extremity; also known as a lap tray.

Mobile arm support—A mechanical device that uses ball-bearing joints, gravity, and possibly rubber bands to support the arm and assist in movement when proximal muscles are weak; may be mounted onto a wheelchair or table; also known as a balanced forearm orthosis, ball-bearing arm support, or ball-bearing feeder.

Orthosis—Any medical device added to a person's body to support, align, position, immobilize, prevent or correct deformities, assist weak muscles, or improve function; also known as a splint, brace, or support.

Serial casting—Applying casts at routine intervals as range of motion improves, with the goal of restoring joint mobility.

Serial static splinting—Remolding or fabricating new static splints as range of motion improves, with the goal of restoring joint mobility.

Static splint—Orthosis that has no moving parts; primarily used to support, stabilize, protect, or immobilize.

Static progressive splint—Orthosis that uses non-dynamic forces; primarily used to regain joint motion.

Wrist-driven wrist–hand orthosis—Flexor hinge orthosis that uses tenodesis to accomplish palmar pinch.

Orthoses are often an integral component of occupational therapy for patients with physical dysfunction. Orthotics entails prescription, selection, design, fabrication, testing, and training in the use of these special devices.

Successful use of orthoses is made possible only through an integrated team approach including the patient, his or her significant others, and health care providers. Several rehabilitation professionals may bring their expertise to different aspects of the orthotic process. The physician typically prescribes the device. The certified orthotist is an expert in the design and fabrication of permanent orthoses, especially complicated spinal, lower extremity, and upper extremity orthoses used to restore function. The rehabilitation engineer is an expert in technical problem solving involving mechanical and/or electrical solutions to unique needs of patients.

The occupational therapist, as an expert in the adaptive use of the upper extremities in occupational performance tasks, has the major responsibility for the recommendation of appropriate orthoses, the testing and training in the use of orthoses for the upper extremities, and the selection, design, and fabrication of thermoplastic splints. Occupational therapists often collaborate with orthotists and rehabilitation engineers to solve problems encountered by patients in performing their occupations and activities of daily life. The therapist presents the parameters of the problem to these professionals in terms of the patient's abilities and limitations and the functional and psychological goals that the prescribed device should meet or allow. The orthotist or engineer then proposes technical solutions, and together they apply them to the patient and evaluate the outcome.

Finally, and possibly most importantly, the patient and caregivers bring key physical, psychological, social, and functional characteristics to the orthotic process and should be considered the primary members of the team. For the orthosis to be successful, all team members must work in close collaboration.

KINDS OF ORTHOSES

The numerous kinds of upper extremity orthoses vary according to the body parts they include, their mechanical properties, and whether they are custom made or prefabricated.

Classification Systems

An **orthosis** is any medical device applied to or around a body segment to address physical impairment or disability (Lunsford & Wallace, 1997). Orthoses may also be called splints; the American Society of Hand Therapists (ASHT) (1992) validated that the two terms may be used interchangeably. *Brace* and *support* are other commonly used terms for orthoses. One challenge when discussing orthoses is the lack of uniform terminology in the medical literature, which makes it difficult to compare and contrast features and outcomes when a single orthosis may be known by many names.

Before the 1970s, there was no standard system for classifying orthoses, and orthoses were identified by proper names or eponyms based on the place of origin or the developer. A classification system was later developed to describe orthoses using acronyms based on the major joints or body parts they include. For example, a thumb carpometacarpal (CMC) support is a hand orthosis (HO); a wrist cock-up splint is a wrist-hand orthosis (WHO); an elbow brace is an elbow orthosis (EO); and a complete support for an arm is a shoulder-elbow-wrist-hand orthosis (SEWHO) (Long & Schutt, 1986; Lunsford & Wallace, 1997). Each classification may contain several types of splints. A wrist cock-up splint and a flexor hinge hand splint are both WHOs, although they serve different purposes.

To simplify, organize, and describe a standardized professional nomenclature, the ASHT developed the ASHT Splint Classification System in 1992. It classifies splints in terms of their function and the number of joints they secondarily affect. According to this system, a wrist cock-up splint is a wrist extension immobilization, type 0, because no other joints are affected. As this system becomes more widely accepted and used, it will likely serve as a universal language for referral, reimbursement, communication, and research.

This chapter uses the traditional or most commonly used names for the splints it describes.

Basic Types of Orthoses

Mechanical splint properties fall into three categories: static, static progressive, and dynamic (Colditz, 2002a; Wilton, 1997). The **static splint**, which has no moving parts, is used primarily to provide support, stabilization, protection, or immobilization. **Serial static splinting** can be used to lengthen tissues and regain range of motion by placing tissues in an elongated position for prolonged periods (Bell-Krotoski, 2002; Colditz, 2002a). With this process, splints are remolded as range of motion increases. Because immobilization causes such unwanted effects as atrophy and stiffness, a static splint should never be used longer than physiologically required and should never unnecessarily include joints other than those being treated.

Static progressive splints use nondynamic components, such as Velcro, hinges, screws, or turnbuckles, to create a mobilizing force to regain motion. This type of splinting, termed inelastic traction mobilization, offers benefits not available with serial static or dynamic splinting because the same splint can be used without remolding, and adjustments can be made more easily as motion improves (Fess et al., 2005).

Dynamic splints use moving parts to permit, control, or restore movement. They are primarily used to apply an intermittent, gentle force with the goal of lengthening tissues to restore motion. Forces may be generated by springs, spring wires, rubber bands, or elastic cords. This type of splinting is termed elastic mobilization (Colditz, 2002a; Fess et al., 2005).

With dynamic splinting to increase range of motion, two concepts are critical. The first is that the force must be gentle and applied over a long time (Brand, 2002; Fess, 1995). Safe force for the hand has been determined to be 100–300 g (Brand, 2002; Fess & McCollum, 1998); parameters for proximal joints are not yet clinically defined. Excessive force results in tissue trauma, inflammation, and necrosis.

The second concept is that, to be effective and prevent skin problems, the line of pull must be at a 90° angle to the segment being mobilized (Brand, 2002). To ensure this, forces are directed by an outrigger, a structure extending outward from the splint.

Outriggers may be high profile or low profile (Fig. 16-1). Each design has distinct advantages and disadvantages. Selection of outrigger design must be based on the specific patient's needs and abilities. High-profile outriggers are inherently more stable and mechanically efficient, require fewer adjustments to maintain a 90° angle of pull, and require less effort for the patient to move against the dynamic force. Low-profile outriggers are less bulky but require more frequent adjustments and greater strength to move against the dynamic force (Fess, 1995; Fess et al., 2005).

By allowing motion in the opposite direction, dynamic splints reduce the risk of joint stiffness from immobility,

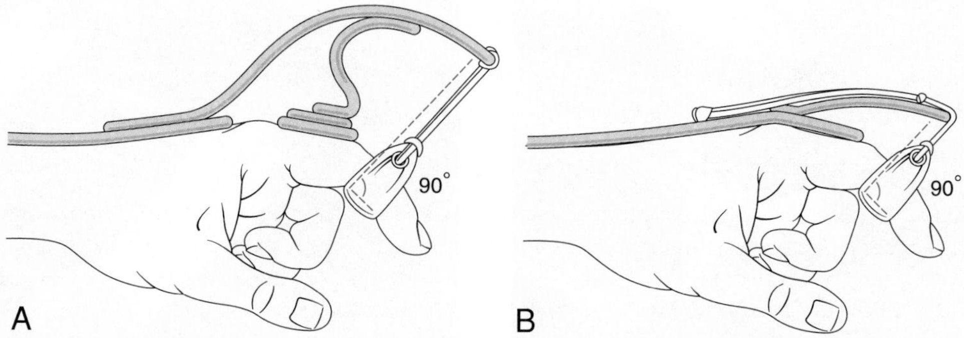

Figure 16-1 Outriggers directing proper 90° line of pull. **A.** High profile. **B.** Low profile. (Adapted with permission from Hunter, J. M., Mackin, E. J., & Callahan, A. D. [Eds.]. [1995]. *Rehabilitation of the hand: Surgery and therapy* [4th ed.]. St. Louis: Mosby.)

as seen with static splinting. If successful, an increase in passive joint mobility can be expected within 2 weeks (Fess & McCollum, 1998).

In addition to gaining motion, dynamic splints can be used to assist weak or paralyzed muscles. These dynamic splints may be intrinsically powered by another body part or by electrical stimulation of the patient's muscles. Extrinsic power sources, including gas-operated devices and battery-powered motors, have also been used (Long & Schutt, 1986). In practice, these externally powered devices proved to be too complex and difficult to maintain, causing their use to decline (Clark, Waters, & Baumgarten, 1997).

ORTHOTIC SELECTION

Splinting is one of the most useful modalities available to therapists when used correctly and appropriately (Fess, 1995). Remember, the end result of splinting should always relate to the patient's function (Figs. 16-2 through 16-5). McKee and Rivard (2004) caution that: "Orthotic intervention may have become an end unto itself in the minds of therapists and clients rather than the means to enable occupational performance." The outcome of successful splinting is that the splint serves its purpose and that the patient accepts and wears it. To meet these ends, the therapist must think critically and often creatively.

The therapist's multifaceted role is to evaluate the need for a splint clinically and functionally; to select the most appropriate splint; to provide or fabricate the splint; to assess the fit of the splint; to teach the patient and caregivers the purpose, care, and use of the splint; and to provide related training as needed. The therapist must take a leadership role to ensure that the treatment team, including the patient and caregivers, work collaboratively in every phase of the orthotic process. A client-centered, occupation-based approach empowers the patient and caregivers to participate actively. This also positions them as the experts in the patient's occupations, lifestyle, values, image, and activity contexts, which complements the expertise that the health care professionals bring. The therapist should clearly explain rationales, make clinically sound recommendations, and offer choices to the patient whenever possible. This helps establish each team member's accountability and increases the likelihood that the patient will actually use the splint.

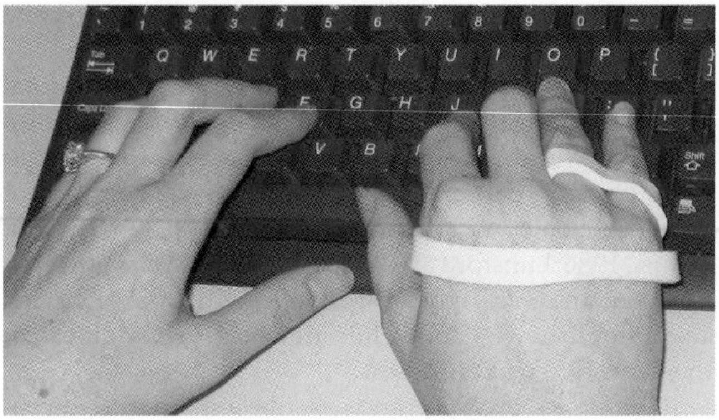

Figure 16-3 Hand splint enabling keyboarding.

A problem-solving approach to splinting directs the therapist to answer several key questions before splinting proceeds:

- What is the primary clinical or functional problem?
- What are the indications for and goals of splint use?
- How will the orthosis affect the problem and the patient's overall function?
- What benefits will the splint provide?
- What limitations will the splint impose?
- What evidence is available related to the splint?

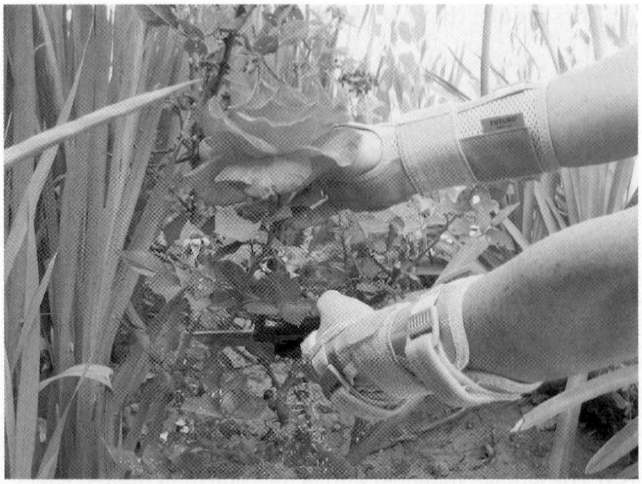

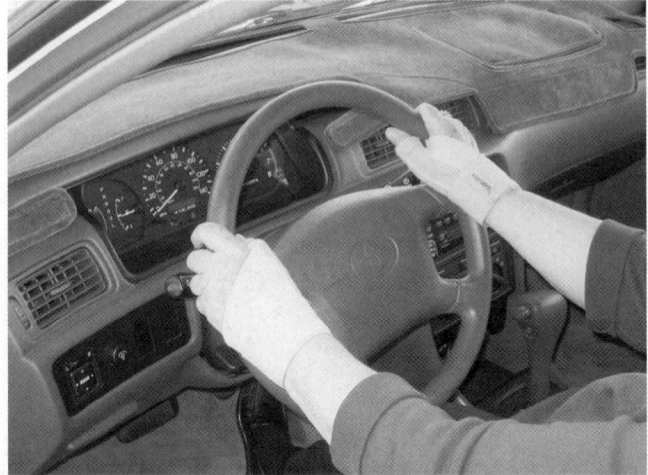

Figure 16-2 Wrist splints enabling gardening.

Figure 16-4 Thumb splints enabling driving.

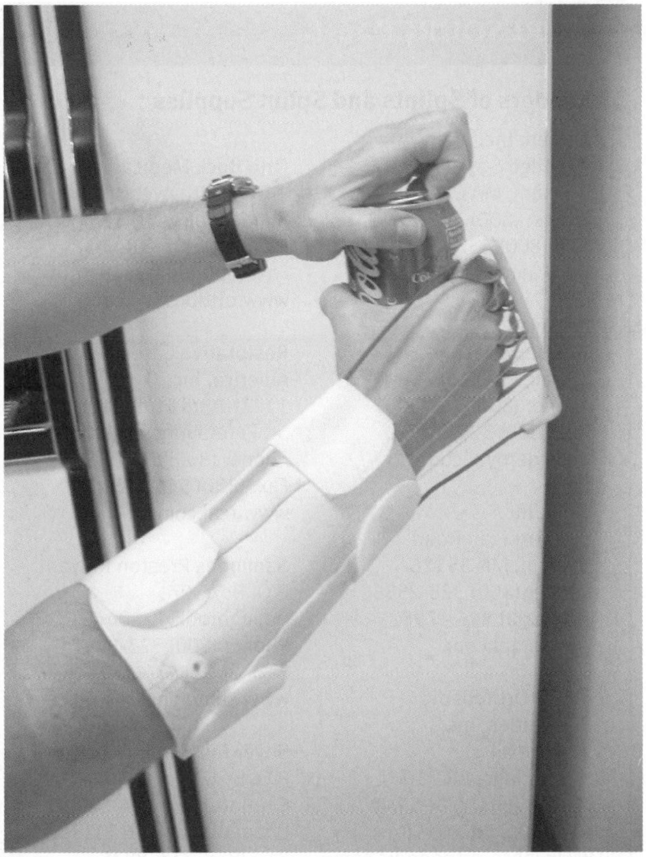

Figure 16-5 Wrist–hand splint enabling function in the kitchen.

Based on these considerations, the therapist must select or design the most appropriate orthosis. In some cases, the best choice is no orthosis at all.

The growing array of commercial products has led to a greater number of choices. The first is whether the orthosis should be custom fabricated or prefabricated. Materials must also be considered. The therapist must be familiar with properties, benefits, and drawbacks of each. Options abound, with rigid, semirigid, and soft materials available (Breger-Lee, 1995; Canelon, 1995).

When making a splint selection, several key factors must be carefully weighed:

- Among the splint-related factors are type, design, purpose, fit, comfort, cosmetic appearance, cost to purchase or fabricate, weight, ease of care, durability, ease of donning and doffing, effect on unsplinted joints, and effect on function.
- Patient-related factors include clinical and functional status, attitude, lifestyle, preference, occupational roles, living and working environments, social support, issues related to safety and precautions, ability to understand and follow through, and financial or insurance status.

Several studies have been done on patients' preferences and factors that contribute to splint wear. They show that the following factors may encourage splint wear: flexibility of the splinting regimen and vigorous teaching to enable patients to understand the purpose and wearing schedule (Pagnotta, Baron, & Korner-Bitensky, 1998); individualized prescriptions focusing on the patient's comfort and preference (Callinan & Mathiowetz, 1996; Stern et al., 1996); strong family support (Oakes et al., 1970); positive attitudes and behaviors exhibited by health care providers (Feinberg, 1992); and benefits that are immediately obvious to the patient (Groth & Wulf, 1995). Rapport, trust, sensitivity to individual patient's learning styles, trial evaluations, and giving patients the opportunity to voice their concerns and frustrations can also greatly enhance the collaborative process and outcome (Collins, 1999). With the relatively small base of literature on orthotics, therapists must continue to put their clinical judgments and experience to the test and strive for evidence-based practice related to outcomes and factors that influence successful orthotic intervention.

SAFETY NOTE 16-1

Orthotic Precautions

The therapist must consider, carefully monitor, and teach the patient and caregiver to report any of these problems related to orthotic use:

- Impaired skin integrity (pressure areas, blisters, maceration, dermatological reactions)
- Pain
- Swelling
- Stiffness
- Sensory disturbances
- Increased stress on unsplinted joints
- Functional limitations

Should problems with splint wear arise (Safety Note 16-1), the therapist should examine both the splint and the wearing schedule. The splint itself may not fit properly or comfortably. The patient's functional demands may outweigh the benefits of splint wearing, or the wearing schedule may be too complex. Actively engaging the patient in the problem-solving process is likely to improve the outcome. Although it is important to strive for the ideal, therapists must remain realistic in the scope of the patient's daily life.

PURPOSES OF ORTHOSES

In this chapter, orthoses are categorized according to several purposes (Definition 16-1). Although a specific orthosis is discussed under the category for which it is most commonly used, that purpose may not be its only one. Also, a single orthosis may fulfill several functions simultaneously. The orthoses presented here are by no means an exhaustive list but

DEFINITION 16-1 *definition*

Purposes of Orthoses

- Support a painful joint
- Immobilize for healing
- Protect tissues
- Provide stability
- Restrict unwanted motion
- Restore mobility
- Substitute for weak or absent muscles
- Prevent contractures
- Modify tone

a representative sampling of commonly used or historically significant orthoses. Inclusion of specific orthoses should not be interpreted as an endorsement of one type over another. Whenever possible, published evidence-based data have been included. As the intent of this chapter is to provide an overview of orthotics, the reader is encouraged to explore the references and resources for more detailed information.

Support a Painful Joint

Pain in a joint or soft tissues can result from a wide variety of causes, including acute trauma (such as sprains and strains), nerve irritation (such as carpal tunnel syndrome and ulnar nerve neuritis at the elbow), inflammatory conditions (such as tendonitis and rheumatoid arthritis), and joint instability (such as degenerative arthritis, ligamentous laxity, and shoulder subluxation). When resting a joint is indicated to relieve pain, protect joint integrity, and/or decrease inflammation, supportive orthoses can be used. These orthoses are often worn all day, all night, or both to provide the maximum benefit; or they may be worn only during selected activities. Unless contraindicated, the orthosis should be removed at least once a day for skin hygiene and gentle range-of-motion exercises to prevent loss of joint mobility. The following are common examples of orthoses used for pain relief.

Support a Painful Shoulder or Elbow

Arm slings have been developed to prevent or correct shoulder subluxation or reduce pain in patients who have subluxation caused by brachial plexus injuries, hemiplegia, and central cord syndrome injuries. Sling designs are numerous, with some commercially available and others fabricated by the therapist.

Certain slings support and immobilize the whole arm. These slings, such as the standard pouch and the double arm cuff sling (Fig. 16-6) restrict motion by keeping the humerus in adduction and internal rotation and the elbow in flexion. Although these slings may take some of the weight off the affected shoulder, downsides are that they place the extremity in a nonfunctional position, reinforce synergy patterns, and fail to provide the patient with the opportunity for motor and sensory feedback (Bobath, 1990; Moodie, Brisbin, & Margan, 1986). Other sling designs support the shoulder but leave the rest of the arm free for function, such as a humeral cuff sling (Fig. 16-7).

RESOURCE 16-1

Vendors of Splints and Splint Supplies

AliMed, Inc.
297 High Street
Dedham, MA 02026
Phone: (800) 225–2610
Fax: (800) 437-2966
www.alimed.com

DeRoyal
200 DeBusk Lane
Powell, TN 37849
Phone: (800) 362-3002
Fax: (800) 327-0340
www.deroyal.com

Empi, Inc.
599 Cardigan Road
St. Paul, MN 55126
Phone: (800) 328-2536
Fax: (800) 896-1798
www.empi.com

JAECO Orthopedic Specialties, Inc.
214 Drexel
Hot Springs, AR 71901
Phone: (501) 623-5944
Fax: (501) 623-0159
www.jaeco-orthopedic.com

Joint Active Systems, Inc.
2600 South Raney
Effingham, IL 62401
Phone: (800) 879-0117
Fax: (217) 347-3384
www.jointactivesystems.com

Kinex Medical Company
1801 Airport Rd., Suite D
Waukesha, WI 53188
Phone: (800) 845-6364
Fax: (888) 845-3342
www.kinexmedical.com

North Coast Medical, Inc.
18305 Sutter Boulevard
Morgan Hill, CA 95037
Phone: (800) 821-9319
Fax: (877) 213-9300
www.ncmedical.com

Otto Bock Medical
14630 28th Ave. North
Minneapolis, MN 53447
Phone: (800) 328-4058
Fax: (800) 962-2549
www.ottobockus.com

Restorative Care of America, Inc.
12221 33rd Street North
St. Petersburg, FL 33716
Phone: (800) 627-1595
Fax: (800) 545-7938
www.rcai.com

Sammons Preston Rolyan
P.O. Box 5071
Bolingbrook, IL 60440
Phone: (800) 323-5547
Fax: (800) 547-4333
www.sammonspreston.com

Silver Ring Splint Company
P.O. Box 2856
Charlottesville, VA 22902
Phone: (800) 311-7028
Fax: (888) 456-8828
www.silverringsplint.com

3-Point Products, Inc.
1610 Pincay Court
Annapolis, MD 21401
Phone: (888) 378-7763
Fax: (410) 349-2648
www.3pointproducts.com

UE Tech
P.O. Box 2145
Edwards, CO 81632
Phone: (800) 736-1894
Fax: (970) 926-8870
www.uetech.com

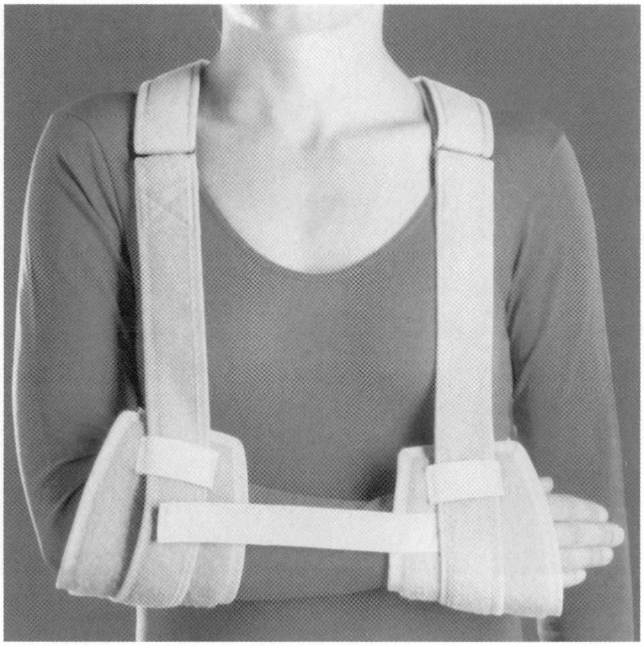

Figure 16-6 Rolyan® Figure-of-8 Sling.

Arm troughs, **lapboards**, and half-lapboards are also used to support the painful shoulder when the patient is seated in a wheelchair. These may be more acceptable to patients than slings, and they allow the arm to be ideally positioned with the scapula pulled forward and the hand supported (Bobath, 1990). It is important to remember that these supports lack the constant relationship between the patient and the support as exists with slings. Any change in postural alignment will alter forces and the support effectiveness (Spaulding, 1999). Lapboards (Fig. 16-8) are generally indicated for patients with poor trunk control or visual field deficits and for those who require greater variability of upper extremity positioning or a

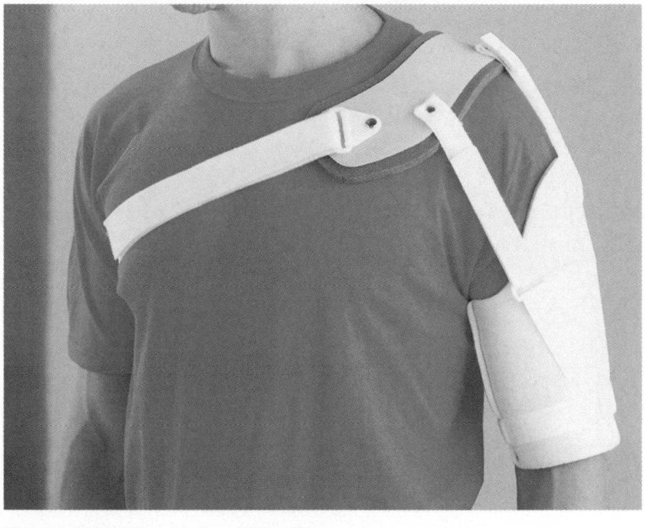

Figure 16-7 Hemi shoulder sling.

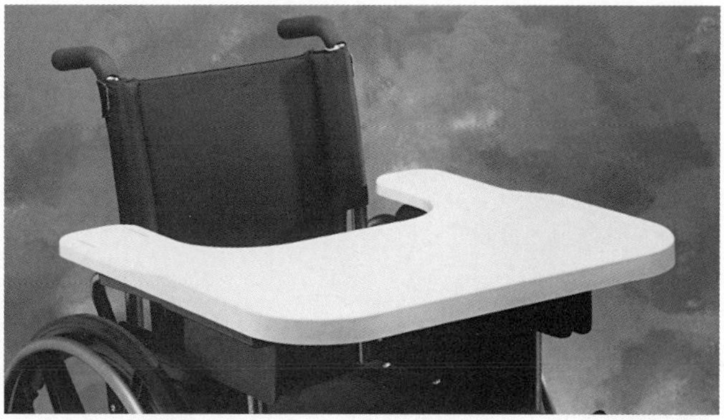

Figure 16-8 Rolyan® Slide-On Adjustable Lap Tray.

work surface. Arm troughs (Fig. 16-9) are used for patients who need a device that does not interfere with wheelchair propulsion or transfer activities (Lange, 1999). The half-lapboard (Fig. 16-10) combines the positive features of both the arm trough and the full lapboard (Walsh, 1987). Full and half-lapboards can be purchased commercially or custom fabricated from acrylic or wood. Some designs allow the half-lapboard to be rotated up and out of the way instead of having to be removed from the wheelchair when the patient needs to transfer. Arm troughs are also commercially available or can be custom made.

The use of supports in reducing shoulder subluxation remains controversial. In addition, whether subluxation has a causal relationship to shoulder pain is in question (Zorowitz et al., 1996). There is no consensus as to which type of support is the best in the treatment of shoulder subluxation or whether a support should be used at all. The effects of various sling and support designs have proved variable in multiple studies over the years as summarized by Zorowitz et al. (1995).

Ultimately, it is agreed upon that, if a support is to be used, several types should be evaluated on the patient to optimize the reduction of shoulder pain, the function of the affected extremity, and the ease of donning and doffing (Zorowitz et al., 1995). Therapists need to consider the different mechanical forces each support produces on

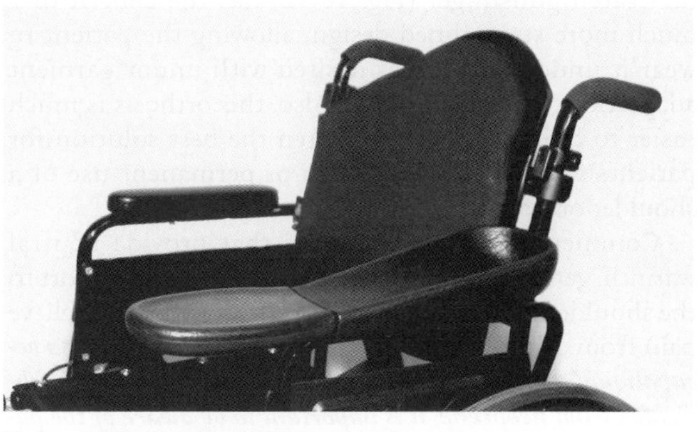

Figure 16-9 Otto Bock™ Arm Trough.

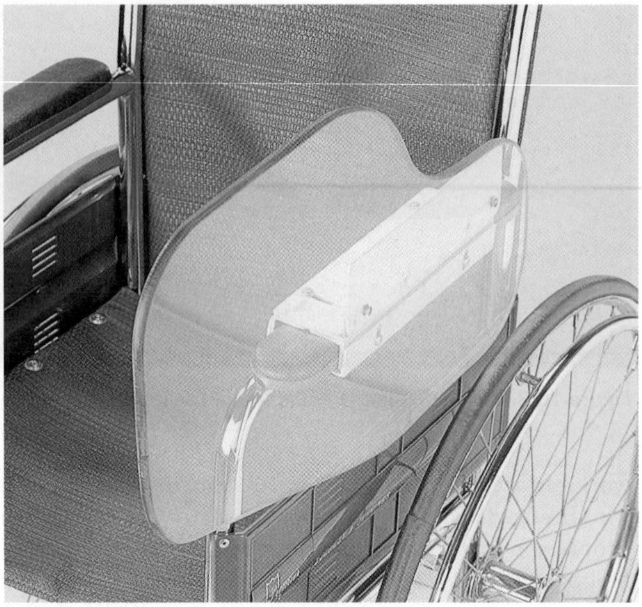

Figure 16-10 Clear Flipaway Armrest in upright position.

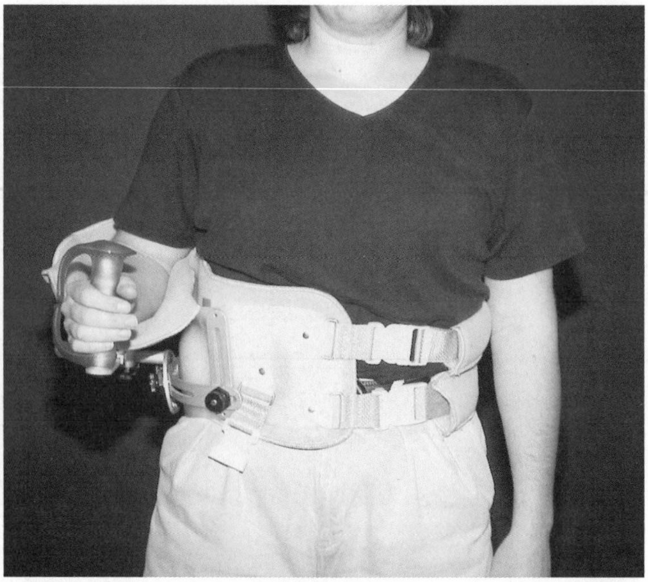

Figure 16-11 Commercial gunslinger orthosis.

the shoulder complex (Spaulding, 1999). Smith and Okamoto (1981) reviewed more than 22 distinctive hemiplegic sling designs and developed a checklist of 19 desirable and 4 undesirable characteristics to guide the therapist in examining and comparing slings for individual patients. The patient's acceptance of the sling also must be considered. Relative ease of donning and doffing the sling is imperative so the limb is not damaged further from improper wearing. More definitive research on the effectiveness of slings and orthoses in the management of the flaccid or subluxed shoulder is needed, and therapists should carefully consider all options before prescribing slings.

A gunslinger orthosis is another means of supporting a painful shoulder, such as from a brachial plexus injury. This type of orthosis is commercially available or can be custom fabricated for the patient. A commercial gunslinger (Fig. 16-11) can be easily adjusted to position the shoulder and elbow for maximal pain relief. A custom-fabricated gunslinger (Fig. 16-12) has the benefit of a much more streamlined design, allowing the patient to wear it under clothing as desired with minor garment adaptations (Lunsford, 1997). Also, this orthosis is much easier to don and doff. It is often the best solution for patients who require long-term or permanent use of a shoulder orthosis.

Commercial neoprene sleeves that provide neutral warmth, gentle compression, and soft dynamic support to the shoulder or elbow (Fig. 16-13) are often used to relieve pain from arthritis, tendinitis, sprains, and strains. ***As occupational therapists are expanding their use of supports fabricated from neoprene, it is important to be aware of the potential for dermatological reactions to the material and to teach patients to discontinue use of the support should symptoms develop (Stern et al., 1998).***

The treatment of lateral and medial epicondylitis often entails the use of orthoses to relieve pain and prevent further stress to affected tissues. In both conditions, pain reduces grip strength and function. Counterforce braces (Fig. 16-14), of which there are several commercial models, are wide, nonelastic bands designed to reduce stresses on the common forearm extensor or flexor musculature origins (Wilton, 1997). These braces can also be custom fabricated from thermoplastic or strapping materials (Jacobs & Austin, 2003). The literature reports wide variation in the success of braces (Borkholder, Hill, & Fess, 2004; Wuori et al., 1998). ***Complications can result from the brace***

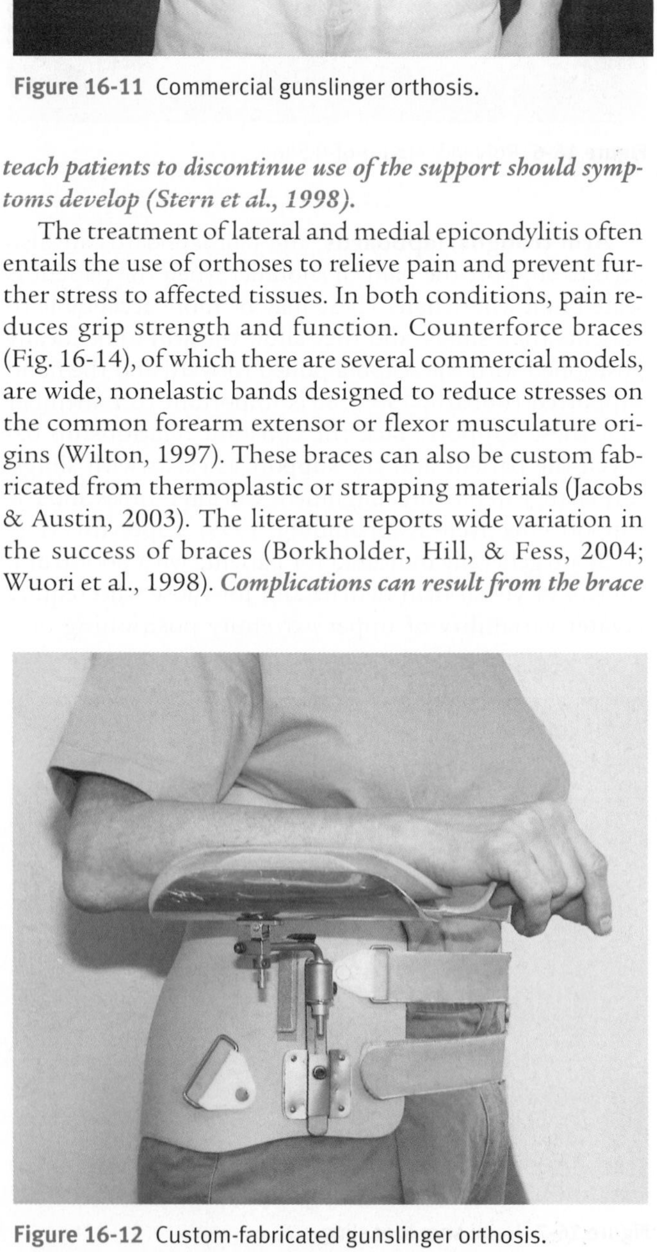

Figure 16-12 Custom-fabricated gunslinger orthosis.

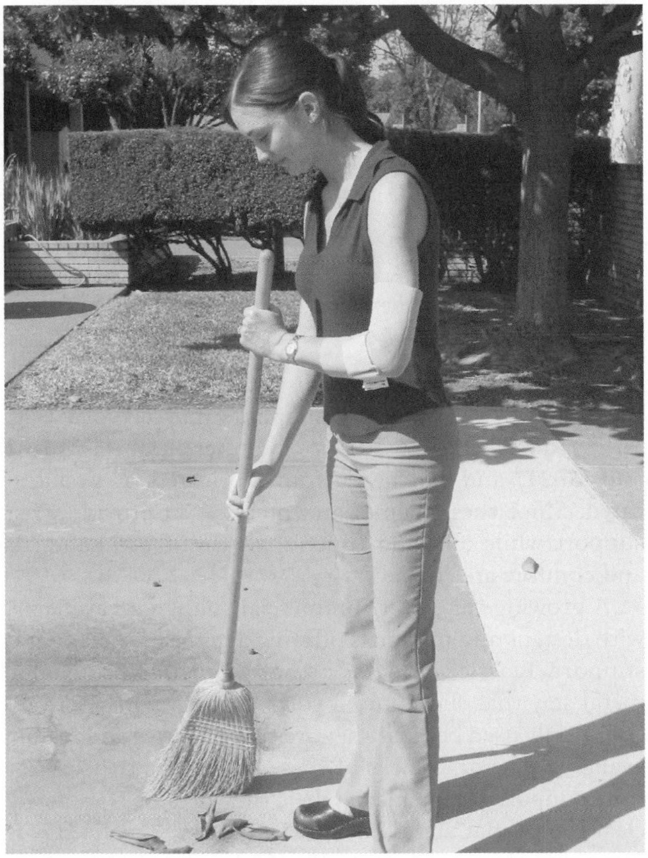

Figure 16-13 Commercial soft elbow support.

being applied too tightly, including nerve compression syndromes. The patient must be carefully taught accordingly.

A wrist splint placing the wrist in 45° of extension and worn in conjunction with a counterforce brace is often prescribed to rest the forearm musculature (Aiello, 1998).

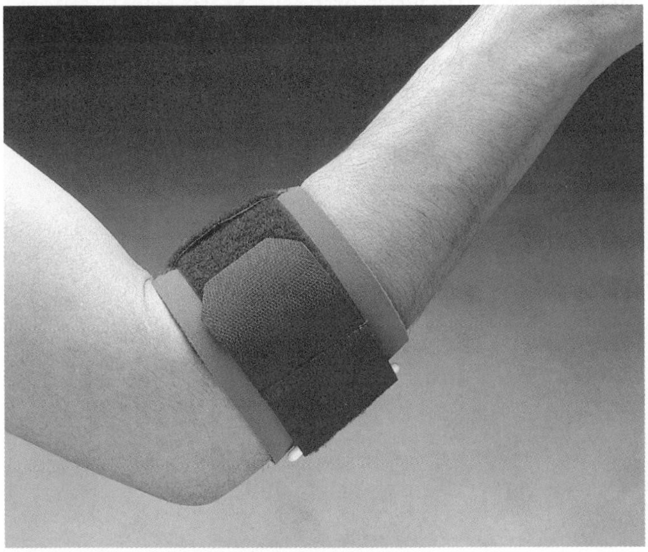

Figure 16-14 VariPad Tennis Elbow Support.

The prescription of orthoses must be based on the patient's symptoms. It is vital that the cause of the problem and the biomechanics of loading forearm musculature are also addressed in relation to vocational or recreational demands (Wilton, 1997).

Support a Painful Wrist or Hand

Resting hand splints are used to support the wrist, fingers, and thumb. The normal resting position of the hand is determined anatomically by the bony architecture, capsular length, and resting tone of the wrist and hand muscles. This is typically 10–20° of wrist extension, 20–30° of metacarpophalangeal joint (MCP) flexion, 0–20° of proximal interphalangeal joint (PIP) flexion, the distal interphalangeal joints (DIPs) in slight flexion, the thumb CMC in slight extension and abduction, and the thumb MP and IP in slight flexion (Wilton, 1997).

A resting hand splint is commonly prescribed for patients with rheumatoid arthritis. Resting splints can reduce stress on joint capsules, synovial lining, and periarticular structures, thereby decreasing pain (Melvin, 1989) (see Chapter 44). With this population, splinting should be in a position of comfort regardless of whether this is the ideal anatomical position (Fess et al., 2005). During an acute exacerbation of the disease, splints are generally worn at night and during most of the day and removed at least once for hygiene and gentle range-of-motion exercises. It is recommended that splint use continue for at least several weeks after the pain and swelling have subsided (Fess et al., 2005; Melvin, 1989).

Resting hand splints can be volar or dorsal, depending on needs and preferences. Commercial splints, such as those fabricated from wire-foam (Fig. 16-15) or a malleable metal frame covered by dense foam padding (Fig. 16-16), may be used if the limited adjustments they allow for can provide the patient with a proper fit. This becomes more difficult if the patient has established joint deformities. Custom-fabricated splints (Fig. 16-17) allow for a precise, individualized fit.

If the thumb or IP joints of the fingers are not painful, a modified resting hand splint (Fig. 16-18) may keep these joints free. This often results in less stiffness related to

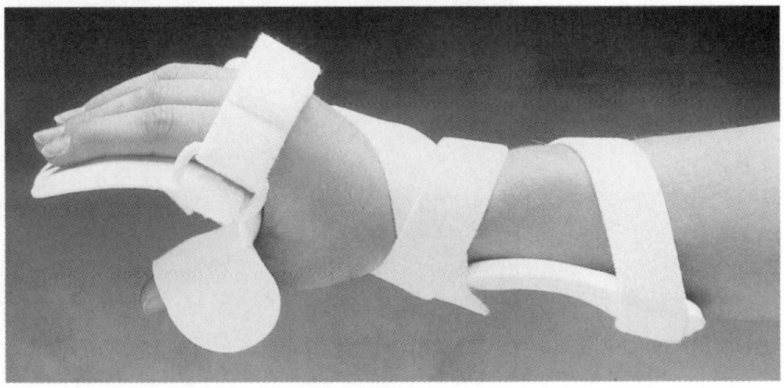

Figure 16-15 LMB Economical Resting Splint.

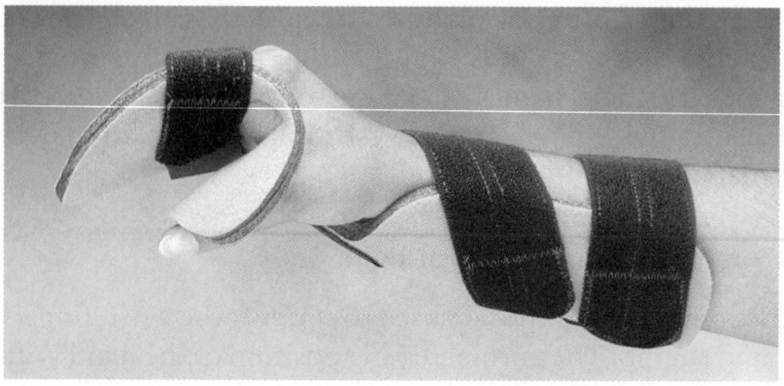

Figure 16-16 Progress™ Functional Resting Splint.

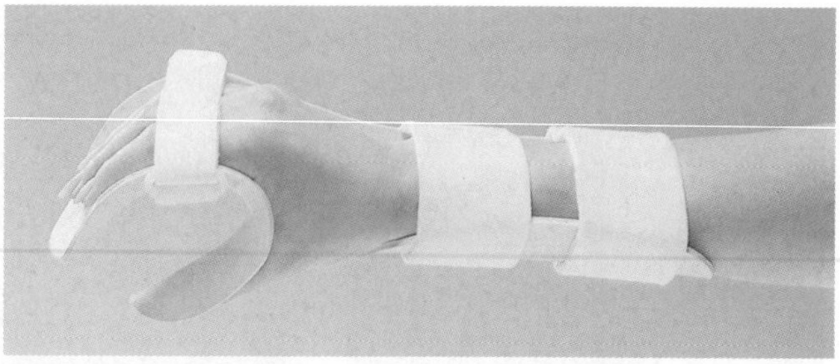

Figure 16-17 Custom thermoplastic resting hand splint.

splint wear, some degree of hand function while the splint is worn, and improved splint wear and comfort.

Although health care professionals generally agree on the benefits of using splints to rest inflamed and painful joints, studies have shown that compliance with wearing resting hand splints as prescribed is less than optimal at approximately 47% (Feinberg, 1992). In a study by Callinan and Mathiowetz (1996), which compared soft versus hard resting hand splints on pain and hand function, results showed that pain was significantly decreased with splint wear and that 57% of patients preferred the soft splint, 33% preferred the hard splint, and 10% preferred no splint. The rate of compliance was greater for the soft splint (82%) than for the hard splint (67%). The authors advocate that therapists provide patients with options relative to comfort and preference to ensure patient satisfaction and improved outcome.

Wrist extension, or cock-up, splints are probably the most commonly prescribed type of orthosis for the upper extremity. Indications for use include sprains, strains, tendonitis, arthritis, carpal tunnel syndrome, wrist fractures following cast removal, and other conditions that cause pain. A wrist splint typically positions the wrist in 10–30° of extension, which is thought to be the best position for hand function (Fess et al., 2005). A well-fitting splint is one that clears the distal palmar and thenar creases to allow for unrestricted mobility of the fingers and thumb and that conforms to the palm to support the arches of the hand. Wrist splints may be volar (Fig. 16-19), dorsal (Fig. 16-20), or circumferential (Figs. 16-2 and 16-21) and can be custom fabricated or prefabricated. Since these splints are intended to provide wrist support while allowing functional use of the hand, fit and comfort are crucial.

A growing variety of commercial splints are available, with designs and materials offering a range of soft to rigid support. Elasticized wrist orthoses with an adjustable metal stay that slides into a volar pocket (Fig. 16-22) are commonly used because they are cost-effective and readily available. The drawbacks of these splints are they do not fully support the palmar arches, they do not completely clear the palmar and thenar creases, and the metal stay is often prepositioned at a 35–45° angle of extension. Therefore, it is critical to fit and adjust the stay to the desired angle before issuing the splint. Other commercial products are made of wire-foam, neoprene, leather, canvas, and other fabric blends, all of which offer features having distinct advantages and disadvantages.

Several studies have been conducted on the effects on hand function of different styles of wrist extension splints. Carlson and Trombly (1983) reported a decrease in hand function when normal subjects were tested without and then with a static wrist orthosis. Stern (1991) studied hand function speed in normal subjects who wore three styles of custom-fabricated wrist splints and a commercial elastic wrist splint. She found that, although all of the

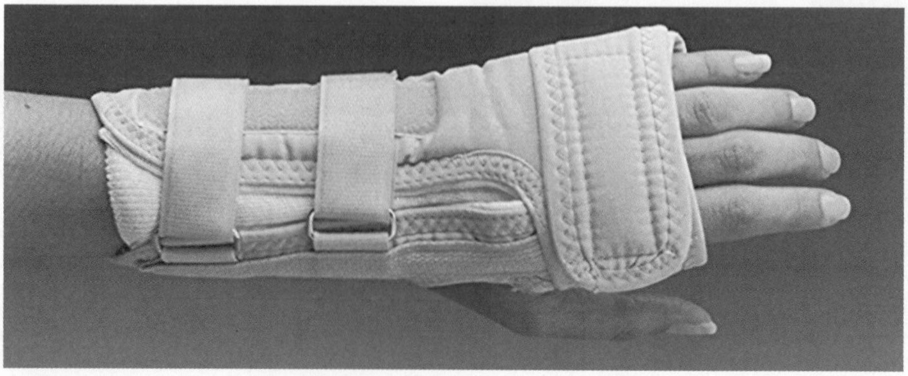

Figure 16-18 Rolyan® D-Ring™ Wrist Brace with MCP Support.

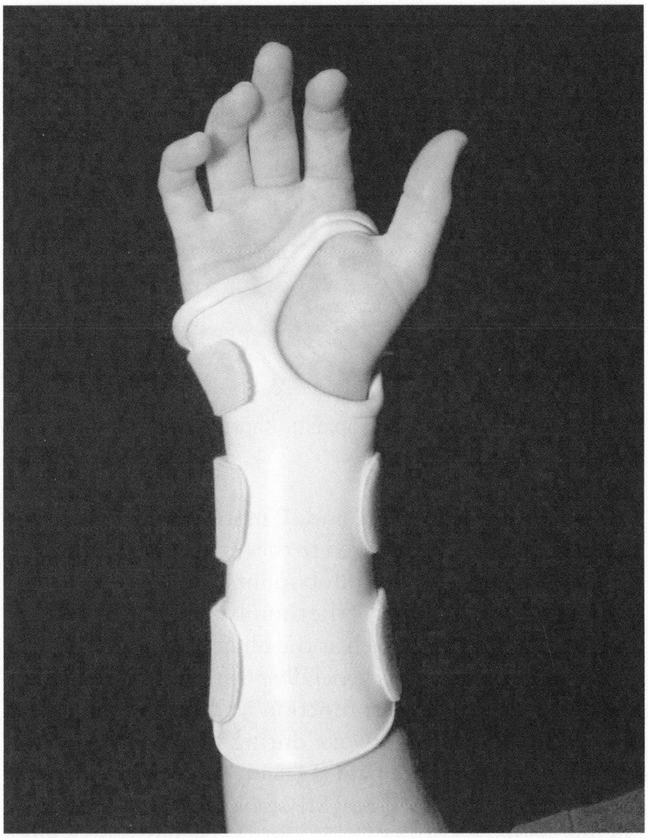

Figure 16-19 Custom thermoplastic volar wrist extension splint.

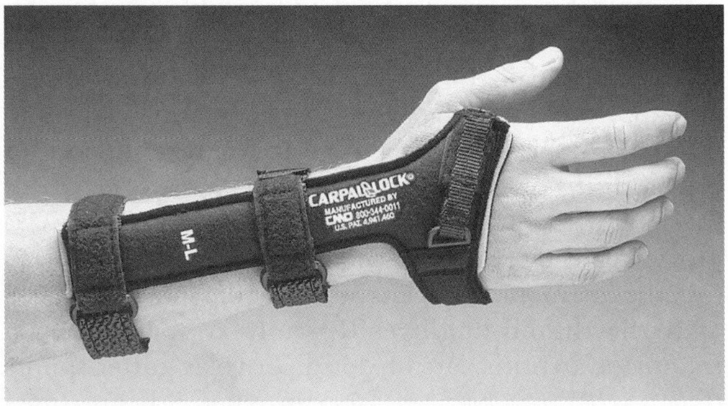

Figure 16-20 Carpal Lock® Splint.

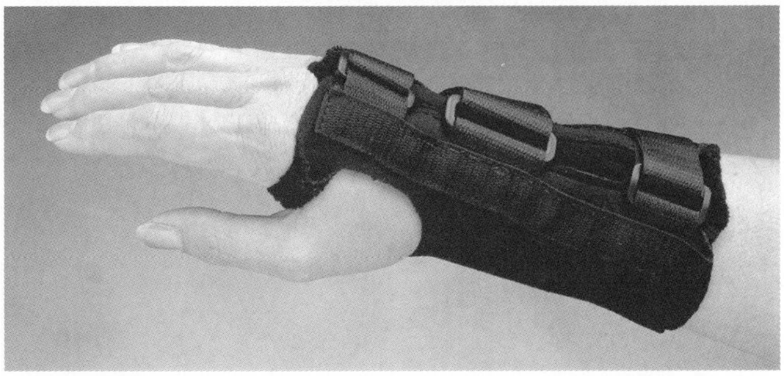

Figure 16-21 Comfort Cool™ D-Ring Wrist Splint.

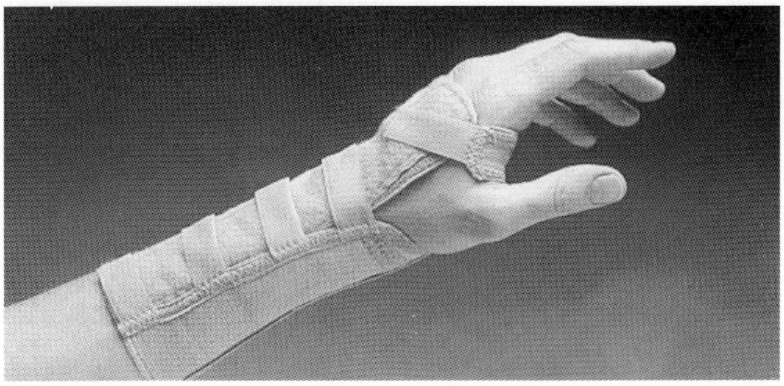

Figure 16-22 Norco™ Wrist Brace.

splints significantly slowed hand speed, the elastic splint allowed for faster speeds and dexterity than the others. A later study on grip strength and dexterity across five styles of commercial wrist splints concluded that each style impeded power grip and dexterity but to different extents (Stern, 1996).

Splints vary in the amount of motion they allow or restrict. Collier and Thomas (2002) compared range of motion at the wrist with three commercial supports and a custom-made volar thermoplastic splint. The commercial splints allowed the same amount of motion (wrist flexion to about neutral and wrist extension to about 26–31°). In contrast, the thermoplastic splint allowed less wrist flexion (not past 14° of wrist extension) and more wrist extension (about 40°). This suggests a custom thermoplastic splint may be more appropriate for conditions where limited wrist flexion is desired.

Elastic wrist orthoses have been widely used in the treatment of arthritis to stabilize wrists, decrease pain, and improve function. Again, studies have shown conflicting results across different styles of orthoses in grip strength, dexterity, hand function, pain reduction, comfort, security during task performance, and adverse effects of stiffness or muscle atrophy due to orthotic wear (Pagnotta, Baron, & Korner-Bitensky, 1998; Stern et al., 1996). In a related study, most of 42 subjects knew their preferred orthosis within a few minutes of wear when given three styles to try (Stern et al., 1997). These studies reinforce the importance of task analysis, having a wide variety of splints to try with each patient, and a careful weighing of the benefits and limitations of splinting.

Another common indication for wrist splinting is carpal tunnel syndrome, a condition caused by median nerve compression, which results in symptoms including pain, sensory disturbances, muscle weakness, swelling, stiffness, and frequent dropping of items. Symptoms often are worse at night or with repetitive activity involving wrist flexion (see Chapter 42). For pain and related symptoms caused by carpal tunnel syndrome, conservative or postoperative treatment often uses wrist splints to prevent the elevation of carpal tunnel pressure by restricting wrist motion (Gelberman et al., 1988).

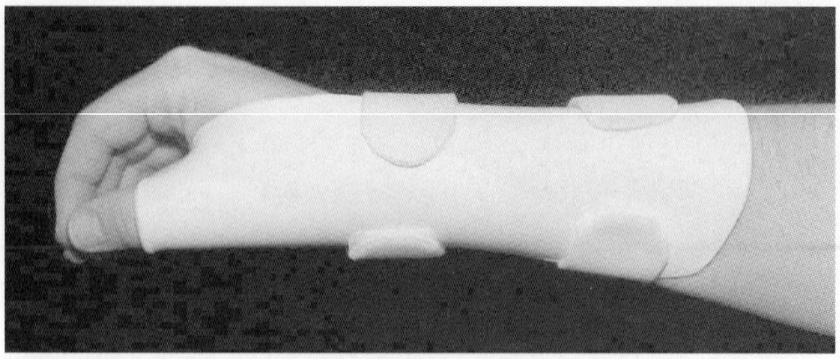

Figure 16-23 Custom thermoplastic long thumb spica splint.

The ideal position of the wrist to minimize pressure in the carpal tunnel varies according to sources from 10–15° of extension (Melvin, 1989) to neutral (Weiss et al., 1995) to slight flexion (Gelberman et al., 1988). There is a consensus that commercial wrist splints, which often place the wrist in excessive extension, may not be of any benefit unless they are modified to a less extended position. Dorsal wrist splints (Fig. 16-20) are often recommended because they do not create external pressure over the volar wrist. A systematic review of splinting for carpal tunnel syndrome showed benefits from splinting across splint types and wrist angles, with evidence suggesting custom splints and full-time splint wear promote better results (Muller et al., 2004).

A long opponens splint (Fig. 16-23), also known as a long thumb spica, can relieve pain from wrist and thumb arthritis or from DeQuervain's tendonitis of the abductor pollicis longus and extensor pollicis brevis. This splint is typically based on the radial aspect of the forearm and extends distally to immobilize the thumb CMC and MP joints. The wrist is generally splinted in slight extension, with the thumb in slight flexion and palmar abduction to enable opposition to the index and middle fingers (Wilton, 1997). If the thumb IP joint or the extensor pollicis longus tendon is involved, the IP joint can be included in the splint as well (Fig. 16-24). Prefabricated splints often provide a softer support, whereas custom-made thermoplastic splints give more rigid immobilization.

A thumb CMC stabilization splint, or a short thumb spica, is a static splint that encompasses the first metacarpal to provide stability, reduce pain, and increase hand function. It restricts motion of the CMC and MP joints but leaves the wrist relatively mobile and the thumb IP free. A static thumb MP splint allows for CMC and IP motion and can be used when the disorder is localized to the MP joint alone.

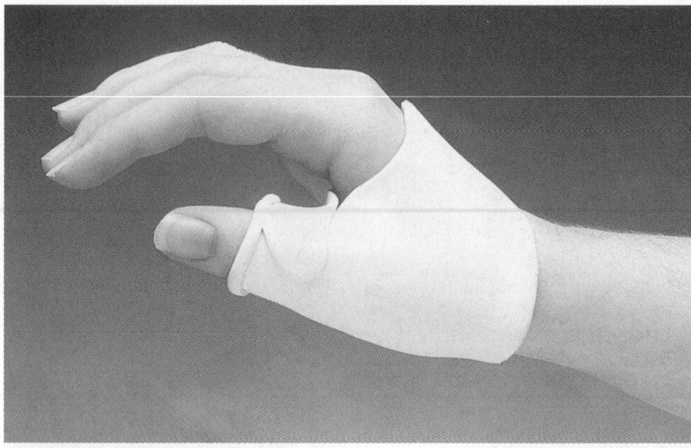

Figure 16-25 Custom thermoplastic short thumb splint.

Indications for short thumb splints include rheumatoid arthritis or osteoarthritis of the thumb CMC or MP joints or trauma to soft tissues, such as the ulnar collateral ligament of the MP. The thumb is generally positioned to enable opposition to the fingers for function while in the splint, and the splint is most often worn during functional activities that cause or aggravate pain (Melvin, 1995). Commercially prefabricated rigid CMC and MP stabilization splints are often ineffectual because they fit poorly (Melvin, 1995). For a precise fit and rigid support, splints can be custom fabricated from thermoplastic materials (Fig. 16-25). Newer commercial products made of soft, breathable elastic material have moldable thermoplastic stays to enable a custom fit, combining comfort and ease of fabrication with the required individualized rigid support (Fig. 16-26). Rigid support may not always be needed. In comparing a custom-made thermoplastic splint and a soft neoprene support for osteoarthritis of the thumb CMC joint, Weiss et al. (2004) found that the prefabricated neoprene splint (Fig. 16-27) provided greater pain relief and function and was preferred over the thermoplastic splint by 72% of the subjects.

If the thumb or finger IP joints are painful from trauma or arthritis, lateral, dorsal, or volar gutter splints (Fig. 16-28) may be used for pain relief. Silicone-lined sleeves or pads (Fig. 16-29) can protect painful joint nodules from external trauma.

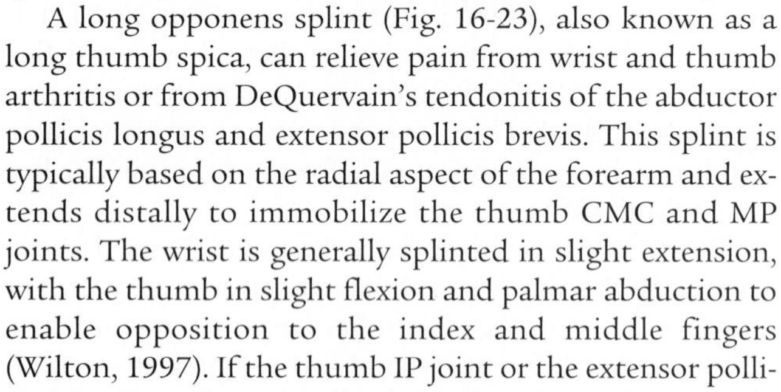

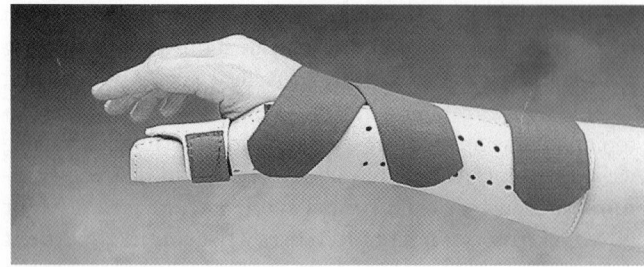

Figure 16-24 Liberty™ Wrist and Thumb Splint.

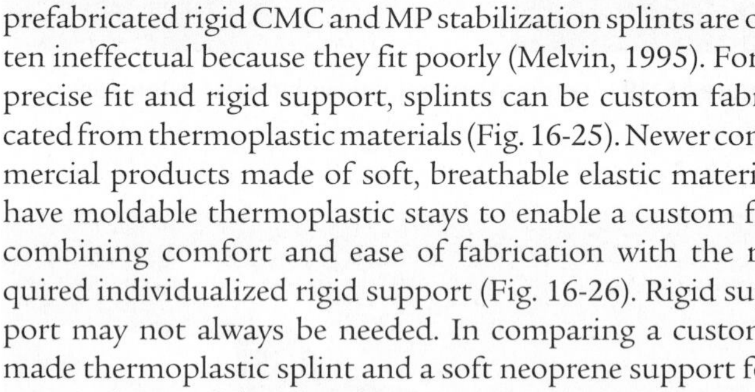

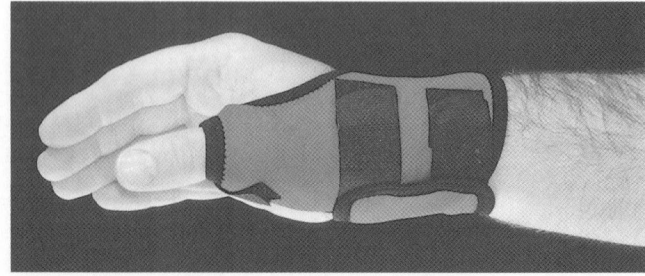

Figure 16-26 Custom-molded thumb splint.

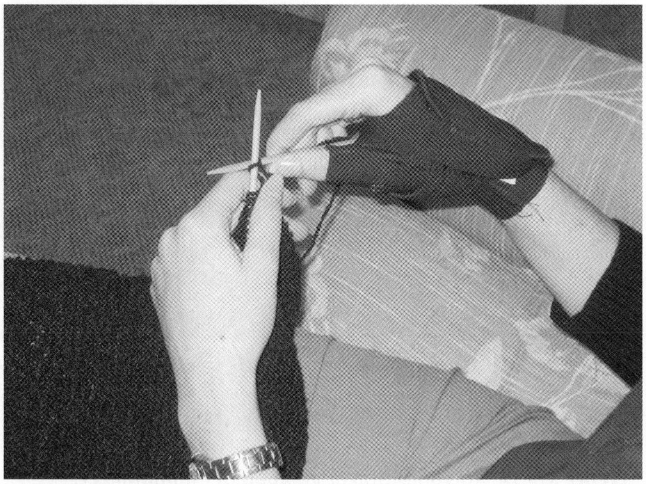

Figure 16-27 Commercial soft thumb splint.

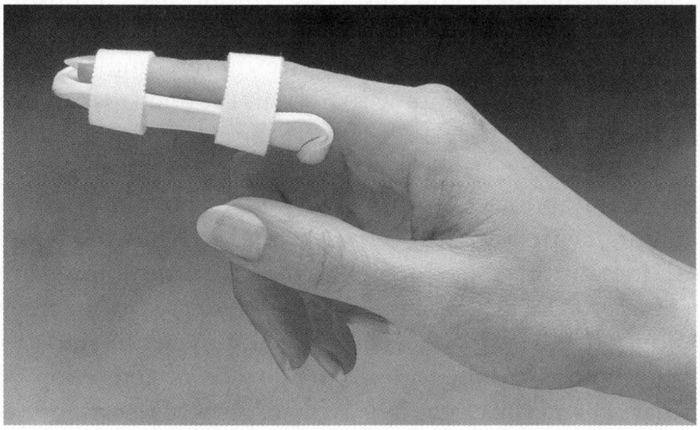

Figure 16-28 Custom thermoplastic volar gutter splint.

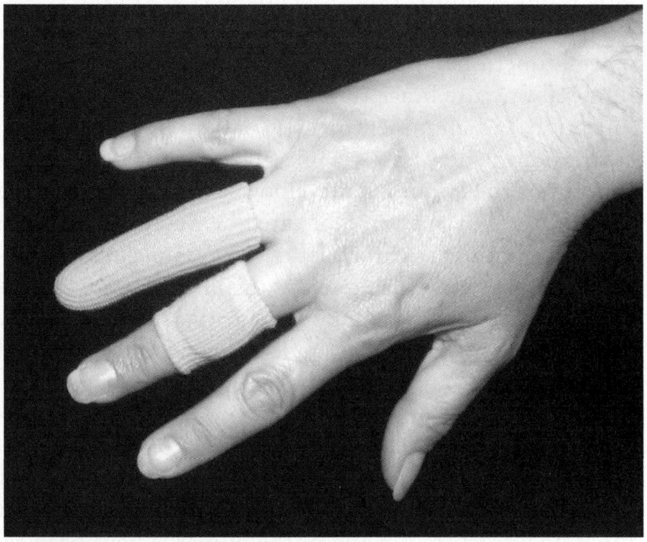

Figure 16-29 Silicone-lined digital sleeve and pad.

Pain, volar subluxation, and ulnar deviation of the MCPs are common sequelae of rheumatoid arthritis. MCP ulnar deviation supports may be used to provide stability, realign joints, reduce joint stress, and relieve pain. They may delay the progression of deformity but do not correct or prevent it (Melvin, 1995; Philips, 1989). These supports may be worn alone or incorporated into a resting hand splint.

Prefabricated and custom-designed orthoses with dividers or straps to align the digits include dynamic and static and soft and rigid. Rigid static splints (Fig. 16-30) used to achieve passive correction of deformity can create focal pressure points on the digits. It is therefore important not to try to achieve ideal alignment at the risk of creating pressure problems (Melvin, 1989).

Despite the variety of splint materials and designs, MCP ulnar deviation supports are reported to be not frequently prescribed or used by patients for a variety of reasons (Rennie, 1996). For some patients, immobilization of the MCPs impairs functional use of the hand and may increase stress and pain on the adjacent PIP joints (Melvin, 1995; Philips, 1989). Additionally, bulky or volar-based splints interfere with palmar sensation and impede the ability to grasp objects. Some patients, however, benefit from the improved digital alignment and pain reduction that supports offer. High patient satisfaction rates have been reported for a custom dorsal-based design (Rennie, 1996). Soft ulnar deviation splints are commercially available (Fig. 16-31) or can be custom fabricated (Gilbert-Lenef, 1994). The prime indicator for use and selection of an MCP ulnar deviation support should be the patient's preference (Melvin, 1995).

Immobilize for Healing or to Protect Tissues

Many of the orthoses previously discussed for pain relief can also be used to immobilize for healing or protection

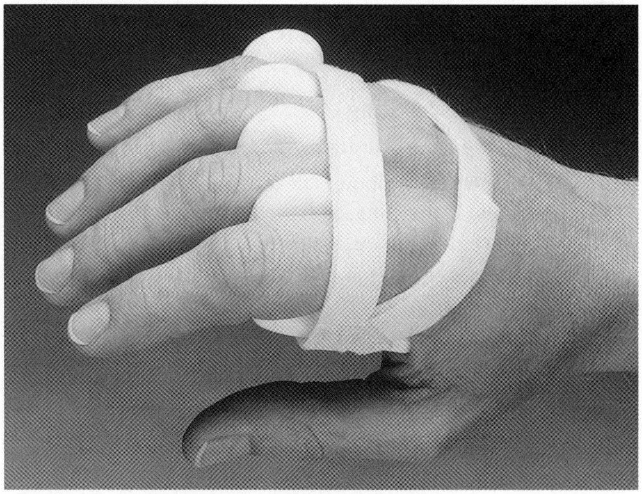

Figure 16-30 LMB Soft-Core™ Wire–Foam™ Ulnar Deviation Splint.

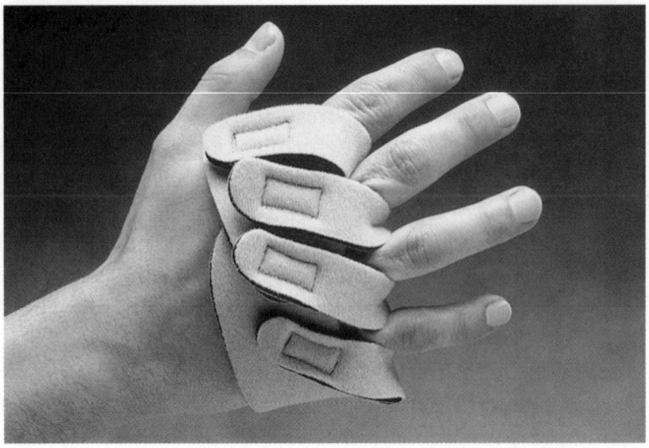

Figure 16-31 Norco™ Soft MP Ulnar Deviation Support.

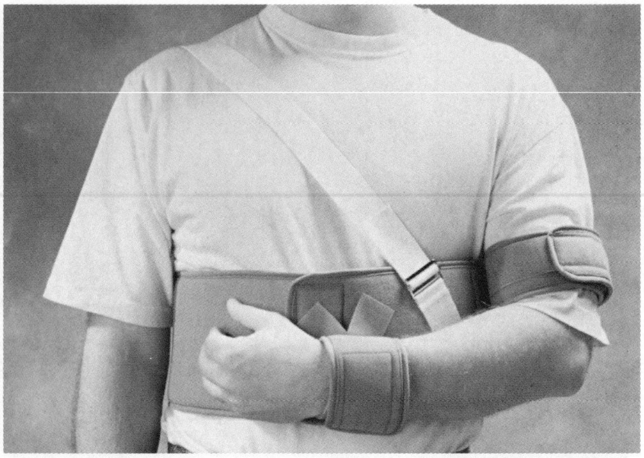

Figure 16-32 Rolyan® Universal Shoulder Immobilizer.

following injury or surgery. For example, a gunslinger orthosis used to relieve traction pain associated with a brachial plexus injury can also protect the nerve structures from overstretching during the healing phase. A thumb MP splint that relieves pain from arthritis may also be used while an acutely injured collateral ligament heals. These orthoses are not discussed in detail again; different ones are reviewed.

Immobilize or Protect the Shoulder, Upper Arm, or Elbow

The sling is the simplest and most commonly used device for the upper extremity when there is a need to limit motion of the shoulder yet allow for some motion of the arm on the thorax. The basic arm sling consists of a forearm pouch or cuffs, a strap, and a mechanism for adjusting and securing the strap. Guidelines for sling adjustment are in Procedures for Practice 16-1.

PROCEDURES FOR PRACTICE 16-1

How to Adjust a Sling

- Place the patient upright.
- Ensure that the elbow is flexed to 90° and is seated properly in the sling, with the hand and wrist also supported as the design allows.
- Adjust the strap or straps so that the arm is comfortably supported.
- Check for comfort.
- Teach patient and caregiver about proper donning and doffing of sling.
- Monitor the axilla and areas where sling straps cross the body for signs of skin breakdown.
- Monitor for signs of edema and joint stiffness.

To further limit mobility, shoulder immobilizers (Fig. 16-32) can be used. These devices, which relatively immobilize the shoulder and elbow, are typically used following shoulder surgical reconstructions, arthroplasty, and rotator cuff repair. Immobilizers are more complex than slings, involving strapping that wraps the body to stabilize the arm against the trunk. Several commercial designs are available.

Foam abduction pillows or wedges may be used to maintain the arm at a certain elevation from the body. Abduction braces, sometimes called airplane splints, are commercially available or custom fabricated from thermoplastics. These devices are based on the trunk and can position the shoulder in varying degrees of abduction or rotation and the elbow in varying degrees of flexion or extension. Commercial braces offer ease of adjustability with the use of wrenches but may need extra padding to prevent skin breakdown. Indications for use include postoperative shoulder repairs, burns, and skin grafts to the axillary region (Long & Shutt, 1986; McFarland et al., 1997).

The treatment of humeral shaft fractures often involves functional fracture bracing (see Chapter 41). A humeral fracture brace (Fig. 16-33) provides external stabilization and alignment of the fracture by compressing surrounding soft tissues while allowing for early mobilization of the shoulder and elbow. These braces may be prefabricated or custom fabricated by the therapist from low-temperature thermoplastics. They are circumferential in design, with D-ring straps to allow for a secure closure and size adjustments as edema subsides. They should be lightweight and made of a perforated material for ventilation.

Whether the brace is prefabricated or custom, the therapist should ensure that its distal end does not block elbow flexion motion and that its proximal end does not unnecessarily limit shoulder motion. Excellent results with the use of functional fracture bracing of the humerus have been reported (Wallny et al., 1997).

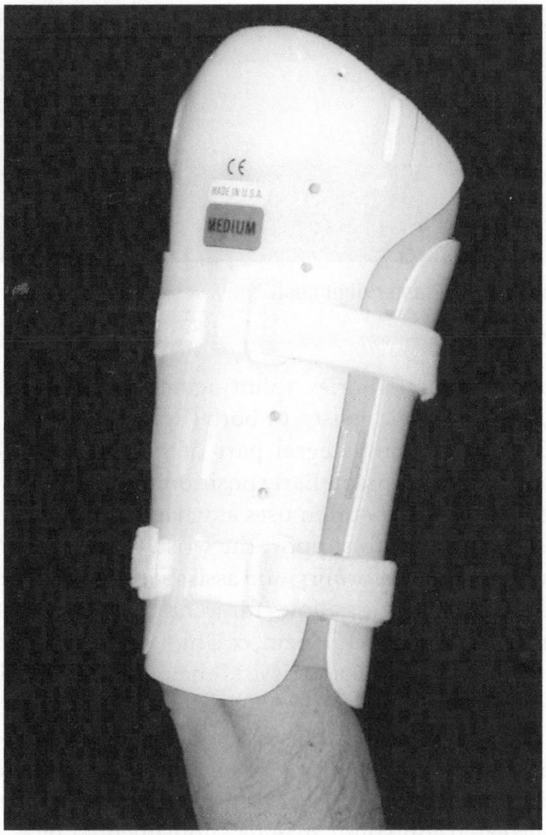

Figure 16-33 Commercial humeral fracture brace.

Casts, splints, and hinged braces can be used to immobilize and protect the elbow following fractures, burns, ligamentous injuries, or surgical procedures. Casts offer rigid immobilization and may be made according to a circumferential, posterior, or anteroposterior bivalve design that allows the cast to be removed for wound care or range of motion. Hinged braces are frequently used to protect healing ligaments while allowing motion of the elbow. Thermoplastic splints may be anterior or posterior and may be secured by Velcro straps or an elastic wrap. Anterior elbow extension splints (Fig. 16-34) are most commonly used to immobilize and position the elbow following skin grafting.

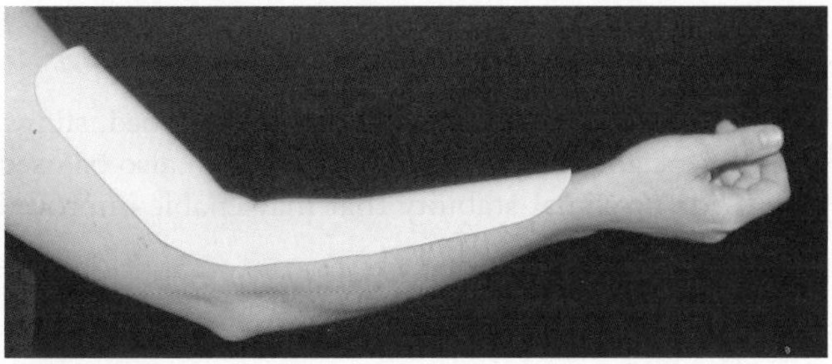

Figure 16-34 Custom thermoplastic anterior elbow extension splint.

Immobilize or Protect the Wrist or Hand

The maintenance of normal hand function requires strong tissue repair with free gliding between neighboring structures. Proper positioning of the wrist and hand is critical to prevent complications caused by injury, edema, and tissue healing. Splinting in the early stages of healing can counteract the typical joint contractures of the injured hand that produce the deformities of wrist flexion, MCP extension, IP flexion, and thumb adduction. It is essential to position joints correctly and keep uninvolved joints moving so that they will not stiffen (Stewart Pettengill, 2002). ***Incorrect application of a splint or improper positioning while in a splint may lead to both joint limitations and tissue damage (Fess, 1995).***

Unless specifically contraindicated, the antideformity, or safe, position of immobilization is with the wrist in 10–30° of extension, the MCPs in 70–90° of flexion, the IPs in 0–15° of flexion, and the thumb in palmar abduction (Fess et al., 2005; Stewart Pettengill, 2002). This is most often accomplished through a volar custom-fabricated low-temperature thermoplastic splint (Fig. 16-35). If edema is present, the splint should be secured by an elastic wrap or gauze wrap to avoid a tourniquet effect from straps. ***It is crucial never to force joints into the ideal position but to position joints as closely as possible to the ideal and serially revise the splint until the optimal position is realized.***

Antideformity splints are integral to the treatment of acute dorsal hand burns (see Chapter 45). An investigation of the literature found an overall lack of consensus on the design of these splints (Richard et al., 1994). The most commonly recommended position for joints is with the wrist in 15–30° of extension, the MCPs in 50–70° of flexion, the IPs in full extension, and the thumb in palmar abduction with the IP in slight flexion (Richard & Staley, 1994). Pre-formed splints are commercially available and may be used if adequate fit can be obtained given the size of the hand and any edema. Custom-fabricated splints, preferably of a perforated material, ensure the best fit. Splints may have to be adjusted daily for optimal fit and maintenance of proper joint positioning. For the grafting

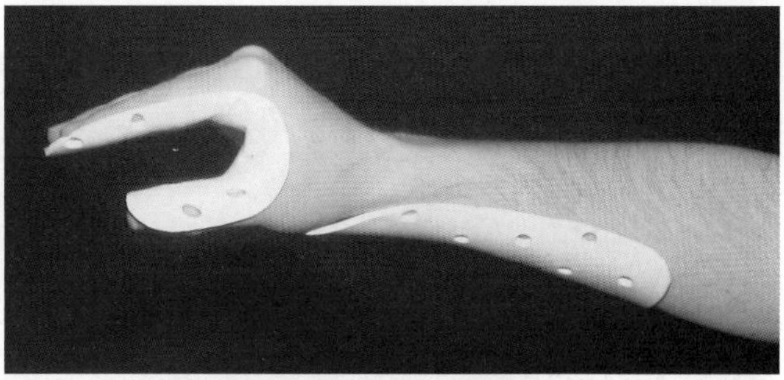

Figure 16-35 Custom thermoplastic "safe position" wrist–hand splint.

and rehabilitation phases of burn treatment, splint design varies with the positions necessary to counteract the contractile forces of the scars.

Wrist splints, as discussed in the previous section, may be used for protection or immobilization of wrists following cast removal or to treat soft tissue injuries. Athletic injuries to the wrist and hand, such as contusions, sprains, strains, fractures, and joint dislocations, often require the use of protective splints to enable the patient to continue participation in sports. As with other splints, selection of material and design should be carefully tailored to the patient's needs. Materials may be thermoplastic, silicone rubber, plaster, fiberglass, cloth tape, or neoprene. Selection should be based on the degree of immobilization required, material durability and breathability, the player's sport position, governing rules of the sport, and the safety of other players (Canelon, 1995).

Treatment of tendon injuries and repairs may involve static positioning to immobilize the tendon for healing or dynamic splinting to protect the tendon while allowing controlled motion to increase tendon repair strength and gliding. Flexor tendon repair protocols vary, but a protective dorsal blocking splint (Fig. 16-36) positioning the wrist and MCPs in flexion and blocking the IP joints in 0° of extension is typically used. Rubber band traction may be added to hold the digits in a flexed position or to enable resistive extension and passive flexion exercises. The splint is usually custom fabricated from low-temperature thermoplastic and is often worn for as long as 6 weeks (Stewart Pettengill & vanStrien, 2002).

Extensor tendon injuries involve treatment and splinting based on the level of injury. For injuries at the DIP level that may result in a mallet finger deformity, the DIP is immobilized for 6–8 weeks in a slightly hyperextended position. The PIP joint is left free. The splints most commonly used are volar based and may be prefabricated or custom fabricated from padded aluminum strips or thermoplastics. Excellent results for the treatment of mallet finger have also been reported with custom-made dorsal splints (Evans, 2002; Foucher et al., 1996). For injuries at the PIP level, treatment includes digital cast (Fig. 16-37) or splint immobilization with the PIP in absolute 0° of extension for 6–8 weeks to prevent boutonniere deformity. For more

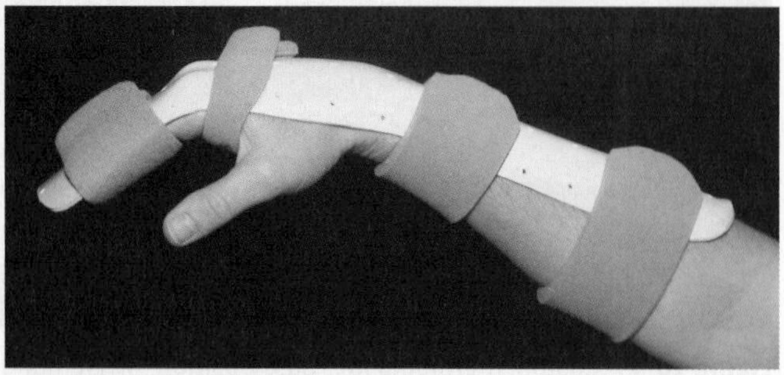

Figure 16-36 Custom thermoplastic dorsal blocking splint.

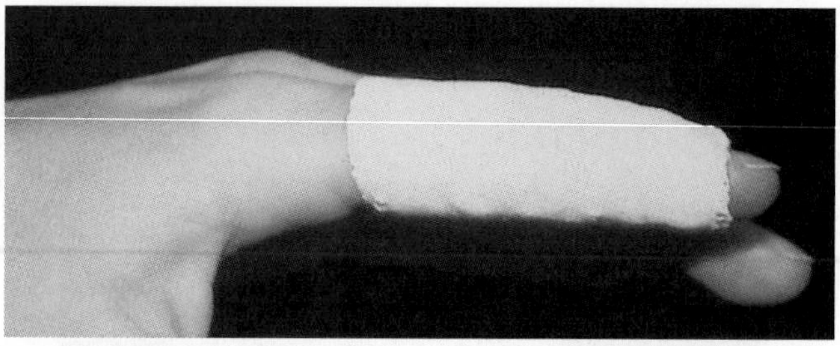

Figure 16-37 Plaster digit cast.

proximal tendon injuries, splinting may involve static positioning, dynamic assists, or both (Evans, 2002).

Splinting is an integral part of postoperative MCP arthroplasty treatment. Early positioning and motion following arthroplasty often uses a dynamic MCP extension assist (Fig. 16-38) to support the wrist, control MCP motion, correct the deformity, and assist with extensor power. This controlled stress allows for joint capsule remodeling over time (Kirkpatrick, Kozin, & Uhl, 1996; Melvin, 1989). Dynamic MCP extension assists may use high-profile or low-profile outrigger designs. They have slings to support the MCPs in neutral extension and deviation and to provide rotatory alignment. Outrigger kits are commercially available, or the outrigger may be hand fabricated. The dynamic extension splint may be supplemented by a static positioning splint at night (Fess et al., 2005).

To protect digits but allow for stabilization or controlled motion of the MCP, PIP, or DIP joints following injury or surgery, buddy straps (Fig. 16-39) (Jensen & Rayan, 1996), buddy sleeves (Bassini & Patel, 1994), or buddy splints (Lamay, 1994), which connect an injured finger to an adjacent finger, can be used. Common indications for these include stable fractures, PIP joint dislocations, collateral ligament injuries, and staged flexor tendon reconstructions.

Provide Stability or Restrict Unwanted Motion

Orthoses can be helpful in stabilizing joints when their integrity has been compromised by an acute injury or a chronic disease such as arthritis. Stabilization or restriction of motion can often greatly facilitate functional use of a limb.

Stabilize or Restrict Motion of the Shoulder or Elbow

In addition to the purposes previously described, slings, gunslingers, and hinged elbow orthoses can also be used to provide proximal stability that may enable improved distal function.

Stabilize or Restrict Motion of the Wrist or Hand

It is essential to determine the position in which a joint is to be supported relative to hand dominance and task

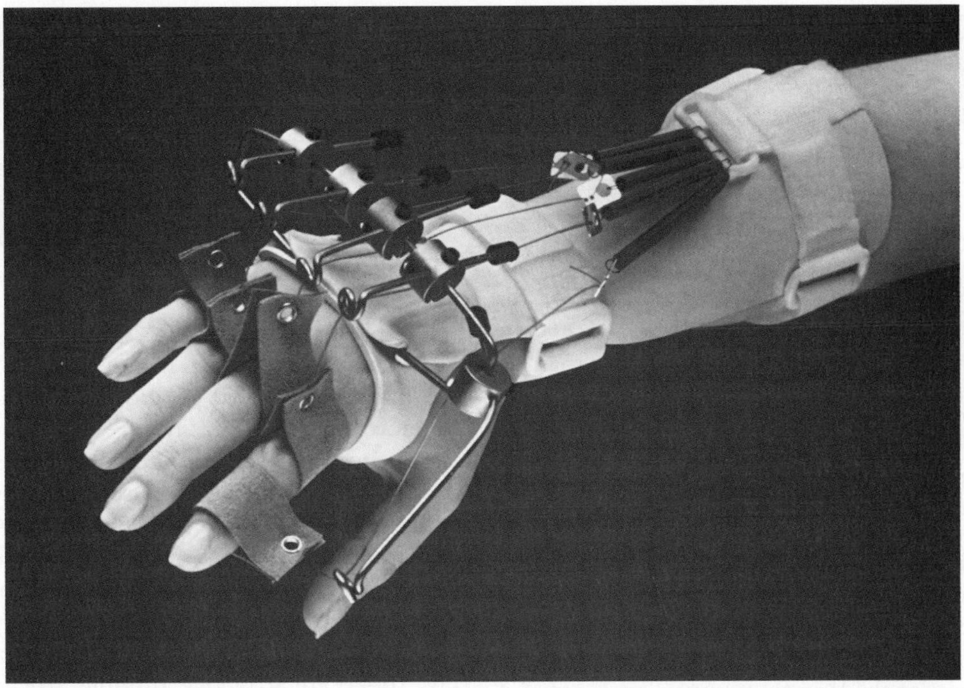

Figure 16-38 Custom thermoplastic low-profile dynamic MCP extension splint using Rolyan® Adjustable Outrigger Kit.

requirements because specific functional demands vary greatly among individual patients. The wrist is considered by many to be the key to ultimate hand function, and wrist splints are commonly prescribed to provide stability. Dorsal wrist splints allow for the greatest palmar sensation but are least supportive; volar wrist splints are most commonly prescribed and provide a moderate amount of stability; and circumferential wrist splints provide the greatest amount of stability (Wilton, 1997).

For optimum mechanical advantage to support the weight of the hand, the forearm portion of the splint should be two thirds the length of the forearm (Fess et al., 2005; Wilton, 1997). Although greater length is believed to add to stability, studies have shown that a longer splint can decrease grip strength, slow finger dexterity, and decrease hand function speeds compared with a shorter wrist splint (Stern, 1996). For smaller or lighter hands and for patients who do not use their hands for high-demand activities, a shorter wrist support (Fig. 16-40) can increase comfort while being less obtrusive than a long splint (Melvin, 1995).

A lumbrical bar is a hand-based orthosis that extends over the dorsal aspect of the proximal phalanges to re-

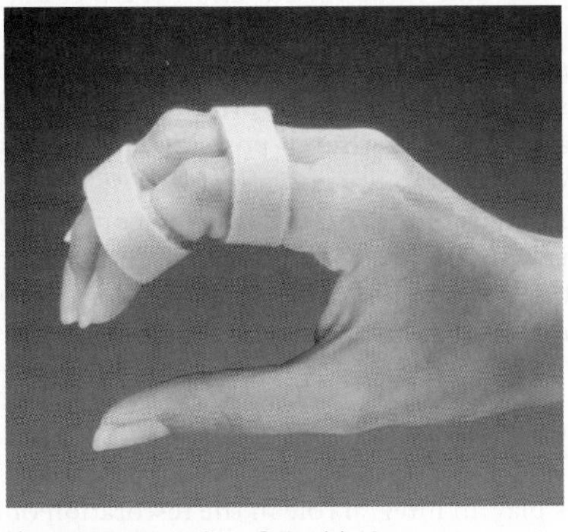

Figure 16-39 Rolyan® Buddy Straps.

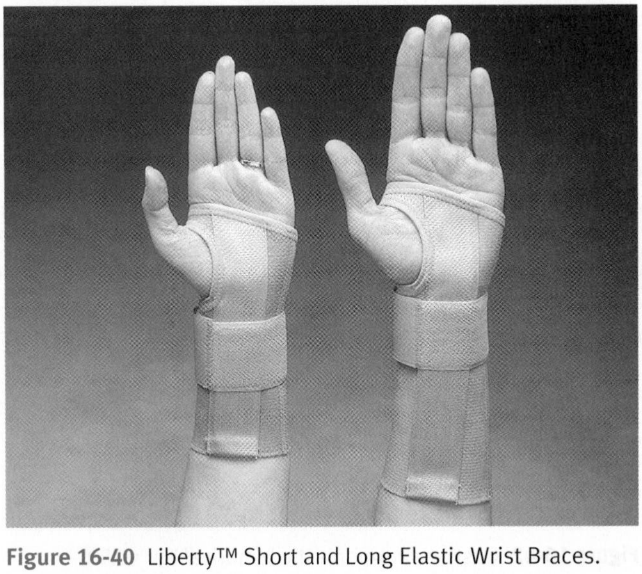

Figure 16-40 Liberty™ Short and Long Elastic Wrist Braces.

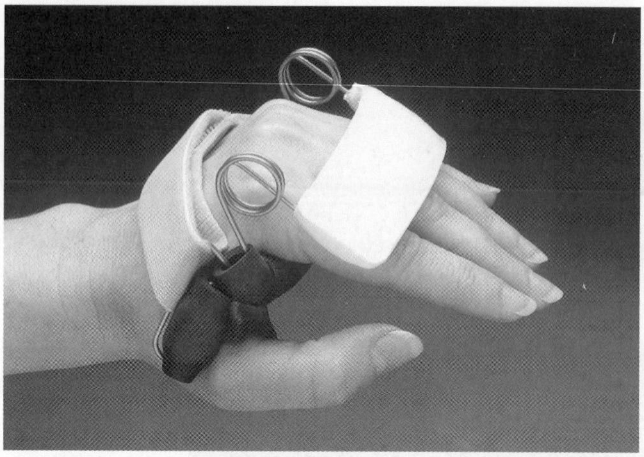

Figure 16-41 LMB MP Flexion Spring.

strict unwanted hyperextension of the MCPs, which can result from an ulnar nerve or combined median and ulnar nerve injury. By blocking this motion, IP flexion contractures can be prevented and functional hand opening improved as the power of the long finger extensors is transferred to the IPs for extension. Lumbrical bar orthoses using spring wire are commercially available (Fig. 16-41), but these tend to be bulky and limit the ability to grasp objects. Custom-fabricated thermoplastic splints (Figs. 16-3 and 16-42) provide for a more intimate and streamlined fit (Colditz, 2002b; Wilton, 1997).

This same principle of restricting undesired motion is used in a PIP hyperextension block, also known as a swan-neck splint. Swan-neck deformities are common sequelae of rheumatoid arthritis and a possible complication following an extensor tendon injury or repair. These deformities often cause difficulty with hand closure, as PIP tendons and ligaments can catch during motion, and the finger flexors have less of a mechanical advantage to initi-

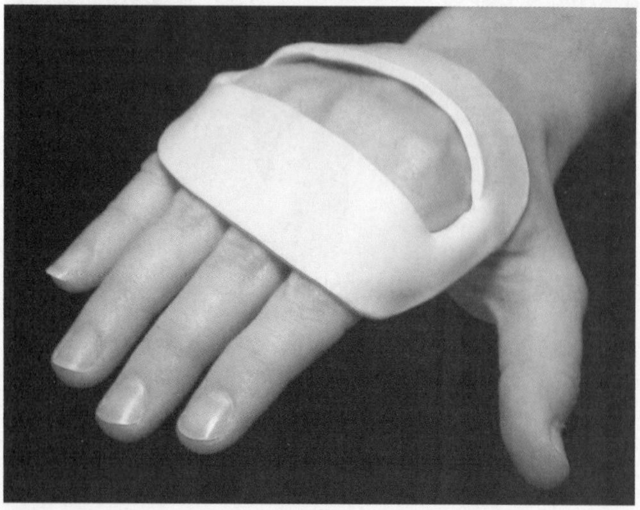

Figure 16-42 Custom thermoplastic lumbrical bar splint.

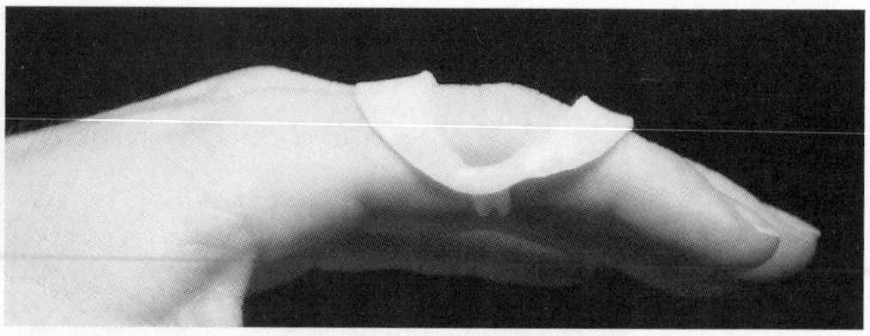

Figure 16-43 Custom thermoplastic PIP hyperextension block.

ate flexion when the PIP is hyperextended. By blocking the PIP in a slightly flexed position, the patient can flex the PIP more quickly and easily.

For short-term use or for trial purposes, custom-fabricated thermoplastic swan-neck splints (Fig. 16-43) may suffice (McKee & Morgan, 1998). For long-term use or for use on adjacent digits, commercial swan-neck splints are often recommended because they are more durable, less bulky, more easily cleaned, and more cosmetically appealing. Custom-ordered ring splints made of silver or gold (Fig. 16-44) are attractive, durable, streamlined, and adjustable for variations in joint swelling, but they are more costly. Prefabricated splints made of polypropylene (Fig. 16-45), also available commercially, offer some of the benefits of silver splints with less cost. Heavy-duty metal splints, such as Murphy ring splints, may benefit patients who use their hands in highly demanding tasks. Swan-neck splints can also be used to provide lateral stability to unstable IP joints of the fingers or thumb.

Flexible boutonniere deformities may benefit from boutonniere splinting to block the PIP in a more extended position to allow for greater functional hand opening. These may also be custom made by the therapist or custom ordered from the companies that fabricate swan-neck splints (Fig. 16-46). Since there is direct pressure over the PIP, the dorsal skin must be carefully monitored for signs of breakdown.

Thumb stability is a requirement of almost all prehensile activities, so splinting of unstable thumb joints may have a particular value for function (Fess et al., 2005). Instability of the CMC often requires a long thumb splint that crosses the wrist because shorter splints may not adequately support the CMC. Short thumb spica splints (Fig. 16-25), also known as thumb posts or opponens splints, can provide MP stability and a stable post for pinching. Although a circumferential design is commonly used, problems with marked MP deformity can make donning and doffing of the splint difficult, and direct pressure over the MP may lead to breakdown of fragile skin.

Restore Mobility

Orthoses play an integral role in the restoration of mobility by correcting soft tissue or joint contractures that can

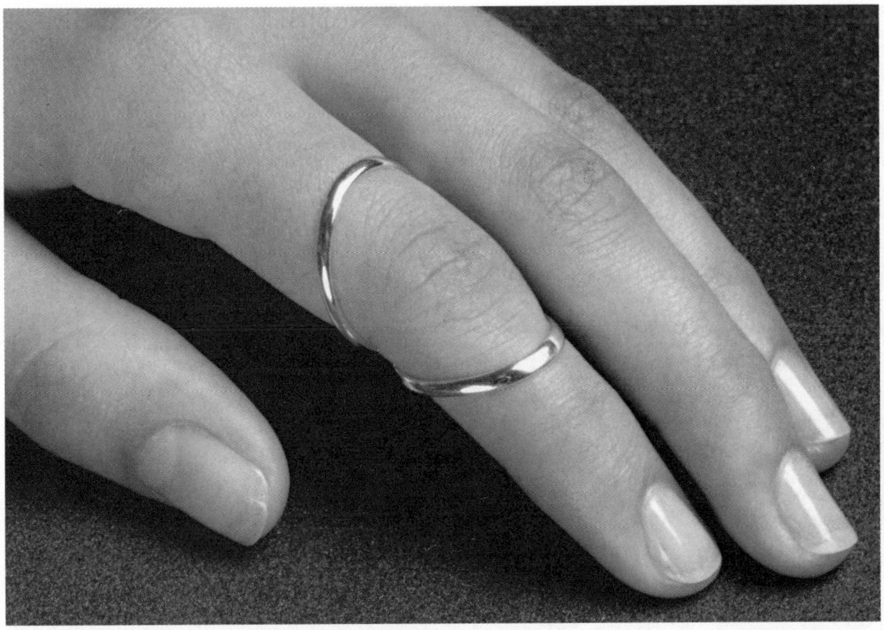

Figure 16-44 Siris™ Silver Swan Neck Splint.

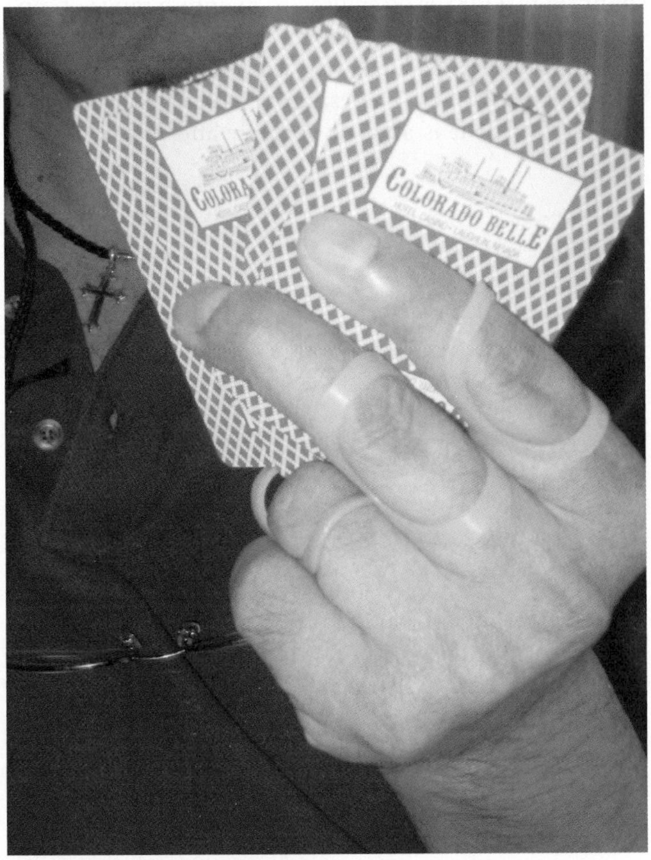

Figure 16-45 Oval-8™ commercial ring splints.

occur as a result of poor positioning, trauma, scarring, or increased muscle tone. Devices providing low-load, prolonged stretch have proven to be effective in the contracture management of patients having a neurological or orthopedic disorder (Hill, 1994; Nuismer, Ekes, & Holm, 1997). As described earlier in this chapter, different types of splinting may be used: serial static plaster or thermoplastic, dynamic, and static progressive.

A therapist implementing a splinting program to regain motion must understand how splints work to effect positive change. Range of motion is gained not by tissue stretching but by actual tissue elongation from new cell growth (Bell-Krotoski & Figarola, 1995; Fess et al., 2005). ***The forces used must be gentle and carefully applied, and the tissue must be closely monitored for signs of excessive stress, such as redness and inflammation, which are indicators to mediate or stop treatment.*** Inelastic mobilization applies constant forces needed to remodel tissues and is the most effective means for gaining motion in chronically stiff joints. Elastic mobilization is most indicated for acute joint stiffness or more supple joints because forces can be more easily controlled and fine adjustments made (Fess et al., 2005).

Fixed contractures and chronically stiff joints often respond best to inelastic mobilization from **serial casting**. Plaster is an ideal material because it conforms intimately and is more rigid than thermoplastics. Casts are changed as motion gains are achieved.

Dynamic splinting is more effective when used for early contractures (Bell-Krotoski & Figarola, 1995). It allows for motion in the opposite direction, which helps prevent unwanted stiffness. Splints can also be removed for hygiene and function. Often dynamic splints are worn at night so

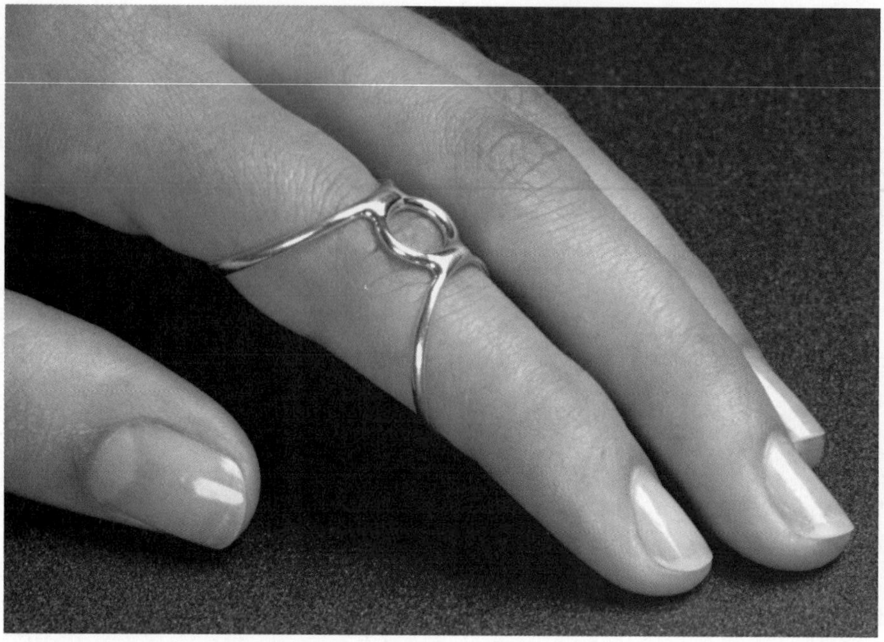

Figure 16-46 Siris™ Silver Boutonniere Splint.

as not to interfere with use of the limb. This decrease in wearing time, however, means that tissues are not kept under constant tension, and less rapid gains may result. The amount and direction of force must be carefully monitored and adjusted as joint angles change.

Static progressive splinting is often indicated for fixed contractures. It has the advantage of being worn for shorter periods throughout the day, allowing for motion and functional use of the limb.

Restore Mobility of the Shoulder, Elbow, or Forearm

A serial static abduction splint can be used to apply pressure to and elongate burn scars in the axilla. The benefits of wearing this type of splint must be carefully weighed against the complete lack of function that it imposes. For flexion contractures of the elbow, thermoplastic anterior elbow extension splints (Fig. 16-34), serial casts or dropout casts, and dynamic elbow extension or static progressive elbow extension splints can be used.

Serial casting, which typically entails changing the cast weekly, is thought to be most effective with contractures that have been present for less than 6 months (Keenan, 1997). When the contracture is a result of increased tone, such as in the patient with a brain injury, casting is often used in conjunction with nerve blocks or surgical procedures. ***Great care must be taken with casting in the presence of severe tone, as pressure areas may develop.***

Dropout casts (Fig. 16-47) use the force of gravity to assist in reducing an elbow flexion contracture. The posterior portion of the cast above the elbow is removed, allowing the forearm to drop into extension. This type of casting is effective only if the patient is upright most of the day.

A bivalved cast, also known as an anteroposterior splint (Fig. 16-48), is often used to maintain range of motion once it is achieved through casting or other means. This splint is well padded, with several straps holding the two halves together. The caregiver must be thoroughly trained so that it is applied properly and in the correct

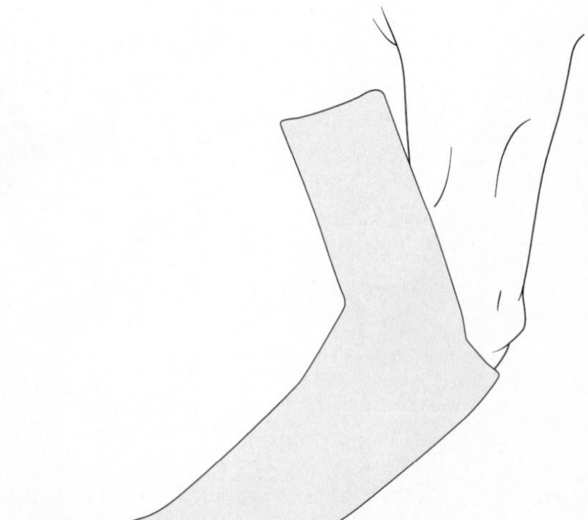

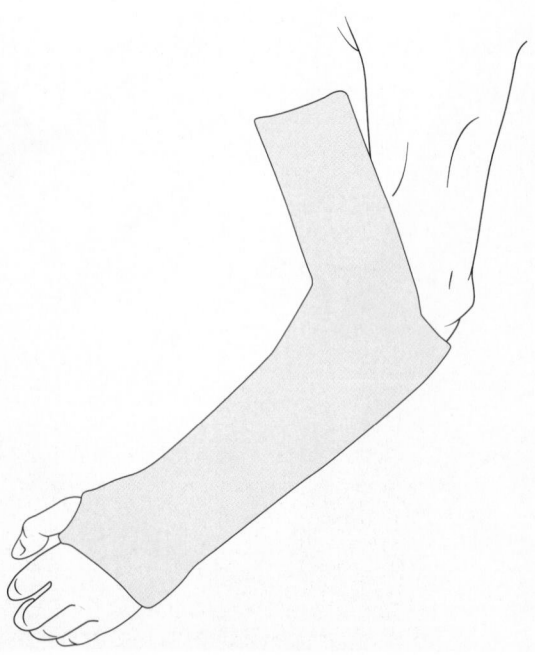

Figure 16-47 Plaster elbow dropout cast.

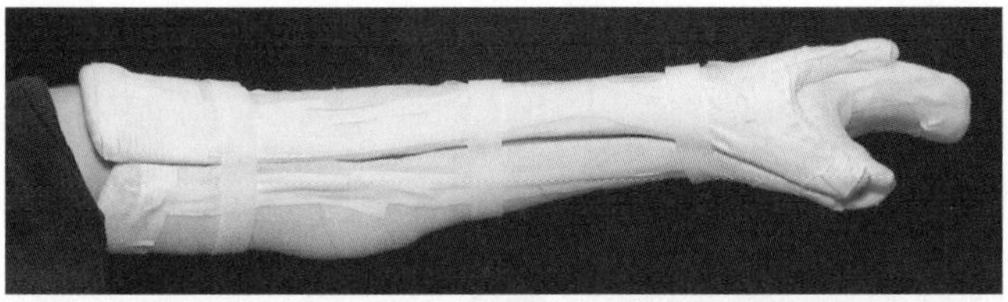

Figure 16-48 Fiberglass anteroposterior elbow splint with wrist and digits included.

alignment to prevent pressure problems and skin breakdown.

Dynamic or static progressive splints (Fig. 16-49) have been reported to be successful in the treatment of elbow burn flexion contractures when static splinting was not effective. An average of 5–10° can be gained per day (Richard, Shanesy, & Miller, 1995). They have also proved to be effective in the treatment of neurological and orthopedic flexion contractures (Nuismer, Ekes, & Holm, 1997).

Elbow extension contractures, which are less commonly seen, can be treated with serial casting into flexion, dynamic flexion splinting, or static progressive splinting.

Loss of forearm rotation, often seen following spinal cord injury, peripheral nerve injury, or fracture, can be treated with dynamic forearm rotation splinting. Splints can be custom fabricated (Collelo-Abraham, 1990) or obtained commercially as a pre-formed product or kit (Fig. 16-50). Altering the direction of force when using these

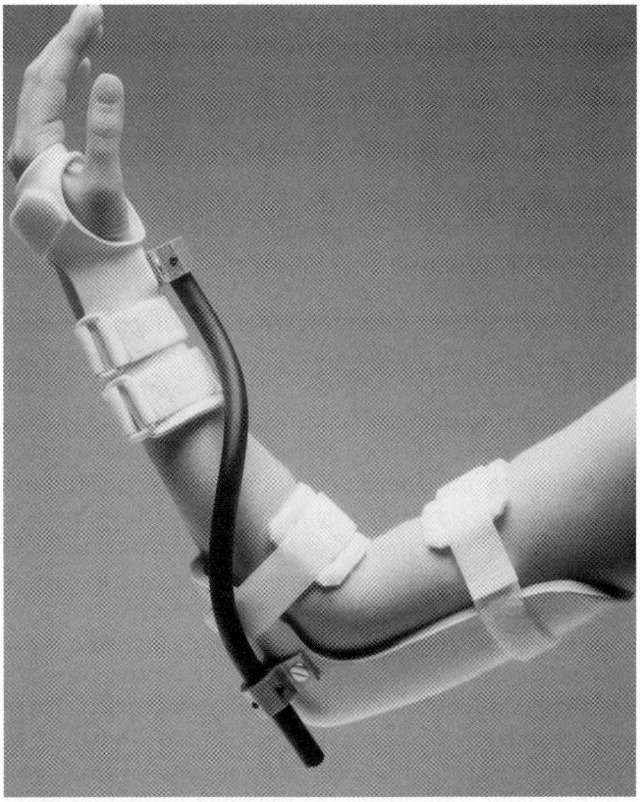

Figure 16-50 Rolyan® Preformed Dynamic Pronation/Supination Splint.

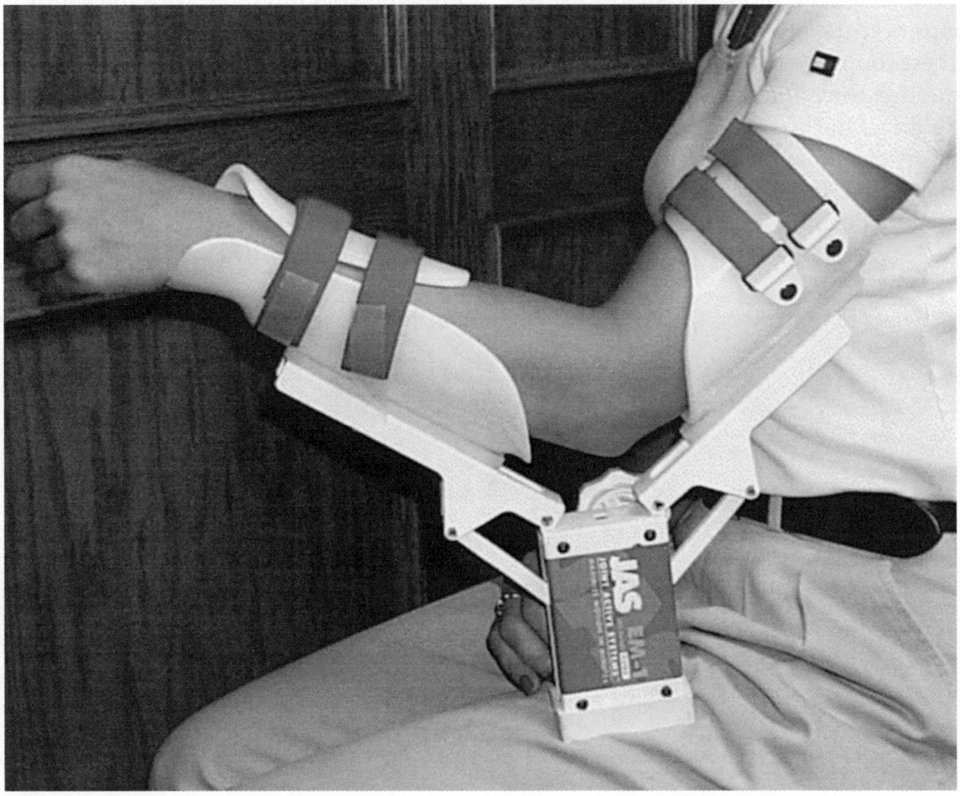

Figure 16-49 JAS Static Progressive Elbow™ Orthosis.

splints can produce supination or pronation. A static progressive supination splint has also been described by Murphy (1990) as achieving favorable results.

Restore Mobility of the Wrist or Hand

Serial short arm casts, with or without the fingers or thumb, can be used in the treatment of flexion or extension contractures related to increased muscle tone. Serial plaster slab splinting (Tribuzi, 2002) can be especially effective in the presence of muscle–tendon unit shortening that can result in the inability to compositely flex or extend the wrist and fingers. Long flexor tightness can develop as a result of the wrist being in a prolonged position of flexion, such as with wrist drop from radial nerve palsy, wrist fracture immobilization, and protective positioning following flexor tendon repair. A plaster slab splint or a volar thermoplastic splint that positions the wrist and fingers in maximum composite extension can help to correct tightness of the long finger flexors.

Serial static thermoplastic wrist splints, dynamic wrist splints (Fig. 16-51), and static progressive wrist splints can be used for limitations in wrist flexion or extension. These may be custom fabricated or pre-formed. Dynamic or static progressive component kits can also be purchased commercially. This allows the therapist to custom mold the splint bases while more easily assembling force units.

Lack of MCP flexion can devastate hand function. Many dynamic splint designs to regain MCP motion are available. Custom-fabricated thermoplastic splints use individual finger loops over the proximal phalanx (Fig. 16-52). Attached to these loops are rubber bands or springs that provide the needed force for sustained tension. An outrigger is used to direct the line of pull at 90°. It is important to clear the distal palmar crease so as not to block full flexion range of motion. These splints may be forearm based or hand based, depending on the mechanical advantage needed, any adhesions, and the patient's wrist strength and stability (Fess et al., 2005).

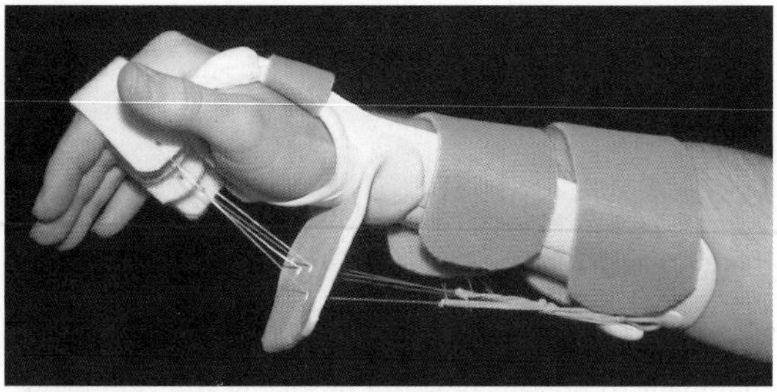

Figure 16-52 Custom thermoplastic dynamic MCP flexion splint.

Commercial hand-based dynamic splints use springs, coiled spring wire (Fig. 16-41), or rubber bands to provide flexion force to the MCPs as a unit. These splints are effective only if all MCPs are uniformly stiff. Some force adjustments can be made, but individual finger force amount or angle adjustments are not possible, as they are with custom-made thermoplastic splints having separate finger loops. Finger flexion gloves (Fig. 16-53), which incorporate rubber band traction, can be used to gain composite flexion of all joints, but they have the most effect on the MCPs.

Limited PIP flexion makes grasp difficult, and limited PIP extension interferes with the ability to open the hand in preparation for grasp or to release objects. PIP flexion contractures are a frequent complication of trauma or poor positioning, and extension contractures can be seen following dorsal hand burns or prolonged immobilization for fracture management.

To address these contractures, forearm- or hand-based dynamic thermoplastic splints similar to those designed

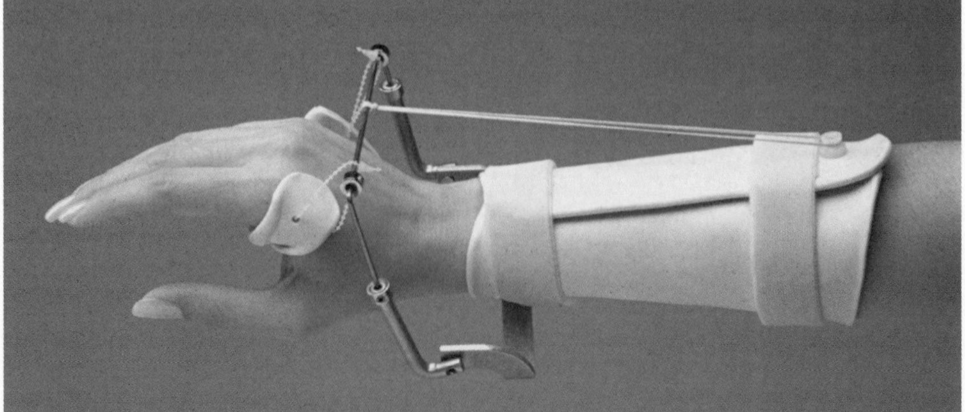

Figure 16-51 Custom thermoplastic dynamic wrist extension splint using Phoenix Wrist Hinge.

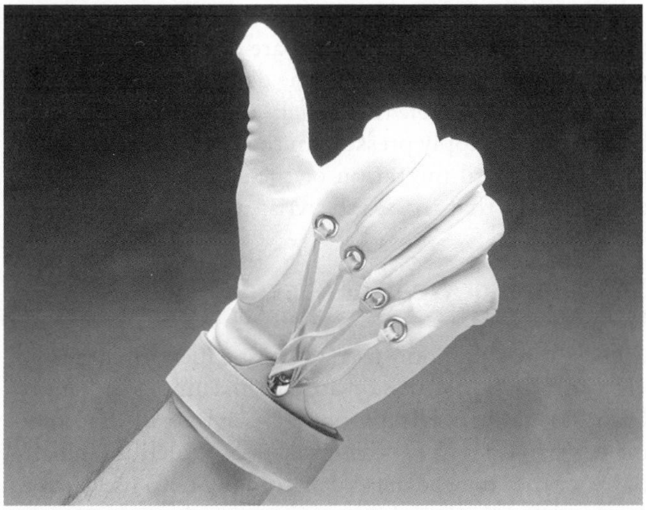

Figure 16-53 Finger flexion glove.

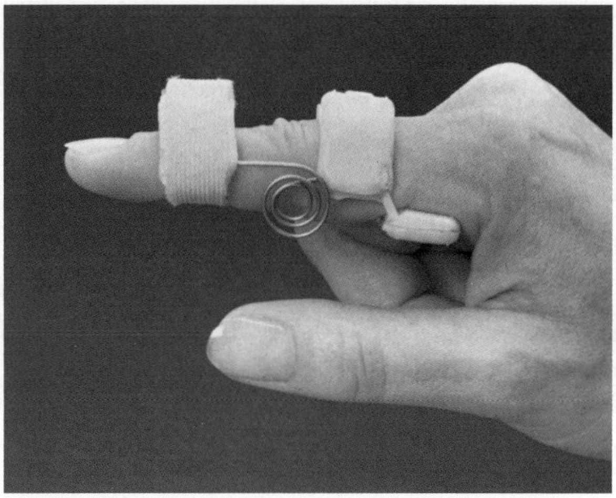

Figure 16-55 Rolyan® Sof-Stretch Coil Extension Splint.

for MCP flexion and extension can be used by extending the distal part of the splint across the MCP to just proximal to the PIP joint. Immobilizing the MCP applies force to the PIP.

Prefabricated spring wire and spring coil splints are also available to gain flexion or extension range of motion. In a study of prefabricated spring wire (Fig. 16-54) and spring coil (Fig. 16-55) extension splints by Fess (1988), exerted forces were found to vary in the same splint design and to vary also according to the degree of joint contracture. Some forces were alarmingly high, well above recommended limits. Callahan and McEntee (1986) found similar results and expressed concern about whether these splints fit accurately and about forces being distributed over small surface areas as compared with custom-fabricated splints. Designs have since been improved so that tension can be somewhat modified. If used, these splints must be carefully monitored to avoid further joint or tissue damage.

Spring coil extension splints, sometimes called Capener splints, may be custom fabricated and are described in the literature (Callahan & McEntee, 1986; Colditz, 1995). A study of dynamic splinting in the management of PIP flexion contractures using Capener and low-profile hand-based outrigger splints found the two to be equally effective, suggesting that the patient may prefer the less bulky Capener splint if offered a choice (Prosser, 1996). Additional findings concluded that the longer the flexion contracture was present, the less it resolved and that splint wearing time was a significant factor affecting outcome.

A commercial neoprene dynamic finger extension tube (Fig. 16-56) provides circumferential pressure and a dynamic force into extension via an angled seam on its volar surface. It may also offer other therapeutic values, such as heat, mild joint distraction, and longer tolerable wearing times (Clark, 1997). PIP extension can also be gained though serial plaster casting or splinting.

Thermoplastic gutter (Fig. 16-28) or circumferential splinting and dynamic traction splinting are useful in the treatment of mild contractures, whereas serial plaster dig-

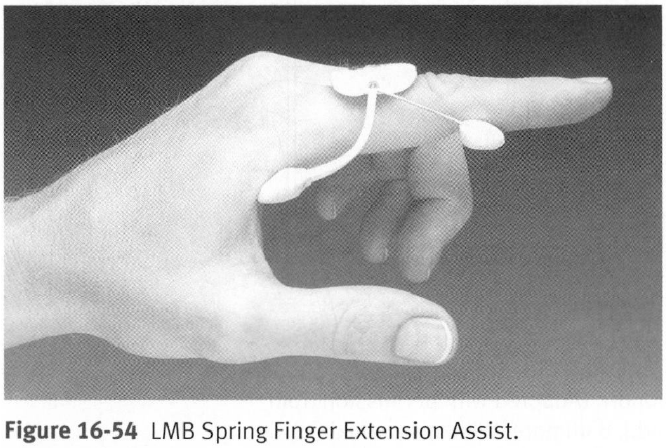

Figure 16-54 LMB Spring Finger Extension Assist.

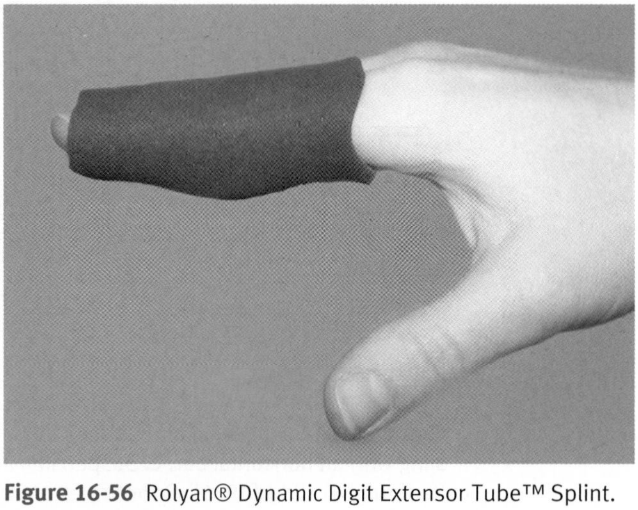

Figure 16-56 Rolyan® Dynamic Digit Extensor Tube™ Splint.

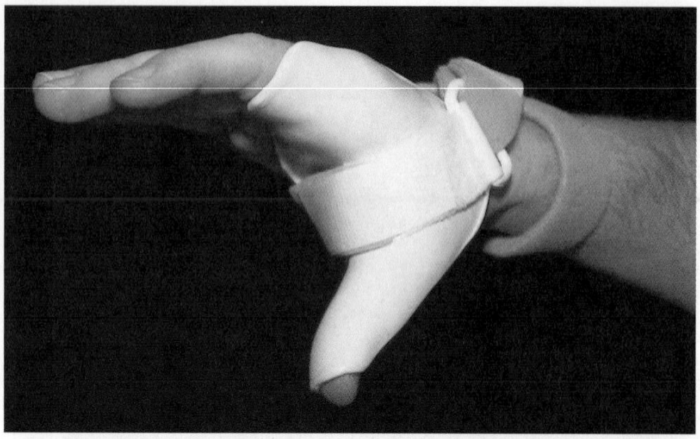

Figure 16-57 Custom thermoplastic thumb abduction splint.

ital casting (Fig. 16-37) has been advocated for moderate to severe contractures (Bell-Krotoski, 2002). Plaster casting offers the advantages of intimate conformity, rigidity, breathability, and uniform distribution of pressure. Casting does require the patient's cooperation in keeping the cast dry, and casts have the disadvantage of not being removable for function or motion. For most effective results, casts should be changed every 2–7 days (Bell-Krotoski & Figarola, 1995) or sooner if they become loose or wet. The DIP joint may be left free if its motion is not limited. It is at times beneficial to involve the DIP in the cast if increased mechanical advantage is desired for PIP extension. Variations of many of these splints can be used for the treatment of DIP contractures or contractures of the thumb MP or IP.

Adduction contractures of the thumb, which are commonly seen in burns and nerve injuries, are most often treated with serial static thumb abduction splints, which conform to the first web space (Fig. 16-57). It is important to ensure that abduction forces are directed to the CMC joint by involving as much of the distal aspect of the first metacarpal as possible (Fess et al., 2005). Strapping must be designed to apply pressure in the proper direction and to prevent distal migration of the splint. This often requires a strap that crosses the wrist.

Substitute for Weak or Absent Muscles

Orthoses are commonly used to assist patients in maximizing the functional use of an affected upper extremity. Orthoses may be used temporarily, as in the case of recovering nerve injuries or neurological diseases such as Guillain-Barré, or they may be prescribed for long-term use, such as in complete spinal cord injury or progressive neuromuscular conditions like postpolio syndrome. They are generally worn only during the day or for specific functional tasks. An orthosis successful in improving the ability to function is often much more accepted and appreciated by the patient than orthoses prescribed for other purposes.

Substitute for Weak or Absent Shoulder or Elbow Muscles

Proximal arm devices can support the shoulder and forearm to encourage motion of weak proximal musculature, allow for distal function, and enable occupational performance as well as prevent loss of motion and provide pain relief.

Suspension arm devices (Fig. 16-58) suspend from above the head, generally on an overhead rod that is

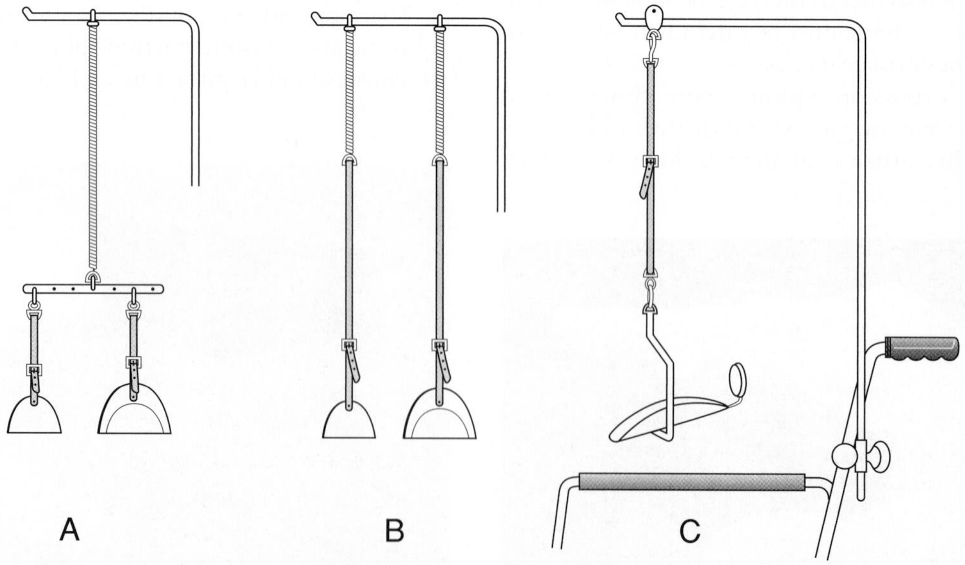

Figure 16-58 Suspension arm devices. **A.** Suspension sling with horizontal bar. **B.** Suspension sling without horizontal bar. **C.** Suspension arm support. (Adapted with permission from Redford, J. B. [Ed.]. [1986]. *Orthotics etcetera* [3rd ed.]. Baltimore: Williams & Wilkins.)

mounted to a wheelchair. The arm swings as in a pendulum from straps attached to the overhead rod. The ease of management and low cost have contributed to the long-standing popularity of these devices (Long & Shutt, 1986). The following variations are commercially available and in current use.

The suspension sling has a single strap suspended from the overhead rod. A horizontal balance bar with multiple holes for adjustment of the fulcrum supports separate wrist and elbow cuffs. The suspension sling without horizontal bar has two straps that originate directly from the overhead rod with cuffs to support the elbow and wrist. The suspension arm support has a forearm trough suspended from a single point on the overhead rod. It can also be easily attached to an overhead frame on the patient's bed. Springs of various tensions may be added to the straps that support the limb, allowing a patient with only slight active motion to produce accelerated shoulder movement by bouncing the arm up and down. Suspension devices can be adjusted to allow for certain motions (Procedures for Practice 16-2) but lack the fine adjustment that extremely weak patients may need.

PROCEDURES FOR PRACTICE 16-2

How to Adjust Suspension Arm Devices

Suspension Arm Sling

- For horizontal abduction, rotate the overhead rod laterally.
- For horizontal adduction, rotate the overhead rod medially.
- For external rotation, move the arm cuffs back on the balance bar to shift weight toward the elbow.
- For internal rotation, move the arm cuffs forward on the balance bar to shift weight toward the hand.
- For elbow flexion, move the point of suspension backward on the overhead rod to put the hand toward the patient's face.
- For elbow extension, move the point of suspension forward on the overhead rod to put the hand away from the patient's face.
- For height adjustments, vary the length of the strap or straps that connect to the overhead rod; or raise or lower the bracket on the wheelchair upright.

Suspension Arm Support

- For horizontal motion and height adjustments, see list under Suspension Arm Sling.
- For elbow flexion, move the rocker arm farther from the trough elbow dial.
- For elbow extension, move the rocker arm closer to the trough elbow dial.

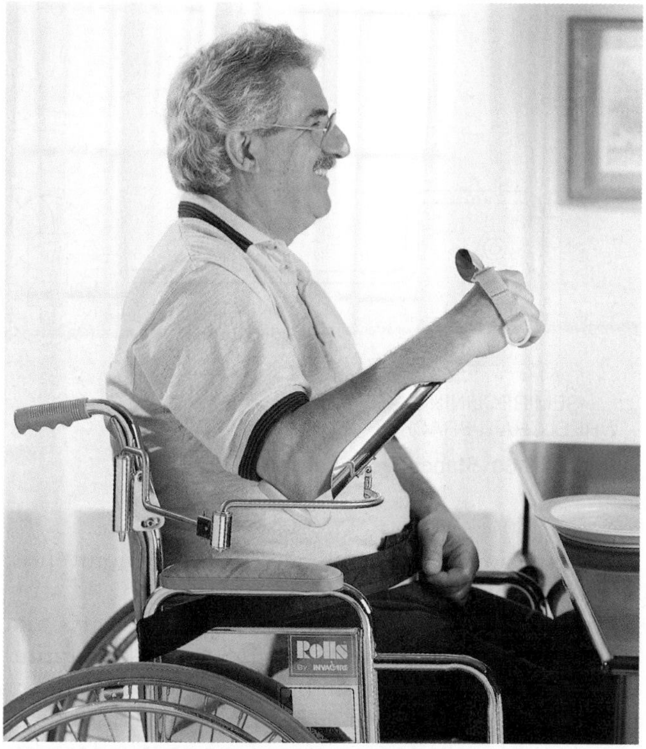

Figure 16-59 Mobile arm support.

A **mobile arm support** (MAS) (Fig. 16-59) is a mechanical device that supports the weight of the arm and provides assistance to shoulder and elbow motions through a linkage of ball-bearing joints (Long & Shutt, 1986; Lunsford, 1997; Yasuda, Bowman, & Hsu, 1986). The MAS is typically mounted to a patient's wheelchair, but it can also be attached to a tabletop. Their mechanical principles are threefold: (1) use of gravity to assist weak muscles, (2) support of the arm to reduce the load on weak muscles, and (3) reduction of friction by using ball-bearing joints. Criteria for use include:

- A defined functional need.
- An adequate source of power from neck, trunk, shoulder girdle, or elbow muscles.
- Adequate motor control such that the patient can contract and relax functioning muscles.
- Sufficient passive joint range of motion, with 0–90° of shoulder flexion and abduction, 0–30° of external rotation, full internal rotation and elbow flexion, and 0–80° of pronation preferred.
- Stable trunk positioning.
- A motivated patient.
- A supportive environment that provides the patient with the opportunity and assistance to use the device.

Patients who may benefit include those with cervical spinal cord injury, muscular dystrophy, Guillain-Barré

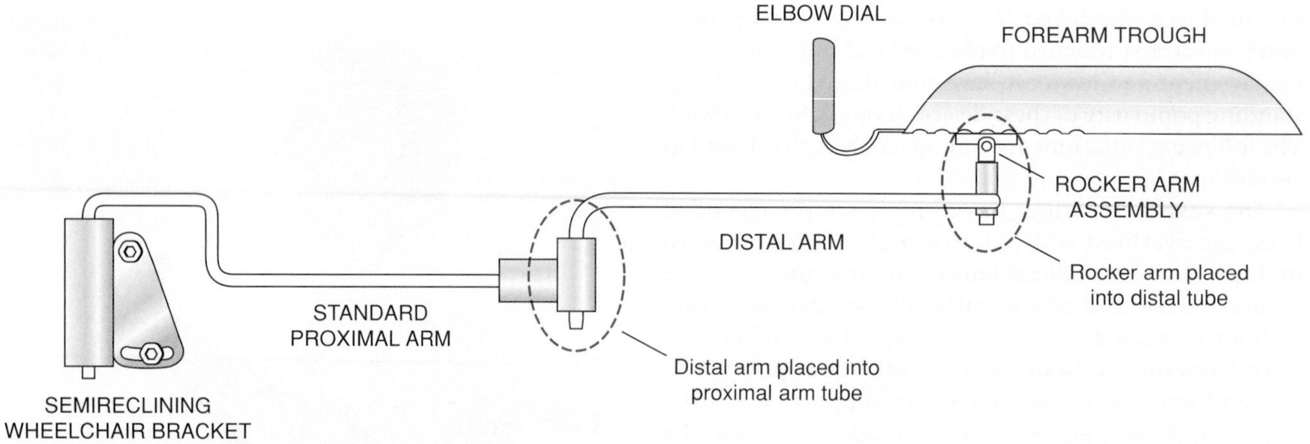

Figure 16-60 Standard components of a MAS.

syndrome, amyotrophic lateral sclerosis, poliomyelitis, and polymyositis.

Selection of MAS components, assembly of parts, and balance and adjustment of the MAS generally requires postgraduate hands-on training. Balance and adjustment principles are presented in Procedures for Practice 16-3 to give the reader a basic overview and appreciation for what is possible. This does not negate the need for additional training or consultation with experienced therapists to ensure that the best possible adjustments are made to give the patient maximal mechanical advantage.

The standard MAS assembly described in this chapter consists of an adjustable arm positioner bracket (also known as a semireclining bracket), standard proximal and distal arms, a standard rocker arm assembly, and a basic forearm trough (Fig. 16-60). The many commonly used special MAS component parts include the outside rocker arm assembly and the elevating proximal arm (Fig. 16-61). The outside rocker arm (or offset swivel) has a ball-bearing joint that allows for greater freedom in vertical motion, thus facilitating hand-to-mouth or hand-to-table movements. The elevating proximal arm is useful for a patient with poor to fair deltoid strength. As the patient initiates the elevating motion, the rubber band assists, allowing the patient to flex and abduct the humerus to a higher level. A less complicated and more user friendly MAS system is also available (Fig. 16-62). It is easier to set up and allows adjustments to be made without any tools.

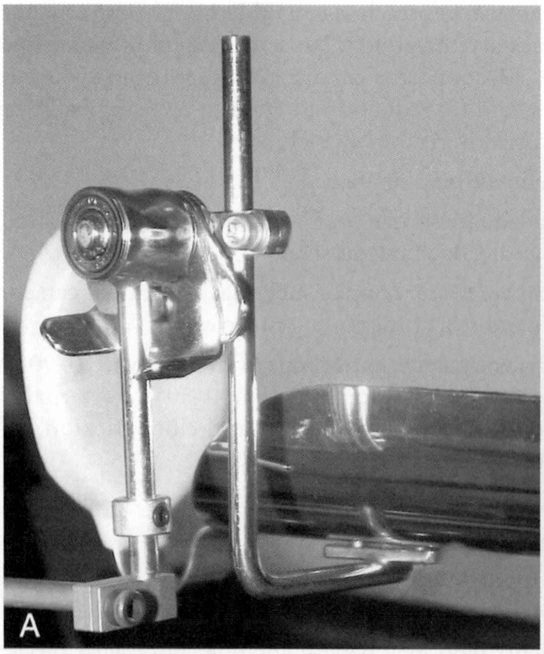

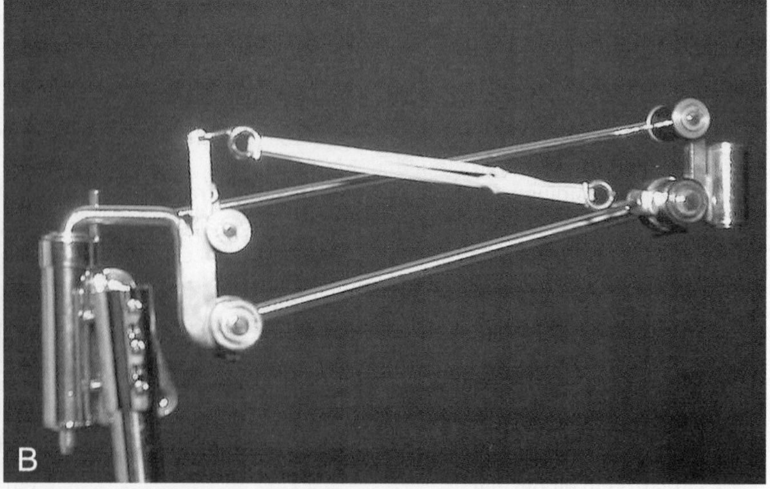

Figure 16-61 Special MAS components: **A.** Outside rocker arm. **B.** Elevating proximal arm.

PROCEDURES FOR PRACTICE 16-3

MAS Assembly and Training Principles

How to Assemble and Balance the Standard MAS Assembly

- Assemble tools (Phillips and flathead screwdrivers, Allen wrenches) and MAS parts (bracket, proximal arm, distal arm, rocker arm, trough).
- Inspect ball-bearing components for smooth operation.
- Ensure that the patient is seated properly in the wheelchair, with pelvis well back in chair and trunk in good vertical alignment.
- Fit the trough to the patient's arm by bending the elbow dial toward the radial side of the trough.
- Attach the rocker arm to the trough by placing the screws in the third and fifth holes from the dial.
- Attach the bracket to the wheelchair at approximately the midhumerus level so that it is neutrally rolled[1] and pitched[2].
- Attach the proximal arm to the bracket.
- Attach the distal arm to the proximal arm.
- Attach the trough to the distal arm.
- Balance the arm support to neutral by adjusting the pitch of the bracket and the distal end of the proximal arm so that the bearing tubes are perpendicular to the floor.
- Place the patient's arm in the trough.
- Observe for abnormal shoulder elevation and adjust the height of the bracket as needed to correct it.

MAS Hand-to-Mouth Movement Pattern

Instructions to Patient

- Push down on the trough dial while adducting your humerus.
- Externally rotate your shoulder.
- Shift your body weight toward the MAS.
- Straighten up or lean back in your chair.
- Rotate your trunk toward the MAS.
- Turn your head toward the MAS.

Equipment Adjustments to Aid this Motion

- Move the rocker arm farther from the trough elbow dial.
- Pitch the MAS at the bracket assembly toward the wheelchair back.
- Raise the bracket assembly on the wheelchair upright.

[1]Roll is the rotation of the bracket assembly on the wheelchair upright governing the side-to-side (horizontal) slope. The name comes from the side-to-side swaying of a ship.

[2]Pitch is the tilt of the ball-bearing tube on the bracket assembly governing the upward-downward (vertical) slope. The name comes from the backward-forward pitch of a ship as it goes over waves.

MAS Hand-to-Table Movement Pattern

Instructions to Patient

- Lift and internally rotate your shoulder to lower your hand.
- Shift your body weight away from the MAS.
- Roll your shoulder forward.
- Rotate your trunk away from the MAS.
- Tilt or turn your head away from the MAS.

Equipment Adjustments to Aid this Motion

- Move the rocker arm closer to the trough elbow dial.
- Pitch the MAS at the bracket assembly toward the patient's feet.
- Lower the bracket assembly on the wheelchair upright.

MAS Horizontal Abduction and Adduction Movement Patterns

Instructions to Patient

- Shift your body weight in the direction you want to move.
- Rotate your trunk toward the direction you want to move.
- Turn your head briskly in the direction you want to move.

Equipment Adjustments to Aid this Motion

- Roll the bracket assembly on the wheelchair upright toward the patient for adduction.
- Roll the bracket assembly on the wheelchair upright away from the patient for abduction.

MAS Controls Training and Use Training

Controls Training

- Teach the patient the effects of head, trunk, and proximal movements on the movement of the MAS.
- If bilateral MASs are used, begin with one side first.
- Begin with horizontal motions by having the patient practice moving the MAS as far as possible from side to side and front to back.
- Proceed with vertical motions by having the patient practice moving the hand to the table and up to the mouth at various points within the horizontal range.

Use Training

- Teach the patient to use the MAS for specific desired functional activities, such as eating, grooming, writing, keyboarding, page turning, and power wheelchair driving.
- Encourage practice and independent problem-solving skills.

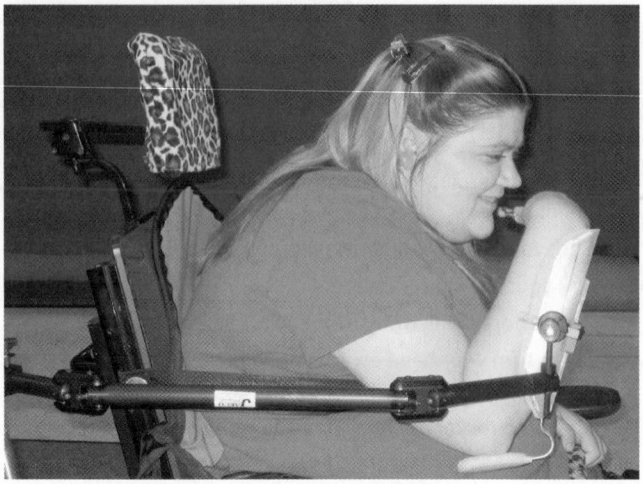

Figure 16-62 JAECO/Rancho MultiLink MAS.

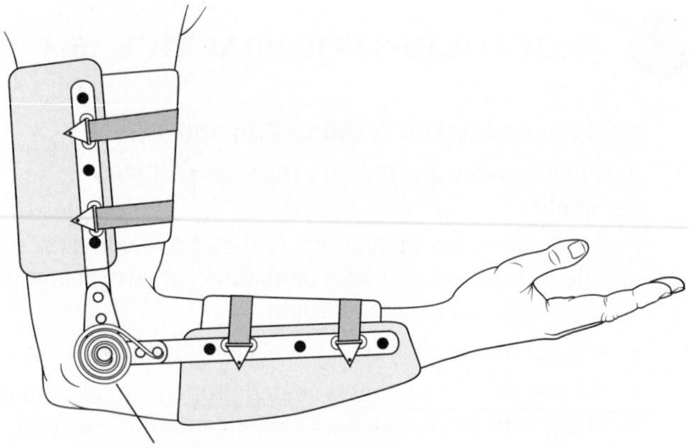

Figure 16-64 Custom dynamic elbow orthosis with flexion assist. (Adapted with permission from Goldberg, B., & Hsu, J. S. [Eds.]. [1997]. *Atlas of orthoses and assistive devices* [3rd ed.]. St. Louis: Mosby.)

An alternative MAS design, the linear MAS (Fig. 16-63), uses linear bearings and straight rods without joints. This streamlines the overall width of the support and lets wheelchairs more easily fit through doorways (Clark, Waters, & Baumgarten, 1997).

For a patient who can walk, a gunslinger orthosis can provide both proximal stability and mobility. This type of shoulder–elbow orthosis consists of a metal forearm trough that is mechanically coupled to a plastic hemigirdle anchored on the patient's pelvis. This device is most useful for patients having good distal function but proximal weakness from brachial plexus injuries, spinal cord injuries, or postpolio syndrome. Prefabricated gunslingers (Fig. 16-11) are commercially available, but for long-term use, a custom-designed orthosis (Fig. 16-12) is indicated (Lunsford, 1997).

Depending on the patient's proximal muscle status and specific functional needs, the coupling between the trough and hemigirdle base can be customized to permit a variety of motions, such as glenohumeral internal–external rotation and flexion–extension. It can also be made to hold a very weak shoulder in a static position for function, which may be with the hand in midline. If the wrist also has weakness, the trough can be extended to support the hand. Usefulness must be determined for each individual case, considering factors such as acceptance by the patient, ease of donning, cost, and especially functional benefit.

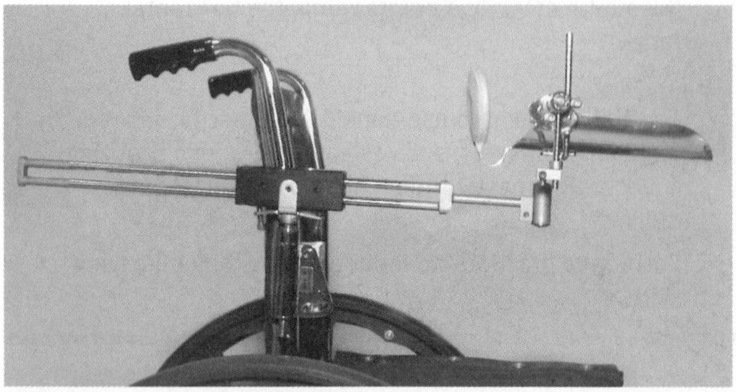

Figure 16-63 Linear MAS.

For patients having selective loss of elbow flexion strength, a dynamic elbow orthosis with an elbow flexion assist (Fig. 16-64) may be used. This functional orthosis typically has a spring-loaded elbow mechanism with a ratchet lock. When the patient initiates flexion using residual muscles or compensatory motions, the spring device assists with elbow flexion. A release button allows the elbow to be repositioned into greater flexion or to drop down into extension (Lunsford, 1997).

Substitute for Weak or Absent Wrist or Hand Muscles

The combination of sensory loss and motor imbalance caused by a peripheral nerve injury greatly impairs normal hand function. As Colditz (2002b) points out, it is impossible to build an external device that can substitute for the intricately balanced muscles that a splint attempts to replace. In splinting nerve palsies, the key concept is to understand the patient's condition and neuromuscular status so as to prescribe or design an appropriate splint to increase function. Splints should keep areas of intact sensibility free if possible, should be as simple as possible, and should not immobilize joints unnecessarily. The splinting program must be closely monitored and altered in response to nerve recovery as the patient's muscle status changes (see Case Example). In a study to assess factors that influenced splint wear in peripheral nerve lesions, the only significant variable was a positive effect as perceived by the patient. Fifty-two percent of patients reported terminating wear because splints hindered their daily life, and 23% reported terminating wear because splints had not been of any use. Interestingly, the highest effectiveness score was for day splints for the dominant hand aimed at replacing function (Paternostro-Sluga et al., 2003).

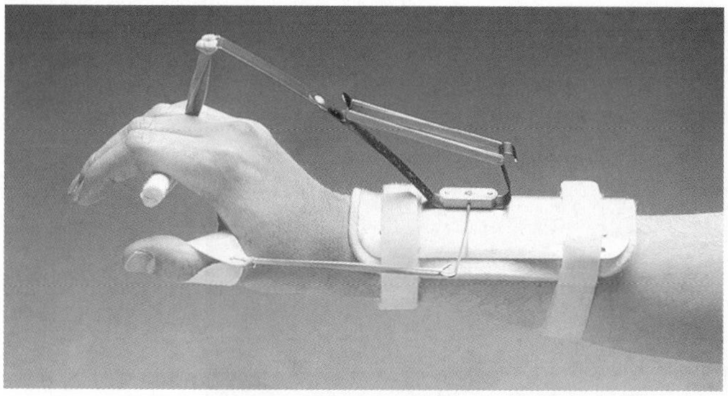

Figure 16-65 Bunnell™ Thomas Suspension Splint.

Radial nerve palsy, commonly associated with humeral fractures, can result in the complete loss or partial weakness of wrist, finger, and thumb extensors and weakness of forearm supination and thumb abduction. The loss of wrist extensor strength devastates hand grasp. Not only is the patient unable to position the hand properly, but the inability to stabilize the wrist in extension impairs normal function of the long finger flexors. Loss of extrinsic finger extension is much less of a functional problem, as the unaffected intrinsic muscles can actively extend the IPs. Supporting the wrist in extension is the primary goal of radial nerve splinting, and the use of a simple static wrist splint may suffice in improving hand function (Fess et al., 2005).

Prefabricated radial nerve splints, such as a Thomas suspension splint (Fig. 16-65) or a wire-foam splint, are designed to dynamically extend the wrist, MCPs, and thumb. It is usually preferable not to include the thumb because of the limitation in intrinsic motion it imposes and the danger of stressing the MP collateral ligament through poorly directed forces. Adding individual finger loops to the palmar bar, thus removing bulk in the palm and allowing individual finger motion, can enhance the Thomas suspension splint. The palmar bulk of the wire-foam splint often impedes the ability to grasp large objects. ***Caution should be used when prescribing a dynamic orthosis because strong unopposed flexors may easily overcome the dynamic forces trying to hold the wrist and hand in extension, negating functional benefits.***

A custom-fabricated radial nerve splint, also known as a Colditz splint, has been designed to allow for partial wrist and full finger motion and a facsimile of a normal tenodesis effect (Fig. 16-66). This splint consists of a low-profile outrigger attached to a dorsal forearm base (Figs. 16-5 and 16-67). Nonelastic cords connect the splint base to finger loops. The cord length is adjusted so that, when the MCPs actively flex, the wrist is brought into extension. Conversely, when the wrist flexes, the cord tension causes the MCPs to extend. Little training is required for the patient to be able to use the splint functionally, and grasp and release of objects is greatly enhanced. Further advantages of this splint are the maintenance of normal hand arches, the absence of splinting material covering the palm, the low-profile design, and the facilitation of wrist extensor strength as return of nerve function occurs (Colditz, 2002b). Pre-formed splints and outrigger kits are commercially available.

Splinting in median nerve palsy is geared toward substituting for weak or absent thenar muscles that render the thumb unable to pull away from the palm and oppose to the fingers. This is most often accomplished through a custom-fabricated thermoplastic opponens splint, which stabilizes the thumb in a position of abduction and opposition to enable pulp-to-pulp pinch (Fig. 16-25). Although such a splint often greatly improves fine motor prehension, this must be individually assessed because substitu-

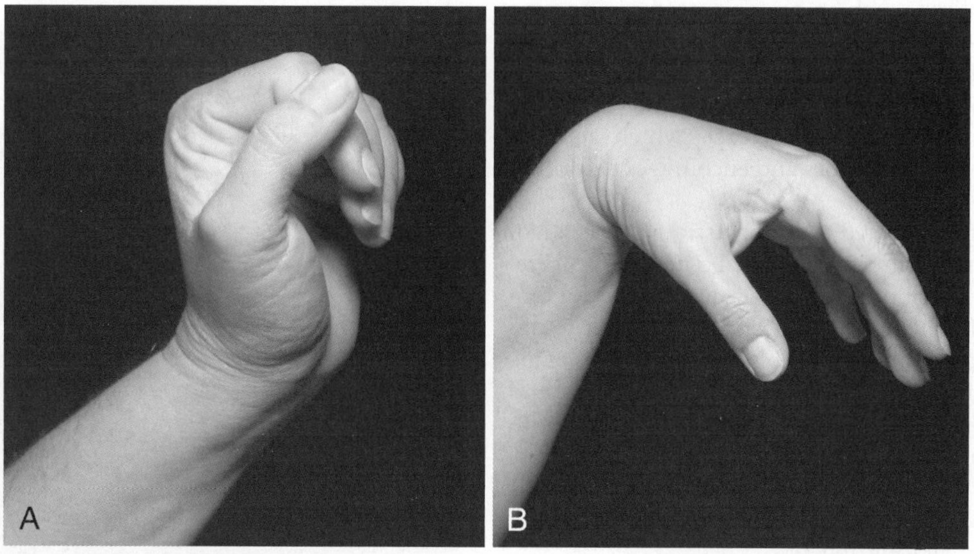

Figure 16-66 Normal tenodesis effect. **A.** When the wrist is extended, the fingers flex. **B.** When the wrist is flexed, the fingers extend.

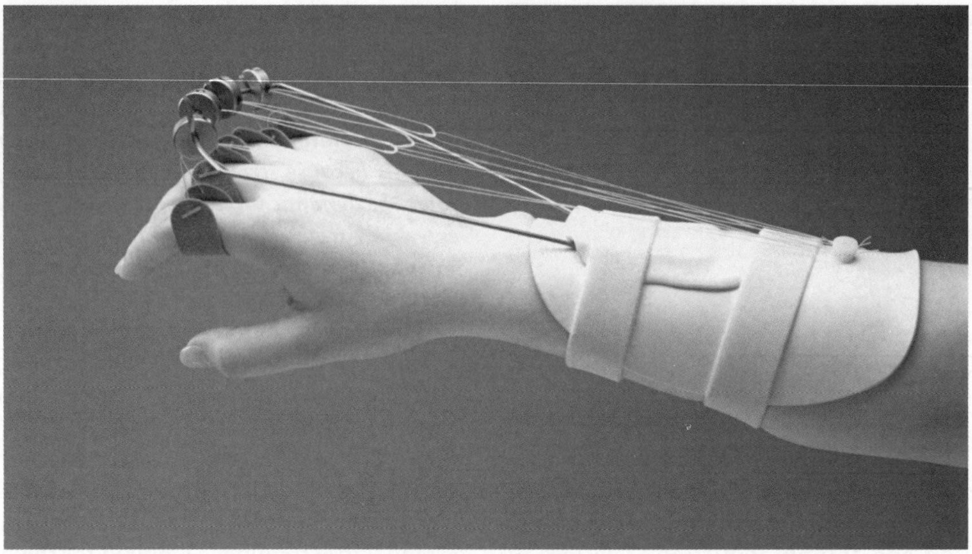

Figure 16-67 Custom thermoplastic radial nerve splint using low-profile Phoenix Extended Outrigger.

tion patterns from unaffected thumb muscles may provide sufficient thumb function (Colditz, 2002b; Fess et al., 2005). Patients may choose to wear an opposition splint for selected activities only.

In the presence of ulnar nerve palsy, the hand assumes a claw position, or intrinsic-minus position, with ring and small finger hyperextension of the MCPs and flexion of the IPs. This is a result of weakness or loss of lumbrical and interossei muscles, which are responsible for MCP flexion and IP extension. The prime splinting objective is to assist in grasp and release of objects by preventing the claw position. This is accomplished by a lumbrical bar splint, which blocks the MCPs in slight flexion, allowing the force of the unaffected long finger extensors to extend the IPs.

Dynamic splints, such as prefabricated spring wire splints (Fig. 16-41), do not work well because the spring tension is usually not sufficient to hold the MCPs in flexion when the patient actively opens the hand. Thus, the MCPs hyperextend against the force, which actually strengthens the long extensors and encourages deformity (Colditz, 2002b).

A static custom-molded thermoplastic splint is advocated as the best solution. It should be non-bulky, carefully molded to distribute pressure evenly over the dorsum of the proximal phalanges, and designed so as not to obstruct full flexion of all joints (Colditz, 2002b; Fess et al., 2005). The splint may include just the affected ring and small fingers (Figs. 16-3 and 16-68) or may include all fingers to distribute pressure more effectively and comfortably (Fig. 16-42). The latter splint is used in the treatment of combined median and ulnar nerve injuries, which result in the clawing of all four fingers.

For a patient who has only radial nerve function, a custom-fabricated RIC (Rehabilitation Institute of Chicago)

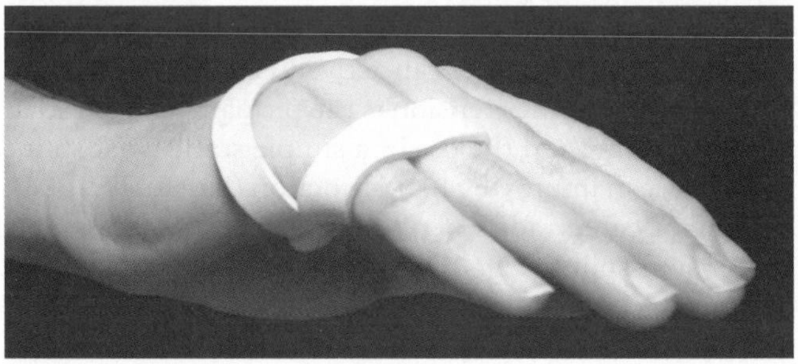

Figure 16-68 Custom thermoplastic lumbrical bar splint for ring and small fingers.

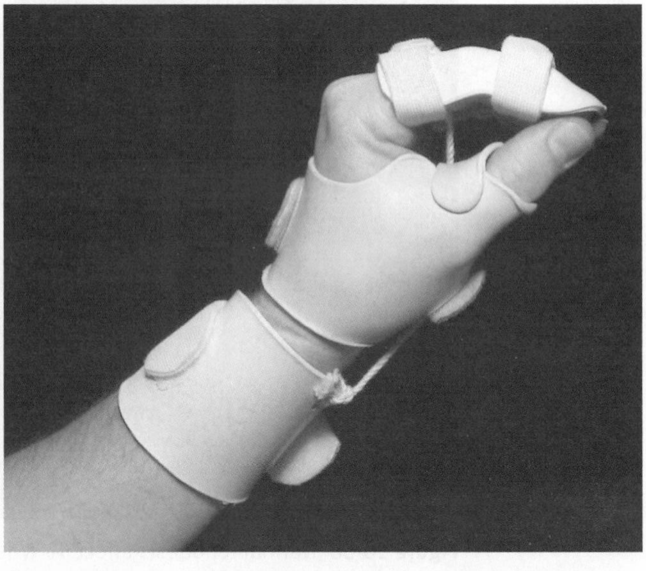

Figure 16-69 Custom thermoplastic RIC tenodesis splint.

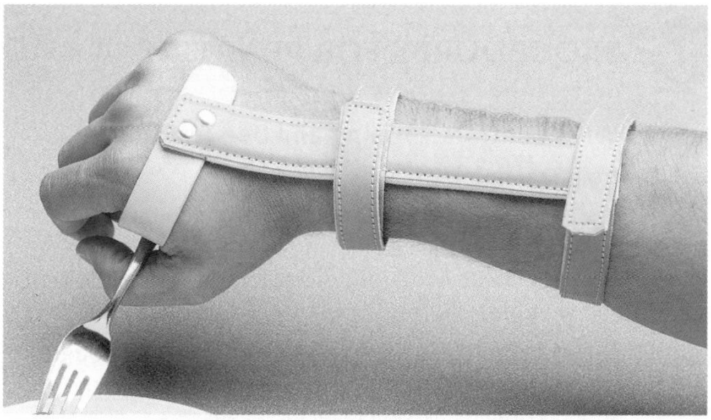

Figure 16-70 Economy Wrist Support with Universal Cuff.

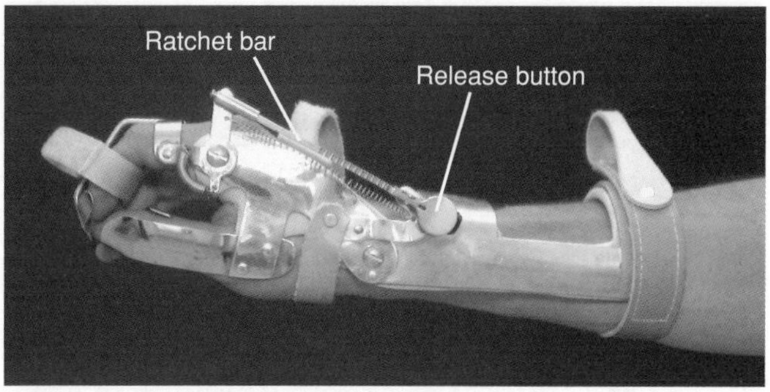

Figure 16-72 Custom metal ratchet wrist–hand orthosis.

tenodesis splint (Fig. 16-69) may be used. This splint can provide minimal hand grasp by harnessing the power of the wrist extensors to bring the thumb, index finger, and long finger into a functional pinch. It has three molded thermoplastic pieces: one to position the thumb, one to position the index and long fingers, and a wrist cuff to serve as the base for connecting a static line from the wrist to the fingers (Colditz, 2002b).

Static orthoses, which allow passive holding of functional implements such as utensils or pens, may also be used in the presence of wrist or hand weakness. Examples include a hand-based universal cuff, an economy wrist support with universal cuff (Fig. 16-70), and a short or long design Wanchik writing splint (Fig. 16-71).

For patients with long-term or permanent loss of muscle function, as is the case in complete spinal cord injury or progressive neuromuscular disease, permanent functional orthoses may be used. These orthoses are fabricated by experienced orthotists from metal and are recommended by occupational therapists for individual patients based on neuromuscular status and specific functional needs. Often these distal orthoses are used in conjunction with proximal ones (such as a MAS) if proximal weakness is also present.

A ratchet wrist–hand orthosis (Fig. 16-72) may be used for patients with weak (below grade 3) wrist extension and finger strength, such as that seen with C5 tetraplegia (see Chapter 43). A thumb post positions the thumb in abduction and in alignment with the index and long fingers, and a finger piece assembly maintains the index and long fingers in a position for pinch. A ratchet system is used to close the hand in discrete increments. Closing is accomplished by manually pushing the finger piece to flex the fingers against the thumb using the contralateral hand, the chin, or the side of a table or chair. Release is accomplished by a spring that is activated by the press of a release button (Clark, Waters, & Baumgarten, 1997; Lunsford, 1997).

For patients with the potential for neurological return at the C6 level, a wrist-action wrist–hand orthosis (Fig. 16-73) can be used as a transition system (Clark, Waters, & Baumgarten, 1997). This orthosis allows for free wrist motion, with stops that can be adjusted to limit motion to a prescribed range. When no wrist extensors are present, the wrist is locked into a set position. As recovery occurs and

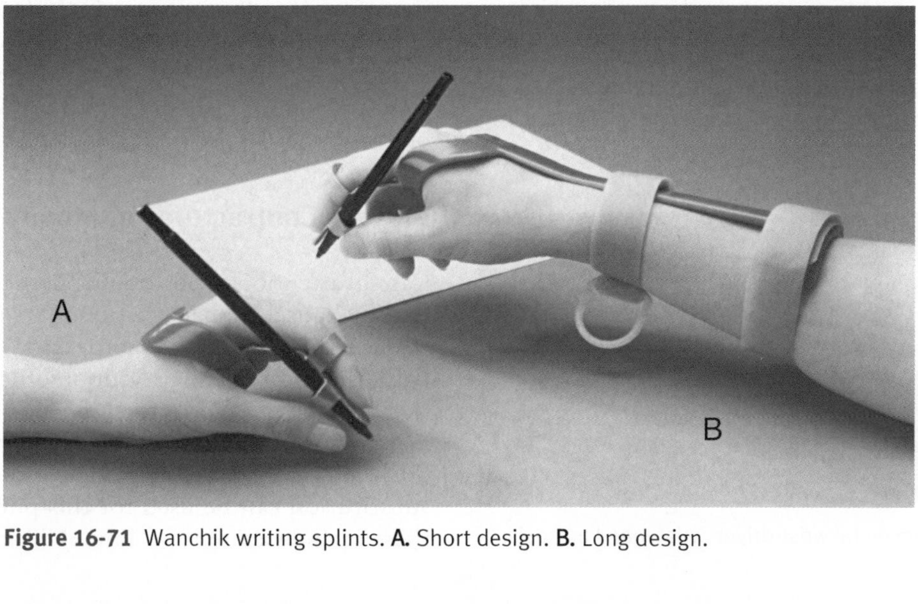

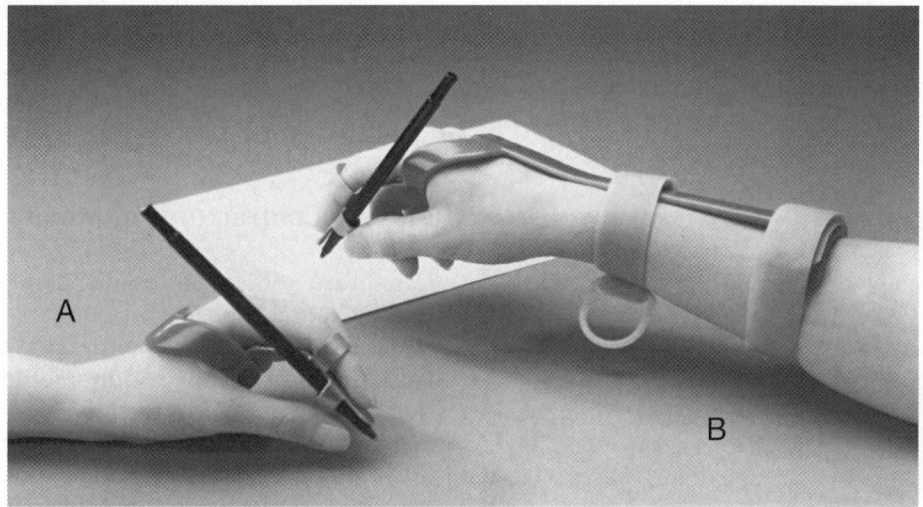

Figure 16-71 Wanchik writing splints. **A.** Short design. **B.** Long design.

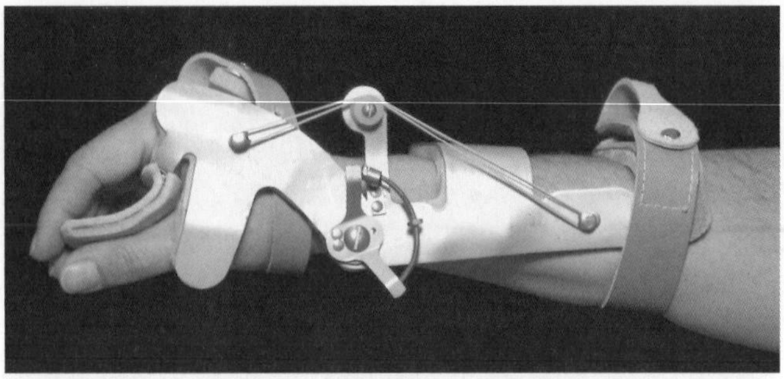

Figure 16-73 Custom metal wrist-action wrist–hand orthosis with rubber band assist.

strength increases, progressive range of motion is allowed. Rubber bands are often attached to provide an extensor assist to weak muscles.

A **wrist-driven wrist–hand orthosis** (WDWHO) (Fig. 16-74) may be indicated for patients having 3+ or greater wrist extensor strength, such as a patient with C6 tetraplegia. Using the principle of tenodesis (Fig. 16-66), this type of flexor hinge orthosis transfers wrist extensor power to the fingers for grasping. Active wrist extension operates a mechanical linkage transferring power to flex the index and long fingers against the thumb. A properly adjusted orthosis allows for 1 pound of pinch for every 2 pounds of wrist extensor force. Gravity-assisted wrist flexion opens the hand for release. An activating lever at the wrist controls the size of the opening and the resultant position of prehension to allow for grasp of various size objects and different pinch forces.

Fitting the patient with bilateral WDWHOs may be tempting, but patients do not typically achieve a higher level of function with two orthoses than with one (Clark, Waters, & Baumgarten, 1997). Bilateral orthoses are difficult to use, requiring a great deal of balance, coordination, and practice to become successful. If the patient has inadequate proximal strength, it may be difficult to bring the arms into midline. If sensation has been lost, the patient must rely on visual compensation, which also makes bilateral orthotic use difficult. A patient generally uses one WDWHO, with the contralateral hand serving as a gross assist. Training principles are listed in Procedures for Practice 16-4.

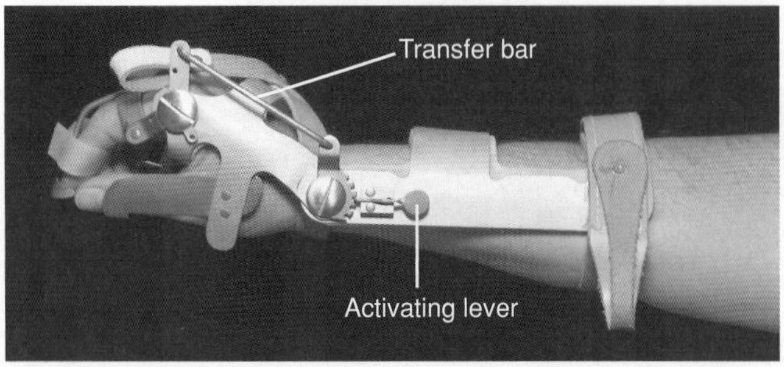

Figure 16-74 Custom metal wrist-driven wrist–hand orthosis.

PROCEDURES FOR PRACTICE 16-4

WDWHO Controls Training and Use Training

Controls Training

- The patient needs to become proficient in basic orthotic skills, such as picking up, placing, and releasing objects of various sizes, textures, densities, and weights.
- Soft medium-sized objects or 1-inch firm, semirough objects are often best to start with; progress to more difficult objects as skill level increases.
- Encourage skills practice from a variety of heights because the patient may have to learn to abduct and internally rotate the shoulder to approach and handle objects appropriately.

Use Training

- Teach the patient to use the WDWHO to perform specific functional tasks, such as writing, eating, and oral hygiene.
- Have the patient practice activities under various conditions to encourage independent problem solving and spontaneous use of the orthosis.

Given the cost and complexity of fabrication and training, follow-up studies have been done to assess whether patients use WDWHOs over the long term after discharge from therapy. Knox, Engel, and Seibens (1971) reported a 51% continued use rate; Shepherd and Ruzicka (1991) reported a 50% rate; and Allen (1971) reported a 43% rate. Factors that were reported to contribute to continued use are education, commitment, and involving the patient in the orthotic decision-making process (Knox, Engel, & Seibens, 1971); the ability to don the orthosis easily (Allen, 1971); and adequate training, acceptance, internal motivation, and strong functional or vocational goals (Shepherd & Ruzicka, 1991). In these same studies, reasons for orthotic discontinuation were stated by subjects to be improvement in muscle strength, use of alternative methods or equipment to perform tasks previously done with the WDWHO, poor fit, bulk, and the orthosis taking too long to put on.

Prevent Contractures or Modify Tone

Careful attention to positioning in the presence of wound healing, muscle imbalance, abnormal muscle tone due to stroke or brain injury, or motor disorders such as cerebral palsy is critical in the prevention of loss of range of motion, which can lead to functional or skin hygiene problems. Many of the static splints, casts, and orthoses previously mentioned for immobilization, stabilization, or substitution can be used for this purpose. Examples of these include acute burn immobilization splints to pre-

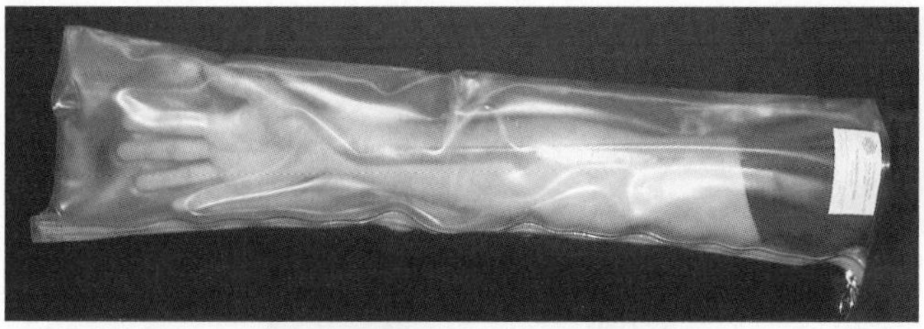

Figure 16-75 Commercial inflatable pressure splint.

vent wrist and digital contractures, wrist extension splints to prevent contractures caused by wrist drop, thumb abduction splints to prevent thumb adduction contractures, and lumbrical bar splints to prevent MCP hyperextension and IP flexion contractures.

Ideally, these splints should not limit function, exert excessive stress to soft tissues, or interfere with movement of uninvolved joints. If splints are not required for functional use, often it is possible for patients to wear static positioning splints at night only. In addition to the prevention of contractures, splints may be used to prevent shortening of the muscle-tendon unit. For example, a volar thermoplastic or plaster splint worn at night to position the wrist and fingers in maximum composite extension can help to prevent tightness of the long finger flexors (Tribuzi, 2002).

Lapboards, arm troughs, and suspension arm slings can help to position the upper extremities properly. Bivalved plaster casts or anteroposterior splints (Fig. 16-48) can be used to maintain range of motion, especially in the presence of increased tone. ***Care must be taken to avoid pressure problems by ensuring that casts are properly padded and the skin is closely monitored.***

An inflatable pressure splint (Fig. 16-75), originally designed as an emergency immobilizer for the limbs, has been adopted for use in patients with abnormal tone. When inflated, it provides deep pressure and warmth, and depending on how it is used, it can either reduce tone in hypertonic extremities or increase tone in hypotonic extremities. It may be worn as a precursor to movement therapy or during weight-bearing activities to help position the limb. A study of 18 patients with CVA who wore the splint for 30 minutes a day, 5 days per week, for 3 weeks found no significant difference in upper extremity sensation, pain, and motor function between the splinted and control groups, leading the authors to suggest further study as to the long-term effects that inflatable splints may have on tone (Poole et al., 1990).

The use of thermoplastic splinting in the modification of tone in the wrist and hand continues to be controversial in the literature and in practice. A survey of occupational therapists clearly demonstrated the conflicting practices in splinting (Neuhaus et al., 1981). Opponents of splinting argue that splinting may lead to increased muscle tone, joint stiffness, and muscle atrophy and may interfere with treatment aimed at facilitation and functional use. Proponents of splinting contend that splinting can reduce tone (McPherson, Becker, & Franszczak, 1985; Neuhaus et al., 1981). In a systematic review of hand splinting to prevent contracture and reduce spasticity following stroke, Lannin and Herbert (2003) found insufficient evidence to either support or refute its effectiveness.

Literature regarding optimal thermoplastic splint designs and wearing times shows no consensus. Static designs may be volar or dorsal, and comparative studies have been done in attempts to determine quantitatively which design is more effective in tone reduction. A study by McPherson et al. (1982) demonstrated no significant difference between the two basic splint designs and encouraged therapists to reexamine the amount of wearing time prescribed so that tonal reduction occurs without unwarranted secondary stiffness.

A design clinically studied by McPherson (1981) used a dorsal forearm base, volar finger and thumb pans, and finger abductors to position the wrist in 30° of extension, the MCPs in 45° of flexion, the IPs in full extension, the fingers fully abducted, and the thumb in extension and abduction. McPherson reported that splint wearing resulted in a reduction of tone related to the length of time that subjects wore the splint and that the effects of splint wearing were not necessarily permanent.

Common static splint designs include resting pan splints, finger spreaders or abduction splints, and cone splints (Coppard & Lohman, 2001; Jacobs & Austin, 2003). Several pre-formed splints are commercially available (Figs. 16-76 and 16-77), but no clinical studies have been done to establish their fit and effectiveness.

Dynamic splint designs have also been developed to reduce tone in the wrist and hand. In a study of eight subjects, the finding was a greater reduction in hypertonus using a dynamic splint as compared with static splints and passive range of motion (McPherson, Becker, & Franszczak, 1985). Scherling and Johnson (1989) studied the effects of their dynamic splint design on 18 subjects, with all subjects achieving varying degrees of tone reduction with a minimum of 4 hours of splint use per day.

Soft splints made of neoprene can be custom fabricated (Casey & Kratz, 1988) or purchased commercially. A hand-based thumb loop can be used to decrease tone and position the thumb out of the palm for function (Fig. 16-78). To position the forearm, a long neoprene strap can be added to the hand splint.

A thermoplastic hand-based inhibitive weight-bearing splint described in the treatment of children with increased flexor tone (Coppard & Lohman, 2001; Kinghorn & Roberts, 1996) can also be used with adult patients having hypertonicity. This volar splint is custom fabricated to hold the fingers in extension and thumb in ra-

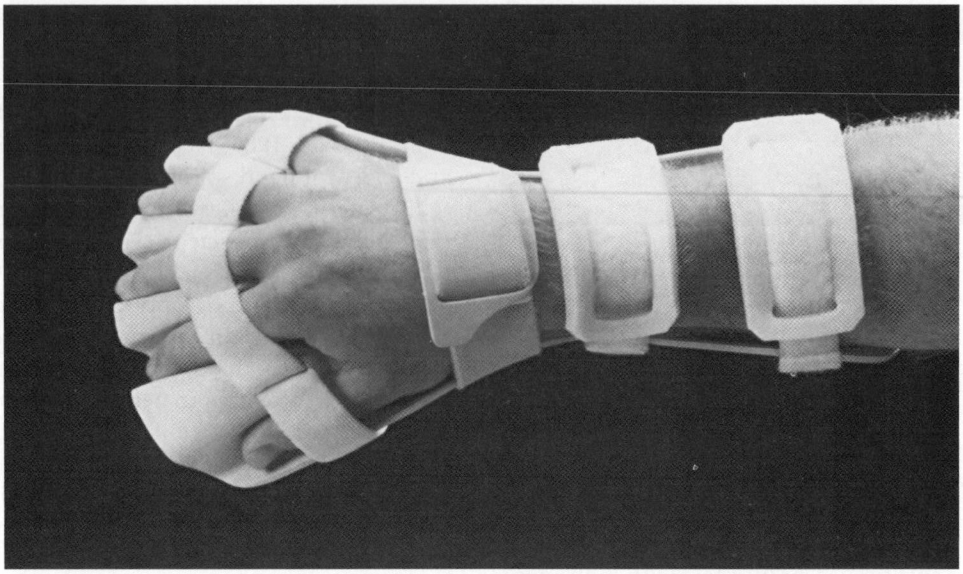

Figure 16-76 Rolyan® Anti-Spasticity Ball Splint with Slot and Loop Strapping.

dial abduction to enable the hand to be in an optimum position for upper extremity weight-bearing activities (Fig. 16-79).

Splinting may be an effective means of providing a low-cost, noninvasive method for decreasing tone in some patients but may not be effective in others (Langlois, Pederson, & Mackinnon, 1991). Continued research on the long-term effectiveness of splinting for tone reduction and the key patient variables that contribute to that effectiveness is needed. Meanwhile, therapists must carefully decide on splint use and monitor outcomes patient by patient.

SPECIALIZED PERMANENT FUNCTIONAL ORTHOSES

Permanent functional orthoses represent a great investment of time, cost, expertise, and commitment to fabrication, fit, training, and use by the patient-therapist-orthotist team. Proper fit, training, and successful functional use are accomplished only through close collaboration and communication among all who participate in the process. As with all orthoses, this process should begin with careful consideration of functional needs, achievable goals, and education of the patient and significant others in orthotic purpose and selection. Providing the patient with opportunities to interact with experienced users of similar equipment can be quite helpful to the patient, both before the prescription and during training.

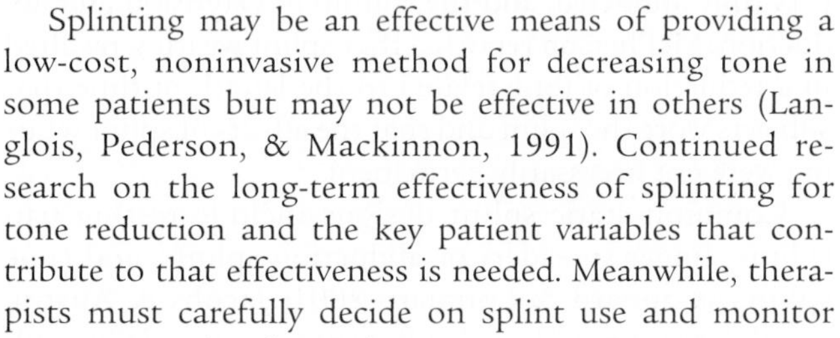

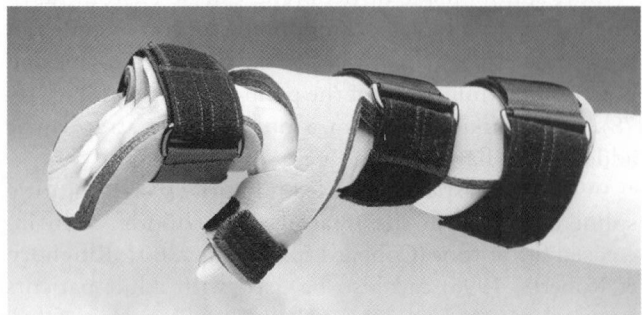

Figure 16-77 Progress™ Dorsal Anti-Spasticity Splint.

A permanent orthosis that is useful to the patient must be valued, accepted, and incorporated into the patient's body image. A prime prerequisite to acceptance is that the orthosis allows the patient to do something meaningful that cannot otherwise be done without it (Long & Shutt, 1986; Yasuda, Bowman, & Hsu, 1986). Since the orthosis will be used over the long term, the patient and caregivers must also be told whom to contact should problems arise after the therapy program has ended.

The principles of orthotic training are similar to those of prosthetics. They include testing of fit and mechanics; teaching the patient the names and functions of component parts; care of the orthosis; donning and doffing of the orthosis; controls training; and functional use training. Intensive practice under various conditions to encourage independent problem solving by the patient and skilled spontaneous use is a key element of training. Following is a closer look at two commonly used permanent functional orthoses.

Mobile Arm Supports

As described earlier in this chapter, the MAS (Figs. 16-59 and 16-60) is a mechanical device prescribed to support the weight of an arm and assist weak proximal muscles for function.

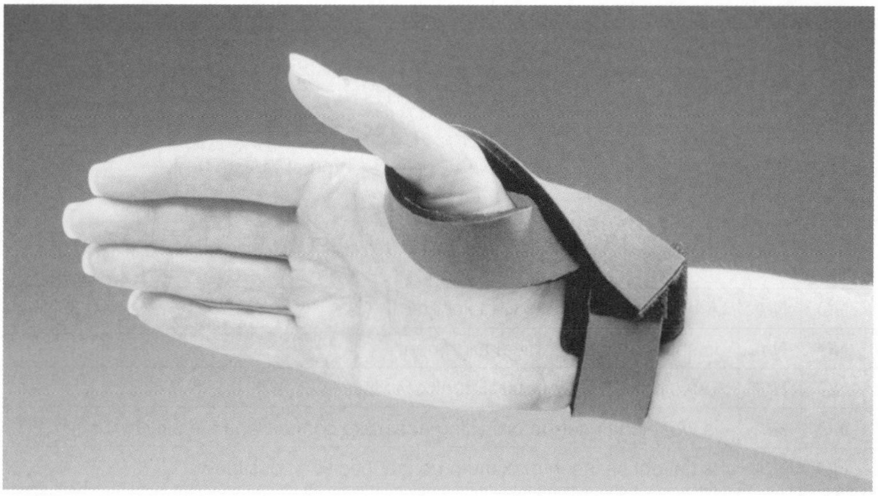

Figure 16-78 Rolyan® Thumb Loop.

Patient and Caregiver Education

If the patient has been actively involved in the decision making, a brief review of the MAS's purpose and capabilities should be sufficient. The patient and caregiver should be oriented to key component names and how they operate. Finally, they should know how to care for and maintain the orthosis.

Assembling and Balancing

Procedures for Practice 16-3 has instructions on how to assemble and balance the standard MAS assembly.

Training and Adjusting

Adaptive equipment or a WHO is commonly used in conjunction with the MAS, and these should be integrated during all phases of MAS training and adjusting. Once the patient is proficient with basic movement patterns, MAS training with all of the activities that the patient is interested in performing should be done. Any of these activities may require various fine component adjustments before final MAS adjustments are completed. Periodic follow-up may be required, especially with a growing child. Procedures for Practice 16-3 has information related to MAS training and adjusting.

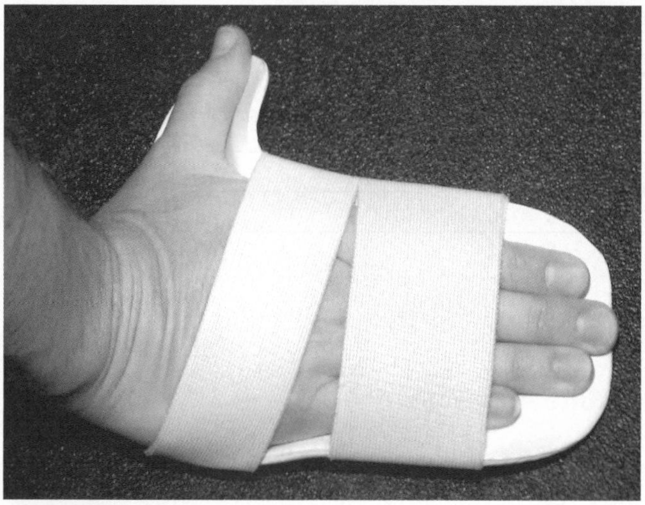

Figure 16-79 Custom thermoplastic hand-based weight-bearing splint.

Orthotic Checkout

Once final adjustments have been completed, bolts and screws should be checked for a secure fit. A MAS appraisal form (Fig. 16-80) can be used to ensure that all important details are assessed.

Wrist-Driven Wrist–Hand Orthosis

A WDWHO (Fig. 16-74), as previously described, is used to enhance hand function in the presence of distal muscle weakness by using wrist extensor power to enable prehension.

Orthotic Checkout

The therapist must begin with a careful inspection of the orthosis both on and off the patient. Optimal fit is crucial for maximum function. Ensuring smooth operation of mechanical parts, proper positioning of the digits for pad to pad prehension, and proper location of splint joint axes at the wrist and second MCP is essential. The strength of pinch should be assessed, and the length of the transfer bar should be changed by the orthotist to increase pinch strength as needed.

Straps should facilitate independent application and removal of the orthosis. Loops added to the ends of

Rancho Los Amigos National Rehabilitation Center — Occupational Therapy Department

MOBILE ARM SUPPORT APPRAISAL

Patient's Name______________________ Type of MAS (L)______________________

Date Fitted__________________________ Type of MAS (R)______________________

I. PATIENT'S POSITION IN WHEELCHAIR

YES	NO	N/A	Are hips well back in wheelchair?
YES	NO	N/A	Is spine in good vertical alignment?
YES	NO	N/A	Does patient have lateral trunk stability?
YES	NO	N/A	Is wheelchair set-up providing adequate comfort and stability?
YES	NO	N/A	Is patient sitting in maximum upright position possible?
YES	NO	N/A	Does patient have needed hand splints on?
YES	NO	N/A	Does patient meet requirements for passive range of motion?

II. MECHANICAL CHECKOUT

YES	NO	N/A	Are all screws tight?
YES	NO	N/A	Is bracket tightly secured on wheelchair?
YES	NO	N/A	Are all MAS arms and joints freely movable?
YES	NO	N/A	Is proximal arm inserted completely in bracket bearing tube?
YES	NO	N/A	Is distal arm inserted completely in proximal arm bearing tube?
YES	NO	N/A	Is bracket at proper height so shoulder is not forced into elevation?
YES	NO	N/A	Does elbow dial clear lapboard when trough is in "up" position?
YES	NO	N/A	Is patient's hand (in "up" position) as close to mouth as possible?
YES	NO	N/A	Can patient obtain maximum active reach?
YES	NO	N/A	Is patient's arm secured in trough?
YES	NO	N/A	Is trough long enough to give maximum support to forearm?
YES	NO	N/A	Is trough short enough to allow wrist flexion if desired?
YES	NO	N/A	Are trough edges rolled so that they do not contact forearm?
YES	NO	N/A	Is elbow secure and comfortable in elbow dial?
YES	NO	N/A	Is trough balanced correctly?
YES	NO	N/A	During vertical motion, is elbow dial free of distal arm?
YES	NO	N/A	Are vertical stops correctly placed for both up and down motions?
YES	NO	N/A	Are rubber band hooks secured?
YES	NO	N/A	Are rubber bands securely attached?

Figure 16-80 Mobile Arm Support Appraisal Form.

III. CONTROL CHECKOUT

YES	NO	N/A	Can patient control motion of proximal arm from either extreme?
YES	NO	N/A	Can patient control motion of distal arm from either extreme?
YES	NO	N/A	Can patient control vertical motion from either extreme?
YES	NO	N/A	Have stops been applied to limit motion, if necessary?
YES	NO	N/A	Does patient accomplish maximum horizontal reach in front of body?
YES	NO	N/A	Can patient easily reach mouth?
YES	NO	N/A	Can patient easily reach tabletop?
YES	NO	N/A	Can patient horizontally adduct arm sufficiently to clear doorways?
YES	NO	N/A	Is performance consistent from day to day?

IV. USE CHECKOUT

YES	NO	N/A	Are fine adjustments necessary to enable patient to perform different activities?
YES	NO	N/A	Are there some tasks that patient can perform better without MAS?
YES	NO	N/A	Is patient able to instruct caregivers in how to assemble MAS components?
YES	NO	N/A	Have patient and caregivers been instructed in care of MAS?

Figure 16-80 *(continued).*

the straps enable the patient to use the thumb of the other hand to fasten and unfasten them with increased ease.

The patient's ability to don and doff the orthosis is strongly related to independence in activities and to the patient's ultimate acceptance of the device. This is true especially if the patient must remove the orthosis to perform other activities such as propulsion of a wheelchair. Removal of the WDWHO is typically easier than application of it. With training, donning the orthosis can be accomplished in less than a minute (Clark, Waters, & Baumgarten, 1997). Initially, the orthosis should be placed on the patient for no more than 30 minutes. Upon removal, the skin should be carefully checked for any areas of redness. These red areas should be reassessed in half an hour, and if they are still present, the orthosis requires adjustment before the patient can use it. Once pressure problems have been resolved, wearing time can be gradually increased.

Patient and Caregiver Education

A brief review of the WDWHO's purpose and capabilities should be provided. The patient and caregivers should be instructed in the importance of skin inspection to prevent excessive pressure and skin breakdown. Accordingly, they should also be taught wearing tolerance and the schedule. They should be oriented to key component names and how the components operate prior to orthotic controls training. Finally, they should know how to care for and maintain the orthosis. Education in these areas should be reinforced throughout the orthotic training process.

Controls Training and Functional Use Training

Procedures for Practice 16-4 shows WDWHO controls training and use training.

EFFICACY AND OUTCOMES

The state of best evidence about upper extremity orthoses is limited at best (Evidence Table 16-1). Most published materials are anecdotal, based on clinical experience, or of varying study quality. Further research is needed to enhance our knowledge of splinting efficacy and variables that lead to optimum outcomes.

Evidence Table 16-1

Intervention	Description of Intervention Tested	Participants	Dosage	Type of Best Evidence and Level of Evidence	Benefit	Statistical Probability and Effect Size of Outcome	Reference
Hand splinting to prevent contracture and reduce spasticity following stroke	Different types of splints and splint designs.	230 patients.	Splint wear for unknown time up to 11 weeks, various wearing patterns.	Meta-analysis of 21 studies.	Insufficient evidence to either support or refute the effectiveness of hand splinting for adults following stroke.	Heterogeneity of study design, methods, splint design and regimen, and outcomes prevented the pooling of data to determine effect size.	Lannin & Herbert, 2003
Splinting for lateral epicondylitis	6 splint designs.	362 participants (277 patients and 85 normal subjects).	Splint wear for test session up to 4 weeks.	Systematic review of 11 studies.	Yes. Early positive, but not conclusive, effectiveness of splinting.	Not reported.	Borkholder et al., 2004
Splinting for carpal tunnel syndrome	Different types of splints and various angles of immobilization.	197 patients (242 hands).	Splint wear for 1–12 weeks, night only or night and day.	Systematic review of 6 studies.	Yes. Significant benefits from splinting across different splint types and wrist angles.	Not reported.	Muller et al., 2004

Splinting for pain relief in thumb arthritis	Soft pre-fabricated CMC/MP splint vs. rigid custom-made CMC splint.	25 patients with stage I or II osteoarthritis of the first CMC.	Randomly assigned to wear one splint for 1 week, followed by the other splint for 1 week.	Randomized controlled trial. IB1b	Yes. Significant decrease in pain. Greater reduction in pain when wearing soft splint. Pinch strength greater wearing soft splint. Higher satisfaction with soft vs. rigid splint. Problematic ADL easier to do using the soft splint.	$p \leq 0.001$, $Z = 3.09$, $r = 0.62$ $p = 0.019$, $Z = 2.075$, $r = 0.41$ $p = 0.012$, $Z = 2.26$, $r = 0.45$ $p \leq 0.001$, $Z = 3.09$, $r = 0.62$; 72% vs. 20% preferred soft splint 48% vs. 26% reported activities easier to do with soft splint	Weiss et al., 2004
Compliance-enhancing approach to resting hand splint wear	Approach emphasizing learning principles, sharing of expectations, positive affect and behaviors by therapist (therapeutic rapport), and patient assumption of responsibility vs. standard approach.	40 outpatients with rheumatoid arthritis and no prior referral for resting hand splints; mean age = 48.8 years.	Initial treatment session plus follow-up call at ~2 weeks. Splint wear for 28–56 days.	Randomized controlled trial. IB1b	Yes. The treated group showed greater compliance with splint wear vs. other group.	$t_{(38)} = -1.97$, $p = 0.056$, $r = 0.30$	Feinberg, 1992

CASE EXAMPLE

Orthotic Intervention in a Patient with Peripheral Nerve Injury

Occupational Therapy Intervention Process	Clinical Reasoning Process: Objectives	Clinical Reasoning Process: Examples of Therapist's Internal Dialogue
Patient Information Ms. N., a 22-year-old woman 8 weeks post motor vehicle collision, was referred to outpatient occupational therapy for evaluation and splinting of her left arm. She had a brachial plexus traction injury and a humeral fracture, treated with a closed reduction and fracture brace (purpose: to immobilize for healing). Prior to her injury, she was right-hand dominant and employed full time as a secretary.	Appreciate the context	"Ms. N. is dealing with a significant injury with an enormous impact on her life. I am concerned not only about the status of her left arm, but also about the disruption of her routines and roles. She is obviously frustrated about not being able to work and having to ask her mother to help with most tasks. I need to help her feel empowered and instill hope for her future."
On initial assessment, the following problems were identified as related to her left upper extremity: (1) poor positioning of the entire arm, with Ms. N. using her right arm to help and support the left arm; (2) absent motor function and impaired sensation throughout; (3) limited passive range of motion of the shoulder in all planes, forearm supination, MCP flexion, and thumb abduction; (4) traction pain in the shoulder; and (5) lack of functional use for any activities.	Develop intervention hypotheses	"I think that poor left arm positioning is the factor contributing most to her lack of occupational functioning. If I can free up her right arm for function, I believe this will go a long way in helping her cope with her injury."
	Select an intervention approach	"Orthoses will be an integral part of Ms. N.'s treatment and will need to be carefully selected based on her clinical and functional status. From reviewing the literature, I know that collaborating with the patient closely throughout the splinting process is crucial to a successful outcome. I also understand that recovery may occur at a slow rate and orthoses will need to be durable."
	Reflect on competence	"I have treated patients having similar peripheral nerve injuries in the past and have seen good functional recovery occur in many cases. These past experiences have also taught me that I have to do what I can to help Ms. N. be patient since recovery time with these types of injury can be frustratingly slow."
Summary of Short-Term Goals and Progress Ms. N. was fitted with a standard pouch sling that was easy to don and doff and supported the weight of her arm with the goals of pain relief and freeing her right arm for functional use (purposes: to support a painful joint and to protect tissues); she was also fitted with a custom-fabricated static wrist extension–thumb abduction splint to prevent the loss of wrist extension and to regain MCP flexion and thumb abduction range of motion (purposes: to prevent contractures and to restore mobility).	Assess the patient's comprehension Understand what he or she is doing Ascertain the patient's endorsement of plan Compare actual to expected performance Know the person Appreciate the context	"I think it is important to begin with an intensive program that will quickly address Ms. N.'s clinical and functional needs. Even though they have to travel a good distance from home, Ms. N. and her mother understand the importance of early therapy intervention to improve the prognosis for recovery. I acknowledge the hardship this causes for them, so I promise to minimize the therapy visits as much as possible."

Next Steps As Ms. N.'s neuromuscular recovery progressed, the following orthoses were used in response to new problems and functional potential identified: **Week 11:** The sling was discontinued, as shoulder and elbow strength had improved to 3 to 3+ and traction pain had resolved. Ms. N. continued to use the wrist extension–thumb abduction splint during the day. At night, Ms. N. wore a custom-fabricated composite wrist and finger extension static splint to prevent long flexor tightness from unopposed finger flexors that had regained 3+ strength (purpose: to prevent contractures). **Week 17:** At night, Ms. N. wore a custom-fabricated serial static elbow extension splint to regain elbow extension range of motion lost to initial positioning from the sling, an ineffective home range-of-motion program, and return of unopposed 3+ elbow flexor strength (purpose: to restore mobility).	Anticipate present and future patient concerns	"I need to be ready to respond to Ms. N.'s unique needs. I need to closely monitor for changes in range of motion, motor function, and sensory function, and be on the lookout for development of deformity that may occur from muscle imbalance. I want to optimize her ability to use her left arm as soon as her clinical status allows. To enable an optimum functional and clinical outcome, I need to discontinue orthoses as soon as they become unnecessary and implement new orthoses as different needs arise."
Week 21: A Colditz radial nerve splint was fabricated to substitute for weak muscles supplied by the radial nerve and to enhance hand function as long finger flexors and wrist flexors recovered to sufficient strength of 3+. Ms. N. wore this splint during the day to allow functional use of the hand during light tasks (purpose: to substitute for weak or absent muscles).	Analyze patient's comprehension	"It is important to continuously educate Ms. N. on her status so she can see her recovery progressing and understand how important the various orthoses are to optimize her functional outcome."
Week 26: The Colditz radial nerve splint was discontinued, as wrist and long finger extensors had regained 3+ strength. A custom-fabricated thermoplastic lumbrical bar splint for the ring and small fingers was issued to address residual weakness of intrinsic muscles innervated by the ulnar nerve, leading to clawing. Ms. N. wore this splint during the day to assist with hand opening and prevent IP flexion contractures (purposes: to restrict unwanted motion and to prevent contractures). **Week 28:** A dynamic forearm rotation splint was fabricated from a commercial kit; Ms. N. wore it at night to regain full supination range of motion initially lost from positioning and an imbalance of forearm rotator muscle strength (purpose: to restore mobility). **Week 36:** No further splinting was required, as Ms. N. had full neuromuscular recovery. Ms. N. was able to return to her previous employment with full functional use of her left arm.	Decide if she should continue or discontinue therapy and/or return in the future	"I also need to give Ms. N. the opportunity to voice her questions, concerns, and preferences so that we can work together to select the most appropriate orthoses and design optimal wearing schedules."

CLINICAL REASONING IN OCCUPATIONAL THERAPY PRACTICE

Selecting the Most Appropriate Orthoses for a Patient

Ms. N. is a young, socially active woman who was living independently. What would the therapist anticipate to be Ms. N's primary concerns in orthotic selection? How could the therapist best engage her in the orthotic selection process while determining priorities for her orthotic needs? What are the clinical and functional components that must be closely monitored to determine specific orthotic needs?

SUMMARY REVIEW QUESTIONS

1. What is the role of the occupational therapist in orthotic rehabilitation?
2. Define orthosis.
3. Name the purposes for which splinting may be used.
4. What are key factors for selecting an orthosis for a particular patient?
5. Discuss factors that may enhance splint wearing and those that may interfere with it.
6. Discuss why a static splint may be chosen and the precautions related to such splints.
7. Describe two dynamic splints and the purposes for which they are used.
8. Select an orthosis to decrease an elbow flexion contracture, discuss the reasons for your choice, and state the principle or principles that it implements.
9. Discuss two types of finger or hand orthoses that assist in restoring function while stabilizing a joint.
10. For which type of patient would you choose a wrist-driven wrist–hand orthosis?
11. Name the basic components of a standard MAS and two diagnostic categories of candidates who may benefit from its use.
12. Describe a treatment session to improve a patient's hand-to-mouth and hand-to-table control of a MAS and basic adjustments that can be made to the MAS to facilitate these motions.
13. What are the pros and cons of various orthoses designed to modify tone?

ACKNOWLEDGMENTS

I thank Y. Lynn Yasuda, MSEd, OTR, FAOTA, and Maura Walsh, OTR/L, CHT, for sharing their clinical expertise and advice; Michele Berro, MA, OTR/L, for assisting with obtaining photographs; Paul Weinreich (in memoriam), former Medical Photographer at Rancho Los Amigos National Rehabilitation Center, for his photography and technical support; and the colleagues and patients who inspire and teach me daily.

I acknowledge the following contributions:

- Figures 16-2–16-5, 16-9, 16-11–16-13, 16-19, 16-23, 16-27, 16-29, 16-33–16-37, 16-42, 16-43, 16-45, 16-48, 16-52, 16-56, 16-57, 16-61–16-63, 16-66, 16-68, 16-69, 16-72–16-75, 16-79, and 16-80 courtesy of Rancho Los Amigos National Rehabilitation Center, Downey, CA.
- Figures 16-6–16-8, 16-10, 16-17, 16-18, 16-32, 16-38, 16-39, 16-50, 16-51, 16-55, 16-59, 16-67, 16-71, 16-76, and 16-78 courtesy of Sammons Preston Rolyan, Bilingbrook, IL.
- Figure 16-4–16-16, 16-20–16-22, 16-25, 16-28, 16-30, 16-31, 16-40, 16-41, 16-53, 16-54, 16-65, 16-70, and 16-77 courtesy of North Coast Medical Center, Inc., Morgan Hill, CA.
- Figure 16-26 courtesy of AliMed, Inc., Dedham, MA.
- Figures 16-44 and 16-46 courtesy of Silver Ring Splint Company, Charlottesville, VA.
- Figure 16-49 courtesy of Joint Active Systems, Inc., Effingham, IL.

References

Aiello, B. (1998). Epicondylitis. In G. L. Clark, E. F. S. Wilgis, B. Aiello, D. Eckhaus, & L. Valdata Eddington (Eds.), *Hand rehabilitation: A practical guide* (2nd ed., pp. 175–179). New York: Churchill Livingstone.

Allen, V. (1971). Follow-up study of wrist-driven flexor-hinge-splint use. *American Journal of Occupational Therapy, 25,* 420–422.

American Society of Hand Therapists. (1992). *Splint classification system.* Chicago: American Society of Hand Therapists.

Bassini, L. B., & Patel, M. R. (1994). Buddy sleeves. *Journal of Hand Therapy, 7,* 257–258.

Bell-Krotoski, J. A. (2002). Plaster cylinder casting for contractures of the interphalangeal joints. In E. J. Mackin, A. D. Callahan, T. M. Skirven, L. H. Schneider, & A. L. Osterman (Eds.), *Rehabilitation of the hand and upper extremity* (5th ed., pp. 1839–1845). St. Louis: Mosby.

Bell-Krotoski, J. A., & Figarola, J. H. (1995). Biomechanics of soft tissue growth and remodeling with plaster casting. *Journal of Hand Therapy, 8,* 131–137.

Bobath, B. (1990). *Adult hemiplegia: Evaluation and treatment* (3rd ed.). London: William Heinemann Medical.

Borkholder, C. D., Hill, V. A., & Fess, E. E. (2004). The efficacy of splinting for lateral epicondylitis: A systematic review. *Journal of Hand Therapy, 17,* 181–199.

Brand, P. W. (2002). The forces of dynamic splinting: Ten questions before applying a dynamic splint to the hand. In E. J. Mackin, A. D. Callahan, T. M. Skirven, L. H. Schneider, & A. L. Osterman (Eds.), *Rehabilitation of the hand and upper extremity* (5th ed., pp. 1811–1817). St. Louis: Mosby.

Breger-Lee, D. (1995). Objective and subjective observations of low-temperature thermoplastic materials. *Journal of Hand Therapy, 8,* 138–143.

Callahan, A. D., & McEntee, P. (1986). Splinting proximal interphalangeal joint flexion contractures: A new design. *American Journal of Occupational Therapy, 40,* 408–413.

Callinan, N. J., & Mathiowetz, V. (1996). Soft versus hard resting splints in rheumatoid arthritis: Pain relief, preference, and compliance. *American Journal of Occupational Therapy, 50,* 347–353.

Canelon, M. F. (1995). Material properties: A factor in the selection and application of splinting materials for athletic wrist and hand injuries. *Journal of Orthopedic Sports Physical Therapy, 22,* 164–172.

Carlson, J. D., & Trombly, C. A. (1983). The effect of wrist immobilization on performance of the Jebsen Hand Function Test. *American Journal of Occupational Therapy, 37,* 167–175.

Casey, C. A., & Kratz, E. J. (1988). Soft splinting with neoprene: The thumb abduction supinator splint. *American Journal of Occupational Therapy, 42,* 395–398.

Clark, D. R., Waters, R. L., & Baumgarten, J. M. (1997). Upper limb orthoses for the spinal cord injured patient. In B. Goldberg & J. D. Hsu (Eds.), *Atlas of orthoses and assistive devices* (3rd ed., pp. 291–303). St. Louis: Mosby.

Clark, E. N. (1997). A preliminary investigation of the neoprene tube finger extension splint. *Journal of Hand Therapy, 10,* 213–221.

Colditz, J. C. (1995). Spring-wire extension splinting of the proximal interphalangeal joint. In J. M. Hunter, E. J. Mackin, & A. D. Callahan (Eds.), *Rehabilitation of the hand: Surgery and therapy* (4th ed., pp. 1617–1629). St. Louis: Mosby.

Colditz, J. C. (2002a). Therapist's management of the stiff hand. In E. J. Mackin, A. D. Callahan, T. M. Skirven, L. H. Schneider, & A. L. Osterman (Eds.), *Rehabilitation of the hand and upper extremity* (5th ed., pp. 1021–1049). St. Louis: Mosby.

Colditz, J. C. (2002b). Splinting the hand with a peripheral nerve injury. In E. J. Mackin, A. D. Callahan, T. M. Skirven, L. H. Schneider, & A. L. Osterman (Eds.), *Rehabilitation of the hand and upper extremity* (5th ed., pp. 622–634). St. Louis: Mosby.

Collelo-Abraham, K. (1990). Dynamic pronation-supination splint. In J. M. Hunter, J. L. H. Schneider, E. J. Mackin, & A. D. Callahan (Eds.), *Rehabilitation of the hand: Surgery and therapy* (3rd ed., pp. 1134–1139). St. Louis: Mosby.

Collier, S. E., & Thomas, J. J. (2002). Range of motion at the wrist: A comparison study of four wrist extension orthoses and the free hand. *American Journal of Occupational Therapy, 56,* 180–184.

Collins, L. (1999). Helping patients help themselves: Improving orthotic use. *Occupational Therapy Practice, 4,* 30–34.

Coppard, B. M., & Lohman, H. (2001). *Introduction to splinting: A clinical reasoning and problem-solving approach* (2nd ed.). St. Louis: Mosby.

Evans, R. B. (2002). An update on extensor tendon management. In E. J. Mackin, A. D. Callahan, T. M. Skirven, L. H. Schneider, & A. L. Osterman (Eds.), *Rehabilitation of the hand and upper extremity* (5th ed., pp. 542–579). St. Louis: Mosby.

Feinberg, J. (1992). Effect of the arthritis health professional on compliance with use of resting hand splints by patients with rheumatoid arthritis. *Arthritis Care and Research, 5,* 17–23.

Fess, E. E. (1988). Force magnitude of commercial spring-coil and spring-wire splints designed to extend the proximal interphalangeal joint. *Journal of Hand Therapy, 1,* 86–90.

Fess, E. E. (1995). Splints: Mechanics and convention. *Journal of Hand Therapy, 8,* 124–130.

Fess, E. E., Gettle, K. S., Philips, C. A., & Janson, J. R. (Eds.). (2005). *Hand and upper extremity splinting: Principles and methods* (3rd ed.). St. Louis: Mosby.

Fess, E. E., & McCollum, M. (1998). The influence of splinting on healing tissues. *Journal of Hand Therapy, 11,* 157–161.

Foucher, G., Binhamer, P., Cange, S., & Lenoble, E. (1996). Long term results of splintage of mallet finger. *International Orthopaedics, 20,* 129–131.

Gelberman, R. H., Rydevik, B. L., Pess, G. M., Szabo, R. M., & Lundborg, G. (1988). Carpal tunnel syndrome: A scientific basis for clinical care. *Orthopedic Clinics of North America, 19,* 115–124.

Gilbert-Lenef, L. (1994). Soft ulnar deviation splint. *Journal of Hand Therapy, 7,* 29–30.

Groth, G. N., & Wulf, M. B. (1995). Compliance with hand rehabilitation: Health beliefs and strategies. *Journal of Hand Therapy, 8,* 18–22.

Hill, J. (1994). The effects of casting on upper extremity motor disorders after brain injury. *American Journal of Occupational Therapy, 48,* 219–224.

Jacobs, M. L., & Austin, N. M. (Eds.). (2003). *Splinting the hand and upper extremity: Principles and process.* Baltimore: Lippincott Williams & Wilkins.

Jensen, C., & Rayan, G. (1996). Buddy strapping of mismatched fingers: The offset buddy strap. *Journal of Hand Surgery, 21,* 317–318.

Keenan, M. A. (1997). Upper extremity orthoses for the brain-injured patient. In B. Goldberg & J. D. Hsu (Eds.), *Atlas of orthoses and assistive devices* (3rd ed., pp. 281–289). St. Louis: Mosby.

Kinghorn, J., & Roberts, G. (1996). The effect of an inhibitive weight-bearing splint on tone and function: A single-case study. *American Journal of Occupational Therapy, 50,* 807–815.

Kirkpatrick, W. H., Kozin, S. H., & Uhl, R. L. (1996). Early motion after arthroplasty. *Hand Clinics, 12,* 73–86.

Knox, C., Engel, W., & Seibens, A. (1971). Results of a survey on the use of a wrist-driven splint for prehension. *American Journal of Occupational Therapy, 15,* 109–111.

Lamay, G. (1994). Buddy splint. *Journal of Hand Therapy, 7,* 30–31.

Lange, M. L. (1999). Positioning the upper extremities. *Occupational Therapy Practice, 4,* 49–50.

Langlois, S., Pederson, L., & Mackinnon, J. (1991). The effects of splinting on the spastic hemiplegic hand: Report of a feasibility study. *Canadian Journal of Occupational Therapy, 58,* 17–25.

Lannin, N., & Herbert, R. (2003). Is hand splinting effective for adults following stroke? A systematic review and methodological critique of published research. *Clinical Rehabilitation, 17,* 807–816.

Long, C., & Shutt, A. (1986). Upper limb orthotics. In J. B. Redford (Ed.), *Orthotics etcetera* (3rd ed., pp. 198–270). Baltimore: Williams & Wilkins.

Lunsford, T. R. (1997). Upper limb orthoses. In B. Goldberg & J. D. Hsu (Eds.), *Atlas of orthoses and assistive devices* (3rd ed., pp. 195–208). St. Louis: Mosby.

Lunsford, T. R., & Wallace, J. M. (1997). The orthotic prescription. In B. Goldberg & J. D. Hsu (Eds.), *Atlas of orthoses and assistive devices* (3rd ed., pp. 3–14). St. Louis: Mosby.

McFarland, E. G., Curl, L. A., Urquhart, M. C., & Kellam, K. (1997). Shoulder immobilization devices: 3. Abduction braces and pillows. *Orthopaedic Nursing, 16,* 47–54.

McKee, P., & Morgan, L. (1998). *Orthotics in rehabilitation: Splinting the hand and body.* Philadelphia: Davis.

McKee, P., & Rivard, A. (2004). Orthoses as enablers of occupation: Client-centered splinting for better outcomes. *Canadian Journal of Occupational Therapy, 71,* 306–314.

McPherson, J. J. (1981). Objective evaluation of a splint designed to reduce hypertonicity. *American Journal of Occupational Therapy, 35,* 189–194.

McPherson, J. J., Becker, A. H., & Franszczak, N. (1985). Dynamic splint to reduce the passive component of hypertonicity. *Archives of Physical Medicine and Rehabilitation, 66,* 249–252.

McPherson, J. J., Kreimeyer, D., Aalderks, M., & Gallagher, T. (1982). A comparison of dorsal and volar resting hand splints in the reduction of hypertonus. *American Journal of Occupational Therapy, 36,* 664–670.

Melvin, J. L. (1989). *Rheumatic disease in the adult and child: Occupational therapy and rehabilitation* (3rd ed.). Philadelphia: Davis.

Melvin, J. L. (1995). Orthotic treatment of the hand: What's new? *Bulletin on the Rheumatic Diseases, 44,* 5–8.

Moodie, N., Brisbin, J., & Margan, A. (1986). Subluxation of the glenohumeral joint in hemiplegia: Evaluation of supportive devices. *Physiotherapy Canada, 38,* 151–157.

Muller, M., Tsui, D., Schnurr, R., Biddulph-Deisroth, L., Hard, J., & MacDermid, J. C. (2004). Effectiveness of hand therapy interventions in primary management of carpal tunnel syndrome: A systematic review. *Journal of Hand Therapy, 17,* 210–228.

Murphy, M. S. (1990). An adjustable splint for forearm supination. *American Journal of Occupational Therapy, 44,* 936–939.

Neuhaus, B. E., Ascher, E. R., Coullon, B. A., Donohoe, M. V., Einbond, A., Glover, J. M., Goldberg, S. R., & Takai, V. L. (1981). A survey of rationales for and against hand splinting in hemiplegia. *American Journal of Occupational Therapy, 35,* 83–90.

Nuismer, B. A., Ekes, A. M., & Holm, M. B. (1997). The use of low-load prolonged stretch devices in rehabilitation programs in the Pacific Northwest. *American Journal of Occupational Therapy, 51,* 538–543.

Oakes, T. W., Ward, J. F., Gray, R. M., Klauber, M. R., & Moody, P. M. (1970). Family expectations and arthritis patients' compliance to a resting hand splint regimen. *Journal of Chronic Diseases, 22,* 757–764.

Pagnotta, A., Baron, M., & Korner-Bitensky, N. (1998). The effect of a static wrist orthosis on hand function in individuals with rheumatoid arthritis. *Journal of Rheumatology, 25,* 879–885.

Paternostro-Sluga, T., Keilani, M., Posch, M., & Fialka-Moser, V. (2003). Factors that influence the duration of splint wear in peripheral nerve lesions. *American Journal of Physical Medicine and Rehabilitation, 82,* 86–95.

Philips, C. A. (1989). Management of the patient with rheumatoid arthritis: The role of the hand therapist. *Hand Clinics, 5,* 291–309.

Poole, J. L., Whitney, S. L., Hangeland, N., & Baker, C. (1990). The effectiveness of inflatable pressure splints on motor function in stroke patients. *Occupational Therapy Journal of Research, 10,* 360–366.

Prosser, R. (1996). Splinting in the management of proximal interphalangeal joint flexion contracture. *Journal of Hand Therapy, 9,* 378–386.

Rennie, H. J. (1996). Evaluation of the effectiveness of a metacarpophalangeal ulnar deviation orthosis. *Journal of Hand Therapy, 9,* 371–377.

Richard, R., Shanesy, C. P., & Miller, S. F. (1995). Dynamic versus static splints: A prospective case for sustained stress. *Journal of Burn Care and Rehabilitation, 16,* 284–287.

Richard, R., & Staley, M. (1994). *Burn care and rehabilitation: Principles and practice.* Philadelphia: Davis.

Richard, R., Staley, M., Daugherty, M. B., Miller, S. F., & Warden, G. D. (1994). The wide variety of designs for dorsal hand burn splints. *Journal of Burn Care and Rehabilitation, 15,* 275–280.

Scherling, E., & Johnson, H. (1989). A tone-reducing wrist-hand orthosis. *American Journal of Occupational Therapy, 43,* 609–611.

Shepherd, C. C., & Ruzicka, S. H. (1991). Tenodesis brace use by persons with spinal cord injuries. *American Journal of Occupational Therapy, 45,* 81–83.

Smith, R. O., & Okamoto, G. A. (1981). Checklist for the prescription of slings for the hemiplegic patient. *American Journal of Occupational Therapy, 35,* 91–95.

Spaulding, S. J. (1999). Biomechanical analysis of four supports for the subluxed hemiparetic shoulder. *Canadian Journal of Occupational Therapy, 66,* 169–175.

Stern, E. B. (1991). Wrist extensor orthoses: Dexterity and grip strength across four styles. *American Journal of Occupational Therapy, 45,* 42–49.

Stern, E. B. (1996). Grip strength and finger dexterity across five styles of commercial wrist orthoses. *American Journal of Occupational Therapy, 50,* 32–38.

Stern, E. B., Callinan, N., Hank, M., Lewis, E. J., Schousboe, J. T., & Ytterberg, S. R. (1998). Neoprene splinting: Dermatological issues. *American Journal of Occupational Therapy, 52,* 573–578.

Stern, E. B., Ytterberg, S. R., Krug, H. E., & Mahowald, M. L. (1996). Finger dexterity and hand function: Effect of three commercial wrist extensor orthoses on patients with rheumatoid arthritis. *Arthritis Care and Research, 9,* 197–205.

Stern, E. B., Ytterberg, S. R., Larson, L. M., Portoghese, C. P., Kratz, W. N. R., & Mahowald, M. L. (1997). Commercial wrist extensor orthoses: A descriptive study of use and preference in patients with rheumatoid arthritis. *Arthritis Care and Research, 10,* 27–35.

Stewart Pettengill, K. M. (2002). Therapist's management of the complex injury. In E. J. Mackin, A. D. Callahan, T. M. Skirven, L. H. Schneider, & A. L. Osterman (Eds.), *Rehabilitation of the hand and upper extremity* (5th ed., pp. 1411–1427). St. Louis: Mosby.

Stewart Pettengill, K. M., & vanStrien, G. (2002). Postoperative management of flexor tendon injuries. In E. J. Mackin, A. D. Callahan, T. M. Skirven, L. H. Schneider, & A. L. Osterman (Eds.), *Rehabilitation of the hand and upper extremity* (5th ed., pp. 431–456). St. Louis: Mosby.

Tribuzi, S. M. (2002). Serial plaster splinting. In E. J. Mackin, A. D. Callahan, T. M. Skirven, L. H. Schneider, & A. L. Osterman (Eds.), *Rehabilitation of the hand and upper extremity* (5th ed., pp. 1828–1838). St. Louis: Mosby.

Wallny, T., Westermann, K., Sagebiel, C., Reimer, M., & Wagner, U. A. (1997). Functional treatment of humeral shaft fractures: Indications and results. *Journal of Orthopaedic Trauma, 11,* 283–287.

Walsh, M. (1987). Half-lapboard for hemiplegic patients. *American Journal of Occupational Therapy, 41,* 533–535.

Weiss, N. D., Gordon, L., Bloom, T., So, Y., & Rempel, D. M. (1995). Position of the wrist associated with the lowest carpal tunnel pressure: Implications for splint design. *Journal of Bone and Joint Surgery, 77-A,* 1695–1699.

Weiss, S., La Stayo, P., Mills, A., & Bramlet, D. (2004). Splinting the degenerative basal joint: Custom-made or prefabricated neoprene? *Journal of Hand Therapy, 17,* 401–406.

Wilton, J. C. (1997). *Hand splinting: Principles of design and fabrication.* Philadelphia: Saunders.

Wuori, J. L., Overend, T. J., Kramer, J. F., & MacDermid, J. (1998). Strength and pain measures associated with lateral epicondylitis bracing. *Archives of Physical Medicine and Rehabilitation, 79,* 832–837.

Yasuda, Y. L., Bowman, K., & Hsu, J. D. (1986). Mobile arm supports: Criteria for successful use in muscle disease patients. *Archives of Physical Medicine and Rehabilitation, 67,* 253–256.

Zorowitz, R. D., Hughes, M. B., Idank, D., Ikai, T., & Johnston, M. V. (1996). Shoulder pain and subluxation after stroke: Correlation or coincidence? *American Journal of Occupational Therapy, 50,* 194–201.

Zorowitz, R. D., Idank, D., Ikai, T., Hughes, M. B., & Johnston, M. V. (1995). Shoulder subluxation after stroke: A comparison of four supports. *Archives of Physical Medicine and Rehabilitation, 76,* 763–771.

LEARNING OBJECTIVES

After studying this chapter, the reader will be able to do the following:

1. Describe the anatomical, biomechanical, and mechanical principles applied to splint construction.
2. Identify the properties, benefits, and limitations of various splinting materials.
3. Recognize factors affecting splint wear compliance.
4. Explain design, pattern making, and construction for three splints.
5. Describe the components of a splint checkout.

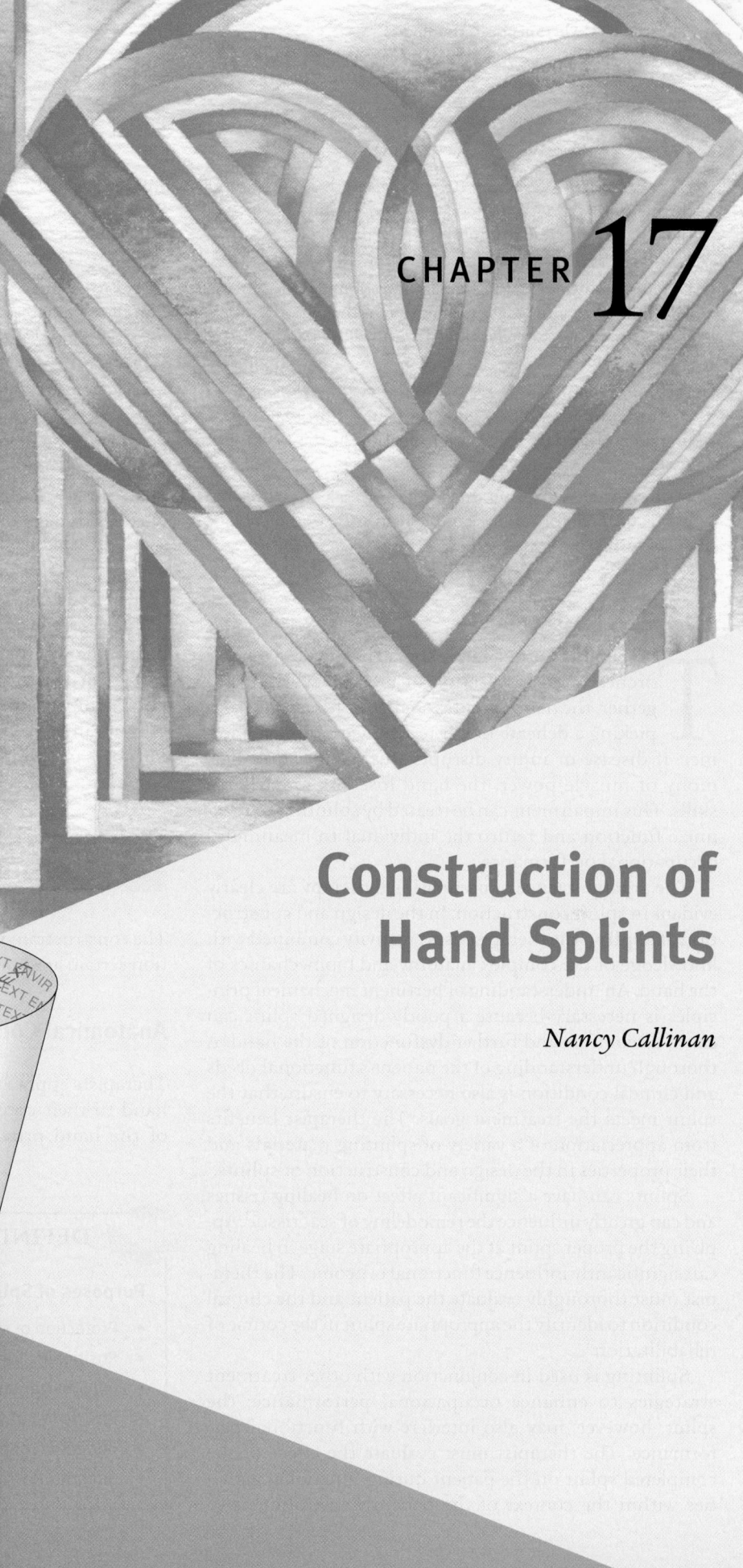

CHAPTER 17

Construction of Hand Splints

Nancy Callinan

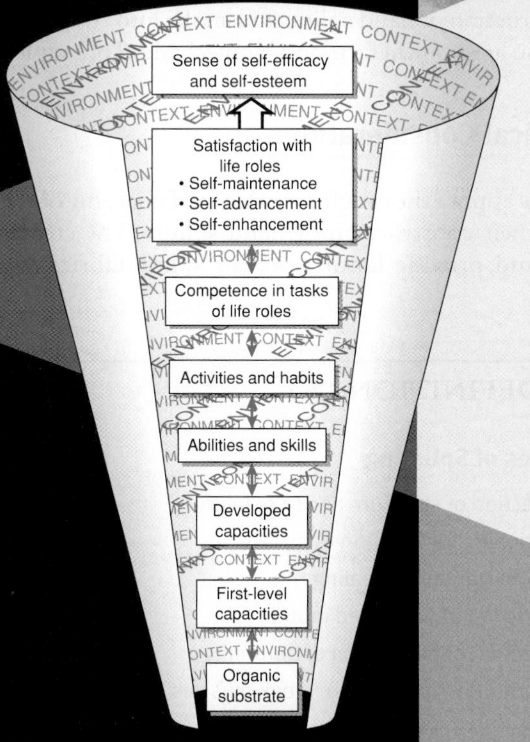

Glossary

Dual obliquity—Variance between the length and height of the metacarpals, with the radial side longer and higher than the ulnar side. These relationships must be considered when splinting the hand.

Dynamic splint—A splint that applies a mobile force in one direction while allowing active motion in the opposite direction. The mobile force is applied with rubber bands, elastic thread, or springs.

Fibroblastic phase—Stage of wound healing that follows the inflammatory phase, during which fibroblasts proliferate and initiate collagen production in the healing of tissues.

Haldex gauge—A spring gauge that precisely measures the grams of force for rubber band dynamic traction or torque angle curves.

Inflammatory phase—Phase of wound healing immediately following injury or surgery; characterized by edema and infiltration of leukocytes and macrophages to begin healing of the injured tissues.

Maturation phase—Stage of wound healing that follows the fibroblastic phase; characterized by wound contraction, remodeling, and maturation of the healed tissues.

Serial static splint—A splint with no moving parts designed to be remolded as a contracture improves.

Splint—A device applied to the body to provide protection, positioning, immobilization, restriction, correction, or prevention of deformity for the splinted part; an orthosis.

Static progressive splint—A splint designed to stretch contractures through the application of incrementally adjusted static force to promote lengthening of contracted tissues.

The hand is an incredible tool. Through a carefully orchestrated integration of muscles working together, the hand executes a range of functions from picking a delicate flower to firmly gripping a hammer. If disease or injury disrupts this balance and harmony of muscle power, the hand loses its remarkable skills. This impairment can be treated by splinting to maximize function and return the individual to meaningful occupational performance.

The art and science of occupational therapy are clearly evident in splint construction. In the design and construction of a **splint**, the therapist uses creativity combined with knowledge of the complex anatomy and biomechanics of the hand. An understanding of pertinent mechanical principles is necessary because a poorly designed splint can cause discomfort and further dysfunction of the hand. A thorough understanding of the patient's functional needs and clinical condition is also necessary to ensure that the splint meets the treatment goals. The therapist benefits from appreciation of a variety of splinting materials and their properties in the design and construction of splints.

Splints can have a significant effect on healing tissues and can greatly influence the remodeling of scar tissue. Applying the proper splint at the appropriate stage in healing can significantly influence functional outcome. The therapist must thoroughly evaluate the patient and the clinical condition to identify the appropriate splint in the course of rehabilitation.

Splinting is used in conjunction with other treatment strategies to enhance occupational performance; the splint, however, may also interfere with functional performance. The therapist must evaluate the effect of the completed splint on the patient during functional activities within the context of the patient's environment to determine whether the splint contributes to the goals of treatment. A splint that impairs performance by causing poor compensatory patterns of movement may necessitate modification of the splint or the wearing schedule. Purposes of splinting are reviewed in Definition 17-1.

ANATOMICAL AND BIOMECHANICAL CONSIDERATIONS IN SPLINTING

The construction of hand splints must take into consideration certain anatomical facts and biomechanical principles.

Anatomical Considerations

Therapists apply a thorough knowledge of anatomy of the hand to their construction of hand splints. The creases of the hand provide landmarks for splint fabrication

DEFINITION 17-1

Purposes of Splinting

- Protection of structure at risk of injury
- Positioning for function
- Immobilization for healing
- Restriction of undesired motion
- Correction or prevention of deformity
- Substitution for absent or weak muscles

(Coppard & Lohman, 1996). These creases identify the axis of motion for the corresponding joint. The distal edge of a splint must not extend beyond a crease if motion at that joint is desired (Fig. 17-1). Bony prominences of the hand and wrist (Fig. 17-2) can create pressure points if the splint does not adequately conform to these areas. Potential pressure points are common on the dorsum of the hand and wrist. The arches of the hand (Fig. 17-3)—the distal transverse (metacarpal) arch, the proximal transverse (carpal) arch, and the longitudinal arch—ensure optimal hand function (Coppard & Lohman, 1996; Tubiana, Thomine, & Mackin, 1996). The splint must conform to these arches to support the functional position of the hand.

The functional position of the hand is 15–30° of wrist dorsiflexion, neutral to slight ulnar deviation, 15–20° of metacarpophalangeal (MCP) flexion, 10° of flexion at the proximal interphalangeal (PIP) and distal interphalangeal (DIP) joints, palmar abduction of the thumb, and extension of the metacarpophalangeal (MP) and interphalangeal (IP) joints of the thumb (Coppard & Lohman, 1996). This position places the muscles, tendons, and ligaments at a resting length and in position for grasp and prehension (Fig. 17-4). The web space of the thumb allows maximal abduction of the thumb for grasp. Every effort is made to preserve the maximum web space because the size of the object that can be grasped depends on the mobility of the thumb web space (Tubiana, Thomine, & Mackin, 1996).

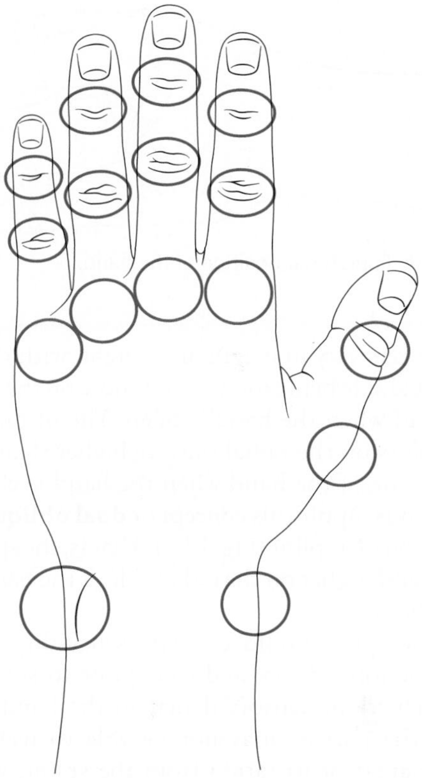

Figure 17-2 Bony prominences can lead to pressure points, especially over the back of the hand. Careful contouring of the splinting material can minimize this problem.

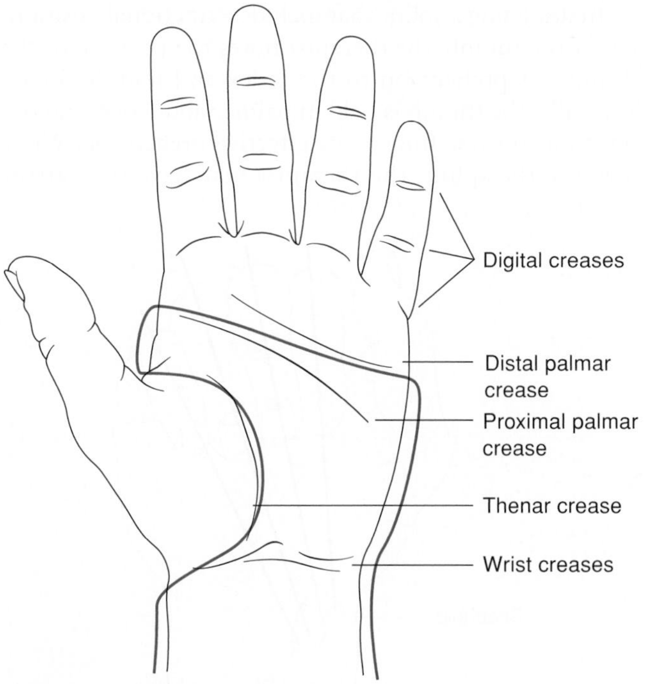

Figure 17-1 Creases of the hand provide landmarks for the distal ends of the splint. For a wrist support splint, the distal end of the splint should not block the thenar eminence or distal palmar crease.

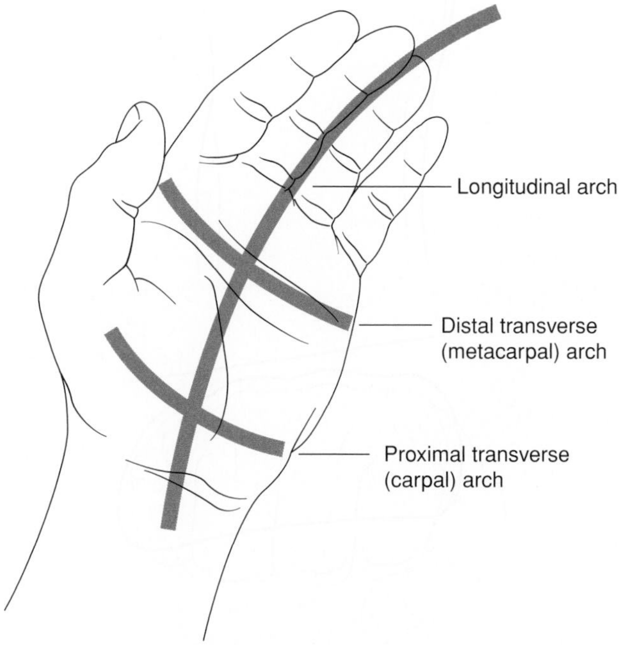

Figure 17-3 Arches of the hand must be supported in splinting.

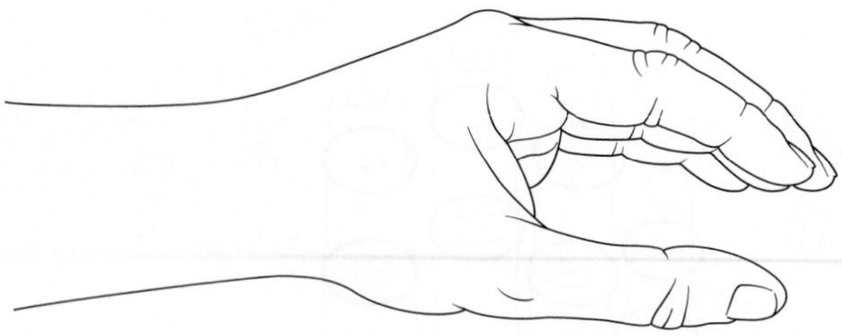

Figure 17-4 Functional position of the hand.

The fingers vary in length and height, with the fingers on the radial side being longer than those on the ulnar side of the hand when the hand is open. The metacarpophalangeal joints on the radial side are higher than those on the ulnar side of the hand when the hand is closed. The therapist must apply this concept of **dual obliquity** to the construction of a splint (Fig. 17-5). That is, the splint must be longer and higher on the radial side of the hand (Fess & Philips, 1987).

The therapist should evaluate sensibility, mobility, motor function, edema, and tone prior to splint design and construction. Sensory deficit in the hand creates a concern: the patient may not be able to feel pressure points or areas of irritation from the splint, which can lead to skin breakdown or injury. In the case of hypersensitivity, the use of a splint can protect the fingertip or hand from unpleasant stimuli. Edema may also indicate the need for close monitoring of splint fit and comfort. As edema diminishes, the splint requires modification or remolding to maintain proper fit. Deficits in mobility may change during the course of splinting, so the splint may have to be modified. Weakness may indicate the need for a dynamic assist splint to prevent muscle imbalance or deformity. As muscle strength improves, the force of the dynamic assist should be adjusted to the patient's needs. Increased or decreased tone may indicate the need for splinting to maintain balance and prevent contracture. As tone changes, the therapist should modify the splint as necessary to meet the goals of treatment. Ongoing assessment helps the therapist identify any need for changes in the splint.

In designing a splint, the therapist must be aware of the natural postures of the hand that affect function. When the hand is held in supination, the wrist is held in neutral to slight radial deviation. When the hand is held in pronation, the wrist assumes a more ulnarly deviated posture. These considerations affect fit: if a splint is fitted in supination for a patient who will be using the hand primarily in pronation, the splint may not fit comfortably. Another consideration is that, normally during flexion, the fingers converge toward the scaphoid bone (Fig. 17-6). Therefore, the application of dynamic or static progressive assists to finger flexion splints must have the direction of pull toward the radial border of the wrist.

In designing a splint that includes functional positioning of the thumb, the therapist notes the position of the thumb for prehension to the index and middle finger. Typically, the thumb is held in palmar abduction and opposition to these fingers for effective prehension. While forming the splint, the therapist may have the patient

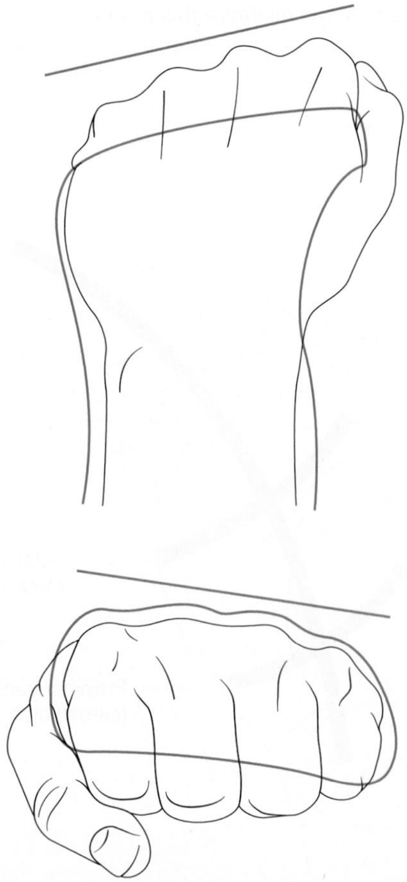

Figure 17-5 Concept of dual obliquity applied to splinting.

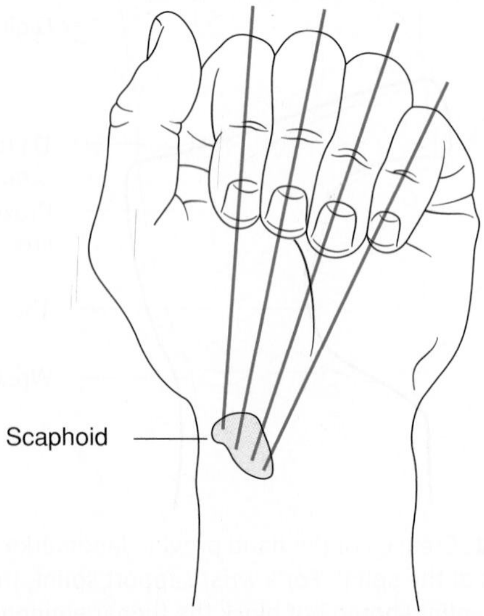

Figure 17-6 Fingers flex toward the scaphoid.

hold a pen or other object in the hand to test the ability of the thumb to achieve functional prehension. When designing a splint for the patient with carpal tunnel syndrome, the therapist should be aware of the position of the wrist that produces the lowest pressure in the carpal canal. The ideal position for the wrist is close to neutral, with 2 ± 9° of dorsiflexion and 2 ± 6° of ulnar deviation (Weiss et al., 1995).

Biomechanical Considerations

Biomechanical considerations include the effects of healing tissue on the biomechanics of hand use and mechanical principles that affect the design of the splint.

Position of Safe Immobilization

Following injury the hand may stiffen in a nonfunctional position. This position typically includes wrist flexion, MCP extension, and PIP and DIP flexion in a claw position (Bunnell, 1996). The distal transverse arch is flattened. If this position is maintained for long, the hand becomes nonfunctional as a result of shortening of the collateral ligaments. The position of safe immobilization (Fig. 17-7) prevents ligamentous shortening and contracture following injury. This position maintains the length of the collateral ligaments by holding the MCP joints in flexion and the PIP and DIP joints in extension while keeping the wrist in dorsiflexion. Specifically, the wrist is held in 30–40° of extension, and the MCP joints are positioned in 70–90° of flexion with full extension of PIP and DIP joints (Coppard & Lohman, 1996; Boscheinen-Morrin & Connolly, 2001). This position is also called intrinsic plus or safe positioning.

Tissue Healing

The therapist should be aware of the phases of wound healing when selecting the splint design for the patient with an injured hand. Splinting applies gentle stress to healing tissues to influence change (Fess & McCollum, 1998). During the **inflammatory phase**, the therapist may use a splint to immobilize and protect the healing tissues. During the **fibroblastic phase** of healing,

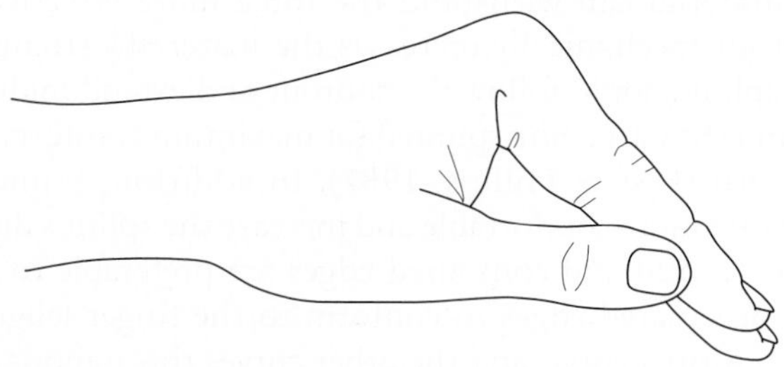

Figure 17-7 Position of safe immobilization.

splints may be used to mobilize healing tissues while protecting them. As the strength of the healing tissues increases and the scar tissue matures in the **maturation phase**, low load force may be applied with splinting. As maturation progresses, the tissues can tolerate an increased amount of stress (Schultz-Johnson, 1996). A splinting program must recognize these changes in healing tissues with appropriate changes in the splint as needed. Exercise programs and functional activity must begin simultaneously with splinting to maximize the benefit.

Influence of Splinting on Scar Remodeling

When mobility is lost to immobilization from casting, injury, or a neurological condition, collagen fibers develop increased intermolecular bonds, which result in dense tissue with relatively little mobility (Bell-Krotoski & Figarola, 1995). This response causes tissues to adapt and shorten, resulting in contracture. Such a limitation in mobility may be treated with splinting. There is some controversy regarding how splinting creates changes in soft tissues (Fess & McCollum, 1998). Is it by stretching existing tissue or the actual production of new tissue? The mechanism of stretching was initially thought to be creep, the elongation of tissues under a prolonged stress over time (Bell-Krotoski & Figarola, 1995; Fess & Philips, 1987). If tissues are stretched excessively, however, they rupture or produce an inflammatory response. Research suggests that ideal tissue remodeling occurs with gentle elongation of tissues. Tissues lengthen and grow if gentle stress is applied. This process is not stretching but rather growth of new tissues to accommodate the stress placed on them (Bell-Krotoski & Figarola, 1995; Brand, 2002). **Dynamic splinting**, **serial static splinting**, and casting are based on this mechanism.

The total end range time (TERT) theory suggests that the amount of increase in passive range of motion of a stiff joint is directly proportional to the amount of time the joint is held at the end of its range (Flowers & LaStayo, 1994). TERT theory states that if a joint is held at the end of its range, the dense connective tissue around the joint grows. This lengthening of tissues increases range of motion. The longer the joint is positioned at its end range, the greater is the gain in mobility. One study (Glasgow, Wilton, & Tooth, 2003) reported that a TERT of 6 hours or more per day resulted in a more effective reduction of contracture at a faster rate than a daily TERT of less than 6 hours over 4 weeks of splinting. Serial static splinting or casting is often used in the application of TERT theory in splinting.

Another theory employs stress relaxation, or static progressive stretch therapy, in splinting (Bonutti et al., 1994). This approach elongates tissues through progressive incremental stretch. The static progressive stretch approach applies 30-minute sessions of splint wear with stretch increased every 5 minutes to the patient's tolerance to increase range of motion. **Static progressive splints** apply this theory by applying a low-load force that can be adjusted incrementally. These splints use methods such as MERiT (maximum end range time) components for gradual advancement of the static stress on the splinted part (King, 1993; Schultz-Johnson, 1996).

Torque angle curves provide a consistent method for measuring changes in soft tissues to determine whether splinting is overcoming joint stiffness (Brand, 2002; Breger-Lee et al., 1993). By using a goniometer and a **Haldex gauge** and plotting the data on a graph, a therapist can evaluate the effectiveness of splinting intervention. The Haldex gauge allows the therapist to apply a precise amount of torque for each measurement (Breger-Lee, Bell-Krotoski, & Brandsma, 1990). The graph displays the joint's response to the force applied with progressive torque on the vertical axis and the range of motion on the horizontal axis. A steep slope of the curve indicates that the joint is less responsive to splinting than a gradually sloped curve (Flowers & Pheasant, 1988).

Flowers (2002) proposed a model for assisting therapists' choice of static, dynamic, or static progressive splinting for a stiff joint based on a formula of the *Modified Weeks Test* (*MWT*). Applying this model, the patient's stiff joint is first tested using standard goniometry. Then the therapist places the patient's involved extremity in a heat modality for 20 minutes. Following heat, stretch is applied for 10 minutes to patient tolerance. A second goniometric reading is taken of the stiff joint and then compared to the first reading. A gain in motion is an indicator of the responsiveness of the joint to stretch. If the gain is 20°, no splint is recommended. If the gain is 15°, a static splint at end range is recommended. If the gain is approximately 10°, a dynamic splint is appropriate, and if the gain is only 5° or less, a static progressive splint is most helpful. The *MWT* provides a useful model for guiding splint selection of any stiff joint.

Casting with plaster of Paris or Quickcast (Sammons Preston Rolyan) is another highly effective method in mobilizing stiff joints. Casting is useful in reducing joint, muscle, or skin tightness and may be used in therapy to enhance tendon glide (Colditz, 2002). Due to its uniform circumferential fit, it is usually well tolerated by the patient and, in addition, can reduce edema.

Mechanical Principles of Splint Design

The following principles concerning force distribution guide splint design.

Increase the Area of Force Application to Disperse Pressure

Splints apply external forces to the splinted part. Pressure is equal to the amount of force divided by the area of force application (Fess & Philips, 1987; Fess, 1995b). The clinical applications of this principle are: (1) a wide, long splint is more comfortable than a narrow, short one; and (2) contoured pressure over a bone or bony prominence is preferable to uneven or point pressure over the prominence. The therapist must be cautious when padding a splint because it may actually increase a point of pressure if the splint is not well molded to the area.

Increase the Mechanical Advantage to Reduce Pressure and Increase Comfort

The mechanical advantage is the application of parallel force systems with the joint as the axis (A), the distal part splinted as the resistance (R), and the proximal part as the force (F), with the splint acting as a first-class lever much like a balanced teeter-totter (Fess & Philips, 1987; Fess, 1995b). Given a constant resistance, the amount of force in the lever system can be decreased by increasing the length of the force arm. In the case of a wrist support splint, the forearm trough is the force arm (FA), and the metacarpal bar serves as the resistance arm (RA) (Fig. 17-8). A longer forearm trough will decrease any pressure caused by the transferred weight of the hand. Mechanical advantage is equal to the FA divided by the RA. In accordance with this principle, the recommended length of the forearm trough is usually two thirds the length of the forearm (Fig. 17-8), although the forearm trough should not be so long as to impede elbow motion.

Ensure Three Points of Pressure

The three parallel forces in a first-class lever system, such as a splint, are in equilibrium. The splint acts as a counterforce proximally and distally to the forces of the forearm and hand, respectively. A strap securing the splint at the axis position provides a reciprocal middle force. These parallel reciprocal forces create the three points of pressure (Fess & Philips, 1987; Fess, 1995b). The concept of three points of pressure guides splint design and directs placement of straps for proper force application (Fig. 17-9).

Add Strength through Contouring

When a force is applied to a flat piece of material, the material bends. If the same material is molded into a curve, the material can withstand the force more effectively. Contour mechanically increases the material's strength. The splint should follow the contour and extend midway around the part being splinted for maximum comfort and strength (Fess & Philips, 1987). In addition, rounded edges are more comfortable and increase the splint's durability. Curved and contoured edges are preferable to angled or squared edges to conform to the finger lengths, which form a curve, and the other curves throughout the hand, wrist, and forearm.

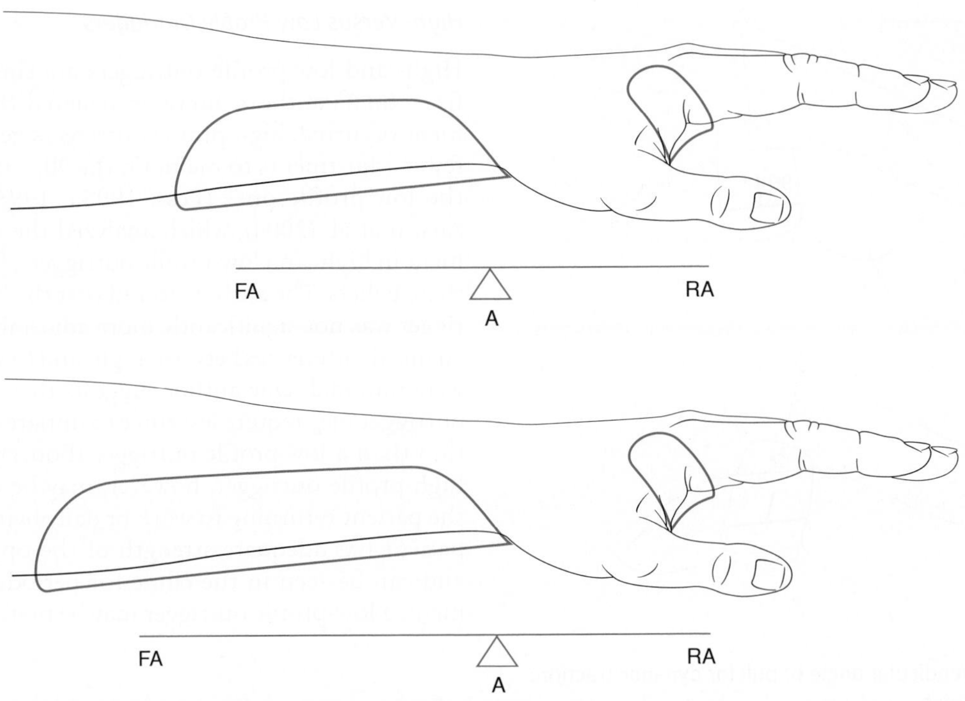

Figure 17-8 Increase the mechanical advantage of the splint by increasing the length of the forearm trough. A, axis; FA, force arm; RA, resistance arm.

Perpendicular Traction for Dynamic or Static Progressive Splinting

To mobilize a joint through dynamic or static progressive splinting, the line of pull must be perpendicular to the long axis of the bone being mobilized. Whether using finger loops with an extension outrigger or nail hooks with a flexion pulley, the therapist must maintain a 90° angle of pull to provide the most effective application of force (Fig. 17-10). The perpendicular force application prevents shearing stress and unwanted traction on the joint. As mobility improves, the therapist must make changes in the outrigger to maintain the 90° angle of pull (Fess & Philips, 1987).

Acceptable Pressure for Dynamic Splinting

Forces in dynamic splinting may be applied with rubber bands, elastic thread, or springs (Gyovai & Howell, 1992). The force must not exceed acceptable limits. Low-load forces of 100–300 g are recommended for dynamic splinting of fingers (Fess, 1995b). Therapists may use lighter forces for the acute stages and heavier forces for treatment of chronic joint contractures (Fess & McCollum, 1998). The therapist must consider the patient's size, condition, and stage of recovery when determining the proper force application. The length and width of the rubber band determine the force of tension. A Haldex gauge (see Resources 17-1) can be used in the clinic to determine the

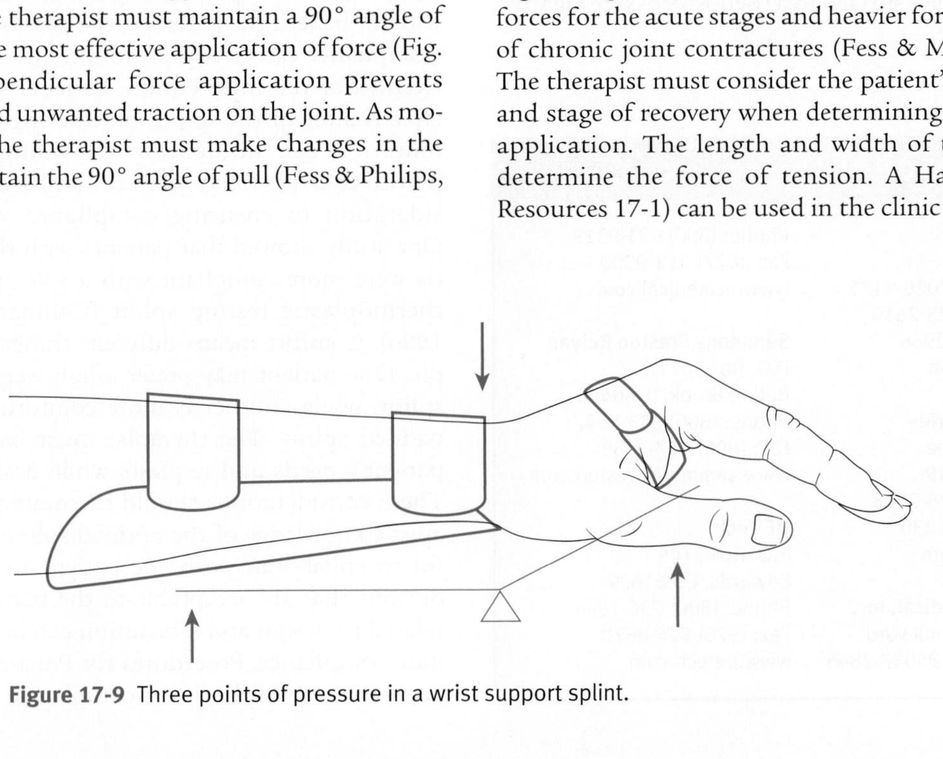

Figure 17-9 Three points of pressure in a wrist support splint.

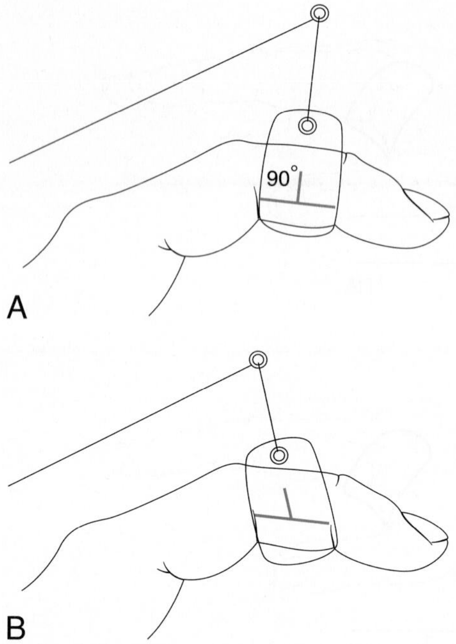

Figure 17-10 Perpendicular angle of pull for dynamic traction: **A.** Correct. **B.** Incorrect.

exact amount of pressure (force) applied by splinting. Eagerness to achieve results quickly may cause the therapist to use excessive force, which may injure tissue. Effective dynamic splinting of a contracture produces a gain of only 10° per week (Brand, 2002). If dynamic splinting is not enough to remodel tissues or if greater pressure is required, serial casting may be preferable. Serial casts contour intimately to the limb and disperse pressure throughout a larger surface area (Bell-Krotoski & Figarola, 1995).

RESOURCE 17-1

Alimed Inc.
297 High Street
Dedham, MA 02026-9135
Phone: (800) 225-2610
Fax: (800) 437-2966
www.alimed.com

DeRoyal Industries
200 DeBusk Lane
Powell, TN 37849
Phone: (888) 938-7828
Fax: (865) 362-1230
www.deroyal.com

North Coast Medical, Inc.
18305 Sutter Boulevard
Morgan Hill, CA 95037-2845
Phone: (800) 821-9319
Fax: (877) 213-9300
www.ncmedical.com

Sammons Preston Rolyan
P.O. Box 5071
Boling Brook, IL 60440
Phone: (800) 323-5547
Fax: (800) 547-4333
www.sammonspreston.com

UE Tech
P.O. Box 2145
Edwards, CO 81632
Phone: (800) 736-1894
Fax: (970) 926-8870
www.uetech.com

High- Versus Low-Profile Outriggers

High- and low-profile outriggers are similar in their effects. Some authors, however, believed that, as improvement occurred, high-profile outriggers generally required fewer adjustments to maintain the 90° angle of pull than the low-profile ones (Fess, 1995a, 1995b). A study by Austin et al. (2004), which analyzed the need for adjustment in high- and low-profile outriggers, failed to support these beliefs. The authors found that the high-profile outrigger was not significantly more adjustable and that mechanical differences between high- and low-profile designs were minimal. One author suggests that the high-profile outrigger may require less force to initiate the allowed motion than a low-profile outrigger (Boozer et al., 1994). A high-profile outrigger, however, may be cumbersome to the patient returning to work or daily living activities. If a patient has adequate strength of the opposing muscles and can be seen in the clinic for periodic splint adjustment, a low-profile outrigger may be preferable.

OTHER CONSIDERATIONS IN SPLINTING

Despite the most beautifully designed and constructed hand splint, the effectiveness of a splinting program depends on two other factors: compliance and education.

Compliance

Even the most expertly designed and constructed splint will not benefit the patient if the patient does not wear it. Compliance can have a profound influence on the effectiveness of the intervention. Patients' perception of the effectiveness of the splint in achieving the goals of rehabilitation can influence their willingness to wear it (Groth & Wulf, 1995). Comfort is also an important consideration in ensuring compliance with splint wear. One study showed that patients with rheumatoid arthritis were more compliant with a soft splint than a hard thermoplastic resting splint (Callinan & Mathiowetz, 1996). Comfort means different things to different people. One patient may prefer a lightweight thermoplastic splint, while another is more comfortable with a softly padded splint. The therapist must be attentive to the patient's needs and requests while designing the splint. These considerations should be combined with the therapist's knowledge of the optimal splint design. It is helpful to collaborate with the patient to identify effective options that are acceptable to the patient. Many factors related to design and fabrication can be adjusted to facilitate compliance. Procedures for Practice 17-1 has strategies to increase splint wear compliance.

PROCEDURES FOR PRACTICE 17-1

Strategies to Increase Splint Wear Compliance

- Offer splint options to the patient if possible.
- Teach the patient about the benefits of splint wear.
- Provide for easy application and removal of the splint.
- Make the splint comfortable.
- Use a lightweight material if possible.
- Immobilize only the joints being treated.
- Make the splint cosmetically pleasing to the patient.
- If feasible, collaborate with the patient on a wearing schedule.

Education

The therapist must provide adequate instruction to the patient regarding wear and care to ensure proper use of the splint. Patients should be taught the goal and purpose of splinting. It may also be helpful to inform the patients of the consequences of failing to comply with splint wear. Provide written instructions on wear and care. If necessary, provide a diagram of proper application. If the patient is a child or has a cognitive deficit, be sure to instruct a caregiver in the proper application of the splint. Include precautions for the patient or caregiver to watch for, including pressure points, edema, and dynamic tension that is too tight. Offer suggestions on adjusting the splint if feasible. Teach the patient how to clean the splint and to keep thermoplastic splints away from heat lest they lose their shape. Make a follow-up visit if you anticipate a change in the patient's status that will necessitate splint modification.

SPLINT CONSTRUCTION

Methods to construct splints from thermoplastic materials are described here. Figures 17-11A and 17-12 to 17-20 pertain to a resting splint. Figures 17-11B and 17-21 to 17-23 pertain to a hand-based thumb splint. Figures 17-11C and 17-24 to 17-31 pertain to a wrist splint serving as a

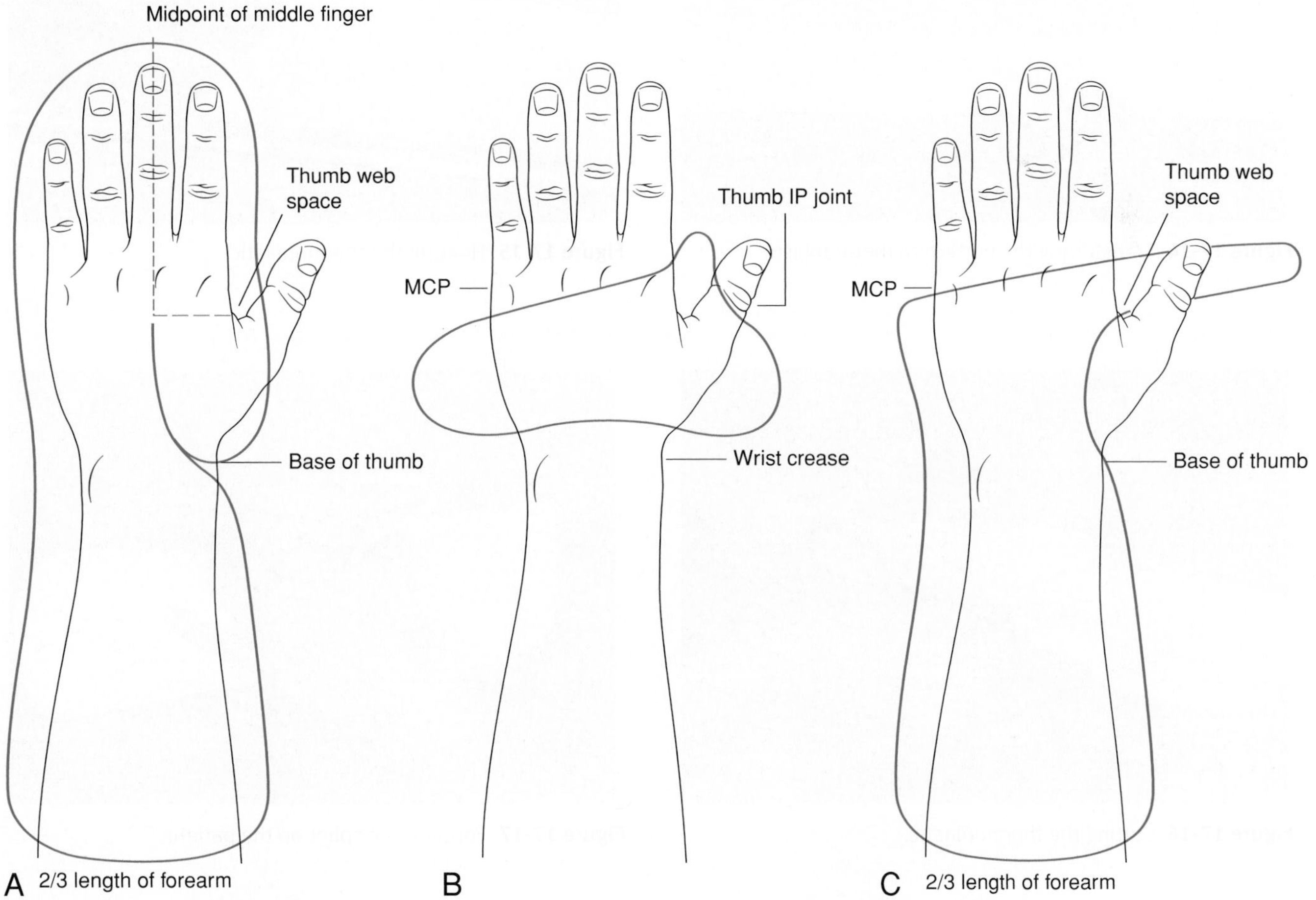

Figure 17-11 Patterns. **A.** Resting splint. **B.** Hand-based thumb splint. **C.** Dorsal wrist splint.

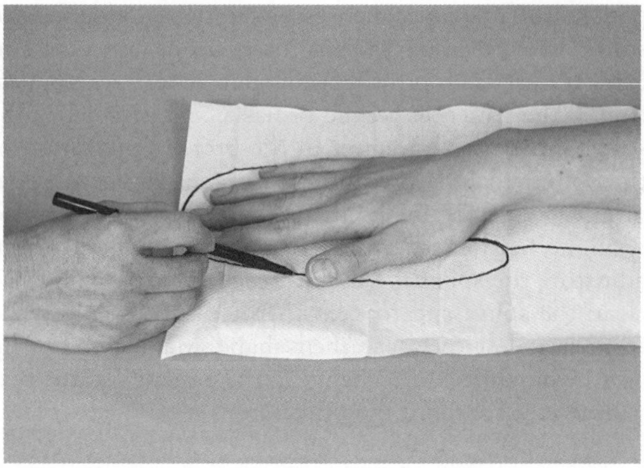

Figure 17-12 Making the pattern for a resting splint on a patient.

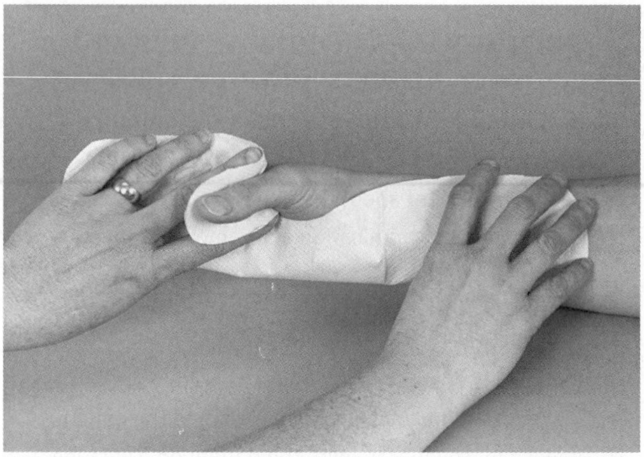

Figure 17-13 Fitting the pattern on the patient.

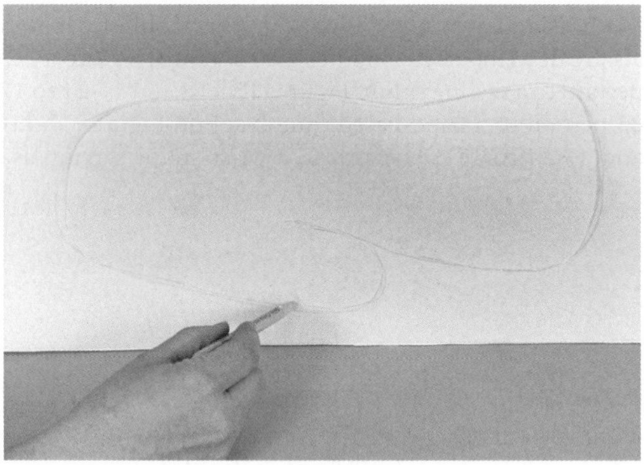

Figure 17-14 Transferring the pattern to thermoplastic.

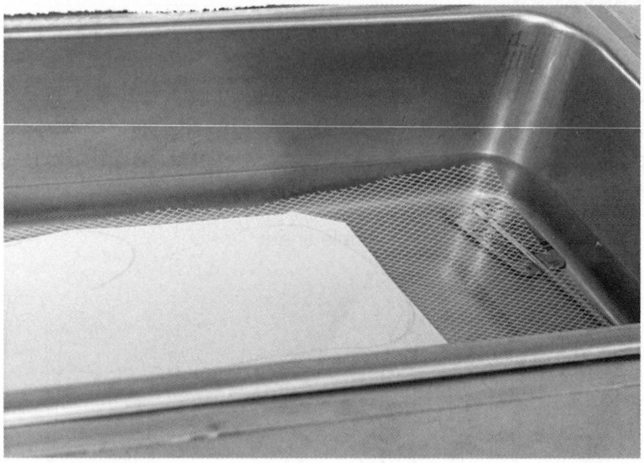

Figure 17-15 Heating the thermoplastic.

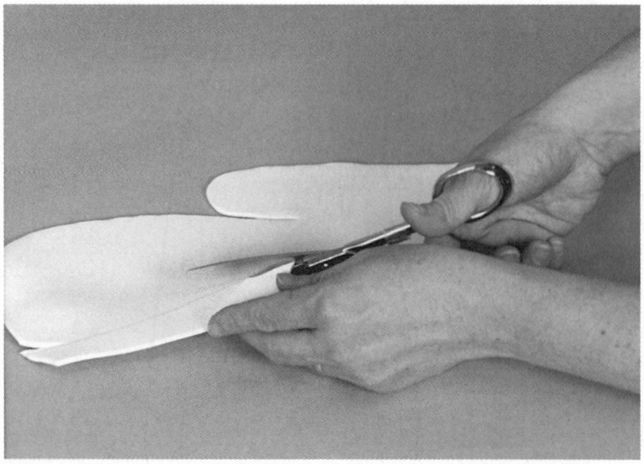

Figure 17-16 Cutting the thermoplastic.

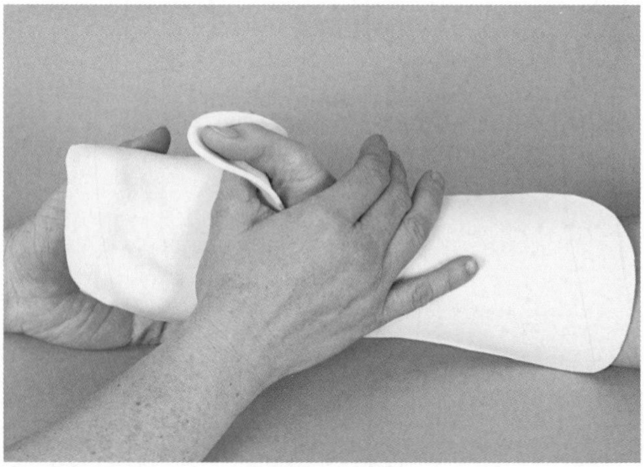

Figure 17-17 Forming the splint on the patient.

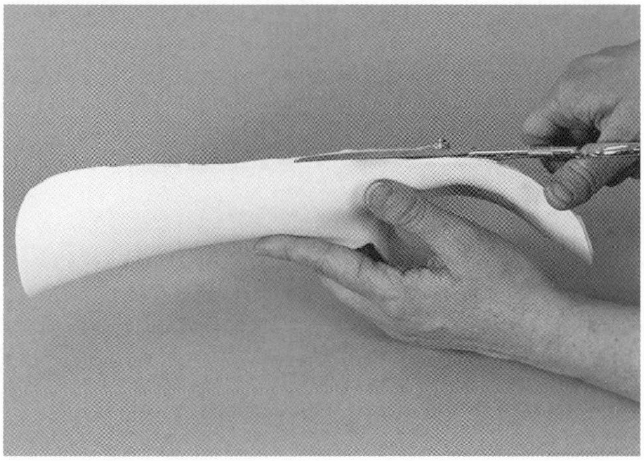

Figure 17-18 Trimming the splint.

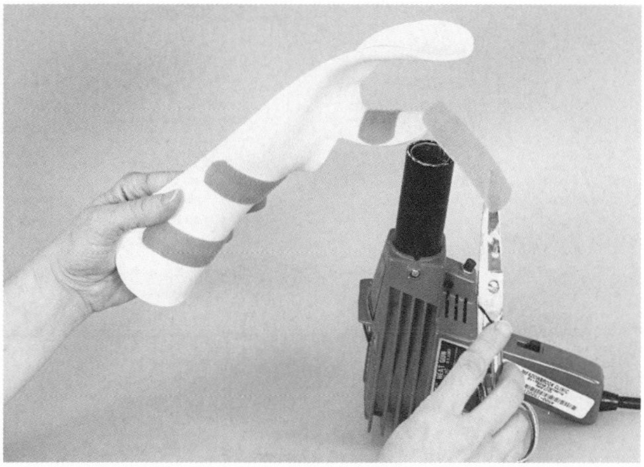

Figure 17-19 Applying straps.

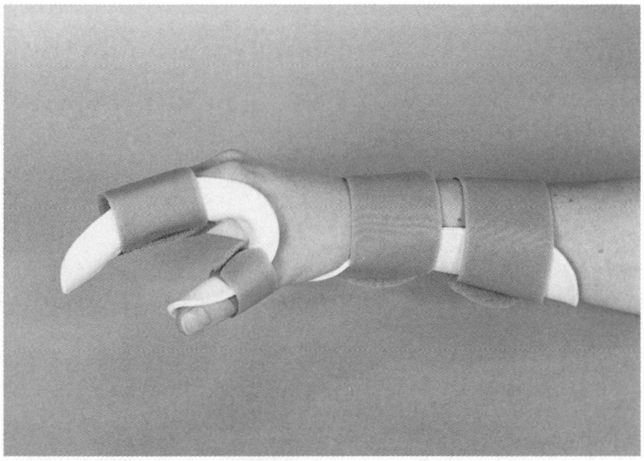

Figure 17-20 Finished resting splint on the patient.

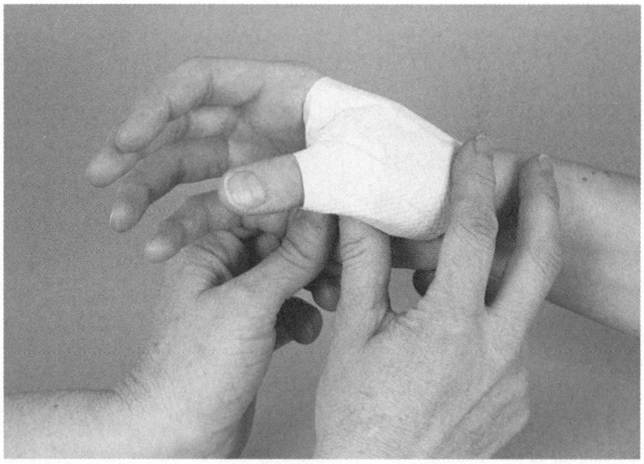

Figure 17-21 Fitting the pattern on the patient for a hand-based thumb splint.

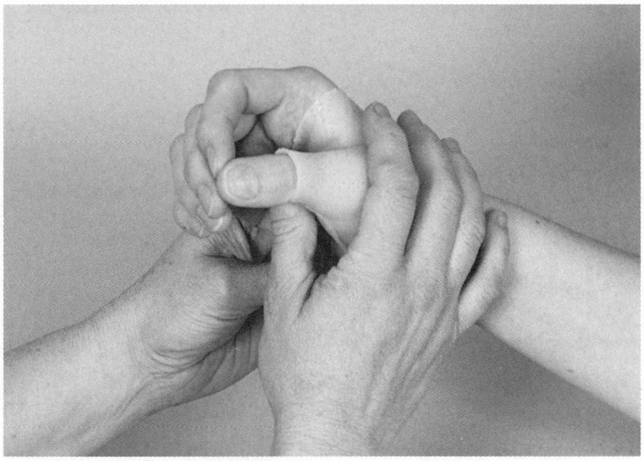

Figure 17-22 Forming the splint on the patient.

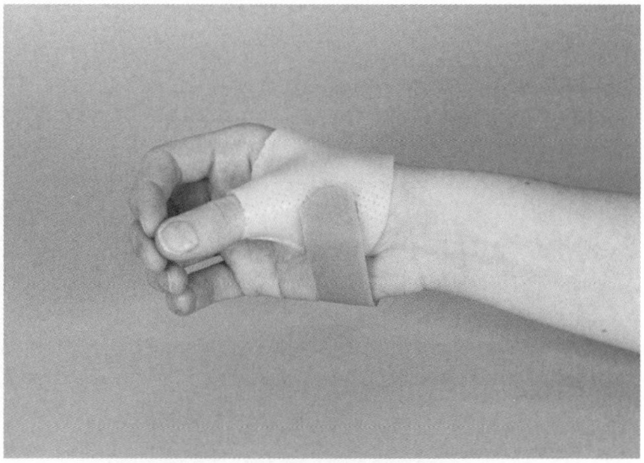

Figure 17-23 Finished splint on the patient.

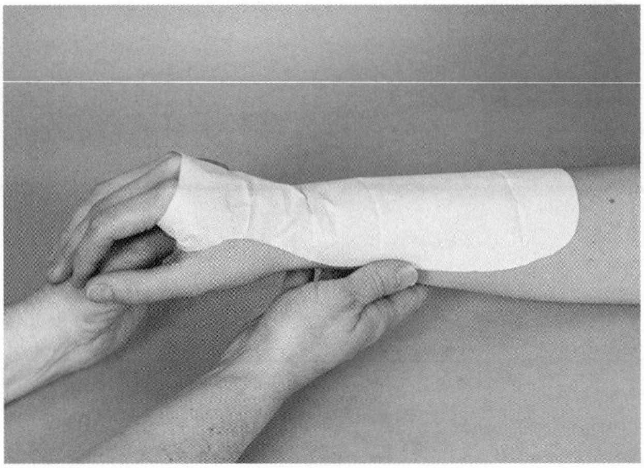

Figure 17-24 Fitting the pattern for the wrist splint base on the patient.

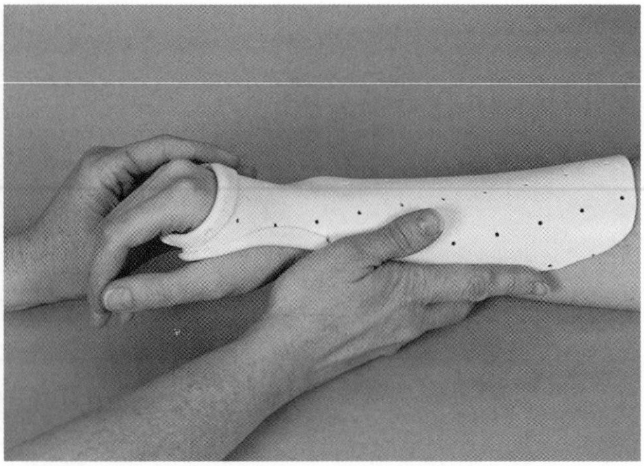

Figure 17-25 Forming the wrist splint on the patient.

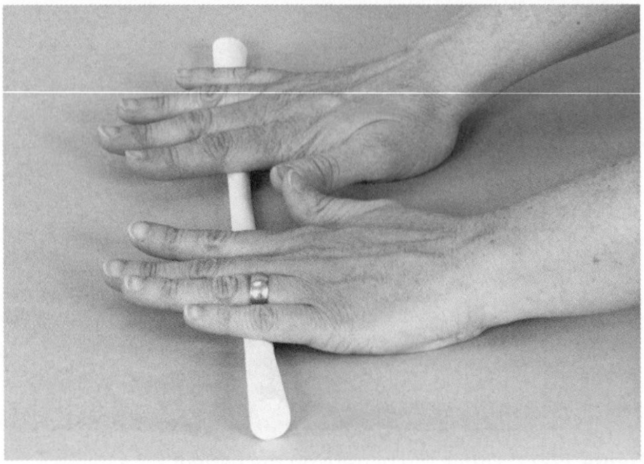

Figure 17-26 Forming the outrigger from splint material scraps.

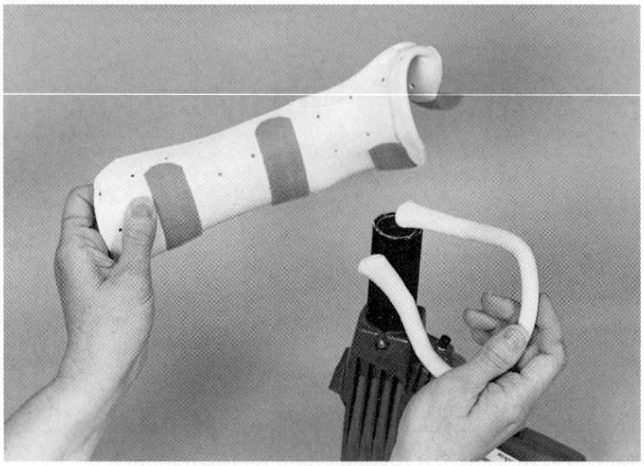

Figure 17-27 Attaching the outrigger to splint base.

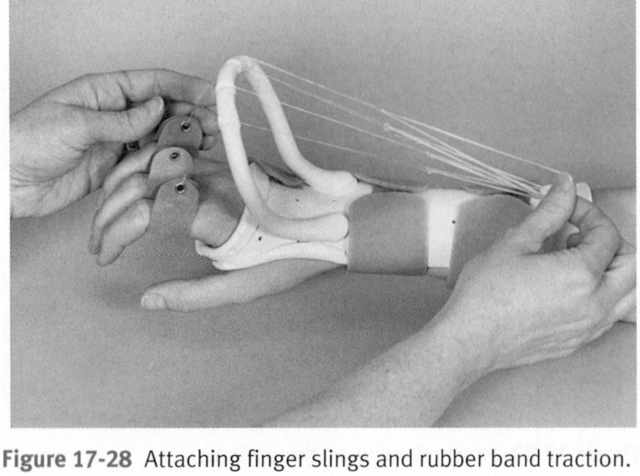

Figure 17-28 Attaching finger slings and rubber band traction.

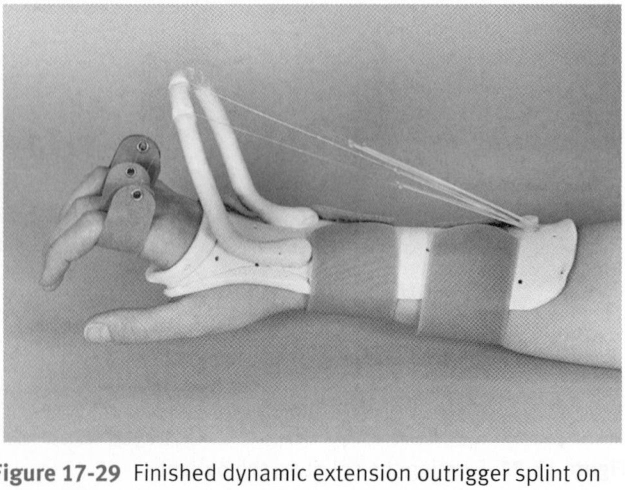

Figure 17-29 Finished dynamic extension outrigger splint on the patient.

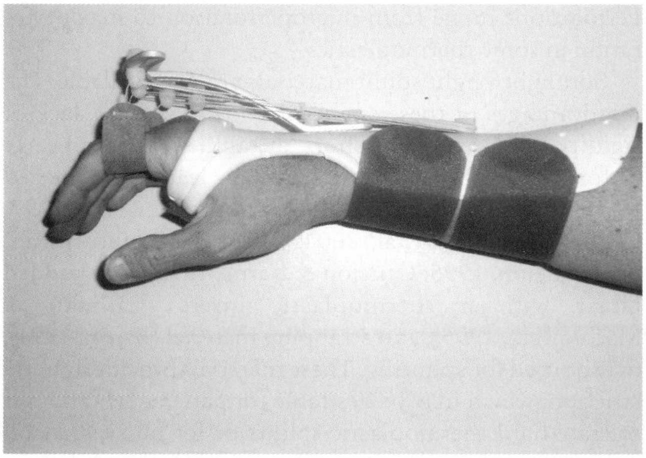

Figure 17-30 Finished dynamic extension splint with commercial outrigger components—side view.

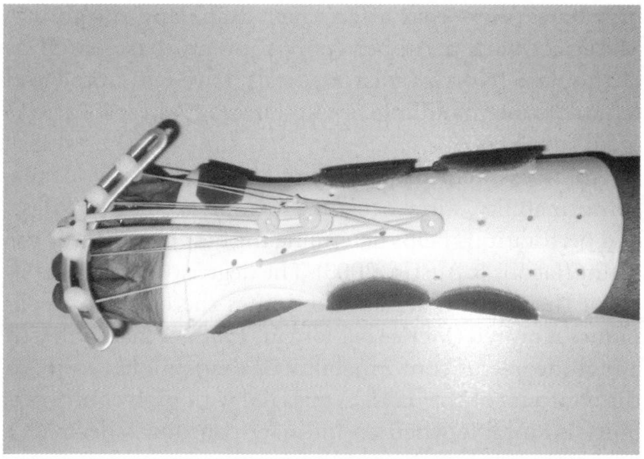

Figure 17-31 Finished dynamic extension splint with commercial outrigger components—overhead view.

base for a dynamic finger extension outrigger. (See Procedures for Practice 17-2.)

Splint Design

Determine the type of splint design by assessing the patient and the clinical condition in reference to the physician's splint order. Consider the goals and purpose of the splint. You can combine this information with an understanding of the patient and any factors that may affect compliance. Also consider relevant cost factors related to custom splint construction. If there is a commercial splint that achieves the same purpose, it may be more cost effective to provide the commercial splint. When time and materials are added up, the custom-made splint is usually more expensive than the commercial splint, but other factors must be considered in this decision and cost should not be the only consideration if effectiveness is an issue. Procedures for Practice 17-3 lists questions to ask when designing the splint.

PROCEDURES FOR PRACTICE 17-2

Steps of Splint Construction

1. Design splint
2. Select material
3. Make pattern
4. Cut splinting material
5. Heat splinting material
6. Form splint
7. Finish edges
8. Apply straps, padding, and attachments
9. Evaluate the splint for fit and comfort

Material Selection

Selecting the proper material for the splint can be a challenge. It is helpful to become familiar with the properties of various thermoplastics so as to apply the most suitable material for the needs of the patient and the purpose of the splint. You may become biased toward certain materials that are relatively easy to work with, but with experience, you will learn to appreciate a variety of materials, each with its own benefits and limitations. Low-temperature thermoplastics have plastic, plastic-like, rubber, or rubber-like bases that give the splinting material its individual characteristics (Breger-Lee, 1995; Breger-Lee & Buford, 1992). Materials with a plastic (polycaprolactone) base, such as Polyform (Sammons Preston Rolyan) and NCM Clinic (North Coast Medical)

PROCEDURES FOR PRACTICE 17-3

Selecting the Splint Design

- How many joints must be immobilized or mobilized?
- What is the best application? Should the splint be volar or dorsal; ulnar, radial, or circumferential; static, static progressive, or dynamic?
- Should the splint be based on the forearm, hand, finger, or thumb to provide the necessary support for the splinted part?
- Is there a cost-effective commercial splint that achieves the goals?
- Will the patient be able to apply and wear the splint as recommended?
- Which material is best to achieve the purpose of the splint? Does the material affect the design of the splint?

may have fillers that affect their drape and durability. Materials with a rubber (polyisoprene) base, such as Orthoplast (North Coast Medical), have less drape and require firmer handling. See Resources 17-1 for locations of all suppliers.

An assessment of properties such as rigidity, drape, conformability, surface texture, memory, color, thickness, and perforations helps determine the best material for the splint (Jacobs & Austin, 2003). The degree of conformability of the splint material determines the handling techniques required (McKee & Morgan, 1998). A material with a high degree of conformability or drape molds easily to the contours of the hand. A material with high conformability is suitable when an intimate contour is desired; a material with less drape is preferable in constructing a long arm splint or a splint requiring firm handling techniques. For example, a resting splint for a patient with spasticity may require a high degree of rigidity with low degree of drape. A material with a rubber-like base, such as Ezeform (Sammons Preston Rolyan) provides the necessary rigidity without drape, allowing the therapist to use firm handling techniques for fabrication.

The surface texture may also be an important consideration. Some materials have a shiny, smooth surface, while others have texture. Some materials are susceptible to fingerprints. Usually the therapist can control fingerprints by using a smooth, gentle, stroking technique during molding. Some materials have a coating on the surface that resists adhesion. This coating must be removed with a solvent or by scraping the surface before attaching straps or other permanent attachments.

Some materials have memory that allows them to stretch and return to their original shape with reheating. These materials are usually translucent and become transparent when heated to the desired temperature. One example is Aquaplast (Sammons Preston Rolyan), which also comes in bright colors.

Many splinting materials are available in a variety of colors. This may be beneficial for ensuring compliance with splint wear in children and teenagers. Allowing patients to select their splint color may improve compliance. Not everybody likes colored splints, however. Many patients prefer a neutral tone. Flesh-tone colors are available in various shades of beige, brown, and black.

Splint materials are also available in a variety of thicknesses. The most commonly used thicknesses are 1/8 inch and 1/16 inch. The 1/8-inch material is preferred for rigid forearm-based splints, while the 1/16-inch material is best suited for hand-based and finger-based splints and circumferential designs. Thinner materials produce lighter weight splints, which may be better tolerated by some patients. Perforations also affect the weight and rigidity of a splint (McKee & Morgan, 1998). Perforations also provide ventilation, which is especially beneficial in warm weather. Perforations range from microperforation to maxiperforation in some thermoplastics.

Soft lightweight splint materials are also available. The disadvantages of these splints may be their bulk, lack of rigidity, and relatively short durability (Breger-Lee & Buford, 1991). Soft materials, such as leather, elasticized fabric (Schultz-Johnson, 1996), neoprene (Clark, 1997; Fillion, 2004; Weiss et al., 2004; Willey, 2004), silicone rubber (Canelon, 1995; Canelon & Karus, 1995), soft padded fabric with a thermoplastic insert (Callinan & Mathiowetz, 1996), and strapping material (Byron, 1994), may be used for splinting. These materials provide light restriction, which may be desirable for patients who do not tolerate hard thermoplastic splints or for musicians and athletes attempting to reduce harmful motion while continuing to play. The therapist should consider the patient's tolerance to any material being used in splinting. Sensitivity to various materials, such as an allergic contact dermatitis to neoprene (Stern et al., 1998), has been reported in the literature.

High-temperature thermoplastics are also available for rigid splinting. They require use of a band saw for cutting and an oven for heating (Fess & Philips, 1987). These high-temperature thermoplastics have high-impact strength and rigidity but do not contour well, which makes them generally not suitable for hand splinting.

Recent technological advances have allowed engineers to incorporate an antimicrobial agent into several splinting materials. Since splints are often worn continuously against the skin, a moist environment can lead to bacteria and an unpleasant smell over time. This antimicrobial protection may make it easier to clean and maintain splints that are worn continuously.

Pattern Making

Once you have decided on the appropriate splint design and material, you will make a pattern. This is an important step because a well-designed splint pattern usually leads to a well-fitting splint. The pattern provides a two-dimensional guide for the three-dimensional splint. The pattern also helps to minimize waste of splint material. Patterns for many commonly prescribed splints are available in splinting textbooks and from splint material manufacturers. Three commonly prescribed splint patterns are demonstrated here (Fig. 17-11). Paper toweling provides an excellent moldable pattern, but any type of paper can be used for the pattern. Place the patient's hand directly on the paper and mark the anatomical landmarks according to the design being used (Fig. 17-12). The pattern must extend beyond the lateral borders of the hand and forearm to allow the splint to form a shallow trough, which will extend halfway around the surface being splinted for adequate support. Extend the forearm trough two thirds of the length of the forearm. Once the pattern is drawn, cut it out and place it on the patient in the design of the splint (see Fig. 17-13 for the resting pan splint, Fig. 17-21 for the thumb splint, and Fig. 17-24 for the dynamic finger extension outrigger splint). If it fits perfectly, transfer it to the splinting material. If it needs modification, modify it by cutting the pattern down or adding a piece of paper for extra length or width as needed. Check the pattern on the patient to see if it blocks any joints unnecessarily. The splint pattern can be cut back to reduce this restriction if necessary. If the patient is unable to lay the hand flat for pattern drawing because of deformity or spasticity, use the uninvolved hand for pattern making and flip the pattern over for the contralateral side. You can adjust the pattern for edema or any other variation before transferring the pattern.

Transfer the pattern to the splinting material by tracing it onto the plastic (Fig. 17-14). A wax pencil is easy to see and erases from the plastic. An awl can also be used to scratch the pattern onto the plastic. If using a pen or pencil, cut away the marks as you cut out the splint.

Cutting

With a full sheet of splinting material, it is best to cut it to a size that will fit the pattern. Cut the full sheet with a utility knife by scoring it and bending it, then turning the sheet over and scoring it again from the other side. This provides a manageable sheet of thermoplastic. Heat the thermoplastic once the splint pattern is marked (Fig. 17-15). When the material is soft, cut the splint out with sharp straight-edge scissors (Fig. 17-16). By cutting the material after heating, you eliminate the rough edges, which saves time in the finishing step. Hold the material horizontally while cutting to avoid overstretching it. Excessive handling of material can cause fingerprinting. To minimize this problem, lightly hold the material on the edges that will be cut away. Curved scissors may help in cutting out hard-to-reach curved areas.

Pre-cut splinting blanks are available for commonly used patterns. Considering the time it takes to trace and cut the pattern out of a full sheet of splinting material and the potential for wasting material, pre-cut materials may be cost effective.

Heating Splinting Material

Electric fry pans, splint pans, and hydrocollators can be used to heat the thermoplastic material (Fig. 17-15). It is recommended that the water be at least 1 inch deep if using a fry pan. If using a hydrocollator, be careful not to let the material overstretch or drop to the bottom. Heat pan liners may be helpful with a hydrocollator. The recommended temperature varies among materials. It is usually best to keep the water at 150–160°F for most materials. Consult the manufacturer's recommendations for specific materials. Use a thermometer in the water to ensure consistent temperature. The heating time for most materials is about 1 minute. The therapist should check the material to make sure it is heated uniformly before forming the splint on the patient. The working time for splinting materials also varies. Some of the thinner thermoplastics (1/16 inch) cool in 1–2 minutes. Most of the thicker materials (1/8 inch) have a 3- to 6-minute working time. Since heat guns do not uniformly soften splinting material, they are recommended only for spot heating, minor adjustments, and edge finishing.

Forming the Splint

Once the entire piece of thermoplastic is heated, carefully remove it from the water with a spatula or tongs. The entire piece should feel soft and easily moldable. Lay the material on a towel to dry briefly. If you are rolling the edges to finish them, do so before forming the splint on the patient. Check the temperature of the plastic before placing it on the patient. If the material is too hot, let it cool slightly for the patient's tolerance and comfort. After placing the patient's hand in the desired position, place the splint material on the patient (Figs. 17-17, 17-22, and 17-25). When using a material with draping qualities, it is best to let gravity assist the positioning. If the splint is based on the volar surface, position the hand in supination or a neutral posture. If the splint is dorsal, place the hand in pronation. Since the wrist posture changes slightly in pronation and supination, check the fit of the splint in both these postures before it cools completely. Using smooth and gentle strokes, contour the splint over the arches and bony prominences of the hand. Try not to grip or squeeze the thermoplastic. Materials with a high degree of drape and conformability, such as Polyform, Polyflex II (Sammons Preston Rolyan), NCM Preferred, and Contour (North Coast Medical), require relatively little handling. Materials with controlled stretch, such as Omega (North Coast Medical), Ezeform, and Synergy (Sammons Preston Rolyan), require a firmer pressure to create contours and maintain their shape. If making a splint on a spastic extremity or an uncooperative patient, you can use an elastic bandage to assist in holding the splint in place while molding.

When splinting the thumb to allow functional use, it is helpful to have the patient hold a pen lightly or hold the thumb in prehension while the splint is being formed (Fig.

17-22). This ensures functional positioning. At this time, it is important to check for any motion that may be unnecessarily restricted. Changes can be made while the splint is forming to reduce any restriction. This is also a good time to check bony prominences for any pressure areas. Light finger pressure can push the material out away from the prominence by rounding out these areas and creating more space for the ulnar styloid or other areas of pressure. You may wish to place a small piece of putty or foam over prominences before splint molding to allow for this enlargement.

While the splint is on the patient, mark the lateral borders if additional material is to be cut away. While the splint is still slightly warm, use your fingernail to mark the trough of the splint so that it extends midway around the forearm. You can also mark distal and proximal edges in this manner and cut away the excess while the material is slightly warm (Fig. 17-18). The warmth facilitates cutting and leaves a nicely finished edge. Flare the proximal edge of the splint away from the skin to prevent a pressure point during wear.

Edge Finishing

Smooth edges are important to prevent pressure points. Cutting the material at the required temperature allows the edges to seal smoothly and not require additional attention. With some perforated materials or rough-cut thermoplastics, however, it may be necessary to smooth the edges. You can achieve a smooth edge by dipping the edge of the splint into the hot water and cutting it to produce a smooth edge or by smoothing it lightly with fingertip pressure after heating it with the heat gun briefly. ***The heat gun produces a very hot stream of dry heat. It should never be directed toward the patient's skin.*** Remember to set the heat gun on a cool setting before turning it off to avoid damage to the motor. You can eliminate the edge finishing step by cutting the edges so they seal or by rolling edges back after heating the thermoplastic before applying it to the patient. If edges remain slightly rough, you can apply a thin piece of moleskin along the edge to seal it for comfort.

Application of Straps

Straps attach the splint to the patient. Their location must be carefully planned to maintain the best contact with the splint and to provide three-point pressure. Apply adhesive-hook Velcro to the splint and attach the soft-brush Velcro or other foam strapping material to hold the splint securely on the patient. Hook Velcro adheres most effectively if the surface of the splint is prepared for adhesion. Remove the non-stick finish on the thermoplastic by applying a solvent or by scraping the plastic with the sharp edge of the scissors. Then briefly spot heat the surface of the splint and the sticky side of the Velcro with a heat gun (Fig. 17-19). It is best to place a full piece of sticky-back Velcro on the splint rather than two small pieces on the edges because repeated pull on the pieces during release of the strap may cause them to peel off. Strapping materials include colored Velcro, durable foam, neoprene, and elastic strapping in a variety of widths. Choose the strapping that best secures the splint to the patient comfortably. It is best to round the corners of the strapping material to avoid bending and dog ears (Fig. 17-20).

Padding

To enhance wearing tolerance, you can pad the splint. When padding a splint, allow extra space at the design and molding phases to contour over a bony prominence, avoiding additional pressure in this area. Some padding is applied before forming the splint, and some is applied afterward. If the padding is applied to the splinting material before heating, the excess water should be squeezed out before applying the material to the patient. Some thermoplastic material is available with a layer of padding already bonded to it. You can use stockinette liners instead of padding if light protection is desired. Prefabricated cotton or synthetic liners are available commercially. The patient may appreciate use of a light, washable stockinette under the splint to absorb perspiration. Sticky-back moleskin is also available for a thin, soft padding material. Padding, however, should never substitute for a well-fitting splint. Silicone gel can be used in splints to reduce slippage and to enhance scar remodeling.

Attachments

Outriggers and pulleys can be attached to splints when the splint base is complete. An outrigger provides a base for positioning the 90° angle of pull for dynamic splints or for directing a static progressive force. It can be made by rolling thermoplastic into a tube (Fig. 17-26), by using prefabricated tubes, or by bending wire to the desired position (Coppard & Lohman, 1996). Commercial outriggers are available in high- and low-profile designs. The therapist should consider the requirements of the outrigger for high or low profile, single or multiple finger, static progressive, or dynamic. Safety pins and paper clips can also be used for finger outriggers or pulleys (Byron, 1997; Saleeba, 2003). Outriggers have also been used for applying traction to a joint (Chinchalkar & Gan, 2003). When attaching an outrigger or pulley, prepare the surface of the splint first for optimal adhesion by scraping the surface or applying solvent. The outrigger or pulley attachment points should be treated similarly. Using dry heat with a heat gun, heat the surfaces and press them together (Fig. 17-27). They must be held together briefly to ensure adequate bonding. They should not be moved at this time unless repositioning is desired. If the pieces need additional reinforcement, heat another piece of thermoplastic and apply it over the outrigger base attachment. Again, prepare surfaces with dry heat and press them together for effective bonding. Some commercial outriggers can be attached with specially designed thumbscrews (Figs. 17-30 and 17-31).

Dynamic splints may be prone to slide distally because of the traction on the splint. You can control this migration by applying a friction surface on the splint that is in contact with the skin. Silicone gel or Microfoam tape (available through Sammons Preston Rolyan), which has a soft padded surface, provides light traction to keep the splint in place.

The tension of a dynamic splint is provided by rubber bands, coil springs, or elastic thread. You can attach these to the splint with Velcro tabs, hooks, thumbscrews, or knobs placed proximal to the outrigger on the splint base. Pulleys or line guides can redirect the line of pull as needed for dynamic or static progressive flexion splinting. Monofilament (fishing line) attached to the rubber band creates a smooth excursion for the rubber band tension as it pulls over the outrigger or under the pulley for dynamic splinting. The monofilament attaches to a finger sling (Figs. 17-28 and 17-30) or fingernail hook or tab to provide the appropriate tension and 90° angle of pull. Dynamic splints may incorporate hinges, which provide a movable axis at a joint. Hinges are available commercially or can be made from rivets (Byron, 1994), crimped thermoplastic tubing, or brass fasteners (Dennys, Hurst, & Cox, 1992). Static progressive splints use locking hinges and various types of inelastic components such as Velcro strips, monofilament line, MERiT components, and ClickStrips (Vazquez, 2002). Hinges and turnscrews may also be used for static progressive splinting to provide adjustable positioning of stiff joints in the optimal position tolerated by the patient. These components then allow adjustments as the patient achieves increased mobility (Schultz-Johnson, 2002).

Evaluating Splint Fit and Comfort

After the splint is finished, have the patient wear it for about 20 minutes and remove it to check for any redness. Redness or blanching of the skin may be an indication that the pressure of the splint is too much (Brand, 1995). Modify the splint if signs of redness or excessive pressure are present. Then reevaluate fit and comfort (Procedures for Practice 17-4).

Orthotic intervention requires a client-centered approach by a skilled therapist. Splinting is not merely the application of a device, but rather it is an important component in the rehabilitation process to meet the occupational performance goals of the patient. McKee and Rivard (2004) suggest that the successful use of this intervention demands the skills of a therapist working closely together with the patient to meet the needs of comfort, cosmesis, and convenience that will ensure wearability of the splint and optimal outcomes.

Technology is changing rapidly. New materials offer new possibilities for the splinting therapist. By combining skill and creativity with knowledge of new technology and the patient's needs, the therapist can meet the challenges of the future by applying principles of splinting to meet the goals of rehabilitation.

PROCEDURES FOR PRACTICE 17-4

Splint Checkout

Review the splint using these questions as guidelines:

- Does the splint achieve the purpose?
- Does the splint maintain the proper position of the joints? Check angles with a goniometer if necessary.
- Does the splint fit the contours of the hand, the arches, and bony prominences?
- Does the splint restrict or immobilize any joint unnecessarily?
- Is the splint long enough to support the splinted part?
- Are all edges smooth and all possible pressure points relieved?
- Does the splint allow functional use of the hand if allowed?
- Can the patient apply and remove the splint?
- Does the patient understand wear and care instructions?
- Is the splint cosmetically acceptable to the patient?

CASE EXAMPLE #1

Construction of a Resting Splint for a Patient with Hemiparesis

Occupational Therapy Intervention Process	Clinical Reasoning Process: Objectives	Clinical Reasoning Process: Examples of Therapist's Internal Dialogue
Patient Information Mr. J is an outpatient who sustained a left cerebral vascular accident (CVA) 3 weeks ago with resulting right hemiparesis. Patient is medically stable. Hypertonicity of finger flexors limit grasp and release of right hand. Limited in full extension passive range of motion (PROM) of fingers due to mild flexor hypertonicity.	Obtain information about the patient	"Hemiparesis may limit patient's full strength and dexterity of right hand, but functional grasp is possible. However, hypertonicity of flexors will affect ability to release objects held in hand." "The patient is highly motivated to retain his current hobbies, though both require functional grasp and release."
Interview: Mr. J. is a 67-year-old right-hand–dominant man who is retired but remains active with hobbies, including golf and bridge. He is married and lives with his wife in their two-story home.		
Interview: Mr. J. plays golf and bridge with a supportive group of friends who encourage his continued involvement and independence. In addition to his role as independent person, Mr. J. values self enhancement roles in his hobbies.	Evaluate to identify the problem(s)	"Mr. J values his role as an independent person, friend and sportsman. His hobbies allow continued socialization and self esteem."
Assessment: The therapist measured Mr. J's grip strength with dynamometer at 10# on right compared to 70# on left. He exhibits slightly increased flexor tone with difficulty fully extending fingers following grip. Passive extension of fingers was only slightly limited, but tone prevented full active extension. Sensation was normal for the right hand. He was able to grasp a golf club and hold cards in his right hand but has difficulty with release.		"He will need to use a resting splint to maintain full extension to counteract the effect of the hypertonic finger flexors."
During occupational therapy, a custom fabricated resting splint from 1/8" Ezeform was made for Mr. J. He tolerated splint wear without difficulty and was instructed in a nighttime wearing schedule.	Implement the intervention	"I will need to monitor splint tolerance as Mr. J. continues to gain strength. Modifications in the splint may be necessary."
Mr. J. gained grip strength on the right to 43# with slight hypertonicity of the finger flexors. He also gained strength in active finger extension. He regained full PROM of fingers. He resumed golf and card playing successfully.	Evaluate the result	"The splint helped to maintain a balance of the flexor spasticity and the weak extensors during the initial stages post-CVA. He used it at night initially, and it didn't seem to interfere with his sleep so he was happy to continue wearing it. He discontinued splint use at 6 months post CVA when he didn't need it anymore."

CASE EXAMPLE #2

Construction of a Hand-Based Thumb Splint for a Patient with CMC Osteoarthritis

Occupational Therapy Intervention Process	Clinical Reasoning Process	
	Objectives	**Examples of Therapist's Internal Dialogue**
Diagnosis: Mrs. O. is an outpatient with carpometacarpal (CMC) osteoarthritis of the right trapeziometacarpal joint of the right hand.	Obtain information about the patient	"She can reduce pain by applying joint protection principles, using a hand-based thumb splint, and modifying her activities."
Interview: Mrs. O. is a 55-year-old, right-hand–dominant woman who is employed part time as a librarian. She is independent in all ADLs but reports pain when grasping books, writing, and turning a key. She also has pain when gardening. She lives alone in her home. She prefers sedentary activities including reading and gardening in her small flower garden.		
Interview: In addition to her role as an independent person, Mrs. O. has the self advancement and self enhancement roles of worker and gardener.	Evaluate to identify the problem(s)	"Mrs. O. values all her roles. She is highly motivated to make changes that will allow her to continue in these roles."
Mrs. O.'s employer at the library is willing to make some changes to help Mrs. O. reduce pain during work if necessary. She is a valued employee, and they have suggested she do less of the shelving and spend more time on check-outs.		"Mrs. O. needs to work with her employer to find ways to manage her demands at work, by rotating tasks and taking mini-breaks during the day."
Mrs. O. loves to garden. She often spends long hours on her projects in the garden on her days off.		"Mrs. O. gets so involved in her gardening that she forgets about her thumb pain until it is quite severe. She may need to find ways to adapt her gardening and manage the time she spends in the garden."
During occupational therapy, Mrs. O. is fitted with a custom-fabricated hand-based thumb splint made from 1/16" Orfit thermoplastic. She is also instructed in gentle active range-of-motion and strengthening exercises for the thumb. Joint protection instruction is provided.	Implement the intervention	"She will benefit from use of the splint during her work day and as needed in the garden. She will try to modify her work day by taking mini-breaks for stretches and alternating tasks that may be more stressful to her thumbs. She would also benefit from setting a timer while in the garden so she remembers to take breaks and listen to her body for any signs of pain. Adaptations like easy-grip pruners may also be helpful in the garden. She will benefit from being shown various methods of joint protection in handling books and writing. She may also want to try a soft pen grip."
Mrs. O. tolerates the splint well. She wears the splint as needed during the day. She is able to write, work at the library, and garden with the splint on.	Evaluate the result	"She may need splint adjustments over time if changes occur in splint fit or comfort. She was given a clinic number to call if problems arise."
She understands the exercise program and is compliant. She enthusiastically applies the joint protection strategies and feels they help her pain.		

CASE EXAMPLE #3

Construction of Dynamic MCP Extension Assist Splint

Occupational Therapy Intervention Process	Clinical Reasoning Process: Objectives	Clinical Reasoning Process: Examples of Therapist's Internal Dialogue
Mrs. D. is a 41-year-old, right-hand–dominant woman who underwent MCP arthroplasties of the left hand for ulnar drift. She has a 12-year history of rheumatoid arthritis with ulnar drift and subluxation of the MCP joints on the left. This deformity has progressed over the past 3 years, and Mrs. D. reports significant loss of function and inability to lay her hand flat, to wash her face, or put her hand in her pocket. She works as a receptionist part time and has significant difficulty using her computer at work. She also experiences difficulty using keys, opening doors, and using a knife in meal preparation. She has become frustrated with her difficulty performing cooking tasks, because cooking is one of her hobbies. She lives in a two-story home with her husband and 3 teenage daughters.	Obtain information about the patient	"Initially Mrs. D. will need assistance with ADLs. She will be limited in use of her left hand. She will need to learn one-hand ADLs and may need to recruit more assistance from her husband and daughters at home. She has taken a medical leave from work to devote the next month to therapy. The surgeon was pleased with surgical result and wants her to follow his standard protocol. She should do well."
Her surgeon performed MCP arthroplasties with rebalancing of the extensor tendons on the left. She is referred to occupational therapy at 5 days post-op for splinting and ADL modifications.		
Interview: In addition to her roles as an independent person and mother, Mrs. D. identifies the self-advancement and self-enhancement roles of worker and cook.	Evaluate to identify the problem(s)	"Mrs. D. values her roles as independent person, mother, worker, and friend. She wants to retain all those roles."
Mrs. D hopes to resume her job, but her leave of absence will allow her to focus on her rehabilitation.		"As she gets further along in her recovery, her job will be reviewed, and modifications will be suggested at that time."
Mrs. D enjoys cooking and baking for her family and hopes to resume these activities. In the meantime, her teenage daughters will help with these tasks at home.		"Mrs. D. will need review of joint protection and may benefit from adaptations for the kitchen."
Assessment: The surgeon has told Mrs. D. that light ADLs can be resumed with the dynamic splint at 3 weeks after surgery.		
Mrs. D. is able to flex fingers in the dynamic splint, and then the rubber bands return her fingers to the extended position.		"She will need to wear the dynamic splint during the day and the resting splint at night per post-operative protocol."

The therapist fabricates a dynamic extension outrigger splint for daytime wear and a resting splint for night use. Mrs. D. is instructed to perform active MCP flexion exercises in the splint 10 times hourly during the day, allowing the rubber bands to return her fingers to full extension. She wears the dynamic splint for 4 weeks. During this time, the therapist also instructs her in joint protection principles and offers suggestions for assistive devices to facilitate occupational performance. She adapts her doorknobs, uses a key holder, and purchases cutlery with enlarged handles. She also enlists her daughters' help in the kitchen.	Implement intervention	"Mrs. D. will follow a standard protocol for post-operative MCP arthroplasty." "Mrs. D. needs review of joint protection and assistive devices. She will be quite open to these suggestions."
Mrs. D. returns to work 4 weeks after surgery to answer phones with the use of a headset. She gradually resumes full duties at 6 weeks after surgery. She continues to use the resting splint at night for 3 months. Mrs. D. achieves an excellent outcome postoperatively. She also achieves a higher level of independence in her occupational performance because of improved hand function and increased awareness of modifications in her daily activities.	Evaluate the result	"Mrs. D. has had a highly successful post-operative recovery and an excellent outcome."

SUMMARY REVIEW QUESTIONS

1. Name the steps of splint making in order.
2. Name the creases of the hand and describe their importance in splint construction.
3. What is the difference between the functional position of the hand and the position of safe immobilization in splinting? Give an example of when you would use each.
4. Describe the concept of dual obliquity as applied to splinting.
5. What does mechanical advantage mean in splinting? How does it apply to the length of the forearm trough?
6. What are some strategies to enhance compliance with splint wear?
7. Which material would be a good choice for a hand-based thumb splint? Why?
8. What does a splint checkout include?

ACKNOWLEDGMENTS

I would like to thank my husband, my family, and my colleagues for their inspiration, support, and encouragement while writing this chapter. I also want to acknowledge my patients who have been my teachers through the years, challenging me in the art and science of splinting.

References

Austin, G. P., Slamet, M., Cameron, D., & Austin, N. M. (2004). A comparison of high-profile and low-profile dynamic mobilization splint designs. *Journal of Hand Therapy, 17,* 335–343.

Bell-Krotoski, J. A., & Figarola, J. H. (1995). Biomechanics of soft-tissue growth and remodeling with plaster casting. *Journal of Hand Therapy, 8,* 131–137.

Bonutti, P. M., Windau, J. E., Ables, B. A., & Miller, B. G. (1994). Static progressive stretch to reestablish elbow range of motion. *Clinical Orthopedics and Related Research, 303,* 128–134.

Boozer, J. A., Sanson, M. S., Soutas-Little, R. W., Coale, E. H. Jr., Pierce, T. D., & Swanson, A. B. (1994). Comparison of the biomechanical motions and forces involved in high-profile versus low-profile dynamic splinting. *Journal of Hand Therapy, 7,* 171–182.

Boscheinen-Morrin J., & Connolly, W.B. (2001). *The hand: Fundamentals of therapy* (3rd ed.). Oxford, UK: Butterworth-Heinemann.

Brand, P. (2002). The forces of dynamic splinting: Ten questions before applying a dynamic splint to the hand. In J. Hunter, E. Mackin, & A. Callahan (Eds.), *Rehabilitation of the hand* (5th ed., pp. 1811–1817). St. Louis: Mosby, Inc.

Breger-Lee, D. (1995). Objective and subjective observations of low-temperature thermoplastic materials. *Journal of Hand Therapy, 8,* 138–143.

Breger-Lee, D., Bell-Krotoski, J., & Brandsma, J. W. (1990). Torque range of motion in the hand clinic. *Journal of Hand Therapy, 3,* 7–13.

Breger-Lee, D. E., & Buford, W. E. Jr. (1991). Update in splinting materials and methods. *Hand Clinics, 7,* 569–585.

Breger-Lee, D. E., & Buford, W. L. Jr. (1992). Properties of thermoplastic splinting materials. *Journal of Hand Therapy, 5,* 202–211.

Breger-Lee, D. E., Voelker, E. T., Giurintano, D., Novick, A., & Browder, L. (1993). Reliability of torque range of motion: A preliminary study. *Journal of Hand Therapy, 6,* 29–34.

Bunnell, S. (1996). Splinting the hand. *Hand Clinics, 12,* 173–178.

Byron, P. (1994). Splinting the arthritic hand. *Journal of Hand Therapy, 7,* 29–32.

Byron, P. (1997). The Rotterdam splint. *Journal of Hand Therapy, 10,* 240–241.

Callinan, N. J., & Mathiowetz, V. (1996). Soft versus hard resting hand splints in rheumatoid arthritis: Pain relief, preference, and compliance. *American Journal of Occupational Therapy, 50,* 347–353.

Canelon, M. F. (1995). Silicone rubber splinting for hand and wrist injuries. *Journal of Hand Therapy, 8,* 252–257.

Canelon, M. F., & Karus, A. J. (1995). A room temperature vulcanizing silicone rubber sport splint. *American Journal of Occupational Therapy, 49,* 244–249.

Chinchalkar, S. J. & Gan, B. S. (2003). Management of proximal interphalangeal joint fractures and dislocations. *Journal of Hand Therapy, 16,* 117–128.

Clark, E. N. (1997). A preliminary investigation of the neoprene tube finger extension splint. *Journal of Hand Therapy, 10,* 213–221.

Colditz, J. C. (2002). Plaster of Paris: The forgotten hand splinting material. *Journal of Hand Therapy, 15,* 144–157.

Coppard, B. M., & Lohman, H. (1996). *Introduction to splinting: A critical-thinking and problem solving approach.* St. Louis: Mosby-Year Book.

Dennys, L. J., Hurst, L. N., & Cox, J. (1992). Management of proximal interphalangeal joint fractures using a new dynamic traction splint and early active motion. *Journal of Hand Therapy, 5,* 16–24.

Fess, E. E. (1995a). Principles and methods of splinting for mobilization of joints. In J. Hunter, E. Mackin, & A. Callahan (Eds.), *Rehabilitation of the hand* (4th ed., pp. 1589–1598). St. Louis: Mosby-Year Book.

Fess, E. E. (1995b). Splints: Mechanics versus convention. *Journal of Hand Therapy, 8,* 124–130.

Fess, E. E., & McCollum, M. (1998). The influence of splinting on healing tissues. *Journal of Hand Therapy, 11,* 157–161.

Fess, E. E., & Philips, C. A. (1987). *Hand splinting: Principles and methods* (2nd ed.). St. Louis: Mosby.

Fillion, F. L. (2004). Ulnar collateral ligament thumb sling. *Journal of Hand Therapy, 17,* 69–70.

Flowers, K. R. (2002). A proposed decision hierarchy for splinting the stiff joint, with an emphasis on force application parameters. *Journal of Hand Therapy, 15,* 158–162.

Flowers, K. R., & LaStayo, P. (1994). Effect of total end range time on improving passive range of motion. *Journal of Hand Therapy, 7,* 150–157.

Flowers, K. R., & Pheasant, S. D. (1988). The use of torque angle curves in the assessment of digital joint stiffness. *Journal of Hand Therapy, 1,* 69–74.

Glasgow, C., Wilton, J., & Tooth, L. (2003). Optimal daily total end range time for contracture: Resolution in hand splinting. *Journal of Hand Therapy, 16,* 207–218.

Groth, G. N., & Wulf, M. B. (1995). Compliance with hand rehabilitation: Health beliefs and strategies. *Journal of Hand Therapy, 8,* 18–22.

Gyovai, J. E., & Howell, J. W. (1992). Validation of spring forces applied in dynamic outrigger splinting. *Journal of Hand Therapy, 5,* 8–15.

Jacobs, M. L. & Austin, N. (2003). *Splinting the hand and upper extremity: Principles and process.* Baltimore: Lippincott Williams & Wilkins.

King, J. W. (1993). Modification of common treatments in hand rehabilitation. *Journal of Hand Therapy, 6,* 214–217.

McKee, P., & Morgan, L. (1998). *Orthotics in rehabilitation.* Philadelphia: Davis.

McKee, P., & Rivard, A. (2004). Orthoses as enablers of occupation: Client-centered splinting for better outcomes. *Canadian Journal of Occupational Therapy, 71,* 306–314.

Saleeba, E. C. (2003). Dynamic flexion splint for the distal interphalangeal joint. *Journal of Hand Therapy, 16,* 249–250.

Schultz-Johnson, K. (1996). Splinting the wrist: Mobilization and protection. *Journal of Hand Therapy, 9,* 165–175.

Schultz-Johnson, K. (2002). Static progressive splinting. *Journal of Hand Therapy, 15,* 163-178.

Stern, E. B., Callinan, N., Hank, M., Lewis, E. J., Schousboe, J. T., & Ytterberg, S. R. (1998). Neoprene splinting: Dermatological issues. *American Journal of Occupational Therapy, 52,* 573–578.

Tubiana, R., Thomine, J.-M., & Mackin, E. (1996). *Examination of the hand and wrist.* St. Louis: Mosby-Year Book.

Vazquez, N. (2002). Introduction to a new method for inelastic mobilization. *Journal of Hand Therapy, 15,* 205–209.

Weiss, N. D., Gordon, L., Bloom, T., So, Y., & Rempel, D. M. (1995). Position of the wrist associated with the lowest carpal tunnel pressure: Implications for splint design. *Journal of Bone and Joint Surgery, 77A,* 1695–1699.

Weiss, S., LaStayo, P., Mills, A., & Bramlet, D. (2004). Splinting the degenerative basal joint: Custom made or prefabricated neoprene. *Journal of Hand Therapy, 17,* 401–406.

Willey, M. (2004). Modification to a pediatric thumb splint. *Journal of Hand Therapy, 17,* 379–380.

CHAPTER 18

Wheelchair Selection

Brian J. Dudgeon and Jean C. Deitz

LEARNING OBJECTIVES

After studying this chapter, the reader will be able to do the following:

1. Describe the factors that should be considered in wheelchair selection and explain how they interrelate.
2. Describe the three basic types of wheelchairs and reasons for each to be chosen.
3. Specify measurements typically taken to determine wheelchair and related seating system configurations for a particular individual.
4. Demonstrate knowledge of the components common to many wheelchairs and describe why each merits consideration in wheelchair selection.
5. Discuss the roles and responsibilities of the occupational therapist in wheelchair selection.
6. Suggest how the occupational therapist can facilitate the user's participation in wheelchair selection.

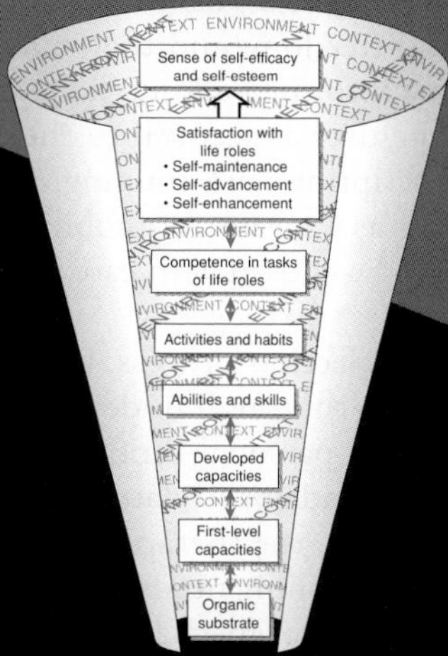

Glossary

Angle in space—Angle of the seat back in relation to the true vertical when the seat and back are rotated counterclockwise as a unit. Sometimes called tilt-in-space or orientation, this position may be altered for postural control.

Camber—The amount of angle on the wheels, creating flare-out at the bottom. A 4–6° camber is recommended for push rim convenience and wheelchair width.

Pelvic rotation—Asymmetrical position of the pelvis with forward position of one side, typically due to low back rotation, muscle asymmetry, or spinal deformity.

Pelvic obliquity—Uneven level of anterior superior iliac spines and ischial tuberosities associated with spinal scoliosis, hip abnormality, and pelvic deformity.

Proximity-sensing devices—Devices or systems that remotely sense the position of a body part (e.g., head) and use that position to control the wheelchair without physical contact between the part of the body used for control and the switch.

Scanning—Control option that presents choices one at a time, grouped or singly, until the desired choice is offered for the user to select by switch activation.

Scoliosis—Abnormal spinal curvature, typically with a lateral curve, S-shaped, or C-shaped pattern creating an unlevel shoulder and pelvic position. Scoliosis deformities may be fixed or flexible.

Seat-back angle—The angle of the seat surface relative to the back surface. This angle is typically 90–100°. Backrest angles and seat plane angles may be designated separately.

Sip and puff—A system typically involving a dual-action switch, in which one action is controlled by the user sipping on a tube held in the mouth and the second action is controlled by puffing on the same tube. (In wheelchair operation, the chair functions can be controlled by patterns of switch closures.)

Snap-secured—A locking mechanism on the frame that holds folding frame parts in place for smoother ride with less frame migration and reduced wheel and caster flutter.

Third-party payer—Individual or organization (i.e., insurance company) other than the person receiving services that pays for services or equipment.

> "Mobility is a fundamental part of living. Being able to move about, to explore, under one's volitional control is a keystone of independence." (Warren, 1990, p. 74)

Mobility is a major part of daily living, facilitating participation in home, work, and community settings. Wheelchairs are a focal point for many people who have mobility challenges. As such, wheelchair selection and training necessitate consideration of the user's preferences and current and anticipated performance needs, capacities, and environments. The process of evaluating and choosing a wheelchair system as part of functional mobility involves the user, an interdisciplinary team, and equipment suppliers or vendors. Also, family members, primary care providers, and others from the user's work and leisure environments may contribute important information useful in choosing an appropriate wheelchair system to meet needs for mobility within and between environments.

Wheelchair selection has a functional orientation and involves multiple factors including the user's (1) needs and goals; (2) home, work, recreational, and other community environments; (3) physical and mental status and anticipated course of impairments; (4) financial and community resources; (5) views about appearance and social acceptability; and (6) needs for interface of the wheelchair system with other assistive technology. A selection process includes issues such as current and changing needs of the user and family, training needs for use and maintenance, and anticipated changes in technology. A wide range of wheelchair options are available, yet funding and community-based resources for training and servicing of mobility devices often limit choices.

Some individuals use wheelchairs only occasionally to meet brief transportation needs, while others use them continuously to meet most day-to-day positioning and mobility demands. Especially in the latter case, the events that lead to the need for a wheelchair may be dramatic. For some, acquiring a wheelchair system may create stress or confusion, and this can hinder their contributions to the assessment of needs and selection of a system. Others view the acquisition of a wheelchair as a positive move toward greater independence and freedom, and they make substantial efforts to become informed about choices. In either case, the needs of the user are central to the overall process of selection, prescription, and training, with the wheelchair viewed not just as a means for mobility but as a highly personal device to be chosen with care and precision (Steins, 1998).

In contributing to the selection process, the occupational therapist must have a thorough understanding of the user's medical needs and personal profile, including environment, daily routines, and goals related to activities and participation. In addition, the therapist should understand the seating and positioning needs of the individual, and wheelchair types, control mechanisms, features, and accessories. Knowledge of product resources and local area vendors is also critical in creating device choice options. Although this information is presented as components, all of these factors inter-relate in comprehensive planning for functional mobility through a clinical reasoning process.

EVALUATION OF THE INDIVIDUAL

During evaluation, primary attention is given to user and family goals for use of the wheelchair as part of a functional mobility system. Further, the therapist evaluates the skills of the user, the user's ability to develop new skills, and changes expected from the diagnosis (e.g., declining sensorimotor skills). How the user plans to transport the system is also an important consideration. Evaluation of needs should include interview, observation, and examination. Trials with seating simulators, trial seating systems, self-propulsion methods, and/or other control systems are often needed to confirm appropriate prescription of these systems. Figure 18-1 outlines evaluation needs; patient-specific information relates to Case Example 1.

The evaluation typically involves both sitting posture and mobility needs. The therapist can best assist in seating and wheelchair selection by understanding the client's personal and medical profiles (Behrman, 1990).

Sample Wheelchair Evaluation: Needs of the Individual

Client information: Lisa, 17-year-old high-school senior with recent C7 level tetraplegia from traumatic SCI in MVC. Attends evaluation with mother. Inpatient stay in acute rehabilitation unit.

Functional Needs and Goals

Environments of use (home, school, work, community at large): Full-time at home, at school, and in other community locations. Has interest in athletics, high school programs.

Seating needs (time, pressure relief, transfers): Postural support needs for trunk and thighs, cushioning for neurogenic skin. Able to perform push-up pressure relief and independent transfers to/from wheelchair.

Control or propulsion methods (attendant, manual needs, power controls): With postural support and seat belt, self-propels using friction push rims and wheel brakes. May benefit from grade aids for propelling up inclines.

Methods of wheelchair transport (car, van, truck; ground travel, air travel): Family owns full-sized truck and minivan. Lisa has driver's license but has not yet explored or been oriented to adaptive driving.

Physical Examination

Head control: No limitations in mobility when trunk is stabilized.

Sitting balance and spinal deformity: Now using TLSO.

Pelvic rotation or obliquity: Symmetrical at this time, mobile pelvis, lumbar support through TLSO.

Lower limb mobility: Full PROM, flaccid at rest with periodic spasms into hip adduction, knee extension and ankle plantarflexion. Neurogenic skin below C8 level.

Upper limb mobility: Full PROM, good to normal strength in shoulder, elbow flexion 5/5, extension 4/5, forearm rotation 4/5, wrist extension 4/5, flexion 3/5, finger extension 3/5. Neurogenic skin lateral hand, 4th and 5th fingers.

Sitting and Balance Needs

Postural support: Now using TLSO for stability, lateral trunk supports for midline positioning. Seat belt and chest harness necessary for support and safety. Explore back cushion contouring when/if TLSO is discontinued.

Cushioning: Solid base of support needed with cushion contour. Tried low-profile Roho and Jay Cushion. Lisa preferred latter for balance, good cushioning effects.

Wheelchair Training Needs

Control or propulsion: Manual propulsion with seating components in place. Enlarged and rubberized friction rim tried and preferred over plain rim or knobs. Wheel camber may assist in hand placement. Needs training for propulsion on level surfaces, maneuvering corners and doorways, all outdoor settings.

Transfers to and from wheelchair and chair, bed, toilet, bathing tub or shower, floor, car: Is beginning transfer training wheelchair to bed using sliding board. Removable armrests and swing-away footrests will enable independence. Will need car transfer training, tub transfer, and floor to wheelchair instruction later.

Wheelchair Maintenance Resources

Lisa expresses interest in learning maintenance routine; father willing to assist as reported by Lisa and her mother. Wheelchair vendor within 15 miles of family home.

Figure 18-1 Evaluation overview. Clinicians address these issues by interview, observation, and physical examination. SCI, spinal cord injury; MVC, motor vehicle collision; TLSO, thoraco-lumbar-sacral orthosis; PROM, passive range of motion.

RESOURCE 18-1

Wheelchairs
The Boulevard
jjMarketing, Inc.
1205 Savoy Street,
Suite 101
San Diego, CA 92107
www.blvd.com

ABLEDATA
8630 Fenton Street,
Suite 930
Silver Springs, MD 20910
www.abledata.com

Ability Magazine
1001 W. 17th Street
Costa Mesa, CA 92627
www.abilitymagazine.com

Assistive Technology, RESNA
1700 N. Moore Street,
Suite 1540
Rosslyn, VA 22209
www.resna.org

Jim Lubin's disABILITY Information and Resources
www.makoa.org

Exceptional Parent
EP Global Communications
65 East Route 4
River Edge, NJ 07661
www.eparent.com

Mainstream Magazine-Online
www.mainstream-mag.com

New Mobility
23815 Stuart Ranch Road
P. O. Box 8987
Malibu, CA 90265
www.newmobility.com

Paraplegia News & Sports 'N Spokes
2111 East Highland Avenue,
Suite 180
Phoenix, AZ 85016
www.pva.org

Rehabilitation Engineering Research Center
University of Pittsburgh
5044 Forbes Tower
Pittsburgh, PA 15260
www.wheelchairnet.org

iBOT™ Mobility System
www.independencenow.com/ibot/index.html

Magic Wheels™
Magic Wheels, Inc.
www.magicwheels.com

ATI
HandMaster Manual Assist
Wheelchair Drive System
www.mycycle.si

Innocom, Ltd
Superwheel Electric
Wheelchair
www.innocom.com.hk/product4.htm

Personal Profile

The client's personal profile includes factors such as age and stature, developmental status, living environment, educational or work routines and plans, recreational pursuits, other assistive technology needs or uses, and future anticipated needs. Special attention is given to seating and operation of the chair in both private and public environments. Specifically, the therapist should consider factors such as floor surfaces, outdoor terrain, climate, doorways, hall spaces, restroom dimensions, workspace design, transportability, and parking. If a client has already used an adaptive mobility device before, it is important for the therapist to determine the user's assessment of pros and cons regarding that mobility method or system. A blending of walking aids and wheelchair use may be planned. Therapists should recognize that uses of adapted mobility systems often conflict with personal spaces and public accessibility. Public accessibility is based in part on human-factors design in which the typical wheelchair user sits at a 19-inch height and propels a manual wheelchair through a 32-inch wide opening and turns around in a 5-foot clear floor space. Many people are served well by environments that accommodate this type of user, but others continue to be constrained by the environment and need individual guidance about making appropriate accommodations. For example, some power mobility devices have a larger turning radius or excessive weight that limits the user's access to some buildings and/or transportation systems.

Medical Profile

A user's medical profile includes review of medical history and physical assessment. The therapist should be aware of the user's diagnosis and prognosis, that is, whether the medical condition is temporary, stable, or progressive. Such factors influence choices related to complexity of options and need for adjustment as well as preferences for rental, lease, or purchase. For example, if a condition is temporary, a chair may be selected with greater concern for cost factors. In contrast, if a client's condition is chronic and stable and necessitates full-time use of a wheelchair, durability and individualization to meet needs are priorities. If a condition is progressive, a chair that permits a range of adjustments for both seating and wheelchair control may be indicated. The physical assessment should focus on neuromuscular status (e.g., muscle tone, postural control, reflexes, and coordination), musculoskeletal status (e.g., range of motion, deformity, strength, and endurance), sensory status (e.g., anesthetic skin and skin integrity), and physiological status (e.g., temperature regulation, respiration, and cardiopulmonary needs).

Total cost over the life of the wheelchair is a consideration for users with chronic disability and everyday use. For manual users, some ultralight models appear to have the greatest longevity, or greater years of expected use, in comparison with standard wheelchairs or other lightweight models (Cooper, Boninger, & Rentschler, 1999).

In recent years, wheelchair products have been evaluated using standards promulgated by the American National Standards Institute (ANSI) and Rehabilitation Engineering and Assistive Technology Society of North America (RESNA), an interdisciplinary association for the advancement of rehabilitation and assistive technologies, and by direct product comparisons regarding features such as stability, safety, durability, and cost (Cooper et al., 1997). These standards are changing and bring new terminology as well as design elements that impact choices regarding seating, wheelchair frame styles, and attachment options.

SEATING AND POSITIONING

Critical to selection of a wheelchair system is the attention given to seating and posture needs of the user. Seating systems have a significant effect on the ability of the user to perform functional activities and on basic decisions about choice of mobility base types and components. Effective seating has several broad goals, including: (1) enhancing posture, comfort, physiological maintenance, and skin protection; (2) preventing injury; (3) accommodating existing deformity; (4) enabling vision readiness and upper limb function; and (5) attending to cosmetic appearance and social acceptance. Evaluation and intervention related to positioning often entail participation by team members such as physical therapists to address postural supports, speech therapists to address augmentative communication, and family members and others to address daily routines and schedules. Occupational therapists may coordinate these concerns by incorporating the needs and goals of the user and family with medical care concerns in making recommendations and by analysis of functional issues so that recommendations optimize the individual's access to activities and participation in various environments. The role of team members varies somewhat in different locations and organizations.

Seating Principles: Solid Base of Support

Seating strategies and particular techniques are both age and diagnosis specific (Letts, 1991), although some principles can be applied to meet a variety of needs (Garber & Krouskop, 1997). One such principle is the need to provide the individual with a solid base of support that begins with appropriate pelvic positioning. The sling seat, common to folding and unlocked wheelchair cross-brace frames, is the seating element most often criticized because it tends to promote pelvic instability and malalignment of the thighs and is often the primary component of seating modification (Krasilovsky, 1993). A solid seating base is accomplished by stabilizing the pelvis on a firm surface with pressure distributed throughout the buttocks and the full length of each thigh.

Postural Supports

Postural control is influenced by the seat and back contact surfaces and by orientation adjustments to the **seat-back angle** and the **angle in space** (Fig. 18-2). There are three commonly used seating position features. First is a sitting position with 90° hip, knee, and ankle positions. Second is a slight anterior tilt to the pelvis to distribute weight through the buttocks and thighs and, for some individuals, to inhibit abnormal reflexive responses (Fig. 18-3). Third is a 95° seat-back angle with a 3–5° angle-in-space recline. Hardware that secures the modular seat and the back components to the frame are often used to adjust these positions.

Seat Surfaces and Cushioning

The seat and back contact surfaces can be planar, precontoured, or custom contoured. Single-plane or flat surfaces are appropriate only for those who need little or no postural support and those who can easily reposition themselves to maintain balance and comfort. Contoured designs are used to provide added contact for postural support and distribution of pressure. Custom contouring is often necessary for individuals who need accommodation for deformity of the pelvis or spine, those with abnormal muscle tone, and those who have discomfort

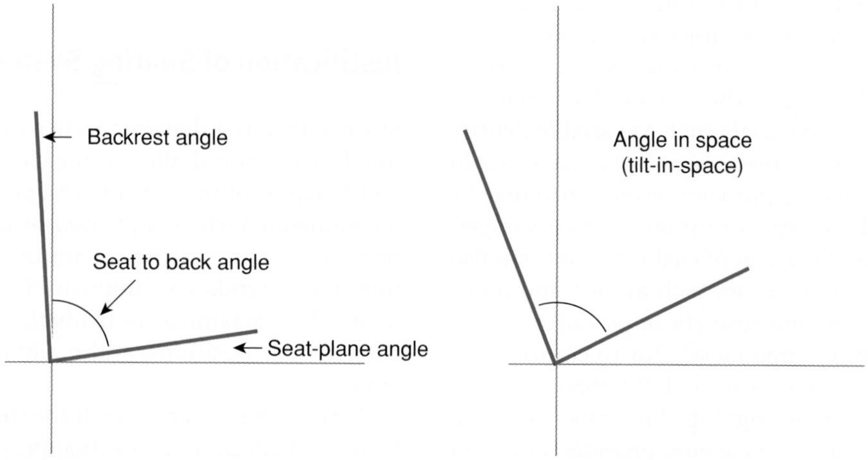

Figure 18-2 Adjustment of seat-back angle and angle in space helps to support posture and provide appropriate pressure distribution.

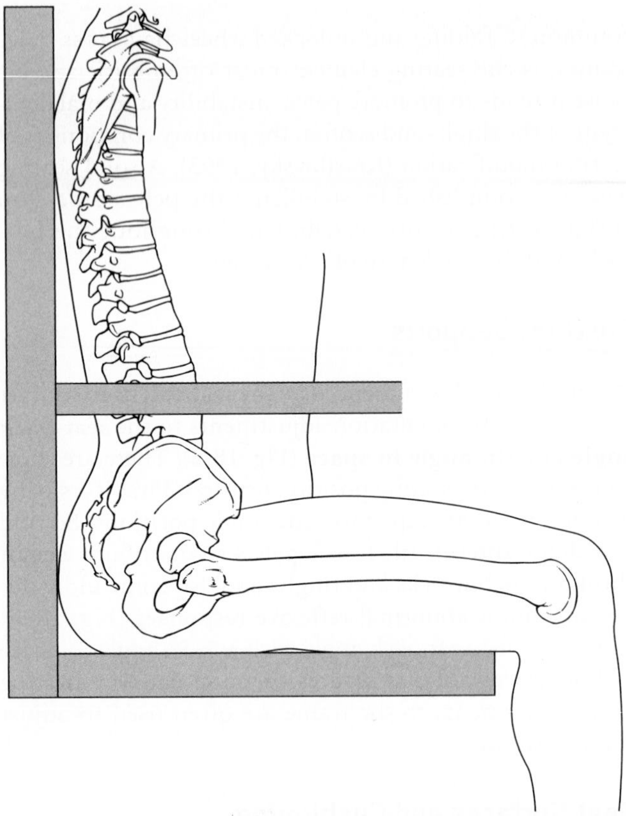

Figure 18-3 Pelvic positioning with slight anterior tilt helps to distribute tissue pressure throughout the buttock and thigh.

from lack of support at the lumbar spine. These cushions are individually fabricated by bead-seat molding, foam-in-place techniques, or other shape-sensing technology (Cooper, 1998).

Cushions are used to reduce peak pressures associated with bony landmarks and to distribute pressure evenly over a large area of skin contact. Shearing forces that compromise circulation also can be reduced by appropriately shaped cushions. Although cushioning relieves skin and soft tissue pressures, factors including postural stability and control, ease of transfers, ability to accommodate deformity, moisture, and maintenance may be as important for some users. Cushioning of the seat and back may call for use of one or more materials such as variable-density foams, gels, air, and honeycomb-shaped plastics. Custom contouring and alternating pressure systems also may be considered. Table 18-1 lists advantages, disadvantages, and examples of each. Selection of cushion coverings also should take into account factors such as heat and moisture, friction, durability, and cosmetic appearance.

Skin should be monitored closely for tolerance when use of any new seat cushion is started. Progressive sitting time schedules along with ongoing skin inspection routines are essential because no cushion provides sufficient pressure relief during regular use. Properties of materials vary, yet no cushion is considered sufficient in relieving pressure enough to preserve capillary blood flow to compressed tissues while a person is seated. Pressure on sitting surfaces is greatest during manual propulsion (Kernozek & Lewin, 1998), and users should be informed about dynamic factors that may threaten the health of skin tissues. Although cushions help to reduce skin pressures (Pellow, 1999), other means of pressure relief are necessary. Assisted or user-performed wheelchair push-ups, side leans, or forward leans may be used for pressure relief needs every 15–30 minutes as required. Alternatively, technologies for pressure relief include tilt-in-space mechanisms, use of alternating pressure cushions that continuously cycle high- and low-pressure segments of a cushion (Burns & Betz, 1999), and custom contouring of cushions (Fig. 18-4). The latter show some promise for reducing static seating pressures (Rosenthal et al., 1996).

Adding Seating System Components

A seatbelt is often recommended because it serves an important role in stabilizing the pelvis as part of a therapeutic positioning in the seating system. This anterior support is typically mounted on the wheelchair frame so that it pulls on the pelvis at a 45° angle to the base of the seat back, fitting just under the anterior superior iliac spines. Additional seating supports should be used as needed to improve posture, restrict abnormal movements, and promote head control and voluntary use of the limbs. For example, if sitting balance and abnormal postures are problematic, lateral trunk and thigh supports may be suggested. In addition, use of anterior supports may be necessary across the upper trunk, knee, or ankle for balance and stabilization. Neck and head supports are used to promote head and neck alignment and are sometimes recommended for safety. Upper extremity positioning also may be a concern, in which case specialized armrests or lap trays can be recommended.

Justification of Seating Systems

Since sitting is a dynamic rather than a static state, seating devices should allow some element of pressure relief and freedom of movement. The principle of *less is more* is recommended when applying specialized seating systems because as more seating apparatuses are used, freedom of movement tends to diminish. Therefore, only components that maximize individuals' abilities to function, correct their positions, and maintain comfort should be applied.

Expense justification with the **third-party payer** must relate to medical necessity. Inappropriate seating and mobility base selection can exacerbate complications and accelerate decline for the user. Functional accessibility and

Table 18-1. Cushion Types and Examples

Classification	Advantages	Disadvantages	Example
Foam	Lightweight	Uneven pressure relief	T-Foam by Alimed
	Easily sized, shaped	Poor durability	
	Low cost	Hard to clean	
Gel-filled	Self-contouring	Heavy to move	Jay Cushion by Jay Medical
	Posture control	Temperature sensitive	
	Sitting balance	Leaking, maintenance	
Air-filled	Lightweight	Reduced control/balance	High or Low Profile by Roho
	Even pressure relief	Requires attention to air-pressure tending	
	Little shear	Potentially requires repair of puncture/air leaking	
Honeycomb	Lightweight	Uneven pressure relief	Supracor Stimulite Contoured
	Easy to clean	Difficult to shape	
	Low maintenance	Excessive thickness	
Custom-contoured foam	Surface area coverage	Expense	Contour U, Pindot by Invacare
	Reduced shearing	Longevity with change	
	Better postural control	Reduced weight shift	
Alternating pressure systems	Scheduled relief cycle	Cost and availability	Dynamic Seating System by Talley Medical
	Reduces user effort	Uneven pressure relief	
	Self contouring	Unsteady sitting balance	

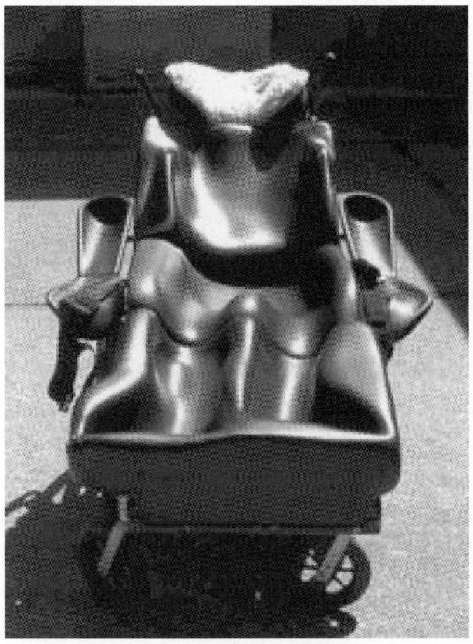

Figure 18-4 Custom contouring. Cushions are molded using a bead-seat system. Molds are then cast for manufacturing of foam core and upholstery. Backs and seats, as well as arm and leg positioning, can be customized.

protection of the user from secondary complications that come with immobility or physiological risks with seating may be cited as part of insurance justifications.

To justify specialized seating with users and families, the experienced therapist can employ clinical observation and literature reviews. Improved motor skills, comfort and participation, physiological supports, and functional independence are widely hoped for as part of specialized seating and wheelchair selection. Some goals should be viewed cautiously, however, because wheelchair and seating configurations can be considered specific to certain diagnostic groups and mostly provide a prosthetic effect, meaning that these benefits are largely limited to the time that the person spends in the seating system. Reid, Laliberte-Rudman, and Hebert (2002) reviewed 46 seating interventions studies with adults and concluded that, although some performance skills and factors have been partially addressed, research has not adequately attended to engagement in occupations and psychosocial issues. Others have reviewed seating needs of specific clinical populations, such as those with spinal cord injury (Krey & Calhoun, 2004; Minkel, 2000) and identify support for some seating strategies while emphasizing the need for more explicit study of outcomes. Although more wheelchair seating research is now being conducted, methodology challenges and studies with small samples have led to calls for a more focused research effort. Geyer et al. (2003) assembled a variety of stakeholders who reviewed existing work addressing wheelchair seating and called for future research efforts aimed to address wheelchair transportation, postural control, comfort, and tissue integrity. See Evidence Table 18-1, which is related to the case examples.

WHEELCHAIR TYPES: MOBILITY BASES

Once the therapist has a full understanding of the user's personal and medical profile and seating needs, it is important to understand the types and uses of wheelchair systems. Wheelchairs used in everyday activity can be divided into three general categories: (1) attendant-propelled chairs, (2) manual chairs, and (3) power mobility devices (Hobson, 1990). Special-use chairs and attachments to standard mobility bases for participation in recreation and sports also can be considered.

Attendant-Propelled Chairs

Attendant-propelled chairs are designed to be pushed by another individual because of the user's inability to propel or operate a wheelchair in a functional or safe manner. This may be necessary for some users on a temporary or circumstantial basis, for example as a means to be mobile as part of community outings. Attendant assistance also may be a full-time need for individuals who have diminished cognitive capacities, severe judgment difficulties, or restricted physical capacities. These chairs may be full size (e.g., those used in skilled nursing facilities) or may be smaller and created for use in limited spaces (e.g., folding stroller types). Attendant-propelled chairs also are used as a substitute for power mobility when the individual's typical mobility system is being repaired or when space constraints preclude power mobility use. When assisting a user in selecting an attendant-propelled chair, it is necessary to consider not only the fit and comfort of the chair for the person who will be seated, but also the sizing needs of the person most likely to be pushing it. As with all wheelchairs, attention to transportation of the user and the wheelchair device between environments needs attention and planning. Besides chairs specifically designed to be attendant propelled, many manual wheelchairs (described next) can be propelled by an attendant.

Manual Chairs

Manual wheelchairs are for those who can propel and brake using the upper limbs (Fig. 18-5). These chairs have a variety of frame types, weights, and transport features. In general, manual wheelchairs have rigid or box frames or folding frames; folding frames are either free or **snap-secured**. Quick-release wheels can also be selected. Folding, snap-secured frames with quick-release wheels and detachable front rigging may offer the greatest flexibility for transporting the wheelchair. Although rigid-frame chairs may provide greater energy efficiency with propulsion, they may be awkward for loading into automobiles.

The conventional manual wheelchair frame has large rear wheels, which are used to propel the chair, with smaller caster wheels in the front. Wheelchairs of this design are highly maneuverable and easy to propel, and they allow freedom for tilting, which is necessary when ascending or descending curbs. Standard designs, sometimes called depot or institutional wheelchairs (Cooper, 1998) weigh at least 50 pounds without specialized seating systems. A distinction can be made between multiuser chairs, often found in health care settings, and single-user or rehabilitation chairs, sometimes designated as lightweight and ultralight chairs. In recent years, sturdy lightweight metals and designs have been adapted from sport wheelchairs, resulting in lightweight and ultra-lightweight wheelchairs ranging from less than 25 pounds to 40 pounds. Lightweight chairs are often used on a full-time basis. Many new designs allow adjustable wheel positions and seat heights, making it possible to optimize biomechanical efficiency for the user (Masse, Lamontagne, & O'Riain, 1992). Along with reduced weight, these changes can enhance propulsion and ease transport (Brubaker, 1990; Parziale, 1991).

Other types of manual wheelchair designs include the amputee frame for the person with loss of or severely reduced weight of the lower limbs. In this design, the rear axle is offset farther behind the seat back than is standard. This concentrates a person's weight farther in front of the rear axle, reducing the risk of the chair tipping backward. Another type of manual wheelchair, although not commonly recommended, is the indoor frame. It has large front wheels, which are used for propulsion, with smaller casters in back. Although this design rolls easily over door sills and rug edges, larger barriers such as curbs are difficult to traverse, and transfers may be awkward because of the forward placement of the large wheels.

Manual propulsion is typically accomplished through hand rims attached to the outside of the large wheels. Optimally, the user is seated so that, with shoulders slightly extended and elbows partially flexed, each hand rests at the 12 o'clock position of each hand rim (Brubaker, 1990). Contact with rims generally occurs between the 11 and 2 o'clock positions on each side. Circular

Evidence Table 18-1
Best Evidence for Occupational Therapy Practice Regarding Wheelchair Selection Based on Case Examples

Intervention	Description of Intervention Tested	Participants	Dosage	Type of Best Evidence and Level of Evidence	Benefit	Statistical Probability	Reference
Manual wheelchair testing using ANSI/RESNA standards	Selected ultra-lightweight wheelchairs were tested and compared to lightweight wheelchairs.	12 models of ultra-light wheelchairs; 4 models receiving greater analysis.	ANSI/RESNA tolerance standards.	Randomization of product testing. IC2b; machine tested vs. consumer use.	Specific products (by Invacare and Kuschall) had better durability characteristics (i.e., life-cycle value).	$p < 0.05$	Cooper, Boninger, & Rentschler, 1999
Pressure distribution using wheelchair seat cushions	Mean and peak pressure mapping with 4 cushion materials/products.	7 adult participants with disability that included **scoliosis**.	Talley pressure monitoring of mean and peak pressures.	Product testing in single-session use by participants. IIIC2b	All cushions relieved peak pressure, although only foam products reduced the mean pressure ratio.	$p < 0.05$	Apatsidis, Solomonidis, & Michael, 2002
Dynamic sitting and reaching by wheelchair users with paraplegia	Displacement of center of pressure (COP) when performing reaching tasks while seated on three types of cushions.	9 adult wheelchair users with SCI.	Reach and COP displacement seated on air, flat foam, and generically contoured seat cushions.	Trials using different cushion types. IC1b	Generically contoured foam resulted in greater reach distance and speed with increased stability.	$p < 0.01$	Aissaoui et al., 2001
Survey completed by individuals with ALS about preferences for use of mobility	Survey about experiences with use of wheelchairs.	42 adult patients with ALS (mean age = 54 years) observed in a neuromuscular clinic who used manual (n = 20) or power (n = 22) wheelchairs.	Naturally occurring accommodations used by individuals.	Survey about clinical course of treatment and change. IIIB3b	Wheelchair use permitted greater community interaction. Focused on comfort and ease of maneuvering. Either manual or motorized beneficial.	Powered wheelchair use had benefit to activity ($p < 0.05$).	Trail et al., 2001

continued

Evidence Table 18-1 Best Evidence for Occupational Therapy Practice Regarding Wheelchair Selection Based on Case Examples (*continued*)

Intervention	Description of Intervention Tested	Participants	Dosage	Type of Best Evidence and Level of Evidence	Benefit	Statistical Probability	Reference
Prospective study of ameliorative and palliative care for ALS	Follow-along regarding receipt of palliative care procedures (e.g., OT) or devices (e.g., adaptive aids).	121 patients with ALS (mean age = 58 years).	Naturally occurring interventions and accommodations, with follow-up every 4 months.	Survey of individuals with ALS (recent and long-term diagnosis). IIIA2b	Use of wheelchair more than doubled in follow-up; use of therapy resources and other accommodations also increased.	Significant increase in wheelchair use from baseline to follow-up with palliative care ($p < 0.001$)	Albert et al., 1999
Description of clinical reasoning by client and physicians	Natural-occurring clinical decision-making process based on client's description and physician's treatment reasoning.	n = 1; Team including 44-year-old woman with ALS and her physicians.	Naturally occurring treatment interventions.	Single case description. VC1c	Psychosocial effects of impaired mobility, with cost challenges leading to recommendation for use of wheelchair for safety and function.	NA	Iezzoni, 2000

SCI, spinal cord injury; ALS, amyotrophic lateral sclerosis; NA, not applicable.

steel tube hand rims are common. For users who have difficulty with grip, hand rims can be covered with vinyl coating; knobs or other projections can be added to the rims so that grip is not required; and/or gloves or mitts can be worn to improve traction. Gloves and mitts also protect the hands. Hand rims vary in size. Small hand rims, often used on racing chairs, result in a slower and more difficult start but provide for a high top speed that is sustainable with relatively little effort (Ragnarsson, 1990).

Manual propulsion by a person with hemiplegia or unilateral upper limb use necessitates additional adaptations. Commonly, the person with hemiplegia uses the more capable side for the hand rim and the leg and foot to steer and provide additional propulsion and braking. This requires removal of the unused footrest and usually requires lowering the seat height or using small-diameter wheels to optimize foot contact with the floor. For the user who plans to propel the wheelchair using only one arm, a chair can be ordered with both hand rims on one side so that each wheel can be controlled independently or together. Learning to maneuver two hand rims on the same side can be perceptually and mechanically difficult. Another option for unilateral control is the single-lever drive. This rare device uses a forward-and-backward motion to propel the chair and rotation of the lever to turn the chair.

Augmentation of manual propulsion and braking systems is available. As an aid to propelling on inclines, hill climbers or grade aid devices restrict the rearward movement of wheels through a friction stop engaged by a lever on each tire. Speed control and braking to a stop simply depend on slowing wheel rotation by use of the arms or legs. New devices that augment propulsion through electrical or mechanical means now also can be considered. Such devices provide supplemental power from an electric motor to amplify the user's effort (e.g., iGlide™ and Superwheel™ electric wheelchair) or mechanical advantage through a two-gear system (e.g., HandMaster™ and Magic Wheels™)

Brakes are used on each large wheel and are engaged through a variable-length single- or dual-action lever, depending on reach and force abilities. Such levers press on the tire to resist rolling and require that tires be fully inflated with periodic tightening after tire wear. Brakes restrict wheel turning when the chair is parked but are not typically recommended for slowing or stopping. In addition, anti-rotation locks also can be used on casters.

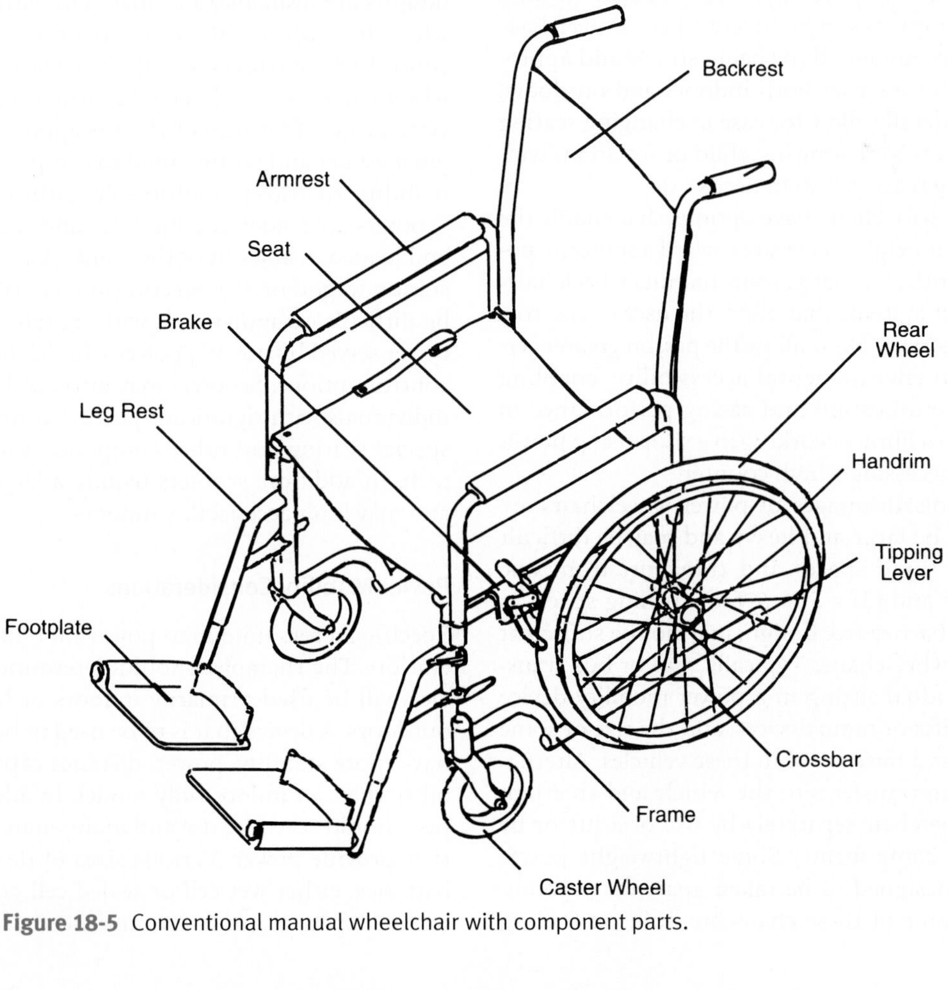

Figure 18-5 Conventional manual wheelchair with component parts.

Power Mobility Devices: Motorized Wheelchairs

Power mobility devices are used by individuals (1) who cannot propel a chair using either the hands or the feet, (2) for whom the energy expenditure required to walk or propel a manual chair is contraindicated, (3) who have musculoskeletal complications, such as arthritis, in upper limb joints, (4) who are prone to repetitive stress injury, and/or (5) who have neuromuscular dysfunction that may cause associated reactions in the lower extremities when the upper extremities are used for manual wheelchair propulsion. There are a number of types of power mobility devices. Selection of power mobility can be a complex task due to the variety of user needs and the many options for wheels, controls, and environmental designs (Field, 1999).

Power Wheelchairs

Most new power wheelchairs have a power-base design so that the wheels are, in effect, independent of the seating components. Such bases may have front-, mid-, or rear-wheel drive, with a variety of wheel diameters. For each type of design, the wheels may be coupled to motors through exposed or concealed chains or gear systems. Mid-wheel–drive chairs generally have a smaller turning radius, which improves maneuverability. Power-base wheelchair designs are noted for being sturdy and appropriate for the full-time user both indoors and outdoors. These designs generally allow for ease in changing seating dimensions, such as for a growing child or for an individual with changing seating system needs.

Several power-base chairs have options that enable the user to change seat height or elevate toward a standing position independently. Similarly, some manual wheelchairs have manual lever systems that allow the user to rise to a near standing position. These allow the person greater vertical flexibility in environmental accessibility, enabling face-to-face communication and easing performance in reaching books in a library, working in a shop using power equipment, and accessing a high counter.

The primary disadvantages of power wheelchairs are that (1) they can be large and heavy and may be difficult to maneuver in small spaces and transport from one place to another; and (2) a 5 × 5–foot turning space, as part of standard barrier-free design, may not be sufficient for some power wheelchairs. Typically, van or bus transport of the individual sitting in a power mobility device requires special lifts or ramp devices, and the size of some chairs necessitates a raised roof in these vehicles. Alternatively, the user can transfer into the vehicle and an attendant can load the chair separately by use of a lift or by breakdown into components. Some lightweight power wheelchairs are designed to be taken apart for automobile transport. Some of these chairs are built on folding frames and/or have low-powered motors, making hill climbing and use on uneven surfaces more challenging. Assistance with taking apart and reassembling the chair often is required.

Manual Wheelchair with Add-On Power Unit

Another option for power mobility is the use of an add-on unit on a manual wheelchair to provide power assistance. Such systems can be engaged and disengaged to switch between manual and power mobility. Since a significant amount of weight is added to the chair and units are not easily taken on and off the frame, this option is most commonly suggested as a trial for a transition to a regular power wheelchair. As previously described, pushrim-activated power-assisted devices (e.g., iGlide™) have also been used to reduce energy demands and the biomechanical strain of manual propulsion (Algood et al., 2004), especially in environmental conditions such as inclined ramps, uneven surfaces, and thick carpet (Algood et al., 2005).

Scooter

A popular type of power mobility device is the scooter. Scooters typically have three wheels, although four-wheeled designs are available, and may have either rear- or front-wheel drive. Most of these designs are characterized by tiller control, wherein users steer the scooter by rotating the front wheel while using a lever-style switch for forward and reverse power. This type of chair is appropriate for the marginal walker and is often used to compensate for a person's inability to travel comfortably within the community. Scooters are sometimes modular and can be disassembled and loaded in and out of the trunk of a car or the back of a station wagon or van. Steering and control of scooters can be difficult, so individuals with marginal control may be better served by use of a power wheelchair with a variety of control options. Scooters may also not be appropriate for individuals with significant posture control needs because special seating and other components are difficult to attach. In addition, scooters require a larger turning radius and may limit accessibility indoors.

Power Mobility Considerations

Specific factors unique to power mobility require consideration. The therapist should determine whether the device will be used primarily indoors or both indoors and outdoors. A device that is to be used in both settings must have more stability, power, distance capability, and durability than an indoor-only model. In addition, the therapist should consider use and maintenance of the batteries that provide power. Various sizes of deep-cycle lead acid batteries, either wet cell or sealed cell gel types, have different expense, longevity, and needs for maintenance.

Other power wheelchair characteristics to consider include noise, braking systems, ride quality, and portability, including ease of assembly and disassembly if appropriate. If the device can be disassembled, the weight and size of each part should be carefully evaluated for transportability. Non-leaking sealed cell or gel batteries are preferred for added safety in airline transportation.

Selection of appropriate controls for driving is critical. Programmable controls are most common and enable careful selection of torque and speed control based on wheeling surface resistance and safety. Power devices are typically driven using one of two types of options: proportional or discrete control. Most commonly, a proportional joystick is used, in which directions and speeds are linked to angle and magnitude of stick displacement. Proportional control also may be achieved through **proximity-sensing devices** that sense the position of the head. The user moves his or her head as a joystick, and the wheelchair's speed and directional control is proportional to the head displacement. An alternative is discrete micro-switch control activated with a joystick, a multiple-switch array, or a single-switch scan. Each switch activation engages a preset or programmed speed and direction. Micro-switch systems require less skilled movement to achieve control, although control of the wheelchair is often less precise than that provided by proportional control. Also, learning to use micro-switch control is not simple. Each direction may be controlled by activating a micro-switch using a body part (i.e., hand, arm, chin, foot, head, mouth, lips, or tongue), and control may be organized through a combination of special techniques such as **sip and puff**, **scanning**, or switches imbedded in headrests (Fig. 18-6). For instance, breath may be used for forward and reverse control, and proximity-sensing switches may be used to activate turning control. When selecting controls, the therapist should consider adjustment options provided by various systems in relation to the needs of the individual. For example, clients with poor motor control may benefit from adjustment of programmable electronics that enable wheelchair speeds to be automatically restricted when turning or that enable several levels of control to be programmed for new learning and training in various environments.

Power wheelchairs and scooters are electronically braked, meaning that drive wheels do not rotate except under power. Gears are then released by levers that allow the chair to roll freely.

Activity- or Environment-Specific Wheelchairs

For everyday use, attendant-propelled, manual, or power wheelchairs are selected. Many users, however, need mobility to overcome unique barriers or for use in recreation and leisure activities that require activity-specific technology (Axelson, 1998). Special power-wheel configurations can be used for ascending or descending stairs (e.g., the iBOT™). Other special designs for wheelchairs, including those for use at the beach and on other soft and uneven surfaces, are available commercially or may be custom made. For recreation, cycling configurations may be requested. Row cycles are large, low to the ground three-wheeled cycles propelled by a rowing action that activates chain-driven rear wheels. Cycling action also can be added to manual wheelchairs (Fig. 18-7) or be configured as a separate chair for outdoor sport. Sport wheelchairs for racing, basketball, and other competitions are commercially available, but often they require customized sizing and expert instruction. For a thorough review of options

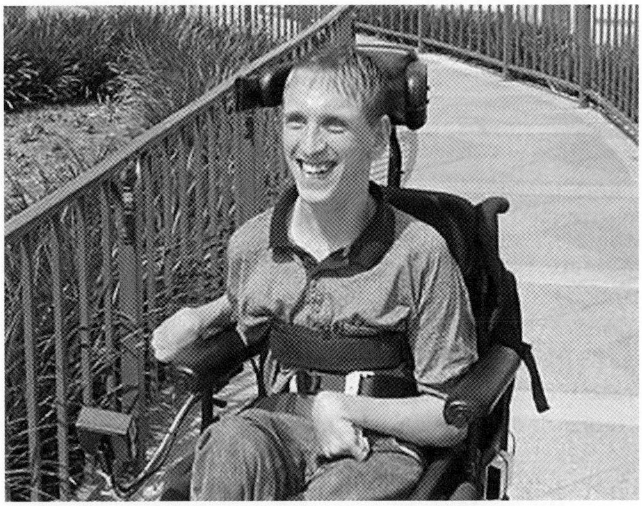

Figure 18-6 College student uses a power wheelchair controlled with proximity switches in a head array. The display in front of right armrest provides feedback regarding drive selection, environmental unit (ECU) functions, and battery level. A switch on the right side of the head array permits selection of drive and ECU functions. (Courtesy of Adaptive Switch Laboratories, Inc., Spicewood, TX.)

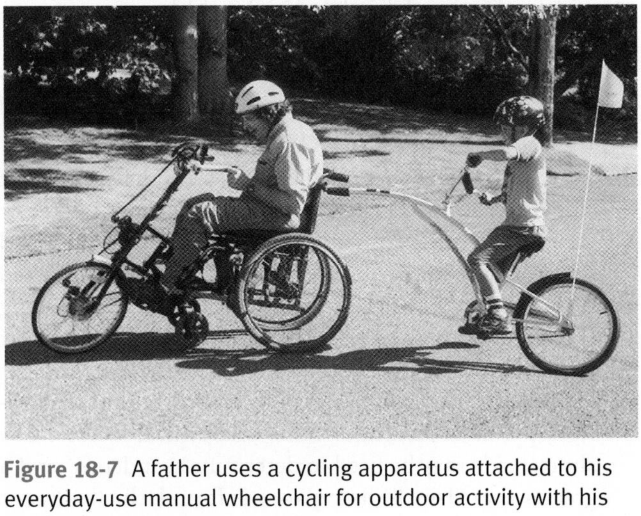

Figure 18-7 A father uses a cycling apparatus attached to his everyday-use manual wheelchair for outdoor activity with his children.

for using activity-specific or sport and recreation chairs, see Cooper (1998).

WHEELCHAIR SIZING AND ERGONOMIC CONSIDERATIONS

Modern wheelchairs are engineered as modular systems and are assembled to match the specific physical dimensions of the user. Measurements of the individual form the basis for determining wheelchair frame size, need for adjustable ranges in component parts, and need for customization to meet special needs.

Sizing

Appropriate size determinations of the wheelchair frame, seat, back, leg rests, and armrests are based on measurements typically taken with the user in an optimally seated position. Alternatively, the therapist can evaluate the individual on a mat in a supine or side-lying position and take careful measurements of distances between key landmarks. These measurements are confirmed for accuracy with the user seated. The user's typical or specialized clothing needs should be considered during measurement. If thoracolumbar bracing or lower limb orthotics and prosthetics are likely to be used in the wheelchair, they should be worn during sizing measurements. Manufacturers of wheelchairs and seating systems have differing standards for measurement and sizing. Typically included are measures of pelvic or hip width; upper and lower leg lengths; mid-back, mid-scapula, and top of shoulder heights; chest and shoulder widths; elbow height; and overall sitting height (Fig. 18-8).

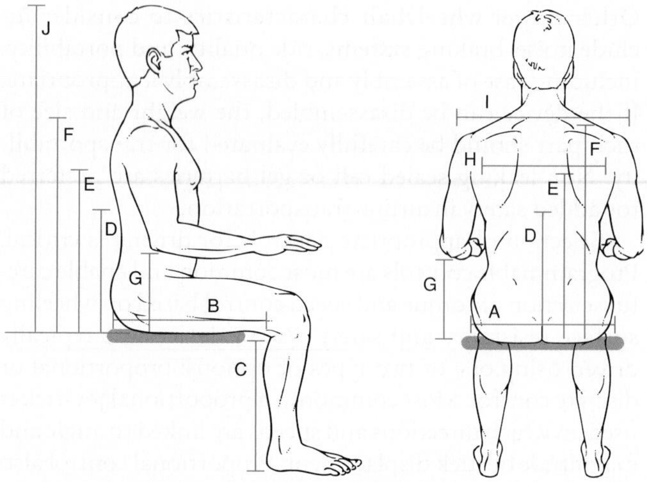

Figure 18-8 Seating measurements. For B to G, all measurements are taken on both right and left sides. A, Hip and thigh width; B, thigh length; C, leg length; D, back height to below scapula; E, back height to mid-scapula; F, back height to top of shoulder; G, elbow and forearm height; H, chest width; I, shoulder width; and J, sitting height.

- Seat width: The therapist determines the widest point across the hips and thighs and typically adds a total of 5 cm (2 inches) for adequate clearance on the sides. Overall wheelchair width may be dictated by the seat width measure. Wheelchairs should be as narrow as possible while allowing for comfort, easy repositioning, clothing needs, and transfers. For manual users, narrower wheelchairs are likely to improve ease of hand rim propulsion and maneuverability.
- Seat depth: The therapist, for both the left and right sides, measures the distance from the most posterior part of the buttocks under the thigh to the popliteal fossa of each knee. About 5 cm (2 inches) is subtracted from the measure. This allows as much weight bearing through the thigh as possible without the front edge of the seat pressing into the back of the knee. Right and left leg length discrepancies can be caused by hip dislocation, **pelvic rotation**, or other anatomical factors. The shorter side may be used to determine seat depth, or if a greater than 1-inch discrepancy is found, the front seat edge may be offset to accommodate the length of each side. Individuals who use their feet to propel or steer will need greater front-edge seat clearance.

Selected seat cushion height should be incorporated into further measures of trunk, arm, and leg.

- Back height and width: The therapist generally takes three measures from the seat surface upward (1) to the mid-back just under the scapula, (2) to the mid-scapula or axilla, and (3) to the top of the shoulder. Back height is affected by seat cushions, which should be considered in sizing decisions. Height of the chair back is based on the need for postural stability and freedom of arm movements for propulsion or other functions. For those who exclusively self-propel, a chair back height of 2–5 cm (1–2 inches) under the tip of the scapula may be preferred. For sporting activities, the optimal back height may be even lower. By contrast, for power wheelchair users, back heights to mid-scapula or the top of the shoulder may be necessary to allow use of postural supports for the upper trunk and the head. Chest and shoulder width should be measured in cases of deformity or to determine the space requirements for lateral trunk supports or other trunk-positioning devices. Alterations of the standard sling back may be necessary for improving trunk posture by using an adjustable or flexible sling back, curved backs, or additions of lateral trunk supports.
- Seat height and leg rests: Seat height is based on positioning of the individual such that footrests have at least a 5-cm (2-inch) clearance from the floor. Use of seat cushions affects this measurement by raising overall seat height. Seat height is determined with the individual's knees and ankles positioned at about 90°.

Measurements are taken from under the distal thigh to the heel of the individual's commonly used footwear or shoe. Several inches of adjustment are typically available in leg rest lengths. Unusual leg lengths or hip or knee deformity may necessitate special ordering.

- Armrest height: The therapist measures from under each elbow to the cushioned seating surface with the shoulder in neutral, the arms hanging at the sides, and the elbows flexed to 90°. Armrests must provide forearm support with neutral shoulder position but should not obstruct reach to hand rims for propulsion or to brake locks.

Common Components

In addition to overall sizing and seat and back surface, the team and user should consider selection of head and neck rests, armrests, leg rests, and other options. Table 18-2 lists options for head, neck, arm, leg, and foot support. Users should consider armrest stability for performing wheelchair push-ups for pressure release. Detachable or swing-away styles may allow greater ease in sliding board and other sideways transfers and improve access to tables and desks. Guards can be used on armrests to keep clothes from coming in contact with wheels. Attachment of lap trays may require use of full-length armrests or other specialized hardware. The front rigging consists of leg rests and foot plates. Options are selected according to needs for elevation of the calf and foot, ankle position, and stabilization of the leg. Flip-down footplates or platforms are common and popular because they can reduce the overall length of the chair. Swing-away or detachable front rigging may enable easy transfers and transportability of the wheelchair in and out of vehicles.

Tires can be either pneumatic (air filled), semi-pneumatic (airless foam inserts), or solid-core rubber and are mounted on spoke or molded wheels. Air-filled tires are lightweight with low rolling resistance, providing a well-cushioned ride and shock absorber function that tends to improve comfort and prolong the life of the chair, but they do require regular maintenance. Semi-pneumatics provide good cushioning and less maintenance, but tire wear may be more of a problem. Solid-core tires are noted for minimal maintenance and approach the weight and low rolling resistance of high-pressure pneumatic tires.

Casters, as either front or rear wheels, vary in diameter, and small ones usually facilitate maneuverability. Pneumatic and semi-pneumatic caster tires provide some shock absorption for use outdoors and on rough surfaces. Solid-core caster tires are best for use indoors and on smooth surfaces. Special designs (e.g., Frog Legs™) for manual wheelchairs and power wheelchairs are promoted for shock absorption and enhanced maneuverability.

Placement of the rear axles can be fixed or adjustable on most manual wheelchairs, especially newer manual lightweight and ultralight styles. Backward placement of the axle tends to increase stability; by contrast, forward placement of the axle decreases stability but increases maneuverability and shortens turning radius. Sometimes rear wheels have a **camber** adjustment. This orients the hand rim for easier propulsion and may slightly widen the wheel base for better stability. Anti-tipping extensions can be used on a wheelchair to prevent the chair from tipping backward or forward. Typically used on the back, these fixed or adjustable extensions can improve safety, particularly during mobility training.

Seatbelts, safety vests, and harnesses vary in design and are used for both safety and positioning. These devices should be considered for individuals who have severe neuromuscular impairments and need control for posture and safety. Restraints may be considered with individuals who have poor judgment, but these should be avoided whenever possible and be regarded separately from seating postural needs. In general, restraint reduction efforts in long-term care facilities are often enhanced by use of appropriate and comfortable seating (Stinnett, 1997).

Frame and upholstery color and material options are numerous. Users can personalize their chair through selections of colors and other styling. Durability, cleaning,

Table 18-2. Head, Arm, and Leg Supports

Component	Attachment to Frame	Adjustment	Style
Head and neck supports	Fixed or removable	Height, depth, and rotation	Flat, winged, lateral, occipital, or wedged
Armrests	Fixed, swing away, and/or removable	Same height or adjustable height	Full length or desk length, rigid or padded
Leg rests	Fixed rigid, swing away, and/or detachable	Fixed or telescoping length	Fixed angle or elevating
Calf pad and foot plate	Rigid or flip up, flip away	Variable sizes in pads or straps	Plate, tubular, rigid, or padded

ease of repair, and compatibility of materials with temperature regulation, friction, moisture, and skin protection also require careful planning.

Recline and tilt-in-space options enable postural changes for rest and pressure relief. In attendant-propelled wheelchairs semi-reclining up to 30° from upright or full reclining up to 90° from upright can be considered. In tilt-in-space systems, the seat and back assembly pivot together. This feature makes the use of postural seating components more stable because the angle between the seat and the back remains unchanged, reducing or eliminating the problem of shear. Power recline systems can be used with conventional or power-base designs. Such systems may involve tilt-in-space and/or low-shear back recline, both of which provide pressure relief and rest positioning (Hobson, 1992). Tilt-in-space chairs that go back 45–60° achieve effective pressure relief under the buttock and thigh and may have other physiological benefits, such as improved respiration (Chan & Heck, 1999). These systems, however, may add costs and increase wheelchair size and weight.

Narrowing devices are available for some non-secured folding frame manual chairs to reduce chair width temporarily for fitting through doorways. These devices mount on one side of the seat and narrow the chair when a crank is turned to shorten a belt wrapped around the frame to narrow the chair.

Other considerations are accessories that optimize use and performance. Lap trays can be used for postural support of the upper limbs and serve a variety of purposes related to function. Other accessories include mounting bags or baskets for storage and carrying, cup or bottle holders for taking fluids, and storage attachments for reacher or walking aids to enhance access and mobility. Some wheelchair users also need other assistive technology, such as communication devices or environmental controls. These devices may be mounted on the wheelchair and operated independently of wheelchair controls or can be integrated with power wheelchair controllers.

MOBILITY TRAINING

Mobility training with the wheelchair system is essential and often involves interdisciplinary team members, such as the physical therapist. Most users benefit from instruction and practice beyond the training provided by vendors. Once the chair has been provided, a check should be conducted, and appropriate training of the user and attendants should commence. This includes review of the user's goals for mobility along with a check of the device for fit and adjustment. Instruction also should be provided regarding (1) use of the chair indoors and outdoors and on a variety of surfaces (e.g., level, carpeted, incline, and uneven); (2) transfers (e.g., bed, toilet, and car); (3) transport of the wheelchair (e.g., cars, trucks, vans, and buses); and (4) maintenance of the wheelchair (e.g., cleaning the chair, lubricating moving parts, monitoring tire pressure and wear, adjusting brakes, and caring for batteries). Troubleshooting with the wheelchair system ultimately becomes the responsibility of the user and equipment supplier or vendor, but the therapist may advise about problem-solving strategies and organization of maintenance routines and schedules. Throughout training, the therapist emphasizes safety issues because accidents during day-to-day wheelchair use, although infrequent, do occur, and some appear to be preventable (Calder & Kirby, 1990).

Manual wheelchair users also benefit from instruction about propelling, braking, and transport. Particular attention to hand placement and trunk lean for effective and efficient wheeling can be explored. General consumer use guidelines are available for the user and trainer (Axelson et al., 1998). Power wheelchair users also need guidance about power functions such as controllers, batteries, and accessory devices. With all wheelchair users, the therapist should provide initial checks; periodic follow-up to address safety issues, fit, and adjustment; and updated information about new options to meet the changing needs of the user.

Transportability of the wheelchair system between environments can be especially challenging. Loading and unloading should be trialed with the vehicle most likely to be used. As noted, car transfers of the user and loading and unloading of the wheelchair need careful planning. Breakdown of the wheelchair for portability or the addition of special lift accessories to vehicles should be considered during selection. Weight of the wheelchair and component parts may be limiting to users as well as care providers who assist with vehicle transfers. Lifts are often used with vans or buses. In these vehicles, wheelchair tie-downs are necessary as safety mechanisms to keep chairs stabilized when traveling. The necessary style may be determined by wheelchair design. Such devices secure the wheelchair to the base of the vehicle; the individual is independently secured in the wheelchair seat or in another seating device within the vehicle.

WHEELED MOBILITY AND PARTICIPATION

As part of the wheelchair selection process, impact of devices on the users' roles and participation needs to be considered relative to home, work, and community contexts. Functionally matching to the environment in terms of access within and between settings, speed of mobility, and positioning may impact interactions. Different routes of travel may be necessary that could detract from feelings of inclusion. Speed of mobility may hinder shopping trips within and between stores or with movements at work. Armrest or other features of the wheelchair may preclude positioning with peers at dinner or meeting room tables. Professional rating tools that address needs (Miller et al., 2004) and consumer rating tools that address satisfaction with wheeled mobility devices are being proposed and address issues and interactions between the person, the technology, and the environment (Mills et al., 2002).

Greater successes in matching devices with environments of participation is needed. Although wheelchair mobility can lead to successful independence, challenges continue regarding integration of wheelchair users in various settings. For example, data on disability and workplace accommodation (http://www.infouse.com/disabilitydata/workdisability/2_1.php) reveal that less than 25% of wheelchair users are employed. Studies involving wheelchair users often indicate that obstacles created by use of wheeled mobility devices are seen as a major reason for lack of community participation and as a source of frustration (Chaves et al., 2004; Hoenig et al., 2003; Reid et al., 2003). Nevertheless, use of wheelchairs, and powered mobility devices in particular, is often credited with enhancing occupational performance and participation (Brandt, Iwarsson, & Stahle, 2004; Buning, Angelo, & Schmeler, 2001; Davies, DeSouza, & Frank, 2003). Although the built environment is a major reason for obstacles, attention also should be given to associated factors such as wheelchair user fitness and health, use of assistants and other assistive technologies, and social interactions in the community (Meyers et al., 2002).

FINAL DETERMINATION

In making a final determination regarding seating components, style, size, and control systems, the user and team take a comprehensive and functional view, simultaneously considering the current and future needs, desires, and resources of the user; environments of participation; and anticipated changes in technology (Batavia, Batavia, & Friedman, 2001).

Decision Making and Justification

Costs and related funding issues are critical components of the decision-making process. Expensive technology and options should not be ordered unless justifiable for increased function, health (e.g., skin protection), user satisfaction, or safety. When expensive choices are being considered, it is important to rule out the feasibility of using less costly alternatives. For example, before selecting power mobility, it is important to rule out the feasibility of using a manual chair because the cost of providing and maintaining a powered system is estimated to be approximately three times that required for a manual system (Warren, 1990). In such cases, appropriate justification must be clearly delineated for users and third-party payers. Some users decide to purchase devices or features on their own or seek funding through other sources.

A comprehensive functional mobility system for an individual often includes more than one means of mobility and selective use in different environments (Hoenig et al., 2002). For example, an individual may use limited walking skills within settings and benefit from a manual chair for traveling short distances, such as at home, and a power chair for traveling longer distances in the community and at work. Funding sources may pay for only one of these options, but with mobility being unique to different activities, negotiation of options may be explored with health insurance as well as educational and vocational support programs.

The Clinician's Responsibilities

Technology design and products are changing rapidly. Therefore, it is a continual challenge for occupational therapists to remain current. Therapists have a responsibility to keep abreast of new technology, new products, and new product evaluation research. They must be able to provide users with current information on the advantages and disadvantages of various wheelchairs, components, and features. In addition, they must have current knowledge of issues related to availability, serviceability, and performance of various wheelchairs and options (Behrman, 1990). Professional and consumer sources of information about wheelchairs, related options, and manufacturers of mobility systems, controls, and seating systems are useful for product information (see Resources 18-1).

Therapists also are encouraged to explore wheelchair standards developed by the American National Standards Institute (ANSI) and Rehabilitation Engineering and Assistive Technology Society of North America (RESNA) and the International Standards Organization (ISO) (http://www.wheelchairstandards.pitt.edu/). These voluntary standards for wheelchair developers and manufacturers provide guidelines for product specifications based on uniform measurements and testing. Use of these standards facilitates product comparisons. Besides being aware of wheelchair standards, the therapist also is responsible, along with the interdisciplinary team, to develop relationships with appropriate vendors of seating and wheelchair systems.

Wheelchairs, selected through a user-led team, can facilitate participation in multiple environments. Selection of an appropriate wheelchair system results from a clinical reasoning process that considers multiple variables, particularly best fit, function, and the user's preferences. Consumers' satisfaction with seating and mobility systems is critical to program evaluation that addresses out-

CASE EXAMPLE #1

Wheelchair Selection for a Student Who Has Tetraplegia

Occupational Therapy Intervention Process	Clinical Reasoning Process	
	Objectives	**Examples of Therapist's Internal Dialogue**
Patient Information Lisa is a 17-year-old high school senior with C7-level tetraplegia from a traumatic spinal cord injury (SCI) that she experienced in an automobile crash. She is expected to be a long-term wheelchair user, and in the hospital, she demonstrates the ability to propel a manual ultralight wheelchair using coated push rims. Lisa previously was active in soccer and other sports and would like to match her school colors with her wheelchair frame. She was intrigued to learn about competitive wheelchair sports but is inexperienced with independent mobility.	Appreciate the context	(See Chapter 43 for review of spinal cord injury rehabilitation).
	Develop intervention hypotheses	"Lisa may not endorse her need for long-term use of a wheelchair but may agree to the interim reality and specific wheelchair choices related to return to home and school." "Ultralight wheelchair styles have good longevity and can be customized in various ways for her size and needs." "A vendor and options for wheelchair choices from such a vendor should be introduced to Lisa and her family."
	Select an intervention approach	"A rehabilitative approach matches her adaptive capacities and skills with training for use of appropriate assistive technology, environmental accommodations, and care providers."
	Reflect on competence	"My own knowledge of wheelchair needs is strong, but my awareness of currently available products will be augmented through the vendor and product representatives. Accessibility needs at home, in school, and in the community will need to be explored specifically for Lisa and her support network."
Recommendations The care team is preparing a wheelchair prescription and considering these features: Wheelchair • Manual ultralight cross-brace folding frame • Purple frame with black upholstery • Adjustable axle position with camber control	Consider the patient's appraisal of performance Consider what will occur in therapy, how often, and for how long	"Lisa may regard the wheelchair as a short-term versus a long-term strategy but seems interested in resuming independent mobility, as seen in her use of a loaner wheelchair. Helping her learn about customization of size, cushioning, colors and other features may encourage her use of the wheelchair."

• Lift-off desk-length tubular armrests • Swing-away fixed-angle foot rests with heel loops on flip-up foot plates • Vinyl-coated push rims with pneumatic tires and non-pneumatic front casters • Grade aids and standard rubber-coated brake levers Seating • Cloth-covered Jay seat cushion with flexible sling back, mid-scapular height • Seat belt and chest strap	Ascertain the patient's endorsement of plan	"Her new wheelchair may not be available until after inpatient hospital discharge." "Options to review with her for selection of chair include frame type, cushioning, armrest and leg rest features, frame and upholstery color, and a variety of hand rim and brake features." "Gel cushion is encouraged for sitting balance and pressure relief. Air demonstrated good pressure relief but can impair sitting balance and necessitates tending to air pressure. Foam or silicone have less even pressure distribution but are lighter weight and do not need regular maintenance. Gel has the precaution of cooling/freezing with low outdoor temperature and could puncture and leak."
Summary of Short-Term Goals and Progress A loaner rehabilitation wheelchair has been provided to Lisa and she makes use of this self-propelled device to go to and from therapy and other appointments. When she is with visitors, she is often pushed to other locations on the hospital campus. Sitting tolerance times have been increasing daily with skin inspection performed by Lisa with nursing or therapy supervision and guidance. Sitting tolerance and travel distances are being staggered and staged to increase time and range of mobility. By discharge, up to 6 hours of wheelchair time is expected before bed-rest relief. Indoor mobility independence is expected including use of doorways and elevators. Outdoor mobility is supervised initially to assure safety with ramps, curb cuts, and cross slopes. Wheelchair-to-bed transfer training is proceeding with use of a lightweight sliding board and standby supervision for safety. Toilet and tub transfer skills are being introduced, and she currently receives moderate assistance. Independence in wheelchair transfers is expected with standby supervision anticipated.	Assess the patient's and family's comprehension Understand what the patient is doing Compare actual to expected performance Know the person Appreciate the context	"Trial use of a loaner wheelchair has Lisa experiencing transfers, self-propulsion, and environmental access on hospital grounds. She is taking responsibility to go to and from therapy sessions but is seen being pushed by family and friends at other times." Staging of wheelchair sitting time is scheduled, and Lisa seems willing to observe this precaution and is accepting of reminders to attempt pressure relief routines. She does not appear to attend to time of day on a regular basis, so she will likely need an external cue of some sort." "Lisa monitors her progress carefully in both occupational and physical therapy with high hopes of regaining strength. Nevertheless, she also is aware of her functional mobility and capacity to self-propel and transfer." "Self-initiated goals for functional mobility in and around the hospital campus are being suggested by her. These are being encouraged with use of appropriate standby supervision."
Next Steps Lisa will be using the wheelchair full time at home, at school, and in other community locations. Her own wheelchair is being ordered and will be available at discharge or soon after her return home. Accessibility at home and school need to be assessed with Lisa and her family.	Anticipate present and future patient concerns Analyze patient's comprehension Decide if patient should continue or discontinue therapy and/or return in the future	"Lisa has become aware and has concerns about accessibility at home and school where stairs are an issue to enter and move between levels." "An accessibility audit of home and school through interview will be conducted and a home visit with Lisa and family members is anticipated before inpatient discharge. School access may be appraised in conjunction with the school therapist." "Lisa continues to hope that she will again be able to walk, but as weeks progress, she has focused increasingly on her wheelchair skills." "Referral to and follow-along in community-based therapy or outpatient visits to the SCI program are anticipated. Goals will be safe mobility and full participation in school and community. Consideration for airline travel and sports participation might be anticipated in coming years."

CLINICAL REASONING IN OCCUPATIONAL THERAPY PRACTICE

Selection of Other Wheelchair Options

Based on Lisa's functional needs, what else should be considered related to wheelchair selection and mobility training? Consider use of other wheelchair accessories, performance in transfers, transportation with the wheelchair, and maintenance of the wheelchair. Under what circumstances might power mobility be considered? What other kinds of activity-specific mobility aids might interest Lisa?

CASE EXAMPLE #2

Dependent Mobility with Amyotrophic Lateral Sclerosis

Occupational Therapy Intervention Process	Clinical Reasoning Process	
	Objectives	**Examples of Therapist's Internal Dialogue**
Patient Information Mr. R. is a 48-year-old husband and father with amyotrophic lateral sclerosis (ALS). He is near the end of his ability to walk safely and has quit driving a car. He teaches in a public school and expects to retire at the end of the month. He coaches his children's youth baseball teams. He lacks sufficient strength in his arms to self-propel a wheelchair. To address his needs now for mobility at home, at work, and in the community, a prescription for a wheelchair is being written. Family financial resources are limited.	Appreciate the context	(See related assessment and intervention in Chapter 40 regarding adults with neurodegenerative disorders.) "Mr. R.'s walking difficulty with upper limb weakness will necessitate power wheelchair mobility and/or dependent wheelchair use. Use of power mobility in homes is problematic for maneuverability and will likely necessitate a dependent wheelchair for function and care."
	Develop intervention hypotheses	"Medicare funding would address wheeled mobility for at-home use and perhaps transportation to and from medical appointments. Other community mobility needs should be addressed separately."
	Select an intervention approach	"A rehabilitative approach will attempt to match devices and environments with abilities to address Mr. R.'s family goals. Wheelchair use will take place along with uses of other assistive devices and environmental accommodations planned for home."
	Reflect on competence	"As a therapist, I am familiar with dependent mobility devices and need to carefully match size and adjustment options for the client's home environment. Loaner equipment or used devices are sometimes preferred for cost savings. The ALS Association or other assistive technology recycling programs could be explored."

Recommendations To address needs within the home, an attendant-propelled wheelchair is needed. A tilt-in-space manual chair that permits full upright position to 45° recline is selected, along with a foam seat cushion and flexible sling back with a winged headrest. A lap tray is added to enable positioning of the arms and for attachment of communication devices. This chair is requested through health insurance, and once Mr. R. is unable to walk safely, it will be used at home and for attending medical appointments. Community mobility may be served by this device, but other options will need to be explored as well.	Consider the patient's appraisal of performance Consider what will occur in therapy, how often, and for how long Ascertain the patient's endorsement of plan	"Mr. R. is knowledgeable about his condition but is reluctant to give up walking. Presenting the wheelchair as an option rather than an exclusive device for mobility might be best." "Selecting, fitting, and brief training are specifically needed with the wheelchair device. Operation of brakes, recline mechanism, and other features should be reviewed with Mr. R. and his care providers." "Mr. R. is in agreement but views the wheelchair as being a further indicator of his decline."
Summary of Short-Term Goals and Progress Mr. R. needs consumer education about wheelchair products and options that he could use. Funding mechanisms need careful review in terms of requirements, dollar allowances, and costs of options. Client and family training in use of the wheelchair is a service goal, with Mr. R. having informed options about wheelchair use.	Assess the patient's comprehension Understand what the patient is doing Compare actual to expected performance Know the person Appreciate the context	"Mr R recognizes his mobility needs and is aware of and concerned about costs and access within his home, such as installation of ramps and widening of doorways." "Adjustable cushioning for comfort and function should be devised. Foam cushions are likely the most cost-effective and flexible option, both for seating and transport. He will likely adjust his position easily on his own at first. With more static seating later on, air cushioning could be considered. This will then necessitate adjustment and tending of the cushion relative to air pressure. Gel cushions could be considered, but they are heavy and may make Mr. R.'s own adjustment of his position more challenging." "Resting and functional settings at home are likely to include his bed, wheelchair, and another chair or couch location. Transfer training with family care providers should take place soon."
Next Steps Mr. R. obtains and uses the mobility devices, which appear to meet his present needs. Occupational therapy is put on hold, with plans for re-assessment in 6 weeks.	Anticipate present and future patient concerns Analyze patient's comprehension Decide if patient should continue or discontinue therapy and/or return in the future	"Monitoring of wheelchair operation and use, along with other assistive devices, should occur as part of outpatient follow-up, perhaps every 6 weeks depending on the speed of Mr. R.'s decline. Coordination with home-health or hospice care also may be considered."

CLINICAL REASONING IN OCCUPATIONAL THERAPY PRACTICE

Selection of Other Mobility Options

Mr. R. and his family also recognize his need for independent mobility outside of the home. His extended family are discussing pooling their resources to purchase another mobility device he can use outdoors for coaching baseball, shopping, and other activities. Given the progressive decline expected with ALS, what might you suggest in terms of power mobility? If financial resources were not an issue, what kind of comprehensive mobility system would you recommend and why?

comes (Weiss-Lambrou et al., 1999). Ragnarsson (1990) stated, "Ultimately, the most important factor in the success of a wheelchair prescription is the user's total level of acceptance and satisfaction with [the] chair as it combines looks, comfort, and function" (p. 8).

SUMMARY REVIEW QUESTIONS

1. Who should participate in the wheelchair selection process?
2. What are the three basic types of wheelchairs, and why would each be selected?
3. What factors should be taken into consideration in wheelchair selection?
4. Describe a situation in which the optimal decision for an individual might involve the selection of more than one mobility device.
5. What are the six broad goals of wheelchair seating and positioning?
6. In determining wheelchair and related seating system sizes for a particular individual, what measurements typically are taken?
7. Contrast benefits and limitations of various manual and power mobility frame types.
8. Name and describe two types of controls for power mobility devices. Which would be preferable for a person with cerebral palsy and extremely poor upper extremity control? Why?
9. How can an occupational therapist keep abreast of new product development and research related to these products?
10. How can the occupational therapist facilitate the client's participation in wheelchair selection?
11. Once the wheelchair and seating system have been selected, what is the role of the occupational therapist?

ACKNOWLEDGEMENTS

We thank and acknowledge the following people for critiquing this manuscript and for contributing their knowledge and expertise: Ken Jelinek, MOT, OTR, Assistive Technology Clinic, University of Washington Hospital and Medical Center, Seattle, WA; and Todd Lefkowicz, Rehab Engr., OTR, Northwest Center, Seattle, WA. We are also grateful to Mike Peterson of Wheelchairs Northwest, Bellevue, WA, for contour seating photographs.

References

Aissaoui, R., Boucher, C., Bourbonnais, D., Lacoste, M., & Dansereau, J. (2001). Effect of seat cushion on dynamic stability in sitting during a reaching task in wheelchair users with paraplegia. *Archives of Physical Medicine and Rehabilitation, 82,* 274–281.

Albert, S. M., Murphy, P. L., Del Bene, M. L., & Rowland, L. P. (1999). Prospective study of palliative care in ALS: Choice, timing, outcomes. *Journal of Neurological Sciences, 169,* 108–113.

Algood, S. D., Cooper, R. A., Fitzgerald, S. G., Cooper, R., & Boninger, M. L. (2004). Impact of a pushrim-activated power-assisted wheelchair on the metabolic demands, stroke frequency, and range of motion among subjects with tetraplegia. *Archives of Physical Medicine and Rehabilitation, 85,* 1865–1871.

Algood, S. D., Cooper, R. A., Fitzgerald, S. G., Cooper, R., & Bonindger, M. L. (2005). Effects of a push-rim activated power-assist wheelchair on the functional capabilities of persons with tetraplegia. *Archives of Physical and Medicine Rehabilitation, 86,* 380–386.

Apatsidis, D. P., Solomonidis, S. E., & Michael, S. M. (2002). Pressure distribution at the seating interface of custom-molded wheelchair seats: effort of various materials. *Archives of Physical Medicine and Rehabilitation, 83,* 1151–1156.

Axelson, P. W. (1998). Problem solving through rehabilitation engineering. In D. B. Gray, L. A. Quatrano, & M. L. Lieberman (Eds.), *Designing and using assistive technology: The human perspective* (pp. 209–228). Baltimore: Paul H. Brooks.

Axelson, P. W., Chesney, D. Y., Minkel, J., & Perr, A. (1998). *The manual wheelchair training guide.* Santa Cruz, CA: PAX Press.

Batavia, M., Batavia, A. I., & Friedman, R. (2001). Changing chairs: Anticipating problems in prescribing wheelchairs. *Disability and Rehabilitation, 23,* 539–548.

Behrman, A. L. (1990). Factors in functional assessment. *Journal of Rehabilitation Research and Development: Clinical Supplement, 2,* 17–30.

Brandt, A., Iwarsson, S., & Stahle, A. (2004). Older people's use of powered wheelchairs for activity and participation. *Journal of Rehabilitation Medicine, 36,* 70–77.

Brubaker, C. (1990). Ergonometric considerations. *Journal of Rehabilitation Research and Development: Clinical Supplement, 2,* 37–48.

Buning, M. E., Angelo, J. A., & Schmeler, M. R. (2001). Occupational performance and the transition to powered mobility: A pilot study. *American Journal of Occupational Therapy, 55,* 339–344.

Burns, S. P., & Betz, K. L. (1999). Seating pressures with conventional and dynamic wheelchair cushions in tetraplegia. *Archives of Physical Medicine and Rehabilitation, 80,* 566–571.

Calder, C. J., & Kirby, R. (1990). Fatal wheelchair-related accidents in the United States. *American Journal of Physical Medicine and Rehabilitation, 69,* 184–190.

Chan, A., & Heck, C. S. (1999). The effects of tilting the seating system position of a wheelchair on respiration, posture, fatigue, voice volume, and exertion outcomes in individuals with advanced multiple sclerosis. *Journal of Rehabilitation Outcome Measures, 3,* 1–14.

Chaves, E. S., Boninger, M. L., Cooper, R., Fitzgerald, S. G., Gray, D. B., & Cooper, R. A. (2004). Assessing the influence of wheelchair technology on perception of participation in spinal cord injury. *Archives of Physical Medicine and Rehabilitation, 85,* 1854–1858.

Cooper, R. A. (1998). *Wheelchair selection and configuration.* New York: Demos.

Cooper, R. A., Boninger, M. L., & Rentschler, A. (1999). Evaluation of selected ultralight manual wheelchairs using ANSI/RESNA standards. *Archives of Physical Medicine and Rehabilitation, 80,* 462–467.

Cooper, R. A., Gonzalez, J., Lawrence, G., Renschler, A., Boninger, M. L., & VanSickle, D. P. (1997). Performance of selected lightweight wheelchairs on ANSI/RESNA Tests. *Archives of Physical Medicine and Rehabilitation, 80,* 1138–1144.

Davies, A., DeSouza, L. H., & Frank, A. O. (2003). Changes in the quality of life in severely disabled people following provision of powered indoor/outdoor chairs. *Disability and Rehabilitation, 25,* 186–290.

Field, D. (1999). Powered mobility: A literature review illustrating the importance of a multifaceted approach. *Assistive Technology, 11,* 20–33.

Garber, S., & Krouskop, T. (1997). Technical advances in wheelchairs and seating systems. *Physical Medicine and Rehabilitation: State of the Art Reviews, 11,* 93–106.

Geyer, M. J., Brienza, D. M., Bertocci, G. E., Crane, B., Hobson, D., Karg, P., Schmeler, M., & Trefler, E. (2003). Wheelchair seating: a state of the science report. *Assistive Technology, 15,* 120–128.

Hobson, D. A. (1990). Seating and mobility for the severely disabled. In R. Smith & J. Leslie Jr. (Eds.), *Rehabilitation engineering* (pp. 193–252). Boca Raton, FL: CRC.

Hobson, D. A. (1992). Comparative effects of posture on pressure and shear at the body-seat interface. *Journal of Rehabilitation Research and Development, 29,* 21–31.

Hoenig, H., Landerman, L. R., Shipp, K. M., & George, L. (2003). Activity restriction among wheelchair users. *Journal of the American Geriatrics Society, 51,* 1244–1251.

Hoenig, H., Pieper, C., Zolkewitz, M., Schenkman, M., & Branch, L. G. (2002). Wheelchair users are not necessarily wheelchair bound. *Journal of the American Geriatrics Society, 50,* 645–654.

Iezzoni, L. I. (2000). A 44-year-old woman with difficulty walking. *Journal of the American Medical Association, 284,* 2632–2639.

Kernozek, T. W., & Lewin, J. E. (1998). Seat interface pressures of individuals with paraplegia: Influence of dynamic wheelchair locomotion compared with static seated measurements. *Archives of Physical Medicine and Rehabilitation, 79,* 313–316.

Krasilovsky, G. (1993). Seating assessment and management in a nursing home population. *Physical and Occupational Therapy in Geriatrics, 11,* 25–38.

Krey, C. H., & Calhoun, C. L. (2004). Utilizing research in wheelchair and seating selection and configuration for children with injury/dysfunction of the spinal cord. *Journal of Spinal Cord Medicine, 27 (Suppl. 1),* S29–S37.

Letts, R. M. (1991). *Principles of seating the disabled.* Boca Raton, FL: CRC.

Masse, L. C., Lamontagne, M., & O'Riain, M. D. (1992). Biomechanical analysis of wheelchair propulsion for various seating positions. *Journal of Rehabilitation Research and Development, 29,* 12–28.

Meyers, A. R., Anderson, J. J., Miller, D. R., Shipp, K., & Hoenig, H. (2002). Barriers, facilitators, and access for wheelchair users: Substantive and methodologic lessons from a pilot study of environmental effects. *Social Science and Medicine, 55,* 1425–1446.

Miller, W. C., Miller, F., Trenholm, K., Grant, D., & Goodman, K. (2004). Development and preliminary assessment of the measurement properties of the Seating Identification Tool (SIT). *Clinical Rehabilitation, 18,* 317–325.

Mills, T., Holm, M. B., Trefler, E., Schmeler, M., Fitzgerald, S., & Boninger, M. (2002). Development and consumer validation of the Functional Evaluation of a Wheelchair (FEW) instrument. *Disability and Rehabilitation, 24,* 38–46.

Minkel, J. L. (2000). Seating and mobility considerations for people with spinal cord injury. *Physical Therapy, 80,* 701–709.

Parziale, J. R. (1991). Standard v. lightweight wheelchair propulsion in spinal cord injured patients. *American Journal of Physical Medicine and Rehabilitation, 70,* 76–80.

Pellow, T. R. (1999). A comparison of interface pressure readings to wheelchair cushions and positioning: A pilot study. *Canadian Journal of Occupational Therapy, 66,* 140–149.

Ragnarsson, K. T. (1990). Prescription considerations and a comparison of conventional and lightweight wheelchairs. *Journal of Rehabilitation Research and Development: Clinical Supplement, 2,* 8–16.

Reid, D., Angus, J., McKeever, P., & Miller, K. L. (2003). Home is where their wheels are: Experiences of women wheelchair users. *American Journal of Occupational Therapy, 57,* 186–195.

Reid, D., Laliberte-Rudman, D., & Hebert, D. (2002). Impact of wheeled seating mobility devices on adult users' and their caregivers' occupational performance: A critical review. *Canadian Journal of Occupational Therapy, 69,* 261–280.

Rosenthal, M. J., Felton, R. M., Hileman, D. L., Lee, M., Friedman, M., & Navach, J. H. (1996). A wheelchair cushion design to redistribute sites of sitting pressure. *Archives of Physical Medicine and Rehabilitation, 77,* 278–282.

Steins, S. A. (1998). Personhood, disablement, and mobility technology. In D. B. Gray, L. A. Quatrano, & M. L. Lieberman (Eds.), *Designing and using assistive technology: The human perspective* (pp. 29–49). Baltimore: Paul H. Brooks.

Stinnett, K. A. (1997). Geriatric seating and positioning within a wheeled mobility frame of reference in the long-term care setting. *Topics in Geriatric Rehabilitation, 13,* 75–84.

Trail, M., Nelson, N., Van, J. N., Appel, S. H., & Lai, E. C. (2001). Wheelchair use by patients with amyotrophic lateral sclerosis: a survey of user characteristics and selection preferences. *Archives of Physical Medicine and Rehabilitation, 82,* 98–102.

Warren, C. G. (1990). Powered mobility and its implications. *Journal of Rehabilitation Research and Development: Clinical Supplement, 2,* 74–85.

Weiss-Lambrou, R., Tremblay, C., LeBlanc, R., Lacoste, M., & Dansereau, J. (1999). Wheelchair seating aids: How satisfied are consumers. *Assistive Technology, 11,* 43–53.

Suggested Readings

Batavia, M. (1998). *The wheelchair evaluation: A practical guide.* Woodburn, MA: Butterworth-Heinemann.

Cooper, R. A. (1998). *Wheelchair selection and configuration.* New York: Demos.

Croteau, C. (1998). *Wheelchair mobility: A handbook.* Worcester, MA: Park Press.

Karp, G. (1998). *Choosing a wheelchair: A guide to optimal independence.* Sebastopol, CA: O'Reilly & Associates.

Mayall, J. K., & Desharnais, G. (1995). *Positioning in a wheelchair: A guide for professional caregivers of the disabled adult* (2nd ed). Thorofare, NJ: Slack.

CHAPTER 19

High-Technology Adaptations to Compensate for Disability

Mary Ellen Buning

LEARNING OBJECTIVES

After studying this chapter, the reader will be able to do the following:

1. Explain the role of assistive technology (AT) as a compensation for loss of occupational function and inability to perform the activities underlying role performance.
2. Describe the basic components of the AT assessment, the participating team members, and the unique contribution of occupational therapy to the process.
3. Use knowledge of unimpaired abilities to determine a client's needed technology interface and ability to use features of AT devices.
4. Recognize an individual who could benefit from an AT evaluation and services and make an appropriate referral.
5. Define primary categories of AT and give examples of AT use to support occupational functioning.

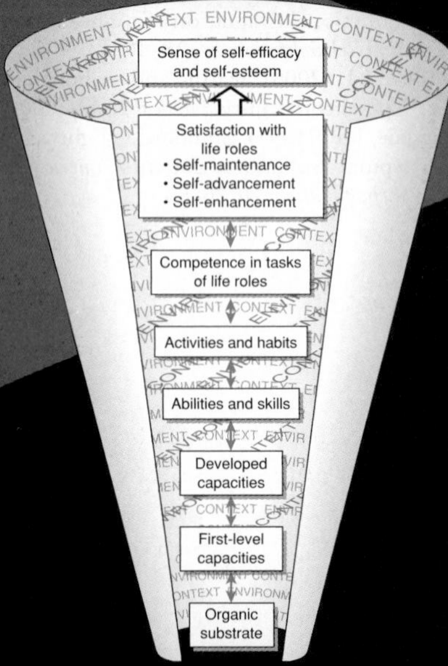

Glossary

Augmentative and alternative communication (AAC)—A communication system that requires use of something external to the body. Examples include pen and paper, letter or picture communication boards, and communication devices. Gestures and vocalizations are often used to enhance communication when using an AAC device. Devices may be manual or electronic. AAC devices use a language representation system, e.g., letters grouped into words or picture symbols.

Abbreviation expansion—Software designed to increase typing speed, decrease keystrokes, and decrease errors. For example, OT is the abbreviation for occupational therapy. The abbreviation is entered instead of the words, and the software expands the abbreviation into the word or phrase it represents.

Array—When indirect selection is used, the array is the set of options that are presented in sequence. The user selects from an array by waiting until the desired item is offered and then activating a switch. Some items in an array may branch to a secondary array, for example when a punctuation array is opened from an alphabet array.

Computer-aided design (CAD)—Software used to design, draft, or lay out technical projects ranging from architecture to manufacturing. CAD makes modifications and estimating construction costs much easier.

Electronic aids to daily living (EADL)—Devices that give consumers control of appliances in their environment. This term is favored over the alternative, Environmental Control Unit (ECU), because it stresses the task (i.e., increased independence, safety, communication, and leisure) rather than the thing being controlled (i.e., television, telephone, and lights). EADL accurately describes the technology and has helped funding, both here and in Europe.

E-Tran board—A non-vocal communication device made of acrylic with an open space in the center to allow a clear view of the consumer's eyes. Communication symbols or letters are placed around the frame, and the consumer indicates choice by eye gaze. Both communication partners must be trained in its use.

Infrared (IR)—Light wave outside of (longer than) the spectrum normally detected by the human eye. Sequences of IR code are interpreted as specific instructions by an IR receiver, which executes a command such as volume up or volume down.

Microprocessor—Miniature piece of integrated circuit board that performs a prescribed operation or set of operations and is common in consumer products and AT devices.

Pixel—Smallest unit of visual display on a computer screen; a dot. These dots combine to form words and images. Pixels per square inch is a measure of resolution or pixel density, e.g., 640 × 480. The larger the number, the more information that can be shown on the display.

Pneumatic—Switch activation by increasing, decreasing, or changing the direction of air pressure. Switches that are commonly called sip and puffs are pneumatic switches.

QWERTY layout—Common layout for computer keyboards in which the letters in the top left row are QWERTY. This layout originated with mechanical typewriters when it was important to slow down typists so that the strike arms that printed each letter had time to avoid each other.

Radio frequency (RF)—Signaling technology that uses nonpublic radio bands to control appliances, open doors, or direct other AT devices.

Scanning—Selection method in which the consumer watches an array and waits for a choice to be offered rather than actively making a choice. Activating a single switch indicates choice.

Speech synthesizer—Computer peripheral (software, hardware, or a combination) that allows a computer to imitate human speech using rules of text pronunciation. Synthesizers are available for many languages.

Ultrasound—Sound outside the frequency detected by the human ear. This signaling technology is occasionally used in AT to control appliances or computer-related devices.

Universal design—Design concept that ensures a built space or a consumer product is accessible or usable by almost all persons. For example, an airport designer considers not only persons using wheelchairs, but also those who are elderly, have visual impairments, or do not speak English.

USB (Universal Serial Bus)—A standard interface updated in 2001 that is commonly used for connections between two or more devices (e.g., mouse, printer, keyboard) connected to a computer. USB II supports high-speed data transfer and works on PC and Apple computers.

Word prediction—Software that uses rules of recency and frequency to anticipate the word the consumer is beginning to type. It is designed to decrease keystrokes and errors but does not increase typing speed. It is used in adaptive word processors and some AAC devices.

Technology, which is now cheaper and more powerful, underlies many of the tasks of modern life. It is difficult to find a school setting or a job that does not use computer-based technology. **Microprocessor** technology controls home appliances, ventilation systems, telecommunications, banking, and transportation. In addition to technology's role in managing the tasks of daily life, it also has the capacity to support the adaptations or alternate access methods used by persons with disabilities. Technology used in this way is called assistive technology.

The goal of assistive technology (AT) is to compensate for absent or impaired abilities and enable occupational performance. Using the concept of occupation-as-end, AT enables a consumer with tetraplegia to use a hands-free interface to perform technology-enabled activities like making phone calls, writing letters, or controlling appliances. AT enables consumers with varied limitations to perform daily living tasks, participate in life as they choose, and make choices based on their abilities and the goals and desired roles that motivate them. As stated in Chapter 1, competent role performance leads to life satisfaction, and this is the goal of AT. Occupational therapists interact with the clients to identify desired life roles and the tasks and activities required to perform these roles. They use their knowledge of the limitations of body structure and function to identify categories of AT solutions and customize control interfaces. They analyze the individual's skills and abilities to build on strengths. They recognize the training as well as the human and environmental supports required to learn to use AT and integrate it into the tasks and activities of life roles. AT devices that match consumers' goals and abilities help them assume or return to meaningful lives in the presence of physical, sensory, or cognitive disabilities.

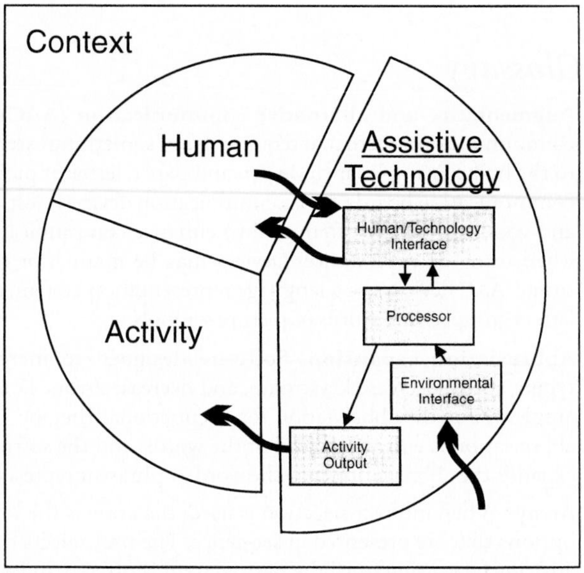

Figure 19-1 The Human Activity Assistive Technology (HAAT) Model shows the interrelationship between components and their interaction with the Assistive Technology System. (Used with permission from Cook, A. M., & Hussey, S. M. [2002]. Assistive technologies: Principles and practice, 2nd Ed. Baltimore: Mosby.)

THE HUMAN ACTIVITY ASSISTIVE TECHNOLOGY MODEL

Models serve as analogies or symbolic representations of difficult-to-visualize elements and interactions within a system and are helpful when planning for AT intervention. The Human Activity Assistive Technology Model (Cook & Hussey, 2002) (Fig. 19-1) represents how AT devices help consumers develop or return to occupational functioning.

The Human Activity Assistive Technology (HAAT) Model, which is widely used by AT practitioners, provides a model for considering AT as part of a system driven by the person or the human. In this model, the human varies based on the skill, ability, and experience it has with its intrinsic enablers, which are categorized as sensors, central processor, and effectors. Activity is understood as daily living tasks categorized as self-care, work/school, and leisure/play. The human, activity, and AT all occur within a context that varies on dimensions of the social, cultural, and physical attributes.

The AT portion of the HAAT Model is also a system with four subsections: the human-technology interface, the processor, the activity output, and the environmental interface. The human-technology interface is the means of interaction between the person and the technology device. This information is relayed to the processor via a mechanical or electrical linkage that interprets or responds to create an activity output. The activity output includes actions for which the device is designed such as opening doors or writing text. The environmental interface adjusts the output of the device in response to input from the environment.

The dynamic nature of the HAAT Model helps identify the needed features of AT devices that will allow them to meet the changing needs of the human. Changing needs occur due to things like progressive impairment, the purpose of activity such as writing for work or for play, and changes in user contexts such as mobility on a sandy beach or on a campus sidewalk. To illustrate, a consumer may choose to take a manual wheelchair and letter board that cannot be damaged by wind and sand to the beach but choose to take a power wheelchair and voice output augmentative communication (AAC) device to a fully accessible college classroom.

AREAS OF AT APPLICATION

Just as occupation infuses all parts of consumers' lives, so also can AT enable accomplishing the activities and tasks of occupations and roles. AT can support self-maintenance, self-advancement, and self-enhancement roles.

Self-Maintenance Roles

Enabling activities of daily living (ADL) performance is a familiar reason for occupational therapy. Technologies such as electric toothbrushes, WaterPics, and electric shavers can increase competence with personal care ADL tasks. However, instrumental activities of daily living (IADLs) clearly benefit from AT. Text telephones (TTY; formerly called telecommunication device for the deaf [TDD]) and hands-free or adapted telephones enable calling paratransit organizations, shopping for groceries, and ordering from catalogs over the telephone (Research Note 19-1). Closed-circuit televisions (CCTV) that enlarge objects help with paying bills and balancing checkbooks for clients with low vision. Even more IADLs are supported with computers, such as banking, shopping, online bill paying, and e-mail, and ATM machines are now equipped with headphone jacks and Braille labels.

RESEARCH NOTE 19-1

Abstract: Hoenig, H., Taylor, D. H., & Sloan, F. A. (2003). Does assistive technology substitute for personal assistance among the disabled elderly? *American Journal of Public Health, 2,* 330–337.

This study examined whether elders who used AT devices (technological assistance) to compensate for limitations in ADLs associated with their disability used fewer hours of help from another person (personal assistance). The investigators conducted a cross-sectional study of 2368 community-living adults older than 65 years who had one or more limitations in basic ADLs. The participants had previously responded to the 1994 National Long-Term Care Survey. The participants were asked further questions to uncover the relationship between technological assistance and personal assistance. Statistical regression was used to locate significant relationships among variables. Findings clearly supported the hypothesis that technological assistance may substitute for at least some personal assistance in coping with disability. Those who did not use equipment reported about 4 more hours of help per week compared with those who did use equipment. Providing personal assistance was associated with increased dependence, whereas use of equipment may have acted to preserve physical conditioning by maintaining a greater level of physical activity, or it may have allowed self-care tasks to be performed more efficiently and, therefore, reduced the need for assistance.

Implications for Practice

- AT device use appears related to maintaining independence or increasing the efficiency in completing ADL tasks and could help elders age in place.
- Through interview, explore the particular value an individual places on independent completion of instrumental ADLs activities.
- Determine which of those activities are associated with meaningful goals or return to a previous environment or life role.
- Determine which AT devices may be most helpful to that individual in compensating for the limitations due to their functional limitations.
- Refer the elder to community AT resources, such as the State Tech Act Project, for more information on AT devices or trial use of AT devices from AT-lending libraries for more specialized devices.

Consumers with significant disabilities can manage their personal space (i.e., control lights, fans, or the volume on a TV or stereo) through the use of **electronic aids to daily living (EADLs)**. These devices modify the typical user interface so that a client can control many devices in the home environment. The signaling technologies used by EADLs are the same as those used in typical controllers: **radio frequency (RF)**, **ultrasound**, and **infrared (IR)** light. Figure 19-2 describes how both simple and complex EADLs may be used.

Mobility is a basic form of self-maintenance that clients give high ratings as a necessity in everyday life (Verbrugge et al., 1997). Self-initiated mobility not only communicates curiosity, interest in participating, or the wish to be alone, but it also gives independent access to basic ADLs like eating, toileting, and bathing. It has been shown to support the activities of role performance, although having access to accessible environments is a key requirement (Buning, Angelo, & Schmeler, 2001). Home modification is usually necessary for using a wheelchair to cook a meal in a kitchen or approach a toilet in the bathroom. **Universal design**, an inclusive design concept, considers the needs of a broad range of users creating people-friendly spaces that are safer and easily modified for more severe impairment (The Center for Universal Design, 1997).

Augmentative and alternative communication (AAC) devices substitute synthetic or digitized speech when consumers are unable to speak or be understood by vocal communication. Some AAC devices provide the capacity to carry on typical conversations; others only relay a few messages. AAC devices allow consumers who have been taught to use them to socialize, call for assistance, direct caregivers, inform health care providers about health issues, initiate plans for activities, and make food and clothing choices.

Self-Advancement Roles: Work, School, or Community Volunteer

Assistive technology can enable self-advancement roles that range from retirees participating in volunteer activities to employees working at jobs or students attending school. Wheelchairs and scooters allow travel on ramped neighborhood sidewalks, commuting on public transportation, and access to schools, stores, and workplaces with level, accessible entrances. Four-wheel drive wheelchairs give mobility on farms, ranches, and the back woods.

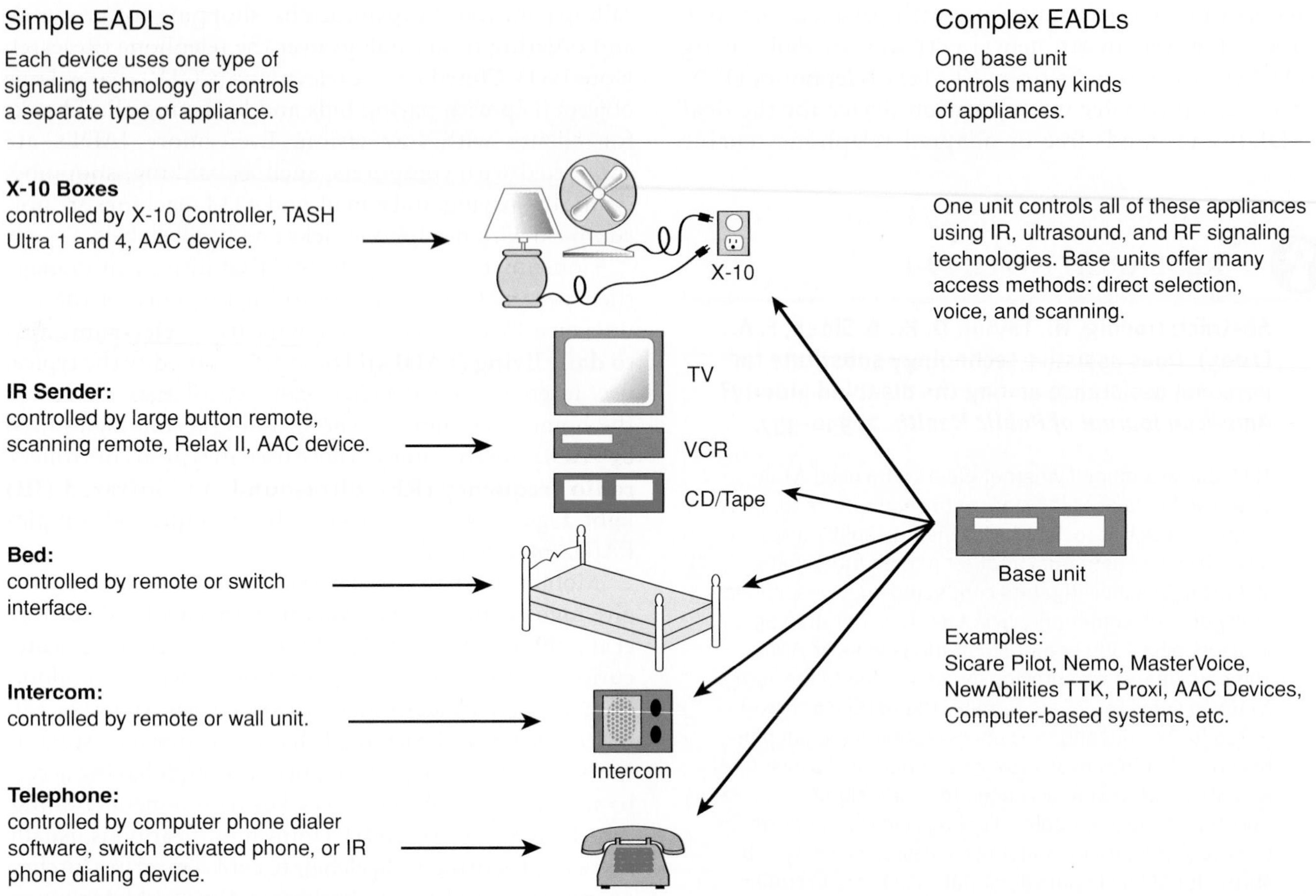
Simple EADLs
Each device uses one type of signaling technology or controls a separate type of appliance.
Complex EADLs
One base unit controls many kinds of appliances.
X-10 Boxes
controlled by X-10 Controller, TASH Ultra 1 and 4, AAC device.
X-10
One unit controls all of these appliances using IR, ultrasound, and RF signaling technologies. Base units offer many access methods: direct selection, voice, and scanning.
TV
IR Sender:
controlled by large button remote, scanning remote, Relax II, AAC device.
VCR
CD/Tape
Base unit
Bed:
controlled by remote or switch interface.
Examples:
Sicare Pilot, Nemo, MasterVoice, NewAbilities TTK, Proxi, AAC Devices, Computer-based systems, etc.
Intercom:
controlled by remote or wall unit.
Intercom
Telephone:
controlled by computer phone dialer software, switch activated phone, or IR phone dialing device.

Figure 19-2 Simple and complex EADLs.

Today's communication technologies make information exchange easier and faster for everyone. When clients with sensory, motor, and language impairments also have access to these technologies they reap huge benefits. Adapted computers enable listening to text, writing, accounting, managing databases, desktop publishing, computer-aided design, searching the Internet, phoning, faxing, and printing. Real-time closed-captioning of a speaker's words, videophones for sign language communication, and captioned multi-media and distance learning software include students and workers with sensory impairment.

AAC devices are an essential part of communication at school and in the workplace. Making choices, demonstrating knowledge, asking questions, forming peer relationships, and getting the job done all occur because of communication.

Self-Enhancement Roles: Recreation and Leisure

Recreational choices often have symbolic meaning and clearly reveal our interests and our tolerance for challenge (Kielhofner, 1997). Recreational choices made for their intrinsic and symbolic qualities allow individuals to take on valued images of self as adventurer, connoisseur, or creator (see Chapter 34). Assistive technology enables activities ranging from alternate controls for video games to adapted reels for one-handed fishing. Recreational AT includes wheelchairs designed for beaches, tennis courts, or mountain trails. Water sit-skis and adaptive snow skis like monoskis allow skill and agility in mainstream recreations.

Children's play is enabled by AT, too. Adaptive mobility devices introduced early to children with motor impairments enable independent play and exploration. Switch-adapted toys teach cause and effect and help children improve their motor control and cognitive skills for more advanced technologies. Video games, whether played on units connected to a TV or a computer, can be controlled with switches as alternatives for triggers. Using EADLs to control home entertainment systems—music, TV, and video—is also a common leisure activity.

Many Americans enjoy using home computers for leisure. Adapted computer access allows browsing sites on the Internet, pursuing interests like genealogy or collecting, and engaging in creative art activities and puzzles. The

Internet allows previewing destinations, finding accessible accommodations, and renting accessible vans. With so many accessible facilities, even traveling is now a form of recreation and play.

THE AT ASSESSMENT PROCESS

The contribution made by a well-chosen and fully used AT device is remarkable. Assistive technology's contribution is the result of a skilled, thoughtful, and thorough assessment. A discussion of the elements of this process follows. (Figure 19-3 is an overview of the AT assessment and intervention sequence.)

Assessments are driven by the consumer's goals and needs (Bain & Leger, 1997; Cook & Hussey, 2002). Family members or caregivers, speaking on behalf of a consumer with communication impairment, may also identify goals and needs. The AT team attempts to understand and address the stated reasons for and expectations of the assessment. It is important to clear up any misunderstandings about the capabilities of the AT team and the types of AT devices available. Clarifying these issues before beginning the assessment creates more realistic expectations for the contribution of AT devices and prevents disappointment.

Consumers, family members, and caregivers come to the assessment with various needs and motivations. For example, a young adult may be transitioning to college and need new computer technology and training to more efficiently complete assignments, search the Internet, participate in online class discussion, and exchange class notes. Parents may be ready to consider powered mobility for their young child while looking for reassurance that they will not inhibit the development of walking with their action. An adult with a newly acquired disability that prevents returning to previous employment may be looking for AT devices to enable retooling for a new type of work or employment.

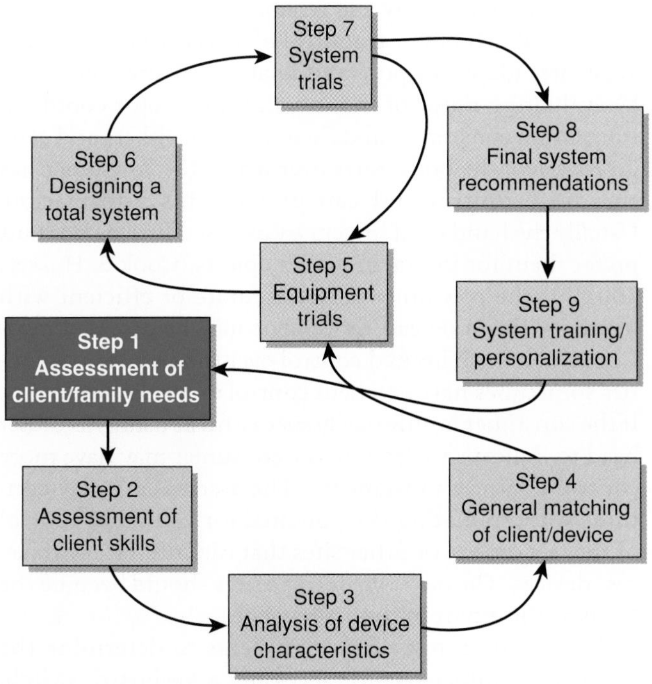

Figure 19-3 Nine steps in the assessment process for AT.

In addition to their goals and priorities, the assessment focuses on consumer and family attitudes toward AT. Some people easily adopt technology and incorporate it into tasks and routines. Others resist and even fear it. Some consumers feel that the latest high-technology equipment is not necessary and prefer simpler, more familiar devices. Consumers' religious and cultural background and personal tastes will also influence their choice of devices. Devices that fit within the personal and cultural context of the consumer and his or her family are more likely to be used than the latest technology innovation that is outside the realm of the consumer's comfort zone. Putting aside personal values, the AT team concentrates on addressing the consumer's goals and preferences.

Team Members

The team consists of a variety of experts and stakeholders. The consumer, family, and caregivers have the key role because they will interact with or use the equipment on a daily basis. Professionals on the team vary according to the consumer's needs.

- The seating and mobility expert may be an occupational or physical therapist who is focused on maximizing function in the seated position. With the consumer's activities in mind, this expert assesses posture and range of motion and specifies seat, back and foot support angles, and cushion type (e.g., support or pressure relief or accommodation to abnormal posture). If the consumer has mobility impairment, assessment includes a review of needs and trial with an appropriate type of wheelchair. The decision to use a manual or powered wheelchair will affect selection and use of other AT devices. See Chapter 18 for information on wheelchairs and assessment.
- The access specialist, typically an occupational therapist, is focused on finding the best possible methods for controlling AT devices including a power wheelchair. The access specialist may work with another team member who knows more about specific devices that might be controlled such as computers, AAC devices, and EADLs.
- The teacher or special educator, if the consumer is a student, describes schoolwork tasks and helps formu-

late solutions to support educational tasks and school participation.

- A vocational rehabilitation counselor, if the consumer works or is preparing for work, will approve AT solutions and help with funding.
- A speech-language pathologist (SLP) with expertise in AAC directs the team when communication is the focus. The SLP evaluates the consumer's verbal and written communication potential, helps determine the types of symbol sets (alphabet, pictures, etc.) that will be most effective, and works closely with the access specialist.
- A rehabilitation engineer may be on the team if the consumer has complex needs and off-the-shelf solutions are not likely to be effective. The engineer may integrate several types of AT when consumers have few options for control. For example, a consumer with reliable control of only a finger would need an integrated control system that allows this small movement to drive a wheelchair, operate a computer, and control an AAC device.
- A social worker may help locate funding sources or provide counseling as consumers and significant others come to terms with disability.
- Rehabilitation technology suppliers (RTSs; previously known as vendors) are the equipment experts. An RTS who sells a device may be able to provide a demo model for the evaluation. The RTS knows product features and can help with selection of components and adjust the product after delivery. Certification for RTS (CRTS) signifies advanced training, expertise with assessment, and commitment to ethical practices.

The AT Assessment

Prior to the AT assessment, the team needs to understand the consumer's goals related to roles and the performance of activities to support roles. This information, captured either through a structured interview or an intake questionnaire (Pollock, 1993), should be coordinated with family members' and caregivers' goals. Once goals are established, the door is open for focusing on a particular area of AT, categories of solutions, and assessing current skills and abilities to determine potential access methods. During this part of the assessment, it is important to gather a realistic picture of the consumer's motor control, social skills, and cognitive and sensory abilities, as well as the environments where the consumer will use the devices. Areas commonly addressed in AT assessments follow.

Seating

Optimal seating is mandatory to achieve the best results during the rest of the assessment. If the client uses a seating system that does not provide adequate support (see Chapter 18), the performance observed during subsequent AT evaluation activities will not accurately show the consumer's ability.

Sometimes it is not possible to address seating issues before the rest of the assessment. When this happens, a seating simulator can be used. A seating simulator has an adjustable back, sides, armrests, lateral supports, pommels, and foot supports and can be set to meet a broad range of postural support needs. The risk is that it may be difficult to duplicate the control the consumer had in the seating simulator. Therefore, whenever possible, the best solution is to assess consumers in their own appropriately fitting seating system and wheelchair.

Another important factor to determine early in the assessment is where and in what positions the consumer spends the most time. Asking these questions at the beginning of the assessment avoids recommending access methods that the consumer can use with accuracy in their wheelchair only to find out that, at home, the consumer spends the most time in bed or a lounge chair. Once seating issues have been resolved, motor control for access is addressed.

Motor Control

Ideally, access methods, such as touch-typing on a keyboard, are effortless. Effortlessness comes after practicing and refining the skill. For a skilled typist, it seems the fingers know the words as they quickly move across the keys. Attention is on the thoughts the typist wishes to enter into the word processor rather than individual keystrokes. To reach effortlessness, it is important to narrow access methods to those that the consumer is able or potentially able to activate consistently and reliably.

To establish physical control of an AT device, the therapist first identifies potential anatomical sites for access by evaluating range of motion and fine motor coordination. Often consumers and their family members and caregivers know the body parts over which the consumer has the most control and can provide this information. Usually the hands and fingers are assessed first, as humans prefer them for interacting with objects (Cook & Hussey, 2002). If the consumer is not accurate or efficient with hands or fingers, head movement may be assessed next. Consumers with limited control over their upper extremities sometimes have excellent control of head movements. If the consumer is only partly successful at using his or her head to indicate a selection, the consumer may have more control over eye movements. The assessment may continue with evaluating the potential for volitional control of the feet, knees, or other sites that can interface with access devices. The best two or three sites should become the focus at this point in the assessment.

Evaluating range of motion helps to determine the range a consumer has for accessing a keyboard, switch, and other input devices. Assessment boards are easily constructed and useful when assessing range of motion and coordination (Procedures for Practice 19-1). The therapist, using an assessment board, can quickly assess range and accuracy. Using one body part, the therapist asks the consumer to point to the squares on the board with a finger, hand, head (using a head pointer), or toe depending on which anatomical site is being evaluated. Using a replica of the grid printed on the assessment form, the therapist indicates the squares the consumer should reach. Assessing range helps the therapist get an idea of the types of access devices the consumer can use successfully. For example, if the consumer easily reaches the perimeter of the assessment board grid, a normal computer keyboard may be useful. Conversely, if the consumer can reach only squares in the middle of the grid and close to the midline, the access method will be limited to this area.

To assess coordination, the therapist asks the consumer to point to specific squares on the perimeter and in the middle of one of the assessment boards. Accuracy in pointing to specific squares gives the therapist an idea of the consumer's coordination. The board with 1-inch squares is used first. If accuracy is sufficient with one or more of the anatomical sites, the therapist proceeds with the assessment. If the accuracy is poor with all anatomical sites, the test is repeated using the 2-inch grid. If the results do not clearly demonstrate pointing ability with at least one anatomical site, the therapist may ask the consumer to try a head pointer or hand-held pointing device to assist with accuracy.

Once pointing trials with three or four anatomical sites are completed with some consistency, compare the results. Comparisons help determine which anatomical site the consumer uses most consistently and accurately. The therapist asks the consumer to point to the same six squares in the same order using each anatomical site being tested. Keeping all the variables identical except for the anatomical site, the therapist determines which anatomical site offers the consumer the best control. The consumer is asked whether he or she agrees with which site provided the most control. If the consumer feels more comfortable using another body part, the therapist and consumer should discuss this and come to agreement on which site should be the primary access site.

Having said all of this, it seems important to note that speech recognition technology has improved greatly in the last few years. This technology creates the possibility that a consumer may need *no* physical interaction with an input device to achieve control. Depending on the consumer's cognitive abilities, motor control issues, and goals, it may be possible to use this constantly improving technology to reduce the amount of time spent searching for a motor control strategy. Even when speech recognition succeeds, however, it is important to have a non-speech control method as back up.

PROCEDURES FOR PRACTICE 19-1

Preparing Range of Motion and Fine Coordination Assessment Boards

Materials needed:

- Two pieces of poster board measuring approximately 11 × 17 inches each
- Permanent marker
- Ruler
- Clear contact paper

Directions:

- Using the permanent marker and ruler, mark off one of the poster boards into a 2-inch grid.
- Mark the other poster board into a 1-inch grid.
- Number the squares on each poster board sequentially.
- Place clear contact paper over each poster board.

The poster boards are now ready to be used during the assessment. The plastic covering protects the boards against moisture. Also, stickers can be placed and removed repeatedly from the poster boards without damaging them.

Some consumers are motivated to touch specific squares with colorful, eye-catching stickers or small food items, such as Cheerios. Consumers whose cognition is intact can point to requested numbers printed in each square. Duplicating a small version of the grid on an assessment form allows the therapist to shade in the squares on the grid with the locations or numbers that the consumer easily reached. This assessment tool is further described in *Assistive Technology for Rehabilitation Therapists* (Angelo, 1997).

Direct Versus Indirect Selection Methods

Once the anatomical site has been determined, the types of access devices can be reviewed. This evaluation determines whether the consumer will use direct or indirect selection (Procedures for Practice 19-2). If a consumer effortlessly uses an anatomical site to point, direct selection is appropriate. The therapist may also need to consider factors such as target size, placement, and other characteristics to reduce effort and improve speed and accuracy. If the consumer cannot accurately and consistently point with any of these anatomical sites, however, it is necessary to consider more sophisticated AT alternatives. Other technologies that use direct selection are speech recognition, head pointing using devices that track head movement, mouth controlled joysticks, eye pointing, and tongue touching keys on a keypad worn in the mouth. These devices will be discussed later.

As a last resort and in absence of motor control that will allow a consumer to accurately point to or select from

PROCEDURES FOR PRACTICE 19-2

Direct and Indirect Selection

In direct selection, all items in the selection set are available at any time. Examples of direct selections are computer keyboards, telephone keypads, and calculators. The advantage of direct selection is that it is intuitive. If an individual presses a K on the keyboard, he or she can expect to get a K on the visual display. The disadvantage is that direct selection requires coordination and some range of motion, depending on the size of each item in the selection set.

At times, trying to press the right key is too difficult for consumers with limited motor control. For example, the A key on a computer keyboard may be too far away, or the consumer may repeatedly press the Q or Z key when trying for the A key.

With indirect selection or **scanning**, only a subset of all possible choices is available at any given time. An example is setting the time on a digital clock and waiting for the correct number to appear. The advantage is that the consumer needs reliable control over only one movement, such as an eyebrow, one finger, or a toe. The disadvantage is that it is much slower to use and more intellectually demanding than direct selection. It requires the ability to remember and sequence steps with a high level of attention.

a set of selection options (i.e., like a keyboard or a number pad), the evaluation moves toward indirect selection. Indirect selection reduces the size of the "selection set," and choices are presented one at a time until the one desired is offered. The consumer indicates choice by activating a switch or sending an electronic signal. The goal when assessing indirect selection is to identify anatomical sites that the consumer can control consistently without doing so unintentionally. The type of switch, its orientation to the body, and method of mounting are determined based on the anatomical site, the consumer's movement patterns, and the durability required. The goal is to ensure optimal accuracy and reliability for the body segment with the best motor control. Table 19-1 describes several commonly used switches along with typical activation methods. As with direct selection, the hands or fingers may be assessed first, followed by the head and other body sites.

Switch Assessment

Switch mounting is critical for success when using single-switch access. Switches must be mounted so they remain in place and in line with the angle of activation. This provides for consistent and reliable switch pressing throughout use. Wheelchair and desk mounts with solid, one-way connections are far more likely to be used correctly than those that are adjustable. A switch mount must also be easily removable so it does not interfere with transfers or eating.

Table 19-1. Common Switches and Activation Method

Category and Specific Switches	Company	Primary Activation Site
No Physical Contact—Requires an external power source (e.g., power wheelchair battery)		
IST switch (infrared)	Words+	Eye blink
Adjustable proximity switch	Adaptive Switch Laboratory	Head, elbow, hand, etc.
Adjustable photoelectric switch	Adaptive Switch Laboratory	Any gross movement capable of interrupting the light beam
Physical Contact, No Pressure		
Pneumatic (also known as sip and puff)	Prentke Romich	Mouth and lips
P-switch	Prentke Romich	Any volitional and consistent muscle contraction
Physical Contact with Pressure		
Single rocking lever	Prentke Romich	Arm, hand, head, foot
Tongue switch	Prentke Romich	Tongue
Wobble	Prentke Romich	Arm, hand, head
Jelly bean switch	Ablenet	Arm, hand, head, foot
Specs switch	Ablenet	Arm, hand, head, foot
Big red	Ablenet	Arm, hand, head, foot
Wobble	Zygo	Arm, hand, head, foot
Bass	Don Johnston	Arm, hand, head, foot

The type of switch depends on the anatomical site chosen to control it. A variety of switches are shown in Figure 19-4. For example, consumers with control over one finger may best use a small, sensitive switch. In contrast, a foot switch mounted on a wheelchair footrest must be rugged to withstand impact from shoes and obstacles when the wheelchair is in motion. For an anatomical site that is bony, such as the back of the hand, a switch with a padded covering is appropriate.

Regardless of the type of switch recommended, it should provide feedback so the consumer knows whether the movement was successful. Usually this feedback is auditory, but it may be visual. Switches activated through head movements should produce quieter auditory feedback because a noisy switch mounted near the ear can be annoying.

Six occupational therapists with expertise in AT participated in a focus group to develop a list of the 10 most important considerations for switch access (Angelo, 2000). In the control category, the therapists indicated that the most important considerations were reliability of response, ability to perform timed responses, ability to activate and deactivate the switch within a given time frame, and endurance (the ability to sustain a force and to apply that force repeatedly over time). In the ease of movement category, therapists said that tasks should be performed volitionally, easily, and efficiently and that past performances with positive outcomes should be considered. Since context was considered important, assessments should occur in the environment where tasks are routinely performed. Finally, switch safety should be considered. Switches should have rounded corners, and all wires should be secured so that they do not become entangled with fingers, pointing devices, or other equipment (Procedures for Practice 19-3).

PROCEDURES FOR PRACTICE 19-3

Switch Assessment

1. Identify the anatomical sites over which the consumer has most control for switch activation. No timing is involved in this step.
2. Evaluate the consumer's ability to wait a specific length of time before activating the switch. This skill is critical for effectively using indirect selection. Errors in selection occur when the switch is released too soon or too late.
3. Evaluate the consumer's ability to maintain contact with the switch and to release the switch on command. This information will help to identify the best scanning mode, e.g., automatic, inverse, or step scanning.
4. When one or more anatomical sites have been identified for accurate switch pressing, the AT team determines which type of switch is most appropriate and how best to mount the switch. This concept is further described in Cook and Hussey, 2002.

Cognition

Cognition is usually evaluated informally during AT assessments (Cook & Hussey, 2002). During the assessment activities and interaction, it is possible to estimate the consumer's attention span, reading level, short- and long-term memory, and ability to follow instructions and sequence tasks. Knowing about these aspects of cognitive functioning helps the AT team determine which devices have the features and performance characteristics that will match the consumer's cognitive ability (see Chapter 9).

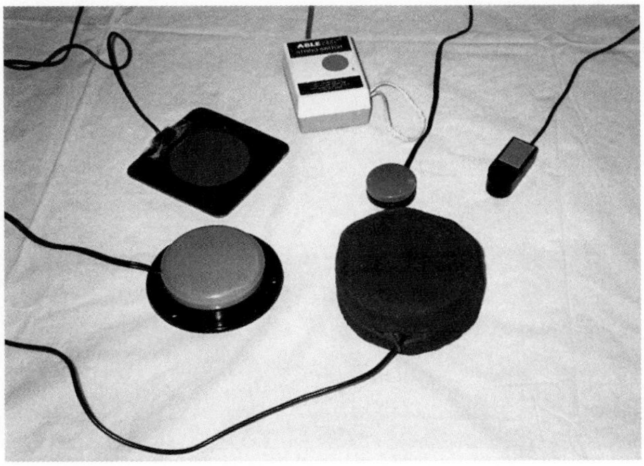

Figure 19-4 Commonly used switches (clockwise from bottom: Soft switch, Jelly Bean, Plate, String, Spec, and Microlite).

Visual Acuity and Visual Perception

Blindness or visual impairment as the primary reason for an AT assessment necessitate a different type of assessment. However, the evaluation team should always consider vision and the possibility of impaired acuity, occulomotor skills, or visual perception. Visual acuity will affect the size of symbols used for communication boards and the size of letters and icons on a computer display. Decreasing the distance from the eye to the display (typically one arm's length) or altering the contrast or magnification helps compensate for poor acuity.

During an AT assessment, eye range of motion, conjugate eye movements, visual field cuts, tracking, and figure-ground discrimination are assessed. Knowing the extent of eye movement and whether the eyes work together is important when consumers are using indirect selection methods. This method requires the eye to track or follow a cursor and scan options to find a specific item. If imbalance is noted, then eye preference should be established and this information used during the assessment and later during equipment set up. Information about a visual field loss helps to determine the location of visual displays and may influence choice of fonts, sizes, or contrast to help compensate.

When the consumer is thought to have a learning disability or cognitive impairment, such as cerebrovascular accident (CVA) or traumatic brain injury (TBI), it may be important to assess visual perception. Knowledge about figure-ground problems helps the team ensure that a visual display is usable. Icons, words, or symbols may need to be placed farther apart or the background simplified to reduce visual stimulation.

Assessments such as the *Motor Free Visual Perception Test* (Colarusso & Hammill, 2002) and the *Test of Visual Perception Skills* (Gardiner, 1993), which directly test visual perception, may help identify the consumer's needs (see Chapter 8). If tracking is impaired, activities to encourage the development of tracking skills, such as simple cause-and-effect software under the control of a single switch, can be helpful.

Finalizing the Match between User and Technology

By this time in the assessment, the AT team has a clear idea of the consumer's motor, cognitive, visual, and visual perception abilities. The AT team should have begun to narrow the range of AT options down to a few AT devices with input method, mounts, and control enhancers that match the consumer's needs and abilities.

Once options have been narrowed to two or three, a more extensive trial of each is conducted. Trials of two to three devices with the control interface and control enhancers allow the consumer to become familiar with the equipment and determine how comfortable he or she feels when using it. As previously mentioned (Angelo, 2000), this trial, if not the entire assessment, should occur in the environment where the consumer will use the equipment. Using the system in the actual or intended environment—home, workplace, or school—uncovers problems that may not emerge during center-based trials. Noise, desks that are too small for devices, tables that are too low for rolling under with a wheelchair, and lights that are too dim or that glare on the display can be addressed and resolved. Trials should occur before making recommendations and submitting a final equipment list because this increases the likelihood that the devices will actually be used and not abandoned. Since the reauthorization of the Tech Act of 1988 now requires each state to develop an AT device-lending library, teams can begin to make use of this resource (United States Congress, 2004). Many states already have such a resource in place.

The AT Intervention Process

The specifics of AT device recommendations are guided by the consumer's skills and abilities, which are broadly guided by their preferences and goals. Broad categories of AT solutions include control enhancers, computer modifications, AAC devices, and EADL, and each of these will be discussed in turn.

Hierarchy of Access

The earlier discussion of the HAAT model established that AT devices are comprised of a user interface, processor, activity output, and environmental interface (see Fig. 19-1) (Cook & Hussey, 2002). Occupational therapists, by their education and interest in human function, are well suited to analyze and recommend solutions for the user interface aspect of this model. When consumers have difficulty with or cannot use standard input devices, a principle called hierarchy of access is used (Schmitt, 1992). When this principle is used, potential solutions are considered based on a range of simple to complex. Solutions that are less complex are also less costly and easier to implement and support. When complexity is reduced, the likelihood for technical conflicts is also reduced. The goal is to create the optimal solution without burdening the consumers with more technology than they need. The following paragraphs will elaborate on this range of solutions.

Control Enhancers

AT devices alone do not usually provide enough support for consumers to engage in the activities of occupational roles. Consumers may also need the help of low-technology aids called control enhancers. The term control enhancer, first used by Cook and Hussey (Cook & Hussey, 1995), refers to aids that enhance or extend a consumer's physical control. Control enhancers include head pointers, hand-held pointing devices (pencils, pointers with built-up handles, and typing sticks), mouth sticks, wrist rests, and arm supports (Fig. 19-5). Control enhancers also include devices that modify placement of user interfaces such as easels, flexible switch mounts, and LCD monitor arms. For example, a lever adjustable keyboard tray can increase keyboarding comfort, or an easel can position a regular keyboard for a consumer using a mouth stick and eliminate the need for a special keyboard. Control enhancers also support using devices efficiently and with reduced fatigue.

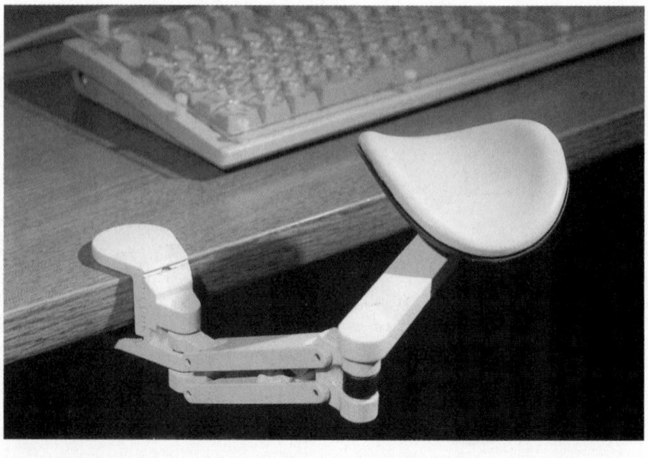

Figure 19-5 Control enhancers, such as a mobile forearm support and key guard, improve direct access.

Comparing several control enhancers helps determine the best fit between the consumer and the AT devices.

Adaptive Computer Access

A discussion on methods for adapting computers to allow use by consumers with disabilities should start with a review of the basic parts and functions of a computer (Definition 19-1). The methods for adapting a computer fall into two categories—modifications to input and to output—based on the two interfaces humans have with computers. Depending on diagnosis or impairment, consumers have difficulty getting information either into or out of computers—and sometimes both.

Any discussion of adapting computers should start with a review of the accessibility options in the computer operating system (OS). Since these options are found on all computers at no additional cost, they are a likely first step in the "hierarchy of access." Accessibility options, which are found in the control panel, allow any user to modify input and output options like setting the size and speed of the mouse, latching modifier keys on the keyboard to aid one-handed typing, reducing keyboard sensitivity to cut errors due to tremors, increasing the contrast or size of fonts on the menus and icons, and controlling basic computer functions with speech. Both Microsoft and Apple websites offer extensive tutorials and step-by-step guides for using these features.

> **DEFINITION 19-1**
>
> **Parts of a Computer**
>
> Central Processing Unit (CPU)—The hardware including circuit boards, microprocessors, timing clocks, disk drives, and a cooling fan. The speed of the computer, measured in gigahertz, and the computing power of the microprocessor dictate how efficiently a computer can sequence instructions and perform calculations.
>
> Application Software—The software that allows people to be productive with computers. It ranges from drawing and early-learning software for children to advanced statistical and mathematical programs for scientists. Common application software includes word processors, spreadsheets, and databases.
>
> Computer Peripherals—Additions to the CPU that enable the computer to meet the user's requirements. Flat monitors, telephone and cable modems, page scanners, plotters for creating technical drawings, trackballs and joysticks, digital cameras, speech recognition microphones, printers, and cameras are just a few examples of computer peripherals.
>
> Operating System (OS)—The underlying software that coordinates with hardware and enables the computer to run applications software. Operating systems now use a graphical user interface (GUI, pronounced *gooey*) to make computers easier for non-technical users. GUIs use the analogy of desktop, pages, file folders, and wastebaskets to represent OS tasks. Windows and Macintosh OS are common, and Unix is used by computer information systems (CIS) professionals.
>
> Random Access Memory (RAM)—Memory that is built into the circuit boards and is used for routine computer tasks. The amount of active memory or RAM required varies with the task. When writing a paper, RAM "remembers" the words and pictures in a document until the user saves them. Information stored in RAM is lost if the computer shuts down before work is saved.
>
> Storage—Computers save or store a user's work so it can be retrieved at another time. Data is stored on floppy disks, internal and external hard drives, remote drives on networks, USB flash drives, memory cards, and read/write optical discs. Digital media (cameras, music, and video) have increased the need for large-capacity storage.

Input

Specialized software and hardware can modify computer input. Input is the means by which a user gives instructions to the computer, usually using a keyboard or mouse.

Alternative Keyboards

Consumers should first try a standard keyboard with an adaptation such as a keyguard to physically reduce unintended key hits. Only then consider alternative keyboards. Most alternative keyboards provide transparent computer access; that is, the computer thinks the input is coming from a standard computer keyboard. Additionally, most of these keyboards are equipped with **USB** connectors so they can be exchanged without rebooting and will work on Windows or Macintosh platforms.

Several commercial products are included in this category. Some are adaptable and can be used in a variety of ways; others have narrow application. One keyboard, Intellikeys (Fig. 19-6), crosses computer platforms. It comes with a set of standard overlays that are instantly detected by the keyboard through bar code readers. The layouts of these overlays range from simple enough for use by early learners to more complex for advanced computer users. Key press acceptance rates are easily adjusted, and keyguards can facilitate key pressing accuracy. The keyboard also allows mouse control to be assumed by arrow keys if the consumer cannot smoothly point with a mouse. Since the keyboard is made from a pressure sensitive membrane rather than mechanical switches, custom overlays with keys that vary in size can easily be created. Additional software designed for this keyboard allows an interface specialist to create overlays for early learning software or beginning writing or to support curriculum modification for students struggling to meet educational objectives.

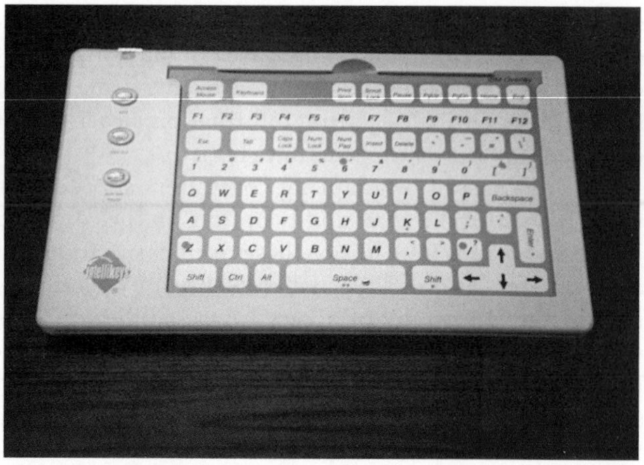

Figure 19-6 Intellikeys stores a user's preferences within the keyboard's memory.

The keyboard is 11 × 17 inches, so good range of motion is needed to reach all of the keys.

For consumers with limited range of motion, smaller keyboards are helpful. Although it looks like a typical keyboard, the Datalux (Fig. 19-7) offers a smaller footprint and a more compact key layout, making it ideal for small hands or mounting for mouth stick use. A very small keyboard that also uses pressure-sensitive membranes is the TASH Mini, sized at 7.25 × 4.24 inches. Fingertips or a mouth stick have only a short reach to press all keys. The TASH Mini keyboard is offered in two permanent layouts, either with the most used keys in the center of the keyboard or in a **QWERTY** layout. Keys also control mouse movements.

Another small keyboard is the Magic Wand. The consumer holds a metal stylus like a pencil and touches the appropriate metal key on the keyboard with this stylus. No force is required. The half-QWERTY keyboard offers another approach in which a one-handed consumer with knowledge of touch-typing simply uses the space bar to create access to the mirror image of QWERTY layout. Software helps to teach the concepts and users quickly relearn touch-typing with one hand. A one-handed typist may prefer the concept of a chordic keyboard like the BAT personal keyboard. The hand stays in a home position and uses multiple finger combinations, as in playing chords on a piano, to enter all of the alphanumeric characters. Macros (small programs that run inside an application) can execute special commands and keyboard shortcuts, although a pointing device such as a mouse or trackball is usually also necessary.

Trackballs

Although a mouse is the most common pointing device, a trackball offers some important advantages because the ball remains stationary in a base. A trackball separates the actions of pointing and clicking, allowing more accurate cursor control and reducing the frustrating movement that can occur when initiating a mouse click. The hand rests on the base of the trackball, thus increasing proximal stability for the fingers. Many consumers with poor coordination who cannot control a mouse can control a trackball. Furthermore, a trackball is sturdy enough for control via elbow or toe movements. Trackballs usually come with software that allows adjusting the ratios between ball movement and cursor speed. Clicks and double clicks can be linked to buttons on the right or left side of the trackball base. Another substitute for mouse use is the 1.5-inch square track pad. Cursor movement happens in response to fingertip movement, and clicks happen in response to finger taps.

Touch Screens

Like the trackball, a touch screen is a mouse substitute or mouse emulator. Selecting or interacting with a touch screen is as simple as touching an icon to select it or dragging a finger to draw in a paint program. Touch screens are used when the cognitive demands for computer tasks must be kept low, such as when working with young children or adults with cognitive impairments. Touch screens are also commonly used in public kiosks where intuitive use is required.

Mouse Emulation

When hands or feet cannot control a mouse or cursor, head movements can be substituted to direct the mouse. Mouse clicks are produced with an external switch or with associated software. One device of this type is HeadMaster Plus, which is worn as a headset. The headset, with its attached **pneumatic** switch that allows clicking and dragging, sends ultrasonic signals to a receiver that sits atop the computer display. The signals are accurately converted into head position and allow the head to precisely direct the mouse. The HeadMaster can be paired with a control box that adds

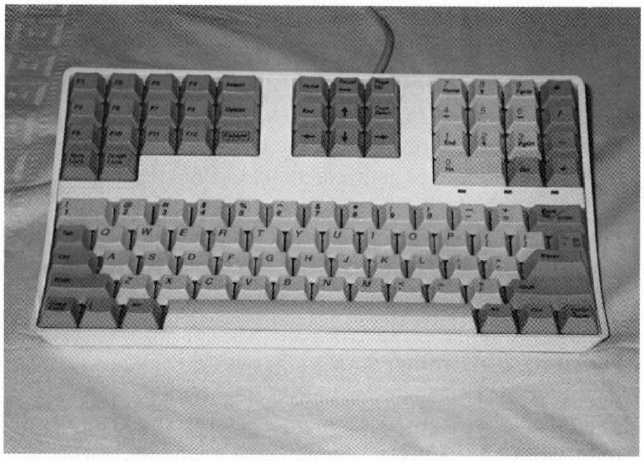

Figure 19-7 Datalux keyboard has a compact key arrangement and a small footprint.

cordless IR communication to the unit. Infrared allows a consumer with a power wheelchair to independently drive-up to a computer and begin to use it without disconnecting wires or headset. Another technology used for head pointing is reflected light. The Tracker Pro, another head mouse, emits light from LEDs around the lens of a 2″ × 2″ × 3″ camera that sits atop the display. Solid-state photo sensors in the camera detect this light when it is returned from a reflective dot worn on the forehead or eyeglasses. An external switch or dwell-activated software is used for mouse clicks. Both of these technologies allow **pixel-to-pixel** accuracy and smooth cursor movement.

Jouse, a joystick mouse operated by mouth, also provides for quick and precise cursor movement. The Jouse sits on an adjustable mount that attaches to the edge of the desktop. Once adjusted, a consumer simply pulls up to the computer and begins computer tasks. A built-in sip/puff switch activates mouse buttons or, in an additional mode, sends Morse code signals. Text entry is achieved via Morse code or through software that creates an on-screen keyboard. All of these head-controlled devices allow use of graphical user interface (GUI)-based programs like computer-assisted drawing (CAD), desktop publishing, and graphic design.

On-Screen Keyboards

To write text with these mouse alternative technologies, consumers need on-screen keyboards. They work with any pointing device and are occasionally used with trackballs. These keyboards are created by software and displayed on the monitor (Fig. 19-8). Virtual keys are activated by clicking on them or by hovering over them with the cursor (called dwell) for a user-defined amount of time. Since the text entry rate is equivalent to one-finger typing, on-screen keyboards are usually packaged with **word prediction** and **abbreviation expansion** software. Word prediction

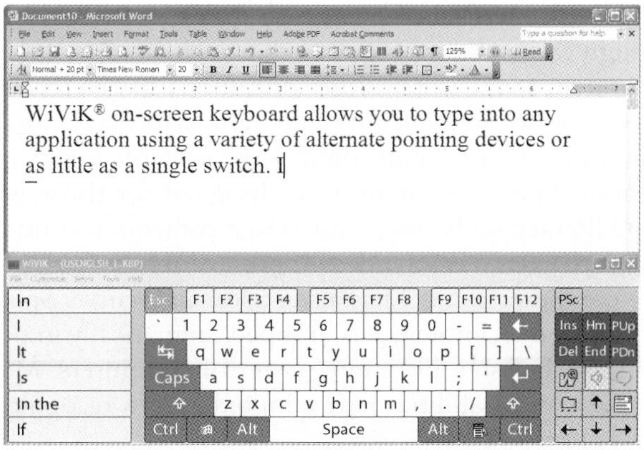

Figure 19-8 WiVik3 is an on-screen keyboard for Windows that allows a consumer to enter text using direct or indirect selection along with word prediction, abbreviation expansion, and synthesized speech feedback.

software uses rules of recency and frequency to guess the word the typist is beginning to spell. Optimally configured, it saves keystrokes. Word prediction works well in this application since the consumer's eyes are already focused on the on-screen keyboard where the predicted words are displayed. A second click or dwell chooses the whole word and enters it into the text document. Abbreviation expansion lets the consumer establish shortcuts to represent frequently used phrases or personal information, such as BTW for "by the way."

Speech Recognition

Speech recognition technology has made rapid advances since its development. Originally a tool for data entry in environments where the hands were busy, its usefulness for those with disabilities was quickly recognized. Consumers with significant motor impairments who had speech, even with mild dysarthria, were able to train voice

CLINICAL REASONING IN OCCUPATIONAL THERAPY PRACTICE

AT Related to Self-Advancement Roles

Eighteen months ago, George had a cervical spinal cord injury at C5–6 secondary to a motor vehicle accident. George's biggest frustration is the limited recovery of motor skills in his hands. He can shrug his shoulders, flex and extend his elbows, and pronate and supinate his forearms. He has limited grasp and release, however, and no independent finger movement. After a significant episode of reactive depression, George is now receptive to ideas about how to manage his limitations. Prior to the injury, he worked as a graphic designer. Currently, he is receiving full disability as a result of the injury. The firm he worked for completely transitioned to **computer-aided design (CAD)** last year. His employer has expressed willingness to make a PC and software available to George at home. The employer's hope is that George might, with adaptations and training, be able to return to his former position at work. George's primary graphics tools will be a computer mouse and digitizing pad. Keyboarding will be used occasionally for correspondence and the textual elements of designs.

1. What AT solutions could help George reengage in computer-aided design?
2. How would control enhancers be useful to George?
3. How much training will be needed to ensure that George will be successful?
4. Where should the training take place?

models and write independently using a computer. Although early versions required that each word be spoken separately, today systems use continuous speech recognition. Sophisticated software and high-performance microphones compare sound input with probable words and phrases. Speech recognition is designed for those with good literacy skills since a user must compare text on the screen to what was intended. At present, its use for hands-free computer control has a steep learning curve. Speech recognition technology has dropped dramatically in price along with faster and more powerful computers. Many people with disabilities have adopted speech recognition technology.

Optical Character Recognition

Optical character recognition (OCR) is a technology that converts pages of print into computer documents. Originally developed to help secretaries avoid retyping documents, OCR is a mainstream technology that offers adaptation for individuals with disability. OCR uses a flatbed page scanner to capture a page image and software to analyze the image and recognize it as alphanumeric characters or text. A technology that converts print into computer text creates a significant compensation for those with visual impairment or learning disability. Computer text can be spoken, converted to large print, or sent to a Braille printer. OCR is available in stand-alone products like the SARA (scanning and reading appliance) or as a component of a personal computer. Special education programs use OCR technology to convert paper worksheets and tests to digital documents. Students then complete digital worksheet using an adaptive computer access method. Naturally, the accuracy of the recognition process is critical for success, but accuracy rates of 99% are achieved with high-quality printed materials.

Eye Gaze

Some consumers with severe motor impairments, such as those with high-level spinal cord injury or brainstem stroke, can only control their eye movement. This control, however, will allow them to use one of several eye gaze technologies. VisionKey uses a small keyboard on an LCD display attached to eyeglass frames. A small camera directed toward the eye reads its position in relation to characters on that keyboard. By focusing on the desired character for a set amount of time, a selection is made and confirmed with a beep. Using this process, the consumer types or selects characters or commands from the keyboard. These inputs are sent to a computer and viewed on its display by the other eye. The advantage of this solution is that the tiny keyboard moves with the consumer's head, which maintains alignment of eye-to-sensor. Another eye gaze approach uses cameras mounted on a computer display and focused on one eye to interpret the eye's movement in relation to the head. Eye Tech and LC Technology both use this approach. Software analyzes the eye movement to determine where the consumer is looking and moves the cursor to that point. This technology is paired with onscreen keyboards, and mouse clicks are performed with dwell, a slow eye blink, or a hardware switch. Computer software supports word processing, **speech synthesizers**, and control of EADLs. The consumer's head must be kept stationary so the eye remains in the sensor's field of view. Recalibration is needed if the head moves outside this range. Eye gaze technology was very expensive in the past, but newer products have brought competition and reduced prices.

Morse Code

When consumers have few motor control sites, Morse code is an option. Although Morse code brings up images of pre-telephone days, it is a physically simple means of sending encoded data to a computer or other device. Users must have control and endurance at a minimum of one motor site (e.g., a finger or eyebrow) and the cognitive ability to learn and recall codes. One or two switches can be used. Consumers with the motor ability to initiate both long and short signals use one switch. Those unable to time switch closure must use two switches, one for dit and one for dah. Once the code is sent, computer software converts signals into alphanumeric characters, keyboard shortcuts, or operating system macros. Using Morse code, consumers compose text, use spreadsheets, and browse the Internet. Using a body part that can be moved quickly as a switch site, it is possible to type at rates of 30 wpm. No other input method for a person with severe motor limitation allows writing at this rate of speed (Anson, 1997).

Tongue-Touch Keypad

Another strategy used when there are few motor control sites is the tongue-touch keypad (TTK). A consumer with good tongue control can use its tip to touch one of nine keys imbedded in an orthodontic appliance worn on the roof of the mouth. A battery-powered ultrasound transmitter in the TTK can send an RF signal to a power wheelchair controller, an EADL, or a computer. Computer software that accompanies the TTK allows total control of the computer operating system and application software. Each switch embedded in the TTK corresponds to a cell in a 3×3 matrix. When one of the nine cells is touched, the computer accepts the input and displays a sub-matrix on the monitor with nine additional choices. In this way, many options are offered with only a small set of keys.

Scanning

Scanning, or indirect selection, is the input method of last resort. When a consumer lacks the ability to accurately choose one item from a set of all options (e.g., a key on a keyboard or push button phone), an **array** with subsets of options is offered. In an array, the subsets are offered in sequence, and the individual signals choice by activating a

DEFINITION 19-2

Basic Scanning Modes

Automatic—The consumer presses the switch to initiate scanning. The cursor highlights items in the selection set one at a time. The consumer presses the switch as the desired item is highlighted.

Inverse—The consumer presses the switch to initiate scanning. The consumer must maintain switch closure for the cursor to move across the selection set. When the desired item is highlighted, the consumer releases the switch, indicating the choice.

Step—The consumer presses the switch to move to the next item in the selection set. The cursor moves to the adjacent item each time the switch is pressed. A selection is made when the cursor dwells on an item and the consumer refrains from pressing the switch.

switch when the desired option is offered. This input method is very inefficient because of the time spent waiting. This delay increases further when the consumer cannot see. In this case, auditory scanning is used, and the consumer listens for an announcement of each choice just before it is available for selection. Scanning arrays can be used to control computers, EADLs, and AAC devices. Information on scanning modes is provided in Definition 19-2.

Output

Once a computer receives input, the central processing unit (CPU) and OS software perform the requested task. CPUs deliver the same output regardless of how the input is delivered to the processor. Output is the result that a computer delivers on the screen, as a printed page or as sound. Output may be a final product, dialog boxes, or alert sounds played as a computer processes data. Individuals with sensory impairment are most affected by computer output because they do not have equal access to it. This leads to the other category of adaptations: adaptations to computer output.

SCREEN

Most computer output is interpreted visually, so most adaptations to output are used by consumers with visual impairments. The range of visual impairments is broad, ranging from field deficits and color blindness to low vision and total inability to perceive light. Thus, there is a broad range of adaptations. Some are as simple as reducing the amount of light coming from the screen, which is accomplished by reversing the screen contrast so that the letters are light on a dark background. This adaptation is possible in the accessibility option in the computer OS. Another simple adaptation is to increase the size of objects on the screen by reducing the monitor resolution. For example, if a 17-inch monitor capable of displaying 1280 × 1024 pixels is set to 640 × 480, everything displayed on the screen is twice as large.

SCREEN ENLARGEMENT

Screen enlargement software more powerfully accommodates visual impairment by magnifying the screen 2 to 16 times. One product, Zoomtext, shown in Figure 19-9, creates a virtual magnifying glass for a particular section of the screen. The user can move between an area that is greatly magnified and the normal display and thus zoom in to see parts of the screen that are of interest, e.g., a radio button or close box. Most enlargement software offers options such as panning through sentences or highlighting words as a speech synthesizer reads them. Listening along with viewing enlarged text allows listening to support weak visual skills. Screen enlargement software also allows users to set up default colors for text and background, which may enhance their remaining vision.

TEXT-TO-SPEECH

When consumers have no usable vision, they need software to completely substitute for seeing, not just in application software, but also in the OS. Adaptive software, generically called a screen reader (e.g., JAWS, WindowEyes), allows a consumer to direct the cursor around the screen while listening to a speech synthesizer read menu choices, text in dialog boxes, and paragraphs in word-processed documents. The cursor and reading functions are controlled either by the keyboard's number pad or by a separate keypad. Consumers can set up preferences (e.g., pronunciation of special words or speech rate).

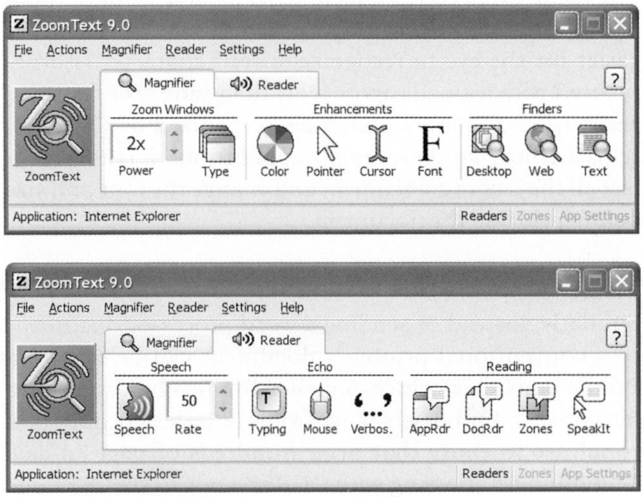

Figure 19-9 Applications now offer both text-to-speech and enlargement of information on the computer monitor. ZoomText control panels are shown.

Refreshable Braille Display

Braille continues to be an important tool for literacy despite the prevalence of audio recordings and speech synthesizers. Currently only about 12% of school-age children with blindness use Braille as their primary reading medium (Raeder, 2005). This concerns many in the blind community, who know that reading Braille is highly correlated with literacy and academic achievement. Refreshable Braille is an innovative adaptation that overcomes several problems associated with Braille documents, such as the bulk of thick paper and the inability to search the documents quickly or correct errors (Cook & Hussey, 2002).

A refreshable Braille display is created with pins that make tactile dots that rise and fall to show changing computer text. A Braille display sits under and extends beyond the lower edge of a computer keyboard so that a consumer using one easily moves their fingers between the keyboard and the display. A 40-character Braille display shows half of the typical 80-character line of text seen on the computer monitor. The consumer controls the line of text that is displayed in Braille and edits by sending the cursor to the intended Braille cell.

As a means of computer output, a Braille display modifies the output for all computer-based tasks. This means the Braille display presents the text in a web page, the numbers in a column, the text in a table, or the notation in a math formula. Additional information is communicated, and consumers using Braille displays have access to more information than they do when using text-to-speech computer output modifications.

Large Print

People commonly take away the products of a computer work session in print form. What adaptations are possible if text printed on paper cannot be read? Consumers with low vision often convert documents to large print or modify the font based on its purpose. Serif fonts are considered easier for the eye to recognize (a serif character is ornamented with a small cap or foot) than sans serif text. Yet, san serif text is more accurately recognized by OCR systems. In most word processing applications, it is easy to select all the text in a document and change the font and size before printing the document.

Braille Embossing

Similarly, instead of sending a word processor document to a conventional printer, a document can be sent to a Braille embosser, which punches Braille characters into heavy paper. Embossers range from those designed for personal use to those that print hundreds of pages a day. Combining embossing with OCR systems to create Braille versions of text documents reduces the work for Braille transcribers who only need to check for errors. Technology makes it easier to produce documents in Braille. New software now combines print and embossing to aid others who do not read Braille.

Auditory Signals

Hearing impairment also creates a need for modifying computer output. Operating systems offer the option of having the menu bar flash as a substitute for alert sounds. Computers, being highly visual tools, do not usually require other adaptations. As the multimedia capacity of computers has developed, however, it has become important to offer captioning or a text description of a sound feature in educational software and on web pages. This is particularly important when sound is part of conveying the full meaning.

Augmentative and Alternative Communication Devices

AAC intervention is the process of facilitating functional communication across all contexts. Communicating with an AAC device is slow, and it is based on hours of work by the augmented communicator and a team of professionals who provide training and support services (United States Society for Augmentative and Alternative Communication [USSAAC], 2005). AAC methods are multimodal and can be divided into two main groups. Unaided communication systems include sign languages, gestures, facial expressions, and looking up for yes and down for no. Aided communication systems use physical objects like picture and letter boards and high-tech and voice output devices to communicate (USSAAC, 2005). Although both types are needed for effective communication, we will focus on aided communication systems.

Non-Electronic Communication Systems

Aided communication systems can be categorized in several ways, non-electronic or electronic, non-vocal or vocal output, and dedicated or non-dedicated devices. Non-electronic devices include devices that function without batteries or electricity. Examples of non-electronic aids are pencil and paper and alphabet, symbol, or picture boards and books. These aids vary in size from those fitting into a shirt pocket to filling a wheelchair tray. They can be used nearly anywhere, since maintenance is minimal and no electricity is required. These devices do not have storage capability, however, so unique messages cannot be prepared ahead of time. When messages can be prepared ahead of time and stored, as in electronic devices, they can be delivered at the convenience of the consumer and the communication partner. Electronic devices also have the advantage of being able to get the attention of others through a sound or voice output. Their disadvantages are increased weight (anywhere from approximately 0.5 pound to 10 pounds) and the need for regular battery charging.

Synthesized or Digitized

Electronic AAC devices have voice output either as digitized or synthesized speech. Digitized devices can record and store human voice recordings on microchips within the device. Usually speakers of the same gender and age make the recordings so that the device sounds like their own voice might sound. Devices using digitized speech can provide anywhere from a few seconds to a few minutes of voice output. A disadvantage of digitized speech is that it requires a lot of memory for storage and only complete phrases or words can be stored, reducing its usefulness for phrases that may change in grammar.

Synthesized speech is more flexible since it will speak whatever text is presented. Microprocessor-based programs in the device follow rules of pronunciation for the language and convert text to vocal output (synthesized speech) following those rules. Exceptions for things like proper names can be created to meet the user's preference. High-quality speech synthesizers at low cost are available, giving consumers choices in vocal personality and gender. Synthesized speech is available in multiple languages. Although most devices come with some stored words and phrases, they are easy to customize and generally allow the consumer to speak whatever sentence they can create. Customization is accomplished by using the keyboard to enter new words and phrases and following a sequence for storing new vocabulary. Synthesized speech offers independence and flexibility. Consumers can add words and sequence them in any combination.

Static or Dynamic

Visual displays for electronic AAC devices are either static or dynamic. Static displays do not change appearance as the consumer uses them. To give the consumer more communication options on static displays, strategies such as page levels (layers) or visually rich icons with multiple meanings are used. With the level strategy, categories, such as words for mealtime, are grouped on a level. The multiple-meaning icon strategy keeps all communication options on one level. A scheme for associating words or phrases with pictures and the sequence in which they are selected allows a consumer to produce both standard and novel utterances. With static displays, commands and icons remain in the same place. This allows the consumer to develop automatic sequences for messages and increases speed. Because AAC device use is slow, speed in generating speech is very important.

Dynamic displays change in response to anticipated communication needs. Imagine that it is lunchtime and a friend asks the consumer, "Where do you want to go for lunch?" The consumer turns to the device, which provides a menu of topics, such as greetings, mealtime, school, and vacation. The consumer selects the mealtime icon. The screen changes to present a different set of choices: foods and restaurants. The consumer selects restaurants. Once again, the screen changes and presents a new set of selections, including Dairy Delight, McDonald's, and Pizza Hut. The consumer selects a restaurant for lunch, and the associated stored sentences or words are displayed.

Dynamic displays offer some advantages, since only a smaller set of options that are closer to the theme of a conversation are presented. This is an excellent strategy for presenting words used infrequently in conversation, although core vocabulary—the words and phrases that are part of all speech regardless of the topic—may be left behind on previous pages. Some devices are designed so that this separation is minimized. The cognitive load of retrieving pages can be high. Therefore, groupings of topics or vocabulary should be logical. Figure 19-10 shows the Dynamo, an augmentative communication device with dynamic display capabilities. Most AAC devices now offer a combination of static and dynamic display. In devices that use both types, static icons are used for core vocabulary because this allows the development of automaticity. Dynamic icons are useful for fringe vocabulary, which is less often used and varies among users (Ballandin, Baker, & Hill, 1999).

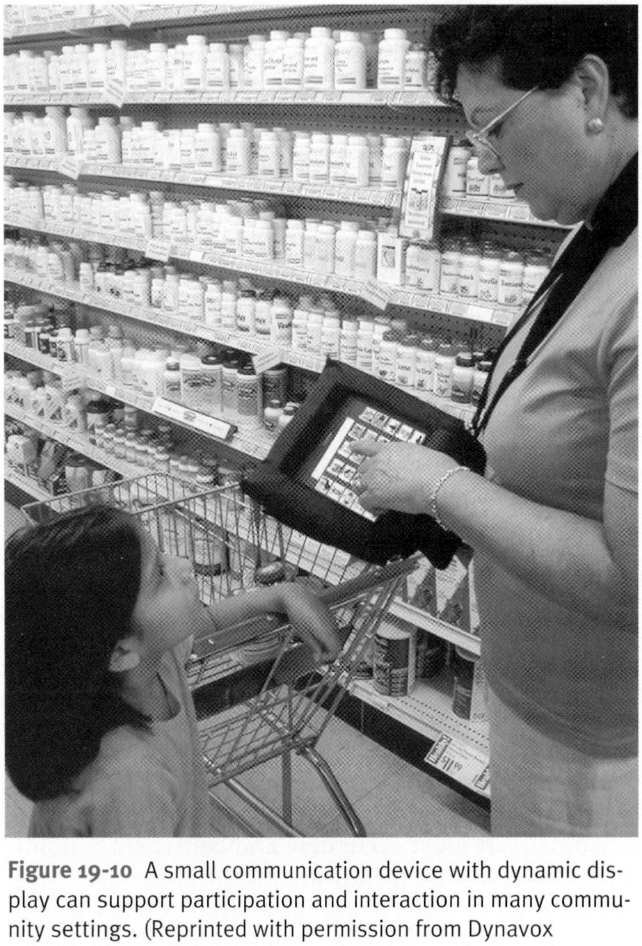

Figure 19-10 A small communication device with dynamic display can support participation and interaction in many community settings. (Reprinted with permission from Dynavox Technologies, Pittsburgh, PA, 1-800-344-1778.)

Dedicated or Non-Dedicated

AAC devices can be dedicated or non-dedicated. Dedicated devices function solely as communication devices. These devices may or may not produce voiced messages, connect to a computer, or print messages. Non-dedicated devices perform other functions while they also serve as communication aids. Most non-dedicated devices are computers loaded with communication software. The advantage is that the consumer has a fully functioning computer that can be used for word processing and other tasks as well as an AAC device. Separation between dedicated and non-dedicated devices was common in the past, but as microprocessors increase in power and speed and decrease in size, most of the more powerful AAC devices offer computer-like functions. Most control EADL devices through an IR port, and they are often used as keyboards for desktop computers too.

Vocal or Non-Vocal

Devices also vary by whether they have non-vocal or vocal output. As with non-electronic devices, when using non-vocal output aids, the consumer must get the attention of the communication partner before beginning the message. The communication partner must be looking at the communication aid before communication can begin. For some non-vocal output devices, communication cannot take place unless the partner understands the system. Examples of non-vocal output devices include alphabet boards, picture boards, drawings, photographs, symbols, and **E-tran boards**. Vocal aids mean that the device speaks the message. These devices are vocal output communication aids (VOCA). VOCAs include digitized and synthesized speech.

Orthography or Representation

When consumers use the alphabet and spell messages to the partner, the alphabet can be arranged in one of several ways, depending on the need. Typical layout arrangements are alphabetical, QWERTY, and frequency. Alphabetical order is used when the team anticipates that the consumer will continue to use cognitively simple devices and not advance to devices with more options. The QWERTY arrangement, the typical alphanumeric keyboard, is appropriate for consumers familiar with keyboarding or expecting to use a computer.

The third strategy is arranging the letters by frequency of use to maximize efficiency or control. Consumers who point to the letters or scan use this strategy. With pointing, the most frequently used letters are placed where the consumer can most accurately and consistently point. Letters used less frequently are placed in the periphery. Placing the most frequently used letters where the consumer has the best accuracy facilitates use of the device and the flow of communication. Scanning arrays should be designed so that the commonly used letters or words are offered as the first or second choice.

Symbol systems are used with both vocal and non-vocal output systems. Symbols may be drawings, icons, or figures specifically developed for communication systems and designed to represent concepts. There is little similarity among representational systems, and each approach has its followers and preferred methods for introduction and use. Examples of published symbol sets are Picture Communication Symbols, PicSyms, MinSpeak, and Blissymbolics. Information on these and other symbol sets can be found in *Augmentative and Alternative Communication* (Beukelman & Mirenda, 1992).

Electronic Aids to Daily Living

EADL provide alternative independent control of the electrical devices in an environment, most often at home. The name has recently changed from environmental control unit (ECU) to EADL as a more accurate description of the function of this technology and to improve reimbursement from funding sources by relating its use to functional outcomes (Lange, 2002). The term environmental control unit emphasizes what is being controlled (i.e., television, telephone) rather than an outcome (i.e., increased independence, safety, communication, leisure). EADLs give access to devices such as lights, telephones, audiovisual or home entertainment appliances, beds, intercoms, thermostats, door locks, and window curtains. Consumers without disabilities increasingly use this type of technology. In new home construction, this technology is called home automation and is marketed as a means to create ease or save money by remotely regulating sprinklers, lights, and thermostats.

EADLs can be activated either through direct (pressing a button on a garage door opener) or indirect (scanning) methods. Most direct-access devices were developed for the mass market and therefore are inexpensive and found in electronics stores. If motor impairment prevents direct selection, a specialized AT product must be used. The same criteria used for determining an access method for computer or AAC device apply to choosing an access method for EADL.

Categories of EADL Control Technology

EADL let the consumer control electrical items without having to move to the appliance or interact with its typical controls. Anyone who has used a TV remote recognizes the convenience and ease of controlling an appliance remotely. Occupational therapists recommend EADL devices to consumers who are unable to control devices due to inability to reach or manipulate knobs, dials, and buttons or who are limited by pain or fatigue.

Appliances vary in complexity of the control signals they require. For example, turning a light on or off requires only an on/off signal, but changing the channel on a television set or reshuffling the songs on the CDs in a 5-disc player requires complex control signals. EADL control signals can be transmitted by several methods, such as through the building's electrical wiring; IR, ultrasound, and RF transmitters and receivers; or a combination of these modes. Certain technologies lend themselves to control of specific kinds of appliances.

Using a building's electrical wiring for control of electrical appliances is convenient for appliances such as lights or fans, which require only simple on/off control signals. Such appliances are plugged into a small coded switch module that is plugged into the wall outlet. A control box, also plugged into an electrical outlet somewhere in the consumer's house, sends a signal with the module code and the on/off signal over the wiring system. The receiver module detects the signals and switches electrical power to the plugged-in appliance. The quantity of codes and variety of modules available make it possible to turn electrical devices off and on throughout a home or apartment. The variety of control boxes ranges from simple hardwired push-button switches to sophisticated computer-controlled interfaces. These devices are known collectively as X-10 modules and controllers.

IR light transmitters are also used to generate control signals. IR light control signals are invisible to the human eye. The control signal is interpreted by an IR receiver and translated into the correct function. Television remote controls use this technology, and their invisible light beam must be pointed directly at the television and have a clear line of sight. Various patterns of IR light are coded to direct the appliance to perform specific functions. IR tends to be used in applications that require multiple adjustments, such as television sets, VCRs, and CD players.

An ultrasound controller works in a similar manner, but control signals are transmitted via inaudible, high-frequency sound waves. Since sound waves disburse readily in home environments, ultrasound controllers do not need a line of sight and can travel farther (up to 200 feet), although walls and other obstacles block them. Ultrasound is used in some simple EADL devices that send on/off signals to IR receiver modules.

Radio frequency (RF) signal transmitters are another option. RF signals are less affected by obstacles such as walls but are sometimes susceptible to interference from other radio frequencies. Devices using RF usually offer the consumer a choice of bands to bypass interference on heavily used channels. That is, the consumer can change the frequency band or channel so as not to turn on devices in the neighbor's house. RF transmitters and receivers are often used to open garage doors and unlatch front doors. They are also frequently the controller of choice to use with an X-10 system that has a RF control box.

Simple EADL

Simple EADLs give simple control over one electrical device. They can contribute to learning cause and effect, increasing personal control, and developing responsibility. Simple EADLs can be set up to work in momentary mode (i.e., work only as long as the switch is activated) or latched mode (i.e., stay on until the switch is pressed again to turn off the device). One simple EADL is the appliance interface, which can be easily incorporated into group participation or fun in the kitchen. Using a single switch, consumers can participate in cooking by turning on small appliances, such as blenders and popcorn poppers. Figure 19-11 shows the Power Link 3 being used with an infrared switch to operate a fan. Therapists can build on this skill and set up other simple switch-controlled EADL interfaces that send ultrasound signals to bedroom lights or fans providing control over personal space. Phones that scan phone numbers or picture phones that combine large buttons and photos with speed dial give modified phone access with simple interfaces. A scanning device like the Relax II is an alternative TV remote control for someone who cannot press small buttons.

Complex EADL

Consumers who have significant impairment or who desire control over more types of appliances within their environment need complex EADL devices with sophisticated functions (see Fig. 19-2). These exist as dedicated EADL devices, as components of a computer-based system, and as a subsystem within AAC devices.

Dedicated devices (e.g., Quartet, Sicare Pilot) perform complex adjustments to multiple systems within a consumer's environment. Some use voice commands; others use scanning input to take commands. They respond and

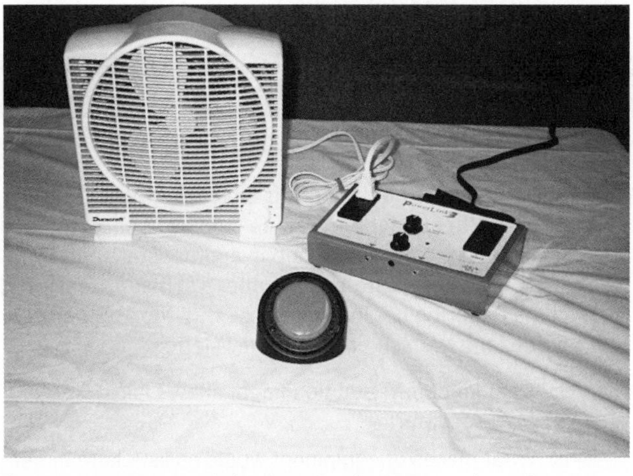

Figure 19-11 Power Link 3 is a simple EADL tool used to operate appliances. Here it is used with a fan.

transmit control signals to systems in the environment using a combination of transmission technologies based on what is best for the appliance being controlled. These systems can activate intercoms, unlock doors, and dial the phone. Consumers should be aware of their vulnerability in power outages and either install uninterruptible power supplies or have a 911 auto-dial backup system.

Systems with similar capacity can be found in computer-based EADLs. Computer software, such as Words+ or MultiMedia Max, transmits a signal to a control box, which sends IR to a phone, appliance, entertainment center, or X-10 module. Computer-based systems are ideal for work settings where consumers are already interacting with their computers. Improvements in speech recognition enable consumers to use voice commands to control EADL software on a computer, although this same feature may be limiting if the consumer must go to the computer to interact with an appliance.

Many top-end AAC devices include EADL control. A subset of icons like the ones the consumer uses in the choosing of words and phrases can activate and send IR signals either directly to an IR-controlled appliance or to an intermediary device that forwards signals on to X-10 modules or telephone dialers. AAC devices can be customized so functions can be added as the consumer gains skill and confidence.

Sensory Accommodations

Many microprocessor-based aids help people with sensory impairments manage their daily living environments.

Closed-Circuit Television

Consumers with low vision and limited interest in computer-based adaptations may consider closed-circuit television (CCTV) systems. A mounted television camera is focused on the item that the user wants to see. This may be a surface where the consumer places the printed material to read (e.g., a recipe, invoice, magazine article, or greeting card) or the writing on the blackboard in the front of the room. The camera sends the image to a TV monitor positioned at the consumer's eye level. Screen magnification and contrast can be set to needs. This technology has become lighter and so much more portable that small handheld units are now available. Now CCTV is being used out in the community and not just at home.

Braille Note Takers

For consumers with visual impairment, portable microprocessor-based note takers function like personal digital assistants (PDAs). Consumers can choose between models with a 6-key Braille keyboard or a full QWERTY keyboard. Some models offer speech feedback via earphone; others offer review through a small refreshable Braille display. Consumers record notes from class or meetings and later upload them to a computer or print them directly to a paper or Braille printer. These devices also contain appointments, contacts, clocks, and reminder systems. With the continued development of technology, they now log on to servers, access e-mail and web pages, and/or operate as cell phones.

Closed Captioning

Real-time closed captioning is an excellent accommodation for consumers with hearing impairments. This system combines a court stenographer's skill for capturing spoken language with a computer for processing the text. This technology projects or displays a speaker's words as readable text. It is often used for keynote speakers at large conferences or in office meetings where participants are gathered around a table.

Environmental Access and Universal Design

AT devices enable participation and control only when the human and non-human environments allow access for consumers and their devices. Independent power mobility

CLINICAL REASONING IN OCCUPATIONAL THERAPY PRACTICE

AT Related to Self-Maintenance Roles

Claire, a 65-year-old widow, is increasingly frustrated in her ADL routines as her macular degeneration worsens. She depends on her daughter, Jean, to stop by her apartment daily to assist her with visual tasks. Claire is upset because Jean's husband has taken a new job in another state and they will be moving soon. Jean has heard that there are low vision aids that might help restore her mother's self-sufficiency and has encouraged her mother to seek assistance. Claire's goals include restoring her independence with food preparation instructions, bill paying, and reading correspondence, the TV guide, and the Senior Activity Newsletter.

1. What kind of AT solution might allow Claire to regain some of her self-sufficiency and ease her daughter's mind about moving away?
2. What pieces of equipment would assist Claire in her environment?
3. What would help ensure a good "fit" between Claire and the equipment?

offers no advantage in places without ramps and rooms where doorways are too narrow to accommodate the wheelchair. Consumers using AAC devices cannot communicate if people will not take the time to interact with them.

Just considering the variability among humans in the design process can eliminate many barriers. Incorporating universal design means that products and environments are designed to be usable by all people, to the greatest extent possible, without the need for adaptation or specialized design (The Center for Universal Design, 1997).

Since people who use AT devices to compensate for impairment are not always given the opportunity to demonstrate their capabilities, the Americans with Disability Act (ADA) supplies the force of federal law to facilitate their opportunities (see Chapters 11 and 36).

Funding

Clearly, AT devices cost money. At times, inexpensive solutions can be found to enhance the consumer's occupational performance, but often the equipment or the training to use it is costly. AT enables consumers to participate in roles that might otherwise be denied to them. Therefore, the consumer's abilities, needs, and specific occupational goals should drive the assessment, not the availability of funding. The compelling need for an AT device or services should drive the search for funding.

AT Should Drive the Funding Process

The consumer's goals may require AT devices that are totally beyond his or her financial resources. When funding drives the assessment, more costly solutions are not reviewed, and the consumer is offered only solutions that are within his or her means. If the best solution facilitates the consumer's occupation but is expensive, the assessment team needs to document that the solution will best meet the consumer's goals and present a strong case to the funding agency.

Legislation and Funding for AT

The Assistive Technology Act of 2004 recently reaffirmed AT devices as valuable tools for individuals with disabilities (United States Congress, 2004). The original law placed AT education and advocacy resources in all states and United States territories (United States Congress, 1988). The new law requires states to increase access to AT devices through lending libraries, recycling programs, and low-interest consumer loan programs.

Congress, recognizing the natural links between people and their societal roles, sought to make paying for AT a responsibility for a range of publicly supported agencies. Therefore, considering an individual's life role leads to good starting points for finding funding for AT.

Workers

Vocational rehabilitation agencies, which are federally funded in each state, are responsible for providing the training, education, services, and AT that working-age consumers need to become employable. Vocational rehabilitation is a major payer for AT evaluations and for the devices and training those evaluations recommend.

The ADA makes it unlawful to exclude persons with disabilities from public services, transportation, telecommunications, and employment. To help pay for reasonable accommodation for an employee or prospective employee with a disability, a business can apply for an Internal Revenue Service (IRS) Business Tax Credit and Deduction or a Department of Labor Work Opportunity Tax Credit to offset their costs. Expenditures to make a workplace accessible include computer adaptations and remodeling bathrooms (Jeserich, 2003; Mendelson, 1996).

Social Security can help a consumer who wants to begin work through a Plan to Achieve Self Support (PASS). Under Social Security rules, any income reduces benefits. With an approved PASS plan, however, that income can be preserved to pay for items such as AT devices or training that are needed to reach a goal or return to work (Social Security Administration, 2004).

The IRS allows workers to take a tax write-off for health care and miscellaneous work expenses. The IRS definition of medical care, "for the diagnosis, care, treatment or prevention of disease or for the purpose of affecting any structure or function of the body," covers the purpose of AT (IRS, 2005). Other tax provisions enable employed consumers with disabilities to deduct work-related expenses, like AT, from their gross income. A tax credit can also be taken when the expenses incurred by a taxpayer for the care of a dependent who has one or more disabilities frees the taxpayer to work (Mendelson, 1996).

Workers with health insurance can use it to fund some types of AT. Since health insurance uses the criterion of medical necessity to decide whether to fund AT devices or services, they are more likely to cover a wheelchair or prosthesis than a computer adaptation. Policies must be reviewed carefully to determine an individual's coverage.

Older Adults and Unemployed Adults

Medicare is the primary insurer for older adults and those on permanent disability. Medicare will pay for durable medical equipment, wheelchairs, and speech-generating devices (i.e., AAC). Medicare only pays for wheelchairs when they are necessary for mobility-related activities of daily living in the home. This need must be well documented in the medical record. Medicare generally pays 80%, and other health insurance pays the remaining 20%, but only if Medicare pays. In early 2001, Medicare expanded coverage to include funding for dedicated AAC devices and services. If a beneficiary can pay for an AT device with private funds, Medicare outpatient services may cover occupational therapists for AT-related services to increase independence in IADL.

Unemployed adults with disabilities are often eligible for Medicaid. Medicaid is administered at the state level and each state interprets the regulations independently, so coverage varies from state to state.

Injury- and Illness-Related Causes

Health insurance can become a source of reimbursement for AT devices and services when the need for AT devices is the result of an injury or illness. Health insurance, at present, is primarily offered by managed care organizations and health maintenance organizations. Many large health organizations hire case managers to coordinate rehabilitation resources in complex cases. It is clear that consumers who have strokes, head or spinal cord injuries, or progressive neurological disease benefit from AT devices and services. Nevertheless, teaching a case manager about the potential of AT to increase independence and enable a return to occupation remains an important function of occupational therapy practice.

When trauma or negligence causes an injury that necessitates the use of AT, a financial settlement or a trust fund can be the source of reimbursement for AT devices and services. In this case, the occupational therapist may direct a letter of justification to a judge or trustee.

Consumer Loans

Loans are a common way to purchase products. Banks and credit unions are required to offer consumers with disabilities loans that take their special financial circumstances into consideration. The Tech Act Project in each state has information on these low-interest loan programs (United States Congress, 2004).

Charity

When all other sources fail, there are still bake sales, raffles, car washes, and appeals to service clubs and civic organizations as a means of funding AT devices.

Justification Letters

With the knowledge gained from the consumer-centered assessment, trial use of a device, interviews with significant others, and possibly a home visit, the occupational therapist is in a strong position to justify the need for AT devices. This document is called a letter of justification or, in some cases, a letter of medical necessity. A physician's prescription is needed for all requests in medical model services and generally accompanies the therapist's letter of justification. With education- or work-related funding sources, another form of "prescription" may be needed.

The occupational therapist uses knowledge gained in clinical assessment, knowledge of product features, and the potential outcomes for the consumer to develop a report. Using clear writing, case data, and sometimes photographs or videotape footage of the consumer using the device, the therapist presents how the cost of AT devices will be offset by an increase in function, engagement in education, employability, and/or greater independence. It is important to tailor the letter to the funding source. For example, requests for funds from Medicaid must justify AT devices and services as medically necessary, whereas services through the Individuals with Disabilities Education Act (IDEA) must emphasize educational necessity.

A letter of denial does not necessarily mean no. Many private and public sources of funding use a system of appeals to weed out groundless requests. First, get the denial in writing; then, prepare for an appeal. The mandate for funding AT is clear, but agencies and organizations still attempt to avoid financial responsibility by raising objections. A clear, logical letter of justification has won many appeals for AT devices and services.

ROLES OF OCCUPATIONAL THERAPISTS IN AT INTERVENTION

Even when occupational therapists can advise about AT for common needs, some consumers with complex problems will need referral to an AT center for integration of multiple solutions to allow them to reach their functional goal. A referral to an expert (probably in a metropolitan area or a larger facility) creates an opportunity for OT practitioners to learn more about AT. In addition to the opportunity to provide input, there is an opportunity to learn more about AT and provide follow-up as the consumer learns to integrate a complex solution into everyday tasks and routines. Specific roles for the professionals within the AT assessment team have already been discussed, and now, possible roles for occupational therapists are presented.

AT Specialist

Occupational therapists with AT service delivery experience usually strive for the assistive technology provider (ATP) credential. This certification, offered through the Rehabilitation Engineering and Assistive Technology Society of North America (RESNA), validates an individual's knowledge and experience in AT and sets a standard for entry-level expertise. RESNA is an interdisciplinary association of professionals united in a desire to improve the potential of people with disabilities to achieve their goals through the use of technology. Professionals with ATP credentials are expected to adhere to a code of ethics, to practice in a consumer-centered manner, and to continue to gain competence in their area of AT specialty.

Consultant

Some occupational therapists have developed consulting practices in which they advise organizations on program development, change issues, quality improvement, and planning (Jaffe & Epstein, 1992). Many educational, rehabilitation, governmental, or private sector organizations need assistance to implement AT service delivery. Occupational therapists with consulting skills and knowledge of AT solutions can offer important services to these organizations.

Product Development Team and Product Testing

With their broad clinical knowledge of the limitations caused by impairment and their comfort with functional tasks and environments, occupational therapists contribute important knowledge to engineering and research teams. Their input is helpful when conceptualizing solutions, developing prototypes, and measuring efficacy with consumers.

CONTINUING EDUCATION

AT is always changing. Any occupational therapist practicing in AT must commit to continuing education. RESNA and other organizations continuously offer education (Resources 19-1). University courses, as well as sessions at annual conferences, weekend workshops, and online courses allow practitioners to pick up the knowledge and skills needed to incorporate AT into a range of practice settings. Listserves, like those offered by the American Occupational Therapy Association, RESNA, and university programs, allow novice practitioners to use the expertise and help of experienced AT practitioners to solve practical problems. Therapy departments can hire staff development expertise to increase their comfort with using AT in their practice setting.

RESOURCE 19-1

Assistive Technology Suppliers

Adaptive Switch Laboratories, Inc.
125 Spur 191, Suite C
Spicewood, TX 78669
Phone: (800) 626-8698
www.asl-nc.com/

Ablenet
2808 Fairview Avenue
Roseville, MN 55113-1308
Phone: (800) 322-0956
www.ablenetinc.com/

Datalux Corporation
155 Aviation Drive
Winchester, VA 22602
Phone: (800) 328-2589
www.datalux.com/

Don Johnston Incorporated
26799 West Commerce Drive
Volo, IL 60073
Phone: (800) 889-5242
www.donjohnston.com/

DynaVox Technologies
2100 Wharton Street
Pittsburgh, PA 15203
Phone: (888) 697-7332
www.dynavoxsys.com/

Freedom Scientific
11800 31st Court North
St. Petersburg, FL 33716-1805
Phone: (800) 444-4443
www.freedomscientific.com/

H.K. Eyecan, Ltd.
36 Burland Street
Ottawa, Ontario, Canada
K2B 6J8
Phone: (800) 356-3362
www.eyecan.ca/

Humanware
175 Mason Circle
Concord, CA 94520
Phone: (800) 722-3393
www.humanware.com/

IntelliTools
1720 Corporate Circle
Petaluma, CA 94954
Phone: (800) 899-6687
www.intellitools.com/

Kensington Technology Group
333 Twin Dolphin Drive
Redwood Shores, CA 94065
Phone: (800) 535-4242
www.kensington.com/

LC Technologies, Inc.
3955 Pender Drive, Suite 120
Fairfax, Virginia 22030
Phone: (800) 393-4293
www.lctinc.com/

Madentec Inc.
4664 99th Street
Edmonton, Alberta, Canada
T6E 5H5
Phone: (877) 623-3682
www.madentec.com/

Matias Corporation
129 Rowntree Dairy Road, Unit #20
Vaughan, Ontario, Canada
L4L 6E1
Phone: (888) 663-4263
www.half-qwerty.com/

Natural Point Incorporated
PO Box 2317
Corvallis, OR 97339
Phone: (541) 753-6645
www.eyecontrol.com/

NewAbilities Systems, Inc.
2938 Scott Boulevard
Santa Clara, CA 95054
Phone: (800) 829-8889
www.newabilities.com/

Prentke Romich Company
1022 Heyl Road
Wooster, OH 44691
Phone: (800) 262-1984
www.prentrom.com/

RJ Cooper & Association
27601 Forbes Road, Suite 39
Laguna Niguel, CA 92677
Phone: (800) 752-6673
www.rjcooper.com/

ScanSoft, Inc
1 Wayside Road
Burlington, MA 01803
Phone: (781) 565-5000
www.scansoft.com/

TASH Inc.
Unit 1, 91 Station Street
Ajax, Ontario, Canada L1S 3H2
Phone: (800) 463-5685
www.tashinc.com/

Words+ Inc.
1220 West Avenue J

(continued)

RESOURCE 19-1 *(continued)*

Lancaster, CA 93534-2902
Phone: (800) 869-8521
www.words-plus.com/

Zygo Industries, Inc.
P.O. Box 1008
Portland, OR 97207
Phone: (800) 234-6006
www.zygo-usa.com/

Research and Development Centers

Center for Applied Special Technology
40 Harvard Mills Square, Suite 3
Wakefield MA 01880
Phone: (781) 245-2212
www.cast.org/

Center for Assistive Technology and Environmental Access
Georgia Institute of Technology
90 10th Street,
Atlanta, GA 30318
Phone: (404) 894-4960
www.catea.org/

Human Engineering Research Laboratory
VAPHS, 7180 Highland Drive, 151R-1
Pittsburgh, PA 15206
Phone: (412) 365-4850
www.herlpitt.org/

Trace Research and Development Center
University of Wisconsin-Madison
5901 Research Park Boulevard
Madison, WI 53719-1252
Phone: (608) 262-6966
www.trace.wisc.edu/

AT and Disability Information Resources

Alliance for Technology Access
304 Southpoint Boulevard, Suite 240
Petaluma, CA 94954
Phone: (707) 778-3011
www.ataccess.org/

American Foundation for the Blind
11 Penn Plaza, Suite 300
New York, NY 10001
Phone: (800) 232-5463
www.afb.org/

American Occupational Therapy Association–Technology Special Interest Section
4720 Montgomery Lane, P.O. Box 31220
Bethesda, MD 20824
Phone: (301) 652-2682
www.aota.org/ (within the member login area)

California State University Northridge Center on Disabilities: CSUN
18111 Nordhoff Street
Northridge, CA 91330-8264
Phone: (818) 677-2578
www.csun.edu/cod/

Closing the Gap
P.O. Box 68, 526 Main Street
Henderson, MN 56044
Phone: (507) 248-3294
www.closingthegap.com/

Council for Exceptional Children
110 North Glebe Road, Suite 300
Arlington, VA 22201-5704
Phone: (888) 232-7733
www.cec.sped.org/

DO-IT: Disabilities, Opportunities, Internetworking and Technology
University of Washington, Box 355670
Seattle, WA 98195-5670
Phone: (888) 972-3648
www.washington.edu/doit/

EASI: Equal Access to Software and Information
P.O. Box 818
Lake Forest, CA 92609
Phone: (949) 916-2837
www.rit.edu/;easi/

Job Accommodation Network
West Virginia University
P.O. Box 6080
Morgantown, WV 26506
Phone: (800) 526-7234
www.jan.wvu.edu/

LD Online
c/o WETA, 2775 South Quincy Street
Arlington, VA 22206
Phone: (703) 998.2600
www.ldonline.org/

National Center for the Dissemination of Disability Resources
211 E. Seventh Street, Room 400
Austin, TX 78701-3281
Phone: (800) 266-1832
www.ncddr.org/

RESNA (Rehabilitation Engineering and Assistive Technology Society of North America)
1700 N. Moore Street, Suite 1540
Arlington, VA 22209-1903
Phone: (703) 524-6686
www.resna.org/

Richard Wanderman
LD Resources
202 Lake Road
New Preston, CT 06777
www.ldresources.com/

World Wide Web Consortium–Web Accessibility Initiative
Web Accessibility Initiative, MIT/CSAIL,
Building 32-G530, 32 Vassar Street,
Cambridge, MA 02139
www.w3.org/WAI/

CASE EXAMPLE

Using High-Technology Adaptations

Occupational Therapy Assessment Process	Clinical Reasoning Process	
	Objectives	**Examples of Therapist's Internal Dialogue**
Patient Information S.S. participated in an AT evaluation. He is a 29-year-old male, left-hand dominant, who is 4 months post TBI with injury to his right motor cortex, sustained in a bicycle collision with a car. He has worked hard in rehab and is eager to return to work as an environmental engineer, resume his active lifestyle, and return to a more balanced relationship with his wife. The following problems were identified: 1) reduced balance and endurance in walking on uneven surfaces; 2) difficulty with handwriting and keyboarding which are essential job skills in his work; 3) mild cognitive impairment in the area of short-term memory and task sequencing; and 4) desire for greater safety and independence in self maintenance activities at home.	Appreciate the context	"I think that SS has nearly maximized the benefits of in and out patient rehab that were focused on motor return. His desire to return to employment is strong and will help to focus the adaptations and AT services needed to help him return to employment and greater self-reliance. His motivation, encouragement from his wife, support from a vocational rehabilitation counselor, and history of physical fitness and active lifestyle are real facilitators to his recovery and return to occupational functioning."
	Develop intervention hypotheses	"I think that the right type of environmental supports and AT devices will enable SS to return to work. His motor limitations seem to be the greatest barrier. His cognitive limitations may be adequately addressed with AT devices. His desire to return to work makes him ideally suited to have AT evaluation and support services paid for by vocational rehabilitation. If he is open to use of adaptive devices and strategies he will be able resume many aspects of his active and independent lifestyle."
	Select an intervention approach	"I want to develop a plan that will focus on **compensation** for motor and cognitive deficits through careful use of AT devices and strategies. I expect there will be **remediation** of cognitive deficits through graded return to familiar work task. The predictable and sequential nature of computer software is often helpful. Using computer applications at work should be in long-term memory. I will work to **change the physical and social environment** around him so that he can return to a level of self-reliance. Mobility aids and grab bars may increase his safety, confidence, and endurance in home and work site locations."
	Reflect on competence	"S.S. reminds me of other young adults with TBI that I have worked with but his intelligence and desire to return to work are particularly striking. I am not sure he will accept mobility aids, so this may lead to a later decision about whether or not he wants to go out on job sites or work primarily in the office. I suspect that a return to sports and physical activities will be highly motivating so I will look up resources on adaptive sports."

Recommendations Developing a computer access strategy is a top priority for both return to work and cognitive support. First, an assessment is needed to determine best compensatory strategy for computer tasks. The amount of training needed to teach strategy and integrate it into daily computer use will be determined as part of that assessment. The OT will also visit both home and workplace to determine their physical and social characteristics with the goal of identifying barriers and recommending modifications for safety and independence. She also will set up a consultation with S.S.'s physical therapist and vocational rehabilitation (VR) counselor to discuss adaptations for increasing mobility in community settings. In collaboration with S.S. and his wife, the OT established the following long-term goals: 1) Return to productive computer use with the help of a computer access strategy; 2) Learn to use personal information management (PIM) software to help organize daily routines and serve as a memory aid; 3) Evaluate the need for modifications to the home and workplace to support safety and independence; and 4) Refer to the mobility team to explore use of a 4-wheel scooter at work and in community or jobsite locations. S.S. and his wife were pleased with this plan as it seemed clearly focused on helping their life return to a more "normal" state.	Consider the patient's appraisal of performance Consider what will occur in therapy, how often, and for how long Ascertain the patient's endorsement of plan	"It seems like S.S. and his wife are pleased with the plan because it is focused on return to work and greater safety and independence in self-maintenance activities. They are grateful for his recovery to this point. Though they expect more recovery they seem willing to accept and compensate for his physical limitations. They are both eager to return to a more balanced relationship." "Computer use is important to them both and seems like a welcome new topic apart from all of the medical interventions. Learning to use PIM software is an opportunity for new learning and the software itself will help S.S. more involved in planning his daily routine." "I think an intensive approach is warranted in order to make return-to-work happen as soon as possible. OT sessions will need to happen about 3 times a week in order to keep parallel processes working, maintain continuity in instruction, and use findings to coordinate intervention among team members." "I'm not sure that S.S. knows what he is facing but at this point he is relieved to be moving beyond medical rehab and into activities that are focus on return to function."
Summary of Short Term Goals and Progress S.S. participated in a 2-hour computer access evaluation and the findings led to an agreement on the usefulness of two strategies: using Half QWERTY ™ software for routine computer tasks and Dragon Naturally Speaking ™ (DNS) speech recognition for writing reports and long text messages. Also, he will begin to use a track ball to compensate for the reduced motor control in his left hand. Because S.S. reported in the assessment that his desk at work was located in a cube environment, it was necessary to consult with S.S.'s company before confirming the DNS recommendation. His supervisor will accommodate S.S. by moving his desk to an enclosed space and IT manager will integrate his software solutions into the networked computer system at the company. With this clear, the recommendation is to have OT training in these adaptations 3 times per week for 4 weeks with follow-up activities for practice and continued learning at home. Loaned devices will be used to start training and confirm their suitability before seeking purchase approval from his VR counselor. 1) S.S. will successfully integrate the 4-button trackball (with settings adjusted to compensate for his impaired fine motor performance skills) into file management and desktop activities with increased accuracy in pointing and clicking as shown by manipulating cards in computer solitaire.	Assess the patient's comprehension Understand what he is doing Compare actual to expected performance Know the person Appreciate the context	"I think the fact that S.S. is an engineer makes him a good problem-solver. He likes the use of technology to solve problems because it is a familiar concept and one that he uses in solving client's problems too." "Because I need to teach S.S. a series of computer access strategies I am going to teach them sequentially and create as much natural motivation to use them as possible. Mousing is essential for computer use and attaching practice to a game will increase the amount of time S.S. spends in mastery of the task." "I want him to get a strategy for writing text so we can use text to work on a software-based reminder strategy. I know that once the basic skill is developed, Half-QWERTY™ is compensatory strategy that relies on practice to develop automaticity. It will rely on his long-term memory and that should be a boost to his self-esteem too. I like how the software provides a visual aid for learning. This strategy will be most useful when he wants to sit down and type a short e-mail message or add an entry to his to-do list." "I am much more confident in the approach of teaching practical new skills as a means of restoring cognitive function. I know the research evidence just doesn't support the notion that repetitive cognitive ex-

S.S. realized immediately the value a trackball adds by separating the actions of pointing and clicking. His earlier efforts at mousing has been unsuccessful because the action of clicking the mouse button with his left index finger caused an involuntary arm movement that pushed the mouse off its target. Correcting miss-selections was annoying and time consuming. Next, he determined that placing the trackball 10-12" in from the edge of the desk gave him space to rest his left forearm and increased his motor control due to proximal stabilization. The therapist had him practice mousing skills in computer solitaire because it required him to select, move and release cards in specific places. As S.S. got comfortable with the new motor skill, the OT observed that it required extra effort for S.S. to isolate his little finger for a button click. Relocating the click and drag function to an upper button on the thumb side of the trackball increased his efficiency. This control parameter was modified in the trackball control panel and S.S. was immediately more successful in moving cards. The OT noted this change and will incorporate it into the set up for S.S.'s own trackball when it is installed. The OT sent S.S. home with a loaner trackball to practice. S.S. planned to also practice the new motor skill with a simple graphics application on his home computer.

2) S.S. will transfer previous knowledge of touch-typing to the Half-QWERTY™ application and will use his right hand alone to type with a goal of achieving 15/wpm in two weeks.

At the second computer training session, S.S. was introduced to formal instruction in half-QWERTY™ software. The OT had confirmed in a timed typing trial that S.S. was able to type 10/wpm using just his right hand. His left hand was only able to assist with holding down the left shift key or (with significant motor planning effort) in holding control+alt. S.S. reported that he had typed about 50/wpm before his injury. (Half-QWERTY™ allows the right hand to type the letter on the key located in the mirror position when the space bar is held down. Users are able to acquire keyboarding rates that are near 2-handed rates.) The OT first used the tutorial that comes with the application to teach S.S. the concept. S.S. worked to relearn the location of letters that had previously been typed by his left hand. S.S. left the session with a demo version of the software to use in the 2 days before the next visit. The goal was to return with two ~100-word paragraphs typed with his right hand alone. At the next visit, S.S. met the goal but reported that it had gone very slow. The next two sessions were spent with a "drill & practice" typing tutor intended to develop proficiency and speed. The OT reminded S.S. to pursue accuracy over speed, assuring him that new motor patterns would develop and speed would return. Each session ended with assignments and homework. On the 4th session, S.S. was able to type 17 wpm and was pleased to have more than met his goal. He reported he was expending less cognitive effort and had started pressing the correct keys without conscious thought.

ercises lead to functional changes. Working on a reminder strategy and developing new motor patterns will be good cognitive rehab for S.S."

"I know that S.S. is going to appreciate having a reminder system. His wife has been really patient and supportive but I know he want to return to a level of self-sufficiency in remembering things. Besides, in our discussion about return to work S.S. he has mentioned that he has to work very hard to remember his rehab schedule. He appears to have developed the insight that returning to work will mean remembering even more things like meeting schedules, client visits and project deliverable deadlines."

"I'm really seeing progress. S.S. has been very focused on the learning each of these adaptive computer strategies. Each time he comes in with an assignment completed, his self-confidence seems to have grown too. He has been very appreciative of my incremental approach and that makes me feel good too. His team recognizes his potential and that is a strong source of support too."

3) S.S. will learn to use Palm Desktop as a means to set up calendar, reminders, contacts, and a to-do list.
The OT knew that S.S. would rely on a small, pocket size reminder in the future. In the short term it was important to teach the concept with free desktop software. At the 5th session, the OT introduced S.S. to the software. He was taught how to set up a daily reoccurring event on his computer and add a reminder. The OT suggested that he use his new keyboarding skill to enter text and set up reminders. At first the software will be used to create a schedule for computer practice and reminders for therapy visits. S.S.'s wife, who accompanied him on that visit, agreed to install the software on their home computer and set up those 2 calendar activities. If S.S. is successful, the OT will request funding for a handheld from the VR counselor and teach the skill of syncing the device with the desktop software.

4) S.S. will successfully train DNS voice files and use a quick start table of speech commands to write 100 words per day in a daily journal about his recovery.
The OT spent the next 4 sessions introducing S.S. to DNS and developing his confidence with using his voice to write. First they created a voice file and then, using a quick-start menu, started writing text using speech and voice commands. The OT had already determined that S.S. would be most successful with DNS if new learning and the memory load were reduced. Because S.S. is able to use his right hand, he did not need to use voice commands except where convenient. Additionally, the trackball provides access to menus and the half-QWERTY™ keyboard gives convenient access to the alphabet for correcting recognition errors. The OT focused direct intervention on training recognition accuracy and building vocabulary. Focus on these skills reduces corrections and actively builds voice files. The next 2 session were focused on developing a speech pattern that emphasizes "preparing to speak" i.e., silently developing an idea before speaking it. During the 3rd session the OT arranged for S.S.'s coworker and friend, Joe, to shadow the 4th DNS training session. The OT wanted to add additional coaching resources into S.S.'s support system. Joe was selected because he already used DNS and only needed to understand more about how S.S. uses the application. By the end of the last DNS training hour, S.S. has written 200 words and had corrected another 4 recognition errors with Joe watching. S.S. has learned to pause and think before speaking and had adopted a speech pattern that was clear and deliberate when using his voice for writing. The plan was made to have a follow up session in 2 weeks. Joe agreed to alert the OT if the progress S.S. had demonstrated was not maintained.

The results of the mobility team consultation with S.S. and his wife led to a decision to rent a 4-wheeled scooter for a 2-week trial. The trial will help to determine if it increases his use of community resources (e.g., going to a community sidewalk festival) or increased S.S.'s potential to visit job sites or meet customers in community locations. This trial will occur approximately 3 weeks before S.S. is scheduled to return to work.

"I am glad that my approach to DNS for S.S. has worked so well. (There are so many ways to teach this application. If I were teaching a client with C-4 quadriplegia my approach would be entirely different.) Since he has the motor skills to use the keyboard and mouse to direct the application, we only need to work on training recognition accuracy. That makes learning for someone with short-term memory deficits just that much easier."

"Learning about Joe and his skills with DNS was a real bonus. Working on this project appears that it will give these friends a means to reconnect after S.S.'s injury. Having Joe as a back-up will help when I am not available and should help him bridge back into the workplace too. It is good to know that some of S.S.'s coworkers also use DNS. That will create a point of camaraderie as S.S. reintegrates back into the workplace."

"I am glad my PT colleague on the department AT team is willing to see the scooter as a good strategy for someone as young as S.S. Most PTs would want to work harder and longer on gait strengthening. I guess our past work together on developing compensatory strategies for clients has taught her that returning to functional environments can provide its own form of intense motivation. She agrees with me that using a scooter won't hinder S.S. in developing endurance and balance in continued outpatient PT. Progress in PT may lead to abandoning the scooter in a year. In my opinion, there may always be some occasions when S.S. is safer and more functional when riding a scooter."

"S.S. and his wife were very open to adding grab bars at home. They recognized that this will ease her mind and allow her to reduce her level of monitoring when he is in the shower or bathroom. She has already asked her dad, who has handyman skills, to install the bars I recommended in the shower and next to the commode."

"They plan to try using the loaned aluminum, folding ramp during the two-week trial. Depending on how that goes they will decide whether or not to make a permanent modification to their minivan. At least the style of ramp that is suggested can be added or removed without permanently defacing the vehicle."

At the end of the 2-week trial, the team met again and agreed that a scooter greatly increased S.S.'s range and frequency of community mobility while increasing his independence because of reduced risk of falls. S.S. is not giving up on his desire to walk but is willing to speed his community and employment re-entry through scooter use. He is willing to accept that even if he walks in most settings, there will still be situations in which fatigue or uneven ground will limit his participation. The VR counselor is willing to purchase the scooter.

With the information from this mobility consult, the OT visited S.S.'s home and workplace and made the following recommendations.

- Shower has a built in bench seat. Install grab bars in the shower to increase safety in enter, exiting, and recovering balance.
- Reinforce use of stool in kitchen for food preparation tasks.
- Electricity in the garage will allow S.S. to store his scooter there. The garage door opener will facilitate entry and exit.
- Adding a power assist ramp to their minivan will allow SS or his wife to drive the scooter up and into the van independently if the scooter is needed at work or for leisure activities.
- At work, handicapped parking and accessible bathrooms are available.
- Recommend the addition of automatic door openers to the office building to facilitate entry by S.S. when in his scooter or by other customers with mobility limitation. (Paid for with help of a ADA-based tax benefit for the small business owner.)

"I do think they will decide on the power-assisted ramp because it will give SS independence with the scooter—which is the purpose of using the scooter. If my experience is any indicator, I think they will quickly discover that unfolding one of those ramps is much more work than it looks like it is."

Next Steps

The final three computer access sessions will be reserved for follow up. They will be needed for setting up the new software on the workplace computer and for checking on successful integration of S.S.'s new software skills into the workplace environment.

The VR counselor will also be checking on S.S. and has agreed to alert the OT if follow-up is needed. S.S. has agreed to schedule a follow up visit in 3 months to discuss the need for modifications to computer access strategies.

Mobility strategies will also be discussed in 3 months to determine if scooter use is supporting community involvement and access to jobsites for S.S.

Anticipate present and future patient concerns

"As we conclude this intense 5-6 weeks of intervention, I am sure that there will be some unexpected 'wrinkles'... there always are. With these 3 approved remaining visits, I know I will be able to provide the follow-up that will insure success."

Analyze patient's comprehension

"This case has been one that really demonstrated the value of an AT team. S.S. must really be a valuable employee because his company really went out of the way to accommodate his needs and reintegrate him into the office."

Decide if he or she should continue or discontinue therapy and/or return in the future

"I look forward to seeing S.S. in 3 months. The knowledge of his success with the adaptations that were recommended will reinforce my confidence as a practitioner and give the information I need to build my AT practice repertoire. I will decide at that time whether any short-term intervention is needed or whether I will encourage S.S. to contact the VR counselor if his needs change."

Clinical Evidence Table 19-1
Best Evidence for Occupational Therapy Practice Regarding Assistive Technology

Intervention	Description of Intervention Tested	Participants	Dosage	Type of Best Evidence and Level of Evidence	Benefit	Statistical Probability and Effect Size of Outcome	Reference
Use of automatic speech recognition (ASR) as a means of computer access	Collected performance data via interview and task measures from experienced ASR users on: (1) computer use, (2) type of ASR, (3) reasons for ASR use, and (4) measures of performance on 6 operationalized ASR tasks (e.g., file management, transcription rate, etc.). For 18 users with choice: comparison between ASR and alternative method.	24 users of ASR with > 6 months experience; 5 participants could use ASR only, and 19 used ASR plus keyboard.	Exploration of the ASR experience for variety of experienced users. Results varied widely due to (1) limitations of the technology and (2) limitations in user's ability to maximize effective use of ASR.	One group, descriptive statistics. IIIC1a	Reasons ASR chosen: (1) reduce pain or fatigue, (2) ease of use, and (3) few alternatives. Of participants with choice, 48% used ASR for ≤25% of computer tasks and 37% used ASR for >50% of computer tasks. 63% reported overall satisfaction with ASR. Text entry rate ranged from 3 to 32 wpm, with accuracy of 72–94%. Best users had best repair strategies. Typists with speed >15 wpm got less benefit from ASR.	Those with higher recognition accuracy had higher satisfaction scores, $p = 0.027$ For non-text entry tasks, ASR plus keyboard was 61% slower, $p < 0.05$. For study participants, more agreed with: (1) I can enter text more quickly with ASR than with any other method, (2) ASR is easy to use, and (3) I can enter text more accurately ($p > 0.05$).	Koester, 2004

SUMMARY REVIEW QUESTIONS

1. Describe the main points of the HAAT model.
2. Define high and low technology.
3. List the steps in an AT assessment.
4. What are the various roles the occupational therapist can play on an AT team?
5. List several input and output devices, other than a keyboard and standard mouse, and describe who might use them.
6. Explain the main methods that EADL use to transmit signals from the input device to the control box.
7. Where could consumers look for funding for AT devices?

References

Angelo, J. (1997). *Assistive technology for rehabilitation therapists.* Philadelphia, F. A. Davis, Inc.

Angelo, J. (2000). Factors affecting single switch efficiency in assistive technology. *Journal of Rehabilitation Research and Development, 37,* 591-598.

Anson, D. (1997). *Alternative computer access: A guide to selection.* Philadelphia: F. A. Davis, Inc.

Bain, B. K., & Leger, D. (1997). *Assistive technology: An interdisciplinary approach.* New York: Churchill Livingstone.

Ballandin, S., Baker, B., & Hill, K. (1999). *Vocabulary: More than a word list.* Paper presented at the 14th Annual CSUN Technology and Disability, Los Angeles, CA, March 15-20, 1999.

Beukelman, D. R., & Mirenda, P. (1992). *Augmentative and alternative communication.* Baltimore: Paul H. Brookes Publishing Company, Inc.

Buning, M. E., Angelo, J. A., & Schmeler, M. R. (2001). Occupational performance and the transition to powered mobility: A pilot study. *American Journal of Occupational Therapy, 55,* 339-344.

Colarusso, R. P., & Hammill, D. (2002). *Motor-free visual perception test* (3rd ed.). Novato, CA: Academic Therapy Publications.

Cook, A. M., & Hussey, S. M. (1995). *Assistive technology: Principles and practice.* St. Louis: Mosby.

Cook, A. M., & Hussey, S. M. (2002). *Assistive technology: Principles and practice* (2nd ed.). St. Louis: Mosby.

Gardiner, M. F. (1993). *Test of visual-motor skills.* Novato, CA: Academic Therapy Publications.

Internal Revenue Service. (2005). Publication 502: Medical and Dental Expenses. Retrieved August 10, 2006 from http://www.irs.gov/publications/p502/index.html.

Jaffe, E. G., & Epstein, C. F. (1992). *Occupational therapy consultation: Theories, principles and practice.* St. Louis: Mosby-Year Book, Inc.

Jeserich, M. (2003). Assistive technology and taxes: Not a perfect fit. *AT Journal 70,* available at http://www.infinitec.org/work/tools/atdeductions.htm.

Kielhofner, G. (1997). *Conceptual foundations of occupational therapy* (2nd ed.). Philadelphia: F. A. Davis Company.

Lange, M. L. (2002). The future of electronic aids to daily living. *American Journal of Occupational Therapy, 56,* 107-109.

Mendelson, S. B. (1996). *Tax options and strategies for people with disabilities* (2nd ed.). New York: Demos Vermande Publications.

Pollock, N. (1993). Client-centered assessment. *American Journal of Occupational Therapy, 47,* 298-301.

Raeder, W. M. (2005). The case for braille. Retrieved August 3, 2005 from http://www.nbp.org/ic/nbp/braille/case_for_braille.html.

Schmitt, D. (1992). *Hierarchy of access.* Paper presented at Closing the Gap, Minneapolis, MN, October, 1992.

Social Security Administration. (2004). Working while disabled: A guide to plans for achieving self-support. Available at http://www.ssa.gov/pubs/11017.html.

The Center for Universal Design. (1997). What is universal design? The principles of universal design. Retrieved October 3, 2005 from http://www.design.ncsu.cud/aboutud/aboutud.htm

United States Congress. (1988). Technology-related assistance for individuals with disabilities act of 1988. Available at http://www.resna.org/taproject/library/laws/techact94.htm.

United States Congress. (2004). Public law 108-364: Assistive technology act of 2004 (Vol. 118 Stat. 1707, pp. 1707-1737): Federal Register. Washington, DC: United States Congress.

United States Society for Augmentative and Alternative Communication [USSAAC]. (2005). What is AAC intervention and what should it include? Retrieved August 1, 2005 from http://www.ussaac.org/.

Verbrugge, L.M., Rennert, C., Maddans, J.H. (1997). The great efficacy of personal and equipment assistance in reducing disability. *American Journal of Public Health, 97,* 384-392.

CHAPTER 20

Physical Agent Modalities

Alfred G. Bracciano

LEARNING OBJECTIVES

After studying this chapter, the student will be able to do the following:

1. Describe the phases of wound healing and types of pain.
2. Identify the professional and regulatory issues related to physical agents.
3. Define and discuss superficial and deep thermal agents.
4. List the precautions and contraindications in the use of physical agents.
5. Describe the clinical application of electrotherapeutic modalities.
6. Describe how superficial EMG biofeedback can be used for muscle reeducation.

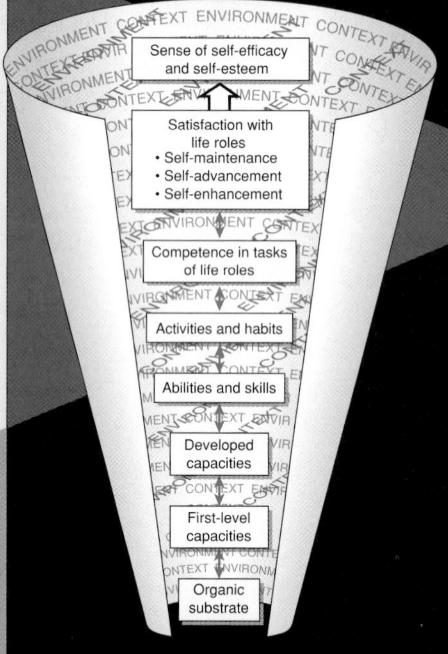

Glossary

Acute pain—Rapid onset of pain relative to a biological function associated with tissue trauma.

Biofeedback—Procedures or techniques that are used to provide an individual with an auditory or visual cue or "feedback" to learn and gain volitional control over a physiological response.

Chronic pain—Recurring or persistent pain, often poorly localized; may be associated with anguish, apprehension, depression, or hopelessness.

Conduction—Exchange of energy (for example heat or cold) when two surfaces are in direct contact with each other.

Convection—Conveyance of heat by the movement of heated particles, such as air or water molecules, across the body part being treated, creating temperature variations.

Cryotherapy—Application of a superficial cold agent to part of the body. Often used for pain relief, reducing edema, and decreasing inflammation following trauma.

Deep thermal agent—Therapeutic application of any modality to the skin and underlying soft tissue structures to cause a temperature elevation in tissue up to a depth of 5 cm.

Dosage—Amount and intensity of heat delivered to selected tissue causing temperature variations; classified as mild, moderate, or vigorous.

Electrotherapeutic agents—Therapeutic application of an electrical current to selected tissue or monitoring of endogenous electrical activity in tissue. Includes biofeedback, neuromuscular electrical stimulation, functional electrical stimulation, transcutaneous electrical nerve stimulation, electrical stimulation for tissue repair, high-voltage galvanic stimulation, and iontophoresis.

Impedance—Resistance of tissue to the passage of electrical current or ultrasound waves.

Inflammation—Cellular and vascular response in affected tissue that follows injury or abnormal stimulation; the initial phase of the healing process; the body's attempt to rid itself of bacteria, foreign matter, and dead tissue and to decrease blood loss.

Pelvic floor—Refers to the pelvic diaphragm, the sphincter mechanism of the lower urinary tract, the upper and lower vaginal supports, and the internal and external anal sphincters.

Physical agent modality—Treatment technique that uses heat, light, sound, cold, electricity, or mechanical devices.

Proliferation—Formation of new collagen tissue and epithelium in the intermediate stage of wound healing.

Referred pain—Pain occurring in an area different from the source of injury or disease.

Remodeling—Third phase of wound healing; dynamic process with maturation of new collagen tissue within the wound.

Superficial thermal agents—Therapeutic application of any modality that raises the temperature of skin and superficial subcutaneous tissue to a depth of 1 cm.

Ultrasound—Deep-heat modality; application of sound waves to soft tissue, causing thermal and non-thermal effects; sound having a frequency greater than 20,000 Hz.

The profession of occupational therapy has a long and colorful history, adapting and changing in response to internal and external issues and challenges. The use of preparatory methods, such as physical agents and **biofeedback**, as a part of clinical practice has become more widely accepted within the profession, with ever-increasing numbers of states adopting regulatory and practice guidelines. This transition has come about in part because of changes in health care delivery, expanded practice specialization, and service delivery in hand therapy and orthopedics. The use of physical agents and biofeedback as a part of clinical practice has been motivated by the need to facilitate outcomes and healing in our patients as quickly and cost effectively as possible. As increasing numbers of occupational therapists use these preparatory methods to facilitate occupational function in their patients, the need for training and education to understand how and why these agents work is crucial.

Physical agent modalities are interventions or technologies that produce a response in soft tissue through the use of light, water, temperature, sound, electricity, or mechanical devices. There are four primary classifications of physical agents: **superficial thermal agents**, **deep thermal agents**, **electrotherapeutic agents**, and mechanical devices. Superficial thermal agents include hydrotherapy/whirlpool, **cryotherapy**, hot packs, paraffin, water, and infrared heating. Deep thermal agents include therapeutic **ultrasound** and phonophoresis. Electrotherapeutic agents include biofeedback, neuromuscular electrical stimulation, functional electrical stimulation, transcutaneous electrical nerve stimulation, electrical stimulation for tissue repair, high-voltage galvanic stimulation, and iontophoresis. Mechanical devices may include vasopneumatic devices and continuous passive motion (CPM) devices (American Occupational Therapy Association [AOTA], 2003).

AOTA (2003) supports the use of physical agents as an adjunctive method of treatment that can be used preparatory to intervention with the intent to enhance engagement in occupation and performance. Physical agents are used to remediate capacities that allow reacquisition of abilities that may enhance participation in activities of daily living and role performance. Use of physical agents without application to functional outcome or occupational performance is not considered occupational therapy treatment. Although other health professions may also use physical agents as part of their treatment protocols, the occupational therapy profession's distinct approach focuses on occupational performance issues at the level of the person and environment.

This chapter provides a broad overview of the physical agents commonly used by occupational therapists. It is important to recognize that physical agents are an additional "tool" that occupational therapists can use as part of their repertoire of interventions preparatory to occupation. Physical agents are most often used as part of the treatment protocol to address pain, edema, muscle weakness or guarding, and loss of function or sensation. This chapter discusses pain theories and wound healing. This information, often overlooked by therapists, is vital to determine which type of agent would be most efficacious and at which point in treatment and healing it should be applied.

This chapter reviews superficial thermal agents, such as hydrotherapy, hot packs, and paraffin; cryotherapy; and deep thermal agents, such as ultrasound, along with their biophysiological effects. A discussion of the principles of electrotherapy and clinical application of neuromuscular electrical stimulation and transcutaneous electrical stimulation are also presented. Surface EMG and biofeedback to decrease pain and improve motor control will also be reviewed. It is beyond the scope of this chapter to present all of the information needed to use physical agents safely and effectively. The intent of this chapter is to provide a basic description of physical agents and their potential for incorporation into clinical practice to facilitate occupational function and performance. The reader is encouraged to continue learning through review of other texts and materials and through further academic preparation and education.

COMPETENCY AND REGULATORY ISSUES

AOTA (2003) revised its position paper on physical agents to ensure that the profession remained current with advances in technology, training, and practice. AOTA (2003) contends that physical agent modalities are considered "preparatory and adjunctive methods" that can only be used or applied by occupational therapists and occupational therapy assistants who have documented evidence through training and education and possess the theoretical background and technical skills necessary for the safe and competent use of physical agents as part of an occupational therapy intervention plan. Skill and training in these interventions can be accomplished through in-service training or professional education, such as continuing education or accredited higher education programs and courses. It is important to note that the training and education should be verifiable and the therapist must demonstrate competence in **physical agent modality** use. AOTA (2003) states that course work should include foundational education and training in biological and physical sciences as well as modality-specific content in the areas of the biophysiological, neurophysiological, and electrophysiological adaptations that occur because of the application of a selected modality. It is also vital that any education in physical agent modalities include indications, precautions, and contraindications to ensure the safe and efficacious application of the modalities as part of the treatment process. Therapists must be critical consumers of continuing education course work, which may be provided by a manufacturer or sales representative during in-service training. (See Resources 20-1 for a list of manufacturers and vendors.) It is important that education and training in physical agents provide the therapist with more depth and breadth of knowledge than the mere technical skill of application. Without a thorough grounding in the fundamentals of physical agents, occupational therapists become mere technicians, applying physical agents incorrectly, at the wrong time in the treatment process, or without regard to facilitating occupational function.

Occupational therapists who use physical agents as part of their clinical practice also need to know local, state, and institutional rules and guidelines, which may restrict or limit the use of physical agents. Many states have adopted new policies and regulations related to the use of physical agents by occupational therapists. California, Montana, Tennessee, New Hampshire, Nebraska, and other states identify specific training and competency standards that are regulated by licensing boards. It is illegal in these states and others to apply physical agent modalities without meeting the licensing criteria and guidelines outlined in their respective laws. Some state guidelines may also regulate or limit specific applications by occupational therapy assistants. It is the responsibility of the occupational therapist to stay up to date concerning any local or state regulatory issues related to practice in their state. All occupational therapists who anticipate using these agents should contact their respective state regulatory board to obtain the most current information and should be able to document and defend their training and expertise to their colleagues and patients in meeting any competency requirements.

RESOURCE 20-1

Physical Agent Modalities and Biofeedback

Amrex Electrotherapy Equipment
641 E. Walnut Street
Carson, CA 90746
Phone: (800) 248-4031

Anodyne Therapy LLC
13570 Wright Circle
Tampa, FL 33626
Phone: (800) 521-6664

Chattanooga Group, Inc.
4717 Adams Road,
P.O. Box 489
Hixson, TN 37343-4001
Phone: (800) 592-7329

Comfort Technologies, Inc.
P.O. Box 7
Pittstown, NJ 08867
Phone: (800) 321-STIM (7846)

Dynatronic
7030 Park Centre Drive
Salt Lake City, UT 84121-6618
Phone: (800) 874-6251

Electromedical Products Intl.
2201 Garrett Morris Parkway
Mineral Wells, TX 76067
Phone: (800) 367-7246

Empi, Inc.
1275 Grey Fox Road
St. Paul, MN 55112
Phone: (800) 328-2536

Erchonia Medical Lasers
4751 E. Indigo Street
Mesa, AZ 85205
Phone: (888) 242-0571

Kinetic Muscles, Inc.
2103 E. Cedar Street, #3
Tempe, AZ 85281
Phone: (480) 557-0448

MedX Health Corp.
3350 Ridgeway Drive, Unit 3
Mississauga, Ontario,
Canada L5L5Z9
Phone: (888) 363-3112

Metler Electronics
1333 S. Claudina Street
Anaheim, CA 92805-6235
Phone: (800) 854-9305

Microlight Laser
2401 Colorado Avenue,
Suite 160 B
Santa Monica, CA 90404
Phone: (866) 575-2737

Neoforma
www.neoforma.com

North Coast Medical
187 Stauffer Boulevard
San Jose, CA 95125-1042
Phone: (800) 821-9319

Sammons Preston
P.O. Box 5071
Bolingbrook, IL 60440-5071
Phone: (800) 323-5547

Smith and Nephew, Inc.
One Quality Drive,
P.O. Box 1005
Germantown, WI 53022-8205
Phone: (800) 558-8633

WOUND HEALING AND PAIN

Physical agents have been defined as treatment techniques that use heat, light, sound, cold, electricity, or mechanical devices. They include electrical therapeutic modalities that induce heat or electrical current beneath the skin to obtain a specific biophysiological effect. In addition to course work related to the properties of light, water, temperature, sound, and electricity, occupational therapists using physical agents should have a thorough understanding of the wound healing process, classification of pain, and physiological effects of these agents so as to apply them in a timely, appropriate, and safe manner.

Normal Wound Healing

An understanding of wound healing and an appreciation for the sequence of events that follows an injury are necessary to determine the appropriate intervention to facilitate healing. Tissue and wound healing is a complex process affected by both physical and psychological components. In the healthy individual, the body's attempt to heal itself in response to an injury is well ordered and sequenced (Fig. 20-1, A–D). The stages of healing and repair may overlap, but they consist of three primary phases: inflammatory, proliferative, and remodeling.

Phase I: Inflammatory

The inflammatory phase is the initial response to an injury; it is both vascular and cellular. The inflammatory response is the body's attempt to rid itself of bacteria, foreign matter, and dead tissue and to decrease blood loss. The inflammatory response may be associated with changes in skin color (red, blue, or purple), temperature (heat), turgor (swelling), sensation (pain), and loss of function. Acute **inflammation** usually lasts for 24–48 hours and is completed within 7 days, although a subacute phase may last for 2 weeks.

Phase II: Proliferative

The proliferative phase of recovery is also known as the fibroplastic, granulation, or epithelialization phase. At this point, the injured area is filled with new connective tissue, and the wound is covered with new epithelium (**proliferation**). The primary components of this stage of healing are granulation, epithelialization, and wound contraction. Wound contraction, which is caused by the forming of red granulation tissue, shrinks the affected area. It begins approximately 5 days after the injury. It is complete approximately 2–3 weeks after injury. Fibroblasts are responsible for fibroplasia and collagen synthesis. Cross-linkages of the collagen tissue provide the wound with its tensile strength and durability, with the fibers becoming more organized (Davidson, 1998). This phase overlaps with the inflammatory phase, continuing until the wound is healed. The proliferative phase is complete when epithelialization has covered the wound, a collagen layer has formed, and initial remodeling is achieved.

Phase III: Remodeling

Remodeling is also known as the maturation phase. This stage begins about 2 weeks after injury and may continue for a year or more. Remodeling is characterized by a

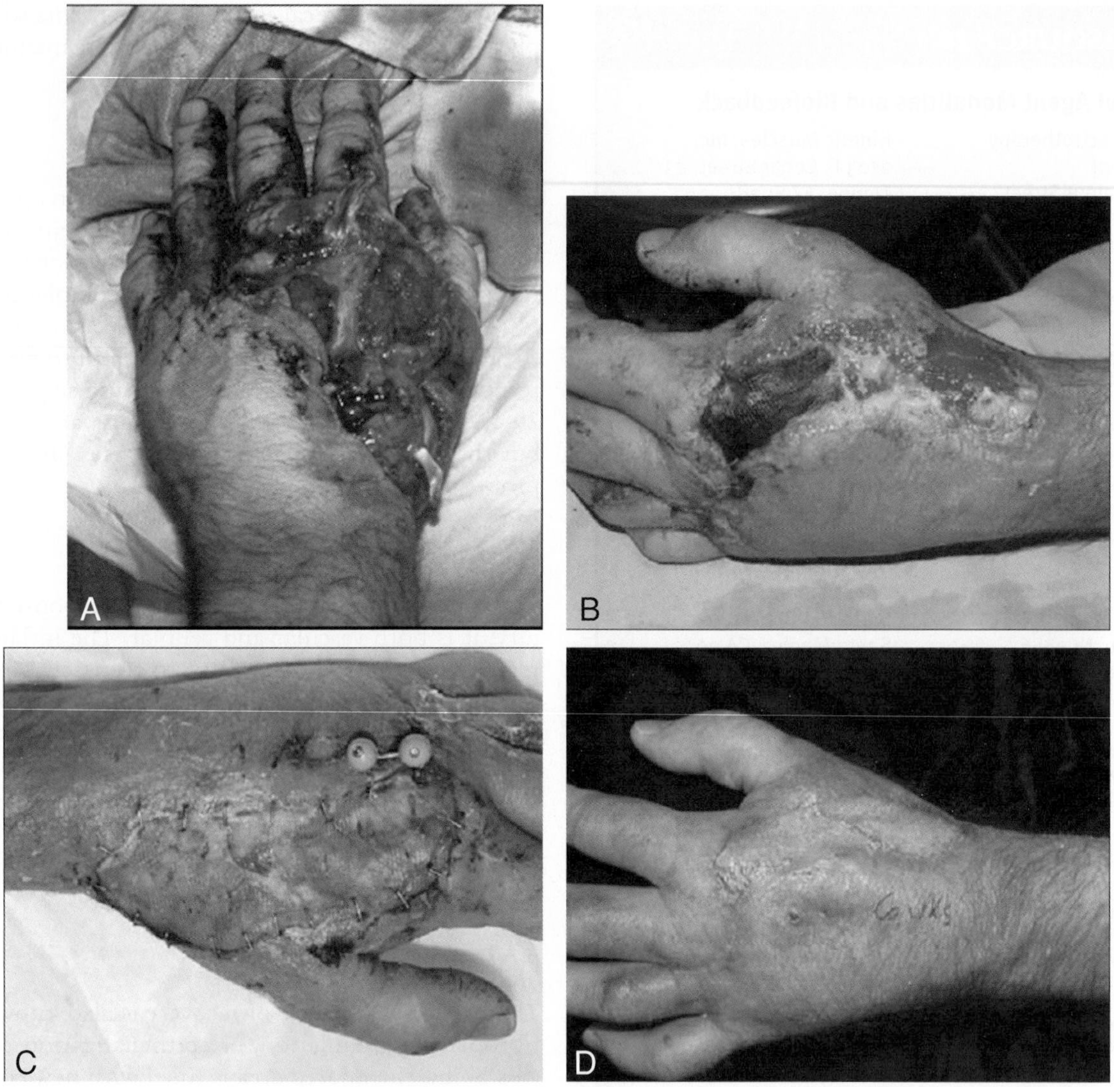

Figure 20-1 **A.** Initial injury. Trauma to right upper extremity hand secondary to motor vehicle accident. Patient's arm went out the window and scraped along the pavement after his vehicle rolled over. Note extensive tissue loss and extensor tendon lacerations. Patient also suffered multiple fractures and radial nerve laceration. **B.** Patient's hand ready for skin grafting. Note tissue colors indicating various stages of healing. "Black" area indicates necrotic tissue, which must be debrided for skin grafting. **C.** Status/post percutaneous pinning and skin graft on dorsal surface of the hand. Note pins in place and staples securing skin graft. **D.** Patient's hand 6 weeks after grafting and occupational therapy intervention. Note pink viable tissue. Some edema remains in the hand. Percutaneous pins have been removed, and fractures are solid.

balance of collagen synthesis and collagen lysis, formation, and breakdown. During this time, the scar becomes more elastic, smoother, and stronger. If collagen synthesis exceeds collagen lysis, hypertrophic scarring or keloids may occur. As remodeling continues, the collagen fibers assume the characteristics of the tissue they are replacing. Internal and external factors, such as presence of foreign objects, infection, nutrition, and medications may slow or affect the healing process; they are most significant in elderly people (Mulder, Brazinsky, & Seeley, 1995). Physical agents applied at the appropriate sequence and phase during wound healing can accelerate healing and resolution of the injury. Appropriate selection of the type and depth of penetration of the thermal agent may significantly affect the healing process at a cellular level.

Wound Assessment

When treating open wounds, therapists should obtain baseline information on the wound's appearance prior to treatment. Documentation should include the anatomical location and area of wound, the size and shape of the wound, the color of any dead or necrotic tissue, a description of the exudate (purulent, with pus or a milky look; serous [clean, yellowish]; or serosanguinous [pinkish]), any granulation tissue or epithelialization, and a description of the surrounding intact skin (erythema, heat, pain, or edema).

Pain Perception

Pain, which may limit participation in occupational tasks, is reported by many of the patients seen by occupational therapists. By using physical agent technologies to treat pain, we may be able to help patients more fully assume their primary roles and activities, improving outcomes and quality of life. Understanding the pain experience informs clinical reasoning and influences our selection of physical agents.

Pain occurs when there is a noxious event, such as injury or inflammation, to an area of the body causing an excitation of the nociceptors in somatic or visceral tissue (Hakim, 1995). Nociceptors (sensory receptors specific to pain), which have variable thresholds, identify potential or actual tissue damage and respond to mechanical distortion, variations in the chemical components, and thermal changes in the tissue fluid. There are several ascending tracts that transmit pain signals to the brain.

Pain is characterized as being acute or chronic and can be referred, that is, felt in an area of the body other than the site of injury.

- **Acute pain** has a biological function; it lasts from seconds to days, acting as a warning that injury has occurred or that something is wrong. Acute pain is closely associated with tissue damage and nociception occurring with a rapid onset. Physical agents are indicated as a part of the treatment approach in patients with acute pain.
- **Chronic pain** recurs or persists for a long time. It may be associated with anguish, apprehension, depression, or hopelessness. Chronic pain is often poorly localized, without an underlying cause being fully identifiable. Chronic pain pervades the individual's life. Chronic pain affects an individual's occupational functioning, affecting society, the economy, employment, and health care systems. Physical agents are usually ineffective in consistently relieving chronic pain.
- **Referred pain** occurs at an area different from the source of the injury or disease, that is, not where the nociceptors were stimulated. These irritable areas, sometimes known as trigger points, can be located through palpation and are electrically active and facilitate current flow into the tissue. Trigger points can also be identified by using TENS to locate and stimulate these areas.

Physical agents such as heat, sound, compression, cold, or electricity may all reduce the effects of pain and can influence healing in soft tissue injuries. Selection of the correct intervention or physical agent is based on a thorough evaluation of the patient and on the diagnosis, treatment goals, clinical experience of the therapist, and the goals of the patient.

INCORPORATING PHYSICAL AGENTS INTO A TYPICAL OCCUPATIONAL THERAPY TREATMENT

Physical agents are used as a precursor to functional activity to facilitate occupational performance. The therapist determines which physical agents will help achieve the patient's goals. For example, a patient with rheumatoid arthritis may have pain and limited movement. Paraffin to both hands and wrists may alleviate the patient's pain and stiffness prior to training with adaptive equipment for self-care activities.

Before administration of any modality, the therapist questions the patient as to any untoward negative response to physical agents applied in previous treatment and reviews whether the patient has any contraindications for the selected agent. Prior to administration of the physical agent, the therapist informs the patient as to the procedure, expected outcome, and subjective sensation that the patient may feel during the treatment. Skin integrity is always evaluated prior to administration of physical agents and immediately following the intervention. Documentation should be clear and concise, stating the modality applied, parameters or settings, sequence in the course of treatment, and patient's response (Procedures for Practice 20-1). Therapists also assess the effectiveness of the modality on a session-by-session basis. If the modality fails to provide the desired outcome or if the patient has discomfort or negative results, the modality should be discontinued.

PROCEDURES FOR PRACTICE 20-1

Documenting Physical Agent Interventions

Documentation of physical agent interventions should include the following:

- Physical agent applied and treatment parameters
- Site of application or placement
- Treatment duration
- Physiological responses elicited from treatment
- Subjective responses from the patient, such as tolerance, reaction, and clinical effectiveness

SUPERFICIAL THERMAL AGENTS

A superficial thermal agent is any modality applied to the skin that can increase or decrease skin and superficial subcutaneous tissue temperature. Thermotherapy is the term used to describe the therapeutic application of heat. The objectives of heating agents are to decrease pain and stiffness, improve range of motion and tendon excursion, improve viscosity of synovia, and promote healing and relaxation. Conditions that may benefit from heat include muscle spasm, subcutaneous adhesion, sympathetic nervous system disorders, contractures, neuromas, chronic arthritis, trauma, wounds, and subacute and chronic inflammation. Superficial heat has a therapeutic effect at depths of up to 1 cm (Kaul, 1994). If a depth greater than 1 cm is desired, ultrasound should be considered.

Treatment Planning

In planning treatment that involves heat, one typically considers general and specific **dosage** guidelines, primary effects, and modality selection.

Dosage Guidelines

Thermotherapy is used when an increase in tissue temperature is the intended goal of treatment. General dosage guidelines provide a starting point for selection of an agent and for application parameters. Dosage refers to the amount of heat applied to the tissue, which then elevates the tissue temperature. When the temperature of soft tissue is increased between the range of 102 and 113°F, it can have a positive therapeutic effect. If the soft tissue is heated to a temperature less than 102°F, cell metabolism may not be stimulated adequately enough to elicit a therapeutic response. If tissue is heated too vigorously, to a temperature greater than 113°F, catabolism and cell death may occur. Physiological response in thermal applications is dependent on the extent of the temperature elevation within the tissue. Elevation of tissue temperature in turn depends on the rate the temperature is applied to the tissue, the duration of the application, and the volume or area of tissue exposed to the heat. Consideration of dosage intensity guides application based on specific characteristics of the patient.

The dosage of a thermotherapy can be described as mild to vigorous. Application of a mild dose of heat implies a minimal elevation in tissue temperature. The primary benefits of a mild application of heat is related to the somatosensation of warmth. Many conservative home remedies provide this mild dosage. A moderate dose causes an increase in tissue temperature of approximately 6°F and a moderate increase in blood flow. A vigorous dose implies a marked increase in blood flow with substantial tissue temperature elevation (up to 14°F). Safety Note 20-1 lists precautions and contraindications of thermotherapy. One should be especially vigilant with moderate and vigorous doses of heat and monitor skin color and respiratory status.

SAFETY NOTE 20-1

Superficial Thermal Agents

Precautions

- Edema
- Diminished sensation
- Compromised circulation
- Use of anti-coagulant medications

Contraindications

- Impaired sensation due to skin graft or scar
- Tumors, cancer
- Advanced cardiac disease (body inadequately dissipates heat)
- Acute inflammation, acute edema
- Deep-vein thrombophlebitis
- Pregnancy (systemic effects of circulating blood on fetus are unclear)
- Bleeding tendencies
- Infection
- Primary repair of tendon or ligament
- Semicoma or impaired cognitive status
- Rheumatoid arthritis: vigorous dosages of heat can exacerbate joint inflammation

Adapted from Schmidt, 1979.

Primary Effects of Thermotherapy

The four primary effects of thermotherapy are analgesic, vascular, metabolic, and connective tissue responses. Each has different dosage guidelines.

- The analgesic effect influences pain symptoms. Heat acts selectively on free nerve endings, tissues, and peripheral nerve fibers, which directly or indirectly reduces pain and elevates pain tolerance (Behrens & Michlovitz, 2005). A mild to vigorous dose is required to obtain an analgesic effect.
- Vascular effects aid in pain relief and in decreasing muscle spasm. At 6°F of tissue temperature elevation, substances such as histamines are released in the bloodstream, resulting in vasodilation. This increased blood flow reduces ischemia, muscle spindle activity, and tonic muscle contractions, decreasing pain. Moderate dosage is needed to obtain these effects.

- Thermal agents affect the components of inflammation and healing due to changes in the rate of circulation and chemical reactions. Metabolic effects influence tissue repair and aid pain relief. Increases in blood flow and oxygen within the tissues bring a greater number of antibodies, leukocytes, nutrients, and enzymes to injured tissues. Pain is reduced by the removal of byproducts of the inflammatory process. Nutrition is enhanced at the cellular level and repair occurs. A mild to vigorous dosage of heat is needed to facilitate the metabolic effects, depending on the acuity of the wound or soft tissue condition.
- Collagen is the primary component protein of skin, tendon, bone cartilage, and connective tissue. Those tissues containing collagen can become shortened due to immobilization or limited range of motion as a result of weakness, injury, or pain. Improvement in the properties of collagen and extensibility of tissues occurs when heat is combined with passive or active mobilization and/or engagement in occupation. This connective tissue response occurs during an 8- to 10-minute window after the application of heat (Norkin & Levangie, 1992). Reduced joint stiffness and increased range of motion also occur. A moderate to vigorous dose is needed to achieve these benefits.

Selection of Superficial Thermal Agents

Regardless of the mechanism of heat application to the tissue (paraffin, hot pack, etc.), the biophysiological effects will be the same. There are three primary mechanisms of heat transfer within the body: **conduction**, **convection**, and radiation. Conduction occurs when there is direct contact between tissue and the heat or cold source. Convection occurs when particles or molecules, such as air or water, move across the body part thereby creating a temperature variation. Radiation occurs when there is a transfer of heat from a warmer source to a cooler source, such as through air in application of infrared lamps.

The choice of modality depends on the treatment objective, the location and surface area of the involved structure, and the desired dosage and tissue temperature. Other considerations include whether moist or dry heat is desired, the positioning of the extremity in a non-dependent or intermittently dependent position, and whether active or passive participation by the patient is desired (Earley, 1999). The acuity or chronicity of the patient's condition is also an important factor. Injuries in the inflammatory or acute phase (24–48 hours) should be treated with cryotherapy, not heat. Wounds in the **remodeling** stage of recovery would be treated with higher dosages of heat to facilitate the remodeling process of collagen alignment and differentiation.

Clinical Use of Thermotherapy

As previously mentioned, superficial heat is primarily transmitted through conduction and convection. Hydrotherapy and fluidotherapy are examples of convection agents, whereas hot packs and paraffin are categorized as conduction agents.

Whirlpool Baths and Hydrotherapy

The whirlpool bath is effective with open wounds, status post fractures, inflammatory conditions, peripheral vascular disease, and peripheral nerve injuries. An advantage for whirlpool use is that the therapist can see and have immediate access to the body part being treated, and the client can actively move the extremity. Water temperature can be set to the desired temperature (100–104°F), and the degree of agitation of the water can be controlled to act as a soft tissue massage or resistance for exercise or to cleanse and debride a wound. With any open wounds or lesions, proper disinfecting of the whirlpool bath is necessary.

Fluidotherapy

Fluidotherapy uses fine particles of ground corn husks suspended in a hot air stream to heat the extremity (Borrell et al., 1980). Temperature is controlled by a thermostat, with most conditions requiring a temperature between 105 and 118°F. Temperature settings depend on the dosage of heat needed and the area of the extremity being treated. The force of the air and particles circulating within the machine can be graded via the blower speed, facilitating mobilization and desensitization through its impact on nerve conduction (Kelly et al., 2005). The advantage of fluidotherapy is the ease of implementation and the therapist's access to the client's extremity while in the unit, allowing for passive or active assistive range of motion or manual therapy.

Hot Packs

Hot packs, or hydrocollator packs, are forms of moist heat that come in a variety of sizes. They heat large areas of the body and adequately cover contoured areas of the body, such as the shoulder. The temperature of the hot pack is typically between 104°F and 113°F. Hot packs are stored in a thermostatically controlled container of hot water kept at approximately 158–167°F. Hot packs are generally easy to use and require minimal maintenance. It is important to ensure that a dry padding is used between the hot pack and the skin to avoid burns, even though it cools as the treatment progresses. Continued use of the hot pack covers between patients during the day will decrease their effectiveness as an insulator and may cause burns. The hot pack should be wrapped in six to eight layers of dry towels or two to three layers of hot pack covers. More layers should be used if the towels or pack covers become worn or damp. Hot packs help to reduce pain and muscle spasms and to improve connective tissue extensibility. The extremity can be placed in a positional sustained stretch of the tissue being treated to facilitate extensibility.

Paraffin

Paraffin is used to provide a high degree of localized heat to smaller joints. The paraffin is mixed with mineral oil in a 6:1 or 7:1 ratio to effectively lower the melting point of the paraffin to between 113 and 122°F. The paraffin is kept in a thermostatically controlled unit, and the temperature of the paraffin should be checked before it is applied to a patient. Paraffin is primarily used to decrease stiffness, improve range of motion, and relieve pain. Healed amputations, arthritis, strains, and sprains are a few conditions that benefit from paraffin. Paraffin allows for an even distribution of heat to the treatment surface, reducing the viscosity of the synovia and, hence, decreasing stiffness and pain associated with arthritis.

The wrap or glove technique is the most popular method of application. **The therapist should always check the temperature of the paraffin before use to ensure a safe temperature and avoid burns.** The client immerses the extremity in the bath and withdraws it to allow the paraffin to harden. This gloving process is repeated approximately 10 times, depending on the client's tolerance to heat. The extremity is then wrapped in a plastic bag followed by a towel to retain the heat and is left on for 20 minutes (Fig. 20-2). At the end of treatment, the paraffin is removed and discarded.

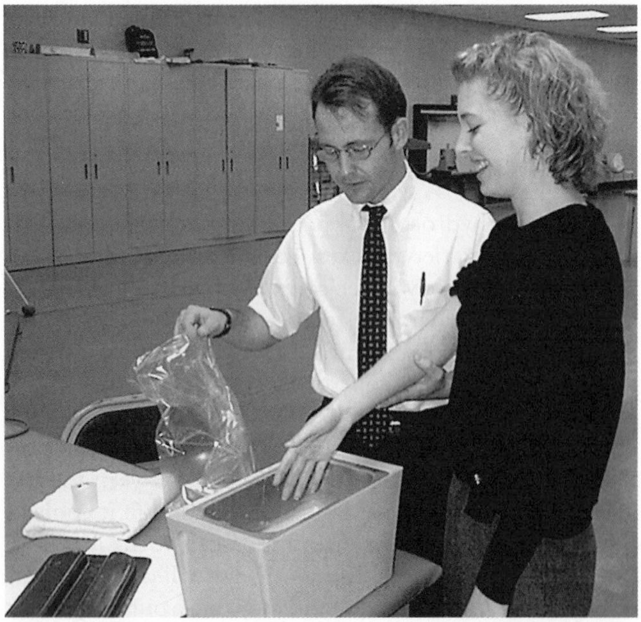

Figure 20-2 Application of paraffin to increase pain-free AROM of the interphalangeal joints. The extremity will be wrapped in a plastic bag and then a towel.

Passive stretching of joints can be accomplished with an elastic wrap or Coban tape, which is secured prior to the dipping. This form of treatment facilitates tissue extensibility and can maximize the benefits of mobilizing and remodeling connective tissue.

CRYOTHERAPY

Cryotherapy is the application of a cold agent to relieve pain and to reduce edema and inflammation following trauma. Cryotherapy involves the application of any substance to the body that results in withdrawal of heat from the body, lowering the temperature of the tissue. Tissue temperature change and biophysical effects of cooling are related to the time of exposure, the method used to cool the tissue, the conductivity of the tissue, and the size or area being treated. Care must be used when determining the length of exposure to the cold agent because changes in skin temperature occur quickly and tissue may be damaged before the desired biophysical effects are achieved.

Purpose and Effects

The clinical use of cold is based on physiological changes resulting from tissue temperature reduction. Cold is used in the management of acute trauma because it affects arteriolar vasoconstriction, reducing bleeding; decreases metabolism and vasoactive agents such as histamine, thereby reducing inflammation and swelling; and elevates the pain threshold. In most acute traumas, cold is used with compression and elevation.

There are four primary methods for administering cold treatment: cold packs, ice cubes, cold baths, and controlled cold-compression units. Application of cold provides an anesthetic or numbing effect, and the patient may initially report a cold, aching, or burning sensation. As with any thermal agent, monitoring of the skin is essential to avoid damage to the tissue, and caution is advised for patients with decreased sensation or mentation.

Indications and Precautions

Cryotherapy is easy to apply and is indicated for a number of treatment conditions. The most common use for cryotherapy is in the treatment of acute injury and inflammation (Fig. 20-3). Other conditions and indications for the use of cold include edema, exercise-induced muscle soreness (combined with compression, exercise, and massage), arthritic exacerbation, acute bursitis or tendinitis, spasticity, and acute or chronic pain secondary to muscle spasm.

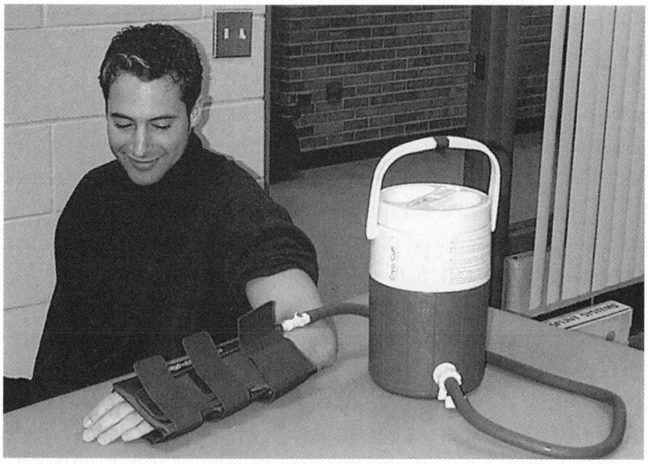

Figure 20-3 Application of cryotherapy for distal extremity edema and inflammation.

The physiological effects of cold can last for several hours. Rewarming of the tissue takes approximately 20 minutes. Care should always be used when applying cold, and the skin condition should be monitored to avoid frostbite and tissue damage. Safety Note 20-2 lists contraindications to cryotherapy.

THERAPEUTIC ULTRASOUND

Therapeutic ultrasound is classified as a deep-heat modality and works via acoustic energy that is inaudible to the human ear. Ultrasound is acoustic energy that is used in medicine for diagnosis and tissue destruction and in rehabilitation to help restore and heal soft tissues. The ultrasound beam in therapeutic ultrasound itself does not transmit heat. Heat accumulates in the tissue because of the conversion of energy absorbed from the sound wave in continuous-mode ultrasound. Therapeutic ultrasound has two primary effects on tissue: thermal and non-thermal (or mechanical). Thermal effects refer to those biophysiological changes produced by cellular heating, while non-thermal, or mechanical, effects refers to biophysiological changes produced by the cellular effects of cavitation, microstreaming, or acoustic streaming. Both can be used to facilitate healing and ultimately improve occupational function (Bracciano, 1999; Bracciano, 2000).

Physical Principles

Standard ultrasound units consist of a power supply, oscillator circuit, transformer, coaxial cable transducer, and ultrasound applicator. The generator uses alternating current as a power source, converting electrical energy into ultrasonic energy. Inside the applicator, a crystal contracts or expands in response to alternating current (Fig. 20-4). The vibration of the crystal generates the sound waves, which are transmitted to a small volume of tissue, causing the tissue molecules to vibrate. Ultrasound travels poorly through air, so a lubricant is used to maintain contact between the transducer and the tissue, ensuring that the energy is dispersed into the tissue (Fig. 20-5).

When the sound waves are generated rapidly and dispersed into the tissue, the molecules in the waves' path are pushed back and forth by the alternating phases of successive waves until the wave runs out of energy. This type of wave, moving in one direction and compressing and decompressing the molecules in its way, is termed a *longitudinal wave.* When the wave encounters bone, the sound energy is transferred along the periosteum and is then deflected up at a right angle causing a *shear wave.* Shear waves occur when the sound energy strikes a solid

SAFETY NOTE 20-2

Cryotherapy

Avoid cryotherapy with patients who exhibit the following:

- Peripheral vascular disease or any circulatory compromised area
- Cold sensitivity, Raynaud's phenomenon
- Multiple myeloma, leukemia, systemic lupus (cryoglobinemia is a disorder of abnormal protein formation that can lead to ischemia in these individuals)
- Cold urticaria/intolerance; can occur with rheumatic diseases or after crush injuries and amputations

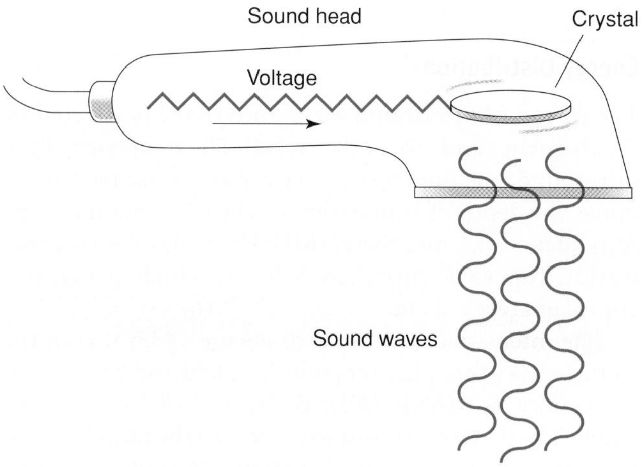

Figure 20-4 Production of ultrasound.

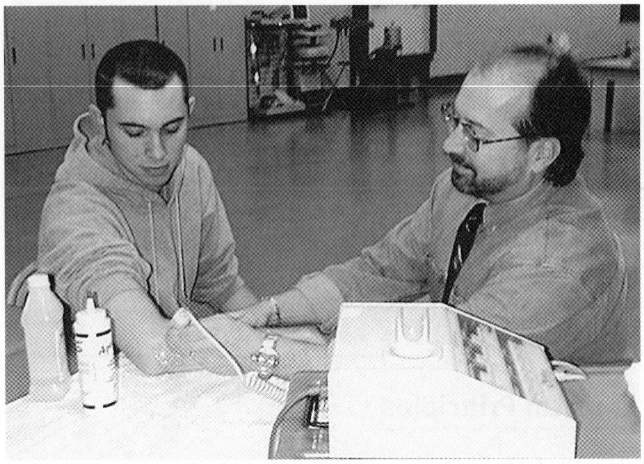

Figure 20-5 Application of non-thermal ultrasound for acute elbow lateral epicondylitis.

substance. This may cause heating of the outer covering of the bone but is negligible in terms of tissue temperature elevation (Bracciano, 1999; Bracciano, 2000; Cameron, 2003). A *standing wave* occurs when the sound head isn't moved adequately enough, and the incoming sound waves encounter the reflected sound waves moving back up toward the surface, creating hot spots and potential overheating of tissue.

Each tissue in the body transmits and absorbs ultrasound energy according to its unique properties, known as absorption coefficients. The rate at which the sound wave travels depends on the density of the molecules of the tissue, with body fluids such as blood and water having the lowest **impedance** (or resistance to ultrasound waves) and lowest acoustic absorption coefficient. Bone possesses the highest impedance and absorption coefficient, making it a good absorber of ultrasound energy (Kimura et al., 1988) along with other protein-dense structures, such as scars, joint capsules, ligaments, and tendons.

Energy Distribution

The spread of ultrasound waves into tissue is affected by the frequency and size of the crystal. The frequency of the ultrasound (the number of wave cycles per second) determines the depth of penetration of the ultrasound energy. A frequency of 1 megahertz (MHz) provides deeper penetration (up to 5 cm) than 3 MHz, which penetrates approximately 1–2 cm.

The intensity of the beam of energy varies within the sound wave; this phenomenon is called the beam nonuniformity ratio (BNR) (Allen & Batye, 1978; Kimura et al., 1988). The BNR of a transducer refers to the ratio between its spatial peak intensity and spatial average intensity. These higher areas of intensity are in part responsible for hot spots, which can be prevented by moving the sound head during treatment. Smaller ratios refer to a more uniform ultrasound beam (Hekkenberg, Reibold, & Zeqiri, 1994). The intensity of the beam of energy is a significant factor in determining tissue response. In general, there is greater tissue temperature elevation with higher intensities. Intensity is documented as watts per square centimeter (W/cm^2).

The duty cycle determines the overall amount of acoustic energy a patient receives and plays a role in determining tissue response (Fig. 20-6). The duty cycle is a percentage or ratio of time that the ultrasound energy is actually being introduced into the body. A 50% duty cycle provides twice as much acoustic energy as a 25% duty cycle because the on-time is twice as long (Kollmann et al., 2005). Consider a hose with a squeeze nozzle as analogous to the ultrasound transducer. If the handle is squeezed and held, water is released in a constant stream from the hose, which is comparable to a constant flow of sound energy. If the handle is squeezed and released rapidly, the water is turned on and off, or pulsed. The same concept holds for ultrasound. When the sound wave is on 100%, the sound wave and energy are constant. When the sound energy is turned on and off rapidly, the sound wave is pulsed and is described in terms of a ratio of the cycle. Whether to use continuous or pulsed ultrasound depends on the pathology, stage of wound healing, and amount of area being treated (Bracciano, 2000; Fyfe & Parnell, 1982).

Effects on Tissue: Thermal Versus Non-Thermal Ultrasound

As previously mentioned, ultrasound has thermal and non-thermal effects on tissue. In the thermal mode, ul-

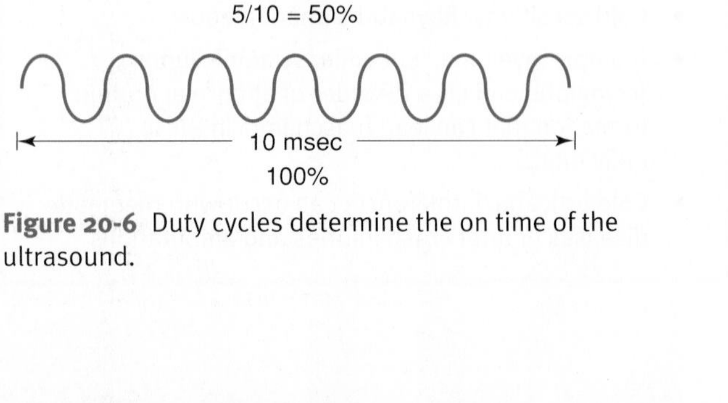

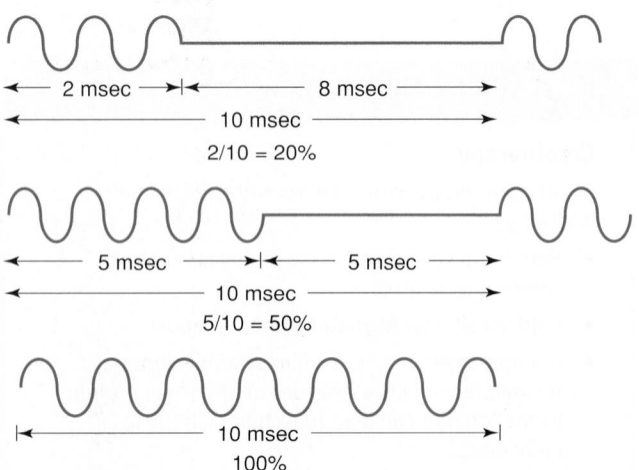

Figure 20-6 Duty cycles determine the on time of the ultrasound.

trasound is a deep-heating agent capable of elevating tissue temperatures to a depth of 5 cm. Thermal effects are typically achieved with continuous sound waves (as in a 100% duty cycle). Non-thermal ultrasound exerts mechanical effects at the cellular level but does not elevate tissue temperature. It typically involves delivering the ultrasound at a 20% duty cycle and provides secondary cellular effects, such as increased cellular permeability and diffusion. Clinicians may use ultrasound to achieve thermal or non-thermal effects and must select the effect considering a patient's given problem and the therapeutic effect that is desired.

A number of physiological effects occur with thermal ultrasound. They include increased metabolic rates, increased blood flow and tissue permeability, increased viscoelasticity of connective tissue, elevation of pain thresholds, and increased enzymatic activity, which may stimulate the immune system. Thermal ultrasound may increase joint range of motion, facilitate tissue healing, decrease muscle spasm and pain, and decrease chronic inflammatory processes (Enwemeka, 1989; Fabrizio, Schmidt, & Clemente, 1996; Gan et al., 1995; Hsieh, 2005).

The heating effects of ultrasound can be decreased by pulsing the sound waves or by decreasing the intensity or strength of the sound wave. Pulsing the ultrasound refers to modification of the ultrasound wave. Rather than the sound waves being produced continuously, the sound wave is intermittently turned on and off (pulsed), leading to a non-thermal effect.

Non-thermal ultrasound causes increased cellular permeability and diffusion and a variety of second-order effects that facilitate tissue repair (Dyson & Pond, 1970; Dyson & Suckling, 1978).

The effects of non-thermal ultrasound on tissue healing occur with short treatment duration along with lower intensities (0.1 and 0.2 W/cm^2 pulsed at 20% duty cycle). Treatment sessions should be repeated every 24–48 hours to facilitate tissue repair.

Non-thermal effects of pulsed ultrasound occur at the cell membrane due to stable cavitation, acoustic streaming, and micromassage (Apfel, 1989). Acoustic streaming occurs with the unidirectional movement of the body fluids that cause currents, which exert force and structural changes in the cell membrane along with increased permeability. Second-order effects of non-thermal ultrasound are due to the destabilization of the cellular membrane. Secondary effects of pulsed ultrasound may include an increase in phagocytic activity; increase in the number and motility of fibroblasts, resulting in enhanced protein synthesis; increased granular tissue; and improved angiogenesis, facilitating wound contraction. Low-intensity pulsed ultrasound may also accelerate fracture healing in tibial and Colles fractures (Doyle, 2004; Lehmann & Guy, 1971).

Clinical Use of Ultrasound

A thorough evaluation of the patient is necessary to identify problems and to set treatment goals prior to using ultrasound. It is essential to determine the location, stage of healing, depth, and anatomical location of the injury and the area and type of tissue to be treated. Superficial conditions, for example epicondylitis, are best treated using a frequency of 3 MHz. If a thermal effect is not needed, such as in a subacute condition or superficial pathology, low intensities can be used with a pulsed sound wave. Acute conditions should be treated for shorter periods than chronic conditions, and smaller areas of tissue require less time than larger areas (Bracciano, 1999).

Acute conditions are best treated with very low-intensity dosages (0.1 to 0.5 W/cm^2); the patient is unlikely to feel any warmth at this low level. Subacute conditions can be treated using a low-intensity dosage (0.5 to 1 W/cm^2); chronic conditions and those requiring a thermal effect require a setting between 1 and 2 W/cm^2. Patients may report some degree of warmth during the treatment but should not report any pain, discomfort, or burning. If these symptoms occur, the intensity should be reduced, the sound head should be moved more quickly, or ultrasound gel should be added if an inadequate amount is causing an uncomfortable tingling, vibration, or burning sensation.

Ultrasound may also be used before functional activity for prophylactic pain-relieving effects. Thermal ultrasound (100% duty cycle, high intensities) can be used to heat tissue and increase its length. Combining thermal ultrasound with positional stretch, splinting, functional activities, or manual therapy may be effective in stretching the heated tissue through a pain-free range of motion following application of ultrasound.

Phonophoresis

Phonophoresis is the use of ultrasound to facilitate the delivery of topically applied drugs or medication to selected tissue. Although it is frequently used, there are questions as to the effectiveness of phonophoresis because of variability in outcomes associated with inconsistent treatment parameters, such as intensity of sound waves and transmission characteristics of the conducting gel. Many hydrocortisone creams commonly used in the clinic (1% or 10% hydrocortisone in a thick, white cream base) do not transmit ultrasound, and this method of delivery is ineffective (Henley, 1991; Masse, 1996). Dexamethasone sodium phosphate mixed with a sonic gel transmits ultrasound effectively and can be formulated by a pharmacist. Following phonophoresis, a dressing can be used to seal the area and prevent moisture from escaping. Intensities of 1.5 W/cm^2 are effective for both the thermal and non-thermal effects of ultrasound as part of phonophoresis. A low intensity (0.5 W/cm^2) may be more effective for treating acute injuries (Bracciano, 2000).

Precautions for Use of Ultrasound

Patients should be monitored during ultrasound, and any pain or discomfort may indicate that the intensity is too high or there is an inadequate amount of gel. Ultrasound should never be applied over the eye, the heart, the pregnant uterus, or the testes. Sonification to malignant tissue should also be avoided. Caution must be used when applying ultrasound over areas of decreased circulation and avoided over areas of thrombophlebitis. High intensities and application over the growth plates in children should also be avoided (Sicard-Rosenbaum, Lord, & Danoff, 1995). When using ultrasound as a thermal agent, one must follow general contraindications and precautions for any thermal modality. Safety Note 20-3 lists precautions and contraindications for ultrasound.

SAFETY NOTE 20-3

Ultrasound

Precautions

- Unhealed fracture sites
- Primary repair of a tendon or ligament
- Marked demineralization/osteoporosis
- Plastic and metal implants

Contraindications

- Suspected deep-vein thrombophlebitis
- Bleeding and edema; areas with tendency to hemorrhage
- Where sensation is reduced or if a person cannot report heat sensations accurately
- In the very old and very young because of compromised body temperature regulation
- Skin or lymphatic cancers; tumors or malignancies
- Over a cardiac pacemaker or surrounding adjacent tissue
- Pregnancy
- Infected areas
- Epiphyses of growing bone
- In conjunction with radium or radioactive isotopes treatment for cancer within 6 months
- Over the heart, eyes, or testes
- Over carotid sinus and cervical ganglion
- Over the spinal column or where there is inadequate protection over the spinal cord, such as after laminectomy

LOW-LEVEL LASER THERAPY

Low-level laser therapy (LLLT) is also known as "cold laser" because it will not increase the thermal temperature of the tissue. Laser is an acronym for light amplification by stimulated emission of radiation (LASER). Low-level laser, although gaining popularity with many clinicians, has been generating an increase in research regarding its overall effectiveness and mechanism of action. Many of the early studies evaluating the use of lasers supported their use with promotion of tissue repair in experimental animals and with human wounds and ulcers, although other studies were less conclusive (Conlan, Rapley, & Cobb, 1996; Reddy, Stehno-Bittel, & Enwemeka, 1998).

Light is another form of radiant energy with wavelengths that vary between 100 and 10,000 nm within the electromagnetic spectrum. Different wavelengths of light have been shown to promote healing of skin, muscle, nerve, tendon, cartilage, bone, and dental and periodontal tissues. These tissues respond to appropriate doses of light, which may vary within 600- to 1000-nm wavelengths. This low-energy light appears to facilitate the stages of healing by accelerating inflammation, promoting fibroblast proliferation, and enhancing revascularization of wounds and bone repair and remodeling (Abergel et al., 1987; Whelen et al., 2001). The mechanism of action appears to be through facilitation of the ATP cycle, the form of energy that cells use to facilitate metabolic processes, and through histochemical changes used to repair and regenerate cell and tissue components (Gum et al., 1997; Reddy, Gum, Stehno-Bittel, & Enwemeka, 1998; Reddy, Stehno-Bittel, & Enwemeka, 1999).

LLLT is a relatively recent addition to the therapeutic tools for occupational therapy and rehabilitation, although it has been used in Europe for the past decade. There are three primary types of laser in use by therapists: HeNE (helium neon), GaAs (gallium arsenide), and gallium-aluminum-arsenide (GaAlAs) lasers. The laser "beam" is produced by electrical or mechanical stimulus to the type of matter in the specific laser. When the stimulation is applied to the matter, there is a change in the position of the electrons of an atom, causing a release of photons. Photons are the energy component of light and are absorbed as energy when they collide with other atoms, which make them "unstable." Within the laser itself, the molecules being stimulated are in an enclosed chamber that has a reflective surface. As the photons continue to collide with other atoms and thus releasing more photons, a chain reaction occurs, causing emission of radiation. As the energy is released from the chamber and directed toward tissue or an object, the laser is emitted as a coherent beam of light. The light wave streams in the same parallel direction and phase (coherence) and possesses the other unique characteristics of monochromaticity (a single wavelength) and collimation (a defined, concentrated beam).

It has been proposed that the mechanism of action of LLLT is due to biostimulation of the tissue. This stimulation is dependent on the dosage of the energy, which can either facilitate or inhibit the biochemical, physiologic, and proliferative activities of cells. The mechanism of action of LLLT appears to be at the cellular level, with the biophysiological effect related to the wavelength, depth of penetration, and dosage. There is an expanding body of evidence that indicates low-energy light may increase the healing process. LLLT may accelerate the inflammatory process, promote fibroplasias (Akai et al., 1997), enhance chondroplasia (Akai et al., 1997), upregulate the synthesis of type I and type III procollagen mRNA (Saperia, Glassberg, & Lyons, 1986), facilitate bone repair and remodeling and revascularization of wounds, and accelerate tissue repair (Houghton et al., 1999). The variable in most studies and the question that needs to be answered relates to determining the appropriate energy density that is needed to facilitate the healing response (Enwemeka et al., 2004).

LLLT uses low-power laser. Thus, it is essentially safe, unless the laser beam is directed toward the eye, where it may cause damage to the retina or cornea. Care should also be used over areas with active bleeding or hemorrhage, over cancerous tissue, during pregnancy, or in individuals with photosensitive skin. Research appears to support the use of LLLT to facilitate tissue healing through the stimulation of collagen formation and vasodilation, to modulate pain through decreased nerve conduction velocity, and to influence the histochemical changes that occur during inflammation (Akai et al.,1997; Chow, 2002; Halevy et al., 1997; Houghton et al., 1999; Ozawa et al., 1998). As research continues in the area of laser therapy, greater acceptance and use of the modality will likely occur.

ELECTROTHERAPY

Electrotherapy has been used since the time of the early Romans. The growth of electrical stimulation in recent years is due to the research of Melzak and Wall (1965) and their gate theory of pain and to advances in technology. Electrotherapy is the application of electrical stimuli to accomplish any of a variety of therapeutic purposes and goals. Frequently used applications include neuromuscular electrical stimulation (NMES), transcutaneous electric nerve stimulation (TENS), electrical stimulation for tissue repair (ESTR), functional electrical stimulation (FES), electrical muscle stimulation (EMS), and iontophoresis. Surface electromyography (sEMG) biofeedback monitors the level of electrical activity in muscles and is often paired with neuromuscular electrical stimulation. (Clinical application of commonly used modalities will be discussed later.)

- NMES uses pulsating, alternating current to activate muscles through stimulation of intact peripheral nerves to cause a motor response. Stimulation of the nerve is used to decrease muscle spasm, for muscle strengthening, and for its effect on muscle pumping, which can reduce edema. NMES stimulation of innervated muscle can also be used for muscle reeducation and to prevent atrophy.
- FES is neuromuscular electrical stimulation to activate targeted muscle groups for orthotic substitution or to facilitate performance of functional activities or movements (Fig. 20-7). FES is often used with individuals who have shoulder subluxation or foot drop after a stroke.
- TENS describes the wide variety of stimulators used for pain control. TENS uses surface electrodes with the goal of sensory analgesia rather than a motor response.
- EMS is electrical stimulation of denervated muscle to facilitate viability and to prevent atrophy, degeneration, and fibrosis of the fibers. EMS may facilitate nerve regeneration and muscle reinnervation while decreasing muscle atrophy.
- Iontophoresis is the use of low-voltage direct current to ionize topically applied medication into the tissue. Iontophoresis is often used in the treatment of inflammatory conditions or for scar formation and management.
- ESTR, also known as high-voltage galvanic stimulation (HVGS) or HVPC, has been used for wound healing. There is a "current of injury" that occurs when the skin is disrupted by injury. Electrical stimulation has been correlated with accelerated healing by stimulating cell processes during the phases of tissue repair, by

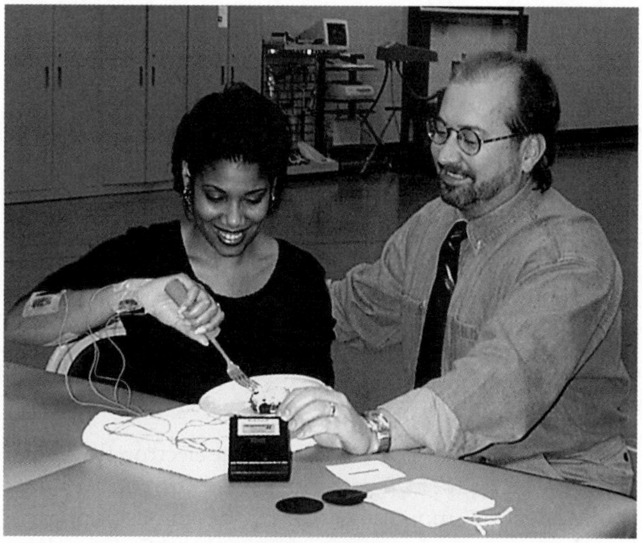

Figure 20-7 FES for the extrinsic flexor and extensor muscle groups to facilitate grasp for self-feeding.

inhibiting bacterial growth, and by increasing oxygen perfusion through localized vasodilation. Due to its complexity for entry-level clinicians, it is not reviewed in this chapter.

Principles of Electricity

To use electrotherapy in occupational therapy practice, clinicians need working knowledge of the principles of current, duration, rise and decay time, frequency, duty cycle, and current modulation and ramp time.

Current

Electric current is the movement of ions or electrons, which are charged particles, from one point to another to equalize the charge. Current, measured in amperes, occurs when there is an imbalance in the number of electrons in two distinct locations. Voltage is the potential or electromotive force that drives the current and is measured in volts. Current flows from an area of high electron concentration (cathode, or negative pole) to an area of less concentration (anode, or positive pole). Opposition or resistance to current flow is measured in ohms. Ohm's law states that voltage is proportional to both current (I) and resistance (R), such that $V = I \times R$. For clinical application, three specific forms of currents, direct current (DC), alternating current (AC), and pulsatile current, are used (Fig. 20-8).

Direct Current

Direct current (DC) is unidirectional, with the electrons moving continuously in one direction and the electrodes maintaining their polarity. DC flow, characterized by the square wave, can cause chemical reactions in the body and facilitate the ionization of medication through the skin.

Alternating Current

Alternating current (AC) is characterized by periodic changes in the direction of the current flow. The current is uninterrupted and bidirectional, without any true positive or negative pole. Household electricity uses AC. Hertz is the number of times the current reverses direction in 1 second (cycles per second).

Pulsatile Current

Pulsed current is the term used when the electron flow is periodically interrupted. These interrupted currents can flow in one direction (monophasic) or two directions (biphasic). In pulsed current, the current is interrupted for very short periods of milliseconds or microseconds. Most stimulators can be classified under one of three wave forms: monophasic, biphasic, or polyphasic.

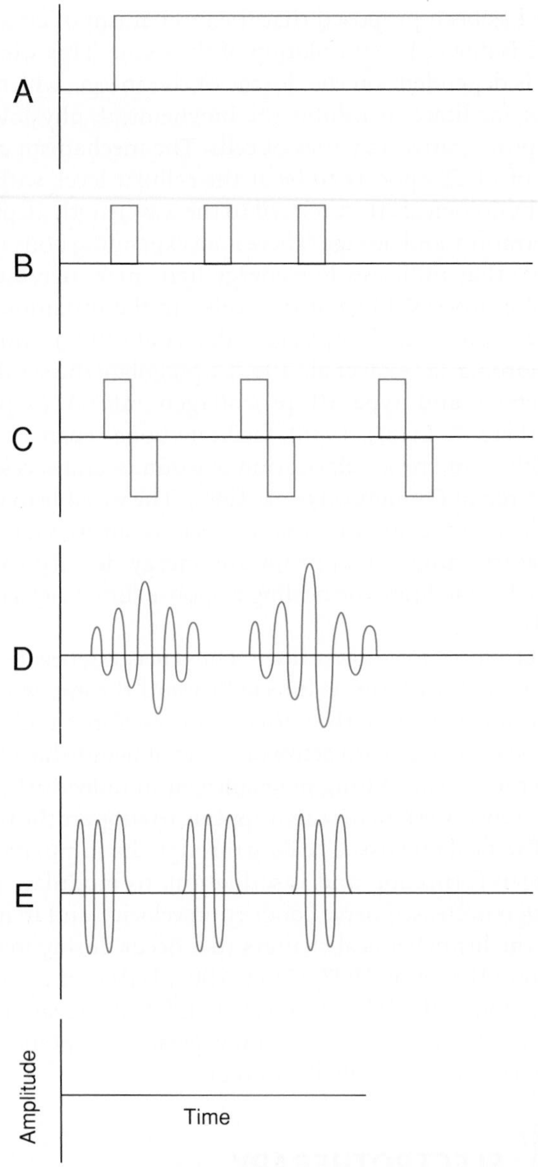

Figure 20-8 Commonly used electrotherapeutic current wave forms. **A.** Direct current. **B.** Monophasic pulsed. **C.** Biphasic pulsed. **D.** Interferential beats. **E.** Russian bursts.

- Monophasic wave forms have a single phase to each pulse, with the current flow being unidirectional and either negative or positive. A monophasic pulse has a pulse duration averaging 40–60 msec.
- Biphasic currents have two opposing phases in a single pulse, with the lead phase of the pulse above the baseline and the final phase below. Biphasic pulses may be symmetrical or asymmetrical and have a phase duration between 25 and 250 sec.

- Polyphasic waveforms consist of a burst of three or more phases, a series of pulses delivered as a single charge. This current is also known as interferential or Russian current. There have been many claims as to the uniqueness of this type of current, although there are no confirmed physiological advantages to this type of waveform.

Duration

For monophasic current, phase and pulse duration are synonymous and refer to the length of time between the beginning and end of one phase of the pulse. For biphasic currents, the pulse duration is equal to the total of the two phase durations, including the intra-pulse interval. As phase duration increases, comfort levels decrease. Shorter pulse and duration result in better conductivity of the current with less impedance (Currier, 1993).

Rise Time and Decay Time

Rise time is the amount of time needed for the amplitude to go from 0 volts to peak. The rate of rise is related to the ability of the amplitude to excite nervous tissue. The depth of current penetration is related to the peak amplitude. With biological tissue, the higher the voltage applied, the larger the current that will be passed through the tissue.

Frequency

The number of pulses or wave forms repeated at regular intervals is the pulse or stimulus frequency. The pulse frequency consists of the number of pulses or cycles per second delivered to the body. The rate of successive electrical stimuli is adjustable and may range from 1–120 stimuli per second (1–120 Hz). Frequency may also be labeled as the pulse rate.

Duty Cycle

Duty cycle is the amount of time between the stimulation period and the rest period. That is, it is the ratio of the time the current is on to the time the current is off. The duty cycle may be expressed as a percentage or a ratio. For example, a treatment protocol in which electrical stimuli are delivered for 10 seconds followed by a 50-second off period is expressed as a 1:5 duty cycle. Duty cycle is important in determining muscle fatigue. As the patient's condition improves, the duty cycle can be gradually increased.

Current Modulation and Ramp Time

Changes to the current or to the pulse characteristics are referred to as modulation. Current can be modulated by modifying the frequency, amplitude, or duration. Ramping is a change of the pulse intensity or duration of the pulse. Ramp time is the time required for successive current stimuli to reach the desired amplitude. Ramp-down, the gradual decrease of the intensity, describes the movement of the peak amplitude back to zero.

Physiology of Nerve and Muscle Excitation

In addition to a working knowledge of electrical principles, clinicians using electrotherapy must understand the physiology of nerve and muscle excitation. The application of electrical current causes physiological changes at both a local and cellular level; these changes can occur segmentally or systemically. The application of electrical current modifies the body's physiological response and physiochemical effects (Hess, Howard, & Attignger, 2000).

Human tissue is either excitable or non-excitable. Excitable tissues, such as nerves and muscles, can initiate and propagate an action potential if the stimulation parameters are sufficient. Stimuli must be sufficiently intense and long lasting to cause the ions to shift across the resting membrane and depolarize the cell. Depolarization of the neural or muscle cell occurs quickly, and the sudden alteration in the cell membrane's electrical potential is known as an action potential. Action potentials are an all-or-none occurrence and, once started, are carried along the cell membrane. Following depolarization, if a membrane becomes hyperpolarized, it may be unable to discharge an action potential, and accommodation occurs.

Propagation

Tissues with high water content, such as muscle and nerve, transmit electricity better than those with lower water content, such as bone, fascia, and adipose tissue. The diameter of the fiber and degree of myelination are also factors affecting the rate of propagation of action potentials. Conduction is faster in myelinated fibers and in large-diameter fibers, which offer less resistance to the conduction of current. More intense stimuli, which are achieved by increasing the stimulus duration and amplitude, are needed to depolarize smaller diameter nerves and denervated muscle membrane (Mehreteab & Weisberg, 1994). Large-diameter nerves are associated with non-noxious cutaneous sensory modalities and motor nerves linked to large motor units. The small-diameter cutaneous sensory nerves are associated with pain pathways. As the amplitude and pulse duration increase, so do the number of nerve fibers recruited. The strength–duration curve in Figure 20-9 describes the relationship between the amplitude and duration of the stimulus needed to depolarize the membranes of various types of nerves to achieve a response (Mehreteab & Weisberg, 1994).

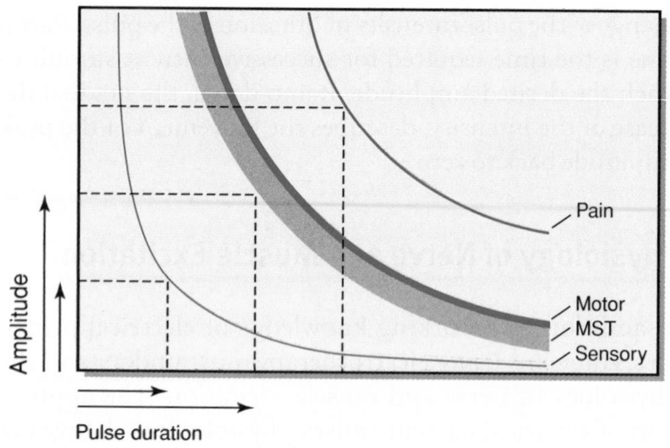

Figure 20-9 Strength–duration curve of an electrical stimulus. MST, maximum sensory threshold.

When the cell membrane or tissue receives an unchanging stimulus over time, the cell membrane begins to adapt to the stimulus and requires higher levels of stimulation to trigger an action potential; this is termed accommodation. Following stimulation and generation of an action potential in a nerve cell membrane, the membrane needs a short period to recover its excitability. This recovery time is known as the absolute refractory period.

Electrically Stimulated Movement

The diameter of the nerve, depth of the nerve, and duration of the pulse affect a nerve's response to electrical stimulation. Sensory nerves are stimulated first, followed by motor nerves, then pain fibers (Fig. 20-9), and finally muscle fibers. Although pain fibers are superficial in relation to motor nerves, they also have a smaller diameter and a greater resistance to electrical current flow. Motor nerves reach threshold, and if there is sufficient intensity, contraction of all muscle fibers attached to that nerve (motor unit) occurs. Stimulation of the skin surface causes an activation of sensory receptors before motor or pain nerves (Baker, Bowman, & McNeal, 1988). Smaller motor units are recruited at varying and slowly increasing frequencies, followed by larger motor units. If the stimulus frequency is sufficient, the muscle twitch contractions become fused in synchronous rapid succession, and the contraction becomes tetanic, leading to a complete contraction of the muscle and movement at the specified joint.

In a voluntary contraction, smaller motor units are recruited first, followed by the larger motor units as contraction strength increases. This gradual, asynchronous sequence allows for fine motor control, with larger fibers recruited as increased strength or speed is needed. This type of recruitment allows smooth, controlled movement. In electrically stimulated movement patterns, however, the reverse occurs, with larger motor units recruited first in a synchronous pattern. This causes electrically stimulated muscle to fatigue more rapidly and limits the finely controlled quality of functional movement.

Treatment Planning Specific to Electrotherapy

Before incorporating electrotherapy into treatment, clinicians make decisions about the type of electrical stimulator to use and placement and size of electrodes.

Parameters of Electrical Stimulation Devices

The many stimulators available are offered with a variety of poorly supported claims by both manufacturers and clinicians. Research has been equivocal, and the clinician must critically evaluate the claims against the research-based outcomes of electrotherapeutic interventions. Prior to use, the therapist should be familiar with the specific capabilities of the available stimulators and their stimulation parameters.

Electrodes

Electrodes are the contact point providing the current flow from the stimulation device to the body. The electrode acts as an interface with the skin surface, the point where the electron–ion conversion occurs. Electrodes should offer little resistance to the current flow. A variety of electrodes are commercially available. Common electrode material includes carbon-rubber electrodes, which are silicon rubber impregnated with small carbon particles; metal- or foil-backed electrodes; sponges over metal plates; karaya gum electrodes; and self-adherent polymer electrodes. The self-adhering electrodes may be reusable and do not require strapping or taping, making them convenient to use. Adequate contact with the skin is crucial, and complete coverage of the electrode with gel, if used, is necessary.

Electrodes should be examined before each use and changed when necessary. Electrodes degrade with use and become unable to conduct the current efficiently. Therapists should look for cracking and worn spots in the carbon-rubber electrodes or excessive dryness in self-adhering electrodes and replace them as needed. With frequent use, carbon-rubber electrodes may develop nonconductive areas because of the absorption of dirt, skin oil, or electrode gel and depletion of the carbon-rubber. This may cause "hot spots," areas of high current density that may be uncomfortable for the patient and cause skin burns. A biting or stinging sensation during electrical stimulation may be caused by uneven conductivity, and the electrodes should be replaced.

Regardless of the type of electrode used, proper skin care and hygiene is necessary to prevent skin irritation or breakdown. This factor becomes critically important for patients who are using the stimulators on a home program or when there is prolonged placement and use of the electrodes.

Electrode Size

Current density is inversely related to the electrode size. As the electrode size decreases or the contact area of the electrode decreases, the current density increases, which can cause "hot spots," as mentioned earlier. As the current density increases, there is a greater perception of the stimulation beneath the electrode along with a greater physiological response due to the charge transfer. Excessive current density under an electrode can lead to discomfort or skin burns.

The inverse relationship between electrode size and current density means that smaller electrodes require less current to stimulate tissue, and large electrodes generally produce a stronger contraction with decreased pain or discomfort. Electrode size is determined by the size of the targeted tissue.

Electrode Placement

As the current density is greater in superficial layers of the skin, the distance between the electrodes also influences the depth of the current flow. When the electrodes are close together, the current passes superficially, and when the electrodes are farther apart, the current penetrates deeper. Location and orientation of electrodes must also be considered when stimulating muscles. Small electrodes can be used to obtain an isolated contraction from smaller muscles, such as those of the hand. Larger electrodes disperse the current into the tissue and are less specific in stimulating isolated muscles. Care should be taken when applying and selecting location of the electrodes because closely spaced electrodes may increase discomfort.

There are two primary methods of electrode placement for electrical stimulation: monopolar and bipolar. Simply put, the terms identify whether one lead and electrode is placed over the targeted tissue or if both leads and electrodes are placed over the area. The monopolar technique uses one stimulating electrode, which is placed over the targeted area. The other lead and electrode are placed over an area that is not affected by stimulation; this is the dispersive, or non-treatment, electrode. In the monopolar technique, only one pole or side of the circuit (active electrode) of the electrical stimulator is used to stimulate the target area. The dispersive electrode completes the electrical circuit and can be placed away from the target area on the same side of the body so as not to affect cardiac conduction. The dispersive electrode is often larger, minimizing the current density and perception of sensory stimulation. Monopolar techniques are most often associated with trigger and acupuncture-point stimulation.

Bipolar techniques consist of both electrodes placed over the target area to cause stimulation of the tissue. Since both electrodes or sides of the circuit are in contact with the targeted area, the current flow is more local, and the stimulation is perceived under both electrodes of the circuit. Most often, the electrodes are the same size, and this technique can be used to stimulate large muscles or muscle groups. Bipolar techniques are often used to activate muscles atrophied because of disuse, for muscle reeducation, or to obtain stronger contraction (neuromuscular facilitation) to increase limited movement.

Clinical Use of Electrotherapy

The unique applications and indications for each type of electrotherapy are discussed in turn.

Electrical Stimulation

Electricity has been advocated in the treatment of a variety of body systems and for a plethora of conditions, including joint swelling and inflammation, joint dysfunction, tissue healing, muscle reeducation, circulatory disorders, postural disorders, **pelvic floor** disorders, fracture healing, and pain management. There are a number of claims for electrical stimulation along with a variety of protocols and applications; some are objective, but many are unsubstantiated or anecdotal. The clinician should take a systematic and objective approach to the use of electrical stimulation.

Neuromuscular Electrical Stimulation

Neuromuscular electrical stimulation (NMES) has a variety of clinical uses as an adjunct to occupational therapy treatment. NMES is defined as the "use of electrical stimulation for activation of muscle through stimulation of the intact peripheral nerve" (American Physical Therapy Association, 1990, p. 29). NMES is often erroneously referred to as "functional" electrical stimulation. Functional electrical stimulation is a subcategory of neuromuscular electrical stimulation and refers to the use of NMES as a substitute for an orthosis to assist with a functional activity, such as standing or holding an object, or as a substitute for a sling. NMES can be used for strengthening and endurance, range of motion, facilitation of muscle function, management of muscle spasms and spasticity, edema reduction, and orthotic substitution (Cahe, Yu, & Walker, 2004). Clinical use of NMES requires a partially intact or intact peripheral nerve, and its use with primary muscle disease or muscular dystrophy is questionable.

CASE EXAMPLE

Biofeedback/NMES

Occupational Therapy Intervention Process	Clinical Reasoning Process: Objectives	Clinical Reasoning Process: Examples of Therapist's Internal Dialogue
Patient Information M.J. is a 36-year-old female who suffered a stroke affecting her left side. The stroke occurred while she was camping with her two sons (ages 12 and 9) and her husband. When her condition stabilized, she was referred to an inpatient rehabilitation program where she stayed for 5 weeks. She was discharged home with the recommendation for outpatient treatment. Prior to the cerebrovascular accident (CVA), she was employed as a nurse. She was right-hand dominant and independent for ADLs. She was accompanied by her husband for the initial evaluation. She was alert and oriented, but somewhat apprehensive and subdued. The following problems were identified during the occupational therapy assessment: (1) decreased initiation of IADL; (2) decreased functional use of the left upper extremity (active shoulder flexion/abduction to 95°); (3) increased tone in the left upper extremity with active grasp and weak release; (4) impairment in sensation, stereognosis, and proprioception in the left upper extremity; and (5) dependent for community mobility on public transportation.	Appreciate the context	"M.J. is a young, vibrant woman whose entire occupational roles have been affected by her CVA. She has gone from total independence to a state of greater dependence on her family and husband. She seems apprehensive and concerned over whether she will regain function in her upper extremity."
	Develop intervention hypotheses	"M.J. seems worried about whether she will be able to return to work and is also concerned about the financial impact her disability will have on the family. Her husband and family seem extremely supportive of her, and I am pleased that they are very engaged in her rehabilitation and in facilitating her independence."
	Select an intervention approach	"I am proposing an intervention plan that emphasizes compensatory techniques but also remediation and neuro-reeducation techniques to facilitate the return of function in the upper extremity. M.J. is anxious to continue to re-learn to use her affected arm and hand. Because of her nursing background, she seems to want to 'try everything and anything to get better.'
	Reflect on competence	"I have to admit that M.J. is a challenging case because she is about my age and extremely active prior to her CVA. She wants to try to return to work and recognizes the fact that she 'has' to get her 'hand and arm to work.' I know that we can use neuromuscular electrical stimulation to facilitate movement and strength in the upper extremity, but we also need a mechanism to provide her with feedback as to the level of volitional activity that she has in the arm and hand. Because of her motivation and progress to date, I recommend the use of biofeedback synchronized with NMES to strengthen the volitional control that she demonstrates and to facilitate the full ROM of the extremity. I do have concerns about safety issues related to ADL independence and am concerned that M.J. could injure her left upper extremity because of impaired upper extremity sensation and proprioception."
Recommendations The occupational therapist recommended three outpatient treatment sessions each week for 4 weeks. In collaboration with M.J. and her family, the occupational therapist established the following long-term treatment goals: (1) M.J. will display full AROM in the left upper extremity; (2) M.J. will display active grasp and release patterns of the upper extremity to manipulate large objects; (3) M.J. will be independent for IADLs; (4) M.J. will return to work; (5) M.J. will drive independently.	Consider the patient's appraisal of performance Consider what will occur in therapy, how often, and for how long Ascertain the patient's endorsement of plan	"M.J. seems highly motivated to attempt to return to work, and her family was supportive of this goal. In addition, because of the school and church activities that her sons were involved in and the fact that public transportation is negligible in the county that she lives in, M.J. really wants to return to driving independently. I know that this goal would strengthen her independence and ability to engage in those IADLs that are so vital to an active and involved family."

Summary of Short-Term Goals and Progress

1. MJ will display full AROM in the left upper extremity.
2. MJ will display active grasp and release patterns of the upper extremity to manipulate large objects.

The therapist began treatment using biofeedback and NMES to isolate shoulder flexion and abduction greater than 110°. The biofeedback parameters were set to register the amount of volitional muscle activity and provide the patient with auditory and visual feedback. She engaged in a variety of reaching activities that initially required active shoulder movement slightly below the point that would stimulate her flexor synergy pattern to override her active extension. When M.J. would volitionally reach this point and "get stuck," the NMES would trigger and stimulate the targeted muscle groups to contract, completing the movement for her. As her strength and control continued, the parameters were adjusted, requiring her to volitionally control more of the movement and to strengthen functional movements. To stimulate shoulder movements, electrodes were placed over the supraspinatus/upper trapezius, the anterior deltoid, and, to ensure elbow extension, the triceps. As greater proximal control developed, the electrodes were placed more distally on the arm, providing feedback and stimulation at the elbow (triceps), the wrist extensors, and then finally, alternating between the wrist extensors and flexors as needed.

Assess the patient's comprehension

Understand what the patient is doing

Compare actual to expected performance

Know the person

"In the initial evaluations and subsequent visits in the first week of therapy, it was clear to me that M.J. was developing active control in the extremity. Due to the strong flexor synergies prevalent, however, when she attempted to move beyond the range of motion she could control, the flexor patterns predominated in the upper extremity. She is anxious to learn how to override the synergy patterns and strengthen the volitional control in her arm and hand. The use of the auditory and visual feedback of the motor activity is reinforcing to her and provides her with the input she needs to determine which muscles are active and which need to relax. When synchronized with the NMES, the electrical stimulation of the weaker extensor patterns is reinforced and provides her with visual and neurological feedback to strengthen the movements. M.J. is a perfect candidate for this kind of intervention. She quickly learns how to use the feedback and stimulation to reinforce the distal control that she needs. I need to keep track of the degree of volitional movement she can demonstrate and monitor fatigue and synergy patterns that seem to vary depending upon M.J.'s emotional and physical state."

Appreciate the context

"I am pleased to see M.J. translate her gains in upper extremity function into expansion of her IADLs. She recently began testing to determine if she could resume driving independently and ultimately succeeded. This will further her independence and resumption of IADLs and eventually enable her to attempt to return to her work."

Next Steps

Continued outpatient occupational therapy for 1 month but with declining contact is recommended. Intervention will focus on weaning M.J. away from the biofeedback and NMES and ensuring that she continues to use the extremity for functional movements. Occupational therapy will incorporate educating the patient's family members and spouse on the returning function and importance of a home program of exercise and movement as crucial to ensure continued strength, independence, and function. The patient will also be assisted in resuming many of her social and religious activities and reintegrating her into meaningful community organizations and activities.

Anticipate present and future patient concerns

Analyze patient's comprehension

Decide if the patient should continue or discontinue therapy and/or return in the future

"Because of the patient's background as a nurse, M.J. seems well aware of challenges and potential limitations based on her initial prognosis. She has always been highly motivated to 'try almost anything' if it would 'work.' But I am impressed at her insight into the possible risks and difficulties she will face returning to her career as a surgical nurse, and she is starting to prepare herself for other options that might require less fine motor dexterity and endurance as her condition improves. I expect that she will work closely with her employer and physicians to adapt her work site and work requirements."

CLINICAL REASONING IN OCCUPATIONAL THERAPY PRACTICE

Identifying Appropriate Therapeutic Goals and Interventions

M.J. was a young, active, healthy individual prior to her devastating stroke. Overnight, her life and roles changed, impacting not only her immediate family but the community in which she lived and her patients and employer. She was highly motivated to return to some semblance of her pre-morbid activities and life. The difficulty she faced was in determining short-term, realistic goals and objectives (which the therapist had to assist her to prioritize) and expanding those into long-term functional goals. As functional return and movement occurred in her upper extremity, refining and strengthening the motor patterns and movements available to the patient became a motivating factor for her. There are a variety of neuromuscular facilitation techniques that can be used as part of neuromuscular reeducation. What other therapeutic techniques and interventions could have been used with this patient? What were the components of NMES and biofeedback that were motivating and intrinsically rewarding to the patient? Could only NMES have been used? What are some of the complications that occur with cerebrovascular accidents in terms of the shoulder and upper quadrant?

Maintain Muscle Mass

NMES can be a successful adjunct to conventional treatment in individuals with limited traumatic or orthopedic injuries. There is a relationship between training intensity and strength gains, and improving muscle strength is based in part on the overload principle. The overload principle refers to the fact that, for strength gains to occur, the body must be subjected to greater levels of stress than it is accustomed to. To accomplish this, the therapist must increase the load, frequency, or duration of the exercise or activity. Patients who are deconditioned or have areas of weakness may benefit from NMES to improve endurance of the targeted muscle. Isometric strengthening using NMES produces better results than conventional isometric exercises alone but is most effective when paired with functional goals and movements (Baker, 1993).

Maintain or Gain Range of Motion

Neurologically impaired patients often develop spasticity as a consequence of their injury. Range-of-motion techniques and positioning are often part of the overall training and education program for family members and caregivers. Unfortunately, patients with moderate to severe spasticity often have difficulty following through on these techniques and can develop limitations affecting their occupational function. Hemiplegic patients with chronic moderate spasticity in the wrist or finger flexors may be appropriate candidates for this intervention (Powell et al., 1999). For these individuals, the stimulus should ramp up and be sufficiently intense to allow for a slow stretch without increasing spasticity due to a quick stretch or jerk (Baker, 1993). Ramp-up times should be extended to 6–8 seconds or longer, and proper positioning or blocking of other muscles should be considered. Serial casting or splinting of the extremity can be an effective adjunct to NMES. The use of NMES is effective as part of a home program because it reduces the spasticity and allows the caregiver to carry out passive range of motion several times daily.

For the orthopedic patient, range of motion may be limited by contractures secondary to immobilization or pain. NMES may be used to improve joint range of motion if the limitation is due to intrinsic soft tissue shortening as opposed to a bony block or biomechanical limitation. The technique should maintain a low-intensity stretch for a few seconds.

Management of Spasticity

The effectiveness of NMES for the treatment of spasticity depends in part on the underlying disease causing the spasticity. The response of NMES in a patient with a spastic spinal cord injury may be different from the response in a patient with a brain injury or multiple sclerosis. The variability of abnormal tone may only result in a temporary interruption of the motor neuron excitability, with short-term treatment effects. Stimulation of a spastic muscle in the neurologically impaired client using a high frequency causes a response similar to fatiguing the muscle (Vodovnik, Bowman, & Hufford, 1984).

NMES also affects spasticity by stimulating the muscle antagonist to the spastic muscle, which inhibits the spastic muscle, allowing range-of-motion exercise (Wang, Tsai, & Chan, 1998). Heat or ice and serial casting or splinting paired with functional movements and activities may enhance the therapeutic response.

Orthopedic patients may have pain–spasm cycles caused by local spasm of a particular muscle or group. Decreasing the pain–spasm cycle through the application of NMES to the area improves and enhances range of motion and occupational performance.

Facilitate Voluntary Control

NMES has been used frequently for muscle reeducation and facilitation, particularly with neurological injuries and orthopedic injuries after surgery. Facilitation and retraining can be effective for patients suffering from disuse atrophy, muscle weakness, and pain (Lewek, Stevens, & Snyder-Maackler, 2001). In neurologically involved patients, the sensory feedback loop becomes distorted or impaired.

The goal of NMES for facilitation and reeducation is to incorporate the stimulation with voluntary contraction, functional movement and activity, and sensory feedback (Bracciano, 2000). The intent of NMES for facilitation and reeducation is to flood the central nervous system with sensory and kinesthetic information linked to an anticipated motor response. A variety of functional activities incorporating the desired motor response should be used to ensure adequate carryover of the response. For example, a stroke patient who is working on grasp and release should be provided with a variety of objects consisting of various shapes, sizes, and weights to hold and release. Placement of the objects should require movements to various heights and locations.

Functional Electrical Stimulation

Functional electrical stimulation (FES), the use of NMES as a replacement for orthoses, has been an effective adjunct in facilitating occupational function, most notably positional stability and mobility. Stimulation of innervated paretic or paralyzed muscles can decrease dependence on slings, splints, or orthotics through the development of increased strength and endurance of the paretic musculature.

FES has been effectively used with hemiparetic patients who display shoulder subluxation during the flaccid phase of recovery and also to facilitate grasp-and-release activities (Eckerson & Axelgaard, 1984; Phillips, 1989). In the hemiplegic patient, gravity stresses the shoulder capsule, stretching the ligamentous capsule. When muscle tone and voluntary control develop at the shoulder, normal glenohumeral alignment may not recur when the arm is at rest because of ligamentous laxity (Yu, Cahe, & Walker, 2001). Slings may be helpful to establish glenohumeral alignment, but stimulation of the posterior deltoid and supraspinatus muscles may be more effective in improving normal shoulder integrity (Lin, Granat, & Lees, 1999; Wang, Chan, & Tsai, 2000). Use of FES for maintaining shoulder integrity by preventing subluxation and reeducating muscles can be an effective adjunct to splinting and facilitate occupational function. Clearly outlining and teaching the client and caregivers in a home program is vital to ensure continuity and carryover.

Transcutaneous Electrical Nerve Stimulation

Pain is one of the most common complaints that cause patients to seek medical care. Adequate pain management facilitates occupational function (Fig. 20-10). Transcutaneous electrical nerve stimulation (TENS) can be used to manage pain in musculoskeletal disorders. The two primary theories on which the modulation of pain with TENS is based are the gate control theory (Low and Reed, 2000) and the endorphin theory (Bonica, 1990).

Treatment applications using electrical stimulation for pain control employ pulsed or alternating current with a variety of stimulation patterns. The type of stimulation is based on the neurological response to the stimulation. The four primary types of stimulation frequently employed include subsensory level, sensory level, motor level, and noxious level. Stimulation sites for electrode placement are based on the problem areas and goals for the patient. Optimal electrode placements should correlate with the structures and sources of pain and include motor points, trigger points, and acupuncture points. TENS units are often used at home, and the therapist should explain the purpose of the equipment and instruct the patient in its operations and precautions, with written and pictorial instructions. Through application of TENS for sensory analgesia, the patient may better perform functional activities and movements that foster independence and function.

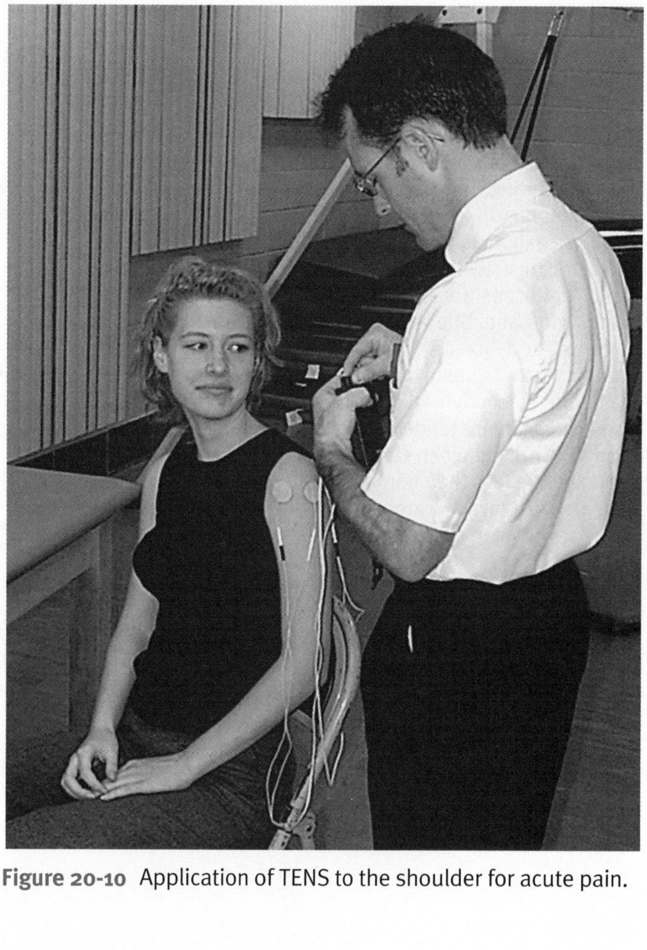

Figure 20-10 Application of TENS to the shoulder for acute pain.

Iontophoresis

Iontophoresis is a method of topically delivering a medication or ionized drug to an area of tissue by using direct electrical current. Iontophoresis is non-invasive, essentially painless, and an effective way to administer medications to local targeted tissues. Occupational therapists frequently use iontophoresis in the treatment of inflammatory conditions such as epicondylitis, carpal tunnel syndrome, glenohumeral bursitis, ulnar nerve inflammation, and wrist tendinitis and tenosynovitis. Therapists using iontophoresis should thoroughly understand the pathophysiology of the condition, the wound healing process, medications being used, and any potential drug interactions. Caution must be used whenever using iontophoresis because medications may cause an allergic or anaphylactic reaction, which is a life-threatening condition and medical emergency. Patients should *always* be asked for a list of current medications and whether they have any known allergies, sensitivities, or reactions to foods or medications. Documented orders should always be obtained from the patient's physician prior to using iontophoresis (Bracciano, 2000).

CASE EXAMPLE

Iontophoresis

Occupational Therapy Intervention Process	Clinical Reasoning Process	
	Objectives	**Examples of Therapist's Internal Dialogue**
Patient Information Laura is an active and athletic 47-year-old female who was referred to occupational therapy by her family physician. She relates that she was "painting her kitchen and family room" in the "new house" they recently purchased. After 3 days of painting, she developed pain in her right elbow (dominant hand), increasing inability to "hold" onto objects such as a gallon of milk, and further difficulty with cooking and self-care activities requiring her to use her right hand in static "hold" positions, along with "tingling and numbness" in her right hand. She reports pain being "constantly a 4–5 out of 10" and increasing to "7–8 out of 10" with use. Cozen's test was positive, with patient displaying pain on the lateral epicondyle with resisted wrist extension. Laura also displays point tenderness over the right lateral epicondyle. Grip and pinch strengths are decreased in the right hand and are less than normal for women her age. The patient also displays an extension lag of 10° and lacks full flexion by 12° (pain in both distal ranges).	Appreciate the context	"It seems that Laura's signs and symptoms are consistent with a diagnosis of lateral epicondylitis. Her symptoms developed quickly after apparently overusing the right upper extremity to paint her house."
	Develop intervention hypotheses	"Because of the rapidity with which her symptoms developed, the quick referral by her physician, and lack of previous difficulties in her right upper extremity, Laura's condition is considered an acute episode. I believe that she will require a multi-faceted approach to treat her condition."
	Select an intervention approach	"Laura's problems and clinical presentation are consistent with a diagnosis of acute lateral epicondylitis. I expect that her physician will recommend some form of NSAIDs or other anti-inflammatory medications. I will be recommending static splinting of the right wrist in neutral, ROM and gradual strengthening of the upper extremity, use of physical agent modalities to facilitate the healing process of the tissue, and modification of her daily activities to avoid further exacerbating her condition."
	Reflect on competence	"There are a number of therapeutic approaches that can be used with lateral epicondylitis. I will need to consistently monitor Laura's response to the interventions used, which will assist in modifying the treatment as needed. I will also want to monitor her level of use of the right upper extremity, compliance with the splint-wearing schedule, and modifications to her daily routine to prevent further exacerbation of her condition."

Recommendations

The occupational therapist recommended three treatment sessions per week for 3 weeks. The following long-term goals were established: (1) decrease pain in the right upper extremity; (2) improve pain-free ROM; and (3) improve pain-free pinch and grip in the right hand.

Consider the patient's appraisal of performance

Consider what will occur in therapy, how often, and for how long

Ascertain the patient's endorsement of plan

"From the beginning, it was apparent that Laura would follow through on all recommendations. She was highly motivated and had been very active and participated in a number of athletic activities prior to her injury. She was anxious to return to her premorbid activities, and there was more concern that she might 'overdo it' as she progressed in treatment and her symptoms began to subside. Because her children were also older, I wasn't concerned with her having to 'lift' any babies or infants. Additionally, she could ask her family members to help her with those activities that required heavy lifting or static hold and release patterns."

"Laura agreed with the goals and was anxious to begin treatment to decrease the pain and loss of function in her right upper extremity. "

Summary of Short-Term Goals and Progress

The treatment approach and intervention included: (1) static splinting of the right hand; (2) iontophoresis with dexamethasone to decrease the inflammatory process and pain (2–3 out of 10); (3) friction massage to the lateral epicondyle, and icing as needed; (4) ROM to the right elbow; (5) and modification of ADLs and movements to prevent exacerbation of her condition.

Laura was instructed in different methods of modifying activities that required her to lift or manipulate objects as part of her daily activities. She was also provided with a static positioning splint for her right hand that she was to wear at night and initially during the day. She was aware of skin and splint care and her wearing schedule.

Laura's condition responded to the iontophoresis, and she reported a decrease in pain by 50% after the fourth treatment (every other day). As she responded to the iontophoresis and her treatment, her dosage was increased from 40 mA/min to 60 mA/min and, for her final three treatments, to 80 mA/min. (Using a gradually increasing 40/60/80 milliamp protocol as the patient improves allows a greater number of ions to be delivered to the underlying tissue and may hasten healing.) All activities and interventions were graded and gradually increased in resistance and/or intensity as her condition and symptoms improved.

Assess the patient's comprehension

Understand what the patient is doing

Compare actual to expected performance

Know the person

Appreciate the context

"I noticed that Laura was apprehensive to ask for assistance at home, but after we talked about the importance of 'resting' the elbow the first 2 weeks or so, her family took an active role in assisting her with her activities and responsibilities. Because she was responding so positively to the treatment interventions, I recommended that she begin wearing her splint only at night but resume wearing the splint during the day if she noticed any return of her symptoms or pain. I know how important it is for me to monitor Laura's condition closely and to note any changes in pain or symptoms during each treatment visit, modifying the treatment and interventions as needed. If she reports a reversal back to earlier levels of pain and symptoms, I'll have to figure out whether or not the interventions are effective or whether she is impacting the injury somehow in the performance of her daily occupations and activities."

Next Steps

Revised short-term goals (2 weeks):

1. Laura will display decreased pain (1–2 out of 10) with use of her hand to lift "light" objects.
2. Laura will display full active ROM in the right elbow (she will be able to fully extend her arm to reach for and manipulate objects).
3. Laura will wear her splint at night.
4. Laura will improve her grip and pinch strength within functional limits without pain.

Anticipate present and future patient concerns

Analyze patient's comprehension

Decide whether the patient should continue or discontinue therapy and/or return in the future

"I am pleased with Laura's response to the initial course of treatment. She was compliant with her splint wearing and modified her routine and activities to avoid using the right upper extremity. She noticed a marked decrease in pain 'by at least 50%' and a decrease in her other symptoms after the fourth treatment using iontophoresis. Because she responded so well to the treatment, I recommend that we continue with the iontophoresis, begin gentle strengthening activities and exercises, and allow her to begin using the right upper extremity in more activities requiring a static hold and release pattern."

CLINICAL REASONING IN OCCUPATIONAL THERAPY PRACTICE

Determining Progress in Physical Agent Modalities

Laura's "injury" occurred following her engagement in a rather normal activity, painting her house. The signs and symptoms that she exhibited, such as pain in her elbow, difficulty holding onto objects and performing routine activities, and numbness and tingling, are all diagnostic clues that an occupational therapist needs to use to determine a differential diagnosis and select an appropriate treatment plan and physical agent. Establishing a realistic "starting point" based on the evaluative and assessment components provides a mechanism for determining progress and efficacy of the therapeutic interventions, guiding modifications to the treatment.

What clues, both subjective and objective, did Laura provide to the therapist to guide him in his thinking and treatment plan? What other physical agents could have been used with Laura to achieve the identified goals and objectives? What was the primary factor that indicated to the therapist that the iontophoresis should be continued?

SURFACE ELECTROMYOGRAPHIC BIOFEEDBACK

Biofeedback is an often overlooked modality that therapists can use for neuromuscular reeducation, relaxation techniques, and behavioral modification. The general term "biofeedback" refers to those procedures or techniques that are used to provide an individual with an auditory or visual cue or "feedback" to learn and gain volitional control over a physiological response. Biofeedback equipment provides the individual with an external mechanism for monitoring a specific physiological function and response and, through instant feedback, allows the individual to attempt to control or modify the behavior or response.

The term biofeedback was first used by researchers to describe procedures that were being attempted to train subjects to alter brain activity, blood pressure, heart rate, and other physiological functions not controlled volitionally. Biofeedback was given its initial impetus by the work of Basmajian and his research on single motor unit training of the neuromuscular system. Clinically, biofeedback techniques and equipment continue to develop and are used to treat a variety of conditions including migraine headaches, tension headaches, pain, disorders of the digestive system, hyper- and hypotension, cardiac arrhythmias, Raynaud's disease, seizures, and paralysis and movement disorders (Foster, 2004; Engel, Jensen, & Schwartz, 2004; Smania et al., 2003; Middaugh et al., 2001). Specialists in a variety of fields use biofeedback to control pain, anxiety, muscle tone, behaviors, and muscle function and movement. Since the primary use of biofeedback in physical medicine and rehabilitation is in the form of sEMG or surface electromyographic feedback for muscle reeducation and training, we will focus on this dimension of biofeedback in this chapter.

Clinical use of sEMG biofeedback for neuromuscular dysfunction was demonstrated to be an effective education method for a variety of conditions, and later research used sEMG to improve function in hemiplegic patients (Booker, Rubow, & Coleman, 1969; Johnson & Garton, 1973). Research using sEMG neuromuscular reeducation has also demonstrated success when compared to traditional methods of treating stroke (Moreland, Thomson, & Fuoco, 1998). sEMG uses electronic instrumentation to measure and display muscle activity. Surface electrodes are placed on the skin over the muscles being retrained or examined. These electrodes and the associated computer electronics sense the electrical activity associated with muscle tension or relaxation and quantify and display the activity. Electromyography can demonstrate asymmetrical muscle activation during symmetrical movements, co-contraction of antagonists during movement, difference in onset or timing of muscle firing during specific movements, and failure of the muscle activity to "shut off" following movement. These can all lead to musculoskeletal pain, spasm, contractures, or loss of functional movement and are considerations for incorporating sEMG as part of the treatment regimen. Using sEMG, a spastic muscle, for example, would be treated with relaxation and "calming" of the targeted muscle. Contractures would be treated with mobilization and stretching. Paralysis would be treated with activation and mobilization, with the patient "attempting" to move the affected muscle to increase biofeedback activity. As the desired control or movement is developed by the patient, he or she should be weaned from the biofeedback with an emphasis on volitional movement and activity being reinforced. Some sEMG equipment can be linked or synchronized with neuromuscular electrical stimulation to facilitate motor unit activity or to increase motor unit recruitment and movement. sEMG and paired NMES can be used for patients who are, for example, unable to fully complete a movement through partial or full range of motion. The therapist can set the threshold so that the patient receives auditory and visual feedback with activation of a selected muscle, which, when achieved, activates the NMES to complete the movement, thereby reinforcing and strengthening the response (Pullman et al., 2000; Seo et al., 2005).

Muscle Reeducation

sEMG enables the therapist and patient to objectively measure and visually determine muscular activity patterns. Depending on the equipment, the therapist is also able to quantify and track changes in motor performance and function. Use of biofeedback for muscle reeducation or strengthening most often uses auditory and visual feedback. Depending on the device, the feedback is set to an all-or-none response or to a specific threshold that the patient must achieve to activate the auditory or visual response. The threshold can be raised or lowered depending on the need and allows the therapist to grade the activity and response, allowing the patient to achieve higher levels of performance based on earlier training sessions. If the goal is muscle inhibition, the threshold is set so that the device will either turn on or turn off when the level of motor activity decreases below the specific setting. One disadvantage to using surface electrodes is that they are susceptible to movement artifacts or electrical noise. Electrodes are placed over the bulk of the targeted muscle belly parallel to the muscle fibers. As with neuromuscular electrical stimulation, placing the electrodes further apart increases the amplitude of the EMG signal.

sEMG is motivating for patients because they are provided instantaneous feedback in the form of visual and auditory modes. With many patients who have suffered a cerebrovascular accident, along with disruption of motor control, there is a concurrent impairment in proprioception and kinesthesia, which impacts functional abilities because of the loss of sensory input and feedback. Incorporating sEMG into the therapeutic mix provides the central nervous system and patient with additional feedback and input. As the patient's condition improves and muscle function and performance are normalized, conditioning and engagement in functional tasks and activities reinforces and strengthens the "learned" movement patterns (Procedures for Practice 20-2 and 20-3).

PROCEDURES FOR PRACTICE 20-2

EMG Biofeedback Session for Muscle Reeducation

- Begin with large, widely spaced electrodes over the muscle belly.
- Initially set the threshold at an attainable level.
- During a 10- to 15-minute treatment session, the patient voluntarily contracts the muscle to reach the threshold level.
- When possible, incorporate purposeful activities to facilitate the muscle activity desired.
- Gradually raise the threshold during the treatment session to challenge the patient to contract the muscle more strongly.

Biofeedback in the Treatment of Incontinence

Biofeedback has also been used in the treatment of pelvic floor disorders (Dannecker et al., 2005; Kielb, 2005). Although men may suffer from pelvic floor disorders, the vast majority of patients with this condition are women because of the anatomy and function of the pelvis in women. Pelvic floor disorders refers to the pelvic diaphragm, the sphincter mechanism of the lower urinary tract, the upper and lower vaginal supports, and the internal and external anal sphincters. This complex of muscles, tissue, and ligaments holds up the organs of the pelvis, the vagina, rectum,

PROCEDURES FOR PRACTICE 20-3

EMG Biofeedback Session to Decrease Spasticity

- Begin with small, closely spaced electrodes over the muscle belly.
- Initially set the threshold at an attainable level.
- Place the limb in midrange, and keep the environment free of distractions.
- During a 10- to 15-minute treatment session, the patient attempts to maintain relaxation of the muscle below the threshold level.
- Gradually decrease the threshold as the patient learns to relax the muscle.
- In subsequent sessions, challenge the patient to maintain relaxation of the spastic muscle while contracting the antagonistic group.

Evidence Table 20-1
Best Evidence for Interventions Used in Physical Agent Modalities Case Examples

Intervention	Description of Intervention Tested	Participants	Dosage	Type of Best Evidence and Level of Evidence	Benefit	Statistical Probability	Reference
Functional Electrical Stimulation (FES)	Use of functional electrical stimulation to wrist and finger extensor muscles to improve grip acquisition and grip processing speed.	38 patients with hemiplegia.	FES to affected extremity 2 times per week for 6 months.	IIIB3b; Pre-post only.	Yes. FES administered twice weekly for 6-month increased grip speed.	Statistically significant improvement in grip speed after treatment ($p = 0.0309$).	Lourencao et al., 2005
Iontophoresis	Iontophoresis of corticosteroids (compared with local corticosteroid injection).	30 patients (48 median nerves) with clinical and electrophysiological evidence of carpal tunnel syndrome.	1 session only. One group received 40 mg of methylprednisolone acetate injected into the carpal tunnel; the second group received iontophoresis of dexamethasone sodium phosphate.	Random assignment of median nerves to 1 of 2 groups; unblinded. IC2b.	Yes. At 2 weeks and 8 weeks after therapy, there was a statistically significant improvement in pain, symptom severity scale, and functional status in both groups compared with baseline ($p < 0.05$). But symptom relief was greater at 2 and 8 weeks with injection of corticosteroids.	Statistically significant ($p < 0.05$).	Gokoglu et al., 2005

uterus, and bladder. This system of support often becomes weak following vaginal delivery of several children or in women who have had perineal or pelvic floor tears during delivery. As they age or reach menopause, these women may develop symptoms of pelvic floor disorders, which are caused, in part, by the organs shifting, bulging, and pushing against each other. This may lead to urinary or fecal incontinence, obstruction, vaginal pain or prolapse, sexual dysfunction, and other difficulties (Jundt & Friese, 2005; Kielb, 2005).

The nature of the pelvic floor musculature provides individuals with voluntary control. These muscles contract and relax with the action becoming automatic. If the normal contract-relax coordination of the pelvic floor muscles becomes disrupted, bowel and bladder disorders may occur. Since these muscles can be controlled voluntarily, however, they can be "retrained" using sEMG. Special EMG sensors are available that can be placed in the anal canal or vagina and measure and display the amount of electrical activity. The therapist can provide instruction and training to assist the patient in regaining control and changing abnormal muscle activity. If the patient is unable to isolate muscle contraction, pelvic floor exercises can be paired with electrical stimulation to provide proprioceptive feedback and strengthen the muscular contraction. Portable electrical stimulation units can be used at home, and a variety of internal and external electrodes are available. Some pelvic floor biofeedback devices are also linked to neuromuscular electrical stimulators; these are called pelvic floor stimulators. These biofeedback-triggered stimulation units provide both active and passive strengthening of the weakened musculature. The patient contracts the pelvic floor muscles to a specific threshold, which, when reached, triggers the electrical stimulation to further strengthen the response. These devices provide the patient with additional assistance in developing volitional control, changing muscle tone, or increasing muscle activity through the administration of electrical current at a specific threshold (Lin et al., 2004; Seo et al., 2005). Treatment of pelvic floor or urogynecological and colorectal systems requires advanced training and clinical practice. There may also be specific requirements related to state practice acts that must be met prior to developing or implementing these programs and interventions, and the clinician is cautioned to review both institutional and state regulatory guidelines before using these techniques.

Physical agents like the ones discussed in this chapter should never be the single method or treatment approach in occupational therapy treatment. When used judiciously after taking into account the diagnosis, healing process, and phase of recovery, physical agents can make a valuable contribution to occupational therapy, facilitating outcomes and occupational performance.

SUMMARY REVIEW QUESTIONS

1. Identify and discuss the three phases of wound healing. Why is the phase of wound healing a significant factor in selection of a specific physical agent modality as an adjunct to treatment?
2. Discuss the types of pain and their effect on occupational function.
3. Define and discuss superficial and deep thermal agents. Identify indications and contraindications for application of deep thermal agents and their effect on occupational function.
4. List the most frequently used applications of electrotherapy.
5. Discuss AOTA's position on physical agents and how physical agent modalities can be incorporated into a comprehensive treatment program.
6. Define and discuss therapeutic ultrasound and its thermal and non-thermal effects.
7. List precautions and contraindications for superficial thermal agents and cryotherapy.
8. Identify indications for use of sEMG biofeedback.

References

Abergel, R. P., Lyons, R. F., Castel, J. C., Dwyer, R. M., & Uitto, J. (1987). Biostimulation of wound healing by lasers: Experimental approaches in animal models and in fibroblast cultures. *Journal of Dermatologic and Surgical Oncolcology, 13,* 127–133.

Akai, M., Usuba, M., Maeshima, T., Shirasaki, Y., & Yasuika, S. (1997). Laser's effect on bone and cartilage: Change induced by joint immobilization in an experimental animal model. *Lasers in Surgery and Medicine, 21,* 480–484.

Allen, K. G., & Battye, C. K. (1978). Performance of ultrasonic therapy instruments. *Physiotherapy, 64,* 174–179.

American Occupational Therapy Association [AOTA]. (2003). Physical agent modalities: Position paper. *American Journal of Occupational Therapy, 57,* 650–651.

American Physical Therapy Association [APTA] (1990). *Electrotherapeutic terminology in physical therapy.* Alexandria, VA: American Physical Therapy Association.

Apfel, R. (1989). Acoustic cavitation: A possible consequence of biomedical uses of ultrasound. *British Journal of Cancer, 45,* 140–146.

Baker, L. L. (1993). *Neuromuscular electrical stimulation: A practical clinical guide* (3rd ed.). Downey, CA: Rancho Los Amigos Research and Education Institute.

Baker, L. L., Bowman, B. R., & McNeal, D. R. (1988). Effects of wave form on comfort during neuromuscular electrical stimulation. *Clinical Orthopedics, 223,* 75–85.

Behrens, B., & Michlovitz, S.L. (2005). *Physical agents: Theory and practice* (2nd ed). Philadelphia: F. A. Davis.

Bonica, J. J. (1990). *The management of pain* (Vol. 1 and 2, 2nd ed.). Malvern, PA: Lea & Febiger.

Booker, H. E., Rubow, R. T., & Coleman, P. J. (1969). Simplified feedback in neuromuscular retraining: An automated approach using EMG signals. *Archives of Physical Medicine, 50,* 621–625.

Borrell, R. M., Parker, R., Henley, E. J, Masley, D., & Repinecz, M. (1980). Comparison of in vivo temperatures produced by hydrotherapy, paraffin wax treatment, and fluidotherapy. *Physical Therapy, 60,* 1273–1276.

Bracciano, A. (1999). Therapeutic ultrasound: Sound information for the occupational therapist. *OT Practice, 4,* 20–25.

Bracciano, A. (2000). *Physical agent modalities: Theory and application for the occupational therapist.* Thorofare, NJ: Slack.

Cahe, J, Yu, D., Walker, M. (2004). Percutaneous, intramuscular neuromuscular electrical stimulation for the treatment of shoulder subluxation and pain in chronic hemiplegia: A case report. *American Journal of Physical Medicine and Rehabilitation, 80,* 296–301.

Cameron, M. (2003). *Physical agents in rehabilitation.* Philadelphia: W.B. Saunders.

Chow, R. (2002). EBM in action: Is laser treatment effective and safe for musculoskeletal pain? *Medical Journal of Australia, 176,* 194–5.

Conlon, M. J., Rapley, J. W., & Cobb, C. M. (1996). Biostimulation of wound healing by low-energy laser irradiation. A review. *Journal of Clinical Periodontology, 23,* 492–496.

Currier, D. (1993). Effects of electrical and electromagnetic stimulation after anterior cruciate ligament reconstruction. *Journal of Orthopedic and Sports Physical Therapy, 17,* 177–184.

Dannecker, C., Wolf, V., Raab, R., Hepp, H., & Anthuber, C. (2005). EMG-biofeedback assisted pelvic floor muscle training is an effective therapy of stress urinary or mixed incontinence: A 7-year experience with 390 patients. *Archives of Gynecology and Obstetrics, 6,* 1–5.

Davidson, J. (1998). Wound repair. *Journal of Hand Therapy, 11,* 80–94.

Doyle, N. D. (2004). Rehabilitation of fractures in small animals: Maximize outcomes, minimize complications. *Clinical Techniques in Small Animal Practice, 19,* 180–192.

Dyson, M., & Pond, J. (1970). The effect of pulsed ultrasound on tissue regeneration. *Physiotherapy, 64,* 105–108.

Dyson, M., & Suckling, J. (1978). Stimulation of tissue repair by ultrasound: a survey of the mechanisms involved. *Physiotherapy, 64,* 105–108.

Earley, D. (1999). Superficial heat agents: A hot topic. *OT Practice, 4,* 26–30.

Eckerson, L. F., & Axelgaard, J. (1984). Lateral electrical surface stimulation as an alternative to bracing in the treatment of idiopathic scoliosis. *Physical Therapy, 64,* 483–490.

Engel, J. M., Jensen, M. P., & Schwartz, L. (2004). Outcome of biofeedback-assisted relaxation for pain in adults with cerebral palsy: preliminary findings. *Applied Psychophysiology and Biofeedback, 29,* 135–140.

Enwemeka, C. (1989). The effects of therapeutic ultrasound on tendon healing. *American Journal of Physical Medicine and Rehabilitation, 68,* 283–287.

Enwemeka, C., Parker, J., Dowdy, D., Harkness, E., Sanford, L. E., & Woodruff, L. D. (2004). The efficacy of low-power lasers in tissue repair and pain control: A meta-analysis study. *Photomedicine and Laser Surgery, 22,* 323–329.

Fabrizio, P. A., Schmidt, J. A., & Clemente, F. R.(1996). Acute effects of therapeutic ultrasound delivered at varying parameters on the blood flow velocity in a muscular distribution artery. *Journal of Orthopedic and Sports Physical Therapy, 24,* 294–302.

Foster, P. S. (2004). Use of the Calmset 3 biofeedback/relaxation system in the assessment and treatment of chronic nocturnal bruxism. *Applied Psychophysiology and Biofeedback, 29,* 141–147.

Fyfe, M., & Parnell, S. (1982). The importance of measurement of effective transducer radiating area in the testing and calibration of therapeutic ultrasonic instruments. *Health Physics, 43,* 377–381.

Gan, B. S., Huys, S., Sherebrin, M. H., & Scilley, C. G. (1995). The effects of ultrasound treatment on flexor tendon healing in the chicken limb. *Journal of Hand Surgery (Edinburgh), 20,* 809–814.

Gokoglu, F., Fndkoglu, G., Yorgancoglu, Z. R., Okumus, M., Ceceli, E., & Kocaoglu, S. (2005). Evaluation of iontophoresis and local corticosteroid injection in the treatment of carpal tunnel syndrome. *American Journal of Physical Medicine and Rehabilitation, 84,* 92–96.

Gum, D. L., Reddy, G. K., Stehno-Bittel, L., & Enwemeka, C. S. (1997). Combined ultrasound, electrical stimulation, and laser promote collagen synthesis with moderate changes in tendon biomechanics. *American Journal of Physical Medicine and Rehabilitation, 76,* 288–296.

Hakim, M. H. (1995). Pain and its measurement. *Hamdard, 38,* 86–90.

Hekkenberg, R. T., Reibold, R., & Zeqiri, B. (1994). Development of standard measurement methods for essential properties of ultrasound therapy equipment. *Ultrasound in Medicine and Biology, 20,* 83–98.

Henley, E. (1991). Transcutaneous drug delivery: Iontophoresis, phonophoresis. *Critical Reviews in Physical Medicine and Rehabilitation, 3,* 139–151.

Hess, C. L., Howard, M., & Attignger, C. (2000). A review of mechanical adjuncts in wound healing: Hydrotherapy, ultrasound, negative pressure therapy, hyperbaric oxygen, and electrostimulation. *Annals of Plastic Surgery, 51,* 210–218.

Houghton, P. E., & Campbell, K. E. (1999). Choosing an adjunctive therapy for the treatment of chronic wounds. *Ostomy-Wound Management, 45,* 43–52.

Hsieh, Y. L. (2005). Reduction in induced pain by ultrasound may be caused by altered expression of spinal neuronal nitric oxide synthase-producing neurons. *Archives of Physical Medicine and Rehabilitation, 86,* 1311–1317.

Johnson, H. E., & Garton, W. H. (1973). Muscle re-education in hemiplegia by use of electromyographic device. *Archives of Physical Medicine and Rehabilitation, 54,* 320–322.

Jundt, K., & Friese, K. (2005). Female urinary incontinence. *MMW Fortschrittle der Medizin, 147,* 26–29.

Kaul, M. P. (1994). Superficial heat and cold. *The Physician and Sports Medicine, 22,* 65–74.

Kelly, R., Beehn C., Hansford A., Westphal, K. A., Halle, J. S., & Greathouse, D. G. (2005). Effect of fluidotherapy on superficial radial nerve conduction and skin temperature. *Journal of Orthopedic and Sports Physical Therapy, 35,* 16–23.

Kielb, S. J. (2005). Stress incontinence: Alternatives to surgery. *International Journal of Fertility and Womens Medicine, 50,* 24–29.

Kimura, I., Gulick, D., Shelly, J., & Ziskin, M. (1988). Effects of two ultrasound devices and angles of application on the temperature of tissue phantom. *Journal of Orthopedic and Sports Physical Therapy, 27,* 27–31.

Kollmann, C., Vacariu, G., Schuhfried, O., Fialka-Moser, V., & Bergmann, H. (2005). Variations in the output power and surface heating effects of transducers in therapeutic ultrasound. *Archives of Physical Medicine and Rehabilitation, 86,* 1318–1324.

Lehmann, J., & Guy, A. (1971). Ultrasound therapy. In J. Reid & M. Sikov (Eds.), *Interaction of ultrasound and biological tissues* (pp. 141–152). DHEW Publication FDA 73-8008. Washington, DC: Government Printing Office.

Lewek, M., Stevens, J., & Snyder-Maackler, L. (2001). The use of electrical stimulation to increase quadriceps femoris muscle force following total knee arthroplasty. *Physical Therapy, 91,* 1565–1571.

Lin, L. S., Song, Y. F., Song, J., & Chen, M. F. (2004). A clinical study of pelvic floor electrical stimulation in treatment of overactive bladder. *Zhoghua Fu Chan Ke Za Zhi, 39,* 801–803.

Lin, S. L., Granat, M. H., & Lees, K. R. (1999). Prevention of shoulder subluxation after stroke with electrical stimulation. *Stroke, 30,* 963–968.

Lourencao, M., Battistella, L. R., Martins, L. C., & Livoc, J. (2005). Analysis of the results of functional electrical stimulation on hemiplegic patients' upper extremities using the Minnesota manual dexterity test. *International Journal of Rehabilitation Research, 28,* 25–31.

Low, J., & Reed, A. (2000). *Electrotherapy explained: Principles and practice* (3rd ed.). Oxford, United Kingdom: Butterworth-Heinemann.

Masse, J. (1996). Phonophoresis. *Sports Medicine, 10,* 4–6.

Mehreteab, T., & Weisberg, J. (Eds.). (1994). *Physical agents: A comprehensive text for physical therapists.* Norwalk, CT: Appleton & Lange.

Melzack, R., & Wall, P. D. (1965). Pain mechanisms: a new theory. *Science, 150,* 971–999.

Middaugh, S. J., Haythornthwaite, J. A., Thompson, B., Hill, R., Brown, K. M., Freedman, R. R., Attanasio, V., Jacob, R. G., Scheier, M., & Smith, E. A. (2001). The Raynaud's Treatment Study: Biofeedback protocols and acquisition of temperature biofeedback skills. *Applied Psychophysiology and Biofeedback, 26,* 251–278.

Moreland, J. D., Thomas, M. A., & Fuoco, A. R. (1998). Electromyographic biofeedback to improve lower extremity function after stroke: a meta-analysis. *Archives of Physical Medicine and Rehabilitation, 79,* 134–140.

Mulder, G., Brazinsky, B. A., & Seeley, J. (1995). Factors complicating wound repair. In J. M. McCulloch & L. C. Kloth (Eds.), *Wound healing alternatives in management* (2nd ed., pp. 45–59). Philadelphia: F. A. Davis.

Norkin, C., & Levangie, P. (1992). *Joint structure and function: A comprehensive analysis* (2nd ed.). Philadelphia: F. A. Davis.

Ozawa, Y., Shimizu, N., Kariya, G., & Abiko, Y. (1998). Low-energy laser irradiation stimulates bone nodule formation at early stages of cell culture in rat calvarial cells. *Bone, 22,* 347–354.

Phillips, C. A. (1989). Functional electrical stimulation and lower extremity bracing for ambulation exercise of the spinal cord injured individual: A medically prescribed system. *Physical Therapy, 69,* 842–849.

Powell, J., Pandyan, A. D., Granat, M., Cameron, M., & Stott, D. J. (1999). Electrical stimulation of wrist extensors in poststroke hemiplegia. *Stroke, 30,* 1384–1389.

Pullman, S., Goodink, D., Marquinez, A., & Tabbal, S. (2000). Clinical utility of surface EMG: Report of the Therapeutics and Technology Assessment Subcommittee of the American Academy of Neurology. *Neurology, 55,* 171–177.

Reddy, G. K., Gum, S., Stehno-Bittel, L., & Enwemeka, C. S. (1998). Biochemistry and biomechanics of healing tendon: part II. Effects of combined laser therapy and electrical stimulation. *Medicine-Science-Sports-Exercise, 30,* 794–800.

Reddy, G. K., Stehno-Bittel, L., & Enwemeka, C. S. (1998). Laser photostimulation of collagen production in healing rabbit Achilles tendons. *Lasers in Surgery and Medicine, 22,* 281–287.

Reddy, G. K., Stehno-Bittel, L., & Enwemeka, C. S. (1999). Matrix remodeling in healing rabbit Achilles tendon. *Wound Repair Regeneration, 7,* 518–527.

Saperia, D., Glassberg, E., & Lyons, R. F. (1986).Demonstration of elevated type I and III procollagen mRNA level in cutaneous wounds treated with helium-neon laser: Proposed mechanism for enhanced wound healing. *Biochemical and Biophysical Research Communications, 138,* 1123–1128.

Schmidt, K. L. (1999). Heat, cold, and inflammation. *Rheumatology, 39,* 301–404.

Seo, J. T., Choe, J. H., Lee, W. S., & Kim, K. H. (2005). Efficacy of functional electrical stimulation-biofeedback with sexual cognitive-behavioral therapy as treatment of vaginismus. *Urology, 66,* 77–81.

Sicard-Rosenbaum, L., Lord, D., & Danoff, J. (1995). Effects of continuous therapeutic ultrasound on growth and metastasis of subcutaneous murine tumors. *Physical Therapy, 75,* 3–13.

Smania, N., Corato, E., Tinazzi, M., Montagnana, B., Fiaschi, A., & Aglioti, S. M. (2003). The effect of two different rehabilitation treatments in cervical dystonia: preliminary results in four patients. *Functional Neurology, 18,* 219–225.

Vodovnik, L., Bowman, B. R., & Hufford, P. (1984). Effects of electrical stimulation on spinal spasticity. *Scandinavian Journal of Rehabilitation Medicine, 16,* 29–34.

Wang, R. Y., Chan, R. C., & Tsai, M. W. (2000). Functional electrical stimulation on chronic and acute hemiplegic shoulder subluxation. *American Journal of Physical Medicine and Rehabilitation, 79,* 385–394.

Wang, R. Y., Tsai, M. W., & Chan, R. C. (1998). Effects of spinal cord stimulation on spasticity and quantitative assessment of muscle tone in hemiplegic patients. *American Journal of Physical Medicine and Rehabilitation, 77,* 282–287.

Whelan, H. T., Smits, R. L., Buchman, E. V., Whelan, N. T., Turner, S. G., Margolis, D. A., Cevenini, V., Stinson, H., Ignatius, R., Martin, T., Cwiklinski, J., Philippi, A. F., Graf, W. R., Hodgson, B., Gould, L., Kane, M., Chen, G., & Caviness, J. (2001). Effect of NASA light-emitting diode irradiation on wound healing. *Journal of Clinical Laser and Medical Surgery, 19,* 305–314.

Yu, D. T., Cahe, J., Walker, M. E., & Fan, Z. P. (2001). Percutaneous intramuscular neuromuscular eletric stimulation for the treatment of shoulder subluxation and pain in patients with chronic hemiplegia: a pilot study. *Archives of Physical Medicine and Rehabilitation, 82,* 20–25.

Supplemental References

American Occupational Therapy Association [AOTA] Commission on Education Physical Agent Modalities Task Force (1993). Educational Preparation for use of physical agent modalities in occupational therapy (report). Rockville, MD: American Occupational Therapy Association.

Armagan, O., Tascioglu, F., & Oner, C. (2003). Electromyographic biofeedback in the treatment of the hemiplegic hand: A placebo-controlled study. *American Journal of Physical Medicine and Rehabilitation, 82,* 856–861.

Arora, D., Cooley, D., Perry, T., Skliar, M., & Roemer, R. (2005). Direct thermal dose control of constrained focused ultrasound treatments: Phantom and in vivo evaluation. *Physics in Medicine and Biology, 50,* 1919–1935.

Michlovitz, S. L. (1996). *Thermal agents in rehabilitation.* Philadelphia: F. A. Davis.

SECTION V: Treatment of Occupational Function

CHAPTER 21

Optimizing Abilities and Capacities: Range of Motion, Strength, and Endurance

Nancy A. Flinn, Jeanne Jackson, Julie McLaughlin Gray, and Ruth Zemke

LEARNING OBJECTIVES

After studying this chapter, the reader will be able to do the following:

1. State the biomechanical and physiological mechanisms that underlie therapeutic exercise and occupation.
2. Apply the methods of movement, positioning, and compression to prevent limitation of range of motion.
3. Apply the principles of the biomechanical approach to increase range of motion, strength, and endurance as needed for occupational performance.
4. Apply these principles to the selection of occupations as a means for treating range of motion, strength, and/or endurance problems.
5. Design treatment goals and therapy for clients who have problems with range of motion, strength, and/or endurance to enhance occupational performance.

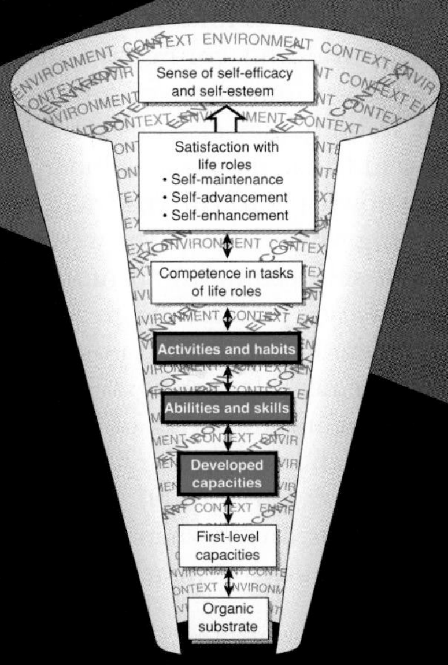

Glossary

Ankylosis—Pathological stiffening of a joint due to fibrotic changes in the bones and/or tissues surrounding the joints.

Concentric contraction—Muscle contraction that moves a limb segment in the direction of the muscle pull.

Contracture—Static shortening of muscle and connective tissue that limits ROM at a joint.

Cross-bridge—ATP segment that moves and reconnects actin and myosin fibrils during muscle contraction.

Eccentric contraction—Muscle contraction that applies a braking force to a movement produced by an opposing force (e.g., gravity) or resistance because the direction of the muscle pull is opposite the actual movement.

Guillain-Barré—An inflammatory disorder in which the body's immune system attacks the peripheral nervous system, resulting in weakness and numbness in the arms, legs, trunk, and face. Most patients make substantial improvements, but about one third of patients still have some residual weakness 3 years after onset.

Heterotopic ossification—Formation of new bone material in an abnormal site, such as adjacent muscle (Salter & Cheshire, 2000).

Kinematics—Study of the form of motion, describing movement paths in terms of the amount and direction of displacement of body segments in meters, velocity or speed in meters per second, and acceleration or rate of change of speed in meters per second squared. Joint angle changes in a given direction are also kinematic characteristics.

Kinetics—Study of forces, including static forces that balance or stabilize and dynamic forces that mobilize.

Parameter—Variable that can be manipulated.

Torque—Product of force × perpendicular distance between the force and the axis of rotation.

According to the Occupational Functioning Model, a goal of occupational therapy is to foster competency and self-esteem through participation in life occupations (see Chapter 1). Biomechanical and physiological principles that relate to movement can provide guidelines for treatment when participation in occupation is threatened because of limitations in the capacities of range of motion, strength, or endurance. For example, occupational therapists use these principles to assist in remediating impairments from acute injuries or compensating for chronic disability to enable occupation. Occupational therapists also use these principles in preventing illnesses and conditions such as cumulative stress trauma and back injuries, which often result from occupations requiring a sustained position or repetitive motions. In this chapter, we will address treatment methods to increase range of motion, strength, and endurance.

MUSCULOSKELETAL SYSTEM

The following is a simple overview of the biomechanical and physiological elements of the musculoskeletal system that underlie range of motion (ROM), strength, and endurance. This basic understanding enables occupational therapists to analyze and prescribe therapeutic occupations and exercise to promote occupational function.

Biomechanical Aspects

The biomechanical aspects of human movement are described in terms of the path of a limb in time or space or the forces that influence that motion, either making it persist or making it cease. These two ways of describing motion are called kinematics and kinetics, respectively.

Kinematic analysis describes the amount and direction of movement, speed, and acceleration of body segments and joint angles (Levangie & Norkin, 2005). Researchers have used these quantitative kinematic descriptors to describe the reaching movements in children with cerebral palsy (Chang et al., 2005), the influence of instructions on reach in adults with and without cerebrovascular accidents (Fasoli et al., 2002), and the effect of wheelchair handrim size on manual wheelchair propulsion (Guo, Su, & An, 2005). Therapists use this information for structuring occupation and designing exercise programs.

Kinetics addresses the forces that cause motion or maintain stability (Hall & Brody, 2005). These forces may be internal to the body, such as muscle contraction or the elasticity of structural and connective tissue, which enable us to engage in our daily occupations. Forces of movement or stability may also be external to an individual, such as wind that moves a sailboat, the friction of grass slowing down a golf ball, the friction of the carpet against a moving wheelchair, or the weight of a spoon, which may limit self-feeding in an individual with muscle weakness. Gravity is perhaps the greatest external force, unnoticeable and constant to most of us, that affects all human movement. It is the gravitational pull on the body, body segments, and other objects that gives them weight and is often the biggest challenge to the patients we treat (Baechle & Earle, 2000). Therapists must be aware of these various forces when developing treatment plans using therapeutic occupations and/or exercise programs.

The following is an example of forces, stability, and motion in occupation. While dining, a person grasps a glass

RESEARCH NOTE 21-1

Abstract: Vuillemin, A., Boini, S., Bertrais, S., Tessier, S., Oppert, J., Hercberg, S., Fuillemin, F., & Briançon, S. (2005). Leisure time physical activity and health-related quality of life. *Preventive Medicine*, 41, 562–569.

Abstract

Background: Intensity, frequency, and duration of physical activity may contribute in various ways to health related quality of life.

Methods: The relationship of frequency and vigorousness of leisure time physical activities and health related quality of life was studied in 2333 male participants aged 45 to 60 years of age, and 3221 female participants aged 35 to 60.

Results: Leisure time physical activity (LTPA) was related to all categories of health related quality of life, including physical functioning, bodily pain, mental health, emotional and physical role performance, social functioning, vitality, and general health. LTPA was divided into four categories: Inactive, Irregular (some activity, but not meeting the next category), Moderate activity (more than 150 minutes/week, but less than the next category), Vigorous activity (more than 60 minutes/week, at high energy cost). Individuals whose leisure time physical activity fell into the "vigorous" category had even better scores in health related quality of life. For all participants, meeting the public health recommendations of 30 minutes of vigorous or moderate activity on a regular basis led to better health related quality of life scores on all dimensions, except for bodily pain in women, which was not affected.

Conclusion: Regular leisure time physical activity of 30 minutes per day, even at a moderate level, can significantly improve health related quality of life.

Implications for Practice

A unique expertise of occupational therapy is the design and prescription of purposeful and meaningful activity (occupation) to enhance and promote health. Along these lines, occupational therapists frequently use therapeutic occupation to improve an individual's ROM, strength, and endurance. This study supports the notion that a variety of daily activities, if performed at moderate or vigorous level, have the potential to improve a client's health-related quality of life.

Occupational therapists should be aware of the variety of activities available for strengthening, endurance building, fitness, and overall health promotion. They should complete a thorough occupational history to learn which activities in the patient's background may provide interest and exercise benefits. Through careful activity analysis and monitoring, occupational therapists can frequently use meaningful and purposeful activity to enhance strength and endurance, achieving the additional cognitive, psychosocial, and spiritual gains these activities may be designed to provide.

filled with a beverage and lifts it to take a sip. This task requires both stability and motion. Initially, muscles in the trunk and shoulder girdle (internal forces) co-contract to provide proximal stability, allowing for controlled distal mobility. To raise the glass, muscle contractions of the elbow flexors act as an internal force that overcomes the weight of the forearm and hand and the glass (external forces). The biceps contraction causes rotary motion, or flexion, of the elbow joint. When rotary motion occurs, each point on the bone segment (ulna and radius) moves through an arc at the same time at a constant distance from the axis (elbow joint) (Levangie & Norkin, 2005). The arc formed by that rotary movement is called the ROM of that joint. To cause rotation, the biceps must have enough strength to overcome the external forces created by gravity.

To analyze the movement in this scenario, one must also consider **torque**. Torque is the effectiveness of a force in causing rotary movement (Levangie & Norkin, 2005). In rotary movements, torque depends on (1) the amount of force applied and (2) the distance of the force from the axis of movement. Thus, in mathematical terms, the torque of a force is equal to the amount of force applied times the perpendicular distance between the line of force and the axis of rotation [$T = (F)(D)$] (Levangie & Norkin, 2005; Neumann, 2002). In relation to the example of taking a sip, the torque of the biceps (effort force) is equal to the force the muscle can produce times the perpendicular distance from its insertion on the radius to the axis of motion or elbow joint (Fig. 21-1A). The torque of resistance force (the glass and forearm) is equal to the resistance force (weight of glass and forearm) times the perpendicular distance between the glass and the axis of movement or elbow joint (Fig. 21-1B). In this case, biceps torque is greater than the torque of the forearm and glass, so flexion can occur.

The concept of torque shows that the placement of an object either closer to or farther from the axis of rotation changes the effort needed to make the movement, even though the object's weight remains constant. Therapists use this concept in a number of situations. For example, a short reacher as opposed to a long one requires less force of the patient's upper extremity muscles to pick up an object. With a long reacher, the object provides more resistance torque because the distance between the object and the person's joint (axis of movement) is greater than with the short reacher. Likewise, when assisting a patient to perform a stand-and-pivot transfer from the wheelchair to bed, a therapist stands close to the patient as they both pivot, and the therapist lowers the patient to a sitting position. The patient provides less resistance torque (the weight of the patient times the perpendicular distance between the patient and the therapist's back) when he or she is close to the therapist. This in turn requires less effort force by the therapist's back muscles for raising, maintaining the position during the pivot, and lowering the patient to the bedside. This body mechanic principle for protecting stress on one's back (i.e., holding objects close

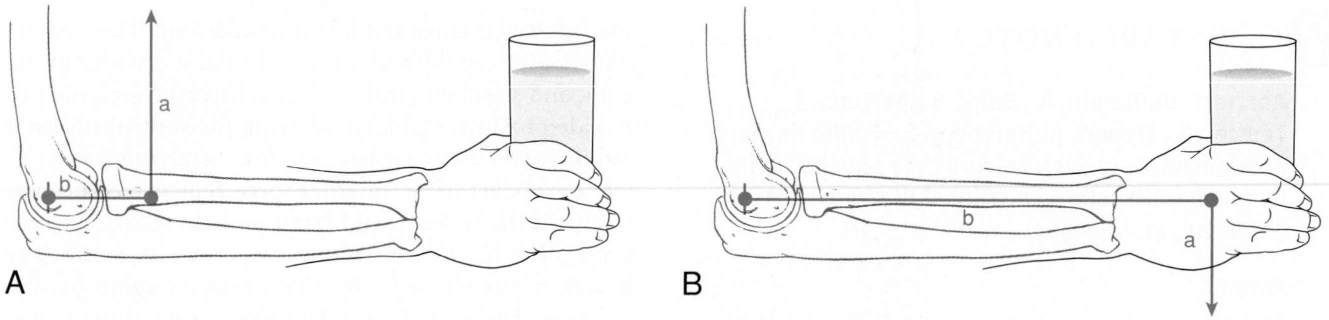

Figure 21-1 **A.** Torque of effort force. *a*, Line of pull of effort force (elbow flexors). *b*, Perpendicular distance between the insertion of the elbow flexors and the axis of rotation. **B.** Torque of resistance force. *a*, Line of pull of resistance force (weight of glass and forearm). *b*, Perpendicular distance between the resistance force and the axis of rotation.

to one's center of gravity when lifting or transporting) can be explained by this principle of torque.

In biomechanical terms, rotary movement is analyzed as one of three types of lever systems. A lever system consists of a rigid bar (such as a bone), an axis of rotation (such as a joint), and two forces, effort and resistance. Effort is the force that causes movement, and resistance is the force that tends to keep the object from moving.

A first-class lever is a system in which the effort and resistance forces lie on either side of the axis of rotation (Levangie & Norkin, 2005). A common example of a first-class lever is the seesaw (Fig. 21-2A). As one can see, a seesaw would remain in balance, with no movement, if two children of the same weight sat the same distance from the axis. This balance, or equilibrium, is maintained because the torque (weight of child 1 times the perpendicular distance from child 1 to the axis of rotation) on one side of the seesaw equals the torque (weight of child 2 times the perpendicular distance from child 2 to the axis of rotation) on the opposite side of the seesaw. In essence, they balance, and there is no movement. If one of the children is heavier, he or she must move closer to the axis to maintain that balance (Fig. 21-2B).

In second- and third-class levers, the effort and resistance force lie on the same side of the axis (Baechle & Earle, 2000). A second-class lever system, such as a bottle opener or a wheelbarrow used to carry compost in a garden, is a system in which the resistance force lies closer to the axis of rotation than does the effort force (Fig. 21-3). With a bottle opener, the resistance force is the force of the cap that is tightly connected to the bottle. The effort force is a person's hand lifting the end of the opener to release the cap. This lever system allows a relatively small amount of force to overcome strong resistance. Second-class lever systems explain the tools used frequently in occupations when mechanical advantage is required, such as an extended handle on a faucet.

In third-class lever systems the effort force lies closer to the axis than does the resistance force (Levangie & Norkin, 2005) (Fig. 21-4, top). The example of bringing a glass to

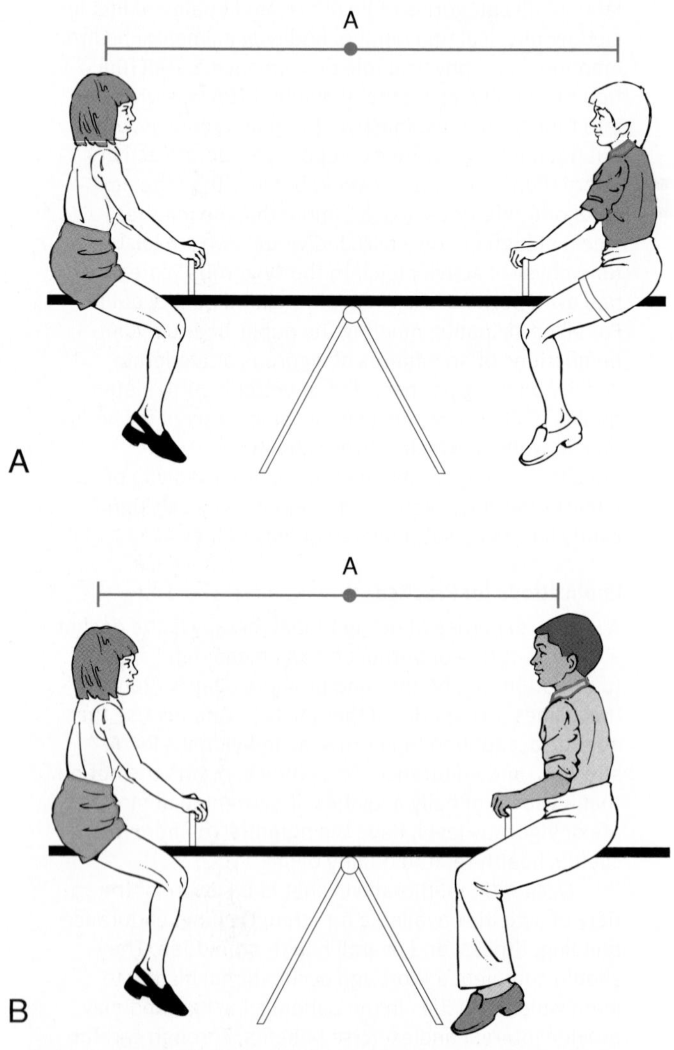

Figure 21-2 **A.** First-class lever system. Balanced equilibrium depicted by children on a seesaw. Both children weigh 60 pounds, and they are equidistant from the axis. **B.** First-class lever system. The heavier child must be closer to the axis of the seesaw to maintain the equilibrium.

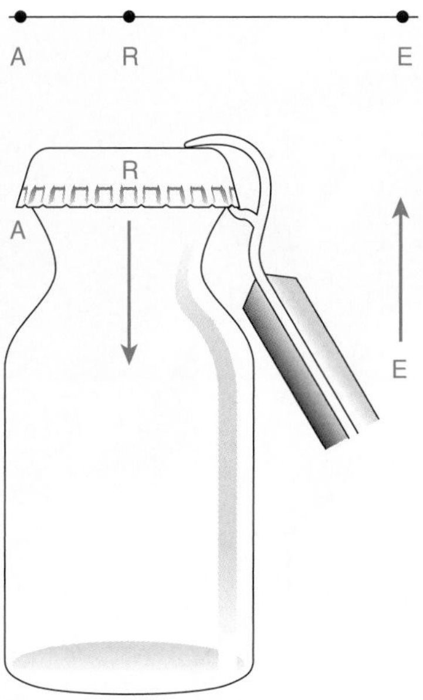

Figure 21-3 Top, Schematic drawing of a second-class lever. Bottom, Second-class lever depicted by using a bottle opener to remove the cap from a bottle. *A,* axis; *R,* resistance force (tightly secured cap); *E,* effort force (force from bottle opener to open cap).

one's mouth represents a third-class lever. The elbow joint is the axis; the biceps is the effort force; and the combined weight of the forearm and glass is the resistance force (Fig. 21-4, bottom). In contrast to the stability of first-class levers and the mechanical advantage of second-class levers, third-class levers produce greater speed and ROM. For this reason, most of the muscles in the human body work in third-class lever systems when they contract concentrically to produce the speed and ROM needed to engage in occupation.

The mechanical aspects of the musculoskeletal system promote both stability and mobility to provide the basis for action in occupation. The potential work capacity of the various muscles of the body also depends on the force they can generate and the distance over which they can shorten. In other words, the resulting work depends not only on biomechanical factors but also on physiological factors.

Physiological Aspects

The contractile portion of skeletal muscle is within the myofibrils of the muscle, where adenosine 5+ triphosphate (ATP) creates **cross-bridges** between the actin and myosin filaments. According to the sliding filament theory, muscle contraction occurs when the ATP cross-bridges are broken, actin is pulled over the myosin, and new cross-bridges are developed (Fig. 21-5) (Levangie & Norkin, 2005; Baechle & Earle, 2000). As this sequence continues, tension is generated, and the muscle shortens **(concentric contraction)**. In a lengthening contraction **(eccentric contraction)**, the opposite process occurs (Definition 21-1).

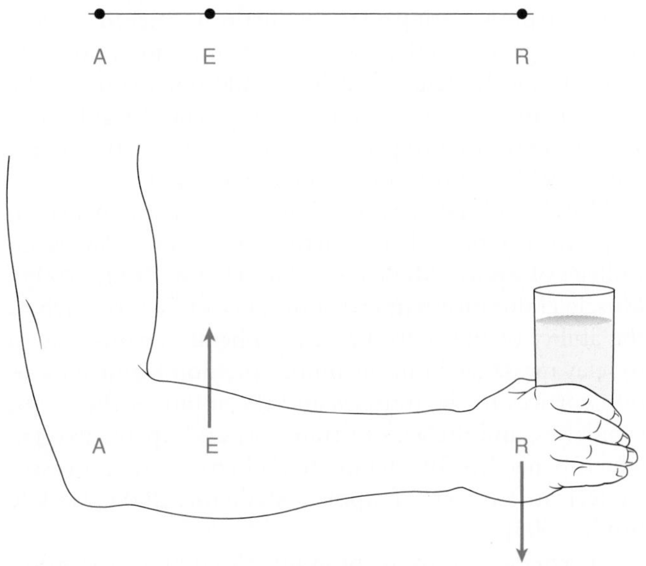

Figure 21-4 Top, Schematic drawing of a third-class lever. Bottom, Third-class lever depicted by lifting a filled glass. *A,* axis; *E,* effort force (elbow flexors); *R,* resistance force (weight of glass and forearm).

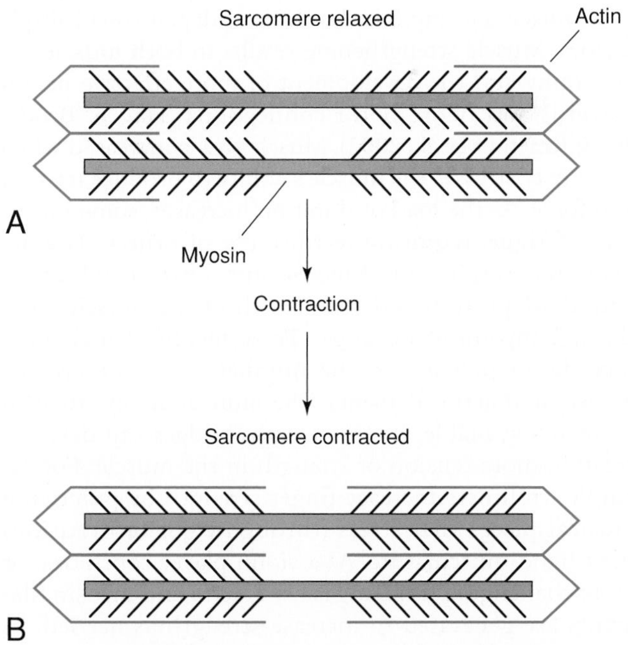

Figure 21-5 Schematic of actin and myosin cross-bridges during muscle relaxation and contraction. **A.** Relaxed muscle. **B.** Contracted muscle. (Adapted with permission from Hall, C. M., & Brody, L. T. [1999]. Functional approach to therapeutic exercise for physiological impairments. In C. Hall & L. Brody [Eds.], Therapeutic exercise: Moving toward function (pp. 45–46). Philadelphia: Lippincott Williams & Wilkins.)

DEFINITION 21-1

Types of Muscle Contractions

Concentric

Muscle shortens to move a limb section in the direction of the muscle pull. In a concentric contraction, the internal force of the muscle overcomes the external resistance.

Eccentric

Contracted muscle lengthens to act as a brake against an external force to allow for a smooth controlled movement.

Isometric

External and internal forces are in equilibrium, and the length of a contracted muscle remains the same.

Example

In Figure 21-6, lowering a filled 10-pound cookie jar from the top of the refrigerator uses an eccentric contraction of the shoulder flexors and, concurrently, of the scapula upward rotators. Returning the cookie jar to the top of the refrigerator before mom finds out you have eaten the cookies requires concentric contractions of the shoulder flexors and, concurrently, the scapula upward rotators. Maintaining a grasp on the cookie jar exemplifies isometric contraction of the shoulder horizontal adductors and the distal upper extremity muscles.

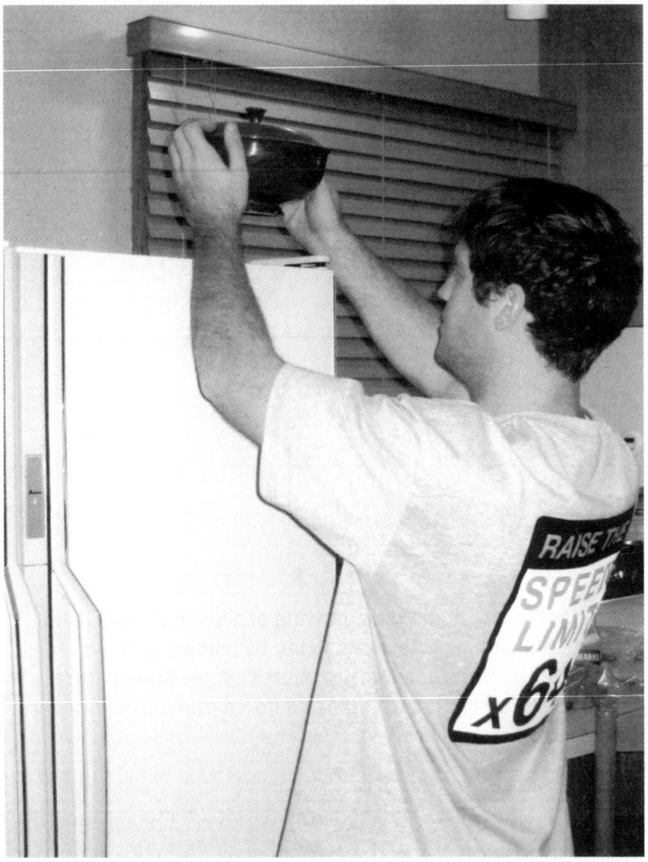

Figure 21-6 Getting a cookie jar down from the top of the refrigerator and putting it back requires eccentric, concentric, and isometric muscle contractions.

A muscle's strength and endurance depend on multiple factors. Muscle strengthening results in both muscle hypertrophy and the development of more effective neural patterns and neuromotor connections (Hall & Brody, 2005; Kraemer et al., 2002). Muscle size is increased when an activity stresses the muscle's ability to produce tension and force. As the load or duration increases, some motor units fatigue, requiring recruitment of others. The demand for recruitment of motor units ultimately leads to neural adaptation and the growth of the muscle fiber through myofibrillar changes. Those myofibrillar changes include an increase in the number of sarcomeres or myosin and actin filaments. The more actin and myosin filaments available, the more cross-bridges can develop, creating more tension or strength in the muscle. For example, violinists increase finger strength by practicing musical pieces that stress (through vigor or duration) their hand musculature. As a violin player continues, or more challenging fingering is used, actin and myosin filaments are generated to increase strength as needed. In contrast, when muscles are not used, myosin and actin filaments are lost, resulting in weakness.

Neural change, namely increased number of motor units activated and increased synchrony of motor unit activation, also contributes to muscle strength (Elbert et al., 1998; Kisner & Colby, 2002; Kraemer et al., 2002). Individual motor units, which make up muscles, fire according to the all-or-none principle of neural propagation. When all of the required motor units of the hand and finger muscles needed to press a string on the violin fire in synchrony, more tension is generated than when those same motor units fire asynchronously. Remember that, in addition to muscle size and synchrony of motor unit firing, psychological factors, such as motivation to perform an occupation, affect effort exerted, which contributes to muscle strength.

Muscle endurance is the ability of a muscle to sustain or perform repeated contractions over time (American College of Sports Medicine, 2000; Hall & Brody, 2005). Muscle endurance relies on a number of factors, such as the ability of the central and peripheral nervous system to relay messages from the limbic, premotor, and association cortices to the muscles and the ability of the lungs, capillaries, and muscles to transport and uptake oxygen, which is needed for metabolic and enzymatic processes (American College of Sports Medicine, 2000; Hall & Brody, 2005).

In general, improvement in muscle endurance requires availability of more oxygen. When heart rate increases, so does the amount of oxygen the person can take in during a given amount of time and dispense to the muscles (VO_2). The muscles require oxygen to break down ATP into the

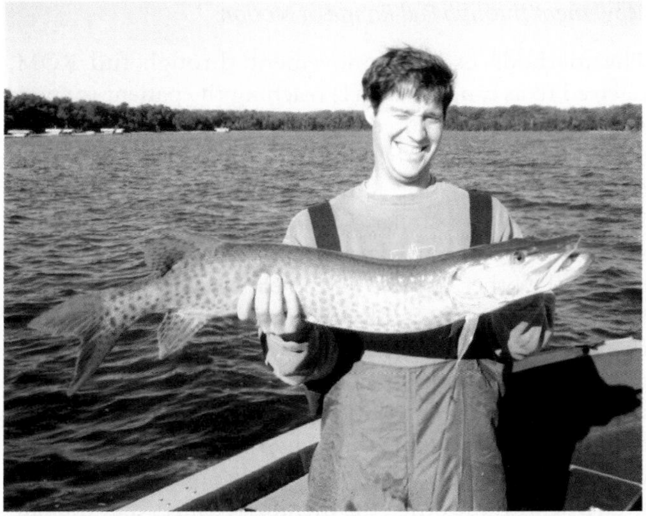

Figure 21-7 Fishing is an occupation that requires both muscular strength and muscular endurance.

chemical energy needed for actin and myosin to form cross-bridges and thus create a muscle contraction (American College of Sports Medicine, 2000; Baechle & Earle, 2000). Local muscle fatigue is often related to impaired capillary systems interfering with the transportation of blood (oxygen) to the muscles, insufficient storage of glycogen, and/or a disruption of the metabolic process that breaks ATP into chemical energy (Hall & Brody, 2005).

Muscle endurance is intricately related to muscle strength. In fact, most occupations that require muscular endurance, such as tennis, also require muscle strength. For example, in Figure 21-7, muscular strength was required to hold up the fish for the picture, but muscular endurance was also required to get the fish into the boat. For many of our clients, endurance and strength are related problems, although some occupations, such as those requiring maintained postural control, require muscle endurance more than muscle strength. (For a more detailed understanding of the cardiac and pulmonary systems, see Chapter 47.)

BIOMECHANICAL APPROACH TO TREATMENT

Based on these biomechanical and physiological principles, occupational therapists can design treatment programs to address ROM, strength, and endurance problems affecting occupation. Ultimately the remediation or prevention of these limitations is aimed at ensuring the individual's occupational functioning.

Maintaining or Preventing Limitation in Range of Motion

ROM assessments provide guidelines for the typical ranges available at various joints in the human body, but an individual's actual ROM at any joint is determined by the physical constitution of the body and the person's typical occupations. For example, a waiter who carries platters of food with one hand throughout the work shift probably has greater wrist extension ROM than most others. Functional ROM is the range necessary to perform daily occupations. Occupational therapists are concerned with preventing ROM limitations that interfere with daily occupations.

Immobilization Reduces Range of Motion

Many ROM limitations can and should be prevented. When a joint remains immobilized, changes in the muscle through loss of muscle fiber, changes in the number and length of sarcomeres, and changes in the connective tissue through disorganized synthesis of new collagen, ligament weakness, and elastic stiffness result in shortening of the muscle itself. These changes, along with disruption of the workings of the synovial fluid, synovial membrane, and articular cartilage, create limitations in ROM (De Deyne, 2001; Hall & Brody, 2005). Tendons and ligaments change biochemically and lose tensile strength in the absence of motion and stress. With immobilization, muscle filaments lose their ability to slide, which is necessary for contraction. Edema and developing viscosity of fluid can increase the circumference of a joint and limit ROM (Hall & Brody, 2005; Kisner & Colby, 2002; Wong, 2002). Prolonged swelling leads to fibrotic changes and adhesions in the edematous tissue that result in **contractures** (Wong, 2002). Changes begin at as early as 24 hours of immobilization. As a result of these underlying changes, a joint maintains only the range through which it is moved on a regular basis.

Patients who cannot move their own joints and for whom motion is not contraindicated need passive ROM exercises and proper positioning to maintain their available ROM. For example, when a patient is in a coma or unable to move because of paralysis, ROM should be maintained to enable a return to occupations when recovery occurs. Also, when an agonist muscle is significantly weaker than its antagonist, the uneven tension between the two muscles may create a contracture. Furthermore, maintaining ROM can prevent discomfort, skin breakdown, hygiene problems, and difficulty in caring for the person. Occupational therapists are ultimately concerned with limitations in ROM that affect a client's ability to perform occupations.

Methods

The methods occupational therapists use to prevent limitations in ROM include compression, positioning, and movement through full ROM.

Compression

Compression is used to prevent ROM limitations secondary to edema. Edema can be controlled by compression with elastic strip or tubular bandages. The occupational therapist must take care to apply these correctly so they do not constrict circulation in the more distal part of the extremity. ***Skin color is observed regularly to confirm that circulation is preserved.*** Coban (3M, St. Paul, MN), a self-adhesive elastic bandage, is wrapped around the part spirally in a distal to proximal direction, and the edges are overlapped by at least 25% of the width of the material so that the fluid can flow evenly back toward the body and not be trapped in pockets of unwrapped tissue (Lowell et al., 2003; Salter & Cheshire, 2000). Tubigrip (Mark One Health Care Products, Philadelphia, PA) is a tubular elastic support bandage that provides graduated constant pressure support when the correct size is applied. Compression is most effective in eliminating edema when combined with positioning and passive or active movement of the limb.

Positioning

When a person's limb is too weak to resist gravity, positioning in a resting or functional position is essential to avoid development of deformities, minimize edema, and maintain ROM gained in treatment. Positions of function are encouraged, and all non-functional positions are avoided throughout the day and night. In particular, positions that are opposite of normal patterns of tightness should be encouraged for at least periods of the day. For example, patients often develop tightness in the shoulder internal rotators after stroke. So, positioning the patient with the arm in at least neutral rotation will help prevent that tightness from developing. In addition, elevating a patient's edematous hand by use of a pillow assists the fluid to drain back to the body.

In spite of prevention, sometimes contractures and consequent **ankylosis** are unavoidable because of the disease process. In these instances, positioning, splinting, and bracing are used to ensure that ankylosis occurs in as nearly a functional position as possible. A functional fixed position is one that allows the person to manage self-care and other functional tasks. For example, the functional position of the hand and wrist is slight (10–30°) extension of the wrist, opposition and abduction of the thumb, and semi-flexion of the finger joints. If a patient's hand contracts in that position, the person can still use it to hold objects. If, however, the hand contracts in a fully flexed position, it not only is non-functional but also presents a hygiene problem. Likewise, a hand that fuses in an extension contracture has no holding capacity. When positioning a patient, the occupational therapist must be vigilant in anticipating eventual outcomes of prolonged immobilization that may compromise occupational performance.

Movement through Full Range of Motion

The methods used for movement through full ROM, referred to as ranging, are (1) teaching the patient to move the joints that are injured, immobilized, or edematous and (2) passively moving the joints if the patient cannot. The ranging technique for active ROM (AROM) and passive ROM (PROM) are similar. Twice daily each involved joint is slowly and gently moved three times from one limit of motion to the other. In AROM, the patient actively performs the desired motion. In PROM, the therapist gently moves the patient's limb through the desired motion, paying particular attention to planes of motion and joint biomechanics. For example, the therapist pays special attention to the scapulohumeral rhythm when ranging the shoulder girdle. By moving the scapula with one hand and the humerus with the other, the therapist ensures that they are moving in synchrony (Fig. 21-8). Attention to this alignment during movement of the scapula and humerus eliminates injury to the glenohumeral joint, bursae, capsule, and ligaments. As previously mentioned, the joint maintains only the range through which it is moved and, therefore, the

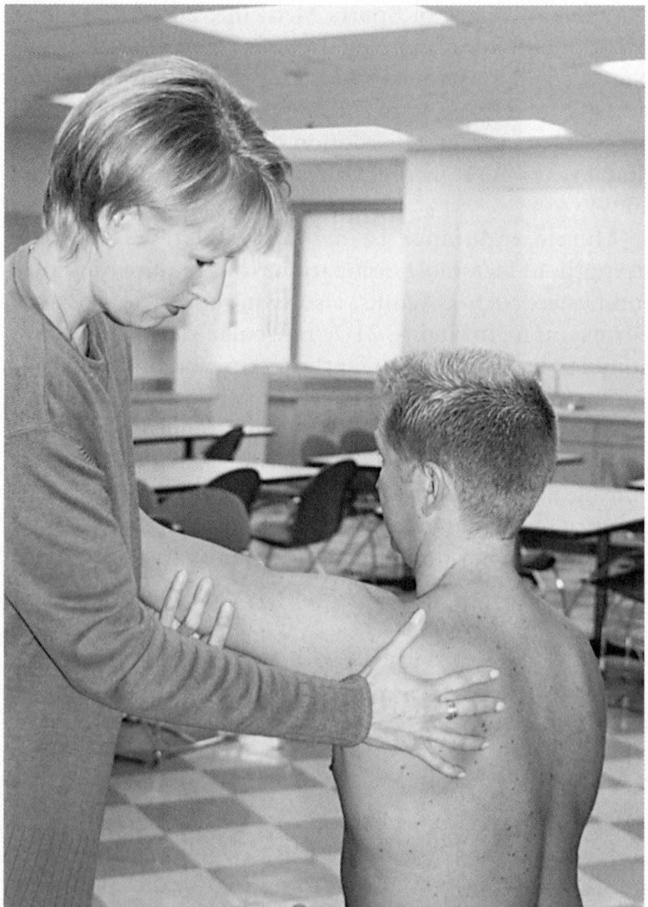

Figure 21-8 Facilitation of glenohumeral rhythm during passive ROM.

therapist or patient must move a limb through the full available range or it will not be maintained. ***Exception: A person who has tetraplegia and will rely on tenodesis action for grasp (see Chapter 43) must be ranged in the following manner to allow finger flexor tendons to develop necessary tightness for grasping. When flexing the fingers, the wrist must be fully extended, and when extending the fingers, the wrist must be fully flexed.***

PROM can also be performed by external devices, such continuous passive motion (CPM) machines. CPM machines are commercial orthoses used to maintain ROM and prevent postoperative swelling by continually moving the joint from one limit of motion to the other (Griggs, Ahn, & Greene, 2002; Salter & Cheshire, 2000). See O'Driscoll and Giori (2000); Michlovitz, Harris, and Watkins (2004); and LaStayo et al. (1998) for additional information on the use of CPM with the upper extremities.

AROM is preferred to PROM for reduction of edema because the contraction of the muscles helps pump the fluid out of the extremity. If AROM is not possible, however, PROM can aid in reducing edema. Positioning of the edematous extremity above the heart during distal PROM is recommended to aid in venous return.

Occupational therapists often structure activities to provide AROM to prevent limitations in ROM. For example, the patient may use his or her hemiplegic upper extremity in weight bearing for balance and postural stability while having to maintain the ROM in wrist and finger extension. Another example is the *ROM Dance Program* devised by Harlowe and Yu, which is a 7-minute movement program modeled after Tai Chi Chuan that incorporates joint motion in all ranges while the dancer listens to a poem that is meant to evoke pleasurable images. Although the ROM dance was developed for people with rheumatoid arthritis, it has been used with other populations, including the well elderly (Mandel et al., 1999).

Increasing Range of Motion

If limitations in ROM impair a patient's ability to function independently in occupations or are likely to lead to deformity, treatment to increase ROM is indicated. Whereas some significant limitations of ROM can be ameliorated or corrected by occupation and exercise, some cannot. Problems that can be changed include contractures of soft tissue, such as skin, muscles, tendons, and ligaments. Problems that cannot be changed through these means include bony ankylosis or arthrodesis, long-standing contractures in which there are extensive fibrotic changes in soft tissue, and severe joint destruction.

Occupational therapists may treat ROM limitations, using the principle of stretch, to help a patient develop the capacities needed to perform occupations. If ROM limitations cannot be reduced, occupational therapy becomes compensatory, focusing on providing techniques and/or equipment to enable participation in life occupations.

Stretching

Stretch is a process by which tissue is lengthened by an external force, usually to eliminate tightness that has the potential to cause a contracture. Stretch produces change only if done to the point of maximal stretch, defined as a few degrees beyond the point of discomfort, and held there for between 15 and 30 seconds (Bandy & Sanders, 2001). The force, speed, direction, and extent of stretch must be controlled (Kisner & Colby, 2002; Salter & Cheshire, 2000). The force must be enough to put tension on the tissue but not enough to rupture it. Different tissues tolerate stretch differently; tight muscles can be stretched more vigorously than tight joints (Kottke, 1990). The speed should be slow to allow the tissue to adjust gradually. The direction of stretch is exactly opposite to the tightness. The stretch is applied to the point of maximal stretch.

Gentle stretching that achieves small increments of gain over time is more effective than vigorous stretching aimed at large, rapid gains. As a protective mechanism, connective tissue resists quick, vigorous stretching, which is therefore ineffective or injurious (Kisner & Colby, 2002; Kottke, 1990; Salter & Cheshire, 2000). The method of moving gently to the point of maximal stretch and holding that position allows connective tissue, which has plasticity, to adapt to new requirements and adjust its length gradually over time. ***Residual pain after stretching indicates that the stretch was too forceful and caused tearing of soft tissues or blood vessels.*** It is clinically recognized that maintained stretching is most effective; however, gains are also noted using a briefly held stretch, usually 15–30 seconds (Bandy, 2001; Kisner & Colby, 2002). A study of healthy subjects found that 30 seconds of passive stretch was as effective as 120 seconds (Ford, Mazzone, & Taylor, 2005).

Methods

There are two types of stretching, active and passive. In active stretching, the muscle contraction is the source of the force, and in passive stretching, an external force is applied.

Active Stretching

An occupational therapist's expertise lies in using occupations for treatment, in this case as a means of reaching the goal of increasing ROM. The use of occupation for stretching is empirically based on the idea that a person involved in an interesting and purposeful activity will gain greater range because he or she is relaxed, is not anticipating pain, is motivated to complete the task, and therefore is likely to move as the activity demands.

The therapist and patient choose a life occupation that has significance to the patient. Occupations can be performed using a number of muscle patterns, thus, the therapist must determine how the patient completed the activity prior to injury. If the activity, as naturally performed by the patient, requires stretching the soft tissues that are shortened, it can be used as a form of active stretching. Occupations used as a means to increase ROM must provide a gentle active stretch by use of slow, repetitive isotonic contractions of the muscle opposite the contracture or by use of a prolonged passive stretched position of the contracted tissue. In both types of stretch, the requirement is that the range be increased slightly beyond the limitations. If the contracture existed before the limb was immobilized, active stretch is not likely to be effective; that is, if the patient was free to move and did not during daily activities, it is unlikely that gains will be made using activity to correct the contracture. People move in individually characteristic ways and frequently compensate by using available range in adjacent joints, so the therapist must carefully monitor the patient's motions. The therapist cannot assume that the activity itself will evoke the desired response in all persons. Reasonable adaptations of the occupation may sometimes be used to elicit the desired motions. Examples of adaptations are adjusting the size of a handle to stretch finger flexors or extensors or placing an object on a higher shelf to increase the amount of shoulder ROM during daily activities (Fig. 21-9). See Evidence Table 21-1 for support for occupationally based range of motion exercises.

Exercises that increase the range of shortened tissue are the proprioceptive neuromuscular facilitation (PNF) techniques called contract-relax (CR) and agonist contraction (AC) (Bonnar, Deivert, & Gould, 2004; Feland, Myrer, & Merrill, 2001) (Chapter 26). CR involves a maximal isometric contraction of the tight muscle, usually performed at the point of limitation. The muscle is contracted maximally for approximately 3–10 seconds against resistance provided by the therapist and then relaxed. During the relaxation phase, the therapist moves the part in the direction opposite to the contraction and holds it. For example, if there is a contracture of elbow flexors, the elbow is extended to its limit. The patient is instructed to contract the flexors isometrically and maximally and then relax, at which moment the therapist smoothly extends the elbow into greater range. The CR is repeated until as many increments of gain as possible are achieved.

Therapists have typically used a variety of stretching techniques, including those described here. Based on a review of studies spanning 20 years, Hall and Brody (2005) concluded that no one technique has been demonstrated to have greater benefit over any other.

Passive Stretching

Although passive stretching is often done by a physical therapist, occupational therapists may have to perform passive stretching prior to engagement in occupation. Techniques for passive stretching may include manual stretch and the use of orthotic devices, such as splints or casts, to provide controlled passive stretching (see Chapter 16). The procedures for manual stretching by the therapist are outlined in Procedures for Practice 21-1. Safety Note 21-1 lists precautions.

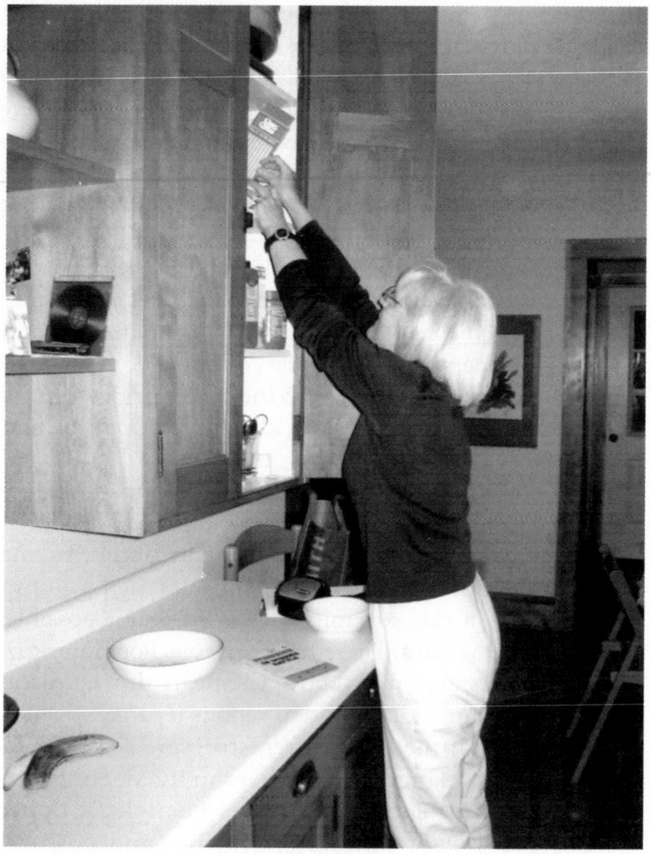

Figure 21-9 Placing an object on a higher shelf can help incorporate greater active range of motion into the daily activity of cooking.

Some patients can perform passive stretching of soft tissue contractures themselves. Activities such as the ROM dance, which includes some passive stretching, can be integrated into their daily occupations. Occupational therapists can modify the ROM dance to provide the necessary active and passive stretches to meet the patient's needs. Therapists must remember that with any method to increase rather than maintain ROM, the patient's limb must move to the point of maximal stretch.

Strengthening

If limitations in a patient's strength prevent participation in occupations or may lead to a deformity, treatment aimed at increasing strength is warranted. Weakness can be deforming if the muscles on one side of a joint are significantly weaker than their antagonists, as in a patient

PROCEDURES FOR PRACTICE 21-1

Manual Stretching Methods

- Provide a relaxing environment for the patient.
- Describe manual stretching, noting that it involves tolerable pain.
- Use motions identical to motions used in ROM evaluation (see Chapter 5).
- Stabilize the bone proximal and distal to the joint that is to be moved to avoid any compensatory movement.
- Move the bone smoothly, slowly, and gently to the point of maximal stretch (mild discomfort indicated verbally or facially by the patient).
- Make sure the movement is in the line of pull of the muscle.
- Encourage the patient to assist in moving the limb if possible.
- Hold the limb at the point of maximal stretch for 15–30 seconds (Kisner & Colby, 2002).
- Relief of discomfort should immediately follow the release of stretch.
- If the patient complains of residual pain, future stretches should be performed more slowly and with less force.

SAFETY NOTE 21-1

Safety Precautions Related to Passive Stretching

- Inflammation weakens the structure of collagen tissues; therefore, those tissues must be stretched cautiously with slow, gentle motion (Kottke, 1990).
- Sensory loss prevents the patient from monitoring pain; thus, the therapist must pay particular attention to the tension of the tissues being stretched.
- Overstretching must be avoided because it causes internal bleeding and subsequent scar formation that may eventually ossify. Overstretching can lead to **heterotopic ossification**.
- Resistance can be provided by weights either held in patient's hand or strapped around the moving part. Resistance can also be provided by tools and materials of activity. The greater the resistance that is provided, the more aggressive the stretch will be, so the therapist must take care that the stretch is slow and gentle.

after a stroke, in whom there is activation of the biceps (elbow flexor) but no activation of elbow extensors. These patients often develop an elbow flexion contracture if stretching is not done. If the weakness prohibits the person from moving the limb or maintaining a functional position, the lack of regular active range of motion will lead to contracture.

Muscle strength increases when the muscle is stressed to the extent that additional motor units are recruited through increased efficiency of the neuromotor system, and the muscle hypertrophies (Hall & Brody, 2005; Kraemer et al., 2002). For muscles to hypertrophy and strengthen they must be stressed to the point of fatigue. Occupation or exercise **parameters** that may be manipulated to increase stress to a muscle include type of contraction, intensity or load, duration of contraction, rate or velocity of contraction, and the frequency of exercise. It is important to realize that strengthening is a very specific process, that muscle will only gain strength within the range of motion that is exercised, and that the speed of contraction is quite specific. Therefore, if there are specific activities that the strengthening is being designed to address, the types of contractions, ranges of motion, and speed of contraction of the strengthening program should be similar to the performance environment. If the patient needs general strengthening, then the types of contractions, ranges of motion, and strength of contraction should be varied (Hall & Brody, 2005; Kraemer et al., 2002).

Methods

Occupations and Exercise

Occupations, exercise, or both can be used to increase strength. Therapists may find that various occupations provide sufficient opportunities for muscle strengthening and are more effective at maintaining the patient's interest and motivation than exercise alone. At other times, therapists may develop an exercise program specifically targeted to strengthen certain muscles needed for occupation. This exercise may also be combined with occupation in a number of ways. Exercise may be used as a warm-up to occupation, or occupation may be introduced to enhance carryover of the strength gained by exercise. Carefully prescribed therapeutic occupations can strengthen muscles in situations closely approximating their intended uses.

For some individuals, an exercise program may be a valued occupation in and of itself. In these cases, exercise can be used as a therapeutic occupation designed to address the individual nature of the performance, the meaning of exercise for that person, and the context in which that person typically exercises. In this instance, the occupational therapist may use the therapeutic occupation of exercise to remediate any performance component. For example, weightlifting can be used with a patient who has a brain injury not only to increase strength but also to enhance attention, memory, and organizational skills (see Chapters 29 and 39).

Grading Muscle Strength Parameters

When prescribing a strengthening program, therapists can manipulate the exercise or occupational parameters. DeLorme (1945) and DeLorme and Watkins (1948) developed exercise programs based on principles of resistance and repetition to increase muscle strength. DeLorme's classic method, progressive resistive exercise, continues to be used today in a modified form. Progressive resistive exercise is a program in which a person lifts 50%, then 75%, and finally 100% of his or her 10-repetition maximum (RM) (Baechle & Earle, 2000). Ten RM is the maximum weight a person can lift with coordination through full ROM 10 times. Each exercise set (50%, 75%, and 100%) is done 10 times, with a rest break between sets. For example, if a client's 10-RM was 10 pounds, the client would repeat 10 repetitions with 5 pounds, 10 repetitions with 7.5 pounds, and 10 repetitions with 10 pounds. Procedures for Practice 21-3 has guidelines for setting up a therapeutic exercise or occupation program. Although these guidelines are for exercise programs, the principles can be used in designing a routine of occupations to be used for strengthening.

More recently, a simplified strengthening protocol has been identified (Rhea et al., 2003.) In this protocol, the patient's 1-repetition maximum (1-RM) is established by determining the maximum weight a warmed-up muscle can move smoothly through the range of motion one time, but not two times. The amount of resistance provided during strengthening is determined by the patient's strength training history. For patients who are untrained or who have not lifted weights consistently in the past year, 60% of 1-RM is moved through the full ROM 10 times, followed by a rest break. For individuals who are considered trained or who have been doing strength training consistently for more than 1 year, 80% of the 1-RM is moved through the full ROM 10 times, followed by a rest break. Four sets of the 10 repetitions are completed for each muscle's strengthening program, regardless of whether the patient is trained or untrained. This strengthening program should be repeated three times a week for untrained individuals and two times a week for trained individuals. The advantage of this simplified strengthening protocol is that there is less changing of weights required and it can be more easily integrated into occupation.

The use of elastic bands for strengthening exercise provides an inexpensive method of strengthening and is often used when patients will be doing strengthening on their own, as in a home program or in community-based programs, where resources are often limited (Gill et al., 2003; Rogers et al., 2002). The elastic bands are color coded for different levels of resistance and have been shown to be an effective method of providing isotonic strengthening (McCann et al., 1993). The elastic bands are cut to length and tied into a loop. The loop is stabilized on one end by one limb of the client, or it can be attached to a stable object in the environment. The occupational therapist designs the exercises so that the joint moves through the full range of motion against the resistance provided by the elastic band. The client is asked to move the joint through the full range of motion against the resistance of the loop. In Figure 21-10, the subject is strengthening her right triceps by holding the loop against her chest with her left hand, while her right arm goes through full elbow extension. In addition, in this case, a small piece of plastic pipe has been added to the loop to provide a handle for the client to use.

The type of contraction—concentric, eccentric, or isometric—is established by the demands of the task and assistance provided by the therapist (see Definition 21-1). Isometric contraction of a muscle at resting length can produce the most forceful contraction. ***When the patient has hypertension or cardiovascular problems, however, isometric contraction should be avoided because isometric contraction of either large or small muscles increases blood pressure and heart rate (Kisner & Colby, 2002; Hall & Brody, 2005) (see Chapter 47).*** More weight can be lowered by a given muscle during an eccentric contraction than can be lifted concentrically or held at any one point. A corollary is that less effort is exerted when lowering a given weight than when lifting it. Regardless, the type of contraction should mirror what is required by the patient's occupations because transfer of ef-

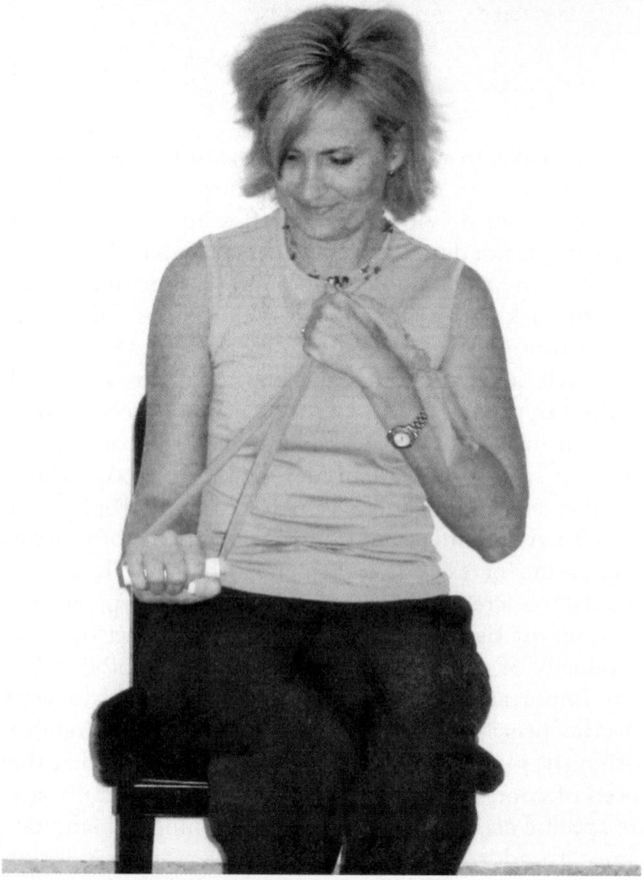

Figure 21-10 The patient is strengthening her triceps by moving her arm from elbow flexion to elbow extension against the resistance of the elastic band.

PROCEDURES FOR PRACTICE 21-3

Guidelines for a Strengthening Program

Type of Exercise	Definition	Muscle Grades	Procedures
Isometric	Exercise in which a weak muscle is isometrically contracted to its maximal force 10 times with rest periods between each contraction	Trace (0) The force of contraction is not sufficient to move the part.	Provide a stimulating environment. Explain procedures. Instruct the patient to contract the weak muscle ("hold"). External resistance applied by the therapist may help the patient isolate the contraction to the weak muscle or muscle group. Patient holds contraction at maximum effort as long as possible while breathing normally. Repeat 10 times with a rest between each contraction. Increase duration of maximal contraction as patient improves. *Maximal isometric contraction is contraindicated for patients with cardiac disease.*
Isotonic Assistive (Active Assistive ROM)	Exercise in which a weak muscle is concentrically or eccentrically contracted through as much ROM as patient can achieve; therapist and/or external device provides assistance to complete motion	Poor minus (2−) Fair minus (3−) The muscle can move only through partial available range in either a gravity-eliminated or against-gravity plane.	Provide a stimulating environment. Explain procedures. For a 2− muscle, position limb to move in a gravity-eliminated plane. For a 3− muscle, position the limb to move against gravity. Patient moves weak muscle through as much range as possible. Therapist provides external force to complete motion. Although this seems similar to PROM, it differs because patient actively attempts to contract weak muscle.
Isotonic Active (Active ROM)	Patient contracts muscle to move part through full ROM.	Poor (2) Fair (3) Muscle can move through full available range in either gravity-eliminated or against-gravity plane.	Provide a stimulating environment. Explain procedures. For a 2 muscle, position the limb to move in a gravity-eliminated plane. For a 3 muscle, position the limb to move against gravity. Patient moves weak muscle through full available ROM. Patient repeats motion for 3 sets of 10 repetitions with rest break between sets.

PROCEDURES FOR PRACTICE 21-3 *(continued)*

Guidelines for a Strengthening Program

Type of Exercise	Definition	Muscle Grades	Procedures
Isotonic Active Resistive (Active Resistive ROM)	Patient contracts muscle to move part through full available ROM against resistance.	Poor plus (2+) Fair (3) Fair plus (3+) Good (4) Good plus (4+)	Provide a stimulating environment. Explain procedures. For a 2+ or 3 muscle, position limb to move in gravity-eliminated plane. For a 3+ or above muscle, position limb to move against gravity. Therapist determines appropriate amount of resistance depending on the strengthening protocol chosen. If the DeLorme protocol is used, the 10-RM is established, which is the maximum weight a patient can lift through 10 repetitions with smooth controlled movement. If the simplified protocol is used, the 1-RM is established, which is the maximal amount of weight the patient can lift one time in a smooth controlled movement. Patient moves weak muscle through full available ROM against resistance.[a] If the DeLorme protocol is used, the patient does 3 sets of 10 repetitions with varying resistance and rest break between sets. If the simplified protocol is used, the patient does 4 sets of 10 repetitions at a set weight with rest breaks between sets.

[a] Resistance can be provided by weights either held in the patient's hand or strapped around the moving part. Resistance can also be provided by tools and materials of activity.

fects of training is unlikely between isometric and isotonic training programs (Hall & Brody, 2005; Kraemer et al., 2002). Occupational therapists commonly use occupation to build strength.

In the context of strengthening, the intensity of occupation or exercise refers to the amount of resistance offered and includes gravity. The intensity or resistance should be increased over time for strengthening. For example, Ms. C. (see Case Example 1), who has poor musculature but needs upper extremity strengthening to accomplish her daily tasks, can begin by washing her face side-lying in bed (reduced effect of gravity) until she can complete the task upright. Ms. C.'s occupational therapist can set up the task to be accomplished in bed and assist Ms. C. to bring her hand to her face so that she washes with her muscles in a gravity-eliminated plane. Ms. C. may next attempt to wash her face sitting upright in a chair in the bathroom, moving the extremity against the resistance of gravity. The therapist can further increase the intensity by adding various weighted tools, such as a light puff, a washcloth, and a washcloth and bar of soap. The therapist can continue to increase the intensity through more resistive occupations, such as dressing, making a bed, washing a car, gardening, or playing basketball, to increase strength gradually.

In this situation, resistance is graded by adding a load to the extremity (i.e., tools such as a washcloth, different textured clothing, or the resistance of dirt on a car) or by changing the plane of movement (i.e., gravity eliminated to against gravity). The duration of occupation can also be graded by increasing the need for muscle contraction through time spent in activity. A patient who is very weak

CASE EXAMPLE #1

Ms. C.'s Experience of Guillain-Barré

Occupational Therapy Assessment Process	Clinical Reasoning Process: Objectives	Clinical Reasoning Process: Examples of Therapist's Internal Dialogue
Patient Information Ms. C. is a 40-year-old woman who was the executive administrator of a large computer company. She lives at home with her partner and her high school–aged son from a previous marriage. Her partner is a lawyer in a small law firm that requires at least 10- to 12-hour work days. Ms. C. is a high-powered, motivated woman who not only enjoyed but was energized by the various people with whom she interacted at her job and the diverse assignments she supervised. When Ms. C. returned home from work, she often used household occupations as a means of changing from her high-energy level to a more relaxed state. Ms. C. shared household tasks equally with her partner and also her son. Relationships are essential in her life.	Appreciate the context	See Chapter 3, 4, 5, 10, and 11 for description of the assessment process and patient's background.
Ms. C. began to complain of tingling in her legs about 3 weeks ago. This progressed to her trunk and then to weakness in her legs and arms about 2 weeks ago. She was admitted to the hospital at that point and was then diagnosed with **Guillain-Barré**. She was in intensive care for about 10 days and has now been admitted to the rehab unit. At this point, she is extremely weak and has poor endurance. She is unable to lift her arms against gravity and has been up in a reclining wheelchair for about 30 minutes before she needs to go back to bed. Following an occupational therapy evaluation that included this history, the following problems were identified by Ms. C. and the therapist: (1) loss of independence in all occupations including all self-care activities and use of the phone and computer; (2) weakness throughout her arms, trunk, and legs, with manual muscle testing scores of 2–3, but very limited endurance, so that she is able to do only 3–4 repetitions of a motion before she is fatigued; (3) depression and anxiety due to an unpredictable future; and (4) inability to communicate with her employees, employer, and her son, which is causing considerable anxiety.	Develop intervention hypotheses	"I think if Ms. C. reestablished some of her more important activities, such as being able to communicate with work, she would feel that she was making progress. In addition, with her endurance and strength both so low, repetition of any movements would help to increase them both."

	Select an intervention approach	"Ms. C. would benefit from remediation to increase strength and endurance in her extremities, which would allow her to regain independence in her occupations. However, I also think she would benefit from compensation through the use of adapted equipment to help her resume some important activities."
	Reflect on therapist's competence	"Ms. C. is really having difficulty being separated from work. I think that if she could communicate with her workplace, she would feel that she was back in some control. In addition, it is difficult for her to see her son because he can only come after school, and at that point, she is usually exhausted. But if she could have some other means to communicate with both work and her son, she might begin to see that she is making progress. I will need to see if she is willing to use adaptive equipment as a bridge to independence; some patients don't tolerate 'gadgets,' so I will have to check that out."
Recommendations The occupational therapist recommended three treatment sessions each day for 4–6 weeks. Ms. C. and the therapist established the following long-term treatment goals: (1) Ms. C. will carry out her hygiene, self-care, dressing, and showering independently, which would prepare her for being at home during the day; (2). Ms. C. will prepare a light meal for lunch, which will also ready her for discharge; (3) Ms. C. will learn skills and develop strategies to be able to work from home when she is discharged, for at least a few hours a day; (4) Ms. C. will be independent in a home exercise program for strengthening and endurance; and (5) Ms. C. will resume an active role as the mother of her son.	Consider the patient's appraisal of performance Consider what will occur in therapy, how often, and for how long Ascertain the patient's endorsement of plan	"I think that Ms. C. is so overwhelmed with what has happened that she really isn't aware. It is such a change from her previous life of being in charge of everything. I think that we will need to start with things that are very important to her and that she can succeed at. Since work and her son are so important, I think that, if we used an overhead sling, she might be able to operate both a speakerphone and email and that would allow her to be involved. My one concern is that she might overdo it, so we will have to talk about that. I will need to maintain her passive range of motion, particularly in those antigravity positions that she cannot move into. Daily PROM will be necessary until she gains enough strength to move herself. In addition, care will need to be taken to ensure that she is not developing imbalances of muscle strength around joints that would lead to contractures. Once she has had some success, we can begin to do other activities such as strengthening activities and self-care."
Summary of Short-Term Goals and Progress 1. Ms. C. will start assisting with hygiene and grooming activities and then advance to independence in daily self-care. Ms. C. was fitted with overhead slings, so that she could move her arms without lifting them against gravity. With that equipment, Ms. C. was able to wash her face and brush her teeth and was able to drive a power wheelchair, which greatly improved her independence.	Assess the patient's comprehension	"Ms. C. seems to understand that any activities she does with her arms will help with strengthening and endurance and is motivated to do more. Now that she can access her email and use the phone and feed herself, she is beginning to think about what she needs to do to be home alone for periods of time after discharge."

2. Ms. C. will access a speakerphone and email to make working from home possible. With the overhead slings, she was able to operate both a speakerphone and her laptop computer in her room. She was able to work for about 25 minutes before she fatigued. 3. Ms. C. will feed herself and get food in and out of the refrigerator. Ms. C. was able to feed herself with a set up using the overhead slings and progressed to feeding herself without equipment. Using the power wheelchair, she was able to get items out of the refrigerator. 4. Ms. C. will develop ways to communicate with her son more frequently. She was able to access her email account and sent an email to her son. She also was able to call him on his cell phone over the noon hour, and he was really excited to talk to her when she was alert and awake. 5. Ms. C. will begin an upper extremity strengthening and endurance program. As she gained endurance, she was able to begin doing resistive exercises to some muscles, as well as assume some responsibility for stretching. She will have to be independent in some parts of the program when she goes home. The therapist and Ms. C. discussed that it was important that she not overdo it, and she seemed to understand that. Her endurance for activity increased considerably over the first week, as she had the opportunity to do things that were important to her on her own schedule.	Understand what the patient is doing Compare actual to expected performance Know the person Appreciate the context	"Ms. C. is accepting of the use of adaptive equipment as a bridge to independence, so that opens up a lot of opportunities. She is doing better than I expected, and she is tolerating all the activity well." "We will continue to advance her to more complex activities, such as meal preparation, and more work-related tasks, such as handling files, organizing a work station, etc." "I need to check with her partner and her son to see how things are going at home. If the partner is working 10–12 hours a day and her son is home alone, we may need to come up with a new plan."
Next Steps We are also going to need to assess the accessibility of her home, since she will probably be using her wheelchair most of the time at home, particularly when she is alone. At some point in the next several weeks, we will remove the overhead slings, progress her to a manual wheelchair, and then begin doing more activities in standing, as she can tolerate. This may be frustrating for her because occupations she is currently doing will become more difficult, so I'll have to be careful of that. We will need to plan out a typical day and make sure that Ms. C. can do all the things she will need to do at home.	Anticipate present and future patient concerns Analyze patient's comprehension Decide if the patient should continue or discontinue therapy and/or return in the future	"Ms. C. is making very good progress and will be able to leave the hospital in several more weeks. Since her partner works and they don't have any family nearby, Ms. C. will need to be home alone for periods of time after discharge. I'm not sure Ms. C. is anticipating how isolating that can be. Although she will probably be walking short distances at that time, she will likely spend most of her time in her wheelchair. I will need to be sure that she has an emergency plan, can operate a cell phone that she has with her, and has anticipated as much as possible what things she needs to be able to do. Home care may be a very feasible option for Ms. C. for a while, and then she can consider outpatient therapy when she is no longer homebound. Transportation to and from rehab will be a challenge. She will also need to check with her doctor about when he might allow her to drive."

CLINICAL REASONING IN OCCUPATIONAL THERAPY PRACTICE

Effects of Endurance and Strength on Performing Occupations

The therapist developed an exercise program to assist Ms. C. in building the strength and endurance needed to carry out her daily occupations. How would the strengthening program differ from the program to build endurance? How could Ms. C. use occupation to build strength? How could Ms. C. use occupation to increase her endurance?

may not even be able to finish washing his or her face in bed. The therapist can manipulate the rest breaks during the activity or complete a portion of the activity to increase the duration of the patient's participation. In this example, the treatment goal may be for the patient to take an entire bath or complete other occupations that take longer.

The rate or velocity of contraction, described as the number of repetitions per period of time, must be gradually increased according to the patient's abilities and comfort. As specified in the literature, the velocity of muscle contraction in training should eventually match the velocity of muscle contraction that is required in the patient's occupational routine (Kraemer et al., 2002). Finally, the frequency of exercise periods can also be graded for added strength benefit.

Increasing Endurance

Exercise programs designed to increase muscle endurance rather than muscle strength require somewhat different design. The following describes the underlying principles and guidelines for those modifications.

Less Than Maximal Resistance Over Time

In ordinary daily occupations that are lightly resistive, motor units are activated asynchronously. After a motor unit ceases activity, the muscle fibers recover to some degree while fellow units take their turn. Fatigue occurs more slowly with light resistive movements than with maximal contraction, in which many more units must contract simultaneously without the opportunity to recover. Doing repetitive concentric or eccentric contractions against less than maximal resistance increases endurance through less glycogen depletion and improved oxidative capacity of muscle fibers. Exercise to increase muscle endurance therefore uses moderately fatiguing activity for increasingly longer periods with intervals of rest to allow metabolic recovery (Kisner & Colby, 2002; Kraemer et al., 2002).

Methods

Grading Occupations to Increase Endurance

One of the most dramatic examples of adaptability of the muscular system is the extent to which muscle endurance can be improved by engaging in mild activity with increased numbers of repetition. To increase endurance, therapists guide patients to engage in longer periods of occupation at 40–60% of their repetition maximum (RM) (Kisner & Colby, 2002; Kraemer et al., 2002). Occupation or exercise used to build muscular endurance is graded by increasing the exercise period, which is done either by raising the number of repetitions of a contraction or by lengthening the time an isometric contraction is held. The occupational therapist can also increase the frequency of engaging in occupation or exercise if patients are not ready to increase duration times.

Occupational therapists provide the patients with interest-sustaining occupations that can be graded along the dimension of time or repetition. For example, patients who are interested in board games, such as backgammon or chess, may increase the number of games they play or the length of time they play. Occupational therapists can also work with patients to schedule their everyday routines so that they gradually increase the amount of time they engage in occupations throughout the day and/or gradually increase the duration of engagement in one particular occupation. For example, in Figure 21-11, increasing the time working in the garden or the amount of muscular effort put forth (picking tomatoes vs. pulling weeds) is an effective way to increase muscular endurance. Remember, to increase muscle endurance, the therapist must increase the number of repetitions of a specific motion. Programming for cardiovascular endurance specifically with patients who have cardiopulmonary problems is discussed in Chapter 47.

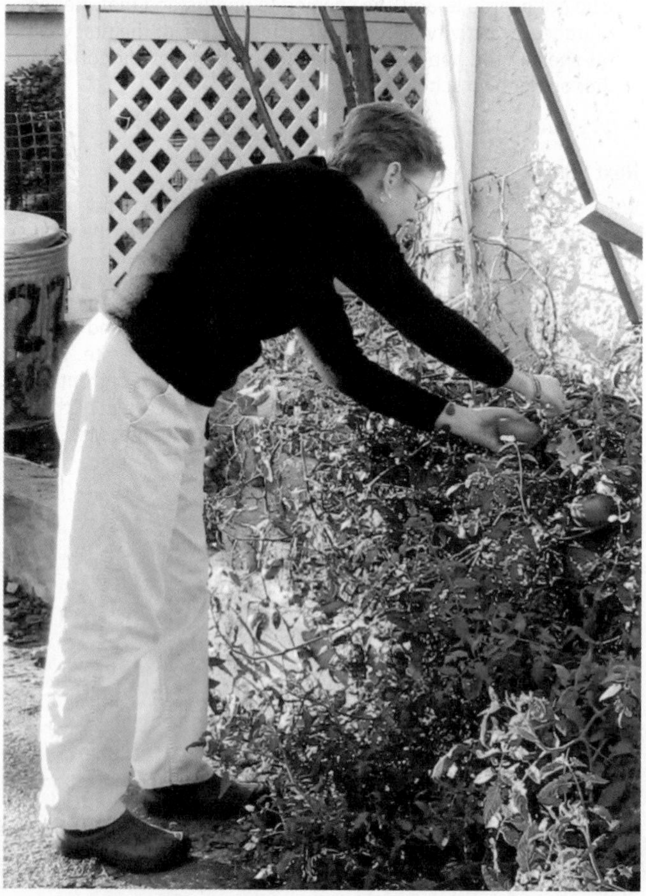

Figure 21-11 Muscular endurance can be increased by adding to the time spent on a task or adding to the resistance of the activity. In gardening, picking tomatoes could advance to weeding the garden.

CASE EXAMPLE # 2

Mr. G.: Back Injury

Occupational Therapy Assessment Process	Objectives	Clinical Reasoning Process: Examples of Therapist's Internal Dialogue
Patient Information Mr. G., a 46-year-old man with a landscaping career, sustained a back injury when he tripped over his 2-year-old son's play lawnmower, lost his balance, and fell on the grass. Initially he had pain in his lower back and a sharp tingling sensation down his leg. Medical examination revealed that he had severely sprained his back muscles in the fall and had exacerbated pain because of previous bone spurs on the lumbar spine and a degenerating disc at L5-S1. Mr. G. was prescribed a brief period of bed rest and given medication for pain and muscle relaxation. Following this medical intervention, Mr. G. was referred to outpatient occupational therapy for exercises and instruction in how to perform his daily occupations so that his back pain would be relieved or minimized and further back injury would be prevented. Mr. G. described two main roles in his life, work (landscaping) and childcare. Mr. G. explained that he and his partner both work outside the home and share the childcare and household responsibilities. Mrs. G. works part time at a travel agency. Although she has a flexible schedule, she usually goes to the office at least two evenings per week, and Mr. G. takes care of their three children, Eliza, aged 4, and Tom and Pat, aged 2. Mr. G. is performing his self-care occupations with moderate assistance from his wife and with severe discomfort. He requires maximal assistance for all home and childcare occupations. He had not performed any other leisure or work occupations at the time of the evaluation. Mr. G. is the sole owner of his landscaping business and has five experienced gardeners working for him. The occupations of his job include the following: (1) manage the finances, which requires sitting at a computer for approximately 5 hours, two to three times per month; (2) design landscapes, which requires sitting at a drawing table for 3–4 hours at a time; (3) consult with the client and nursery personnel to design the landscape and buy the plants; these tasks require driving, creativity, communicating, and, at times, bending and lifting heavy pots; and (4) supervise the gardeners, which often entails working with them to plant or lay down cement, stones, birdbaths, and other heavy garden fixtures. Mr. G.'s evening schedule consists of cooking dinner, changing diapers, bathing the children, dressing them for bed, playing with them, and emotionally supporting them. The children love to play rough-and-tumble with their daddy. Multiple piggy-back and horsey rides are an expected part of playtime. Furthermore, each parent has developed a special bedtime activity. Mrs. G. reads a book and Mr. G. pulls them on a cardboard train around the house and deposits each child in his or her bed.	Appreciate the context	See chapter 3, 4, 5, and 10 for description of the assessment process and patient's background. Mr. G.'s therapist conducted an interview and observed him to determine which occupations were particularly significant in Mr. G.'s life, which occupations created pain, and how he performed the occupations.

Develop intervention hypotheses	"Mr. G. has a very physically demanding life; landscaping is hard physical work, and picking up and playing with 3 small children is demanding, too. I wonder how much flexibility he has at work. To decrease his symptoms, he will need to make changes in body mechanics in both his home and work life."
Select an intervention approach	"Mr. G. will need to learn how to apply body mechanic principles on his own so that he can solve problems as they arise. This will involve compensation by using equipment and adapted movement techniques. I can use situations with his children as teaching tools and make some specific suggestions about his work, but he will need to learn the principles and be able to apply them on his own. I wonder if Mr. G. can make some changes at work to reduce the physical demands. I know that we can work out some changes in handling his children at home, but the work situation may be more difficult."
Reflect on therapist's competence	"Mr. G. is like a lot of other patients I've worked with, and his success will depend on how well I teach him to adopt the principles of body mechanics. I also don't know a lot about the landscaping business, and although I assume there is a lot of hard work, I'm not very sure about the specifics. I will need to learn more about landscaping and also about equipment that might be helpful for him to use."

Recommendations

The occupational therapist recommended two treatment sessions per week for 5 weeks. In collaboration with his wife and the therapist, Mr. G. set the following long-term goals: (1) change or delete certain daily occupations to prevent further injury; (2) learn proper body mechanics during daily occupations to relieve strain on his back; and (3) perform self-care, home, childcare, and landscaping occupations independently without pain.

Consider the patient's appraisal of performance	"I think that Mr. G. knows that he needs to make changes to get better. He seems very motivated to make changes, and his wife is very supportive of those changes."
Consider what will occur in therapy, how often, and for how long	"Mr. G. and I, and his wife if she can come to the sessions, will spend each session reviewing the principles of body mechanics and why they work and then apply them to a variety of daily activities. At the end of each session, I will give him homework to do before he comes back to the next session so he can evaluate how it is working and we can continue problem solving."
Ascertain the patient's endorsement of plan	"Mr. G. seems optimistic about the plan and so does his wife. I think they are both willing to make the changes that are going to be needed to make this work."

Summary of Short-Term Goals and Progress

Mr. G. will explore his options for avoiding some of the physically stressful occupations at his landscaping business and will enact a reasonable plan. The therapist and Mr. G. discussed various scenarios about his business. The most feasible option was to increase the responsibilities of two of the gardeners and give them a pay raise so that he would no longer purchase or carry heavy plants or help with planting. By eliminating these tasks and using proper body mechanics for the other tasks, Mr. G. can maintain his landscaping business. Mr. G. will pick up his children, incorporating good body mechanics 75% of the time. Initially, Mr. G. stopped his childcare and household responsibilities. The therapist taught Mr. G. the principles of body mechanics, such as holding objects close to the body when lifting, keeping the back straight and using the leg muscles to lift, and avoiding simultaneous bending and twisting when moving items from one place to another. Mr. G. practiced and was successful with these techniques with various items around the house. He applied these principles to lifting his children, paying close attention to facing his child, being close to his child, and lifting with his legs. Although this technique worked, Mr. G. also taught his children to climb up on his lap, where he could position them well and use his leg muscles to stand up.	Assess the patient's comprehension Understand what the patient is doing Compare actual to expected performance Know the person Appreciate the context	"Mr. G. has been very good at following through on his homework. He is learning the principles of body mechanics very well and has been creative about coming up with solutions to avoid problematic movements. Mr. G. seems to be pleased and relieved that he is able to care for his children and run his business with decreased pain and that he is in control of the situation. Being able to resume his work and taking care of his children are the most important things for Mr. G."

Next Steps

Mr. G. will analyze his body movements and change them to reflect good body mechanics during cooking, diapering, and playing with the children. Mr. G. will perform his computer work and landscape designing independently, incorporating proper body mechanics, pacing, energy conservation, and joint protection.	Anticipate present and future patient concerns Analyze patient's comprehension Decide if the patient should continue or discontinue therapy and/or return in the future	"Mr. G. has been able to anticipate activities that might be problems and avoid them, which is an indication that he's really learning the principles and techniques. Even when he had a flare up of pain last week, he was able to identify the activity that had probably increased his pain, and that seemed to help him manage the situation. I think that one concern might be that he will follow the movement adaptations while his back is flared up but may revert to old habits if they don't cause him pain. We've discussed his desk arrangement in addition to all the activities at work and home, so I think it is time to discharge him. I do want him to know that he should return to therapy if he gets into trouble again or if his activities change and he needs information about equipment or techniques."

CLINICAL REASONING IN OCCUPATIONAL THERAPY PRACTICE

Prevention of Back Injuries While Lifting

While alone at work, Mr. G. had to lift a large, heavy box of office supplies from the floor to his desk. How might a therapist instruct Mr. G. to position the box to lessen the force on his back when lifting the box? Using the concept of torque, how might the therapist justify the positioning of the box?

Evidence Table 21-1
Best Evidence for Occupational Therapy Practice Regarding Strengthening, Stretching, and Endurance Training

Intervention	Description of Intervention Tested	Participants	Dosage	Type of Best Evidence and Level of Evidence	Benefit	Statistical Probability and Effect Size of Outcome	Reference
Resistive exercise program for muscle strengthening	Experimental groups received general conditioning, resistance training, and isokinetic exercise program.	52 healthy, inactive elderly persons were randomly assigned to groups (control, n = 10; isokinetic strengthening, n = 12; resistance training, n = 15; and general conditioning, n = 15).	45–55 minutes of exercise 3 times a week for 10 weeks.	Randomized controlled study. 1C1b	Yes. The resistance training group improved the most on the strength tests of the target muscles.	Concentric contractions of the knee extensors: $p < 0.05$, $r = 0.63$.	Malliou et al., 2003
Stretching to increase joint ROM	5 different groups of students received stretch of different lengths of time to the hamstrings.	35 healthy college students randomly assigned to 30-, 60-, 90-, or 120-second stretch treatment groups or a no-treatment control group.	One self-administered stretch daily for the prescribed period, 7 days a week, for 5 weeks.	Randomized controlled study. 1C1b	Yes. All stretching groups improved range; no differences between lengths of stretch.	Increase in knee extension range of motion: $p < 0.005$, $r = 0.24$.	Ford, Mazzone, & Taylor, 2005
Effect of occupationally embedded exercise for bilaterally assisted supination	Participants practiced assisted pronation under two conditions, one that was occupationally embedded and one that was rote.	28 stroke survivors were randomly assigned to 2 groups (mean age, 68.4 years; mean time since stroke, 53.5 days; ratio of left hemiplegia to right hemiplegia, 15:11.	20 trials of the activities in 1 day.	Randomized controlled study. 1C1a	Yes. Participants in the occupationally embedded condition had more bilaterally assisted supination than the control group.	Increased range of motion in bilaterally assisted supination: $p < 0.016$, $r = 0.40$.	Nelson et al., 1996

Efficacy of the ROM Dance Program for adults with rheumatoid arthritis	ROM Dance Program is a 7-minute exercise and relaxation program.	34 adults with rheumatoid arthritis were assigned to the ROM Dance Program or control group.	8-week ROM Dance Program, followed by 1 month of self-administered ROM Dance Program, or control group that was not given any specific instructions for ROM or relaxation.	Randomized controlled study. 1C3a	Yes. ROM Dance Program participants had greater ROM in shoulder flexion, shoulder internal and external rotation, and total upper extremity ROM combined at 4-month follow-up.	Improvement in shoulder flexion, $p = 0.02$, $r = 0.21$; improvement in shoulder internal and external rotation, $p = 0.03$, $r = 0.21$; total upper extremity ROM combined, $p = 0.048$, $r = 0.16$.	Van Deusen & Harlowe, 1987
Effect of Tai Chi exercise on physical function in inactive older persons	Tai Chi exercise group of 60 minutes.	94 inactive older adults were assigned to a Tai Chi exercise group or wait-list control group.	60 minute exercise sessions twice a week for 6 months.	Randomized controlled study. 1B2b	Yes. Tai Chi group improved in physical functioning.	Improvement in composite score of physical function of SF-20, $p = 0.008$, $r = 0.62$.	Li et al., 2001

SUMMARY REVIEW QUESTIONS

1. What are the physiological aspects of muscle contraction?
2. Give an example of a third-class lever system in the body. What is the force arm (effort force)? What is the resistance arm (resistance force)?
3. Explain lifting a handled shopping bag in terms of torque.
4. Analyze the forces, stability, and motions required to put a can of soup on the shelf at nose height.
5. How should passive stretching treatment be modified if the patient acknowledges residual pain after treatment?
6. What parameters can be manipulated to alter stress on the muscle to increase strength?
7. What are the necessary characteristics of exercise or occupation required to increase muscle endurance?
8. Plan a therapeutic occupation program to strengthen a patient who has generalized poor (grade = 2) upper extremity musculature. Revise the program to accommodate changes in the patient's musculature from poor (grade = 2) to fair (grade = 3).
9. Differentiate between a therapeutic occupation program designed to strengthen muscles and one designed to increase muscle endurance.
10. Following replacement of the PIP joint of the ring finger, the patient's finger and hand are edematous. What treatment choices does the occupational therapist have?

ACKNOWLEDGEMENTS

Nancy Flinn thanks James Polga and other unnamed family and friends for volunteering to be photographed for this chapter.

Resources

Harlowe, D., & Yu, P. (1993). ROM dance: seated version. Distributed by Tai Chi Health, 408 South Baldwin Street, Madison, WI. www.taichihealth.com.

References

American College of Sports Medicine. (2000). *Guidelines for exercise testing and prescription* (6th ed.). Baltimore: Williams & Wilkins.

Baechle, T. R., & Earle, R. W. (Eds.). (2000). *Essentials of strength training and conditioning; National Strength and Conditioning Association* (2nd ed.). Champagne, IL: Human Kinetics.

Bandy, W. D., & Sanders, B. (2001). *Therapeutic exercise: Techniques for intervention.* Philadelphia: Lippincott Williams & Wilkins.

Bonnar, B. P., Deivert, R. G., & Gould, T. E. (2004). The relationship between isometric contraction durations during the hold-relax stretching and improvement of hamstring flexibility. *Journal of Sports Medicine and Physical Fitness, 44,* 258–261.

Chang, J., Wu, T., Wu, W., & Su, F. (2005). Kinematical measure for spastic reaching in children with cerebral palsy. *Clinical Biomechanics, 20,* 381–388.

De Deyne, P. G. (2001). Application of passive stretch and its implications for muscle fibers. *Physical Therapy, 81,* 819–827.

DeLorme, T. (1945). Restoration of muscle power by heavy resistance exercises. *Journal of Bone and Joint Surgery, 27,* 645–667.

DeLorme, T., & Watkins, A. L. (1948). Technics of progressive resistance exercise. *Archives of Physical Medicine and Rehabilitation, 29,* 263–273.

Elbert, T., Candia, V., Altenmuller, E., Rau, H., Sterr, A., Rockstroh, B. P., Pantev, C., & Taub, E. (1998). Alteration of digital representations in somatosensory cortex in focal hand dystonia. *NeuroReport, 9,* 3571–3575.

Fasoli, S. E., Trombly, C. A., Tickle-Degnan, L., & Verfaellie, M. H. (2002). Effect of instructions on functional reach in persons with and without cerebrovascular accident. *American Journal of Occupational Therapy, 56,* 380–390.

Feland, J. B., Myrer, J. W., & Merrill, R. M. (2001). Acute changes in hamstring flexibility: PNF versus static stretch in senior athletes. *Physical Therapy in Sports, 2,* 186–193.

Ford, G. S., Mazzone, M. A., & Taylor, K. (2005). The effect of four different durations of static hamstring stretching on passive knee-extension range of motion. *Journal of Sports Rehabilitation, 14,* 95–107.

Gill, T. M., Baker, D. I., Gottschalk, M., Gahbauer, E. A., Charpentier, P. A., de Regt, P. T., & Wallace, S. J. (2003). A prehabilitation program for physically frail community-living older persons. *Archives of Physical Medicine and Rehabilitation, 84,* 394–404.

Griggs, S. M., Ahn, A., & Greene, A. (2000). Idiopathic adhesive capsulitis: A prospective functional outcome study of nonoperative treatment. *The Journal of Bone and Joint Surgery, 82-A,* 1398–1407.

Guo, L., Su, F., & An, K. (2006). Effect of handrim diameter on manual wheelchair propulsion: Mechanic energy and power flow analysis. *Clinical Biomechanics, 21,* 107–115.

Hall, C. M., & Brody, L. T. (2005). *Therapeutic exercise: Moving toward function* (2nd ed.). Philadelphia: Lippincott Williams & Wilkins.

Kisner, C., & Colby, L. A. (2002). *Therapeutic exercise: Foundations and techniques* (4th ed.). Philadelphia: Davis.

Kottke, F. J. (1990). Therapeutic exercise to maintain mobility. In F. J. Kottke & J. F. Lehmann (Eds.), *Krusen's handbook of physical medicine and rehabilitation* (4th ed., pp. 436–451). Philadelphia: Saunders.

Kraemer, W. J., Adams, K., Enzo, C., Dudley, G. A., Dooly, C., Fiegenbaum, M. S., Fleck, S. J., Franklin, B., Fry, A. C., Hoffman, J. R., Newton, R. U., Potteiger, J., Stone, M. H., Ratamess, N. A., & Triplett-McBride, T. (2002). Progression models in resistance training for healthy adults: Position stand. *Medicine and Science in Sports and Exercise, 34,* 364–380.

LaStayo, P. C., Wright, T., Jaffe, R., & Hartzel, J. (1998). Continuous passive motion after repair of the rotator cuff: A prospective outcome study. *Journal of Bone and Joint Surgery, 80-A,* 1002–1011.

Levangie, P. K., & Norkin, C. C. (2005). *Joint structure and function: A comprehensive analysis* (4th ed.). Philadelphia: F. A. Davis Company.

Li, F., Harmer, P., McAuley, E., Duncan, T. E., Duncan, S. C., Chaumenton N., & Fisher, K. J. (2001). An evaluation of the effects of tai chi exercise on physical function among older persons: A randomized controlled trial. *Annals of Behavioral Medicine, 23,* 139–146.

Lowell, M., Pirc, P., Ward, R. S., Lundy, C., Wilhelm, D. A., Reddy, R., Held, B., & Bernard, J. (2003). Effect of 3M Coban self-adherent wraps on edema and function of the burned hand: A case study. *Journal of Burn Care Rehabilitation, 24,* 253–258.

Malliou, P., Fatouros, I., Beneka, A., Gioftsidou, A., Zissi, V., Godolias, G., & Fotinakis, P. (2003). Different training programs for improving muscular performance in healthy inactive elderly. *Isokinetics and Exercise Science, 11,* 189–195.

Mandel, D., Jackson, J., Zemke, R., Nelson, L., & Clark, F. (1999). *Lifestyle redesign: Implementing the well elderly program.* Bethesda, MD: American Occupational Therapy Association.

McCann, P. D., Wootten, M. E., Kadaba, M. P., & Bigliani, L. U. (1993). A kinematic and electromyographic study of shoulder rehabilitation exercises. *Clinical Orthopaedics and Related Research, 288,* 179–188.

Michlovitz, S. L., Harris, B. A., & Watkins, M. P. (2004). Therapy interventions for improving joint range of motion: A systematic review. *Journal of Hand Therapy, 17,* 118–131.

Nelson, D. L., Konosky, K., Fleharty, K., Webb, R., Newer, K., Hazboun, V. P., Fontane, C., & Licht, B. C. (1996). The effects of an occupationally embedded exercise on bilaterally assisted supination in persons with hemiplegia. *American Journal of Occupational Therapy, 50,* 639–646.

Neumann, D. A. (2002). *Kinesiology of the musculoskeletal system: Foundations for physical rehabilitation.* St. Louis: Mosby.

O'Driscoll, S. W., & Giori, N. J. (2000). Continuous passive motion (CPM): Theory and principles of clinical application. *Journal of Rehabilitation Research and Development, 37,* 179–188.

Rhea, M. R., Alvar, B. A., Burkett, L. N., & Ball, S. D. (2003). A meta-analysis to determine the dose response for strength development. *Medicine and Science in Sports and Exercise, 35,* 456–464.

Rogers, M. E., Sherwood, H. S., Rogers, N. L., & Bohlken, R. M. (2002). Effects of dumbbells and elastic band training on physical function in older inner-city African-American women. *Women and Health, 36,* 33–41.

Salter, M., & Cheshire, L. (Eds.). (2000). *Hand therapy: Principles and practice.* Oxford, United Kingdom: Butterworth Heinemann.

Van Deusen, J., & Harlowe, D. (1987). The efficacy of the ROM Dance Program for adults with rheumatoid arthritis. *American Journal of Occupational Therapy, 41,* 90–95.

Vuillemin, A., Boini, S., Bertrais, S., Tessier, S., Oppert, J., Hercberg, S., Fuillemin, F., & Briançon, S. (2005). Leisure time physical activity and health-related quality of life. *Preventive Medicine, 41,* 562–569.

Wong, J. M. W. (2002). Management of stiff hand: An occupational therapy perspective. *Hand Surgery, 7,* 261–269.

CHAPTER 22

LEARNING OBJECTIVES

After studying this chapter, the reader will be able to do the following:

1. Name the treatment principles of the Occupational Therapy (OT) Task-Oriented Approach.
2. Discuss personal and environmental factors that may be major influences on occupational performance.
3. Define the terms unique to the OT Task-Oriented Approach.
4. Explain the roles of the client and the therapist in the OT Task-Oriented Approach.

Optimizing Motor Behavior Using the Occupational Therapy Task-Oriented Approach

Julie Bass-Haugen, Virgil Mathiowetz, and Nancy Flinn

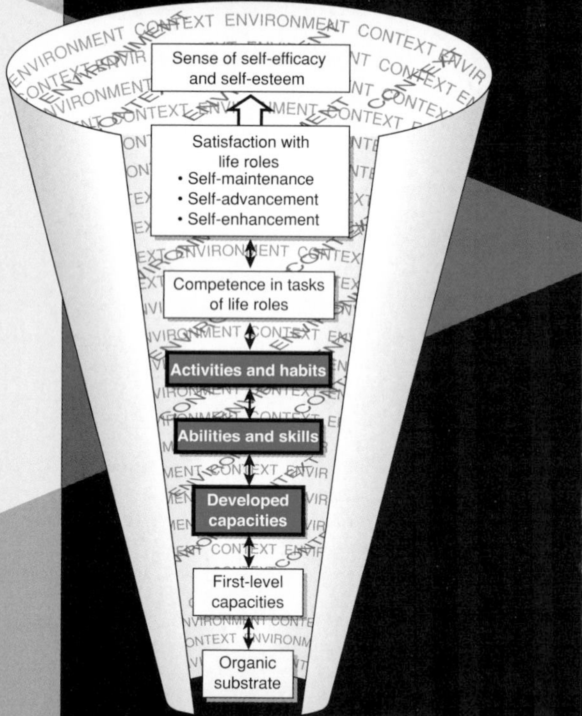

Glossary

Attractor—Preferred but not obligatory pattern of motor behavior that emerges from the interaction of a unique person with a particular task and environment.

Blocked practice—Practice that consists of drills and requires many repetitions of the same task in the same way (Schmidt, 1991).

Closed task—A task with stable environmental conditions and consistency from one trial to the next.

Collective variable—Fewest number of variables or dimensions that describe a unit of behavior quantitatively.

Continuous task—Repetitive task without a clear beginning or end.

Control parameter—Variable that shifts behavior from one preferred pattern to another and does not control the change but acts as agent for reorganization of behavior (Heriza, 1991).

Degrees of freedom—Elements that are free to vary.

Discrete task—Task involving movements with a recognizable beginning and end.

Motor learning—Acquisition of general strategies for solving movement problems in a variety of contexts.

Open task—Task in which some features of the environment are in motion or unstable and there is variation from one trial to the next.

Part learning—Practice of separate steps of a task.

Phase shift—Transition, often nonlinear, from one preferred qualitative coordinated pattern to another (Heriza, 1991).

Random practice—Practice of tasks that vary randomly within the session (Schmidt, 1991).

Serial tasks—Tasks with connected discrete movements.

Whole learning—Practice of a task in its entirety.

The OT Task-Oriented Approach emerges from a systems model of motor behavior and is influenced by recent developmental and motor learning (skill acquisition) theories. Two primary bodies of knowledge serve as the basis for the approach: task-oriented approaches that have been discussed in the physical therapy and exercise science literature (e.g., Davis & Burton, 1991; Horak, 1991) and OT models that are occupation based and client centered (Christiansen & Baum, 1997; Law et al., 1997; Trombly, 1995). In particular, the model of occupational functioning (Trombly, 1995) contributes to an emphasis on roles and tasks in the OT Task-Oriented Approach. The model of occupational functioning clearly influences the occupational therapy systems model of motor behavior depicted in Figure 6-2.

Before reading further, review the model, theories, assumptions, and basic evaluation ideas related to this approach in Chapter 6 and principles of learning in Chapter 14. This chapter examines specific treatment strategies related to the assumptions of this approach (Procedures for Practice 22-1).

Although many ideas (e.g., occupational performance, person, environment) presented as part of the OT Task-Oriented Approach are as old as occupational therapy itself, recent motor behavior literature provides a stronger theoretical basis for using purposeful and meaningful tasks as the primary treatment modality. The development of this approach is still evolving. The motor behavior, physical therapy, and adapted physical education literature is examined for identification of principles and key concepts related to task-oriented approaches. Similarly, the OT literature on client-centered, occupation-based models is used to frame the task-oriented approach in an OT context. There is limited but growing empirical support for the assumptions and treatment principles of this approach. Further development of the OT Task-Oriented Approach and empirical research will provide direction for future practice.

This approach suggests that the client have active involvement in treatment and may have limited applications in acute settings and for clients with significant cognitive impairments. Some aspects of the OT Task-Oriented Approach (e.g., use of real objects and natural environments, focus on meaningful tasks and functional goals), however, are appropriate even in these situations.

PROCEDURES FOR PRACTICE 22-1

Assumptions for the OT Task-Oriented Approach

- Functional tasks help organize motor behavior.
- Occupational performance emerges from the interaction of multiple systems that constitute the unique characteristics of the person and environment.
- After central nervous system damage or other changes in personal or environmental systems, clients' behavioral changes reflect attempts to achieve functional goals.
- Practice and active experimentation with varied strategies and in varied contexts are needed to find the optimal solution for a motor problem and develop skill in performance.

TREATMENT PRINCIPLES AND PRACTICES

The treatment principles and general treatment goals are listed in Procedures for Practice 22-2 and are described next. Procedures for Practice 22-3 summarize general indicators used to determine when to discontinue treatment.

Client-Centered Focus

A client-centered focus is an integral aspect of the OT Task-Oriented Approach.

Adopt a Client-Centered Focus in Treatment

Many therapists refer to the art and science of OT. The art of the OT Task-Oriented Approach is the identification of interventions for the unique needs of each client, taking into account unique personal and environmental systems and roles that have importance and meaning for the individual. Thus, treatment planning cannot be prescriptive. This may seem overwhelming when trying to process a lot of new information, but these challenges in practice can be the very things that make OT so exciting and rewarding.

In the OT Task-Oriented Approach, assessment and the planning of treatment should look different for each client. Although this may seem obvious, it has been shown that, in practice assessment, documentation and treatment activities often do not reflect the priorities and meaningful occupations identified by clients (Neistadt, 1995a, 1995b) and that perceptions of collaboration during goal setting differ for therapists and patients (McAndrew et al., 1999).

Elicit Active Participation of the Client During Treatment

Clients should have an active role in treatment. They should guide selection of tasks for treatment and contribute to finding solutions for occupational performance problems. Clients who are actively engaged in their treatment show achievement in self-identified goals (Trombly, Radomski, & Davis, 1998), greater participation in the rehabilitation process (Wressle et al., 2002), increased functional independence at discharge, and discharges to less restrictive environments (Gibson & Schkade, 1997).

PROCEDURES FOR PRACTICE 22-2

Treatment Principles of a Task-Oriented Approach

Client-Centered Focus

- Adopt a client-centered focus in treatment.
- Elicit active participation of the client during treatment.

Occupation-Based Focus

- Use functional tasks as the focus in treatment.
- Select tasks that are meaningful and important to the client's roles.
- Analyze the characteristics of the tasks selected for treatment.
- Describe the movements used for task performance.
- Determine whether the movement patterns are stable or in transition.
- Analyze the movement patterns and functional outcomes of task performance.

Person and Environment

- Identify the personal and environmental factors that serve as major influences on occupational performance.
- Anticipate that the personal and environmental variables influencing occupational performance will change.
- Address critical personal and environmental systems to cause change in occupational performance.
- Treat neural and non-neural factors of the sensorimotor system that interfere with optimal occupational performance.
- Adapt the task or broader environment to promote optimal occupational performance.
- Use natural objects and natural environments.

Practice and Feedback

- Structure practice of the task to promote motor learning.
- Design the practice session to fit the type of task and learning strategies.
- Provide feedback that facilitates motor learning and encourages experimentation with solutions to occupational performance problems.
- Optimize occupational performance given the constraints on the person and environment.

General Treatment Goals

- Discover the optimal movement patterns for task performance.
- Achieve flexibility, efficiency, and effectiveness in task performance.
- Develop problem-solving skills with clients so they can identify their own solutions to occupational performance problems in home and community environments.

PROCEDURES FOR PRACTICE 22-3

Discontinuing Treatment

The therapist looks for one or more of these indicators to assist in determining when it is appropriate to discontinue treatment:

- The client is satisfied with performance of occupations and related roles.
- The client spontaneously uses efficient and effective movements that are stable but flexible in functional tasks.
- The client has developed independent and effective skills for solving occupational performance problems in the home and community.
- The client uses movement patterns and demonstrates functional outcomes of task performance that are optimal given the constraints on the person and environment.
- The client easily reverts to long-standing obligatory or irregular movement patterns after an intervention is withdrawn.
- The client does not demonstrate more optimal movement patterns or improved task performance after critical personal or environmental systems have been systematically modified.

There are several ways to facilitate active participation in treatment. Provide user-friendly instructions on how to practice tasks outside of the therapy session and structure clients' environments to facilitate this practice (Ada, Canning, & Westwood, 1990). Create therapeutic environments that are conducive to active learning by attending to both organizational and physical structures of the setting. An environmental analysis can assist in determining whether the broader environment promotes passivity or active involvement in treatment. Characteristics of an active learning environment are summarized in Definition 22-1.

Teach clients the principles of task analysis (Higgins, 1991) and how to evaluate their own performance in terms of the outcomes of their efforts and the efficiency and effectiveness of their movement patterns. Involve clients in graphing their results and recording progress toward functional goals (Ada, Canning, & Westwood, 1990). A goal of therapy is to help clients understand the movement patterns and the performance contexts that contribute to optimal performance for given tasks (Burton & Davis, 1992). The therapist promotes understanding of personal capabilities and limitations and encourages exploration of modifiable environmental resources (Higgins, 1991). These strategies assist clients in developing skills needed for solving motor problems in their home and community.

Give skilled clients permission to solve their own motor problems and to use movement patterns that are the most functional for them, regardless of how these strategies are perceived by others (Burton & Davis, 1992; Latash & Anson, 1996). When clients become skilled in task analysis and solving motor problems, the therapist can celebrate their participation in various tasks and autonomy in learning (Higgins, 1991). This is true even when clients' solutions are not traditional or identical to the strategies therapists would recommend. For example, Mattson, a wheelchair racer with a C6-7 spinal cord lesion, found he could propel faster using a backhand stroke that maximized use of his remaining muscle groups (Burton & Davis, 1992). This technique was unconventional, but Mattson's performance dramatically improved, and soon afterward, many other wheelchair racers were using the same technique. Thus people may use unique movement patterns because they require the least amount of energy and are an efficient means of achieving a functional goal (Kamm, Thelen, & Jensen, 1990).

Occupation-Based Focus

The intervention plan for the OT Task-Oriented Approach is occupation based.

DEFINITION 22-1

Characteristics of an Active Learning Environment

- Create an environment that encompasses the common challenges of everyday life.
- Develop learning contracts that describe shared rehabilitation goals.
- Develop a cohesive team that is committed to active learning.
- Require clients to communicate their need for help in specific tasks to staff.
- Give clients control over when and where they are to be transported.
- Give able clients responsibility for routine housekeeping.
- Arrange chairs in small circles in reception and common areas.
- Provide opportunities for practice outside of therapy.
- Provide written instructions, audiotapes, videotapes, and diagrams for practice.
- Organize the environment to match the level of performance.
- Illustrate progress to clients.

Ada, L., Canning, C., & Westwood, P. (1990). The patient as active learner. In L. Ada & C. Canning (Eds.), Key issues in neurological physiotherapy (pp. 99–124). Boston: Butterworth Heinemann.

Use Functional Tasks as the Focus in Treatment

The goal of treatment for motor behavior problems is to enable clients to do the things they want to do now and in the future. Thus, at each point from the initial evaluation to recording progress to discharge to follow-up, the determination of the effectiveness of interventions is performance on functional tasks. The interventions themselves also emphasize the practice of real functional tasks.

There is renewed interest in functional tasks and goals in clinical and basic research. Neurological recovery from central nervous system (CNS) dysfunction supports task-related training and experiences (Dobkin, 1998, 2005), and functional disability is one of the most important predictors of discharge outcomes (Inouye et al., 2000). Thus, recently developed evaluations in OT emphasize measures of functional task performance. Treatment protocols for motor behavior problems emphasize using functional tasks (Burton & Davis, 1992; Carr & Shepherd, 1998) as both the means and ends in the treatment process (Gray, 1998; Trombly, 1995).

Many studies have examined the effect of functional goals on motor behavior. Thelen and Fisher (1983) studied kicking behavior in 3-month-old infants. They found that kicking increased when a mobile was tied to the leg by way of a control line. Adults with hemiplegia have demonstrated more repetitions of movement patterns when an occupation-based activity was used rather than rote exercise (Hsieh et al., 1996). Research is also beginning to support the idea that occupation-based interventions are more effective than other interventions in addressing impaired performance components such as coordination (Flinn, 1999; Neistadt, 1994; Trombly & Wu, 1998). Finally, performance efficiency improves when personal preferences and higher level functional goals are incorporated into treatment activities (Wu et al., 2001).

The results of these studies support the idea that therapists' interventions for motor behavior problems should revolve around meaningful occupations and functional goals. The functional goals of interest in OT are broad. Basic activities of daily living (ADLs) tasks are important. The functional goals, however, should also relate to other self-maintenance, self-advancement, and self-enhancement roles because the longer term reported limitations are often more significant for instrumental activities of daily living (IADLs) and community activities (Mayo et al., 2002).

RESEARCH NOTE 22-1

Liepert, J., Bauder, H., Miltner, W. H. R., Taub, E., & Weiller, C. (2000). Treatment-induced cortical reorganization after stroke in humans. *Stroke*, 31, 1210–1216.

Abstract

The purpose of this study was to evaluate reorganization of the motor cortex in individuals with stroke who had received constraint-induced movement therapy. Thirteen subjects with stroke in the chronic stage participated in a 12-day period of constraint-induced movement therapy. They used the affected arm exclusively in a variety of tasks during the therapy period. Focal transcranial magnetic stimulation was used to map the cortical motor output area of a hand muscle on both sides before and after treatment. Results showed that before treatment, the affected hand muscle had a significantly smaller cortical representation area than the contralateral side. After treatment, the cortical representation of the affected hand muscle was significantly enlarged. There was also a corresponding improvement in motor performance of the affected limb. In follow-up studies to 6 months after treatment, motor performance remained improved, and the cortical area sizes in the two hemispheres became almost identical and close to the normal condition. This study supports a therapy-induced improvement in movement and long-term alteration in brain function after stroke.

Implications for Practice

- Individuals use whatever movements are possible and needed to achieve functional goals. In constraint-induced movement therapy, individuals use the affected arm for task performance when the unaffected arm is not available.
- The motor cortex demonstrates neuronal plasticity after stroke even in the chronic stage.
- Constraint-induced movement therapy programs that incorporate a variety of tasks may influence cortical reorganization after stroke and improve movements and performance.

Select Tasks That Are Meaningful and Important to the Client's Roles

The importance of many functional tasks is unique to the individual. What is important to one person may not be important to another. So how do therapists determine the key tasks for a given individual? They should consider a client's occupational roles and the meaning of these roles to the person (see Chapter 4). Life satisfaction is not determined by successful completion of a random set of functional tasks (e.g., changing a diaper and taking out the garbage). Satisfaction or reward comes from the feeling that roles are fulfilled (e.g., parent and homemaker). Roles are defined by the client in terms of the tasks and related activities that are interesting or important (Fisher & Short-DeGraff, 1993; Pollock, 1993; Trombly, 1993, 1995). For example, two clients may view the role of parent differently. One may identify washing a child's clothing as a key functional task, whereas another may view playing touch football as more important. These two functional tasks vary greatly in their environments and in the motor behaviors required to achieve the functional goals.

The consideration of roles also helps the occupational therapist tap into the personal motivations of clients for performing particular tasks. When a client is motivated to change motor behaviors, it usually reflects an internal desire to perform, acquire, or accomplish something (Crutchfield & Barnes, 1993). This motivation may occur because the degree of skill in performance is not personally satisfactory (Higgins, 1991) or because of other intrinsic and extrinsic factors, including perceptions regarding the chance of success, importance of the goal, and the costs in terms of barriers and access as well as inclinations to continue current task performance (Phillips, Schneider, & Mercer, 2004). In summary, select tasks that are within the realm of capabilities, are goal oriented, have meaning for the clients, and motivate them.

Analyze the Characteristics of the Tasks Selected for Treatment

After a specific task has been selected for treatment, a task analysis is necessary because clients' capabilities vary and different tasks require different skills. Task analysis entails an examination of the task requirements and the personal capabilities to determine whether there is a match that permits task performance (see Chapter 13). If there is no match, the occupational therapist plans interventions that address the problems of the client or the characteristics of the environment or both. The outcome of a task analysis helps the therapist design appropriate **motor learning** experiences and select practice and feedback strategies that fit the nature of the task. Several classification schemes may be useful in task analysis (Davis & Burton, 1991; Gentile, 1987; Schmidt, 1988).

In Schmidt's (1988) classification, tasks and the required movements for tasks are described as discrete, serial, or continuous. Skilled performance in a **continuous task** is generally retained even when there are periods when practice is impossible (Crutchfield & Barnes, 1993). For example, most people learn to ride a bike when they are quite young. As an adult, they may go through long periods when there is no opportunity to practice this skill, but once they have learned to ride a bike, they easily remember it later after only brief practice. On the other end of the continuum are tasks requiring discrete movements. Many skilled movements used in sports with balls (e.g., hitting, slam dunking, and pitching) are discrete; they have a definite beginning and end. Frequent practice of the movements is required to maintain skill at a high level. Neither discrete nor continuous tasks are easily broken into steps, as **serial tasks** are.

Gentile (1987) proposed a taxonomy of tasks based on characteristics of the environment and a person's actions during task performance. The environment is described in terms of its characteristics and variability in these characteristics from one performance to the next. The environment, which includes objects, supporting surfaces, and other people, may be stationary or in motion during a given task. In addition, there may be variation or consistency in these environmental characteristics from trial to trial. When the environment is stationary during performance and does not change from one trial to the next, the task is a **closed task**. Signing your name on a check at a desk is a closed task because the environment is generally stable and unchanging. In an **open task**, some features of the environment are in motion and vary from one performance to the next. These tasks are complex and place many demands on the person because the performance context is unstable and changes for different trials. Driving a car is an example of an open task (Poole, 1991) because the driver must process the motions of other cars, pedestrians, and the broader performance context (e.g., snow or rain). Furthermore, these features of the environment vary dramatically from one trip to another.

The function of a person's actions is the second dimension in Gentile's (1987) taxonomy. This dimension consists of the person's actions during task performance and includes body orientation and object manipulation. In a given task, body orientation might require stabilization or transport. For example, during a word processing task, the trunk and lower extremities primarily provide stability. In a tennis match, however, the trunk and lower extremities move or transport toward the ball. Actions are also analyzed in terms of whether the upper extremities provide stability or manipulate objects. For example, the upper extremities help maintain balance and are part of the postural support system when a person walks on a wet kitchen floor. In this situation, there is no object manipulation. In washing the floor, however, arms and hands are used for object manipulation (e.g., mop or sponge). The complete taxonomy proposed by Gentile combines the environmental context and the function of the action dimensions and results in 16 categories of tasks.

Describe the Movements Used for Task Performance

A description of the preferred movement patterns that emerge for a given task in a given context helps guide treatment. Preferred movement patterns, or **attractors**, are ordinarily stable and the optimal way to achieve a functional goal because they are efficient and effective (Kamm, Thelen, & Jensen, 1990). A preferred movement pattern can be illustrated by how a marble moves on different surfaces (Fig. 22-1). The wells in the figure depict the stability of the patterns (Thelen, 1989). The marble on a surface with a shallow well (Fig. 22-1A) illustrates optimal movement patterns used for everyday tasks. The movements tend to be stable, just as a marble would tend to fall into the same well. This well is shallow enough, however, that the marble can move out of it, signifying how a person can modify

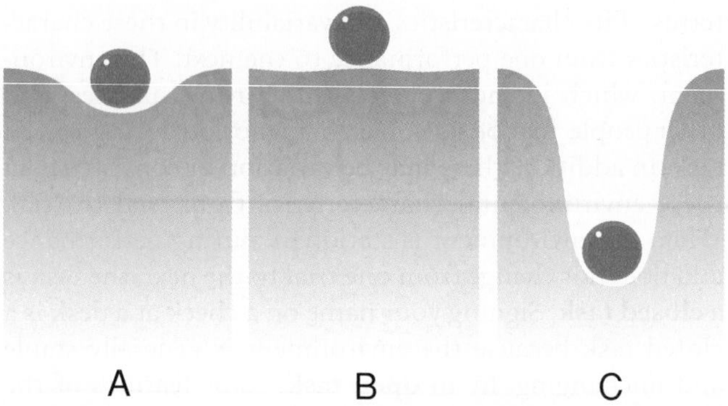

Figure 22-1 Various attractor states. **A.** Shallow well, stable and flexible attractor state. **B.** No well, no attractor state. **C.** Deep well, stable and inflexible attractor state.

movements or use a new movement pattern if there is a change in the person or environment. For example, how would you describe movements used to write your name? One characteristic is that there is a fair amount of consistency in the way a person moves as he or she writes. These preferred movements are usually the best movements for a given situation (e.g., writing on paper with a pencil at a desk). There may be some variations in the ways people move in this situation, but the movements do not vary widely. There is also some flexibility in movements, however, so that if a need arises (e.g., one has a blister on a finger or wants to use a stick to write in the sand), a person can temporarily or permanently change the movements used to complete the task. Many clients with CNS damage show good motor recovery and resumption of movement patterns similar to this example. They resume stable but flexible performance of tasks in their daily lives (Fig. 22-1A).

Clients in the acute stage of recovery often use movement patterns that show little stability (Fig. 22-1B). Their performance is similar to the movement patterns represented by a marble on a flat or bumpy surface—very irregular and unpredictable. It may appear that there is no preferred movement pattern. Every time they do a task, they do it in a different way. As a result, task performance is not efficient or effective. This is similar to the movement patterns seen the first few times a new sport is tried.

Other clients seem obligated to perform a task in only one way (Fig. 22-1C). In this situation, the well is so deep that a large perturbation or disturbance would be needed to dislodge the marble or to change the preferred movement pattern. Performance is likely to revert to this pattern soon after treatment. This movement pattern may be effective for task performance in one context, but the person may be unable to achieve functional goals in varied contexts because there is no flexibility in movement patterns. For example, a client may use a flexor pattern for all tasks that require reaching. This pattern may be effective when the arm is only an assist in some bilateral reaching tasks; most reaching tasks, however, require complex and varied motor skills. For these tasks, the client may be unable to adapt movements and thus be unable to achieve the functional goals. These obligatory patterns are often observed in people years after CNS damage.

Determine Whether the Movement Patterns Are Stable or in Transition

The next step is to determine whether the movement patterns are stable or in transition. This information is important because it helps the therapist identify the optimal times to provide treatment and the strategies necessary to produce a change in the preferred movement patterns (Kamm, Thelen, & Jensen, 1990; Scholz, 1990). The beginning of a transition period may coincide with aging, CNS damage, a new environment, or many other factors. Data on movement patterns are gathered by analyzing task performance and by constructing an individual developmental profile of previous changes in motor behavior (Thelen, 1989). The therapist observes performance of the same task several times in the same context and then in different contexts. Intervention is not needed if the preferred movement pattern is relatively efficient and effective for a given task and is stable but flexible so that it can be modified for different contexts. On the other hand, if there is no preferred movement pattern or if the pattern is fixed, the therapist may consider treatment to facilitate change in movement patterns and occupational performance.

If the movement patterns are in transition, there is increased variability in the movements used to complete a task and increased susceptibility to change or perturbation by the influence of some personal or environmental systems. In addition, movement patterns take longer to return to a stable state if perturbed (Heriza, 1991). These findings mark a potential transition period or **phase shift** and may be characterized as a marble on a smooth or bumpy surface (Fig. 22-1B). When the movement patterns are unstable or in transition, therapists are generally more likely to facilitate a change to different patterns—ones, it is hoped, that are more efficient and effective in achieving the task goal. Remediation of motor behavior problems should begin before the movement patterns fall into obligatory, stereotyped patterns (Kamm, Thelen, & Jensen, 1990).

If the movement patterns are stable in a particular performance context, it may be more difficult to produce a change in the way the task is performed in that context. In this scenario, change in movement patterns is less likely, and the person is apt to return easily to the preferred pattern, even if it is possible to produce a temporary change. This stability may be characterized as preferred but flexible (Fig. 22-1A) or obligatory (Fig. 22-1C). For example, neuromotor synergy patterns may represent the stable, obligatory movement patterns of a damaged system. If the movement patterns have been obligatory or irregular for a long time, interventions may not effect a change to other movement patterns. In this case, perhaps only a trial period of therapy is warranted.

Analyze the Movement Patterns and Functional Outcomes of Task Performance

An analysis of movement patterns will help estimate stability and flexibility, understand changes, and prevent fixation of movement patterns (Kamm, Thelen, & Jensen, 1990; Scholz, 1990). Scholz used an example to illustrate two strategies for evaluating the stability of movement patterns. Consider the gait of a child with cerebral palsy. The preferred pattern for this child may be a bunny hop, and a goal of therapy may be to move toward a reciprocal pattern of walking. One quantitative measure of movement patterns may be the relative phase of the hip motions as measured by videography. That is, are the hip motions in the same phase (both in flexion) or in opposite phases (one in flexion and the other in extension)? The therapist analyzes the fluctuations in the relative phase when the child is using the preferred pattern, the bunny hop. Next, this pattern is perturbed by slowing the locomotion or by imposing a physical restraint on one lower extremity. The therapist learns the child's movement patterns for this task by analyzing how much slowing or restraint is needed to change to a reciprocal pattern and how long it takes to return to a bunny hop after the critical factors are removed.

The first strategy is to look at fluctuations in one or more quantitative measures of movement patterns during task performance. The second strategy is to determine what happens when the therapist tries to disturb or perturb the movement patterns by changing some critical personal or environmental factors. Therapists ask themselves how much change is necessary to disturb the pattern and how long it takes for the movement pattern to return to the previous state. The quantitative measures of movement patterns are **collective variables**, and the critical factors influencing behavior are **control parameters**.

One of the challenges in the OT Task-Oriented Approach is identification of collective variables, the measures of movement that can describe in simple terms all of the systems that cooperate to produce movements (Clark, 1997; Heriza, 1991; Thelen & Ulrich, 1991). These variables are a way of objectively measuring motor behavior and changes in motor behavior. Therapists continue to discover new ways to measure the outcomes of functional performance. Sometimes, however, OT interventions are not intended to result in a substantial change in the outcome. For example, a client may have achieved moderate independence in bathing but still not have optimal performance. The goal in OT may be to help change the movement patterns used for getting out of the tub so that performance is more safe and efficient. Thus, measures are needed to document progress in motor performance as well as levels of independence.

Motor behavior research may help to identify these potential measures of occupational performance. Slow reaction times, slow movement times, performance variable variance, movement trajectories with discontinuities, absolute error, and rate or speed limitations have been noted in disorders of movement (Campbell, 1991; Corcos, 1991; Reisman & Scholz, 2003). One measure that is easy to use in treatment is time (time to begin the task, time to complete the task, and time until movement patterns regress to previous patterns after being perturbed). As videography and movement analysis become more accessible in clinical settings, occupational therapists may measure the relative timing of one motion with respect to another (relative phase), the curvature or straightness of movements (trajectories), the distance and direction of movement (displacement), and the speed or constancy of speed (velocity, accelerations, and decelerations) (Corcos, 1991; Fetters, 1991; Heriza, 1991; Rice & Newell, 2004; Scholz, 1990).

Person and Environment

The interventions used in the OT Task-Oriented Approach address personal and environmental systems to enable optimal occupational functioning.

Identify the Personal and Environmental Factors that Serve as Major Influences on Occupational Performance

The therapist begins treatment planning by examining tasks that were difficult for the person to perform and describing the preferred movement patterns for these tasks. The therapist then identifies the personal and environmental systems that support optimal functional performance and those that contribute to ineffective performance (Letts et al., 1994). The interactions of these systems are also important (Shepherd, 1992) (see Chapter 6). Part of the OT process, then, is making systematic changes in personal characteristics (e.g., attention and positioning) and environmental context (e.g., size of object and stability of base of support) and observing the effect on occupational performance. This process can help identify one or several critical factors (control parameters) that can cause a shift in motor behavior.

A qualitative analysis (observation and description) also may be used to describe the interactions of person and environment on task performance. For example, VanSant (1991) identified the personal systems used for activities requiring righting (e.g., rising from a bed and getting up from a chair or the floor). She found that the preferred movement patterns for these activities are influenced by body dimensions (e.g., ratio of leg length to body length; size of body relative to bed or chair; height; weight; body build and topography), age, gender, and activity level. Thelen (1989) studied treadmill stepping in infants and found that neurological and morphological maturation and the postures of the leg were the critical factors influencing the movements used. Velocity has been identified as a control parameter in the locomotion patterns used by people and animals (Scholz, 1990). If a horse is forced to increase its speed, changes in movements associated with a walk, trot, and gallop can be observed (Crutchfield & Barnes, 1993). Studies to determine control parameters of common motor behaviors are important to help occupational therapists identify the critical systems inherent in performing particular tasks.

Although it may seem impossible to identify only a couple of critical systems from the multiple systems and subsystems that influence motor performance, occupational therapists already do this, using quantitative and qualitative analysis. Consider the task of placing items on a shelf above shoulder level. Now imagine or, better yet, actually try placing various items on the shelf. Consider the different movement patterns used to lift an empty paint can and a full paint can to a high shelf. What is the critical factor that explains the change in movement patterns when lifting an empty can versus a full can? It is the weight of the can relative to arm strength. What is the critical factor that explains the change in movement patterns when lifting a tennis ball versus a beach ball in the same task (assuming weight is held constant)? In this situation, it is the size of the object relative to hand size. Both of the critical factors in these examples are performer-scaled variables (Davis & Burton, 1991), or parameters that link a characteristic of the person (e.g., strength or hand size) to a characteristic of the object that is used in the task (e.g., weight or size).

Thelen (1989) stated that it is also important to consider non-obvious and distantly related factors as possible critical factors. She described studies showing that the onset of crawling, a motor skill, is an influential factor in cognitive, affective, and social changes in children. The ability to move to another environment is a critical factor that can cause a dramatic change in the problem-solving, communication, and play behaviors of children.

One last clinical example suggests that other systems might serve as critical factors. In one long-term care setting, health care professionals were wondering why older men who had experienced cerebrovascular accidents were not achieving independence in dressing. One therapist hypothesized that it was loss of automatic reactions and postural control. Other therapists proposed that motor planning problems or general loss of strength and endurance explained the performance deficit. Although all of these systems did indeed influence motor behavior, a family member revealed that the critical factor for the motor behaviors related to dressing was the culture of the residents. That is, most residents in this setting were members of a culture that did not place value on independence in self-care for older adults, especially men who had disease-related impairments. In fact, it was an expectation that women in the extended family would come to the residence every day to complete ADLs.

There are several purposes in relating these examples. One is to challenge therapists to use creativity and common sense in treatment. For given individuals with given tasks, the critical factors may be neural or non-neural sensorimotor components (e.g., soft tissue contracture, muscle weakness, and abnormal muscle tone). Occupational therapists, however, sometimes neglect important factors such as a different culture and look only at performance components that seem directly related to the motor behaviors. No system automatically deserves more attention than any other system unless research indicates otherwise.

Anticipate that the Personal and Environmental Variables Influencing Occupational Performance Will Change

The critical variables influencing motor behavior change over time. CNS damage affects each system differently relative to occupational performance. This idea is illustrated in Figures 22-2 and 22-3, which depict hypothetical changes in systems and subsystems over time for a unique person. The *y* axes represent the system's degree of positive or negative influence on occupational performance, and the *x* axes represent these changes over time from onset of CNS damage to the rehabilitation stage to discharge or home. Some systems are highly affected immediately after CNS damage, while other systems become more important later. For example, the physical environment in Figure 22-2 may become a more important variable when the person returns home. The home may or may not support performance of previous occupational roles and tasks. In rehabilitation settings, the physical environment is designed for persons with physical disabilities and thus may not be as important because the setting is so unlike the natural environment. Systems that influence occupational performance at one time may not be the critical systems at other times. Figure 22-3 shows the effects of neural and non-neural components of muscle tone at different points in time. Based on our clinical experience, neural factors (e.g., spasticity) are important immediately after the onset of CNS damage but have less of an effect on performance later. The influence of non-neural factors (e.g., soft tissue contracture), however, is almost the reverse.

A client's occupational performance at any one time reflects the interaction of all of these systems. The critical variables at a given time may vary greatly depending on the characteristics of the person and environment. What is effective for one client may not be effective for the next client with similar CNS dysfunction. In addition, systems that enhance performance at one time may interfere with

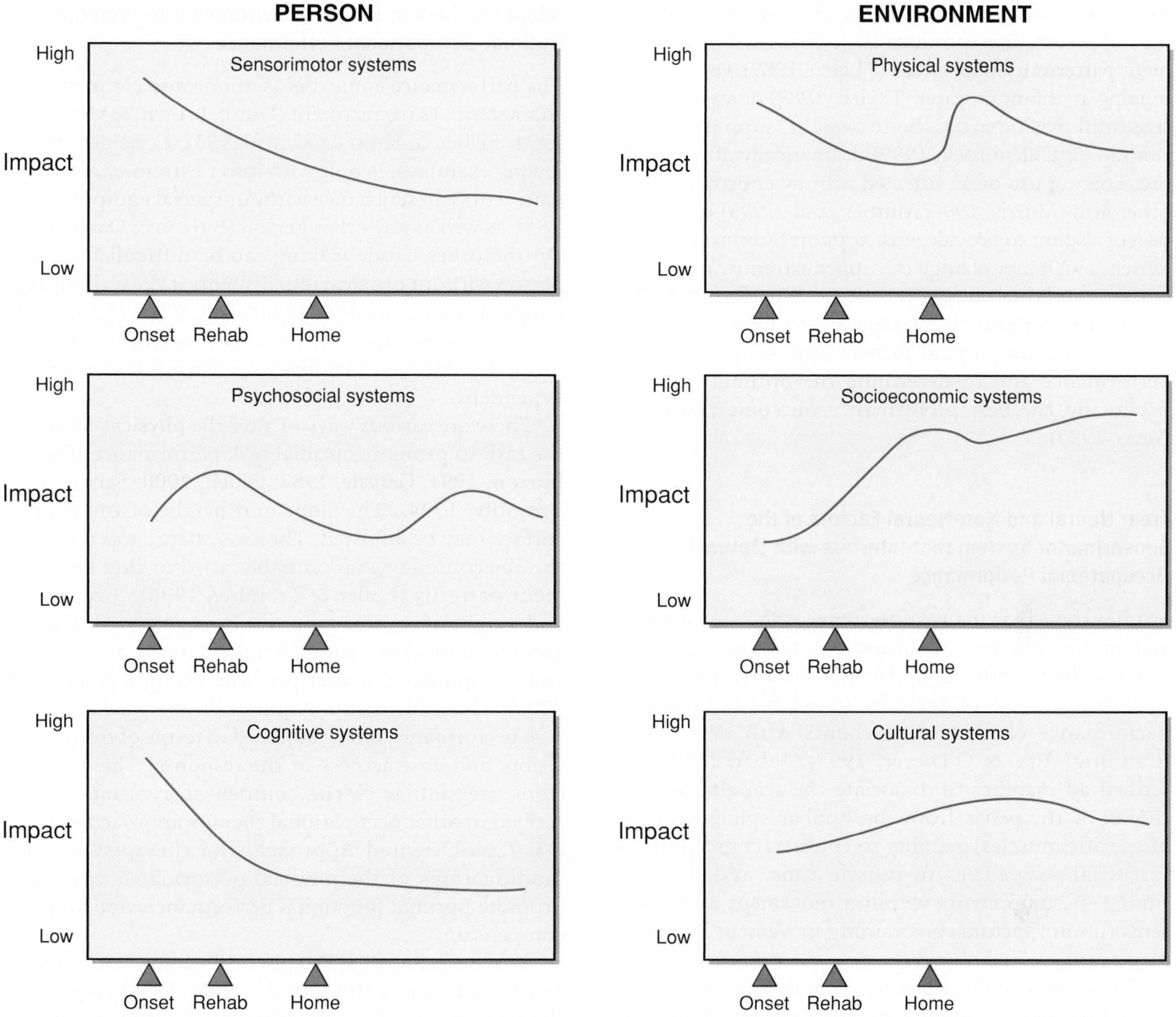

Figure 22-2 Hypothetical influences of personal and environmental systems on occupational performance for a unique person at different times (at onset, during rehabilitation, and at home).

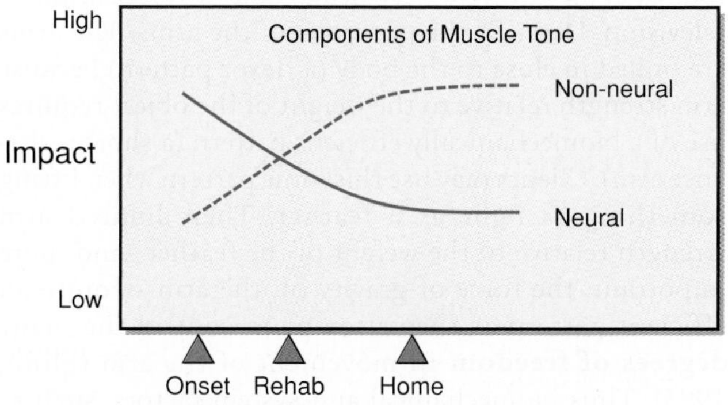

Figure 22-3 Hypothetical influences of neural and non-neural components of muscle tone on occupational performance at different points in time (at onset, during rehabilitation, and at home).

it later (Kamm, Thelen, & Jensen, 1990). What is effective early in treatment may not be effective later. Therapists must identify the major influences on motor behavior at a specific time for a specific person and anticipate changes in the critical variables.

Address Critical Personal and Environmental Systems to Change Occupational Performance

After a critical personal or environmental factor is identified, the therapist alters this personal or environmental characteristic until a shift in motor behavior is observable.

Relatively small changes in a critical personal or environmental system may produce large changes in the movement patterns used for a task (Thelen, 1989). For example, putting an infant in water (Thelen, 1989) or an adult on a treadmill with partial body weight support (Hesse, Konrad, & Uhlenbrock, 1999) dramatically affects walking. Forcing use of an affected arm by constraining the other arm (Morris, 1997; Miltner et al., 1999) or application of a splint to provide wrist support (Kamm, Thelen, & Jensen, 1990) may change the upper extremity movement patterns and thus change occupational performance. The goals of occupational therapy are to help individuals identify and use critical factors that support optimal performance and to determine the optimal value for producing the best performance outcome (Burton & Davis, 1992).

Treat Neural and Non-Neural Factors of the Sensorimotor System that Interfere with Optimal Occupational Performance

Studies show that many subsystems of the sensorimotor system, not just neural subsystems, may have a role in motor behavior after CNS damage. For example, muscle weakness and loss of dexterity are related to functional performance challenges in clients with hemiparesis (Canning, Ada, & O'Dwyer, 1999). Sabari (1991) described an inability to dissociate the scapula from the thorax or the pelvis from the lumbar spine, weakness of specific muscles, inability to counteract gravitational forces, abnormalities in muscle tone, and incorrect timing of components within a movement as possible sensorimotor factors constraining movement in a hemiplegic arm.

These sensorimotor factors offer alternative explanations for the movement patterns used by clients. For example, a client with hemiparesis may use a flexor pattern for reaching or lifting because of muscle weakness; a person without CNS damage, however, uses this pattern, too. Imagine lifting a very heavy object, for example, a television. Describe the positions of the arms. The arms are pulled in close to the body (a flexor pattern) because arm strength relative to the weight of the object requires use of a biomechanically efficient pattern (a short resistance arm). Clients may use this same pattern when lifting something as light as a feather. Their limited arm strength relative to the weight of the feather—and more important, the force of gravity on the arm—require an efficient pattern as they attempt to control the many **degrees of freedom** in movement of the arm (Flinn, 1995). Thus biomechanical and system factors, such as those described by Spaulding (1989) for prehension and those discussed in other chapters, are an important part of treatment approaches for clients with CNS dysfunction.

Adapt the Task or Broader Environment to Promote Optimal Occupational Performance

The performance context is as important as the personal characteristics in treatment (Dunn, Brown, & McGuigan, 1994; Fisher & Short-DeGraff, 1993). Consider the following examples. People with lower extremity motor impairments can scuba dive without special equipment and do so as well as any other person (Burton & Davis, 1992). On the other hand, walking can be difficult for even a person without physical impairments if the walking is attempted at an altitude of 15,000 feet. What factors influence motor behavior in these two examples? In both cases, the ability or inability to perform a task is context dependent.

There are various ways to alter the physical context of the task to promote optimal task performance (Davis & Burton, 1991; Gentile, 1987; Gillen, 2000; Sabari, 1991; Trombly, 1994). The slope and height of the support surface may be adjusted. The size, shape, and texture of the object used in a task may be varied to alter the movement patterns (Fuller & Trombly, 1996). Size, length, and weight of equipment or tools may be modified. The accuracy and speed requirements for a task as well as the task complexity can alter performance (Ma & Trombly, 2004). The information required or provided as part of task performance can be adjusted in terms of timing, precision, and abstractness of the response. These adaptations are similar to the compensatory strategies described in other occupational therapy approaches. In the OT Task-Oriented Approach, the therapist explores modifications of the physical performance context to promote optimal functional performance, not simply to compensate.

Systems other than the physical context must also be considered. Heriza (1991) and Thelen (1989) emphasized the importance of social influences on motor behavior. They reviewed studies that show that infants' locomotion changes and develops faster when there is social reinforcement of the behaviors. Therapists themselves are part of the broader environment affecting occupational performance (Newell, 1998). They coach clients to help them discover and adopt optimal patterns of task performance (Scholz, 1996). They structure the learning activities and provide feedback to help clients achieve reliable, stable, and efficient performance without prohibiting clients from identifying their own optimal movement patterns (Masters & Polman, 1996). A summary of the roles of the therapist is provided in Procedures for Practice 22-4. The role of environmental systems on motor behavior continues to be explored.

Use Natural Objects and Natural Environments

Use natural objects for practice of the task. Simulations and rote exercise do not produce the same movement

PROCEDURES FOR PRACTICE 22-4

Roles of Therapist

Many roles for the therapist are proposed in the literature (Burton & Davis, 1992; Gentile, 1992; Heriza, 1991; Higgins, 1991; Kamm, Thelen, & Jensen, 1990). All are important in helping the client to become autonomous in solving motor problems.

- Collaborate with the client in selecting a variety of tasks for practice.
- Modify the task initially so the learner can succeed.
- Teach task analysis, structure learning opportunities, provide feedback, and facilitate understanding of unique personal and environmental systems that promote optimal performance.
- Provide non-generalizable solutions that the client can memorize if the client cannot learn a more flexible approach.
- Coach the client during learning by directing the focus to the functional outcome, suggesting movements to try, recording progress, and assisting with decision making when new challenges arise.
- Alter the personal and environmental factors and identify optimal times to change movement.
- Provide manual guidance if necessary, but allow some elements to vary so that the client can experiment with movement patterns.
- Fade assistance provided through handling as soon as possible.

patterns as tasks using real objects. Studies of persons with stroke showed more efficient, direct, smooth, and planned movements in reaching tasks enriched with natural objects than in the condition without objects (Trombly & Wu, 1998; Wu et al., 1998, 2000). Other research supports the idea that the greater the number of real objects and the greater the symbolic information, the more performance is improved (Lin, Wu, & Trombly, 1998; Lin et al., 2001; Mathiowetz & Wade, 1995; Wu et al., 1998).

Use natural environments to help clients develop stable but flexible movement patterns for the tasks and contexts in their home and community (Burgess, 1989; Gillen & Wasserman, 2004). The rehabilitation unit should simulate the real-life setting as much as possible if interventions cannot be provided in the actual situation (Mulder, 1991; Poole, 1991). Therapeutic modules (Stahl, 1993) simulate community-based environments. Many rehabilitation units have apartments with ordinary home furniture. Other resources of the institution can also simulate community settings (e.g., gift shop, cafeteria, and chapel).

Practice and Feedback

The design of practice sessions and characteristics of feedback are important in interventions based on the OT Task-Oriented Approach.

Structure Practice of the Task to Promote Motor Learning

Until recently, motor learning, or the outcome of practice, was primarily measured in terms of observable changes in performance during or immediately after practice. Our goal for the outcome of practice, however, is that clients can perform better once they leave treatment. Research in motor learning (Schmidt, 1991) shows that measurement outcomes of the performance during practice are not the same as later performance. If the goal is to improve motor performance over the long term, the effectiveness of the practice must be evaluated in terms of later performance.

Blocked practice includes drills that require clients to perform many repetitions of the same task in the same way (Schmidt, 1991). For example, for dressing, the client is presented a series of steps that must be practiced again and again in the same manner. Some studies have examined the type of practice that is most beneficial for changing the capability for later performance. These studies (Hanlon, 1996; Schmidt, 1991) suggest that practice of tasks should vary randomly (**random practice**); that is, therapists should ask clients to try a variety of dressing tasks within one session. One thing to remember when adopting a random practice approach is that performance during the practice session may actually look worse than performance after blocked practice. This is acceptable because the goal is to enhance motor learning or the capability for later performance rather than change observable behaviors during a practice session.

Variation of the context within a task is also an important component of practice (Jarus, 1994; Keshner, 1991; Lee, Swanson, & Hall, 1991; Mulder, 1991; Sabari, 1991; VanSant, 1991). Manipulation of task dimensions such as support surfaces, objects, equipment, task demands, and required information are examples of strategies to vary the context (Davis & Burton, 1991). The contexts for mobility include distance, temporal characteristics, ambient conditions (light and weather conditions), terrain characteristics, physical load, attentional demands, postural transitions, and density (number of people and objects in immediate environment) (Shumway-Cook et al., 2003). Varied contexts promote development of preferred movement patterns for specific contexts and flexibility in movement patterns for different contexts (Heriza, 1991; Thelen, 1989). The client who practices only in a narrow context learns only a limited number of solutions. The client who practices the task in many contexts, however, learns many solutions and can vary performance (Higgins, 1991). Bernstein (1967) summarized this principle by stating that people need repetition without repetition.

Design the Practice Session to Fit the Type of Task and Learning Strategies

Research shows that different types of tasks require different types of practice sessions to facilitate learning (Winstein, 1991). Practice may require the client to practice the task in its entirety (**whole learning**), in separate steps (**part learning**), or in some combination of whole and part learning. Winstein (1991) studied weight shifting with part learning to improve locomotion, a continuous task, in persons with hemiparesis. She found that persons in the treatment group using part learning did improve in the symmetry of standing posture but showed no significant improvement over a control group in actual locomotion. Ma and Trombly (2001) compared performance of elders on a signature task for part and whole task conditions. They found that the whole task condition produced movements that were more smooth, efficient, and forceful. Whole learning rather than part learning is generally recommended for both continuous and **discrete tasks** (Crutchfield & Barnes, 1993). Separate practice (i.e., part learning) of the discrete components of a serial task is beneficial. Kerr (1982) stated that the complexity of the task should also be taken into consideration. When the task is relatively simple, whole learning is recommended. Part learning is suggested for more complex tasks.

The stages of learning have been described as discovery (cognitive), mastery (associative), and generalization (autonomous) (Fitts & Posner, 1967; Higgins, 1991). Many clients are in the discovery stage as they develop an understanding of the task, identify the performance problems, and find a general solution for their new capabilities. This stage is characterized by slow performance, clumsiness, and self-imposed rigidity or freezing of body parts to control all degrees of freedom that are normally free to vary in high levels of skill. In this stage, clients attempt to exert control over some parts of the body to learn the influence of changes in their personal systems and relationships to the environment (Higgins, 1991). In later stages of learning, the client refines the solutions identified in the discovery stage and generalizes these solutions to other tasks. The behaviors in these later stages are more consistent, more accurate, faster, and better coordinated (see Chapter 14).

Therapists must also consider the type of learning that the practice session will elicit (Gentile, 1998). Explicit (declarative) learning requires conscious learning of the rules for task performance and is more generalizable because it is not very context dependent. Implicit (procedural) learning requires learning how to do the task on an unconscious level. This type of learning is facilitated by structuring the environment and practice of the task. Chapter 14 provides additional detail on these aspects of learning.

Provide Feedback that Facilitates Motor Learning and Encourages Experimentation with Solutions to Occupational Performance Problems

If the goal is to have clients rely on intrinsic feedback for task performance in the future, careful planning of the extrinsic feedback during treatment is important. Lee, Swanson, and Hall (1991), Schmidt (1991), and Winstein (1991) reviewed results of studies on appropriate feedback strategies related to the knowledge of results or the outcome of performance. Studies of people without motor problems suggested that feedback should be less frequent, scheduled randomly or intermittently, faded over time, and given as summary information or when performance is outside a given error range. These feedback strategies resulted in better retention of motor skills over time than frequent, immediate, and consistent feedback. Preliminary studies indicate that reduced frequency of feedback may improve generalization when learning difficult tasks for elders (Rice, 2003) and performance consistency but not accuracy for individuals post stroke (Merians et al., 1995). Further research on feedback with subjects having motor problems is needed. Therapists should carefully analyze the effect of their feedback on an individual client's performance.

Optimize Occupational Performance Given the Constraints on the Person and Environment

"Optimization in the process of therapeutic intervention should be directed at a functional outcome rather than a peripheral motor pattern to promote learning in a functionally significant context so that adaptive solutions are developed and optimized by the CNS with respect to a certain activity" (Latash & Anson, 1996, p. 98).

After CNS damage, clients may have to learn strategies for task performance given personal limitations. When clients understand the idea of the task, their personal limitations and capabilities, environmental resources, and a basic solution to the problem, they may begin to practice the task. The inefficient and ineffective movements sometimes seen at this time are consistent with the limited understanding and control one has during the early stages of learning and at the lower levels of skill (Higgins, 1991). Perhaps the client simply needs further practice and time to develop skill. Therapists, however, must identify ineffective movement patterns that are hindering optimal task performance or contributing to future problems in personal and environmental systems. Mulder (1991) added one more caution regarding the analysis of preferred patterns: The achievement of functional outcomes is probably more important to the client and family than the therapist's goal of "normal" movement patterns. Again, a client-centered approach focused on meaningful occupations and roles is important.

LIMITATIONS AND FUTURE DIRECTIONS

A consideration of limitations and future directions is important in the discussion of any occupational therapy approach.

Limitations

There are some limitations to the OT Task-Oriented Approach. It is not yet fully developed or refined, and efficacy studies are needed. It is also difficult to simulate natural environments or some work and leisure tasks in many clinical settings. As therapy clinics are remodeled and new clinics are designed, the potential exists to create more natural environments in the hospital. This limitation suggests that therapy interventions should ideally occur in clients' home, school, leisure, and work settings whenever possible. The increased pressure to shorten hospital stays and the increased development of community-based treatment programs should support this trend. Another limitation of this approach relates to communication problems when using concepts that originate outside of occupational therapy and the testability of an approach based on abstract, complex ideas (Horak, 1991).

Future Directions

All treatment approaches evolve over time. Clinical practice and research will continue to test the assumptions and treatment principles of this approach. Some assumptions and principles will be supported and developed further. Others will not be supported and may be dropped or modified. The OT Task-Oriented Approach offers occupational therapists new ideas about the remediation of motor behavior problems. Basic and clinical research is needed. Development of evaluation tools and measures of change is critical. Identification of critical factors influencing occupational performance and measures of motor behavior will lead to more effective treatment strategies. Further testing of the assumptions and treatment principles with persons having CNS dysfunction and other motor behavior problems will provide additional support for its use in practice.

CASE EXAMPLE

Mr. B.: Application of the OT Task-Oriented Approach

Occupational Therapy Intervention Process	Clinical Reasoning Process: Objectives	Clinical Reasoning Process: Examples of Therapist's Internal Dialogue
Patient Information Mr. B., a 55-year-old man, had a left cerebral vascular accident with resultant right hemiparesis 6 months ago. He is on disability status from his job as an administrator at a junior college. His goal in outpatient rehabilitation is to participate in a trial of the student counseling aspect of his administrative job to determine whether he has potential to return to work. Mr. B.'s medical and social histories are further described in Chapter 6.	Appreciate the context	"I believe Mr. B.'s right hemiparesis is a significant barrier to his occupational functioning at the college. In addition, I assume his current job requires efficient and effective performance. I wonder about current features of the environment that support and limit current task performance. I think that Mr. B. has accurately identified critical tasks that are important in his role as worker."

Patient Information (cont'd)	Develop intervention hypotheses	"I hypothesize that targeted remediation interventions, compensation strategies, and modification of the physical and social contexts will assist Mr. B. in achieving optimal task performance."
	Select an intervention approach	"I will develop an intervention plan that emphasizes both compensation and remediation to improve task performance. I know from the evidence that he is at risk for learned non-use of his right upper extremity and that he may have muscle weakness that interferes with performance. I will provide Mr. B. with opportunities to practice the actual tasks important in his job and related tasks that may improve strength in targeted muscle groups. I will also want to examine the physical and social contexts to determine their influence on task performance."
	Reflect on competence	"I have a lot of ideas already about intervention strategies I want to explore with Mr. B. I realize I don't have very much information on expectations for performance in his job or the college's support for gradual resumption of his duties. I will also need more information on ADA policies and to refer Mr. B to his human resources department."
Recommendations The occupational therapist recommended three 1-hour treatment sessions at the college. The first session was to take place immediately. The second session would take place after supplies and furniture arrived, and the third session would take place about a week after the second session. (Separate recommendations were developed for other tasks related to his role as mediator.) OT will work on tasks related to Mr. B.'s role as mediator in student issues. The following tasks were identified as important for success in this role: contact student to gather information and set up meeting; review documentation; meet the student in a conference room; discuss issue with student; document discussion; return to office; and write, copy, and send report on the outcome to student and others as needed. It was agreed that documenting the discussion during the meeting was a critical component of the role and had to be addressed. During a simulation of a meeting, a number of problems related to performance of this task were evident: slow movement in bringing his chair close to the table; slow movement in bringing his arm to rest on top of the table; slow movement and limited endurance in grasping a regular pen; and decreased speed and accuracy and increased variation in cursive writing. Critical factors impairing performance were the weight of the conference room furniture, decreased strength (power) in shoulder flexion, and decreased strength (power) and endurance in palmar pinch. Critical factors suggesting improved future performance were adequate budget for needed supplies and furniture, Americans with Disabilities Act support for return to work, desire to appear capable to handle the task, good cognitive skills, and supportive secretary.	Consider the patient's appraisal of performance Consider what will occur in therapy, how often, and for how long Ascertain the patient's endorsement of plan	"I think that Mr. B. can make significant progress toward his goals within a short period of time. He seems highly motivated to improve task performance so he can go back to work. I have hope that occupational therapy will make it possible for Mr. B. to return to work at least on a part-time basis. At this point, the primary unknown is the level of performance that is necessary to meet expectations of the job."

Summary of Short-Term Goals and Progress

The occupational therapist and Mr. B. established the following short-term goals. At the end of two sessions, Mr. B. will independently (1) adjust furniture in the conference room to prepare for task performance; (2) use a tape recorder to record the discussion; and (3) record notes during a 5-minute discussion with sufficient completeness and accuracy for development of a report.

During the first session, a conference room chair with adjustable height, wide armrests, and swivel seat was ordered. A tape recorder with voice activation, adjustable speed, and an internal microphone was requisitioned. Felt-tip pens with a textured grip were acquired. Several adapted pens and pen holders were lent to Mr. B. for a trial period. A practice session of writing using various pens and grasps was conducted. Mr. B. also helped design a home program of additional tasks that would strengthen targeted muscle groups in the right hand. The tasks included reaching for the spices needed for each meal, organizing cupboards, buttering bread, and writing down recipes.

During the second session, Mr. B. practiced a variety of ways to position himself for efficient writing. He learned to adjust the chair and use the swivel feature to position the chair close to the table before sitting. When moving from standing to sitting, Mr. B. could use his right arm as an assist by placing it on the table as he lowered himself. Mr. B. was instructed in and practiced operation of the tape recorder. Use of the left hand was better for manipulation of the small buttons on the recorder when efficiency in performance was needed. The occupational therapist observed Mr. B.'s right-handed writing using different devices and timed (1) bringing right arm from lap to table, (2) picking up pen, and (3) completing specified writing task. Summary feedback was provided after each performance. The home program was adjusted to promote practice of positioning self and operating the recorder and to increase the task demands related to targeted muscle groups. Finally, the occupational therapist worked with Mr. B. and the secretary to develop a template and some codes for recording discussions and reducing the writing requirements during the discussion.

During the third session, Mr. B. demonstrated all components of the task. He practiced variations in task performance. Mr. B. was instructed in strategies for analyzing his own performance. Increased speed in bringing the right arm from the lap to the table was noted. Movement time for picking up the pen was still slow. It was agreed that the left hand would pick up the pen and hold it vertical to allow an easier and quicker grasp by the right hand. The right palmar pinch had increased in strength and endurance sufficiently to enable completion of a 10-minute writing task with the felt-tip pen. The home program was adjusted to promote practice of use of codes in simulated discussions and to continue work on tasks related to targeted muscle groups.

Assess the patient's comprehension

Understand what the patient is doing

Compare actual to expected performance

Know the person

Appreciate the context

"I think Mr. B. didn't fully realize the environmental supports that were available to improve his task performance. He had been frustrated with his speed of writing and didn't think he could adequately record information during a meeting. We talked about the combinations of strategies he could use to continue to work on improving his motor performance and, in the mean time, 'get the job done.' His interest in finding related tasks to perform at home made it easy to develop a home program."

"By the end of the second session, I could tell that Mr. B. was pleased to have smoother movements and successful strategies during a simulated meeting task. Mr. B. was also fortunate to have a supportive secretary who knew his responsibilities and communication style. They seemed eager to try working with the template and codes and had some of their own ideas on possible practice scenarios before a real meeting."

"I really felt that Mr. B. was more confident about resuming this important task of his job. The college was very supportive of Mr. B. working a few hours a day on selected tasks as a trial. Mr. B. seemed ready to resume responsibility for general student meetings that were routine in nature. I was glad he was taking it slow at work. I think that engaging in a variety of tasks will help Mr. B. discover his potential for movement in all his life roles."

Next Steps Within 4 weeks, Mr. B. will independently record notes during a 15-minute discussion with sufficient completeness and accuracy for development of a final report.	Anticipate present and future patient concerns Analyze patient's comprehension Decide if the patient should continue or discontinue therapy and/or return in the future	"Mr. B. has learned some effective strategies for one of his tasks at work. More importantly, he is more engaged in learning about his own movement capabilities and performance as well as developing plans to improve performance in others tasks. I would like to meet with Mr. B. on a periodic basis to help him solve problems he encounters in different situations and reevaluate his motor performance."

CLINICAL REASONING IN OCCUPATIONAL THERAPY PRACTICE

Application of the OT Task-Oriented Approach

What information could you use to determine whether Mr. B.'s optimal performance of the writing task is with his left or right hand?
What other personal or environmental factors might influence Mr. B.'s performance in a discussion with a real student (see assessment of Mr. B. in Chapter 6)?
What might be some future changes in the personal or environmental factors influencing performance given what you know about Mr. B.?
How would you determine when performance is optimal and when to discontinue treatment for this particular goal?

SUMMARY REVIEW QUESTIONS

1. What are the treatment principles of the OT Task-Oriented Approach?
2. What does *attractor* mean? Describe the characteristics of the different movement patterns illustrated by Figure 22-1 in terms of attractor states. Give examples of these patterns that might be observed in clients who are attempting to achieve functional goals.
3. What are optimal and less than optimal times for producing a change in motor behavior?
4. What are some strategies for making the treatment process more client centered and unique to the characteristics of the person and environment?
5. What is the role of the client in the OT Task-Oriented Approach? What is the role of the therapist?
6. How is change in motor behavior measured?
7. What are some possible measures of performance, and how are they important in determining whether optimal performance is achieved?
8. What are critical variables (i.e., control parameters) or systems of the person and environment, and how should they be used in treatment to facilitate optimal performance?
9. What are the characteristics of skilled and optimal performance, and how can therapists facilitate development of these characteristics in their clients?
10. Describe feedback that facilitates development of skill in performance and an optimal solution to a motor problem.
11. Why are natural objects and environments important to use in finding the optimal solution for a motor problem and developing skill in performance?

Evidence Table 22-1
Best Evidence for Occupational Therapy Practice Regarding Aspects of the OT Task-Oriented Approach

Intervention	Description of Intervention Tested	Participants	Dosage	Type of Best Evidence and Level of Evidence	Benefit	Statistical Probability and Effect Size of Outcome	Reference
Use of real objects	Condition 1: reach to scoop coins off table; condition 2: reach forward without object present; setting: laboratory.	14 subjects with stroke: 8 with chronic LCVA, 5 with RCVA, 1 with other; 24 healthy subjects. Mean age was 61.8 years for stroke subjects and 63.2 years for healthy subjects.	10 trials/condition within 1 day.	IC1c	Yes. Better reaching movements when objects present on 4/5 kinematic variables ($p < 0.01$).	Mean effect over 5 variables: $r = 0.63$. Speed: $r = 0.70$; directness of movement: $r = 0.72$; smoothness: $r = 0.66$; preorganization of movement: $r = 0.75$.	Wu et al., 2000
Use of natural objects with functional information	Condition 1: enriched affordance (reach to food chopper to chop mushroom); condition 2: impoverished affordance (reach to disguised food chopper and push handle down); setting: laboratory.	14 subjects with stroke: 8 with chronic LCVA, 5 with RCVA, 1 with other; 24 healthy subjects. Mean age was 61.8 years for stroke subjects and 63.2 years for healthy subjects.	10 trials/condition within 1 day.	IC1c	Yes. Better reaching movement for enriched affordance on 3/5 kinematic variables ($p < 0.05$).	Mean effect over 5 variables: $r = 0.44$. Speed: $r = 0.54$; directness of movement: $r = 0.47$; smoothness: $r = 0.58$.	Wu et al., 1998
OT in natural environment	Experimental group: OT in home; patients practice between OT visits; leisure activities encouraged. Control group: Routine, existing services.	N = 185 acute, not hospitalized subjects (LCVA: 80; RCVA: 85; other: 20). Mean age = 74.3 years; attrition = 12%.	1–15 visits (mean = 5.8); 24–90 minutes per visit (mean = 52 minutes) for 5 months.	IA2b	Yes. Experimental group had better ADL and IADL ratings on 3 scales ($p < 0.01$) than the control group.	Nottingham EADL Scale: $\varphi = 0.18$; Handicap scale: $\varphi = 0.15$; Barthel Index: $\varphi = 0.22$.	Walker et al., 1999

LCVA, left cerebral vascular accident; RCVA, right cerebral vascular accident; OT, occupational therapy; ADL, activities of daily living; IADL, instrumental activities of daily living; EADL Scale, Extended Activities of Daily Living Scale.
Evidence Table Studies from: Trombly, C. A., & Ma, H.-I. (2002). A synthesis of effects of occupational therapy for persons with stroke. Part I: Restoration of roles, tasks, and activities. *American Journal of Occupational Therapy, 56*, 250–259 and Ma, H.-I., & Trombly, C. A. (2002). A synthesis of the effects of occupational therapy for persons with stroke, part II: Remediation of impairments. *American Journal of Occupational Therapy, 56*, 260–274.

References

Ada, L., Canning, C., & Westwood, P. (1990). The patient as active learner. In L. Ada & C. Canning (Eds.), *Key issues in neurological physiotherapy* (pp 99–124). Boston: Butterworth Heinemann.

Bernstein, N. (1967). *The coordination and regulation of movements.* Oxford, United Kingdom: Pergamon.

Burgess, M. K. (1989). The issue is: Motor control and the role of occupational therapy: Past, present, and future. *American Journal of Occupational Therapy, 43,* 345–348.

Burton, A. W., & Davis, W. E. (1992). Optimizing the involvement and performance of children with physical impairments in movement activities. *Pediatric Exercise Science, 4,* 236–248.

Campbell, S. K. (1991). Framework for the measurement of neurologic impairment and disability. In M. J. Lister (Ed.), *Contemporary management of motor control problems: Proceedings of the II STEP Conference* (pp. 143–154). Alexandria, VA: Foundation for Physical Therapy.

Canning, C., Ada, L., & O'Dwyer, N. (1999). Slowness to develop force contributes to weakness after stroke. *Medical Rehabilitation, 80,* 66–70.

Carr, J. H., & Shepherd, R. B. (1998). *Neurological rehabilitation: Optimizing motor performance.* Oxford, United Kingdom: Butterworth-Heinemann.

Christiansen, C., & Baum, C. (1997). *Occupational therapy: Enabling function and well-being.* Thorofare, NJ: Slack.

Clark, A. (1997). The dynamical challenge. *Cognitive Science, 21,* 461–481.

Corcos, D. (1991). Strategies underlying the control of disordered movement. *Physical Therapy, 71,* 25–38.

Crutchfield, C. A., & Barnes, M. R. (1993). *Motor control and motor learning in rehabilitation.* Atlanta: Stokesville.

Davis, W. E., & Burton, A. W. (1991). Ecological task analysis: Translating movement behavior theory into practice. *Adapted Physical Activity Quarterly, 8,* 154–177.

Dobkin, B. (1998). Activity-dependent learning contributes to motor recovery. *Annals of Neurology, 44,* 158–160.

Dobkin, B. (2005). Rehabilitation after stroke. *New England Journal of Medicine, 352,* 1677–1684.

Dunn, W., Brown, C., & McGuigan, A. (1994). The ecology of human performance: A framework for considering the effect of context. *American Journal of Occupational Therapy, 48,* 595–607.

Fetters, L. (1991). Measurement and treatment in cerebral palsy: An argument for a new approach. *Physical Therapy, 71,* 244–247.

Fisher, A., & Short-DeGraff, M. (1993). Nationally speaking: Improving functional assessment in occupational therapy: Recommendations and philosophy for change. *American Journal of Occupational Therapy, 47,* 199–201.

Fitts, P. M., & Posner, M. I. (1967). *Human performance.* Belmont, CA: Brooks/Cole.

Flinn, N. (1995). A task-oriented approach to the treatment of a client with hemiplegia. *American Journal of Occupational Therapy, 49,* 560–569.

Flinn, N. (1999). Clinical interpretation of effect of rehabilitation tasks on organization of movement after stroke. *American Journal of Occupational Therapy, 53,* 345–347.

Fuller, Y., & Trombly, C. (1996). Effects of object characteristics on female grasp patterns. *American Journal of Occupational Therapy, 51,* 481–487.

Gentile, A. M. (1992). The nature of skill acquisition: Therapeutic implications for children with movement disorders. In H. Forssberg & H. Hirschfeld (Eds.), *Movement disorders in children* (pp. 31–40). Basel, Switzerland: S. Karger.

Gentile, A. M. (1987). Skill acquisition: Action, movement, and neuromotor processes. In J. H. Carr, R. B. Shepherd, J. Gordon, A. M. Gentile, & J. M. Held (Eds.), *Movement science: Foundations for physical therapy in rehabilitation* (pp. 93–154). Rockville, MD: Aspen.

Gentile, A. M. (1998). Implicit and explicit processes during acquisition of functional skills. *Scandinavian Journal of Occupational Therapy, 5,* 7–16.

Gibson, J. W., & Schkade, J. (1997). Occupational adaptation intervention with patients with cerebrovascular accident: A clinical study. *American Journal of Occupational Therapy, 51,* 523–529.

Gillen, G. (2000). Improving activities of daily living in an adult with ataxia. *American Journal of Occupational Therapy, 54,* 89–96.

Gillen, G., & Wasserman, M. (2004). Mobility: Examining the impact of environment on transfer performance. *Physical and Occupational Therapy in Geriatrics, 22,* 21–29.

Gray, J. M. (1998). Putting occupation into practice: Occupation as ends, occupation as means. *American Journal of Occupational Therapy, 52,* 354–364.

Hanlon, R. E. (1996). Motor learning following unilateral stroke. *Archives of Physical Medicine and Rehabilitation, 77,* 811–815.

Heriza, C. (1991). Motor development: Traditional and contemporary theories. In M. J. Lister (Ed.), *Contemporary management of motor control problems: Proceedings of the II STEP Conference* (pp. 99–126). Alexandria, VA: Foundation for Physical Therapy.

Hesse, S., Konrad, M., & Uhlenbrock, D. (1999). Treadmill walking with partial body weight support versus floor walking in hemiparetic subjects. *Archives of Physical Medicine and Rehabilitation, 80,* 421–427.

Higgins, S. (1991). Motor skill acquisition. *Physical Therapy, 71,* 123–139.

Horak, F. B. (1991). Assumptions underlying motor control for neurologic rehabilitation. In M. J. Lister (Ed.), *Contemporary management of motor control problems: Proceedings of the II STEP Conference* (pp. 11–27). Alexandria, VA: Foundation for Physical Therapy.

Hsieh, C., Nelson, D., Smith, D., & Peterson, C. (1996). A comparison of performance in added-purpose occupations and rote exercise for dynamic standing balance in persons with hemiplegia. *American Journal of Occupational Therapy, 50,* 10–16.

Inouye, M., Kishi, K., Ikeda, Y., Takada, M., Katoh, J., Iwahashi, M., Hayakawa, M., Ishihara, K., Sawamura, S., & Kazumi, T. (2000). Prediction of functional outcome after stroke rehabilitation. *American Journal of Physical Medicine & Rehabilitation, 79,* 513–518.

Jarus, T. (1994). Motor learning and occupational therapy: The organization of practice. *American Journal of Occupational Therapy, 48,* 810–816.

Kamm, K., Thelen, E., & Jensen, J. L. (1990). A dynamical systems approach to motor development. *Physical Therapy, 70,* 763–775.

Kerr, R. (1982). *Psychomotor learning.* New York: CBS.

Keshner, E. (1991). How theoretical framework biases evaluation and treatment. In M. J. Lister (Ed.), *Contemporary management of motor control problems: Proceedings of the II STEP Conference* (pp. 37–47). Alexandria, VA: Foundation for Physical Therapy.

Latash, M. L., & Anson, J. G. (1996). What are "normal movements" in atypical populations? *Behavioral and Brain Sciences, 19,* 55–106.

Law, M., Cooper, B. A., Strong, S., Stewart, D., Rigby, P., & Letts, L. (1997). The person-environment-occupation model: A transactive approach to occupational performance. *Canadian Journal of Occupational Therapy, 63,* 9–23.

Lee, T., Swanson, L., & Hall, A. (1991). What is repeated in a repetition? Effects of practice conditions on motor skill acquisition. *Physical Therapy, 71,* 150–156.

Letts, L., Law, M., Rigby, P., Cooper, B., Stewart, D., & Strong, S. (1994). Person-environment assessments in occupational therapy. *American Journal of Occupational Therapy, 48,* 608–618.

Lin, K. C., Tang, F. T., Wu, C. Y., & Shen, I. H. (2001). Effects of contextual constraints on reaching performance in adults without disabilities: A kinematic study. *Occupational Therapy Journal of Research, 21,* 168–184.

Lin, K.C., Wu, C.-Y., & Trombly, C. (1998). Effects of task goal on movement kinematics and line bisection performance in adults without disabilities. *American Journal of Occupational Therapy, 52,* 179–187.

Ma, H., & Trombly, C. A. (2001). The comparison of motor performance between part and whole tasks in elderly persons. *American Journal of Occupational Therapy, 55,* 62–67.

Ma, H., & Trombly, C. A. (2002). A synthesis of the effects of occupational therapy for persons with stroke, part II: Remediation of impairments. *American Journal of Occupational Therapy, 56,* 260–274.

Ma, H., & Trombly, C. A. (2004). Effects of task complexity on reaction time and movement kinematics in elderly people. *American Journal of Occupational Therapy, 58,* 150–158.

Masters, R. S. W., & Polman, R. C. J. (1996). What are normal movements in any population? *Behavioral and Brain Sciences, 19,* 81–82.

Mathiowetz, V. G., & Wade, M. (1995). Task constraints and functional motor performance of individuals with and without multiple sclerosis. *Ecological Psychology, 7,* 99–123.

Mayo, N. D., Wood-Dauphinee, S., Cote, R., Durcan, L., & Carlton, J. (2002). Activity, participation, and quality of life 6 months post stroke. *Archives of Physical Medicine and Rehabilitation, 83,* 1035–1042.

McAndrew, E., McDermott, S., Vitzakovitch, S., Warunek, M., & Holm, M. (1999). Therapist and patient perceptions of the occupational therapy goal-setting process: A pilot study. *Physical and Occupational Therapy in Geriatrics, 17,* 55–63.

Merians, A., Winstein, C., Sullivan, K., & Pohl, P. (1995). Effects of feedback for motor skill learning in older healthy subjects and individuals post-stroke. *Neurology Report, 19,* 23–25.

Miltner, W., Bauder, H., Sommer, M., Dettmers, C., & Taub, E. (1999). Effects of constraint-induced movement therapy on patients with chronic motor deficits after stroke. *Stroke, 30,* 586–592.

Morris, D. M. (1997). Constraint-induced movement therapy for motor recovery after stroke. *Neurorehabilitation, 9,* 29–43.

Mulder, T. (1991). A process-oriented model of human motor behavior: Toward a theory-based rehabilitation approach. *Physical Therapy, 71,* 157–164.

Neistadt, M. (1994). The effects of different treatment activities on functional fine motor coordination in adults with brain injury. *American Journal of Occupational Therapy, 48,* 877–882.

Neistadt, M. (1995a). Methods of assessing clients' priorities: A survey of adult physical dysfunction settings. *American Journal of Occupational Therapy, 49,* 428–436.

Neistadt, M. (1995b). Treatment activity preferences of occupational therapists in adult physical dysfunction settings. *American Journal of Occupational Therapy, 49,* 437–443.

Newell, K. M. (1998). Therapeutic intervention as a constraint in learning and relearning movement skills. *Scandinavian Journal of Occupational Therapy, 5,* 51–57.

Phillips, E. M., Schneider, J. C., & Mercer, G. R. (2004). Motivating elders to initiate exercise. *Archives of Physical Medicine and Rehabilitation, 85 (Suppl. 3),* S52–S57.

Pollock, N. (1993). Client-centered assessment. *American Journal of Occupational Therapy, 47,* 298–302.

Poole, J. L. (1991). Motor control. In C. B. Royeen (Ed.), *AOTA self-study series: Neuroscience foundations of human performance* (Monograph 11, pp. 1–31). Rockville, MD: American Occupational Therapy Association.

Reisman, D., & Scholz, J. (2003). Aspects of joint coordination are preserved during pointing in persons with post-stroke hemiparesis. *Brain, 126,* 2510–2517.

Rice, M. (2003). Motor learning strategies for well elderly: A pilot study. *Physical and Occupational Therapy in Geriatrics, 21,* 59–74.

Rice, M., & Newell, K. M. (2004). Upper-extremity interlimb coupling in persons with left hemiplegia due to stroke. *Archives of Physical Medicine and Rehabilitation, 85,* 629–634.

Sabari, J. S. (1991). Motor learning concepts applied to activity-based intervention with adults with hemiplegia. *American Journal of Occupational Therapy, 45,* 523–530.

Schmidt, R. A. (1991). Motor learning principles for physical therapy. In M. J. Lister (Ed.), *Contemporary management of motor control problems: Proceedings of the II STEP Conference* (pp. 49–63). Alexandria, VA: Foundation for Physical Therapy.

Schmidt, R. A., (1998). *Motor control and learning: a behavioral emphasis* (2nd ed.). Champaign, IL: Human Kinetics.

Scholz, J. (1990). Dynamic pattern theory: Some implications for therapeutics. *Physical Therapy, 70,* 827–843.

Scholz, J. (1996). How functional are atypical motor patterns? *Behavioral and Brain Sciences, 19,* 85–86.

Shepherd, R. B. (1992). Adaptive motor behaviour in response to perturbations of balance. *Physiotherapy Theory and Practice, 8,* 137–143.

Shumway-Cook, A., Patla, A., Stewart, A., Ferrucci, L., Ciol, M., & Guralnik, J. (2003). Environmental components of mobility disability in community-living older person. *Journal of American Geriatric Society, 51,* 393–388.

Spaulding, S. (1989). The biomechanics of prehension. *American Journal of Occupational Therapy, 43,* 302–306.

Stahl, C. (1993). Rehab in the rain or in a rowboat: New environments bring the outdoors indoors. *Advance for Occupational Therapists, 9,* 14–15.

Thelen, E. (1989). Self-organization in developmental processes: Can systems approaches work? In M. R. Gunnar & E. Thelen (Eds.), *Systems and development* (pp. 77–117). Hillsdale, NJ: Lawrence Erlbaum.

Thelen, E., & Fisher, D. M. (1983). The organization of spontaneous to instrumental behavior: Kinematic analysis of movement changes during very early learning. *Child Development, 54,* 120–140.

Thelen, E., & Ulrich, B. D. (1991). Hidden skills. *Monographs of the Society for Research in Child Development, 56,* 1–98.

Trombly, C. A. (1993). The issue is: Anticipating the future: Assessment of occupational function. *American Journal of Occupational Therapy, 47,* 253–257.

Trombly, C. A. (1994). Purposeful activity. In C. Trombly (Ed.), *Occupational therapy for physical dysfunction* (4th ed., pp. 237–254). Baltimore: Williams & Wilkins.

Trombly, C. A. (1995). Occupation: Purposefulness and meaningfulness as therapeutic mechanisms. *American Journal of Occupational Therapy, 49,* 960–972.

Trombly, C. A., & Ma, H.-I. (2002). A synthesis of effects of occupational therapy for persons with stroke. Part I: Restoration of roles, tasks, and activities. *American Journal of Occupational Therapy, 56,* 250–259.

Trombly, C., Radomski, M. V., & Davis, E. S. (1998). Achievement of self-identified goals by adults with traumatic brain injury: phase I. *American Journal of Occupational Therapy, 52,* 810–818.

Trombly, C., & Wu, C.-Y. (1998). Effect of rehabilitation tasks on organization of movement after stroke. *American Journal of Occupational Therapy, 53,* 333–344.

VanSant, A. (1991). Life-span motor development. In M. J. Lister (Ed.), *Contemporary management of motor control problems: Proceedings of the II STEP Conference* (pp. 77–83). Alexandria, VA: Foundation for Physical Therapy.

Winstein, C. J. (1991). Knowledge of results and motor learning: Implications for physical therapy. *Physical Therapy, 71,* 140–149.

Wressle, E., Eeg-Olofsson, A.-M., Marcusson, J., & Henriksson, C. (2002). Improved client participation in the rehabilitation process. *Journal of Rehabilitation Medicine, 34,* 5–11.

Wu, C.-Y., Trombly, C., Lin, K.-C., & Tickle-Degnen, L. (1998). Effects of object affordances on reaching performance in person with and without cerebrovascular accident. *American Journal of Occupational Therapy, 52,* 447–456.

Wu, C., Trombly, C., Lin, K.-C., & Tickle-Degnen, L. (2000). A kinematic study of contextual effects on reaching performance in persons with and without stroke: Influences of object availability. *Archives of Physical Medicine and Rehabilitation, 81,* 95–101.

Wu, C., Wong, M., Lin, K., & Chen, H. (2001). Effects of task goal and personal preference on seated reaching kinematics after stroke. *Stroke, 32,* 70–76.

CHAPTER 23

Optimizing Motor Skill Using Task-Related Training

Joyce Shapero Sabari

LEARNING OBJECTIVES

After studying this chapter, the reader will be able to do the following:

1. Identify key concepts and principles from movement science that have influenced the use of task-related training, as described by Carr and Shepherd.
2. Describe the key factors that contribute to optimal movement and explain how therapeutic interventions can influence each of these key factors.
3. Interpret scores from the *Motor Assessment Scale* and practice using this tool to assess motor performance.
4. Analyze movement during functional task performance to determine occupational therapy treatment goals.
5. Develop individualized treatment plans to assist patients in reaching their optimal motor function in the areas of balance, walking, standing up and sitting down, and reach and manipulation.

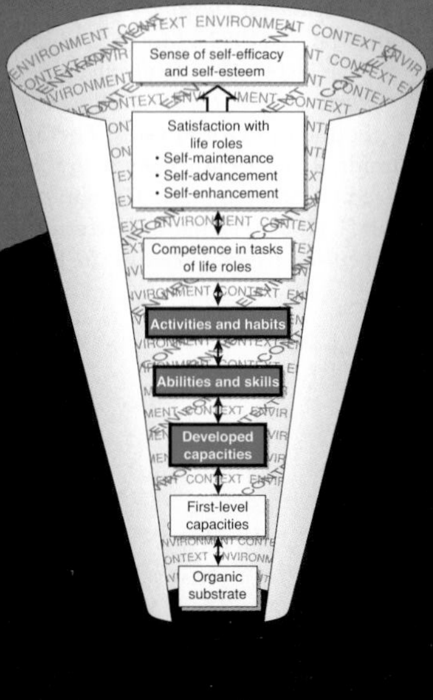

Glossary

Adaptive features—Physiological, mechanical, and functional changes that develop as a person's neuromuscular system attempts to function within the constraints of negative features associated with CNS dysfunction.

Attractor state—Preferred pattern of organization within a system.

Control parameter—Variable that, when changed, will influence changes in a system's pattern of organization. The term *regulatory condition* is used to describe control parameters within the task or environment.

Degrees of freedom—Number of elements that are free to vary within a system and hence must be controlled.

Kinematics—Description of movement in terms of direction, speed, and position of body segments.

Kinetics—Description of movement in terms of forces required.

Negative features—Losses in motor function directly attributable to CNS pathology.

Positive features—Exaggerations of normal phenomena after CNS pathology due to release of primitive centers from inhibitory hierarchical control.

Practice—Opportunity to develop skill through engagement in tasks that require problem solving and implementation of effective motor strategies.

Postural adjustments—Automatic, anticipatory, and ongoing muscle activation that enables individuals to maintain balance against gravity, optimal alignment between body parts, and optimal orientation of the head, trunk, and limbs in relation to the environment.

Skill—Goal-directed patterns of movement that efficiently address the spatiotemporal demands of a task.

Motor impairments are significant obstacles to the desired achievement of occupational and role performance in many individuals who have sustained disease or damage to the central nervous system (CNS). Occupational therapists provide intervention to assist these people in (1) optimizing their motor function and (2) integrating their improved motor skills into enhanced performance of functional activities that provide independence and meaning to their daily lives.

Research literature in neuroscience (Nudo, 2003; Pascual-Leone, 2001) and movement science (Schmidt & Lee, 2005; Shumway-Cook & Woollacott, 2000) provides consistent support for the efficacy of task-oriented **practice** in promoting motor skill and neural plasticity in humans with and without movement impairments due to CNS dysfunction. A core, historical assumption of occupational therapy practice, that engagement in specially designed therapeutic activities can improve motor function, is now embraced by every rehabilitation discipline. Carr and Shepherd, Australian physical therapists with doctoral degrees in movement science, have articulated and tested a coherent approach to task-related training in neurorehabilitation for the past 25 years (Carr & Shepherd, 1980, 1983, 1987, 1998, 2003). Their goal, along with others who advocate evidence-based rehabilitation, is to break away from the mid-20th century practice of offering a smorgasbord of treatment methods, from which therapists might choose the approach that personally appeals to them. Rather, Carr and Shepherd base their treatment model on published theoretical and outcomes evidence and present specific guidelines to direct patient treatment. Not all of Carr and Shepherd's treatment suggestions are new. Rather, it is the coherent organization of their presentation and their ongoing modifications in response to theoretical and outcomes research that make their published work so valuable to occupational therapy and physical therapy practitioners. Carr and Shepherd's ideas are entirely compatible with the Occupational Functioning Model and the OT Task-Oriented Approach, presented in Chapter 22. A major difference is that Carr and Shepherd provide specific guidelines for assessing and treating deficits in motor performance but do not discuss guidelines for enhancing individuals' participation in occupations or social roles.

Carr and Shepherd's specific strategies for helping individuals reach optimal potential in motor control provide a foundation for a critical component of occupational therapy intervention. These strategies are particularly applicable to individuals who are coping with residual motor impairments after stroke (Carr & Shepherd, 2003) but may also be useful in interventions with clients who face challenges presented by traumatic brain injury, multiple sclerosis, or Parkinson's disease (Carr & Shepherd, 1998).

Clients who demonstrate potential to improve motor control deserve the opportunity to learn to perform motor tasks with efficiency, fluidity, and versatility. Carr and Shepherd's work provides occupational therapists with practical guidelines for the following:

- Assessment of motor function during task performance
- Analysis of motor performance to determine key limiting factors that are amenable to change through therapeutic intervention
- Prevention or reduction of these key limiting factors through direct intervention and client education
- Design of activities to be used as therapeutic challenges that stimulate development of effective movement strategies

- Adaptation of the physical environment to promote maximum function by each individual
- Assistance for individuals in developing strategies for approaching and mastering the motor challenges of new activities they may wish to perform in the future.

THEORETICAL FRAMEWORK

The framework for task-related training includes the dynamical systems theory of motor control, plasticity of the CNS, and the maladaptive biomechanical changes that occur after CNS injury. Principles of motor learning and biomechanics guide the therapist in structuring the therapeutic environment to maximize patients' recovery of motor function.

Dynamical Systems Theory and CNS Plasticity

A principle of dynamical systems theory, described in Chapter 6, is that organisms demonstrate an inherent tendency to self-organize throughout life (Perry, 1998). Plasticity (Boller, 2004) is a system's capacity to reorganize after disruption and to adapt to functional demands. Although damaged neural tissue does not structurally regenerate, plasticity in the mammalian CNS has been well documented (Ward, 2004). Neuroscience research (Calautti & Baron, 2003; Chen, Cohen, & Hallett, 2002) has shown that functional improvements after brain lesions are associated with changes in metabolic activity or patterns of neural connections in brain regions that were previously inactive during performance of the function under study. A critical factor common to all situations in which CNS plasticity has been observed is the presentation of environmental opportunities for animal or human research participants to attempt to perform functional tasks previously mediated by the impaired system (Briones, Klintsova, & Greenough, 2004; Johansson, 2003). Environmental challenges serve as the impetus for dynamic reorganization of an injured CNS.

Carr and Shepherd assume that therapeutic challenges have the potential to influence how a person's neuromuscular system will reorganize itself after injury to the CNS. Furthermore, they recognize that voluntary movements are initiated by functional task goals (Willingham, 1998) and influenced by the spatial and force characteristics of goal objects (Trombly & Wu, 1999; Wu et al., 2000). Therefore, functional task demands are used instead of exercise to provide graded motor challenges.

Dynamical Systems Theory: Attractor States and Control Parameters

Chapters 6 and 22 introduce the term **attractor state**, which refers to a preferred pattern. People develop preferred movement patterns for various categories of motor performance. Attractor states for activities ranging from handwriting to a golf swing cast a unique and identifiable imprint on each individual's style of performance.

The flexibility of an attractor state is characterized, in a schematic presentation, by the depth of its well (see Fig. 22-1). Movement patterns with shallow wells are extremely unstable. They are inconsistent; they vary each time the task is performed. Movement patterns with deep wells are extremely stable. Deep well patterns make it difficult for the person to achieve versatility in task performance. Neither shallow nor deep attractor wells allow for optimal motor function. When one's neuromuscular system is functioning efficiently, the preferred patterns are characterized by attractor wells that are deep enough to allow for consistent performance but shallow enough to allow sufficient flexibility to deal with varying task and environmental demands.

Control parameters are variables that, when changed, influence changes in motor behavior (Perry, 1998). External control parameters, such as task requirements or features in the environment, frequently elicit variations in performance. In the case of efficient handwriting, the type of pen and the writing surface influence a person's motor strategies for executing the task. Internal control parameters, such as body alignment, muscle length, and muscle strength, also influence motor behavior. Postural asymmetry or mobility limitations impose constraints that limit a person's choices regarding motor performance. Although Carr and Shepherd do not typically use the terms *attractor states* and *control parameters,* Figure 22-1 illustrates how these concepts are critical to understanding and implementing their approach. Early in the intervention, internal control parameters for each individual are identified as obstacles to efficient movement. Interventions for preventing or reducing these obstacles to efficient movement are discussed later in this chapter.

Impairments of Interest to Rehabilitation Professionals

Typically, neuroscientists, physicians, and therapists have categorized the motor characteristics of CNS dysfunction as **positive features** or **negative features**. Positive features are exaggerations of normal phenomena due to release of spinal or brainstem reflexes from hierarchical inhibitory control. Positive features of stroke and brain injury include spasticity and hyperreflexia. In the latter decades of the 20th century, medical and therapy professions had considered positive features to be the major obstacle to improved clinical function, but no clinical or experimental evidence supports this view (Carr, Shepherd, & Ada, 1995). Furthermore, research findings are increasingly supporting the view that negative features of brain dysfunction are more important than positive features in causing motor disability. Negative features, which include weakness, fatigability, slowness, and impaired dexterity, are due to impairments in recruitment and firing rate modulation of motor neurons (Ada et al., 1996).

Carr and Shepherd introduced a third category of features associated with upper motor neuron dysfunction. **Adaptive features** are physiological, mechanical, and functional changes in muscle and other soft tissues that develop in response to immobility, disuse, and attempts to move within the constraints of weakness. For occupational therapists, who typically use the term *adaptive* to connote behaviors that are effective in coping with environmental demands, Carr and Shepherd's term may seem misleading. *Secondary impairment,* which indicates areas of dysfunction that are not directly caused by the neurological pathology (Sabari, 2004), is synonymous with Carr and Shepherd's term *adaptive features.* When muscles are immobilized in their shortened position, physiological changes include the loss of sarcomeres and remodeling of connective tissue (Carr, Shepherd, & Ada, 1995; O'Dwyer, Ada, & Neilson, 1996). Subsequently, muscles undergo mechanical changes of shortening and stiffening. As illustrated in Figure 23-1, abnormal movement patterns are not necessarily manifestations of spasticity or reflex disinhibition. Rather, they can be explained as functional adaptations to movement demands in the presence of negative symptoms.

Carr and Shepherd advocate early therapeutic intervention after stroke or brain injury to prevent or minimize the adaptive features of CNS dysfunction. It is particularly essential to prevent muscle stiffness and shortening through early passive and active mobilization.

The Rehabilitation Environment

Above and beyond the actual therapeutic procedures that are employed, environmental factors play a critical role in determining the effectiveness of interventions. Carr and Shepherd suggest practical ways to structure the rehabilitation environment for enhanced efficacy in improving motor skill. These factors include the therapeutic relationship between patient and therapist, the therapist's effectiveness at focusing a patient's attention on the most salient features of motor performance, and the type and amount of ongoing practice.

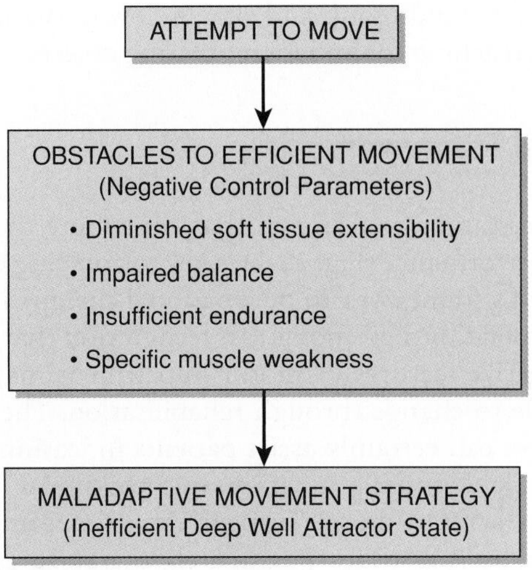

Figure 23-1 Development of maladaptive strategies.

Therapist as Coach

The patient–therapist relationship in task-related training is an active, collaborative mentorship with regard to motor performance. Therapists must have extensive knowledge about the **kinetic** and **kinematic** features of movement, both as performed by individuals with intact neuromuscular systems and as frequently observed in people demonstrating specific motor dysfunction, such as hemiparesis or ataxia. Therapists apply this knowledge when assessing performance, setting goals, structuring practice sessions, and providing feedback and instruction. The therapist's critical goals as coach are (1) to encourage performance of the most important mechanical features within a given category of motor tasks and (2) to discourage behavioral adaptations that have limited effectiveness.

Focusing Attention

As coach, a therapist's goal is to structure the practice sessions so that the patient focuses attention on those features of the task that are most salient for learning. An early step in the process of learning a motor skill is to identify the key components of the action. At this stage, demonstration and instructions, which focus on one or two salient points, are important in directing the patient's efforts. Learning proceeds most smoothly when the patient has a clear idea of the motor goal and which strategies are appropriate or inappropriate for reaching that goal. Carr and Shepherd recommend that therapists routinely ask patients to describe or demonstrate, with another body segment if necessary, the specific movements required to achieve a task. This allows therapists to understand what patients think they are being asked to do. Instructions can then be modified to ensure that each patient and therapist is actually working toward the same goal.

Once an individual has internalized this "model" of an action, however, research indicates that the focus of attention shifts away from the details of the action to the external goals of the current activity (Fasoli et al., 2002; Wulf et al., 2000). At this stage, it may actually be detrimental to focus a patient's attention on the details of performance or to the way the movement "feels." Rather, reflecting a traditional occupational therapy tenet, Carr and Shepherd suggest that the task goal and control parameters inherent within the task objects be used to shape the intended kinematics of a movement sequence. This textbook provides many examples of applying this principle.

Addressing members of the physical therapy profession, Carr and Shepherd caution against an over-reliance on focusing patients' attention on abstract movements, such as shifting weight or moving one's arm through a specific trajectory. Rather, consistent with occupational therapy practice and research (Hsieh et al., 1996; Ma et al., 1999; Nelson et al., 1996), they recommend the creative, individualized organization of control parameters within each task environment to focus a patient's practice of intended movement sequences. Similarly, Carr and Shepherd caution against excessive physical handling as a technique to teach patients the model of an action. Instead, they advocate the use of temporary adaptive aids designed to allow for practice with less need for physical support and manipulation by the therapist. Carr and Shepherd refer to this approach as "modifying the task or environment." Occupational therapists have long been familiar with this component of therapeutic intervention, which Trombly (see Chapter 1) terms "occupation-as-means." Occupational therapists must use, and report outcomes of, our skills in modifying the task and environment to elicit optimal practice opportunities for clients' emerging capacities and skills.

Practice

Theories about motor skill acquisition emphasize the active problem-solving aspects of learning (Schmidt & Lee, 2005). Correspondingly, Carr and Shepherd view the individual as an active participant whose major goal in rehabilitation is to relearn effective strategies for performing functional movement.

Instead of learning specific movements, participants in Carr and Shepherd's program learn general strategies for solving motor problems. Rather than performing exercises without functional goals, patients practice tasks that require mild variations in movement patterns during successive repetitions. Furthermore, limb movements and **postural adjustments** are always learned simultaneously and in the context of task performance. Whole task performance is emphasized, rather than practicing component parts of tasks.

Carr and Shepherd believe that practice is a critical component to motor skill development. Patients learn what they practice, so it is important that they not revert to compensatory movement strategies during daily activities outside of therapy. Carr and Shepherd emphasize that significant motor improvements are achieved only if patients practice movement according to the therapist's guidelines throughout each day. Therefore, the therapist structures a practice program for each patient to reinforce activities performed during therapy sessions. Friends and relatives learn effective ways to assist the patient in this program. The therapist provides clear written directions, photographs, drawings, and/or performance checklists to ensure that the additional practice is consistent with the motor strategies promoted during therapy. Group circuit training classes can be an effective way to increase the amount of training and practice, while also adding both competitive and cooperative components to the training situation (McNevin, Wulf, & Carlson, 2000). Carr and Shepherd (2003) provide extensive guidelines and photographs from the outpatient circuit training classes for upper and lower limb rehabilitation they developed with colleagues at New South Wales Hospital in Australia.

Treatment is task specific and based directly on movement analysis of the patient's performance of that task. The therapist continues to reevaluate and analyze the patient's performance throughout each treatment session to make ongoing decisions about intervention. If performance does not improve, the therapist checks the original analysis of the patient's problems and considers whether the training approach should be modified. Finally, therapy includes opportunities for task analysis and motor problem solving through the introduction of novel activities that require application of a particular motor strategy the person has learned in a different context.

Self-care and leisure activities provide logical opportunities for task-based practice. Too often, occupational therapists prescribe universal methods for activities of daily living that contradict our goals for optimum motor performance. Unless balance and limb function are routinely challenged during daily activity performance, there are no environmental challenges to stimulate brain plasticity. Unless patients have opportunities for routine practice of motor skills required for balance and functional use of their affected limbs, time spent during therapy sessions will have little impact. Therefore, occupational therapists must design safe, individualized methods for *each* patient that continually include that person's emerging capacities into daily self-care and leisure performance.

INTERVENTION

The next section presents the general framework for intervention using task-related training and more specific information for treatment of four key areas of functional movement: standing up and sitting down, balance, walking, and reaching for and manipulating objects.

General Framework

An understanding of factors that contribute to optimal motor performance (Fig. 23-2) is key to applying Carr and Shepherd's framework to occupational therapy intervention. Implicit in their model is a recognition that positive and negative features of motor impairment may not be amenable to change through rehabilitation. Therapeutic challenges can certainly assist patients in learning to use their available muscle function, but no known interventions can facilitate muscle firing in the absence of required physiological substrates. Fortunately, therapists can play a critical role in preventing and reducing the adaptive features associated with CNS motor dysfunction. In addition,

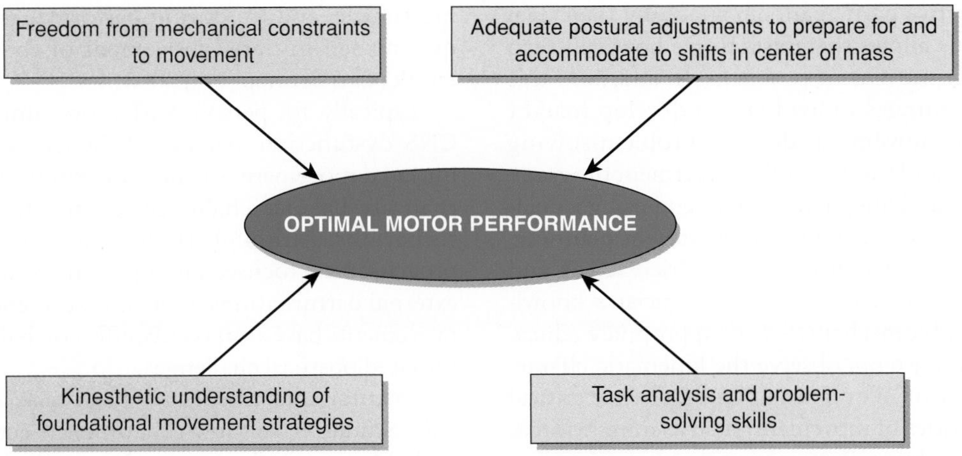

Figure 23-2 Contributing factors to optimal motor performance.

in our role as coaches, we can assist patients in developing cognitive skills that will enable them to optimize their available levels of motor control.

Carr and Shepherd (2003) present a framework for assessing and improving four general categories of motor performance: balance, walking, standing up and sitting down, and reaching and manipulation. For each of these areas, they provide these guidelines for therapists:

- Anticipate, prevent, and reduce mechanical constraints that are likely to interfere with performance.
- Understand the kinematics and kinetics that research has shown to accompany typical performance by individuals with intact musculoskeletal function.
- Understand how research has shown the kinematics and kinetics of performance to differ in individuals with CNS dysfunction.
- Understand how postural adjustments are integrated into efficient task performance.
- Structure activities to provide graded challenges to anticipatory and ongoing postural adjustments.
- Structure activities that help patients develop a kinesthetic understanding of fundamental movement strategies.
- Structure activities that help patients develop motor task analysis and problem-solving skills.

Evaluation and Treatment Planning

As with the OT Task-Oriented Approach, clinical evaluation is a detailed analysis of the patient's performance of selected tasks in each of the four categories of motor performance. Therapists observe patients as they perform functional activities and compare performance with critical kinematic features that are associated with these tasks (Procedures for Practice 23-1). This observation enables therapists to develop individualized treatment plans that include the following:

- Stretching exercises to lengthen shortened muscles and enhance mobility at body segments where limitations were noted
- Environmental modifications or coaching to improve postural alignment
- Exercises and activities designed to strengthen muscles that are innervated but weak
- Verbal and kinesthetic instruction about key foundational strategies to improve performance
- Practice of key strategies in a variety of other tasks
- Practice of the observed task in varying conditions, incorporating newly acquired mobility, muscle strength, and foundational strategies

PROCEDURES FOR PRACTICE 23-1

Assessment

During task observation, the therapist assesses performance for the following:

- Evidence of mobility impairments at specific joints
- Missing or limited components (e.g., lack of anterior pelvic tilt, hip flexion, ankle dorsiflexion when rising to stand)
- Incorrect timing of components within a movement pattern (e.g., inappropriate interplay among extrinsic and intrinsic finger muscles during attempts at grasp)
- Evidence of weakness or paralysis of specific muscles (e.g., weakness in quadriceps on attempts to stand up)
- Compensatory motor behavior (e.g., elevation of the entire shoulder girdle on attempts to reach forward)

Patients are active participants in analyzing their own performance. This allows therapists to see how well each person can detect movement problems. In addition, this self-analysis encourages individuals to develop insight about their own movement, develop problem-solving skills, and understand the goals of the treatment program.

Although Carr and Shepherd recommend using a qualitative assessment style as a guide to treatment planning, they caution that the validity of these observations and subsequent analysis is dependent on a clinician's knowledge of normative biomechanics. With appropriate educational background, we *can* observe the kinematic characteristics of movement. We *cannot,* however, observe critical kinetic characteristics of movement, such as muscle forces or ground reaction force. Recognizing that kinetic assessments are not available in clinical environments, Carr and Shepherd developed a quantitative scale, based on kinematic observations. The *Motor Assessment Scale* (*MAS*) (Carr et al., 1985, revised: J. Carr & R. Shepherd, personal communication, 1994) consists of eight movements: supine to side-lying, supine to sitting on the edge of the bed, balanced sitting, sitting to standing, walking, upper arm function, hand movements, and advanced hand activities (Procedures for Practice 23-2). As indicated in Procedures for Practice 23-2 and discussed in Chapter 6, each motor activity is scored on a 7-point ordinal scale ranging from 0 to 6. A score of 6 indicates optimal behavior. The *MAS* has been successfully used as an outcome measure in published efficacy studies of clinical intervention (Ada & Westwood, 1992; Dean & Mackey, 1992; Monger, Carr, & Fowler, 2002; Nugent & Schurr, 1994; Thickbroom et al., 2004). Positive aspects of the tool include its ease of administration, high reliability (Poole & Whitney, 1988), high concurrent validity with selected items on the *Fugl-Meyer Assessment* (Poole & Whitney, 1988), and its emphasis on functional task performance. In addition, occupational therapists have found that use of the *MAS,* with its structured format of task observation, is helpful in focusing and sharpening their observational skills (Kieran, Lim, & Sabari, 1999). A study of the upper limb items, using Rasch analysis, provides support for the scoring criteria hierarchy on the upper arm item but indicates a need for revising the scoring criteria hierarchies for the two items of the *MAS* that assess hand function (Sabari et al., 2005).

Balance

Balance is the ability to maintain an upright posture against the dynamically changing effects of gravity on our body segments. Postural control mechanisms enable us to maintain balance by ensuring that our body's center of mass remains within the base of support. During daily activities, a person's center of mass can be displaced in three ways: (1) by an external force applied to the body, as occurs during contact sports; (2) by external movement of the support surface, as occurs when we sit or stand in a moving vehicle; and (3) during performance of activities requiring self-initiated movement of the head, limbs, or trunk (Carr & Shepherd, 2003).

Typically, for persons with motor impairments due to CNS dysfunction, balance challenges arising from self-initiated movement are more important to daily function than are balance challenges arising from external perturbations. Although traditional neurobehavioral approaches have focused on improving postural reactions to external perturbations, there is no evidence that these improvements have any positive effect on balance during self-initiated postural challenges.

Postural adjustments are both task and context specific. Studies have shown that muscle activation patterns for balance control vary according to (1) the position of the person, (2) the task being performed, (3) the context in which the activity occurs, and (4) the person's perception of which body part is in contact with the more stable base of support (Dean, Shepherd, & Adams, 1999a, 1999b; Nashner & McCollum, 1985). Therefore, Carr and Shepherd advocate that postural adjustments be learned only in the context of task performance. Furthermore, balance training in one position or during performance of one task is not likely to generalize to improved postural control in other contexts (Shepherd, 1992).

Essential Features of Performance

Effective balance requires adequate function in sensory and motor systems (Procedures for Practice 23-3). Sensory processing of visual, vestibular, tactile, and proprioceptive information allows a person to maintain continuous and dynamic awareness about the body's center of mass and alignment between body segments. Muscle contractions of appropriate amplitude and timing allow for predictive and ongoing force production to match the changing influence of gravity during motor performance. Sufficient joint mobility and muscle length allow the necessary movements to be generated through their full ranges of motion.

Individuals with impairments in these areas are likely to develop adaptive strategies that may seem effective in the short run but that have long-term maladaptive influence on balance and other motor function (Procedures for Practice 23-3). When people feel unable to maintain their balance in posturally threatening situations, one such strategy is to constrain movement at selected body parts and thus decrease the number of motor elements, or **degrees of freedom**, the CNS must control. Individuals with postural adjustment deficits as a result of CNS dysfunction may feel insecure about their ability to maintain balance, even in routine sitting or standing positions. The strategy of fixating one's pelvis on the lumbar spine or the scapula on the thorax has short-term benefits for enhancing the person's sense of postural security. A negative consequence is that these patterns lead to soft tissue shortening and difficulty disassociating the scapula and pelvis

PROCEDURES FOR PRACTICE 23-2

Abridged Criteria for Scoring *MAS*

The score assigned on each item is the highest criterion met on the best performance of three. A 0 score is assigned if the patient is unable to meet the criteria for a score of 1.

Supine to Side-Lying to Intact Side

1. Pulls self into side-lying with intact arm, moving affected leg with intact leg.
2. Moves leg across actively and lower half of body follows. Arm is left behind.
3. Lifts arm across body with other arm. Moves leg actively; body follows in a block.
4. Actively moves arm across body; rest of body follows in a block.
5. Rolls to side, moving arm and leg; overbalances. Shoulder protracts and arm flexes.
6. Rolls to side in 3 seconds. Must not use hands.

Supine to Sitting on Edge of Bed

1. After being assisted to side-lying, lifts head sideways; cannot sit up.
2. Side-lying to sitting on edge of bed with therapist assisting movement.
3. Side-lying to sitting on edge of bed with standby help assisting legs over side of bed.
4. Side-lying to sitting on edge of bed with no standby help.
5. Supine to sitting on edge of bed with no standby help.
6. Supine to sitting on edge of bed within 10 seconds with no standby help.

Balanced Sitting

1. Sits only with support after therapist assists.
2. Sits unsupported for 10 seconds.
3. Sits unsupported with weight well forward and evenly distributed.
4. Sits unsupported with hands resting on thighs; turns head and trunk to look behind.
5. Reaches forward to touch floor 4 inches in front of feet and returns to starting position.
6. Sitting on stool, reaches sideways to touch floor and returns to starting position.

Sitting to Standing

1. Gets to standing with help (any method).
2. Gets to standing with standby help.
3. Gets to standing with weight evenly distributed and with no help from hands.
4. Gets to standing; stands for 5 seconds, weight evenly distributed, hips and knees extended.
5. Stands up and sits down with no help; even weight distribution; full hip and knee extension.
6. Stands up and sits down with no help 3 times in 10 seconds; even weight distribution.

Walking

1. Stands on affected leg with hip extended; steps forward with other leg (standby help).
2. Walks with standby help from one person.
3. Walks 10 feet alone. Uses any walking aid but no standby help.
4. Walks 16 feet with no aid in 15 seconds.
5. Walks 33 feet, picks up small sandbag from floor, turns around, walks back in 25 seconds.
6. Walks up and down four steps with or without an aid three times in 35 seconds. May not hold rail.

Upper Arm Function

1. Supine, protracts shoulder girdle. Tester places arm in 90° flexion and supports elbow.
2. Supine, holds shoulder in 90° flexion for 2 seconds. (Maintains 45° external rotation and 20° elbow extension.)
3. From position in level 2, flexes and extends elbow to move palm to forehead and back.
4. Sitting, holds arm in 90° shoulder flexion with elbow extended, thumb pointing up, for 2 seconds. No excess shoulder elevation.
5. Achieves position in level 4; holds for 10 seconds; lowers arm. No pronation allowed.
6. Standing, arm abducted 90°, with palm flat against wall. Maintains hand position while turning body toward wall.

Hand Movements

1. Sitting, lifts cylindrical object off table by extending wrist. No elbow flexion allowed.
2. Sitting, forearm in midposition. Lifts hand off table by radially deviating wrist. No elbow flexion or forearm pronation allowed.
3. Sitting, elbow into side, pronates and supinates forearm through three quarters of range.
4. Sitting, reaches forward to pick up 5-inch ball with both hands and puts ball down. Ball placement requires elbow extension. Palms stay in contact with ball.
5. Sitting, picks up plastic foam cup from table and puts it on table across other side of body.
6. Sitting, continuous opposition of thumb and each finger more than 14 times in 10 seconds.

Advanced Hand Activities

1. Reaches forward arm's length; picks up pen top; releases it on table close to body.
2. Picks up a jellybean from teacup with eight jellybeans and places it in another cup. Cups are at arm's length.
3. Draws horizontal lines to stop at a vertical line 10 times in 20 seconds.
4. Makes rapid consecutive dots with a pen on a sheet of paper. (Picks up and holds pen without assistance; at least 2 dots per second for 5 seconds; dots, not dashes).
5. Takes a dessert spoon of liquid to the mouth, without spilling. (Head cannot lower toward spoon).
6. Holds a comb and combs hair at back of head. (Shoulder is externally rotated, abducted at least 90°; head is erect.)

Used with permission from J. Carr & R. Shepherd, personal communication, 1994.

PROCEDURES FOR PRACTICE 23-3

Impairments Underlying Balance Dysfunction

Negative Features Affecting Balance Dysfunction

- Impairments in muscular force and timing
- Impairments in sensory processing (visual, tactile, proprioceptive, vestibular)

Adaptive Features Affecting Balance Dysfunction

- Avoiding all shifts in center of mass
- Shifting weight away from a paretic limb
- Using hands for support
- Stiffening the body
- Soft tissue shortening

PROCEDURES FOR PRACTICE 23-4

Graded Task Demands to Improve Balance

Position of the Person

- Size and shape of base of support (foot placement, seating or standing surface)
- Initial alignment of body segments

Object Placement

- Position determines direction of weight shift; moving laterally more difficult than moving forward
- Distance

Object Characteristics

- Weight
- Size; greater challenge to balance when both hands must be used

Temporal Demands

- Stationary object—increasing demands on speed of performance
- Moving object—increasing the speed at which the object moves

from adjacent proximal structures. This lack of sufficient mobility at the limb girdles subsequently limits the normal kinematics of upper and lower extremity movement. Figure 23-3 illustrates how immobility and muscle shortening interact in a self-perpetuating cycle.

The strategies of shifting weight away from a paretic leg, unnecessarily widening the base of support, or using one's hands excessively for support present further obstacles to using and improving available muscle strength and sensory processing skills. In addition, they contribute to additional problems in gait and in using the upper limbs to their maximum potential. Task-related training seeks to prevent the development of these maladaptive strategies through the early introduction of techniques to enhance balance and postural security.

Assessment and Treatment

Balance is assessed through observational analysis as the person performs self-initiated movements in sitting and standing. These include the following:

- Looking in a variety of directions (e.g., up at the ceiling, behind oneself)
- Reaching forward, sideways, and down to the floor to pick up objects
- Walking in various conditions

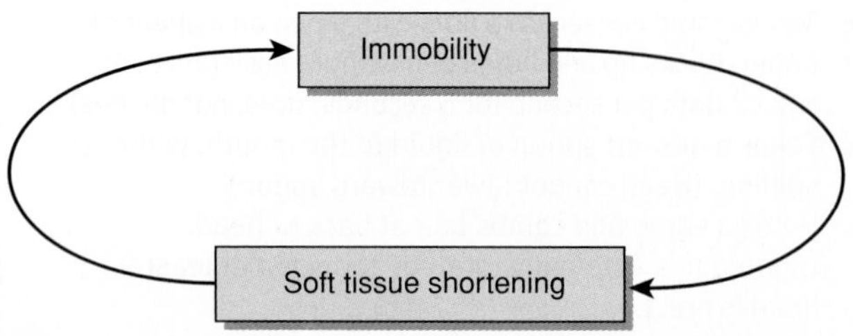

Figure 23-3 Cycle of immobility and soft tissue shortening.

Balance training overlaps with each of Carr and Shepherd's three other areas of functional performance. Patients are presented with activities that offer graded challenges to their ability to shift their center of mass over the base of support. Prior to activity engagement, the therapist ensures that joint mobility and postural alignment are maximized. Procedures for Practice 23-4 lists the critical activity elements that therapists manipulate in structuring activity-based balance training. These general guidelines provide occupational therapists with limitless possibilities for creative activity synthesis based on each patient's interests, goals, and level of function. The outcomes study (Dean & Shepherd, 1997) highlighted in this chapter's Research Note provides support for the clinical efficacy of these interventions.

Walking

Walking, a critical component of daily task engagement, is a reasonable expectation for many individuals with CNS dysfunction. Occupational therapists work with patients who wish to improve their performance in kitchen and bathroom activities and in leisure or work pursuits. In each of these contexts, the occupational therapist must help patients reach their optimal walking potential.

Essential Features of Performance

Successful walking requires production of a basic locomotor rhythm, support and propulsion of the body in the desired direction, dynamic balance control of the moving

RESEARCH NOTE 23-1

Abstract: Dean, C. M., & Shepherd, R. B. (1997). Task-related training improves performance of seated reaching tasks after stroke: A randomized controlled trial. *Stroke, 28,* 722–728.

After a stroke, the ability to balance in sitting is critical to independence. Although impairments in sitting balance are common, little is known about the effectiveness of rehabilitation strategies designed to improve it. The purpose of this randomized placebo-controlled study was to evaluate the effect of a 2-week task-related training program aimed at increasing reaching distance and the contribution of the affected lower leg to support and balance.

Twenty subjects, at least 1 year after stroke, were randomized to an experimental or control group. The experimental group participated in a standard training program involving practice of reaching beyond arm's length. The control group received sham training, which involved completion of cognitive-manipulative tasks within arm's length. Reach while sitting was measured before and after training using electromyography, videotaping, and two force plates. Variables tested were movement time, distance reached, vertical ground reaction forces through the feet, and muscle activity. Subjects were also tested on sit-to-stand, walking, and cognitive tasks. Nineteen subjects completed the study.

After training, experimental subjects could reach significantly faster and farther, significantly increase load through the affected foot, and increase activation of the affected leg muscles compared with the control group ($p < 0.01$). The experimental group also improved in sit-to-stand. The control group did not improve in reaching or sit-to-stand. Neither group improved in walking. This study provides strong evidence of the efficacy of task-related motor training to improve the ability to balance during seated reaching activities after stroke.

Implications for Practice

- After a stroke, sitting balance can be improved through opportunities to practice reaching to grasp objects with the unaffected hand under variable conditions.
- Providing patients with task-related challenges to use self-initiated balance adjustments is an effective method for improving sitting balance and performance in rising to stand.
- When self-initiated balance adjustments are not challenged, patients do not improve sitting balance or sit-to-stand.
- Individuals recovering from stroke need opportunities to sit without external supports and to challenge self-initiated balance adjustments by reaching to grasp objects, with variations in object location and weight, seat height, movement speed, and extent of thigh support on the seat.

body, and the ability to adapt movement to changing environmental demands and goals (Carr & Shepherd, 1998, 2003).

Research on individuals with no musculoskeletal impairments has revealed remarkable consistency among people in the kinematic aspects of gait. Patterns of muscle use, however, vary widely. Besides differing between subjects, the kinetics of gait may vary within a single subject, depending on walking speed and fatigue. Furthermore, a natural redundancy in the motor system for walking readily allows for compensation by stronger muscles when specific muscles are weak.

Walking forward in a uniform direction is achieved through repetitive performance of sequential gait cycles. Each cycle begins when the heel of one foot makes contact with the ground. As that leg supports the body weight, it rocks forward until its only ground contact is at the toes. Simultaneously, the other leg swings forward until its heel makes contact with the ground. Double support is the brief period when both feet are on the ground. Immediately after double support, the first leg swings forward while the second leg supports the body weight. One gait cycle is completed when the heel of the first foot touches the ground once again.

For purposes of description, the gait cycle for each leg is divided into a stance phase and a swing phase. Definition 23-1 shows the subdivision of these phases of the gait cycle. Basic knowledge about the motor requirements during each phase of the gait cycle guides therapists in their interventions for patients with CNS dysfunction.

The essential components of motor activity during the stance phase include extensor muscle activity at the hip, knee, and ankle; smooth alternation of eccentric and concentric muscular activity in knee and ankle muscles; muscle activity in the gluteus medius at midstance to prevent excessive downward tilt of the pelvis on the side of the swing-

DEFINITION 23-1

The Gait Cycle

Stance Phase

- Weight–load acceptance: from heel contact to foot flat on ground
- Midstance: from foot flat on ground to heel off of ground
- Push-off: weight moving forward onto toes and foot preparing to leave ground

Swing Phase

- Liftoff (early swing): leg swings forward with foot clearing the ground.
- Reach (late swing): leg decelerates and prepares for heel contact.

ing leg; and ongoing postural adjustments to balance the body mass over a dynamically changing base of support.

Since the goals of the swing phase are (1) to clear the foot from contacting the ground as the leg swings forward and (2) to prepare the leg to assume a stance position as it reaches the end of its swing forward in space, the essential components of motor activity during the swing phase are fluid pelvic mobility, including lateral pelvic tilt as weight is shifted from the current leg onto the other leg and pelvic rotation to allow the swinging leg to advance forward; sufficient hip, knee, and ankle (dorsi) flexion to shorten the leg for foot clearance as the leg swings forward; and knee extension and ankle dorsiflexion just prior to heel contact to ensure that the heel, rather than the flat foot or the toes, will strike the ground to initiate the stance phase.

Assessment and Treatment

Gait problems in stroke patients and others with neurological diagnoses are caused by impairments associated with the lesion as well as by secondary cardiovascular and musculoskeletal consequences of disuse, physical inactivity, and aging. Physical therapists determine initial walking goals based on observation and comparison of each patient's performance against the critical kinematic features of walking that have been determined through descriptive research. Although observational analysis cannot provide information about the kinetics of a person's gait, spatiotemporal and kinematic variables provide clues about the underlying kinetic dynamics.

Treatment goals are to prevent soft tissue shortening; improve muscle strength and control for support, propulsion, balance, and toe clearance; and improve rhythm and coordination during functional walking. Treatment methods include soft tissue stretching; active exercises to lengthen shortened muscles; strength training to improve force generation and speed of muscle contraction; step-up, step-down, and side-stepping exercises; and actual walking practice. Carr and Shepherd advocate early walking training using treadmills and, when necessary, harnesses providing partial body weight support (Carr & Shepherd, 2003; Shepherd & Carr, 1999). Treadmill training provides opportunities for practice at walking velocities that foster more efficient gait parameters than walking at slow speeds (Hesse et al., 2003; Visintin et al., 1998).

Consistent with their emphasis on training in a variety of environmental contexts, Carr and Shepherd advocate walking and stair climbing practice on a variety of surfaces, slopes, and naturalistic settings. Occupational therapists play a critical role in maximizing walking **skill** during our interventions that require the simultaneous performance of walking with carrying or pushing, as is inherent in naturalistic activities within home, work, and leisure environments. In addition, we can incorporate sideways, forward, and backward walking, as well as step-up and step-down practice into task-based training activities designed to challenge upper limb and balance skills.

Standing Up and Sitting Down

Carr and Shepherd argue that the stand pivot transfer is typically overemphasized in neurorehabilitation. For patients who demonstrate potential to walk, learning how to stand up and sit down has greater functional implications and is more natural to learn than traditional transfer techniques.

Treatment to enhance a patient's ability to stand up and sit down improves that person's sitting posture, sitting and standing balance, functional reach, and gait. Each of these aspects of motor performance demands ability to appreciate how one's own body alignment and dynamic movement affect one's center of mass. In addition, each of these categories of functional activity demands a balance of mobility and stability in the pelvis, trunk, and limbs.

Essential Features of Performance

There are two phases to the normal kinematics of standing up. During the pre-extension phase, or forward phase, the hips flex to move the center of mass forward (Shepherd & Gentile, 1994). The extension phase, or upward phase, begins at "thighs off" (TO). During this phase, the hips and knees extend to move the center of mass upward to final standing alignment. Each phase is characterized by kinematic and kinetic requirements. Force requirements are most important during the extension phase. These are met via contractions in the extensors of the ankle, knee, and hip. The kinetic requirements of standing up are similar to those of the stance phase during gait. To ensure that the limb does not collapse, a decrease in force at one joint can be compensated for by an increase at the other joints.

Several kinematic features during the pre-extension phase influence the amount of force needed during the extension phase. Forward foot placement has been found to interfere with both phases of standing up (Khemlani, Carr, & Crosbie, 1999; Shepherd & Koh, 1996). Therefore, Carr and Shepherd recommend that people with CNS movement dysfunction prepare for standing by placing their feet behind an imaginary perpendicular line drawn down from the knees, with the ankles at approximately 75° of dorsiflexion (Carr & Shepherd, 1998, 2003). Trunk position during pre-extension, determined by flexion at the hips, significantly affects the kinematics and kinetics of the extension phase. In subjects with normal movement, failure to flex forward at the hips lengthens the extension phase, increases muscle force requirements during the extension phase, and changes the order of movement during the extension phase from knee-hip-ankle to hip-knee-ankle (Shepherd & Gentile, 1994). Therefore, forward flexion at the hips is emphasized in treatment as a key element to standing up and sitting down.

Arm movement and speed of performance also affect the mechanics of rising to stand. Active arm flexion naturally accompanies the onset of leg extension and contributes to maximizing available extensor force in the lower limb (Carr & Gentile, 1994). Forward motion of the arms and upper body assists in establishing momentum prior to the extension phase. This momentum decreases the amount of lower limb force required to lift the body up against gravity to the erect standing posture. Research evidence (Carr, Ow, & Shepherd, 2002) indicates that slower speed of performance, as measured by hip flexion velocity, decreases the potential effect of this momentum. To capitalize on this momentum, Carr and Shepherd recommend that patients learn to complete the task of standing up with no pause between the pre-extension and extension phases. Therefore, unless there are safety considerations, they advise that patients practice the task in its entirety.

Finally, Carr and Shepherd caution against using the common strategy of teaching patients to push down with their arms to assist themselves in standing up. Although this may be useful in the short run as a compensatory technique to reduce force requirements at the hip, knee, and ankle, it denies patients the opportunity to improve their muscle strength. Instead, Carr and Shepherd recommend raising seat height for individuals with weak hip and knee extensors to practice standing up and sitting down. As strength increases, lowering the seat height will provide progressive strength training to lower limb extensors (Carr & Shepherd, 2003).

Assessment and Treatment

Procedures for Practice 23-5 provides the essential factors of Carr and Shepherd's program for developing the ability to stand up. Passive muscle lengthening may be necessary if patients demonstrate mobility limitations in ankle dorsiflexion, knee flexion or extension, hip flexion or extension, or sagittal-plane pelvic motion. Whole-task practice is important to assist patients in developing necessary sequencing and timing during functional performance.

Sitting down from standing has several similarities to standing up but is a different activity that must be practiced as well. No momentum to reduce force requirements is present, so additional muscle strength (particularly in knee extensors) is needed just before the body mass is lowered onto the seat. Carr and Shepherd recommend that, when learning to stand, patients should be instructed to stop the movement and reverse their direction for a few degrees. This will help them develop control over changing from concentric to eccentric muscle activity.

PROCEDURES FOR PRACTICE 23-5

Sit-to-Stand

Strategic Movement Components

- Initial foot placement (knee and ankle <90°)
- Forward motion of upper body (requires sufficient ankle dorsiflexion and hip flexion; trunk remains erect)
- Sequential extension at the knee, hip, and ankle
- Relatively equal contributions by both lower limbs

Environmental Modifications

- Raise seat to decrease lower limb force requirements.
- Grade seat to lower heights as strength in leg extensors improves.
- Use chair without arms if patient shows over-reliance on using hands for push-off.
- Select chair that allows for placing the feet back (knee and ankle flexed to less than 90°).

Reach and Manipulation

The arm and hand function as a single unit in reach and manipulation, with the hand beginning to open for grasp at the start of a reaching action (Hoff & Arbib, 1993). In many activities, the upper body, or even the entire body, is an integral component of this single coordinated unit. Clearly, reach and grasp are not exclusively upper limb activities. All reaching actions from sitting or standing are preceded and accompanied by postural adjustments. When objects are beyond the arm's reach, shifts in total body alignment contribute to functional performance.

Essential Features of Performance

Forward reach in sitting entails (1) anterior movement of the pelvis, (2) flexion of the trunk at the hips, and (3) active use of the legs to aid in balancing by creating an active base of support. Reaching sideways while sitting is more challenging than reaching forward, since the base of support is smaller. Reaching while standing requires (1) establishment of an appropriate base of support with one's feet and (2) shifting body weight and center of mass toward the direction of the goal object.

Therapeutic interventions for individuals with CNS dysfunction must inherently combine evaluation and treatment of balance with assessment and training of reach and manipulation. Carr and Shepherd caution against waiting until patients achieve a certain level of balance before introducing therapeutic tasks to improve reach and manipulation. Similarly, they caution against waiting until patients demonstrate a specified level of shoulder function before assessing for and providing treatment to improve hand skills.

Current Perspective for Conceptualizing Therapeutic Intervention

Traditionally, upper limb function after serious stroke or traumatic brain injury has been associated with poor outcomes (Nakayama et al., 1994). Carr and Shepherd suggest that several factors, in addition to the direct extent of neural pathology, have limited the effect of rehabilitation interventions on functional recovery of reach and grasp. They agree with Taub and Wolf (1997) that, during the flaccid period immediately after brain injury, patients learn to rely exclusively on the unaffected arm for performing one-handed activities. This "learned nonuse" (Taub et al., 1993), combined with inappropriate therapeutic intervention for the upper limb, results in insufficient practice opportunities for the paretic arm. In addition, the effects of immobility on soft tissue extensibility limit active motor function even further. Finally, Carr and Shepherd debunk some common beliefs that prevail among rehabilitation professionals. They recommend that therapists shed unsubstantiated beliefs about recovery of motor control after brain injury and replace them with the following guidelines:

1. Recovery does not necessarily proceed in a proximal to distal sequence. Rather, therapists and patients should consistently monitor emerging muscle strength in all segments of the upper limb.
2. There is no reason to wait until patients demonstrate shoulder stability and control before presenting therapeutic challenges to hand function. Rather, the presentation of activities requiring limited grasp may provide valuable therapeutic challenges that can help organize emerging shoulder function.
3. Therapeutic challenges to active limb use need not be postponed until spasticity is inhibited. In fact, evidence indicates that the hypertonus, or resistance to passive movement, that many clinicians associate with spasticity is, in most patients, typically due to muscle shortening and increased stiffness (Carr, Shepherd, & Ada, 1995). Therefore, Carr and Shepherd do not advocate the use of any procedures aside from those that preserve or enhance soft tissue extensibility for reducing spasticity as a means to enhancing active, functional use of the upper limb.
4. There are no universal patterns of muscle linkages associated with recovery of motor function after brain injury. Rather, research has shown that abnormal patterns of motor performance are related to each patient's distribution of muscle weakness combined with the mechanical demands of each task (Trombly, 1992, 1993). For example, the pattern of shoulder elevation combined with retraction of the shoulder girdle, which is often seen when individuals attempt to flex or abduct a hemiparetic shoulder, is not directly linked to the neural pathology. Rather, it is an adaptive use of available muscle strength against gravitational force. Thus, interventions to improve motor patterns are based on individualized analyses of each patient's abilities, and activities are presented as graded challenges to provide opportunities for developing motor skills.
5. Conventional slings and splints that immobilize the affected shoulder or hand contribute to the development of learned non-use. The current approach is to provide shoulder supports (Shepherd & Carr, 1998) and splints that provide necessary stabilization and to use these devices to promote active use of the upper limb during task-based training. Occupational therapists are developing these functional orthoses for clinical practice, but, to date, have rarely reported them in the published literature.
6. Traditional rehabilitation efforts at improving upper limb function have previously focused on those patients with the most severe paralysis of arm and hand muscles. Aside from providing preventive intervention to minimize secondary impairments of muscle shortening and postural misalignment, restorative treatments are most applicable to those stroke survivors with mild to moderate impairment levels (Duncan et al., 1998).

The Degrees of Freedom Problem

Of the four categories of motor performance addressed by Carr and Shepherd's approach, reach and manipulation are characterized by the greatest number of degrees of freedom. This provides us with exceptional flexibility in tailoring reach and manipulation to the contextual demands of different tasks and environments. At the same time, this freedom of choice increases the complexity of motor demands during upper limb activities (Latash & Latash, 1994). Many people with stroke or head injury demonstrate a capacity to perform singular motions of a paretic upper limb when assisted by a therapist. Their inability to control multiple degrees of freedom, however, results in an inability to use the arm for functional reach or grasp.

One effective strategy observed in people who move with ease is to reduce the degrees of freedom by linking some elements together in synergistic combinations. The kinesiology of normal movement is characterized by several synergistic combinations in the upper limb and trunk (Levangie & Norkin, 2005). Some examples are:

- Combined action of rotator cuff muscles to assist the deltoid during glenohumeral (GH) flexion and abduction
- Upward rotation of the scapula that accompanies GH flexion and abduction (scapulohumeral rhythm)
- Shifts in body weight and pelvic orientation that accompany reaching motions of the upper limb
- Synergistic combinations between GH and forearm rotators for efficient positioning of the hand in space
- Synergistic contraction of the wrist extensors during grasp patterns requiring forceful finger flexion

After stroke or head injury, many persons lose their ability to implement these synergistic linkages automatically. The critical goals of intervention to improve reach and manipulation skills are:

- Minimize movement obstacles presented by weakness and immobility.

- Teach foundational movement combinations that underlie efficient reach and grasp.
- Provide graded opportunities to practice controlling an increasing number of degrees of freedom during exercise and activity performance.

Assessment and Treatment

Like other evaluations in Carr and Shepherd's approach, clinical assessment of reach and manipulation is achieved through detailed observation of each patient's attempts to perform selected functional tasks. Therapists use their knowledge about the kinetics and kinematics of upper limb function to develop hypotheses as to which deficits may be serving as control parameters in limiting the versatility or efficiency of motor strategies. Most motor dysfunction can be attributed to specific muscle weakness, muscle stiffness and length changes, and/or adaptive strategies developed to compensate for these impairments. Shoulder pain may also be a significant control parameter to efficient reach. (Safety Note 23-1 lists ways to prevent secondary impairments at the shoulder.) Therapists test their hypotheses through direct assessment of muscle strength and length and through patients' responses to interventions designed to modify adaptive strategies.

Training is individualized and based on the hypotheses developed during observation of functional task performance. Early control of weak muscles is facilitated by finding an optimal length for muscle contraction, by providing early opportunities for eccentric exercise, and by positioning the limb so that gravity assists rather than resists the muscle. An example also used in the neurodevelopmental treatment (NDT) approach is to elicit early contraction of the deltoid with the person lying supine with the shoulder flexed to 90°. In this position, gravity provides a stabilizing force on the shoulder. Therefore, activation of fewer motor units is required for the individual to hold the arm and move it slightly from this position. Shortened muscles are lengthened by slow, passive stretch by the therapist, family members, or patients themselves. Therapists make patients aware of inefficient adaptive strategies and provide them with opportunities to perform a variety of reach and grasp activities using alternative movement strategies. Definition 23-2 summarizes the motor components essential to reach and manipulation. Therapists consider these components when synthesizing and grading therapeutic tasks.

Carr and Shepherd recognize that many patients with hemiparesis may rely excessively on one-handed perform-

SAFETY NOTE 23-1

Preventing Secondary Impairments at the Shoulder

- Prevent muscle shortening of adductor and internal rotator muscles; provide stretch through positioning or passive motion.
- Minimize downward gravitational force on soft tissue around glenohumeral joint.
- Avoid passive humeral flexion or abduction without appropriate concomitant scapular motion.
- Avoid any passive movement of the arm by individuals unfamiliar with scapulohumeral interactions.

Shepherd & Carr, 1998.

DEFINITION 23-2

Essential Components to Functional Arm Use

Reaching (Forward, Diagonally, Upward, Sideways, Backward)

- Appropriate scapular motion (upward rotation and abduction for forward, sideways, and upward reach; downward rotation and adduction for backward and downward reach)
- Elbow extension and varying amount of shoulder external rotation
- Opening of hand aperture between thumb and fingers
- Extension of wrist
- Pronation and supination appropriate to object orientation

Grasping

Preparation to grasp:

- Extension of wrist and fingers
- Abduction and opposition at thumb carpometacarpal joint
- Finger abduction for large objects

Grasp: Closure of thumb and fingers around object

Holding

- Flexion and extension of wrist while holding object
- Lifting, placing, and rotating objects of various sizes, shapes, and weights

Manipulating

- Flexion and extension of fingers
- Flexion and opposition at carpometacarpal joints of thumb and fifth finger
- Independent finger flexion and extension (e.g., keyboard depression)

Adapted with permission from Carr, J. H., & Shepherd, R. (2003). *Stroke rehabilitation: Guidelines for exercise and training to optimize motor skill.* London, United Kingdom: Butterworth-Heinemann.

ance of daily tasks, even when they demonstrate potential to use their affected arm and hand. They support the use of constraint-induced movement therapy (Mark & Taub, 2004; Wolf et al., 2002) when appropriate. In addition, they recognize that bimanual tasks provide a natural framework for encouraging active use of available hand function.

Actual training in grasp and manipulation is achieved through varied task-related practice of both unilateral and bilateral activities. Sensory training is provided naturalistically through opportunities to manipulate objects with various shapes, sizes, and textures in the context of task performance. Carr and Shepherd suggest a variety of interventions to augment training, including specialized feedback, functional electrical stimulation, mental practice, and the use of functional orthoses. Intensity of practice can be increased through constraint-induced movement therapy (Mark & Taub, 2004), access to computer-driven games, and teaching friends and family to serve as training coaches. Dean and Mackey's (1992) study provides research support for the efficacy of Carr and Shepherd's approach in improving upper limb and hand function.

Occupational therapists are particularly qualified to synthesize activities designed to provide graded challenges to reach and manipulation. In addition, occupational therapists excel at designing individualized orthotic and environmental adaptations to facilitate task performance while providing opportunities to develop functional skill to each person's maximal potential. In their most recent textbook about stroke rehabilitation, Carr and Shepherd (2003) acknowledge this in their references to studies conducted by occupational therapists.

SUMMARY

Carr and Shepherd's approach to optimizing motor control is well suited for use and adaptation in occupational therapy. Occupational therapists who apply these ideas use their skills in analyzing the kinematic and kinetic requirements of specific activity performance to develop individualized goals and treatment. In addition, occupational therapists structure tasks and environments to assist patients in developing efficient motor strategies and motor problem-solving skills. Finally, occupational therapists provide meaningful practice that enables individuals to use their available motor function to its fullest potential in daily activity performance.

CASE EXAMPLE

Mr. M.: Optimizing Motor Skill Using Task-Related Training According to Carr and Shepard Guidelines

Occupational Therapy Intervention Process	Clinical Reasoning Process	
	Objectives	**Examples of Therapist's Internal Dialogue**
Patient Information Mr. M. is a 70-year-old man who sustained an infarct to his left middle cerebral artery 4 weeks before his referral for home-based occupational therapy. After hospitalization and inpatient rehabilitation, he returned home to his apartment in a building with an elevator. After occupational therapy assessment in his home, the following problems were identified: • Mild difficulties with bed mobility and sitting balance because of limitations in thoracolumbar dissociation and pelvic mobility. • Need for contact guard and occasional minimal assist in rising to stand from sitting because of limitations cited above. • Insecure balance in standing.	Appreciate the context	"Enhancing thoracolumbar and pelvic mobility will enable Mr. M. to use more effective movement kinematics during functional task performance." "Enhancing Mr. M.'s knowledge of movement kinematics and his ability to monitor his own performance will contribute to improving his motor skills."
	Develop intervention hypotheses	"Opportunities for practice of available movements, with increasing number of degrees of freedom, will help Mr. M. develop enhanced arm motor skill."
	Select an intervention approach	"I will implement task-related training, with specific guidelines suggested by Carr and Shepherd."

- Inability to use his dominant right arm for any task. Testing revealed intact proprioceptive and tactile sensation and ability to perform all active movements of the shoulder, elbow, forearm, and wrist with therapist support and positioning. All individual movements required great effort, however, and he could not combine movements at multiple arm segments to meet the demands of functional tasks. Although he could perform finger flexion and extension, he was unable to achieve functional grasp and could not oppose his thumb to his other fingers.

- Inability to independently perform self-care activities requiring advanced skills in sitting or standing balance, standing up or sitting down, or use of both arms. He relied on assistance from a home health attendant to perform toileting activities in sitting or standing, get on to and off a tub seat, dress himself, cut meat, shave himself to his own high expectations, and prepare any food.

Initial *MAS* scores are indicated in Figure 23-4.

Reflect on competence

"I have sufficient knowledge of kinesiology and skill in analyzing control parameters when observing Mr. M.'s movement patterns during functional task performance."
"I am knowledgeable about the findings of research literature describing efficient kinematics during performance of a variety of tasks."
"I am knowledgeable about findings of research studies identifying common control parameters of inefficient movement patterns demonstrated by stroke survivors."

Motor Assessment Scale

Patient's Name: Mr. M.

	Pre-treatment Score	Re-evaluation Score
1. Supine to side lying	4	6
2. Supine to sitting over side of bed	5	6
3. Balanced sitting	4	6
4. Sitting to standing	3	5
5. Walking	3	5
6. Upper arm function	1	6
7. Hand movements	3	5
8. Advanced hand activities	0	3

Figure 23-4 Mr. M.'s *MAS* scores.

Recommendations
The occupational therapist recommended two treatment sessions each week for 6 weeks and, in collaboration with Mr. M., established the following long-term treatment goals: (1) Mr. M. will safely and independently stand up and sit down from a variety of seating surfaces and will perform functional tasks while standing. (2) Mr. M. will use his right arm and hand during task performance. (3) Mr. M. will safely and independently perform all activities in which he engaged prior to the stroke and will have sufficient motor and task analysis skills to attempt performing new activities.

Consider the patient's appraisal of performance

Consider what will occur in therapy, how often, and for how long

Ascertain the patient's endorsement of plan

"Mr. M.'s motor, cognitive, and perceptual skills are sufficient for his success with task-related training. He follows directions well and shows the ability to participate as an active collaborator in the treatment process. He shows potential to apply his improvements in motor flexibility to improved functional performance. He has expressed willingness to follow the therapist's recommendations for practice outside of therapy sessions."

Summary of Short-Term Goals and Progress

Mr. M. will achieve full, fluid, active motion at the right scapula, the thoracic and lumbar spine, and the pelvis.

Treatment focused on teaching Mr. M. exercises in lying supine and sitting that provided soft tissue stretch to improve mobility in scapular protraction and upward rotation, thoracolumbar dissociation, and pelvic mobility. The OT taught Mr. M. to appreciate which planes of motion should be available in his scapulae, trunk, and pelvis and encouraged Mr. M. to design activities that would elicit movements at each body segment in all available planes of motion. Mr. M. also learned to determine optimal alignment of body segments for various body postures and functional tasks. Achievement of this goal enabled Mr. M. to attain full independence in bed mobility and facilitated his performance in tasks requiring sitting balance, standing balance, sit-to-stand, and right upper arm control.

Assess the patient's comprehension

Understand what the patient is doing

Compare actual to expected performance

Know the person

Appreciate the context

"Mr. M. showed full understanding of his own body's potential for optimal alignment and full flexibility of his scapula, spinal column, and pelvis. He understood the therapist's rationale for the exercises and task-related practice opportunities. Mr. M.'s part-time attendant is available to help him during practice after therapy sessions to ensure safety."

Mr. M. will maintain sitting balance during activities requiring self-initiated movements of his head, limbs, and trunk and will independently stand up and sit down from a variety of seating surfaces.

Mr. M. improved his balance by using his improved mobility at the trunk and pelvis and practicing unilateral and bilateral reach and grasp in sitting and standing. He improved his ability to stand up and sit down from a variety of seating surfaces in his home after the OT identified the major control parameters influencing his initial performance (Figs. 23-5 and 23-6) and helped him improve his performance strategy (Figs. 23-7 and 23-8).

Mr. M. will use his right arm and hand as an assist to his left during a variety of functional tasks. He will achieve this by improving his control over increasing numbers of degrees of freedom at the right shoulder, elbow, forearm, and hand.

Mr. M. began by practicing holding his shoulder at 90° flexion while supine, with decreasing external support from the therapist. As soon as he demonstrated ability to hold his shoulder in this position, the therapist added one new movement demand at a time, while Mr. M. maintained his shoulder in this position. Examples of new movement demands included scapular motions, elbow motion, wrist motion, lateral pinch to grasp a tissue, and rotational movements at the GH (glenohumeral) joint. Mr. M. practiced varying movement combinations as homework, and he progressed to controlling these combined motions while sitting, a position with greater gravitational demands. Mr. M. accomplished his earliest hand activities while resting his right hand in his lap and reaching down and forward or down and to the side. He practiced a variety of bimanual tasks, such as ripping paper, operating a vacuum cleaner (Fig. 23-9A), buckling a belt, and holding his face in position while shaving. Unilateral tasks included grasping tissues (Fig. 23-9B), operating a television remote control, applying lotion to his left forearm, and using cylindrical grasp to pick up a variety of items in his home. On reevaluation, he could achieve lateral pinch and pad-to-pad pinch. He developed active control of thumb flexion and began to demonstrate thumb opposition.

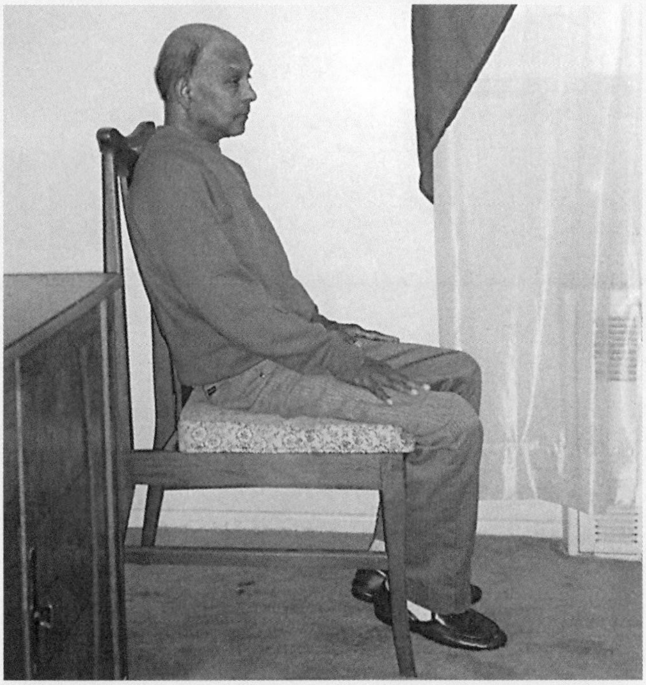

Figure 23-5 Early pre-extension phase of standing up: Mr. M.'s initial evaluation.

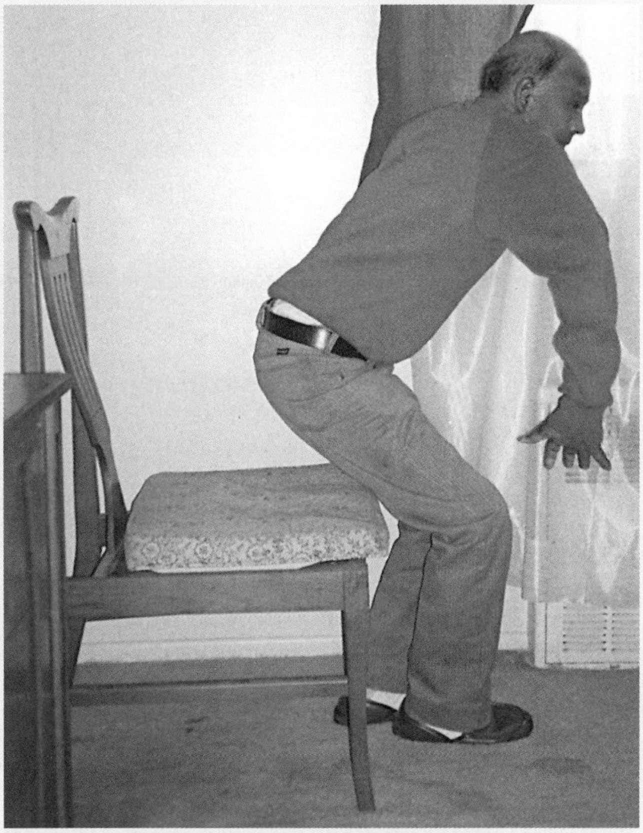

Figure 23-6 Extension phase of standing up: Mr. M.'s initial evaluation.

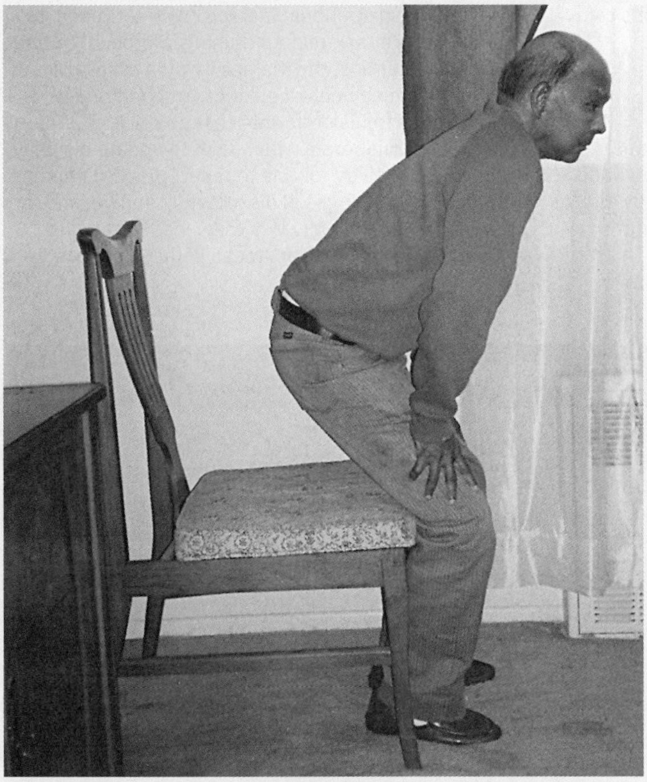

Figure 23-7 Pre-extension phase of standing up: Mr. M.'s reevaluation.

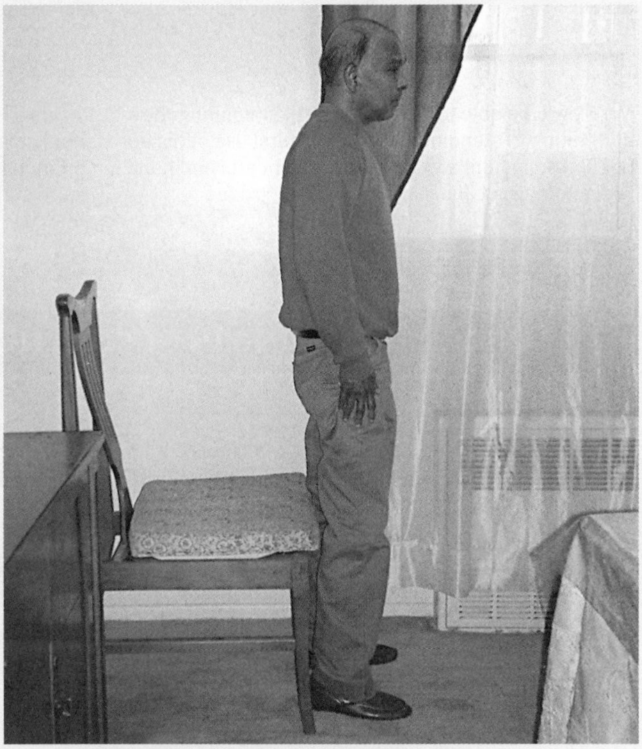

Figure 23-8 Extension phase of standing up: Mr. M.'s reevaluation.

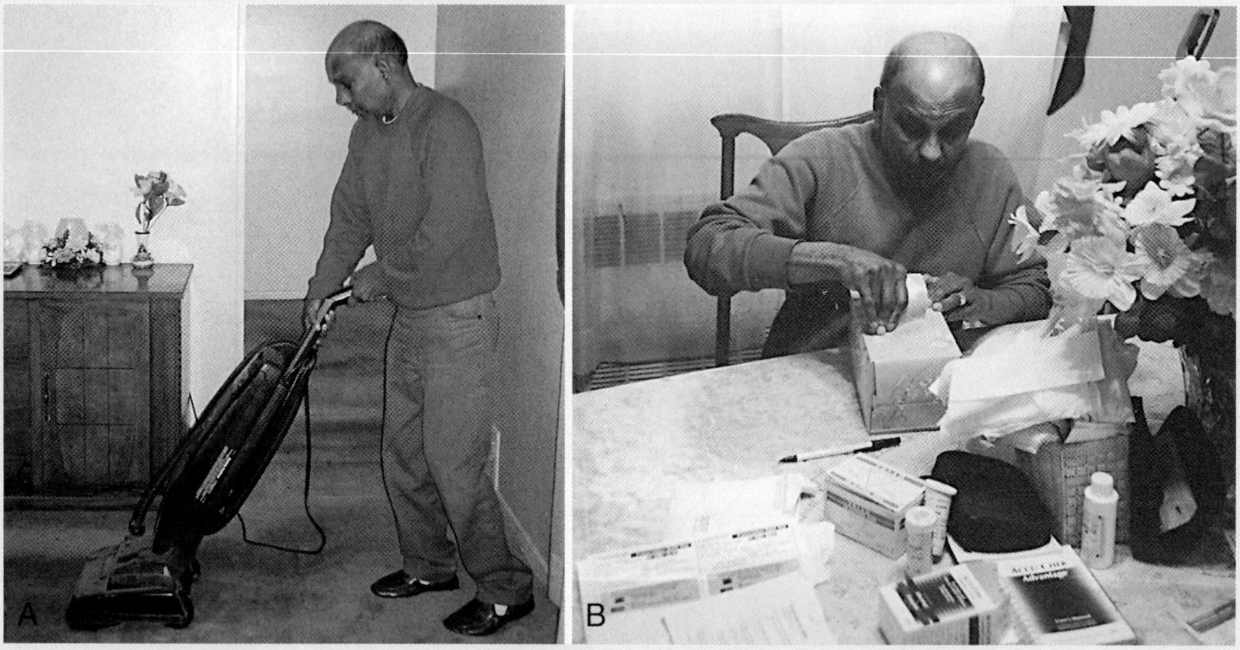

Figure 23-9 Functional task practice during occupational therapy sessions: **A.** Standing. **B.** Seated.

Next Steps		
Mr. M. will be able to perform activities requiring right thumb opposition and individual finger movements. He will be able to perform all hand activities, regardless of what shoulder position is required for a given task.	Anticipate present and future patient concerns Analyze patient's comprehension	"Mr. M. understands that continued practice is essential to maintain the new motor skills he has developed. Occupational therapy sessions will be discontinued. Ideally, Mr. M. should have access to periodic reevaluations by an occupational therapist who is trained in implementing a task-related training approach. During these reevaluations, the therapist would assess Mr. M.'s safety, movement kinematics, and addition of new activities to his performance repertoire. The therapist would collaborate with Mr. M. to update his daily exercise and activity routine to reflect practice needs determined by changes in his motor, cognitive, and/or perceptual status. In Mr. M.'s case, Medicare would not provide reimbursement for such reevaluations."
Mr. M. will be able to perform activities requiring the integration of standing balance, bilateral use of his upper limbs, and unilateral use of his right arm and hand while holding a cane in his left hand.	Decide if the patient should continue or discontinue therapy and/or return in the future	

CLINICAL REASONING IN OCCUPATIONAL THERAPY PRACTICE

Assessing Sit to Stand

Analyze Mr. M.'s performance in Figures 23-5 and 23-6 to determine which factors contributed to his difficulty in rising to stand. What interventions would you use to assist him in improving his ability to rise to standing to the level of function illustrated in Figures 23-7 and 23-8?

Evidence Table 23-1
Best Evidence for Efficacy of Task-Related Training in Improving Motor Skill in Patients with CNS Dysfunction

Intervention	Description of Intervention Tested	Participants	Dosage	Type of Best Evidence and Level of Evidence	Benefit	Statistical Probability and Effect Size of Outcome	Reference
Task-related training	Treatment group: home-based program of reaching tasks while seated; control group: no motor intervention.	9 stroke survivors >1 year post stroke, randomized to group.	10 sessions over a 2-week period	IC1b	Yes. This treatment resulted in increased distance reached. Ipsilateral reach: Treatment group (TG) gained an average of 80 mm; control group (CG) lost 20 mm. Forward reach: TG gained 90 mm; CG lost 30 mm. Across reach: TG gained 120 mm; CG lost 30 mm. And a significant increase in load through affected foot when reaching forward. Peak vertical ground reaction force (by % of body weight) improved by 5.9% for TG; in CG, it decreased by 1.9%.	Ipsilateral reach, $p = 0.042$, $r = 0.39$. Forward reach: $p = 0.005$, $r = 0.59$. Across reach: $p = 0.028$, $r = 0.44$. Increase in load through affected foot: $p = 0.004$, $r = 0.61$.	Dean & Shepherd, 1997

continued

Evidence Table 23-1 (*continued*)

Intervention	Description of Intervention Tested	Participants	Dosage	Type of Best Evidence and Level of Evidence	Benefit	Statistical Probability and Effect Size of Outcome	Reference
Task-related circuit training	Treatment group: exercise class to strengthen the affected lower limb and to practice functional tasks involving the affected limb; control group: practice of upper limb tasks.	9 stroke survivors >3 months post stroke; able to walk 10 m with or without assistive device. Randomized to group (treatment group, n = 5; control group, n = 4)	1-hour class 3×/week for 3 weeks.	IC2c	Yes. The treatment resulted in immediate and retained (2-month follow-up) improvement in walking distance, walking speed without assistive devices, and standing balance. No significant changes in upper limb (unpracticed) strength or dexterity.	Statistical results were not reported; the change scores on which the statistical analyses were done were also not reported; therefore. effect size could not be calculated.	Dean, Richards, & Malouin, 2000
Task-related training (TRT) vs. progressive resistive exercise (PRE)	TRT = reaching to contact or grasp objects placed across work space. PRE = whole arm pulling against resistive therapeutic tubing in planes and distances similar to that in TRT. Home-based training (testing in laboratory).	12 stroke survivors >5 months after rehabilitation, randomly assigned to 1 of 2 treatment conditions and subsequently categorized at high or low functional level based on speed of reach movement.	4 weeks; 12 sessions.	IC2c	Yes. TRT was significantly more effective in improving straightness of hand path (better coordination of elbow-shoulder motion) for the more impaired group but not for the less impaired group whose hand paths were already relatively straight. However, PRE was more effective in decreasing compensatory use of the trunk during reach in the less impaired group, although it had no effect on the more impaired group.	Hand path: $F_{(1,8)} = 5.60$, $p < 0.05$, $eta^2 = 0.41$. Rivermead Stroke Assessment (arm section): $F_{(2,16)} = 6.8$, $p < 0.03$, $eta^2 = 0.46$. *MAS*: not significant. Arm motion (without trunk motion): $F_{(2,16)} = 5.40$, $p < 0.02$, $eta^2 = 40$.	Thielman, Dean, & Gentile, 2004

Task-related training	Home-based program to improve sit-to-stand (STS). Exercise protocol consisted of 10 repetitions of sit-stand-sit (using graded chair heights) and two exercises in standing (step-ups and calf-stretches).	6 stroke survivors >1 year post stroke evaluated before and after treatment.	3×/week for 3 weeks.	IIIc1c	Yes. This treatment resulted in increase in *MAS* score for STS; a significant improvement in timing of thigh-off, which approximated that seen in able-bodied subjects; and an increase in walking speed (mean change of 0.24 m/sec).	*MAS* score: $p = 0.04$, $r = 0.71$. Timing of thigh-off: $p = 0.01$, $r = 0.95$. Increase in walking speed: $p = 0.03$, $r = 0.77$.	Monger, Carr, & Fowler, 2002
Occupationally embedded exercise to improve active forearm supination	Treatment group: adapted dice game requiring bilaterally assisted supination of hemiparetic forearm; control group: repeated performance of bilaterally assisted supination of the hemiparetic forearm.	6 stroke survivors with pronator spasticity, full PROM in supination after brief stretching, and no active supination. Randomized to group.	2 sets of 10 repetitions; 1 treatment session.	IC2c	Yes. Treatment resulted in significantly more bilaterally assisted forearm supination (as measured by degrees of rotation of the measurement handle). Treatment mean = 95.3°; control mean = 81.9°.	$t_{(24)} = 2.28$, $p <$ 0.05 (one tailed), $r = 0.42$.	Nelson et al., 1996
Occupationally embedded exercise to improve forward arm reach	Treatment group: engagement in Simon, a computer-controlled game, positioned to promote forward arm reach; control group: repeated exercise in forward reach, with no embedded task. Counterbalanced design: each subject experienced each condition 1 week apart.	20 young adults after traumatic brain injury with mild to moderate upper limb spasticity.	Single session with 10 movement repetitions for each condition.	IIC2c	Yes. The occupationally embedded condition resulted in significantly greater arm reach (based on video analysis of distance from hip to wrist). Treatment mean = 71.6 cm; control mean = 59.4 cm.	$t_{(19)} = 5.77$, $p <$ 0.001, $r = 0.80$.	Sietsema et al., 1993

SUMMARY REVIEW QUESTIONS

1. What are the relationships between control parameters, adaptive features of CNS dysfunction, and attractor states?
2. How are the principles of activity analysis and synthesis applied when implementing task-related training?
3. Why do Carr and Shepherd lay greater emphasis on assessing and intervening to improve postural adjustments than postural reactions?
4. What are the essential components of the stance phase and swing phase of the gait cycle? How can occupational therapists structure interventions to assist patients in walking to their optimal potential?
5. Which kinematic features of the pre-extension phase of standing up influence the ease with which a person will perform the extension phase?
6. How can occupational therapists structure interventions to assist patients in controlling increasing numbers of degrees of freedom when performing reach and manipulation tasks?
7. What specific mechanical constraints are likely to affect a person's ability to maintain balance during activity performance? To stand up and sit down? To walk during activity performance? To perform activities requiring reach, grasp, and manipulation?
8. What foundational movement strategies are likely to assist a person's ability to maintain balance during activity performance? To stand up and sit down? To walk during activity performance? To perform activities requiring reach, grasp, and manipulation?
9. Provide specific examples of postural adjustments that are likely to assist a person's ability to stand up and sit down, to maintain balance during activity performance, to walk during activity performance, and to perform activities requiring reach, grasp, and manipulation.
10. How can occupational therapists assist patients in developing their task analysis and problem-solving skills in the context of functional movement?

References

Ada, L., O'Dwyer, N., Green, J., Yeo, W., & Neilson, P. (1996). The nature of the loss of strength and dexterity in the upper limb following stroke. *Human Movement Science, 15,* 671–687.

Ada, L., & Westwood, P. (1992). A kinematic analysis of recovery of the ability to stand up following stroke. *Australian Physiotherapy, 38,* 135–142.

Boller, F. (2004). Rational basis of rehabilitation following cerebral lesions: A review of the concept of cerebral plasticity. *Functional Neurology, 19,* 65–72.

Briones, T. L., Klintsova, A. Y., & Greenough, W. T. (2004). Stability of synaptic plasticity in the adult rat visual cortex induced by complex environment exposure. *Brain Research, 1018,* 130–135.

Calautti, C., & Baron, J. C. (2003). Functional neuroimaging studies of motor recovery after stroke in adults: A review. *Stroke, 34,* 1553–1566.

Carr, J. H., & Gentile, A. M. (1994). The effect of arm movement on the biomechanics of standing up. *Human Movement Science, 13,* 175–193.

Carr, J. H., Ow, J., & Shepherd, R. B. (2002). Some biomechanical characteristics of standing up at three different speeds: Implications for functional training. *Physiotherapy Theory and Practice, 18,* 47–53.

Carr, J. H., & Shepherd, R. B. (1980). *Physiotherapy in disorders of the brain.* Rockville, MD: Aspen.

Carr, J. H., & Shepherd, R. B. (1983). *A motor relearning program for stroke.* Rockville, MD: Aspen.

Carr, J. H., & Shepherd, R. B. (1987). *A motor relearning program for stroke* (2nd ed.). Rockville, MD: Aspen.

Carr, J. H., & Shepherd, R. (1998). *Neurological rehabilitation: Optimizing motor performance.* Oxford, United Kingdom: Butterworth-Heinemann.

Carr, J. H., & Shepherd, R. B. (2003). *Stroke rehabilitation: Guidelines for exercise and training to optimize motor skill.* London, United Kingdom: Butterworth-Heinemann.

Carr, J. H., Shepherd, R. B., & Ada, L. (1995). Spasticity: Research findings and implications for intervention. *Physiotherapy, 81,* 421–429.

Carr, J. H., Shepherd, R. B., Nordholm, L., & Lynne, D. (1985). Investigation of a new motor assessment scale for stroke patients. *Physical Therapy, 65,* 175–180.

Chen, R., Cohen, L. G., & Hallett, M. (2002). Nervous system reorganization following injury. *Neuroscience, 111,* 761–773.

Dean, C.M., & Mackey, F. (1992). Motor assessment scale scores as a measure of rehabilitation outcome after stroke. *Australian Physiotherapy, 65,* 175–180.

Dean, C. M., Richards, C. L., & Malouin, F. (2000). Task-related circuit training improves performance of locomotor tasks in chronic stroke: A randomized, controlled pilot trial. *Archives of Physical Medicine and Rehabilitation, 81,* 409–417.

Dean, C. M., & Shepherd, R. B. (1997). Task-related training improves performance of seated reaching tasks after stroke: A randomized controlled trial. *Stroke, 28,* 722–728.

Dean, C., Shepherd, R., & Adams, R. (1999a). Sitting balance I: Trunk-arm and the contribution of the lower limbs during self-paced reaching in sitting. *Gait and Posture, 10,* 135–144.

Dean, C., Shepherd, R., & Adams, R. (1999b). Sitting balance II: Reach direction and thigh support affect the contribution of the lower limbs when reaching beyond arms' length in sitting. *Gait and Posture, 10,* 147–153.

Duncan, P. W., Richards, L., Wallace, D., Stoker-Yates, J., Pohl, P., Luchies, C., Ogle, A., & Studenski, S. (1998). A randomized controlled pilot study of a home-based exercise program for individuals with mild and moderate stroke. *Stroke, 29,* 2055–2060.

Fasoli, S. E., Trombly, C. A., Tickle-Degnen, L., & Verfaellie, M. H. (2002). Effect of instructions on functional reach in persons with and without cerebrovascular accident. *American Journal of Occupational Therapy, 56,* 380–390.

Hesse, S., Werner, C., von Frankenberg, S., & Bardeleben, A. (2003). Treadmill training with partial body weight support after stroke. *Physical Medicine and Rehabilitation Clinics of North America, 14,* S111–S123.

Hoff, B., & Arbib, M. A. (1993). Models of trajectory formation and temporal interaction of reach and grasp. *Journal of Motor Behavior, 25,* 175–192.

Hsieh, C. L., Nelson, D. L., Smith, D. A., & Peterson, C. Q. (1996). A comparison of performance in added-purpose occupations and rote exercise for dynamic standing balance in persons with hemiplegia. *American Journal of Occupational Therapy, 50,* 10–16.

Johansson, B. B. (2003). Environmental influence on recovery after brain lesions: Experimental and clinical data. *Journal of Rehabilitation Medicine, 41 (Suppl.),* 11–16.

Khemlani, M. M., Carr, J. H., & Crosbie, W. J. (1999). Muscle synergies and joint linkages in sit-to-stand under two initial foot positions. *Clinical Biomechanics, 14,* 236–246.

Kieran, O. P., Lim, A. L., & Sabari, J. S. (1999). Using the MAS to measure functional recovery of the hemiplegic arm. Academic Annual Assembly Abstracts. *Archives of Physical Medicine and Rehabilitation, 80,* 1138.

Latash, L. P., & Latash, M. L. (1994). A new book by N. A. Bernstein: "On Dexterity and Its Development." *Journal of Motor Behavior, 26,* 56–62.

Levangie, P. K., & Norkin, C. C. (2005). *Joint structure and function: A comprehensive analysis* (4th ed.). Philadelphia: F. A. Davis.

Ma, H., Trombly, C.A., & Robinson-Podolski, C. (1999). The effect of context on skill acquisition and transfer. *American Journal of Occupational Therapy, 53,* 138–144.

Mark, V. W., & Taub, E. (2004). Constraint-induced movement therapy for chronic stroke hemiparesis and other disabilities. *Restorative Neurological Neuroscience, 22,* 317–336.

McNevin, N. H., Wulf, G., & Carlson, C. (2000). Effects of attentional focus, self-control, and dyad training on motor learning: Implications for physical therapy. *Physical Therapy, 80,* 373–385.

Monger, C., Carr, J. H., & Fowler, V. (2002). Evaluation of a home-based exercise and training programme to improve sit-to-stand in patients with chronic stroke. *Clinical Rehabilitation, 16,* 361–367.

Nakayama, H., Jorgensen, H. S., Raaschou, H. O., & Olsen, T. S. (1994). Recovery of upper extremity function in stroke patients: The Copenhagen Stroke Study. *Archives of Physical Medicine and Rehabilitation, 75,* 852–857.

Nashner, L. M., & McCollum, G. (1985). The organization of human postural movements: A formal basis and experimental synthesis. *The Behavioral and Brain Sciences, 8,* 135–172.

Nelson, D. L., Konosky, K., Fleharty, K., Webb, R., Newer, K., Hazboun, V. P., Fontane, C., & Licht, B. C. (1996). The effects of an occupationally embedded exercise on bilaterally assisted supination in persons with hemiplegia. *American Journal of Occupational Therapy, 50,* 639–646.

Nudo, R. J. (2003). Adaptive plasticity in motor cortex: Implications for rehabilitation after brain injury. *Journal of Rehabilitation Medicine, 41 (Suppl.),* 7–10.

Nugent, J. A., & Schurr, K. A. (1994). A dose-response relationship between amount of weight-bearing exercise and walking outcome following cerebrovascular accident. *Archives of Physical Medicine and Rehabilitation, 75,* 399–402.

O'Dwyer, N. J., Ada, L., & Neilson, P. D. (1996). Spasticity and muscle contracture following stroke. *Brain, 119,* 1737–1749.

Pascual-Leone, A. (2001). The brain that plays music and is changed by it. *Annals of the New York Academy of Science, 930,* 315–329.

Perry, S. B. (1998). Clinical implications of a dynamic systems theory. *(American Physical Therapy Association) Neurology Report, 22,* 4–10.

Poole, J. L., & Whitney, S. L. (1988). Motor assessment scale for stroke patients: Concurrent validity and interrater reliability. *Archives of Physical Medicine and Rehabilitation, 69,* 195–197.

Sabari, J. (2004). Activity-based intervention in stroke rehabilitation. In G. Gillen & A. Burkhardt (Eds.), *Stroke rehabilitation: A function-based approach* (2nd ed., pp. 75–92). St. Louis: Mosby.

Sabari, J., Lim, A. L., Velozo, C., Lehman, L., Kieran, O., & Lai, J. S. (2005). Assessing arm and hand function after stroke: A validity test of the hierarchical scoring system used in the Motor Asssessment Scale for stroke. *Archives of Physical Medicine and Rehabilitation, 86,* 1609–1615.

Schmidt, R. A., & Lee, T. D. (2005). *Motor control and learning: A behavioral emphasis* (4th ed.). Champaign, IL: Human Kinetics.

Shepherd, R. B. (1992). Adaptive motor behaviour in response to perturbations of balance. *Physiotherapy Theory and Practice, 8,* 137–143.

Shepherd, R. B., & Carr, J. H. (1998). The shoulder following stroke: Preserving musculoskeletal integrity for function. *Topics in Stroke Rehabilitation, 4,* 35–53.

Shepherd, R. B., & Carr, J. H. (1999). Treadmill walking in neurorehabilitation. *Neurorehabilitation and Neural Repair, 13,* 171–173.

Shepherd, R. B., & Gentile, A. M. (1994). Sit to stand: Functional relationship between upper body and lower limb segments. *Human Movement Science, 13,* 817–840.

Shepherd, R. B., & Koh, H. P. (1996). Some biomechanical consequences of varying foot placement in sit-to-stand in young women. *Scandinavian Journal of Rehabilitation Medicine, 28,* 79–88.

Shumway-Cook, A., & Woollacott, M. (2000). *Motor control: Theory and practical applications* (2nd ed.). Baltimore: Williams & Wilkins.

Sietsema, J. M., Nelson, D. L., Mulder, R. M., Mervau-Scheidel, D., & White, B. E. (1993). The use of a game to promote arm reach in persons with traumatic brain injury. *American Journal of Occupational Therapy, 47,* 19–24.

Taub, E., Miller, N. E., Novack, T. A., Cook, E. W., Fleming, W. C., Nepomuceno, C. S., Connell, J. S., & Crago, J. E. (1993). Technique to improve chronic motor deficit after stroke. *Archives of Physical Medicine and Rehabilitation, 74,* 347–354.

Taub, E., & Wolf, S. L. (1997). Constraint induced movement techniques to facilitate upper extremity use in stroke patients. *Topics in Stroke Rehabilitation, 3,* 38–61.

Thickbrook, G. W., Byrnes, M. L., Archer, S. A., & Mastaglia, F. L. (2004). Motor outcome after subcortical stroke correlates with the degree of cortical reorganization. *Clinical Neurophysiology, 115,* 2144–2150.

Thielman, G. T., Dean, C. M., & Gentile, A. M. (2004). Rehabilitation of reaching after stroke: Task-related training versus progressive resistive exercise. *Archives of Physical Medicine and Rehabilitation, 85,* 1613–1618.

Trombly, C. A. (1992). Deficits of reaching in subjects with left hemiparesis: A pilot study. *American Journal of Occupational Therapy, 46,* 887–897.

Trombly, C. A. (1993). Observations of improvement of reaching in five subjects with left hemiparesis. *Journal of Neurology, Neurosurgery, and Psychiatry, 56,* 40–45.

Trombly, C. A., & Wu, C. Y. (1999). Effect of rehabilitation tasks on organization of movement after stroke. *American Journal of Occupational Therapy, 53,* 333–344.

Visintin, M., Barbeau, H., Korner-Bitensky, N., & Mayo, N. E. (1998). A new approach to retrain gait in stroke patients through body weight support and treadmill stimulation. *Stroke, 29,* 1122–1128.

Ward, N. S. (2004). Functional reorganization of the cerebral motor system after stroke. *Current Opinions in Neurology, 17,* 725–730.

Willingham, D. B. (1998). A neuropsychological theory of motor skill learning. *Psychological Review, 105,* 558–584.

Wolf, S. L., Blanton, S., Baer, H., Breshears, J., & Butler, A. J. (2002). Repetitive task practice: A critical review of constraint-induced movement therapy in stroke. *The Neurologist, 8,* 325–338.

Wu, C.-Y., Trombly, C. A., Lin, K.-C., & Tickle-Degnen, L. (2000). A kinematic study of contextual effects on reaching performance in persons with and without stroke: Influences of object availability. *Archives of Physical Medicine and Rehabilitation, 81,* 95–101

Wulf, G., McNevin, N. H., Fuchs, T., Ritter, F., & Toole, T. (2000). Attentional focus in complex skill learning. *Research Quarterly in Exercise and Sport, 71,* 229–239.

CHAPTER 24

Optimizing Motor Behavior Using the Bobath Approach

Kathryn Levit

LEARNING OBJECTIVES

After studying this chapter, the reader will be able to do the following:

1. Identify the major problems that result from stroke according to Bobath and Bobath.
2. Describe the major principles underlying the Neuro-Developmental Treatment (NDT)/Bobath approach to stroke rehabilitation.
3. Discuss the role of muscle tone and postural control in the production of normal movement, and describe how problems in these areas contribute to impaired occupational functioning.
4. Integrate NDT/Bobath concepts and techniques with the occupational functioning model.
5. Develop an OT treatment plan for a patient with acute stroke using NDT/Bobath principles and techniques.

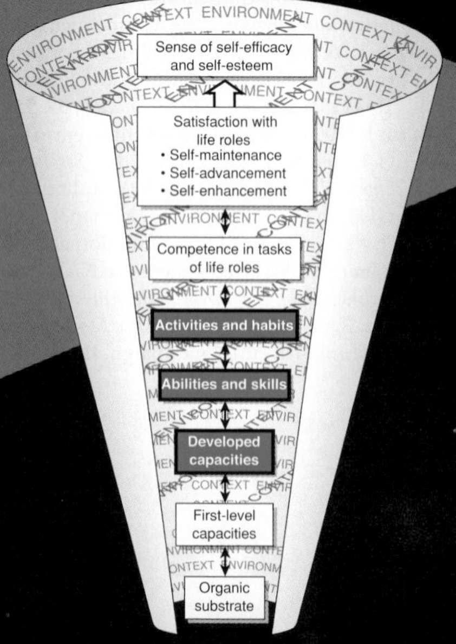

Glossary

Abnormal coordination—Patterns of muscle activation, timing, and sequencing that deviate from normal, resulting in inefficient, stereotyped movement patterns.

Abnormal tone—Muscle tone that is higher or lower than normal.

Associated reactions—Involuntary and non-functional changes in limb position and muscle tone associated with difficult or stressful activities.

Facilitation—Manual techniques and other processes including tactile and verbal feedback used to help the patient achieve a more normal quality of movement.

Flaccidity—Muscle tone that is lower than normal. Also known as hypotonicity.

Handling—Manual techniques designed to change muscle tone and normalize movement. Handling includes inhibition and facilitation.

Inhibition—Manual techniques and positions used to decrease or eliminate the effects of spasticity and abnormal coordination.

Key points of control—Hand placements used to influence the quality of posture and movement.

Loss of postural control—Inability to use automatic patterns of muscle activation to maintain the body within a stable base of support at rest and during movement.

Placing response—Part of the normal system of postural adjustments to changes in position, characterized by automatically maintaining a position when support is removed.

Reflex-inhibiting pattern (RIP)—A position that is used to inhibit spasticity by lengthening shortened muscles.

Spasticity—Muscle tone that is higher than normal and resists passive stretching; also known as hypertonicity.

K. Bobath and B. Bobath developed a treatment approach designed to increase normal movement patterns in children with cerebral palsy and adults with acquired hemiplegia. Their treatment is known as the Bobath approach or Neuro-Developmental Treatment (NDT). NDT/Bobath treatment focuses on eliminating abnormal movements and restoring normal movements. The occupational functioning model usually describes this type of treatment as preparatory because it is directed toward establishing sensorimotor performance components that are prerequisites for function while minimizing the impairments that interfere with functional behavior. This chapter introduces the NDT/Bobath approach to the treatment of adults with hemiplegia. A complete description of the treatment approach and its techniques can be found in Bobath (1990) and Davies (1985). Eggers (1984) provides information on using the approach to improve occupational functioning. Current theoretical foundations and principles of clinical practice are described in Howle (2002).

INTRODUCTION

NDT is one of the classic neurophysiological treatment approaches that were developed to address the impairments associated with damage to the central nervous system. This section briefly reviews the history of the NDT approach and provides an overview of principles of treatment and methods for integrating this treatment into occupational therapy for individuals with stroke and brain injury.

History and Principles

Bobath and Bobath began to develop their treatment approach in England in the 1940s. B. Bobath, trained in Germany as a gymnast and remedial movement specialist, went to England to avoid persecution and found work as a physical therapist. When treating adults with hemiplegia, she noted the abnormal stiffness in their affected extremities, their asymmetrical body postures, and the non-functional stereotyped patterns of movement in their involved side. B. Bobath tried to help her patients regain functional use of their hemiplegic side. She assumed that the abnormal patterns of muscle tone and motor control were the major impairments interfering with normal motor control of the trunk, arm, and leg. Through trial and error, B. Bobath developed techniques for decreasing abnormal reflex activity and muscle tone and for increasing control of normal patterns of movement on the hemiplegic side of the body. These techniques were based on her knowledge of normal kinesiology, not the developmental sequence.

B. Bobath discovered that she could help her patients with hemiplegia move more freely and function with less compensation by decreasing the abnormal tone in their affected side. She also found that, when spasticity decreased, her patients could acquire improved control of posture and movement on their affected side and could use these new patterns for function. Based on these clinical findings, B. Bobath developed a new model for treating adults with hemiplegia. Her approach involved the use of manual techniques to eliminate abnormal tone and dysfunctional movement and to retrain normal patterns of coordination in the affected trunk, arm, and leg.

Since her goal was to restore normal movement and function on the affected side, she specifically rejected compensatory approaches that neglected the potential for function in the hemiplegic side and other neurophysiological approaches that encouraged abnormal movement and reflex activity.

As B. Bobath developed the treatment techniques, neurologist K. Bobath reviewed research in neurology and neurophysiology to develop a scientific basis for his wife's treatment. B. Bobath's claims that her treatment could change spasticity and restore normal movement responses were controversial, and K. Bobath used research findings to support her discoveries. Since the clinical techniques developed first, K. Bobath presented his scientific rationale in hypothetical terms, describing it as an explanation for, not the basis of, intervention.

Bobath and Bobath called their treatment approach a living concept because they expected it to change and develop over time. They made many changes to the treatment over the years to make it more active and functional. They also made an effort to update their theory by adding new scientific explanations for certain aspects of their treatment. Although controversial when first introduced, many of the assumptions of Bobath and Bobath are now an accepted part of stroke rehabilitation, and the approach is widely used throughout the world (Rast, 1999). The theoretical models that K. Bobath proposed as a basis for treatment are now out of date, however, and the NDT/Bobath approach has been the target of criticism (Howle, 2002; Gordon, 1987). For the past 15 years, the Neuro-Developmental Treatment Association (NDTA) in the United States and similar groups in other countries have been working to update the theoretical basis for NDT/Bobath treatment (Definition 24-1). The NDTA Theory Committee has recently published an updated account of theoretical foundations and principles of treatment as they apply to adults with hemiplegia and children with cerebral palsy (Howle, 2002).

DEFINITION 24-1

NDT Philosophy

The NDTA website (www.ndta.org) contains the following statement about Neuro-Developmental Treatment:

"The Neuro-Developmental Treatment (NDT)/Bobath approach was developed by Berta and Karel Bobath as a 'living concept.' The approach is intended to grow and develop over time as new information is gained from clinical experience and scientific research. NDT is used for the treatment and management of individuals with movement dysfunction resulting from central nervous system (CNS) pathophysiology. The individual's strengths and impairments are identified through an in-depth analytical process and addressed in relation to functional abilities and limitations. NDT is an interactive process which includes individuals, caregivers and members of the interdisciplinary team in assessment, treatment planning and application.

The overall goal of treatment and management is to enhance the individual's capacity to function, minimize impairments, and prevent disabilities. To achieve this goal, the therapist addresses the quality of movement utilizing principles of movement science. Intervention involves direct handling including facilitation, and inhibition to optimize function. The application of NDT contributes to the individual's increased independence and an enhancement of the quality of life."

Definitions of Terms and Constructs

Bobath and Bobath developed their approach to address the motor problems associated with **hemiplegia**, or loss of muscular control on one side of the body. They believed that hemiplegia is associated with two categories of motor problems: the loss of normal movement responses and the development of abnormal tone and movement. B. Bobath hypothesized that these two problems cause the abnormal patterns of coordination and functional limitations common following stroke. She also believed that treatment that addressed these problems would improve movement control on the hemiplegic side and, hence, increase the possibilities for occupational performance. These assumptions are discussed separately in the sections that follow.

Movement Control Problems after Stroke

Bobath and Bobath described the loss of normal movement responses as the first type of motor impairment associated with hemiplegia. Patients with hemiplegia may demonstrate **loss of postural control**, or inability to activate muscles automatically to maintain the body in balance at rest and during movement, and **loss of selective movement control** of the muscles controlling movement of the hemiplegic arm and leg. Loss of postural control is associated with difficulty shifting weight, maintaining a stable body position against gravity, and activating equilibrium responses when balance is challenged. These problems interfere with the performance of life roles and lead patients to rely on adaptive equipment to substitute for poor balance (Fig. 24-1). Loss of selective movement control prevents patients from using the hemiplegic arm, resulting in reliance on one-handed techniques for task performance. B. Bobath suggested that patients who adopt these asymmetrical compensations learn to neglect the potential for functional performance on the hemiplegic side even when the necessary sensory-motor components are present.

Bobath and Bobath identified **abnormal tone** as the second major problem interfering with movement control and function in hemiplegia. Abnormal tone refers to alterations in muscle tension and resistance to passive stretch. After a stroke, muscle tone on the hemiplegic side may be

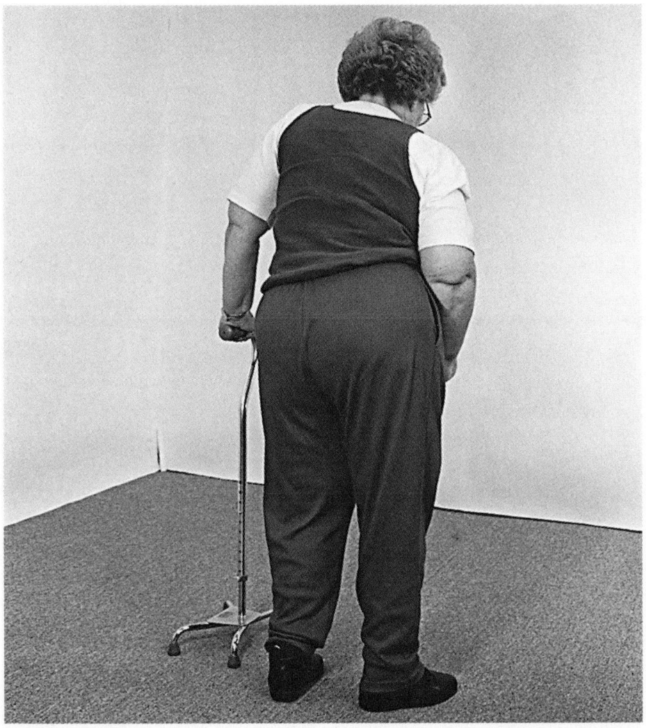

Figure 24-1 Patient showing poor postural control while walking with a cane.

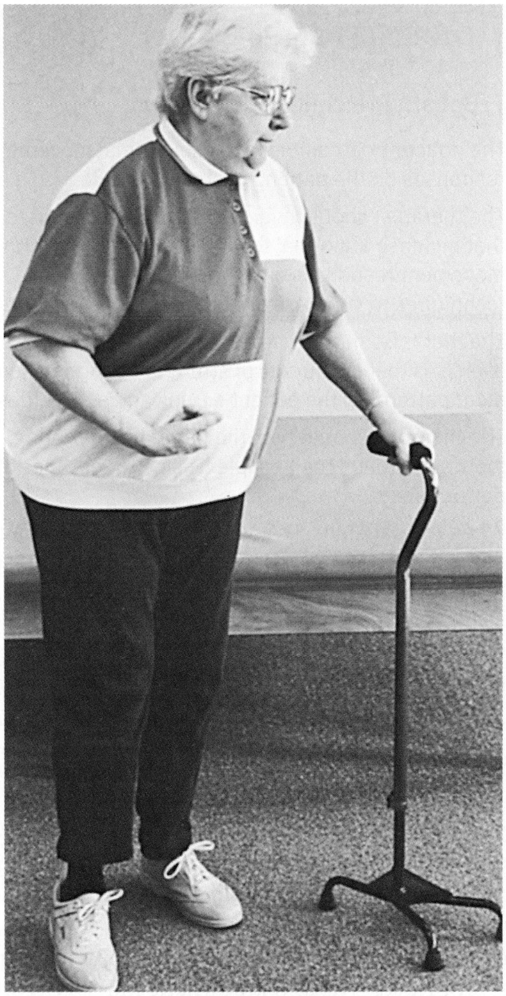

Figure 24-2 Patient showing associated reaction in the hemiparetic arm while walking.

higher or lower than normal. Patients demonstrate **flaccidity**, or hypotonia, when muscle tone is lower than normal. Flaccidity is generally present immediately after the stroke. **Spasticity**, or hypertonia, develops gradually in selected muscles of the affected trunk, arm, and leg and is characterized by excessive muscle stiffness and slow effortful movements. Spasticity is often accompanied by **associated reactions**, which are involuntary, nonfunctional changes in limb position associated with the performance of difficult or stressful activities. For example, the hemiplegic arm may assume a flexed position when the patient walks (Fig. 24-2). According to Bobath and Bobath, spasticity interferes with selective muscle activity on the hemiplegic side, contributing to abnormal patterns of coordination and loss of functional use.

Bobath and Bobath believed that these two categories of motor impairment result in the stereotyped non-functional movement patterns and functional limitations associated with hemiplegia. In their writings, the Bobaths also emphasized that sensory disturbances may contribute to abnormal coordination and decreased motor control. They hypothesized that patients with hemiplegia have forgotten how to move in normal patterns of coordination and suggested that this sensory disturbance may result in loss of normal movement responses, even when muscles are sufficiently strong to support movement. The loss of the sensory memory for movement may also contribute to abnormal patterns of coordination by causing patients to initiate and sequence muscle activity inappropriately. Thus, although their treatment approach was designed to address problems with tone and movement, Bobath and Bobath recognized that sensation was necessary for motor coordination and motor learning, and their treatment techniques use sensory information as part of the process of reeducating normal movement.

Neuro-Developmental Treatment of Patients with Stroke

NDT/Bobath treatment uses manual techniques to address the problems of tone and movement control and to provide sensory messages about how movement is organized and executed. These techniques have the goals of preventing or eliminating abnormal tone and coordination, retraining normal movement responses, and increasing functional use of the hemiplegic side (Definition 24-2). B. Bobath used her hands on the patient's body to produce therapeutic changes in tone and movement. She called this treatment **handling** to reflect the hands-on quality of her treatment. Initially, handling was relatively static, requiring the use of reflexes and passive positioning to produce changes in muscle tone.

DEFINITION 24-2

NDT/Bobath Principles of Treatment

- The goal of treatment is to retrain normal movement responses on the patient's hemiplegic side.
- The therapist should avoid activities and exercises that increase abnormal tone or strengthen abnormal movement responses and should use treatment techniques to suppress or eliminate these patterns.
- The therapist should use treatment activities and exercises that encourage or strengthen normal movement patterns in the patient's trunk and extremities.
- The therapist should help the patient use existing motor control on the hemiplegic side for occupational performance.
- When the patient lacks adequate strength and control of the affected arm and leg for normal occupational performance, the therapist should develop compensations and adaptations that encourage use of the affected side and decrease the development of abnormal movements and asymmetrical postures.

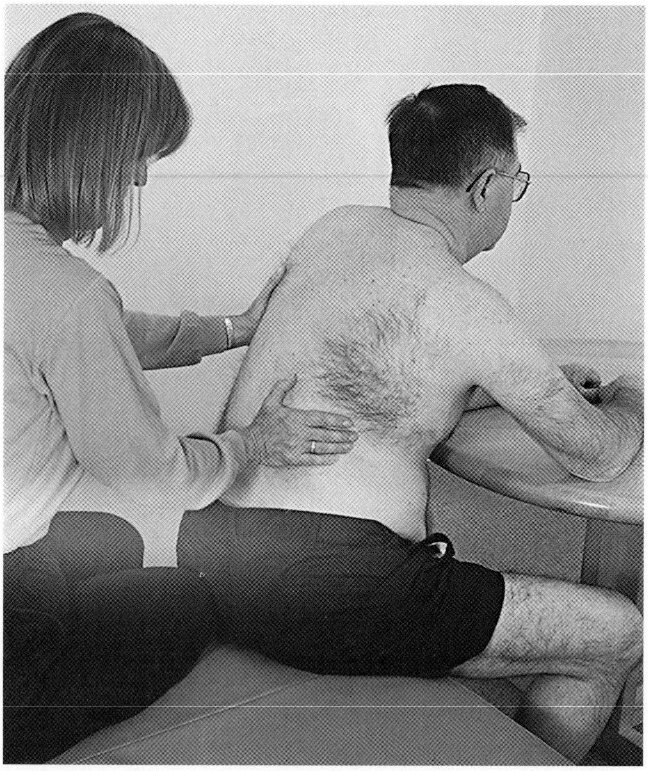

Figure 24-3 Therapist's hands showing key points of control on the trunk.

As the approach evolved, handling became a more dynamic process used to activate movement responses to decrease abnormal tone and coordination and reeducate normal movements.

The NDT therapist uses handling to provide specific tactile, proprioceptive, and kinesthetic messages that help organize the quality of the patient's movement and influence the status of relevant impairments, such as spasticity and flaccidity. Although B. Bobath did not specifically identify impairments such as subluxation and contracture as contributing to abnormal coordination, these secondary impairments may present mechanical blocks to normal movement and are also addressed through handling (Howle, 2002). B. Bobath found that certain hand placements, which she called **key points of control**, are most effective for controlling the patient's movement. During treatment, the therapist selects key points that give maximal control over the patient's problems and the movement pattern the therapist wishes to influence. Proximal key points are used to influence posture and movement of the trunk, shoulder girdle, and hip, and distal key points are used to control the position of the distal extremities (Fig. 24-3).

Handling incorporates two types of techniques: inhibition and facilitation (Procedures for Practice 24-1). **Inhibition techniques** are used for problems of abnormal tone and abnormal coordination. The NDT therapist uses inhibition to decrease spasticity and block or eliminate abnormal patterns of movement. B. Bobath believed that therapists should not attempt to retrain normal move-

PROCEDURES FOR PRACTICE 24-1

NDT Handling Techniques

Inhibition techniques are used to:

- Decrease abnormal muscle tone that interferes with passive and active movement.
- Restore normal alignment in the trunk and extremities by lengthening spastic muscles.
- Stop unwanted movements and associated reactions from occurring.
- Teach methods for decreasing the abnormal posturing of the arm and leg during task performance.

Facilitation techniques are used to:

- Provide the sensation of normal movement on the hemiplegic side.
- Provide a system for relearning normal movements of the trunk, arm, and leg.
- Stimulate muscles directly to contract isometrically, eccentrically, or isotonically.
- Allow practicing movements while the therapist maintains some constraints.
- Teach ways to incorporate the involved side into functional tasks and occupations.

ment responses until spasticity is minimized through inhibition because spasticity blocks the patterns of reciprocal muscle activation needed for optimal motor and functional performance. For this reason, treatment often begins with the use of inhibition techniques to reduce spasticity. Inhibition techniques often use **reflex-inhibiting patterns (RIPs)**, a term for patterns that counteract the pull of tight or spastic muscles. Spasticity may also be inhibited by using weight bearing and trunk rotation to lengthen shortened muscles.

When muscle tone is normalized through inhibition or when spasticity is not a major impairment, the NDT therapist uses **facilitation techniques** to train normal movement patterns. Facilitation techniques are used to activate automatic postural responses and trunk control and to reeducate weight-bearing and non–weight-bearing movements in the arm and leg. The assumption is that facilitation will minimize the learning of abnormal movements by allowing the patient to practice normal patterns of movement and coordination from the earliest days of rehabilitation. Occupational therapists may also use facilitation techniques to introduce and practice new strategies for performing functional activities in occupation-as-means or occupation-as-end. During facilitation, the therapist establishes light contact with appropriate key points of control and manually assists the patient's movement patterns. The therapist initially controls the quality and characteristics of the movement, while the patient follows these manual cues and moves with assistance. As the patient learns to perform the desired movements, the therapist gradually decreases the amount of assistance provided until the patient moves without input from the therapist.

Relationship to Occupational Functioning

Bobath and Bobath assumed that most of the disability associated with hemiplegia is related to impairments in posture and movement (Bobath, 1990; Howle, 2002). Thus, they believed that treatment directed toward improving the status of sensorimotor performance components would result in improved occupational performance. They noted that, when patients learn new movements, they often spontaneously use these movements functionally without further treatment. For example, when NDT facilitation techniques are used to increase postural control in sitting, patients may spontaneously use their improved trunk control to lean forward to adjust the foot pedals on the wheelchair or to stay erect while putting on a shirt. Since remediation of lower level functional prerequisites may not, however, automatically result in improved occupational performance (Dijkers, 1999; Trombly, 1995), NDT therapists must also use aspects of occupation-as-means and occupation-as-end to ensure that improvements in tonal state and movement control are incorporated into occupational functioning.

In occupation-as-end, the patient is directly engaged in learning an activity or task. After a stroke, occupational therapists use occupation-as-end to teach self-care skills, such as dressing and bathing, or mobility activities, such as rolling, transfers, and wheelchair propulsion. NDT therapists have developed compensatory occupation-as-end techniques for activities such as dressing, grooming, and bed mobility. These techniques are designed to maintain symmetry and bilaterality and to encourage patients to activate their trunk muscles and incorporate their involved extremities into task performance. The NDT/Bobath approach rejects the use of one-sided compensations, emphasizing instead that patients should perform tasks in ways that use the hemiplegic side. Examples of the use of NDT/Bobath techniques in occupation-as-end are discussed later in the chapter.

In occupation-as-means, the therapist uses activities therapeutically to influence impairments and provide opportunities for motor learning and practice. The NDT therapist frequently uses actual tasks or parts of tasks in occupation-as-means treatment to increase postural control or improve strength and coordination in the hemiplegic arm. For example, in the sitting position, the therapist may use activities that require weight shifts over the body's base of support to increase control of the postural muscles of the trunk and the lower extremity (Fig. 24-4). Similarly, the therapist may structure cooking or grooming tasks to practice weight support in the hemiplegic arm or to train the use of the hemiplegic arm in bilateral grasp. Occupation-as means should incorporate movement patterns that the patient can perform independently without asymmetry or excessive use of the uninvolved side. Activities that are too difficult or that result in increased tone or compensation should be avoided, although the NDT therapist may use facilitation to help the patient practice an activity that cannot be performed independently. Some examples of NDT occupation-as-means activities are in-

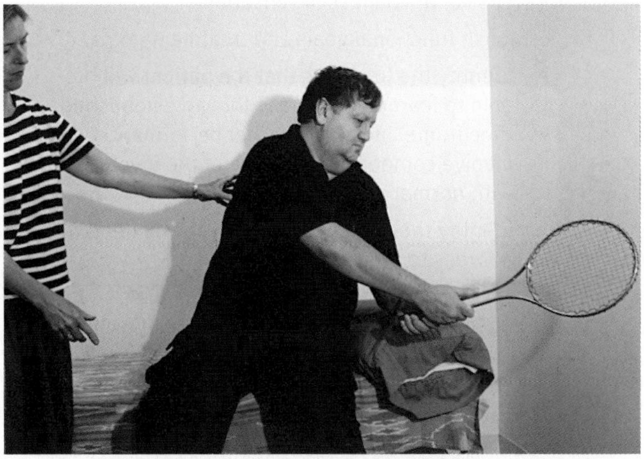

Figure 24-4 Patient swinging a tennis racquet to increase control of trunk.

cluded in the treatment section of this chapter. Eggers (1984) provided a complete description for using occupation-as-means within an NDT framework.

EVALUATION AND TREATMENT PLANNING

The NDT/Bobath approach uses assessment to gather information about the patient's movement control and functional status, the problems interfering with functional use of the hemiplegic side, and the patient's response to handling (Procedures for Practice 24-2). This information is used to set treatment goals and plan treatment activities. This section reviews the important components of this system of evaluation and treatment planning.

PROCEDURES FOR PRACTICE 24-2

NDT/Bobath Evaluation and Treatment Planning

1. Identify abilities and functional capabilities. Include movements of both the arm and leg, postural patterns of the trunk, and functional independence in life skills. How does the patient accomplish these functions?
2. Identify functional limitations, including functions that the patient cannot perform that are necessary for improved independence and quality of life.
3. Determine what problems interfere with movement control and functional performance, such as:
   - Abnormal tone
   - Abnormal coordination
   - Loss of postural control
   - Loss of selective movement control
   - Loss of or changes in sensation
4. Establish functional goals and treatment goals.
   - Identify the functions that the patient will be able to learn to perform within an established time frame. Indicate whether performance will involve compensation or use of the involved side with normal coordination.
   - Identify the impairments that you will need to address to meet the functional goal.
5. Based on the patient's response to handling, determine where to begin treatment. What techniques of inhibition and facilitation will be used?

Adapted with permission from Bobath, B. (1990). *Adult hemiplegia: Evaluation and treatment* (3rd ed.). London: Heinemann; and from Ryerson, S., & Levit, K. (1997). The shoulder in hemiplegia. In R. Donatelli (Ed.), *Physical therapy of the shoulder* (3rd ed., pp 205–228). New York: Churchill Livingstone.

Assessment in the NDT/Bobath Approach

The NDT therapist gathers assessment information through a variety of procedures. During the initial contact with the patient, the therapist observes the patient's behavior to gather information about typical posture, preferred movement patterns, and spontaneous use of the hemiplegic side. The therapist also observes how the patient performs activities of daily living (ADL), transfers, and bed mobility and notes whether the patient spontaneously uses the affected side or relies on compensations that reflect asymmetry and neglect. The therapist also watches to see whether the patient demonstrates abnormal tone and coordination on the hemiplegic side. Although these initial observations yield important information, the most important aspect of the NDT assessment is the evaluation of motor patterns and the patient's response to being moved. These tests are described briefly next. A more detailed description of the tests can be found in Bobath (1990).

The NDT therapist uses handling to identify the normal patterns of movement that are present on the hemiplegic side and the abnormal patterns that are contributing to the patient's movement problems and functional limitations. To assess movement control, the therapist moves the patient into postures and movement sequences that are important for occupational performance. For example, the therapist tests postural control by facilitating trunk movements, equilibrium reactions, and protective responses (Fig. 24-5) with the patient sitting and standing. The therapist also uses handling to test selective control of arm and leg movements by moving proximal and distal limb segments in varying combinations of joint movement. The therapist uses information about the patient's balance and spontaneous movements gained in the observational stage of assessment and the goals of treatment identified by the patient to select the movement patterns to be assessed via handling.

During assessment, handling provides the therapist with specific sensory information about the quality and strength of the patient's movements. When movement control is present on the hemiplegic side, the patient actively assists with the movement, and the movement seems effortless and flowing. If the therapist stops the movement briefly and lightens manual support, the patient will briefly hold the position. B. Bobath referred to this as the **placing response** (Fig. 24-6). Facilitation is easy and placing is possible when muscle tone is in the normal range and muscle strength is available to support movement. Facilitation and placing are not possible, however, when muscle tone on the hemiplegic side is too high or too low. When the therapist facilitates movements that require spastic muscles to lengthen, the therapist feels resistance while movements that go in the direction of

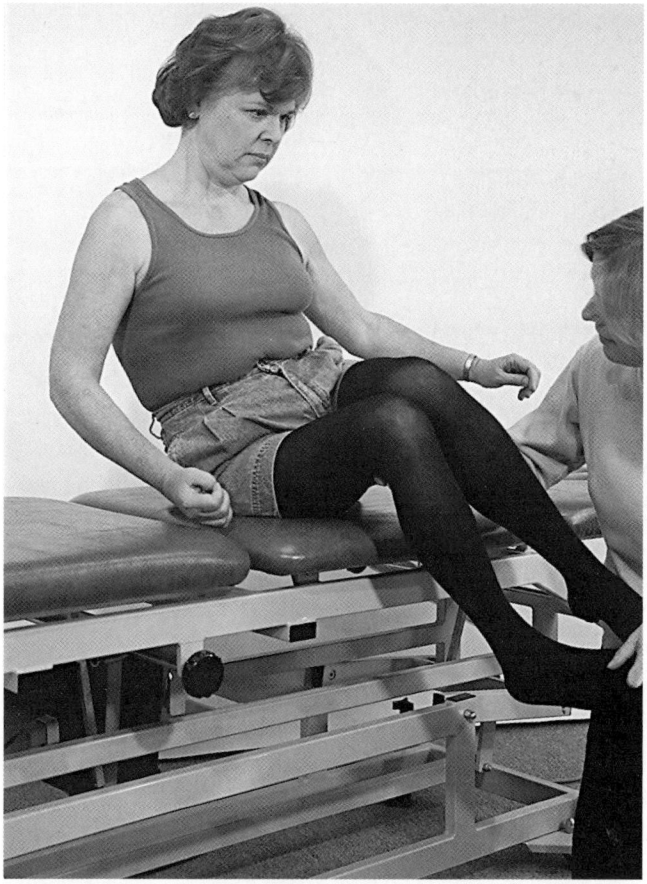

Figure 24-5 Therapist using handling to test equilibrium reactions.

spastic activity are performed with excessive assistance. Similar problems with facilitation arise when muscle tone is hypotonic. Patients with flaccidity do not assist movements or show the placing response. Their limbs feel heavy and floppy during handling.

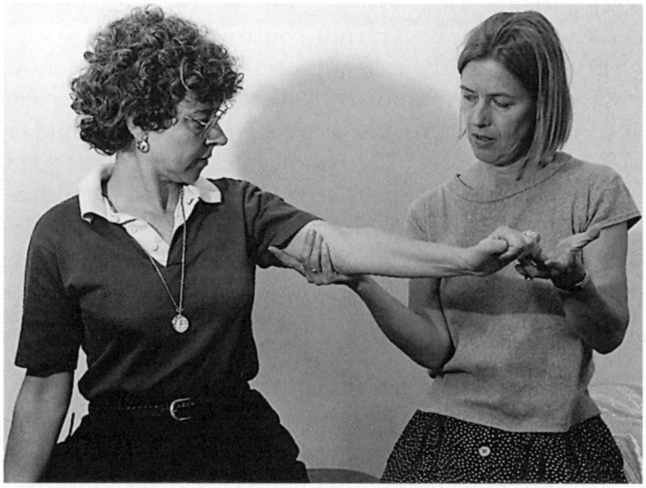

Figure 24-6 Therapist using placing to assess control of the hemiparetic arm.

Treatment Goals for the Stages of Recovery

The NDT/Bobath therapist uses the information about muscle tone and movement control gathered in the evaluation to establish treatment goals. NDT therapists establish several types of goals. The therapist sets functional goals to be achieved through practice of occupation-as-means or occupation-as-end. These goals address limitations in ADL and IADL. The therapist also establishes treatment goals for impairments in basic abilities and capacities in the trunk and arm and identifies problems that may benefit from inhibition and facilitation. These treatment goals depend on the patient's problems, level of functional independence, movement control, and reasons for seeking treatment. Treatment goals will also vary according to where the person is in the process of recovery and his or her prognosis.

In acute-care or inpatient rehabilitation settings, most patients have impairments such as weakness, low tone, and loss of muscle control and are dependent in most self-care activities. NDT goals focus on increasing independence in self-maintenance roles, preventing the development of abnormal tone and abnormal movements, and increasing motor control on the hemiplegic side. To accomplish functional goals, the NDT/Bobath therapist introduces and practices adapted techniques for ADL, bed mobility, transfers, and wheelchair management designed to increase occupational performance and level of independence while preventing learned neglect, postural asymmetry, and associated reactions. For example, the therapist may train the patient to sit up in bed from lying on the hemiplegic side to introduce weight bearing on the hemiplegic arm and leg (Fig. 24-7). The therapist also uses positioning and inhibitory treatment techniques, such as supine scapula mobilization and weight bearing on the hemiplegic arm, to maintain muscle length and prevent spasticity. Facilitation is used to increase muscle control in postural adjustments and selective movements of the arm as preparation for skilled use.

As patients recover from strokes, a new set of treatment goals is necessary. Although some patients remain flaccid on their hemiplegic side or recover motor control without developing abnormal tone, many develop spasticity in some muscles of the affected side. Spasticity first appears as an associated reaction in conjunction with patients' efforts to become more independent in self-care activities and walking. Over time, the spastic muscles develop increased resistance to passive stretch. The hemiplegic side of the trunk may appear shortened or rotated posteriorly, and the arm assumes a flexed position during movement and at rest. Patients with spasticity typically use compensatory patterns for gross motor patterns like rolling and sitting up and for ADL activities. Although they are usually able to sit and stand without loss of balance and walk with a brace and cane, their

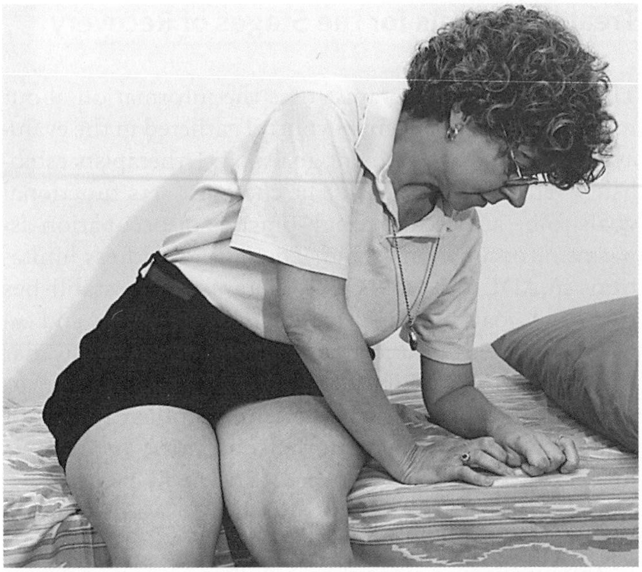

Figure 24-7 Patient practicing sitting up using the hemiparetic arm for support.

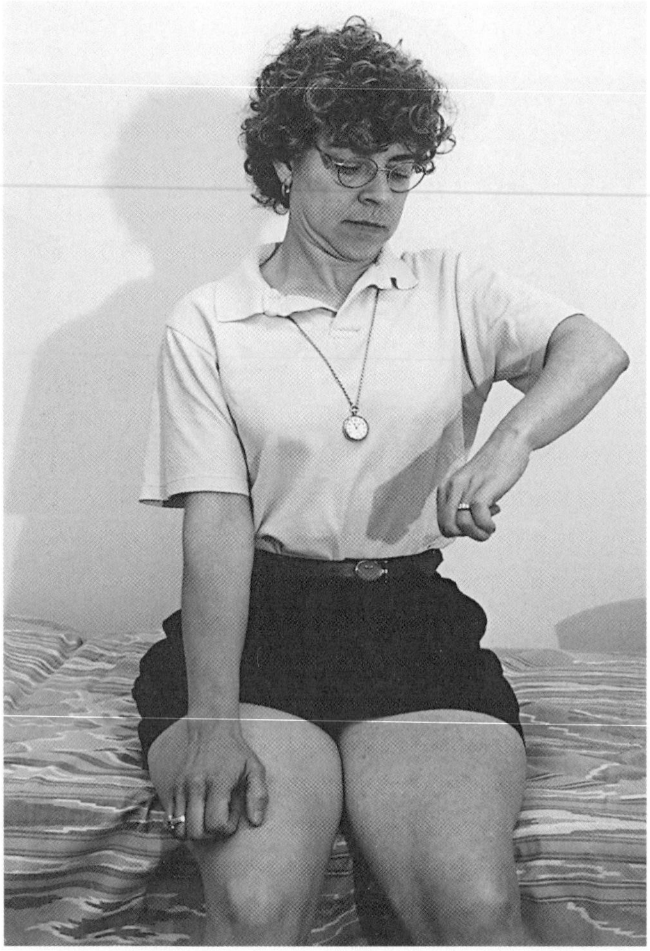

Figure 24-8 Patient moving arm that demonstrates abnormal pattern of coordination.

trunk posture is often asymmetrical, with less weight taken on the hemiplegic leg and a flexed arm posture during most activities. The patient with spasticity may also have regained sufficient muscle control in the hemiplegic arm to move it, but abnormal coordination and excessive stiffness prevent skilled functional use (Fig. 24-8).

NDT treatment goals for the patient with spasticity include inhibiting abnormal tone and movement, increasing normal movement responses, and improving occupational performance by incorporating the hemiplegic side into task performance. The therapist uses inhibition techniques to address problems with abnormal tone, abnormal coordination, and associated reactions, followed by facilitation to increase postural control in sitting and standing and to develop selective movement control in the hemiplegic arm and hand. Patients at this stage of recovery are functionally independent in many tasks, thus, functional goals may include training of new tasks, decreasing compensations in tasks that are performed independently, and increasing functional use of the hemiplegic arm and hand. For example, to increase functional independence for a patient who shaves with his uninvolved hand while sitting, the therapist may either teach him to perform this task while standing or train him to use the hemiplegic hand to apply shaving cream.

Many patients with hemiplegia do not progress beyond the problems associated with spasticity and fail to develop normal movement control in their hemiplegic side, some patients never develop spasticity in the involved side, and other patients recover movement control. These higher level patients walk well without postural asymmetry because they have better trunk control and are able to support weight on their hemiplegic leg. They also show improvements in motor control of the hemiplegic arm and may be able to use the arm for weight support and to hold objects that are placed in the hand. Despite the good motor recovery, problems opening the hand to initiate grasp and release and maintaining good elbow extension during reaching may persist. These patients may also complain of problems with the accuracy and speed of movement that make it difficult to use the arm for function. NDT goals for higher level patients focus on improving coordination of the hemiplegic arm and hand, especially in the patterns necessary for reach, grasp, and manipulation; increasing functional use of the arm and hand; and decreasing compensation in life tasks. The therapist may use facilitation, occupation-as-means, and occupation-as-end to achieve these goals.

TREATMENT TECHNIQUES: INTEGRATING NDT/BOBATH INTO OCCUPATIONAL THERAPY PRACTICE

The NDT/Bobath approach is most effective when nurses; physical, occupational, and speech therapists; and family members all use a similar approach to management. Occupational therapists can have a significant effect on tone and movement, however, by integrating NDT principles and techniques into OT practice, even when other professionals use different treatment approaches. The next section describes ways to integrate NDT concepts and techniques into rehabilitation of the hemiplegic arm and into ADL. The Neuro-Developmental Treatment Association (NDTA) offers postgraduate training courses for physical and occupational therapists interested in learning more about this approach to treatment (Resource 24-1).

Treatment of the Hemiplegic Arm

The NDT/Bobath approach to treatment of the hemiplegic arm is designed to address impairments, such as abnormal tone, pain, subluxation, and the loss of movement control, that are related to deficits in capabilities and occupational performance. Specific impairments are treated using inhibition techniques such as reflex-inhibiting patterns, scapula mobilization, trunk rotation, and weight bearing. NDT therapists also use facilitation to reeducate selective arm movements, to teach the patient to use the arm for weight bearing, and to increase skilled use of the hand. Although inhibition of abnormal responses is generally done before facilitation of normal movements, the line between inhibition and facilitation is often indistinct because techniques such as weight bearing can be used for both inhibition and facilitation. The amount of treatment time devoted to inhibition versus facilitation varies according to severity of problems and treatment goals, but both techniques are generally used in every treatment session so that changes in tone and muscle length are immediately translated into motor and functional performance.

RESOURCE 24-1

Neuro-Developmental Treatment Association (NDTA)
A resource for NDT continuing-education courses and literature about the NDT/Bobath approach for adults and children.

NDTA
1550 S. Coast Highway, Suite 201
Laguna Beach, CA 92651
E-mail: ndta@alderdrozinc.com
www.ndta.org

Use of Inhibition

Inhibition is an important part of the NDT approach to movement reeducation because normal movements cannot be facilitated in the presence of abnormal tone and reflex activity. NDT therapists use inhibition with patients who have spasticity to decrease the amount of tension in the muscle, restore normal resting lengths to muscles that are habitually shortened, and stop excessive or unwanted muscle contraction. B. Bobath described inhibition of spasticity as the process of "normalizing tone" because, after treatment, the spastic arm feels flexible and light rather than stiff and heavy. This reduction in spasticity allows the patient to follow guided movement more easily and to initiate arm movements outside of synergy.

Reflex-inhibiting patterns (RIPs) are one of the main techniques for inhibiting spasticity in the hemiplegic arm. Since flexor spasticity in the arm is concentrated in shoulder elevators and internal rotators and elbow, wrist, and finger flexors, the tension in these muscle groups can be systematically decreased or "inhibited" by gradually moving the arm into a position that includes shoulder girdle depression and shoulder external rotation, elbow and wrist extension, and an open hand (Fig. 24-9). Spastic muscles resist lengthening, and the therapist must use handling to gradually lengthen the affected muscles and bring the arm into the full RIP (Procedures for Practice 24-3). Rather than passively stretching the spastic muscles into the RIP, B. Bobath (1990) described the use of trunk rotation and shoulder mobilization in the supine position and weight bearing to inhibit flexor spasticity in the hemiplegic arm. Once spasticity in the arm has decreased, the therapist immediately begins to retrain selective movements using facilitation, as the purpose of decreasing muscle tone is always to allow the patient to experience normal movement. The process of facilitation, including using weight bearing to increase muscle contraction in the arm, is described in the next section.

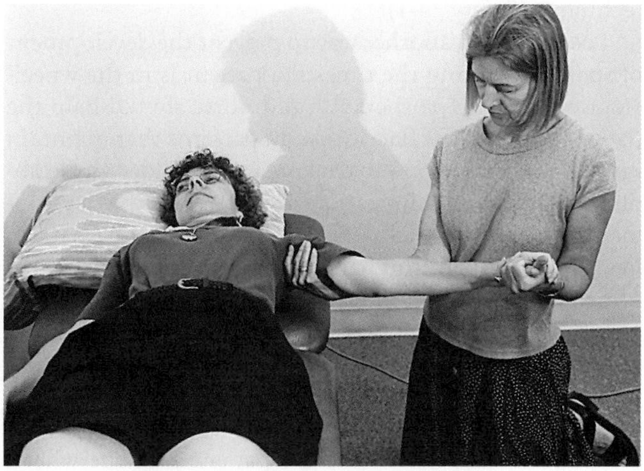

Figure 24-9 Therapist using a reflex-inhibiting pattern (RIP) to inhibit flexor spasticity.

PROCEDURES FOR PRACTICE 24-3

Inhibition of Spasticity in the Hemiplegic Arm using RIP

1. Position patient in sitting.
2. Place hands on the hemiplegic arm using proximal and distal key points of control. Patient's arm will be in a flexed, adducted position.
3. Correct adduction of the humerus first, leaving the elbow in flexion.
4. Maintain the humerus in neutral rotation by the side of the body and use pressure on top of the forearm to extend the elbow gradually. If the forearm is supinated, pronate it first.
5. When the tension in the biceps has decreased, slide your hand from the top of the forearm to the wrist and hand. Extend the wrist to neutral first, leaving the fingers flexed.
6. When tension in the wrist flexors has decreased, open the fingers, keeping the wrist in a neutral position.
7. Maintain the arm in an extended position and proceed to weight bearing or guided movement.

SAFETY NOTE 24-1

Avoiding Overstretch of the Flaccid Hand and Wrist

The therapist must be careful to avoid overstretching the flaccid muscles of the hand and wrist during inhibition, facilitation, and upper extremity weight bearing. Precautions include:

- Avoid positioning the wrist in maximal extension or flattening the palm of the hand.
- Do not pull the hemiplegic thumb into hyperextension or hyperextend the metacarpal joints of the fingers because this may result in hypermobility of these small joints.
- Use a distal grip that maintains the wrist joint in neutral or slight extension and supports the transverse arches of the palm. The therapist may let the patient's fingers flex when the palm and wrist are supported.

In acute rehabilitation, most patients exhibit low tone and weakness rather than spasticity. In this setting, inhibition techniques are used to maintain muscle length and normal joint mechanics in the arm and to prevent the development of spasticity and abnormal coordination as the patient learns to function more independently. For example, the therapist may maintain the affected arm in an extended position while the patient practices moving from sitting to standing to prevent an associated reaction in the arm during this difficult movement. If the hemiplegic arm has little or no flexor spasticity, it does not resist movements into extension, so the therapist must be careful not to overstretch the elbow, wrist, and hand while using this technique (Safety 24-1).

Positioning is another way to prevent the development of spasticity during the times the patient is in the wheelchair or in bed. The therapist and nurse should help the patient position the flaccid arm in patterns that maintain muscle length in elbow extension and shoulder girdle abduction and external rotation to counteract the development of flexor spasticity. For example, when the patient lies supine in bed, the hemiplegic arm should be positioned with the elbow in extension, the shoulder and forearm in neutral rotation, and the hand and wrist supported so that they do not fall into flexion (Fig. 24-10). This position is preferable to allowing the patient to rest the arm in flexion across the chest since this flexed position may increase muscle tone. While the patient is in the wheelchair, lap boards or pillows should support the hemiplegic arm. These wheelchair aids help prevent both shoulder subluxation and spasticity. Positioning techniques are used less frequently as the patient is more active or recovers motor control in the hemiplegic arm.

Facilitation in Arm Treatment

Facilitation techniques are designed to restore normal movement responses. In treating the arm, facilitation includes teaching the patient to support weight on the hemiplegic arm, teaching the patient to perform selective movements of the hemiplegic arm and hand, and providing opportunities to practice functional use of the arm in occupation-as-means. Facilitation in occupation-as-end is discussed separately in the next section.

Facilitation of Weight Bearing

Weight bearing is one of the most important aspects of treating the hemiplegic arm because it can be used to maintain muscle length, normalize tone, and increase activity in the muscles of the trunk and arm (Ryerson & Levit, 1997b). In the NDT/Bobath approach, weight bear-

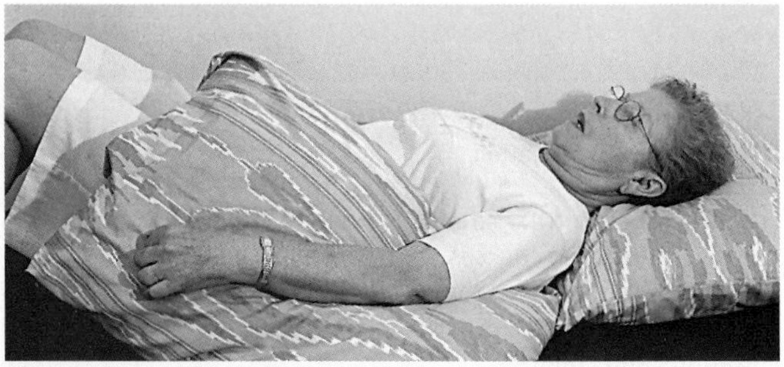

Figure 24-10 Hemiplegic arm correctly positioned for sleeping.

ing is a dynamic process. Rather than statically propping on a rigid arm, the patient is taught to activate muscles in the trunk by moving body weight over the stable arm. The movements of the trunk cause muscles in the arm and hand to lengthen and shorten and contract to maintain the arm on the support surface. Since use of the arm for weight support does not require fine motor control, even patients with severe weakness and loss of motor control can learn to use their hemiplegic arms to support body weight. Thus, weight bearing is used both to facilitate muscle activity in the hemiplegic arm and to increase functional use of that arm.

The NDT therapist generally begins by teaching the patient to accept weight on the hemiplegic arm with forearms on a table (Ryerson & Levit, 1997a). This pattern is important for activities that are commonly performed at a table, such as eating, reading, and writing (Fig. 24-11). Weight bearing on an extended arm is more difficult for the patient because it requires control of the elbow and wrist joints as well as control of the trunk and shoulder girdle. It is used with patients who have more selective control of the arm. NDT therapists often train extended-arm weight bearing with the hemiplegic arm by the side of the body when the patient is sitting. As the patient improves balance control in standing, the therapist may also train extended-arm weight bearing in standing, so that the patient learns to use the hemiplegic arm for support while working in the kitchen or bathroom.

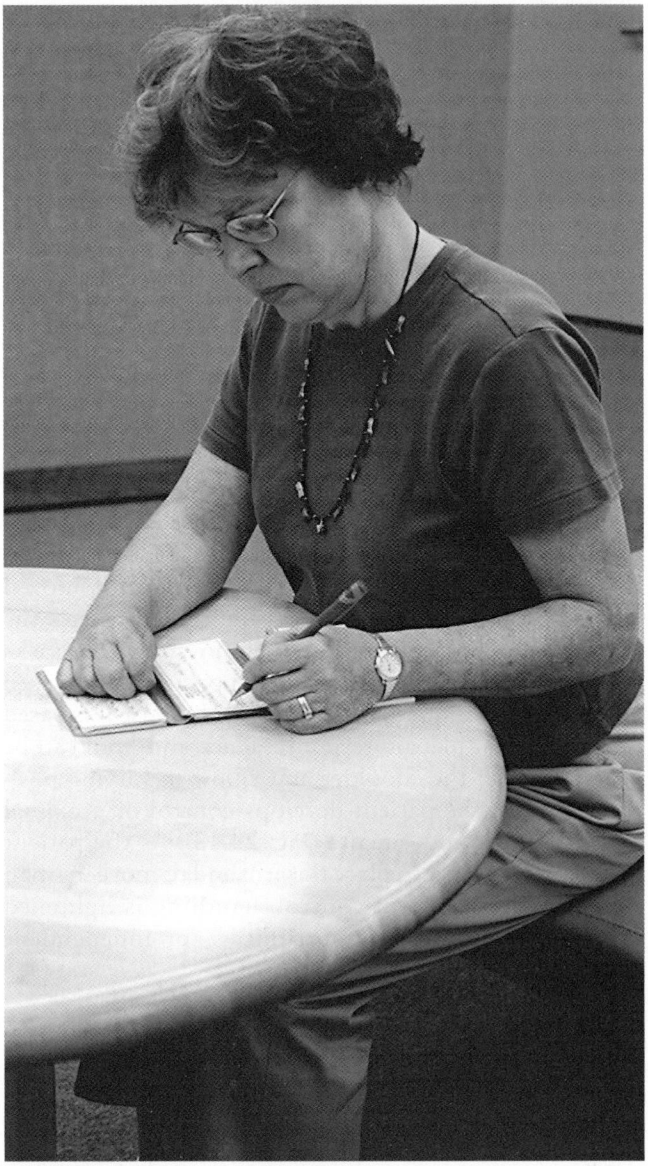

Figure 24-11 Patient using hemiparetic arm to support weight and provide stability while writing.

Facilitation of Arm Movement

Facilitation of arm movements is another important part of arm treatment (Procedures for Practice 24-4). The NDT therapist uses this aspect of facilitation to give the patient the sensation of normal movement, teach normal patterns of initiation and sequencing, and reeducate and strengthen normal movements to be used for function (Ryerson & Levit, 1997a). Facilitation is really a system of guided movement or active-assistive exercise. The therapist uses proximal and distal key points to establish normal alignment in the arm and maintains this control while moving the patient's arm in patterns that are important for functional use. This handling provides sensory messages about how movements are sequenced. The patient is encouraged to assist with the movement when possible. As the patient begins to participate, the therapist decreases the assistance, giving the patient partial control of arm movement. The NDT therapist uses

PROCEDURES FOR PRACTICE 24-4

The Process of Facilitation

1. Restore alignment of the segments to be moved using key points of control.
2. Assist the desired movement using light hands.
3. Proceed slowly and feel for the patient's response. The arm will feel lighter and movement easier when the patient is assisting.
4. Repeat movements until patient can actively assist and you feel the patient is active.
5. Lighten messages of your hands so that the patient moves with less assistance. Give verbal feedback during this phase.
6. Gradually withdraw control. The patient's movement control may decline but should not produce an abnormal response.
7. Provide practice opportunities through use of activities (occupation-as-means) or home exercises.

sensory information from handling to decide where and when to let go, so that the quality of movement stays relatively consistent when the therapist withdraws control. The active-assistive quality of facilitation also helps to decrease the excessive effort that many hemiplegic patients use to initiate movements of their involved side.

Facilitation is used to reeducate or strengthen movements that are difficult for the patient to perform without assistance. The movements of shoulder flexion or shoulder abduction with elbow extension are usually the most difficult because they go against the pattern of muscle return. The therapist facilitates extended arm movements to establish this difficult pattern of coordination and to prevent the patient from learning to use flexor spasticity to move the arm. To use the arm for function, however, the patient must initiate arm movements with different combinations of shoulder and elbow movements. To do this, the therapist uses facilitation of elbow flexion and extension so that the patient gains control of elbow movements outside the pattern of mass flexion.

During facilitation of arm movements, the therapist must make sure that the humerus is correctly positioned in the glenoid fossa and the scapula can rotate on the thorax. Patients feel pain in the hemiplegic shoulder during facilitation when the humerus is not seated in the fossa or when normal scapulohumeral rhythm is not available. Therefore, the therapist must correct shoulder joint alignment and maintain normal joint mechanics while facilitating arm movements in any position to avoid traumatizing the shoulder joint. This is described further in Procedures for Practice 24-5. As the muscles of the shoulder girdle become more active, the therapist may decrease control of joint alignment and mechanics.

PROCEDURES FOR PRACTICE 24-5

Restoring Normal Joint Mechanics to the Subluxed Shoulder

The therapist must reposition the subluxed shoulder joint before active or passive movements of the arm are attempted. Correcting the subluxation entails moving the scapula into neutral or slight upward rotation and lifting the humerus so that it rests in the glenoid fossa. The therapist should maintain the shoulder joint in this corrected position during treatment of the arm. To restore normal joint mechanics, the therapist should follow these steps:

1. Place one hand under the axilla to support the inferior portion of the shoulder joint and the other hand on the patient's scapula. The therapist uses this hand placement to correct the position of the upper trunk and to rotate the scapula upward.
2. Hold the corrected shoulder position with one hand, and move the other hand to the distal humerus. Gently lift the humerus up into the glenoid fossa.
3. If the humerus is internally rotated, move the humerus into neutral or slight external rotation.
4. Check that the scapula can rotate on the thorax before moving the arm above 60° of forward flexion or abduction. If the scapula cannot rotate freely, scapular mobility should be restored before moving the humerus into elevation.
5. Maintain correct scapulohumeral rhythm during active and passive arm movements.

Arm Treatment in Supine

The NDT therapist often begins to inhibit abnormal tone and facilitate normal patterns of arm movement with the patient lying supine. Supine is the easiest position for patients with loss of postural control and weakness to practice moving their arms because the bed or mat provides postural stability. The stable position of the patient's trunk also makes it easier for the therapist to maintain normal scapulohumeral rhythm while lifting the hemiplegic arm into flexion and abduction. To facilitate arm movements in supine, the therapist uses proximal and distal key points on the arm to extend the hemiplegic elbow and bring the patient's shoulder into flexion (Fig. 24-12). The therapist should make sure that the scapula rotates easily before elevating the arm above 60° of shoulder flexion. If spasticity or muscle tightness is blocking scapula movement, it is important to use inhibition to restore normal joint mechanics before bringing the arm into elevation.

When the hemiplegic arm can be moved without pain or resistance, the therapist begins to use facilitation to increase muscle activity. The extended arm is moved slowly through small ranges. As the therapist feels the patient begin to assist or follow her movements, she asks the patient to try to hold the arm in position. B. Bobath called this technique "place and hold" because it is based on the normal placing response. Place and hold can be practiced with the shoulder and elbow in varying positions so that the patient develops control of proximal and distal arm movements (Fig. 24-13). As the patient develops the ability to place the arm and to move in small ranges without loss of control, handling is lightened or removed to allow opportunities for independent practice.

Arm Movement in Sitting

As soon as the patient begins to assist with facilitated movements in supine, the therapist should begin to practice guided movements of the arm with the patient in sitting. Subluxation of the glenohumeral joint is more common in sitting than supine because the muscles of the

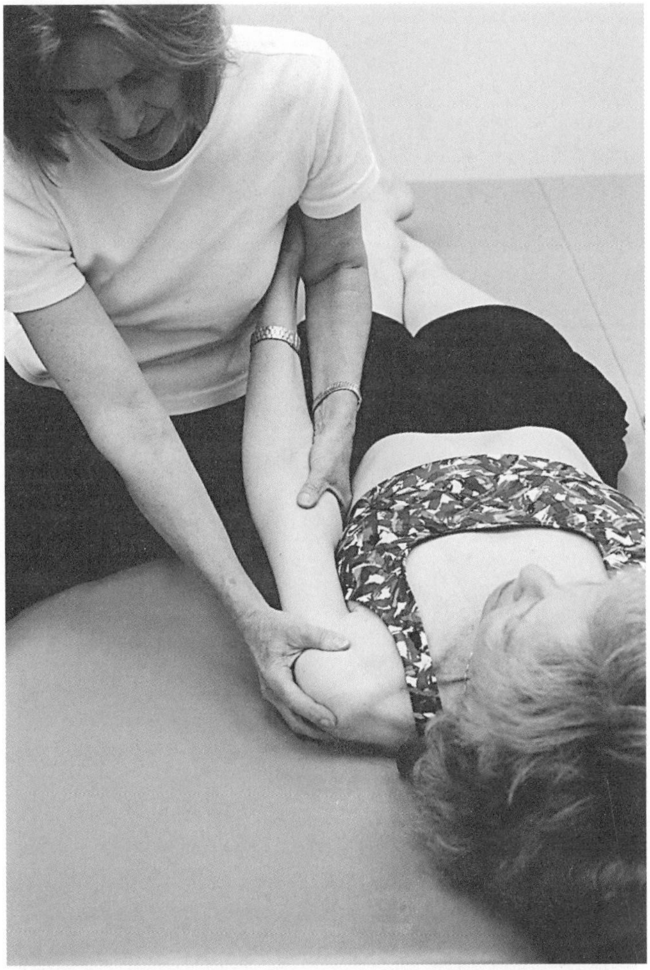

Figure 24-12 Therapist corrects position of hemiparetic arm prior to facilitating arm movements.

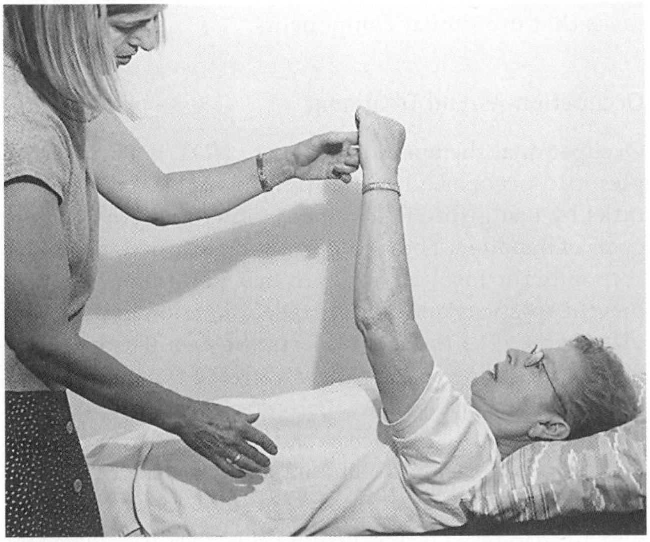

Figure 24-13 Placing and holding for the hemiparetic arm.

hemiplegic arm are too weak to hold the scapula in the correct position on the trunk and because the loss of trunk control also affects scapula alignment (Ryerson & Levit, 1997a, 1997b). The therapist must reduce the subluxation before beginning facilitation and maintain this corrected position during arm treatment. (Figs. 24-14 to 24-16). Initially, the therapist controls the position of the shoulder girdle during guided movements of the arm to strengthen normal patterns of coordination and prevent pain. As strength and control increase in the hemiplegic arm, the therapist gradually withdraws this control, and the patient attempts to move the arm in the same patterns and ranges.

Using Occupation-As-Means in Arm Treatment

The NDT therapist uses occupation-as-means activities to practice and strengthen movement control in the hemiplegic arm. The therapist uses handling to introduce these activities but should withdraw this control as quickly as possible, letting the patient practice without assistance. Occupation-as-means activities can be set up with the hemiplegic arm in weight bearing. For example, the patient may play checkers on the treatment mat while weight bearing on the hemiplegic arm or rinse dishes in the sink

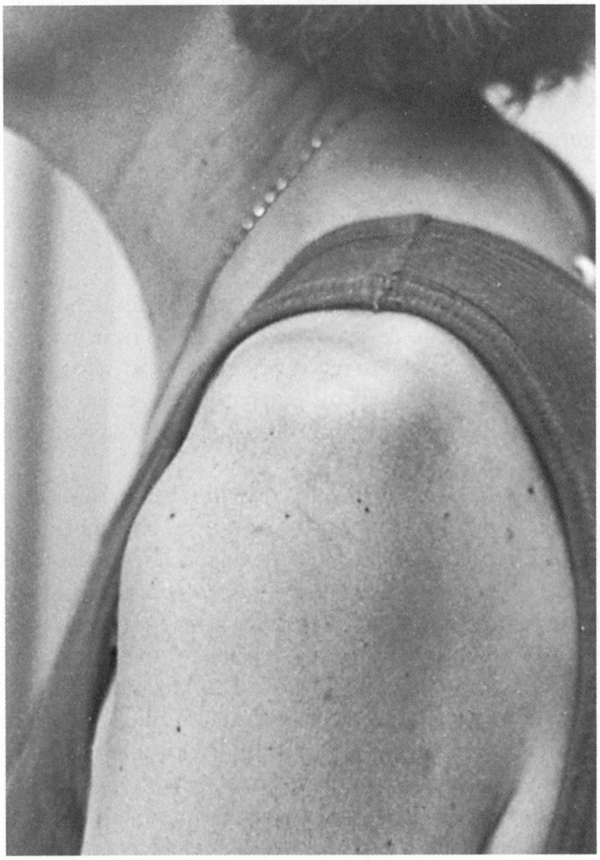

Figure 24-14 Close-up of shoulder showing glenohumeral subluxation.

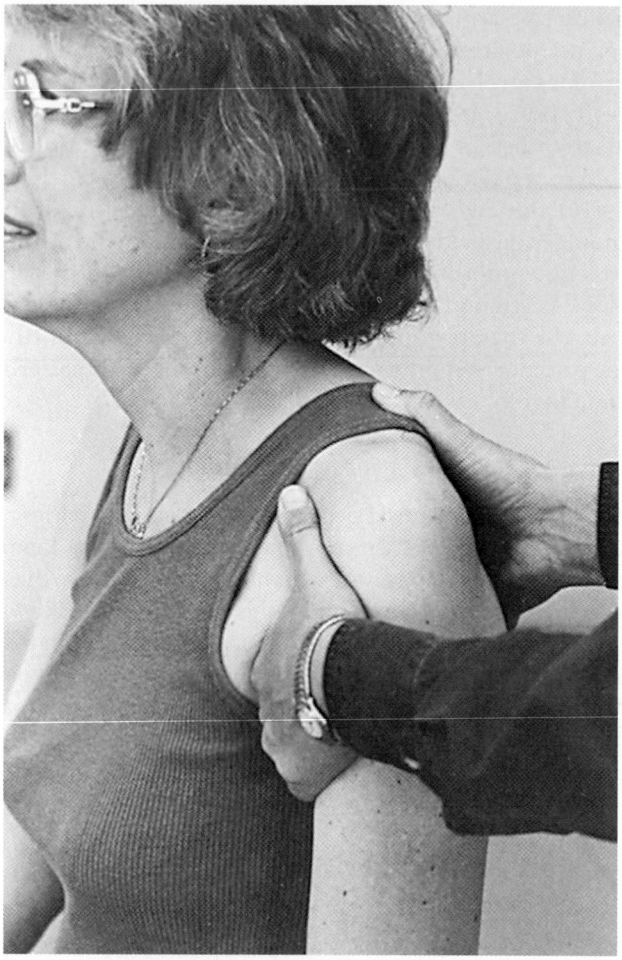

Figure 24-15 Therapist correcting subluxation.

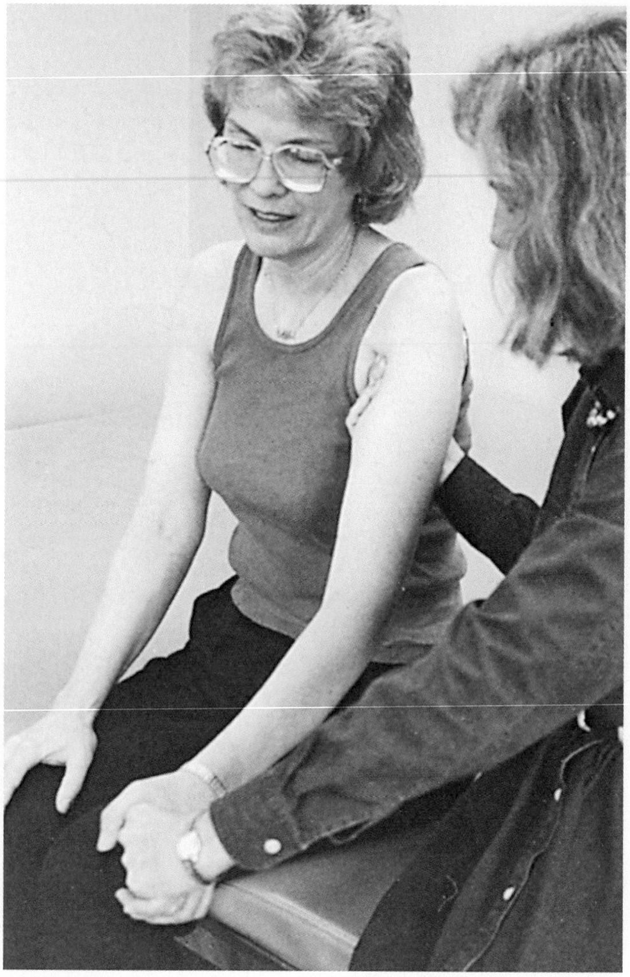

Figure 24-16 Therapist controlling subluxation while facilitating arm movement.

with the unaffected hand while maintaining the hemiplegic arm on the counter (Fig. 24-17). These activities help the patient learn to use the hemiplegic arm to provide support and assist balance. The patient may also practice using weight bearing to inhibit associated reactions during dressing (Fig. 24-18).

Occupation-as-means also provides opportunities for practice moving the hemiplegic arm or coordinating use of both hands in bilateral patterns of coordination. For example, the patient may strengthen reaching patterns of the hemiplegic arm by practicing wiping the table or washing a window. To practice control of elbow movements, the therapist may facilitate arm movements while the patient holds an object in the hemiplegic hand and practices bringing it to the body or face (Fig. 24-19). Bilateral coordination is reinforced by tasks such as carrying a tray or pushing a vacuum cleaner. The therapist selects tasks for occupation-as-means according to the movement components embedded in them. The practice of these meaningful activities is expected to generalize to increased functional use of the hemiplegic arm in other tasks that use similar components.

Occupation-As-End Treatment

Occupational therapists incorporate NDT/Bobath principles into occupation-as-end training of ADL and other tasks by using specific compensations that support the goals of handling. These compensations are designed to incorporate the involved arm into task performance and to prevent spasticity and abnormal coordination in the hemiplegic arm. The therapist selects the occupations to be trained according to the patient's level of functioning and the goals for independence. Early treatment may focus on retraining basic ADLs, such as bathing, dressing, and toileting, and tasks such as rolling in bed and transfers. As patients regain their independence in these tasks, therapists may incorporate NDT principles into occupation-as-end training of vocational tasks, such as using a computer mouse, or leisure activities, such as golf or swimming.

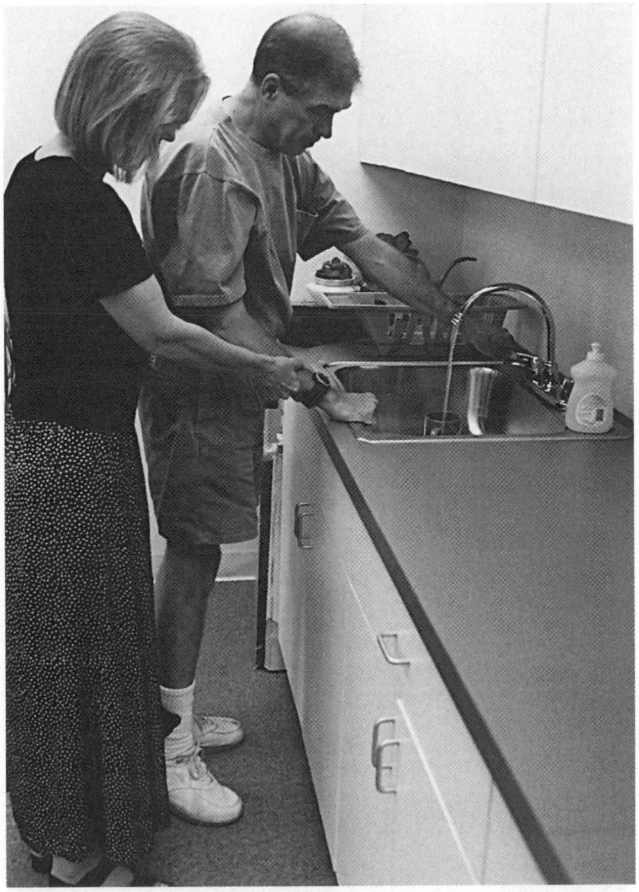

Figure 24-17 Therapist helps maintain the hemiparetic arm in weight bearing while the patient rinses the dishes at the sink.

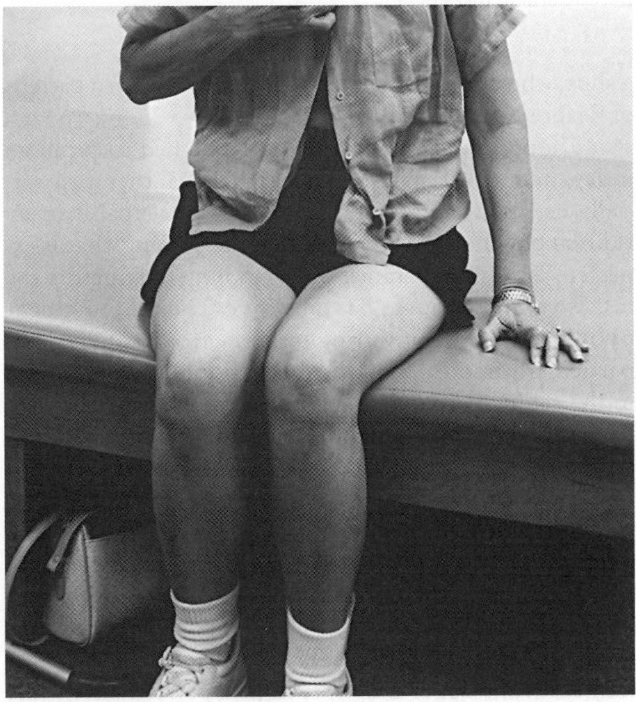

Figure 24-18 Patient uses hemiparetic arm in weight bearing while dressing.

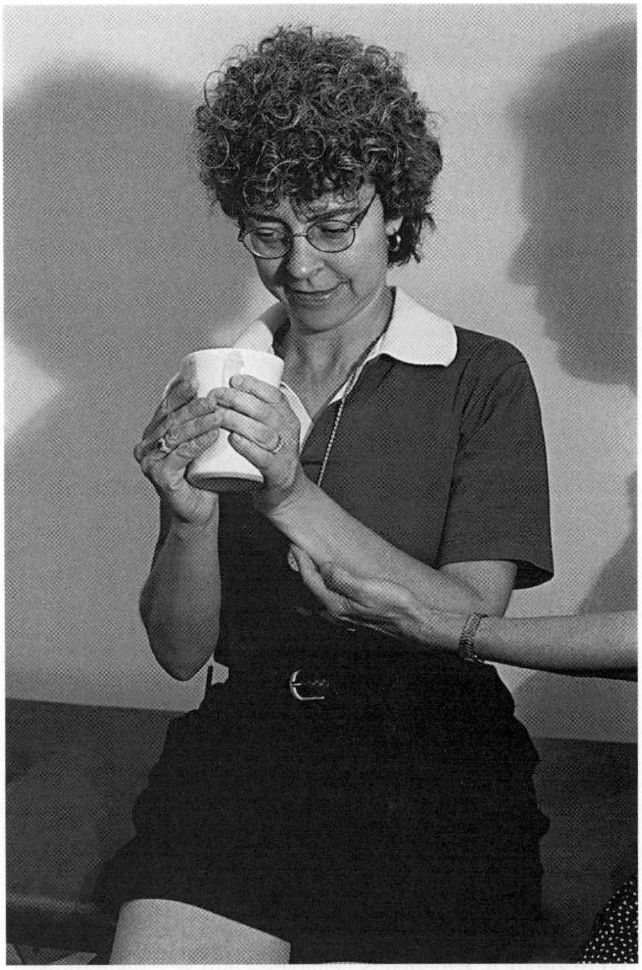

Figure 24-19 Therapist facilitates elbow flexion while the patient grasps the cup with both hands and brings it to the mouth.

Gross motor activities, such as rolling in bed, sitting up, and standing up, are important functional tasks that are introduced in acute treatment. When the patient cannot move the hemiplegic arm, the NDT therapist trains specific compensations designed to promote symmetry, prevent neglect of the hemiplegic arm, and inhibit abnormal tone and movement. For example, the patient may be taught to interlace the fingers of both hands, keeping palms together and thumbs facing up, when it is necessary to move the arm. This clasped-hand grip helps patients to maintain the hemiplegic forearm in an extended position during self-range of motion and during movements such as rolling and standing up. The therapist may teach rolling to the uninvolved side by having the patient clasp the hands, reach both hands toward the ceiling with extended elbows, and then initiate rolling by turning the head and reaching both arms across the body (Fig. 24-20, A & B). This technique ensures that the hemiplegic arm does not get left behind the body and that the patient will actively use her trunk muscles to initiate rolling rather than turning in bed by pulling on the bed rails. Similarly, having the

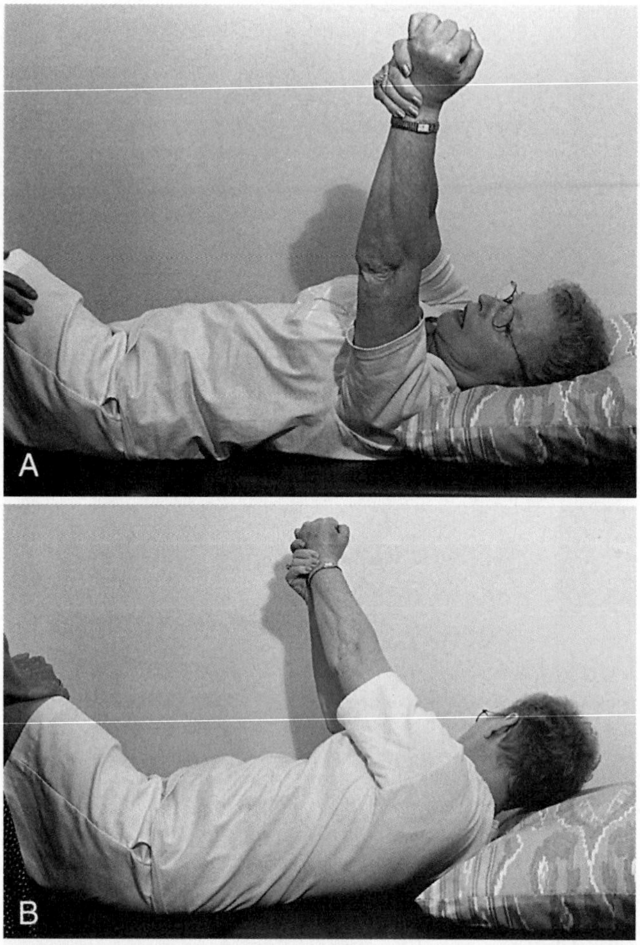

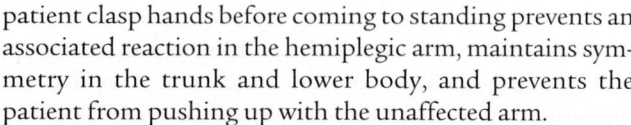

Figure 24-20 A. Patient lifts hemiplegic arm. **B.** Patient turns the arms and upper trunk to roll to the uninvolved side.

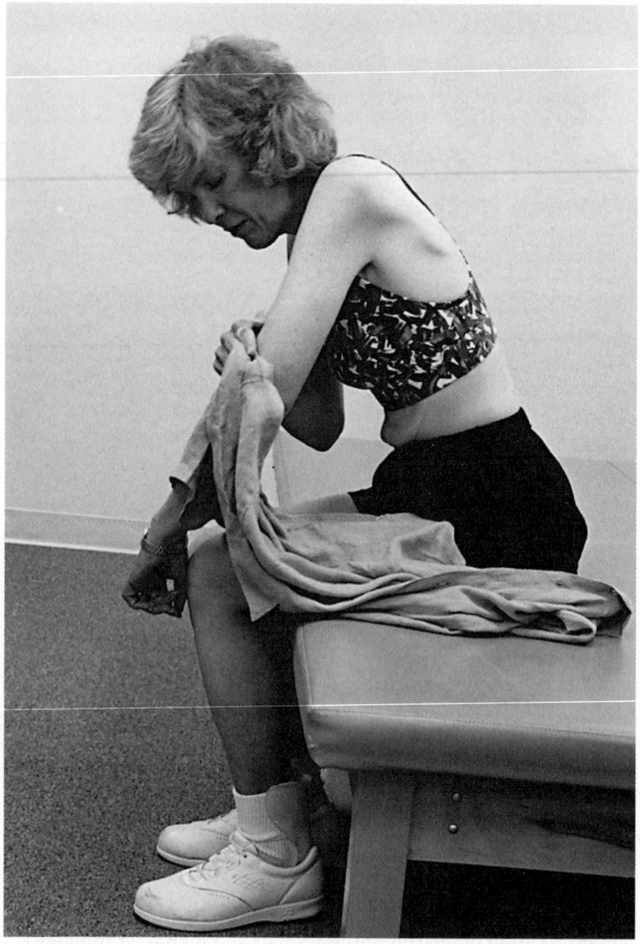

Figure 24-21 Patient using compensation to put the hemiparetic arm in the sleeve.

patient clasp hands before coming to standing prevents an associated reaction in the hemiplegic arm, maintains symmetry in the trunk and lower body, and prevents the patient from pushing up with the unaffected arm.

The NDT therapist also uses compensatory techniques to incorporate the hemiplegic arm into activities such as dressing and grooming. Flexor posturing of the arm during task performance is a major problem for some patients, particularly when the patient is struggling or using excessive effort. After the task is complete, the arm may remain in this flexed position. The NDT therapist introduces compensations during life tasks to maintain symmetry in the trunk and maintain the hemiplegic arm in extension. For example, to prevent posturing of the hemiplegic arm while the patient puts on a shirt, the patient may be taught to flex the trunk forward and reach the hemiplegic arm to the floor before putting it into the shirt sleeve (Fig. 24-21) (Davis, 1990). This technique passively maintains extension in the arm during this difficult movement. As control of the arm improves, the patient may learn to place the hemiplegic arm in a position of extended weight bearing on the bed during tasks such as buttoning a shirt, when the arm is most likely to posture in a pattern of flexor spasticity.

Although functional training is designed to promote independent task performance, the NDT therapist initially uses handling in combination with verbal instructions and demonstrations to teach the patient what is expected. The NDT therapist uses handling to structure the task, so that the patient has only to control the movement of one body segment during task practice. Handling is a particularly important part of occupation-as-end training in the acute phase, since patients at this stage of recovery have problems controlling both trunk and arm position (Van Dyck, 1999).

For patients with poor sitting balance, the NDT therapist may assist the movement of the trunk during task practice. For example, the therapist may use his or her hands on the patient's trunk to provide stability and maintain weight on the hemiplegic hip while the patient leans forward to don shoes (Fig. 24-22). Or the therapist may assist the upper extremity in task performance while the patient performs the necessary trunk movements independently. For example, the therapist may facilitate the

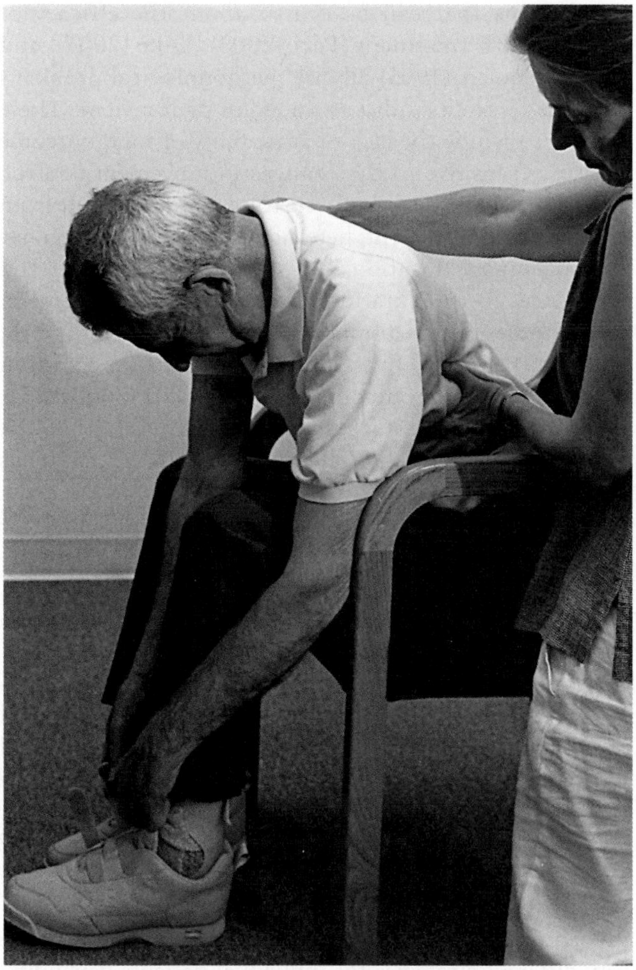

Figure 24-22 Therapist using handling techniques to provide trunk stability while the patient fastens his shoes.

correct shoulder and elbow movements while the patient holds the deodorant stick in the hemiplegic hand and applies it to the uninvolved side. As the patient's movement control increases and task performance becomes more automatic, the therapist withdraws physical assistance. At this point, verbal feedback may be offered to help improve the patient's performance.

Contributions to Psychosocial Adjustment

The emphasis that the NDT/Bobath approach places on functional recovery in the hemiplegic side has potential psychosocial as well as physical benefits to patients who have had strokes. In traditional rehabilitation approaches, the emphasis is on compensatory use of the uninvolved side. This may suggest that the hemiplegic side will not recover. In contrast, the NDT/Bobath approach, with its emphasis on treating the hemiplegic side, offers stroke patients a very different message. From the early days of rehabilitation, NDT therapists help stroke patients relearn functional tasks in ways that make use of the existing motor patterns in the trunk, arm, and leg. They also use treatment to increase control of movement in the affected side and to minimize or eliminate secondary impairments that affect quality of life. These treatment activities give the patient realistic hopes of functional recovery in the affected side of the body and may contribute to a more positive attitude toward the disability and a sense of self-efficacy.

EFFICACY AND OUTCOMES RESEARCH

Since NDT/Bobath treatment is widely used in many countries, research documenting the efficacy of this approach is an extremely important component of evidence-based practice. A literature search identified a small number of recent studies examining the efficacy of the NDT/Bobath approach in stroke rehabilitation. The majority of these studies compare treatment outcomes of patients receiving the Bobath approach to the outcomes of patients receiving other therapeutic interventions with the goal of determining which approach is most effective for remediating impairment and improving general functional outcomes. Although this literature suggests that the NDT/Bobath approach is effective for improving physical and functional outcomes, no strong evidence supports the superiority of NDT/Bobath over other treatment approaches following stroke. Methodological limitations and inadequate outcome measures, however, may limit the conclusions that can be drawn from these research studies (Luke, 2004; Paci, 2003), and the nature of this approach may make it difficult to devise standardized treatment interventions for research study.

Systematic literature review and meta-analysis provide the highest level of scientific evidence. Two recent studies used systematic literature search to investigate the clinical effectiveness of NDT/Bobath in the treatment of stroke. Paci (2003) reviewed the literature in English, French, and Italian and identified 15 studies where Bobath treatment was used in either experimental or control groups. Outcome measures included effectiveness of general treatment, effectiveness of treatment of lower extremity and gait, and effectiveness of treatment of the arm. Although the groups receiving NDT/Bobath treatment showed an improvement in some or all measures in most studies, the majority of studies found no significant differences between treatment groups. Luke (2004) performed a similar literature search and identified eight articles that compared the effectiveness of Bobath treatment in upper limb disability with similar findings. Like Paci, Luke concluded that NDT/Bobath is not superior to other treatment approaches at improving tone and movement in the upper limb, addressing activity limitation, or increasing participation in life roles. Since Hiraoka (2001) and Hafsteinsdottir (1996) reported similar results after reviewing a slightly older group of studies, it seems safe to conclude that the bulk of existing research does not demonstrate any advantage for NDT as a clinical intervention over other methods of neurological rehabilitation.

The evidence from recent randomized, controlled studies is more ambiguous. Langhammer and Stanghelle (2000) performed a randomized, controlled study of 61 acute stroke patients, half of whom were treated with NDT/Bobath and half of whom received treatment based on Motor Relearning Program (MRP). During the acute phase of rehabilitation, patients treated with MRP had shorter hospital stays and showed significantly greater improvements on two tests of motor function. The authors concluded that these results demonstrate that MRP is preferable to Bobath in the rehabilitation of acute stroke. When the same patients were reassessed at 1 and 4 years post stroke (Langhammer & Stanghelle, 2003), however, both groups showed a large decrease in function, and no significant differences were present between the two groups on measures of arm function and ADL independence. In other words, the type of treatment patients received in the acute phase did not have a differential effect on long-term recovery because the patients treated with NDT did not have significantly lower functioning than those who had been treated with MRP.

A second series of studies presents evidence of positive benefits associated with NDT treatment for the hemiplegic arm. Feys et al. (1998) performed a single-blind, randomized, controlled study in which 100 stroke patients were assigned to a control group that received standard rehabilitation or an experimental group that received 6 weeks of sensorimotor treatment based on NDT/Bobath concepts to the arm in addition to standard rehabilitation. The experimental treatment involved 30 minutes of active or active-assisted exercise with the hemiplegic arm positioned in an RIP in an air splint. Feys et al. found that, although both groups improved significantly over time and there were no group differences on the *Barthel Index,* the experimental group showed a greater improvement in the hemiplegic arm as measured by the *Brunnstrom-Fugl-Meyer Motor Assessment* at the 6- and 12-month follow-ups. In addition, when subjects were re-assessed 5 years later (Feys et al., 2004), patients in the experimental group scored significantly higher on the *Brunnstrom-Fugl-Meyer Motor Assessment* and *Action Research Arm Test.* As in the earlier study, the groups did not differ significantly on the *Barthel Index.* These studies suggest that the sensorimotor stimulation provided by the supplemental NDT/Bobath intervention was highly effective in improving arm function in the acute phase and that the benefits of this intervention were long lasting.

In considering the evidence, it is important to note that several problems with the existing research may limit the conclusions that can be drawn about the efficacy of NDT/Bobath treatment. Paci (2003), Luke (2004), and Hafsteinsdottir (1996) all cite methodological problems with the research studies included in their reviews. These concerns include the lack of availability of valid outcome measures sensitive to the changes in movement control, postural responses, and muscle tone that may result from NDT/Bobath treatment; heterogeneous samples with few controls on age, location, and severity of the stroke; and differences in the duration and dosage of treatment. In many studies, small sample size also resulted in low power to detect treatment effects. These problems have also been noted in relation to outcome research on NDT/Bobath for children with cerebral palsy (Butler & Darrah, 2001). Existing research on the effectiveness of NDT/Bobath has also focused almost exclusively on intervention for acute hemiplegia. As the studies of Langhammer and Stanghelle indicate, this focus may not adequately reflect the long-term benefits of a given intervention.

A second problem with the existing research is related to the nature of NDT/Bobath treatment and the problems inherent in standardizing and measuring motor interventions for a treatment intervention that is evolving and individualized. NDT/Bobath treatment principles and techniques have changed over time and are taught mainly through post-graduate continuing-education courses. For this reason, the Bobath text (1990), cited in many of the studies as the source of the techniques used, does not adequately reflect the current practice of NDT. The NDT approach is individualized, so that NDT therapists may use very different strategies for individual patients depending on the problems identified during assessment. Since the procedures and techniques used in research must be standardized, the NDT delivered in the treatment protocol may not reflect the true benefits of the technique. Finally, the effectiveness of NDT and other motor interventions depends largely on the experience and skill of the therapist and specific goals of the treatment session (Butler & Darrah, 2001). Although the skill level of the therapists delivering the treatment is rarely mentioned and is difficult to quantify, it is clear that most research studies do not use therapists with expertise in the NDT/Bobath approach. This suggests that the research outcomes may underestimate the true efficacy of the approach. Given these problems, research studies in which operationally defined and current NDT/Bobath treatment is delivered by experienced therapists with clinical education in this approach will be needed to accurately evaluate the efficacy of this approach in the future.

Barriers to Effectiveness

The NDT approach and NDT handling has been criticized by motor learning theorists as too passive and lacking in opportunities for independent practice (Gordon, 1987). This criticism may be valid. Although B. Bobath stressed that handling should involve active participation by the patient, she also stressed that the therapist should prevent abnormal tone and movement. Her emphasis on movement quality has resulted in a perception among NDT therapists that patients should not move independently until they are able to use normal patterns of muscle activation. Research on motor learning suggests that this restriction may limit the patient's functional recovery and affect both functional performance and use of the involved arm (Langhammer & Stanghelle, 2000). For example, Langhammer and Stanghelle (2000) performed a randomized double-blind study comparing motor function and functional level of patients treated with Bobath with motor function and functional level of patients receiving the Motor Relearning Program (MRP), which is a treatment stressing independent practice. They found that motor function in the arm was significantly better in the MRP group at discharge, although this did not remain true at 5-year follow-up. NDT therapists and clinical instructors are aware of this problem and are changing the practice of handling to incorporate opportunities for independent practice (Ryerson & Levit, 1997a; see Howle, 2002 for a complete discussion of this problem).

CASE EXAMPLE

Mr. R.: Optimizing Motor Behavior Using the Bobath Approach

Occupational Therapy Intervention Process	Clinical Reasoning Process: Objectives	Clinical Reasoning Process: Examples of Therapist's Internal Dialogue
Patient Information Mr. R., a 64-year-old retired economist 2 months post stroke, was referred to outpatient occupational therapy after treatment in a rehabilitation center and at home. Mr. R. had a severe stroke that resulted in flaccidity in the muscles of the left trunk, arm, and leg and loss of balance in sitting and standing. At the time of the evaluation, the patient and his wife were living with a daughter and her family because of the demands associated with his care. The occupational therapy assessment identified the following problems: (1) dependence in ADLs and IADLs due to loss of postural control; (2) severe pain in left shoulder and edema of the left hand; (3) failure to attend to the left side of the body or to position the left arm for safety or comfort; (4) non-functional left arm and hand due to flaccidity and weakness; and (5) mild depression.	Appreciate the context	"Mr. R was an active person with a challenging and important job before his stroke. He was forced to retire because of his physical limitations, and he and his wife have left their own home to live with their daughter because he is too much for his wife to manage independently. These dual losses must be hard on this proud man and disruptive to his sense of self-efficacy. His depression seems appropriate to these changes in life roles. He is also discouraged because he remains so dependent after 2 months of intensive rehabilitation and home therapy. It is clear that he has begun to doubt that he will ever get better."
	Develop intervention hypotheses	"I believe that Mr. R.'s poor trunk control and his shoulder pain are the two major causes of his inability to care for himself. He seems afraid to touch or move his left arm because it may hurt, and he knows he is likely to fall over when he tries to dress himself or transfer to the wheelchair. Sleeping at night is also difficult because of arm and hand pain, and he cannot find a comfortable position or turn easily. Therefore, reducing his pain and making him safer during daily activities are important priorities. Improvements here should give him hope."

Summary of Short-Term Goals and Progress

Goal 1: Mr. R. will be able to sit unsupported on a firm chair and initiate trunk weight shifts in anteroposterior, lateral, and rotational planes without loss of balance. The therapist determined that Mr. R. lacked sufficient control of trunk movements in sitting to dress safely. During treatment, she worked to increase control of trunk movements in the patterns necessary for upper and lower body dressing and grooming. She also used upper extremity weight bearing at a table to increase trunk control so that Mr. R. would learn to support weight on his affected left arm and activate muscles in his trunk and shoulder girdle. The therapist taught Mr. R. and his daughter how to practice these trunk movements at home. She also changed the way the daughter helped Mr. R. transfer to increase weight bearing on the left leg and appropriate activity in trunk extensor muscles. As trunk control improved, Mr. R. could use his uninvolved right arm to put on his shirt while sitting without loss of balance. He also could independently manage his wheelchair locks and foot pedals. Visual neglect of the left side decreased, as he was able to turn his head to the left without loss of balance.	Assess the patient's comprehension Understand what he is doing	"Mr. R. is able to follow directions in therapy and to repeat the directions and goals on command. I think his cognitive abilities will be a strength—he has more difficulty with execution because his body doesn't always behave the way he wants. He is able to get set up for his home exercises independently but needs some physical assistance from his daughter to get his sling and splint on correctly." "The daughter reports that he is motivated to do things the way we practiced in therapy. Transfers are easier, as are ADLs. Both are pleased with the program."
Goal 2: Mr. R. will wear the prescribed shoulder support and hand splint while he is out of bed and perform edema massage and shoulder exercises three times a day. The therapist removed the elevated arm trough from the patient's wheelchair because it increased shoulder pain. She showed the patient's daughter how to use a pillow to position the arm in the wheelchair. Mr. R. was fitted with a commercial shoulder brace for use during walking. This brace supported the subluxation but did not position the elbow in flexion. The therapist also fabricated a wrist splint that supported the wrist in neutral. The patient and daughter were instructed to stop all exercises that caused pain. They were taught how to massage the hand to decrease edema. In addition, the therapist taught Mr. R. how to move his arm in small ranges, supporting the left hand in the right using the modified clasped hand grasp and how to position the arm in bed. The treatment was successful. Hand edema began to decrease immediately, and the hand was no longer painful to the touch after three treatments. The therapist also could passively move the arm below 60° of shoulder elevation without pain in supine when supporting the shoulder joint. The therapist changed the massage and passive exercise program to reflect these improvements. She also introduced transfers and rolling using the clasped-hand technique to incorporate the left arm into the activity.	Compare actual to expected performance Know the person Appreciate the context	"Mr R is starting to come into each therapy session with a list of questions or problems. He is able to see a difference in the edema in his hand and has been using the positioning techniques in the wheelchair and in bed. He reports that he is able to fall asleep more easily now that he knows where to put his arm, but he still wakes up with shoulder pain, which shows that we are making progress but have more work to do." "Daughter is extremely concerned and follows through well. His success with his home exercises is due to her. She is a real asset to him."
Goal 3: Mr. R. will actively assist with dressing. Mr. R.'s daughter dressed her father while he lay in bed. The therapist recommended that they start dressing with Mr. R. seated in a straight chair with arms. One treatment session was devoted to teaching Mr. R.'s daughter how to assist dressing while encouraging her father to be active and assist the task. The daughter initially supported the left arm and assisted trunk weight shifts. As her father grew more confident, she provided less physical assistance but continued to give verbal cues. The therapist introduced occupation-as-end dressing when Mr. R. had sufficient trunk control to perform necessary weight shifts without loss of balance and when pain no longer limited passive movements of the left arm. The slow approach gave Mr. R. time to learn and fostered confidence in his own abilities.		

Select an intervention approach	"I will develop a treatment plan based on NDT principles and techniques to treat his trunk control and attempt to change the pain and increase function in the left arm. I believe that improving his trunk control and restoring pain-free shoulder movements in the left arm will make it possible for Mr. R. to dress and bathe himself. I know that there is no evidence that NDT is more effective than compensatory training, but Mr. R. has already had 2 months of compensatory training without results, and focusing on his motor impairments will represent a new approach to his loss of independence. I will also work with his daughter to develop more consistent ways to perform ADLs, transfers, and arm exercise."
Reflect on competence	"Mr. R. is very similar to other stroke survivors that I have worked with, and I believe he will respond well to my treatment plan. I expect that we can decrease his pain fairly quickly, which should make therapy/home exercises less stressful. I also believe that his depression will lighten when he starts to see progress, but if not, he may require a medical evaluation and medication."

Recommendations

The occupational therapist recommended 2 therapy sessions per week for 8 weeks. Mr. R.'s insurance company authorized 16 30-minute sessions. In consultation with Mr. R. and his daughter, the occupational therapist established the following treatment goals, which were motivated by the patient's desire to return to his own home: (1) Mr. R. will bathe his upper and lower body and dress himself with assistance and verbal cues using compensations that increase the use of the left side; (2) Mr. R.'s daughter will be able to move his left arm through 120° of shoulder elevation without pain; (3) Mr. R. will transfer with contact guarding to and from wheelchair to bed and toilet; (4) Mr. R. will position his left arm on the table during meals and speech therapy and shift weight over this arm; (5) the left arm will be properly positioned in wheelchair with hand splint on 75% of the time; and (6) hand edema will be eliminated.

Consider the patient's appraisal of performance	"I think that continued therapy is warranted despite the lack of improvement in previous treatment programs. Mr. R. is anxious to be more independent so that he can move back to his own home and participate in more of his former life roles. His cognitive abilities do not seem to be affected, and he has a realistic sense of what he can do now and what is needed to return to his own home with his wife. He seems afraid to be too optimistic for fear of failure, but I expect that if he can see progress he will want to keep going."
Consider what will occur in therapy, how often, and for how long	
Ascertain the patient's endorsement of the plan	"Mr. R. is extremely happy with the goals we have set and our new methods. His daughter is rather protective but interested in helping her father with his therapy and pleased with our goals. Because of her physical limitations, Mrs. R. is not likely to assume much of a role in direct care. But she is supportive of her husband and watches each therapy session."

Next Steps Revised Short-Term Goals (after 16 treatments) • Mr. R. will perform upper body and lower body dressing activities independently while sitting in a straight chair. • Mr. R. will attend to the position of his left arm at all times and will position the arm appropriately without verbal reminders. • Mr. R. will support weight on the left forearm while sitting at a table and use this pattern functionally in activities such as eating, reading, and writing. • Mr. R. will transfer independently from the wheel chair using the clasped-hands technique.	Anticipate present and future patient concerns Analyze the patient's comprehension Decide if the patient should continue or discontinue therapy and/or return in the future	"Mr. R. has made good progress on all our goals but still requires assistance for most life roles. He is beginning to realize that, while he may achieve his goals, therapy is likely to last several more months. He has been talking with his wife and daughter about moving back to their own house with a live-in aide to assist with his care and exercises. I think this is probably a good solution but encouraged him to continue to work on the program we have set up to see if we can accomplish our new goals. He agrees that continuing treatment is important no matter where he is living."

CLINICAL REASONING IN OCCUPATIONAL THERAPY PRACTICE

Effects of Physical Impairments on ADL Performance

At the time of his evaluation, Mr. R. could not dress himself and his daughter was dressing him. The occupational therapist wanted to start dressing training immediately because independent self-care was a major long-term goal. Her plan was to develop a system for Mr. R. and his daughter to use at home. The daughter would provide support and assistance initially and gradually withdraw her assistance as Mr. R. developed better control of the movement components necessary for independence.

What impairments contributed to Mr. R.'s loss of functional performance? What types of support and assistance are most important during the first dressing sessions? How do you teach Mr. R.'s daughter to assist upper body dressing during the early phase of treatment? How could she position the hemiplegic arm during lower extremity dressing?

Evidence Table 24-1
Best Evidence for Occupational Therapy Practice Regarding NDT/Bobath

Intervention	Description of Intervention Tested	Participants	Dosage	Type of Best Evidence and Level of Evidence	Benefit	Statistical Probability and Effect Size of Outcome	Reference
NDT for stroke survivors	Effectiveness of NDT in 3 areas: general treatment, upper limb recovery, and lower limb and gait.	726 acute stroke survivors; age range, 15–95 years; mean age cannot be calculated.	Ranged from 2–15 weeks.	Systematic review of 15 trials: 6 randomized controlled trials, 6 non-randomized controlled trials, and 3 case studies.	Of general effectiveness studies (n = 6), 1 found more improvement in NDT group, and 5 found no difference or more gains in alternate group; 1 of 3 studies of upper extremity effectiveness found greater benefit with NDT.	$p < 0.001$ set as statistical significance level for all studies included. Effect sizes were not reported.	Paci, 2003
NDT for upper limb post stroke	Effectiveness of NDT in improving impairment (tone, strength, pain), activity limitation, and participation.	374 stroke survivors 6 weeks to 2 years post cerebrovascular accident; age range, 35–95 years; mean age cannot be calculated.	Ranged from 1 session to 20 weeks of daily 45-minute sessions.	Systematic review of 8 studies: 5 randomized controlled trials, 1 single-group cross-over design trial, and 2 single case studies.	NDT more effective than proprioceptive neuromuscular facilitation but not more than general rehab at reducing muscle tone. No significant effects of NDT on motor control, upper extremity function, or participation.	Improvement in upper extremity tone using RIPs, $d = 0.46$.	Luke, 2004

SUMMARY REVIEW QUESTIONS

1. What do Bobath and Bobath say are the major problems after stroke?
2. Define the following terms: facilitation, inhibition, and handling. How are these procedures used to treat adult hemiplegia?
3. How do Bobath and Bobath define postural control, and what problems are associated with loss of postural control?
4. Explain why abnormal tone is a major problem requiring occupational therapy treatment.
5. List several ways to control spasticity.
6. What is the overall goal of NDT/Bobath treatment for stroke patients? How does this goal relate to the practice of occupational therapy?
7. Describe several ways occupational therapists may incorporate NDT/Bobath concepts into ADL training.
8. How do the goals of treatment differ for patients with low tone and patients with spasticity?
9. Why is weight bearing on the arm important for function? List several ways to use upper extremity weight bearing in treatment.
10. Describe a treatment program to increase movement and function in the hemiplegic arm if the patient has flexor spasticity.

References

Bobath, B. (1990). *Adult hemiplegia: Evaluation and treatment* (3rd ed.). London, United Kingdom: Heinemann.

Butler, C., & Darrah, J. (2001). Effects of neurodevelopmental treatment (NDT) for cerebral palsy: An AACPDM evidence report. *Developmental Medicine and Child Neurology, 43,* 778–790.

Davies, P. (1985). *Steps to follow.* New York: Springer-Verlag.

Davis, J. (1990). The Bobath approach to the treatment of adult hemiplegia. In L. Williams Pedretti & B. Zoltan (Eds.), *Occupational therapy practice skills for physical dysfunction* (pp. 351–362). St. Louis: Mosby.

Dijkers, M. (1999). Correlates of life satisfaction among persons with spinal cord injury. *Archives of Physical Medicine and Rehabilitation, 80,* 867–876.

Eggers, O. (1984). *Occupational therapy in the treatment of adult hemiplegia.* Rockville, MD: Aspen.

Feys, H., De Weerdt, W., Selz, B., Steck, G., Spichiger, R., Vereeck, L., Putnam, K., & Van Hoydonck, G. (1998). Effect of a therapeutic intervention for the hemiplegic upper limb in the acute phase after stroke. *Stroke, 29,* 785–792.

Feys, H., De Weerdt, W., Verbeke, G., Steck, G., Capiau, C., Kiekens, C., Dejaeger, E., Van Hoydonck, G., Vermeersch, G., & Cras, P. (2004). Early and repetitive stimulation of the arm can substantially improve the long-term outcome after stroke: A 5-year follow-up study of a randomized trial. *Stroke, 35,* 924–929.

Gordon, J. (1987). Assumptions underlying physical therapy intervention: Theoretical and historical perspectives. In J. Carr, R. Shepherd, J. Gordon, A. Gentile, & J. Held (Eds.), *Movement science: Foundations for physical therapy in rehabilitation* (pp. 1–30). Rockville, MD: Aspen.

Hafsteinsdottir, T. (1996). Neurodevelopmental treatment: Application to nursing and effects on the hemiplegic stroke patient. *Journal of Neuroscience Nursing, 28,* 36–47.

Hiraoka, K. (2001). Rehabilitation effort to improve upper extremity function in post-stroke patients: A metaanalysis. *Journal of Physical Therapy Science, 13,* 3–9.

Howle, J. (2002). *Neuro-developmental treatment approach: Theoretical foundations and principles of clinical practice.* Laguna Beach, CA: Neuro-Developmental Treatment Association.

Langhammer, B., & Stanghelle, J. (2000). Bobath or motor relearning programme? A comparison of two different approaches of physiotherapy in stroke rehabilitation: A randomized controlled study. *Clinical Rehabilitation, 14,* 361–369.

Langhammer, B., & Stanghelle, J. (2003). Bobath or motor relearning programme? A follow-up at one and four years post stroke. *Clinical Rehabilitation, 17,* 731–734.

Luke, C. (2004). Outcomes of the Bobath concept on upper limb recovery following stroke. *Clinical Rehabilitation, 18,* 888–898.

Paci, M. (2003). Physiotherapy based on the Bobath concept for adults with post-stroke hemiplegia: A review of effectiveness studies. *Journal of Rehabilitation Medicine, 35,* 2–7.

Rast, M. (1999). NDT in continuum: Micro to macro levels in therapy. *American Occupational Therapy Association Developmental Disabilities Special Interest Section Quarterly, 2,* 1–3.

Ryerson, S., & Levit, K. (1997a). *Functional movement re-education.* New York: Churchill Livingstone.

Ryerson, S., & Levit, K. (1997b). The shoulder in hemiplegia. In R. Donatelli (Ed.), *Physical therapy of the shoulder* (3rd ed., pp. 205–228). New York: Churchill Livingstone.

Trombly, C. (1995). Occupation: Purposefulness and meaningfulness as therapeutic mechanisms. 1995 Eleanor Clark Slagle Lecture. *American Journal of Occupational Therapy, 49,* 960–972.

Van Dyck, W. (1999). Integrating treatment of the hemiplegic shoulder with self-care. *OT Practice, 4,* 32–37.

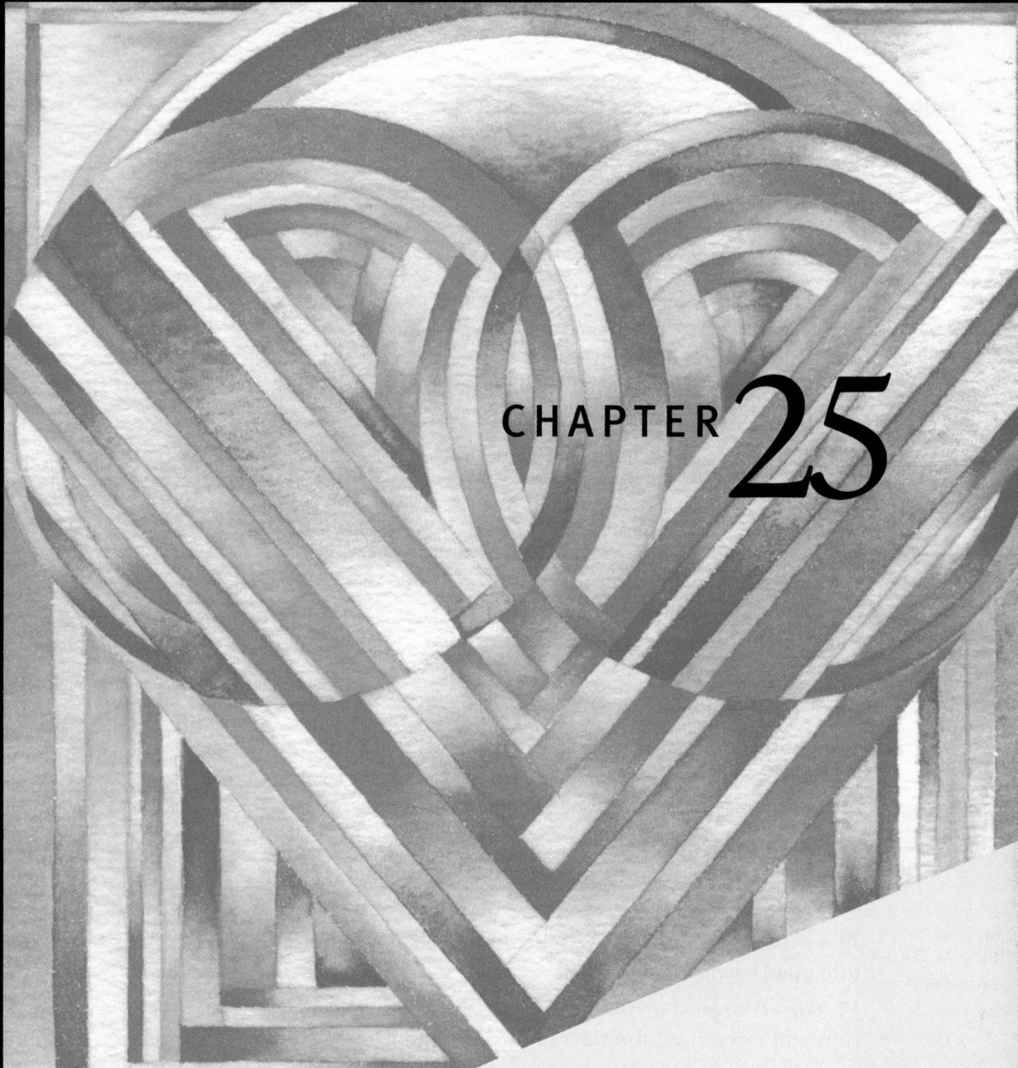

CHAPTER 25

LEARNING OBJECTIVES

After studying this chapter, the reader will be able to do the following:

1. State the assumptions that underlie the Brunnstrom Movement Therapy approach.
2. List the six stages of recovery for the upper extremity and for the hand.
3. State the treatment principles of this approach.
4. Describe the treatment procedures to facilitate movement control in the trunk and upper extremity of hemiparetic patients using this approach.
5. Suggest functional activities suitable to encourage practice of movement behavior at various stages of recovery.

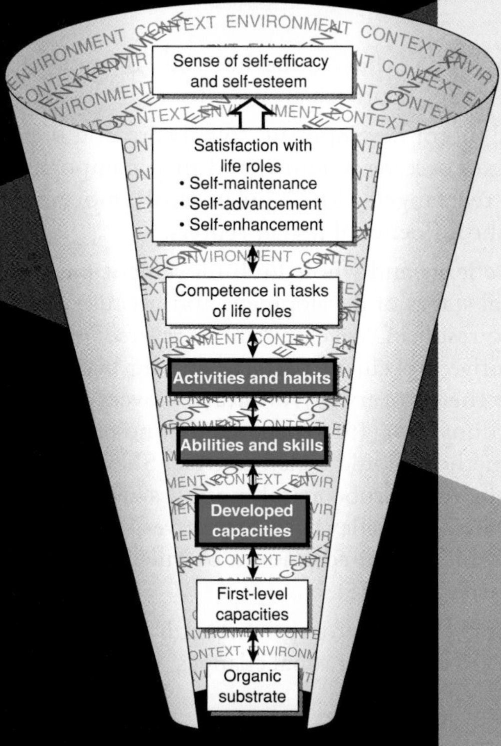

Optimizing Motor Behavior Using the Brunnstrom Movement Therapy Approach

Catherine A. Trombly Latham

Glossary

Associated reaction—Involuntary movement or patterned, reflexive increase in muscle tone and limb position on the hemiplegic side that occurs in stressful situations. An associated reaction is commonly seen when movement is resisted, when the patient exerts effort, or when the patient fears loss of balance.

Assumption—Supposition that something is true, although not proved; component of a theory.

Extensor synergy—For the upper extremity: scapular protraction, shoulder horizontal adduction and internal rotation, elbow extension, and forearm pronation. For the lower extremity: hip extension, adduction, and internal rotation; knee extension; plantar flexion and inversion of the ankle; and plantar flexion of the toes.

Facilitate—To make easier.

Facilitation—State of readying neurons to depolarize and propagate an impulse or to make contraction of a muscle or a reflex response more likely.

Facilitation techniques—Manual treatment techniques and hand placements used to increase muscle tone and to produce movement responses.

Flaccidity—State of lacking tone; limb feels limp and falls into place when not supported.

Flexor synergy—For the upper extremity: scapular elevation and retraction, shoulder abduction and external rotation, elbow flexion, and forearm supination. For the lower extremity: hip flexion, abduction, and external rotation; knee flexion; ankle dorsiflexion and inversion; and dorsiflexion of the toes.

Inhibit—To restrain; to make more difficult.

Inhibition—State of hyperpolarization of neural cell membranes decreasing the likelihood of propagating an impulse or to make contraction of a muscle or a reflex response less likely.

Inhibition technique—Manual treatment techniques and movement patterns used to decrease spasticity and stop abnormal movement patterns.

Practice—Repetition with the intent to improve.

Rasch analysis—A mathematical procedure that compares how an individual with a specific ability responds to assessment items of various difficulties. Rasch analysis produces tables and graphs that place "person ability" and "item difficulty" on the same continuum (Woodbury & Velozo, 2005).

Spasticity—State of excess tone and hyperactive response to stretch. If moderately to severely spastic, the limb feels tight and is difficult to move into position.

Synergy—Patterned movements of the entire affected limb in response to a stimulus or to voluntary effort.

Brunnstrom, a physical therapist, was particularly concerned with remediation of impaired motor control following stroke to enable everyday activities. Her method of developing this treatment approach gives therapists insight into the behaviors of a master clinician. Brunnstrom created movement therapy procedures after reading studies on recovery of motor control in animals and humans and observing the natural recovery of her patients post stroke. She experimented with trial-and-error application of these procedures and observed the patients' responses. She paid careful attention to the patients' motor and verbal reactions to each procedure, interpreted those reactions in light of her knowledge of motor control and development, and adjusted the procedure accordingly. Successful procedures were replicated patient to patient, until an integrated treatment approach was created. Brunnstrom's Movement Therapy is an example of augmented maturation treatment because it facilitates the recovery of abilities from first-level or developed capacities and organic substrate.

The principles of movement therapy and the evaluation and treatment procedures presented here are summarized and adapted from Brunnstrom (1970). This publication describes her approach in detail. No further development of the approach has occurred since then.

ASSUMPTIONS AND PRINCIPLES OF BRUNNSTROM MOVEMENT THERAPY

The **assumptions** that underlie the Brunnstrom Movement Therapy approach are as follows:

- In normal motor development, spinal cord and brainstem reflexes become modified and their components become rearranged into purposeful movement through the influence of higher centers.
- Because reflexes and whole-limb movement patterns are normal stages of development and because stroke appears to result in "development in reverse," reflexes and primitive movement patterns should be used to **facilitate** the recovery of voluntary movement post stroke. Brunnstrom (1956) believed that no reasonable training method should be left untried. She stated, "It may well be that a subcortical motion synergy which can be elicited on a reflex basis may serve as a wedge by means of which a limited amount of willed movement may be learned" (p. 225).
- Proprioceptive and exteroceptive stimuli can be used to evoke desired motion or tonal changes.

PROCEDURES FOR PRACTICE 25-1

Principles of the Brunnstrom Movement Therapy Approach

- Treatment progresses developmentally from evocation of reflex responses to willed control of voluntary movement to automatic functional motor behavior.
- When no motion exists, facilitate it using reflexes, associated reactions, proprioceptive facilitation, and/or exteroceptive facilitation to develop muscle tension in preparation for voluntary movement.
- Elicit reflex responses and associated reactions in combination with the patient's voluntary effort to move, which produces semi-voluntary movement; this allows the patient to feel the sensory feedback associated with movement and the satisfaction of having moved to some degree voluntarily.
- Proprioceptive and exteroceptive stimuli also assist in eliciting movement. Resistance, a proprioceptive stimulus, promotes a spread of impulses to other muscles to produce a patterned response (associated reaction), whereas tactile stimulation (exteroceptive) and muscle or tendon tapping (proprioceptive) facilitate only the muscles related to the stimulated area.
- When voluntary effort produces a response, ask the patient to hold (isometric) the contraction. If successful, ask for an eccentric (controlled lengthening) contraction and finally a concentric (shortening) contraction.
- Even when only partial movement is possible, stress reversal of movement from flexion to extension in each treatment session.
- Reduce or drop out facilitation as quickly as the patient shows evidence of volitional control. Drop out facilitation procedures in order of their stimulus-response binding. Reflexes, in which the response is stereotypically bound to a certain stimulus, are the most primitive and are dropped out of treatment first. Responses to exteroceptive stimulation are least stereotyped, and therefore, tactile stimulation is eliminated last. No primitive reflexes, including associated reactions, are used beyond stage III.
- Place emphasis on willed movement to overcome the linkages between parts of the synergies. Willed movement means that the patient is trying to accomplish it. Patients may be more successful if you ask them to do familiar movements involving a goal object (Trombly & Wu, 1999; Wu et al., 2000).
- Have the patient repeat correct movement, once elicited, to learn it. Practice should involve functional activities to increase the willed aspect and to relate the sensations to goal-directed movement.

- Recovery of voluntary movement post stroke proceeds in sequence from mass stereotyped flexor or extensor movement patterns to movements that combine features of the two patterns and, finally, to discrete movements of each joint at will. The stereotyped movement patterns are called limb synergies. **Synergy** in this sense refers to patterned movements of the entire limb in response to a stimulus or to voluntary effort.
- Newly produced correct motions must be practiced to be learned.
- **Practice** within the context of daily activities enhances the learning process.

The principles of this approach derive from these premises and are listed in Procedures for Practice 25-1.

EVALUATION

Evaluation using the Brunnstrom Movement Therapy approach is appropriate for persons who have had a stroke and who have occupational dysfunction secondary to sensorimotor impairments. If the occupational therapist determines that the patient cannot carry out activities and tasks that are important to the roles that the patient wants, needs, or is expected to do, the therapist observes the patient's attempts and, if it is indicated, assesses the patient's sensorimotor status (Procedures for Practice 25-2).

Sensation

The sensory evaluation precedes the motor evaluation. The patient's ability to recognize movements of the affected arm and to localize touch in the hand without looking are especially noted because they are associated with better eventual recovery of voluntary movement of the arm and hand, respectively. See Chapter 7 for evaluation procedures. The results of the sensory evaluation guide the therapist's choice of **facilitation** modalities to improve movement or alert the therapist to encourage the patient to substitute visual feedback for lost movement or position senses.

Tonic Reflexes

Tonic reflexes are assessed to determine whether they can be used in early treatment to initiate movement when none exists. The primitive tonic brainstem reflexes that may be present include the symmetrical and asymmetrical tonic neck reflexes, tonic labyrinthine reflexes, and tonic

PROCEDURES FOR PRACTICE 25-2

Evaluation in the Brunnstrom Movement Therapy Approach

Determine the following:

1. Proprioceptive and exteroceptive sensory status
2. Effect of tonic reflexes on the patient's movement
3. Effect of associated reactions on the patient's movement
4. Level of recovery of voluntary motor control

lumbar reflexes. The evaluation of these reflexes is described in Procedures for Practice 25-3. The complete reflex response may not be manifest; however, a change in tone does occur if the patient's movement is under reflex control. A change in tone is gauged by comparing the amount of resistance to passive stretch in the test condition to that in a neutral condition.

Associated Reactions

Associated reactions are involuntary movements or patterned, reflexive increases of tone in muscles that would be expected to contract to cause the movement. Associated reactions are triggered by effortful voluntary movement (Boissy et al., 1997). They are seen in the involved extremities of stroke patients when other parts of the body are resisted during movement or when the patient makes an effort to move. Associated reactions are evaluated to determine which can be used to facilitate movement when no voluntary movement exists.

Basic Limb Synergies

Limb synergies are instances of associated reactions. They may occur reflexively or as early stages of voluntary control when **spasticity** is present. When the patient initiates a movement of one joint, all muscles that are linked in synergy with that movement automatically contract, causing a stereotyped movement pattern.

In the upper extremity, the **flexor synergy** is composed of scapular retraction and/or elevation, shoulder abduction and external rotation, elbow flexion, and forearm supination (Fig. 25-1; see Fig. 24-8). Position of the wrist and fingers is variable. Elbow flexion is the strongest component of the flexor synergy and the first motion to appear or to be facilitated. Shoulder abduction and external rotation are weak components. Shoulder hyperextension may be seen when abduction and external rotation are weak, although it is not considered part of the flexor synergy. Flexor synergy can be evoked when no movement exists by applying resistance to shoulder elevation or elbow flexion of the uninvolved upper extremity.

The **extensor synergy** of the upper extremity is composed of scapular protraction, shoulder horizontal adduction and internal rotation, elbow extension, forearm pronation, and variable wrist and finger motion, although wrist extension and finger flexion may be seen (Fig. 25-2). The pectoralis major is the strongest component of the extension synergy; consequently, shoulder horizontal adduction and internal rotation are the first motions to appear or to be facilitated. Pronation is the next strongest component. Elbow extension is a weak

PROCEDURES FOR PRACTICE 25-3

Evaluation of Brainstem Reflexes

Reflex or Reaction	Stimulus	Response
ATNR	Turn head 90° to one side; repeat to the other side.	Increase in extensor tone of limbs on the face side and flexor tone on the skull side.
STNR	1. Flexion of the head	1. Flexion of arms and extension of legs.
	2. Extension of the head	2. Extension of arms and flexion of legs.
TLR	1. Prone position	1. Increased flexor tone in arms and legs.
	2. Supine position	2. Increased extensor tone in arms and legs.
Tonic lumbar	Rotate upper trunk in relation to the pelvis	Increased flexor tone in the upper extremity and increased extensor tone in the lower extremity on the side toward which the trunk is turned. Tone increases in the opposite way on the side opposite to the direction of rotation.

ATNR, asymmetrical tonic neck; STNR, symmetrical tonic neck; TLR, tonic labyrinthine.

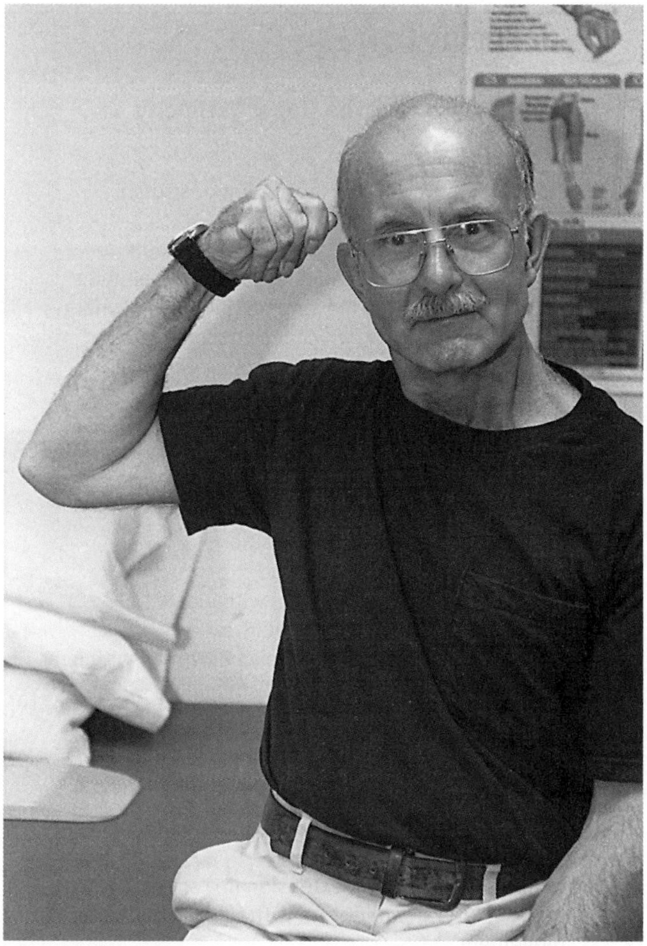

Figure 25-1. Flexor synergy. This patient lacks the supination component of the flexor synergy.

component. Extensor synergy can be evoked when no movement exists by applying resistance to horizontal adduction of the uninvolved upper extremity.

Upper extremity flexor synergy usually develops before extensor synergy. When both synergies are developing and spasticity is marked, the strongest components of the flexion and extension synergies sometimes combine to produce the typical upper extremity posture in hemiplegia: the arm is adducted and internally rotated, with the elbow flexed, forearm pronated, and the wrist and fingers flexed.

The lower extremity flexor synergy is composed of hip flexion, abduction, and external rotation; knee flexion; dorsiflexion and inversion of the ankle; and dorsiflexion of the toes. In this synergy, hip flexion is the strongest component; hip abduction and external rotation are weak components. The lower extremity extensor synergy is composed of hip extension, adduction, and internal rotation; knee extension; plantar flexion and inversion of the ankle; and plantar flexion of the toes. Hip adduction, knee extension, and plantar flexion of the ankle with inversion are all strong components. Weak components of this synergy are hip extension, hip internal rotation, and plantar flexion of the toes. Ankle inversion occurs in both lower extremity synergies.

The lower extremity extensor synergy is dominant when the person is standing because of the strength of this synergy combined with the influences of the positive supporting reaction and stretch forces against the sole of the foot that elicit plantar flexion.

Other Associated Reactions Identified by Brunnstrom

The brainstem reflexes listed in Procedures for Practice 25-3 are associated reactions that Brunnstrom used to evoke some movement when no movement existed but spasticity was present in hemiparetic limbs. In addition to these brainstem reflexes and to the basic limb synergies, Brunnstrom identified other associated reactions that she used in the early stages of treatment:

- Resistance to flexion of the uninvolved leg causes extension of the involved extremity, and resistance to extension of the uninvolved leg causes flexion of the involved extremity. This has been verified electromyographically (Fujiwara, Hara, & Chino, 1999).

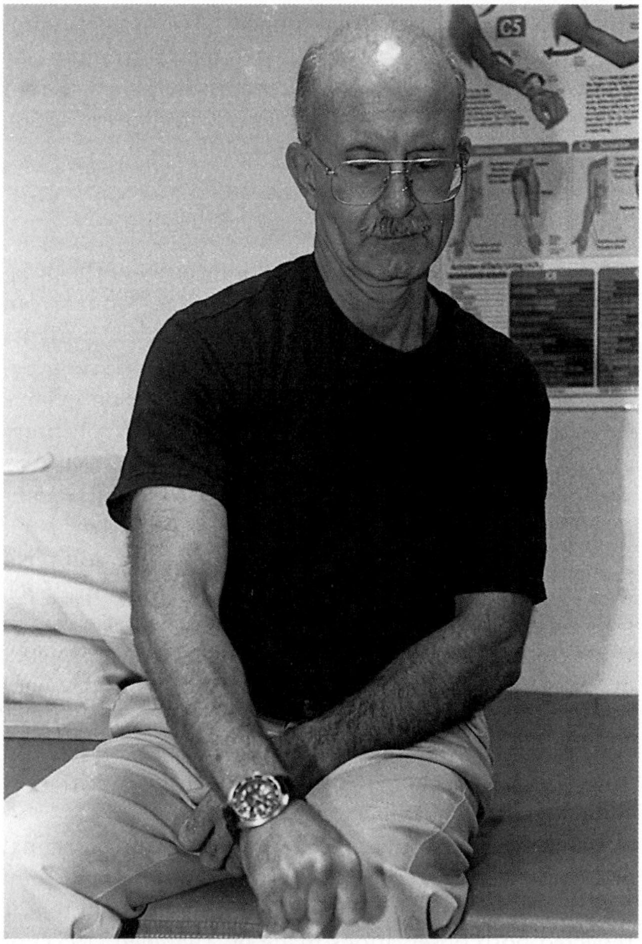

Figure 25-2. Extensor synergy.

- Resisted grasp by the uninvolved hand causes a grasp reaction in the involved hand. This is an example of mirror synkinesis.
- Attempt to flex the involved leg or resistance to leg flexion causes a flexor response in the involved arm. This reaction is called homolateral synkinesis.
- Actively or passively raising the affected arm above the horizontal causes the fingers to extend and abduct. This is Souque's phenomenon.
- Resistance to abduction or adduction of the unaffected lower limb results in a similar response in the opposite affected leg. This is Raimiste's phenomenon.

Level of Recovery of Voluntary Movement

The level of motor recovery is evaluated using an instrument that sequences motor performance after stroke from reflex to full voluntary control. In preparation for evaluation, the patient is made physically and psychologically comfortable. Each motion is demonstrated to the patient, who does it with the unaffected extremity before attempting to do it with the affected one. That allows the therapist to be certain that the person understands the request. Instructions should be given in functional terms. For example, to test the flexor synergy of the upper extremity, say "Touch your ear" and, for the extensor synergy, say "Reach out to touch your [opposite] knee" (Brunnstrom, 1966). No facilitation is used during the evaluation.

The Brunnstrom Stages

Definition 25-1 lists the six stages of recovery of the proximal upper extremity and the hand that Brunnstrom (1970) identified. Although, on average, stroke patients proceed through these stages, recovery of a particular patient may stop at any stage. To date, there are no reliable ways to predict which patients will recover voluntary movement.

Brunnstrom stages I to VI are useful to designate summarily the status of voluntary control. The patient is reported to be in the stage at which he or she can accomplish all motions specified for that stage (Definition 25-1). Because progress is gradual, sometimes the patient is in transition between stages. If the patient has completed one stage but is just beginning to be able to do the motions of the next stage, many therapists report the level as II going on III, III going on IV, and so on. The upper and lower extremities and the hand may all be in different stages of recovery at a given time.

The stages were quantified in Brunnstrom's original evaluation, the *Hemiplegia Classification and Progress Record* (Brunnstrom, 1966). That instrument was valid in that it reflected both observations made by Twitchell (1951) of

DEFINITION 25-1 *definition*

Stages of Recovery of the Upper Extremity

Arm

I. Flaccidity: no voluntary movement or stretch reflexes
II. Synergies can be elicited reflexively; flexion develops before extension; spasticity developing
III. Beginning voluntary movement, but only in synergy; increased spasticity, which may become marked
IV. Some movements deviating from synergy:
   a. Hand behind back
   b. Arm to forward horizontal position
   c. Pronation and supination with the elbow flexed to 90°; spasticity decreasing
V. Independence from basic synergies
   a. Arm to side horizontal position
   b. Arm forward and overhead
   c. Pronation and supination with elbow fully extended; spasticity waning
VI. Isolated joint movements freely performed with near normal coordination; spasticity minimal

Hand

I. Flaccidity
II. Little or no active finger flexion
III. Mass grasp or hook grasp; no voluntary finger extension or release
IV. Semi-voluntary finger extension in a small range of motion; lateral prehension with release by thumb movement
V. Palmar prehension
   a. Cylindrical and spherical grasp (awkward)
   b. Voluntary mass finger extension (variable range of motion)
VI. All types of prehension (improved skill).
   a. Voluntary finger extension (full range of motion).
   b. Individual finger movements

CLINICAL REASONING IN OCCUPATIONAL THERAPY PRACTICE

Planning Treatment According to the Brunnstrom Stages of Recovery

It is useful for therapists to think ahead of need about what occupations could and could not be used to reinforce particular levels of recovery. To that end, list homemaking activities that a patient in stage IV of upper limb recovery and stage V of hand recovery can be expected to do. What are some activities the patient won't be able to do?

the recovery process of 118 patients with acute and chronic strokes and Brunnstrom's (1970) own observations of 100 patients. However, a preliminary cross-sectional study in which **Rasch analysis** was applied to the scores of the upper extremity subtest of 100 subjects calls into question the underlying sequence proposed by Brunnstrom on which the *Fugl-Meyer Motor Assessment* is based (Woodbury & Velozo, 2005). More extensive analysis and longitudinal study of recovery sequence are needed. No data exist concerning the reliability of the *Hemiplegia Classification and Progress Record*, but it can be assumed to be low because the rating scales were not operationally defined.

The Fugl-Meyer Assessment of Motor Function

The *Fugl-Meyer Motor Function Assessment* (*FMA*) (Fugl-Meyer et al., 1975), sometimes called the *Brunnstrom-Fugl-Meyer Motor Function Assessment*, is a widely used adaptation of Brunnstrom's *Hemiplegia Classification and Progress Record*. This assessment is used by researchers as well as clinicians, even when Brunnstrom's approach to therapy is not used.

Fugl-Meyer et al. (1975) defined 50 details of movement across Brunnstrom's six levels of recovery. The patient's ability to do the requested movement is scored according to the degree of completion. The *FMA* uses an ordinal-level scoring system in which each detail is rated 0, cannot be performed; 1, can be partly performed; or 2, can be performed faultlessly. For example, when asked for a flexor synergy response, if the patient can bring the hand only as far as the mouth rather than to the ear, the score is 1. When the patient's response is incomplete, as in this example, it is necessary to observe the patient's repeated attempts to determine the specific weak areas of the synergy or movement pattern.

Total score ranges from 0, flaccidity, to 100, normal motor function, for the upper and lower extremities. The subtests may be used independently; Table 25-1 shows the upper extremity subtest. The total score for the upper extremity is 66. The score can also be recorded as percentage of recovery (score obtained ÷ total score × 100%) (Duncan et al., 1994).

Both intra-rater and inter-rater reliability of the upper extremity subtest of the *FMA* (33 items) were determined to be strong ($r = 0.96$) (Duncan, Probst, & Nelson, 1983; Sanford et al., 1993). The *FMA* is more discriminative than the *[Carr & Shepherd] Motor Assessment Scale* (Malouin et al., 1994). The *FMA* correlates strongly ($r = 0.97$) with the *Arm Function Test*, which uses tasks for evaluation; however, the *FMA* is more responsive because it does not exhibit the ceiling and floor effects that the *Arm Function Test* does (Berglund & Fugl-Meyer, 1986). A preliminary study that applied **Rasch analysis** to the *Upper Extremity Subtest* of the *FMA* indicates that the underlying sequence may not be as Brunnstrom and Fugl-Meyer described (Woodbury & Velozo, 2005); more extensive analysis is needed.

TREATMENT

Rehabilitation of trunk control precedes treatment of the limbs.

Rehabilitating Trunk Control

Some patients with hemiplegia have poor trunk control and require training to enable them to bend over to retrieve an object from the floor or to dress their lower extremities. To elicit balance responses, the patient is gently pushed forward, backward, and side to side. Reaching for objects in various locations while seated demands dynamic trunk balance responses (Dean & Shepherd, 1997) and seems to be a better, more natural approach to improve balance than simply pushing the patient. Brunnstrom, had she known about the newer research that documents the importance of goal and context on the organization of movement (Ma, Trombly, & Robinson-Podolski, 1999; Trombly & Wu, 1999; Wu et al., 2000), in all likelihood would have incorporated task-oriented movement into her approach.

Brunnstrom emphasized promoting contraction of trunk muscles on the uninvolved side first by pushing the patient off balance toward the involved side (today we would place an object to be touched or grasped on the involved side), while guarding in case of poor response. Then, once it is determined that the person has that skill, recovery from a push toward or reach toward the uninvolved side is sought. This requires contraction of the trunk muscles on the involved side. The patient is pushed or asked to reach only to the point at which he or she can hold the position and regain upright posture. ***The patient is guarded throughout.*** Training then progresses to promote trunk flexion, extension, and rotation.

Practice in forward flexion of the trunk is assisted. The patient crosses the arms with the uninvolved hand under the involved elbow and the uninvolved forearm supporting the involved forearm. The therapist, sitting facing the patient, supports the patient under the elbows and assists in trunk flexion forward, avoiding any pull on the shoulders (Fig. 25-3). Some pain-free shoulder flexion is accomplished during this forward movement. While the patient is concentrating on trunk control, shoulder movement occurs without conscious awareness.

Return from trunk flexion is performed actively by the patient. Then, while sitting without back support and with the involved arm supported as described, the patient is pushed backward and encouraged to regain upright posture actively. Forward flexion in oblique directions is done next, not only to promote regaining balance but also to incorporate more scapular motion with the shoulder flexion already achieved.

Table 25-1. Fugl-Meyer Assessment of Motor Function: Upper Extremity Subtest

Patient Name *Mrs. G ** **Date** *6/27/05* *8/10/05*

Shoulder/Elbow/Forearm

Stage	Instruction	Response	Scoring Criteria	8/10/05
I & II: Reflex activity	Tap the biceps and finger flexor tendons	2 Stretch reflex at elbow and/or fingers	0 = no reflex can be elicited	2
	Tap the triceps tendon	2 Stretch reflex	2 = reflex can be elicited	2
III: Voluntary movement within synergy	Flexor synergy "Turn your affected hand palm up and touch your ear."	Flexor synergy 2 Shoulder retraction	(for each of 9 details) 0 = cannot perform 1 = can perform partly 2 = can perform faultlessly	2
		2 Shoulder elevation		2
		2 Shoulder abduction to 90°		2
		1 Shoulder external rotation		2
		2 Elbow flexion		2
		1 Forearm supination		2
	Extensor synergy "Turn your hand palm down and reach to touch your unaffected knee."	Extensor synergy 1 Shoulder adduction and internal rotation		2
		0 Elbow extension		2
		1 Forearm pronation		2
IV: Voluntary movement mixing flexor and extensor synergies	"Show me how you would put a belt around you [or tie an apron]."	0 Affected hand moves to lumbar spine area	0 = cannot perform 1 = hand must actively pass anterior-superior iliac spine 2 = faultless	1
	"Reach forward to take [object held in front of patient]."	0 Reaches into 90° of shoulder flexion	0 = elbow flexes or shoulder abducts immediately 1 = if these occur later in motion 2 = faultless	0
	"Put your arm to your side and bend your elbow. Turn your palm up and down."	0 Pronates and supinates forearm with elbow at 90° and shoulder at 0°	0 = if cannot position arm or cannot pronate or supinate 1 = shoulder and elbow joints correctly positioned and supination seen 2 = faultless	0
V: Voluntary movement outside of synergies	"Turn your palm down and reach over here to touch [object held out to side]."	NT Abducts shoulder to 90° with elbow extended to 0° and forearm pronated	0 = initial elbow flexion or loss of pronation 1 = partial motion or elbow flexes and forearm supinates later in motion 2 = faultless	NT
	"Reach as high as you can toward the ceiling."	NT Flexes shoulder from 90–180° with elbow in 0°	0 = elbow flexes or shoulder abducts immediately 1 = if these occur later in motion 2 = faultless	NT

*See the case example at the end of this chapter.

(continued)

Table 25-1. *(continued)*

Stage	Instruction	Response	Scoring Criteria	
	"Reach your arm directly forward and turn your palm up and down."	NT Flexes shoulder to 30–90°; extends elbow to 0°; and supinates and pronates	0 = if cannot position arm or cannot rotate 1 = correct position and beginning rotation 2 = faultless	NT
VI: Normal reflex activity (tested if patient scores 6 in stage V tests)	Tap on biceps, triceps, and finger flexor tendons	NT Normal reflex response	0 = 2 reflexes are markedly hyperactive 1 = 1 reflex hyperactive or 2 reflexes lively 2 = no more than 1 reflex lively and none hyperactive	NT
Upper Arm Subtotal Score (36 points)		Mrs. G.'s score = 16 (44%)	Mrs. G.'s re-evaluation score = 23 (64%)	
Wrist				
Wrist stability with elbow flexed	Put the shoulder in 0°, elbow in 90° flexion, and forearm pronated. "Lift your wrist and hold it there."	1 Patient extends wrist to 15°. Therapist can hold upper arm in position.	0 = cannot extend 1 = can extend, but not against resistance 2 = can maintain against slight resistance	2
Wrist stability with elbow extended	Put the elbow in 0°. "Lift your wrist and hold it there."	1 As above	As above	2
Active motion with elbow flexed and shoulder at 0°	"Move your wrist up and down a few times."	0 Patient moves smoothly from full flexion to full extension. Therapist can hold upper arm.	0 = no voluntary movement 1 = moves, but less than full range 2 = faultless	1
Active motion with elbow extended	"Move your wrist up and down a few times."	0 As above	As above	1
Circumduction	"Turn your wrist in a circle like this [demonstrate]."	NT Makes a full circle, combining flexion and extension with ulnar and radial deviation.	0 = cannot perform *o* 1 = jerky or incomplete motion 2 = faultless	
Wrist Subtotal Score (10 points)		Mrs. G.'s score = 2 (20%)	Mrs. G.'s re-evaluation score = 6 (60%)	
Hand				
III: Mass flexion:	"Make a fist."	2 Patient flexes fingers.	0 = no flexion 1 = less than full flexion as compared to other hand 2 = full active flexion	2
III: Hook grasp	"Hold this shopping bag by the handles."	2 Grasp involves MCP extension and PIP and DIP flexion.	0 = cannot perform 1 = active grasp, no resistance 2 = maintains grasp against great resistance	2

(continued)

Table 25-1. *(continued)*

Stage	Instruction	Response	Scoring Criteria	
IIIB–VI: Finger extension	"Let go of the shopping bag." "Open your hand wide."	1 From full active or passive flexion, patient extends all fingers.	0 = no extension 1 = partial extension or able to release grasp 2 = full range of motion as compared to other hand	1
IV: Lateral prehension	"Take hold of this sheet of paper [or playing card]."	1 Patient grasps between thumb and index finger.	0 = cannot perform 1 = can hold paper but not against tug 2 = holds paper well against tug	2
V: Palmar prehension	"Take hold of this pencil as if you were going to write."	o Therapist holds pencil upright and patient grasps it.	Scoring as above	1
V: Cylindrical grasp	"Take hold of this paper cup [or pill bottle]."	o Therapist holds the object and patient grasps with 1st and 2nd fingers together.	Scoring as above	o
VI: Spherical grasp	"Take hold of this tennis ball [or apple]."	o Patient grasps with fingers abducted.	Scoring as above	o
Hand Subtotal Score (14 points)		Mrs. G.'s score = 6 (43%)	Mrs. G.'s re-evaluation score = 8 (57%)	
Coordination/Speed				
VI: Normal movement	"Close your eyes. Now, touch your nose with your fingertip. Do that as fast as you can 5 times."	Patient does finger-to-nose test NT Tremor NT Dysmetria o Speed	*Tremor:* 0 = marked 1 = slight 2 = none	o o 1
			Dysmetria: 0 = pronounced or unsystematic 1 = slight and systematic 2 = none	
		(Compare to unaffected side)	*Speed:* 0 = > 6 sec slower 1 = 2–5 sec slower 2 = < 2 sec slower	
Speed and Coordination Subtotal Score (6 points)		Mrs. G.'s score = 0	Mrs. G.'s re-evaluation score = 5 (83%)	
TOTAL UPPER EXTREMITY SCORE (66 points)		Mrs. G.'s score = 24 (36%)	Mrs. G.'s re-evaluation score = 42 (63%)	

Adapted from Fugl-Meyer et al., 1975.

NOTE: The scores pertain to the person described in the case example.

NT, not tested. Because recovery is sequential, more advanced movements are not tested if the patient fails the movements in the earlier stage.

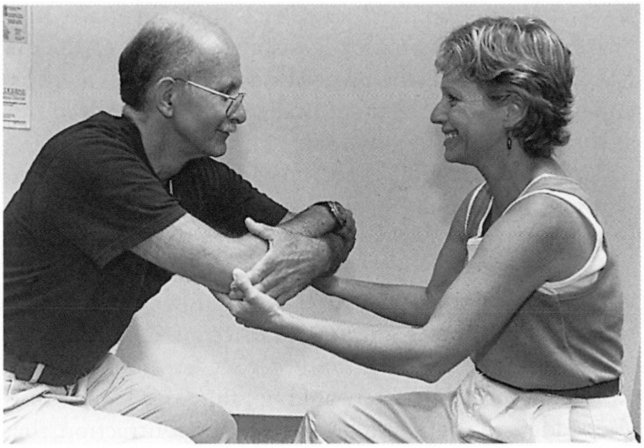

Figure 25-3 Therapist supporting the patient's arms to assist forward flexion of the trunk. The shoulders become more flexed as the patient leans forward.

Next, trunk rotation is practiced with the patient supporting the involved arm and the therapist guiding trunk motion. Trunk rotation can be combined with head movements in the opposite direction of the trunk rotation, so that the tonic neck and tonic lumbar reflexes can be used to begin to elicit the shoulder components of the upper extremity synergies. The arms and trunk move in one direction, and the head turns in the opposite direction (Fig. 25-4). Head and trunk movements are combined with increasing ranges of movement of the shoulder, enabling pain-free shoulder and scapular abduction and adduction during trunk rotation.

Retraining Proximal Upper Extremity Control

The focus of treatment is the recapitulation of normal movement developmentally from its reflexive base to voluntary control of individual motions that can be used functionally. The general format for treatment is listed in Procedures for Practice 25-4. Because recovery proceeds sequentially, once the stage of recovery is identified, the short-term goal is the next step in the sequence.

Stages I to III

The goal of treatment is to promote voluntary control of the synergies and to encourage their use in functional activities. In these stages, all movements occur in synergy patterns but with increasing voluntary initiation and control of these patterns.

To move the patient from stage I (**flaccidity**) to stage II (beginning synergy), the basic limb synergies are elicited at a reflex level, using as many reflexes, associated reactions, and facilitation procedures as are necessary to elicit a response. The effects of these procedures are additive and combine to produce a stronger response. The patient tries to move (willed movement) as these facilitation techniques are used.

The flexor synergy is the first to develop. Elbow flexion, the strongest component of that synergy, is the first motion to be elicited. Once the elbow flexes, the therapist turns concentration from elbow flexion to the proximal components of the synergy with the goal of enabling the patient to "capture the synergy," that is, bring it under voluntary control (stage III). Efforts to achieve voluntary control of the flexor synergy begin with scapular elevation. Lateral flexion of the neck toward the involved side can be used to initiate scapular elevation because the upper trapezius does both motions, although it may have "forgotten" how to elevate the scapula. With the patient's arm supported on a table in shoulder abduction with elbow flexion, the therapist simultaneously gives resistance to the head and shoulder while the patient is asked to hold the head and not let it move away from the shoulder. When the trapezius is felt to respond, both the patient's effort and the therapist's resistance emphasize shoulder elevation when lateral flexion of the neck is repeated. Once elevation begins, active contraction may be promoted by an

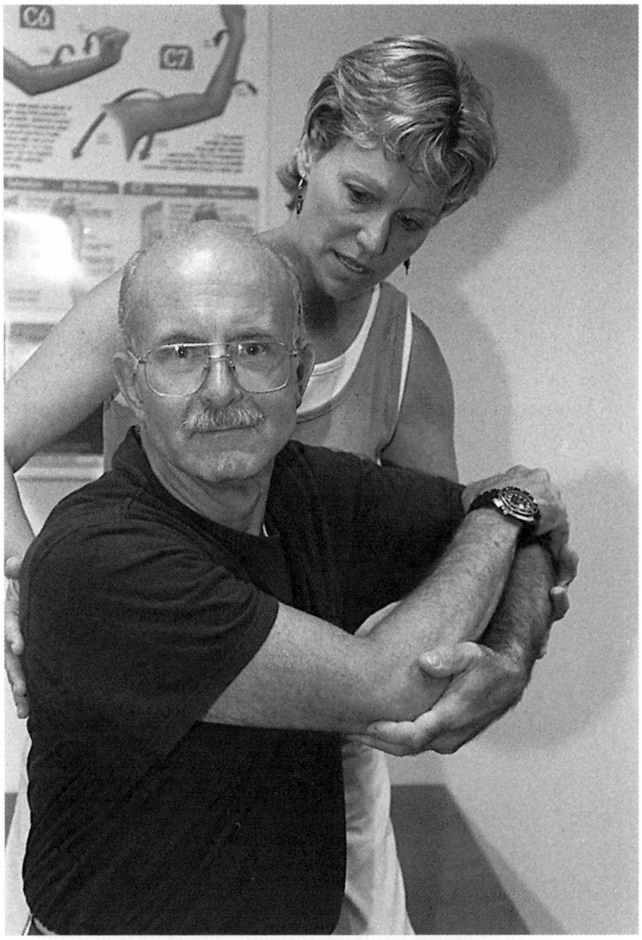

Figure 25-4 Through manual guidance, the therapist helps direct the patient to carry out trunk rotation while keeping the head forward or looking in the opposite direction.

PROCEDURES FOR PRACTICE 25-4

General Treatment Sequence to Achieve Movement Control Within Brunnstrom's Movement Therapy Approach

1. Gain some movement through sensory facilitation and reflexes, including associated reactions.
2. Resist the movement and ask for a holding (isometric) contraction.
3. If the patient can produce an isometric contraction, ask for a lengthening (eccentric) contraction.
4. If the patient can produce a controlled lengthening contraction, ask for a shortening (isotonic) contraction.
5. Once the patient can voluntarily move the limb to some degree, ask the patient to reverse the movement repeatedly.
6. Provide opportunities for use of the targeted movement and the reversing movement functionally.
7. Provide suggestions of functional situations that would allow practice of the newly acquired movements in daily life.

associated reaction. For example, as the patient attempts bilateral scapular elevation, resistance is given to the uninvolved scapula. If the involved scapula elevates as an associated reaction, resistance is added on the involved side as the patient is asked to hold.

Unilateral scapular elevation of the involved arm is attempted next; it may be achieved as a result of the previous procedures. If the patient cannot do the motion, the therapist supports the patient's arm and assists the patient to elevate the scapula. Percussion or stroking over the upper trapezius facilitates muscle contraction. The therapist tells the patient to hold and "Don't let me push your shoulder down." After repeated holding with some resistance added, the patient does an eccentric contraction, that is, lets the shoulder down slowly. Then a concentric, or shortening, contraction is attempted when the person is told, "Pull your shoulder up toward your ear."

Active scapular elevation evokes other flexor components and tends to **inhibit** the pectoralis major. The patient repeats scapular elevation and relaxation as the therapist gently abducts the shoulder in increasing increments. Because many patients with hemiplegia have shoulder pain and/or shoulder subluxation, the shoulder is given special care, and the correct scapulohumeral orientation is maintained. Once shoulder elevation and some active abduction have been achieved, external rota-

PROCEDURES FOR PRACTICE 25-5

Procedures to Develop Elbow Extension

"Rowing"

1. Sit facing the patient.
2. Cross your arms so that your right hand grasps the patient's right hand and your left hand grasps the patient's left hand.
3. Resist as the pronated, uninvolved extremity moves toward the involved knee (Fig. 25-5). This elicits elbow extension in the involved arm through an associated reaction.
4. At the same time, assist the involved arm into extension toward the uninvolved knee.
5. Still holding the patient's hands, guide movements into flexion combined with supination (Fig. 25-6).
6. Repeat steps 3 to 5 until you feel the affected limb actively extending.
7. Then, offer resistance bilaterally.
8. Then, reinforce voluntary effort of the involved extremity by asking the patient to hold against resistance to that limb only.
9. Facilitate the extensors by lightly and repeatedly pushing the involved arm back toward elbow flexion, which causes quick stretches to the triceps.

Weight Bearing

When the extensor synergy is seen to come under some active control, it is further developed through use of bilateral weight bearing.

1. Have the patient lean forward onto extended arms supported by a low stool or cushions placed in front (Fig. 25-7). To make it comfortable for the patient, place a sandbag, pillow, or towel on the stool.
2. Stroke the skin over the triceps vigorously or tap over the triceps tendon while the patient attempts to bear weight on both outstretched arms (Fig. 25-8).
3. Once this is successful, have the patient shift weight so that the involved extremity bears more of the weight of the upper trunk.
4. Again, tap the tendon and apply tactile stimulation to the triceps.
5. In the unilateral weight-bearing position, have the patient do functional tasks such as holding down objects with the affected arm while working on them with the other hand, such as holding a piece of wood while sawing, hammering, or painting it; holding a package steady while opening it, addressing it, or fastening it; or supporting body weight while polishing or washing large surfaces with the uninvolved arm.

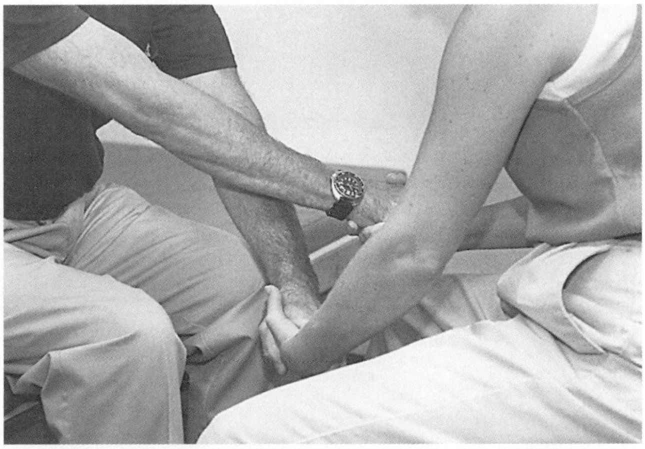

Figure 25-5 "Rowing." The therapist resists the pronated uninvolved (left) extremity while guiding the involved (right) extremity into extensor synergy.

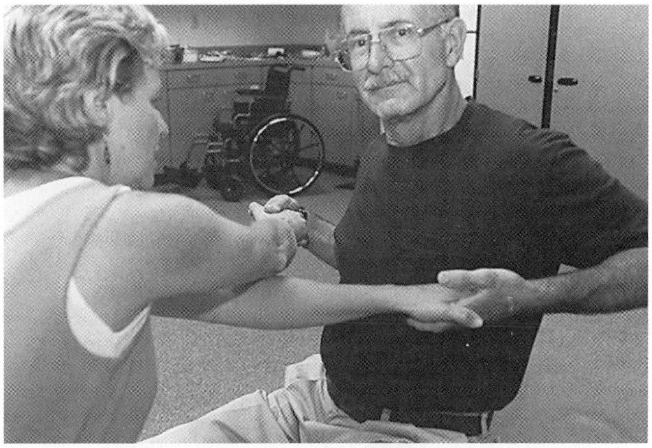

Figure 25-6 "Rowing." The therapist guides the patient into the reverse motion of flexion and supination.

tion and forearm supination are included in the movement. Reversal of movements to the opposite direction is done from the start, and this begins to develop some components of the extensor synergy.

The extensor synergy tends to follow the flexor synergy but may have to be assisted in its initiation. Contraction of the pectoralis major, a strong component of the extensor synergy, can be elicited by the associated reaction in which the therapist supports the patient's arms in a position between horizontal abduction and adduction, instructs the patient to bring his arms together, and resists the uninvolved arm just proximal to the elbow. As bilateral contraction occurs, the patient is instructed, "Don't let me pull your arms apart." Then the patient attempts to bring the arms together voluntarily.

Because of the predominance of excess tone in the elbow flexors and relative weakness of elbow extensors, elbow extension is usually more difficult to obtain, but it can be assisted by the methods in Procedures for Practice 25-5. Other means that may be used to facilitate extension movement include use of supine position (tonic labyrinthine reflex); having the patient watch the extremity, which requires head turning and pulls in the asymmetrical tonic neck reflex; working with the forearm pronated, which is a strong component of the extensor synergy; and rotating the trunk toward the uninvolved side to facilitate extension of the involved arm via the tonic lumbar reflex.

After the patient achieves elbow extension in weight bearing, the goal is to encourage active elbow extension free of weight bearing. Unilateral manual resistance is offered to the patient's attempts to move into an extension synergy pattern. Resistance gives direction to the patient's effort and facilitates a stronger contraction.

As the synergies come under voluntary control, they should be used in functional activities. The extensor synergy can be used to stabilize an object to be worked on by the other arm, to push the arm into the sleeve of a

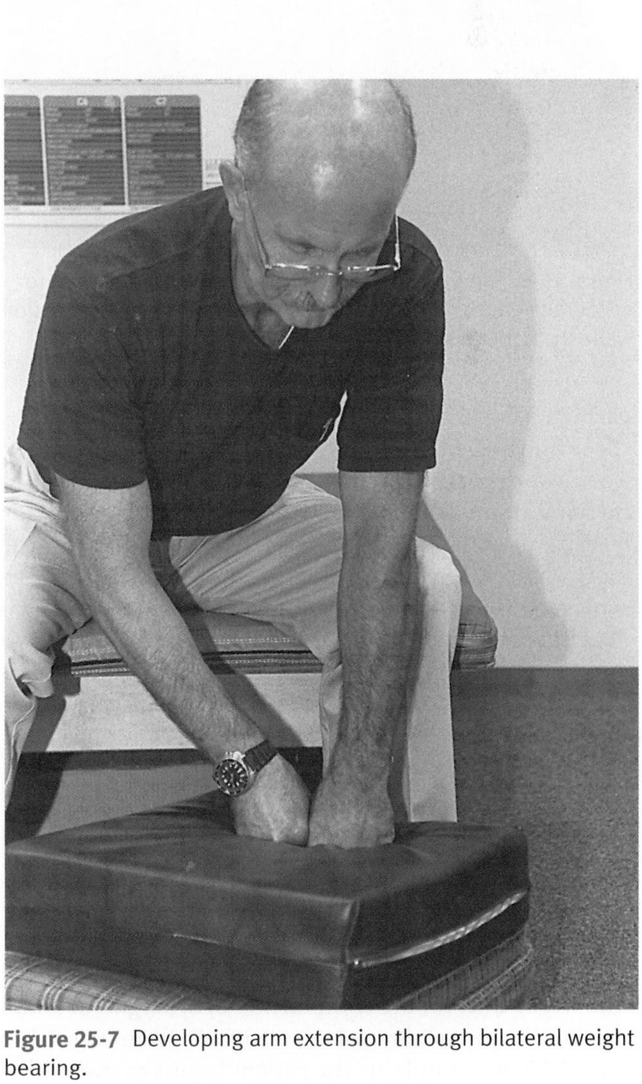

Figure 25-7 Developing arm extension through bilateral weight bearing.

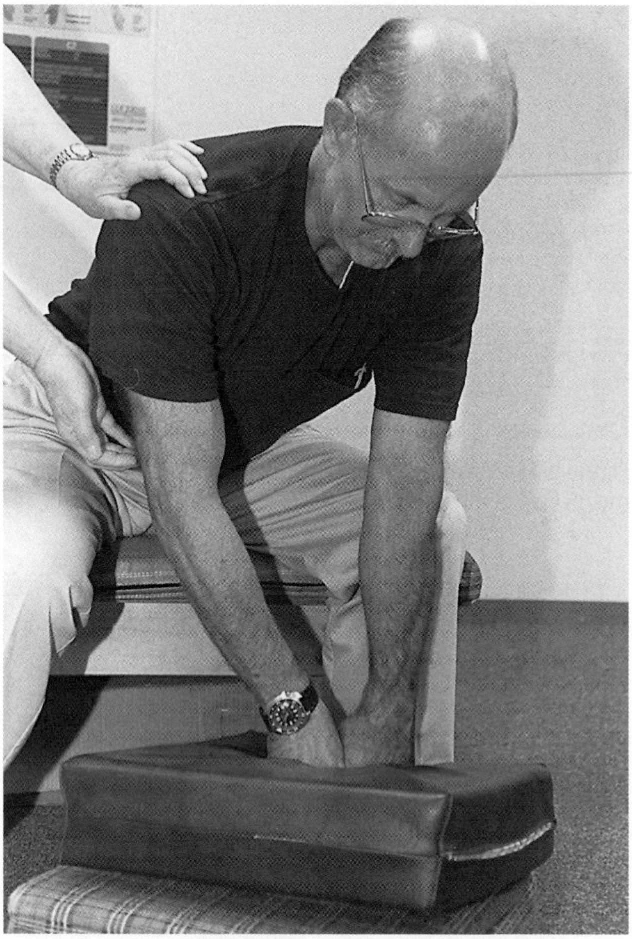

Figure 25-8 The therapist taps on the skin over the triceps to encourage greater muscle contraction and better arm extension while the patient is bearing weight on the outstretched arm.

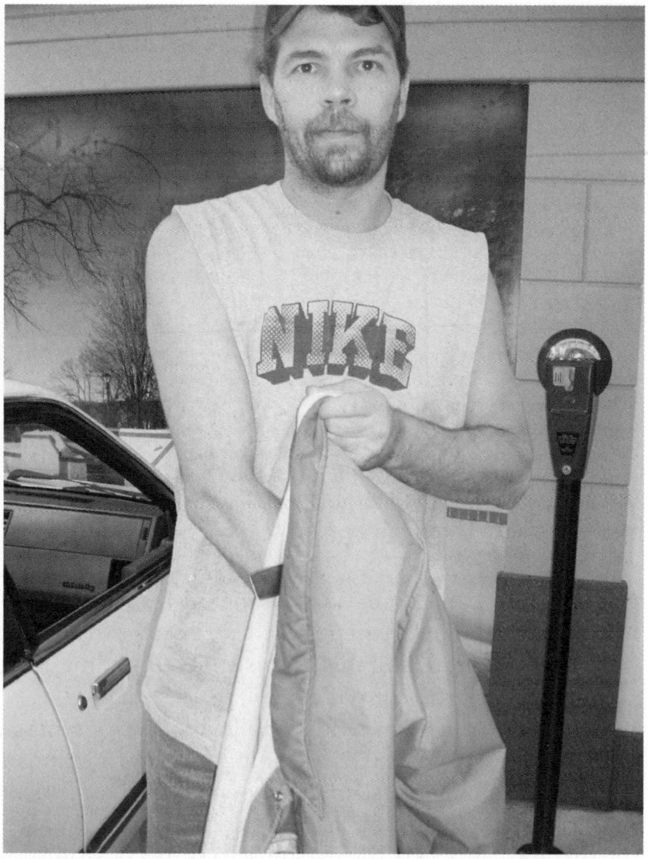

Figure 25-9 The patient practices extensor synergy functionally when putting his arm through the sleeve of garments.

garment (Fig. 25-9; see also Fig. 24-21), to smooth out a sheet on the bed, or to sponge off the kitchen counter. The flexor synergy can be used functionally to assist in carrying items (such as a coat, handbag, or briefcase); feeding oneself; putting on glasses; and combing the hair. Bilateral pushing and pulling reinforce both synergies. Bilateral identical movements performed independently (i.e., no ball or stick connecting the two limbs) were observed to improve movement of the hemiplegic arm when that arm was tested unilaterally. The improvement was limited to the practiced movement patterns but was maintained over time (Mudie & Matyas, 2000). Sanding, weaving, ironing, and polishing (Fig. 25-10) use the flexor and extensor synergies alternately and repeatedly.

Stages IV to VI

To promote movement deviating from synergy, motions that begin to combine components of synergies in small increments are encouraged as a transition from stage III to stage IV. For example, as the patient begins to extend the

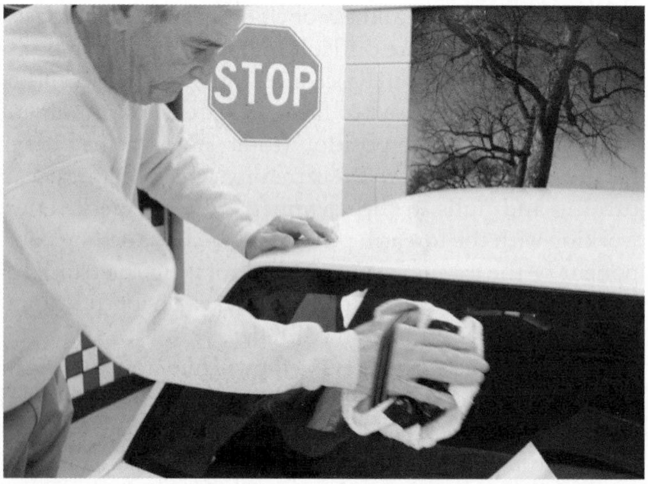

Figure 25-10 Polishing the car window functionally alternates between flexion and extension. The adapted polisher assists the patient who lacks grasp. This photograph was taken at Independence Square inside of Sister Kenny Institute in Minneapolis; the patient was not polishing the car in the street at a stop sign!

arm consistently in response to the unilateral manual resistance that the therapist provides, the therapist guides the direction of movement away from the extensor synergy pattern and toward greater shoulder abduction in conjunction with elbow extension. This breaks up the synergistic relationships of shoulder adduction with elbow extension and shoulder abduction with elbow flexion. The therapist directs the patient to push the hand into the therapist's hand and moves the hand in small increments away from the patient's midline. When the triceps and pectoralis major are disassociated, the synergies no longer dominate.

In stages IV and V, the goal of treatment is to "condition the synergies," that is, to promote voluntary movement combining components of the two synergies into increasingly varied combinations of movements that deviate from synergy. Proprioceptive and exteroceptive stimuli are still used in this phase of training, but tonic reflexes and associated reactions, appropriate in the earlier stages when reflex behavior was desirable, are no longer used. Willed movement with isolated control of muscle groups is the desired goal.

The first out-of-synergy motion of stage IV is hand behind the body (see Definition 25-1), which combines relative shoulder abduction (flexor synergy) with elbow extension and forearm pronation or internal rotation (extensor synergy). This motion requires that the strongest components of each synergy be subdued. A swinging motion of the arm combined with trunk rotation helps to get the hand behind the body. If balance is good, this can be done more easily when standing. As the hand reaches the back of the patient, the patient strokes the dorsum of the hand against the body to complete the sensory awareness of the movement. Stroking the dorsum of the hand on the back is thought to give direction to the attempted voluntary movement. If the patient cannot do the full motion actively, the therapist passively moves the patient's arm into final position and strokes the dorsum of the patient's hand against the sacrum. The patient, while attempting to do the movement independently, is assisted into and out of the pattern, which gradually becomes voluntary with practice. Practice, using functional tasks as much as possible, continues until the motion can be freely accomplished. Examples of functional tasks include putting a belt on when the patient is standing, swimming using the crawl stroke, and tucking a shirt into trousers (Fig. 25-11).

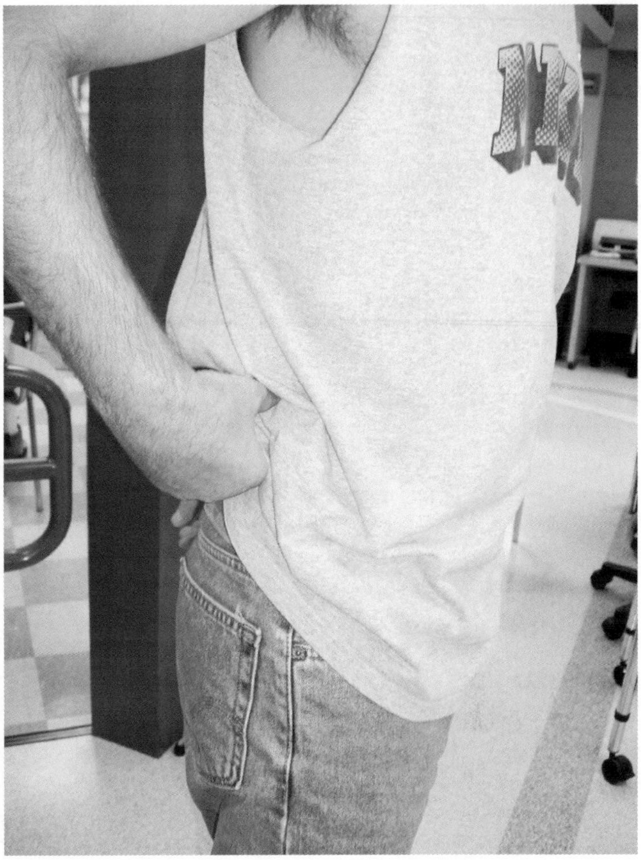

Figure 25-11 The patient attempting to tuck his shirt into his trousers uses arm-behind-the-back motion functionally.

The second out-of-synergy motion is shoulder flexion to a forward horizontal position with the elbow extended. If the patient cannot flex the shoulder forward actively, even with the therapist providing local facilitation and guidance of movement, the arm is brought passively into position. While tapping over the anterior and middle deltoid muscles, the therapist asks the patient to hold the position. If the patient can hold after positioning, active motion in small increments is sought, starting with lowering of the arm followed by active shoulder flexion. This continues until the full forward flexion motion can be done. Stroking and rubbing of the triceps are used to help the patient keep the elbow straight as the arm is raised. Repetitive non-resistive activities are used to motivate this action. Raising the arm to forward horizontal is involved in any vertically mounted game, such as tic-tac-toe or checkers (using Velcro tabs to secure the pieces), or in reaching for objects in a cupboard (Fig. 25-12), for example.

The third motion sought in stage IV is pronation and supination with the elbow flexed to 90°. Supination would not be expected to be a problem unless the pronators retained some spasticity. The problem would be to combine pronation of the extensor synergy with elbow flexion of the flexor synergy. Initially, pronation can be resisted with the elbow extended, and gradually, the elbow can be brought into flexion as the resistance to pronation is repeated. Block printing is an activity to consider when resistance to pronation is wanted. It can be positioned to resist pronation, with gradual changes in the amount of elbow flexion. This motion has been achieved when resistance is no longer required and the patient can supinate and pronate with the elbow near the trunk. Practice should include activities that require turning objects,

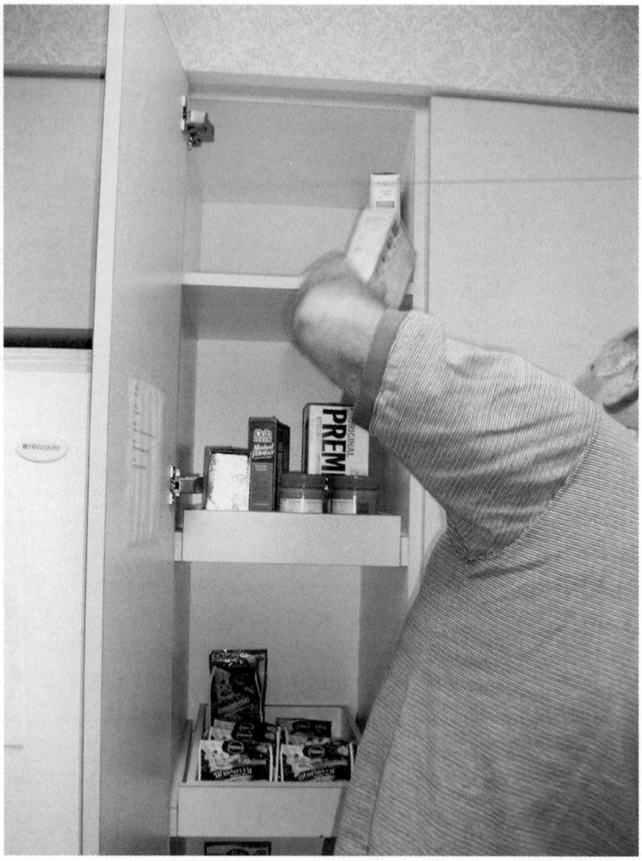

Figure 25-12 Attempting to reach for objects in the cupboard offers opportunities to practice forward (and overhead) reach.

such as a knob, a screwdriver, or a dial, to reinforce it. Some games, such as skittles, are knob operated and require rotary motions, as do card games that require turning the cards over and the adapted dice game described by Nelson et al. (1996).

Once the patient is confident of these stage IV movements and performance is fairly consistent, stage V training commences. Movement in stage V entails active attempts by the patient to move in patterns increasingly away from synergy. Excess effort is avoided, however, so that the limbs will not revert to stereotyped movements. The attempts are bolstered by use of quick stretch and tactile stimulation. Each new motion is incorporated into functional activities. Although it is Brunnstrom's approach to regain motion through exercise and then introduce functional activities to practice the motion, recent research indicates that goal is a powerful organizer of movement, including that of stroke patients (Ma, Trombly, & Robinson-Podolski, 1999; Trombly & Wu, 1999; Wu et al., 2000); therefore, functional activities should be introduced earlier in treatment.

The first motion sought in stage V is arm raised to side horizontal, which combines full shoulder abduction with

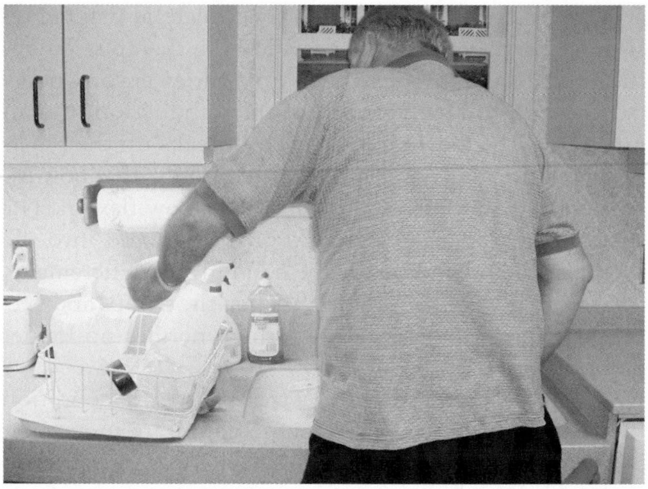

Figure 25-13 By arranging the dish drainer on the patient's hemiparetic side, he practices arm to the side motion when putting the clean dishes into the drainer.

elbow extension. When this can be accomplished, disassociation of components of the synergies has occurred. No longer will the arm drift toward horizontal adduction when the elbow is extended or the elbow flex when the shoulder is abducted, as they would when the muscles are still under the influence of the synergies. Again, practice with functional tasks assists learning. Activities that have game pieces or materials that can be placed on a high table to the side of the patient to encourage side horizontal movement to play the game or do the project are useful in encouraging this motion. The table can be gradually moved to require more and more horizontal abduction and elbow extension. Other activities that could be used to encourage this motion include weaving on a floor loom, table tennis, driving golf balls, hitting a baseball, and washing dishes (Fig. 25-13).

The second motion of stage V is arm overhead. To achieve it, the scapula must upwardly rotate. The serratus anterior must be specifically retrained to do this. If the scapula is bound by spastic retractor muscles, passive mobilization may be necessary before seeking an active protraction response. Passive mobilization of the scapula is done by grasping the vertebral border and repeatedly and *slowly* rotating it as the arm is passively moved into an overhead position. Once the scapula is mobilized, the serratus is activated in its alternative duty of scapula protraction by placing the arm in the forward horizontal position and asking and assisting the patient to reach forward. ***Do not put traction on the patient's glenohumeral joint.*** It is helpful to rehearse this motion with the patient using the uninvolved extremity. Apply quick stretches by pushing backward into scapular retraction to activate the serratus. Once the serratus is activated, seek a holding contraction of the serratus. These procedures continue, with the therapist moving the arm incrementally overhead. Once the movement has been achieved, practice with functional activities reinforces it. Sanding on an inclined plane is an example of an activity requiring a forward push with an increasing range of movement in scapular protraction and rotation and shoulder flexion. Bilateral sanding will allow the stronger uninvolved arm to help the weaker one. Table tennis would still be useful, as would shooting baskets and putting on overhead garments every day. Washing a wall or painting it with a roller requires repeated reversal of movement up overhead and down.

The third motion sought in stage V is supination and pronation (external and internal rotation) with the elbow extended. To improve supination, the elbow is at first kept close to the trunk and gradually extended. Brunnstrom had no special treatment recommendations to assist in developing disassociation of supination and elbow flexion. The best way to achieve control of supination and pronation with the elbow extended is to have the patient use both hands in activities of interest that entail supination and pronation in various arm positions. One such activity is grasping a beach ball with the arms outstretched and rotating it so the affected arm is on top (pronated) and the unaffected arm is on the bottom (supinated) and vice versa. The patient can graduate to handling a smaller ball, such as a basketball. Adapted games, such as an adapted dice game, that capture the patient's attention and interest have been found to be more effective than exercise (Nelson et al., 1996).

Patients who recover comparatively rapidly after a stroke may spontaneously achieve stage VI; however, many patients do not achieve full recovery after stroke. Twitchell (1951) stated that patients who reached stages III and IV within 10 days after stroke recovered completely; however, this observation has never been verified in the literature. In Twitchell's sample, patients who failed to respond to proprioceptive facilitation did not recover willed movement at all. He observed, and it is generally accepted, that the longer the flaccid stage lasts, the less likely recovery will occur. Duncan et al. (1994) verified that patients with a severely impaired upper extremity did not regain full voluntary use of that extremity.

Retraining Hand and Wrist Control

Training techniques for return of function in the hand are presented separately from the rest of the upper extremity because the hand may be at a different stage of recovery from that of the arm. If the patient cannot initiate active finger flexion (hand stage I) or mass grasp (hand stage II), the traction response in which stretch of the scapular adductors produces reflex finger flexion or an associated reaction of resisted grasp by the unaffected hand may be used in combination with voluntary effort.

In hemiplegia, wrist flexion usually accompanies grasp initially, so stability of the wrist in extension must be developed. It is easier for the patient to stabilize the wrist in extension when the elbow is extended; therefore, training starts with the elbow extended and the wrist supported by the therapist. The wrist extensor muscles are facilitated, and the therapist directs the patient to do a forceful grasp by saying, "Squeeze!" That grasp should promote normal synergistic contraction of the facilitated wrist extensors. This is repeated until the wrist extensors are felt to respond, allowing the therapist to remove support from the wrist with the command, "Hold." Tapping on the wrist extensor muscles facilitates holding. Once wrist extension and grasp with the elbow extended are possible, the process of positioning, percussion, and hold is repeated in increasing amounts of elbow flexion. Emphasis in this stage of training is on wrist stability, although wrist flexion, extension, and circumduction may also be practiced.

To move from hand stage III (flexion) to hand stage IV (semi-voluntary mass extension) spasticity of the finger flexors must be relaxed using a series of manipulations listed in Procedures for Practice 25-6. The second motion sought at hand stage IV is lateral prehension and release. The patient attempts to move the thumb away from the index finger to gain release of lateral prehension while the therapist percusses or strokes over the extensor pollicis longus and abductor pollicis longus tendons to facilitate this motion. Once the patient has some active release, functional use of lateral prehension is encouraged. Activities include holding a book while reading, holding or dealing cards, using a key, and dressing.

Once the patient can extend the fingers voluntarily to release objects, advanced prehensile patterns (hand stage V) are encouraged through activities. As the patient progresses, activities are chosen to reinforce particular prehensions at more precise levels. Holding a pencil or paintbrush encourages palmar prehension. Spherical grasp is used to pick up or hold round objects such as containers (Fig. 25-15) or an orange. Cylindrical grasp is used to hold the handles of tools.

Individual finger movements (hand stage VI) may be regained in rare instances. The patient should be given a home program of activities to encourage more and more individual finger use and to increase speed and accuracy of finger movements but should also be cautioned about expecting full recovery. One stroke survivor published a workbook of his exercises for hand recovery that may be incorporated into the home program of a patient with determination to recover hand function (Smits & Smits-Boone, 2000). It advocates many repetitions of simple activities. Intensive repetitive movement has been shown to improve the particular movements practiced (Barreca et al., 2003; Butefisch et al., 1995; Kawahira et al., 2004).

Brunnstrom also described gait patterns, principles used in preparation for walking, and training to walk.

PROCEDURES FOR PRACTICE 25-6

Procedures to Develop Finger Extension

1. Release the patient's grasp by holding the thumb into extension and abduction.
2. Still holding the thumb, *slowly* and rhythmically supinate and pronate the forearm.
3. Apply cutaneous stimulation over the dorsum of the hand while the forearm is supinated.
4. With the forearm still supinated, apply rapid, repeated stretch to the extensors of the fingers by repeatedly rolling them toward the palm (Fig. 25-14).
5. Continue these manipulations until flexion relaxes.
6. Slowly pronate the forearm and elevate the arm above horizontal to evoke a finger extensor response (Souque's phenomenon).
7. Stroke over the dorsum of the fingers and forearm as the patient attempts extension. To avoid a buildup of flexor tension, do not allow the patient to exert more than minimal effort. Imitation synkinesis, in which the normal side performs a motion that is difficult for the involved side (Boissy et al., 1997), may be observed when the patient attempts finger extension.
8. After the fingers can be voluntarily extended with the arm raised, gradually lower the arm.
9. If there is a decreased range in extension, repeat all above manipulations to again inhibit flexion and facilitate extension.
10. Provide opportunities for the patient to reach and pick up large, lightweight objects and to release them. Putting bagels, apples, or oranges into a basket is one example of an activity to practice finger extension. The larger the object, the greater the extension required. Other extensor-type activities require the hand to be used flat, such as smoothing out a garment while ironing or a sheet while making the bed.

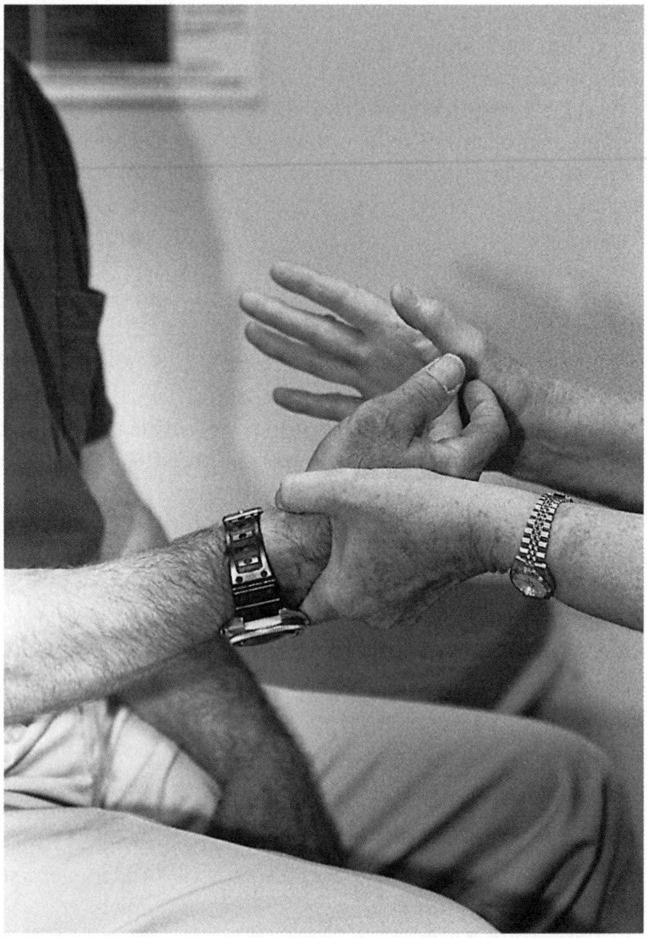

Figure 25-14 The therapist applies rapid repeated stretches to the extensors of the fingers by rolling the fingers toward the palm.

These procedures are the primary responsibility of the physical therapist.

EFFECTIVENESS

The only study of the effectiveness of this approach compared the relative effectiveness of Brunnstrom's movement therapy to Bobath's neurodevelopment treatment (Wagenaar et al., 1990). Seven selected post-stroke patients were randomly assigned to one treatment for 5 weeks and then to the other for 5 more weeks; this was repeated using a B-C-B-C design. Functional recovery of activities of daily living (ADLs), upper limb function, and

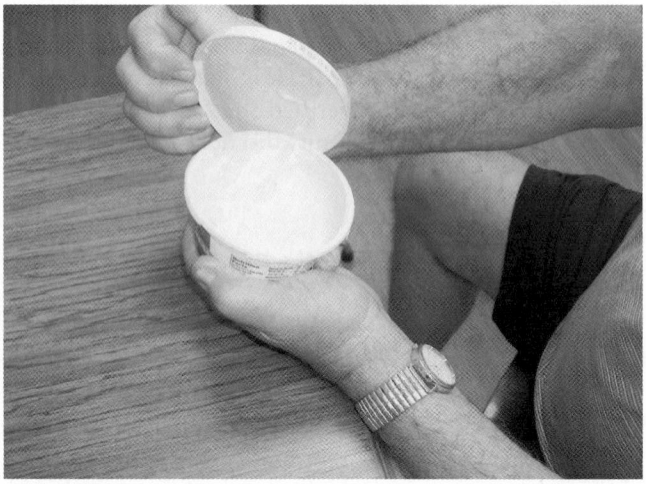

Figure 25-15 Holding a round container demands spherical grasp.

Evidence Table 25-1
Best Evidence Regarding the Brunnstrom Movement Therapy Approach

Intervention	Description of Intervention Tested	Participants	Dosage	Type of Best Evidence and Level of Evidence	Benefit	Statistical Probability and Effect Size of Outcome	Reference
Movement Therapy Approach vs. Bobath NDT therapy	One treatment (randomly assigned) applied during the 5-week B phases and other treatment applied during the alternate 5-week C phases. Treatments adhered to published principles and were applied by specially trained therapists.	7 persons 5–9 days post stroke. Age 40–77 years. Ischemic stroke in area of MCA; 5 patients with right cerebrovascular accidents; 2 with left cerebrovascular accidents. No severe memory or understanding deficits. No medical complications.	30 minutes per weekday while inpatient; 30 minutes 3–4 times per week after discharge for a total of 20 weeks (10 weeks each treatment).	Single-subject experimental design (BCBC) across subjects. Level IV. (Lacked control for many threats, especially spontaneous recovery and the design of alternating two opposing treatments.)	No, neither treatment was better than the other. All patients improved, but that may be due to spontaneous recovery. No difference in ADL (*Barthel Index*); arm function (*Action Research Arm Test*); or gait quality. One patient improved significantly in gait speed during the Brunnstrom weeks compared with the Bobath weeks.	Not reported.	Wagenaar et al., 1990

MCA, middle cerebral artery.

CASE EXAMPLE

Mrs. G.: Moving from Brunnstrom's Stage III to Stage IV

Occupational Therapy Intervention Process	Clinical Reasoning Process	
	Objectives	Examples of Therapist's Internal Dialogue
Patient Information Mrs. G. is a 38-year-old right-hand dominant woman who was employed as a clerk in a local department store prior to June 2005, when she suffered an embolytic stroke of the left middle cerebral artery. She was an accomplished amateur artist who did oil portraiture. She lives with her husband, a plumber, and 16-year-old son in a ranch-style house. This young woman identified several roles important to her: self-maintenance roles of independent person, mother, and homemaker; self-advancement role of worker, and self-enhancement role of artist. At admission to inpatient rehabilitation, she had no voluntary movement of the right upper extremity and impaired kinesthesis of that limb. She was wheelchair dependent. She was discharged to outpatient rehabilitation after 15 days, independent in ambulation and in self-care ADL using the unaffected arm. At admission to outpatient occupational therapy, Mrs. G. is dependent in her valued roles of homemaker and artist because of weakness and poor motor control of the dominant upper extremity. However, she did score 24 (36%) on the *Fugl-Meyer Motor Assessment* (see Table 25–1). The problem list concerning upper limb motor control includes: • Unable to do extensor synergy movement, although the strongest components are active (stage III). • Able to maintain wrist extension in any elbow position but cannot take resistance. • Able to hold a playing card put between her thumb and index finger but not against resistance (stage IV). • Unable to do other types of grasp, other than mass grasp, or to extend the fingers, other than release of mass grasp (stage III).	Appreciate the context	"Gosh, she is young; she's only 10 years older than I am. I wonder how I would react if this had happened to me? I think I will discuss my feelings of vulnerability and vicarious anger with my supervisor so that I can offer Mrs. G. the best therapy I can." "Mrs. G. will be returning to good, enabling physical and social environments." "She is making rapid recovery. Restoration of some useful motor control in the upper extremity seems feasible."
	Develop intervention hypotheses	"Spontaneous recovery can be enhanced through neurodevelopmental therapies such as Brunnstrom's Movement Therapy. Repetitive practice of motor activities with the unaffected upper extremity will enhance occupational performance. This approach does not contradict Brunnstrom's Movement Therapy."

Recommendations The patient's long-term goals are to use both upper extremities to recover IADL related to self-care, preparation of meals, and other household tasks and to resume oil painting. Therefore Mrs. G. agrees to the three focuses of therapy: 1. Brunnstrom's Movement Therapy 2. Compensatory methods of accomplishing IADL 3. Practice to improve motor skill of the unaffected limb	Select an intervention approach	"Although there is no published evidence of the effectiveness of Brunnstrom's Movement Therapy, I will use that approach because I have had success with other patients similar to Mrs. G. in age, diagnosis, and pace of recovery. Concurrently, I will teach compensatory methods for meal preparation and other household tasks important to her so she can resume that role more quickly than if we wait for restoration of motor control. I will also engage her in occupations to improve dexterity of the unaffected non-dominant upper extremity."
	Reflect on competence	"I have used these approaches numerous times before. I am competent to administer these therapies."
	Consider the patient's appraisal of performance	"Mrs. G. has decided to take an extended leave of absence from her job because of the continuing excessive effort required for all tasks. This is a sensible decision to allow for concentration on the work of rehabilitation."
	Consider what will occur in therapy, how often, and for how long Ascertain the patient's endorsement of the plan	"Constrained by limited insurance coverage, I recommend treatment 3 times weekly for 6 weeks with intensive home practice between therapy visits. Then, there is enough insurance coverage for an additional 6 visits if warranted. Mrs. G. agrees and is eager to begin the work of therapy."
Summary of Short-Term Goals and Progress 1. Increase dexterity of the left, unaffected hand to accelerate engagement in instrumental self-care and homemaking activities. Dexterity of the unaffected hand increased through Mrs. G.'s efforts to accomplish tasks of her self-maintenance roles that naturally demanded dexterous responses. She is now able to apply make-up, crack and separate eggs, and write shopping lists. 2. Develop elbow extension (stage III). Voluntary control of the extensor synergy was achieved using rowing and weight-bearing maneuvers listed in Procedures for Practice 25-5. Between therapy appointments, Mrs. G. practiced using whatever extensor movement she had to do activities like sponging off the table and kitchen counters after meals, putting her arms into the sleeves of sweaters and jackets, and vacuuming with a self-propelled vacuum cleaner. She interspersed these activities with weight bearing on the affected arm with the elbow extended while working with the other hand. 3. Develop the first motion of stage IV: hand behind back. After repeated attempts in therapy to swing the hand behind the back, with tactile facilitation of the latissimus dorsi, posterior deltoid, and triceps, Mrs. G. was successful in bringing her hand past the anterior superior iliac spine. Encouraged, she continued to practice at home and to use the motion functionally in pulling on her underpants and slacks.	Track progress	"Mrs. G. is progressing nicely. She is particularly pleased that we have related each improvement to important functional activities."

4. Improve wrist stability against mild and moderate resistance. Wrist stability was encouraged during mass grasp and lift of increasingly heavy objects by tapping the wrist extensors during the lift. At home, she practiced lifting weighted shopping bags. 5. Strengthen lateral pinch (stage IV) and develop release to enable primitive use of paintbrushes, paint tubes, and other artist tools. Therapy to develop release of lateral pinch consisted of tapping of the extensor pollicis longus and the abductor pollicis longus tendons. Once release was enabled, resistance to pinch was gradually increased and alternated with active release. The patient was given a home program of activities to encourage lateral prehension. She resumed painting with the canvas on the table and used lateral pinch to squeeze the paint tubes and hold the brushes. 6. Develop palmar pinch (stage V) to enable more normal use of a paintbrush and other artist tools. In the process of using various brushes, Mrs. G. redeveloped palmar prehension without specific treatment.		
	Anticipate present and future patient concerns	"Although Mrs. G. is making good progress in recovering use of her affected arm and hand, I must be sure that she understands that recovery can stop at any time and that it is unlikely that she will regain 100% normal use of her limb. I must keep a balance between encouraging her to work for greater improvement and having realistic expectations."
Next Steps **Revised Short-Term Goals (6 weeks)** 1. Develop arm forward flexion (second motion of stage IV) to enable painting on an easel. 2. Develop cylindrical grasp (stage V) to enable use of a toothbrush, broom, mop, large spoons, etc.	Decide if the patient should continue or discontinue therapy and/or return in the future	"Based on the progress made after 6 weeks of therapy (refer to the column labeled 8/10/2005 in Table 25-1) and her faithful practice at home, Mrs. G. and I formulated new goals for 6 more weeks of once-a-week therapy."

walking ability were assessed weekly. The treatment program included occupational therapy, physical therapy, and nursing. All members of the treatment team adhered strictly to the written protocol for each treatment developed from primary sources. The only significantly different outcome was greater improvement of gait speed by one patient in the Brunnstrom condition compared with the Bobath condition. The lack of difference detected in other subjects and for other assessments may be the result of alternating short periods of each treatment for each subject; that is, no subject received a full treatment program that followed one method. This is an important limitation because these methods have opposite views concerning the use of associated reactions. The recovery graphs for each patient showed steady recovery regardless of treatment, indicating that either (1) both methods were effective or (2) the subjects were recovering spontaneously. The actual interpretation cannot be made, however, because the study did not include a control condition (i.e., a period when no treatment was given) to determine the effects of spontaneous recovery alone. In a critical review of studies of interventions aimed at improving the paretic upper limb of stroke survivors, no significant difference was found among various "sensorimotor" treatment approaches, although these did not include the Brunnstrom approach, per se (Barreca et al., 2003).

SUMMARY REVIEW QUESTIONS

1. What are the assumptions of the Brunnstrom Movement Therapy approach?
2. What is an associated reaction and how is it elicited?
3. Describe the flexor synergy of the upper extremity and state which component or components are strongest.

4. Describe the extensor synergy of the upper extremity and state which component or components are strongest.
5. List in order the six recovery stages of the proximal upper extremity.
6. List in order the six stages of hand recovery.
7. Name the treatment principles of the Brunnstrom Movement Therapy approach.
8. How is the flexor synergy initiated in the upper extremity when the patient is flaccid?
9. How is elbow extension developed?
10. How is finger extension developed?

ACKNOWLEDGEMENT

Photography by Robert Littlefield and Catherine Trombly. Thanks are extended to the Sister Kenny Institute in Minneapolis, MN, for facilitating some of the photography. I especially acknowledge the participation of Alan Berg, Michelle Brown, M.Ed., OTR/L; Tim Carle; Larry R. Chaney; Susan Fasoli, Sc.D., OTR/L; Robb Miller, OTR/L; and Mary Vining Radomski, M.A., OTR/L.

References

Barreca, S., Wolf, S. L., Fasoli, S., & Bohannon, R. (2003). Treatment interventions for the paretic upper limb of stroke survivors: A critical review. *Neurorehabilitation and Neural Repair, 17,* 220–226.

Berglund, K., & Fugl-Meyer, A. R. (1986). Upper extremity function in hemiplegia: A cross-validation study of two assessment methods. *Scandinavian Journal of Rehabilitation Medicine, 18,* 155–157.

Boissy, P., Bourbonnais, D., Kaegi, C., Gravel, D., & Arsenault, B. A. (1997). Characterization of global synkineses during hand grip in hemiparetic patients. *Archives of Physical Medicine and Rehabilitation, 78,* 1117–1124.

Brunnstrom, S. (1956). Associated reactions of the upper extremity in adult patients with hemiplegia. *Physical Therapy Review, 36,* 225–236.

Brunnstrom, S. (1966). Motor testing procedures in hemiplegia. *Journal of the American Physical Therapy Association, 46,* 357–375.

Brunnstrom, S. (1970). *Movement therapy in hemiplegia.* New York: Harper & Row.

Butefisch, C., Hummelsheim, H., Denzler, P., & Mauritz, K-H. (1995). Repetitive training of isolated movements improves the outcome of motor rehabilitation of the centrally paretic hand. *Journal of Neurological Sciences, 130,* 59–68.

Dean, C. M., & Shepherd, R. B. (1997). Task related training improves performance of seated reaching tasks after stroke. *Stroke, 28,* 722–728.

Duncan, P. W., Goldstein, L. B., Horner, R. D., Landsman, P. B., Samsa, G. P., & Matchar, D. B. (1994). Similar motor recovery of upper and lower extremities after stroke. *Stroke, 25,* 1181–1188.

Duncan, P. W., Propst, M., & Nelson, S. G. (1983). Reliability of the Fugl-Meyer Assessment of sensorimotor recovery following cerebrovascular accident. *Physical Therapy, 63,* 1606–1610.

Fujiwara, T., Hara, Y., & Chino, N. (1999). The influence of nonparetic leg movements on muscle action in the paretic leg of hemiplegic patients. *Scandinavian Journal of Rehabilitation Medicine, 31,* 174–177.

Fugl-Meyer, A. R., Jaasko, L., Leyman, I., Olsson, S., & Steglind, S. (1975). The post-stroke hemiplegic patient: I. A method for evaluation of physical performance. *Scandinavian Journal of Rehabilitation Medicine, 7,* 13–31.

Kawahira, K., Shimodozono, M., Ogata, A., & Tanaka, N. (2004). Addition of intensive repetition of facilitation exercise to multidisciplinary rehabilitation promotes motor functional recovery of the hemiplegic lower limb. *Journal of Rehabilitation Medicine, 36,* 159–164.

Ma, H.-I., Trombly, C. A., & Robinson-Podolski, C. (1999). The effect of context on skill acquisition and transfer. *American Journal of Occupational Therapy, 53,* 138–144.

Malouin, F., Pichard, L., Bonneau, C., Durand, A., & Corriveau, D. (1994). Evaluating motor recovery early after stroke: Comparison of the Fugl-Meyer Assessment and the Motor Assessment Scale. *Archives of Physical Medicine and Rehabilitation, 75,* 1206–1212.

Mudie, M. H., & Matyas, T. A. (2000). Can simultaneous bilateral movement involve the undamaged hemisphere in reconstruction of neural networks damaged by stroke? *Disability and Rehabilitation, 22,* 23–27.

Nelson, D. L., Konosky, K., Fleharty, K., Webb, R., Newer, K., Hazboun, V. P., Fontane, C., & Licht, B. C. (1996). The effects of occupationally embedded exercise on bilaterally assisted supination in persons with hemiplegia. *American Journal of Occupational Therapy, 50,* 639–646.

Sanford, J., Moreland, J., Swanson, L. R., Stratford, P. W., & Gowland, C. (1993). Reliability of the Fugl-Meyer Assessment for testing motor performance in patients following stroke. *Physical Therapy, 73,* 447–454.

Smits, J. G., & Smits-Boone, E. C. (2000). *Hand recovery after stroke: Exercises and results measurements.* Boston: Butterworth Heinemann.

Trombly, C. A., & Wu, C.-Y. (1999). Effects of rehabilitation tasks on organization of movement after stroke. *American Journal of Occupational Therapy, 53,* 333–344.

Twitchell, T. (1951). The restoration of motor function following hemiplegia in man. *Brain, 74,* 443–480.

Wagenaar, R. C., Meijer, O. G., van Wieringen, P. C. W., Kuik, D. J., Hazenberg, G. J., Lindeboom, J., Wichers, F., & Rijswijk, H. (1990). The functional recovery of stroke: A comparison between neuro-developmental treatment and the Brunnstrom method. *Scandinavian Journal of Rehabilitation Medicine, 22,* 1–8.

Woodbury, M. L., & Velozo, C. (2005). Potential for outcomes to influence practice and support clinical competency. *OT Practice, 10,* 7–8.

Wu, C.-Y., Trombly, C. A., Lin, K.-C., & Tickle-Degnen, L. (2000). A kinematic study of contextual effects of reaching performance in persons with and without stroke: Influences of object availability. *Archives of Physical Medicine and Rehabilitation, 81,* 95–101.

CHAPTER 26

Managing Deficit of First-Level Motor Control Capacities Using Rood and Proprioceptive Neuromuscular Facilitation Techniques

Kathy Longenecker Rust

LEARNING OBJECTIVES

After studying this chapter the reader will be able to:

1. Use knowledge of controlled sensory input for making treatment choices to reduce first-order motor impairments and prepare patients with orthopedic and central nervous system conditions for successful participation in occupational performance.
2. Delineate treatment strategies for improving mobility and stability.
3. Analyze the diagonal components of functional activities and use this knowledge to utilize optimal movement patterns and positions in treatment.
4. Perform the proprioceptive neuromuscular facilitation diagonal patterns of the head, neck, trunk, and upper extremities.

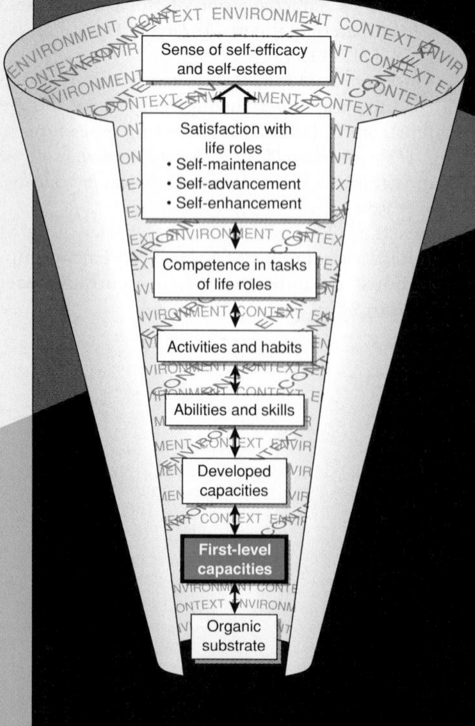

Glossary

Balance of antagonists—Normal mobility and strength of both agonist and antagonist muscles to allow successful motor function for activity to occur.

Chopping—Bilateral asymmetrical D1 extension. One arm performs the chop and the other hand is placed on the lateral-extensor surface of the distal forearm. The reversal of this pattern is the reverse of the chop.

Contracture—Fixed posture secondary to shortening or loss of elasticity of ligaments, joint capsule, tendons, and muscles (Preston & Hecht, 1999).

Controlled sensory stimulation—Concept that the neural component of tone can be affected by sensory stimuli applied in a specific manner to increase or reduce the electrical charge of interneurons or motor neurons, making them more or less likely to fire when they receive additional goal-specific stimulation from supraspinal centers.

Controlled mobility—The ability to perform fluid reversing motions necessary to perform skilled activity.

D1 extension—The final position of D1 extension is shoulder extension, abduction, and internal rotation; elbow extension; and pronation so that the hand passes the hip on the same side of the body. The wrist, fingers, and thumb extend, and fingers and thumb abduct. During range of motion exercises, D1 extension is combined with its reciprocal, D1 flexion.

D1 flexion—The final position of D1 flexion is shoulder flexion, adduction, and external rotation; elbow flexion; and supination so that the hand passes close to the ear on the opposite side of the head. Wrist, fingers, and thumb flex, and fingers and thumb adduct.

D2 extension—The final position of D2 extension is shoulder extension, adduction, and internal rotation; elbow extension; and pronation so that the hand moves past the opposite hip. Wrist flexes; fingers flex and adduct; and thumb opposes. During range of motion exercises, D2 extension is combined with its reciprocal, D2 flexion.

D2 flexion—The final position of D2 flexion is shoulder flexion, abduction, and external rotation; and supination so that the hand comes close to the ear on the same side of the head. Wrist extends, and fingers and thumb extend and abduct.

Lifting—Bilateral asymmetrical D2 flexion. One arm performs the lift, while the other arm maintains contact on the lateral flexor side of the forearm. The opposite of this pattern is called reverse of lift.

Normalization of tone—Process of changing excessive tone (hypertonia) or insufficient tone (hypotonia) to a state of normal tone needed for normal motor responses.

Overflow—The neuromuscular response to increasing resistance where the electrical activity of the interneuronal pool continues to rise with more and more motor units recruited to fire. Muscles are recruited in a predictable manner.

Reciprocal inhibition—The mechanism whereby contraction of an agonist muscle produces inhibition of its antagonist.

Vital functions—Respiration, facial motions, tongue motions, swallowing, and bowel and bladder control.

Without movement, occupational functioning is jeopardized. The organic substrate that supports movement includes the skeleton, muscles, sensory and motor nerves, heart, lungs, and skin. Therapists who developed the neurophysiological treatment approaches in the 1950s and 1960s presented clinical solutions to improve motor function for individuals who had impairments of these structures. In a seminal publication of the *American Journal of Physical Medicine* (1967), the proceedings of a 4-week conference on therapeutic exercise were detailed. One objective of the conference was to explore the thesis that an understanding of normal motor behavior is essential to the use of therapeutic exercise as a rehabilitative procedure and that exercise is bound to motor learning (Wood, 1967). Another important objective was to identify common denominators among the various approaches to treatment. Both of these objectives were met, and today there is a growing body of scientific evidence that supports many of the assumptions of the presenters. Chapters 24 and 25 describe the history and evolution of two of the approaches from this conference, the Bobath and Brunnstrom approaches. This chapter presents the methods of two additional approaches that have directed our understanding of how neuromuscular function affects occupational functioning. Both the Rood and proprioceptive neuromuscular facilitation (PNF) approaches share the commonality of using reflex arcs to elicit particular types of motor responses by supplying sensory stimulation in a controlled way. Another interesting similarity is that both of these approaches address **vital functions**. Understanding these mechanisms and using the techniques provide the occupational therapist with skills to affect first-level motor control capacities for patients with both orthopedic and neurological problems and for patients with muscle weakness secondary to primary illness or disuse. Facilitation and inhibition of muscle function along with the concepts of **stability** and **mobility** are basic to the application of **controlled sensory stimulation** used in both approaches.

DEVELOPED CAPACITIES OF STABILITY AND MOBILITY THAT SUPPORT MOVEMENT

When planning treatment and considering the goal of an activity, technique, or exercise to improve motor function, the first question that needs to be answered is whether the patient's limitation is due to a stability problem or a mobility problem. If both problems exist, then it is usually best to start with reestablishing stability. Stability is both dynamic and static. An individual must be able to maintain a posture and, when disturbed from a position, be able to recover the posture.

Mobility has two components. First of all, an individual needs adequate functional range of motion to engage in activity. The second aspect of mobility is the ability to initiate and sustain active range of motion (AROM) in activity. Patients with central nervous system (CNS) damage may lack this ability due to abnormal tone such as spasticity with concomitant weakness of the antagonist, flaccidity, loss of sensory input, and loss of voluntary control as is seen in conditions such as Parkinson's disease. Non-CNS conditions also exhibit muscle weakness.

The Rood approach addresses these components of motor function in Margaret Rood's classification of light-work or heavy-work muscles, her sequence for development of motor control, her ontogenic skeletal muscle sequence, and the techniques she identified for muscle facilitation and inhibition (Trombly, 1995). The PNF approach employs a similar model that addresses the progressive stages of movement control and also relies heavily on techniques for facilitation and inhibition of movement. The PNF approach, however, applies a broader scope of techniques, using additional applications of vision, sound, and normal reflex activity.

ABNORMAL TONE FOLLOWING CNS INJURY

After CNS injury, the basic first-level capacity of movement, muscle tone, changes (see Definition Box 6-2). Tone is a constant state of mild tension in the muscle. It is the characteristic of muscle that resists passive elongation or stretching (Gilman & Newman, 1992). Movement is superimposed on normal postural muscle tone (Carpenter, 1996; Gilman & Newman, 1992) and is difficult or impossible when tone is low or excessive. For persons with abnormal tone, the goal is **normalization of tone** to enable the patient to engage in and benefit from therapies and to accomplish the activities and tasks of daily life.

Hypertonicity, or high tone, is more than normal resistance to passive elongation. An arm that displays high tone requires effort from the therapist to move it in the direction opposite to the high tone, yet in its most frequent manifestation, it moves easily into the other direction. It was once believed that it was necessary to reduce excessive tone before voluntary movement could develop. Although current research indicates that that is not so (Ada et al., 1998; Malouin et al., 1997; O'Dwyer, Ada, & Neilson, 1996; Teixeira-Salmela et al., 1999), it is still important to decrease excessive tone. With abnormally high tone, malalignment of trunk and limbs occurs quickly because of shortening of spastic muscles on one side of a joint. If prolonged malaligned positioning is allowed, the outcome is a **contracture** with subsequent deformity and/or interference with basic activities of daily living (BADL) and increased caregiver burden. For example, an individual with end-stage multiple sclerosis may be confined to bed. Washing under the arm or the palm of the hand may be very difficult for the caregiver if the areas have high tone. These sequelae of hypertonicity should be prevented with daily stretching (Braddom, 1996).

Hypotonicity (low tone, or flaccidity) is less than normal resistance to passive elongation of the muscle. When a flaccid arm is moved, it feels heavy, and the muscles feel soft. If dropped, the arm falls because it cannot hold the position against gravity. For persons with low tone, the goal is to increase muscle response through sensory input and to blend this with the effort to move to accomplish goal-directed actions (Fig. 26-1). Even if movement is not achieved, it is important to increase tone to counteract joint subluxation, overstretching of muscles, edema, pain, and contracture. Normalization of muscle action is facilitated within the context of attempted goal-directed movement or maintained posture (Huss, 1971; Voss, 1967). Application of facilitation techniques alone is inadequate therapy. Even though the patient may not be able to do any activity, the effort to accomplish a simple goal is powerful and should be an integral part of every therapy session. Because attempting to accomplish a goal enhances neurological integration, facilitation is always done within an occupational context.

FACILITATION AND INHIBITION TECHNIQUES DEVELOPED PRIMARILY BY ROOD (1954, 1956, 1962)

Facilitation Techniques

Techniques to facilitate muscle activation include application of tactile, thermal, and proprioceptive stimuli, and stimuli to the special senses. These various techniques may be combined to produce a greater response.

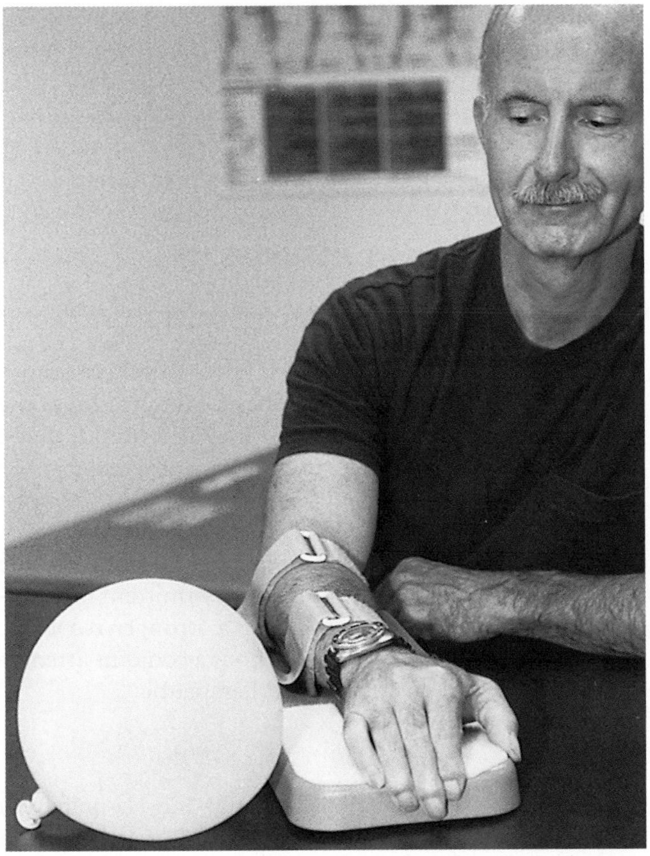

Figure 26-1 Patient's arm is supported on a therapeutic skate, a rectangular board supported by easily movable ball-bearing casters at the corners. With the slightest effort, the patient can move the arm at the shoulder and elbow on a smooth surface. The patient should concentrate on an activity goal rather than the movement per se. (Photo by Robert Littlefield, Scientific and Technical Photography, Dorchester, MA.)

Tactile Stimuli

Tactile stimulation is done using light touch (A-brushing) or fast brushing (C-brushing).

Light Touch

Light touch or stroking of the skin activates the low threshold A-size sensory fibers to activate a reflex action of the superficial phasic or mobilizing muscles (Rood, 1956, 1962; Stockmeyer, 1967). Light stroking of the dorsum of the webs of the fingers or toes, or of the palms of the hands or the soles of the feet elicits a fast, short-lived withdrawal motion of the stimulated limb (Rood, 1962). The stroking is done at a rate of twice per second for approximately 10 seconds (Rood, 1956). After a rest period, this procedure can be repeated 3–5 more times. When the reflex response occurs, resistance to the movement in activity is usually given to reinforce it and to help develop voluntary control over it (Stockmeyer, 1967).

Brushing

Fast brushing involves brushing the hairs or the skin over a muscle with a soft camel hair paintbrush that has been substituted for the stirrer of a hand-held battery-powered cocktail mixer to produce a high-frequency, high-intensity stimulus (Harris, 1969; Rood, 1962; Stockmeyer, 1967). The revolving brush, which is held sideways to avoid catching and pulling the hair, is applied on each skin area to be stimulated (Rood, 1956, 1962). Fast brushing is thought to stimulate the C-size sensory fibers, which discharge into polysynaptic pathways that influence the background activity of muscles involved in the maintenance of posture (Harris, 1969; Matyas & Spicer, 1980; Rood, 1962). Spindles so biased respond more readily to added external or internal stretch (Rood, 1962).

Rood (1962) proposed that the effect of fast brushing was non-specific, had a latency of 30 seconds, and reached its maximum facilitative state 30–40 minutes after stimulation because of the enhancement of the reticular activating system into which the C fibers feed. In controlled studies of fast brushing applied to normal and poststroke individuals, however, it was demonstrated that, although fast brushing produced a significant immediate facilitatory effect, the effect lasted only 30–45 seconds (Mason, 1985; Matyas & Spicer, 1980; Spicer & Matyas, 1980). Moreover, in normal subjects, the facilitatory effect was seen only in the lower extremity and not in the upper extremity.

Precautions necessary for controlled and appropriate fast brushing are listed in Safety Note 26-1.

Thermal Stimuli

Icing is thought to have similar effects as stroking and brushing through the same neural mechanisms (Harris, 1969; Rood, 1962). Icing, however, has been found to be significantly less effective than fast brushing for recruitment of motor units in hemiplegic patients (Matyas & Spicer, 1980). Two types of icing, A and C (referring to the size of the sensory fibers), are used.

A-Icing

A-icing is the application of three quick swipes of an ice cube to evoke a reflex withdrawal, similar to the response to light touch, when the stimulus is applied to the palms or soles or the dorsal webs of the hands or feet (Rood, 1962). The water is blotted up after every swipe. A-icing of the upper right quadrant of the abdomen in the dermatomal representation for T7-9 (along the rib cage) stimulates the diaphragm and inspiration. Touching the lips with ice opens the mouth (a withdrawal response). But ice applied to the tongue and inside the lips closes the mouth (Rood, 1962). Swiping the ice upward over the skin of the sternal notch promotes swallowing.

SAFETY NOTE 26-1

Precautions Necessary for Appropriate Application of Afferent Stimuli

- Fast brushing of the pinna of the ear stimulates the vagal parasympathetic fibers, which influence cardiorespiratory functions (Rood, 1962). Activation of these fibers slows the heart, constricts the smooth muscles of the bronchial tree, and increases bronchial secretions (Gilman & Newman, 1992). Fast brushing or scratching of the skin over the back at the level of S2-4 may cause bladder emptying (Gilman & Newman, 1992).
- In the application of C-icing, the distribution of the posterior primary rami along the back is avoided because it may cause a sympathetic nervous system fight or flight protective response (Rood, 1962; Huss, 1971).
- Icing of the pinna causes vagal responses, including cardiovascular reactions such as low blood pressure (Umphred, 1995). Ice to the back at the level of S2-4 may cause voiding (Rood, 1962).
- Prolonged icing is contraindicated for patients with Raynaud's phenomenon or circulatory disorders, including hypertension.
- Vibration applied on tendons can be conducted to adjacent muscles via the bone, and this possibility must be attended to and prevented (Dobkin, 1996; Preston & Hecht, 1999).
- Vibration should not be maintained longer than 1–2 minutes in any one place because of the heat that develops from the friction and potential for tearing thin skin. Vibration over areas previously immobilized can dislodge a blood clot and cause an embolism (Umphred, 1995).
- Scapulohumeral rhythm must be adhered to during all upper extremity range of motion (UE ROM) movements to prevent damage to the shoulder muscles and development of pain syndromes.
- Isometric contractions may produce the Valsalva maneuver, resulting in tachycardia and increased blood pressure, followed by reflexive bradycardia. Patients with cardiac conditions must be closely monitored.
- Application of quick stretch (QS) in diagonal patterns must be carefully applied. If a muscle is very near its full anatomical range (see D2 flexion example), application of too great a stretch may damage the muscle. Neck muscles are also close to their full anatomical range at the beginning of patterns.

C-Icing

C-icing is a high-threshold stimulus used to stimulate postural tonic responses via the C-size sensory fibers (Rood, 1962). Icing to activate the C fibers is done by holding the ice cube in place for 3–5 seconds, then wiping away the water. The skin areas to be stimulated are the same as for fast brushing, with one exception. ***The distribution of the posterior primary rami along the back is avoided because it may cause a sympathetic nervous system fight or flight protective response (Rood, 1962; Huss, 1971).*** Other precautions about icing are similar to those for brushing, see Safety Note 26-1.

Proprioceptive Stimuli

Quick Stretch

Quick, light stretch of a muscle is a low-threshold stimulus that activates an immediate phasic stretch reflex of the stretched muscle and inhibits its antagonist (Rood, 1962). Stretch is applied in the form of quick movement of the limb or tapping over the muscle or tendon. The therapist uses fingertips to vigorously tap the skin over a muscle or tendon while the patient is attempting to contract the muscle (see Fig. 25-8). This provides intermittent mechanical stretch to the muscle to evoke a stronger response. Evocation of the stretch reflex without a conjoint attempt to move or hold a position is not therapeutic.

Vibration

High-frequency (100–300 Hz, with 100–125 Hz preferred) vibration, delivered by an electric vibrator that has an excursion of 1–2 mm, to the belly or tendon of the slightly stretched muscle is an additional form of stretch (Umphred, 1995) (Fig. 26-2). The action of the vibrator pro-

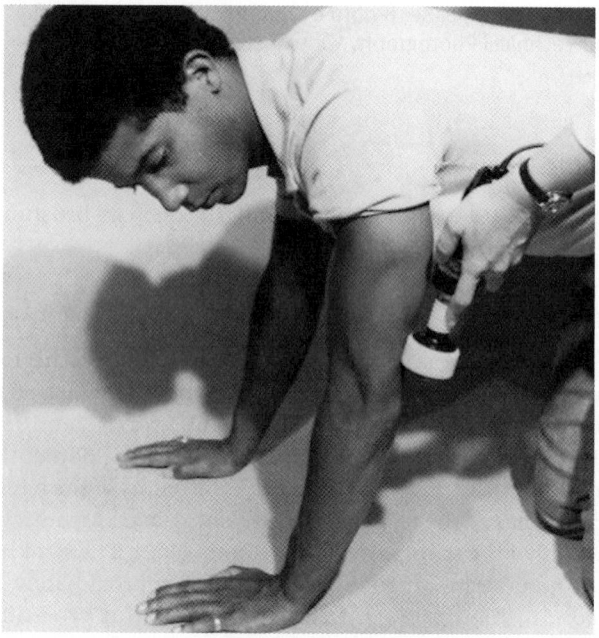

Figure 26-2 An electrical vibrator is applied to the triceps tendon to elicit a sustained elbow extensor response while the patient is weight bearing in quadruped.

vides a rapidly repeated mechanical stretch to the muscle, which increases the number of motor units recruited. This is the tonic vibratory reflex (TVR). Tension within the muscle increases over 30–60 seconds and is sustained for the duration of the application of the vibrator (Umphred, 1995). The stronger response is obtained from application over the tendon. Vibration evokes a tonic holding contraction and adds to the strength of an already weakly contracting muscle.

Stretch to Finger Intrinsics

Stretch to the intrinsic muscles of the hand is used to facilitate co-contraction of the muscles around the shoulder joint (Ayres, 1974; Stockmeyer, 1967). Forcefully grasping handles of tools obtains this response, especially if the handles have been modified to be spherical or conical, with the widest part of the cone at the ulnar border of the hand, both of which increase intermetacarpal stretch. This treatment is used for patients who have distal movement but proximal weakness.

Heavy Joint Compression

Heavy joint compression facilitates co-contraction of muscles around a joint, thereby facilitating the stability component of movement in activity. Heavy compression refers to resistance greater than body weight that is applied so that the force is through the longitudinal axes of the bones whose articular surfaces approximate each other (Ayres, 1974; Rood, 1962). Resistance greater than body weight is resistance that is more than the weight of the body parts usually supported by the joint. One method by which heavy joint compression can be achieved during activity is to have the patient, who is in a weight-bearing position, lift one limb off the supporting surface. The arm still in contact with the surface now has more than the usual weight. Other methods include compression delivered by the therapist or the addition of weights, for example, having the client wear a weighted cap.

Resistance

Resistance to an ongoing movement or maintained posture is a form of stretch in which many or all of the spindles of a muscle are stimulated (Umphred, 1995). The muscle spindle, of course, cannot know whether the discrepancy between itself and the extrafusal muscle fibers is due to stretching by a moving force or by resistance that is preventing extrafusal muscle fibers from shortening as the spindle continues to shorten as programmed. The discrepancy causes the spindle to fire. The electrical activity of the interneuronal pool is consequently high, and more and more motor units are more easily recruited to fire; this phenomenon is called **overflow**.

Inhibition Techniques

Hypertonicity is treated with general inhibition techniques or by applying tactile, thermal, or proprioceptive stimulation either to the muscle itself or to the antagonists of the spastic muscle in the context of goal-directed activity. It is hypothesized that, when stimulation is applied to the antagonist, the relaxation effect in the agonist spastic muscle occurs through **reciprocal inhibition**. The reciprocal inhibition mechanism of persons post stroke, however, has been found to be disturbed and may result in unexpected outcomes (Okuma & Lee, 1996). Therefore, application of these techniques in this population must be monitored carefully.

Some of the following methods are aimed at the neural component of hypertonicity, and others, such as prolonged stretching, address the viscoelastic component. The therapist determines which component needs treatment and chooses appropriate techniques.

Tactile Stimuli

Slow stroking over the distribution of the posterior primary rami produces general relaxation. It involves rhythmical moving touch instead of maintained touch. The person lies prone or sits unsupported in a quiet environment with his or her back exposed. The therapist uses the palm or extended fingers of one hand to apply firm pressure along the vertebral musculature from occiput to coccyx, at which time the therapist's other hand starts at the occiput and progresses likewise to the coccyx. One hand is always in contact with the patient. This slow, rhythmical stroking using alternating hands is done until the patient relaxes or for about 3–5 minutes (Rood, 1956; Farber, 1982).

Thermal Stimuli

Both warming and cooling can be inhibitory.

Neutral Warmth

Neutral warmth refers to maintaining body heat by wrapping the specific area to be inhibited or the area served by the posterior primary rami for a general effect. A cotton flannel or fleece blanket or a down comforter is used for 10–20 minutes (Ayres, 1974; Huss, 1971). Neutral heat, rather than heat greater than body temperature, is used to avoid a rebound effect in 2–3 hours. The rebound effect manifests as facilitated or even superfacilitated muscles (Rood, 1962). Elastic bandages and air splints (see Fig. 16-75) can be used also. They not only maintain neutral warmth but also offer sustained pressure, both of which are inhibitory (Preston & Hecht, 1999).

Prolonged Cooling

Sustained cooling of the skin to 50°F (10°C) decreases the monosynaptic stretch reflex excitability (Preston & Hecht, 1999). A cold pack applied for 20 minutes achieves this effect (Braddom, 1996).

Proprioceptive Stimuli

Several proprioceptive techniques to inhibit one or both components of hypertonicity are described next.

Prolonged Stretch

Prolonged manual stretch is used to inhibit a specific spastic muscle so that the patient may move more easily (Carey, 1990). The limb is held so that the muscle is *steadily* kept at its greatest length for more than 20 seconds, until letting go is felt as the muscle adjusts to the longer length. As a special case of this inhibitory procedure, prolonged holding of the thumb in abduction and extension may relax a tight grasp.

Prolonged stretch by splinting or positioning the limb so that the hypertonic muscles are maintained in stretch over several hours to several weeks allows growth of additional sarcomeres and makes the muscle less sensitive to stretch during movement (O'Dwyer, Ada, & Neilson, 1996). The mechanical lengthening also changes the viscoelastic configuration of muscle by disrupting crossbridges between myosin and actin filaments and/or by reducing the stiffness of periarticular connective tissue (Carey, 1990). See serial casting in Chapter 16.

Joint Approximation

Light joint compression, also called joint approximation, can be used to inhibit specific spastic muscles. This procedure is commonly used to relieve shoulder pain due to spastic muscles in hemiplegic patients. The method is to grasp the patient's elbow and, while holding the humerus abducted to about 35–45°, gently move the head of the humerus into the glenoid fossa and hold it there (Fig. 26-3) until the spastic muscles relax (Ayres, 1963, 1974).

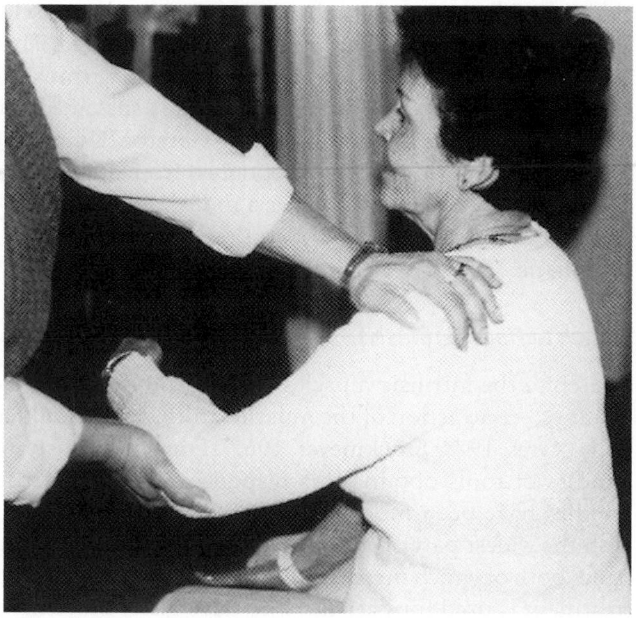

Figure 26-3 Light joint compression, or joint approximation, is used to inhibit spastic muscles and to allow range of motion.

Tendon Pressure

Pressure on the tendinous insertion of a muscle inhibits that muscle (Ayres, 1974; Huss, 1971; Stockmeyer, 1967). The extrinsic flexors of the hand may be inhibited by applying constant pressure over the length of the long tendons (Stockmeyer, 1967) through grasp of enlarged, hard handles of tools or utensils or via splints.

Vestibular Stimuli

Slow, rhythmical movement is inhibiting (Huss, 1971). Slow rolling is done by the therapist holding the patient at the hip and shoulder and slowly rolling him or her from supine to side-lying (Fig. 26-4). The patient should be lying comfortably, with a pillow under the head and between the knees if necessary for comfort. A decrease in hypertonicity should be seen within minutes.

Stimuli for the Special Senses

Rood (1962) used stimulation to the special senses to facilitate or inhibit the skeletal musculature generally. Auditory and visual stimuli can be used deliberately.

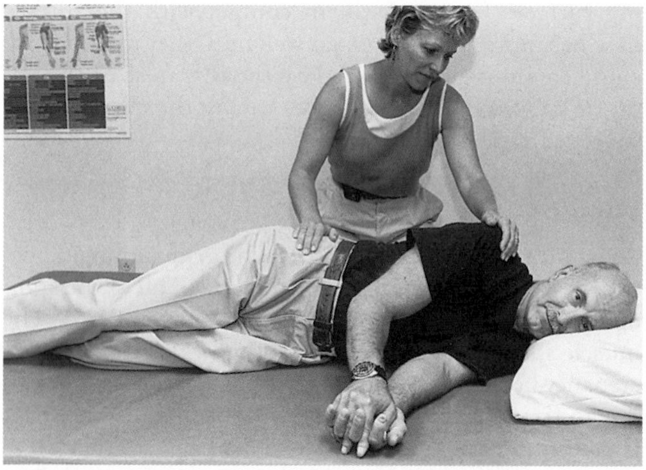

Figure 26-4 Slow rolling inhibits spastic or tense muscles. The therapist holds the patient at the hip and shoulder and *slowly* rolls him from supine to side-lying and back again. (Photo by Robert Littlefield, Scientific and Technical Photography, Dorchester, MA.)

However, auditory and visual stimuli also occur incidental to treatment, a fact of which the therapist needs to be aware. Music with a definite beat is facilitatory. A noisy, raucous clinic is stimulating and may affect the performance of the patient with CNS dysfunction. A colorful, bright multistimulus environment has a general facilitatory effect. The therapist's voice and manner of speech (fast and staccato vs. slow and calming) may also affect the patient's performance. A loud, sharp command yields a quick response and recruits more motor units (Voss, 1967).

Olfactory and gustatory stimuli are facilitating or inhibiting through their influence on the autonomic nervous system. Unpleasant or dangerous stimuli (like ammonia smell) elicit a sympathetic fight or flight reaction, and pleasant stimuli (like vanilla) evoke a parasympathetic response that inhibits the sympathetic response (Rood, 1962). These stimuli, especially olfactory, produce an emotional response as well as a motor response.

Moving from Muscle Contraction to Movement

As noted earlier, facilitation and inhibition techniques are used in conjunction with attempts at goal-directed action for the purpose of enabling development of movement-related capacities and abilities. Rood (1962) identified a sequence regarding the development of movement that is useful in guiding activity choices. She stated that movement first appears as phasic, reciprocal shortening and lengthening contractions of the muscles that cause movement subserving a protective function. Such movements might be facilitated using A-brushing or A-icing. In these phasic movements, muscles contract to cause movement through range, which produces reciprocal inhibition of the antagonists (Ayres, 1974; Rood, 1962). The movement of an infant waving his or her extremities back and forth when shown a desired object typifies phasic movement. Movement to touch an object or bat away a lightweight object, such as a balloon or bubble, is the first voluntary movement to aim for in patients beginning to develop tone and movement.

After phasic movements begin, tonic holding contractions are next to develop, according to Rood. Stability is obtained through co-contraction, such as occurs during heavy joint compression (Ayres, 1974; Stockmeyer, 1967). A goal-directed action, such as leaning on the desk with the affected arm while writing with the unaffected hand, is again sought.

PNF APPROACH AS TAUGHT BY VOSS

Proprioceptive neuromuscular facilitation (PNF) has been defined as "a method of promoting or hastening the response of the neuromuscular mechanism through stimulation of the proprioceptors" (Voss, Ionta, & Myers, 1985, p. xvii). To take the name of the approach literally, however, is to do disservice to the comprehensive theory proposed by the originators of the approach. As we see with the techniques outlined in the Rood approach, clinical reasoning considering the beneficial aspects of the application of controlled sensory input leads to the application of multisensory afferent input. The PNF approach uses these sensory tools additively after evaluating the functional problem and identifying the necessary diagonal patterns of movement in the appropriate positions. Also, the clinical reasoning to enhance first-level motor control capacities considers the patient's breathing, pain, and general arousal level congruent with motor performance. Treatment sessions start with attention to therapeutic applications for breathing. Controlled sensory input and the effects of reflex activity are superimposed on movement patterns to provide as many favorable influences as possible to affect motor function that is the basis for skills and abilities. Baum et al. (1998) published a case study that demonstrates some of these multiple applications in an exercise protocol for a patient with acute C5 quadriplegia. The approach as described in this chapter presents basic knowledge and techniques directed toward the entry-level occupational therapist.

The Rotational Requirement for Developed Movement Capacities

The PNF approach is based on patterns of motion identified in 1951 by Kabat, a neurophysiologist and physician, while working with the other developers of the approach, Maggie Knott and Dorothy Voss, physical therapists (Myers, 1995). All parts of the body, head and neck, trunk, limbs, and even facial muscles have two diagonal patterns based on normal motor activity, and the motor pattern itself is a method of facilitation. The stronger muscles in the diagonal patterns influence weaker ones, which is in keeping with the axiom that the brain knows nothing of individual muscle action but knows only of movement (Voss, Ionta, & Myers, 1985). The skeletal, ligamentous, and muscular systems of the body support these patterns. Muscle alignment is spiral and diagonal. Shimura and Kasai (2002) investigated the effect of starting a movement pattern from a neutral position of the wrist versus starting with the wrist in the PNF-prescribed position. The initiation of voluntary wrist movement was operationalized in terms of the electromyographic reaction time (EMG-RT) and the excitability of the motor cortex as measured by motor-evoked potentials (MEPs). The PNF group performed significantly better. The authors concluded that the amount of sensory input coming from the periphery was greater in the PNF position. Also, the PNF position improved movement efficiency by inducing changes in the sequence in which the muscles were activated.

The PNF diagonal patterns are combinations of the cardinal plane movements of flexion or extension, abduction or adduction, and internal or external rotation. The inclusion of a rotary component in all movement patterns is the unique aspect of the approach. Therapeutic applications, as we see in analysis of normal human movement, are not performed in cardinal planes of movement. In this approach, all movement patterns are reversing. If you reach up to install a light bulb, you need to be able to bring your arm back down. To perform these functional reversing patterns of the diagonal movements, a **balance of antagonists** is required. If a patient does not have this balance, treatment must start with techniques that focus on the agonist.

A significant body of literature from the disciplines of exercise physiology, sports medicine, athletic training, and physical education purports to investigate many of the PNF stretching techniques. Most of these studies, however, implement exercise in only one plane of motion. PNF patterns are performed in all three planes of movement (sagittal, frontal, and horizontal) simultaneously. Although the research generally substantiates the hypotheses that the techniques tested achieve increased ROM, two major problems preclude any generalization of findings to the clinical practice of PNF. The first major problem with the studies that focus on hamstring tightness to demonstrate effectiveness of PNF stretching (Bonnar, Deivert, & Gould, 2004; Carter et al., 2000; Feland & Marin, 2004; Feland, Myrer, & Merril, 2001; Ferber, Osternig, & Gravelle, 2002; Funk et al., 2003; Rowlands, Marginson, & Lee, 2002; Spernoga et al., 2001; Stopka et al., 2002) is that passive range of motion (PROM) and isometric and isotonic contractions are used with only the hamstrings and their antagonists applied in the position of a straight leg raise from the hip. Movement occurs only in the sagittal plane, and not in the diagonal patterns of a PNF approach. Similarly, a study testing the effects of contract-relax (CR) on the soleus muscle involved only sagittal plane movement (Etnyre & Abraham, 1986). Without rotation, these are not PNF techniques.

The second major problem with "PNF" research from the athletic sciences is the manner in which these studies define and apply their techniques. The use of hold-relax (HR) and CR are very common in athletic training. Unfortunately, they are not using the techniques as they were originally developed. For example, Young and Elliott (2001) described their CR procedure as a maximal isometric contraction against resistance, relaxation, and passive stretch by the examiner "where the participant held the stretch for 15 s [seconds]" (p. 275). Compare this to the definition in Procedures for Practice 26-1, which summarizes the PNF relaxation techniques as developed by Knott and Voss.

The Two Diagonal Patterns of Movement for Each Body Part

Note that vision is always combined with diagonal patterns.

Head and Neck, Trunk

- Flexion [of head and neck, or head, neck, and trunk] with rotation [of head and neck, or head, neck, and trunk] to the right (reversing, extension with rotation to the left)
- Flexion [of head and neck, or head, neck, and trunk] with rotation [of head and neck, or head, neck, and trunk] to the left (reversing, extension with rotation to the right)

Head and neck patterns may be performed specifically, but they are generally combined with the patterns of the trunk and extremities. Beazell (1998) published a case study of the use of the head and neck patterns for a patient who incurred two incidents of cervical trauma. Trunk patterns will naturally include the head and neck patterns when the patient is upright.

Upper Extremity

- Diagonal one (D1): **D1 flexion** combines flexion + adduction + external rotation at the shoulder (Fig. 26-5). It reverses as **D1 extension**, which combines the shoulder movements of extension + abduction + internal rotation (Fig. 26-6).
- D1 extension, when performed in a bilateral asymmetrical pattern, is called **chopping**, and D1 flexion is called **reverse of chop**.
- Diagonal two (D2): **D2 flexion** combines flexion + abduction + external rotation at the shoulder (Fig. 26-7). It reverses as **D2 extension**, combining extension + adduction + internal rotation of the shoulder (Fig. 26-8).
- D2 flexion, when performed in a bilateral asymmetrical pattern is called **lifting**, and D2 extension is called **reverse of lift**.

The upper extremity patterns are named by the direction of movement at the shoulder joint. A flexion pattern occurs when the patient moves his or her arm upward to retrieve an object from a high shelf. As the arm moves in a downward direction, as it does when we put on socks, this is an extension pattern. Again, patients are always directed to look at their hand while they move. In this manner, the movements of the head, neck, and trunk reinforce limb movements. The movements of the forearm and hand are delineated in the Glossary. It is important to note that some joints do not

PROCEDURES FOR PRACTICE 26-1

PNF Relaxation Techniques

Understand before you start:

- The techniques are based on reciprocal inhibition.
- "Any technique which demands or makes possible a gain in range of motion in one pattern has achieved relaxation of its antagonist" (Knott & Voss, 1968, p. 98).
- Contract = isotonic contraction.
- Hold = isometric contraction.
- The agonist is the pattern that has limited motion.
- The antagonist is the muscle or muscles that are shortened, limiting the range of the agonist pattern.

Technique	Method
Contract–Relax (CR)	1. Passive or active-assisted movement in the agonist pattern until limit is felt
Indication: When agonist is weak	2. Isotonic contraction of antagonist pattern ("Turn and pull" or "Turn and push") and resist 3. Relaxation 4. Passively move through new available range; repeat
Hold–Relax (HR)	1. An isometric contraction of the antagonist
Indication: Muscle spasm with pain	2. Relaxation 3. Active movement of the agonist by the patient
Slow Reversal–Hold–Relax (SRHR)	1. Isotonic contraction of the agonist
Indication: When the patient has the ability to move the agonist	2. Isometric contraction of the antagonist 3. Relaxation 4. Active movement of the agonist
Rhythmic rotation (Rro)	1. Perform PROM until resistance is met
Indication: Hypertonicity	2. Slowly and gently repeat and reverse rotation of all limb segments 3. Continue PROM and repeat

These principles have been derived from the writings of Myers (1995).

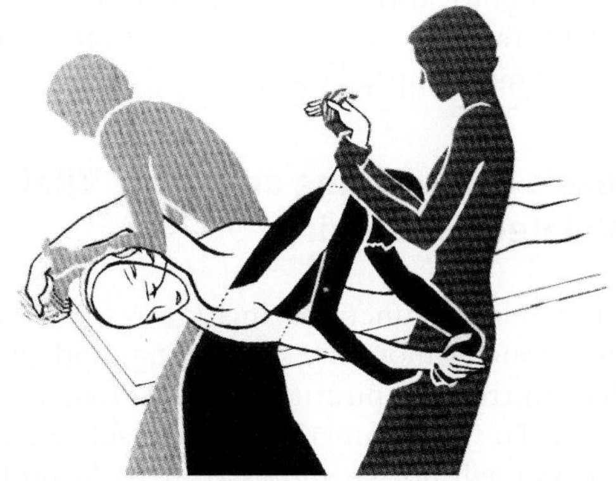

Figure 26-5 D1 flexion. Starting position is represented by the darkest drawing of the therapist. Manual contacts: The therapist's left hand is in patient's palm (thumb to thumb), and her right arm wraps under to contact the flexor tendons of the forearm. Patient's head is drawn to demonstrate how the head and neck turn while the patient watches his or her hand during the movement. Note the therapist's movement as the pattern progresses (progressively lighter drawings). Note: Figures 26-5, 6, 7, and 8 are used with permission from: Voss, D.E., Ionta, M.K., & Myers, B.J. (1985). *Proprioceptive Neuromuscular Facilitation: Patterns & Techniques* (3rd ed.). New York: Harper & Row.

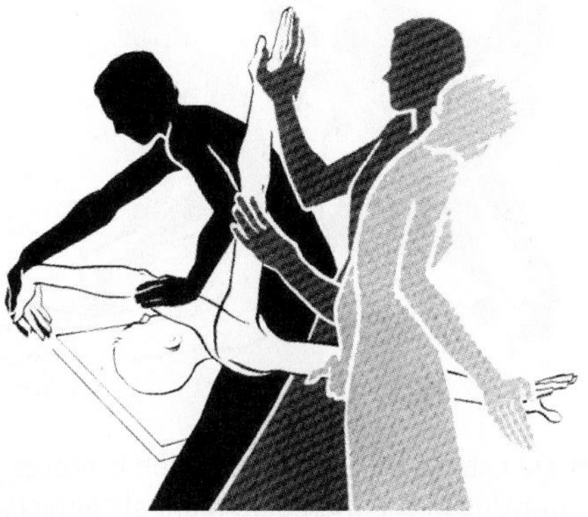

Figure 26-6 D1 extension. Starting position is represented by the darkest drawing of the therapist. Manual contacts: Therapist's right hand is over the dorsum of the patient's hand, while the therapist's left hand cradles the triceps.

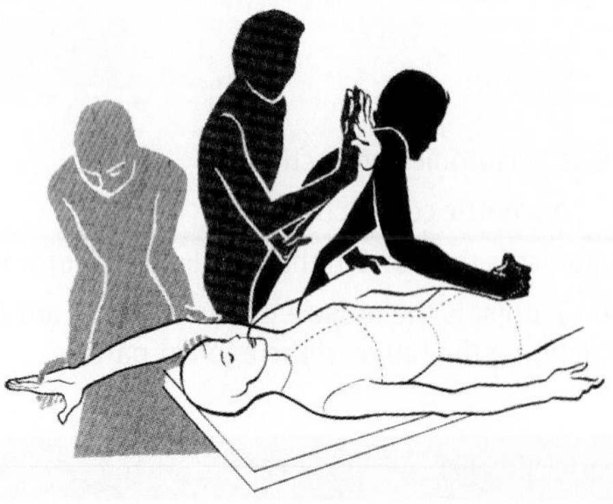

Figure 26-7 D2 flexion. Starting position is represented by the darkest drawing of the therapist. Manual contacts: Therapist's right hand is over the dorsum of the patient's hand, and her left hand is over the triceps.

move through their full anatomical ranges in diagonal patterns. The PNF patterns represent functional range of motion.

Another attribute of the diagonal patterns is that each upper extremity muscle is a prime mover in one of the patterns. Sullivan and Portney (1980) demonstrated this in a study that electromyographically recorded muscle activity during diagonal patterns of shoulder musculature in 29 healthy adults. Therefore, the therapist selects the optimum pattern for particular muscles (see example of radial nerve injury, below).

As the arm starts in a pattern, all of the muscles are in their lengthened range. As the pattern continues, the muscles of the pattern contract, and when the movement is completed, the muscles are now in their shortened range. This distinction between shortened range and lengthened range is important because the muscles respond differently in the application of quick stretch (QS) based on their length.

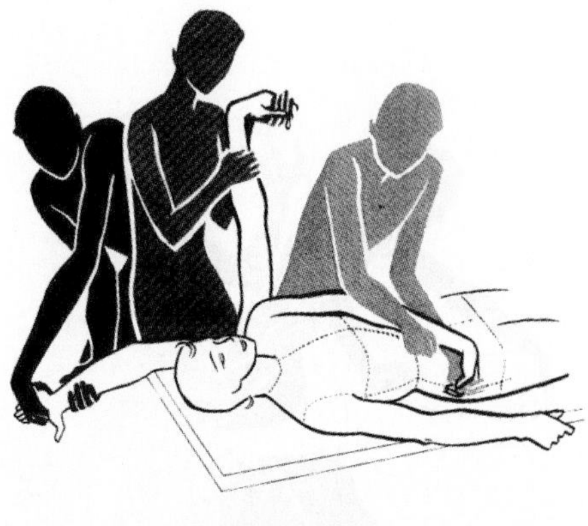

Figure 26-8 D2 extension. Starting position is represented by the darkest drawing of the therapist. Manual contacts: The therapist's left hand is in the palm of the patient's left hand, and her right hand is over the finger and wrist flexors in the forearm.

It is easiest to learn the upper extremity patterns as unilateral or bilateral symmetrical patterns. In treatment though, for the majority of applications, attention is always given to how to use the upper extremities in contact, that is, when one hand contacts the opposite forearm and wrist with the patient facilitating their own flexion or extension pattern with manual contact (see below) over the muscle that is acting in the pattern. These patterns are technically bilateral asymmetrical patterns but are most commonly called *chopping* and *lifting*. Keeping both upper extremities in contact is referred to as self-touch, and Voss, Ionta, and Myers (1985) described the spontaneous appearance of self-touch during development, during daily activity, and in the patient in pain. The facilitatory effect of self-touch is frequently described as "closing the sensory loop."

The PNF approach also uses two other upper extremity patterns called thrusting patterns, but they are not included in this chapter because they add an additional level of complexity when learning the basic D1 and D2 movements.

Lower Extremity

There are two diagonal patterns in the lower extremities as well, but they will not be discussed here. The advanced occupational therapy PNF practitioner may use these patterns to facilitate functional ambulation or to retrain bowel and bladder control (Voss, Ionta, & Myers, 1985). Yigiter et al. (2002) compared traditional prosthetic training versus PNF resisted gait training in patients with transfemoral amputations. Although both groups improved significantly on all measures ($p < 0.05$), the group who received intervention based on the PNF approach had more improvement.

Emphasis on Breathing and Other Vital and Related Functioning

Vital and related functions include respiration, facial motions, tongue motions, swallowing, and bowel and bladder control. Respiration is addressed in all PNF treatment. The other functions are considered advanced practice and will not be addressed here. Stimulation of the intrinsic muscles of respiration and increased AROM of the chest and diaphragm is achieved by directing facilitory techniques toward motions of the lateral chest walls, upper chest, sternum, and diaphragm (Voss, Ionta, & Myers, 1985). Nitz and Burke (2002) performed a randomized double-blind study of PNF breathing techniques and found that the combined techniques of PNF were the main contributor to improvement in arterial oxygen saturation for subjects

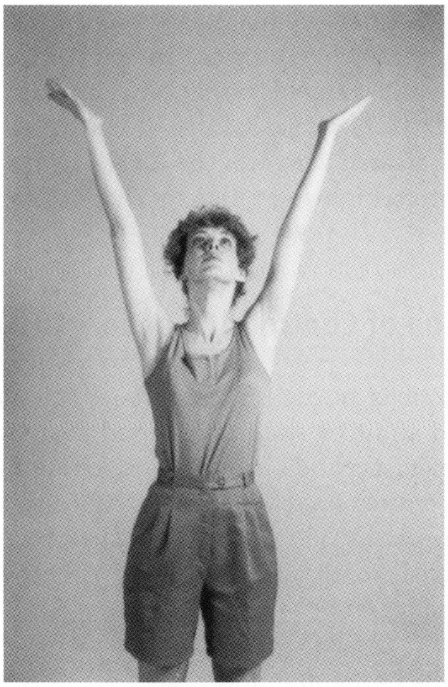

Figure 26-9 Bilateral symmetrical D2 flexion, shortened range; bilateral symmetrical D2 extension, lengthened range. Shoulders flex, abduct, externally rotate; elbows extend (as the intermediate joint, the elbow, may flex or extend); forearms supinate; wrists extend toward radial side; fingers extend and abduct; and thumbs extend and adduct.

with myotonic dystrophy. Two methods to facilitate breathing are as follows.

Bilateral Symmetrical (BS) D2 Pattern of the Upper Extremities Combined with Trunk Movements

To facilitate breathing, patients are placed in upright positions or in supine. Both arms do the D2 pattern, combined with trunk flexion and extension. Quick stretch (QS, described below) is added by the therapist, along with an appropriate tone of voice and manual contacts (MC) in the direction of trunk flexion, shoulder extension, or both. The bilateral symmetrical D2 flexion pattern of the extremities facilitates trunk extension and expands the chest (Fig. 26-9). If a patient lacks upper extremity strength or ROM to complete the full D2 pattern, the therapist may actively assist the patient or the patient may move only through partial ROM or perform the pattern with elbows bent. Bending the elbow reduces the resistance of the arm, which reduces the effort necessary to perform the movement.

Facilitation of the Chest Wall Muscles in Side-Lying or Supine

In side-lying or supine positions, the therapist applies manual contacts on the chest walls using quick stretch (QS) at the end of exhalation to enhance the inspiratory response. The muscles of the chest attach so that their placement relative to the ribs is diagonal. MCs are applied directly over the muscles of the chest wall considering their diagonal orientation. This method is used with patients in acute care who cannot be moved from supine.

Positions and Movement between Postures

Treatment planning considers the best position for the patient and the need to move between postures. These postures are combinations of the patterns of the head, neck, trunk, and extremities, as necessary, to accomplish the motor aspects of occupational performance. Positions include side-lying, prone on elbows, hands-knees, plantigrade, kneeling, half-kneeling, long sitting, short sitting (knees flexed from long sitting position), tailor sitting (sitting with knees bent and legs crossed), heel sitting, side-sitting, and chair sitting (Myers, 1981). Modified plantigrade is a frequently used position where the client is standing or sitting with both arms in contact with a surface such as a table. Having clients bear weight on their elbows can further modify this. Consider the balance requirement of each position. Are there different demands for the head and neck; for the trunk; for the upper extremity; or for the lower extremity?

Several factors influence the choice of postures in therapy. For more involved patients, treatment is started in the position in which the client is most stable. Frequently this is side-lying, although patients in acute care may need to start supine in bed. The progression toward the use of the arm and hand in activities considers basic mobility (adequate ROM), stability, **controlled mobility**, and finally skill. Stability is comprised of two sequential skills: tonic holding, where muscles can perform an isometric contraction in their shortened range; and co-contraction, where muscles are able to maintain isometric contractions in their midrange. Controlled mobility is the ability to use a limb in a smooth and regulated movement against gravity. Once a patient demonstrates stability in a bilateral weight-bearing position and demonstrates the ability to perform isometric contractions in the midrange, tasks are presented where one arm leaves the contact surface to engage in activity (Fig. 26-10). As controlled mobility improves, patients will be able to move their arm through greater arcs of active range of motion (AROM). When one arm is stationary and the other arm is moving, PNF terms this position simultaneous static dynamic (SSD).

Another consideration when choosing postures is the activity of the client. If the activity that the client is performing is difficult, then the postural demand is lowered. Conversely, if the activity is not challenging, then the postural demand may be increased. For example, a patient who has the goal of signing his or her

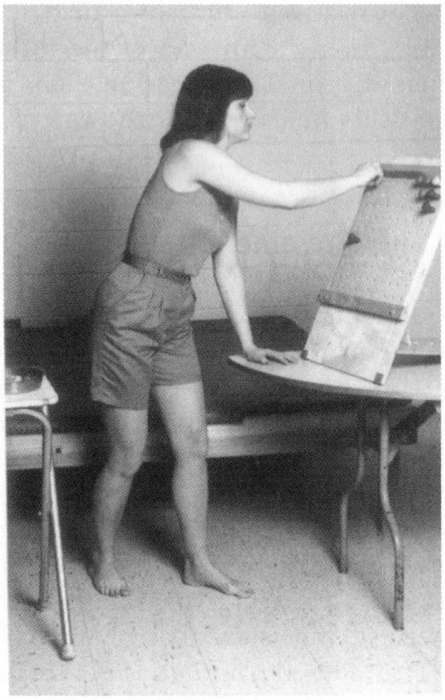

Figure 26-10 Bilateral reciprocal D1 in a palmar prehension activity. Note the simultaneous static and dynamic position, with the left arm weight bearing (static) in D1 extension and the right arm moving (dynamic) in D1 flexion.

name (difficult activity) may work on writing activities in prone on elbows (lowered postural demand). If a patient is performing a surface contact activity like washing a counter (easy), standing may be the posture of choice (high demand).

Finally, movement between postures is an essential skill. Patients may start a treatment session in side-lying, progress to side-sitting and then to kneeling, and then return to a less demanding posture such as heel sitting as they fatigue. A progression beginning with bilateral weight bearing, moving to an activity performed in a simultaneous static dynamic (SSD) position, and then moving back again to weight bearing demonstrates an upper extremity-based progression between postures. In these sequences, by asking patients to look at their hands or in the direction of the activity, reflex support (see below) reduces conscious effort (Voss, 1967).

The Influence of Reflex Activity

A basic tenet of the PNF approach is that the reflex mechanisms underlying normal movements are potent forces for influencing movement and posture (Voss, Ionta, & Myers, 1985). The tonic neck reflexes and righting reflexes (see Chapter 6) are used to influence movement. For example, in assisting a patient who is lying supine in bed to roll to side-lying, a very important functional movement, the facilitory effects of the asymmetric tonic neck reflex (ATNR) and optical righting reflex are used as the therapist simultaneously slaps the surface of the bed and uses a sharp tone of voice in the command "Look over here" while using his or her other arm at the scapula or hip to actively assist rolling. Looking at where the therapist indicated activates the ATNR by neck rotation and the optical righting reflex by change in position of the head.

Application of Controlled Sensory Input

As was described in the Rood approach, tactile, proprioceptive, and auditory systems are used in treatment. The PNF approach expands proprioceptive input to include inner ear receptors (in reflex support) and also includes an essential emphasis on visual input. The procedures that follow are basic to the approach and part of the treatment of every patient.

Proprioceptive Stimuli

The proprioceptive input as applied in PNF has many similarities to the manner in which it is used in the Rood approach. For example, the physiology that supports the use of quick stretch (QS) is the same; however, in the PNF approach, the therapist administers QS with his or her manual contacts to muscles in their lengthened range.

Traction and Approximation

Traction, or separation of joint surfaces, promotes mobility by stimulating the joint receptors that are sensitive to stretch (Knott & Voss, 1968). Approximation, or compression of the joint surfaces, promotes joint stability.

Quick Stretch (QS)

Muscles respond with greater force after stretch, particularly when they are in their lengthened positions. Stretch increases feedback from muscle and joint receptors and enhances the response. Specific to PNF, however, is the precept that QS is always applied to all three components of the diagonal pattern with an emphasis on the rotational components (Voss, Ionta, & Myers, 1985). As mentioned earlier, the PNF diagonal patterns do not require full anatomical range of motion. The difference between the PNF position and full anatomical range allows for the safe application of stretch to a muscle. For example, if you want to facilitate the D2 flexion pattern for an overhead reaching activity, the patient's arm begins in the lengthened range of D2 flexion (shortened range of D2 extension), and the therapist places manual contacts to the back of the hand and to the dorsal surface of the scapula. Then, the therapist quickly leans a slight bit more into the D2 extension pattern and administers QS at the same time giving the verbal command for movement. ***Avoid excessive stretch to the wrist extensors. In this starting position, the wrist extensors are close to their end range anatomical position.*** In the PNF approach, the therapist's entire body is involved in the application of QS, not just his or his hands and arms. This is a much smoother and safer application. Study the beginning position in Figure 26-7. To facilitate the movement with QS, the therapist moves very slightly but quickly into the D2 extension pattern and commands the patient to execute the movement. Immediately, the patient responds and performs the D2 flexion pattern.

Resistance

Resistance is used to improve muscle contraction. Padua et al. (2004) used a PNF intervention as one of three shoulder exercise protocols on 57 physically active college-age men and women. Although all three exercise protocols resulted in significant improvement ($p < 0.05$) on measures of strength, active angle reproduction, and single arm balance, only the PNF group demonstrated significant improvement in functional performance (throwing). The PNF group actively performed D1 and D2 patterns against maximal resistance offered manually by the investigator. From a PNF perspective, we resist the patient's effort while, at the same time, we are part of the movement. The therapist moves at the same time as the patient. If the therapist does not move, the pattern will be blocked. As was described for QS, graded resistance is applied by the therapist using whole-body movements. Although pulleys or weights may provide resistance as the client works independently, manual resistance through manual contacts (MCs) and the therapist's use of his or her body is integral to the approach. Resistance can be provided in many different ways depending on the goal, such as only at the end of ROM in a pattern; intermittently as the patient moves through the pattern (this is called repeated contractions, or RC); or continuously throughout the range. Figures 26-6 and 26-8 demonstrate how the therapist applies resistance with one choice of placement for manual contacts in the extension patterns. Understanding how resistance is applied in these patterns is important because the muscles of the extension patterns will not be fully activated without resistance. In most positions, the effect of gravity will cause the muscles of the flexion pattern to work in an eccentric contraction. Certainly there are instances where working on the ability to perform eccentric contractions is the goal, but if your goal is to activate the muscles of the extensor patterns, you must consider the effects of gravity.

"Maximal resistance" is the term that has historically been used to describe the application of resistance in PNF. This is misleading, however, because resistance is always graded in relation to the patient's capabilities. Although the term appears in older textbooks, the current thinking is to drop the word "maximal." The amount of resistance you would use to facilitate movement in a healthy young adult is very different from what you would use with a 55-year-old patient with Guillain-Barré syndrome who is still in acute care. With isotonic contractions, the appropriate amount of resistance is the amount that can be applied allowing full AROM to occur. For isometric contractions, it is the amount of resistance that the patient can manage in a stable position. Resistance is never used to "break" the effort of the patient. The goal is to cause irradiation to other muscles, which increases as resistance increases. Irradiation causes muscle groups other than the ones originally excited to take part in the response. This spread of facilitation is not haphazard but occurs in synergistic muscles. This effect is also referred to as overflow. As applied in PNF, resisting stronger movements to facilitate weaker muscle groups is termed reinforcement. Research supports the use of resistance to one extremity to increase the response in the opposite extremity for orthopedic patients with unilateral lower extremity impairment (Arai et al., 2001) and in healthy women at the shoulder (Pink, 1981) and elbow (Kamplain, 1986).

Tactile Stimuli

The therapist's manual contacts and the patient's use of self-touch are the two primary methods of providing tactile afferent input. Temporal and spatial discriminations occur with MCs and help patients understand the direction of the anticipated movement (Knott & Voss, 1968). Cold or vibration, as described in the Rood approach, may be used adjunctively (Myers, 1995).

The therapist places his or her hands on the skin overlying the muscles or tendons responsible for the pattern. There are no absolutes as to which segments of the body are to be facilitated with MCs. You can vary MCs, shifting the emphasis. For example, with an upper extremity pattern you may choose contacts at the wrist and upper arm or at the scapula and forearm. When facilitating rhythmic stabilization (RS) of the trunk, you may place MCs on one shoulder and the opposite hip, or on both shoulders, or on both hips. For a patient with significant weakness or pain, however, the therapist must support the limb and is not able to use MCs over the muscles in the patterns. As mentioned earlier, it is crucial that therapists place themselves in the diagonal pattern and move with the patient for successful completion of the range of the pattern. When the goal is stability, the therapist must be in a stable position for techniques to be successful.

Auditory Stimuli

Auditory input takes two primary forms. Tone of voice is the first. Sharp commands are used for maximum stimulation. Moderate tone of voice is used when the patient is responding with their best effort. A soft tone of voice is used when a patient has pain or when they are in an aroused state.

Commands are the second. Commands both prepare the patient for what is going to happen and are timed to provide maximum stimulation. For example to achieve D1 flexion you may first explain, "You are going to close your hand, turn it, and pull up and across your face." Then, with appropriate manual contacts, you simultaneously apply the quick stretch and say, "Squeeze, turn, pull up and across [your face]!"

Visual Stimuli

Visual input is used to facilitate movement. In diagonal patterns, the clients are always instructed to look at their hand (or object in their hand) when performing the unilateral or bilateral upper extremity patterns or to look at a specific place (e.g., "Look at the corner of the room" or "Look back at me") when working specifically on head and neck patterns or trunk patterns. In moving between postures, the optical righting reflexes are harnessed by directing the patient's gaze in the direction of movement, which is timed congruently with other facilitory stimuli at the initiation of movement.

Basic Techniques

Slow Reversal (SR)

The diagonal patterns were described earlier. The reversing nature of the diagonal pattern reflects how we all move in activity. In treatment, whether the direction of the pattern is named agonist or antagonist will vary. For example, if you are working with a client following a radial nerve repair and your objective is to strengthen the extensor carpi radialis longus (ECRL), the extensor carpi radialis brevis (ECRB), and the supinator, the focus would be on these muscles, and they would be designated the agonist muscles. All three of these muscles are prime movers in the D2 flexion pattern, so it would be considered the agonist pattern. D1 extension becomes the antagonist pattern.

In addition to irradiation, described earlier, two additional physiological principles are active during slow reversal (SR). Reciprocal inhibition is one principle. As explained in the Rood approach, when voluntary or reflexive contraction of a muscle occurs, the antagonist simultaneously relaxes. Successive induction is the second principle. According to this principle, the stronger antagonist becomes a source of proprioceptive facilitation for the weaker agonist. One action lowers the threshold for the opposite action. Successive induction causes a greater motor response because of the increased synaptic activity (Knott & Voss, 1968). Therefore, it is not uncommon to perform the antagonist pattern first to use the facilitating mechanism of successive induction.

Rhythmic Initiation (RI)

Rhythmic initiation (RI) is a technique used with patients who have trouble initiating movements, such as is seen in patients with Parkinson's disease. It involves a sequence of voluntary relaxation followed by therapist-assisted isotonic contraction and then unassisted movement by the patient. Tone of voice is slow, soothing, and repetitive. The therapist starts the movement, "Relax and let me move you" (PROM). The therapist repeats the movement with reversal several times. Then the patient is instructed, "Now do it with me" (active-assisted range of motion). Finally, the therapist removes his or her manual contacts while saying, "Now you do it," and the patient then performs the motion in activity (AROM). Components of feeding, washing, and dressing are examples of some of the activities that this technique facilitates. Wang (1994) studied the effects of RI on the gait patterns of patients with both long- and short-duration hemiplegia and found that the cumulative effects (treatment over time) were more beneficial than the immediate effects (at initial treatment session) and that patients with hemiplegia of short duration respond to training sooner than those with hemiplegia of long duration, although the cumulative effect for both groups was similar.

Rhythmic Stabilization

Rhythmic stabilization (RS) is a primary method for developing stability. This technique involves a midrange isometric contraction of the agonist that is followed by an isometric contraction of the antagonist with no movement occurring (co-contraction). It may be used in all positions. Joint approximation may be added and is administered on the "1, 2, 3" command. Establishing trunk stability is practiced with the therapist using manual contacts at both shoulders, both hips, or at the contralateral hip and shoulder. There will be no movement of the patient or therapist involved in this technique, but both are working to maintain stability (Fig. 26-11). Commands are the same regardless of position or contacts. Preparation involves the instruction, "On the count of three, I am going to push you from side to side. Don't let me move you." The action commands are, "1, 2, 3, hold! [sharp]. And hold [moderate, drawn out], and hold [same], and relax." The use of "hold" in PNF always means an isometric contraction. See Case Example #2, which elucidates this process.

RS involves only three reversals to avoid the potential for the patient to hold their breath. It is not infrequent to have to provide reminders to the patient to maintain a normal breathing pattern. Especially for patients with

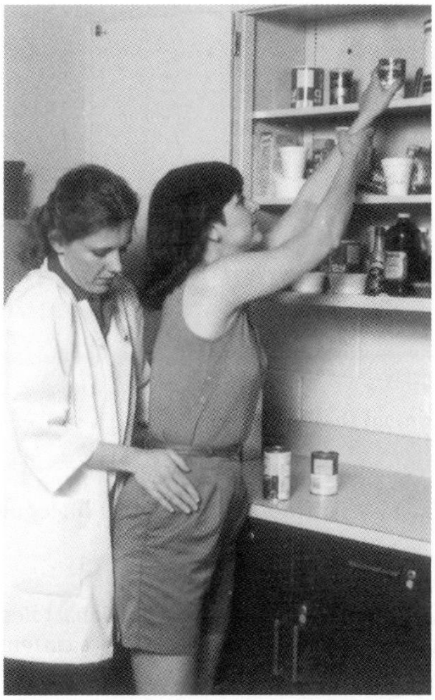

Figure 26-11 Lifting to the left. The therapist approximates at the pelvis. Before fatigue is evident, the patient would place both hands on the countertop, and both the patient and the therapist would perform rhythmic stabilization.

cardiac precautions, the relationship between isometric contractions and the Valsalva maneuver must be monitored (see Safety Note 26-1).

RS is also used with patients experiencing pain. Pain typically causes muscles in the area to be tightly contracted, a protective mechanism. Breathing, rhythmic stabilization, and reciprocal reversing movements of other body parts are what PNF refers to as indirect approaches to reduce muscle guarding and reestablish the balance of antagonists necessary for functional movement. For example, RS is performed on a part of the body that is not compromised by pain. Irradiation, or overflow, starts to break up the protective muscle contractions in the painful area. For patients with upper extremity pain, this is frequently performed with the patient lying supine with knees bent (hook-lying) with the therapist sitting along side of the patient. The therapist encircles the patient's legs with both arms and uses body weight to provide resistance in one direction and then the other. Again, if you are observing this procedure, you will not see any movement but the patient and therapist are working very hard. This is an instance where diagonal movement is not used.

If the patient is unable to perform rhythmic stabilization, it is necessary to develop the precursor muscle contractions by facilitating shortened-range isometric contractions.

Recuperative Motion

PNF takes a novel approach to fatigue. At the earliest sign that the patient is beginning to tire, rather than resting, the patient is guided into the use of a new combination of movements to reduce or circumvent fatigue produced by repetitive activity against resistance. In treatment focusing on improving upper extremity function, this may mean activity in the other diagonal. When working with patients on trunk stability, this may mean reducing the postural demand by changing the position that the client is working in. Temporarily stopping the activity and engaging in RS may also reduce the fatigue. For example, working with a client on morning ADLs (activities of daily living), activity may start with the patient sitting to apply toothpaste to a brush (skill) and then standing to brush the teeth. Brushing would be performed using the chopping pattern or in a simultaneous static dynamic (SSD) position. If standing for this part of the activity appears to be getting more difficult for the patient, a modified plantigrade position may be used while the patient rinses his or her mouth and the therapist performs RS. Alternatively, the patient would sit to finish the activity.

CASE EXAMPLE #1

K.S.: PNF Treatment of Limitations of Occupational Functioning Because of Pain and Limited Shoulder Range of Motion

Occupational Therapy Intervention Process	Clinical Reasoning Process	
	Objectives	**Examples of Therapist's Internal Dialogue**
Patient Information K.S. is a 46-year-old married mother of two who works full time as an operating room technician. She presents with a diagnosis of adhesive capsulitis of her left (L) dominant shoulder. An outpatient occupational therapy assessment identified the following problems: (1) decreased ability to perform ADL and BADL activities taking place above shoulder level secondary to PROM limitations, muscle spasms, and pain with active movement and decreased muscular endurance; (2) decreased overall systemic endurance, and (3) increased irritability in work and home situations secondary to pain disturbing sleep.	Appreciate the context	"K.S. has a multitude of occupational roles. All of them are affected by the problems she is currently experiencing with her shoulder. "
	Develop intervention hypotheses	"Frustration with her inability to use her dominant arm in her very busy lifestyle is wearing on this client. We need to develop some compensatory strategies and pain control measures that she can manage independently right away while we work to gain PROM and then concurrent strength and endurance of her dominant arm in activities."
	Select an intervention approach	"A PNF approach should work well for her pain. In addition to starting with breathing techniques, teaching the use of the unaffected arm in diagonal patterns with left arm in contact as able will lay the foundation for reestablishing normal motor function on her dominant side."
	Reflect on competence	"I can adapt many of the bilateral asymmetrical arm patterns to help her move within her pain-free range. She can use her unaffected arm to provide support to the affected one when she needs to perform skilled activities."
Recommendations The occupational therapist recommended two treatment sessions per week for 6 weeks. In collaboration with the patient, the following long-term goals were developed: client will return to competent pre-morbid occupational task performance, family, and job roles using strategies to prevent recurrence of pain and ROM limitations.	Consider the patient's appraisal of performance Consider what will occur in therapy, how often, and for how long Ascertain the patient's endorsement of plan	"I feel we have a very good chance of remediating symptoms and regaining occupational functioning objectives without the client undergoing an invasive orthopedic procedure. She appears motivated and agrees with the plan. There do not appear to be any cognitive issues precluding her participation in a home program. Her employer is willing to allow her to reduce her work days by 40%, and the family has discussed the ramifications of this temporary decrease in her salary."

Summary of Short-Term Goals and Progress 1. For relaxation and/or pain control during daily activities, K.S. will demonstrate performance of breathing technique: bilateral D2 trunk and arm pattern in sitting, elbows flexed initially. K.S. learned the pattern during her first outpatient session. The therapist used quick stretch, soothing tone of voice, and active assist strategies until the pattern was learned. K.S. said it was a little more difficult to perform this pattern by herself at home. 2. K.S. will demonstrate performance of non-painful, weight-bearing, modified plantigrade postures to perform occupational tasks, alternating arms as able. Diagonal patterns superimposed on this posture will initially support laundry activities, loading and unloading the dishwasher, and placement and retrieval of items in drawers. K.S. participated in many modified plantigrade postures during initial therapy sessions. She was quick to learn how to use these movement patterns around home and work. 3. K.S. will demonstrate active-assisted use of affected arm in bilateral asymmetrical diagonal patterns in skilled activities. In therapy, K.S. learned unilateral D1 and D2 with her right upper extremity (RUE) in activity. Chopping and lifting were demonstrated by the therapist, and then she learned modified chopping and lifting performed with the left arm, modifying the placement of the right hand to provide active-assisted movement to use her dominant hand in activities without increasing shoulder pain. 4. K.S. will gain left shoulder PROM, AAROM (active-assisted range of motion) and AROM in flexion, abduction, and external rotation by participation in therapy sessions and home exercise program. Rhythmic stabilization in various supportive postures will follow breathing techniques. After manual techniques by the therapist, K.S. participated in AAROM activities, which she continued in her home program. She kept an active log given to her by her therapist, and the two of them discussed her comments and reactions to the program, usually while they were doing icing.	Assess the patient's comprehension Compare actual to expected performance Know the person Appreciate the context	"One of K.S.'s strongest habits was 'pushing through' to complete activities, no matter what. She felt that she needed to do this to complete all tasks of her many life roles. I had to do a lot of patient education about that. Many of the therapeutic techniques during treatment gave us time to talk. Rhythmic stabilization in hook lying position helped break up muscle spasms. As she was experiencing less pain and starting to sleep better, she was more willing to accept my suggestions for at least slowing down and taking breathing breaks. Learning the active-assisted diagonal patterns helped her immensely when she had to perform fine motor tasks with her dominant hand. K.S. told me that she had never had anyone explain the use of breathing patterns for this kind of problem. Sure, she had done it during labor, but, 'that was a different story.'"
Next Steps Initial short-term goals were modified throughout the 6-week period by increasing the movement demands. Initially, diagonal patterns were performed with the elbow flexed as she lifted her arm against gravity and with her elbow extending on the reversals. Gradually, gentle manual resistance was added to the eccentric contractions. She maintained gains in range of motion between treatment sessions by using diagonal movements in activity and exercise. As strength returned, K.S. continued to increase repetitions, improve muscular endurance, and avoid potential reinjury during activities requiring eccentric contractions of shoulder muscles.	Anticipate present and future patient concerns Analyze patient's comprehension Decide if the patient should continue or discontinue therapy and/or return in the future	"At the end of 6 weeks, K.S. 'graduated' from OT. The protective techniques that she learned throughout her therapy interventions and that she incorporated into her daily habits served her well. By the end of treatment, she was a real 'pro' at knowing when she might be overdoing it with her arm, but more importantly, she knew how to change the task before overdoing became a problem."

CLINICAL REASONING IN OCCUPATIONAL THERAPY PRACTICE

Modified Upper Extremity Diagonal Patterns

With pain and limited active range of motion, movement through the full range of either diagonal pattern was not possible for K.S.

1. Why would you instruct the client to do diagonal plane movements when she cannot complete the patterns instead of instructing her in one-plane shoulder exercises?
2. How is the client's use of self-touch different than what is typically done in chopping and lifting?
3. What else would you teach her to do while working in the patterns?

CASE EXAMPLE # 2

M.G.: PNF Treatment to Develop Postural Control

Occupational Therapy Intervention Process	Clinical Reasoning Process: Objectives	Clinical Reasoning Process: Examples of Therapist's Internal Dialogue
Patient Information M.G. is a 24-year-old male, former Marine, who is 20 months post closed-head injury and right (dominant) humeral fracture with subsequent peripheral nerve damage following a motor vehicle injury while on active duty in Iraq. He was in a coma for nearly 2 months. He has gone through extensive inpatient rehabilitation. He received an honorable discharge from the military. Four months ago, surgeons performed a triple tendon transfer to restore hand function, replacing muscle function that was lost because peripheral nerve regeneration was not occurring. Subsequently, he received extensive hand therapy at a VA hospital near his home. Currently, he is returning to college to complete his final year of studies and is referred as an outpatient to this local VA hospital in the city where he will be studying. The objective is to complete rehabilitation following tendon transfers while he is in school. He participated in an occupational therapy assessment, and in addition to RUE impairments with resulting functional deficits, he has an ataxic gait. Upon further evaluation, problems related to the ataxia included: (1) inability to maintain midrange isometric contractions of the right shoulder girdle in seated position; and (2) limited control of trunk midrange isometric contractions in side-lying secondary to abdominal muscle weakness.	Appreciate the context	"M.G. presents in an upbeat manner. He acknowledges the important role his parents have played in his rehabilitation process but appears to be glad to be out from 'under their wings.' He talks in an animated manner about the therapists he worked with and identifies things he liked about rehab and things that he did not like. His frustration with not being able to use his right hand appears appropriate; however, he does not demonstrate a lot of affect when talking about his initial injury."
	Develop intervention hypotheses	"M.G. needs significant work to reestablish postural muscle control and strength, not only at the shoulder, but also the trunk."

	Select an intervention approach	"We will be using PNF diagonals and thrusting patterns extensively to meet objectives for restoring RUE control. The approach also offers techniques to effect trunk stability."
	Reflect on competence	"Despite his enthusiastic manner (or perhaps because of it), M.G. is going to be a challenge. I will need to restrain myself from getting into a "parent" role. He accomplished so much so quickly in rehab so far that I am going to have to gradually inform him that this stage of his rehab is not going to move as quickly."
Recommendations The client's physician referral was for "upper extremity/hand rehabilitation, 2 times per week." Following assessment, the therapist contacted the physician to increase frequency of therapy to 3 times per week. Sessions were scheduled for 30–45 minutes, with potential use of modalities being the consideration for increasing the time of some visits. Therapy was approved until maximum benefit was achieved. M.G.'s identified long-term goal was to be able to throw a baseball. In addition to the long-term hand function goals related to this task, the long-term goals related to his ataxia were identified as: (1) M.G. will demonstrate postural control adequate to pitch slow-pitch softball; (2) M.G. will demonstrate postural control adequate to support throwing a ball from second base to home plate.	Consider the patient's appraisal of performance Consider what will occur in therapy, how often, and for how long Ascertain the patient's endorsement of plan	"M.G. is back on campus, but all of his former friends have graduated. He is very personable and motivated; however, he states that he is pretty bored and doesn't know how much this will change once school starts in 10 days. Due to the poor fine motor skills in his dominant hand, he is taking a reduced load of 9 credits each semester, then 6 credits the following summer, at the end of which he will graduate. Because of his long rehabilitation, he is familiar with therapies and has seen improvement. He states, 'I always liked OT.' Due to the scope of issues related to his return to college with the extent of his rehab needs, 3 times per week seemed the appropriate frequency of treatment, and M.G. agreed. We also agreed that we could be flexible with this scheduling if school tasks were more demanding than he anticipated. He also agreed to use a tape recorder in lieu of note taking at the beginning of the fall semester."
Summary of Short-Term Goals and Progress (Specific to Ataxia) 1. M.G. will perform midrange isometric contractions of trunk muscles in side-lying, as evidenced by successful rhythmic stabilization (RS) side-lying right and side-lying left. Following breathing exercises, therapy started with hold-relax active motion (HRAM) in side-lying and was eventually graded to slow reversal-hold (SR-H) in side-lying. When RS was successful in side-lying, we started a progression of movements from side-sitting to kneeling, to half-kneeling, to standing, moving back and forth between the positions, decreasing the skill requirement during the most challenging postures and increasing the skill of hand and arm activities in the less demanding postures. RS was performed multiple times in all positions, and the less demanding positions and activities were performed at initial signs of fatigue. 2. M.G. will demonstrate strengthened abdominal muscles by performing 10 sets of sit-ups, arms across chest, in a sequence of left diagonal sit-up, straight sit-up, and right diagonal sit-up (1 set). This is an ex-Marine. When the weakness of his abdominal muscles became apparent, he appeared to be fairly devastated by this. We had to work at this very carefully because this was one area where he was prone to overdo it. The progression of sit-ups was performed until he could do 15. Then the number decreased as we made the task harder by moving his arms behind his head (increasing the lever arm). Lower abdominal exercises were gradually introduced and graded as well.	Assess the patient's comprehension Understand what he is doing Compare actual to expected performance Know the person Appreciate the context	"When the patient is unable to perform isometric contractions, the patient must be taught to 'hold.' One approach is to have him perform slow reversal-hold (SR-H) through decreasing ranges of motion until no motion occurs (Voss, Ionta, & Myers, 1985). Another approach is hold-relax active motion (HRAM). This is probably the approach we need to start with because it is more appropriate when there is an imbalance of antagonists. We will try both to see which is easier to begin with." "It was interesting that, despite all of the limitations he has endured and overcome, the weakness of his abdominal muscles affects him so deeply. However, this was his first real-time experience of being out of the military. He is exhibiting no other signs that might be indicative of post-traumatic stress syndrome (PTSS); however, this strong reaction led to the discussion of many of his feelings about being injured so early in his tour of duty. His father was a retired military man (served in Vietnam), and while his dad was available for him during his extensive rehab, he said that they never talked about combat experiences." "He worked diligently at all of his home program activities and exercises. Frequency of therapy was reduced to two times per week after normal gait was reestablished."

3. M.G. will perform midrange isometric contractions of right shoulder girdle in reversal of both D1 and D2 patterns as demonstrated by successful rhythmic stabilization (RS) efforts in these patterns both from sitting and side-lying on left side.

Work toward this goal started with SR-H in sitting and side-lying, monitoring arm position for biomechanical load and modifying as appropriate. As he was able to perform RS at the shoulder, he began spending a lot of time in prone on elbows while practicing fine motor abilities and skills. He took a liking to the fine felt-tipped marker drawing kits of relatively small and complex designs and initially did these in prone on elbows. Eventually, we would tape these to the wall, and he would work on them from a standing position with his elbows in contact with the wall.

Next Steps M.G.'s improvement in gait foreshadowed his improvements with hand function and provided the necessary support for skilled movement of his affected arm. M.G. was performing a controlled underhand and overhand throw with a nerf ball before hand strength was adequate to advance to a heavier ball.	Anticipate present and future patient concerns Analyze patient's comprehension Decide if the patient should continue or discontinue therapy and/or return in the future	"M.G. made excellent progress and eventually internalized the need to take things at a rate a bit slower than he really thought he could perform at. He was discontinued from OT at the point when he was able to perform his own note taking during lectures. The following spring, he invited the OT staff to his first slow-pitch baseball game. It appeared that he was developing some good friendships in this activity."

CLINICAL REASONING IN OCCUPATIONAL THERAPY PRACTICE

Facilitating Trunk Control in Side-Lying

M.G. is unable to perform rhythmic stabilization (RS), so you must build the ability to perform isometric contractions of the muscles in their shortened range.

1. How should you start the session?
2. What should the therapist be doing?
3. For stability techniques in side-lying, where are your manual contacts?
4. When and how do you use resistance?
5. Describe how you use quick stretch (QS) and resistance.
6. What tone of voice do you use?
7. What else must you do?

Evidence Table 26-1
Best Evidence for Occupational Therapy Practice Regarding Restoration of First-Level Motor Control Capacities

Intervention	Description of Intervention Tested	Participants	Dosage	Type of Best Evidence and Level of Evidence	Benefit	Statistical Probability and Effect Size of Outcome	Reference
Soft tissue mobilization plus PNF in patients with musculoskeletal disorders	PNF group vs. control group	20 persons, aged 21–83 years with orthopedic shoulder pathology of 1 year or less. (No significant difference in age between groups).	10 minutes, one-time treatment.	Randomized controlled study. IB1a	Yes, soft tissue mobilization combined with PNF intervention was found to be effective both in gaining external rotation at the shoulder and in overhead reach as compared with no treatment.	Significant gain in external rotation ($p < 0.0005$; $r = 0.74$). Significant gain in overhead reach ($p < 0.009$; $r = 0.53$)	Godges et al., 2003
Prosthetic training for individuals receiving first prosthesis following unilateral transfemoral amputation	PNF group vs. traditional prosthetic training group.	50 persons with unilateral transfemoral amputations, 20–40 years old.	30 minutes daily for 10 treatments.	Randomized controlled study. IA1a	Yes. PNF intervention was an effective way to achieve balance, symmetrical weight acceptance, and gait in this population.	Weight acceptance and gait parameters, $p < 0.05$.	Yigiter et al., 2002
Effects of 3 shoulder exercise protocols	PNF vs. closed kinetic chain vs. open kinetic chain vs. control.	54 college-aged persons with no history of upper extremity injury.	3 times per week for 5 weeks.	Randomized controlled study. 1C1a	Yes. Shoulder strength, proprioception, and neuromuscular control improved; however, only the PNF group improved in functional performance.	All three groups significantly improved on all 3 measures ($p < 0.05$). *Functional Throwing Performance Index* was significantly greater for the PNF group compared with the other groups ($p < 0.05$).	Padua et al., 2004

SUMMARY REVIEW QUESTIONS

1. What specific parameters must be considered in the application of appropriate sensory stimulation to enhance motor performance?
2. Describe how general hypertonicity, such as seen in some patients after traumatic brain injury, may be inhibited.
3. How does abnormal tone affect occupational functioning?
4. How does flaccidity contribute to contracture development? How does spasticity contribute?
5. What are the unique characteristics of the PNF approach that distinguish it from other approaches to therapeutic exercise?

ACKNOWLEDGEMENT

The author wishes to thank Beverly Myers, OT, and Sharon Mukayama, OT, PT, for their enthusiasm, patience, and knowledge as PNF instructors.

References

Ada, L., Vattanasilp, W., O'Dwyer, N. J., & Crosbie, J. (1998). Does spasticity contribute to walking dysfunction after stroke? *Journal of Neurology, Neurosurgery, and Psychiatry, 64,* 628–635.

American Journal of Physical Medicine. (1967). *46,* 1–1191.

Arai, M., Shimizu, H., Shimizu, M. E., Tanaka, Y., & Yanagisawa, K. (2001). Effects of the use of cross-education to the affected side through various resistive exercises of the sound side and settings of the length of the affected muscles. *Hiroshima Journal of Medical Sciences, 50,* 65–73.

Ayres, A. J. (1963). Occupational therapy directed toward neuromuscular integration. In H. S. Willard & C. S. Spackman (Eds.), *Occupational therapy* (3rd ed., pp. 358–459). Philadelphia: Lippincott.

Ayres, A. J. (1974). Integration of information. In A. Henderson, L. Llorens, E. Gilfoyle, C. Meyers, & S. Prevel (Eds.), *The development of sensory integrative theory and practice: A collection of the works of A. Jean Ayers* (pp. 63–82). Dubuque, IA: Kendall-Hunt.

Baum, M., Nicholas, S., Stock, C., & Lee, R. (1998). A proprioceptive neuromuscular facilitation shoulder progression for patients with spinal cord injury resulting in quadriplegia. *Physical Therapy Case Reports, 1,* 296–300.

Beazell, J. R. (1998). Dysfunction of the longus colli and its relationship to cervical pain and dysfunction: A clinical case presentation. *Journal of Manual and Manipulative Therapy, 6,* 12–16.

Bonnar, B. P., Deivert, R. G., & Gould, T. E. (2004). The relationship between isometric contraction durations during hold-relax stretching and improvement of hamstring flexibility. *Journal of Sports Medicine and Physical Fitness, 44,* 258–261.

Braddom, R. L. (Ed.). (1996). *Physical medicine and rehabilitation.* Philadelphia: Saunders.

Carey, J. R. (1990). Manual stretch: Effect on finger movement control and force control in stroke subjects with spastic extrinsic finger flexor muscles. *Archives of Physical Medicine and Rehabilitation, 71,* 888–894.

Carpenter, R. H. S. (1996). *Neurophysiology* (3rd ed.). New York: Oxford University.

Carter, A. M., Kinzey, S. J., Chitwood, L. F., & Cole, J. L. (2000). Proprioceptive neuromuscular facilitation decreases muscle activity during the stretch reflex in selected posterior thigh muscles. *Journal of Sport Rehabilitation, 9,* 269–278.

Dobkin, B. H. (1996). *Neurologic rehabilitation.* Philadelphia: Davis.

Etnyre, B. R., & Abraham, L. D. (1986). H-reflex changes during static stretching and 2 variations of proprioceptive neuromuscular facilitation techniques. *Electroencephalography and Clinical Neurophysiology, 63,* 174–179.

Farber, S. (1982). *Neurorehabilitation.* Philadelphia: WB Saunders.

Feland, J. B., & Marin, H. N. (2004). Effect of submaximal contraction intensity in contract-relax proprioceptive neuromuscular facilitation stretching. *British Journal of Sports Medicine, 38,* E18.

Feland, J. B., Myrer, J. W., & Merrill, R. M. (2001). Acute changes in hamstring flexibility: PNF versus static stretch in senior athletes. *Physical Therapy in Sport, 2,* 186–193.

Ferber, R., Osternig, L. R., & Gravelle, D. C. (2002). Effect of PNF stretch techniques on knee flexor muscle EMG activity in older adults. *Journal of Electromyography and Kinesiology, 12,* 391–397.

Funk, D. C., Swank, A. M., Mikla, B. M., Fagan, T. A., & Farr, B. K. (2003). Impact of prior exercise on hamstring flexibility: A comparison of proprioceptive neuromuscular facilitation and static stretching. *Journal of Strength and Conditioning Research, 17,* 489–492.

Gilman, S., & Newman, S. W. (1992). *Manter and Gatz's essentials of clinical neuroanatomy and neurophysiology* (8th ed.). Philadelphia: Davis.

Godges, J. J., Mattson-Bell, M., Thorpe, D., & Shah, D. (2003). The immediate effects of soft tissue mobilization with proprioceptive neuromuscular facilitation on glenohumeral external rotation and overhead reach. *Journal of Orthopaedic and Sports Physical Therapy, 33,* 713–718.

Harris, F. (1969). Control of gamma efferents through the reticular activating system. *American Journal of Occupational Therapy, 23,* 403–408.

Huss, A. J. (1971). Sensorimotor approaches. In H. L. Hopkins & H. D. Smith (Eds.), *Willard and Spackman's occupational therapy* (5th ed., pp. 125–134). Philadelphia: J.B. Lippincott.

Kamplain, B. (1986). Proprioceptive neuromuscular facilitation: Contralateral effects of combined isotonics using resisted concentric and eccentric phases. *Physical Therapy, 66,* 796–796.

Knott, M., & Voss, D. E. (1968). *Proprioceptive neuromuscular facilitation techniques.* New York: Harper & Row.

Malouin, F., Bonneau, C., Pichard, L., & Corriveau, D. (1997). Non- reflex mediated changes in plantar flexor muscles early after stroke. *Scandinavian Journal of Rehabilitation Medicine, 29,* 147–153.

Mason, C. R. (1985). One method for assessing the effectiveness of fast brushing. *Physical Therapy, 65,* 1197–1202.

Matyas, T. A., & Spicer, S. D. (1980). Facilitation of the tonic vibration reflex (TVR) by cutaneous stimulation in hemiplegics. *American Journal of Physical Medicine, 59,* 280–287.

Myers, B. J. (1981). *Assisting to posture and application in occupational therapy activities.* Videotape. Chicago: Rehabilitation Institute of Chicago.

Myers, B. J. (1995). Proprioceptive neuromuscular facilitation (PNF) approach. In C. A. Trombly (Ed.), *Occupational therapy for physical dysfunction* (4th ed., pp. 474–495). Baltimore: Williams & Wilkins.

Nitz, J., & Burke, B. (2002). A study of the facilitation of respiration in myotonic dystrophy. *Physiotherapy Research International, 7,* 228–238.

O'Dwyer, N. J., Ada, L., & Neilson, P. D. (1996). Spasticity and muscle contracture following stroke. *Brain, 119,* 1737–1749.

Okuma, Y., & Lee, R. G. (1996). Reciprocal inhibition in hemiplegia: Correlation with clinical features and recovery. *Canadian Journal of Neurological Sciences, 23,* 15–23.

Padua, D. A., Guskiewicz, K. M., Prentice, W. E., Schneider, R. E., & Shields, E. W. (2004). The effect of select shoulder exercises on strength, active angle reproduction, single-arm balance, and functional performance. *Journal of Sport Rehabilitation, 13,* 75–95.

Pink, M. (1981). Contralateral effects of upper extremity proprioceptive neuromuscular facilitation patterns. *Physical Therapy, 61,* 1158– 1162.

Preston, L. A., & Hecht, J. S. (1999). *Spasticity management: Rehabilitation strategies.* Bethesda, MD: American Occupational Therapy Association.

Rood, M. S. (1954). Neurophysiological reactions as a basis for physical therapy. *Physical Therapy Review, 34,* 444–449.

Rood, M. S. (1956). Neurophysiological mechanisms utilized in the treatment of neuromuscular dysfunction. *American Journal of Occupational Therapy, 10,* 220–225.

Rood, M. S. (1962). The use of sensory receptors to activate, facilitate, and inhibit motor response, autonomic and somatic, in developmental sequence. In C. Sattely (Ed.), *Approaches to the treatment of patients with neuromuscular dysfunction* (Study Course VI, 3rd International Congress WFOT, pp. 26–37). Dubuque, IA: W. C. Brown.

Rowlands, A. V., Marginson, V. F., & Lee, J. (2002). The effect of isometric contraction time on flexibility gains after training using proprioceptive neuromuscular facilitation. *Journal of Sports Sciences, 20,* 57.

Shimura, K., & Kasai, T. (2002). Effects of proprioceptive neuromuscular facilitation on the initiation of voluntary movement and motor evoked potentials in upper limb muscles. *Human Movement Science, 21,* 101–113.

Spernoga, S. G., Uhl, T. L., Arnold, B. L., & Gansneder, B. M. (2001). Duration of maintained hamstring flexibility after a one-time modified hold-relax stretching protocol. *Journal of Athletic Training, 36,* 44–48.

Spicer, S. D., & Matyas, T. A. (1980). Facilitation of the tonic vibration reflex (TVR) by cutaneous stimulation. *American Journal of Physical Medicine, 59,* 223–231.

Stockmeyer, S. (1967). An interpretation of the approach of Rood to the treatment of neuromuscular dysfunction. *American Journal of Physical Medicine, 46,* 900–956.

Stopka, C., Morley, K., Siders, R., Schuette, J., Houck, A., & Gilmet, Y. (2002). Stretching techniques to improve flexibility in Special Olympics athletes and their coaches. *Journal of Sport Rehabilitation, 11,* 22–34.

Sullivan, P. E., & Portney, L. G. (1980). Electro-myographic activity of shoulder muscles during unilateral upper extremity proprioceptive neuromuscular facilitation patterns. *Physical Therapy, 60,* 283–288.

Teixeira-Salmela, L. F., Olney, S. J., Nadeau, S., & Brouwer, B. (1999). Muscle strengthening and physical conditioning to reduce impairment and disability in chronic stroke survivors. *Archives of Physical Medicine and Rehabilitation, 80,* 1211–1218.

Trombly, C. A. (1995). Managing deficit of first-level motor control capacities. In C. A. Trombly & M. V. Radomski (Eds.), *Occupational therapy for physical dysfunction* (5th ed., pp. 571–584). Baltimore: Lippincott Williams & Wilkins.

Umphred, D. A. (1995). Classification of treatment techniques based on primary input systems. In D. A. Umphred (Ed.), *Neurological rehabilitation* (3rd ed., pp. 118–178). St. Louis: Mosby.

Voss, D. E. (1967). Proprioceptive neuromuscular facilitation. *American Journal of Physical Medicine, 46,* 838–898.

Voss, D. E., Ionta, M. K., & Myers, B. J. (1985). *Proprioceptive neuromuscular facilitation: Patterns and techniques* (3rd ed.). New York: Harper & Row.

Wang, R.Y., (1994). Effect of proprioceptive neuromuscular facilitation on the gait of patients with hemiplegia of long and short-duration. *Physical Theraphy, 74*(12), 1108-1115.

Wood, E. C. (1967). The objectives of the project. *American Journal of Physical Medicine, 46,* 25.

Yigiter, K., Sener, G., Erbahceci, F., Bayar, K., Ulger, O. G., & Akdogan, S. (2002). A comparison of traditional prosthetic training versus proprioceptive neuromuscular facilitation resistive gait training with trans-femoral amputees. *Prosthetics and Orthotics International, 26,* 213–217.

Young, W., & Elliott, S. (2001). Acute effects of static stretching, proprioceptive neuromuscular facilitation stretching, and maximum voluntary contractions on explosive force production and jumping performance. *Research Quarterly for Exercise and Sport, 72,* 273–279.

Supplemental References

Bobath, B. (1990). *Adult hemiplegia: Evaluation and treatment.* Oxford, United Kingdom: Butterworth Heinemann.

Munih, M., Obreza, P., Sega, J., Bajd, T., & Savrin, R. (2004). Proprioceptive neuromuscular facilitation in combination with electrical stimulation: Combined treatment in comparison to each treatment alone. *Neuromodulation, 7,* 48–55.

Klein, D. A., Stone, W. J., Phillips, W. T., Gangi, J., & Hartman, S. (2002). PNF training and physical function in assisted-living older adults. *Journal of Aging and Physical Activity, 10,* 476–488.

CHAPTER 27

Optimizing Sensory Abilities and Capacities

Karen Bentzel

LEARNING OBJECTIVES

After studying this chapter, the reader will be able to do the following:

1. Select appropriate sensory treatment for a patient or description of a patient.
2. Explain the rationale for sensory reeducation and desensitization.
3. Demonstrate a variety of sensory reeducation and desensitization strategies for patients following peripheral nerve injury and stroke.
4. Name several mechanisms of damage to areas of skin with diminished protective sensation and describe related compensatory strategies to prevent injury.

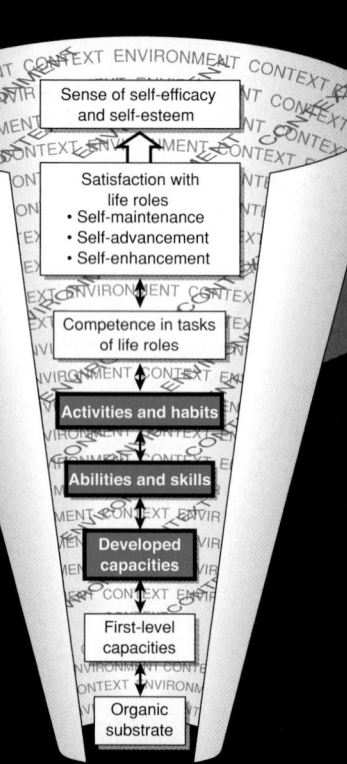

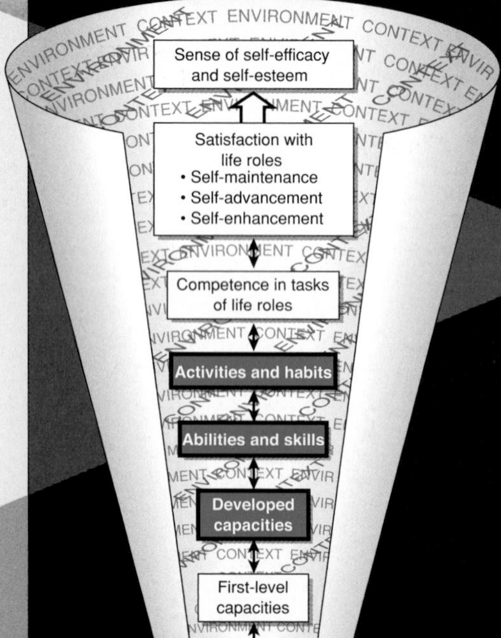

Glossary

Allodynia—Condition in which non-painful stimuli produce painful sensations.

Decubitus ulcer—Open sore caused by pressure, friction, and moisture. These factors lead to reduced blood flow to the area and consequent tissue death. The most common sites for decubitus ulcers are over bony prominences.

Hyperesthesia—Condition in which there is increased sensitivity to somatosensory stimuli

Hypersensitivity—Condition in which ordinary stimuli produce an exaggerated or unpleasant sensation.

Learned non-use—Loss of capacity in an impaired extremity because of a tendency to avoid using that extremity and to use other body parts instead.

Protective sensation—Painful sensation evoked by potentially damaging sensory stimuli, such as excessive temperature, pressure, or tissue stress.

Graphesthesia—The ability to identify numbers or letters traced on the skin.

Tactile sensation is considered by many people to be less important than visual and auditory sensations (Manske, 1999). Most would be surprised to find the extent and number of difficulties resulting from loss of tactile and proprioceptive information. The story of Ian Waterman, who lost all tactile and proprioceptive sensations from the neck down as a result of a rare neurological illness, was introduced in Chapter 7. As Waterman tried to explain to others what was wrong with him, he found that they could not begin to understand the severe difficulties he faced as a result of his sensory loss. His family and friends failed to find the connection between his sensory loss and his inability to move and complete activities of daily living. Even those in the medical community did not comprehend the extent of his difficulties. A detailed account of Waterman's struggle to compensate for his lost sensation is provided in Cole's book (1991), *Pride and a Daily Marathon*.

Touch is a developed capacity that supports abilities and skills such as grasping and releasing objects. These abilities and skills are necessary for competence in self-maintenance, self-enhancement, and self-advancement. Biologist Geerat Vermeij (1999), who is blind, states that, in general, people neglect the role of the hand as a source of information about the world around us. Handling and manipulating objects enhances learning and helps human beings appreciate the world. Touch is also a means of communication and a source of pleasure.

Without sensation in the hand, there is a greater risk of injury to the hand and decreased ability to manipulate small objects. There is also a tendency not to use the hand in functional activities, which adds to the phenomenon of **learned non-use**, loss of function that results from not using the hand (Carr & Shepherd, 1998). Because of the role of tactile sensation in learning, exploring, and communicating and because loss of hand sensation is particularly disabling, occupational therapists should provide treatment or education in compensatory strategies for patients with lost or diminished sensation.

CHOOSING AN INTERVENTION STRATEGY

Chapter 7 addresses assessment of sensation and describes types of sensory losses. The choice of interventions for sensation is based on the diagnosis, prognosis, and evaluation findings. Diminished or lost **protective sensation**, the inability to feel pain in response to stimuli that are potentially damaging, suggests a need for teaching the patient and/or caregiver compensatory strategies to prevent injury. Findings of discomfort associated with touch (hypersensitivity) suggest a need for desensitization. Sensory reeducation is provided for patients who have some sensation and potential for better sensation or better interpretation of sensory information.

All of the sensory interventions described in this chapter are learning experiences for the patient. Strategies of learning (see Chapter 14) should be applied. Dellon (1997) describes sensory retraining strategies based on learning principles. Each patient should practice within the natural context of activities. Tailor training and training materials to the interest and ability of the patient. Grade the activity so that the patient can meet the expectations for improved performance. The patient must attend to the stimuli and information provided and perceive them as important and relevant.

COMPENSATION FOR IMPAIRED OR ABSENT PROTECTIVE SENSATION

Protective sensations are sensations of pain and temperature extremes that signal the threat of tissue damage. When the brain receives this message, the normal response is to move the body part away from the source of the stimulus. Without this message, tissue damage can quickly occur. The goal of treatment for the patient with diminished or absent protective sensation is to avoid injury. Treatment consists of teaching the patient and/or the caregiver precautions necessary to prevent injury to any body part with compromised protective sensations. The loss of sensation could be due to diagnoses such as stroke, head injury, spinal cord injury, or peripheral nerve injury.

Rationale for Compensation

In a classic 1969 article in the *American Journal of Occupational Therapy*, Helen Wood described the role of the occupational therapist in preventing injury and deformity in hands that lacked sensitivity. She stated that, when hands are used in activities without protective sensory feedback, there is a high frequency of burns, cuts, lacerations, and bruises. Damage or injury to an insensitive limb is the result of external forces that are normally avoided by people who are able to feel pain, which acts as a warning mechanism. Sensations of pain warn us when we are gripping an item too tightly or sitting in one position for too long. Therefore, pain has been considered the most valuable sensation that humans have (Brand, 1979).

Brand (1979) described five mechanisms of damage to insensitive limbs: continuous low pressure, concentrated high pressure, excessive heat or cold, repetitive mechanical stress, and pressure on infected tissue (Definition 27-1). Prevention principles evolve from an understanding of these mechanisms of damage.

DEFINITION 27-1

Mechanisms of Damage Secondary to Loss of Protective Sensation

- Continuous low pressure: With sustained pressure as light as 1 pound per square inch, capillary flow is blocked; this can cause tissue necrosis, leading to pressure sores (**decubitus ulcers**).
- Concentrated high pressure: Sudden high force that is accidental and/or a high force applied over a very small area, so that the force is inadequately distributed. This may result in tearing of skin and/or soft tissue or tissue necrosis as a result of insufficient blood supply.
- Excessive heat or cold: Temperature extremes that lead to burn or frostbite injuries.
- Repetitive mechanical stress: Repetitive motions or shearing of skin against clothing or objects that causes inflammation of the tendons or skin. Blistering of skin can also occur.
- Pressure on infected tissue: Continued use and pressure on infected tissue can hinder or prevent the natural healing process.

Adapted from Brand, P. (1979). Management of the insensitive limb. *Physical Therapy, 59,* 8–12.

Compensation Techniques

Brand et al. (1999), Skirven and Callahan (2002), and Eggers (1984) recommend the following content for patient education sessions, based on the five mechanisms of damage to insensitive skin. Skin areas over bony prominences are particularly prone to pressure ulcers because the cutaneous tissue is trapped between the unyielding bone and the external pressure. Frequent position changes are necessary for patients with decreased or absent protective sensation to avoid damage due to continuous low pressure. Cushions for seating and shoe insoles help to distribute forces over larger areas.

Instruct patients to avoid concentrated high pressure by careful handling of sharp tools and by using enlarged handles on suitcases, drawers, and keys. Patients may need to become consciously aware to use only as much force as necessary to grasp objects. Excessive pressure can also result from splint straps that are too narrow and splints that are too tight; therefore, therapists must carefully construct splints to prevent injury.

Teach patients to increase their awareness of potential sources of extreme heat or cold and to protect themselves from contact with them. Insulated coffee mugs are recommended. Oven mitts or quality pot holders are necessary for cooking. Utensils with wooden or plastic handles are better than metal ones. Patients using wheelchairs should insulate exposed hot water pipes under sinks. In cold weather, gloves or mittens are necessary protection for insensate hands.

Instruct patients to avoid repetitive motions and excessive friction between skin and objects. Decrease repetitions by working for shorter periods, resting, using a variety of tools, or alternating hands or type of grip. Methods to reduce friction include wearing gloves and using enlarged or padded handles on tools.

Educate patients who have lost protective sensation regarding special care for blisters, cuts, and bruises necessary to avoid infection. If infection occurs, the infected part should be completely rested to keep it free from pressure and overuse, allowing healing to occur.

Additional techniques of compensating for absent sensation incorporate reliance on other senses. For example, vision may be used to prevent contact with sharp objects. Using a body part with intact sensation to test water temperature before immersion of any body part without sensation is recommended. Auditory cues may also help to prevent injury. For instance, a person with paraplegia might hear the rubbing of the wheelchair caster against the foot if it slips from its proper position on the leg rest.

Finally, patients should be instructed in good skin care. Applying lotion or oil daily enhances skin hydration. Well-hydrated skin is more elastic and pliant and less prone to injury. Skin needs to be visually inspected daily. A warm or reddened area indicates a possible site of tissue breakdown, which will lead to a decubitus ulcer, and extreme care must be taken to relieve pressure totally from this area until the color returns to normal. ***If the time for the skin to recover its normal color exceeds 20 minutes, it is absolutely essential to discover the cause of the skin irritation and correct it. Modification of position, schedule, procedure, equipment, or orthotics is necessary.*** If the patient cannot inspect and care for the skin properly, instruct a care provider to perform these tasks every day.

Effectiveness of Compensatory Techniques

A review of the literature reveals no research studies that confirm the effectiveness of instructing patients to avoid injury. These compensatory techniques have face validity in that they evolved out of evidence that patients lacking protective sensation had incurred injuries, many of which could have been prevented. Anecdotal evidence of effectiveness includes Wood's (1969) description of a patient who had a series of hand injuries prior to occupational therapy and none following instruction and fitting of gloves to be worn in his electronics repair work.

Widespread acceptance of compensatory techniques is further evidence of reliance on their assumed effectiveness. The American Diabetes Association (2004) recommends sensory testing of the feet of all people with diabetes so that foot ulcers and amputations can be prevented in those with sensory loss. Techniques of testing and education for patients with diabetes appear in the nursing and physical therapy literature (Sloan & Abel, 1998; Thompson, Medley, & Motts, 2002).

DESENSITIZATION

Desensitization is chosen when the sensory evaluation reveals an area of **hypersensitivity**, in which ordinary stimuli produce exaggerated or unpleasant sensations (Yerxa et al., 1983). The term hypersensitivity includes **allodynia**, which is the perception of pain as a result of a non-painful stimulus, and **hyperesthesia**, which is a heightened sensitivity to tactile stimuli (Venes, Thomas, & Taber, 2001). Desensitization is an intervention designed to decrease the discomfort associated with touch in the hypersensitive area. A program of desensitization generally includes repetitive stimulation of the hypersensitive skin with items that provide a variety of sensory experiences, such as textures ranging from soft to coarse.

Rationale for Desensitization

Hypersensitivity is observed in some but not all patients following nerve trauma, soft tissue injuries, burns, and amputation (Waylett-Rendall, 1995; Yerxa et al., 1983). Patients with hypersensitivity tend to avoid using the affected part in functional activities (Waylett-Rendall, 1995) and typically hold the affected part protectively (Hardy, Moran, & Merritt, 1982). Hypersensitivity can lead to disability through non-use of the involved body part (Robinson & McPhee, 1986).

Desensitization is based on the idea that progressive stimulation will allow progressive tolerance. The origin of the concept of desensitization is unknown. Civil War veterans with amputations were known to tap silver spoons on their residual limbs to improve their tolerance of artificial limbs, which, in those days, were constructed from wood (Hardy, Moran, & Merritt, 1982). Dellon (1997) considers desensitization a form of sensory retraining during which the patient learns accurate, less painful perception of sensory input. The desensitization program should use principles that enhance learning, such as structured practice within the context of functional activities.

Desensitization Techniques

Initially, a patient may have to compensate for hypersensitivity by wearing a splint or padding over the affected area. The patient must be weaned gradually from the protective device as improvement occurs (Anthony, 1998). In the treatment program, the patient develops progressive tolerance to a hierarchy of sensory stimuli, although several different hierarchies of desensitization materials exist.

The hierarchy described by Hardy, Moran, and Merritt, (1982) includes five levels:

- Level 1. Tuning fork, paraffin, massage
- Level 2. Battery-operated vibrator (Fig. 27-1), deep massage, touch pressure with pencil eraser
- Level 3. Electric vibrator, texture identification
- Level 4. Electric vibrator, object identification
- Level 5. Work and daily activities

Patients advance to the next level after they demonstrate tolerance of the current level without signs of irritation. Work simulation is believed to be extremely important to ensure that the patient is using the painful site. Activities must be tailored to the patient's interest and occupation.

Table 27-1 shows the Downey Hand Center hierarchy of textures and vibration (Barber, 1990; Yerxa et al., 1983). Commercial dowel and immersion textures (Resources 27-1) are similar to this hierarchy. Patients arrange the dowel textures and immersion textures (Fig. 27-2) according to their own perception, in the order of least to most irritating. They select the dowel texture, immersion texture, and vibration level that are uncomfortable but tolerable for 10 minutes three or four times daily. Advancing to the next level of treatment depends on tolerance of lower levels. Documentation includes the patient's initial

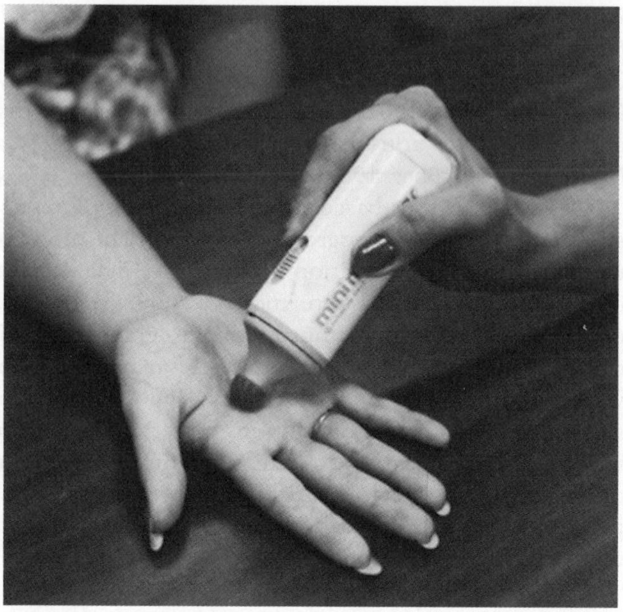

Figure 27-1. The small head of this battery-powered vibrator is useful for desensitization of specific areas of the hand.

RESOURCE 20-1

Sensory Treatment Equipment Suppliers

North Coast Medical
(three-phase desensitization kit, portable desensitization kit, vibrators, stereognosis kit)
18305 Sutter Boulevard
Morgan Hill, CA 95037-2845
Phone: (800) 821-9319
Fax: (877) 213-9300
www.ncmedical.com

Sammons Preston Rolyan
(multi-phase desensitization kit, sensory reeducation wands, sensory reeducation home program kit, tactile activity kit, stereognosis kit, vibrators)
270 Remington Boulevard, Suite C
Bolingbrook, IL 60440-3593
Phone: (800) 323-5547
Fax: (800) 547-4333
www.sammonspreston.com

hierarchy and progress for each of the three modalities (Waylett-Rendall, 1995).

Other clinical activities thought to decrease hypersensitivity include weight-bearing pressure, massage, transcutaneous electrical stimulation, fluidotherapy, and therapy putty. Use of the affected body part in leisure, work, and daily occupations is believed to facilitate desensitization. Typing, hair washing, macramé, and assembling leather link belts are examples of activities used to decrease hypersensitivity in the hand or fingers (Anthony, 1998; Dellon, 1997; Waylett-Rendall, 1995).

Effectiveness of Desensitization

Evidence of the effectiveness of desensitization techniques in therapy is limited to a small number of studies. Barber (1990), using descriptive statistics, reported effectiveness following a chart review of intervention. Additional evidence of the success of desensitization includes a narrative single-case study (Robinson & McPhee, 1986) and a small-sample, non-randomized trial (Hardy, Moran, & Merritt, 1982).

Despite the lack of evidence, desensitization techniques are generally accepted as effective in clinical practice. Experts in the field of hand therapy describe patient improvement and promote use of desensitization techniques (Skirven & Callahan, 2002; Walyett-Rendall, 1995). In a

Table 27-1. Hierarchy of Texture and Vibration Used in Desensitization

Level	Dowel Textures	Immersion Textures	Vibration (cps)
1	Moleskin	Cotton	83 cps near area
2	Felt	Terry cloth pieces	83 cps near area, 23 cps near area
3	QuickStick[a]	Dry rice	83 cps near area, 23 cps intermittent
4	Velvet	Popcorn	83 cps intermittent, 23 cps intermittent
5	Semirough cloth	Pinto beans	83 cps intermittent, 23 cps continuous
6	Velcro loop	Macaroni	83 cps continuous, 53 cps intermittent
7	Hard foam	Plastic wire insulation pieces	100 cps intermittent, 53 cps intermittent
8	Burlap	Small BBs, buckshot	100 cps intermittent, 53 cps continuous
9	Rug back	Large BBs, buckshot	100 cps continuous, 53 cps continuous
10	Velcro hook	Plastic squares	No problem with vibration

[a] A closed-cell, firm splint padding material.

Adapted from Barber, L. (1990). Desensitization of the traumatized hand. In J. Hunter, L. Schneider, E. Mackin, & A. Callahan (Eds.), *Rehabilitation of the hand* (3rd ed., pp. 721–730). St. Louis: Mosby.

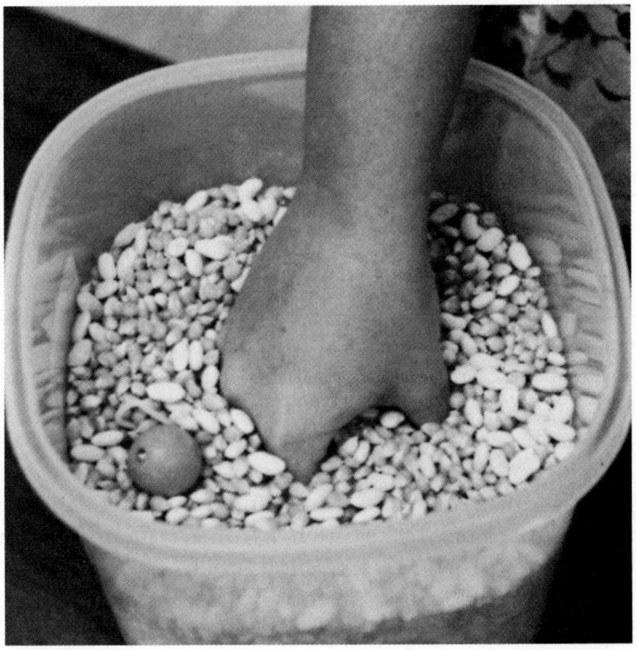

Figure 27-2. Immersion of the hand into a container filled with popcorn kernels and pinto beans facilitates desensitization. Patients use touch to find objects hidden in the immersion particles.

large study of hand therapy practice, all of the therapists surveyed used desensitization techniques on at least some of their patients, and more than half of the therapists elected to use the techniques for 26–50% of their patient caseload (Muenzen et al., 2002).

SENSORY REEDUCATION

Sensory reeducation is a combination of techniques that helps the patient with a sensory impairment learn to reinterpret sensation (Dellon, 1997). Dellon (1988), a hand surgeon, related his experience in 1970 with nerve-injured patients who could feel fingertip stroking, pinprick, and pressure but could not correctly identify a nickel and a quarter using only touch sensation. These patients could feel a difference between the coins, but they could not identify them, and the coins did not feel the same as before the injury.

Dellon concluded that the sensibility was recovered but that there was a mismatch of the new sensory profile with past profiles in the association cortex. Within a few minutes, he could train patients to tell the difference between the two coins. With the patient's vision shielded, he placed a nickel in the hand, said what it was, and explained that it did not feel the way a nickel used to feel but that what the patient was feeling should thereafter be called a nickel. After repeating the process with a quarter, the patient could correctly identify both coins. The sensation had been reeducated.

In daily activities, cutaneous information from the fingers, palm, and toes is most important because it is generally these skin surfaces that interact with the external environment (Dannenbaum & Dykes, 1988). The focus of sensory reeducation is usually to regain the use of sensation of the hand. Ninety-nine percent of hand therapists surveyed reported using sensory reeducation techniques (Muenzen et al., 2002). Sensory reeducation is an appropriate and commonly used treatment for patients with a variety of peripheral nerve injuries, including nerve lacerations and neural compressions and injuries resulting in replantation, toe-to-thumb grafting, and skin grafting (Dellon, 1997).

Sensory reeducation is also sometimes used for patients who have had cerebral vascular accidents (CVA). In a study of occupational therapists treating patients with CVA, Neistadt and Seymour (1995) asked the therapists to rank 10 categories of treatment activities according to frequency of use. Sensory reeducation was ranked ninth, indicating that sensory retraining following CVA has low priority in many clinical settings. Despite evidence that recovery of motor function depends on sensation, the focus of treatment following CVA seems to be motor rather than sensory deficits (Dannenbaum & Jones, 1993).

Rationale for Sensory Reeducation after Peripheral Nerve Injury

Cortical maps have been found to change as a result of peripheral nerve injuries. Loss of sensory input from the peripheral nerve causes the associated areas of the sensory cortex to begin to serve sensory inputs from adjacent areas. After nerve repair, when the peripheral nerve regrowth leads to reinnervation of sensory receptors, the corresponding area of the somatosensory cortex reorganizes to allow interpretation of incoming stimuli from the affected area (Dellon, 1997; Merzenich & Jenkins, 1993). In children, this reorganization is sufficient for return of normal sensory interpretation without sensory retraining. In adults, the neural reorganization may be facilitated by sensory reeducation (Rosen et al., 1994).

The return of sensation following hand injury is an extremely complex event. Recovery is not just a process of altering the cortical representation; it also depends on reinnervation. Following nerve laceration and surgical repair, some sensory fibers, given sufficient time, regenerate and reinnervate the tactile receptors. Return of sensation is limited by scar tissue that blocks sensory fiber regrowth and atrophy of sensory receptors prior to reinnervation. Sensory return is also limited by malalignment of axonal sheaths that allows misdirection of regrowing fibers, meaning that fibers do not usually regrow to innervate the same sensory receptors that they innervated before the injury (Callahan, 1995).

As a result of scar tissue, atrophy of sensory receptors, and the misdirection of fibers, there is an inevitable change in the profile of neural impulses reaching the sensory cortex. A previously well-known stimulus initiates a different set of neural impulses from that elicited by the same stimulus before the injury. When this altered profile reaches the sensory cortex, the patient cannot match it with patterns previously encountered and remembered (Callahan, 1995; Dellon, 1997) and, hence, cannot identify or recognize the stimulus (Fig. 27-3). The purpose of sensory reeducation in patients with peripheral injuries is to help them learn to recognize the distorted cortical impression (Skirven & Callahan, 2002).

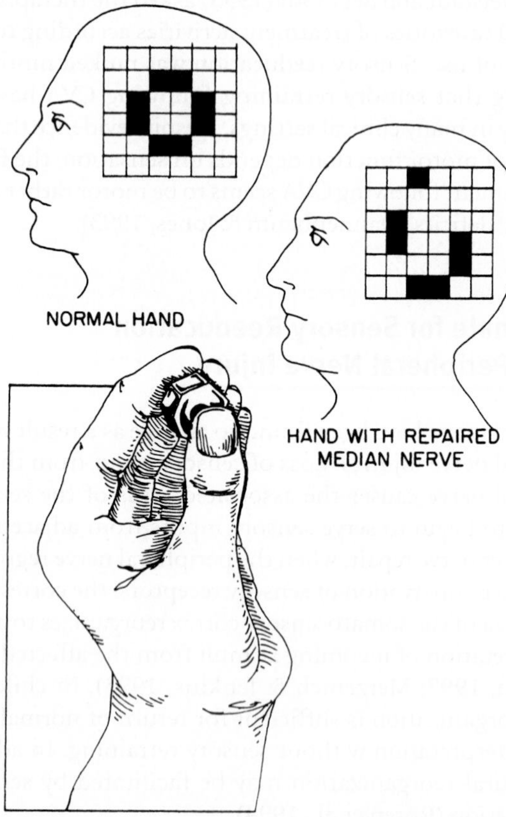

Figure 27-3. In the normal hand, a stimulus, such as this gripped bolt, elicits a profile of neural impulses that reaches the sensory cortex and ultimately is perceived, as represented by the checkerboard pattern. After a nerve repair, the same stimulus elicits an altered profile of impulses that reaches the sensory cortex. The new perception, the altered checkerboard pattern, may be so different from the previous one that object recognition is at first impossible. (Reprinted with permission from Dellon, A. [1988]. *Evaluation of sensibility and re-education of sensation in the hand.* Baltimore: Lucas.)

Sensory Reeducation Techniques after Peripheral Nerve Injury

After peripheral nerve injury, axonal regeneration and reinnervation are necessary for improvement in sensation. Dellon (1997) cautions that implementation of sensory reeducation before adequate axonal regeneration has no benefit and causes frustration. Because of varying rates of axonal sprouting and growth, sensory receptors are reinnervated over time. Sensory reeducation can begin when the patient first can appreciate deep, moving touch. In the early phase of intervention, the patient concentrates on learning to match the sensory perception of stimuli with the visual perception. After time, when reinnervation allows for perception of light non-moving touch with good touch localization, the focus of intervention changes to more functional tasks, such as object identification through touch (Fig. 27-4) (Dellon, 1988).

Sensory reeducation protocols differ among facilities, even those treating patients with similar diagnoses. Dellon (1997) shares protocols for sensory reeducation after peripheral injury from five institutions. A summary of the protocol he presents from the Raymond M. Curtis Hand Center of Union Memorial Hospital, which is based on Dellon's earlier work, is given in Procedures for Practice 27-1.

Skirven and Callahan (2002) describe similar procedures. They begin each moving and constant touch sequence with eyes closed, followed by eyes open, and concluding with eyes closed. They recommend using a smaller and lighter stimulus as the patient improves, with a goal of localization of a touch that is near the light-touch threshold. Touch localization continues throughout the sensory reeducation process, and more tasks are added to the training program. Discrimination of similar and different textures using sandpaper, fabrics, and edges of

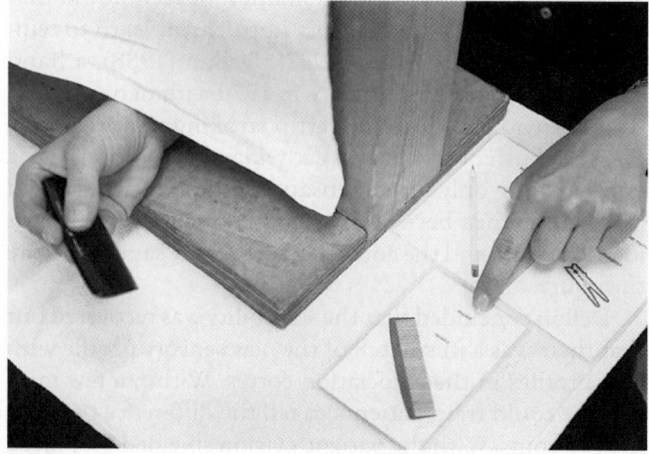

Figure 27-4. Late-phase sensory reeducation after peripheral nerve injury includes identification of various objects by touch.

PROCEDURES FOR PRACTICE 27-1

Sensory Reeducation Principles

- Choose a quiet environment that will maximize concentration.
- Sessions should be brief, approximately 5–15 minutes.
- Three or four practice or homework sessions per day are recommended.
- Instruct the patient and/or family in techniques to be used during practice.
- Monitor patient's home program and progress during therapy sessions.

Prerequisites for Early-Phase Sensory Reeducation

- Patient must be able to perceive 30 cycles per second vibration and moving touch in the area.
- Patient must be motivated and able to follow through with the program.

Techniques for Early-Phase Sensory Reeducation

- Use the eraser end of a pencil.
- Apply moving strokes to the area.
- Use enough pressure for the patient to perceive the stimulus but not so much that it causes pain.
- Ask the patient to observe what is happening first and then to close the eyes and concentrate on what is being felt.
- Instruct the patient to put into words (silently) what is being felt.
- Instruct the patient to observe the stimulus again to confirm the sensory experience with the perception.
- When perception of constant touch returns to the area, use a similar process for constant touch stimuli.
- Test the patient by requiring localization of moving and constant touch without seeing the stimulus.

Prerequisites for Late-Phase Sensory Reeducation

- Patient must be able to perceive constant and moving touch at the fingertips.
- Patient must demonstrate good localization of touch.

Techniques for Late-Phase Sensory Reeducation

- Use a collection of common objects that differ in size and shape.
- Instruct the patient to grasp and manipulate each item with eyes open, then with eyes closed, and then with eyes open for reinforcement.
- The patient should concentrate on the tactile perception.
- Test the patient by timing correct identification of each object without vision.
- Grade the practice by introducing objects of similar size but different texture and then small objects that vary in size and shape but are similar in texture.

Adapted from Dellon, A. L. (1997). *Somatosensory testing and rehabilitation.* Bethesda, MD: American Occupational Therapy Association.

coins are introduced early. Patients practice identification of shape or letter blocks and **graphesthesia**, which is the ability to identify a letter or number drawn on the skin. In the later stages of training, patients pick objects from containers filled with sand or rice and practice identification of common objects. Finally, patients practice daily living activities with vision occluded. Skirven and Callahan state that a variety of activities, including games or puzzles, are more engaging and therefore more beneficial than simply practicing with various objects.

Nakada and Uchida (1997) described a five-stage sensory reeducation program that was useful for a patient with very limited sensation in her left hand as a result of peripheral neuropathy secondary to leprosy. She also had total impairment of vision, so that sensory feedback was critical to occupational performance. Following reeducation, the patient regained hand function for activities of daily living such as drying dishes, putting on socks, and holding dentures while brushing them. The reeducation program included the following five stages:

- Stage 1. Object recognition using feature detection strategies. Objects that varied greatly in shape, material, and weight were used. The patient was encouraged to handle each object and identify the object characteristics.
- Stage 2. Prehension of various objects with refinement of prehension patterns. In this stage, grasping objects that varied in size and shape was emphasized. The patient needed to maximize the contact between the object and the hand to develop the ability of the hand to closely contour to objects, which is seen in normal grasp.
- Stage 3. Control of prehension force while holding objects. Feedback regarding excessive force that was used to maintain grasp was provided through the use of a strain gauge and therapy putty.
- Stage 4. Maintenance of prehension force during transport of objects. While holding an object, the patient moved the shoulder, elbow, and wrist into varying positions of flexion and extension.
- Stage 5. Object manipulation. The patient practiced grasp and release of objects and moved objects in the hand into various positions.

Appropriate grading of sensory reeducation activities is important to optimize patient motivation and progress.

Choose activities that provide a challenge but allow for success. During stimulus localization tasks, progress from firm pressure to lighter pressure. When working with objects, progress from larger items to smaller items and from dissimilar items to more similar items. Progress from differentiation of a few objects to selecting, sequencing, or organizing many objects (Skirven & Callahan, 2002).

As daily training is necessary for successful sensory reeducation, teach patients techniques appropriate for a home program. Patients can be involved in assembling their own collection of objects for use in their program. Include objects with varying size, shape, texture, weight, and temperature (Fess, 2002).

Effectiveness of Sensory Reeducation after Peripheral Nerve Injury

Dellon (1997) reviewed a large number of studies of the effectiveness of sensory reeducation following peripheral nerve injury, replantation, and innervated skin graft. Study designs included: (1) comparison of patients who today routinely receive sensory reeducation with those in the past before widespread acceptance of the technique, and (2) assessment of the results of sensory reeducation provided long after spontaneous recovery is likely. Dellon concluded that sensory reeducation clearly improves sensory and functional recovery in a shorter period than without training and indicates that the techniques have been globally accepted as necessary following peripheral nerve injury.

The best evidence in the therapy literature for the effectiveness of sensory reeducation is the study by Cheng et al. (2001) described in Evidence Table 27-1. Sensory reeducation effectiveness following digital replantation and revascularization has also been demonstrated in a small, randomized control trial (Shieh et al., 1995).

Rationale for Sensory Reeducation after CVA

Sensory reeducation after CVA is based on the concept of neural plasticity. Carr and Shepherd (1998), in their review of the scientific evidence for the ability of the brain to reorganize following brain lesions, stated that reorganization seems to be related to frequency of use. They suggested that enlargement of sensory receptive areas within the cortex is a result of increased participation of the body part in activities requiring tactile sensations. Therapists may alter the cortical map by directing the sensory experiences of the patient. Therefore, the goal of sensory reeducation after CVA is to gain a larger cortical representation for the areas of skin from which sensory feedback is crucial to performance of daily tasks.

The rationale for sensory reeducation following CVA is also based on the premise that functional use of a body part with reduced sensation is possible but that spontaneous use is limited. Without training, there is a tendency not to use the extremity, and learned non-use leads to further loss of sensory and motor abilities (Dannenbaum & Dykes, 1988). Sensory reeducation has the potential to facilitate increased functional use of the hand and prevent loss of function due to learned nonuse.

Sensory Reeducation Techniques after CVA

Sensory reeducation after CVA is less well defined than the protocols described for peripheral injuries. Carr and Shepherd, in their book, *A Motor Relearning Programme for Stroke* (1982), and in their more recent work (1998), emphasize the need for sensory learning concurrent with motor learning. They advocate the use of meaningful and relevant sensory and motor experiences very early in rehabilitation. Use of the more involved hand in bimanual tasks such as opening jars and using eating utensils is advocated. They suggest that the patient can be cued to attend to the tactile aspects of the task and that practice of object identification without vision may be helpful.

Dannenbaum and Jones (1993) give detailed goals and proposed methodology for sensory intervention following CVA. They believe that appreciation of some form of tactile stimulation and some basic motor skills are prerequisite to success in sensory reeducation. To establish that a patient with severe sensory loss can perceive some stimuli, they recommend testing and early training using 100-Hz electrical stimulation. Patients identify which finger was stimulated, first with vision and then with eyes closed. Patients with better sensation perform a similar task, first with textured moving stimuli followed by non-moving stimuli.

In addition, Dannenbaum and Jones suggest early incorporation of the hand into functional activities and prevention of abnormal patterns of grasp and movement. Add textures to handle surfaces to increase the friction and support weak grasping ability. Enlarge or modify handles to facilitate both tactile contact and tactile feedback. Patients should practice modulation of grip forces in response to the objects and maintenance of appropriate grip force during forearm movements.

Yuketiel and Guttman's (1993) research protocol included the following sensory reeducation activities:

- Identification of the number of touches
- Graphesthesia tests
- "Find your thumb" without looking
- Identification of shape, weight, and texture
- Passive drawing and writing: the patient identifies a letter, number, or drawing made by the therapist passively moving the patient's hand while it holds a pencil

These sensory treatment activities are just a few examples of a wide variety of techniques that can be used in clinical treatment for patients after CVA. Therapists working with this population use creativity, patients' interests, and

Evidence Table 27-1
Best Evidence for Occupational Therapy Practice Regarding Sensory Reeducation

Intervention	Description of Intervention Tested	Participants	Dosage	Type of Best Evidence and Level of Evidence	Benefit	Statistical Probability and Effect Size of Outcome	Reference
Early tactile stimulation for digital nerve injuries	In-clinic stimulation of digital sensation by pressing injured finger against rotating disc with raised and lowered segments. Home program of rubbing finger over rows of raised staples on a plastic card.	49 subjects with a total of 65 digital nerve injuries following surgical repair.	Clinical program required 20 minutes twice weekly; home program completed daily, as much as patient desired. Clinic program averaged 11 weeks in duration; home program averaged 16 weeks.	Randomized control trial, using ordinal measures and nonparametric statistics. IB2a	More participants in the experimental group recovered touch threshold measuring 0.217 g or less, and static and moving two-point discrimination of 6 mm or less.	$p = 0.097$, $r = 0.22$ for touch threshold; $p = 0.0023$, $r = 0.48$ for static two-point discrimination; and $p = 0.0144$, $r = 0.36$ for moving two-point discrimination.	Cheng et al., 2001; Cheng, 2000
Training of somatosensory discrimination after stroke	Training in discrimination of textures and joint motion, using training principles of high intensity, repetition, graded progression, intermittent feedback, and comparison with visual feedback or contralateral hand.	10 subjects with a diagnosis of stroke and tactile or proprioceptive discrimination impairment	Ten treatment sessions, scheduled three times per week, lasting 40-60 minutes each.	Single case, multiple baseline experiments with meta-analysis of intervention effects. IC2b	Yes. Discrimination of textures and joint position improved from baseline following initiation of training.	Meta-analysis $p<.001$. Average effect size 0.52	Carey & Matyas, 2005

theoretical understanding to develop programs of sensory intervention since no one protocol has been widely accepted or thoroughly researched.

Effectiveness of Sensory Reeducation after CVA

The number of research studies of the effectiveness of sensory retraining after CVA is limited, and the results of these studies have not been strong enough for the technique to be recommended in the *Clinical Practice Guideline: Post-Stroke Rehabilitation* (United States Department of Health and Human Services, 1995) or in the Veterans Affairs/Department of Defense Clinical Practice Guidelines (Bates et al., 2005).

Improved proprioception, touch localization, two-point discrimination, and tactile discrimination following training have been demonstrated in several small, non-randomized studies (Carey, Matyas, & Oke, 1993; Dannenbaum & Dykes, 1988; Yekutiel & Guttman, 1993). Increased cerebral blood flow and changed cerebral activation in the somatosensory cortex following proprioceptive input has been demonstrated experimentally (Nelles et al., 1999). Additional sensory input was associated with improved grip-force modulation in one small non-randomized controlled trial (Aruin, 2005). The best evidence of effectiveness of sensory reeducation following cortical injury is the study by Carey and Matyas described in Evidence Table 27-1, which showed good learning of texture discrimination and joint position with a systematic program that heavily incorporated principles of learning.

Teasell and Kalra (2004) described six emerging trends in stroke rehabilitation, two of which relate to sensory reeducation. There is increasing use of robotic-assisted sensorimotor training, in which repetitive passive or active-assistive motion provides proprioceptive stimulation and leads to improved motor recovery. Another trend is the increased understanding of the importance of sensory stimulation in facilitating stroke recovery. Both of these trends are likely to increase research in treatment of somatosensory dysfunction after cortical injury.

CASE EXAMPLE

Mr. T.: Sensory Remediation after Median Nerve Laceration

Occupational Therapy Intervention Process	Clinical Reasoning Process	
	Objectives	**Examples of Therapist's Internal Dialogue**
Patient Information Mr. T., a 25-year-old appliance repairman with a laceration of the median nerve, was reassessed approximately 6 weeks after his injury. The outpatient occupational therapy reassessment identified the following sensory problems: • Absent and decreased protective sensation in the thumb, index and middle fingers, and radial palm • Mislocalization of touch sensations in the radial portion of the palm • Hypersensitivity in the area of the scar • Decreased ability to pick up and manipulate objects • Decreased use of the right hand in functional activities	Appreciate the context	(See Chapter 7 for description of the assessment process and patient's background.)
	Develop intervention hypotheses	"While a good bit of time in therapy will be spent on Mr. T.'s motor deficits, I know that good sensation is needed for hand coordination and for return to full function at work."
	Select an intervention approach	"Because Mr. T. has multiple sensory issues, he will need multiple approaches. A compensatory approach will be needed for lost protective sensation and a remedial approach is needed to decrease hypersensitivity and relearn touch localization and object identification."
	Reflect on competence	"As I work with Mr. T., I may need to discuss ideas with a colleague, particularly for creative sensory retraining strategies to increase the variety of activities."

Recommendations

At the time of the reassessment, the occupational therapist recommended outpatient occupational therapy twice a week for 6 additional weeks and then reassessment, with reduction to one session per week likely at that time. Mr T. has demonstrated quick learning of therapy instructions and will be responsible for an intensive home program. Because recovery of the ability to differentiate small objects at the fingertips will probably not occur until 10–12 months after the nerve repair, therapy would ideally continue for that length of time. In collaboration with Mr T., the occupational therapist established the following long-term goals for sensory intervention: (1) Mr. T. will correctly interpret sensory stimuli throughout the right hand, as demonstrated by correct tactile identification of objects; and (2) Mr. T. will demonstrate good use of the right hand in work simulation activities that rely on touch sensation.

Consider the patient's appraisal of performance	"Mr. T. has demonstrated quick learning of therapy instructions so far. He doesn't seem to fully understand the connection between sensation exercises and his eventual hand function, so I may need to give him more examples of how he uses sensory feedback in his work and daily activities."
Consider what will occur in therapy, how often, and for how long	"During therapy, I will definitely need to focus on teaching Mr. T. what he needs to do at home. He will be completing an extensive home program. Experts in the field of hand therapy suggest the home program should be completed three to four times daily. During therapy sessions, I will need to provide evaluation of progress, grading of sensory activities for the home program, and motivational strategies."
Ascertain the patient's endorsement of plan	"Mr. T. seems eager to complete therapy tasks right now, and if he follows through with his home program, that should further indicate his agreement with the plan of care."

Summary of Short-Term Goals and Progress

1. Mr. T. will avoid injury to the right hand by demonstrating compensatory protective strategies during functional activities. The therapist instructed Mr. T. about risk of injury from sharp and hot objects and gripping forces. Mr. T. and the therapist discussed an appropriate routine for skin care and implementation of precautions in his daily routine. By the end of the second session, Mr. T. demonstrated good understanding of these techniques during home and simple work simulation activities.
2. Mr. T. will tolerate touch of all textures over and around his scar area so that hypersensitivity does not interfere with functional hand use. Mr. T. ranked the 10 dowel textures from least to most irritating. At that time, he easily tolerated the first four textures as they were rubbed by the therapist over the scar area. He disliked touch from the fifth texture and was unable to tolerate textures 6 through 10. The therapist provided textures for a home desensitization program, beginning with textures 5 and 6. Mr. T. used these textures three or four times a day for scar desensitization. During therapy sessions, massage and vibration were provided around and over the scar area. At the end of 3 weeks, Mr. T. tolerated all textures and no longer reported discomfort from sleeve cuffs or inadvertent touch during functional activities.
3. Mr. T. will demonstrate touch localization below 10 mm in the right palm to improve interpretation of tactile sensations during work activities. The therapist initiated a sensory reeducation program for touch localization using moving and static touch stimuli in the palm. Instructions were provided, and Mr. T. faithfully followed through with this program at home, four sessions per day. At the end of 3 weeks, localization in the palm measured 12–14 mm. The therapist initiated graphesthesia and texture discrimination activities in the palmar area. After 6 weeks of sensory reeducation, localization measured 9–10 mm, and Mr. T. could identify 50% of the letters and shapes drawn in his palm and 40% of the textures.

Assess the patient's comprehension	"Mr. T. not only understands his home program, but he is also learning when to progress to the next dowel texture without me needing to tell him."
Understand what he is doing	
Compare actual to expected performance	"Mr. T. is progressing even faster than I expected he would in his desensitization program. His sensory reeducation is proceeding at the expected rate, consistent with the typical rate of neural regrowth."
Know the person	"Mr. T. demonstrated such good learning of techniques that, after these first 3 weeks, I could consider decreasing the frequency of therapy for his sensory deficits to once weekly. He will need to continue his home program at the same intensity of three to four sessions daily. Whether or not to decrease frequency of therapy will also depend on how his motor recovery is progressing."
Appreciate the context	

Next Steps Revised Short-Term Goals (1 month): To improve interpretation of tactile sensations during work activities, (1) Mr. T. will demonstrate 100% correct graphesthesia and texture identification in his right palm; and (2) Mr. T. will demonstrate touch localization below 10 mm in the proximal phalanges of the right thumb, index, and middle fingers.	Anticipate present and future patient concerns	"Mr. T. has made exceptional progress over the past 6 weeks and is eager to return to work, which will make attendance at therapy and completion of his home exercise program more difficult."
	Analyze patient's comprehension	"Mr. T. continues to need extensive home program activities to improve his sensation. He has learned his home program well and knows how to advance it."
	Decide if the patient should continue or discontinue therapy and/or return in the future	"Because recovery of the ability to differentiate small objects at the fingertips will probably not occur until 10–12 months after the nerve repair, he will require ongoing sensory reeducation for at least a year or more. It would be advisable to follow up with reassessment and program revision every 2–3 months during that time period. This will also help Mr. T. to be more motivated to continue his home program throughout this long time period."

CLINICAL REASONING IN OCCUPATIONAL THERAPY PRACTICE

Transition of Sensory Reeducation Program from Early Phase to Late Phase

Mr. T. will begin the second phase of sensory reeducation at the fingertips approximately 6–8 months after his surgery to repair the median nerve. What reassessment findings will indicate the appropriate time for Mr. T. to begin late-phase sensory reeducation? What treatment activities and home program activities would be appropriate for Mr. T. as he begins this phase? What work simulation activities could be incorporated into his therapy program during sensory reeducation?

SUMMARY REVIEW QUESTIONS

1. What is the rationale for sensory reeducation after peripheral nerve injury and CVA?
2. What are the differences and similarities between early-phase and late-phase sensory reeducation for patients with peripheral nerve injury?
3. Describe or demonstrate intervention techniques for a patient with hypersensitivity after a fingertip amputation.
4. List five mechanisms of injury for skin areas with absent or diminished protective sensation. For each of the five mechanisms of injury, describe appropriate preventive education and/or adaptive strategies.
5. What should be done if a patient with sensory loss develops an area of skin redness?

ACKNOWLEDGMENT

I extend my appreciation to Paul Petersen and Melanie Seltzer for their assistance with some of the photography for this chapter.

References

American Diabetes Association. (2004). Position statement: Preventive foot care in diabetes. *Diabetes Care, 27,* S63–S64.

Anthony, M. (1998). Desensitization. In G. L. Clark, E. F. Shaw Wilgis, B. Aiello, D. Eckhaus, & L. Valdeta Eddington (Eds.), *Hand rehabilitation* (pp. 77–91). New York: Churchill Livingstone.

Aruin, A. S. (2005). Support-specific modulation of grip force in individuals with hemiparesis. *Archives of Physical Medicine and Rehabilitation, 86,* 768–775.

Barber, L. (1990). Desensitization of the traumatized hand. In J. Hunter, L. Schneider, E. Mackin, & A. Callahan (Eds.), *Rehabilitation of the hand* (3rd ed., pp. 721–730). St. Louis: Mosby.

Bates, B., Choi, J. Y., Duncan, P. W., Glasberg, J. J., Graham, G. D., Katz, R. C., Lamberty, K., Reker, D., & Zorowitz, R. (2005). Veterans Affairs/Department of Defense clinical practice guidelines for the management of adult stroke rehabilitation care: Executive Summary. *Stroke, 36,* 2049–2056.

Brand, P. (1979). Management of the insensitive limb. *Physical Therapy, 59,* 8–12.

Brand, P. W., Hollister, A. M., Giurintano, D., & Thompson, D. E. (1999). External stress: Effect at the surface. In P. W. Brand & A. M. Hollister (Eds.), *Clinical mechanics of the hand* (3rd ed., pp. 215–232). St. Louis: Mosby.

Callahan, A. D. (1995). Methods of compensation and reeducation for sensory dysfunction. In J. M. Hunter, E. J. Mackin, & A. D. Callahan (Eds.), *Rehabilitation of the hand: Surgery and therapy* (4th ed., pp. 701–713). St. Louis: Mosby.

Carey, L. M., & Matyas, T. T. (2005). Training of somatosensory discrimination after stroke. *American Journal of Physical Medicine and Rehabilitation, 84,* 428–442.

Carey, L. M., Matyas, T. A., & Oke, L. E. (1993). Sensory loss in stroke patients: Effective training of tactile and proprioceptive discrimination. *Archives of Physical Medicine and Rehabilitation, 74,* 602–611.

Carr, J. H., & Shepherd, R. B. (1982). *A motor relearning programme for stroke.* Oxford, United Kingdom: Butterworth-Heinemann.

Carr, J. H., & Shepherd, R. B. (1998). *Neurological rehabilitation: Optimizing motor performance.* Oxford, United Kingdom: Butterworth-Heinemann.

Cheng, A. S. (2000). Use of early tactile stimulation in rehabilitation of digital nerve injuries. *American Journal of Occupational Therapy, 54,* 159–165.

Cheng, A. S., Hung, L., Wong, J. M., Lau, H., & Chan, J. (2001). A prospective study of early tactile stimulation after digital nerve repair. *Clinical Orthopedics and Related Research, 384,* 169–175.

Cole, J. (1991). *Pride and a daily marathon.* Cambridge, MA: MIT.

Dannenbaum, R., & Dykes, R. (1988). Sensory loss in the hand after sensory stroke: Therapeutic rationale. *Archives of Physical Medicine and Rehabilitation, 69,* 833–839.

Dannenbaum, R. M., & Jones, L. A. (1993). The assessment and treatment of patients who have sensory loss following cortical lesions. *Journal of Hand Therapy, 6,* 130–138.

Dellon, A. L. (1988). *Evaluation of sensibility and re-education of sensation in the hand.* Baltimore: Lucas.

Dellon, A. L. (1997). *Somatosensory testing and rehabilitation.* Bethesda, MD: American Occupational Therapy Association.

Eggers, O. (1984). *Occupational therapy in the treatment of adult hemiplegia.* Rockville, CO: Aspen.

Fess, E. E. (2002). Sensory reeducation. In: E. J. Mackin, A. D. Callahan, T. M. Skirven, L. H. Schneider, A. L. Osterman, & J. M. Hunter (Eds.), *Rehabilitation the hand and upper extremity* (5th ed., pp. 635–639). St. Louis: Mosby.

Hardy, M., Moran, C., & Merritt, W. (1982). Desensitization of the traumatized hand. *Virginia Medical Journal, 109,* 134–137.

Manske, P. R. (1999). The sense of touch. *Journal of Hand Surgery, 24A,* 213–214.

Merzenich, M. M., & Jenkins, W. M. (1993). Reorganization of cortical representations of the hand following alterations of skin inputs induced by nerve injury, skin island transfers, and experience. *Journal of Hand Therapy, 6,* 89–104.

Muenzen, P. A., Kasch, M. C., Greenberg, S., Fullenwider, L., Taylor, P. A., & Dimick, M. P. (2002). A new practice analysis of hand therapy. *Journal of Hand Therapy, 15,* 215–225.

Nakada, M., & Uchida, H. (1997). Case study of a five-stage sensory reeducation program. *Journal of Hand Therapy, 10,* 232–239.

Neistadt, M. E., & Seymour, S. G. (1995). Treatment activity preferences of occupational therapists in adult physical dysfunction settings. *American Journal of Occupational Therapy, 49,* 437–443.

Nelles, G., Spiekermann, G., Jueptner, M., Leonhardt, G., Muller, S., Gerhard, H., & Diener, C. (1999). Reorganization of sensory and motor systems in hemiplegic stroke patients: A positron emission tomography study. *Stroke, 30,* 1510–1516.

Robinson, S., & McPhee, S. (1986). Case report: Treating the patient with digital hypersensitivity. *American Journal of Occupational Therapy, 40,* 285–287.

Rosen, B., Lundborg, G., Dahlin, L. B., Holmberg, J., & Karlson, B. (1994). Nerve repair: Correlation of restitution of functional sensibility with specific cognitive capacities. *Journal of Hand Surgery (British), 19B,* 452-458.

Shieh, S. J., Chiu, H. Y., Lee, J. W., & Hsu, H. Y. (1995). Evaluation of the effectiveness of sensory reeducation following digital replantation and revascularization. *Microsurgery, 16,* 578–582.

Skirven, T. M., & Callahan, A. D. (2002). Therapist's management of peripheral-nerve injuries. In E. J. Mackin, A. D. Callahan, T. M. Skirven, L. H. Schneider, A. L. Osterman, & J. M. Hunter (Eds.), *Rehabilitation of the hand and upper extremity* (5th ed., pp. 599–634). St. Louis: Mosby.

Sloan, H. L., & Abel, R. J. (1998). Getting in touch with impaired foot sensibility. *Nursing, 28(11),* 50–51.

Teasell, R. W., & Kalra, L. (2004). What's new in stroke rehabilitation. *Stroke, 35,* 383–385.

Thompson, M., Medley, A., & Motts, S. (2002). Foot sensations measured by Semmes-Weinstein monofilaments in persons newly diagnosed with diabetes. *Journal of Geriatric Physical Therapy, 25,* 42.

United States Department of Health and Human Services. (1995). *Clinical Practice Guideline: Post-Stroke Rehabilitation* (AHCPR Publication 95-0662). Rockville, MD: United States Department of Health and Human Services.

Venes, D., Thomas, C. L., & Taber, C. W. (Eds.). (2001) *Taber's cyclopedic medical dictionary* (19th ed.). Philadelphia: F.A. Davis.

Vermeij, G. J. (1999). The world according to the hand: Observation, art, and learning through the sense of touch. *Journal of Hand Surgery, 24A,* 215–218.

Waylett-Rendall, J. (1995). Desensitization of the traumatized hand. In J. M. Hunter, E. J. Mackin, & A. D. Callahan (Eds.), *Rehabilitation of the hand: Surgery and therapy* (4th ed., pp. 693–700). St. Louis: Mosby.

Wood, H. (1969). Prevention of deformity in the insensitive hand: The role of the therapist. *American Journal of Occupational Therapy, 23,* 488–489.

Yekutiel, M., & Guttman, E. (1993). A controlled trial of the retraining of the sensory function of the hand in stroke patients. *Journal of Neurology, Neurosurgery, and Psychiatry, 56,* 241–244.

Yerxa, E., Barber, L., Diaz, O., Black, W., & Azen, S. (1983). Development of a hand sensitivity test for the hypersensitive hand. *American Journal of Occupational Therapy, 37,* 176–181.

CHAPTER 28

Optimizing Vision, Visual Perception, and Praxis Abilities

Lee Ann Quintana

LEARNING OBJECTIVES

After studying this chapter, the reader will be able to do the following:

1. Identify and describe specific treatments for low vision and oculomotor dysfunction.
2. Identify and describe five treatment approaches for unilateral neglect.
3. Identify and describe specific treatment for apraxia, including limb, constructional, and dressing apraxia.

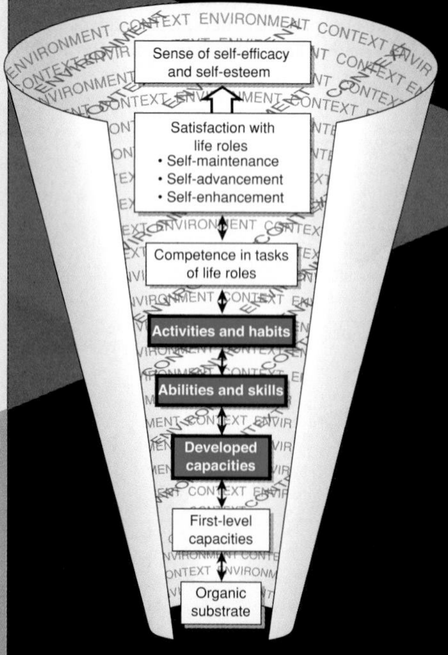

Glossary

Anchoring—Method of providing a cue on the side contralateral to the brain damage, in the presence of unilateral neglect.

Chaining—Method by which a task is broken down into steps. The client learns the first step, then the next, and then puts the two together, after which he or she then learns the third step and puts them all together, and so on. In backward chaining, the therapist completes the task except for the last step, which the client does; then the therapist completes all except the last two steps, which the client does; and so on.

Extinction—Phenomenon of neglect that occurs when stimuli are presented in both visual fields or both sides of space at one time and only one stimulus is reported, whereas if presented to either side individually, the client reports the stimulus.

Fresnel prism—Temporary prism used with a client with hemianopsia or unilateral neglect; applied to the client's glasses, it shifts the visual field toward the intact side.

Low vision—Any condition in which a person's vision is not adequate for his or her needs.

Occlusion—Covering part or all of the visual field of the eye.

Prism—Type of lens that is thicker on one side than the other; the purpose is to bend the light and move the image coming onto the fovea.

Vision therapy—Intervention generally prescribed and carried out by or under the supervision of the eye care professional.

Occupational therapists working with adults with brain injury have traditionally emphasized evaluation and treatment of perceptual dysfunction (Abreu & Toglia, 1987; Warren, 1993a). Although the literature on the identification and evaluation of perceptual dysfunction is extensive, information on the effectiveness of treatment is limited. Much of the research on diagnosis and evaluation has been carried out by psychologists and neuropsychologists who have only recently begun to focus on function. Unfortunately, occupational therapists, who see the effects of perceptual dysfunction on a person's daily living skills, have been slow to generate research and hence support for their treatment.

Remediation of perceptual deficits generally falls under the realm of cognitive rehabilitation, which is provided by occupational therapists, speech and language pathologists, neuropsychologists, and psychologists (Harley et al., 1992). Historically, occupational therapists have emphasized the area of perception, whereas speech and language pathologists and psychologists have emphasized cognition.

Rather than focus on high-level perceptual skills, this chapter discusses specific treatment for visual foundation skills including low vision and ocular motor dysfunction, unilateral neglect, and apraxia, including limb, constructional, and dressing apraxias (see Chapter 8 for detailed descriptions and definitions). Treatment approaches and general treatment principles specific to optimizing cognitive function are discussed in Chapter 29.

VISUAL FOUNDATION SKILLS

Warren (1993a) developed a hierarchy of visual perception (see Fig. 8-1). The base of this hierarchy consists of the visual foundation skills, which include acuity, visual fields, and oculomotor function. Following a screening of these skills, clients may then be referred to an eye care specialist for further evaluation and diagnosis of deficits. These specialists diagnose the problem and may recommend medical treatment, such as medication, surgery, optical changes, use of assistive devices, and/or **vision therapy** to improve the visual function of the client.

With the aging population, vision loss is the third most common chronic condition requiring assistance with activities of daily living (ADL) (Colenbrander & Fletcher, 1995). At the same time, people may not be aware of or complain about their difficulty and just accept it as a part of aging. Some age-related changes and diseases increase the likelihood of vision loss (Table 28-1). As a result, occupational therapists work with many clients who have a vision loss of one kind or another and who may or may not be labeled as having low vision.

Low Vision

"Low vision can be considered any condition in which a person's visual function is not adequate for his or her visual needs" (Kern & Miller, 1997, p. 495). Based on acuity, low vision (LV) covers anywhere from 20/80 vision to total blindness, which denotes *no* residual vision at all (Definition 28-1) (Colenbrander & Fletcher, 1995; Kern & Miller, 1997).

The focus of occupational therapy in LV rehabilitation is "training the patient to use remaining vision as efficiently and effectively as possible to complete daily activities and includes training in use of optical devices" (Warren, 1995, p. 877). Occupational therapy treatment includes environmental adaptation, compensatory techniques, assistive devices, and client/family education (Warren, 1999b).

Table 28-1. Age-Related Changes in Vision

Condition	Definition
Cataracts	A cloudiness of the lens of the eye that dulls color and visual detail (Mogk, 2000). Acuity can improve with increased contrast. Surgical treatment is typically successful.
Glaucoma	Causes increased pressure in the eye, which damages the optic nerve and results in decreased peripheral vision, or tunnel vision. It is generally treated medically with eye drops and laser treatment.
Diabetic retinopathy	Bleeding from small blood vessels in retina can lead to serious vision loss. A person can develop scotomas, decreased contrast sensitivity and color discrimination, decreased night vision, and fluctuations in vision (due to fluctuations in blood glucose levels) (Mogk, 2000).
Age-related macular degeneration (ARMD)	Results in loss of central vision. Two types: dry ARMD is the most common type (90%), it develops gradually, and there is no effective medical or surgical treatment; wet ARMD has a rapid onset, and treatment consists of laser surgery.
Lens tends to yellow	Changes color perception; glare may be a problem.

DEFINITION 28-1

Low Vision Definitions

Normal Vision

Normal—20/12, 20/16, 20/20, 20/25; able to read a standard letter size at a standard distance (e.g., approximately 8-point print at 40 cm)

Near-normal—20/30 to 20/60; generally able to read newsprint by bringing the print closer (may need stronger reading prescription)

Low Vision

Moderate low vision—20/80 to 20/160; must bring the print very close, which isn't comfortable for prolonged use, but can maintain nearly normal reading speeds with assistive devices (i.e., base in prisms, reading glasses, magnifiers).

Severe low vision—20/200 to 20/400 or visual field of 20° or less; must bring print so close that binocularity is no longer possible and must use the best eye to read; as a result, reading is slower than normal and vision substitution (i.e., listening to the radio rather than reading) comes into use. 20/200 is considered legally blind, but a person still has usable vision.

Profound low vision—20/500 to 20/1000 or visual field of 10° or less; must bring print to within less than 2 inches, so reading is limited to essential materials; use of video magnification may be mandatory as well as use of vision substitution.

Blindness

Near blindness—20/1250 to 20/2500; vision is unreliable and is used as an adjunct to other senses; emphasis is on vision substitution techniques and devices.

Total Blindness—no residual vision at all (Colenbrander & Fletcher, 1995; Freeman, 2002; Warren, 2000).

Low Vision Specialists

Rehabilitation Teacher	Emphasis on effect of visual impairment on ADL, patient, and family. Teach techniques, technology, and use of devices for persons with low vision or blindness.
Orientation and Mobility (O & M) Specialist	Teach orientation techniques (use of sensory information to determine position in space relative to the environment) and mobility skills (use of canes, sighted guides, travel aids, dog guides) for safe and independent travel.
Rehabilitation Counselor	Provide counseling related to occupation and employment, provide career guidance, assist with job placement (from teaching interviewing skills to adjusting to the workplace).
Certified Low Vision Therapist (CLVT)	Teach clients to use their vision more efficiently, with and without optical devices, environmental modification, and visual skills training.

From Kern & Miller, 1997; Studebaker & Pankow, 2004; and Sokol-McKay & Michels, 2005.

Table 28-2. Environmental Factors and Adaptations

Environmental Factor	Adaptation
Lighting	Control glare: Window coverings; cover shiney surfaces; positioning and type of lamp used. Special lenses or sunshield may be prescribed by low vision specialist. Decrease the distance between the light and the task. Increase wattage of light bulb. Try alternate types of bulbs (florescent, incandescent, halogen). Task lighting: Position the light opposite the writing hand or nearest to best-seeing eye (Fig. 28-1).
Contrast	Change the background to increase contrast: A solid color rather than a busy pattern; light against dark and vice versa. For example, use a dark cutting board to cut up an egg and a white cutting board to cut up broccoli (Fig. 28-2).
Color	Bright colors are easiest to see. They can be used to highlight points of interest (e.g., mark a certain temperature on a toaster oven) or to provide a warning (e.g., bright tape on the leading edge of a step).
Pattern	Keep the environment uncluttered and simple.
Print size	Enlarge print, increase contrast, increase print quality.
Working distance	Important for both near and far activities, but especially with bifocal and trifocal lenses, which are distance specific. Normal working distance is about 16 inches.

From Sokol-McKay & Michels, 2005; and Watson, 2001.

Most occupational therapists do not specialize in treating LV per se but, instead, encounter LV as a complication in clients with other functional impairments and medical conditions (Kern & Miller, 1997). Occupational therapists are in a unique position to aid LV specialists (Definition 28-1) by providing input on the client's functional impairment and how this may affect the selection and use of assistive devices. For example, the client with tremors may not benefit from a hand-held magnifier or may require certain positioning before using the device. Occupational therapists should have supervision and/or specialized training to recommend and train clients in use of prescribed LV aides (Kern & Miller, 1997).

Many basic self-care activities can be completed with minimal vision, but LV becomes more of a problem with such ADL activities as meal preparation, managing finances, and community activities. Generally, when working with clients who have LV, we should consider both the functional implications and environmental factors involved (Lampert & Lapolice, 1995). For example, clients with poor contrast sensitivity require increased contrast and lighting and have difficulty with curbs, stairs, and finding objects in a low light, while a person with visual field loss will have more difficulty in a busy, moving environment. Environmental factors (Table 28-2) can be manipulated to improve the person's ability to perform a task. For example, with the client who is having difficulty with meal preparation, consider changing the lighting, marking the controls with bright contrasting colors, organizing the kitchen and keeping items in their assigned places, and marking containers with large-print labels.

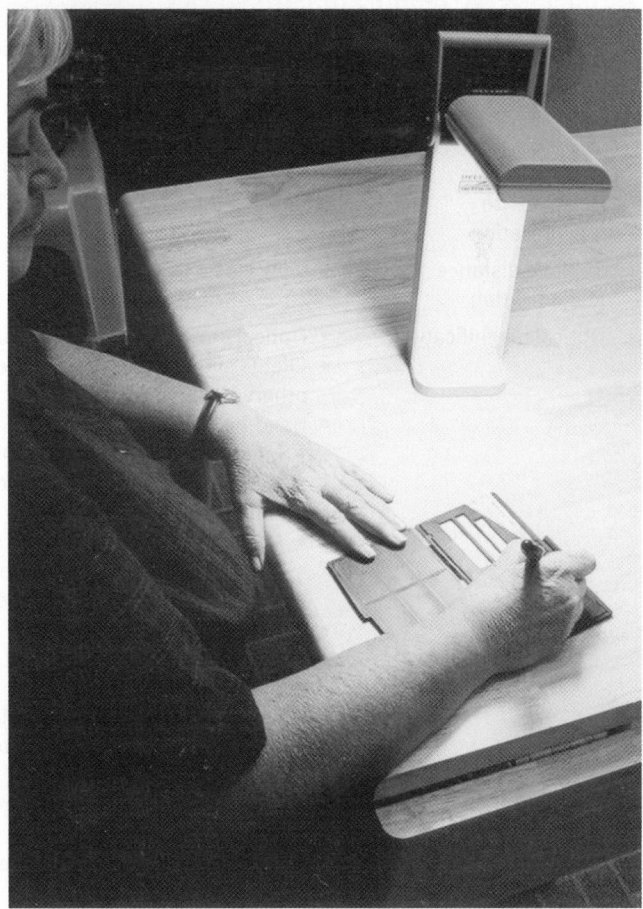

Figure 28-1 The use of task lighting and a check guide to facilitate check writing.

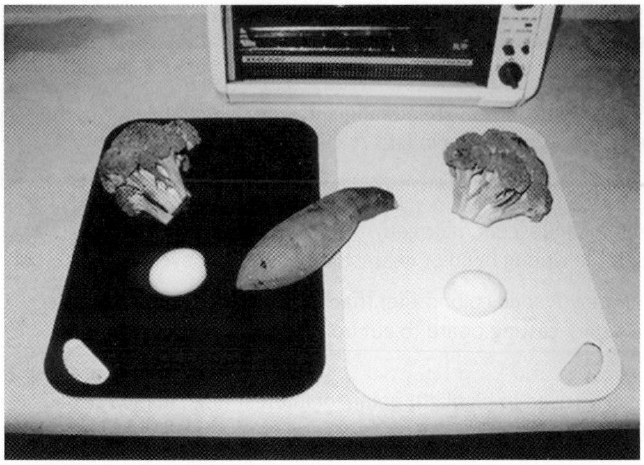

Figure 28-2 Changing the color of the cutting board to increase contrast with the item that is to be cut.

In addition to manipulation of the environment, compensatory techniques include use of optical devices, such as lenses and telescopes, and non-optical devices, such as large print, contrasting tape to mark stair steps, felt tip pen, and a computer (Beaver & Mann, 1995). Magnification (Table 28-3) is a fundamental means of improving vision by making an object larger and thus more visible (Nowakowsi, 2000). The client and family should be taught what the limitations are and how to compensate and manipulate the environment so that they can transfer the techniques to new situations as they arise.

Ocular Motor Dysfunction

Ocular motility refers to the ability of the eyes to move smoothly and with coordination through full range of motion. Ocular motor dysfunction includes problems with binocular vision, accommodation, scanning, and saccades. Problems with binocular vision typically result in diplopia or double vision. Treatment includes lenses, **prisms**, or **occlusion**. Lenses are used to treat a variety of refractive, accommodative, and binocular disorders. In most cases, they are used as a means of compensation to allow the person to function despite the disorder (Scheiman, 1997). A prism is a type of lens that is thicker on one side than the other. Its purpose is to bend the light coming into the eye, moving the image onto the fovea, allowing single vision. Lenses and

Table 28-3. Magnification

Principles	• Does not necessarily make vision clearer, it enlarges the object of regard, which is then more recognizable. • The stronger the magnification, the smaller the field of view and the closer the magnifier is held to the eye. • Special training is usually required by a low vision therapist.
Relative size magnification	Increasing the size of the object: large-print book, large-number measuring cups.
Relative distance magnification	Moving closer to an object makes it relatively larger, for instance, holding a book closer to the face.

Optical magnification	• Optical devices are generally prescribed by an optometrist or ophthalmologist.
	• Clients should wear their own eyeglasses while using the optical device unless instructed otherwise by the doctor.
	• Hand-held magnifiers:
	  • Must be held at a predetermined distance from what is being read.
	  • If wearing bifocals, client should look through the top part of the glasses.
	• Stand magnifiers:
	  • Magnifier rests on a surface while the hand guides it (better choice for a client with tremors).
	  • Must hold the lens a specified distance from the eye.
	  • If wearing bifocals, client should look through the bottom part of the glasses.
	• Microscopic glasses:
	  • Can be a half-eye, bifocal, or full lens.
	  • Allows the hands to be free.
	  • Object of regard must be held close to the face.
	  • Usually involve only the better eye.
	• Telescopes:
	  • Primarily used to view distant objects.
	  • Usually a monocular device.
	  • May be hand held or mounted on eyeglasses.

Electronic	Closed-circuit television (CCTV): • Allows greatest amount of magnification and field of view. • Disadvantages: not portable, cost.

From Nowakoski, 2000; and Sokol-McKay and Michels, 2005.

CLINICAL REASONING IN OCCUPATIONAL THERAPY PRACTICE

Effects of Low Vision on a Functional Task

Based on an optometrist's report for a patient, J.K., his best corrected acuity is 20/160. He has a cataract in the right eye and glaucoma in both eyes, for which he is receiving medication.

How might this affect his ability to complete his self-care activities, meal preparation, and financial activities? What modifications could be made to his environment? What assistive devices could he use?

prisms are recommended by the eye care professional, who is responsible for the strength of the lenses and prisms and any exercise programs. The occupational therapist assists the client with follow-through of the eye care professional's recommendations and encourages compliance with the wearing schedule.

Occlusion should be carried out in consultation with the eye care professional. It may be either total or partial. Total occlusion is achieved by means of a patch or opaque tape on the client's glasses (Fig. 28-3). Compliance with this method is often poor for the following reasons: (1) total occlusion can cause clients to feel off balance because of loss of peripheral and central vision input to the central nervous system, and it reduces depth perception; (2) monocularity can cause discomfort, especially when the dominant eye is occluded (Warren, 1999a). The recommendation is to avoid total occlusion if at all possible (Hellerstein & Fishman, 1997) and, if it is necessary, to alternate occlusion between the eyes every hour (Warren, 1999a). Partial occlusion appears to have better compliance. In this case, an opaque material added to the client's glasses blocks input to the central visual field, leaving the peripheral field unobstructed (Fig. 28-4). Since diplopia in the central visual field is the most bothersome, the tape is applied to the nasal portion of the glasses of the non-dominant eye (Warren, 1999a). As the client focuses on a target, the tape is applied as far centrally as the client reports diplopia. As the muscles get stronger, the occluded area is decreased. When using occlusion, the client should do range-of-motion exercises to prevent contractures to the unaffected eye. Warren (1999a) recommends that exercises first be done with the unaffected eye covered and then with both eyes together.

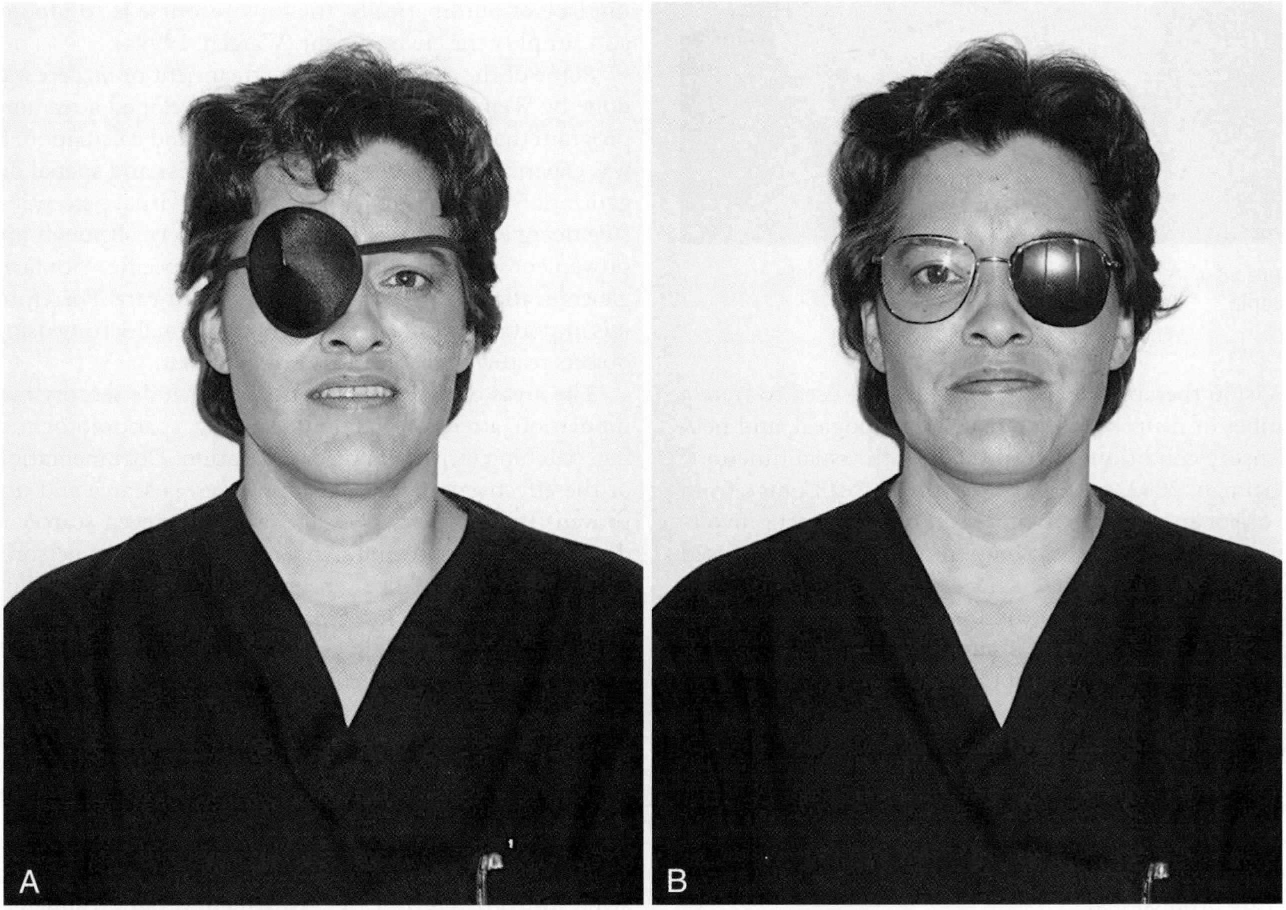

Figure 28-3 Total occlusion. **A.** Pirate patch. **B.** Opaque material covering lens of glasses.

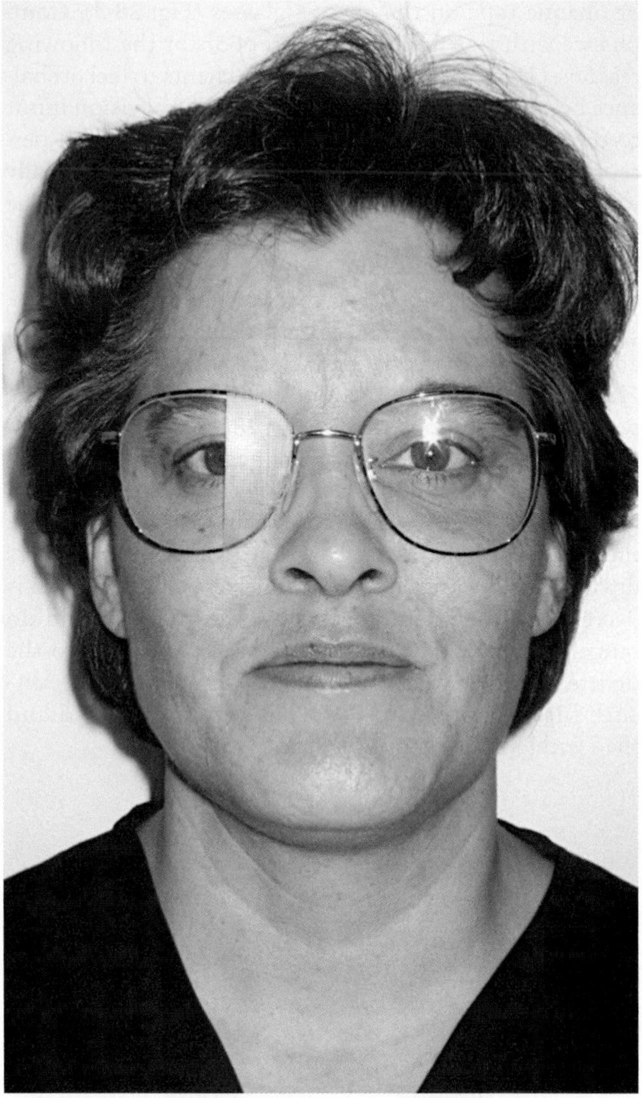

Figure 28-4 A method of partial occlusion to alleviate diplopia.

Vision therapy "is an organized regime used to treat a number of neuromuscular, neurophysiological, and neurosensory conditions that interfere with visual function" (Scheiman, 2002, p. 129). Vision therapy can range from the use of an eye patch to more complex treatment involving instrumentation and computers and is generally used to treat disorders of binocular vision, accommodation, ocular motility, strabismus, and visual information processing (Scheiman, 2002). The occupational therapist who has not been trained in prescribing and training clients with lenses, prisms, and occlusion should not provide vision therapy unless supervised by an eye care professional (Hellerstein & Fishman, 1999). The occupational therapist can work closely with the eye care professional to provide input as to the client's functional needs and situation and then follow through with training that is set up by the eye care professional.

UNILATERAL NEGLECT

Unilateral neglect (UN) is referred to by a variety of names, including hemi-inattention, hemispatial neglect, and unilateral spatial agnosia. It is manifested by a failure to respond or orient to stimuli presented contralateral to a brain lesion (Heilman, Watson, & Valenstein, 1993). It is observed functionally in the client who eats the food on only half of the plate, shaves only one side of the face, and walks into objects on the side contralateral to the brain lesion. It has been suggested (Bisiach et al., 1990; Coslett et al., 1990; Tegner & Levander, 1991) that there are two types of neglect: motor or output neglect (impaired initiation or execution of movement into contralateral hemispace by either limb) and sensory or input neglect (awareness of stimuli on one side of the body or one side of space). The presence of UN has a negative effect on the rehabilitation of right brain-damaged (RBD) patients (Gillen, Tennen, & McKee, 2005; Paolucci et al., 2001).

The treatment of unilateral neglect can be approached in a variety of ways. First, the client must be aware of the problem. If aware that they have a problem, many of these clients can voluntarily orient, even though they have difficulty with automatically orienting (Ladavas, Carletti, & Gori, 1994). If they are unaware and unable to orient voluntarily or automatically, the only recourse is to modify and simplify the environment (Warren, 1999a).

Some of the early work on the treatment of neglect was done by Weinberg et al. (1977), who developed a training program that included reading, writing, and calculation. It was expanded to include sensory awareness and spatial organization and tasks to increase complex visual perception (Weinberg et al., 1979, 1982). Unfortunately, although improvement was seen, it tended to be task specific, with little generalization to other tasks or areas of self-care. Therefore, it is important to train persons in a functional setting using objects readily available in the environment.

The areas of treatment for neglect include sensory manipulation, attention training, scanning, spatiomotor cueing, patching, prisms, and compensation. Documentation of the effectiveness of these approaches is scarce and unproven (Bowen, Lincoln, & Dewey, 2002); even scarcer is documentation of the influence of treatment on a person's functional ability. Since sensory manipulation, including caloric stimulation, optokinetic stimulation, and use of medication, is not within the scope of occupational therapy practice and the effects so far are transitory and without carryover, this area is not addressed.

Attention Training

One theory of UN is that the problem is due to a deficit in attention. If this is the case, a treatment program aimed at increasing attention and general level of alertness should improve UN. Robertson et al. (1995) trained patients with RBD and UN to self-alert during activities. With 5 hours of training, they could mentally tell themselves to pay attention frequently during tasks. Improvement in UN and sustained attention lasted 1–14 days.

In another study, Robertson et al. (1998) found that providing a warning tone as a means of alerting the patient that something was going to happen prior to a task increased perceptual processing and shifting of spatial attention to the left. This was developed further with a limb-activation device (Robertson et al., 2002) that is programmed to emit a tone if there is no movement within a set period of time (2–120 seconds) and can attach to the arm, leg, or shoulder. They found a significant effect on motor function of the arm and leg, which persisted for 18–24 months.

Another method of self-activation is the patient's use of the contralateral extremity as a cue (e.g., to mark the left side of the page while reading or to move the extremity while walking to increase attention to that side). Robertson et al. (1994) found that patients who moved their contralateral hand when walking through a doorway exhibited a decrease in neglect.

Scanning

Visual scanning training is frequently used in treatment for UN. This can include paper and pencil tasks; computer programs; scanning in a functional setting, such as a grocery store; and use of the Dynavision (Fig. 28-5). Research supports improvement on visual perceptual tasks, reading, and academic work with this type of training, but it does not generalize to gross motor tasks (Wagenaar et al., 1992).

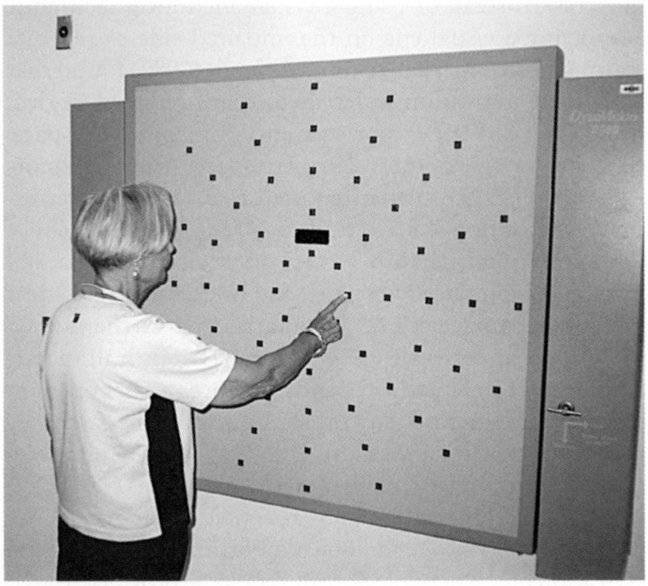

Figure 28-5 Dynavision.

The literature indicates that the effects of scanning training are specific to the situation. If the goal is to improve the client's ability to read or scan at tabletop, tabletop scanning training is appropriate; but if the therapist wants to improve a client's ability to scan in the community, practice in the community is needed. Warren (1993b) provided guidelines for selection of treatment activities for clients with deficits in visual attention and visual scanning (Table 28-4).

Niemeier (1998) developed a visual imagery technique called the lighthouse strategy in which clients are taught to visualize themselves as a lighthouse and use the eyes to sweep the environment. This method was found to increase attention to the neglected side of space. Paolucci et al. (1996) used a training program for neglect that included scanning, copying, and description of scenes in addition to a rehabilitation approach and found that there was an improvement not only on tests of neglect, but also on function. On the other hand, although Bailey, Riddoch, and Crome (2002) found an improvement with scanning and cueing, no generalization to functional activity was present. It seems that scanning tasks and cueing should be included in functional activities whenever possible to facilitate transfer to functional tasks.

Clients who are being trained to scan must learn to take in the information in an organized manner, such as left to right. **Anchoring** (supplying a cue on the impaired side to indicate starting position) can be used to help the client bring attention back to the neglected side

Table 28-4. Training Guidelines for Visual Attention and Visual Scanning

Train patients to reorganize their scanning strategy.	Use of anchoring techniques and scanning devices (Weinberg et al., 1979).
Broaden visual field that patient must scan.	Use of activities that require the patient to turn the head or change body positions to complete the task (e.g., scanning items on a kitchen shelf).
Reinforce visual experience with sensorimotor experiences.	Use of activities in which the patient is required to manipulate what is seen (e.g., reach for or touch items scanned).
Emphasize conscious attention to detail and careful inspection of objects.	Use of matching tasks in which the patient may be encouraged to slow down and double-check interpretation of what is seen.
Practice the skill in context to ensure carryover.	Treatment may begin in the clinic, but strategies must be practiced in a variety of real-life situations.

Reference: Warren, M. (1993b). A hierarchical model for evaluation and treatment of visual perceptual dysfunction in adult acquired brain injury, part 2. *American Journal of Occupational Therapy, 47*, 55–66.

(Table 28-5). During practice of scanning using cancellation tasks, a structured array (symbols arranged in neat, straight rows across the page) should be used at first because patients with RBD have difficulty with organized search (Weintraub & Mesulam, 1988). This array can be made increasingly more complex (e.g., requesting two target letters, decreasing the spacing between letters, or decreasing the size of the letters) as the client progresses (Cooke, 1992). Scanning tasks must be practiced in a variety of settings because clients can improve on a task without an improvement in neglect. An excellent therapeutic intervention is the use of Toglia's (1991) multicontext treatment approach. An example of levels of transfer for a letter, consisting of crossing out a specific letter on a page of four rows of random letters, can be seen in Table 28-6.

Table 28-5. Anchoring Technique

Sequence of Cueing	Task Demand
1. A vertical anchoring line is used on the left side; the beginning and ending of the line are sequentially numbered.	Patient uses the vertical line to find the beginning and the numbers to avoid skipping lines.
Example: 1 | The law was passed to allow the 1 2 | state to conduct a national FBI 2 3 | criminal records check before 3 4 | certifying teachers. 4	
2. A vertical anchoring line is used on the left side, only the beginning of the line is sequentially numbered.	Patient uses the vertical line and numbers on the left; the number cue on the right has been eliminated.
Example: 1 | Family members, followed by 2 | coworkers, are the most 3 | frequent targets of 4 | anger.	
3. A vertical anchoring line is used on the left side.	Patient uses only the vertical line to find left side.
Example: | Environmental groups hope to | minimize the divisiveness and | avoid mistakes made in the | Pacific Northwest.	
4. No cues are provided.	Patient must read without any cues.
Example: The state distributes its lottery proceeds without regard to which communities generate the revenue.	

Reference: Quintana, L. A. (1995). Remediating perceptual impairments. In C. A. Trombly (Ed.), *Occupational therapy for physical dysfunction* (4th ed., pp. 529–537). Philadelphia: Williams & Wilkins.

Table 28-6. Levels of Transfer for a Letter Cancellation Task

Transfer Distance	Task
Near	Patient is instructed to cross out the number 5 (number cancellation task).
Intermediate	Four horizontal rows of various coins are presented. Patient is instructed to place a marker over all the nickels (tabletop task).
Far	Patient is presented with a spice rack and is asked to pick out all of the jars that need to be refilled (standing and reaching at kitchen cabinets).
Very far	Patients is evaluated on the ability to initiate spontaneously left-to-right scanning in the context of simple, everyday life tasks (reading four lines in a large print magazine or locating an item in the medicine cabinet or on a shelf).

Spatiomotor Cuing

If there are two types of neglect, as has been suggested (Bisiach et al., 1990; Coslett et al., 1990; Tegner & Levander, 1991), it is reasonable to expect that each has its own form of treatment. For a client with primarily a motor or output neglect, encouragement of left-hand activation may reduce neglect to a greater extent than visual perceptual cuing. An example might be having the client move the left hand (whatever movement is available) while performing a scanning task instead of using a visual anchoring technique (supplying a visual cue on the impaired side to indicate starting position). Robertson and North (1992) found that left motor activation in left hemispace reduced neglect more than did left motor activation in right hemispace, right motor activation in left hemispace, or visual cuing. Robertson (1992) further reported that (1) left lower extremity activation reduced neglect, (2) passive movement of the left extremity had no effect on neglect, (3) bilateral movements produced no effect, and (4) there was no effect if the movement became automatic. In a further study, Robertson and North (1994) found that simultaneous activation of right and left hands produces a phenomenon similar to **extinction**, such that the advantage gained by activating the left hand is lost. Only single left-hand movement produced a large reduction in neglect. This could have implications for use of bilateral activities, such as those used in the Bobath technique. Opportunity for unilateral activation of the hemiplegic arm should be provided as well as bilateral activation (Robertson & North, 1994).

If the client has more of a sensory or input neglect, he may benefit from visual cuing such as anchoring (Table 28-5) or reminders to look to the left. Training the client to use the left upper extremity as an anchor during functional activities provides both a perceptual anchor and a means of left-limb activation (Robertson, North, & Geggie, 1992).

Patching

Eye patching techniques for UN include single-eye patching (Fig. 28-3) and half-field patching (Fig. 28-6). For the client with neglect, either the entire eye ipsilateral to the lesion is covered or the hemifield of both eyes is covered (i.e., in the case of left UN, the right eye or right hemifields of both eyes).

Patching one eye is believed to influence the central nervous system by way of the superior colliculus (Posner & Rafal, 1987), increasing eye movements to the contralateral side and decreasing neglect. Patching the ipsilateral hemifield is felt to increase activation of the involved hemisphere, resulting in increased attention to the contralateral side.

Butter and Kirsch (1992) found that patching the right eye of patients with left neglect decreased the patients' left neglect score. When lateralized visual stimulation was added, the relative benefits were larger. The beneficial effects, however, were present only when the eye patch was on, and the study did not include generalization to functional tasks.

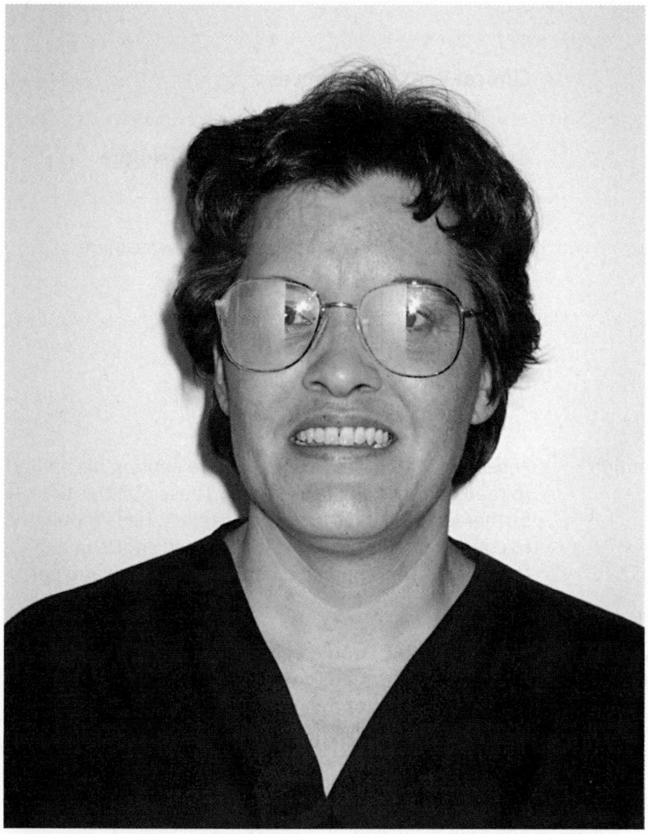

Figure 28-6 Right hemifield patching for left visual neglect.

Beis et al. (1999) followed 22 patients with UN: 7 wore glasses with patches covering the right eye, 7 wore glasses with right half-field patches, and 8 controls had no patching. The patches were worn up to 12 hours a day for 3 months. The results of the patients with the right half-field glasses were significantly different from those of the controls, with the right half-field patients exhibiting an increase in total *Functional Independence Measure* score (Uniform Data System for Medical Rehabilitation, 1997) and increased time looking to the left.

Arai et al. (1997) also looked at the effects of half-field patching with 10 RBD patients. They found a decrease in neglect, improvement on pencil and paper tasks, and good functional return in one patient. Harrell, Kramer-Stutts, and Zolten (1995) also found an improvement of neglect in patients wearing goggles with half-field glasses.

In summary, patching has many benefits. It can be used throughout the day during a variety of functional activities and does not rely on memory and training. Patching is simple, inexpensive, and usable by a variety of disciplines.

Prisms

In the case of UN or heminopsia, the prisms used are called yoked because the base of the prisms are on the same side for each eye (Scheiman, 2002). They function by shifting the visual field toward the intact side and thereby providing the patient with the ability to see things on the involved side. These prisms may involve the whole visual field or partial field. They can be the more temporary **Fresnel prism**, which is a flexible plastic sheet with small ridges that can be cut to shape and stuck to the patient's glasses, or a more permanent prism that is part of the patient's prescription. Advantages of the Fresnel prism are that it is inexpensive and temporary and can be applied and removed easily. The disadvantages are that it may distort visual acuity and tends to bubble and increase distortion (Gianutsos & Suchoff, 2002; Hellerstein & Fishman, 1997).

Gianutsos and Suchoff (2002) recommend the use of the Fresnel prisms as a temporary or diagnostic device. They have found that the partial Fresnel prisms (covering half of the patient's glasses) are not as beneficial as yoked prisms ground into the patient's prescription.

Rossetti et al. (1998) used prisms to shift the visual field (VF) to the right in 16 RBD patients with left UN. Initially the patients exhibited a shift to the left when pointing straight ahead. Following adaptation, patients were given tasks including line bisection, line cancellation, copying, drawing from memory, and reading. Patients in the experimental group exhibited an improvement in neglect, which was maintained for 2 hours. Frassinetti et al. (2002) expanded this and found that the prism adaptation was maintained for at least 5 weeks and, for some subjects, was maintained for up to 17 weeks.

Rossi, Kheyfets, and Reding (1990) found that the use of Fresnel prisms improved visual perception in stroke patients with homonymous hemianopsia or unilateral visual neglect. Another study found that, although prisms improved exploration of space, the information obtained may still be neglected or less salient (Morris et al., 2004).

The advantages of using prisms include: effects can be obtained within a short period of time, they do not require voluntary orientation of attention to the involved side, and they are non-invasive and can be used anywhere (Frassinetti et al., 2002).

Compensation

Compensation can be environmental or cognitive. Adaptation of the environment includes such things as arranging the client's bed so that the uninvolved side is toward the activity in the room and always interacting with the client on the uninvolved side. Although this might be a good idea initially to evaluate clients and to keep them from harming themselves, it does nothing to help them overcome the deficit. It is recommended that both the remedial and adaptive approaches be used.

Cognitive compensation includes metacognitive training (Toglia, 1991), use of video feedback (Soderback, et al, 1992), and teaching the client a routine to complete a specific activity (i.e., donning a shirt) with clients cognitively cueing themselves through each step. Clients must be aware that there is a problem before they can use compensatory techniques (Crosson et al., 1989; Tham, Borell, & Gustavsson, 2000). These techniques must be practiced, and eventually, if the client becomes an active problem solver, the techniques can be generalized to new situations.

CASE EXAMPLE

S.D.: Occupational Therapy Intervention to Address Problems with Visual Scanning

Occupational Therapy Intervention Process	Clinical Reasoning Process: Objectives	Clinical Reasoning Process: Examples of Therapist's Internal Dialogue
Patient Information S.D., a 21-year-old man who is 15 months post right cerebrovascular accident, participated in an outpatient occupational therapy assessment, and the following problems were identified: (1) decreased ocular motor skills including decreased convergence, decreased accommodation, and inefficient saccades and smooth pursuits; and (2) unilateral neglect.	Appreciate the context	See Chapter 8 for description of the assessment process and patient's background.
	Develop intervention hypotheses	"I believe that S.D.'s visual skills are limiting his ability to read and participate in school. These abilities are further limited by his unilateral neglect. He is motivated to continue in school and participate in sports in a different way. This should facilitate his learning and participation in therapy."
	Select an intervention approach	"I think that S.D. would benefit from visual scanning training, using various compensatory techniques, which, according to the research, is successful although task specific. He will probably need to learn compensatory techniques that he can apply to various functional situations. Participation of his family and personal care attendant (PCA) will be very important in follow through with the program."

	Reflect on competence	"I'm afraid that S.D. is going to have to learn to compensate cognitively and may continue to require environmental compensations. Clients I've had with his degree of denial in the past either required a large increase in time to complete a task correctly or continued to require cues."
Recommendations The occupational therapist recommended 1-hour treatment sessions twice a week for 8 weeks. In collaboration with S.D., the occupational therapist established the following long-term goals: (1) S.D. will read his homework with accuracy and good speed; (2) S.D. will demonstrate the ability to maneuver throughout familiar and unfamiliar environments independently; and (3) S.D. will independently use appropriate compensatory strategies for unilateral neglect as needed during functional activities.	Consider what will occur in therapy, how often, and for how long	"I feel that S.D. would benefit from therapy 2 times a week, but his family and PCA will be instrumental in assisting him to follow through with compensatory techniques. Hopefully, they will be able to attend some of the therapy sessions."
Summary of Short-Term Goals and Progress 1. S.D. will demonstrate improved use of scanning strategies such that he is able to copy information from 5 feet away to a sheet of paper at near distance with 80% accuracy. S.D. is having difficulty with accommodation, which interferes with participation in his college classes because he is unable to copy information from the chalkboard. The task was varied by the size and location of the information on the board; by the density of the information; and by the organization of the information (he was a math major and math problems do not tend to be presented in as organized a manner on the board). Goal of 80% was met. 2. S.D. will maneuver his wheelchair through an unfamiliar environment with minimal verbal cues. Since S.D. was having difficulty maneuvering his wheelchair without running into objects on the left side and locating items in the kitchen, it was decided to work on a task that involved both, namely, maneuvering down a hallway or in a room while at the same time being asked to locate items/numbers placed at various height/locations around the room. Upon recommendation of the optometrist, partial occlusion was used as one means of compensation for the left neglect. Although he was usually able to find 90–100% of the objects, it took him a very long time to do so; therefore, he was taught to use the lighthouse strategy. He met the goal, requiring minimal verbal cues to locate items on the floor to his left side, and in addition, his scanning strategy improved, as evidenced by increased speed of locating objects.	Assess the patient's comprehension Understand what he is doing Compare actual to expected performance Know the person Appreciate the context	"When he first started, S.D. had difficulty because he tended to move his head rather than his eyes. We spent some time working on visual tracking exercises without moving his head, and he can now use the glasses to a better advantage. I am encouraged that this has worked for him." "S.D. was able to use the partial occlusion glasses at home as well as during therapy. At first, the family was hesitant, but they have been working with him and gradually been able to decrease assistance and verbal cues." "After observing activities done in therapy, the PCA was able to follow through and encourage use of the lighthouse strategy throughout the day and in many different functional situations."
Next Steps Revised short-term goals (1 month): 1. S.D. will demonstrate improved use of scanning strategies such that he is able to copy words from one sheet of paper to another with 90% accuracy. 2. S.D. will initiate scanning strategies with no more than general cues while navigating in a community setting. 3. S.D. will be able to maneuver his wheelchair in unfamiliar environments with 2–3 verbal cues and independently in familiar environments.	Anticipate present and future patient concerns Analyze patient's comprehension Decide if the patient should continue or discontinue therapy and/or return in the future	"S.D. has made progress over the past month. His accuracy and use of scanning strategy have improved, but they will need to improve more if he is to continue with his classes. He is also managing his wheelchair mobility better in familiar settings, but he needs to be challenged by new situations. I'd like to start working with him in the community, gradually increasing the amount of distraction." "I feel that S.D. is progressing and would benefit from continued therapy."

Evidence Table 28-1
Best Evidence for Occupational Therapy Practice Regarding Unilateral Neglect

Intervention	Description of Intervention Tested	Participants	Dosage	Type of Best Evidence and Level of Evidence	Benefit	Statistical Probability and Effect Size of Outcome	Reference
Prisms	Adaptation to base left wedge prisms (causing a 10° shift of the visual field to the right); 18 straight-ahead pointing trials before and after adaptation.	12 RBD patients with neglect: prism and control groups.	One 2- to 5-minute session of prism exposure.	Randomized controlled study. IC2b (small sample size)	Yes. Following adaptation, patients with neglect showed shifts to the left that lasted 2 hours after the prisms were removed.	$p < 0.05$	Rossetti et al., 1998
Lighthouse strategy (LS)	Patients were taught to visualize themselves as a lighthouse whose lights (eyes) are required to sweep from left to right. The LS was used by the rehab team and family.	31 stroke patients with RBD or LBD: treatment group, n = 16; control group, n = 15.	Four 30-minute training sessions, and then the LS was used as an adjunct in other therapy sessions over average length of stay of 25 days.	Non-randomized controlled study. IIC2b (small sample size)	Yes. Those in the treatment group significantly increased attention to the right or left.	$p < 0.007$ on attention rating scale. $p < 0.002$ on reduction of error on tests of neglect.	Niemeier, 1998

Right hemisphere activation approaches	Reviewed studies related to (1) lateral task approach, (2) controlled sensory stimulation, and (3) limb activation.	Single-subject design to small groups.	Varied.	Meta-analysis of 9 group design studies and 22 single-subject studies.	Yes. Unilateral neglect appears to be amenable to change by way of activation of the right hemisphere.	Mean effect size for group design studies, r = 0.77; for single subject studies, r = 0.89.	Lin, 1996
Table top scanning activities	Exercises included visual scanning, reading and copying, copying of line drawings, and descriptions of scenes.	59 RBD patients: 23 had neglect (12 received training for neglect; 11 received the treatment after a delay), and 36 had no neglect. All participated in a rehabilitation program.	Specific training for 5 1-hour sessions/week for 8 weeks alternated with cognitive stimulation 3 times a week for 1 hour for 8 weeks.	Not randomly assigned to the groups. IIB2b (effect of involvement in rehabilitation program was not controlled)	Yes. Improvement of motor skills and function.	Statistically significant pre-post improvement: Barthel Index ($p < 0.001$) and tests of neglect, $p < 0.001$.	Paolucci et al., 1996

APRAXIA

Apraxia is the inability to carry out purposeful movement in the presence of intact sensation, movement, and coordination (Heilman & Rothi, 1993). Three types of apraxia are addressed: limb, constructional, and dressing. Although there are volumes of literature describing apraxia, little is written on treatment.

Limb Apraxia

Clients with limb apraxia can often complete daily activities, but they tend to be clumsy and/or produce action, tool, or sequencing errors. This is the person who tries to eat soup with a knife or has difficulty opening a soft drink can. Treatment recommendations are just beginning to be tested in controlled research to determine outcome. The lack of research on treatment is most likely a result of the following (Maher & Ochipa, 1997):

- Many patients are often unaware of the deficit (involvement of the non-dominant extremity) or do not complain (often associated with aphasia).
- Many treatment personnel believe that patients will recover spontaneously.
- The method of identification of apraxia is usually by pantomime (which we do not use on a day-to-day basis), and praxis usually improves with tool use. Therefore, many believe that it will have little impact on the patient's life.

The therapist should ask whether the client's clumsiness and/or difficulty with gestures interferes with daily living skills. If so, then this area should be addressed. In the case of the client who has difficulty with actual tool use, the need for treatment is more obvious. Manipulation of the clients' environments or their interaction with the environment is one means of managing apraxia. Usually these changes are related to tool use and/or clumsiness (Table 28-7).

Table 28-7. Management of Apraxic Deficits

If tool use is a problem: • May need to limit patient's access to tools that may be dangerous (e.g., power tools). • Have patient involved in tasks requiring no tools or a minimum of tools. • Limit the number of tools for a given task. • Avoid series of tasks. • Have the patient perform tasks with which they are most familiar.
If clumsiness or accuracy of production is an issue: • Use proximal movement whenever possible. • Decrease the complexity of the required movement.

From Maher & Ochipa, 1997.

Suggested treatment activities include gross motor activities involving interpretation and use of tactile, kinesthetic, and proprioceptive stimulation to influence motor patterns; manual contact or guiding of the apraxic extremity through the task; and **chaining** techniques (Farber, 1993; Zoltan, 1996). The therapist should keep verbal commands to a minimum and ask the client to perform activities in the environment in which they would normally be done. Furthermore, the client can be asked to visualize the movement before attempting to carry it out (Zoltan, 1996). The therapist may have to break down the activity into component parts and teach each part separately; then, as each is learned, the parts are integrated into more complex activities.

In a study using physical manipulation and verbalization of task elements, improvement was noted in areas trained but did not generalize to other tasks (Pilgrim & Humphreys, 1994). Maher and Ochipa (1997) looked at the effects of treatment (verbal instructions, practice, and feedback) on specific error types (external configuration, movement, and internal configuration) and found that the treatment was task specific. An improvement in one error type did not generalize to another error type, and treatment of a specific error type did not improve across gestures.

Current research supports gestural or strategy training for apraxia following left brain damage (LBD) (Cicerone et al., 2005). Smania et al. (2000) developed a training program consisting of gesture-production exercises. Experimental subjects were trained in production of transitive gestures (those involving objects), intransitive symbolic gestures (wave goodbye), and intransitive non-symbolic gestures (put your hand under the chin). The control subjects received an equal amount of aphasia training. They found a significant improvement on tests of ideational apraxia and ideomotor apraxia that indicated a generalization to untrained tasks. It was thought that their positive results were possibly due to the extensive training, which was aimed at a wide range of gestures and error types. How this training generalized to daily life was not addressed in this study and should be researched further.

Van Heugten et al. (1998) developed a program in which patients were taught strategies to compensate for their apraxia. ADL activities are broken down into three phases (initiation, execution, and control), and the patient may have difficulties in any of these areas. The therapist provides instruction, assistance, and feedback (Table 28-8). The therapist may provide instruction if the person is having difficulty initiating an activity. If more assistance is needed, the therapist can hand the object to the client or provide verbal assistance. If clients are unaware of problems with their performance, the therapist can provide feedback (e.g., verbally

Table 28-8. Sample Interventions for Apraxia

Stage	Intervention
Instructions	• Start with verbal instruction • Use gestures, point to the object • Demonstrate part of the task • Show pictures • Write instructions • Adjust task to make it easier for the patient

Assistance	• Verbal assistance to:
	  • Stimulate verbalization of the steps of the activity
	  • Name objects
	  • Direct attention to the task at hand
	• Use gestures and vary intonation of your speech
	• Show pictures of correct sequence of steps
	• Physical assistance can include:
	  • Guiding of the limb
	  • Positioning of the limb
	  • Use of sensory or neurodevelopmental treatment to provoke movement

Feedback	• Verbal feedback:
	  • In terms of the result
	  • To encourage the patient to consciously evaluate the results (see, hear, feel, smell, taste)
	• Physical feedback as to:
	  • Posture of the patient
	  • Support of the limbs
	  • Pointing or handing the object to the patient
	• Verbal and physical feedback to assist patient's knowledge of performance:
	  • Place a mirror in front of the patient
	  • Video record performance and then review together.

Adapted from van Heugten et al., 1998.

or by use of a mirror to show them what is happening). The researchers found that patients improved on all ADL measures. Donkervoort et al. (2001) incorporated this strategy training into a patient's usual occupational therapy rehabilitation program and compared this with a group that received just the usual occupational therapy program. They found that occupational therapy and strategy training was more effective in improving ADL than usual occupational therapy alone. They did not find a long-term effect in favor of strategy training but felt that this was due to patients in the usual occupational therapy group requiring more therapy to reach a similar level of independence.

Constructional Apraxia

Clients with constructional apraxia (CA) cannot "correctly draw or assemble parts to form a unitary structure" (Sunderland, Tinson, & Bradley, 1994, p. 916). The client with constructional apraxia has difficulty with drawing and constructing designs or objects in two and three dimensions and, therefore, demonstrates difficulty putting together a puzzle or a child's bicycle and following a map. This may be caused by any number of problems (e.g., executive, perceptual). Little can be found in the literature on the treatment of CA, possibly because treatment should be based on function and focus on the underlying cause.

Neistadt (1992) compared the effects of adaptive training (preparing snacks and beverages) and remedial training (using parquetry blocks) on head-injured patients' performance. She found that those patients who received training with parquetry blocks improved most on the parquetry block test and least on the food preparation task, whereas those who received the functional training improved more on the food preparation task. The results suggested that learning in adult head-injured men, at least 6 months after injury, is task specific; this supports the use of the functional approach.

Information can be found in the literature on how to improve performance on drawing tasks and construction tasks (Hecaen & Assal, 1970; Neistadt, 1989; Warrington, James, & Kinsbourne, 1966; Zoltan, 1996), but because these are not based on function, they appear not to be useful in today's health care environment. Some of the ideas, such as practice, use of a model, use of cues and landmarks, and progressing from simple to complex, can be applied to performance of functional tasks.

Dressing Apraxia

Dressing apraxia refers to an inability to dress oneself despite adequate motor skills and know-how. Little is written specifically regarding treatment. Treatment generally consists of teaching the patient a pattern of dressing. Cognitive cues, such as using the label to tell front from back and talking through the steps of putting on each item of clothing, are used, and the patient eventually learns through practice (Zoltan, 1996). Cook, Luschen, and Sikes (1991) described the use of an audiotape and a specific method of stacking (sequencing) clothing to improve dressing in an elderly woman with cognitive and perceptual impairments. If the basis for the dressing apraxia is found to be constructional apraxia, unilateral neglect, or body scheme disturbances, treatment is aimed at ameliorating those deficits.

Evidence Table 28-2
Best Evidence for Occupational Therapy Practice Regarding Apraxia

Intervention	Description of Intervention Tested	Participants	Dosage	Type of Best Evidence and Level of Evidence	Benefit	Statistical Probability and Effect Size of Outcome	Reference
Gesture production exercises	Study group received treatment in: transitive, intransitive-symbolic, and intransitive-nonsymbolic gestures. Control group received conventional treatment for aphasia.	13 patients with unilateral LBD and the presence of limb apraxia of at least 2 months duration (range 2–36 months). Study group: n = 6. Control group: n = 7.	50 minute sessions 3 times per week for a maximum of 35 sessions.	IC2b	Yes. Study group demonstrated significant improvement on performance of tests of ideational and ideomotor apraxia, which included gestures not practiced. The control group did not show improvement.	Ideational apraxia: $p = .039$, Ideomotor apraxia: $p = .043$.	Smania et al., 2000.
Strategy training	Patients were taught strategies to compensate for their apraxia. The occupational therapist used instruction, assistance, and feedback, which were varied depending upon the patient.	33 stroke patients with apraxia.	Seen 30 minutes 3 to 5 times a week for 12 weeks	IIIB2a	Yes. Improvement was seen on all ADL measures.	For ADL observations, Barthel Index, and ADL questionnaire $p < 0.001$. Effect size: strong in ADL observations (.92), Barthel Index (.86)	van Heugten et al., 1998
Strategy Training	Study group received training in use of internal and external compensations for apraxic movements during ADLs. They received strategy training and occupational therapy. Control group received conventional OT only.	113 LBD patients with apraxia. Strategy training: n = 56; Usual treatment: n = 57.	15 to 19 hours of treatment over 8 weeks.	IA2b	Yes. Patients in the strategy training group improved more on ADL observations than those in the usual treatment group.	$p = .03$ Effect size = .37 (medium, which the authors felt was good since this intervention was only a part of the total rehabilitation process).	Donkevoort et al., 2001

SUMMARY REVIEW QUESTIONS

1. List three compensatory techniques for use with clients with low vision and give two examples of each.
2. You have a client with double vision. What should you do first?
3. Based on an optometrist's report, your client's best corrected acuity is 20/160. He has a cataract in the right eye and glaucoma in both eyes, for which he is receiving medication. How might his low vision affect his ability to do self-care, meal preparation, and money management?
4. Summarize guidelines for visual scanning training.
5. How does the use of occlusion for diplopia differ from that used for unilateral neglect?
6. Your client with left unilateral neglect is having difficulty finding things in the kitchen cabinets during meal preparation. What activities might you plan for your therapy session?
7. Describe four activities to use with limb apraxia.
8. Your client is a 40-year-old dentist who has apraxia. He can use tools but is clumsy. How would your treatment of this client differ from the treatment of a 70-year-old retired man with the same clumsiness?
9. Deficits in what areas can cause dressing apraxia? Indicate how intervention may differ according to the hypothesized underlying cause of this problem.
10. Why is it important for occupational therapists to become involved in research?

ACKNOWLEDGMENT

Thanks to Liz Stuewe, MS, OTR, for her assistance with preparation of the case study and to Sheri Riggs for her assistance with the photographs.

References

Abreu, B. C., & Toglia, J. P. (1987). Cognitive rehabilitation: A model for occupational therapy. *American Journal of Occupational Therapy, 41,* 439–448.

Arai, T., Ohi, H., Sasaki, H., Nobuto, H., & Tanaka, H. (1997). Hemispatial sunglasses: Effect on unilateral spatial neglect. *Archives of Physical Medicine and Rehabilitation, 78,* 230–232.

Bailey, M., Riddoch, M. J., & Crome, P. (2002). Treatment of visual neglect in elderly patients with stroke: A single-subject series using either a scanning and cueing strategy or a left-limb activation strategy. *Physical Therapy, 82,* 782–797.

Beaver, K. A., & Mann, W. C. (1995). Overview of techniques for low vision. *American Journal of Occupational Therapy, 49,* 913–921.

Beis, J.-M., Andre, J.-M., Baumgarten, A., & Challier, B. (1999). Eye patching in unilateral spatial neglect: Efficacy of two methods. *Archives of Physical Medicine and Rehabilitation, 80,* 71–76.

Bisiach, E., Geminiani, G., Berti, A., & Rusconi, M. L. (1990). Perceptual and premotor factors of unilateral neglect. *Neurology, 40,* 1278–1281.

Bowen, A., Lincoln, N. B., & Dewey, M. E. (2002). Spatial neglect: Is rehabilitation effective? *Stroke, 33,* 2728–2729.

Butter, C. M., & Kirsch, N. (1992). Combined and separate effects of eye patching and visual stimulation on unilateral neglect following stroke. *Archives of Physical Medicine and Rehabilitation, 73,* 1133–1139.

Cicerone, K. D., Dahlber, C., Malec, J. F., Langenbahn, D. M., Felicetti, T., Kneipp, S., Ellmo, W., Kalmar, K., Giacino, J. T., Harley, J. P., Laatsch, L., Morse, P. A., & Catanese, J. (2005). Evidence-based cognitive rehabilitation: Updated review of the literature from 1998 through 2002. *Archives of Physical Medicine and Rehabilitation, 86,* 1681–1692.

Colenbrander, A., & Fletcher, D. C. (1995). Basic concepts and terms for low vision rehabilitation. *American Journal of Occupational Therapy, 49,* 865–869.

Cook, E. A., Luschen, L., & Sikes, S. (1991). Dressing training for an elderly woman with cognitive and perceptual impairments. *American Journal of Occupational Therapy, 45,* 652–654.

Cooke, D. (1992). Remediation of unilateral neglect: What do we know? *Australian Occupational Therapy Journal, 39,* 19–25.

Coslett, H. B., Bowers, D., Fitzpatrick, E., Haws, B., & Heilman, K. M. (1990). Directional hypokinesia and hemispatial inattention in neglect. *Brain, 113,* 475–486.

Crosson, B., Barco, P. P., Velozo, C. A., Bolesta, M. M., Cooper, P. V., Werts, D., & Brobeck, T. C. (1989). Awareness and compensation in post acute head injury rehabilitation. *Journal of Head Trauma Rehabilitation, 4,* 46–54.

Donkervoort, M., Dekker, J, Stehmann-Saris, F. C., & Deelman, B. G. (2001). Efficacy of strategy training in left hemisphere stroke patients with apraxia: A randomized clinical trial. *Neuropsychological Rehabilitation, 11,* 549–566.

Farber, S. (1993). OT intervention for individuals with limb apraxia. Paper presented at the American Occupational Therapy Association Neuroscience Institute, Baltimore, MD.

Frassinetti, F., Angeli, V., Meneghello, F., Avanzi, S., & Ladavas, E. (2002). Long-lasting amelioration of visuospatial neglect by prism adaptation. *Brain, 125,* 608–623.

Freeman, P. B. (2002). Low vision: Overview and review of low vision and treatment. In M. Scheiman (Ed.), *Understanding and managing vision deficits: A guide for occupational therapists* (2nd ed., pp. 265–285). Thorofare, NJ: Slack Inc.

Gianutsos, R., & Suchoff, I. B. (2002). Visual fields after brain injury: Management issues for the occupational therapist. In M. Scheiman (Ed.), *Understanding and managing vision deficits: A guide for occupational therapists* (2nd ed., pp. 247–263). Thorofare, NJ: Slack Inc.

Gillen, R., Tennen, H., & McKee, T. (2005). Unilateral spatial neglect: Relation to rehabilitation outcomes in patients with right hemisphere stroke. *Archives of Physical Medicine and Rehabilitation, 86,* 763–767.

Harley, J. P., Allen, C., Braciszeski, T. L., Cicerone, D. K., Dahlberg, C., Evans, S., Foto, M., Gordon, W. A., Harrington, D., Levin, W., Malec, J. F., Millis, S., Morris, J., Muir, C., Richert, J., Salazar, E., Schiavone, D. A., & Smigielski, J. S. (1992). Guidelines for cognitive rehabilitation. *Neurological Rehabilitation, 2,* 62–67.

Harrell, E. H., Kramer-Stutts, T., & Zolten, A. J. (1995). Performance of subjects with left visual neglect after removal of the right visual field using hemifield goggles. *Journal of Rehabilitation, 61,* 46–49.

Hecaen, H., & Assal, G. (1970). A comparison of constructive deficits following right and left hemispheric lesions. *Neuropsychologia, 8,* 289–303.

Heilman, K. M., & Rothi, L. J. G. (1993). Apraxia. In K. M. Heilman & E. Valenstein (Eds.), *Clinical neuropsychology* (3rd ed., pp. 141–163). New York: Oxford University Press.

Heilman, K. M., Watson, R. T., & Valenstein, E. (1993). Neglect and related disorders. In K. M. Heilman & E. Valenstein (Eds.), *Clinical neuropsychology* (3rd ed., pp. 279–336). New York: Oxford University Press.

Hellerstein, L. F., & Fishman, B. I. (1997). Visual rehabilitation for patients with brain injury. In M. Scheiman (Ed.), *Understanding and managing vision deficits: A guide for occupational therapists* (pp. 249–281). Thorofare, NJ: Slack, Inc.

Hellerstein, L. F., & Fishman, B. I. (1999). Collaboration between occupational therapists and optometrists. *Occupational Therapy Practice, 4,* 22–30.

Kern, T., & Miller, N. W. (1997). Occupational therapy and collaborative interventions for adults with low vision. In M. Gentile (Ed.), *Functional visual behavior: A therapist's guide to evaluation and treatment options* (pp. 493–536). Bethesda, MD: American Occupational Therapy Association, Inc.

Ladavas, E., Carletti, M., & Gori, G. (1994). Automatic and voluntary orientating of attention in patients with visual neglect: Horizontal and vertical dimensions. *Neuropsychologia, 32,* 1195–1208.

Lampert, J., & Lapolice, D. J. (1995). Functional considerations in evaluation and treatment of the client with low vision. *American Journal of Occupational Therapy, 49,* 885–890.

Lin, K. (1996). Right-hemisphere activation approaches to neglect rehabilitation poststroke. *American Journal of Occupational Therapy, 50,* 504–515.

Maher, L. M., & Ochipa, C. (1997). Management and treatment of limb apraxia. In L. J. G. Rothi & K. M. Heilman (Eds.), *Apraxia: The neuropsychology of action* (pp. 75–92). Hove, United Kingdom: Psychology Press.

Mogk, L. G. (2000). Eye conditions that cause low vision in adults. In M. Warren (Ed.), *Low vision: Occupational therapy intervention with the older adult* (lesson 2). Bethesda, MD: American Occupational Therapy Association.

Morris, A. P., Kritikos, A., Berberovic, N., Pisella, L., Chambers, C. D., & Mattingley, J. B. (2004). Prism adaptation and spatial attention: A study of visual search in normals and patients with unilateral neglect. *Cortex, 40,* 703–721.

Neistadt, M. E. (1989). Normal adult performance on constructional praxis training tasks. *American Journal of Occupational Therapy, 43,* 448–455.

Neistadt, M. E. (1992). Occupational therapy treatments for constructional deficits. *American Journal of Occupational Therapy, 46,* 141–148.

Niemeier, J. P. (1998). The Lighthouse strategy: Use of a visual imagery technique to treat visual inattention in stroke patients. *Brain Injury, 12,* 399–406.

Nowakowski, R. W. (2000). Basic optics and optical devices. In M. Warren (Ed.), *Low vision: Occupational therapy intervention with the older adult* (lesson 4). Bethesda, MD: American Occupational Therapy Association.

Paolucci, S., Antonucci, G., Grasso, M.G., & Pizzamiglio, L. (2001). The role of unilateral spatial neglect in rehabilitation of right brain-damaged ischemic stroke patients: a matched comparison. *Archives of Physical Medicine and Rehabilitation, 82,* 743–749.

Paolucci, S., Antonucci, G., Guariglia, C., Magnotti, L., Pizzamiglio, L., & Zoccolotti, P. (1996). Facilitatory effect of neglect rehabilitation on the recovery of left hemiplegic stroke patients: a cross-over study. *Journal of Neurology, 243,* 308–314.

Pilgrim, E., & Humphreys, G. W. (1994). Rehabilitation of a case of ideomotor apraxia. In M. J. Riddoch & G. W. Humphreys (Eds.), *Cognitive neuropsychology and cognitive rehabilitation* (pp. 271–285). Hove, United Kingdom: Lawrence Erlbaum Assoc.

Posner, M. I., & Rafal, R. D. (1987). Cognitive theories of attention and the rehabilitation of attentional deficits. In M. J. Meier, A. L. Benton, & L. Diller (Eds.), *Neuropsychological rehabilitation after brain injury* (pp. 182–201). New York: Churchill Livingston.

Robertson, I. (1992). Treatment of neglect. Paper presented at the conference for Evaluation and Treatment of Disorders of Memory, Attention and Visual Neglect, Philadelphia, PA.

Robertson, I. H., Mattingley, J. B., Rorden, C., & Driver, J. (1998). Phasic alerting of neglect patients overcomes their spatial deficit in visual awareness. *Nature, 395,* 169–172.

Robertson, I. H., McMillan, T., MacLeod, E., Edgeworth, J., & Brock, D. (2002). Rehabilitation by limb activation training reduces left-sided motor impairment in unilateral neglect patients: A single-blind randomized control trial. *Neuropsychological Rehabilitation, 12,* 439–454.

Robertson, I. H., & North, N. (1992). Spatio-motor cueing in unilateral left neglect: The role of hemispace, hand and motor activation. *Neuropsychologia, 30,* 553–563.

Robertson, I. H., & North, N. T. (1994). One hand is better than two: Motor extinction of left hand advantage in unilateral neglect. *Neuropsychologia, 32,* 1–11.

Robertson, I. H., North, N. T., & Geggie, C. (1992). Spatiomotor cueing in unilateral left neglect: Three case studies of its therapeutic effects. *Journal of Neurology, Neurosurgery, and Psychiatry, 55,* 799–805.

Robertson, I. H., Tegner, R., Goodrich, S. J., & Wilson, C. (1994). Walking trajectory and hand movements in unilateral left neglect: A vestibular hypothesis. *Neuropsychologia, 32,* 1495–1502.

Robertson, I. H., Tegner, R., Tham, K., Lo, A., & Nimmo-Smith, I. (1995). Sustained attention training for unilateral neglect: Theoretical and rehabilitation implications. *Journal of Clinical and Experimental Neuropsychology, 17,* 416–430.

Rossetti, Y., Rode, G., Pisella, L., Farne, A., Li, L., Boisson, D., & Perenin, M. T. (1998). Prism adaptation to a rightward optical deviation rehabilitates left hemispatial neglect. *Nature, 395,* 166–169.

Rossi, P. W., Kheyfets, S., & Reding, M. J. (1990). Fresnel prisms improve visual perception in stroke patients with homonymous hemianopsia or unilateral visual neglect. *Neurology, 40,* 1597–1599.

Scheiman, M. (1997). *Understanding and managing vision deficits: A guide for occupational therapists.* Thorofare, NJ: Slack, Inc.

Scheiman, M. (2002). Management of refractive, visual efficiency and visual information processing disorders. In M. Scheiman (Ed.), *Understanding and managing vision deficits: A guide for occupational therapists* (2nd ed., pp. 117–162). Thorofare, NJ: Slack Inc.

Smania, N., Girardi, F., Domenicali, C., Lora, E., & Aglioti, S. (2000). The rehabilitation of limb apraxia: A study in left-brain-damaged patients. *Archives of Physical Medicine and Rehabilitation, 81,* 379–388.

Soderback, I., Begtsson, I., Ginsburg, E., & Eleholm, J. (1992). Videofeedback in occupational therapy: Its effect in patients with neglect syndrome. *Archives of Physical Medicine and Rehabilitation, 73,* 1140–1146.

Sokol-McKay, D. A., & Michels, D. (2005). Facing the challenge of macular degeneration: Therapeutic interventions for low vision. *OT Practice, 10,* 10–15.

Studebaker, J., & Pankow, L. (2004). History and evolution of vision rehabilitation: Parallels with rehabilitation medicine, geriatric medicine, and psychiatry. *Topics in Geriatric Rehabilitation, 20,* 142–155.

Sunderland, A., Tinson, D., & Bradley, L. (1994). Differences in recovery from constructional apraxia after right and left hemisphere stroke? *Journal of Clinical and Experimental Neuropsychology, 16,* 916–920.

Tegner, R., & Levander, M. (1991). Through a looking glass. A new technique to demonstrate directional hypokinesia in unilateral neglect. *Brain, 114,* 1943–1951.

Tham, K., Borell, L., & Gustavsson, A. (2000). The discovery of disability: A phenomenological study of unilateral neglect. *American Journal of Occupational Therapy, 54,* 398–405.

Toglia, J. P. (1991). Generalization of treatment: A multicontext approach to cognitive perceptual impairment in adults with brain injury. *American Journal of Occupational Therapy, 45,* 505–516.

Uniform Data System for Medical Rehabilitation. (1997). *Guide for the uniform data set for medical rehabilitation.* Buffalo, NY: State University of New York.

van Heugten, C. M., Dekker, J., Deelman, B. G., van Dijk, A. J., Stehmann-Saris, J. C., & Kinebanian, A. (1998). Outcome of strategy training in stroke patients with apraxia: A phase II study. *Clinical Rehabilitation, 12,* 294–303.

Wagenaar, R. C., Van Wierignen, P. C. W., Netelenbos, J. B., Meijer, O. G., & Kuik, D. J. (1992). The transfer of scanning training effects in visual inattention after stroke: Five single-case studies. *Disability and Rehabilitation, 14,* 51–60.

Warren, M. (1993a). A hierarchical model for evaluation and treatment of visual perceptual dysfunction in adult acquired brain injury, part 1. *American Journal of Occupational Therapy, 47,* 42–54.

Warren, M. (1993b). A hierarchical model for evaluation and treatment of visual perceptual dysfunction in adult acquired brain injury, part 2. *American Journal of Occupational Therapy, 47,* 55–66.

Warren, M. (1995). Providing low vision rehabilitation services with occupational therapy and ophthalmology: A program description. *American Journal of Occupational Therapy, 49,* 877–883.

Warren, M. (1999a). Evaluation and treatment of visual perceptual dysfunction in adult brain injury, Part 1. Presented at the Conference of visABILITIES Rehabilitation Services, Inc., Nashville, TN.

Warren, M. (1999b). *Occupational therapy practice guidelines for adults with low vision*. Bethesda MD: American Occupational Therapy Association.

Warren, M. (2000). An overview of low vision rehabilitation and the role of occupational therapy. In M. Warren (Ed.), *Low vision: Occupational therapy intervention with the older adult* (lesson 1). Bethesda, MD: American Occupational Therapy Association.

Warrington, E. K., James, M., & Kinsbourne, M. (1966). Drawing disability in relation to laterality of cerebral lesion. *Brain, 89,* 53–82.

Watson, G. R. (2001). Low vision in the geriatric population: Rehabilitation and management. *Journal of the American Geriatric Society, 49,* 317–330.

Weinberg, J., Diller, L., Gordon, W. A., Gerstman, L. J., Liberman, A., Lakin, P., Hodges, G., & Ezrachi, O. (1977). Visual scanning training effect on reading-related tasks in acquired right brain damage. *Archives of Physical Medicine and Rehabilitation, 58,* 479–486.

Weinberg, J., Diller, L., Gordon, W. A., Gerstman, L. J., Liberman, A., Lakin, P., Hodges, G., & Ezrachi, O. (1979). Training sensory awareness and spatial organization in people with right brain damage. *Archives of Physical Medicine and Rehabilitation, 60,* 491–496.

Weinberg, J., Pcasetsky, E., Diller, L., & Gordon, W. (1982). Treating perceptual organization deficits in nonneglecting RBD stroke patients. *Journal of Clinical Psychology, 4,* 59–75.

Weintraub, S., & Mesulam, M. M. (1988). Visual hemispatial inattention: Stimulus parameters and exploratory strategies. *Journal of Neurology, Neurosurgery and Psychiatry, 51,* 1481–1488.

Zoltan, B. (1996). *Vision, perception and cognition: A manual for the evaluation and treatment of neurologically impaired adult* (3rd ed.). Thorofare, NJ: Slack, Inc.

CHAPTER 29

Optimizing Cognitive Abilities

Mary Vining Radomski and Elin Schold Davis

LEARNING OBJECTIVES

After studying this chapter, the reader will be able to do the following:

1. Compare and contrast remedial and adaptive therapy specific to optimizing a client's cognitive abilities.
2. Describe how remedial cognitive retraining can be incorporated into an occupational therapy intervention plan.
3. Analyze how changes in the physical or social context contribute to improved cognitive function.
4. Outline methods for helping clients reestablish routines and habit sequences.
5. Discuss how various compensatory cognitive strategies can be used to override cognitive impairments and inefficiencies.

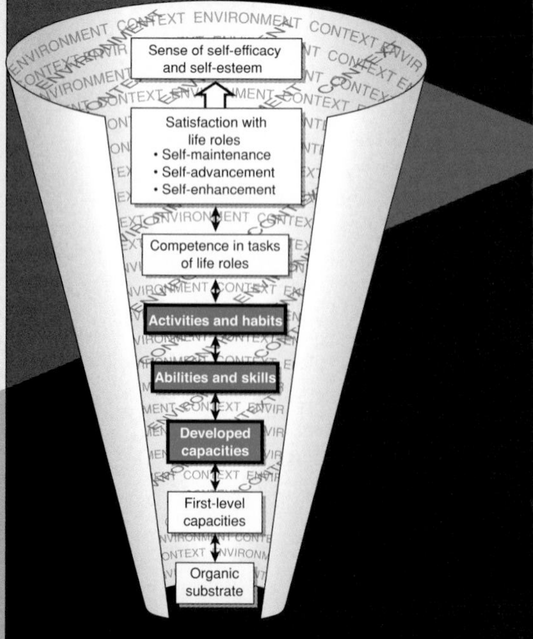

Glossary

Cognitive compensatory strategies—Array of techniques, devices, and aids that people use to circumvent cognitive limitations.

Cognitive rehabilitation—Multidisciplinary field and a broad category of intervention methods aimed at improving cognitive function.

Cognitive retraining—Remedial therapy aimed at restoring cognitive capacities through practice, exercise, and stimulation.

Habits—A continuum of automatic physical, emotional, and social behaviors that become increasingly effortless with repetition within the same context.

Routines—Habit behavior that takes the form of semiautomatic clusters of activities that are prompted by physical context and are fairly consistent for each individual on a day-to-day basis.

A person's ability to concentrate, remember, and solve problems is central to the ability to fulfill valued self-maintenance, self-advancement, and self-enhancement roles. Many people who are referred to occupational therapy services have organic cognitive impairments or short-term cognitive inefficiencies related to illness, injury, pain, or emotional distress. These impairments and inefficiencies are often the primary barriers to occupational functioning and therefore are the primary targets of occupational intervention. This chapter presents a working definition of cognitive rehabilitation, discusses linkage with occupational therapy, and describes specific approaches used in occupational therapy to optimize cognitive abilities.

COGNITIVE REHABILITATION AND LINKS WITH OCCUPATIONAL THERAPY

The term **cognitive rehabilitation** describes both a multidisciplinary field and a broad category of intervention methods aimed at improving cognitive function. Many rehabilitation disciplines, including occupational therapy, speech-language pathology, special education, and neuropsychology, attempt to help patients optimize cognitive abilities, with occupational therapy and speech therapists most often providing cognitive rehabilitation services (Stringer, 2003). With many parallels to occupational therapy treatment planning, contemporary cognitive rehabilitation practice places less emphasis on the drill and practice models of its beginnings and more emphasis on human cognition and its interfaces with health, emotion, individual differences, and context (Sohlberg & Mateer, 2001; Toglia, 2005). For occupational therapists, a client's problems with cognition are always incorporated into a broader treatment plan that may also address motor, perceptual, social, or emotional issues. Whether occupational therapists characterize their efforts to optimize cognitive function as cognitive rehabilitation, occupational therapy, or both, the aim is the same: to help clients fulfill their own role aspirations with minimal interference from cognitive limitations.

The development of cognitive rehabilitation has been and continues to be plagued by the lack of standard, agreed-upon definitions (Carney et al., 1999). In general, the term cognitive rehabilitation simply means the rehabilitation of people with cognitive deficits (Sohlberg & Mateer, 2001). The Commission on Accreditation of Rehabilitation Facilities (CARF) provides a useful working definition for this chapter. CARF suggests that cognitive rehabilitation is a systematic intervention that is directed to achieve functional changes by reinforcing, strengthening, or reestablishing previously learned patterns of behavior or establishing new patterns of cognitive activity or mechanisms to compensate for impaired neurological systems (CARF, 2004).

TREATMENT APPROACHES IN OCCUPATIONAL THERAPY TO OPTIMIZE COGNITIVE FUNCTION

Occupational therapists use the same broad approaches described in Chapters 1 and 3 to optimize clients' cognitive abilities—remedial therapy and adaptive therapy—which are further characterized as changing the context, establishing habits and behavioral routines, and acquiring compensatory skills and strategies. In selecting a primary treatment approach to optimize cognitive abilities, therapists ask themselves a number of questions about the client and the anticipated outcomes of therapy including the following:

- Who is considered the primary recipient of occupational therapy intervention: the patient, the client-family team, or the significant other? What social or cultural factors have a bearing on the outcome of intervention?
- What is the nature of the client's cognitive problems? Are the client's problems attributed to organic impairments in primary cognitive abilities or characterized as a shorter term cognitive inefficiency? Is the client in the

process of recovering, or is his or her condition likely to result in progressive deterioration?

- How are other systems, such as motor, visual, and perceptual systems, functioning? (Schwartz, 1995)
- Is the client aware of the cognitive problems and motivated to improve function in this area?
- Does the client appear to have the capacity to transfer skills learned in therapy to new situations? Does he or she have the resources (e.g., time, financial, emotional) to participate in therapy for the length of time necessary to achieve transfer of training?

Each approach to improving cognitive function is described in detail (Table 29-1). In practice, however, it is almost impossible to separate these approaches (Ben-Yishay & Diller, 1993). Consider a client who is learning to use a day planner to compensate for memory impairment. Although the primary treatment approach centers on acquiring compensatory skills and strategies, successful outcome depends on teaching the individual's family to provide the right prompts and reinforcement (changing the social context) and creating a daily planning routine in which the person reviews and adds notes to the planner (establishing behavioral routines). Furthermore, it is possible that the learning process challenges the attentional and memory systems in such a way as to stimulate neuroanatomical and physiological changes (remediation).

Remediate Deficits

Remedial therapy for cognitive problems, or **cognitive retraining**, is the therapeutic effort to restore cognitive capacities through practice, exercise, and stimulation (Wilson, 1997) with the expectation that these gains will translate to improvements in the tasks and activities to which these capacities and abilities relate (Radomski, 1994; Sohlberg & Mateer, 2001). In this approach, the therapist identifies impaired cognitive domains, such as attention, visuospatial, or memory, and provides graded activities that challenge the weakened process. Cognitive exercises, typically pencil and paper, tabletop, or computer-based exercises, are a means of attacking the deficient cognitive capacity but may have little inherent value in and of themselves (Sohlberg & Mateer, 1989). The therapist collects data on the patient's performance, such as percent correct and speed of performance. As the patient masters therapy tasks or meets criterion levels, the therapist raises the complexity or difficulty of the cognitive exercises, still challenging the original weakened process or capacity (Sohlberg & Mateer, 1989). This progression culminates with rehearsal of a naturalistic activity supported by the previously weakened cognitive capacity (Sohlberg & Mateer, 2001). This intervention sequence is founded on the premise that one cognitive capacity may be treated in isolation from other dimensions of cognition.

Table 29-1. Using Multiple Treatment Approaches to Help a Client with Cognitive Impairment to Optimize His Cognitive Abilities (see Case Example)

Treatment Approaches Described in Chapter 1	Remedial Therapy	Adaptive Therapy		
Intervention method	Remediate the impairment	Change the context	Establish behavioral routines and habits	Learn cognitive compensatory strategies
Treatment fraction (see Chapter 3)	10% of therapy efforts devoted to this approach	25% of therapy efforts devoted to this approach	35% of therapy efforts devoted to this approach	30% of therapy efforts devoted to this approach
Example	Given D.B.'s interest in "fixing" his memory and the recency of his injury, the therapist used paper and pencil activities as part of his homework that were geared toward challenging and improving his attentional system.	The therapist helped D.B. determine how to change the physical environment to optimize his attention and concentration. The therapist also attempted to change the social context by teaching D.B.'s brother appropriate ways to provide cues.	Checklists were developed specific to key self-maintenance tasks (initially ADLs and use of the planner) in the hopes that, with enough consistent repetition, D.B. would maintain these habits and routines without cues.	D.B. was assisted in selecting a number of memory prostheses including day planner, alarm watch, and medication container. The therapist provided numerous opportunities for D.B. to rehearse use of these strategies in increasingly novel situations.

CASE EXAMPLE

D.B.: Using Multiple Approaches to Optimize Cognitive Functioning after Traumatic Brain Injury

Occupational Therapy Intervention Process	Clinical Reasoning Process: Objectives	Clinical Reasoning Process: Examples of Therapist's Internal Dialogue
Patient Information D.B., a 26-year-old man who is 3 months post traumatic brain injury, participated in an outpatient occupational therapy assessment, and the following problems were identified: (1) decreased initiation of ADL and IADL; (2) decreased productivity due to poor stamina and limited appropriate avocational outlets; (3) memory impairment and inadequate repertoire of memory compensation strategies; and (4) decreased awareness of cognitive deficits interfering with compensatory strategy use.	Appreciate the context	See Chapter 9 for description of the assessment process and client's background.
	Develop intervention hypotheses	"I believe that D.B.'s cognitive problems are the most salient barriers to his occupational functioning at present, specifically, his limited awareness of his cognitive deficits. I think that he could better adapt to his physical limitations if he employed an array of strategies to compensate for his cognitive limitations. His motivation and family support are real facilitators of his occupational functioning and recovery."
	Select an intervention approach	"I will develop an intervention plan that emphasizes compensation for deficits because, given the severity of his brain injury, D.B. will likely have long-term cognitive challenges. I will provide D.B. with drill and practice cognitive activities to fill some of his free time and use them to help him gain insight about his cognitive functioning (remediation). D.B. will no longer need assistance from his brother if I help him reestablish an ADL routine. I know that I will also want to work with D.B.'s family to change the social context so that they are not providing him more cues and assistance than is really necessary."
	Reflect on competence	"D.B. reminds me of 3 or 4 other clients I've worked with in recent years. I'm a little concerned that I may not be able to satisfactorily address emotional or adjustment issues that might emerge as he gains insight, and so I need to start thinking about a counselor I might refer him to later."
Recommendations The occupational therapist recommended 3 treatment sessions each week for 8 weeks. In collaboration with D.B. and his brother, the occupational therapist established the following long-term treatment goals: (1) D.B. will independently initiate and carry out all self-care and selected light housekeeping tasks (through use of external memory aids); (2) D.B. will increase his level of productive activity at home such that he initiates avocational activities at least 3 times per week; (3) D.B. will follow through on intended tasks at least 85% of the time through use of external memory aids and strategies. D.B.'s brother indicated a willingness to provide transportation to appointments and to attend at least weekly.	Consider the client's appraisal of performance Consider what will occur in therapy, how often, and for how long Ascertain the client's endorsement of plan	"I think that a fairly intensive outpatient program is warranted because of the scope of our goals and D.B.'s motivation and potential to make progress. I have real hope for D.B.'s recovery for many reasons, including his level of cooperation, his cognitive strengths, and his brother's commitment to the therapy process. D.B. seems agreeable to the plan, but I really don't know how much he truly understood what I'm proposing and why."

Summary of Short Term Goals and Progress

1. D.B. will independently initiate notetaking when presented with occupational therapy homework (at least 60% of the time) and thereby improve his follow-through on intended tasks.

The therapist ascertained that D.B. would be most likely to carry a memory aid if it was highly portable. Therefore, she assisted D.B. in selecting a commercially-available, pocket-sized week-at-glance planner. The therapist created opportunities for D.B. to practice filing and locating information in function-specific planner sections. The therapist used an event record to log each of the three to four homework assignments she presented to D.B. during all treatment sessions, taking note of the extent to which D.B. required cues to initiate notetaking. Any level of notetaking initiation was verbally reinforced. Progress in this realm was reviewed at each session, graphing both notetaking initiation and homework completion as reinforcement and to improve insight. During the last week of this period, D.B. averaged a 65% independent notetaking rate and a 70% homework completion rate.

2. D.B. will initiate and employ consistent routines for self-care tasks (including medication management) through use of checklists and alarm cueing devices.

Based on the therapist's recommendation, D.B. purchased a container for medications taken each week as well as an alarm watch. The therapist set the alarm to sound at 5:00 p.m. as a prompt to refer to his medication checklist and take medications. D.B. required cueing and supervision with this system for 2 weeks but by the end of the month, took medications on schedule, once his brother filled the medication container. A "morning checklist" (D.B.'s hygiene sequence) was posted in D.B.'s bathroom and after 1 month, he progressed to the point that he required his brother's cueing to initiate these activities only 1–2 times per week.

3. D.B. will improve his attention to detail such that he has an error rate of less than 10% on pencil-paper tasks.

D.B. was highly motivated to "fix" his memory and eager to carry out any exercises that might help. To that end, he agreed to work on various attention-concentration worksheets as part of his homework while experimenting with various strategies that might help him focus on the task. For example, he tracked and compared his performance under various conditions: while watching television versus sitting in a quiet room; in the morning when rested versus after dinner; working in a space crowded with many papers and belongings versus a corner of his bedroom from which his "stuff" was not visible.

Assess the client's comprehension Understand what he is doing Compare actual to expected performance	"At first when I started giving D.B. homework, he simply sat and nodded his head as if to confirm that he understood and would remember. It was hard for me to say nothing and 'let the chips fall where they may'. It was uncomfortable for a while when he would argue with me at our next session, telling me that I had never assigned him anything. But as I showed him my log and how to use his planner, he seemed to realize that it's o.k. to write things down rather than trying to memorize everything. I'm seeing progress."
Know the person	"I am so glad that D.B.'s brother is part of the team. Ordinarily I like to allow patients to go ahead and make forgetting errors as a means of helping them improve awareness but I simply can't allow that when it comes to remembering to take medications on schedule."
Appreciate the context	"D.B. would rather 'fix' his memory than learn to compensate for memory problems but the research evidence just doesn't support the notion that repetitive cognitive exercises lead to functional changes. I don't want to create any false hope but have tried to both give him some activities to fill his time at home and create a structure in which he can think about his thinking. He still needs a lot of help to understand the circumstances under which he performs at his best but he seems to feel that these activities give him something important to do during his days off from therapy."

Next Steps

Revised short term goals (1 month):

1. D.B. will use his daily planner and planning checklists in order to schedule and carry-out at least two housekeeping tasks and three avocational activities each week.

2. D.B. will be able to use compensatory strategies to independently take medications on schedule (once his brother sets up the medication box each week).

3. D.B. will demonstrate improved awareness of his current problems with memory by independently initiating notetaking to the presentation of homework at least 85% of the time and at least 75% of the time when his brother provides instructions.

Anticipate present and future client concerns Analyze client's comprehension Decide if he or she should continue or discontinue therapy and/or return in the future	"D.B. has made great progress over the past month but is not yet ready to be living on his own, which remains his primary goal. He really needs to be able to handle self care tasks (including medications) and perform critical household tasks in order to do so. I would like to help D.B. prepare himself to do some sort of volunteer work within the next couple of months and he has indicated at least preliminary interest in doing so. He'll need to be quite proficient with his planner to be a successful volunteer."

CLINICAL REASONING IN OCCUPATIONAL THERAPY PRACTICE

Influence of Awareness on Treatment Approach

D.B. appeared to have limited awareness of his cognitive deficits and the implications of these problems on his functioning and future.

How might the "treatment fraction" (see Table 29-1) have been different if D.B. was keenly aware of cognitive impairments and highly motivated to minimize their influence on his life?

Many factors are believed to explain and influence recovery based on a remedial therapy. The emerging understanding of brain plasticity and neural reorganization suggests a greater degree of plasticity in the adult brain than was previously believed (Sohlberg & Mateer, 2001). The successful outcome of the remediation approach is predicated on the therapist's ability to select the foundational skills likely to respond (Cicerone et al., 2005).

Graded Cognitive Exercises

To optimize cognitive capacities, Abreu and Toglia (1987) recommended that therapists present targeted exercises and activities that "gradually increase demands on the information processing system" (p. 443). They described three phases of activity presentation in an effort to illustrate the progression from simple to complex and automatic to effortful and the ability to respond to the external environment versus the ability to manipulate the internal environment. Blundon and Smits (2000) surveyed Canadian occupational therapy programs and found the most common cognitive rehabilitation activities to be pencil and paper tasks, such as mazes and work sheets; computer-based activities; and board games.

Pencil and Paper and Tabletop Activities

Therapists often use activities such as mazes, math, or seek-and-find work sheets to challenge weakened cognitive capacities. The following is an example of using a worksheet to address attention and concentration. The patient is presented with a worksheet consisting of random symbols and letters spread across the page in rows. The patient is instructed to find and circle a specific target, such as a triangle. The therapist encourages the patient to work as quickly as possible while maintaining accurate performance. The therapist times the activity and episodes of off-task behavior, and together, the patient and therapist score the worksheet for accuracy (Fig. 29-1). Since a remediation approach requires a great deal of repetition and rehearsal to be effective (Chen et al., 1997), the patient performs attention-challenging exercises and activities at home as well as at subsequent sessions. The Attention Process Training (APT) exemplifies cognitive exercises that are designed to remediate and improve attentional systems (Sohlberg & Mateer, 2001). These treatment activities are "drill and practice" oriented and targeted to stimulating isolated components of attention (Sohlberg & Mateer, 2001). Table 29-2 lists other examples of using worksheets and tabletop tasks to improve attention.

Computer-Based Exercises

Computer-based cognitive remediation optimizes the ability to provide repetition and consistency of administration of cognitive stimuli (Fig. 29-2) (Goldstein et al., 1996; Lynch, 2002). Computer-based activities can serve as an effective adjunct to the clinic-based intervention by

Task description: Check writing worksheets		
Session date: 10/20	**Time of day:** 10 a.m.	**Location:** O.T. clinic
Target behavior	**Tally: The frequency of behaviors**	**Comments/observations: Describe performance antecedents or patterns**
♦ **Off Task – a break in ability to maintain attention (internal)**	3	Occasionally D.B. simply stopped working + didn't restart until therapist offered specific cues
♦ **Off Task – in response to an interruption (external source)**	5	Pt chose to sit near entrance to clinic — looked away from work every time someone entered
♦ **Accuracy rate**	62 %	Accuracy improved mid-task p̄ therapist reinstruction
♦ **Performance time**	Total work time - 18 minutes	

Figure 29-1 A work sheet is used to record observations during performance of cognitive retraining activities.

Table 29-2. Examples of Ways to Circumvent Cognitive Impairment and Inefficiency

Technique or Strategy	Description of Its Use	Means by Which It Minimizes Demands on Internal Information Processing
Establish a behavioral routine	Tien proceeds down her checklist of hygiene activities each morning, confident that she has not forgotten an important step.	As consistent repetitions of this sequence accrue, the activities become increasingly automatic, placing less demands on attention and memory.
Change the context	Anton's mother sets out his clothing each evening so that he can easily determine what to put on the next morning.	Removes need to locate clothing and make determinations about what to wear, what articles match, and how recently the combination has been worn.
Learn compensatory strategies: day planner	Kara writes down all of her appointments and tasks in function-specific sections of the planner. She brings the planner with her and then places it in a consistent location at home for easy access. She carries out a formal planning procedure each day to add information and review previous entries.	Allows for reliable storage and retrieval of information while placing minimal demands on memory.
Learn compensatory strategies: alarm watch	As part of her daily planning routine, Maya sets her alarm watch as a prompt to carry out time-specific tasks. For example, by setting the alarm to go off 30 minutes before she needs to leave for an appointment, Maya finds that she is no longer late.	Minimizes need for ongoing attention to the passage of time by prompting the individual to take action (such as checking his or her planner) at a specific time.
Learn compensatory strategies: "divide and conquer"	James often avoided unstructured projects because he felt overwhelmed without an obvious sequence of steps. However, by using a "divide and conquer" worksheet, he is able to create and then follow his own written step-by-step instructions.	Provides a means by which a person can "dump" all of his or her ideas out of working memory onto paper rather than trying to internally manipulate information.

extending training into the home. Specialized or commercially available software offer the opportunity for structured, monitored, and engaging home repetition (Lynch, 2002). Specialized cognitive remediation software, such as Captains Log (Resources 29-1), offers evaluation and treatment modules that target underlying cognitive capacities, such as attention and memory. They use a combination of graded, game-style, attention-friendly activities. One activity, for example, requires the patient to scan the screen from left to right and top to bottom and respond each time a target that is the same color as the border appears. The speed and length of presentation progress as the patient improves task performance. Specialized cognitive rehabilitation software often collect data on patient performance, such as speed of response and accuracy over trials. This may be a desired feature for tracking progress and offering feedback and may not be available with commercially available computer games. It is advisable to select software with an option for independent practice. Commercial computer games also stimulate attention, memory, and processing speed at a more affordable price

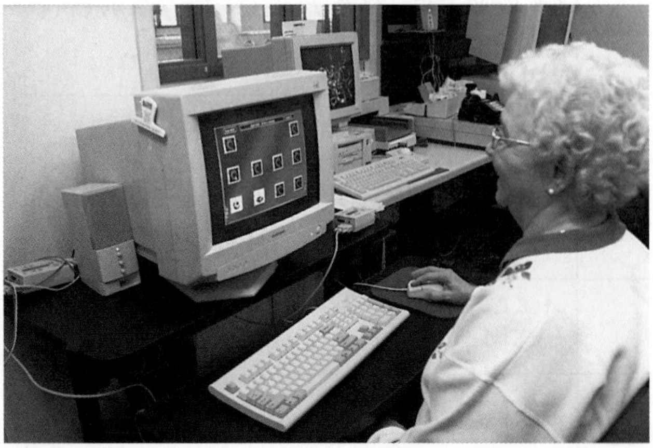

Figure 29-2 Computer-based cognitive remediation allows for extensive rehearsal and repetition.

Effectiveness of Cognitive Remediation

Proponents of this approach suggest that remediation that targets specific cognitive deficits enhances the biological recovery mechanisms during acute recovery from brain injury and facilitates functional reorganization of the brain regardless of the time post injury (Sohlberg & Mateer, 1989). Unfortunately, neither claim has been well supported empirically, and a definite link has not been established between improvements in specific cognitive capacities and functional performance (Carney et al.,

RESOURCE 29-1

Optimizing Cognitive Function

Remediate the Deficit

Captain's Log®
(Computerized cognitive training programs)
www.braintrain.com

Brainwave-Revised: Cognitive strategies and techniques for brain injury rehabilitation (consists of pen-and-paper–based cognitive rehabilitation program divided into five hierarchically graded modules: attention, visual processing, memory, information processing, and executive functions)
www.proedinc.com

Attention Processing Training (APT-I and APT II)
Authors: McKay Moore Sohlberg, PhD, and Catherine Mateer, PhD
http://www.nss-nrs.com/cgi-bin/WebObjects/NSS.woa/wa/Products/detail?id=1000113

A wide variety of board games, such as Master Mind, Simon, Connect Four, or a deck of cards.

Change the Physical Context

Automatic appliance shut-off devices such as the StoveGuard.

An array of devices can be found on the Able Data website at: http://www.abledata.com/ or the AT Network at www.atnet.org.

Choose commercially available small appliances with automatic shut-off features (coffee pots, curling irons) or plug the item into a timer (check that the device you are plugging in does not exceed the AMP or Watt limits for the timer).

Exit alarms can be a standard feature on security systems. Chair and bed exit alarms are also available.
http://www.abledata.com/

Learn Compensatory Cognitive Strategies

Day Planners (essential features are predated pages and defined notebook sections)
- FranklinCovey
www.franklincovey.com
- DayTimer
www.daytimer.com

Alarms and Cueing Devices that Support Scheduling and Time Management

The Catalog of Portable Electronic Devices for Memory and Organization can be located at http://www.biausa.org/Pages/AT/

Watches with features that offer programmable alarms, digital reminders, and vibrating and audible prompts. One example is the Timex Data Link watch that offers alarms, text messages, phone numbers; some models allow wireless download from computer scheduling program.
www.timex.com or www.casio.com

MotivAider® (vibrates at preset intervals) Behavioral Dynamics
www.habitchange.com/motivaider.php

IQ Voice Organizer (can record message to be played at prompt of alarm, letting client receive audible reminder in familiar voice and with explicit detail)
www.voiceorganizer.com

Palm-held (PDA) computer scheduling devices:
- Palm Pilot
www.palm.com
- Psion hand-held computer
www.psionusa.com

Medication Boxes with or without Alarms

Available from medication aisle in the pharmacy section of stores such as Walgreen's, Kmart, or from specialized equipment vendors such as:
www.sammonspreston.com
www.abledata.com

Web-Based Activities

The University of Alabama at Birmingham's Traumatic Brain Injury Clinic created a NIDRR-funded resource of home-based cognitive stimulation activities, games, and exercises. The menu can be accessed by therapists and clients over the internet.
http://main.uab.edu/tbi/show.asp?durki=9968

Resources for Professionals

Brain Injury Association
www.biausa.org (also check for state chapters)

Society for Cognitive Rehabilitation (membership offers access to education, resources, and specialty certification)
http://www.cognitive-rehab.org.uk/

A growing number of internet sites are devoted to providing information, resources, and devices for persons with cognitive disabilities. Examples include:
- http://www.bindependent.com/
- http://www.heath.gwu.edu/links/general_organization_Links.htm
- http://www.familyvillage.wisc.edu/index.htmlx

1999; Malec & Basford, 1996). Some evidence, however, correlates drill and practice in areas of attention and memory with improvement in these areas on neuropsychological testing (Carney et al., 1999).

Based on their review of studies of outcomes after acute brain injury, Malec and Basford (1996) suggested that there may be secondary benefits from a remedial approach. They posited that it may facilitate the patient's initial acceptance that a problem exists and promote improved awareness of deficits (Procedures for Practice 29-1). Similarly, Gianutsos (1992) suggested that therapy should begin with remediation as the goal "even if that goal is remote" (p. 27) because, if the patient is satisfied that every attempt was made to restore function, he or she may be more inclined to work on compensating for the deficit.

Adaptive Therapy

As previously mentioned, adaptive therapy is characterized as intervention aimed at circumventing impairments and inefficiencies through changes in context, habits and routines, and strategies. These three synergistic focuses of intervention are based on what we describe as cognitive ergonomics, that is, use of human information-processing principles to decrease the demands on working memory.

Change the Context

When intervention centers on changing the context, the therapist or family makes changes that lower the cognitive demands placed on the patient to optimize his or her suc-

PROCEDURES FOR PRACTICE 29-1

Helping Patients Improve Self-Awareness

Occupational therapists use a variety of techniques to help patients become more aware of their cognitive strengths and weaknesses:

- Appreciate the different contributions of organically based unawareness and adjustment-based denial. Anticipate that sometimes, as patients become more aware of impairments, they may feel emotional distress, including depression and anxiety (Fleming & Strong, 1995).
- Recognize levels of awareness and focus intervention on helping the patient move up the hierarchy (see Chapter 9). For example, therapists try to help patients who are unaware of their cognitive impairments first to develop intellectual awareness of the problem and then to progress toward emergent or anticipatory awareness (Crosson et al., 1989).
- Create opportunities for the patient to monitor and judge his or her own performance, analyze the results, and determine what to continue or do differently next time. Dougherty and Radomski (1993) recommended a graded approach to performance analysis that consisted of three levels: (1) using an answer key to self-correct, (2) answering multiple choice questions about various aspects of performance after performing the task, and (3) making predictions about performance ahead of time, comparing actual performance to predictions, and determining how to modify performance in the future.
- Introduce therapeutic structured failure when appropriate. That is, do not interfere with the natural consequences of the cognitive impairment during selected supervised activities. For example, if the patient fails to initiate a cognitive compensatory strategy in response to general or specific cues, do not provide further instruction but rather create an opportunity for the patient to observe what happens when the strategy is not used.
- Collaborate with family members to provide feedback. Some family members should focus on maintaining harmony in the household and appropriately prefer that the therapist assume the responsibility of providing any negative feedback to the patient. In other cases, family members or coworkers are so afraid of offending or discouraging the patient that they insulate the patient from any and all challenges or avoid mentioning errors and, as a result, deprive him or her of information that might improve self-awareness.
- Respect the patient's readiness to participate in therapy. Avoid badgering the patient into improved awareness of deficits by maintaining a therapeutic partnership so that he or she will want to return for services in the future.

cess in carrying out tasks (Procedures for Practice 29-2). That is, the client is not expected to change, but the physical properties of the context or social expectations do. This strategy is particularly appropriate for persons suffering from a dementia.

Physical Context

In manipulating the physical context, the therapist looks for ways to use the physical properties of the space to provide information or cues. For example, needed items are strategically placed so as to attract the patient's attention. Drawers can be labeled to help the patient locate items, or important information is positioned so that the patient will see it often (Fig. 29-3). The physical space may also be altered to minimize its stimulus-

PROCEDURES FOR PRACTICE 29-2

Changing the Context

Suggestions for changing the physical context include the following:

- Place the notebook open to today's page in a consistent spot on the counter.
- Use a large wall calendar so all family members can check for needed information.
- Place items in consistent places by using hooks or baskets as receptacles.
- Install a range timer set at a 30-minute delay. The stove will automatically turn off after 30 minutes, eliminating the risk of forgetting to turn a burner off.
- Remove clutter to minimize the stimulus arousal properties of work space.

Suggestions for changing the social context include helping family members do the following:

- Shift roles. The spouse may fill out the schedule each day before leaving for work. The patient's responsibility may be to refer to the schedule regularly and retrieve the information at the correct time. The expectation that the patient will record information on the schedule has been eliminated.
- Simplify tasks so that the patient can participate. For example, setting out supplies for an activity decreases the memory and problem-solving demands on the patient.
- Wait to pass on schedule or to-do information until the patient is seated with paper and pen in hand to maximize the opportunity for the patient to initiate note taking. Sometimes family members benefit from recognizing their contribution to a forgetting error, such as passing on the time of an appointment to the patient who is cooking dinner.

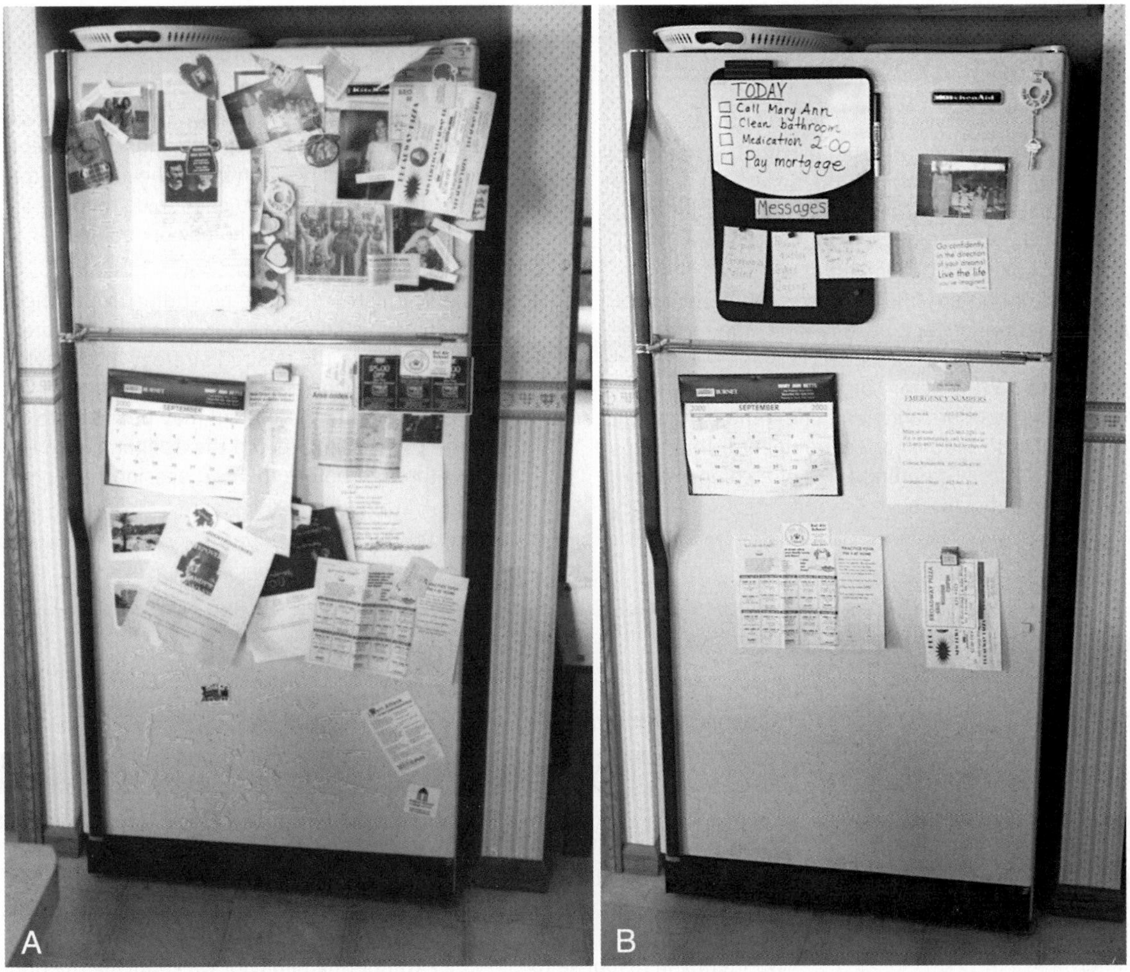

Figure 29-3 **A, B.** Simple changes in the kitchen let a person with cognitive limitations easily find important information.

arousal properties. Items that provoke distraction or worry, such as the mail or unpaid bills, are stored so that the patient will not see them when attempting to concentrate on other tasks. Finally, demands of the physical context can be lowered through use of tools and appliances that eliminate memory requirements by, for example, turning themselves off.

Social Context

Therapists also focus on teaching the family members to set the stage for the client's success. This may mean temporarily or permanently changing roles and responsibilities in the family and learning to capitalize on the client's strengths. Consider the patient who loves to cook but whose memory and judgment problems make this an unsafe activity. The family members understand the patient's limitations and adapt their approach to cover what is difficult, such as remembering to gather the correct ingredients, but facilitate what the patient can do, such as measure and mix. The patient's cognitive abilities are also optimized as families learn appropriate ways to offer prompts and cues (Procedures for Practice 29-3). See Procedures for Practice 29-4 for examples of how changing the context can be used along with other approaches.

Establish Behavioral Routines and Habit Sequences

Automatic **habits** and **routine** enable us to carry out many of our everyday tasks with little or no mental energy, freeing us to think and react to new events in the environment (Jog et al., 1999). For example, we employ consistent and specific procedures for frequently performed activities such as showering, brushing our teeth, and shoe tying, rendering them effortlessly accurate as we deploy our mental resources for mulling over the events of the day ahead. Illness, disability, aging, and life changes disrupt long-standing habits and routines (Dyck, 2002; Wallenbert & Jonsson, 2005). As a result, previously simple activities become taxing and time consuming. The loss of effortless predictability in one's performance has a

PROCEDURES FOR PRACTICE 29-3

Graded Cues

Graded or vanishing cues are used in cognitive rehabilitation to enable the patient to perform tasks with the least amount of cueing (Dougherty & Radomski, 1993). The following terms (from Sohlberg & Mateer, 1989) are useful when writing goals and documenting progress.

- A general or non-specific cue alerts the patient to monitor performance. It usually takes the form of a statement such as, "You'll need to make sure you remember to do this before our next session." The therapist or family offers a general cue if the patient fails to recognize situational or environmental conditions that might otherwise prompt use of a compensatory strategy or behavior.
- A specific cue, which is presented if the patient does not respond to a general cue, reminds the patient he or she must act. It often takes the form of a question such as, "What do you need to do to make sure you remember to do your homework before our next session?"
- An explicit instruction, the most directive of the graded cues, is sometimes provided if the patient does not initiate the desired strategy or behavior upon first receiving a general cue and then a specific cue. For example, the patient may be asked to take out the planner and record the assignment to ensure follow-through before the next session.

PROCEDURES FOR PRACTICE 29-4

Using Multiple Approaches for Persons with Dementia

Problem to Address	Considerations	OT Approach and Interventions
Family is concerned with safety at home. Client with acute dementia wanders and he may leave the house even when others are at home.	Client is living at home with 24-hour care. Family wishes to continue home-based care. Through situational analysis, therapist observes wandering in response to the cue of the door in the kitchen.	Change the context (Silverstein, Flaherty, & Tobin, 2002): Change the environmental context. Wallpaper the door to match the walls, to eliminate the cue of the exit. This recognizes that the stimulus for the wandering behavior was noticing the door and not seeking an exit.
Early complaints of forgetting (mild dementia, early intervention). The client with early dementia frequently has decreased knowledge of new or recent events or acquaintances (Gitlin & Corcoran, 2005).	Research indicates potential benefit from cognitive rehabilitation to optimize remaining memory capacity at the early stages of the disease process (Clare et al., 2003; Gitlin & Corcoran, 2005).	Remediate: Teach a name recollection strategy to recall names of importance such as card club members. The mnemonic strategy described in Table 29-4 involves association and repetition. Encourage cognitively challenging activities such as crossword puzzles or Sudoku.
Client forgets aspects of morning hygiene routine, and others complain of offensive odor.	Developing a hygiene routine can be a strategy for creating successful caregiver interaction in harmony with the performance pattern of self-care.	Routines: Establish a morning routine supported with physical cues (such as a checklist) and set-up ritual (basket on counter for supplies) for consistent hygiene routine.
Client describes a desire to arrive at meals without others needing to remind him.	Cuing devices offer an external prompt to recall information. An alarm requires access to internal recollection to be effective. A cuing device relying only on external information would pair the alarm with a recorded message or written note.	Compensation: Caregiver programs wrist watch to ring 15 minutes before meal time. In addition to the alarm, the digital watch displays "Dining room." The single purpose for this cue is associated with meals.

profound impact on an individual's energy level and sense of continuity, competence, and self (Charmaz, 2002).

Although the occupational therapy profession has its roots in "habit training" (Taylor, 1929; Zemke, 1994), habits and routines have only recently resurfaced as a focus of theory development and in the profession's official terminology (American Occupational Therapy Association [AOTA], 2002). Despite the reemergence of scholarly and clinical interest in habits in a number of academic disciplines, the concepts of habits and routines have not been clearly defined (Clark, 2000), and there are no evidence-based guidelines for how habits and routines are measured or reestablished in clinical practice.

Terminology

The term "habit" denotes a continuum of automatic physical, emotional, and social behaviors that become increasingly effortless with repetition within the same context (Camic, 1986; Kielhofner, 1995; Rogers, 2000). This continuum represents the spectrum of automatic human responses ranging from distinct motor sequences prompted by concrete, localized environmental stimulus cues at one extreme to less observable attitudinal or dispositional responses prompted by abstract, situational triggers at the other extreme (Bargh, 1997; Camic, 1986).

Habits and routines appear to be exemplars of the same phenomenon: goal-directed human behavior that, with enough repetition in the same context, occurs with little or no mental effort. Both are acquired through frequent repetition and activated by consistent goals, anticipated outcomes, or end states and stimulus characteristics of the context or environment (Aarts & Dijksterhuis, 2000; Wood, Quinn, & Kashy, 2002) and are regulated and influenced by culture (Ludwig, 1998). The constructs of micro-habit and routine appear to differ in terms of degree rather than substance. Micro-habits, such as the precise mechanics and sequence used to tie shoes, tend to be comprised of smaller sequences of actions (Rogers, 2000) that may be so automatic as to appear involuntary. Routines take the form of semi-automatic, context-specific scaffolding that provides order and consistency to the typical flow of tasks and activities in a person's daily life (Kielhofner, 1995) and extend through a considerable portion of time (Seamon, 2002). Consider the distinction and overlap between the following two types of habit behavior. Mr. R. always hangs his car keys on a hook near the door as he enters his home, doing so with no conscious awareness whatsoever. Even if the hook is temporarily removed, Mr. R. reaches for the hook upon entering the home despite his best intention to set the keys elsewhere. This micro-habit is embedded in his coming home from work routine, a sequence of semi-automatic tasks comprising letting out the dog, checking the answering machine, and thumbing through the mail.

Habit Learning

As discussed in Chapter 14, learning is believed to be built on two different memory systems: one is the basis of knowledge and expectation (explicit memory), and the other is the basis of non-cognitive habits and skills (implicit memory) (Mishkin & Appenzeller, 1987). Implicit memory (sometimes called non-declarative or procedural memory) refers to an unconscious change in behavior that results from previous experience (Eldridge, Masterman, & Knowlton, 2002) and is closely tied to the original learning situation and, hence, less flexibly applied to novel contexts (Reber, Knowlton, & Squire, 1996). Habit learning is a form of implicit learning (Squire, Knowlton, & Musen, 1993).

Habit learning appears to be independent of the brain structures that underlie explicit learning (medial temporal lobe and hippocampus) (Eldridge, Masterman, & Knowlton, 2002) but instead relies on the basal ganglia, a collection of nuclei deep in the white matter of the cerebral cortex. It is widely accepted that the basal ganglia are involved in motor programming, execution, and control (Krebs et al., 2001; Wu, Kansaku, & Hallett, 2003). Findings from recent animal and human research, however, suggest that the basal ganglia also mediate the formation of habits through stimulus-response associations that are incrementally acquired (Packard & Knowlton, 2002).

Mechanism Underlying the Automaticity of Habits and Routines

The term "automaticity" refers to the ability to perform a skilled task with minimal or no processing resources (Brown & Bennett, 2002). It describes the phenomenon that accounts for the fact that, with enough practice in a consistent setting, features of the environment trigger habits without any mediation by conscious choice or reflection (Bargh, 1997; Logan, 1988a). Instance theory (Logan, 1988a, 1998b; Logan, Taylor, & Etherton, 1999) suggests that each encounter with a stimulus is encoded, stored, and retrieved separately. That is, each processing episode consists of the goal the person is trying to achieve, stimuli encountered in pursuit of the goal, interpretation of the stimuli, and the responses made to the stimuli (Logan, 1988a), and each episode results in a new trace stored in memory (Logan, Taylor, & Etherton, 1999). Instance theory suggests that, when the person subsequently encounters the stimulus, his or her response will be the result of a race between memory retrieval and algorithmic computation and whichever "wins" controls the response (Logan, 1988a). As more and more processing episodes are encountered, stored, and activated, performance is less often controlled by algorithmic computation (whose finishing time remains fixed) and increasingly based on single-step direct access retrieval of prior solutions from memory (whose finishing time decreases with repetition) (Logan, Taylor, & Etherton, 1999). Single-step retrieval, the hallmark of automatization, likely involves few resources compared with multistep algorithms, accounting for increasing ease and speed of performance with practice (Logan, 1988b). Automatization, then, is a relative phenomenon in that, while it may occur after only a few trials, it may never be complete (Logan, 1988a). Memory strengthens automaticity progressively with practice (by virtue of additional representations in memory), thus, performance may be more automatic after 100 repetitions than after 50.

Automatic behaviors such as habits are triggered and constrained by contextual features (Aarts & Dijksterhuis, 2000; Bargh & Chartrand, 1999; Gallimore & Lopez, 2002; Logan, 1988b). Ease of retrieval is a function of the similarity between encoding and retrieval contexts—the more similarity there is, the greater the ease and speed of retrieval (Logan, 1988b). The context at encoding becomes associated with the processing episode and resultant memory trace while context at retrieval serves as an important cue. That is, context- and task-relevant information are encoded together, and contextual consistencies should be strengthened with practice (Logan, 1988b). Performance of the same task in different contexts may inhibit retrieval of task-relevant information, explaining why, for example, one's morning hygiene routine is more effortful and time consuming when performed in a hotel room rather than at home.

Guidelines for Establishing Habits and Routines

Numerous case examples and single-subject research studies in the rehabilitation literature describe the use of applied behavioral analysis to establish or reestablish self-care and/or home-management routines and habit sequences for persons with cognitive impairment (Giles & Clark-Wilson, 1988; Giles & Shore, 1989a; Giles et al., 1997; Katzmann & Mix, 1994; Kime, Lamb, & Wilson, 1996; O'Reilly, Green, & Braunling-McMorrow, 1990; Schwartz, 1995; Zanetti et al., 1997). The following principles of applied behavioral analysis frame occupational therapy intervention to establish routines and habit sequences.

- With input from the patient and caregiver, the therapist selects a key behavioral sequence that becomes the target of intervention (Giles, 1998). Giles emphasized the importance of selecting behaviors and prospective routines with clinical and personal significance. Be sensitive to client readiness to address habits and routines. Wallenbert and Jonsson (2005) reported that stroke survivors may be reluctant to create new habits that they believe will preclude continued physical recovery.
- The therapist analyzes the physical and social context in which the routine or sequence is expected to occur to identify built-in cues or determine where to create them (Schwartz, 1995). At a minimum, significant others participate in the selection of target behavioral sequences and appreciate the methods and benefits of intervention. Since routines and habit sequences are thought to be context specific, training is most effective if it occurs in the environment in which the routines will ultimately be performed (Giles, 1998).
- A task analysis is performed on the target behavioral routine or sequence (Giles, 1998; O'Reilly, Green, & Braunling-McMorrow, 1990). Task analysis involves examining each step of the task as well as the setting, stimulus events, and consequences (Gelfand & Hartmann, 1984).
- The therapist and patient decide on an optimal sequence of steps and use chaining, prompting, and reinforcement each time the sequence is performed (Giles et al., 1997). Giles et al. suggested that "[routine] tasks can be thought of as complex-stimulus-response chains in which the completion of each activity acts as the stimulus for the next step in the chain" (1997, p. 257). They also recommended the use of the whole-task method, in which each step of the chain is trained on each presentation. The therapist often creates a checklist that outlines each component of the task so that the desired sequence of steps remains invariant (Davis & Radomski, 1989) (Fig. 29-4).

For some patients, prompts and reinforcers are established. The checklist itself may be both a prompt if placed in an obtrusive location and a reinforcer as the patient checks each completed step. Technology may also be employed. Schwartz (1995) reported use of a daily tape-recorded message activated by an automatic timer that prompted initiation of a self-care routine. Wilson et al. (1997) described how NeuroPage, a time- and task-specific vibrating prompt that is described later, appeared to facilitate establishing routines related to taking medication and checklist use. Family members may also be enlisted to provide prompts and reinforcement, typically social praise. In our practice, the final step on many patients' checklists requires that they call and leave a voicemail message stating they completed the sequence as an incentive and a reinforcer of the routine.

The therapist facilitates consistent repetition of the behavioral routine or sequence beyond mastery to promote overlearning (Giles, 2005). As discussed in Chapter 14, full automaticity requires at least 200 trials of a task but begins with as few as 10 consistent repetitions (Sternberg, 1986). As the patient frequently and consistently performs the behavioral sequence, steps begin to prompt one another and may be removed from the checklist (Katzman & Mix, 1994). The therapist tracks ongoing compliance with the target behavioral sequence; monitors the patient's perceptions of ease, accuracy, and speed (evidence of increasing automaticity); and, with the

Morning planning checklist

Directions: Check-off each step after it is completed.

	M	T	W	Th	F	Sa	Su
1) After breakfast, open planner to yesterday's page.							
2) Check off all of the tasks you completed yesterday.							
3) Draw an arrow in front of undone or incomplete tasks							
4) Re-write these tasks on today's page.							
5) Move the bookmark to today's planner page.							
6) Review your schedule.							
7) Ask your wife if there are any tasks or appointments that you should write down for today.							
8) Write down at least 3 tasks you intend to complete today.							

Wind-down routine

Directions: Check-off each step after it is completed.

	M	T	W	Th	F	Sa	Su
1) When your MotivAider vibrates at 9:00 p.m, discontinue your current activity.							
2) Make notes where you left off on your project.							
3) Put on your pajamas.							
4) Brush your teeth.							
5) Wash your face.							
6) Gather your magazines and go to your recliner.							
7) Set the MotivAider for 30 minutes and peruse your reading material.							
8) When cued by the MotivAider, retire to bed.							

Figure 29-4 Checklists like these are used to help patients reestablish routines and habit sequences.

patient, determines when applied behavioral analysis methods should be employed to make another important task routine.

Whether because of damage to neural pathways or as a consequence of lack of daily consistency, many persons with cognitive impairment or inefficiency benefit from intervention focused on establishing behavioral routines or habit sequences. Most adults, however, are embarrassed to admit that they make frequent errors on tasks that are supposed to be easy and may be reluctant to bring these problems to the attention of the therapist. In our clinical practice, patients are often relieved that these errors in everyday tasks can not only be explained but also addressed.

In summary, the goal of establishing automatic behavior is to return frequently performed self-management tasks to their status as background activities in everyday life, as described so eloquently by a man with brain injury:

> "Routine is a constant reference as to when and where I am. . . .Routine allows me to compensate for my lack of initiative. I may not notice that the house needs vacuuming, but I know that on Mondays I vacuum. . . .Many people view routine as boring. 'Boring as compared to what?' I ask. 'Boring as compared to being confused and inactive?'. . .I get my variety because routine keeps the distractions at bay." (Strand, 2000, p. 9)

Learn Compensatory Strategies

In addition to context-specific habits and routines, many recipients of occupational therapy services need new strategies that allow them to compensate for cognitive impairments or inefficiencies in a variety of settings. As previously mentioned, the client's awareness of his or her propensity for forgetfulness, however superficial, is prerequisite to occupational therapy aimed at teaching the client to use compensatory strategies (Dirette, 2002). People will not bother to enter information into a memory aid for events that they expect to remember (Wright et al., 2001). If the client denies having cognitive problems, he or she will likely be unable to muster the effort and resolve that learning compensatory strategies requires.

Implicit in this approach is the expectation that the client will use compensatory cognitive strategies, such as aids, devices, and thinking techniques, in multiple contexts, and so intervention is designed to promote the likelihood of generalization. Toglia's multicontext approach (1991, 2005) informs the intervention model adapted from Sohlberg and Mateer's (1989) memory notebook training protocol.

Multicontext Approach

Toglia's (2005) Dynamic Interactional Model of Cognition is based on the premise that cognition is a product of the dynamic interaction between the person, the activity at hand, and the environment in which the activity occurs. According to this model, cognitive dysfunction results from a mismatch among personal (such as cognitive capacities or cognitive strategies), task, and environmental variables. This approach emphasizes the facilitation of client self-awareness, acquisition of new information-processing strategies, establishment of transfer criteria, and practice in the context of varied activities and environments (Table 29-3). Client-specific processing strategies are selected or designed and then practiced in a variety of graded tasks and settings. The therapist guides the transfer of learning by asking the client to employ the new strategy first on similar tasks and then in the context of those that are increasingly dissimilar (Toglia, 1991).

A General Model for Learning Cognitive Compensatory Strategies

Schmitter-Edgecombe et al. (1995) adapted Sohlberg and Mateer's (1989) schema for memory notebook training, and this model applies to helping clients acquire and use any **cognitive compensatory strategy**. Intervention is organized around four training phases, which are anticipation, acquisition, application, and adaptation, and in addition to learning new skills, intervention is typically aimed at improving self-awareness (see Procedures for Practice 29-1).

- Anticipation—Through the use of homework, feedback, and possibly structured failure, clients with low insight experience the consequences of cognitive deficits to heighten motivation for treatment. Patients receive information about human information processing and possible solutions for cognitive problems.
- Acquisition—Through drill and practice exercises, clients learn the mechanics of using the compensatory tool or strategy. For example, with coaching and written instructions from the therapist, clients rehearse setting their alarm watches or practice filing and finding information in function-specific sections of their planners.
- Application—Clients use the compensatory strategy during clinic-based simulated work tasks. These tasks are designed to require use of the targeted strategy. In our practice, they consist of clerical or clinic maintenance projects or crafts. With guidance from the therapist, clients also directly apply the compensatory strategy to real-life problems at home or work.
- Adaptation—Once the client has experience with the strategy in simulations and real-life tasks, the strategy may be further adapted to the client's personal preferences and the demands of additional areas of application in daily life.

Table 29-3. Components of the Multicontext Treatment Approach

Component	Definition	Example
Consideration of personal context	Gaining understanding of the client's pre-morbid personality characteristics, beliefs, valued occupations, and previous lifestyle	Interviewing the client about his or her pre-morbid everyday routines and exploring how those routines have changed after injury or illness and using this information to inform occupational therapy assessment and intervention
Awareness training	Methods designed to enhance the client's understanding of his or her strengths and limitations that are incorporated into every treatment session	• Asking the client to anticipate and identify specific challenges or obstacles that might occur in performance of a therapy task • Instructing the client to watch the therapist perform a task during which client-relevant errors are demonstrated (such as distractibility). Asking the client to identify problems and recommend strategies
Processing strategies	Small units of behavior that reflect internal or external cognitive techniques that contribute to the effectiveness of performance	• Mental repetition, visual imagery (examples of internal processing strategies) • Memory notebooks, alarm cuing devices, use of checklists (examples of external processing strategies)
Activity analysis	Identifying, manipulating, and/or stabilizing salient activity parameters (e.g., physical features, number of items, number of steps or choices involved in the task)	As part of her therapy, a homemaker who has difficulty attending to visual details locates the soup spoons in a drawer of unsorted spoons, forks, and knives. As she progresses, she will locate a set of soup spoons in a drawer of unsorted spoons of different sizes (teaspoons, soup spoons, serving spoons). Note how differentiating between spoons of different sizes requires greater visual attention than differentiating between spoons, forks, and knives.
Establishment of criteria for transfer	Identify series of tasks that decrease in degrees of physical and conceptual similarity to the original task	Task: Donning a pullover T-shirt in the therapy area
	Near transfer: only one or two surface characteristics changed	Donning a pullover sweater (color and texture different from tee shirt)
	Intermediate transfer: 3–6 surface characteristics change; tasks share some physical similarities	Donning a button-down cotton shirt in the client's room (type of clothing, color and texture, fine motor requirements, and environment changed)
	Far transfer: tasks are conceptually similar; surface characteristics are different or only one surface characteristic is similar	Donning outerwear (coat, jacket), pajamas, undershirt or camisole (different types of upper body clothing)
	Very far transfer: generalization, spontaneous application of what is learned to everyday life	Donning pants (strategy of dressing affected side first remains the same for lower body dressing)
Practice in multiple environments	Strategies are used in a variety of situations (e.g., tasks and locations) to demonstrate their applicability and utility to the client	The strategy of left-to-right scanning is practiced on letter cancellation tasks and then used to locate items in a medicine cabinet or to count books on a shelf.

Sources: Toglia, J. P. (1991). Generalization of treatment: A multi-contextual approach to cognitive perceptual impairment in the brain-injured adult. *American Journal of Occupational Therapy*, 45, 505–516; and Toglia, J. P. (2005). A dynamic interactional approach to cognitive rehabilitation. In N. Katz (Ed.), *Cognition and occupation across the life span* (pp. 29–72). Bethesda, MD: American Occupational Therapy Association.

An exhaustive review of all possible methods to circumvent cognitive impairments or inefficiencies is beyond the scope of this chapter. Instead, we provide an overview of three categories of compensatory cognitive strategies: internal information-processing strategies, memory prostheses, and problem-solving schemas.

Internal Information-Processing Strategies

Occasionally occupational therapists teach patients to use mental strategies that facilitate the encoding and storage of information (Parenté & DiCesare, 1991). Theoretically, the techniques outlined in Table 29-4 enable the client to keep information in working memory and thereby facilitate encoding. Given the extensive rehearsal involved in learning these techniques, intervention based on internal information-processing strategies has similar features to a remedial approach. Most people find internal information-processing strategies time consuming to learn and inconvenient to employ. Rather than concocting a first-letter mnemonic to make sure that one purchases everything one needs at the grocery store, one simply makes a list. Internal information-processing strategies may be helpful, however, when the client needs to memorize frequently used, rarely changing information such as his or her social security number or a personal identification number.

Memory Prostheses: Day Planners

Many persons with and without memory problems use day planners to help them keep track of information. Routine use of prosthetic memory aids such as day planners, also known as diaries or memory notebooks, is frequently cited in the rehabilitation literature as a means of circumventing memory impairments and inefficiencies. For example, in a small study in which persons with severe brain injury were randomly assigned to one of two conditions, patients receiving memory notebook training reported significantly fewer observed everyday memory failures at discharge than those receiving supportive treatment (Schmitter-Edgecombe et al., 1995). Seventy-five percent of the patients in the notebook condition were using the notebooks at 6 months of follow-up (Schmitter-Edgecombe et al., 1995). Zenicus, Wesolowski, and Burke (1990) compared the effectiveness of three memory strategies (written rehearsal, verbal rehearsal, and acronym) with notebook use in terms of clients' assignment completion rates. They found the notebook condition to be the clearly superior technique for assignment completion. In another multiple-baseline study, Zenicus et al. (1991) examined the effectiveness of memory notebook training on the ability to remember assignments and appointments in four survivors of severe brain injury. The results suggested that all four participants demonstrated improved follow-through on assignments with notebook use compared to baseline.

To use a day planner effectively to compensate for cognitive impairment or inefficiency, the user must religiously record important information in the appropriate notebook sections, carry the planner about, and look at it regularly during the day. Despite the appearance of an easy, straightforward method to compensate for memory problems, successful intervention is often time consuming. Schmitter-Edgecombe et al. (1995) described an 8-week protocol of 16 sessions, and Donaghy and Williams (1998) used a 9-week protocol of 27 sessions for patients with brain injury to learn to use memory aids of this nature. Good outcome also appears to be linked to patient characteristics, such as strong motivation, some degree of insight, and absence of aphasia and motor deficits that interfere with handwriting (Donaghy & Williams, 1998).

Table 29-4. Internal Compensatory Strategies

Technique	Description
Rehearsal	Patient repeats the information to be remembered out loud or to self.
Visual imagery	Patient consolidates information to be remembered by making a mental picture that includes the information (e.g., to remember the name *Barbara,* the patient pictures a barber holding the letter A).
Semantic elaboration	Patient consolidates information by making up a simple story (e.g., patient who has to remember the words *lawyer, game,* and *hat* develops a sentence such as "The lawyer wore a hat to the game").
First-letter mnemonics	Parenté's NAME mnemonic adds rules to observing features and drawing associations when remembering names: **N**otice the person with whom you speak, **A**sk the person to repeat his or her name, **M**ention the name in conversation, and **E**xaggerate some special feature.
PQRST rehearsal method	Patient: (1) **P**reviews (skims the material for general content), (2) **Q**uestions (asks questions about the content), (3) **R**eads (actively reads to answer the questions), (4) **S**tates (rehearses or repeats the information read), and (5) **T**ests (tests self by answering the questions).

Information from Malec & Questad, 1983; Milton, 1985; Wilson, 1982; Parenté & Herrmann, 2002.

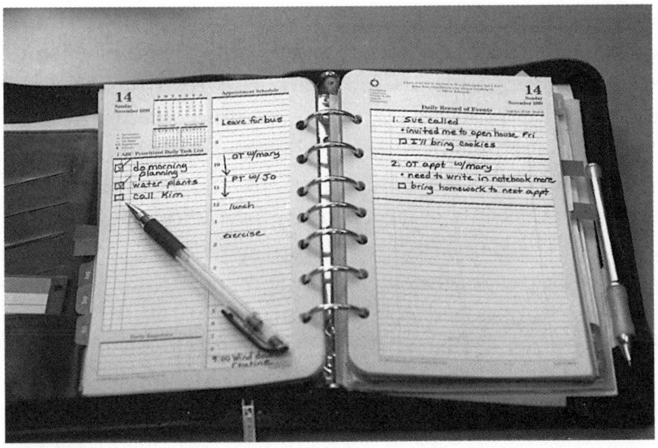

Figure 29-5 Use of function-specific portions of the planner page helps the patient organize notes about the day.

Patients may purchase commercial day planners or obtain them from clinicians who create computer-generated forms and calendars (Fig. 29-5). Day planners are composed of a limited number of function-specific sections such as daily log, assignments and appointments, current work, and long-term information (Dougherty & Radomski, 1987). Table 29-5 summarizes the treatment protocol used at the Brain Injury Clinic at Sister Kenny Rehabilitation Services in Minneapolis. Treatment addresses only learning objectives that are appropriate for the individual and incorporates other compensatory cognitive strategies, such as use of alarm cueing devices, checklists, and problem-solving schemas.

Table 29-5. Example of a Compensatory Strategy Training Protocol Used in the Outpatient Brain Injury Clinic at Sister Kenny Rehabilitation Institute

Sample Long-Term Goals

1. The client will be able to accurately and efficiently file and locate information in his or her planner.
2. The client will be able to get to appointments and complete intended tasks on time through use of compensatory cognitive strategies (such as planner, daily/weekly planning checklists, and alarm watch).
3. Through use of compensatory cognitive strategies, the client will be able to carry out routine personal, household, and work tasks accurately and efficiently without omissions or repetitions.
4. The client will initiate note taking at such times and in such ways that information stored in and retrieved from the planner is accurate and meaningful upon later reference.
5. The client will be able to carry out novel, multistep tasks through employment of compensatory cognitive strategies.

Training Hierarchy and Sample Short-Term Goals

Learning objective	*Client learns to:*
Information retrieval	Select and obtain an appropriate planner, with assistance of therapist. Locate information in function-specific notebook sections. Use written instructions to set an alarm cueing device. Refer to time-specific entries in the planner in response to the alarm. Use asterisk recorded by therapist to prompt reference to other sections of the planner.
Basic planning	Use a checklist to regularly engage in daily and weekly planning. Create daily to-do lists that reflect realistic scheduling and prioritization. Recognize situations in which time-specific prompts would be of help and initiate alarm settings that are pertinent to daily schedule.
Basic information entry	Record appointments, to-do's, and lists in the correct sections of the planner. Initiate use of an asterisk on daily planner pages to cross reference to other planner sections. Routinely use the following note taking mechanics: include date and topic, organize notes by steps or points, check off completed steps or tasks, orally verify accuracy after recording notes.
Complex information entry	Use "People Logs" to record information pertaining to conversations with significant people. Use the main idea/example mnemonic as a means of keeping track of what he or she wants to say during a discussion. Use a tape recorder in conjunction with note taking and identify situations when use of this combination would be most appropriate. Use customized forms to record information pertaining to specific work or household situations.
Complex planning	Analyze long-term projects or tasks in terms of a breakdown of sequential steps. Incorporate project plans and goals into the weekly planning process.

Memory Prostheses: Devices

Alarm watches, pagers, and palm-top computers are often used in conjunction with or as an alternative to day planners (Lynch, 1995). A variety of devices may also be used to minimize cognitive burden (see Resources 29-1), including those that help individuals manage their medications (Fig. 29-6). Giles and Shore (1989b) described the successful use of a Psion Organizer, a palm-top computer, by a woman with acquired brain injury. Among other features, this device provides time-specific prompts for information related to schedule, appointments, and tasks. With 4 hours of therapy and 6 hours of supervised practice with family, this patient with memory impairment but normal intelligence could independently program the device, and she preferred it to a day planner because of its alarm functions. Kim et al. (1999) also used a Psion Organizer but with an inpatient with severe cognitive impairments. Staff programmed the schedule and alarms into the device; it improved the patient's punctuality at therapy sessions and, after 5 days, was effective in prompting the patient to take medications. Wilson et al. (1997) conducted a study using NeuroPage, more recently called LifeMinder, with 15 neurologically impaired subjects, all of whom had significant everyday memory impairment or problems with planning and organization. NeuroPage is a simple portable paging system with a screen that can be attached to a belt (Hersh & Treadgold, 1994). It uses micro-computers linked to conventional computer memory and a paging company. Information about the patient's schedule is entered into the computer, and on the appropriate date and time, NeuroPage accesses the user's data files, determines the reminder to be delivered, and transmits the information (Wilson et al., 1997). These researchers reported that all 15 subjects benefited from the pager and showed significant improvement on task follow-through. Furthermore, even when the pager was removed after 3 months, some subjects were able to maintain the routines initially prompted by the device, such as taking medication on time and using checklists. Wilson et al. (2001) found similar benefits of Neuropage in the completion of everyday tasks in a larger study involving 143 participants with memory and planning deficits (ages 8–83 years). Pre-programmed electronic memory aids have also been demonstrated to help outpatients with mild to moderate dementia remember to do time-specific tasks, significantly more so than use of written lists or trying to recall without any memory aid (Oriani et al., 2003).

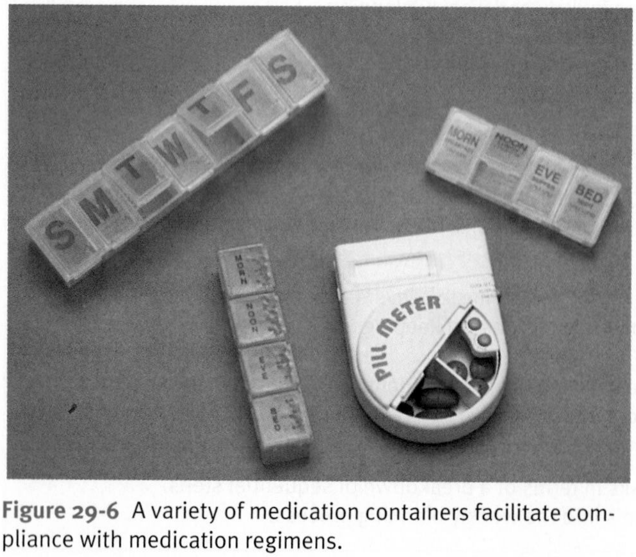

Figure 29-6 A variety of medication containers facilitate compliance with medication regimens.

Considerations for Selecting Client-Specific Memory Aids

Clinician preferences and competence seem to influence the type of memory aid that therapists recommend for their clients. In a study of 94 people with brain injury, Evans et al. (2003) found that most subjects used calendars, wall charts, and notebooks, but only 7.4% used an electronic device as a memory aid. Many experts suggest that despite clients' motivation to use high-tech devices (Wright et al., 2001), electronic memory aids may be under used because clinicians do not have a good working knowledge of these devices (Evans et al., 2003) and lack confidence in guiding clients to use them (Hart, O'Neil-Pirozzi, & Morita, 2003).

Client factors, not clinician preferences, are the most important determinants in the selection of the memory aid. In addition to at least superficial awareness of deficits, premorbid use of memory aids is predictive of effective use of memory aids after acquired brain injury (Evans et al., 2003). In their study of 101 people with acute brain injury, Evans et al. also found that age, time since injury, and attentional ability were important predictors. The younger the person was, the more likely they were to use memory aids, possibly because of their necessity relative to return to work. In this study, the longer the time since injury, the less memory aids were being used. Finally, attention and speed of information processing proved to have a strong relationship with the use of memory aids, possibly because of the importance of attention in the process of learning to compensate for persisting deficits.

The use of electronic aids may place even greater demands on learning than low-tech aids such as day planners. Giles and Shore (1989b) recommended that good candidates have average or nearly average intelligence, retained or mildly impaired reasoning skills, insight into deficits, adequate ability to initiate behavior, and some form of functional disorder resulting from significant memory impairment. Many electronic memory aids require that clients carefully follow multistep instructions for inputting information, and clients may be at risk of losing information because of error or system shutdown. Electronic memory aids, however, typically offer one important feature not available in low-tech (notebook) alternatives—time-specific auditory or vibrating prompts. An alarm watch, for example, can be set to remind the client to take his medication, check his day planner, or leave home for an appointment. Therefore, many clients benefit from a memory aid system involving both a day planner and some sort of time-specific alarm prompt, especially when caregivers or family members of persons with severe impairment assume responsibility for programming the device.

Problem-Solving and Decision-Making Schemas

The enterprise of human problem solving is thought to be comprised of the situation (a conglomeration of task, environment, and person variables) and process (problem definition, evaluation of alternative solutions, determining and implementing a plan, and evaluating the results) (Radomski, 1998). The demands on problem solving can sometimes be minimized by changing the environment, establishing consistent routines, or employing problem-solving schemas. Means-ends analysis and the IDEAL Problem Solver (Bransford & Stein, 1984) are examples of these schemas.

Means-ends analysis, which is known to our patients as divide and conquer, is used to organize multistep, unstructured projects—those that have no obvious first steps and that can be carried out in any number of ways. It entails a four-step process:

1. List the major task components.
2. Under each component, write down all the substeps you can think of (in no particular order).
3. Number the substeps.
4. Decide on deadlines if desired (Fig. 29-7).

The IDEAL Problem Solver was developed for a college course in which students learned problem-solving techniques, learned about the process of solving problems, and uncovered their own strengths and weaknesses in this realm (Bransford & Stein, 1984). The IDEAL acronym stands for the five steps of problem solving: I, Identify the problem; D, Define the problem; E, Evaluate all possible solutions; A, Act; and L, Look back.

Although problem-solving schemas are useful because they are applicable to a wide range of situations, they place much greater demands on patients' metaprocessing abilities (executive functions and metacognition) and require much more training time than simply changing the environment or establishing a routine (Radomski, 1998). Sternberg (1987) questioned whether a program of less than a semester would be adequate for teaching college students to learn and use problem-solving schemas, and therefore, occupational therapists are advised to be selective in using this approach in treatment.

EVIDENCE AND GUIDELINES IN COGNITIVE REHABILITATION

As an emerging, multidisciplinary practice area, cognitive rehabilitation has been praised and criticized (Ylvisaker, Hanks, & Johnson-Greene, 2002). Questionable practices involving unsystematic exposure of clients to video games, cognitive retraining software, or workbooks have prompted skepticism and ethical questions about the efficacy of cognitive rehabilitation intervention (Ylvisaker, Hanks, & Johnson-Greene, 2002). Recent systematic reviews of cognitive rehabilitation research, however, enable clinicians to use evidence to shape intervention plans (Cappa et al., 2003; Cicerone et al., 2000, 2005).

The Brain Injury Interdisciplinary Special Interest Group of the American Congress of Rehabilitation Medicine (ACRM) conducted two evidence-based reviews involving cognitive rehabilitation research published through 2002 (Cicerone et al., 2000, 2005). Based on the strength of the research design and study findings, Cicerone et al. developed practice standards (interventions with *substantive* evidence of effectiveness), practice guidelines (interventions with evidence of *probable* effectiveness), and practice options (interventions with evidence of *possible* effectiveness). A panel of experts from the European Federation of Neurological Societies conducted a similar review with findings consistent with that of ACRM (Cappa et al., 2003). Clinicians who serve clients with cognitive impairments are advised to read these important reviews in detail, but here are some of the central findings:

- Strategy training to address attentional deficits is recommended for outpatients in the post-acute phase of recovery (Practice Standard), but there is insufficient evidence to support it during the acute or inpatient phases (Cappa et al., 2003; Cicerone et al., 2000, 2005).
- Compensatory training is recommended in which the use of notebooks, electronic devices, and internal strategies are directly applied to functional situations (Practice Standard) (Cappa et al., 2003; Cicerone et al., 2000, 2005).
- Training in which problem-solving strategies are applied to functional situations is recommended during post-acute rehabilitation (Practice Guideline) (Cicerone et al., 2005).
- There is no evidence for effectiveness of intervention to restore memory function in persons with severe impairment (Cappa et al., 2003).

Project title: Clean the garage

ORDER	STEPS	COMPLETION DATES
	Remove the debris	
4	Collect items for recycling	9/4
5	Bring to recycling center	9/4
2	Collect trash	9/1
1	Purchase large trash bags	9/1
6	Bring unwanted items to thrift store	9/4
	Clean the floor	
12	Get everything off the floor	9/10
13	Sweep	9/10
14	Rinse down the floor	9/10
15	Put everything back	9/10
	Organize storage	
3	List the items I plan to store	9/1
7	Decide on what add'l storage is needed	9/5
8	List supplies needed + measurements	9/5
9	Purchase supplies	9/5
10	Install	9/5
11	Put items away	9/5

Figure 29-7 Means–ends analysis (also known as divide and conquer) helps patients break large, unstructured projects into a sequence of steps: (1) List major task components (shaded boxes). (2) Write down substeps under each task component in no particular order. (3) Number the substeps. (4) Set completion dates if desired.

- Sole reliance on repeated exposure and practice on computer-based and workbook tasks without involvement of the therapist is not recommended (Cicerone et al., 2000, 2005).

In summary, when planning intervention to optimizing clients' cognitive function, occupational therapists develop intervention plans involving multiple approaches. Ylvisaker, Hanks, and Johnson-Greene (2002) describe this as a "contextualized approach" to cognitive rehabilitation. This paradigm up-ends the traditional intervention sequence (reduction of impairments followed by compensation training) by either using remedial and adaptive approaches simultaneously or in reverse. Clinicians may begin with intervention aimed at enabling participation by changing the environmental or social supports followed by reducing disability through compensatory training and ultimately reduce the cognitive impairment with internalization of well-rehearsed strategies and behaviors (Ylvisaker, Hanks, & Johnson-Greene, 2002).

Evidence Table 29-1
Best Evidence for Interventions Used in Cognitive Rehabilitation

Intervention	Description of Intervention Tested	Participants	Dosage	Type of Best Evidence and Level of Evidence	Benefit	Statistical Probability and Effect Size of Outcome	Reference
Computer-aided retraining of memory and attention	All participants received individualized intervention based on a computer training program entitled, RehaCom. The experimental group performed memory and attention procedures; the control group performed visuoconstructional and visuomotor retraining procedures.	77 adult outpatients with multiple sclerosis who had complaints of poor attention and memory, which were confirmed by neuropsychological testing (mean age = 44 years).	All subjects participated in training for 45 minutes, twice a week for 8 consecutive weeks.	Randomized double-blind controlled trial. Level IB1a (moderately sized groups)	Negligible benefit. No group differences in any of the 8 neuropsychological measures of attention or memory except for word list generation.	Word list generation at 8 weeks ($p = 0.016$, $r = 0.24$) and 16 weeks ($p = 0.035$, $r = 0.20$).	Solari et al., 2004

continued

Evidence Table 29-1 *(continued)*

Intervention	Description of Intervention Tested	Participants	Dosage	Type of Best Evidence and Level of Evidence	Benefit	Statistical Probability and Effect Size of Outcome	Reference
Change the context (social, environmental)	All participants received OT assessment within the home. Treatment group received a second home visit, at which time OT recommendations regarding caregiving and environmental modification strategies were reviewed with caregiver. A written report was also provided. Control group received no further contact during the study but received a copy of written recommendations after the study was over.	40 adults diagnosed with possible or probable Alzheimer's disease and their 40 caregivers (mean age = 77.08 years for those with Alzheimer's disease).	2 at-home sessions (1 assessment, 1 30-minute session to review recommendations).	Pre-test–post-test control group design (random assignment). Level IB2a (small number of subjects per group, unblinded)	Yes. The persons in the treatment group realized improvements in quality of life.	Significant MANCOVA main effect for caregiver burden, positive affect, activity, and self-care status for treatment group. $F_{(4,31)} = 7.34, p < .001$, effect size (eta squired) = .49.	Dooley & Hinojosa, 2004
Learn cognitive compensatory strategies	The treatment group received memory notebook training; subjects in the comparison group participated in supportive group therapy.	8 participants who were at least 2 years post traumatic brain injury (4 subjects per group); mean age = 28 years.	Two 60-minute sessions per week for 8 weeks.	Pre-test–post-test control group with randomized assignment. Level IC2a (small numbers of subjects in groups, unblinded)	Yes. Decrease in observed everyday memory failures for treatment group at post-test (but not at 6-month follow-up).	Observed everyday memory failures ($F_{(1,5)} = 7.15$, $p < 0.05, r = 0.77$)	Schmitter-Edgecombe et al., 1995

SUMMARY REVIEW QUESTIONS

1. Describe diagnoses of patients who are likely to have organically based cognitive impairments. What types of circumstances or conditions result in cognitive inefficiency?
2. Analyze the relative costs and benefits of a remedial approach to cognitive problems versus an adaptive approach.
3. How would your efforts to optimize cognitive function be different for a person with Alzheimer's disease compared with a patient in acute recovery from a traumatic brain injury?
4. Write down the steps to one of your daily routines or habit sequences. Now change the order of steps and, next time, try to follow this revised sequence. How do the attentional requirements change? How do these changes impact your speed of performance?
5. Describe three changes you could make to your own living environment to decrease its cognitive demands.
6. What cognitive compensatory strategies, if any, are a part of your information-processing repertoire?
7. Consider practices or habits that optimize your memory performance and ability to concentrate, plan, and problem solve. How might these same strategies be used by an individual with cognitive impairment?

ACKNOWLEDGEMENT

We appreciate Cathy Trombly's assistance in calculating the effect sizes included in Evidence Table 29-1 in this chapter.

References

Aarts, H., & Dijksterhuis, A. (2000). Habits as knowledge structures: Automaticity in goal-directed behavior. *Journal of Personality and Social Psychology, 78,* 53–63.

Abreu, B. C., & Toglia, J. P. (1987). Cognitive rehabilitation: A model for occupational therapy. *American Journal of Occupational Therapy, 41,* 439–448.

American Occupational Therapy Association [AOTA]. (2002). Occupational therapy practice framework. *American Journal of Occupational Therapy, 56,* 609–639.

Bargh, J. A. (1997). The automaticity of everyday life. In R. S. Wyer (Ed.), *Advances in social cognition* (pp. 1–61). Mahwah, NJ: Lawrence Erlbaum Associates.

Bargh, J. A., & Chartrand, T. L. (1999). The unbearable automaticity of being. *American Psychologist, 54,* 462–479.

Ben-Yishay, Y., & Diller, L. (1993). Cognitive remediation in traumatic brain injury: Update and issues. *Archives of Physical Medicine and Rehabilitation, 74,* 204–213.

Blundon, G., & Smits, E. (2000). Cognitive rehabilitation: Pilot survey of therapeutic modalities used by Canadian occupational therapists with survivors of traumatic brain injury. *Canadian Journal of Occupational Therapy, 67,* 184–196.

Bransford, J. D., & Stein, B. S. (1984). *The IDEAL Problem Solver: A guide for improving thinking, learning, and creativity.* New York: W. H. Freeman.

Brown, S. W., & Bennett, E. D. (2002). The role of practice and automaticity in temporal and nontemporal dual-task performance. *Psychological Research, 66,* 80–89.

Camic, D. (1986). The matter of habit. *American Journal of Sociology, 91,* 1039–1087.

Cappa, S. F., Benke, T., Clarke, S., Rossi, B., Stemmer, B., & van Heugten, C. M. (2003). EFNS guidelines on cognitive rehabilitation: Report of an EFNS Task Force. *European Journal of Neurology, 10,* 11–23.

Carney, N., Chestnut, R. M., Maynard, H., Mann, N. C., Patterson, P., & Helfand, M. (1999). Effect of cognitive rehabilitation on outcomes for persons with traumatic brain injury: A systematic review. *Journal of Head Trauma Rehabilitation, 14,* 277–307.

Charmaz, K. (2002). The self as habit: The reconstruction of self in chronic illness. *Occupational Therapy Journal of Research, 22 (Suppl. 1),* 31S–41S.

Chen, S. H. A., Thomas, J. D., Glueckauf, R. L., & Bracy, O. L. (1997). The effectiveness of computer-assisted cognitive rehabilitation for persons with traumatic brain injury. *Brain Injury, 11,* 197–209.

Cicerone, K. D., Dahlberg, C., Kalmar, K., Langenbahn, D. M., Malec, J. F., Bergquist, T. F., Felicetti, T., Giacino, J. T., Preston Harley, J., Harrington, D. E., Herzog, J., Kneipp, S., Laatsch, L., & Morse, P. A. (2000). Evidence-based cognitive rehabilitation: Recommendations for clinical practice. *Archives of Physical Medicine and Rehabilitation, 81,* 1596–1615.

Cicerone, K. D., Dahlberg, C., Malec, J. F., Langenbahn, D. M., Felicetti, T., Kneipp, S., Ellmo, W., Kalmar, K., Giacino, J. T., Preston Harley, J., Laatsch, L., Morse, P. A., & Catanese, J. (2005). Evidence-based cognitive rehabilitation: Updated review of the literature from 1998 through 2002. *Archives of Physical Medicine and Rehabilitation, 86,* 1681–1692.

Clare, B., Wilson, G., Carter, G., & Hodges, J. (2003). Cognitive rehabilitation as a component of early intervention in Alzheimer's disease: A single case study. *Aging and Mental Health, 7,* 15–21.

Clark, F. A. (2000). The concepts of habit and routine: A preliminary theoretical synthesis. *Occupational Therapy Journal of Research, 20 (Suppl. 1),* 123S–137S.

Commission on Accreditation of Rehabilitation Facilities [CARF]. (2004). *1999 medical rehabilitation standards manual.* Tucson, AZ: Commission on Accreditation of Rehabilitation Facilities.

Crosson, B., Barco, P. P., Velozo, C. A., Bolesta, M. M., Cooper, P. V., Werts, D., & Brobeck, T. C. (1989). Awareness and compensation in postacute head injury rehabilitation. *Journal of Head Trauma Rehabilitation, 4,* 46–54.

Davis, E. S., & Radomski, M. V. (1989). Domain-specific training to reinstate habit sequences. *Occupational Therapy Practice, 1,* 79–88.

Dirette, D. (2002). The development of awareness and the use of compensatory strategies for cognitive deficits. *Brain Injury, 16,* 861–871.

Donaghy, S., & Williams, W. (1998). A new protocol for training severely impaired patients in the usage of memory journals. *Brain Injury, 12,* 1061–1076.

Dooley, N. R., & Hinojosa, J. (2004). Improving quality of life for persons with Alzheimer's disease and their family caregivers: Brief occupational therapy intervention. *American Journal of Occupational Therapy, 58,* 561–569.

Dougherty, P. M., & Radomski, M. V. (1987). *The cognitive rehabilitation workbook.* Rockville, MD: Aspen.

Dougherty, P. M., & Radomski, M. V. (1993). *The cognitive rehabilitation workbook* (2nd ed.). Gaithersburg, MD: Aspen.

Dyck, I. (2002). Beyond the clinic: Restructuring the environment in chronic illness experience. *Occupational Therapy Journal of Research, 22 (Suppl. 1),* 52S–60S.

Eldridge, L. L., Masterman, D., & Knowlton, B. J. (2002). Intact implicit habit learning in Alzheimer's disease. *Behavioral Neuroscience, 116,* 722–726.

Evans, J. J., Wilson, B. A., Needham, P., & Brentnall, S. (2003). Who makes good use of memory aids? Results of a survey of people with acquired brain injury. *Journal of the International Neuropsychological Society, 9,* 925–935.

Fleming, J., & Strong, J. (1995). Self-awareness of deficits following acquired brain injury: Considerations for rehabilitation. *British Journal of Occupational Therapy, 58,* 55–60.

Gallimore, R., & Lopez, E. M. (2002). Everyday routines, human agency, and ecocultural context: Construction and maintenance of individual habits. *Occupational Therapy Journal of Research, 22 (Suppl. 1),* 70S–77S.

Gelfand, D. M., & Hartmann, D. P. (1984). *Child behavioral analysis and therapy.* Needham Heights, MA: Allyn & Bacon.

Gianutsos, R. (1992). The computer in cognitive rehabilitation: It's not just a tool anymore. *Journal of Head Trauma Rehabilitation, 7,* 26–35.

Giles, G. M. (1998). A neurofunctional approach to rehabilitation following severe brain injury. In N. Katz (Ed.) *Cognition and occupation in rehabilitation* (pp. 125–147). Bethesda, MD: American Occupational Therapy Association.

Giles, G. M. (2005). A neurofunctional approach to rehabilitation following severe brain injury. In N. Katz (Ed.), *Cognition and occupation across the life span* (pp. 139–165). Bethesda, MD: American Occupational Therapy Association.

Giles, G. M., & Clark-Wilson, J. (1988). The use of behavioral techniques in functional skills training after severe brain injury. *American Journal of Occupational Therapy, 42,* 658–665.

Giles, G. M., Ridley, J. E., Dill, A., & Frye, S. (1997). A consecutive series of adults with brain injury treated with a washing and dressing retraining program. *American Journal of Occupational Therapy, 51,* 256–266.

Giles, G. M., & Shore, M. (1989a). A rapid method for teaching severely brain injured adults how to wash and dress. *Archives of Physical Medicine and Rehabilitation, 70,* 156–158.

Giles, G. M., & Shore, M. (1989b). The effectiveness of an electronic memory aid for a memory-impaired adult of normal intelligence. *American Journal of Occupational Therapy, 43,* 409–411.

Gitlin, L., & Corcoran, M., (2005). *Occupational therapy and dementia care: The home environmental skill-building program for individuals and families.* Bethesda, MD: American Occupational Therapy Association.

Goldstein, G., Beers, S. R., Longmore, S., & McCue, M. (1996). Efficacy of memory training: A technical extension and replication. *Clinical Neurologist, 10,* 66–72.

Hart, T., O'Neil-Pirozzi, T., & Morita, C. (2003). Clinician expectations for portable electronic devices as cognitive-behavioral orthoses in traumatic brain injury. *Brain Injury, 17,* 401–411.

Hersh, N., & Treadgold, L. (1994). NeuroPage: The rehabilitation of memory dysfunction by prosthetic memory aid cueing. *Neurorehabilitation, 4,* 187–197.

Jog, M. S., Kubota, Y., Connolly, C. I., Hillegaart, V., & Graybiel, A. M. (1999). Building neural representations of habits. *Science, 286,* 1745–1749.

Katzmann, S., & Mix, C. (1994). Improving functional independence in a patient with encephalitis through behavior modification shaping techniques. *American Journal of Occupational Therapy, 48,* 259–262.

Kielhofner, G. (1995). Habituation. In G. Kielhofner (Ed.), *A model of human occupation: Theory and application* (2nd ed., pp. 63–82). Baltimore: Williams & Wilkins.

Kim, H. J., Burke, D. T., Dowds, M. M., & Georges, J. (1999). Utility of a microcomputer as an external memory aid for a memory-impaired head injury patient during inpatient rehabilitation. *Brain Injury, 13,* 147–150.

Kime, S. K., Lamb, D. G., & Wilson, B. A. (1996). Use of a comprehensive programme of external cueing to enhance procedural memory in a patient with dense amnesia. *Brain Injury, 10,* 17–25.

Krebs, H. I., Hogan, N., Hening, W., Adamovich, S. V., & Poizner, H. (2001). Procedural motor learning in Parkinson's disease. *Experimental Brain Research, 141,* 425–437.

Logan, G. D. (1988a). Toward an instance theory of automaticity. *Psychological Review, 95,* 492–527.

Logan, G. D. (1988b). Automaticity, resources, and memory: Theoretical controversies and practical implications. *Human Factors, 30,* 538–598.

Logan, G. D., Taylor, S. E., & Etherton, J. L. (1999). Attention and automaticity: Toward a theoretical integration. *Psychological Research, 62,* 165–181.

Ludwig, F. M. (1998). The unpackaging of routine in older women. *American Journal of Occupational Therapy, 52,* 168–175.

Lynch, B. (2002) Historical review of computer-assisted cognitive retraining. *Journal of Head Trauma Rehabilitation, 17,* 446–457.

Lynch, W. J. (1995). You must remember this: Assistive devices for memory impairment. *Journal of Head Trauma Rehabilitation, 10,* 94–97.

Malec, J., & Basford, J. (1996). Postacute brain injury rehabilitation. *Archives of Physical Medicine and Rehabilitation, 77,* 198–207.

Malec, J., & Questad, K. (1983). Rehabilitation of memory after craniocerebral trauma: Case report. *Archives of Physical Medicine and Rehabilitation, 64,* 436–438.

Milton, S. B. (1985). Compensatory memory strategy training: A practical approach for managing persistent memory problems. *Cognitive Rehabilitation, 3,* 8–15.

Mishkin, M., & Appenzeller, T. (1987). The anatomy of memory. *Scientific American, 256,* 80–89.

O'Reilly, M. F., Green, G., & Braunling-McMorrow, D. (1990). Self-administered written prompts to teach home accident prevention skills to adults with brain injuries. *Journal of Applied Behavior Analysis, 23,* 431–446.

Oriani, M., Moniz-Cook, E., Binetti, G., Zanieri, G., Frisoni, G. B., Geroldi, C., De Vreese, L. P., & Zanetti, O. (2003). An electronic memory aid to support prospective memory in patients in early stages of Alzheimer's disease: A pilot study. *Aging and Mental Health, 7,* 22–27.

Packard, M. G., & Knowlton, B. J. (2002). Learning and memory functions of the basal ganglia. *Annual Review of Neuroscience, 25,* 563–593.

Parenté, R., & DiCesare, A. (1991) Retraining memory theory, evaluation and applications. In J. S. Kreutzer & P. H. Wehman (Eds.), *Cognitive rehabilitation for persons with traumatic brain injury: A functional approach* (pp.147–162). Baltimore: Paul H. Brooks.

Parenté, R., & Herrmann, D. (2002) *Retraining cognition: Techniques and applications.* (2nd ed.). Austin, TX: Pro-ed.

Radomski, M. V. (1994). Cognitive rehabilitation: Advancing the stature of occupational therapy. *American Journal of Occupational Therapy, 48,* 271–273.

Radomski, M. V. (1998). Problem solving deficits: Using a multi-dimensional definition to select a treatment approach. *Physical Disabilities Special Interest Section Quarterly, 21,* 1–4.

Reber, P. J., Knowlton, B. J., & Squire, L. R. (1996). Dissociable properties of memory systems: Differences in the flexibility of declarative and nondeclarative knowledge. *Behavioral Neuroscience, 110,* 861–871.

Rogers, J. C. (2000). Habits: Do we practice what we preach? *Occupational Therapy Journal of Research, 20 (Suppl. 1),* 119S–127S.

Schmitter-Edgecombe, M., Fahy, J. F., Whelan, J. P., & Long, C. J. (1995). Memory remediation after severe closed head injury: Notebook training over supportive therapy. *Journal of Consulting and Clinical Psychology, 63,* 484–489.

Schwartz, S. M. (1995). Adults with traumatic brain injury: Three case studies of cognitive rehabilitation in the home setting. *American Journal of Occupational Therapy, 49,* 655–667.

Seamon, D. (2002). Physical comminglings: Body, habit, and space transformed into place. *Occupational Therapy Journal of Research, 22 (Suppl. 1),* 42S–51S.

Silverstein, N., Flaherty, G., & Tobin, T. (2002). *Dementia and wandering behavior.* New York: Springer Publishing Company.

Sohlberg, M. M., & Mateer, C. A. (1989). *Introduction to cognitive rehabilitation.* New York: Guilford.

Sohlberg, M. M., & Mateer, C. A. (2001). *Cognitive rehabilitation.* New York: Guilford Press.

Solari, A., Motta, A., Mendozzi, L., Pucci, E., Forni, M., Mancardi, G., & Pozzilli, C. (2004). Computer-aided retraining of memory and attention in people with multiple sclerosis: A randomized, double-blind controlled trial. *Journal of the Neurological Sciences, 222,* 99–104.

Squire, L. R., Knowlton, B. J., & Musen, G. (1993). The structure and organization of memory. *Annual Review of Psychology, 44,* 453–495.

Sternberg, R. J. (1986). *Intelligence applied: Understanding and increasing your intellectual skills.* New York: Harcourt Brace Jovanovich.

Sternberg, R. J. (1987). Questions and answers about the nature and teaching of thinking skills. In J. B. Baron & R. J. Sternberg (Eds.), *Teaching thinking skills: Theory and practice* (pp. 251–259). New York: W.H. Freeman.

Strand, M. (2000). A routine gift. *Headlines (Brain Injury Association of Minnesota), Winter,* 1–14.

Stringer, A. Y. (2003). Cognitive rehabilitation practice patterns: A survey of American Hospital Association Rehabilitation Programs. *The Clinical Neuropsychologist, 17,* 34–44.

Taylor, M. (1929). Occupational therapy in industrial inquiries. *Occupational Therapy and Rehabilitation, 8,* 335–338.

Toglia, J. P. (1991). Generalization of treatment: A multi-contextual approach to cognitive perceptual impairment in the brain injured adult. *American Journal of Occupational Therapy, 45,* 505–516.

Toglia, J. P. (2005). A dynamic interactional approach to cognitive rehabilitation. In N. Katz (Ed.), *Cognition and occupation across the life span* (pp. 29–72). Bethesda, MD: American Occupational Therapy Association.

Wallenbert, I., & Jonsson, H. (2005). Waiting to get better: A dilemma regarding habits and daily occupations after stroke. *American Journal of Occupational Therapy, 59,* 218–224.

Wilson, B. A. (1982). Success and failure in memory training following a cerebral vascular accident. *Cortex, 18,* 581–594.

Wilson, B. A. (1997). Cognitive rehabilitation: How it is and how it might be. *Journal of the International Neuropsychological Society, 3,* 487-496.

Wilson, B. A., Emslie, H. C., Quirk, K., & Evans, J. J. (2001). Reducing everyday memory and planning problems by means of a paging system: A randomized control crossover study. *Journal of Neurology, Neurosurgery, and Psychiatry, 70,* 477–482.

Wilson, B. A., Evans, J. J., Emslie, H., & Malinek, V. (1997). Evaluation of NeuroPage: A new memory aid. *Journal of Neurology, Neurosurgery, and Psychiatry, 63,* 113–115.

Wood, W., Quinn, J. M., & Kashy, D. A. (2002). Habits in everyday life: Thought, emotion, and action. *Journal of Personality and Social Psychology, 83,* 1281–1297.

Wright, P., Rogers, N., Hall, C., Wilson, B., Evans, J., Emslie, H., & Bartram, C. (2001). Comparison of pocket-computer memory aids for people with brain injury. *Brain Injury, 15,* 787–800.

Wu, T., Kansaku, K., & Hallett, M. (2003). How self-initiated memorized movements become automatic: A functional MRI study. *Journal of Neurophysiology, 91,* 1690–1698.

Ylvisaker, M., Hanks, R., & Johnson-Greene, D. (2002). Perspectives on rehabilitation of individuals with cognitive impairment after brain injury: Rationale for reconsideration of theoretical paradigms. *Journal of Head Trauma Rehabilitation, 17,* 191–209.

Zanetti, O., Binetti, G., Magni, E., Rozzini, L., Bianchetti, A., & Trabucchi, M. (1997). Procedural memory stimulation in Alzheimer's disease: Impact of a training programme. *Acta Neurologica Scandinavica, 95,* 152–157.

Zemke, R. (1994). Habits. In. C. B. Royeen (Ed.), *The practice of the future: Putting occupation back into therapy* (pp. 1–24). Bethesda, MD: American Occupational Therapy Association.

Zenicus, A., Wesolowski, M. D., & Burke, W. H. (1990). A comparison of 4 memory strategies with traumatically brain injured clients. *Brain Injury, 4,* 33–38.

Zenicus, A., Wesolowski, M. D., Krankowski, T., & Burke, W. H. (1991). Memory notebook training with traumatically brain injured clients. *Brain Injury, 5,* 321–325.

CHAPTER 30

Restoring the Role of Independent Person

Anne Birge James

LEARNING OBJECTIVES

After studying this chapter, the reader will be able to do the following:

1. Describe the use of occupation-as-end as a therapeutic medium.
2. Distinguish between basic activities of daily living and instrumental activities of daily living.
3. State principles to restore adapted function to persons with various functional limitations.
4. Modify tasks and the environment to promote independence.
5. Prescribe and evaluate the use of assistive devices to promote safe independence.
6. Guide problem solving and implementation of solutions to unique situations for persons with a variety of functional limitations.

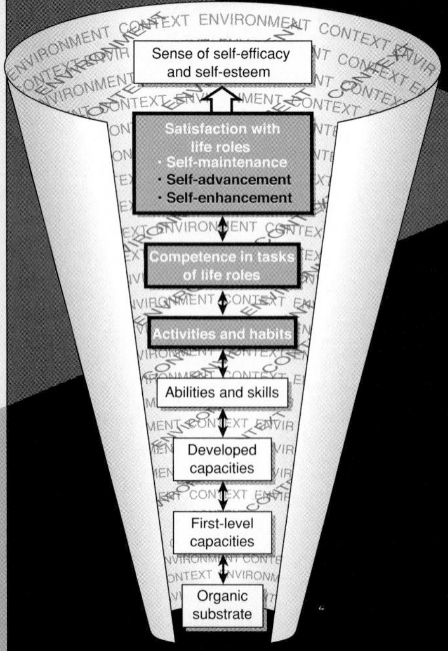

Glossary

Active learning—A process in which a learner is engaged physically and/or cognitively in a learning task. Learners are engaged in finding a solution to a problem (for example, identifying three ways cooking can be modified to save energy) and/or engaging in actual practice of the solution (for example, practicing putting on a sock with a sock aid).

Adaptation—Process of learning to function in an environment. Occupational therapists enable that process by modifying a task, the method of accomplishing the task, and/or the environment to promote independence in occupational functioning.

Blocked practice—Practice consisting of drills that include many repetitions of the same task performed in the same way (Schmidt & Lee, 2000).

Random practice—Practice of several related tasks within one session; sequence of tasks varies randomly (Schmidt & Lee, 2000).

Self-efficacy—The judgments people have of their capabilities to do or learn a task (Gage & Polatajko, 1994). Self-efficacy is task specific and is dependent, in part, on an individual's past experience with a task or similar tasks.

Shaping—A behavior modification technique in which, at first, any approximation of the desired behavior is rewarded. As the person is able to produce the behavior consistently, only the next higher level of performance is rewarded and so forth until the desired behavior is performed consistently well. Rewarding feedback is then faded.

Task parameter—A property or characteristic of a task that can be measured and addressed in treatment. Independence is the most commonly used parameter, but other parameters might include duration of task, quality of performance, and level of fatigue resulting from task performance.

People who are satisfied with their life roles have the resources and capabilities needed to accomplish their everyday tasks, whether or not they actually perform the task themselves. Self-maintenance roles include participation in activities of daily living (ADLs) (Trombly, 1995). The occupational therapist is the rehabilitation specialist responsible for teaching the patient to accomplish these tasks. The assumption is that people want to care for themselves to the best of their ability. This may include directing and/or delegating to others tasks that are beyond the person's capabilities.

The term *basic activities of daily living* (BADLs) is synonymous with self-care. BADL include feeding, grooming, dressing, bathing, toileting, bowel and bladder management, personal device care, sexual activity, functional mobility, sleep/rest, and eating (chewing, swallowing) (American Occupational Therapy Association [AOTA], 2002). These universal tasks are necessary to maintain health. The first eight BADLs are included in this chapter. Functional mobility, including bed mobility, transfers, and wheelchair mobility, is addressed in Chapter 31 and chewing and swallowing are addressed in Chapter 48. Although every human engages in most or all BADLs to some degree, the way that each is done and the importance attached to each differs culturally. BADL is the focus of most insurance coverage for rehabilitation. Baseline measures and examination of progress is documented by such evaluative measures as the *Functional Independence Measure (FIM)* (see Chapter 4).

Suggesting that a person is independent in self-maintenance if they can complete their BADLs gives a false impression of independence. People can be independent in BADL but unable to live without assistance. True independence also requires participation in *instrumental activities of daily living* (IADLs), including but not limited to management of one's own medications, food, shelter, and finances; caring for other people or pets; communication device use; and community mobility (AOTA, 2002). IADLs include a range of diverse tasks that often require greater interaction with the physical and social environments and may have more demanding physical and/or cognitive demands than BADLs (Rogers & Holm, 2003).

OCCUPATION-AS-END

When remedial therapy can correct performance skills/patterns or client factors that interfere with ADLs, patients are often able to resume meaningful tasks and activities as they become able. Intervention that targets ADLs directly is necessary for those who do not regain full capabilities or prefer not to engage in remedial therapy. Occupation-as-end is an intervention focused on learning how to accomplish the activities and tasks that constitute roles in an adapted way (Trombly, 1995). The therapist can employ a modification approach that enables patients to accomplish their everyday tasks by changing the task and/or environment and providing appropriate patient and/or caregiver education (Holm, Rogers, & James, 2003). The modifications recommended by the therapist may be aimed at the patient and/or the caregiver (Chen et al., 2000). Intervention is frequently aimed at improving independence in ADL, that is, the person's ability to complete the task without assistance from others. Intervention, however, may also be used to address other important **task parameters**, including safety and adequacy conditions, such as perceived difficulty or ease of performance, pain, fatigue or dyspnea precipitated by activities, length of time to complete a task, and the ability to complete tasks in a way that meets personal and societal expectations (Holm, Rogers, & James, 2003). For example, a patient with rheumatoid arthritis may be independent in cooking but may experience significant pain that makes her unwilling to engage in the task. The therapist may instruct her in the use of adapted methods of cooking that protect painful joints to help her cook both independently and without pain.

The extent and focus of services offered to a particular patient depends on the person's motivation and the level of independence he or she needs. The patient's perceptions of ADL capabilities may differ from those of staff (Atwood, Holm, & James, 1994) and affect the patient's investment in treatment. Use of an instrument such as the *Canadian Occupational Performance Measure* (*COPM*) or the *Melville-Nelson Self-Identified Goals Assessment* (http://www.meduohio.edu/allh/ot/melville/siga.html) can identify patients' perceptions, values, and goals. Independence in BADL may be sufficient for a person returning to a sheltered and supportive living situation in which IADL needs are few and willingly assumed by others, but it is never enough for a person who expects to reintegrate into community life. This person not only must learn solutions to BADL and common IADL tasks but also must learn to identify and solve problems that prevent accomplishment of unique tasks. On the other hand, independence in only one activity, such as transferring or toileting, may determine whether discharge is to home or an institution. Therefore, full effort should concentrate on achievement of this goal for a person who has otherwise limited potential for full independence.

Intervention by occupation-as-end, then, is a compensatory approach that uses education of adapted methods, assistive technology, and **adaptation** of physical and/or social contexts to enable people to participate in desired roles with a permanent or temporary disability.

EDUCATION

In the modify approach, the therapist is teacher, and patient and caregivers are learners. Both teaching and learning are active processes. The patient must be motivated to learn and must be able to learn. Assessing a client's readiness to learn can help the therapist select appropriate tasks and educational methods to maximize client outcomes.

Readiness to Learn

Patients' **self-efficacy** can have a significant impact on learning and can be evaluated and addressed in the context of ADL intervention. Self-efficacy is defined as the judgments people have of their capabilities to do or learn a task (Gage & Polatajko, 1994). Self-efficacy has been demonstrated to be positively related to actual performance and helps people to persist in tasks, even when faced with tasks that are difficult or new (Gage & Polatajko, 1994). Persons with a new disability may have low self-efficacy for engaging in ADL because they lack experience with their limitations in the context of familiar tasks. Self-efficacy can be measured by asking patients to predict their performance on a given task using a Likert-type scale (e.g., 1 = very unlikely to learn this task, 5 = very likely to learn this task). A baseline self-efficacy measure can be used to determine the need for intervention to address self-efficacy along with the ADL skills training to enhance goal achievement.

Depression is another factor that can impede learning and occurs concurrently with a wide variety of physical disabilities. Depression has been demonstrated to have a negative relationship with functional outcomes for clients with varied physical disabilities, e.g., stroke (Herrmann et al., 1998) and Parkinson's disease (Weintraub et al., 2004). Depression may impact functional outcomes in clients by reducing self-efficacy needed for learning. Identifying depression in clients and referring them to physicians for prescription of anti-depressant medications may facilitate functional outcomes in patients engaged in ADL programs. Reducing depressive symptoms can have a direct positive impact on functional performance (Lin et al., 2003). In addition, structuring occupational therapy treatment that addresses the client's needs related to the depression (e.g., providing structure that helps clients initiate participation in ADL or selecting tasks that challenge clients, while also enabling them to experience success) will increase self-efficacy for future performance.

Several additional factors may interfere with patient learning. Learning is more difficult for patients with cognitive deficits (see Chapters 9 and 29). Persons with severe cognitive deficits may not be candidates for ADL training. The caregiver should be taught appropriate methods for assisting the patient and told to seek reevaluation if the patient's cognitive status improves. Patients with severe receptive aphasia or who speak a different language from the therapist have communication limitations that may impact learning. Therapists should use demonstration for patients who do not understand verbal instructions. A translator can be used to support learning for patients who speak another language. Pain may interfere with learning and should be addressed directly or by selecting adaptive methods that minimize pain. Patients with low literacy will not be able to use written materials to supplement learning, so other methods must be explored that support carry-over of new skills outside of therapy. See Chapters 10 and 14 concerning ways to reduce the effects of low literacy.

Clients may require adaptive equipment to maximize independence in ADLs; however, attitudes toward using adaptive equipment can impede learning and performance.

Some people do not want to use a special tool to do a task most people do without such a tool. Persons with disabilities have reported that assistive devices have both positive and negative connotations (Lund & Nygård, 2003; McMillen & Söderberg, 2002). People value a device if the task is important and cannot be done any other way (McMillen & Söderberg, 2002; Parker & Thorslund, 1991; Rogers & Holm, 1992; Tyson & Strong, 1990; Wielandt & Strong, 2000), but they dislike the stigma associated with device use. Disabled persons who participated in a study by McMillen and Söderberg reported that they not only had to learn to use the device, but they also had to "learn" to go out in public with it. Assessing a client's "gadget tolerance" can help therapists tailor their approach to clients when presenting adaptive equipment as an option. Patients with a low tolerance for "gadgets" may need to have a higher trust in their therapist before they are willing to consider equipment. Building this trust may become an important component of the therapeutic intervention for maximizing independence.

Finally, the motivation to learn is influenced by the learner's values, which guide actions and effort (Trombly, 1995). Therefore, therapists must collaborate with patients to identify those tasks that will be within their capabilities and are also consistent with their values and goals. Attending to the many factors that may impact a client's ability to learn helps the therapist select the most appropriate learning strategies to enhance a patient's performance of ADL.

PROCEDURES FOR PRACTICE 30-1

Effective Teaching

1. Identify and address barriers to learning.
2. Determine what the learner knows.
3. Identify the patient's learning needs.
4. Use active learning strategies.
5. Engage the patient and/or caregivers in a collaborative learning process.
6. Select learning activities that present the "just right challenge."
7. Adapt the presentation to the learner's capabilities.
8. Provide opportunities for practice, considering context and schedule.
9. Facilitate the learner's use of internal feedback and provide appropriate external feedback.
10. Test the learner in the appropriate context(s) to confirm that learning has occurred.
11. Discuss progress toward goals with the patient and revise teaching–learning strategies, as indicated.

Teaching Strategies for Effective Learning

Points of effective teaching are noted as follows and summarized in Procedures for Practice 30-1.

1. Identify potential barriers to learning and develop teaching and learning strategies to minimize them.
2. Determine what routines and skills the learner has retained and whether he or she does them safely, including the ability to figure out adapted methods independently.
3. Identify patients' goals and what they must learn to reach their goals (Shotwell & Schell, 1999). These become learning objectives, which are goals expressed in behavioral terms, such as "The patient will brush his teeth independently in fewer than 5 minutes." Although patients vary, toileting is often a priority for patients because dependence on others has a negative impact on self-esteem (Clark & Rugg, 2005).
4. Present the material in a way that requires patients to be active in the learning process (Shotwell & Schell, 1999). Verbal or written instructions and demonstration are passive learning strategies and are often insufficient for mastering a new task. **Active learning** requires learners to apply new knowledge to real-life problems. For example, patients learning principles of energy conservation may be asked to describe a typical day, identify ways that they could conserve energy, and then practice strategies in an actual task, e.g. cooking. Active learning is vital when the patient is learning a motor task, such as putting on a shirt with one paralyzed arm, and should be guided by motor learning principles (see Chapter 14).
5. Use a collaborative approach, recognizing that each participant in the learning process (therapist, patient, and/or caregiver) has experience and expertise to contribute to the learning task. Many techniques commonly in use have been developed by therapist–patient collaboration. Engaging patients and caregivers in the intervention process helps improve problem-solving skills and increases "ownership" of their functional gains, which enhances self-efficacy. Allowing patients to participate in the selection of equipment appears to have a positive influence on compliance (Wielandt & Strong, 2000).
6. Select the "just right challenge." When first learning an activity, the challenge should be kept low to enhance self-efficacy by reducing anxiety and promoting success (Gage & Polatajko, 1994). For example, if the patient is learning to eat with adapted utensils, begin training with sticky foods that do not easily slide off of the spoon and progress to more difficult foods, such as spaghetti and peas.

7. Adapt the presentation to the particular learner, given his or her abilities and deficits. For patients without brain damage and with average intelligence and literacy, teaching methods can include discussion, demonstration, and printed instructions (Schemm & Gitlin, 1998). Printed materials should be written simply and directly because over 50% of the U.S. population has moderate to severe difficulty understanding simple written content, although this is not detectable through conversation (Thomas, 1999). Persons with intact cognition should be taught strategies and trained in varied contexts and situations so that they become independent problem solvers. Effective problem solvers have an accurate awareness of their abilities and limitations and the ability to identify and define problems. They can select appropriate solutions to a problem from past experience or create a new solution when prior strategies are inadequate. Finally, effective problem solvers assess the outcome of the problem solving, which helps them organize the learning experience so that it is accessible for solving problems in the future.

   Patients with brain damage require a different approach to the teaching–learning process. If the patient cannot do the task automatically using old habit programs, he will be learning a new skill. Behavior modification, including a step-by-step structure, **shaping**, verbal cues, physical cues, and social praise after completion of the whole task, is effective for patients with cognitive deficits (Giles et al., 1997; Katzman & Mix, 1994). For example, a step-by-step program that subjects had to memorize and verbalize was effective for patients with Parkinson's disease (Kamsma, Brouwer, & Lakke, 1995). Brain-damaged patients often have difficulty processing abstract information or large chunks of information at a time, so instructions should be reduced to one- or two-word concrete cues. Given consistently over the course of practice sessions, these key word cues help the patient chain the task from beginning to end. For tasks that can be easily broken into isolated subtasks, it may be helpful for the patient to practice one step at a time, combining steps as learning progresses, e.g., begin brushing teeth with the toothpaste already on the brush. For some tasks and some patients, however, performance of the whole task will enhance learning (see Chapter 14). Use a variety of contexts for practice (Katzman & Mix, 1994). Even with this kind of practice, the learning may or may not transfer to other tasks or contexts; therefore, the patient must practice each task until it is learned within all the contexts in which it will be required.

   Patients with brain damage may not become problem solvers, and their prognosis for independence outside of a sheltered or familiar environment may be limited. ADL tasks that may result in injury if precautions are not practiced, such as cutting with a sharp knife or standing to pull up pants, require supervision for as long as judgment is impaired.

   Some profoundly brain-damaged yet teachable patients benefit from backward chaining, an adaptation of Skinner's (1938) Law of Chaining: One step acts as the stimulus for another. In backward chaining of dressing skills, for example, assistance is given to do the task until the last step of the process is reached. The patient performs this one step independently and gets the satisfaction of having completed the task. Once the patient has mastered the final step, the therapist assists only to the next to the last step, and the patient completes the two remaining steps. This process continues until the patient can do the entire task from start to finish independently. Progress in learning ADL for those with brain damage is slow (Schwartz, 1995). Given the economic constraints, it is unrealistic to expect to teach such patients in the brief period of treatment authorized. The therapist should teach the caregiver how to help the patient learn some ADL skills at home.

   Patients with damage to their dominant hemispheres usually have difficulty processing verbal or written language but may benefit from demonstrated or pictorial instruction. Those with damage to their non-dominant hemisphere may have difficulty with spatial relationships that make it difficult to interpret pictures and demonstrations but be able to process step-by-step verbal instruction.

8. Arrange appropriate practice schedules. Motor skills are learned only through practice. Motor skills learned with contextual interference (**random practice**) were retained better than when practiced in repetitive drill (**blocked practice**) (Hanlon, 1996). Chapter 14 has a discussion of practice schedules.

9. Provide opportunities for internal feedback and use appropriate external feedback. External feedback comes from a source other than the patient, typically the therapist, and can be provided in many forms. Motivational feedback ("Looks good!"; "Keep trying!") has some benefit, but specific feedback about what was correct and what was not correct during a particular trial has more definitive benefit. Occasional feedback concerning the performance ("keep your elbow straighter next time") offered immediately after a trial is helpful. Persons who are not aware of the outcome of their efforts benefit from external feedback so that they gain knowledge of the results of their efforts, which is a requirement for learning (Schmidt & Lee, 2000). Although external feedback from the therapist is an effective teaching method, patients must eventually respond to internal and task feedback, that is, feedback from their own sensory system or the outcome of task performance ("my pants are on, but are twisted and uncomfortable"). Asking patients to

articulate internal feedback before providing external feedback can support their ability to rely on internal feedback when faced with novel tasks outside of therapy when external feedback is unavailable.

10. Test whether the learner has acquired the knowledge or skill by requiring that it be done independently at the appropriate time and place.
11. Discuss progress toward goals and revise teaching strategy or goal as indicated (Shotwell & Schell, 1999). Gagné and Hoppes (2003) found that patients in a rehabilitation center who regularly discussed and updated their goals with their therapists made greater gains in ADL than patients whose treatment did not emphasize goal attainment.

ADAPTATION

Adaptation is the process by which a person maintains a useful relationship to the environment (Thoren Jonsson, Moller, & Grimby, 1999). It is a cumulative process that evolves over time (Spencer et al., 1999). Therefore, older people have a rich repertoire of adaptive strategies based on personal experience that may be helpful in dealing with disability.

Adaptive therapy refers to modifying the task, the method of accomplishing the task, and/or the environment to promote independence in occupational functioning. Examples of modifying the task are to switch to loafers instead of tie shoes or to order from catalogs instead of going to the shops. Adapted methods of dressing for persons with loss of the use of one side of the body or weakness of all four extremities (discussed later) are examples of modifying the method of accomplishing a task. Installation of grab bars in the bathroom to enable safe transfers and storing often-used items within easy reach are examples of modifying the physical environment. Teaching wheelchair users ways of interacting with individuals who are not disabled so that they present themselves as self-assured, capable people is an example of adapting the social environment.

Prescription of and training in the use of assistive devices or adapted tools and utensils to enable occupational performance by persons who are physically disabled is a primary function of occupational therapy. Examples are use of a buttonhook to button a shirt and adding extensions to keys and door handles to extend the force arm and reduce the force required to turn the key or knob (Figs. 30-1 and 30-2). Grasp, a problem for many patients, can be helped by using enlarged handles (Fig. 30-3). A therapist may experiment with adaptations to utensils by wrapping a washcloth, foam rubber, or other material around the handle and securing it with a rubber band. If enlarging the handle improves performance, permanent adaptation is prescribed and purchased or, if necessary, custom built. Low-tempera-

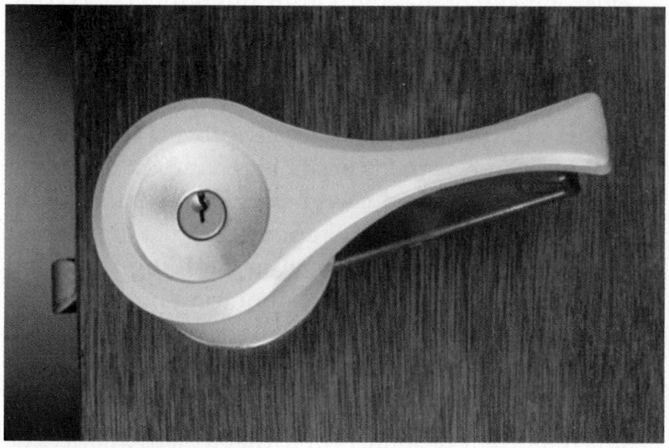

Figure 30-1 Doorknob extension. (Courtesy of Sammons Preston, Bolingbrook, IL.)

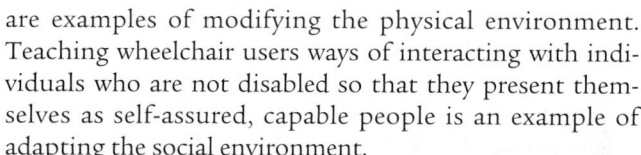

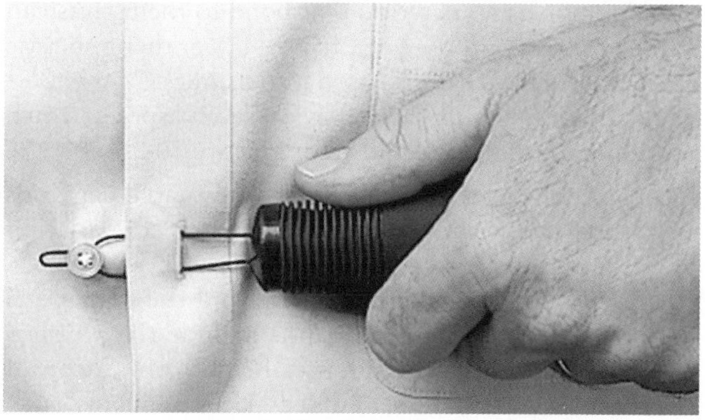

Figure 30-2 Good Grips button hook. (Courtesy of North Coast Medical, Morgan Hill, CA.)

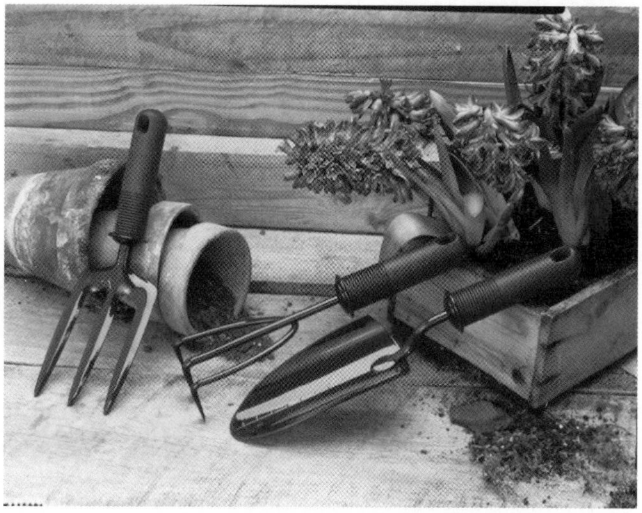

Figure 30-3 Good Grips garden tools with large handles. (Courtesy of Sammons Preston, Bolingbrook, IL.)

ture thermoplastic materials that bond to themselves can be used for this purpose (see Chapter 17), or thermoplastic pellets can be heated and shaped into handles.

Adaptation entails the following seven aspects, which are summarized in Procedures for Practice 30-2:

1. Analyze the activity. Determine the essential demands of the activity. The activity demands are a combination of the performance requirements of a task, such as lifting, reaching, and manipulating, and the contextual demands. Contextual demands include the physical environment, such as counter height or location of faucets in the bathtub, as well as social demands, such as the ability to communicate with others, and temporal demands, such as the need to complete a morning care routine within 45 minutes to get to work on time. Performance requirements must be quantified: What is the weight to be lifted? How high must it be lifted? and so on. Examination of these objective dimensions of the activities suggests how the environment and equipment can be adapted to meet the capabilities of the person (Clark, Czaja, & Weber, 1990). Studies are beginning to appear that evaluate specific performance requirements of particular ADL tasks, such as the minimal wrist ranges of motion needed to accomplish ADL (Ryu et al., 1991), pinch and grasp strength requirements to open containers (Rice, Leonard, & Carter, 1998), and the effect of reacher length on muscle strength needed to lift objects (Pinkston, Boersma, & Spaulding, 2005).
2. Identify the problem. Why can't the person do what the task demands? It is helpful to consider the problem from two perspectives, patient limitations and contextual features. For example, the patient is unable use the left hand, but toothpaste with a screw cap requires the use of two hands. Or, the patient has precautions against bending over, but pots needed for cooking stored in low cabinets cannot be reached. Linking the performance limitations with contextual features helps the therapist identify appropriate solutions.
3. Know the principles of compensation. Principles of compensation for common functional limitations are presented in Procedures for Practice 30-3.
4. Propose solutions. Consider creative ways that the principles of compensation can be applied to a particular task to enable the particular person to do it. Collaboration with the patient or a group of similarly involved patients often generates solutions and increases compliance with assistive devices (Wielandt et al., 2001).
5. Know the resources for implementing the solution. For example, it is important to know what reliable and safe equipment is available to solve the problem. Sources of equipment are rehabilitation supply stores, mail-order or web-based businesses, and gadget stores (Resource 30-1). The occupational therapist needs to know and evaluate each piece of equipment being recommended. The fact that a piece of equipment is sold does not mean that it is effective or safe (Conine & Hershler, 1991). The therapist must know construction techniques needed to implement the solution when environmental modification is needed (e.g., anchor grab bars in studs) and should be familiar with local contractors who provide quality home modifications.
6. Check it out. The assistive device or environmental modification should be checked out for reliability (always works as it should), durability (can withstand repeated use at the force levels the person will apply to it), safety, effectiveness, and patient satisfaction.
7. Train the person. The person must understand and be able to implement the safe use of the assistive device, environment, or method. Gitlin and Burgh (1995) suggest five aspects to device training: develop an activity in which to introduce the device; choose a site for instruction; determine the best time in the rehabilitation process to introduce the device; provide instruction that meets the patient's needs; and reinforce device use with the patient and caregivers. Guidetti and Tham (2002) reported that therapists also use important over-arching strategies, such as building trust and motivating their clients, collaborating on goals, and selecting training methods uniquely suited to each client, so that the therapists adapt themselves "like a chameleon" to meet their clients' needs.

It is important to some people that assistive devices be transparent (McCuaig & Frank, 1991), that is, not call attention to the person as disabled or reveal the extent of

PROCEDURES FOR PRACTICE 30-2

Adaptation Process

1. Analyze activity demands, including performance and contextual requirements.
2. Identify the problem: what performance and/or contextual requirements prevent the person from accomplishing the task?
3. Know principles of compensation for the given limitation.
4. Creatively apply principles of compensation to solve the problem.
5. Select appropriate adapted methods, assistive devices, and specify environmental adaptations to implement the solution.
6. Check out all modifications to verify that they solve the problem.
7. Train in safe use of the assistive devices or modified environment.

PROCEDURES FOR PRACTICE 30-3

Compensation Principles for Particular Impairments

Weakness

- Use lightweight objects, utensils, and tools.
- Let gravity assist.
- Provide external support, e.g., sit if trunk or lower extremities are weak or splint a weak wrist.
- Use assistive devices or methods to replace lost functions such as grasp.
- Use power tools and utensils.
- Use biomechanical principles of levers (e.g., lengthen the force arm in relation to the resistance arm) and friction (e.g., increase friction to decrease power required for pinch or grasp).
- Use two hands for tasks ordinarily done with one hand.

Low Endurance

- Use energy conservation methods (see Procedures for Practice 30-4).
- Pace work to prevent fatigue.
- Use principles listed for weakness that reduce workload, such as lightweight utensils and power equipment.
- Match activity demands to ability.
- Avoid stressful positions and environmental stressors.

Limited Range of Motion

- Use long-handled tools and utensils to increase reach and/or eliminate the need for bending over.
- Build up handles to compensate for limited grasp.
- Store frequently used things within easy reach.
- Use joint protection techniques for rheumatoid arthritis (see Chapter 44).

Incoordination

- Stabilize the object being worked on.
- Stabilize proximal body parts so that need to control is reduced to the distal body parts.
- Use assistive devices that reduce slipperiness or provide stability.
- Use heavy utensils, cooking equipment, tools, and so on.
- Use adaptations that substitute for lack of fine skill.

Loss of the Use of One Side

- Provide assistive devices that substitute for the stabilizing or holding function of the involved upper extremity.
- Teach one-handed methods for activities ordinarily done with two hands.
- Provide assistive devices that change the few truly bilateral tasks into unilateral tasks.
- Improve dexterity of the uninvolved upper extremity if the dominant arm is the involved one.

Limited Vision

Blindness

- Organize the living space so that there is a place for everything and stress the importance of putting everything in its place after use (e.g., in the pantry cabinets, on refrigerator shelves, and in the medicine cabinet).
- Use Braille labels or optical scanners to distinguish canned goods, medications, clothing colors, etc.
- Use devices that operate through voice commands.
- Use assistive devices that provide auditory, tactile, or kinesthetic feedback to compensate for low vision and blindness.
- Eliminate environmental clutter.
- Expect tasks to require extra time.

Low Vision

Some of the principles for blindness are useful for those with low vision. Others include:

- Provide high color contrast (e.g., white mug for coffee, colored towels in a white bathroom).
- Increase the light on a task by bringing the light closer, increasing wattage, or changing the background to increase contrast (Lampert & Lapolice, 1995).
- Use techniques and devices that magnify type or images.
- Reduce visual clutter.
- Use organized scanning techniques (e.g., left to right, top to bottom) when functioning in a stationary environment.

Decreased or Absent Sensation

- Protect the anesthetic part from abrasions, bruises, cuts, burns, and decubiti.
- Develop habit of using areas with intact cutaneous sensation to test temperature (e.g., test bath water temperature with the forearm if finger sensation is impaired).
- Substitute vision for poor awareness of limb position and limb movement or to detect texture.
- Develop habits of directing attention to the affected part.

Poor Memory and/or Organizational Skills

- Use assistive devices that substitute for memory or poor organizational skills (e.g., pill minders, day books, electronic reminder devices, sticky notes, watches with programmable multiple alarm systems, palm-size computers and organizers).
- Teach strategies such as writing memos to self, making to-do and other lists, and placing objects together and at the point needed ahead of time.
- Develop habits regarding time use and how activities are to be accomplished.
- Teach self-awareness strategies to improve carry over of adapted methods or devices.

Low Back Pain

- Teach body mechanics for moving and lifting (e.g., hold objects close to the body, squat to lower the body rather than bending over).
- Use long-handled or bent-handled equipment or sit to substitute for bending over.
- Change position frequently.
- When standing, put one foot up on a step to rotate the pelvis.
- Rest before fatigue results in awkward, careless movements.
- Avoid twisting the trunk.

disability. Use of conventional devices or gadgets that are sold to the general public qualify as transparent. Examples are felt-tipped pens, slip-on shoes, lightweight pots and pans, and magnifying makeup mirrors. They become adaptive because of their specific application. This perception of transparency and its importance are unique to the individual. Transparency is becoming easier because the principles of universal design have been found to be profitable by manufacturers of personal care and home products (One Shape Serves All, 1998).

ACTIVITIES OF DAILY LIVING

This chapter describes methods and devices suggested by occupational therapy practitioners and former patients to enable independence in BADL and IADL. These suggestions are presented according to the problem. Many patients have more than one problem. For example, persons with rheumatoid arthritis have weakness as well as limited range of motion. Persons with spinal cord injury have decreased sensation as well as weakness. The therapist will have to use information from pertinent sections for a patient with particular combinations of impairments. Procedures to enable BADL are presented. Although the need to do these activities and the task demands of each are fairly universal. However, each person has unique constellations of IADL that describe their roles (Trombly, 1993, 1995); thus, only representative IADL can be included as examples of solutions for particular problems.

All tasks that the patient expects to perform independently after discharge must be practiced as they will be done. For example, if a patient will bathe in a tub at home, it is inadequate to practice only sponge bathing while he or she is hospitalized. It is also crucial to address the more intermittent activities inherent in ADL, such as nail care, ear care, and menstrual care, and those ADL that are not universally engaged in, such as managing contact lenses, handling catheters, or flossing teeth. Do not assume that all self-care tasks that a particular person may need to learn are listed on an evaluation checklist.

Techniques and equipment for self-care presented in this chapter are not the only methods of accomplishing these particular tasks. This presentation is meant to provide the student therapist with a repertoire of basic skills with which to approach patients with confidence. The principles of compensation for each problem are key pieces of information that allow the student to evaluate other techniques or equipment to meet the needs of the patient. For many tasks not mentioned here, either no adaptation is required or the adaptation can be extrapolated from the examples cited.

As each task is taught, all equipment should be close at hand. For early training in dressing, clothing that is a size too large should be used because it can be managed more easily. The patient's attention should be called to design details of clothing, as persons with certain disabilities find it difficult to don some designs. The details to be considered are the cut of the garment, sleeve style, type of fabric, and type of closure or fasteners (Dallas & White, 1982). Clothing especially designed for people with disabilities is now commercially available (see Resource 30-1).

PROCEDURES FOR PRACTICE 30-4

Energy Conservation Methods

- Plan ahead. Organize work.
- Eliminate unnecessary tasks.
- Sit to work when possible.
- Have all required equipment and supplies ready before starting the task.
- Combine tasks to eliminate extra work.
- Use electrical appliances to conserve personal energy.
- Use lightweight utensils and tools.
- Work with gravity assisting, not resisting.
- Rest before fatiguing.

Weakness (Procedures for Practice 30-3)

For other information and suggestions see Chapters 13, 19, 40, and 43.

Suggestions for BADL

When muscle weakness affects all four extremities, the techniques and devices are extensive; therefore, this section focuses on compensation for involvement of all four extremities. If the patient is paralyzed in the lower extremities but has normal upper extremities, many of the techniques or devices are unnecessary. Some of the principles apply to limited weakness as well, such as weak pinch secondary to osteoarthritis of the carpometacarpal joint.

When paralysis is extensive, a personal care assistant is needed to carry out BADL. The patient must learn to hire, supervise, instruct, compensate, set limits for, and terminate personnel (Personal Care Assistant, 1994; also see Resource 30-1).

Feeding

The problem with feeding is the inability to grasp and/or bring the hand to the mouth. A universal cuff can be used

RESOURCE 30-1

The Internet has supported an explosion of online resources for persons with disability and the professionals who work with them. This section is organized by topic area. Books that are included in this section can all be purchased through an online book vendor, such as www.amazon.com or www.barnesandnoble.com.

General Online Resources

AARP—American Association of Retired Persons.
http://www.aarp.org/

ABLEDATA—Database funded by the U.S. Department of Education National Institute on Disability and Rehabilitation Research. It lists 17,000 products from 2,000 companies and 8,000 items no longer commercially available, customized devices, and non-commercial prototypes.
www.abledata.com

The Boulevard—Quarterly online magazine (previously *Accent on Living*) that addresses all aspects of living a full life with a disability and makes good suggestions for solving problems of persons with physical disabilities.
www.blvd.com/accent

disABILITY Information and Resources—Offers a wide range of links to information, vendors, and services. Maintained by Jim Lubin, a man with C2 quadriplegia.
http://www.makoa.org/index.htm

NARIC (National Rehabilitation Information Center, formally REHABDATA)
1010 Wayne Avenue, Suite 800
Silver Spring, MD 20910
Phone; (800) 34-NARIC
A bibliographical database of documents on rehabilitation that includes journals, unpublished documents, audiovisual materials, commercial publications, and government reports.
http://www.naric.com/search/

Consumer Information Catalogue—U.S. Government Publications, Pueblo, CO 81009.
www.pueblo.gsa.gov

American Occupational Therapy Association—AOTA's *Occupational Therapy Buyer's Guide*, a yearly supplement in OT Practice.
www.aota.org

Adaptations and Specialized Equipment for ADL for Physical Disabilities

General Information

Greenstein, D. B. (1997). *Easy things to make things easy: Simple do-it-yourself home modifications for older people and others with physical limitations.* Cambridge, MA: Brookline Books.

Online Vendors for Persons with Disabilities

Most vendors offer a wide array of products. Specialty vendors are indicated with a brief description.

Active Forever
http://www.activeforever.com/home.asp

Alimed, AliMed, Inc.
http://alimed.com

Andicap.com
http://www.andicap.com

DynamicLiving.com
Range of daily living needs for people with varied disabilities and needs.
http://www.dynamic-living.com/gadgets.htm

EnableMart
http://www.enablemart.com/default.aspx?store=10

Extensions for Independence: The Mouthstick Connection
Modular mouthsticks with adjustable lengths, varied tips, and mouthstick stands.
http://www.mouthstick.net/

Independent Care Needs
http://independentneeds.com

Invacare
Source for bathroom and other equipment for people weighing over 200 pounds.
www.invacare.com

North Coast Medical, Inc.
www.ncmedical.com

Sammons Preston Roylan
Enrichments catalog, P. O. Box 5071, Bolingbrook, IL 60440-5071. Phone: (800) 323-5547.
www.sammonspreston.com

Self-Wipe Toilet Aids
Sells a toilet aid for limited reach and grasp.
http://www.selfwipe.com

SeniorShops.com
Online store with adaptive equipment for BADL and IADL for a range of disabilities.
http://www.seniorshops.com

Online Vendors with Devices for the General Public

Several vendors are selling items aimed at making life easier for the general population. These products tend to be more "transparent" than those sold by medical vendors, and they are often less expensive because they cater to a much larger population.

Oxo International
Maker of "Good Grips" and many other products.
http://www.oxo.com/

The Wright Stuff
http://store.wrightstuff.biz/index.html

Comfort House
http://www.comforthouse.com/

Carol Wright Gifts
http://www.carolwrightgifts.com

Adaptations and Specialized Equipment for ADL for Specific Limitations

Resources and Products for Persons with Low Vision

Access-USA
Supplier of Braille stickers (salt, pepper, food, beverage, spice tags) and other Braille products, such as menus and maps.
http://www.access-usa.com

Optelec
On-screen magnifier for low vision.
www.optelec.com

The Lighthouse Catalogue
www.lighthouse.org

Independent Living Aids, Inc.
http://www.independentliving.com

Sight Connection
http://www.sightconnection.com

(continued)

RESOURCE 30-1 *(continued)*

Resources and Products for Persons Doing ADL with One Hand

Mayer, T.-K. (2000). *One-handed in a two-handed world* (2nd ed.). Boston: Prince-Gallison. P.O. Box 23, Hanover Station, Boston, MA 02113-0001.

Richardson, N. K. (n.d.) *Type with one hand.* Retrieved from www.ncmedical.com. North Coast Medical.

The Left Hand
Products designed to work effectively with the left hand.
www.thelefthand.com

Resources for People of Exceptional Size

See also companies that provide durable medical equipment because they often carry a line of products for bariatric care.

Amplestuff
A range of products, except for clothing.
http://www.amplestuff.com

Baritric Hospital Beds
http://bariatricbeds.com/

Big John Toilet Seats
http://bigjohntoiletseats.com/

Dynamic Living
Has a section for the "generously sized."
http://www.dynamic-living.com

Seatbelt Extenders
www.extend-it.com

Management of Personal Care Assistants

Birdsall, D. L. (n.d.). *Hiring and management of personal care assistants for individuals with spinal cord injury.* Santa Clara, CA: Spinal Cord Injury Project at Santa Clara Valley Medical Center. Available online at http://www.tbi-sci.org/pdf/pas.pdf.

Personal care assistants: How to find, hire, and keep them. Educational brochure from Craig Rehabilitation Hospital.
Available at http://www.craighospital.org/SCI/METS/personalCareAssist.asp.

Personal care assistance: How much help should I hire? Educational brochure from Craig Rehabilitation Hospital. Available at http://www.craighospital.org/SCI/METS/careAssistHire.asp.

Resources on Sexuality and Disability

Amador, M. J., Lynne, C. M., & Brackett, N. L. (2000). *A guide and resource directory to male fertility following spinal cord injury/dysfunction.* Miami: Miami Project to Cure Paralysis, University of Miami. Available at http://www.themiamiproject.org/documents/mfpguide.pdf.

DuCharme, S. H., & Gill, K. M. (1997). *Sexuality after spinal cord injury: Answers to your questions.* Baltimore: Paul H. Brookes.

Kroll, K., & Levy Klein, E. (1992). *Enabling romance.* Bethesda, MD. Woodbine House, Inc. 6510 Bells Mill Rd, Bethesda, MD 20817; phone: (800) 843-7323.

Neistadt, M. E., & Freda, M. (1987). *Choices: A guide to sex counseling with physically disabled adults.* Melbourne, FL: Krieger Publishing.

Sipski, M., & Alexander, C. (1997). *Sexual function in people with disabilities and chronic illness: A health professional's guide.* Gaithersburg, MD: Aspen.

Service Dogs

Canine Companions for Independence
Six regional centers in the United States train and supply service dogs.
www.caninecompanions.org

Delta Society
A non-profit organization committed to promoting the human-animal health connection, with a wide range of resources on service animals.
http://www.deltasociety.org/home.htm

NEADS: National Education for Assistance Dog Services
http://www.neads.org/index.shtml

Wolf Packs Service Dogs Directory
Lists national service dog training centers, as well as smaller, local organizations that are listed by state.
http://wolfpacks.com/serviced.htm

Organizations for Persons with Specific Diagnoses

The following organizations provide information for regaining independence for the professional and consumer and offer support groups and free brochures.

American Foundation for the Blind
www.afb.org

American Heart Association
www.americanheart.org

American Stroke Association
www.strokeassociation.org

Arthritis Foundation
www.arthritis.org

Brain Injury Association of America
www.biausa.org

National Multiple Sclerosis Society
www.nmss.org

National Parkinson Foundation, Inc
www.parkinson.org

National Spinal Cord Injury Association
www.spinalcord.org

National Stroke Association
www.stroke.org

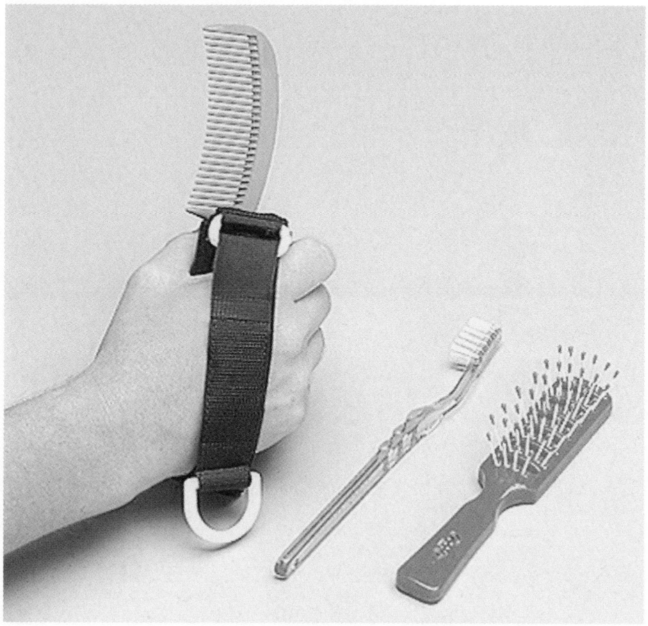

Figure 30-4 Universal cuff. (Courtesy of North Coast Medical, Morgan Hill, CA.)

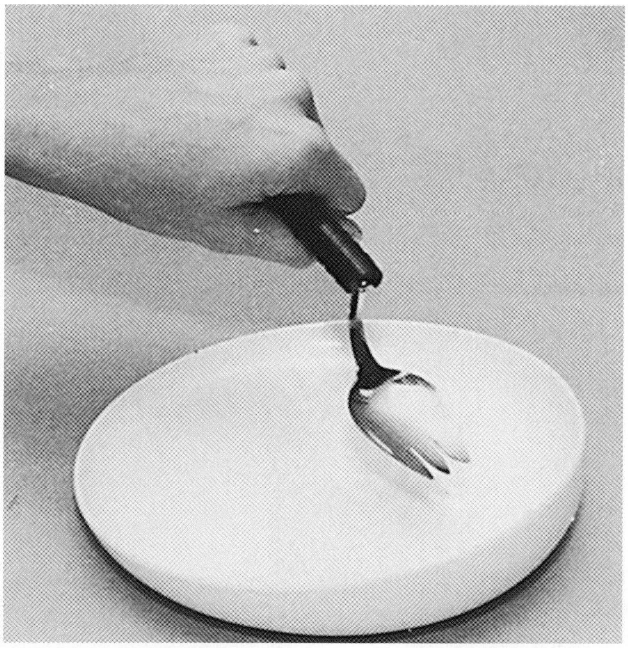

Figure 30-5 Spork (combination fork and spoon). This one also swivels.

to hold the utensil if grasp is absent (Figs. 13-12 and 30-4). This cuff fits around the palm and has a pocket for insertion of the handle of a utensil. Some universal cuffs include a wrist support if wrist extensors are weak. Alternatively, the handle can be woven through the fingers, with the index and ring fingers on top and middle and little fingers under, and held in place passively. A spork, a utensil that combines the bowl of a spoon with the tines of a fork (Fig. 30-5), can be used with the cuff to eliminate the need to change utensils. Some of these have a swivel feature to substitute for the inability to supinate. Gravity and weight of the food keep the bowl level on the way to the mouth. If the patient has weak grasp, lightweight enlarged handles can be used. The patient may use a wrist-driven wrist–hand orthosis to increase the strength of grasp (see Chapter 16). For cutting, a sharp serrated knife is used because less force is needed and it is less likely to slip. L-shaped rocker knives enable patients with weak grasp to apply force for cutting with stronger, larger proximal muscles.

An attachable open-bottomed handle can be added to a glass or soft drink can to permit picking it up in the absence of grasp. A mug with a T-shaped handle (Fig. 30-6) or a handle that allows all four fingers to be inserted provides leverage and stabilizes the fingers around the mug, allowing pick-up with a tenodesis grasp. A foam can insulator can be used for a glass to provide friction to assist weak grasp. A long straw can be used to eliminate the need for lifting the cup to the mouth for drinking. Using a cup with a lid, such as a commuter mug, minimizes the risk of spills in the event that the cup slips, reducing the risk of injury and mess for people with weak grasp, especially when drinking hot liquids. Commuter mugs have the added benefit of being a transparent device.

A mobile arm support or suspension sling (see Chapter 16) may be required to enable patients with very weak proximal upper extremities to feed themselves. A table placed at axilla height offers support for the arm and eliminates the pull of gravity, allowing the patient with elbow flexors graded 3 or 3+ to bring the food to the mouth. As strength increases, the surface can be lowered. For pa-

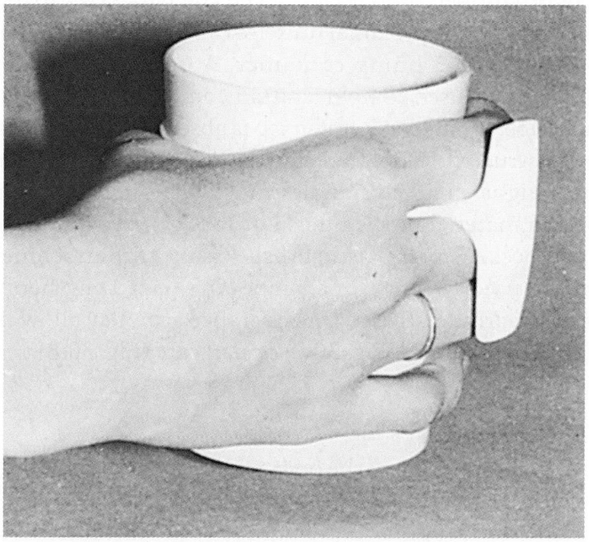

Figure 30-6 Cup with T-shaped handle assists drinking when grasp is weak.

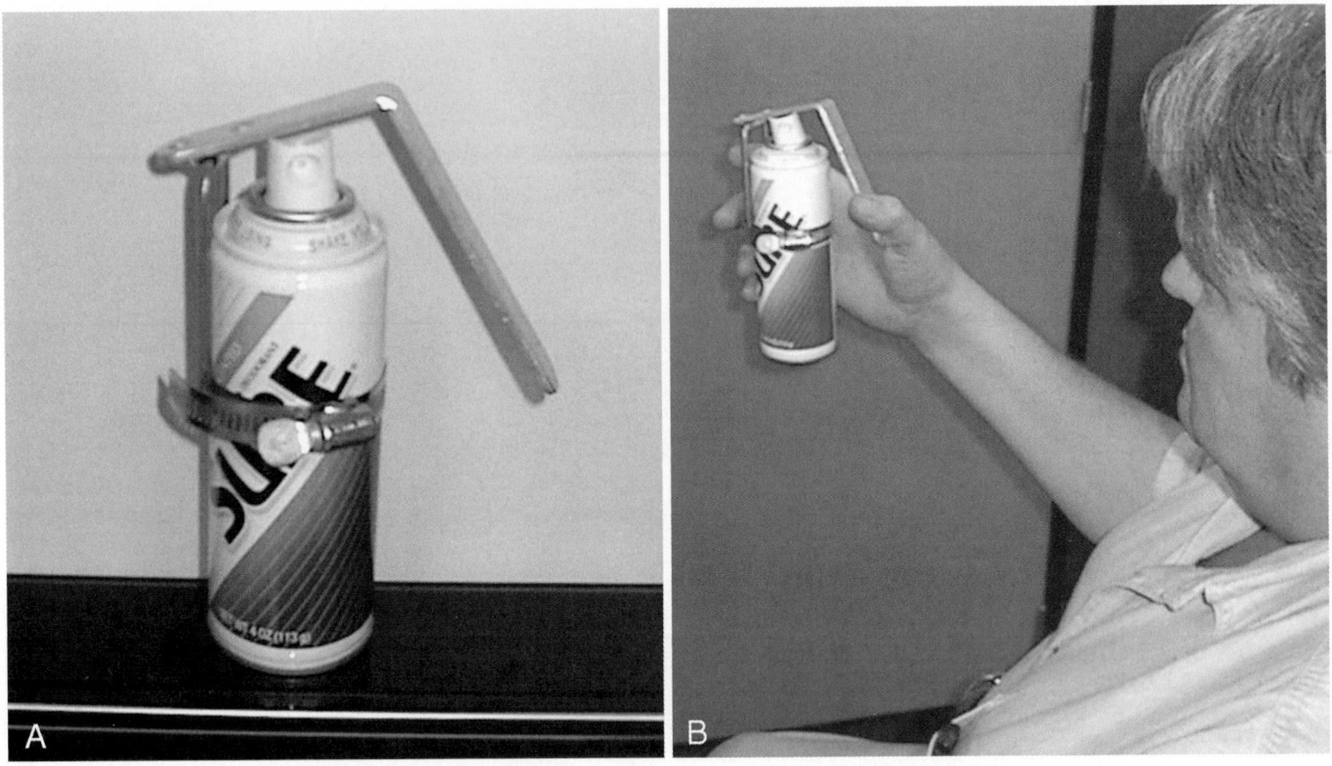

Figure 30-7 **A.** Aerosol can adapter that reduces the force needed to operate the spray. **B.** Operation of the adapter.

tients who lack active upper extremity movement, electronic feeders are available that are operated with a head or sip-and-puff switch (Hermann et al., 1999).

Grooming

Weakness in grasp and pinch are the most common barriers to grooming. Adaptations for makeup jars, tubes, and applicators have been suggested (Hage, 1988). Jar openers can be used to open twist-off caps or products can be selected that open more easily, given the patient's capabilities, for example proximal muscles can be used to dispense toothpaste in a pump container. A universal cuff or a splint can be used to hold a rattail comb, toothbrush, lipstick tube, or safety razor if grasp is absent. A handcuff can be constructed to hold an electric razor. If grasp is weak, lightweight enlarged handles may be enough. Applying friction material to the utensil or tool can provide added assistance. A small plastic brush with a cuff attachment may be used to assist in shampooing hair. Lengthening the force arm relative to the resistance arm may allow use of spray deodorant (Fig. 30-7) or nail care (Fig. 30-8).

Toileting

Transfers, handling of the body while raising and lowering clothing, and weak pinch and grasp are problems. For patients with spinal cord injury, concomitant loss of bowel and bladder control requires special procedures, including bladder irrigation, use of a catheter, or intermittent catheterization (Medline Plus, 2004). Generally, the patient can push down the pants while in the wheelchair by leaning from side to side. If the patient cannot stand or has precarious standing balance, it is necessary to transfer back to the wheelchair before raising the clothing after toi-

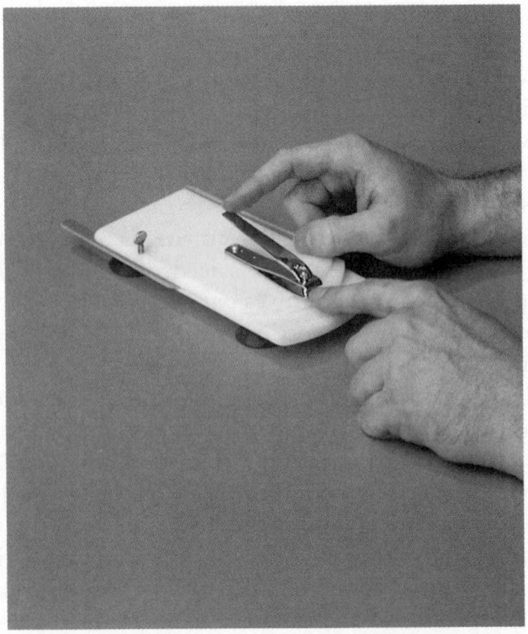

Figure 30-8 Nail clipper and emery boards stabilized to allow one-handed use and with elongated handle to reduce force required. (Courtesy of Sammons Preston, Bolingbrook, IL.)

leting. If the patient uses an indwelling catheter or external drainage device, the collection bag can be emptied into the toilet without transfer or removal of clothing. Usually nurses or enterostomal therapists teach clean intermittent self-catheterization, but the occupational therapist should be aware of the process of this ADL:

1. Assemble the equipment.
2. Wash hands and penis or vulva and urethral opening.
3. Men lubricate the catheter tip with water-soluble lubricant, hold penis at sides, and insert catheter with firm, gentle pressure. Women separate labia, palpate meatus, and insert catheter into the bladder.
4. The patient pushes catheter in 2.5 cm (1 inch) after urine starts to flow.
5. The person allows urine to flow until it stops and then slowly removes the catheter, holding catheter tip as it is removed to prevent spilling.
6. Discard disposable catheters or clean reusable catheters with soap and water, rinse, dry, and store in a plastic bag.
7. Wash hands with soap and water (Medline Plus, 2004). Knee spreaders with a mirror help hold weak or paralyzed lower extremities in abduction and enable people with limited trunk control to see the urethral opening.

Patients on a bowel program may use suppositories or digital stimulation to initiate a bowel movement. Suppositories may be inserted while the patient is in the bed or on the toilet. When patients do digital stimulation or insert suppositories while on the toilet, a raised toilet seat with a space between the seat and toilet bowl rim is needed to allow them to reach the rectum. Suppository inserters for those with weak or absent pinch are commercially available and can be adapted with cuffs for patients who lack grasp. Some inserters have a spring ejector that releases the suppository after it is properly positioned in the rectum. An inspection mirror is needed if the patient lacks anal sensation. Bowel stimulators are available for patients who lack adequate digit control. Patients with weak grasp and pinch can wrap toilet tissue around the hand for use. For patients with very limited hand function, bidets can be fit to the toilet to clean and dry the perianal area. Menstrual needs can be met by adaptations to positioning, pants, pads versus tampons, and aids such as mirrors and knee spreaders (Duckworth, 1986).

Bathing

The problems with bathing include the transfer, dynamic sitting balance, lack of lower extremity movement (Shillam, Beeman, & Loshin, 1983), and lack of pinch and grasp. Transfer tub seats (Fig. 30-9) that have two legs in the tub and two legs outside the tub provide a safe means to transfer from the wheelchair to tub. Patients prone to decubiti need padded seats. Each patient's requirements

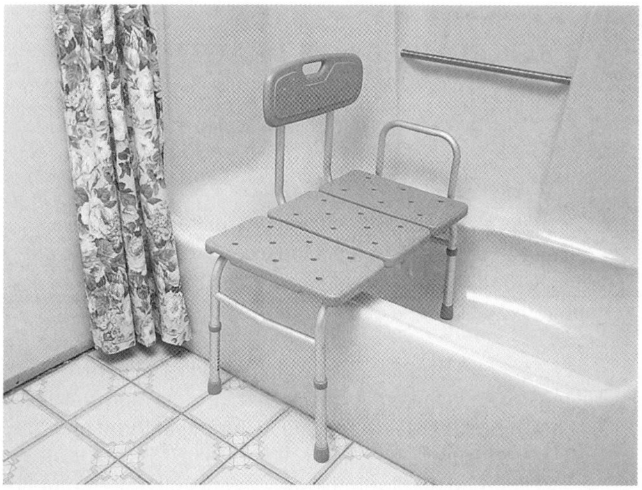

Figure 30-9 Transfer bath bench. (Courtesy of S&S, Colchester, CT.)

should be evaluated and a seat selected to fit them. Users of bath seats (both patients and caregivers) have reported that safety, adequate support, stability of equipment, and comfort are some of the most important considerations in selecting appropriate equipment (Pain & McLellan, 2003). The bath seat must be placed so that the faucets are within reach. Grab bars help during the transfer and while the patient is seated (Procedures for Practice 30-5). Non-slip material is used in the bottom of the tub. The faucets must have lever handles for ease in tapping them off and on with the fist. A hand-held shower that is adapted with a hook handle is used. No-scald faucets and shower heads should be used, but if they are unavailable, water temperature should be regulated by turning on the cold water first and then adding the hot water, which prevents scalding desensitized skin. Soap on a string or in a dispenser is helpful. A bath mitt is used if grasp is weak or absent. The person dries off before transferring back to the wheelchair. A towel placed in the wheelchair seat will dry the perianal area and can be removed when the patient transfers to the bed for dressing. Bathing and drying the feet and legs are particular problems for patients with poor trunk balance; such patients may prefer to do foot hygiene while in bed (Shillam, Beeman, & Loshin, 1983).

A custom-made shower stall and shower wheelchair provide the easiest bathing solution for a person with tetraplegia; however, it typically requires an expensive home modification. The shower area should have a raised slope to prevent the water from running out but allow the person to enter the shower on a shower wheelchair. Plans for such bath enclosures are shown in books on the Resources list. Shower wheelchairs have commode seats and can be positioned over the toilet for bowel programs, reducing the number of transfers required for morning care. For patients who prefer a bath, a number of electronic bath lifts are available that enable patients to transfer onto

PROCEDURES FOR PRACTICE 30-5

Grab Bars

Selection

Grab bars can be purchased from rehabilitation supply houses and some plumbing supply centers. Towel bars are not safe for use as a grab bar. Grab bars must be able to accept 200–250 pounds of force (more if the patient weighs more).

Horizontal bars are for pushing up; vertical bars are for pulling up. An L-shaped grab bar that includes both vertical and horizontal legs is a good choice for the bathtub or shower enclosure.

A clamp-on bathtub-mounted safety grab rail cannot be used on fiberglass tubs because those tubs cannot tolerate the stress.

The optimum diameter for grab bars is 1.25–1.5 inches for adults. The distance between the wall and the bar should be 1.5 inches. A wider space is dangerous because, if the arm slips, it may get caught between the wall and the bar and/or the person may fall (Salmen, 2000).

Placement

Locate bathtub grab bars where a person may be off balance, such as going into or out of the tub, turning in the tub or shower, or standing up from or sitting down on a bench or seat. One vertical bar outside the tub and one horizontal or diagonal bar on the wall along the length of the tub are recommended as basic installations. An L-shaped bar can be substituted for the bar on the wall along the length of the tub. If an L-shaped bar is used, locate the horizontal bar 16 inches above the tub rim and the vertical bar approximately 32 inches from the corner of the tub or as the placement suits the height and transfer and bathing process of the user.

Although the most common site for grab bars is in or near the bathtub enclosure, bars near the toilet (Fig. 30-10) are often necessary. Bars that look like armrests attach to the toilet; those that have legs that extend to the floor are most stable and safe.

Installation

Grab bars must be mounted to the wall with 2-inch stainless steel screws driven into the wall studs. Use a stud finder to locate the studs. It may be necessary to locate the studs

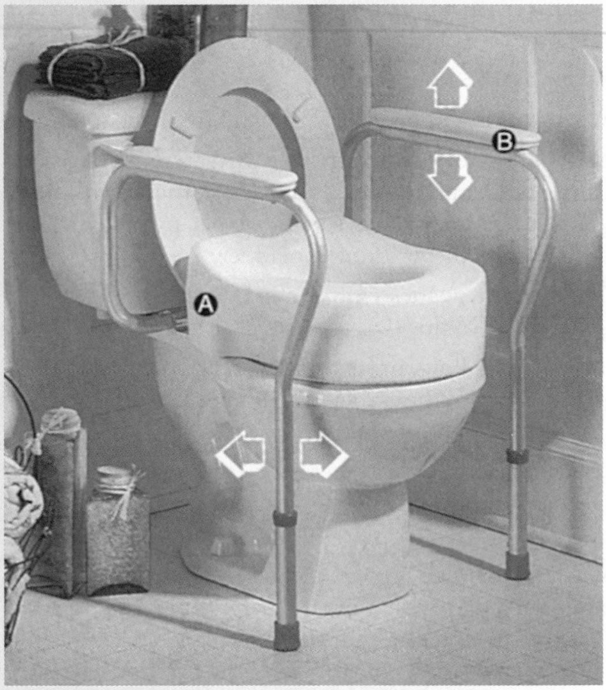

Figure 30-10 The Invacare Toilet Safety Frame and CareGuard by Invacare Raised Toilet Seat make the bathroom a safer environment for those with special needs. These products are recommended for combined use. (Courtesy of Invacare.)

from the other side of the wall if the bathroom walls are tiled. The typical mounting flange has three holes for three screws. Drill a small pilot hole before drilling holes in ceramic tile, using an eighth-inch masonry bit to drill three holes for the mounting screws. Only two screws will actually fit into the stud. Therefore, use a toggle bolt for the third screw. Grab bars from Invacare (see Resource 30-1) have screw holes that are oriented so that they all line up with the stud.

In new construction, double the studs and/or fasten half-inch plywood between the studs flush with the studs where grab bars are to be fastened. Some people cut into existing walls to add the necessary reinforcement and then replace the wall board.

a seat and then be lowered into the tub for independent or assisted bathing, depending on their needs.

Dressing

Dressing in less than an hour is considered reasonable for persons with tetraplegia (Weingarden & Martin, 1989); however, individuals must decide if this time frame is functional or if a personal care assistant is a better option. Problems with dressing include moving the paralyzed limbs to dress them, decreased sitting balance, and the need to compensate for the lack of pinch and grasp. While in bed, patients with spinal cord injuries at C6 and below can pull the knees up to dress the lower extremities by using their wrist extensors and elbow flexors. A dressing stick (Fig. 30-11) with a loop that goes around the wrist attached to the end opposite the hook can help. The person pulls against the loop, using wrist extension and leverage, to stabilize

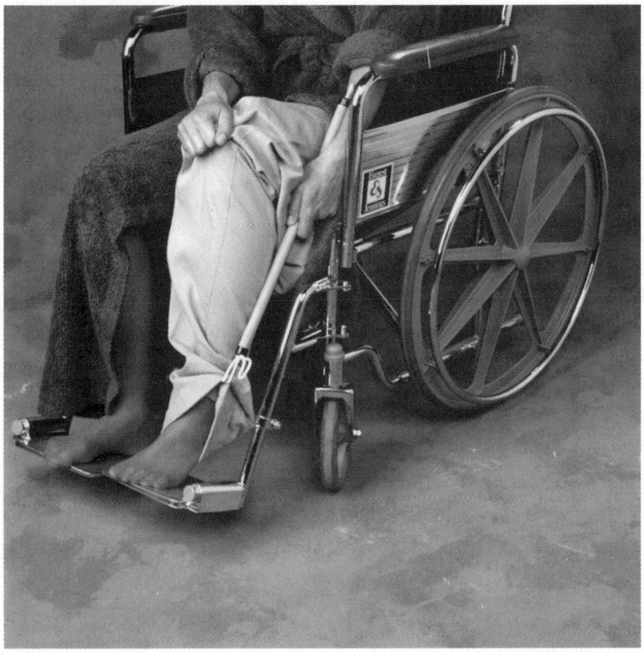

Figure 30-11 Dressing stick. (Courtesy of the Rehabilitation Division of Smith & Nephew, Germantown, WI.)

tenodesis grasp of the stick. Loops of twill tape can be added to the cuffs of socks to facilitate pulling them on by hooking the thumb in the loop when pinch is absent.

A buttonhook attached to a cuff or with a built-up handle is used when fingers are unable to manipulate buttons (Fig. 30-2). The hook is inserted through the buttonhole to hook the button and pull it through the buttonhole. The other hand is used to hold the garment near the buttonhole. A loop of string or leather lacing may be attached to the zipper pull of pants or other garments so that, in the absence of pinch, the thumb can be hooked in the loop to close the zipper. Alternatively, a zipper hook can also be used.

Adaptation of clothes should also be considered to facilitate dressing, undressing, and toileting; to regulate temperature; to increase comfort; and to increase feelings of self-confidence (Kratz et al., 1997; see Resource 30-1). For business people who are wheelchair users, suit jackets, pants, and skirts tailored to accommodate the sitting position look better than off-the-rack suits.

Runge (1967) describes the following methods of dressing for persons with tetraplegia:

Pants and Underwear

1. Have the patient sit in bed with the back against the head of an elevated hospital bed or against the wall. Pants are positioned with the front up and legs over the bottom of the bed. The patient can position pants by tossing them or using a dressing stick with a wrist loop.
2. One leg is lifted by hooking the opposite wrist or forearm under the knee, and the foot is put into the pants leg. The thumb of the other hand hooks a belt loop or pocket to hold the pants open. Working in a cross-body position aids stability for those with poor balance.
3. The other foot is inserted.
4. The palms of the hands are used to pat and slide the pants onto the calves and to get the trouser cuffs over the feet. The wrist or wrists are hooked under the waistband or in the pockets to pull the pants up over the knees.
5. The patient continues to pull on the waistband or pockets while returning to supine position to pull the pants up onto the thighs. This may have to be repeated. Hooking the wrist or thumbs in the crotch helps pull up the pants.
6. In a side-lying position, the thumb of the top arm is hooked in the back belt loop, and the pants are pulled over the buttocks. Then the patient rolls to the other side and repeats the process until the pants are on.
7. In a supine position, the pants can be fastened using a zipper pull loop and Velcro tab closing or buttonhook.
8. The pants are removed by reversing the procedures and pushing the pants off.

An alternative method for getting the pant legs over the feet may be useful for patients with limited forward reach. The pants are positioned parallel to the patient's legs. The first leg is lifted and crossed over the opposite leg so the pant leg can be slid all the way over the foot, up to the knee. The leg is uncrossed, and the second leg is slid in (Regional Spinal Cord Injury Center of Delaware Valley, 2001). To pull the pants over the hips, use the method described above.

Socks. Socks with tight elastic should be avoided. While sitting in the wheelchair or bed, the patient crosses one leg over the other and uses tenodesis grasp to put on the sock and the palms of the hands to help pull it on. If the patient cannot cross his or her legs, the foot can be placed on a stool or chair. Socks are removed by pushing them off with a dressing stick, long shoehorn, or the thumb hooked over the sock edge.

Shoes. Loafers that are a half to one size larger are most practical for patients who cannot walk. Shoes are put on by crossing one leg at a time as for putting on socks. The shoe is pulled onto the foot by balancing the sole of the shoe in the palm of the hand. Then with the foot moved to the floor or to the foot pedal of the wheelchair, the foot is pushed down into the shoe by pushing on the knee. A long shoehorn may be helpful for getting the heel into the shoe. Shoes can be removed by pushing them off with the shoehorn.

Cardigan Garments: Shirts and Blouses

1. Shirts may be donned in either the wheelchair or bed. The shirt is positioned with the brand label of the shirt facing down and the collar toward the knees.

2. The patient puts his or her arms under the shirt and into the sleeves and pushes them up over the elbows.
4. The shirt is gathered up by using wrist extension and by hooking the thumbs under the shirt back.
5. The shirt is placed over the head.
6. The patient shrugs to get the shirt down across the shoulders and hooks the wrists into the sleeves to free the axillae.
7. The patient leans forward and reaches back with one hand to rub on the shirt back to pull it down.
8. The shirt fronts are lined up, and buttoning begins from the bottom button up, using a buttonhook. Alternatively, shirts can be adapted with Velcro fasteners.

A cardigan garment is removed by pushing first one side and then the other off the shoulders and then alternately elevating and depressing the shoulders to allow gravity to assist in lowering the shirt down the arms. Then, one thumb is hooked into the opposite sleeve to pull the shirt over the elbow, and the arm is removed from the shirt.

With the exception of buttons, an overhead garment is put on in a similar manner and removed by hooking one thumb in the back of the neckline and pulling the shirt over the head. The sleeves are pushed off each arm.

Bra. Either a front- or back-closure bra can be used. Velcro can replace hooks for fastening, but some patients can manage the standard hook fastener if it is hooked in front at waist level. After the bra is hooked, it is positioned with the cups in front, and the arms are placed through the shoulder straps. Then, by hooking the opposite thumb under a strap, one strap at a time is pulled over the shoulder.

Sexual Activities

Many persons have concerns about their sexuality early after spinal cord injury, although they may not be ready to learn about the particulars of resuming sexual activities or procreation. Early on, they appreciate acknowledgment of their concerns and sources of information for when they are ready (McAlonan, 1996).

In a pioneering book, *Sexual Options for Paraplegics and Quadriplegics,* Mooney, Cole, and Chilgren (1975) explicitly described methods of sexual expression for people with spinal cord injury. They illustrated the process of getting ready for sex (emptying the bladder, washing). They addressed how to handle a catheter that is left in place during sex (bend the catheter and fold it over along the shaft of the penis where it will be out of the way, but do not anchor it until the erection has taken place to avoid pulling out the balloon of the Foley catheter; be sure the tubing and collection bag are not leaned on to prevent the flow of urine). They presented positions for genital and orogenital sexual expression, alternative means of sexual expression (vibrators, touch, and talking), and how to achieve and maintain a reflex erection of the penis. They discussed fertility of men: ability to ejaculate depends on the level of the lesion, and production of sperm depends on healthy testicles. They pointed out that women remain fertile, and therefore, pregnancy is as possible as for able-bodied women. Although this book is out of print, it is available in many university libraries, and used copies are available through online booksellers, such as amazon.com and barnesandnoble.com. Also, other books have become available as sexuality for the disabled is fully acknowledged (see Resource 30-1).

Suggestions for Selected IADLs

For the persons with severe paralysis, high-tech adaptations, as described in Chapter 19, offer opportunities to engage in communication, leisure, and work activities. Some low-tech adaptations are suggested here.

Handling a Book

The person with tetraplegia encounters problems with holding a book and turning the pages, with writing or recording notes in business or school, and possibly in telephoning. Some book holders support a book on a table, whereas others are designed to hold a book when reading supine in bed. If a person is reading while supine and the book is not held directly above, prism glasses are needed to direct the vision to a 90° angle so that the book may be seen.

To turn pages, some solutions are as follows: (1) when wearing a splint, the patient can use a rubber thimble or finger cot on the posted thumb; (2) a pencil with the eraser end down can be used in a universal cuff (typing stick) or hand splint; (3) electric page turners automatically turn pages when activated by a microswitch or other means of control; and (4) a mouthstick with a friction tip end may be useful (Fig. 30-12). Mouthsticks with flat mouthpieces can be purchased commercially, and custom-molded mouthpieces that conform to the patient's dentition are also available (Regional Spinal Cord Injury Center of Delaware Valley, 2001). The mouthpiece has a lightweight plastic or aluminum rod to which an eraser or other type of end piece, such as pencil, pen, or paintbrush, can be added.

An alternative is books on tape or CD, which can be obtained from libraries and bookstores. The Library of Congress has a large collection of tapes, including many current issues of magazines, and tape players that are available to the blind and the physically disabled for no charge (see Resource 30-1).

Writing

Extensive writing is usually done with computerized word processing. Manual typing can be done with typing sticks or a mouthstick for hitting the keys. Voice recognition

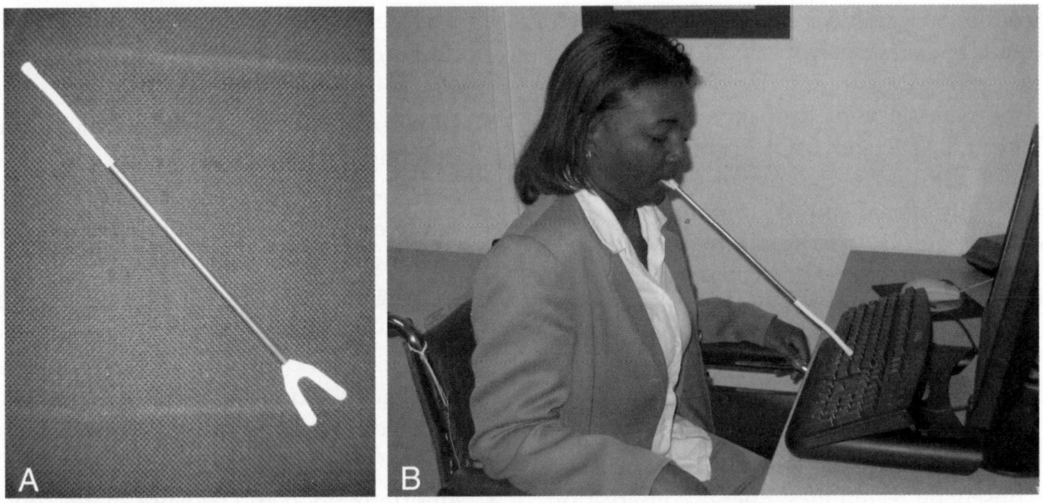

Figure 30-12 **A.** Mouthstick. **B.** Patient using mouthstick on a computer keyboard.

software is a better option for people who need to regularly create large amounts of text. If speed is important, as in taking notes in the classroom or in business, a tape recorder can be used.

Handwriting is important for legal documents and personalizing cards and typed notes. Splints that provide pinch can be used to hold a writing instrument. If pinch is absent and the patient does not use a splint, a pencil holder (Fig. 30-13) that encircles the pencil, thumb, and index finger can be made of thermoplastic materials. Pens with textured grips provide friction to make a weak grip more effective. Felt-tipped pens require little pressure and are therefore easier to use than other types of pens. If the arms cannot be used, with practice, a mouthstick with a pencil attached can become an effective writing tool.

Telephoning

A person whose spinal cord was injured at C6 or below can pick up a traditional telephone receiver and bring it to his or her ear. An executive shoulder rest attached to the receiver holds it there until the conversation is finished.

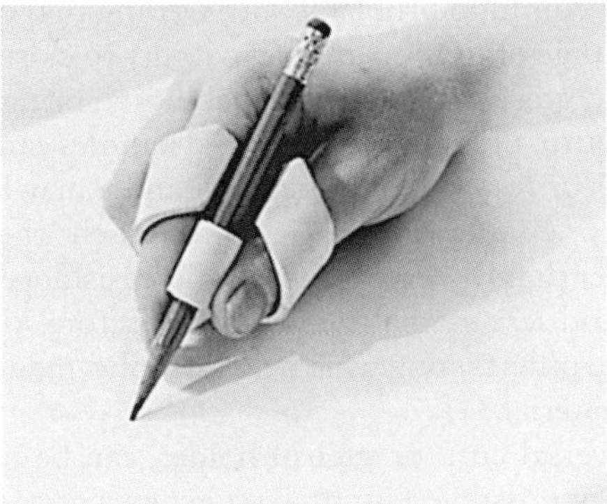

Figure 30-13 Pencil holder made of thermoplastic material.

Persons with higher level injuries can wear headsets or use a speaker phone that precludes the need to hold the phone.

Push buttons can be depressed with a mouthstick or typing stick. Speed dial or memory dial reduces the number of buttons to depress. Many phones are now available with voice recognition dialing options.

Turning Electrical Appliances On and Off

The burgeoning field of electronic aids to daily living (EADLs), formerly known as environmental control units, includes remote control devices for TV, entertainment centers, VCR and DVD players, lights, door openers, electric beds, and appliances. Voice-activated remote controls are available in specialty stores for operating the TV, VCR, and DVD player. See Chapter 19 for a discussion of high-tech assistive devices that are useful for persons with severe weakness or paralysis resulting from a spinal cord injury or degenerative disease such as amyotrophic lateral sclerosis.

Low Endurance (Procedures for Practice 30-3)

For other information and suggestions, see Chapter 47.

Suggestions for ADLs

Patients of various diagnoses and circumstances (e.g., after bed rest) have low endurance, which may be temporary or chronic. Many disorders (e.g., cardiac and pulmonary disease, multiple sclerosis, rheumatoid arthritis, and chronic fatigue syndrome) cause a more or less permanent reduction of endurance to which patients must adapt. Patients with cardiac and pulmonary disorders have reduced ability to use oxygen needed for muscle, including cardiac muscle, and brain functions. If oxygen deprivation is severe enough, neuropsychological changes involving memory, perception, and information processing occur, affecting the teaching and learning process as well as performance.

Adaptations for BADL and IADL involve awareness and reduction of the metabolic cost of activities and working within limits of cardiac and pulmonary capacity. Cardiac patients are cautioned to stop activity when they have angina or shortness of breath (SOB). Patients with pulmonary disease may need to have oxygen blood saturation levels monitored with a pulse oximeter (see Chapter 47) during initial ADL training to establish levels of activity that do not reduce blood oxygen to harmfully low levels. All patients with reduced endurance are taught to take rest periods throughout the day and use other energy-conserving techniques. Energy conservation methods are listed in Procedures for Practice 30-4 and elaborated on in Chapter 32.

Some activities require higher levels of energy than do others. One way to guide activity selection is to use metabolic equivalent (MET) tables. Most self-care activities require less than 3 METs; however, showering, tub bathing, toileting, sexual activity, and washing and setting hair require higher levels (Ainsworth et al., 1993, 2000). It should be remembered that MET charts are averages and do not account for particular circumstances and, therefore, cannot be used without also monitoring the patient's breathing, heart rate, blood pressure, and/or oxygen saturation levels. Dyspnea (SOB) signals the patient that the activity he or she is doing is beyond his or her capacity. Angina or excessive increase in heart rate (20 beats over resting rate) signals the cardiac patient that he or she has reached his or her limit. Activity restrictions and precautions vary depending on the nature and severity of the cardiac disorder (Goodman, 2003). Adapted methods may be used to compensate for activity restrictions, e.g., prolonged bending over may be avoided with long-handled utensils (described in this chapter in the section on limited range of motion). Patients with chronic obstructive pulmonary disease should learn to modify ADL methods to coordinate diaphragmatic and pursed lip breathing into activity routines to minimize dyspnea (Migliore, 2004).

Suggestions offered for persons with low endurance are as follows (Cristy & Sarafconn, 1990):

- Get sufficient sleep. Strategies for the patient who is having trouble sleeping include developing a bedtime routine and schedule; practicing relaxation techniques, such as visualization, listening to soothing music, progressive relaxation technique, and meditation; and avoiding upsetting or exciting activities just before bedtime.
- Consider your energy budget. Identify essential tasks and eliminate nonessential ones. Spread the performance of tasks that must be done throughout the day or week and delegate the rest to others.
- Do preventive maintenance and cleaning. A small chore left undone becomes an energy-consuming one later on.
- Organize work space. Organize to allow sitting without reaching, stretching, or bending while working.
- Use labor-saving products and techniques. Examples of ways to save energy include soaking dishes before washing them, paying bills online to eliminate writing and mailing checks, and purchasing pre-washed and cut vegetables.
- Organize work and errands. Organize tasks to eliminate backtracking and extra steps or trips and to allow planned rest periods. Keep commitments within manageable limits.
- Emotions, good and bad, use energy too. Consider the emotions when budgeting energy.

Sexual Activities

The American Heart Association (1999) booklet *Sex and Heart Disease* discusses the cardiovascular changes that occur during sexual intercourse, when the patient can resume sex after myocardial infarction or heart surgery, how other factors affect sex interest and capacity, guidelines for resuming sex, what to do if symptoms arise during sex, Viagra, and myths and misconceptions. The booklet can be helpful to both the patient and the health professional and can be ordered online at www.americanheart.org. Diaphragmatic breathing is facilitated in supine (Migliore, 2004), so pulmonary patients may find dyspnea is easier to manage when lying supine during sexual activities.

Limited or Restricted Range of Motion (Procedures for Practice 30-3)

For other information and suggestions, see Chapters 41, 42, 44, and 45.

Suggestions for BADLs

Feeding

The most common problems with feeding that occur with limited range of motion are the inability to close the hand enough to grasp the utensil or inability to bring the hand to the mouth. Enlarged or elongated handles can be added to spoons or forks. The elongated handle may have to be angled to enable the patient to reach the mouth. Remember that the longer the handle (resistance arm), the heavier and less stable the device; therefore, the handle should be only as long as is necessary and made of lightweight material.

A universal cuff, or utensil holder, can be used when grasp is not possible (Fig. 30-4). For some patients, such as those with arthrogryposis, independent eating may only be possible with electric feeders. The device must be set up and cleaned up by an assistant, however, and some insurance carriers will not pay for both device and assistant. Another factor to be considered when prescribing this device is that, for an institutionalized person, being fed by another may be an opportunity for social contact that the device would eliminate (Hermann et al., 1999).

Grooming

The problems with grooming are the same as for feeding. Enlarged or extended handles can be attached to a comb (Fig. 30-14), brush, toothbrush, shampoo brush, lipstick tube, or safety razor. Aerosol deodorant, hair spray, powder, and perfume can be used by those with limited range. An assistant may be needed to wash and style hair if the person cannot reach the head to do it independently. A simple hairstyle may eliminate the need for blow drying and styling. For patients who have had hand surgery and are prohibited from getting the incision wet, a waterproof plastic mitten allows the patient to use the hand as much as possible during self-care and kitchen activities (Fig. 30-15).

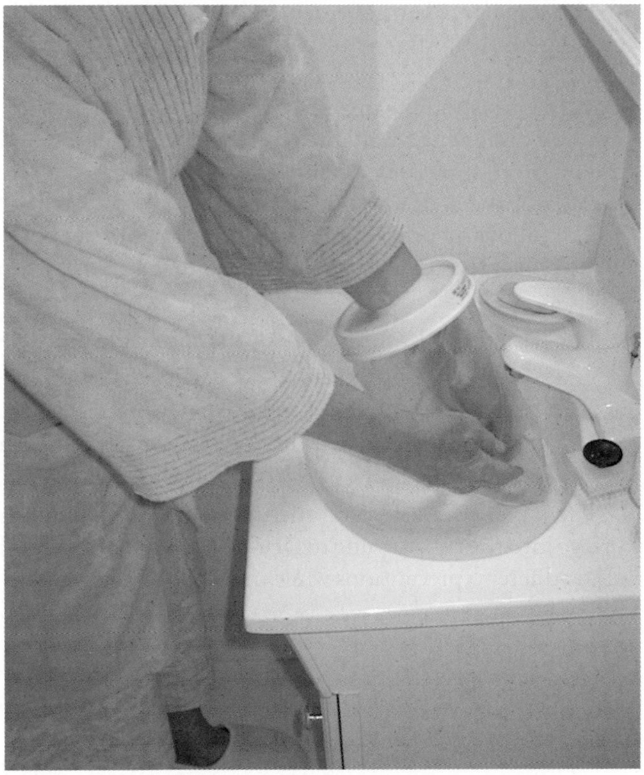

Figure 30-15 Plastic glove prevents operated hand from getting wet during washing of the other hand.

Toileting

The problem with toileting is the inability to reach. The toilet tissue dispenser should be within reach. Wiping tongs can extend reach when using toilet tissue. If grasp is poor, the tissue can be wrapped around the hand. A bidet eliminates the need for wiping by hand. Gravity assists in pulling clothes down; loose clothes slide off easily. A dressing stick can be used to pull up the clothing (Fig. 30-11). Sanitary napkins with adhesive strips can be used more easily than tampons; the protective wrapper can be removed with the teeth. If limited range or movement precautions prevent the patient from using a low commode, a raised toilet seat may solve the problem (Fig. 30-10).

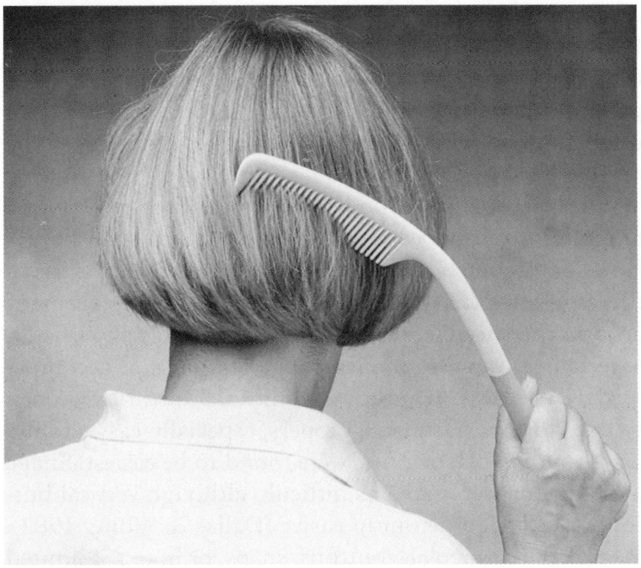

Figure 30-14 Long-handled comb. (Courtesy of North Coast Medical, Morgan Hill, CA.)

Bathing

Tub transfers are facilitated by grab bars (Procedures for Practice 30-5). Non-slip material should be placed on the bottom of the tub. A tub seat is used when the patient is unable or not allowed to get down into the tub or up from the bottom of the tub (Mann et al., 1996). Different heights and styles of tub benches are available, and it is important to select the right one for each patient in terms of stability, ease of transfer, need for padding or back support, access to perianal area, and position of hips and knees (Fig. 30-9). A hand-held shower hose is used for rinsing if a tub seat is required. It is essential to provide practice of strategies to bathe the back, feet, and perianal area when bathing on a tub seat. Lever handles on faucets are recommended because they do not require grasp and they allow better leverage for turning on and off. For patients with hip precautions, it is important to position the tub seat so that faucets can be reached without excessive hip flexion. It is helpful if the soap is on a string, or use soap and shampoo dispensers that can be fixed to the wall in easy reach.

The same problems of reach and grasp encountered in dressing also interfere with bathing. When grasp is limited, a sponge or terry cloth bath mitt works well. A long-handled bath sponge can be used to reach the feet or back; some are designed to hold the soap inside the sponge, and others are designed especially for cleaning feet. A terry cloth bathrobe is effective for drying.

The following procedure is used for patients who cannot step over the edge of the tub and require a transfer tub seat (Fig. 30-9).

1. The patient walks to the side of the tub using assistive devices and weight-bearing precautions, as prescribed, and turns to face away from the tub.
2. The patient reaches for the back of the tub bench with one hand and the edge of the tub seat with the other.
3. The patient sits down on the tub bench and lifts both legs into the tub, turning to face the faucet, being careful to adhere to precautions while moving the involved leg.

Dressing

Lack of ability to reach and grasp and limited shoulder, back, hip, or knee range of motion are limitations that cause problems in dressing. For 2 months after hip replacement, patients will need to follow hip precautions. Most commonly, patients have a cemented total hip arthroplasty via a posterolateral surgical approach. Postoperatively, they are typically weight bearing as tolerated but must avoid flexing the hip past 90°, adducting the leg past midline, or externally rotating the leg (van Stralen, Struben, & van Loon, 2003). Other surgical techniques or complications may necessitate different precautions, so therapists must always confirm activity precautions prior to treatment (see also Chapter 41).

A dressing stick can be used to pull clothing over the feet or to reach hangers in the closet. Reachers can be used to remove clothes from shelves, to start clothes over parts of the body, and to pick up objects from the floor (Fig. 30-16).

Dressing the lower extremities is a particular problem. People who cannot reach their feet or who are not allowed to flex the hip can dress the lower extremities using a sock or stocking aid (Fig. 30-17). To use, the cone is inserted into the foot of the stocking; the top of the stocking is pushed down below the top edge of the cone. While the strings are held, the stocking aid with stocking in place is tossed over the toes, and the person's foot is moved into the foot of the stocking. The cone is then removed by pulling the strings, bringing it out of the stocking behind the heel. This brings the stocking within reach, and it can be pulled up the leg. One study found that patients identified the sock aid as the most useful device at the 2-week follow-up interview at home, but it was the most rejected aid at the time of dispensing in the hospital (Finlayson & Havixbeck, 1992).

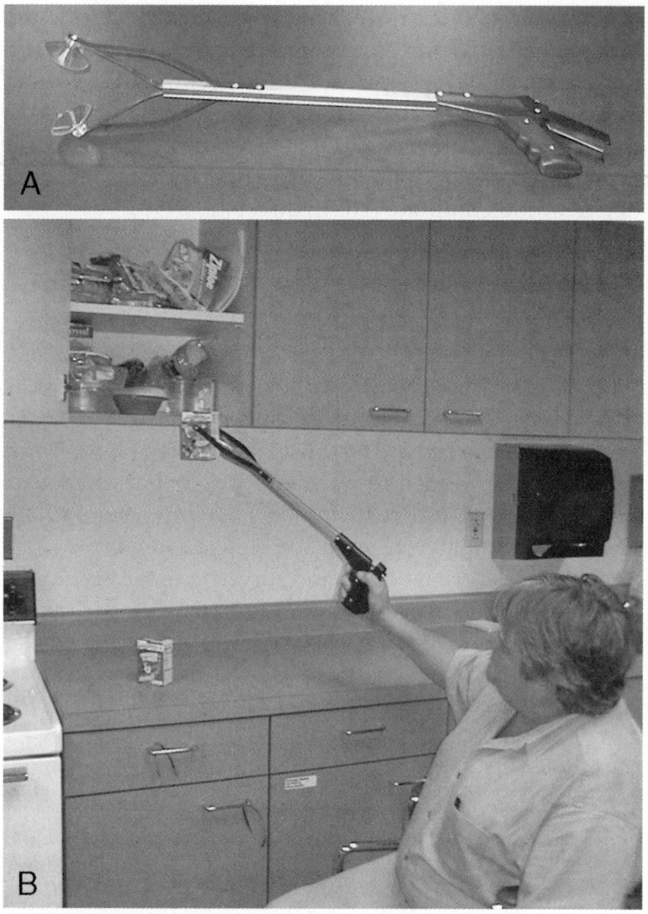

Figure 30-16 A. Reacher with a pistol grip and suction cup tips. **B.** Reacher in use.

A long shoehorn assists in putting on shoes when the feet cannot be reached. Some long shoehorns have a hook on the opposite end that may be used as a dressing stick. Positioning the shoehorn between the legs, rather than on the lateral aspect of the foot, reduces the chance that the patient will move the hip into internal rotation when donning shoes. Slip-on shoes and elastic shoelaces avoid the need to tie shoelaces.

Dressing the upper body with limited upper extremity range of motion is easier when using button- or zipper-front garments rather than over-the-head garments. A dressing stick or reacher is used to bring the garment around the shoulders. Fasteners are particularly difficult, especially if limitation in the range of motion is accompanied by weakness. In a study of ability of 97 arthritic women to use clothing fasteners, zippers, especially easy-sliding, large-toothed plastic ones, were found to be easiest. Snaps and buttons were rated as difficult, although vertical buttonholes made buttoning easier (Dallas & White, 1982). Velcro tabs can replace buttons, snaps, or hooks if limited mobility in the fingers prevents buttoning or fastening. Since few clothes come with this type of fastener, the pa-

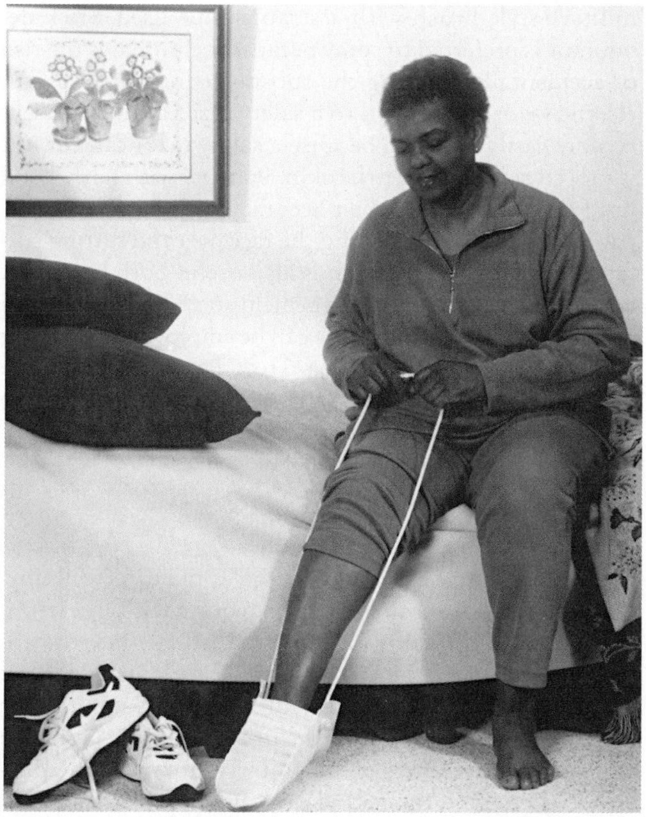

Figure 30-17 Stocking aid in use. (Courtesy of the Rehabilitation Division of Smith & Nephew, Germantown, WI.)

tient's clothing must be adapted. To preserve the look of a buttoned garment, the buttonhole is sewn closed and the button is attached over the hole. The hook-and-pile Velcro tabs are sewn to replace the buttons. Iron-on Velcro button taps, complete with shirt buttons are available to simplify the process (www.easystreetco.com).

Sexual Activities

Intercourse should be planned for the time of day of highest energy level, and the patient should time pain relief medication so its effects are greatest during intercourse. A warm bath may reduce joint stiffness as well as serving as a part of foreplay. Satisfying sex includes romance and intimacy, even though engaging in intercourse may be too exhausting or painful. Patients should explore options for skin-to-skin contact that do not cause pain. The patient and partner can use a trial-and-error process of working out new, comfortable, and biomechanically safe positions for intercourse. For example, both partners may lie on their sides with the man entering from behind for a woman with hip problems; both partners may lie on their sides facing each other with the woman providing most of the hip movement, for a man with back problems (Houtchens, 1998).

Sexual activities such as touching, holding hands, and caressing can be resumed immediately after total joint replacement. Patients with total hip replacement can generally resume intercourse 6–8 weeks post-operatively or according to the surgeon's guidance. Whether male or female, the patient should take the passive position. After 4–6 weeks, patients with unilateral knee replacement no longer have restrictions on resumption of sexual activities except to avoid kneeling positions (Spica & Schwab, 1996).

Suggestions for Selected IADLs

Writing

Use rollerball pens that glide easily. If pinch is limited, the size of the writing instrument can be increased by using sponge rubber, passing it through the holes in a practice golf ball, using commercially available grips that slip on the instrument, or using a comfort-grip pen (Schwarz, 1997).

Telephoning

Cordless phones near where the person is sitting or working are useful, as is one-button automatic dialing. Speaker phones are helpful for patients who cannot hold the phone or hold it to their ear.

Shopping

Shop-at-home services by phone or computer are becoming more common, convenient, and economical. If the patient goes to the shops, he or she should go at off-hours so that clerks are available to get out-of-reach items too heavy to be obtained by use of a reacher.

Opening Containers

Jar openers, including rubber sheets, clamp style, and mounted style, or pliers can be used to open jars, bottles, and pill bottles. Pliers are also useful in other tasks that require pinch, such as weeding or sewing thick fabric. In one study, a pop-off lid was found to require approximately 13 pounds of force to open, and medicine bottles required 2 to 6 pounds (Rice, Leonard, & Carter, 1998). To avoid struggling with pill bottles, medications should be received from the pharmacy in easy-open, not childproof, containers.

Gardening

Choose low-maintenance perennial plants. Use seedlings rather than seeds. Wear a carpenter's apron with pockets for tools. Use tools with ergonomic grips (Fig. 30-3). Use a rolling or stationary stool to sit while working. Wear gloves to protect the skin and joints. Keep pruners sharp to make cutting easier. Use a sprinkler rather than a watering can (Arthritis Foundation, 1997).

Incoordination and Poor Dexterity (Procedures for Practice 30-3)

For more information and suggestions, see Chapter 40.

Suggestions for BADLs

The patient is taught to use the body in as stable a posture as is possible, to sit when possible, and to stabilize the upper extremities by bearing weight on them against a surface or by holding the upper arms close to the body, or both (Gillen, 2000). Stabilizing the head may improve a person's ability to control the upper extremities. Friction surfaces, weighted utensils, or weighted cuffs (see Fig. 13-15) added to the distal segments of the extremities and the use of larger and/or less precise fasteners all contribute to increasing independence by lessening the effects of the incoordination (McGruder et al., 2003). For involuntary movements, such as intention tremors or ataxia, splints may be used to stabilize selected joints, reducing the degrees of freedom that must be controlled by the patient during an activity (Gillen, 2000).

Feeding

The plate can be stabilized on a friction surface, such as a wet towel, wet sponge cloth, or non-skid mat. A plate guard or scoop dish can be used to prevent the food from being pushed off the plate. The utensil may be weighted for stability, may have an enlarged handle to facilitate grasp, and may be plastic coated to protect the person's teeth. Sharp utensils are to be avoided. A weight cuff on the wrist is often chosen rather than a weighted utensil because the cuff can be heavier; also, the cuff makes it unnecessary to weight each item that the patient will use. Weighted cuffs may improve food-to-mouth time, decrease spills, and diminish tremor during eating (McGruder et al., 2003) compared with feeding with no weight. The person may successfully drink from a covered glass or cup with a sipping spout or opening. Some may use a long plastic straw that is held to the side of the cup or glass by a straw holder attachment; the patient moves the head to the straw but does not touch it or the cup or glass with the hand.

Grooming

Weighted cuffs on the wrists may help some patients gain greater accuracy while grooming. Standing in a corner enables patients to stabilize their trunk and head on the wall to the side, and their forearms on the wall in front for activities involving the face, such as brushing teeth, shaving, and applying make-up (Gillen, 2000). Large lipstick tubes are easier to use than small ones. The arms must be stabilized to use lipstick. A simple hairstyle is the best choice. For a patient who has difficulty holding a large comb, a military-style brush with a strap can be used. Stick deodorant is preferred to spray because it eliminates the risk of accidentally spraying the substance into the eyes. An electric razor is preferred to a safety razor both because it is more easily held and because a safety razor can cut if it is moved sideways over the skin. Patients with fairly good head control improve their accuracy by holding the electric razor steady and moving the face over the cutting surface. An electric toothbrush is also useful both because it is heavier and because it can be held steady while the head is moved. This same principle can be employed when filing the nails: fasten the emery board to a flat surface and move each nail over the emery board. Cutting the nails may be unsafe for incoordinated patients, so filing is recommended.

Toileting

Principles described above can be applied to toileting. Patients with incoordination who require self-catheterization may have difficulty inserting the catheter into the urinary meatus. For women, the Asta-Cath female catheter guide helps spread the labia and helps the patient guide the catheter accurately into the urinary meatus (available at www.aplusproducts.biz). Sanitary napkins with adhesive strips to hold them in place may be easier to use than tampons.

Dressing

Clothes that facilitate independent dressing are front-opening, loosely fitting garments with large buttons, Velcro tape closures, or zippers. Wrinkle-resistant and stain-shedding materials enable the person to look well groomed throughout the day. To overcome difficulty with buttoning, a buttonhook with an enlarged and/or weighted handle, if necessary, can be used. A loop of ribbon, leather, or chain can be attached to the zipper pull so that the person can hook it with a finger instead of pinching the zipper pull. Velcro can be substituted to eliminate the need to fasten hooks on a bra. To don the bra, it is easier for the patient to put it around her waist, which is thinner and puts less tension on the garment, and then fasten it in front where she can see what she is doing, turn it around, put her arms in, and pull it up into place. Elastic straps or elastic inserts sewn into the straps make this relatively easy.

Shoe style should eliminate tying. Tie shoes can be adapted using a variety of lacing aids. If a man wears a tie, he may choose to slide the knot down and pull the tie off over his head without undoing the knot.

Bathing

The patient may bathe independently but must adhere closely to safety precautions. Non-slip material is used in the bottom of the tub, and a non-skid mat is placed outside the tub to stand on while transferring. Safety grab bars should be placed where they would be most useful to the particular person's needs. A tub bench or seat can eliminate the difficulty of sitting in and getting up from the bottom of the tub and provides a stable position for the patient who is washing the feet. If a seat is used, a handheld shower spray is necessary.

If the patient chooses to shower instead of bathe, the non-slip material, grab bars, and seat also must be provided. In either case, the water should be drawn once the patient has transferred in and is seated; a mixer tap is ideal, but if it is unavailable, the cool water should be turned on first with the hot water added progressively to prevent scalding. Soap on a string keeps the soap retrievable, or a bath mitt with a pocket to hold the soap is useful. The water should be drained before the person attempts to stand to transfer out of the tub. An extra large towel or large terry wrap-around robe facilitates drying.

Suggestions for Selected IADL

Communication

Writing and speech are problems for some persons with coordination deficits. See Chapter 19 for alternative communication systems and adaptations for computers that are appropriate for these patients. If the patient speaks understandably, the use of large-button phones reduces the fine motor requirements of dialing the telephone, or a speaker phone can be used.

Playing Games

Board game pieces can be weighted or turned into pegs for stability. Game boards can be reproduced to enlarge the squares. Card holders and card shufflers are useful. Computer games that use keyboarding or switches rather than a mouse or joystick are appropriate.

Loss of Use of One Side of the Body or One Upper Extremity (Procedures for Practice 30-3)

For other information and suggestions, see Chapters 38, 42, and 46.

Suggestions for BADLs

The methods described here pertain to the hemiplegic patient who has lost the use of one side of the body. Although most stroke patients can be independent in their BADL, some are prevented from developing independence, especially of the less automatic tasks, such as one-handed upper extremity dressing, by cognitive-perceptual impairments (Edmans & Lincoln, 1990; Walker & Lincoln, 1991; Walker & Walker, 2001). Motor planning deficits, such as ideomotor apraxia, may make learning new skills more difficult; however, patients have been able to learn a new motor process, such as one-handed shoe tying (Poole, 1998).

The methods and equipment described here may also be used by a person with a unilateral upper extremity amputation or temporary or permanent upper extremity limitations resulting from trauma. Patients with upper extremity amputation or injury, however, need fewer adaptations because they have normal trunk and lower extremity function and normal perception and cognition.

Feeding

Feeding is essentially a one-handed task, except for cutting meat and spreading condiments on bread, and these tasks can be done with assistive devices. Food can be simultaneously stabilized and cut by use of a rocker knife, a knife with a sharp curved blade that cuts when rocked over the food (Fig. 30-18). Bread can be spread if stabilized on a non-slip surface or trapped in the corner of a spike board and spread toward the corner (Fig. 32-2). Soft spreads facilitate this process.

Grooming

Difficulties with grooming include care of the unaffected extremity and completing two-handed activities. Spray deodorant for the unaffected arm is easier to use than other types of applicators. Fingernails of the unaffected hand are cleaned by rubbing them on a small suction cup brush attached to the basin (Fig. 30-19). Fingernails of the affected hand can be trimmed with a stabilized nail clipper (Fig. 30-8), and those of the unaffected hand can be trimmed with an emery board fastened down to stabilize it. The fingernail is moved back and forth over the emery board. Toothpaste in pump bottles or a toothpaste dispenser can be used with one hand. A floss holder or disposable flossers enable patients to floss teeth with only one hand.

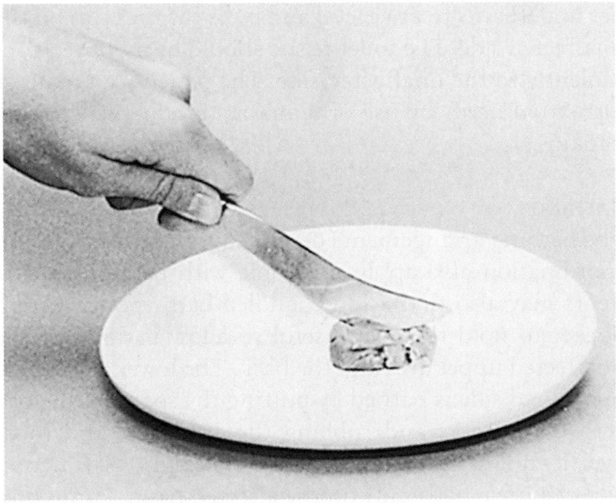

Figure 30-18 Rocker knife for one-handed cutting.

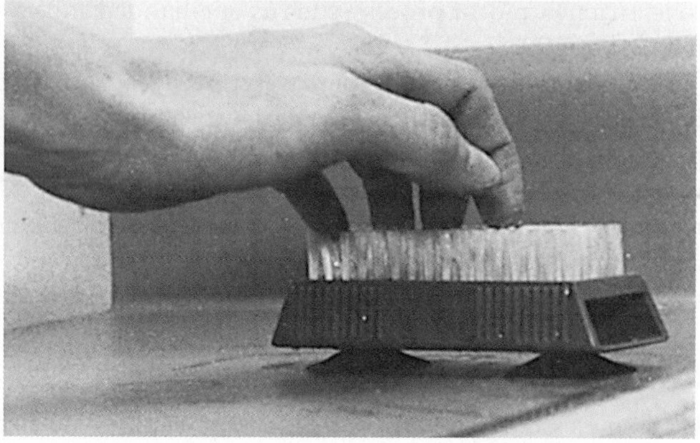

Figure 30-19 Suction cup brush for cleaning nails or dentures with one hand.

Using another suction cup brush fastened to the inside of the basin, the person can scrub dentures by rubbing them over the brush. Partially filling the basin with water and laying a face cloth in the bottom cushions the dentures if they are dropped. An electric razor is recommended for shaving for patients post stroke because accidents are possible with a safety razor.

Toileting

The primary difficulty with toileting is managing clothing, which is normally done with two hands. A grab bar mounted on the wall beside the toilet and/or a frame mounted on the toilet (Fig. 30-10) will assist transfers and maintaining standing balance. Once standing, pants are unfastened, and gravity takes them down. If the patient's standing balance is impaired, pants should be unfastened before standing, and the affected hand should be placed in the pocket, which prevents the pants from sliding below the knees where they are difficult to retrieve. A woman in a dress can raise her dress on the affected side and tuck it between her body and the affected arm. Then she lowers her underpants to knee level and pulls the dress up on the unaffected side. The toilet tissue should be mounted conveniently to the unaffected side. The patient can manage menstrual needs by use of tampons or adhesive sanitary napkins.

Bathing

The bathing arrangements described for patients with incoordination also apply to people with hemiplegia. Patients may also find a long-handled bath sponge with a pocket to hold the soap useful to allow bathing of the unaffected upper arm and the back. The lower arm of the unaffected side is bathed by putting the soapy washcloth across the knees and rubbing the arm back and forth over it, unless the patient has some return of function and can use a bath mitt on the affected hand. Pump bottles of liquid soap and shampoo are useful, as is soap on a rope. If sensory impairment exists, extra precautions should be taken to be certain of water temperature. Patients with hemiplegia should dry off as much as possible while still seated on the bath seat before transferring out of the tub.

A person with a unilateral upper extremity amputation can bathe using similar strategies. A bath bench enables patients to place a washcloth on one leg to enable them to wash the unaffected arm without balancing on one leg, which may present a safety risk for patients who lack excellent balance.

Dressing

Certain prerequisite abilities are considered important for successful dressing. These are ability to reach each foot, stand unsupported for 10 seconds, and maintain sitting balance when reaching down. The most difficult tasks for both men and women were found to be pulling pants up, putting the shoe on the affected foot, and lacing shoes (Walker & Lincoln, 1990, 1991). Many people can manage fasteners with one hand. Patients who have difficulty with one-handed fastening may prefer Velcro fasteners, which are easier to use (Huck & Bonhotal, 1997).

Patients with hemiplegia should dress while seated on a stable surface, with both feet on the floor to increase stability (Ryan & Sullivan, 2004). As a general rule, the affected limb is dressed first and undressed last.

Shirt or Cardigan Garment: Over-the-Shoulder Method (Ryan & Sullivan, 2004)

The over-the-shoulder method is the most similar to the customary method of dressing, and garments are less likely to get twisted than when using the overhead method that follows.

1. Put the shirt on the lap, label facing up, collar toward the knees, with the sleeve for the affected arm hanging between the knees (Fig. 30-20A)
3. Put the affected hand into the sleeve and lean forward to let gravity extend the elbow and to slide the sleeve onto the arm (Fig. 30-20B).
4. Use the unaffected arm to slide the shirt over the affected shoulder.
5. Grasp the collar at the point closest to the unaffected side (Fig. 30-20C).
6. Hold tightly to the collar, lean forward, and bring the collar and shirt around the affected side and behind the neck to the unaffected side (Fig. 30-20C).
7. Put the unaffected hand into the other armhole. Raise the arm out and up to push it through the sleeve (Fig. 30-20D).
8. To straighten the shirt, lean forward, work the shirt down over the shoulders, reach back and pull the tail

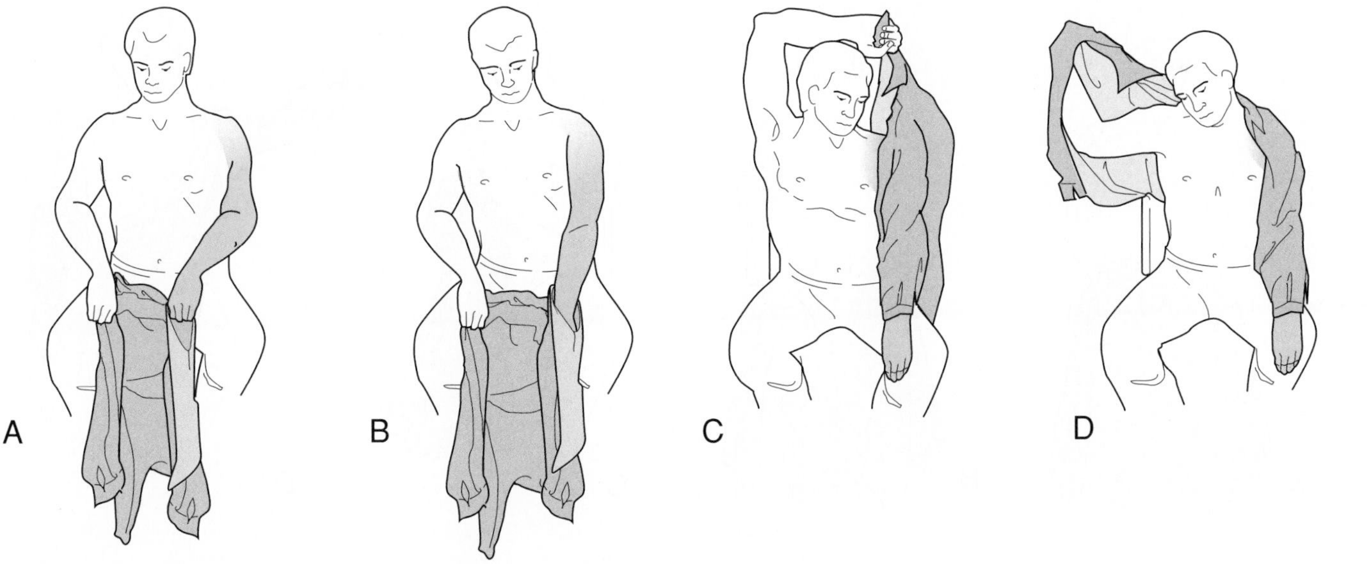

Figure 30-20 Patient with left hemiplegia putting on a shirt. **A.** Position the shirt with the collar toward the knees and the sleeve for the affected arm hanging between the legs. **B.** Guide the affected arm into the sleeve, lean forward, and pull the sleeve up to the shoulder. **C.** Hold the collar tightly. Lean forward and bring the shirt up, around, and behind toward the unaffected arm. **D.** Put the unaffected arm into the armhole. Extend the arm out and up to push it through the sleeve. Straighten the shirt and button it.

down, and then straighten the sleeve under the affected axilla.

9. To button, line up the shirt fronts and match each button with the correct buttonhole, starting with the bottom button.

To remove the shirt, unbutton it and use the unaffected hand to throw the shirt back off the unaffected shoulder. Work the shirt sleeve off the unaffected arm, pressing the shirt cuff against the leg to pull the arm out. Lean forward. Use the unaffected hand to pull the shirt across the back. Take the shirt off of the affected arm.

Shirt or Cardigan Garment: Overhead Method (Brett, 1960)

The overhead method for putting on and removing front-opening tops may be less confusing for a patient with perceptual impairments. This method is not suitable for coats.

1. Put the shirt on the lap, label facing up, and the collar next to the abdomen; drape the shirttail over the knees (Fig. 30-21A).
2. Pick up the affected hand and put it into the sleeve (Fig. 30-21B).
3. Pull the sleeve up over the elbow (Fig. 30-21C). If the sleeve is not pulled past the elbow, the hand will fall out when continuing.
4. Put the unaffected hand into the armhole. Raise the arm and push it through the sleeve as far as possible (Fig. 30-21D).
5. Gather the back of the shirt from tail to collar (Fig. 30-21E).
6. Hold the gathered shirt up, lean forward, duck the head, and put the shirt over the head (Fig. 30-21F).
7. To straighten the shirt, lean forward and work the shirt down over the shoulders. Often the shirt gets caught on the affected shoulder and must first be pushed back over the shoulder. Then reach back and pull the tail down (Fig. 30-21G).
8. To button, line up the shirt fronts and match each button with the correct buttonhole, starting with the bottom button.

To remove the shirt, the patient unbuttons it, leans forward, and uses the unaffected hand to gather the shirt up in back of the neck. He or she ducks the head, pulls the shirt over the head, and then takes the shirt off the unaffected arm first.

Pullover Garment (Brett, 1960)

The following steps are used for putting on a pullover garment.

1. Position the garment on the lap, bottom toward chest and label facing down.
2. Using the unaffected hand, roll up the bottom edge of the shirt back, all the way up to the sleeve on the affected side.
3. Spread the armhole opening as large as possible. Using the unaffected hand, place the affected arm into the armhole and pull the sleeve up onto the arm past the elbow. Alternatively, the sleeve may be positioned between the legs, as described earlier for the cardigan over-the-shoulder method.

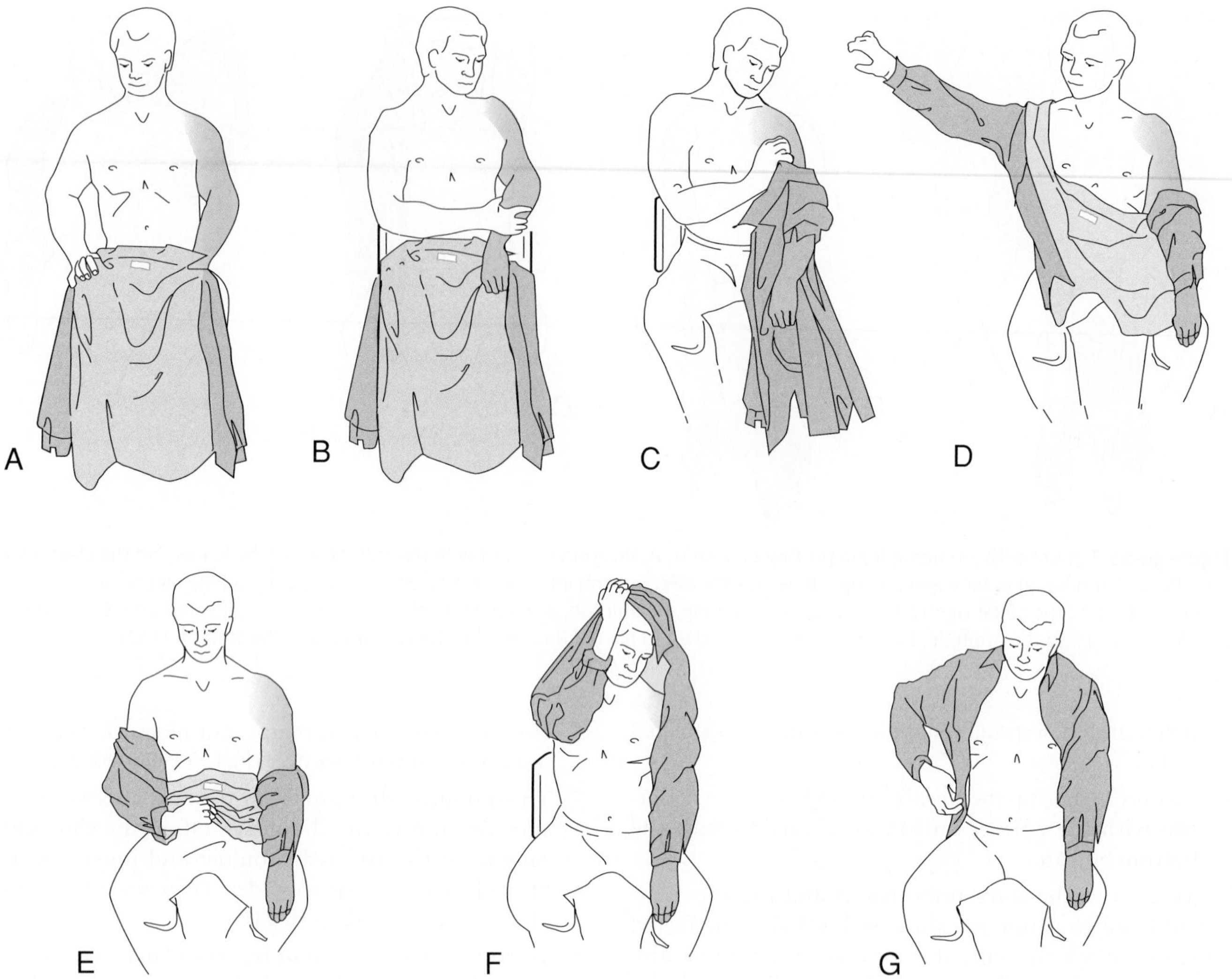

Figure 30-21 Patient with left hemiplegia putting on a shirt using the overhead method. **A.** Put shirt on the lap, with label facing up, collar next to abdomen, and shirttail draped over knees. **B.** Pick up the affected arm and put it into the armhole. **C.** Pull the sleeve well over the elbow. **D.** Put the unaffected hand into the armhole and raise the arm to push it through the sleeve. **E.** Gather the back of the shirt from the tail to the collar. **F.** Hold the gathered shirt up. Lean forward and duck the head to put the shirt overhead. **G.** To straighten the shirt, lean forward and work the shirt over the shoulders. Reach back and pull the tail down and the front sides forward. Button it.

4. Insert the unaffected arm into the other sleeve.
5. Gather the shirt back from bottom edge to neck, lean forward, duck the head, and pass the shirt over the head.
6. Adjust the shirt on the involved side up and onto the shoulder and remove twists.

To remove, starting at top back, gather the shirt up, lean forward, duck the head, and pull the shirt forward over the head. Remove the unaffected arm and then the affected arm.

Bra (Brett, 1960)

The bra is placed around the waist and hooked in front, where the patient can see what she is doing. One end can be tucked into the waistband of panties or under the affected arm until the other end is brought around. It is fastened and rotated to the proper position; the affected arm is placed through the shoulder strap; and the unaffected arm is placed through the other shoulder strap. The bra is pulled up into place. It is removed by reversing the process.

A plump patient may need an adapted front-closing bra if she cannot approximate the two edges of the bra to fasten it. The bra is adapted with a D-ring on the side of the bra opening on the involved side and a pile Velcro strap on the opposite side. After the bra is around the waist, the strap is threaded through the D-ring and pulled to bring the two ends of the bra together. Hook Velcro must be stitched onto the bra so the strap can be fastened.

PANTS (BRETT, 1960)

The following steps describe how to put on pants. Modifications of the following method are used for men's and women's underclothing and pantyhose.

1. Sit. If a wheelchair is used, the brakes should be locked and the footrests should be up and/or swung out of the way. Move the unaffected leg beyond the midline of the body for balance.
2. Grasp the ankle or calf of the affected leg. Lift and cross the affected leg over the unaffected leg (Fig. 30-22, A & B). Alternatively, cup the affected knee in clasped hands to lift and cross the leg.
3. Pull the pants onto the affected leg up to but not above the knee (Fig. 30-22C).
4. Uncross the legs.
5. Put the unaffected leg into the other pant leg.
6. Remain sitting. Pull the pants up above the knees as far as possible (Fig. 30-22D).
7. To prevent the pants from dropping when standing, put the affected hand into the pant pocket or the thumb into a belt loop (Fig. 30-22E). Alternatively, use a pant clip to attach the pants to the shirt so they do not slide down (Ryan & Sullivan, 2004). Pants with

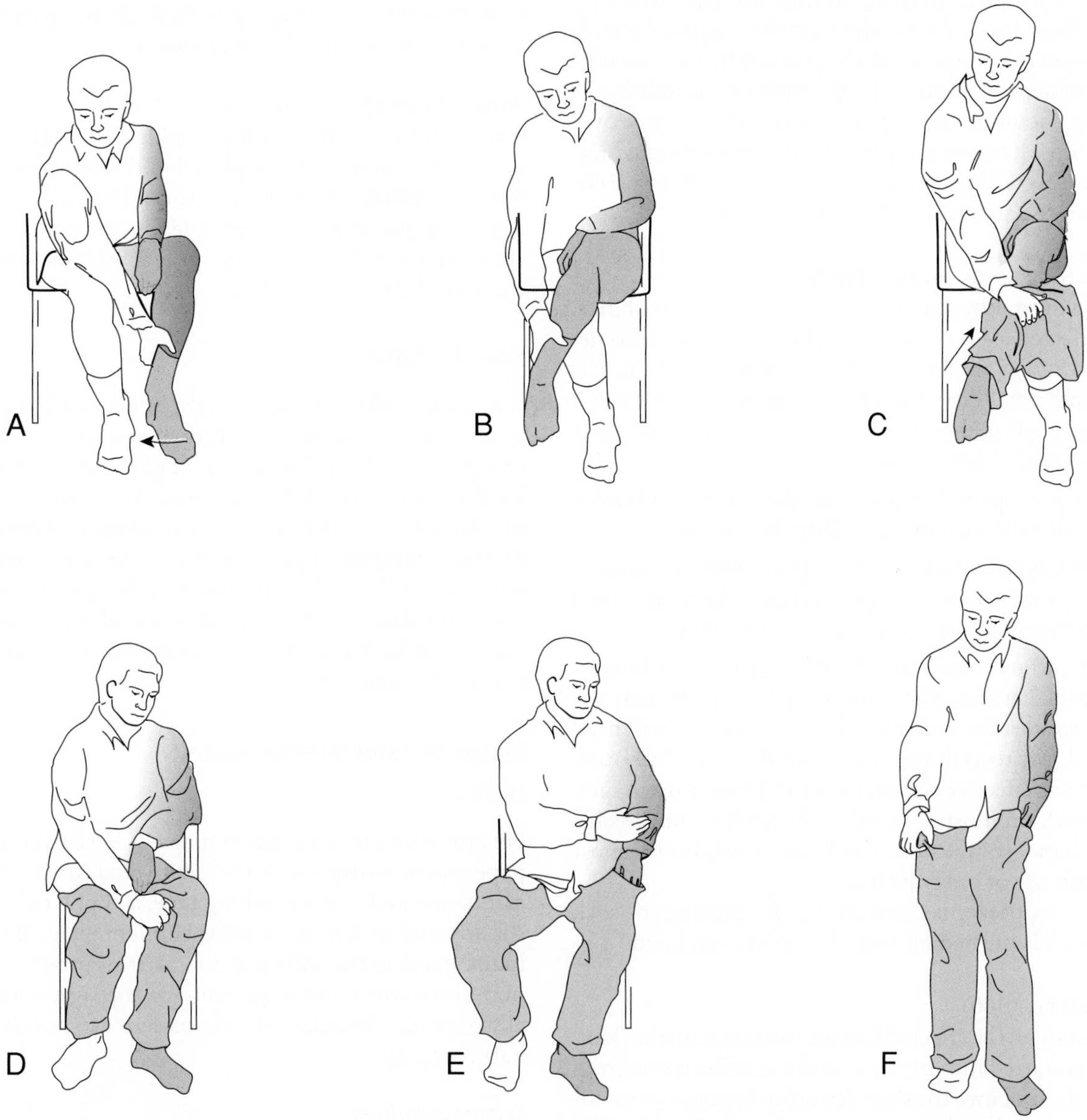

Figure 30-22 Patient with left hemiplegia putting on pants while sitting. **A.** With knees bent, move the unaffected foot across the midline of the body toward the unaffected side. **B.** Grasp the ankle of the affected leg, lift it, and cross it over the unaffected leg. **C.** Pull the pants onto the affected leg up to but not above the knee. **D.** Uncross the legs, put the unaffected leg into the pants, and pull them up above the knees. **E.** To prevent the pants from dropping when the person stands up, put the affected hand into the pocket. **F.** Stand up. Pull the pants over the hips and fasten, or sit to fasten if balance is not good enough to do it while standing.

elastic waistbands are also less likely to slide when standing up.

8. Stand up. Pull the pants up over the hips (Fig. 30-22F); button and zip pants while standing. Persons with poor balance may remain seated and pull the pants up over the hips by shifting from side to side; they should button and zip the pants while seated.

To remove, unfasten the pants in sitting. Stand and let the pants drop past the knees or push down if wearing elastic waist garment. Sit. Remove the pants from the unaffected leg. Cross the affected leg over the unaffected leg. Remove the pants from the affected leg. Uncross the legs.

People with poor balance should use the following method. Place locked wheelchair or chair against a wall. Sit. Unfasten the pants. Work the pants down on the hips as far as possible by shifting weight from side to side in the chair. Use the uninvolved arm to work the pants down past the hips. Remove the pants from the unaffected leg. Cross the affected leg over the unaffected leg. Remove the pants from the affected leg. Uncross the legs.

Socks or Stockings (Brett, 1960)

The following method is used to put on socks or stockings.

1. The affected leg is crossed over the unaffected leg as described earlier for donning pants. Or, if the patient has adequate flexibility, crossing the ankle over the thigh (like men sit) makes the foot easier to reach. The same process is used for the unaffected foot.
2. The sock is opened by inserting the thumb and index finger into the top and spreading the fingers.
3. The sock is put on the foot by slipping the toes into the opening made under the spread hand. The sock is then pulled into place, and wrinkles are smoothed.

Patients who cannot cross their legs can rest the heel on a small stool. Patients who cannot reach their feet may use a reacher to start the sock over the toes, but they will need to reach down to pull the sock over the heel. Although sock aids are effective for overcoming limited reach, getting the sock on most sock aids is difficult or impossible with one hand, so this device will not be helpful for most people with use of only one hand.

To remove, the leg is positioned as for putting the sock on. The sock is pushed off with the unaffected hand.

Shoes (Brett, 1960)

A loafer is put on the affected foot with the shoe on the floor. The foot is started into the shoe, and a shoehorn is used to help ease the foot into the shoe. A tie shoe is put onto the affected foot after the leg is crossed over the unaffected one to bring the foot closer. If the laces have been thoroughly loosened, the person often can work the shoe on while the leg is crossed over by grasping the heel of the shoe with the unaffected hand and working it back and forth over the heel until it goes on completely. Sometimes it is necessary to insert a shoehorn while the leg is crossed over and then carefully lower the foot with the shoe half on and shoehorn in the shoe and finish putting on the shoe by repeatedly pushing down on the knee and adjusting the shoehorn.

Tying the shoes is a problem. It is possible to tie a conventional bow one-handed, but it requires fine dexterity and normal perception. The patient with an amputation may prefer to do this or use loafers. The patient with hemiplegia can use adapted shoe closures or learn a simple, effective one-handed shoe tie as illustrated in Figure 30-23. Putting the lace through the last hole from the outside of the shoe toward the tongue lets the tension of the foot against the shoe hold the lace tight while the bow is being tied. One-hand shoe tying is difficult for patients with cognitive-perceptual deficits to learn.

Ankle–Foot Orthosis

The posterior shell or molded ankle–foot orthosis (AFO) is usually easiest to don if placed in the shoe first (Ryan & Sullivan, 2004). The shoe laces should be quite loose to allow the maximum room possible for getting the foot into the orthosis and shoe. The orthosis acts like a shoehorn, as the foot slides into the shoe.

Sexual Activities

A helpful booklet, *Sex after Stroke* (American Heart Association, 2000), is available online (www.strokeassociation.org/presenter.jhtml?identifier=9065) or in print from the local affiliate of the American Heart Association/American Stroke Association. It discusses sexuality and body image, fears about resuming sex, specifics of sexual intimacy after stroke (bowel and bladder control, change of position to accommodate paralysis, birth control, pregnancy, and ways to make love other than intercourse) and contains a list of additional resources.

Suggestions for Selected IADLs

Writing

Persons with only one functional arm have to stabilize the paper when writing with the unaffected hand. The paper can be secured using masking tape, a clipboard, a weight, the affected extremity, or other similar means. If the dominant hand is the affected one, writing practice for the non-dominant hand, especially for the signature, is usually required. Alternatively, the patient can purchase a signature stamp.

Leisure Activities

Many devices for leisure activities are available for people who have lost the use of one hand, including devices for knitting, crocheting, embroidery, playing cards, and fishing. Resource 30-1 includes sources where devices can be explored and purchased.

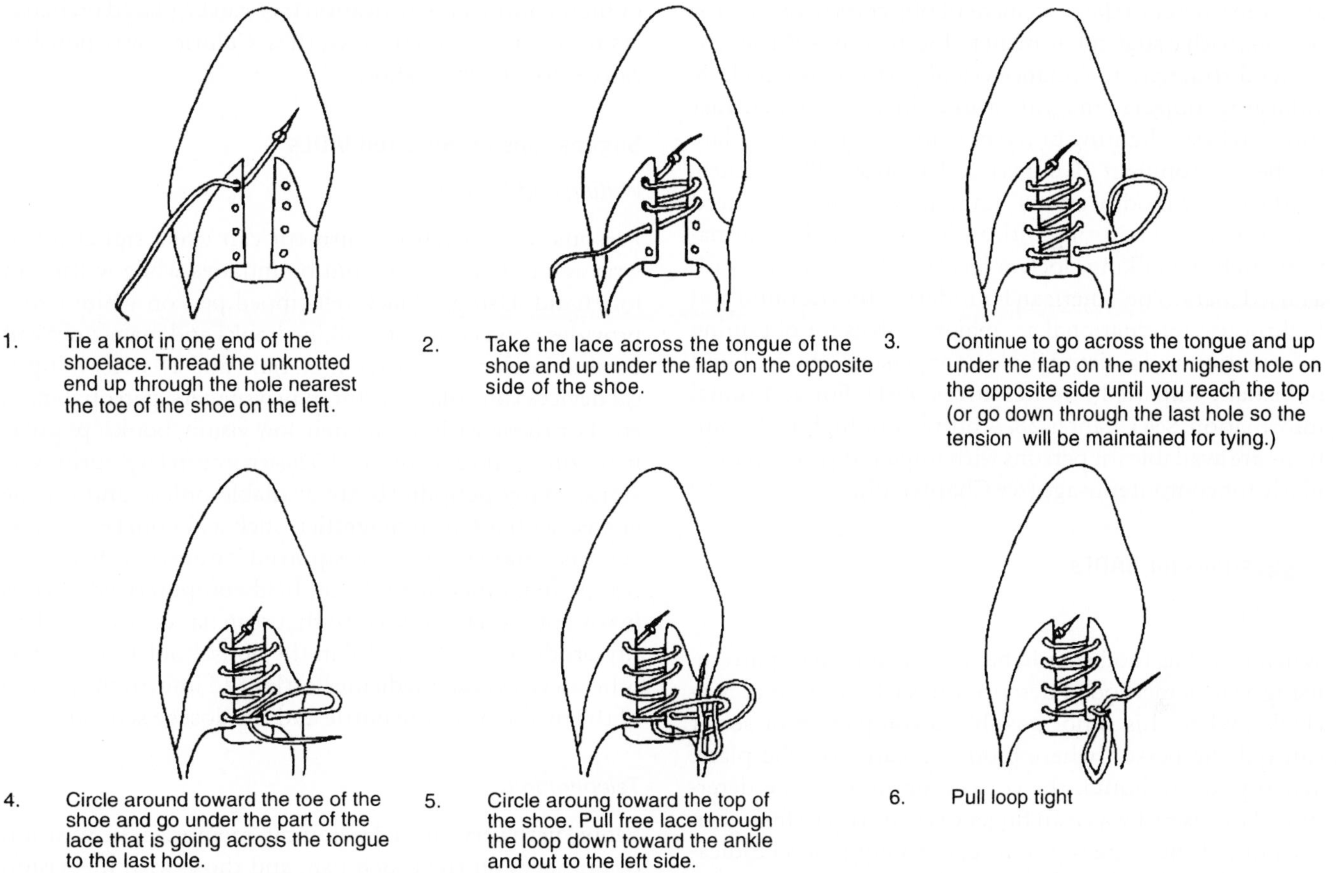

1. Tie a knot in one end of the shoelace. Thread the unknotted end up through the hole nearest the toe of the shoe on the left.
2. Take the lace across the tongue of the shoe and up under the flap on the opposite side of the shoe.
3. Continue to go across the tongue and up under the flap on the next highest hole on the opposite side until you reach the top (or go down through the last hole so the tension will be maintained for tying.)
4. Circle around toward the toe of the shoe and go under the part of the lace that is going across the tongue to the last hole.
5. Circle aroung toward the top of the shoe. Pull free lace through the loop down toward the ankle and out to the left side.
6. Pull loop tight

Figure 30-23 One-handed shoe tie for a left hemiplegic patient. For a right hemiplegic patient, start the lace on the right side of the shoe so that the lace ends on the left side at the top.

Lower Extremity Amputation with Prosthesis

Persons with lower extremity amputations can benefit from many of the adaptations described for people with limited mobility due to weakness or decreased range of motion; however, lower body dressing for prosthetic users presents a unique challenge not previously addressed. Prior to dressing, patients should change the shoe and/or sock on the prosthesis to match the day's clothing. Patients with a transtibial (below knee) amputation with pants wide enough to pull up to the knee should dress while seated using the following steps:

1. Place pants over unaffected leg and amputated leg, pulling pants up as far as possible.
2. Patients who are stable standing on one leg can stand to pull the pants up and then sit down to don the residual limb stocking and prosthesis, exposing the area by sliding the pant leg up over the knee.
3. Patients who are not stable standing on one leg should remain seated and don the prosthesis before standing to pull up their pants so that they have the stability of both lower extremities when standing to complete the task.

Patients with a transfemoral (above knee) amputation or those with a below knee amputation who wish to wear fitted pants that cannot be slid up over the knee should dress as follows:

1. Slide the end of the pant leg for the amputated limb down over the top of the prosthesis so that the prosthesis is dressed first. The shoe and limited ankle mobility will prevent the pants from being slid over the prosthetic foot.
2. Don the stocking and the prosthesis.
3. Place the unaffected leg into the pants.
4. Stand to pull up and fasten the pants.

Limited Vision (Procedures for Practice 30-3)

The suggestions listed here pertain to blindness (20/1250 to worse than 20/2500) and to low vision (20/80 to 20/1000) (Colenbrander & Fletcher, 1995). Organization and consistency in the placement of objects is necessary for persons with visual impairment to locate things efficiently. General strategies to enhance visual performance include enlarging objects, magnification, increasing contrast through better lighting or use of color, and reducing glare in the environment (Lampert & Lapolice, 1995; Smith, 2001). Other modifications eliminate or reduce the need for vision by substituting with auditory or tactile information, such as a talking clock or locating dryer settings with a raised mark. The American Foundation for the Blind and Lighthouse International are major sources for obtaining information and assistive devices for persons who are blind or visually impaired (see Resources 30-1). For additional information, see Chapter 28. A number of high-tech solutions are available for persons with impaired vision, particularly for computer usage (see Chapter 19).

Suggestions for BADLs

Feeding

When possible, food should be set in a consistent pattern, using a clock method of description, such as "meat at 3 o'-clock." When this is not possible, a companion or server can tell the person where food is located on the plate. When pouring liquid, the correct amount can be determined by inserting a clean finger over the rim to feel when the liquid is near the top or by using a liquid level indicator, which is placed on the rim of the cup and gives an auditory signal when the cup is full. Food is cut by finding the edge of the food with the fork, moving the fork a bite-size amount onto the meat, and then cutting the food, keeping the knife in contact with the fork. For those with low vision, the plate, glass, and utensils should be a color that contrasts with both the table covering and the food.

Grooming

A major problem is identification of objects. This can be done through the use of taste, touch (size, shape, and texture), location, and Braille or bar code labels. The application of cosmetics or toiletries is another problem; fingers of the assistive hand can be guides, such as when shaving sideburns or applying eyebrow pencil. Aerosol sprays should be avoided because persons who have low vision cannot see the extent of the spray.

Dressing

Limited vision creates no difficulty with the physical aspects of dressing, but persons with impaired vision need a system to coordinate colors of clothes and compatibility of style. One system is to store clothes of like color together. Clothes should always be hung properly to prevent wrinkles. Wrinkle-free, stain-resistant, no-iron fabrics are desirable. Clothing selection can be done with the assistance of a sighted person who can describe colors and style. Tactile or high-contrast identification tags can be placed on hangers to denote the color of clothes. Colorless wax polishes can be used to shine shoes.

Suggestions for Selected IADLs

Writing and Reading

Persons with visual impairment can use a signature or writing guide to stay within boundaries while writing in longhand. Using a black felt-tipped pen on white paper provides good contrast. Talking books and magazines can be used in place of written materials, and a variety of optical devices can enlarge print in newspapers, personal mail, etc. For those with moderately low vision, books, popular magazines, and *The New York Times* come in large-print versions. Many periodicals are available online and can be viewed with a screen magnifier, such as ZoomText (www.synapseadaptive.com/aisquared/zoomtext_9/zoomtext_9_magnifier.htm). Hand-held computerized devices (www.envisionamerica.com) that scan bar codes and identify products can be useful in the household and at work; other devices scan medicine bottles and inform the person of the medicine in the bottle and the dosage schedule.

Telephoning

People with very limited vision can memorize the position of numbers on the touch pad, and those with low vision can use phones with large buttons. A phone with one-button automatic dialing is very useful, as are voice-activated phones.

Time

The person can tell time using a Braille or talking watch or clock.

Shopping

Much shopping by persons with low vision can be done through catalogs, read by use of closed-circuit television (CCTV) or online with screen magnifiers. Portable CCTV that can be taken out and used in the community is becoming available.

Handling Money

Tactile discrimination enables the person to identify coins. Paper money is discriminated by the way it is folded after its denomination has been identified previously by someone else or viewed by magnification.

Playing Games

Braille versions of popular games, such as Monopoly, Bingo, and playing cards, are available. Large-numbered cards are also available for those with low vision.

Decreased Sensation (Procedures for Practice 30-3)

For additional information, see Chapter 27.

Suggestions for BADL

Problems of absent, decreased, or disturbed sensation affect performance of ADL whenever a possibly dangerous situation is encountered and because the automatic knowledge of limb movement and touch may be missing.

Bathing

With bathing, there is danger of scalding. When turning water on, the cold is turned on first, and then the hot is added gradually. Mixer valves should be installed to compensate when decreased sensation is a permanent condition. If the patient has intact areas of sensation, they can learn to test water temperature with those areas.

Dressing

Wrinkles, seams, or bands on clothing that are sufficient to cause tissue damage may not be felt by patients with impaired sensation and can cause decubitus ulcers within a short time. Clothing should be selected that is snug enough to prevent bunching but loose enough to avoid binding or excessive pressure. Persons with insensitive skin should inspect clothing visually or with an area of intact sensation to avoid wrinkles. They must dress warmly in cold weather to prevent frostbite.

Suggestions for Selected IADLs

Poor sensation does not allow graduated pinch and grip on tools and utensils to meet the demands of the task. The person grips with excessive pressure (Johansson & Westling, 1984). Prolonged, excessive grip or pinch can cause bruising and decubiti. Poor sensation also results in letting go, when the attention is directed away from the object being held. Devices discussed early for poor grip may help persons with impaired sensation for activities requiring sustained grip.

Activities that involve using hot objects, such as a riding mower or cooking at an outdoor barbecue, pose a threat because anesthetic lower extremities can be burned if allowed to rest against the hot engine cover or bottom of the barbecue. Objects should be insulated when possible, and patients should be trained to be extra vigilant in positioning themselves near hot items.

Cognitive-Perceptual Impairments (Procedures for Practice 30-3)

See Chapters 28 and 29 for information concerning methods to compensate for cognitive or perceptual impairments in activities of daily living.

Pain, Including Low Back Pain (Procedures for Practice 30-3)

See Chapters 32 and 41 for information concerning body mechanics to be used during occupational functioning for persons with low back pain.

Considerations in Bariatric Care

Occupational therapists are treating increasing numbers of patients who are exceptionally large. Obesity is associated with a number of health problems (Foti & Littrell, 2004). Additionally, persons who are exceptionally large often have movement limitations that result directly from their size, so these patients often require occupational therapy (Foti, 2005). Several considerations warrant discussion regarding adaptations for these individuals. Excessively large individuals with a medical condition may have more occupational performance deficits than are typically seen because of pre-existing limitations in strength relative to body mass, limited reach, and decreased endurance. A thorough functional assessment is needed to ensure all problems are identified (Foti & Littrell, 2004). Adaptive equipment must be carefully evaluated to make sure that it has been approved to handle the patient's weight and that it is sized appropriately to meet the patient's needs. For example, many tub seats are approved to handle up to 300 pounds and cannot be used safely by a heavier person. Traditional sock aids may be too small to accommodate the patient's foot or calf, and a soft variety may need to be used (Foti, 2005). The typical home environment may present a number of obstacles for persons of exceptional size, including narrow doorways or pathways that prevent the person from entering a room. Bathrooms are commonly too small to be functional for persons who are exceptionally large, and they may find themselves confined to one or two rooms in their homes (Foti & Littrell, 2004). Caregivers may be limited in the tasks they can assist a person with because of risk of physical injuries. Psychosocial issues may complicate the clinical picture.

Adaptive strategies described earlier for persons with weakness, limited reach, and/or endurance may all be effective in treating persons of exceptional size. A number of companies have equipment especially designed for the bariatric population that can help the therapist select appropriate and safe adaptations for these patients (see Resources 30-1; also, additional resources are included in the references by Foti, 2005 and Foti & Littrell, 2004).

Service Dogs: An Adaptation Option for a Range of Performance Limitations

Service dogs are specially trained to meet the needs of persons with limitations in mobility and/or ADL due to loss of vision, hearing, and physical impairments. Service dogs are trained collaboratively with the owner so that they learn skills suited to meet the individual's unique needs. The training is extensive and, therefore, expensive, so service dogs are appropriate only for persons with permanent disabilities.

Service dogs can assist people with a variety of tasks. Dogs for people with visual impairment are primarily used for mobility by acting as a guide. Hearing dogs alert their owners to auditory stimuli that require a response, e.g., doorbells, alarm clocks, oven timers, and smoke detectors. Other physical disabilities vary significantly, and the range of activities that service dogs can assist with is very large. Dogs at Canine Companions for Independence (see Resources 30-1) learn about 40 commands, which can be adapted to individual circumstances. For instance, the tug command is normally used on doors and drawers but can be used to remove socks or other clothes (Fig. 30-24). The most common activities include help with wheelchair and floor transfers, mobility in home and community, carrying items, operating switches (e.g., lights, elevator buttons), retrieving and moving items, and opening doors, drawers, and cabinets (Allen & Blascovich, 1996; Fairman & Huebner, 2000).

Service dogs are an adaptive tool; however, they do not seem to carry the same stigma as assistive devices and may even support social participation. Service dog owners have reported increased interactions with friends and people out in public, increased confidence, and enhanced feelings of safety (Camp, 2001; Fairman & Huebner, 2000; Valentine, Kiddoo, & LeFleur, 1993). Allen and Blascovich (1996) conducted a randomized controlled study to examine the impact of service dogs on a number of variables, comparing an intervention group that received a service dog and a wait-list control group with no dog. The service dog group had higher scores on psychosocial variables (including self-esteem and community integration), increased participation in school and work, and a decrease of 68% in both paid and unpaid assistance hours. The wait list group showed a similar pattern of improvement 18 months later when they received their dogs. Although the cost of training a service dog was estimated at $10,000, the researchers estimated that savings in personal care attendants would reach $60,000 after 8 years, the average working life of the dog (Allen & Blascovich, 1996).

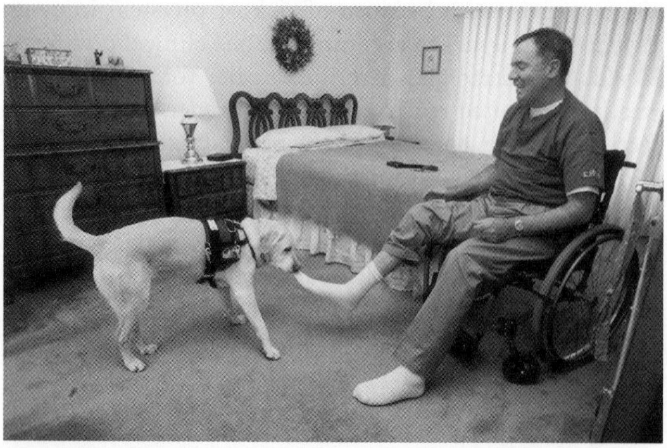

Figure 30-24 Service dog is given the "tug" command to help remove his owner's sock (Courtesy of Canine Companions for Independence, Santa Rosa, CA.)

EFFECTIVENESS OF THERAPY TO RESTORE THE ROLE OF INDEPENDENT PERSON

Evidence from meta-analyses and randomized controlled trials that demonstrate occupational therapy has a positive effect on client functional outcomes in BADLs and IADLs is summarized in Evidence Table 30-1. Additional studies, although less rigorous in design, also offer insight into occupational therapy intervention strategies aimed at increasing occupational performance in adults with physical disabilities through modifying the task and/or environment.

One study examined the effect of occupational therapy on BADL, IADL, and quality of life in 43 patients post stroke in an inpatient rehabilitation center in Australia. All patients received specific BADL training, and 79% received specific IADL training. Significant increases were seen in BADL, IADL, and quality of life. Improvement in BADL and IADL was the most common theme in a follow-up interview of participants who demonstrated an increase in quality of life from admission to discharge (Unsworth & Cunningham, 2002). Although this study lacked a control group, it identified an important link between ADL performance and quality of life that warrants further study.

A study of changes in patients' self-care ability following a 1-week rehabilitation stay was conducted with patients with multiple sclerosis (Mathiowetz & Matuska, 1998). Self-care ability was measured on admission, at discharge, and 6 weeks after discharge. Occupational therapy primarily used a compensatory approach, including adaptive equipment and techniques, as well as energy conservation strategies. Self-care ability for all BADL items from initial assessment to discharge increased significantly. Surprisingly, self-care ability continued to improve, and there were also significant improvements between discharge and 6 weeks later for all activities except feeding. This finding may suggest that participants learned to problem solve in the context of ADLs that enabled them to continue progress even after discharge, although other explanations exist, and this hypothesis should be studied further.

Assistive devices and adapted methods reduced the difficulty in doing daily activities by 42% among women aged 29–54 years who had rheumatoid arthritis (Nordenskiold,

Evidence Table 30-1
Best Evidence for Occupational Therapy Practice Regarding ADL

Intervention	Description of Intervention Tested	Participants	Dosage	Type of Best Evidence and Level of Evidence	Benefit	Statistical Probability and Effect Size of Outcome	Reference
Task-specific practice of client-chosen BADL	Practice of specific tasks in a familiar context	403 stroke survivors (189 LCVA, 194 RCVA, 20 other). Mean age = 72.7 years.	Ranged from 1–15 visits over a period of 2 weeks to 5 months.	Meta-analysis of 4 studies.	Yes. The treated groups improved in BADL as measured by varied ADL assessments.	Mean weighted effect size was $r = 0.30$, equivalent to a 30% success rate over control treatment.	Trombly & Ma, 2002
Follow-up OT in the home after rehabilitation.	Home OT visits for review of assistive devices for bathing introduced in hospital.	53 adults with stroke who were discharged home with bathing equipment. Mean age = 72.1 years.	Control and treatment groups got inpatient instruction. Treatment group got 2–3 home visits.	Single-site randomized controlled trial. IB2a	Yes. The treated group improved more in BADL as measured by the *Functional Independence Measure (FIM)* than the control group.	$t(51) = 2.002$; $p = 0.051$; effect size, $r = 0.27$, equivalent to a 27% success rate over control treatment.	Chiu & Man, 2004
Home-based OT	In-home OT to clients with a diagnosis of stroke. "Home" included own home or residential or nursing homes.	965 stroke survivors. Mean age = 70.0 years.	Ranged from 10 sessions to up to 5 months of intervention.	Meta-analysis of 5 studies. Outcome measure focused on IADL.	Yes. The treated group showed small improvement on *Nottingham Extended ADL Scale.*	$Z = 2.97$; $p = 0.0003$; effect size, $r = 0.10$.	Walker et al., 2004
Home-based OT	Control: Conventional outpatient follow-up. Treatment: Conventional follow-up plus 6 weeks of home OT.	138 adults with stroke.	Client-centered intervention. Approximately 10 30- to 45-minute visits over 6 weeks.	Single-site randomized controlled trial. IA2a	Yes. Treated group reported higher performance scores on the *Canadian Occupational Performance Measure.*	Group differences measured with Mann-Whitney U, $p = 0.0006$; $Z = 3.25$; effect size, $r = 0.27$.	Gilbertson & Langhorne, 2000

continued

Evidence Table 30-1 *(continued)*

Intervention	Description of Intervention Tested	Participants	Dosage	Type of Best Evidence and Level of Evidence	Benefit	Statistical Probability and Effect Size of Outcome	Reference
Joint protection educational-behavioral program	Control: Standard program, including education on joint protection. Treatment: Joint protection including strategies to increase adherence.	127 adults with rheumatoid arthritis (<5 years since diagnosis).	Both programs included 4 2-hour weekly meetings.	Two-site randomized controlled trial. IA1a	Yes. At a 48-month follow-up, the treated group had significantly better ADL scores compared with the control group.	Group differences measured with Mann-Whitney *U*, $p = 0.04$; $Z = 1.75$; effect size, $r = 0.15$.	Hammond & Freeman, 2004
Assistive devices and environmental adaptations	Control: Usual care services. Treatment: Comprehensive assessment, prescription, training, and follow-up in assistive devices and home modifications.	104 home-based frail older adults. Mean age = 73 years.	Treatment group received, on average (means), 14.2 devices, 8.9 OT visits, and 2.4 visits from a home-modification technician.	Randomized controlled trial. IA2a	Yes. Although both groups had declined in BADL and IADL at the 18-month follow-up, the treatment group had declined significantly less than the control group in BADL. The difference in IADL was not significant ($p = 0.13$).	BADL, measured by the *FIM*: $F = 7.02$; $p = 0.01$; effect size, $r = 0.17$.	Mann et al., 1999
Service dog	Control: No dog (wait list for 13 months). Treatment: Received service dog 1 month into the study.	48 individuals with severe, chronic ambulatory disabilities requiring wheelchair use. Mean age = 25 years.	Dog training was 6–12 months. Training with participants was not specified.	Randomized controlled trial. IB1a	Yes. Self-reported biweekly hours of both paid and unpaid assistance were significantly less in the treatment group, suggesting more independence in ADL and IADL performance compared with the control group.	Effect of a service dog on assistance was very large: $r = 0.98$ for paid assistance and 0.96 for unpaid assistance.	Allen & Blascovich, 1996

CASE EXAMPLE

A.C.: Adaptation and Training for Basic Activities of Daily Living

Occupational Therapy Intervention Process	Clinical Reasoning Process: Objectives	Clinical Reasoning Process: Examples of Therapist's Internal Dialogue
Patient Information A.C. is a 50-year-old woman who was admitted to an inpatient rehabilitation unit 1 week after a decompression laminectomy with fusion of T5–T6 secondary to a metastatic spinal tumor with resulting paraparesis. The primary tumor was breast cancer, which was diagnosed and treated 3 years ago, and she was cancer free until the spinal tumor. The inpatient OT assessment revealed the following primary problems: (1) minimal to maximal assistance with bathing, dressing, toileting, bowel and bladder management, and transfers; (2) limited reach secondary to spinal orthosis (TLSO), which restricts trunk and hip flexion (worn whenever upright for 8 weeks post-operatively); (3) significant trunk and lower extremity weakness (2–/5), leading to poor sitting balance; (4) persistent pain in the mid-thoracic area; (5) fatigue; and (6) possible depression. A.C. is in a stable and supportive marriage and has 2 teenage children living at home. She works as an elementary school nurse. Her husband works full time. She lives in a 2-story home. All bedrooms are on the second floor. There is a half-bath on the first floor and a full bath on the second. A.C. sought out both Western and complementary health care when treating her breast cancer, including acupuncture and yoga. Her immediate goal is to be able to return home without having to rely heavily on her family for assistance and to be able to cook for her family. Eventually, she wants to return to work.	Appreciate the context	"A.C. has an incomplete spinal cord injury, and it is hard to predict what her sensorimotor function will ultimately be. She will probably be discharged from inpatient rehabilitation within about 3 weeks, though, which means she will almost certainly still be relying on a wheelchair and will be wearing her brace for the first month she is home. Her home has some environmental barriers that will need to be looked at." "Being diagnosed with metastatic cancer after being cancer free for 3 years must be very difficult for A.C. It appears that she might have a reactive depression. I wonder if she is being treated for that. I wonder what her prognosis is. I should remember to look in her chart to find out the tumor grade and check my pathology books for a refresher on prognosis for metastatic cancer. Her active involvement in her prior treatment, such as using alternative treatments, suggests she might be anxious to work collaboratively in the rehab process." "I wonder how her kids and husband are responding to all this. A.C.'s goals suggest that she wants to return some level of 'normalcy' to their family routines as soon as possible."
	Develop intervention hypotheses	"I think that the things interfering most with A.C.'s ability to be independent in BADL are her limited reach (due to brace, lower extremity weakness, and impaired sitting balance), fatigue, and back pain. I am wondering if depression might be exacerbating her pain and fatigue. The home environment also presents some obstacles. A.C.'s background as a nurse will support the rehabilitation process. Her prior routines, which included healthy exercise and yoga, have left her with excellent upper extremity strength that she can use to compensate for her paraparesis. Her family is supportive, and her desire to return to roles as wife and mother seem to be powerful motivators for participation in treatment."
	Select an intervention approach	"At this point, I will primarily rely on an approach that **compensates** for A.C.'s deficits because her inpatient rehabilitation stay will be fairly short and it is important to her to minimize dependence on her family when she returns home. Additionally, it is likely she will be using a wheelchair at discharge, and her home is not currently accessible. **Modifying the physical environment** will require some time and should be started right away. Although fatigue can be approached with a **remediation** approach to increase the physical component, I think that the level of activity required for learning compensatory strategies will be enough to increase activity tolerance without using a rote exercise program."

	Reflect on competence	"I have worked with many patients who are limited by a back brace, but I haven't worked with many who also have paraparesis. I'll need to think more about how to combine methods to help A.C. reach her feet for dressing and bathing that will work with lower extremities that lack functional movement. I'm also not sure how to address the prognosis issue. Is she worried about her life expectancy? Should I invite her to talk about this, or would that be upsetting to her?"
Recommendations The occupational therapist will see A.C. twice a day for 45-minute treatment sessions. The following long-term goals were established for A.C. to reach prior to her discharge home: (1) A.C. will be independent in all BADL except donning shoes and socks and washing feet; (2) A.C. will be independent in sliding board transfers, wheelchair to and from bed, upholstered chair, toilet, transfer tub seat, and car; (3) A.C. will be independent in planning and preparing simple, hot meals with a maximum of a 10 on the *Borg Rating of Perceived Exertion* at the completion of the task; (4) A.C. will be able to access necessary facilities in her home, including bed, toilet, shower, kitchen appliances, and electronics (telephone, computer, TV, etc.); and (5) A.C. will be independent in wheelchair mobility on smooth level surfaces and appropriately graded ramps.	Consider the patient's appraisal of performance	"A.C. seems to have a realistic view of her abilities and limitations. If anything, she seems to underestimate what she can do, for example, she feels she can't do anything herself, but she can feed herself, complete grooming, and bathe her face, arms, and thighs."
	Consider what will occur in therapy, how often, and for how long	"I'm going to bring up the issue of depression in the team meeting. I think she should be evaluated because, if she is clinically depressed, antidepressants might help with pain management and reduce fatigue, which would allow her to participate more actively in treatment. Right now, it is hard to make the most of the 90 minutes I have allotted for treatment each day. In the meantime, I need to make sure I use the right balance of physically challenging tasks and those that rely on more of her cognitive abilities, like making plans to improve the accessibility of her home. That way, I can utilize all the valuable treatment time without over-taxing her."
	Ascertain the patient's endorsement of plan	"A.C. strongly agrees with the goals, although she seems to doubt whether all this can be accomplished in just 3 weeks. Her sense of self-efficacy seems pretty low right now and will need to be addressed in treatment. It might help to also involve her family in this aspect of care so they can help her see her progress, no matter how small the steps seem to be at first."
Summary of Short-Term Goals and Progress 1. A.C. will require minimal assistance to don underwear and pants using adaptive equipment. The therapist thought that donning the elastic stockings that A.C. is required to wear and donning shoes would be very difficult to master while the back brace had to be worn. The therapist explained the challenges these tasks presented, and A.C. agreed that it would be okay to have her husband help with shoes and socks until the brace was removed and she could reach her feet without adaptive equipment. A.C. positioned herself in long sitting, resting against the elevated hospital bed. She was able to use a dressing stick to get her pants over her feet with minimal assistance and verbal cues to increase her effectiveness with the dressing stick. 2. A.C. will be independent in self-catheterization. A.C. couldn't see her urinary meatus because the back brace prevents trunk flexion. She was given a leg abductor with a mirror that enabled her to see.	Assess the patient's comprehension Understand what the patient is doing Compare actual to expected performance Know the person Appreciate the context	"A.C. follows instructions well and remembers strategies that are taught to her (for example, the steps to doing a sliding board transfer), but she still requires help to initiate problem solving. For example, she needed prompting to come up with ways to apply energy conservation principles to a cooking task. Again, this might be related to depression. She was diagnosed with clinical depression and started on medication, but we can't really expect to see a change for 3 weeks or so, and by that time, she'll be home. So, I just continue to use treatment that I hope will be extra motivating. She loves to be able to transfer to the couch with her family where they can sit close on the couch and visit or watch TV without the wheelchair as a barrier between them. She said she was also glad to be able to make a snack for her kids 'just like a mom!'" "A.C. is actually progressing a little faster than I expected with physical tasks such as transfers and lower body dressing. Maybe her experience with the difficult and controlled postures of yoga helps her adapt her movements to her "new" body. She also isn't afraid to experiment with movement and that might be why she progressed so quickly with transfers and maneuvering the dressing stick for lower body dressing. Maybe I can push her a little more with the physical activities, as long as I watch her fatigue level."

3. A.C. will require supervision for sliding board transfers from wheelchair to and from bed and level, firm, upholstered surfaces.

A.C. progressed quickly with sliding board transfers because her upper extremity strength was excellent and helped her both maintain her balance and move her body along the board. The therapist now just provides supervision in case A.C. loses her balance and pitches forward during the transfer. The therapist instructed A.C.'s husband and children how to "guard" A.C. during transfers, which enabled A.C. to transfer onto the couch in the lounge when her family visited.

4. A.C. will prepare brownies from a box mix with verbal cues and stand-by assistance with a maximum of 13 on the *Borg Rating of Perceived Exertion*.

A.C. was instructed in energy conservation techniques prior to the cooking task and identified 3 strategies she could use to reduce the energy demands of the task with 4 verbal cues from the therapist. She used reachers, a rolling cart, and long oven mitts to complete the task. She reported her perceived exertion was a 12. She shared her brownies with her family when they came in later to visit.

5. A.C.'s husband will bring in a layout of the first floor of their home with measurements, as requested by the OT in preparation for home modifications to increase wheelchair accessibility.

Initially, A.C. and her husband preferred to wait on the home modifications, hoping that A.C. might be able to walk with a walker upon discharge. When A.C. got into her second week, they realized that significant changes needed to be made at home, and the husband brought in the requested information. A.C. was especially upset to learn that the bathroom door was 1″ narrower than her wheelchair.

"Funny, I didn't really expect the resistance to bringing in home plans and measures. I guess those kinds of changes drive the reality of A.C.'s disability home for both her and her husband. A.C. seems especially upset about the bathroom. I wonder if her husband or a friend is handy enough to reframe the door so she can get to the toilet. We're also going to have to address the issue of the bed. I think she'd be better off with a hospital bed until the brace is off because it helps with bed mobility and sitting balance for dressing, but this might be a 'hard sell' for both A.C. and her husband."

Next Steps

- Continue to modify short term goals to progress patient toward BADL, mobility, and cooking using adaptive equipment and methods.
- Make preliminary recommendations for home assessment, collaborating with A.C. and her husband to determine the "best" solution and provide a home program to support follow through with recommendations (Fig. 30-25).
- Complete a home visit with A.C. and her husband to examine accessibility and make final recommendations.
- Provide training to husband and children (as appropriate—determined collaboratively with A.C.) in any areas that required assistance or supervision.
- Examine options for home-based occupational therapy and write a referral.

Anticipate present and future patient concerns

Analyze patient's comprehension

Decide if the patient should continue or discontinue therapy and/or return in the future

"I think A.C. will progress well with independence in occupational performance. I expect the home modifications will be a bigger challenge. She wants to be able to access the full bathroom and her bedroom upstairs, but this would require an expensive stairglide, which may be premature (and A.C. has also said she doesn't want 'such an eyesore' in her house). Intellectually, I think A.C. understands the problems. Emotionally, the choices are hard. The temporary 'fixes' make her feel more disabled (changing the living room to her bedroom, replacing the bathroom door with a curtain so she can get to the toilet, etc.). This is an issue that she will continue to deal with after discharge."

"I think home-based therapy would be best for A.C. after discharge. She certainly has a lot of skilled occupational therapy needs because we had little time to address a host of IADLs, as well as work and leisure tasks. She would qualify for home OT because she is home bound. Additionally, it would be helpful to work with her in her actual environment where she might feel more comfortable problem solving. Once she is out of the brace, she'll become more mobile and should switch to outpatient therapy, which might include a driving evaluation and treatment and possibly return to work training."

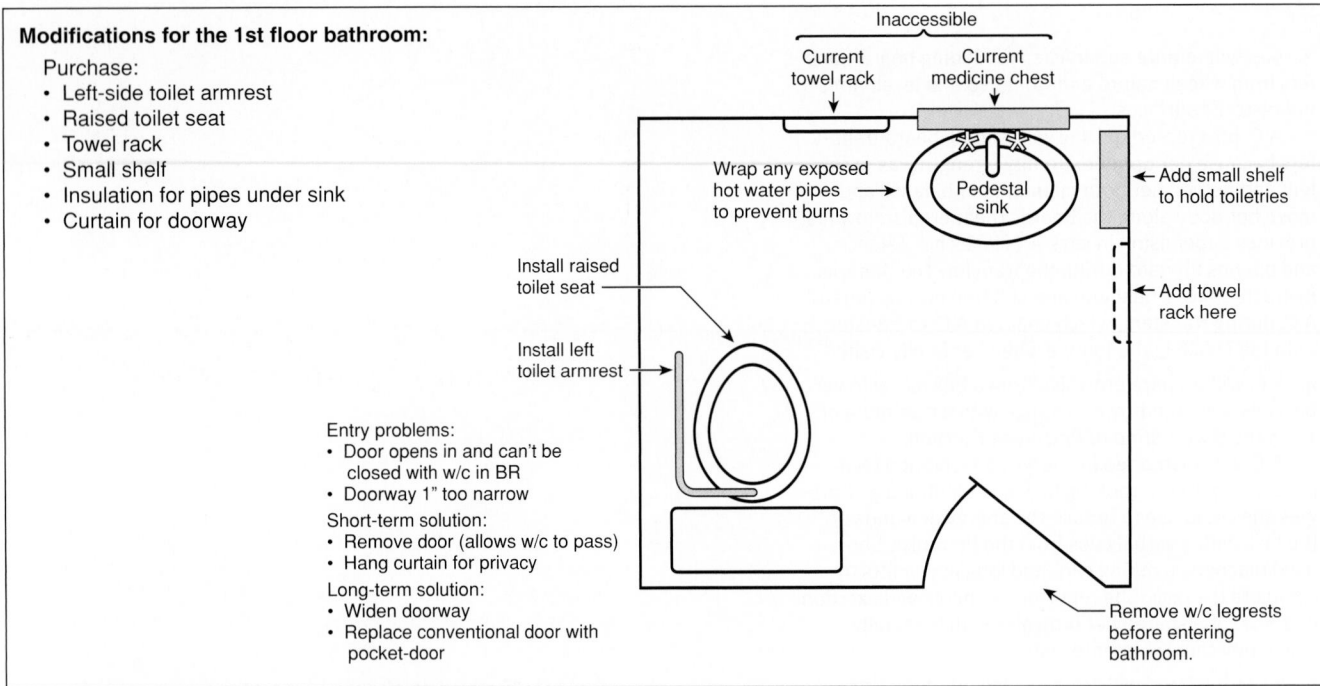

Modifications for the 1st floor bathroom:

Purchase:
- Left-side toilet armrest
- Raised toilet seat
- Towel rack
- Small shelf
- Insulation for pipes under sink
- Curtain for doorway

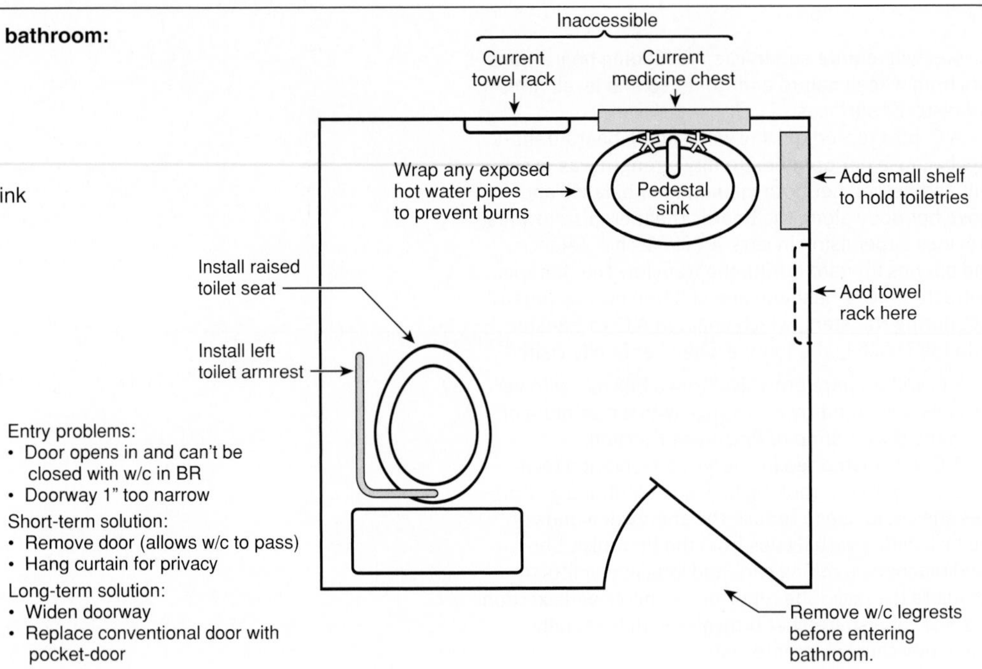
Inaccessible
Current towel rack
Current medicine chest
Wrap any exposed hot water pipes to prevent burns
Pedestal sink
Add small shelf to hold toiletries
Add towel rack here
Install raised toilet seat
Install left toilet armrest
Entry problems:
• Door opens in and can't be closed with w/c in BR
• Doorway 1" too narrow
Short-term solution:
• Remove door (allows w/c to pass)
• Hang curtain for privacy
Long-term solution:
• Widen doorway
• Replace conventional door with pocket-door
Remove w/c legrests before entering bathroom.

Modifications for living room (temporary bedroom for A.C.):

- The existing family room will remain available for visiting, watching TV, etc.
- This arrangement allows A.C. privacy while retaining space for quiet visiting.
- The current plan is for the arrangement to be temporary until it is possible for A.C. to access the 2nd story where her bedroom and full bath is.
- Purchases and modifications:
  - 1 or 2 privacy screens to reduce visability of the bedroom portion of the living room.
  - Empty the existing bookshelf to use for everyday clothing.
  - Bring a nightstand down from the upstairs bedroom.
  - Purchase a touch-lamp for the bedside table.

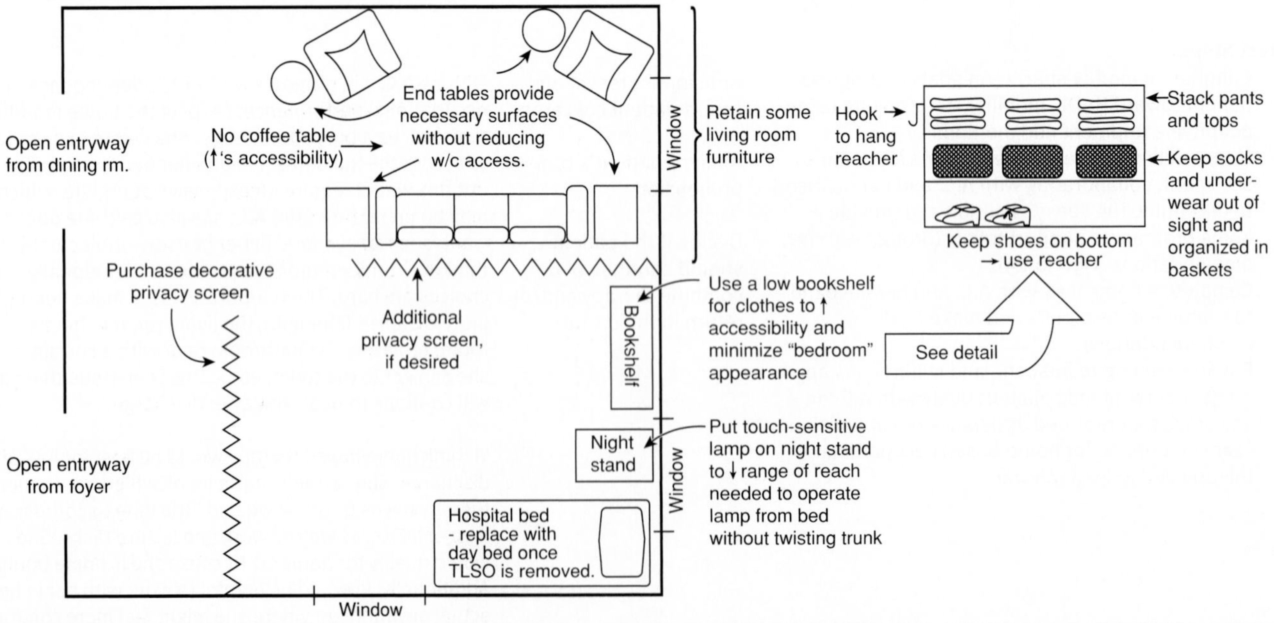
Open entryway from dining rm.
No coffee table (↑'s accessibility)
End tables provide necessary surfaces without reducing w/c access.
Window
Retain some living room furniture
Hook to hang reacher
Stack pants and tops
Keep socks and under-wear out of sight and organized in baskets
Keep shoes on bottom → use reacher
Purchase decorative privacy screen
Additional privacy screen, if desired
Bookshelf
Use a low bookshelf for clothes to ↑ accessibility and minimize "bedroom" appearance
See detail
Open entryway from foyer
Night stand
Put touch-sensitive lamp on night stand to ↓ range of reach needed to operate lamp from bed without twisting trunk
Window
Hospital bed - replace with day bed once TLSO is removed.
Window

Figure 30-25 Home Program for A.C.: Modifications to maximize independence in the home upon discharge.

CLINICAL REASONING IN OCCUPATIONAL THERAPY PRACTICE

Interdisciplinary Treatment in Rehabilitation

During A.C.'s inpatient rehabilitation, the occupational therapist worked as a member of an interdisciplinary team. How would the occupational therapist interact with the following disciplines to facilitate A.C.'s care?

- Physical therapy
- Social work
- Nursing
- Psychology
- Medicine

What avenues of communication might the occupational therapist use?

Grimby, & Dahlin-Ivanoff, 1998). The researchers found that eating, cooking, and toileting were most improved by assistive devices or methods, and dressing, clothes care, cleaning, outdoor mobility, and shopping were least improved. This study suggests that occupational therapists should pay special attention to those ADL least improved by devices when working with patients with rheumatoid arthritis to make sure that their needs are being met.

Shillam, Beeman, and Loshin (1983) used a pre-test/post-test design and found that subjects who participated in occupational therapy, including task-specific training and prescription of assistive devices, had a significant improvement in bathing ability. The greatest barrier to full independence for those who failed to reach independence was the wheelchair to tub transfer. Washing and drying the feet and legs were also problems for many due to limited sitting balance. Additional modifications or practice in transfers and bathing the feet and legs may help to improve outcomes in bathing.

A pre-test/post-test study addressed an occupational therapy program of 12 weeks in which 33 patients in 16 occupational therapy departments were taught strategies to compensate for apraxia during ADL. After statistically controlling for the apraxia score, motor functioning score, and spontaneous recovery, the results indicated large improvements in ADL. Effect sizes were large: $r = 0.75$ for the *Barthel Index;* $r = 0.80$ for ADL observation, and $r = 0.77$ on ADL questionnaire (patient perception) (van Heugten et al., 1998).

In a randomized crossover design, 15 subjects who had trouble dressing at home for 6 months after discharge from hospital post stroke received 3 months of dressing training in the home followed by 3 months of no treatment. Another 15 similar subjects first received no treatment and then received dressing training. Both groups showed significant improvement during the treatment phase, but neither group improved during the no-treatment phase. The group that received treatment during the first 3 months maintained their gains (Walker, Drummond, & Lincoln, 1996). This study is important because it suggests that gains in ADL post stroke can be made many months after the typical rehabilitation period is over.

Consideration of the findings of this research may help occupational therapists develop more effective intervention and provides preliminary evidence that should be studied through more rigorous clinical research.

SUMMARY REVIEW QUESTIONS

1. How is occupation-as-end used to improve occupational functioning?
2. Define and contrast IADL and BADL.
3. What conditions interfere with the patient's ability to learn ADL methods?
4. What principle of compensation is implemented when a patient with limited or restricted range of motion uses a sock aid?
5. What device can enable use of utensils when a patient lacks grasp?
6. What modifications may be necessary to enable a person with C6 tetraplegia to complete the tasks required of a college student majoring in journalism?
7. What principles of compensation are used for problems of incoordination?
8. State the steps a stroke patient can use to put on and remove a cardigan-type garment.
9. Name five energy conservation techniques and give an example of each that could be used by a patient with cardiac disease.
10. Describe how a person with low vision can decorate and arrange the bathroom to facilitate efficient independence.

References

Allen, K., & Blascovich, J. (1996). The value of service dogs for people with severe ambulatory disabilities: A randomized controlled trial. *Journal of the American Medical Association, 275,* 1001–1006.

Ainsworth, B. E., Haskell, W. L., Leon, A. S., Jacobs, D. R., Montoye, H. J., Sallis, J. F., & Paffenbarger, R. S. (1993). Compendium of physical activities: Classification of energy costs of human physical activities. *Medicine and Science in Sports and Exercise, 25,* 71–80.

Ainsworth, B. E., Haskell, W. L., Whitt, M. C., Irwin, M. L., Swartz, A. M., Strath, S. J., O'Brien, W. L., Bassett, D. R., Schmitz, K. H., Emplaincourt, P. O., Jacobs, D. R., & Leon, A. S. (2000). Compendium of physical activities: An update of activity codes and MET intensities. *Medicine and Science in Sports and Exercise, 32,* S498–S504.

American Heart Association. (1999). *Sex and Heart Disease.* Dallas: American Heart Association.

American Heart Association. (2000). *Sex after Stroke.* Dallas: American Heart Association.

American Occupational Therapy Association [AOTA]. (2002). Occupational therapy practice framework: Domain and process. *American Journal of Occupational Therapy, 56,* 609–639.

Arthritis Foundation. (1997). *Gardening and Arthritis.* Atlanta: Arthritis Foundation.

Atwood, S. M., Holm, M. B., & James, A. (1994). Activities of daily living capabilities and values of long-term care facility residents. *American Journal of Occupational Therapy, 48,* 710–716.

Brett, G. (1960). Dressing techniques for the severely involved hemiplegic patient. *American Journal of Occupational Therapy, 14,* 262–264.

Camp, M. M. (2001). The use of service dogs as an adaptive strategy: A qualitative study. *American Journal of Occupational Therapy, 55,* 509–517.

Chen, T.-Y., Mann, W. C., Tomita, M., & Nochajski, S. (2000). Caregiver involvement in the use of assistive devices by frail older persons. *Occupational Therapy Journal of Research, 20,* 179–199.

Chui, C. W. Y., & Man, D. W. K. (2004). The effect of training older adults with stroke to use home-based assistive devices. *The Occupational Therapy Journal of Research: Occupation, Participation, and Health, 24,* 113–120.

Clark, J., & Rugg, S. (2005). The importance of independence in toileting: The views of stroke survivors and their occupational therapists. *British Journal of Occupational Therapy, 68,* 165–171.

Clark, M. C., Czaja, S. J., & Weber, R. A. (1990). Older adults and daily living task profiles. *Human Factors, 32,* 537–549.

Colenbrander, A., & Fletcher, D. C. (1995). Basic concepts and terms for low vision rehabilitation. *American Journal of Occupational Therapy, 49,* 865–869.

Conine, T. A., & Hershler, C. (1991). Effectiveness: A neglected dimension in the assessment of rehabilitation devices and equipment. *International Journal of Rehabilitation Research, 14,* 117–122.

Cristy, D., & Sarafconn, C. A. (1990). *Pacing yourself: Steps to help save your energy.* Bloomington, IL: Cheever.

Dallas, M. J., & White, L. W. (1982). Clothing fasteners for women with arthritis. *American Journal of Occupational Therapy, 36,* 515–518.

Duckworth, B. (1986). Overview of menstrual management for disabled women. *Canadian Journal of Occupational Therapy, 53,* 25–29.

Edmans, J. A., & Lincoln, N. B. (1990). The relationship between perceptual deficits after stroke and independence in activities of daily living. *British Journal of Occupational Therapy, 33,* 139–142.

Fairman, S. K., & Huebner, R. A. (2000). Service dogs: A compensatory resource to improve function. *Occupational Therapy in Health Care, 13,* 41–52.

Finlayson, M., & Havixbeck, K. (1992). A post-discharge study on the use of assistive devices. *Canadian Journal of Occupational Therapy, 59,* 201–207.

Foti, D. (2005). Caring for the person of size. *OT Practice,* 9–13.

Foti, D., & Littrell, E. (2004). Bariatric care: Practical problem solving and interventions. *Physical Disabilities Special Interest Section Quarterly, 27,* 1–3.

Gage, M., & Polatajko, H. (1994). Enhancing occupational performance through an understanding of perceived self-efficacy. *American Journal of Occupational Therapy, 48,* 452–461.

Gagné, D. E., & Hoppes, S. (2003). Brief Report: The effects of collaborative goal-focused occupational therapy on self-care skills: A pilot study. *American Journal of Occupational Therapy, 57,* 215–219.

Gilbertson, L., & Langhorne, P. (2000). Home-based occupational therapy: Stroke patients' satisfaction with occupational performance and service provision. *British Journal of Occupational Therapy, 63,* 464–468.

Giles, G. M., Ridley, J. E., Dill, A., & Frye, S. (1997). A consecutive series of adults with brain injury treated with a washing and dressing retraining program. *American Journal of Occupational Therapy, 51,* 256–266.

Gillen, G. (2000). Case report: Improving activities of daily living performance in an adult with ataxia. *American Journal of Occupational Therapy, 54,* 89–96.

Gitlin, L. N., & Burgh, D. (1995). Issuing assistive devices to older patients in rehabilitation: An exploratory study. *American Journal of Occupational Therapy, 49,* 994–1000.

Goodman, C. C. (2003). The cardiovascular system. In C. C. Goodman, W. G. Boissonnault, & K. S. Fuller (Eds.), *Pathology: Implications for the physical therapist* (2nd ed., pp. 367–476). Philadelphia: Saunders.

Guidetti, S., & Tham, K. (2002). Therapeutic strategies used by occupational therapists in self-care training: A qualitative study. *Occupational Therapy International, 9,* 257–276.

Hage, G. (1988). Makeup board for women with quadriplegia. *American Journal of Occupational Therapy, 42,* 253–255.

Hammond, A., & Freeman, K. (2004). The long-term outcomes from a randomized controlled trial of an educational-behavioural joint protection programme for people with rheumatoid arthritis. *Clinical Rehabilitation, 18,* 520–528.

Hanlon, R. E. (1996). Motor learning following unilateral stroke. *Archives of Physical Medicine and Rehabilitation, 77,* 811–815.

Hermann, R. P., Phalangas, A. C., Mahoney, R. M., & Alexander, M. A. (1999). Powered feeding devices: An evaluation of three models. *Archives of Physical Medicine and Rehabilitation, 80,* 1237–1242.

Herrmann, N., Black, S. E., Lawrence, J., Szekely, C., & Szalai, J. P. (1998). The Sunnybrook stroke study: A prospective study of depressive symptoms and functional outcome. *Stroke, 29,* 618–624.

Holm, M. B., Rogers, J. C., & James, A. B. (2003) Interventions for activities of daily living. In: E. B. Crepeau, E. S. Cohn, & A. A. B. Schell (Eds.), *Willard and Spackman's occupational therapy* (10th ed., pp. 491–533). Philadelphia: Lippincott Williams & Wilkins.

Houtchens, C. J. (1998). A guide to intimacy with arthritis. In: *Arthritis Today.* Atlanta: Arthritis Foundation.

Huck, J., & Bonhotal, B. H. (1997). Fastener systems on apparel for hemiplegic stroke victims. *Applied Ergonomics, 28,* 277–282.

Johansson, R. S., & Westling, G. (1984). Roles of glabrous skin receptors and sensorimotor memory in automatic control of precision grip when lifting rougher or more slippery objects. *Experimental Brain Research, 56,* 550–564.

Kamsma, Y. P. T., Brouwer, W. H., & Lakke, J. P. W. F. (1995). Training of compensational strategies for impaired gross motor skills in Parkinson's disease. *Physiotherapy Theory and Practice, 11,* 209–229.

Katzmann, S., & Mix, C. (1994). Case report: Improving functional independence in a patient with encephalitis through behavior modification shaping techniques. *American Journal of Occupational Therapy, 4,* 259–262.

Kratz, G., Soderback, I., Guidetti, S., Hultling, C., Rykatkin, T., & Soderstrom, M. (1997). Wheelchair users' experience of non-adapted and adapted clothes during sailing, quad rugby, or wheel walking. *Disability and Rehabilitation, 19,* 26–34.

Lampert, J., & Lapolice, D. J. (1995). Functional considerations in evaluation and treatment of the client with low vision. *American Journal of Occupational Therapy, 49,* 885–890.

Lin, E. H. B., Katon, W., Von Korff, M., Tang, L., Williams, J. W., Kroenke, K., Hunkeler, E., Harpole, L., Hegel, M., Arean, P., Hoffing, M., Della Penna, R., Langston, C., & Unutzer, J. (2003). Effect of improving depressive care on pain and functional outcomes among older adults with arthritis: A randomized controlled study. *Journal of the American Medical Association, 290,* 2428–2434.

Lund, M. L., & Nygård, L. (2003). Incorporating or resisting assistive devices: Different approaches to achieving a desired occupational self-image. *The Occupational Therapy Journal of Research: Occupation, Participation, and Health, 23,* 67–75.

Mann, W. C., Hurren, D., Tomita, M., & Charvat, B. (1996). Use of assistive devices for bathing by elderly who are not institutionalized. *Occupational Therapy Journal of Research, 16,* 261–286.

Mann, W. C., Ottenbacher, K. J., Fraas, L., Tomita, M., & Granger, C. V. (1999). Effectiveness of assistive technology and environmental interventions in maintaining independence and reducing home care costs for the frail elderly. *Archives of Family Medicine, 8,* 210–217.

Mathiowetz, V., & Matuska, K. M. (1998). Effectiveness of inpatient rehabilitation on self-care abilities of individuals with multiple sclerosis. *NeuroRehabilitation, 11,* 141–151.

McAlonan, S. (1996). Improving sexual rehabilitation services: The patient's perspective. *American Journal of Occupational Therapy, 50,* 826–834.

McCuaig, M., & Frank, G. (1991). The able self: Adaptive patterns and choices in independent living for a person with cerebral palsy. *American Journal of Occupational Therapy, 45,* 224–234.

McGruder, J., Cors, D., Tiernan, A. M., & Tomlin, G. (2003). Weighted wrist cuffs for tremor reduction during eating in adults with static brain lesions. *American Journal of Occupational Therapy, 57,* 507–516.

McMillen, A.-M., & Söderberg, S. (2002). Disabled persons' experience of dependence on assisted devices. *Scandinavian Journal of Occupational Therapy, 9,* 176–183.

Medline Plus Encyclopedia. (2004). *Clean intermittent self-catheterization.* Retrieved November 6, 2005, from http://www.nlm.nih.gov/medlineplus/print/ency/article/003972.htm.

Migliore, A. (2004). Case report: Improving dyspnea management in three adults with chronic obstructive pulmonary disease. *American Journal of Occupational Therapy, 58,* 639–646.

Mooney, T. G., Cole, T. M., & Chilgren, R. A. (1975). *Sexual Options for Paraplegics and Quadriplegics.* Boston: Little, Brown.

Nordenskiold, U., Grimby, G., & Dahlin-Ivanoff, S. (1998). Questionnaire to evaluate the effects of assistive devices and altered working methods in women with rheumatoid arthritis. *Clinical Rheumatology, 17,* 6–16.

One Shape Serves All (1998). *Modern Maturity, 41,* 28.

Pain, H., & McLellan, D. L. (2003). The relative importance of factors affecting the choice of bathing devices. *British Journal of Occupational Therapy, 66,* 396–401.

Parker, M. G., & Thorslund, M. (1991). Use of technical aids among community-based elderly. *American Journal of Occupational Therapy, 45,* 712–718.

Personal care assistant: Special people for your special care. (1994). *Pushin' On Newsletter, 12.* Retrieved November 6, 2005 from http://www.spinalcord.uab.edu/show.asp?durki=21451

Pinkston, N. E., Boersma, A. M., & Spaulding, S. J. (2005). The impact of reacher length on EMG activity and task. *Canadian Journal of Occupational Therapy, 72,* 89–95.

Poole, J. (1998). Effect of apraxia on the ability to learn one-handed shoe tying. *Occupational Therapy Journal of Research, 18,* 99–104.

Regional Spinal Cord Injury Center of Delaware Valley. (2001). *Spinal cord injury patient-family teaching manual.* Retrieved November 4, 2005 from http://www.spinalcordcenter.org/manual/index.html.

Rice, M. S., Leonard, C., & Carter, M. (1998). Grip strengths and required forces in accessing everyday containers in a normal population. *American Journal of Occupational Therapy, 52,* 621–626.

Rogers, J. C., & Holm, M. B. (1992). Assistive technology device use in patients with rheumatic disease: A literature review. *American Journal of Occupational Therapy, 46,* 120–127.

Rogers, J. C., & Holm, M. B. (2003) Evaluation of areas of occupation: Activities of daily living and instrumental activities of daily living. In: E. B. Crepeau, E. S. Cohn, & A. A. B. Schell (Eds.), *Willard and Spackman's occupational therapy* (10th ed., pp. 315–339). Philadelphia: Lippincott Williams & Wilkins.

Runge, M. (1967). Self dressing techniques for patients with spinal cord injury. *American Journal of Occupational Therapy, 21,* 367–375.

Ryan, P. A., & Sullivan, J. W. (2004). Activities of daily living adaptations: Managing the environment with one-handed techniques. In G. Gillen & A. Burkhardt (Eds.), *Stroke rehabilitation: A function based approach* (2nd ed., pp. 614–632). St. Louis: Mosby

Ryu, J., Cooney, W. P., Askew, L. J., An, K.-N., & Chao, E. Y. S. (1991). Functional ranges of motion of the wrist joint. *Journal of Hand Surgery, 16A,* 409–419.

Salmen, J. P. S. (2000). *The do-able renewable home: Making your home fit your needs.* Washington, DC: American Association of Retired Persons.

Schemm, R. L., & Gitlin, L. N. (1998). How occupational therapists teach older patients to use bathing and dressing devices in rehabilitation. *American Journal of Occupational Therapy, 52,* 276–282.

Schmidt, R. A., & Lee, T. (2000). *Motor control and learning: A behavioral emphasis* (3rd ed.). Champaign, IL: Human Kinetics.

Schwartz, S. M. (1995). Adults with traumatic brain injury: Three case studies of cognitive rehabilitation in a home setting. *American Journal of Occupational Therapy, 49,* 655–667.

Schwarz, P. S. (1997). *250 tips for making life with arthritis easier.* Atlanta: Longstreet Press.

Shillam, L. L., Beeman, C., & Loshin, P. M. (1983). Effect of occupational therapy intervention on bathing independence of disabled persons. *American Journal of Occupational Therapy, 37,* 744–748.

Shotwell, M. P, & Schell, B. A. (1999). Occupational therapy practitioner as health educator: A framework for active learning. *Physical Disabilities Special Interest Section Quarterly, 22,* 1–3.

Skinner, B. F. (1938). *The behavior of organisms.* New York: Appleton-Century-Crofts.

Smith, B. E. (2001). Occupational therapy's role in low vision rehabilitation. *Physical Disabilities Special Interest Section Quarterly, 24,* 1–3.

Spencer, J., Hersch, G., Eschenfelder, V., Fournet, J., & Murray-Gerzik, M. (1999). Outcomes of protocol-based and adaptation-based occupational therapy interventions for low-income elderly persons on a transitional unit. *American Journal of Occupational Therapy, 53,* 159–170.

Spica, M. M., & Schwab, M. D. (1996). Sexual expression after total joint replacement. *Orthopaedic Nursing, 15,* 41–44.

Thomas, J. J. (1999). Enhancing patient education: Addressing the issue of literacy. *Physical Disabilities Special Interest Section Quarterly, 22,* 3–4.

Thoren Jonsson, A.-L., Moller, A., & Grimby, G. (1999). Managing occupations in everyday life to achieve adaptation. *American Journal of Occupational Therapy, 53,* 353–362.

Trombly, C. A. (1993). Anticipating the future: Assessment of occupational function. *American Journal of Occupational Therapy, 47,* 253–259.

Trombly, C. A. (1995). Occupation: Purposefulness and meaningfulness as therapeutic mechanisms: 1995 Eleanor Clarke Slagle Lecture. *American Journal of Occupational Therapy, 49,* 960–972.

Trombly, C. A., & Ma, H. (2002). A synthesis of the effects of occupational therapy for persons with stroke. Part I: Restoration of roles, tasks, and activities. *American Journal of Occupational Therapy, 56,* 250–259

Tyson, R., & Strong, J. (1990). Adaptive equipment: Its effectiveness for people with chronic lower back pain. *Occupational Therapy Journal of Research, 10,* 111–121.

Unsworth, C. A., & Cunningham, D. T. (2002). Examining the evidence base for occupational therapy with clients following stroke. *British Journal of Occupational Therapy, 65,* 21–29.

Valentine, D. P., Kiddoo, M., & LaFleur, B. (1993). Psychosocial implications of service dog ownership for people who have mobility or hearing impairments. *Social Work in Health Care, 19,* 109–125.

van Heugten, C. M., Dekker, J., Deelman, B. G., vanDijk, A. J., Stehmann-Saris, J. C., & Kinebanian, A. (1998). Outcome of strategy training in stroke patients with apraxia: A phase II study. *Clinical Rehabilitation, 12,* 294–303.

van Stralen, G. M. J., Struben, P. J., & van Loon, C. J. M. (2003). The incidence of dislocation after primary total hip arthorplasty using posterior approach with posterior soft tissue repair. *Archives of Orthopedic Trauma Surgery, 123,* 219–222.

Walker, M. F., Drummond, A. E. R., & Lincoln, N. B. (1996). Evaluation of dressing practice for stroke patients after discharge from hospital: A crossover design study. *Clinical Rehabilitation, 10,* 23-31.

Walker, M. F., Leonardi-Bee, J., Bath, P., Langhorne, P., Dewey, M., Corr, S., Drummond, A., Gilbertson, L., Gladman, J. R., Jongbloed, L., Logan, P., & Parker, C. (2004). Individual patient data meta-analysis of ran-

domized controlled trials of community occupational therapy for stroke patients. *Stroke, 35,* 2226–2232.
Walker, M. F., & Lincoln, N. B. (1990). Reacquisition of dressing skills after stroke. *International Disability Studies, 12,* 41–43.
Walker, M. F., & Lincoln, N. B. (1991). Factors influencing dressing performance after stroke. *Journal of Neurology, Neurosurgery, and Psychiatry, 54,* 699–701.
Walker, C. M., & Walker, M. F. (2001). Dressing ability after stroke: A review of the literature. *British Journal of Occupational Therapy, 64,* 449–454.
Weingarden, S. I., & Martin, C. (1989). Independent dressing after spinal cord injury: A functional time evaluation. *Archives of Physical Medicine and Rehabilitation, 70,* 518–519.
Weintraub, D., Moberg, P., Duda, M., Katz, I., & Stern, M. (2004) Effect of psychiatric and other nonmotor symptoms on disability in PD. *Journal of the American Geriatrics Society, 52,* 784–788.
Wielandt, T., McKenna, K., Tooth, L., & Strong, J. (2001). Post discharge use of equipment prescribed by occupational therapists: What lessons to be learned? *Physical and Occupational Therapy in Geriatrics, 19,* 49–65.
Wielandt, T., & Strong, J. (2000). Compliance with prescribed adaptive equipment: A literature review. *British Journal of Occupational Therapy, 63,* 65–75.

Supplemental References

Andrews, K., & Stewart, J. (1979). Stroke recovery: He can but does he? *Rheumatology and Rehabilitation, 18,* 43–48.
Diller, L., Buxbaum, J., & Chiotelis, S. (1972). Relearning motor skills in hemiplegia: Error analysis. *Genetic Psychology Monographs, 85,* 249–286.
Gibson, J. W., & Schkade, J. K. (1997). Occupational adaptation intervention with patients with cerebrovascular accident: A clinical study. *American Journal of Occupational Therapy, 51,* 523–529.
Walker, M. F., Gladman, J. R. F., Lincoln, N. B., Siemonsma, P., & Whiteley, T. (1999). Occupational therapy for stroke patients not admitted to hospital: A randomised controlled trial. *Lancet, 354,* 278–280.

CHAPTER 31

Restoring Mobility

Susan Lanier Pierce

LEARNING OBJECTIVES

After studying this chapter, the reader will be able to do the following:

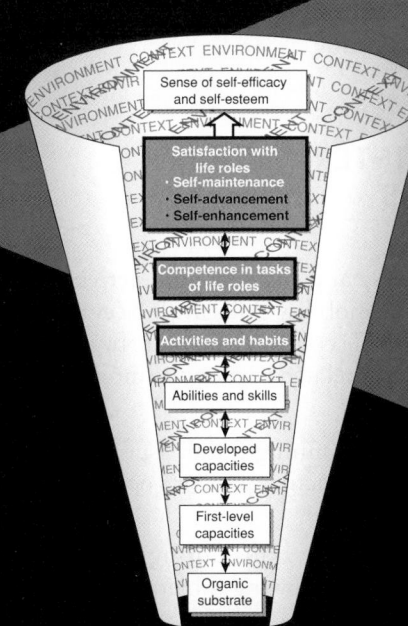

1. Define the terms functional mobility and community mobility and identify issues in each area of mobility that an occupational therapy intervention plan should include.
2. Identify aids and devices used to restore mobility.
3. State the hierarchy of mobility skills used to plan intervention.
4. Describe various transfer techniques and strategies for achieving mobility for persons with physical dysfunction.
5. Describe the roles of the occupational therapy generalist and occupational therapy driver rehabilitation therapist in assisting with community mobility goals.

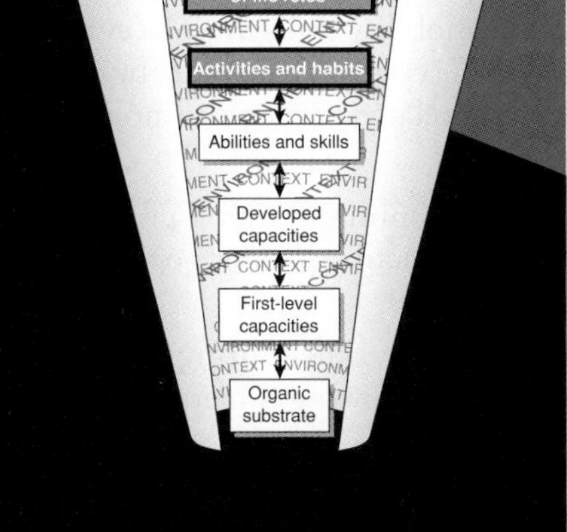

Glossary

Community mobility—"Moving self in the community and using public or private transportation, such as driving, or accessing busses, taxi cabs, or other public transportation systems" (AOTA, 2002, p. 620).

Driver rehabilitation therapist—Allied health professional with advanced knowledge and specialized training, skills, and experience in driver rehabilitation services, including the evaluation and training of persons with disabilities in driving or safe transportation.

Ecological validity—Treatment that reflects a person's actual home and living environment.

Functional mobility—"Moving from one position or place to another (during performance of everyday activities), such as in-bed mobility, wheelchair mobility, transfers (wheelchair, bed, car, tub, toilet, tub/shower, chair, floor). Performing functional ambulation and transporting objects" (AOTA, 2002, p. 620).

Hemiwalker—A one-handed walker with four legs and a wider base than a quad cane. It is held by the strong upper extremity. This device gets its name because it looks like half a walker and is typically used by persons with one-sided weakness, such as those with hemiplegia.

In-home assessment—Objective evaluation of a patient's living environment that takes place at the home. The size of the rooms and doorways, placement of the furniture, and so on are observed and measured (see Chapter 11).

Leg lifter—Device usually made of soft material that a person can use to lift a leg from one place to another or from one surface to another; usually has a large loop on one end that can be placed around one foot or thigh and a loop or handle on the other end.

Mobility—The ability to move about in the home and community.

Quad cane—Straight cane with four short legs in a wide base for stability.

Rope ladder—Ladder device with two long parallel pieces of strapping connected by "rungs." One end of the rope ladder is attached to the foot of the bed. A person pulls up gradually to a sitting position by pulling on the rungs in progression.

Transfer—Movement of one's body from one surface to an adjacent surface. A transfer may be performed independently or with the assistance of one or two persons.

Transfer belt—Wide belt with handles that is wrapped snugly around a client's waist to provide a handhold for another person to pull the client to a standing position and/or to assist the client's balance during transfers or walking.

Transfer board—Device made of hard material, such as wood or fiberglass; placed under the buttocks to bridge the space between two surfaces during transfer.

Wheelchair and occupant restraint system—A crash-tested restraint system for a vehicle that secures a wheelchair and the occupant separately and appropriately for safe transportation.

Wheelchair wheelie—Maneuvering a manual wheelchair onto its rear tires and balancing in this position in order to raise the front casters off the ground.

A person's skill in **mobility** in the home and community can be a key component to the ability to be independent and/or functional in basic and instrumental activities of daily living; therefore, restoring competence in mobility is a key intervention goal for occupational therapy. For persons to participate in the activities and tasks of their life roles, they must be able to move about in their surroundings. This may entail moving around in bed to dress or moving out of bed to go into the bathroom to use the sink or toilet or moving about the community to a workplace, grocery store, theater, or church. During the initial occupational therapy evaluation, the therapist assesses clients' occupational functioning while understanding their occupational role(s) and contextual factors. Initial intervention goals will include mobility in immediate space such as movement in bed, transferring out of bed, and moving onto a treatment mat or onto a toilet. As successful outcomes are obtained in these areas of basic mobility, the intervention plan is reassessed to include more complex mobility skills that enhance basic and instrumental activities of daily living such as moving about the kitchen for cooking or bathroom for personal hygiene and tasks. The occupational therapist may use assistive devices, assistive technology, or compensatory strategies to assist clients to restore their mobility and occupational functioning.

MOBILITY INTERVENTION PRINCIPLES

Mobility affects all basic and instrumental activities of daily living and, as such, mobility skills must be evaluated and treated throughout the continuum of care by occupational therapy. Guidelines related to mobility intervention include:

- Consider intervention planning for all aspects of mobility that influence a particular patient's occupational functioning
- Improve a client's mobility skills during activities of daily living training by following a hierarchy of skill building

- Understand how performance in mobility is influenced by a client's contextual factors
- Be knowledgeable about adaptations and compensatory strategies to enhance mobility skills
- Co-plan with other disciplines or specialists in the total care plan for successful outcomes for individual mobility goals.

Definitions of Mobility

The Occupational Therapy Practice Framework defines two areas of mobility: **Functional Mobility** and **Community Mobility**. Functional mobility is "moving from one position or place to another (during performance of everyday activities), such as in-bed mobility, wheelchair mobility, transfers (wheelchair, bed, car, tub, toilet, tub/shower, chair, floor), performing functional ambulation and transporting objects" (AOTA, 2002, p. 620). Community mobility is "moving self in the community and using public or private transportation, such as driving, or accessing buses, taxi cabs, or other public transportation systems" (AOTA, 2002, p. 620) Both aspects of mobility must be addressed by occupational therapy throughout the evaluation and intervention process.

Each area of mobility requires a certain skill level. Accomplishment in each area of mobility builds a foundation of skills for the next higher level of mobility; therefore, a hierarchy of skills guides the order in which each area of mobility is addressed. Mobility needed in basic activities of daily living (BADL) is followed by mobility needed in instrumental activities of daily living (IADL) (Fig. 31-1). Occupational therapy goals for performance skills and for mobility must be achieved prior to intervention training in BADL. For example, the person with quadriplegia must be able to maneuver his or her body in bed for changing postures and/or sitting up before learning to dress in bed. A person learns to sit on a hard surface without support, such as a mat, before sitting on a soft surface, such as a bed, in order to learn to transfer to and from the bed.

Transfers to bed must be mastered before transfers to a car. A car transfer is more difficult because the wheelchair seat height is different from the car seat height and there is a space gap between the two seats. The client must handle his legs through the cramped space of a car door. Since the task demands for driving are higher than for any other IADL, driving should be the last IADL addressed; however, training and practice in mat, bed, and toilet transfers prepares the person for car transfers.

Every mobility task requires a certain amount of strength, coordination, and range of motion, as well as visual and cognitive abilities. A patient may have more than one area of deficit in occupational functioning that may hinder mobility functioning. A person with rheumatoid arthritis may have range of motion deficits as well as

DRIVING
↑
CAR TRANSFER
↑
TOILET & TUB TRANSFERS
↑
BED TRANSFERS
↑
MAT TRANSFERS
↑
BED MOBILITY

Figure 31-1 Hierarchy of mobility skills illustrates the order of accomplishing mobility skills.

weakness and problems with fatigue. A person with a spinal cord injury may have decreased sensation as well as paralysis or weakness. A person who has had a stroke or traumatic brain injury may have physical as well as visual and cognitive deficits that must be carefully considered in the more complex areas of mobility needed for instrumental activities of daily living.

Mobility Intervention Is Individualized

Each patient has unique methods of doing activities of daily living (ADL); therefore, customization of techniques and equipment is necessary. With a patient- or client-centered approach, the person must have input into the intervention plan for the outcomes in mobility to be successful. The therapist must be an active listener to the patient's thoughts and opinions and be willing to modify techniques and strategies as needed.

Occupational performance skill deficits may affect mobility differently in particular environments of the individual, so the therapist must consider the patient's mobility skills and activities in all relevant environments. For example, one person who has had a stroke may require a wheelchair outside the home but be able to get around at home with the assistance of an orthotic device such as a cane, whereas another requires the wheelchair both in and out of the house.

Strive for Ecological Validity

The first phase of training in functional mobility takes place in the accessible environment of the therapy clinic.

The second phase addresses functional mobility in the patient's home, and the third phase addresses community mobility in the patient's own environment. The occupational therapist should strive for **ecological validity** throughout the intervention process, which means that the intervention and final outcome take into consideration the actual environment to which the patient will be returning. The environment includes the home, yard, and community where the person lives, shops, works, plays, and/or goes to school or other public places.

Assessment of patients' personal environments must be made so that realistic training in the second phase can take place. The training can first use the mock environment of the therapy clinic or simulated environments. Once the therapist is familiar with the client's home and community, they can seek environments in or around the treatment facility that best simulate these environments. A comprehensive **in-home assessment** is crucial for discharge planning (see Chapter 11). The patient's real world may not consist of the level floors, low-pile carpet, easy curb cuts, or nicely ramped entrances of rehabilitation facilities. The outdoor terrain may be soft dirt, sand, or bumpy grass. Wheelchair maneuverability in the home may be through narrow hallways and doorways. The patient may have to transfer onto a waterbed or soft mattress rather than the adjustable-height surface of a firm hospital bed. There may not be a roll-in shower, so the patient may have to learn to use a regular tub with a tub bench. Even if the patient will be discharged to an assisted-living environment, maximum independence in mobility for that environment should be sought. Whether the patient can walk or use a wheelchair and has an ideal situation or not, it is crucial to know the real-world environment for that person so the intervention plan for mobility and the final outcomes will be of real value and meaning to the patient.

Because inpatient rehabilitation is so brief, the level of mobility an inpatient achieves on discharge may not be the same level that the person can achieve 6 or 8 months post discharge. The inpatient therapist should plan long-term post-discharge goals for mobility with the patient and the family so that he or she can work on continued goals for maximum independence and mobility after discharge as an inpatient. Independence in community mobility will more than likely be achieved during or even after outpatient rehabilitation and intervention. Educating the client and family of this fact will prevent the client from becoming discouraged and empower the family to assist in transportation until the client is ready to tackle the goal of returning to driving.

Interdisciplinary Team Approach

Teamwork between occupational therapy and physical therapy is important for intervention planning in mobility so that the two disciplines can share a vision of how each other's treatment relates to planning for future goals in functional and community mobility. Communication between team members eliminates unnecessary duplication and promotes carryover of skills. The direction the occupational therapist takes in pursuing BADL should be influenced by the patient's achievements in physical therapy with lower extremity functioning and ambulation. Conversely, independence in bed mobility achieved in occupational therapy may influence balance and transfer training in physical therapy.

Achievement of physical therapy goals that are precursor skills for mobility training may take several weeks, so during this time, the occupational therapist works on BADL that do not demand a high level of lower extremity strength, trunk balance, and endurance. For example, a patient who will walk first learns to brush her teeth and wash dishes sitting down. When the patient has achieved standing tolerance and balance in physical therapy, the occupational therapist can incorporate standing in activities such as brushing teeth and washing dishes while standing at a sink. When it is determined that the patient will be using a wheelchair, the occupational therapist works on propelling a wheelchair and performing activities from the chair, such as dressing and cooking. If the patient will be a functional but limited walker with an orthotic device, the occupational therapist must incorporate the device into the BADL and IADL intervention goals, including functional and community mobility. For example, a person who uses a cane has to learn to maneuver in the kitchen with this device while cooking.

Intervention planning for community mobility requires the occupational therapist to seek the expertise of a **driver rehabilitation therapist** in order to complete the final outcome for community mobility goals. These experts have advanced knowledge and skill in driving and community mobility, have an allied health background to understand diagnosis and implications, and are able to provide specific evaluation and intervention services for driver evaluation, driver rehabilitation, driver training, assessment for use of community mobility alternatives, and safe transportation. These experts may be on staff in the inpatient or outpatient facility or may be found in private practice.

FUNCTIONAL MOBILITY INTERVENTION PLANNING AND TREATMENT

This section will discuss areas of functional mobility and describe strategies, methods, and adaptive equipment suggested by therapists and former patients that can be used in restoring functional mobility for persons with a variety of performance skill deficits. The occupational therapist would assess and develop an intervention plan for the following areas of functional mobility:

- Bed mobility
- Wheelchair mobility including wheelchair propulsion
- Transfer methods for the person who is ambulatory, has limited ambulation, or is non-ambulatory
- Functional ambulation with or without orthotic devices

Bed Mobility

Bed mobility is the ability to roll from side to side, to roll over from supine to prone position, to sit up in bed, and to handle the upper and lower extremities during these maneuvers. These skills are necessary for dressing in bed, transferring in and out of bed, or changing positions for sleep. Gillen and Burkhardt (1998) suggest that one of the most common movement strategies in rolling from supine to prone is a lift and reach pattern. To begin rolling over, the person throws the arms in the direction he or she wants the body to go. Because of momentum, the upper trunk, hips, and legs follow.

A person with paralysis in the lower extremities and trunk may need a device to pull on in order to turn over. Examples are a **rope ladder**, an overhead trapeze, a bed rail, or a wheelchair positioned near the bedside. The first three devices mentioned are designed specifically to give a person something to grasp with the hand(s) or forearm(s) to assist in pulling to a seated position in a long- or short-leg position in bed (Fig. 31-2). Good scapular, shoulder, and elbow strength is the minimum requirement for using these devices. Wrist flexion and extension and hand grasping capability are helpful in using these devices.

The rope ladder (Fig. 31-2A) is two long parallel pieces of strapping connected by "rungs." One end of the ladder is attached to the foot of the bed. The person pulls up gradually using each rung in progression until he is at the desired sitting level. The overhead trapeze bar can assist a person in rolling over or in coming to a long-leg seated position. The various configurations of bedrails can assist a person in rolling over, in getting positioned for sleep or in coming to a short-legged seated position on the side of the bed. A person can also use a wheelchair by grasping the armrest or push handles to pull against if the wheelchair is close to the bed with the brakes locked. A person with weak grasp can use the same devices by hooking the forearm or extended wrist around the device handle or a part of the wheelchair.

For rolling, the person first holds the bedrail or wheelchair part with the arm closest to the side of the bed toward which he is rolling. The momentum for rolling the upper trunk is gained by flinging the other arm across the body and grasping the device or wheelchair part with that extremity. Pulling with both arms should now turn the hips and legs. If not, the person can use an extended wrist or hand to push the knee or thigh to get the leg moving. A **leg lifter** is a device for moving one leg at time. This device has a large loop at one end that can be placed around the foot or thigh and a smaller loop or handle at the other end that a person can grasp to pull or lift a leg with (Fig. 31-2B). The leg lifter works well for persons who have hip flexion limitations that limit their ability to reach their legs or persons who have balance difficulties when in a long-leg sitting position and must maintain their balance by using one upper extremity. A hospital bed with powered head and knee controls can also assist a person with bed mobility and can be helpful for lower extremity dressing in bed. By raising the head and upper trunk, both hands are freed from holding one's balance to perform the task at hand. Internal contextual factors may influence this choice because not every patient can afford a hospital bed or chooses to use a hospital bed once home.

Figure 31-3 illustrates the sequence a person with C7 quadriplegia uses for bed mobility without the use of orthotic devices. Good strength in the deltoid, pectoralis major and minor, biceps, wrist extensors, and scapula muscles is key, so strengthening these muscle groups in therapy is preparatory to learning this technique. Even without trunk muscles, a sense of balance is important and must be developed prior to performing this technique.

A person who cannot perform bed mobility tasks requires one or two persons to assist with rolling the upper and lower body in the proper sequence or using a log roll technique that moves the entire body at once. Figure 31-4 shows a person with incomplete quadriplegia and proximal weakness in the shoulders and hips performing bed mobility tasks with the assistance of his wife. Figure 31-5 shows mechanical and powered devices that assist the caregiver in moving a dependent person into or out of bed. The mechanical and hydraulic lifts can be on a movable frame, on a freestanding frame that hangs over the bed, or on a moving track that runs on the ceiling. Some lift systems can move the person from one room to another.

The occupational therapist must assess sitting balance for bed mobility and activities of daily living. Balance in long- and short-leg sitting should be assessed. Long-leg sitting is the posture in which the legs are extended straight out in front of the person on a flat surface and the hips are flexed to at least 90°. A position beyond 90° of hip flexion must be achieved to maintain balance in a long-leg sitting position when trunk and hip musculature are weak. Short-leg sitting is the posture in which a person sits with the hips flexed at least to 90° and the knees are flexed over the edge of the surface. The feet may or may not touch the floor, but stability is aided if they do.

Achieving sitting balance on a flat, hard mat precedes working on balance on a soft bed mattress. Upper extremity activities, such as throwing and catching a large ball, can be used to challenge the patient's balance. Balance improves either because weak trunk muscles get stronger or because

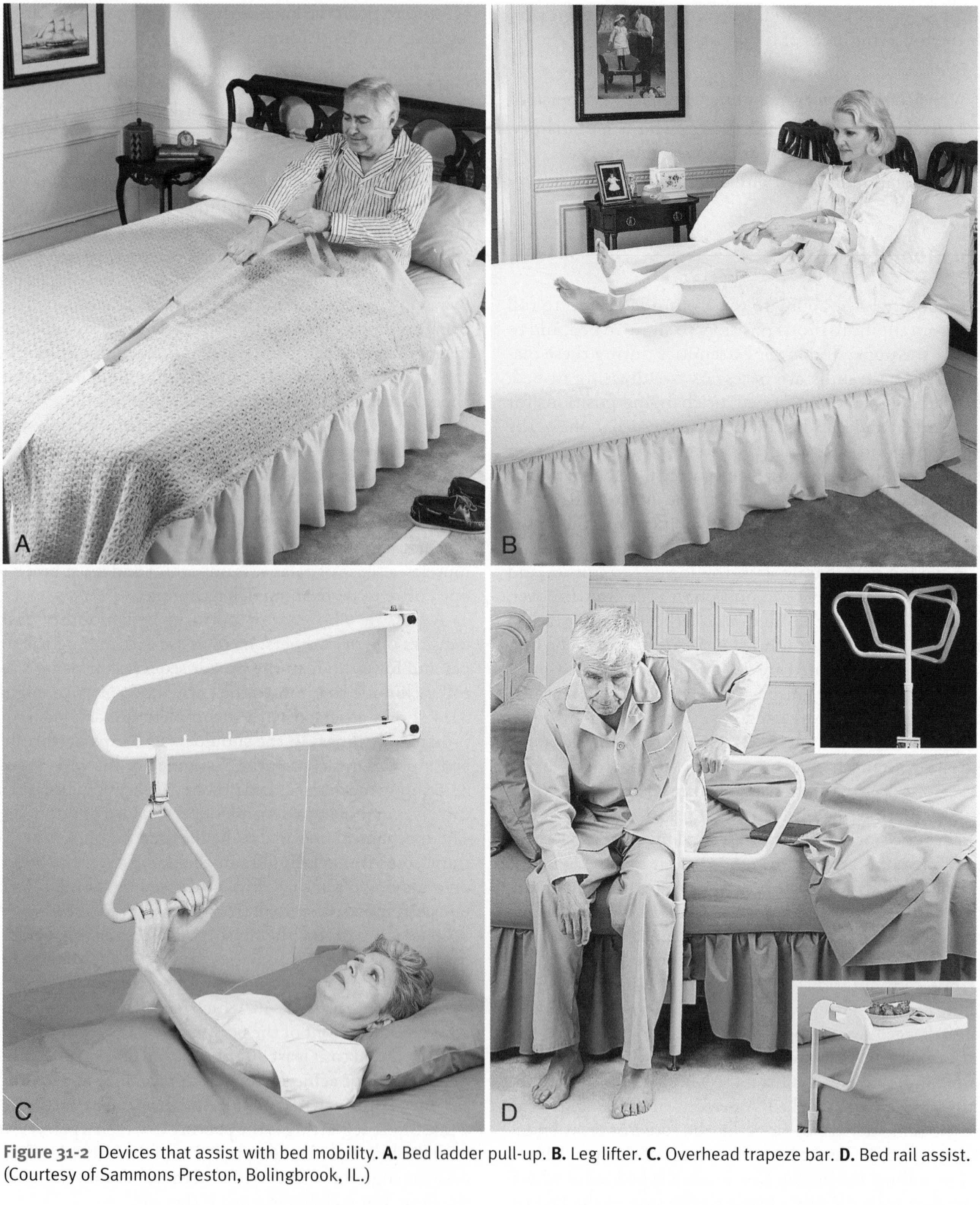

Figure 31-2 Devices that assist with bed mobility. **A.** Bed ladder pull-up. **B.** Leg lifter. **C.** Overhead trapeze bar. **D.** Bed rail assist. (Courtesy of Sammons Preston, Bolingbrook, IL.)

the patient learns to balance by lowering the center of gravity and using the neck muscles to right the body. ***While the person is working on improving balance on the mat or in bed, the therapist must maintain close supervision and contact and be ready to catch the person if balance is lost in any direction.***

A person who has good trunk balance may wish to dress while sitting on the edge of the bed. If the lower extremities are paralyzed, the person must manually move the legs over the side of the bed. For the dependent person, another individual swings the person's legs off the edge of the bed.

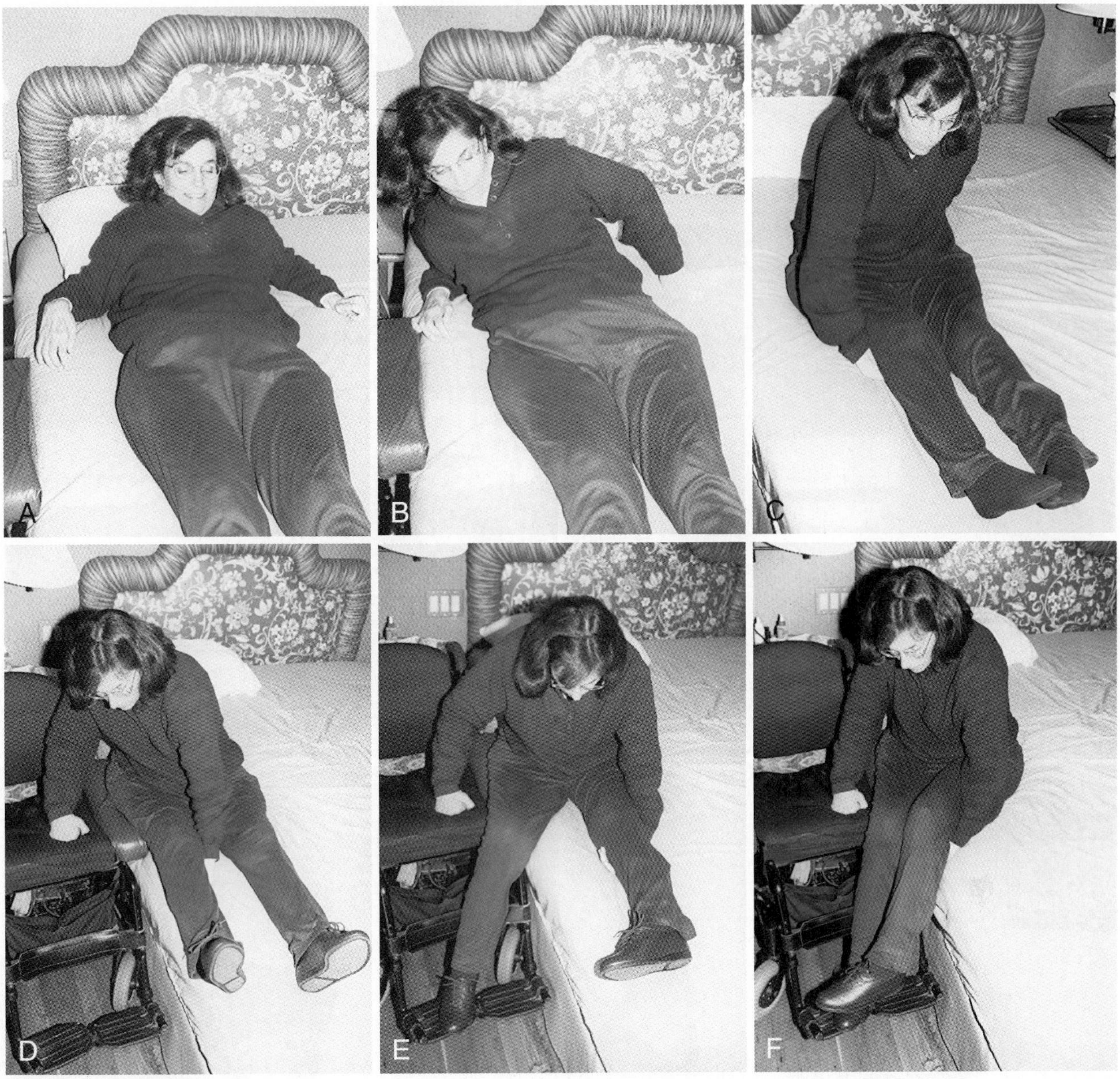

Figure 31-3 A person with C7 quadriplegia illustrates the steps for coming to a sitting position in bed without the use of assistive devices. **A.** The woman uses shoulder and scapula muscles to move to resting on elbows. **B.** She uses the triceps in one arm to lift her upper trunk while balancing on the other bent elbow. Using the triceps in the bent arm, she pushes the whole trunk upright until she is in the long-leg sitting position. **C.** She can hold her balance with one arm behind her while using the other arm to reposition the legs as needed. **D.** Once she is close to the edge of the bed, she can lean on one arm, which is pressing into the wheelchair seat, to hold her balance while she moves the outside leg off the side of the bed. **E.** She then moves the inside leg off the side of the bed. **F.** Now, in a short-legged sitting position, she can prepare for a sliding transfer into her wheelchair.

Performing Activities of Daily Living in Bed

Persons with lower extremity or trunk paralysis may need to perform dressing, skin inspection, self-catheterization, and/or a bowel program while in bed. While dressing in bed, it is necessary to reach one's feet by flexing the hips and knees so that the feet are closer to the hands for preparing to don pants, socks, and/or shoes. Independence in rolling from side to side and reaching one's buttocks are important for performing manual bowel stimulation and clean up or using a long-handled mirror for inspecting potential pressure sore areas.

Wheelchair Mobility

For a person who cannot walk or has limited walking ability, a wheelchair can assist with necessary mobility in and

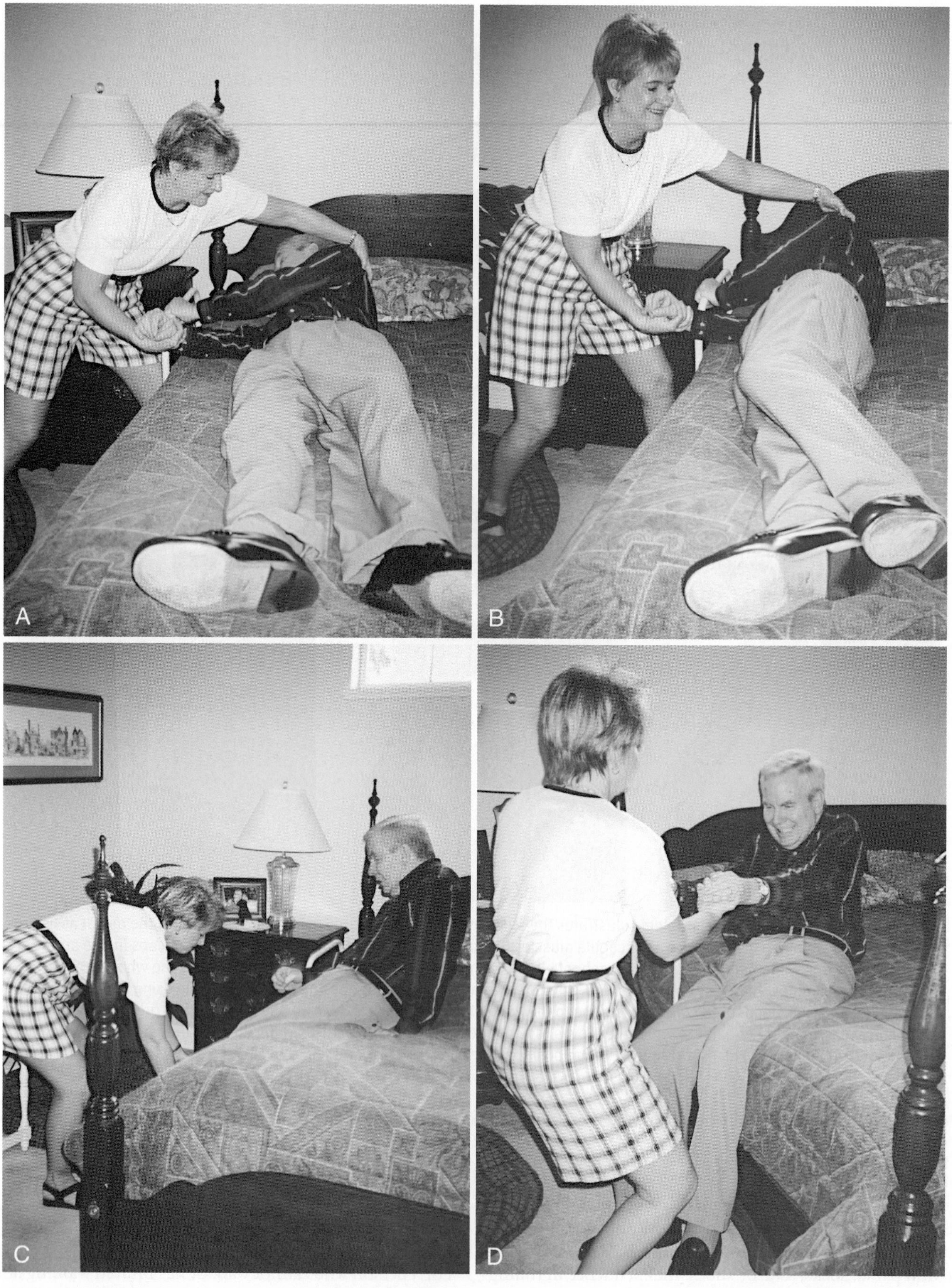
A
B
C
D

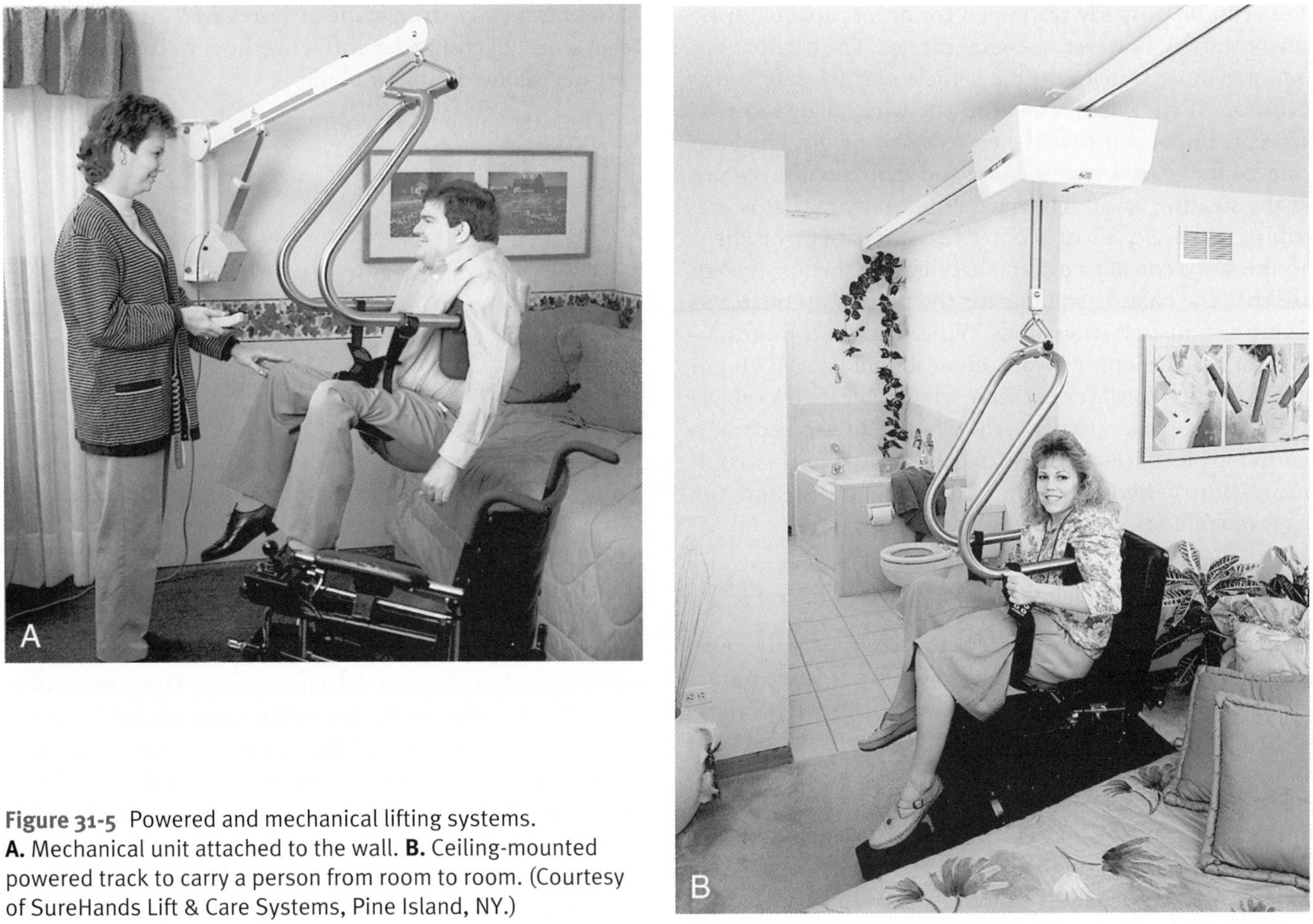

Figure 31-5 Powered and mechanical lifting systems. **A.** Mechanical unit attached to the wall. **B.** Ceiling-mounted powered track to carry a person from room to room. (Courtesy of SureHands Lift & Care Systems, Pine Island, NY.)

outside the home. A manual wheelchair is appropriate for a person who can propel the wheelchair using two arms, one arm, the feet, or a foot and an arm together. A powered wheelchair or motorized scooter is appropriate for the person who does not have the physical capability to propel a manual chair or has limited walking due to low physical endurance or lower extremity weakness. The scooter is popular with individuals with multiple sclerosis or cerebral palsy or the well elderly who have limited capacity for long-distance walking. Personal requirements for a scooter are the ability to transfer, good trunk balance, and an ability to maintain an upright posture with little support. There are persons who are totally dependent and unable to operate a power wheelchair who will require a manual wheelchair that will be propelled by another person. There are many models and styles of wheelchairs and scooters with a variety of standard and optional features from which to choose (see Chapter 18).

The patient's home and community must be considered when assisting him or her in choosing the most appropriate wheelchair. For example, a person who lives in a rural environment with sandy or grassy terrain may require a four-wheel scooter or a more powerful motor on a powered wheelchair. Of great importance in wheelchair selection is the client's means of vehicle transportation. If the person can transfer or will be dependently transferred into a vehicle, then the wheelchair or scooter must break down and fit into the vehicle or onto an appropriate carrier. If the person will use the wheelchair or scooter to ride on while entering a vehicle on a lift or ramp, then it must be determined whether the person can transfer onto another vehicle seat while being transported. Most manual or power wheel-

Figure 31-4 A wife assists her husband in bed mobility. **A.** Using proper body mechanics, the wife assists her husband to roll over by first pulling his left shoulder toward her. **B.** The husband can assist by using his hip and knee flexors and pulling against the half bed rail. **C.** The wife swings his legs off the bed and lowers his feet to the floor while the husband uses the stronger left arm to push against the bed to hold his balance in a half-sitting position. **D.** Again, using proper body mechanics and allowing her legs and arms to do the work, the wife helps her husband come to a full sitting position.

chairs can be properly restrained for an occupant during transportation; however, a scooter cannot. The occupant of a scooter must transfer into a vehicle seat for safe transportation. If the client will sit in the wheelchair to drive, then it is important that the correct seat height has been achieved for good driver visibility and for maneuvering under the steering wheel. The rehabilitation team that is prescribing a wheelchair or scooter for any patient or client should *always* consult a driver rehabilitation therapist to ensure that the chair is suitable for the person's vehicle and driving or transportation needs. "Wheelchairs promote mobility for many people who are physically challenged. But in attempting to interface that same wheelchair with a vehicle to enable the person to drive, the wheelchair can become a stumbling block" (Pierce, 1992, p. 20). To prevent this, communication between the prescribing therapist and the driver rehabilitation therapist is paramount.

Intervention for Wheelchair Mobility

Environmental and/or architectural barriers will most likely affect a person's wheelchair mobility at some point, and he or she should be taught to deal with such barriers. When a patient receives a new wheelchair, indoor and outdoor mobility training is important so that he or she learns to handle and maneuver the chair in whatever circumstances he or she may encounter, such as tight spaces, a curb or ramp, and rough and uneven terrain. A program graded toward independent mobility should be a team effort among the physical, occupational, and recreational therapists, with the practice of skills incorporated into all rehabilitation activities. For example, the occupational therapist may take the person to the grocery store to shop for food in preparation for cooking a meal during therapy. This experience gives the person an opportunity to explore wheelchair mobility in this environment while also carrying items or pushing a shopping cart.

The initial stages of wheelchair training take place inside the rehabilitation facility. In the first phase, the patient learns how to propel the wheelchair on a smooth, uncluttered surface. The patient learns to manipulate the wheelchair and all of the removable parts as well as how to transfer in and out of the wheelchair. The second phase is learning to use the wheelchair outside. The patient learns to maneuver on various terrains, such as uneven sidewalks, gravel, and sand. Then the patient learns to negotiate obstacles such as curbs and steps. Once the patient can traverse outdoor surfaces, public buildings, such as grocery stores and shopping malls, can be used to teach the person to handle the wheelchair in crowded, narrow spaces.

Negotiating Ramps

A ramp enables a person using a wheelchair to overcome steps or a height discrepancy in a doorway or entrance. Ramps come in many shapes, sizes, and dimensions. Ramps can be custom built or purchased and assembled from a kit. Factors that influence how well a wheelchair user negotiates a ramp include:

- The user's upper extremity strength and coordination, including grip strength
- The user's trunk balance
- The length and slope of the ramp
- The surface of the ramp (non-slip vs. slippery)
- The stability of the wheelchair (may require anti-tipping wheels)
- The need for hillclimbers or grade-aids on the wheelchair to prevent the chair from rolling backwards

Federal guidelines specify how ramps in public places should be constructed in terms of length, slope, texture, and so on. For example, for every inch of rise, the ramp must have 12 inches of length (1:12 slope). To overcome a 4-inch step, the ramp must be 48 inches long. A ramp in a public place must have a surface with a detectable texture for persons with visual impairments. It must have sides that are not vertical but slope at 1:10 maximum. There must be 4 feet of level landing at the top of the ramp (Americans with Disabilities Act [ADA], 1990). For private construction, a ramp that is longer and therefore has less slope (1:20) is more satisfactory for a person who uses a manual wheelchair and has upper extremity weakness because it is easier for that person to propel up or down the ramp.

The popular minivan conversions for wheelchair users with the 10-inch lowered floor modifications have ramps measuring 53 inches long by 29 inches wide for entering and exiting the vehicle. Before a person in a manual wheelchair purchases this type of vehicle, particularly for independent driving, his or her ability to ascend and descend the ramp safely should be evaluated (Fig. 31-6). This task is much more difficult than it first

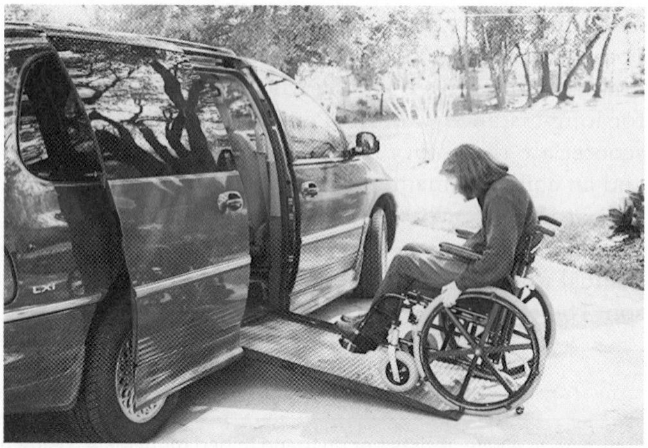

Figure 31-6 A person with quadriplegia in a manual wheelchair attempts to push up the ramp into a minivan whose floor has been lowered 10 inches. This task is easy in a powered wheelchair but difficult in a manual wheelchair.

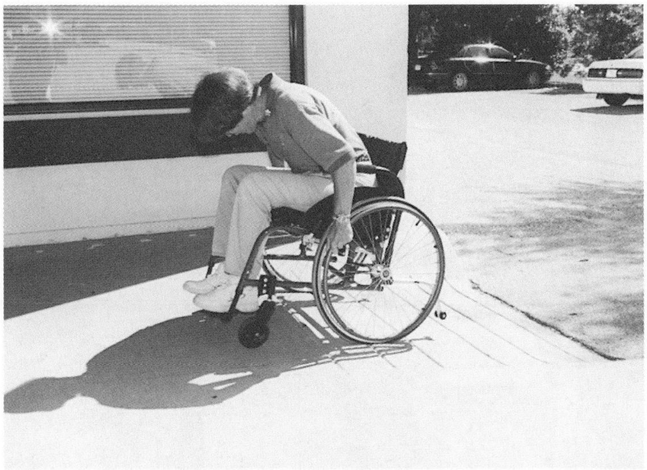

Figure 31-7 A therapist demonstrates how a person with good arm and trunk strength can safely negotiate a steep ramp by moving backward down the ramp. Leaning forward to shift the center of gravity prevents the chair from tipping backwards.

may appear because of the short ramp length and the steep slope. Upper extremity strength, good hand power, and trunk mobility and balance are necessary for safety of a manual wheelchair user while descending or ascending a minivan ramp.

One safe technique to use in descending any steep ramp is to orient the chair backward and lean forward to place most of the weight over the front caster wheels as the chair slowly descends the ramp (Fig. 31-7). If the wheelchair has a tendency to tip backward easily, a helper should stand behind the wheelchair and walk with the person to catch the chair should it begin to tip backward.

Wheelchair Wheelie

An advanced manual wheelchair skill called a **wheelchair wheelie** can be used to elevate the caster wheels so that objects on the floor, sidewalk, or ground can be cleared or a curb or step can be managed (Pierson, 1999). For this complex task, a person must have the following:

- Good basic wheelchair skills
- Upper extremity strength
- Good hand function with a strong grip
- Bilateral upper extremity coordination
- Understanding of the steps to perform the task and the safety issues involved
- Ability to maintain dynamic balance while performing this task

The patient must practice the wheelchair wheelie many times on level surfaces before attempting curbs and steps. In the clinic, a mat can be placed behind the wheelchair or the therapist can stand behind the chair ready to catch the wheelchair should it tip too far backward. ***Because of the danger of losing balance and falling backward, the therapist must be attentive and within close proximity of the wheelchair when the patient is practicing this advanced skill.*** A length of rope attached to the push handles and running through a ceiling pulley can also be used to protect the person from falling and allow him or her to practice without a person behind him (Nixon, 1985).

The first step in performing a wheelie is to grasp the front portion of the wheel rims and quickly pull back equally on both hand rims. This places the hands in a rearward position on the hand rims. Another quick forward thrust on the wheels and then an abrupt stop rotates the chair frame backward with the rear axle acting as a fulcrum. The caster wheels rise, and the wheelchair balances on the rear wheels only. Small movements of the rear wheels control the balance of the chair (Deusterhaus-Minor & Deusterhaus-Minor, 1999).

Negotiating Curbs

In today's world and particularly since passage of the ADA in 1990, curbs on sidewalks at street intersections are becoming less of a problem as curb cuts proliferate. At times, however, the wheelchair user still has to negotiate a curb. Although some power wheelchairs can negotiate curbs well, ascending and descending a curb or step in a manual wheelchair will require good wheelchair skills. Usually the person who can perform a wheelchair wheelie independently can use that same technique for jumping over a curb or step. First the person approaches the curb or step, facing it. Once the wheelie position has been obtained, the casters are placed on the curb. The person leans forward to balance the chair and redistribute the weight and propels the large rear wheels up the curb or step with a hearty push. A person must have good balance and hand function to perform this maneuver.

To go down a curb or a step, the person approaches it backward, leans forward in the chair, and rolls the rear wheels over the step or curb. An alternative method for going down a curb is to approach the curb facing it, move into the wheelie position, and roll off the curb using the back wheels. The person must have an excellent sense of balance and control to perform this technique safely.

If a wheelchair user cannot move up or down a curb or step or roll through grass or over uneven surfaces, another person can provide assistance. In an assisted wheelchair wheelie, the helper pushes the wheelchair once the wheelchair is in the wheelie position (Fig. 31-8).

Negotiating Steps

Ascending or descending multiple steps in a scooter or power wheelchair is impossible except for a newly designed power wheelchair that is designed specifically for climbing stairs. A strong manual wheelchair user may be

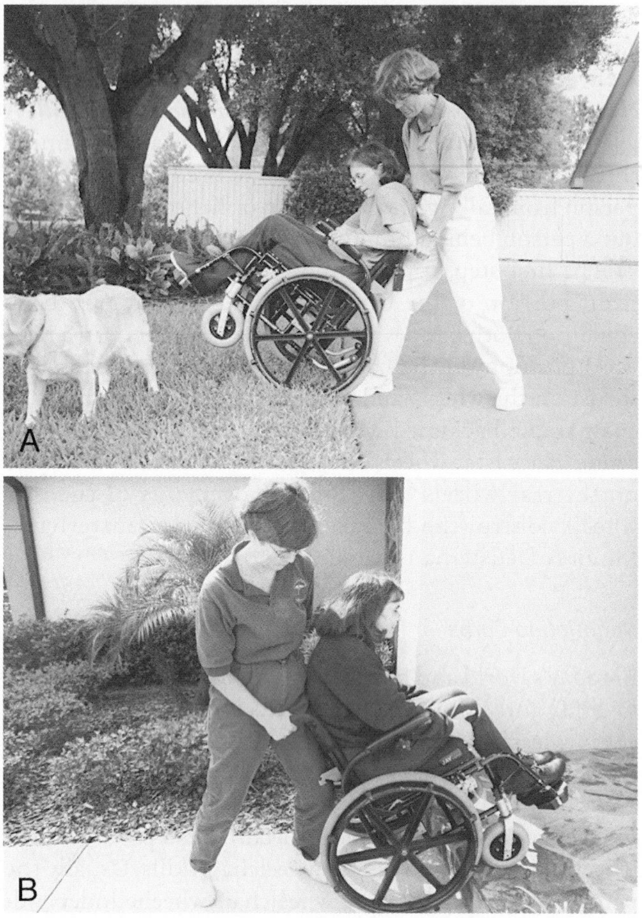

Figure 31-8 **A.** A therapist performs an assisted wheelchair wheelie so the wheelchair can easily be moved through grass and uneven terrain. **B.** An assisted wheelie is also used to move a person in a manual wheelchair up a step or curb.

able to descend a couple of steps safely by performing a wheelie while moving down the steps. A person who can perform a wheelchair-to-floor transfer may be able to get out of the wheelchair in an emergency and "bump" up or down the steps while pulling the chair along. Skin protection during this task must be understood and practiced. ***Training to do this should occur before an emergency arises.***

Moving a manual wheelchair and its dependent occupant up and down steps safely requires the assistance of two people. The back of the wheelchair should be positioned against the steps with one person standing behind the chair and the other person in front of it. The chair is tipped backward, with one person holding the push handles and the other person holding the front of the chair by its frame or leg rests. While the person in front maintains balance of the chair, the person behind pulls the chair up step by step. That person should take care to keep his or her back straight and use leg strength to move the chair. To take a person down the steps, approach the steps forward with the wheelchair tipped and balanced. The procedure is reversed, with the person in front of the chair holding onto the chair

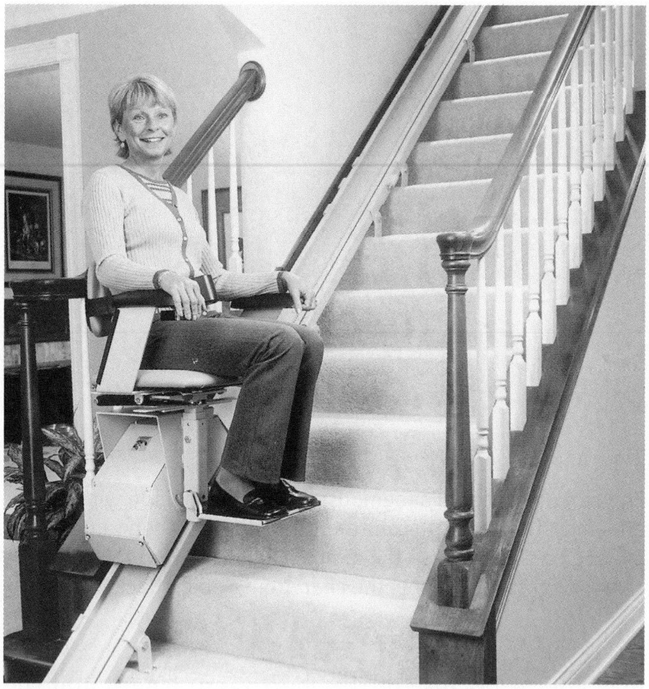

Figure 31-9 A battery-powered stair lift makes going up and down stairs easy.

while guiding and controlling the speed of the chair down each step. Moving a power wheelchair in this manner is impossible and not safe due to the weight of the chair.

For individuals who must negotiate multiple steps in a home, there are various configurations of stair lifts that can be installed on a staircase for straight or curved stairs (Fig. 31-9). The person must be able to transfer onto the seating device and balance himself on the seat while the seat moves up or down the staircase. If the person has no ambulation ability, a second wheelchair must be available at the top of the staircase for the person to transfer into. Another viable but expensive option is a small elevator that can be installed in a commercial or private building that meets the space and structural requirements for installation.

Intervention Planning for Transfers

A **transfer** is the means by which a person moves one's body from one surface to an adjacent surface. The method can be simple or complex depending upon the performance skill level of the person performing the transfers. There are various techniques and methods for safely performing a transfer, and the occupational therapist working in conjunction with the physical therapist must determine the best method for each client. The technique chosen depends upon the patient's disability, upper and lower extremity strength, physical endurance, trunk balance, body type, orthotic devices, and/or wheelchair style (Definition 31-1). A graded training program for transfers

DEFINITION 31-1

Various Levels of Transfers

Dependent Transfer

Person requires maximum assistance of one or more persons using a special technique or device to assist in moving from one surface to another.

Sliding Board Transfer

Person cannot bridge the gap between two surfaces without the use of a sliding board.

Standing Pivot Transfer

Person can stand up, then pivot the feet and turn the trunk, and then sit down on the transferring surface.

Independent Transfer

Person can perform all steps of a transfer with no physical assistance of another person. A device may or may not be used.

is necessary as a patient progresses through the rehabilitation process. A dependent transfer may be necessary until the person can begin learning assisted or independent transfers. The level of the transfer that is ultimately determined to be appropriate for the patient must reflect his or her physical and functional status.

The occupational therapy intervention should include family training so that the family member learns to perform each step of a transfer. The family member should practice with the therapist and patient in a protected, supervised environment. Proper body mechanics must be taught and practiced throughout any transfer to protect the helper as well as the person being transferred. To prevent back injury, the helper should keep the back and spine straight so that the physical lift or rotation of the transfer is done using the stronger muscles of the arms and legs.

Dependent Transfer

A person who is too weak to move requires another person or persons to lift or move him or her in a dependent transfer. A one-person technique entails standing in front of the patient and placing him or her in a forward flexed position with the chest lying on the thighs. This method cannot be used for the patient with limited hip flexion, for example, those with a hip fracture, post-hip replacement surgery, or heterotopic ossificans. This position shifts the patient's body weight over the knees and ankles rather than on the buttocks, which allows the buttocks to be picked up and moved more easily. This method has proven worthy to teach family members because it enables the helper to control the movement of the patient's body while lessening the probability of hurting his or her own back (Fig. 31-10).

For the patient with limited hip flexion, this technique can be modified to sliding the buttocks toward the edge of the wheelchair and placing the patient's knees between the assistant's knees. Using proper body mechanics, the assistant squeezes the knees of the patient with his or her own knees while rocking the patient forward slightly and simultaneously pulling on the patient's pants or belt and rotating the hips to the surface being moved to.

For a two-person dependent transfer using a similar method, the second person stands behind the patient and moves the buttocks to the transfer surface while the first person moves the legs. A **transfer board**, sometimes called a sliding board, can be used to bridge the gap if the buttocks cannot easily be picked up. A dependent transfer can be performed by one or two helpers using a mechanical-hydraulic or powered body lifter (Fig. 31-5).

Sliding Board Transfers

A person who cannot stand but can perform a sliding board transfer can use the transfer board to slide the buttocks and bridge the gap between the two transfer surfaces. There are a wide variety of shapes, lengths, weights, and styles of transfer boards available from various manufacturers (Fig. 31-11). A long transfer board may be needed to bridge the large gap between a wheelchair and a car seat, but a smaller board can be used for transfer to the toilet or bed as the gap is smaller. A cutout on one end of the board may be needed to allow someone with a weak grasp to pick up the board. An angled or notched board may be best for maneuvering around the rear wheel of the wheelchair while transferring. A board made of high-density polished polyethylene plastic provides a slippery surface for bare skin, and a board with a moving center disc may allow easy sliding of the body. Off-the-shelf boards do not always meet specific needs of clients. Figure 31-12 shows a variety of custom transfer boards made by an occupational therapist to meet a specific client's needs when off-the-shelf boards were not useful. The client required various lengths, widths, and shapes of transfer boards to accommodate all of the different transfers that this person was able to perform.

Most transfer boards are positioned with one end under the patient's buttocks and thighs and the other end on the surface to which the person is transferring. Level surfaces greatly aid in the transfer, although one can use gravity to assist when sliding to a lower surface. For an independent transfer, the patient performs shoulder depression with the elbows extended and locked to raise and/or slide the buttocks along the surface of the board (Fig. 31-13). The person must also be able to handle his or her own legs to put them

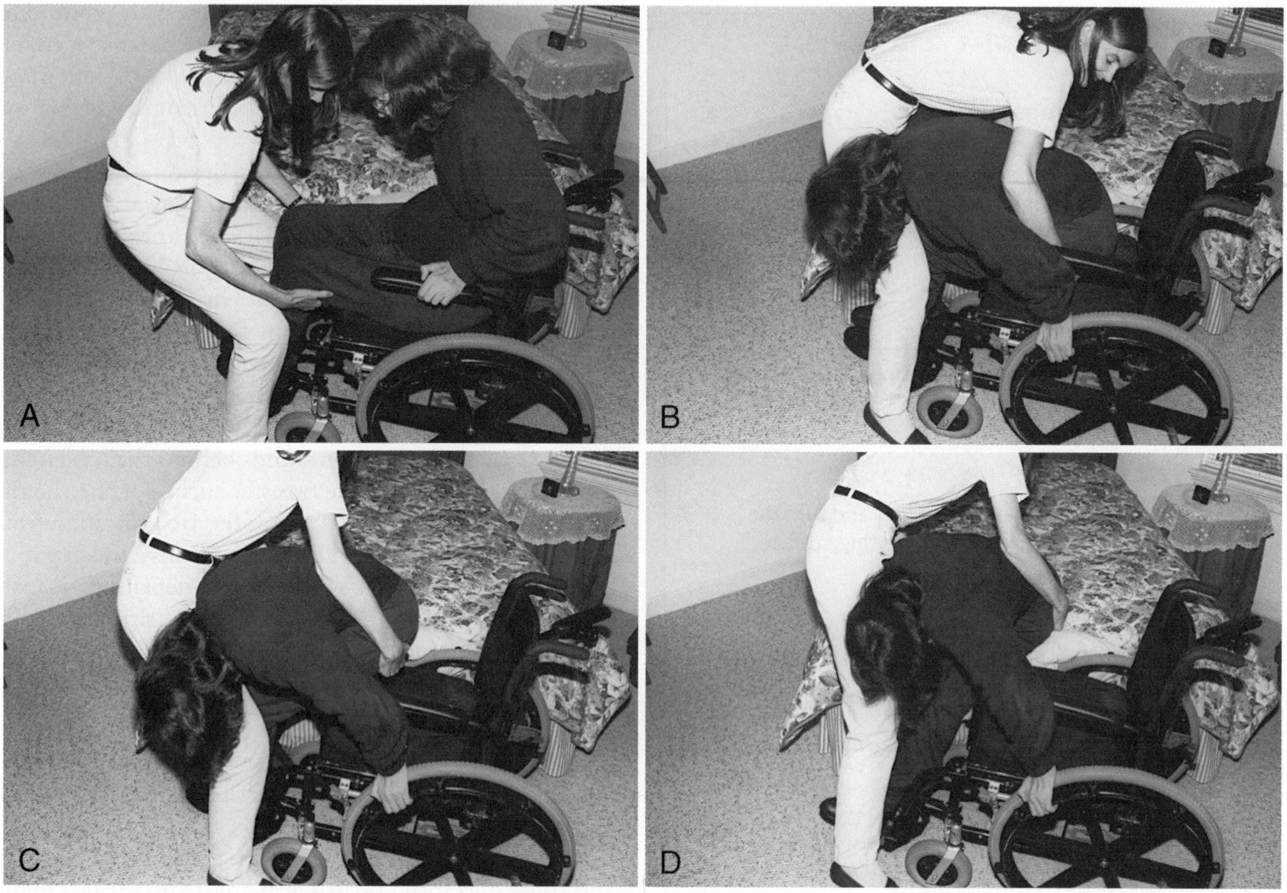

Figure 31-10 A therapist demonstrates one type of dependent wheelchair to bed transfer that can be performed by one person. **A.** The therapist readies the patient by sliding the buttocks forward in the seat to avoid bumping into the rear wheel during the transfer. **B.** The patient is leaned forward onto the therapist's right thigh. If able, the patient can assist with the left hand on the wheelchair tire. The therapist has her legs around the patient's legs and readies herself with proper body alignment. **C.** The therapist uses the strength in her arms and legs to rock the client forward, lift the patient's buttocks, and rotate the patient to the bed. **D.** Since the patient's weight is shifted forward, there is little weight to pick up.

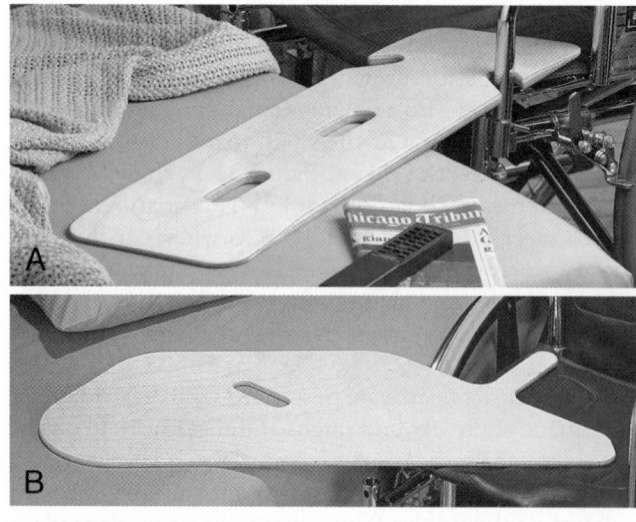

Figure 31-11 Two styles and shapes of transfer boards available through suppliers. **A.** Transfer board with hand holes and notches allows transfers from either side. **B.** Offset transfer board fits around the wheel of the wheelchair when the armrest is removed. (Courtesy of Sammons Preston, Bolingbrook, IL.)

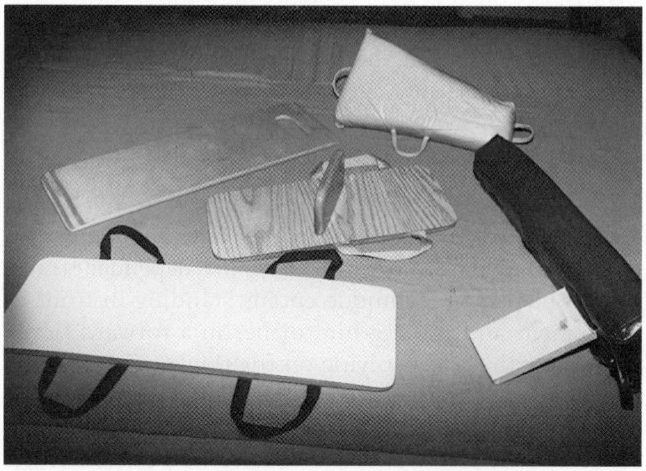

Figure 31-12 An occupational therapist designed and built these specialized transfer boards to meet various clients' needs.

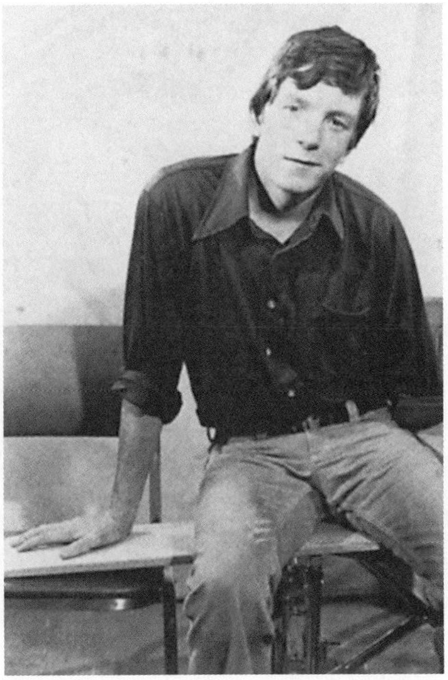

Figure 31-13 Independent sliding board depression transfer.

in place during or after the transfer. Factors that can impede this type of transfer include:

- Poor trunk balance
- Spasticity
- Excessive body weight or large, heavy legs
- Inadequate upper extremity strength
- Inability to lock elbows into extension
- Joint contractures or tightness in the elbows or wrists that prevent full elbow extension and/or full wrist extension
- A low ratio of arm length to trunk length

The same principles apply to tub, shower, and toilet transfers. Equipment, such as grab bars, a raised toilet seat, and tub bench, can make these transfers easier and safer. Car transfers are difficult because of the large gap between the car seat and wheelchair as well as the seat height discrepancy. A person may require a transfer board for this transfer but not for other transfers in the home (Fig. 31-14).

Stand-Pivot Transfer

A person with lower extremity deficits, who can support his or her weight on one or both legs, may be able to perform an independent or assisted stand-pivot transfer. An assisted stand-pivot transfer is performed with the helper standing in front of the patient and the transfer surface as close as possible. Generally it is best to transfer the patient toward his or her stronger side. The patient should first be slid toward the edge of the surface from which the transfer is taking place, with care to protect the person from slipping off the edge completely, especially if there is lower extremity or trunk spasticity. The patient is assisted to a standing position (Fig. 31-15). The helper places his or her knees in front of one or both of the knees of the patient to prevent the patient's knees from buckling upon standing. The patient wraps his or her arms around the helper's body or neck, but only for support, not to pull up. The helper bends his or her knees, keeps the back straight, and grabs the waist or belt of the patient's pants or a **transfer belt**. This belt with handles is wrapped snugly around the patient's waist and provides a handhold for the helper. The helper rocks the person back and forth several times and then, using momentum, pulls the person to a standing position. A patient who can assist uses leg strength to stand or can use upper body strength to push off a wheelchair or chair armrest or bed rail to come to standing. By pressing against the weak knee or knees, the helper assists the patient to swivel or slide the heels toward the transfer surface while standing. The helper can then guide the patient's hips over and down to the transfer surface.

Independent Transfers

Patients with adequate strength to push up and move the trunk and to handle the lower extremities can transfer without assistive equipment. Figure 31-16 illustrates an independent transfer from wheelchair to bed by a person with C7 quadriplegia. This individual desired to live alone and not to have a hospital bed. She accomplished independence in this difficult transfer after discharge as an outpatient from therapy while working with an occupational therapist in her home. A special soft-surfaced transfer aid was custom built for her to bridge the gap between the wheelchair and bed yet protect her skin by preventing her buttocks from sliding over the wheelchair wheel or getting stuck in this gap (Fig. 31-16, B and C).

Orthotic Devices and Aids for Walking and Standing

A person with balance difficulties or weakness in one or both lower extremities may require some type of orthotic mobility device for stability and support while walking. Canes and walkers come in various styles and shapes (Fig. 31-17). The type of cane chosen by the physical therapist depends on the person's balance and gripping ability, with personal preference considered. A straight cane is selected for a person with good strength, coordination, and balance who nevertheless requires a device for support. The four-prong or **quad cane** is chosen for a person who is weak on one or both sides, has increased muscle tone or ataxia, and needs a wider, more stable base than a straight cane provides. The **hemi-walker**, so called because it is often used by persons with hemiplegia, provides the greatest stability for a one-handed orthotic device and can also serve to assist with standing (Fig. 31-17B).

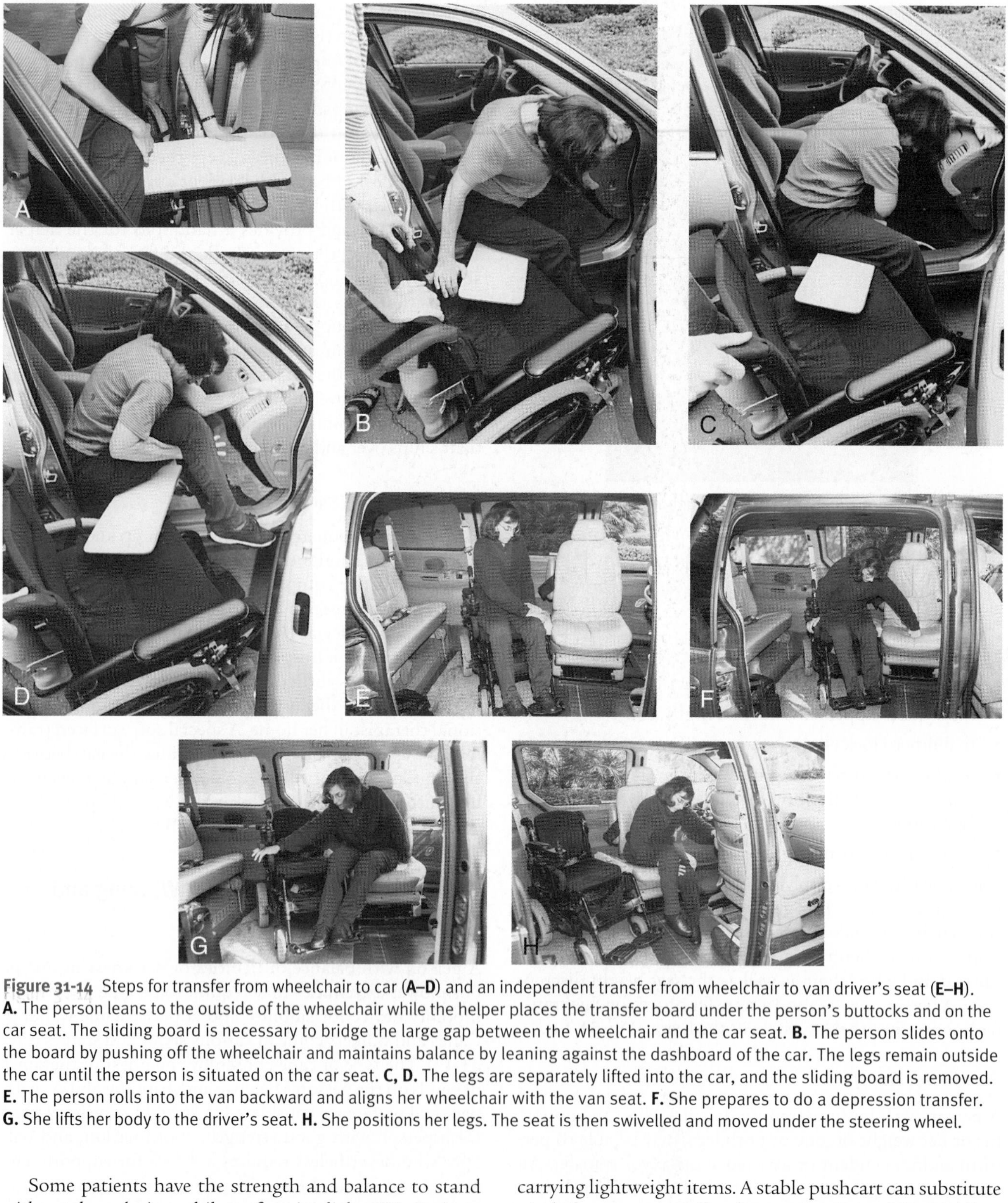

Figure 31-14 Steps for transfer from wheelchair to car (**A–D**) and an independent transfer from wheelchair to van driver's seat (**E–H**). **A.** The person leans to the outside of the wheelchair while the helper places the transfer board under the person's buttocks and on the car seat. The sliding board is necessary to bridge the large gap between the wheelchair and the car seat. **B.** The person slides onto the board by pushing off the wheelchair and maintains balance by leaning against the dashboard of the car. The legs remain outside the car until the person is situated on the car seat. **C, D.** The legs are separately lifted into the car, and the sliding board is removed. **E.** The person rolls into the van backward and aligns her wheelchair with the van seat. **F.** She prepares to do a depression transfer. **G.** She lifts her body to the driver's seat. **H.** She positions her legs. The seat is then swivelled and moved under the steering wheel.

Some patients have the strength and balance to stand without these devices while performing light ADL. Patients who do not have the standing balance or strength to stand at a work surface and use both hands may have to sit or perform ADL with one hand while standing. These individuals have limited ability to carry things while walking, so small carrying bags can be strapped to their assistive device for carrying lightweight items. A stable pushcart can substitute nicely for a cane or walker for carrying items (Fig. 31-18).

A full size walker gives the person bilateral support for balance and stability while walking (Fig. 31-19A). A full-size or rolling walker requires the partial use of both upper extremities. A rolling walker with four small plastic wheels is effective for individuals with an ataxic gait, such as is

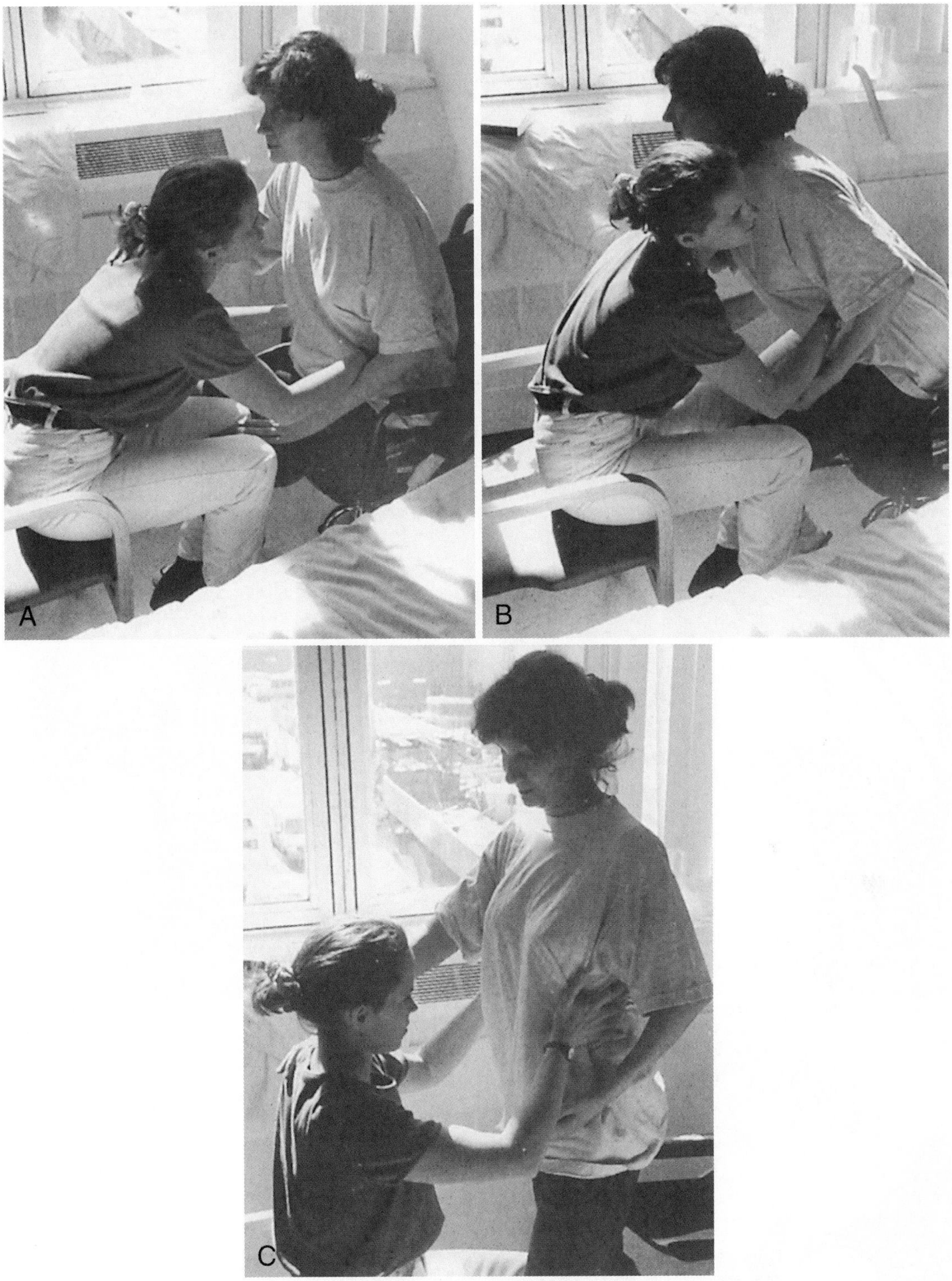

Figure 31-15 A patient with left hemiplegia is assisted in a sit-to-stand position. **A.** The patient places her unaffected hand on the therapist's shoulder for support. The therapist supports the patient's weak left knee by placing her knee against the patient's knee. **B.** The patient leans forward to move the center of gravity forward. **C.** The patient uses the strength of the unaffected side, with the help of the therapist, to stand. (Reprinted with permission from Gillen, G., & Burkhardt, A. [Eds.]. [1998]. *Stroke rehabilitation: A function-based approach* [p. 231]. St. Louis: Mosby.)

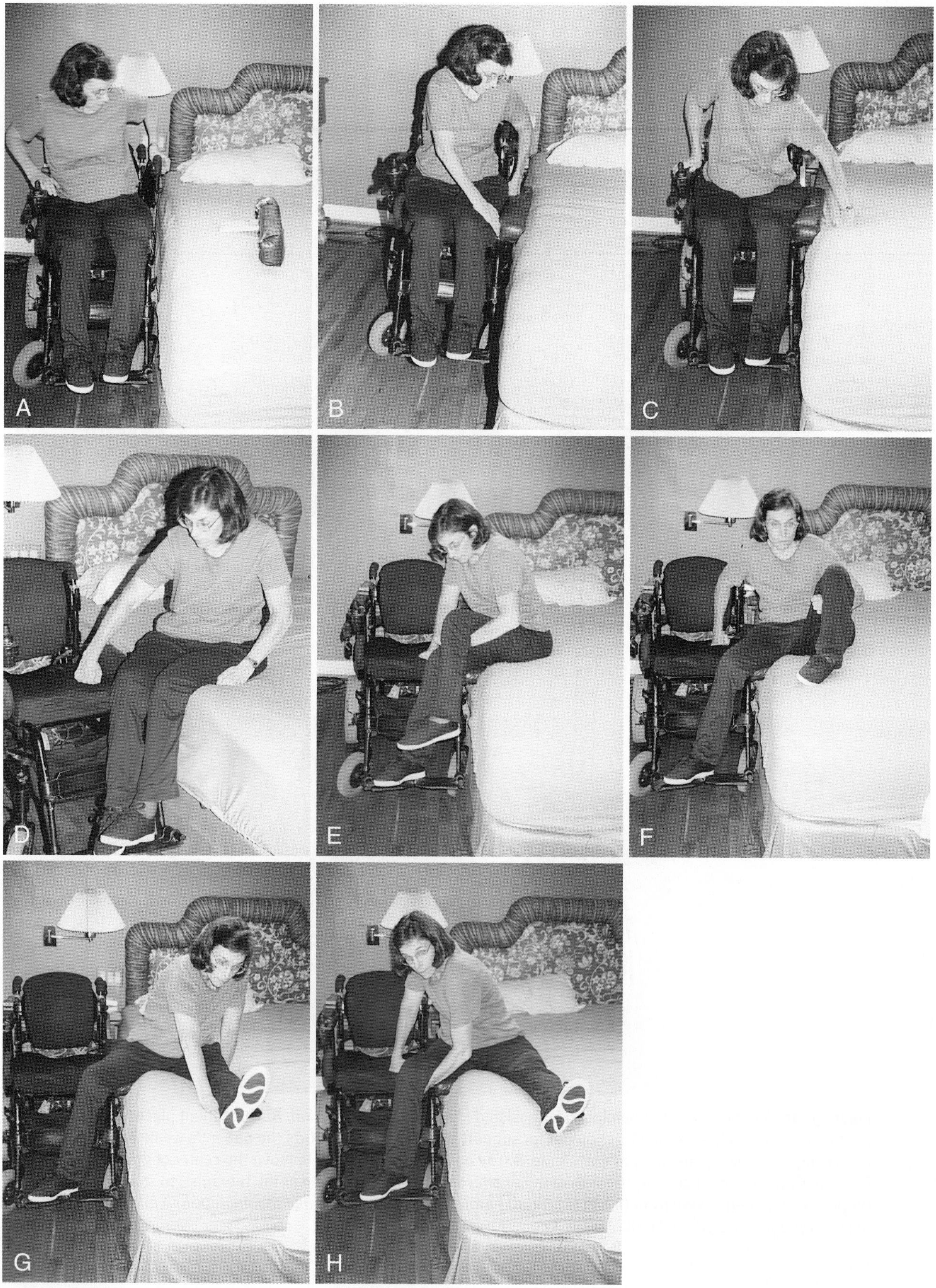
A
B
C
D
E
F
G
H

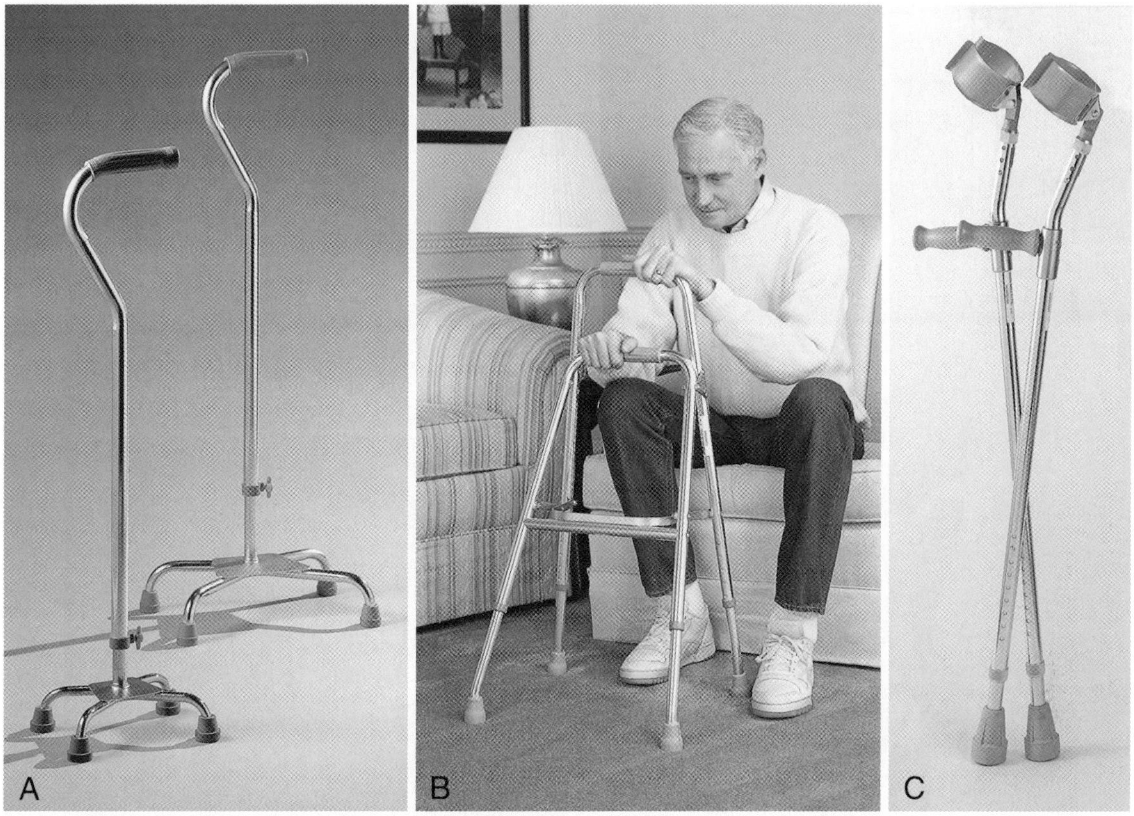

Figure 31-17 Various orthotic devices for walking. **A.** Quad cane has wide base with four points of contact to the ground to provide stability. **B.** Sidestepper cane/walker is typically used by a person with hemiplegia who requires more stability than the quad cane supplies. **C.** Forearm crutches allow a wide base of support for those who have leg weakness but good balance. (Courtesy of Sammons Preston, Bolingbrook, IL.)

seen in cerebral palsy or Frederick's ataxia, since it is easier to push the walker while walking rather than to pick it up for each step. It can be difficult for the person using a rolling walker to pivot to turn corners or prepare to sit down. With the full-size walker, the user can simply rotate around the axis of the body and carry the walker during the turn. Some walkers can be fitted with a fold-down seat for resting or a pouch or basket for carrying items. Folding-frame walkers are easy to store in a car's back seat or trunk or on the back of a scooter. Also, a lightweight, rotating handle can be installed on the walker for a person to push down on when standing from a bed, chair, or a car (Fig. 31-19B). The handle rotates 180° and locks onto the walker frame when not in use.

A three-wheel walker has the advantage of larger pneumatic wheels for a more stable base and hand brakes for safety (Fig. 31-19C). This type of walker can carry heavier items and can have a fold-down seat for individuals who fatigue easily, such as those with multiple sclerosis or arthritis. This type of walker is not indicated for a person who leans on the walker for support. The width and turning radius of these walkers is greater than those of standard walkers and may affect the user's maneuverability where space is limited. Loading the device into a vehicle must be solved if it is to be used in the community.

Patients who can walk only short distances with or without an orthotic device may also require the use of a

Figure 31-16 Steps for an independent transfer from wheelchair to bed by a person with lower extremity paralysis. **A.** The patient positions the wheelchair close to the side of the bed and removes the left armrest. **B.** A custom-made transfer board between the wheelchair and bed fills the gap and prevents skin damage by bumping the wheel. **C.** Shoulder, triceps, and wrist extensor muscles allow the client to lean on her left arm for balance. She pushes off with the right arm, using her triceps and latissimus dorsi, to move her buttocks from the wheelchair to the bed. **D.** She steadies her balance once on the edge of the bed. **E.** Having moved her right hand to the wheelchair seat for balance, she picks up the left leg with her left arm. **F.** The left leg is placed on the bed. **G.** She straightens the leg. **H.** She repeats the process to move the other leg up onto the bed. Maintaining balance is the key to performing this move independently and without assistive devices.

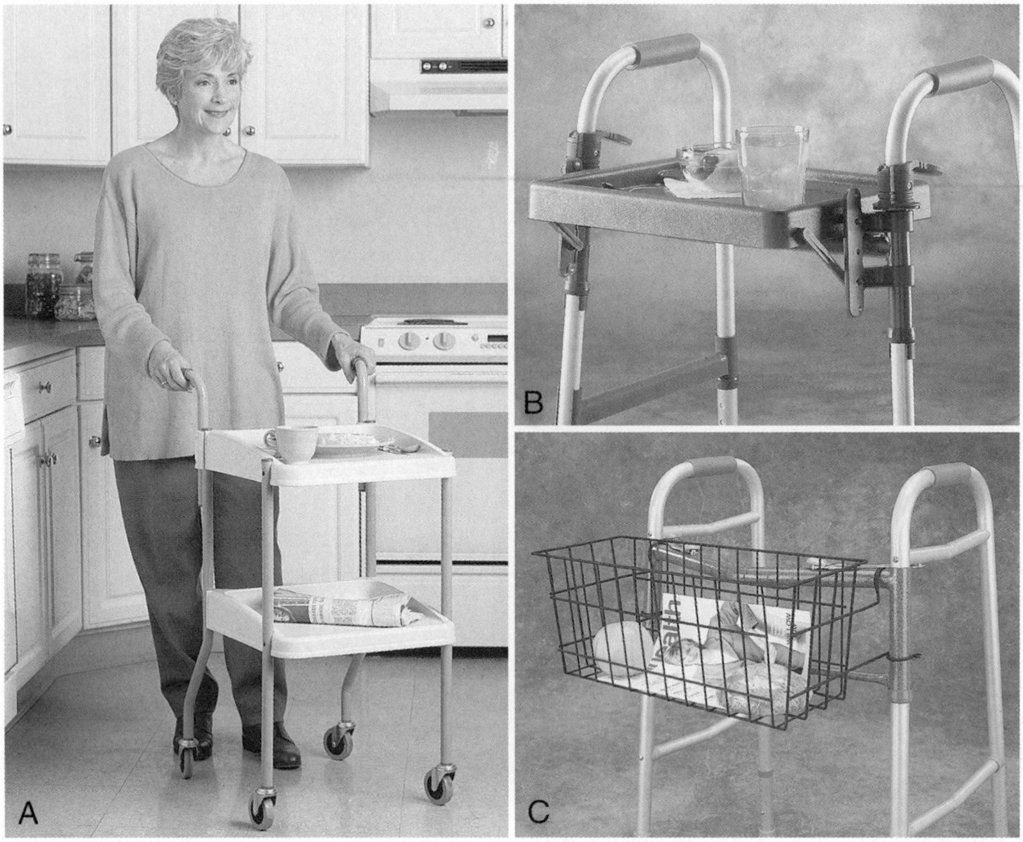

Figure 31-18 Carrying items on orthotic walking devices. **A.** Rolling cart with push handles for carrying many or heavy items. **B.** Tray for walker. **C.** Basket attached to walker. (Courtesy of Sammons Preston, Bolingbrook, IL.)

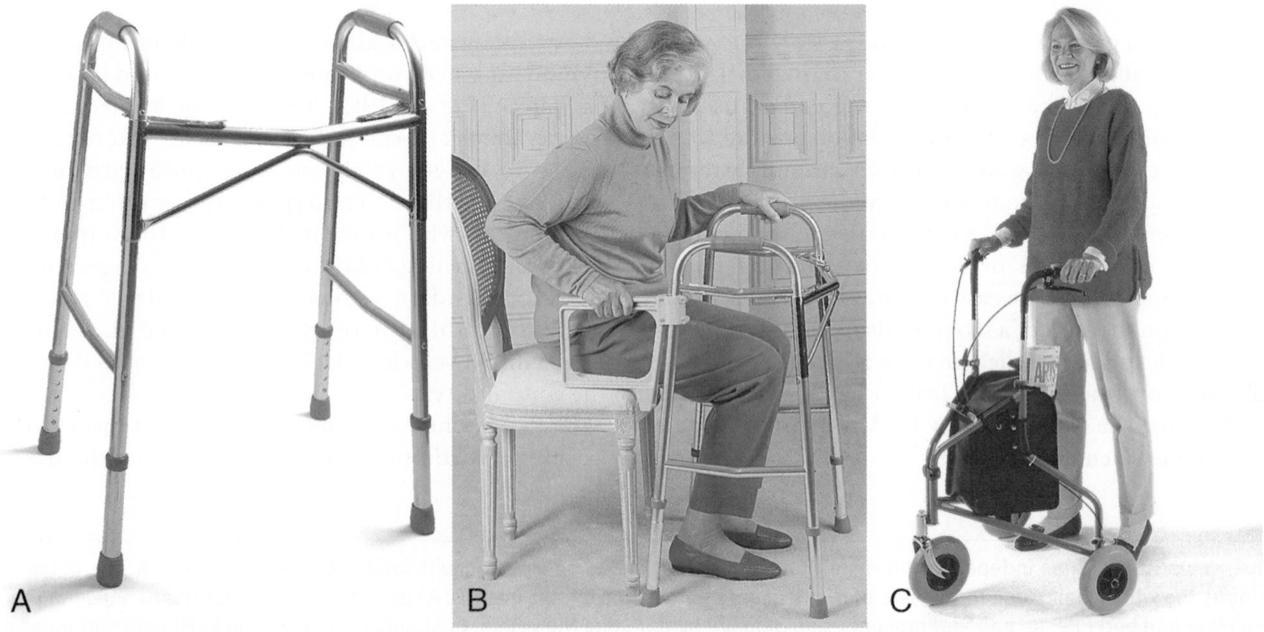

Figure 31-19 Walkers. **A.** Standard walker for child or adult. Small roller wheels can be provided on the front legs to assist with moving the walker. **B.** Easy-Up™ handle for walkers provides leverage for persons who can rise unassisted. The lightweight handle folds into the walker frame when not in use. **C.** Rolling three- or four-wheel walker can be used by child or adult who needs support to walk but has good balance. The large wheels travel over outdoor terrain easily. Hand brakes allow for safe slowing. A pack can be added to transport things. (Courtesy of Sammons Preston, Bolingbrook, IL.)

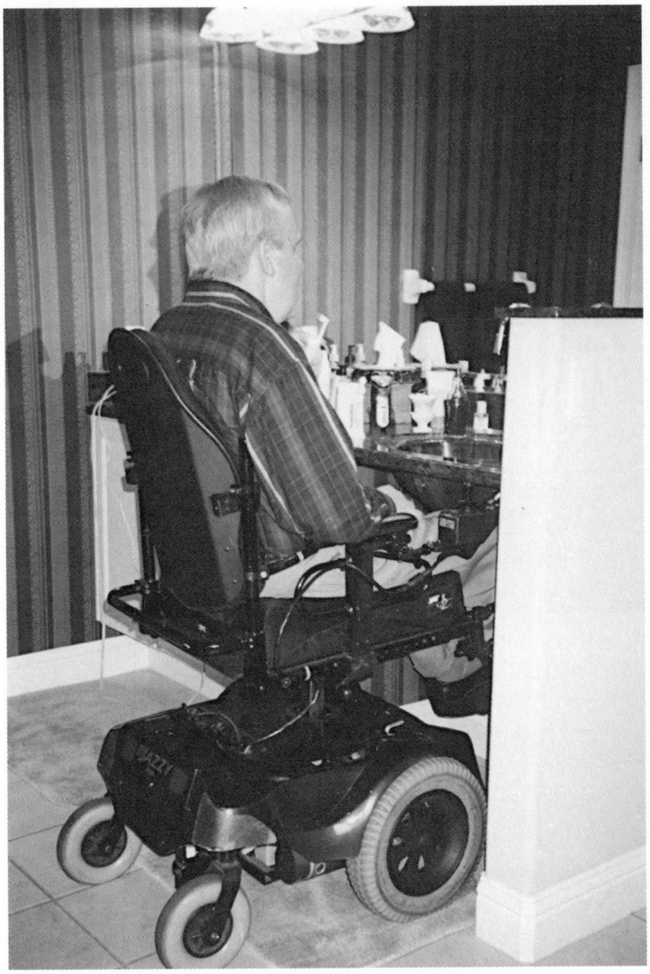

Figure 31-20 Use of a powered vertical up/down seat on a powered wheelchair to allow near approach to the sink for grooming.

manual wheelchair or scooter for longer distances. Using the wheelchair may be a more practical solution to enable performing tasks that require two hands, balance, and/or stability. By sitting in a wheelchair, the person frees up both hands for activities. A person who has good trunk balance may be able to use a stool for working at counter surfaces. Some persons can use a powered up/down seat on a wheelchair or scooter to reach high work surfaces or tall cabinets (Fig. 31-20).

Various mechanical and electric devices are available to assist a person in standing up or rotating and swiveling preparatory to standing. The powered lift wheelchair or the powered lift lounge chair (Fig. 31-21) is popular for persons with a variety of disabilities because the chair raises the person totally supported to a partial standing position. Also, some devices, such as the swivel disk or lift seat, can be placed in a regular chair or vehicle seat to help the person move his or her legs or start the momentum for standing upright. Electric seats for vans and cars similarly assist a person but tend to be expensive and have strict vehicle requirements (Fig. 31-22).

Standing can improve circulation and renal and bowel functions, reduce lower extremity spasticity, and prevent effects of prolonged immobilization. If a person has a job that requires standing, such as a beautician or a schoolteacher, there are various styles of wheelchairs available to assist this person in coming to a supported standing position or to increase her seated height. There is a stand-up manual wheelchair, a stand-up powered wheelchair, or a powered wheelchair with a powered up/down seat. These wheelchairs can provide a great means of mobility as well as meet the task demands of the person's job, including freeing both hands. The person using a powered chair that has this capability can move around in a standing or elevated seated position (Fig. 31-23). The manual wheelchairs with this capability are heavier than standard manual wheelchairs and not conducive to outdoor mobility so an active person may need a second lighter-weight wheelchair to use away from work.

COMMUNITY MOBILITY

Occupational therapy is involved with instrumental activities of daily living (IADLs), which are defined as "activities that are oriented toward interacting with the environment and that are often complex—generally optional in nature" (AOTA, 2002, p. 620). Community mobility is listed as one of the instrumental activities of daily living. Occupational therapy supports "engagement in occupations and in activities that allow desired or needed participation in home, school, workplace, and community life situations" (AOTA, 2002, p. 611). In other words, community mobility allows one to engage in life outside the home and, as an IADL, should be addressed in occupational therapy.

Occupational therapy must consider community mobility as an occupation that has value and meaning for each person. The topic should be treated as important and unique for each person and should be viewed in its entirety. The occupational therapist should understand how each client values community mobility, including driving, and be knowledgeable about how external and internal contextual factors will influence participation in this occupation. Today most people go into the community for almost everything they need. Although the internet and mail order provide extensive resources for persons to purchase drugs, supplies, and clothes without store shopping, these resources are inaccessible to some and can be unsatisfying in terms of social interaction. Therefore, community mobility is an important goal for most patients in occupational therapy. The feasibility, safety, and personal control of mobility are affected by (1) the socioeconomic status of the person (income may limit the type of transportation available), (2) physical characteristics of the site, and (3) transportation technology (Carp, 1988).

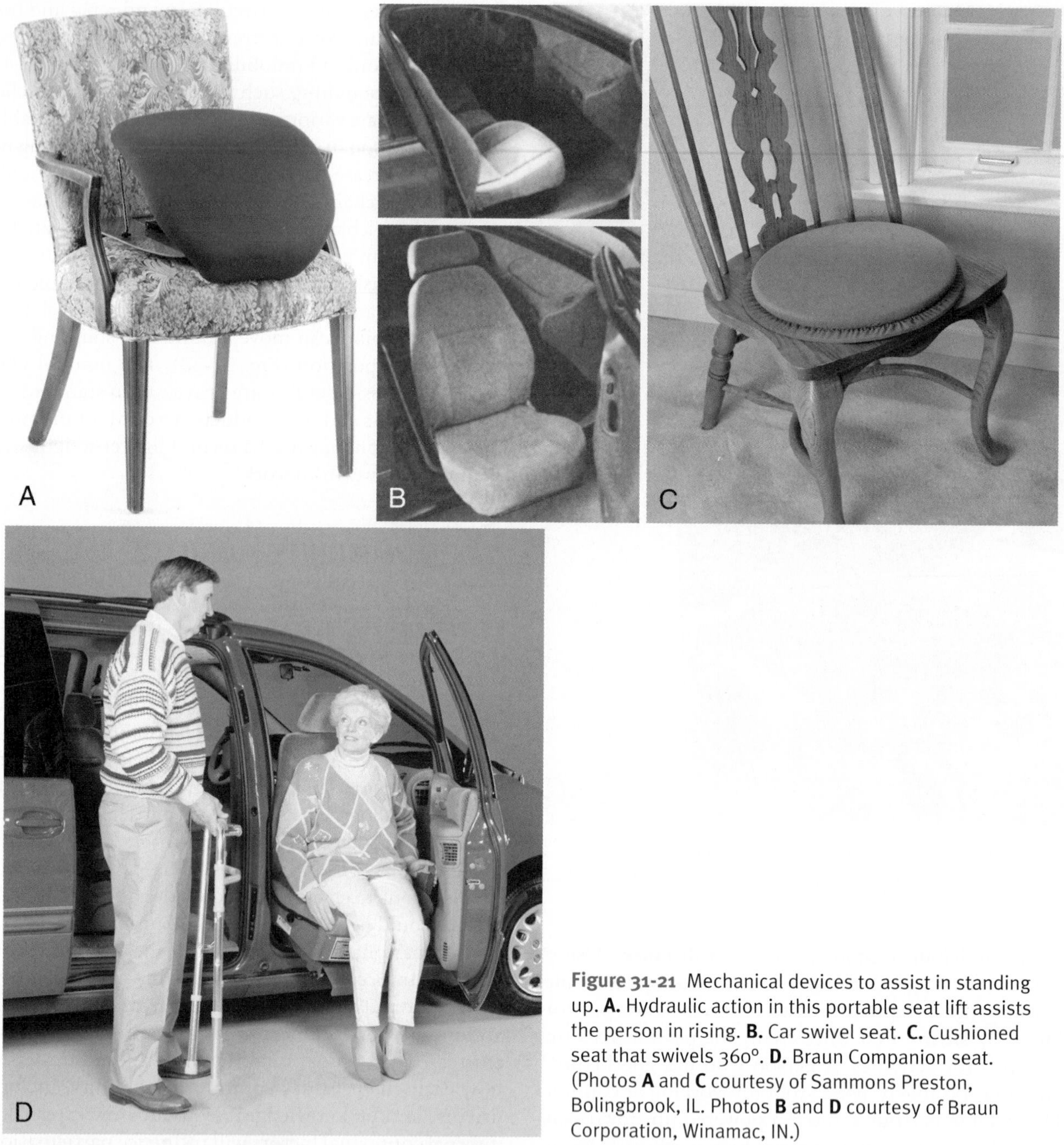

Figure 31-21 Mechanical devices to assist in standing up. **A.** Hydraulic action in this portable seat lift assists the person in rising. **B.** Car swivel seat. **C.** Cushioned seat that swivels 360°. **D.** Braun Companion seat. (Photos **A** and **C** courtesy of Sammons Preston, Bolingbrook, IL. Photos **B** and **D** courtesy of Braun Corporation, Winamac, IN.)

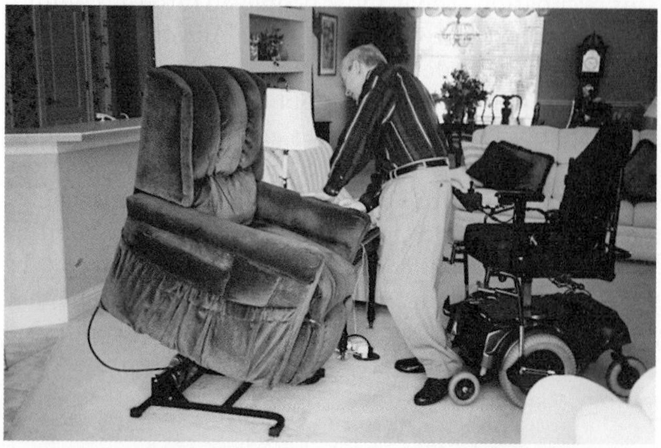

Figure 31-22 Use of a powered lift wheelchair and lounge chair to stand from and sit in both chairs.

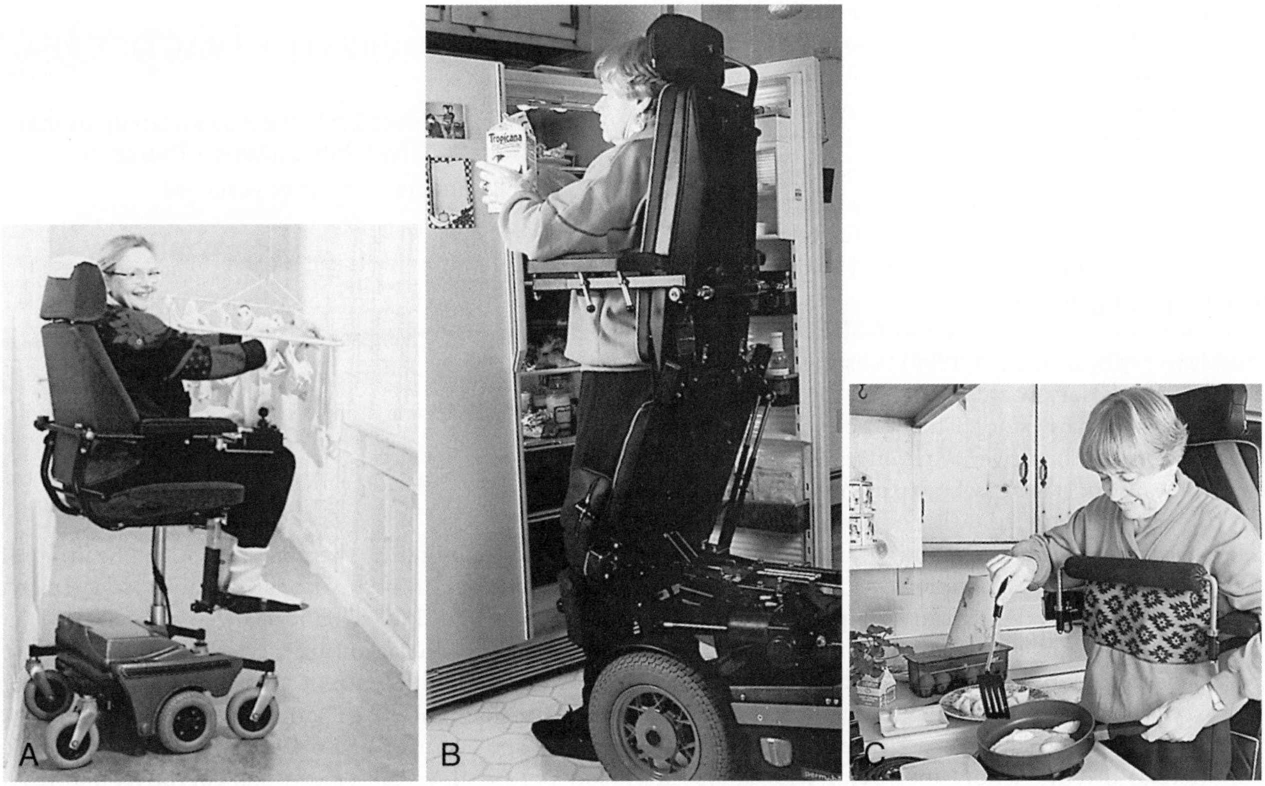

Figure 31-23 Permobil wheelchair options allow for many adjustable sitting and standing positions for activities and tasks at work and at home. (Courtesy of Permobil Company, Woburn, MA.)

Driving Is an Instrumental Activity of Daily Living

Driving a personal vehicle is the main form of transportation for most persons in our society today. Independence in driving can be key for a person to feel a sense of personal well-being and satisfaction through leisure, play, or work activities. Every occupational therapist, no matter the setting, should be addressing driving as an IADL. However, because of its complexity, driving should be one of the last ADLs resumed during rehabilitation (Pierce, 1996). Driving is the most complex IADL for most persons because it requires good physical, visual, perceptual, psychological, and cognitive skills and an integration of these skills. Consequently, most patients are not ready for a driving evaluation before discharge from the inpatient facility. Procedures for Practice 31-1 provides guidelines to determine when a person with a disability is ready for a driving evaluation.

If the patient is driving before he or she is ready, the therapist has an obligation to protect the public welfare by reporting the person to the appropriate licensing authority in the manner dictated by the state of residency. In 2003, the American Medical Association published *The Physician's Guide to Assessing and Counseling Older Drivers* (Wang et al., 2003). The role of the physician in addressing

PROCEDURES FOR PRACTICE 31-1

Guidelines to Determine When a Person with a Disability Is Ready for a Driving Evaluation

A patient or client who has all of the following can be referred for a driving evaluation:

- Maximum independence in basic activities of daily living
- Independent ambulation or wheelchair mobility
- Good strength, sensation, and coordination in at least one or, ideally, two extremities
- 20/40 visual acuity in at least one eye*
- 140° of total field of vision with both eyes*
- No double vision with or without compensation*
- No seizures for 6 months*
- Spasticity under control with or without medication
- Good visual-perceptual functioning, such as depth and figure ground perception
- Good cognitive functioning; short-term memory can be minimally to moderately affected
- Valid driver's license or learner's permit

* Requirements vary among states.

driver safety and the legal and ethical responsibilities of the physician are discussed, and there are also chapters describing the role of the driver rehabilitation specialist. Every occupational therapist should have a copy of this publication, which is available free in hard copy or CD-ROM at www.nhtsa.dot.gov or www.ama-assn.org/go/olderdrivers. Although it is written with older drivers in mind, the material can apply to all age and disability groups.

Every occupational therapist should know the procedure for reporting impaired drivers in his or her state and which functions a therapist is authorized, obligated, or responsible to perform (Kaplan, 1999). A listing of individual state Medical Advisory Board regulations for reporting can be found at www.aamva.org. The occupational therapist should also know the driver rehabilitation therapists in their community or state, to whom patients can be referred when this service is needed. A list of driver rehabilitation specialists nationwide can be found on the website of the Association of Driver Rehabilitation Specialists (ADED) at www.aded.net or on the American Occupational Therapy Association's older driver microsite at www.aota.org/olderdriver. When looking for a driver rehabilitation therapist to assist your patient, consider the diagnosis of the patient and the background and experience of the specialist. A commercial driving school instructor who is also a driver rehabilitation specialist may not have the necessary medical background to understand your client's deficits and their implications for the driving task. If you are referring the client to a driving school instructor, a driver rehabilitation therapist should still be performing an occupational profile and performance skill assessment prior to the person having the road test with the driving school instructor (Pierce, 1993).

During the inpatient stay, the client may be allowed home visits on the weekends in preparation for discharge. It is important to work on community mobility while the person is still in rehabilitation so that feelings of isolation will not develop during these visits or after discharge. Transportation needs, particularly for the wheelchair user, may have to be addressed long before driving because the person may not be ready for a driving evaluation until 8–12 months after discharge. A referral to the driver rehabilitation therapist for "determination of transportation needs only" may be appropriate before discharge so that the patient, family, and funding source can be guided toward the appropriate vehicle and modifications. If the driver rehabilitation therapist can determine that the patient may be able to drive later, vehicle selection and modifications for transportation can be made with future driving needs taken into consideration.

A Driver Rehabilitation Therapist

Driver rehabilitation or driver evaluation programs throughout the United States are housed in hospitals, rehabilitation facilities, private practices, and state agencies.

PROCEDURES FOR PRACTICE 31-2

Steps for a Driver Evaluation by an Occupational Therapy Driver Rehabilitation Therapist

The following areas should be evaluated:

1. Occupational profile
2. Performance skills and client factors
3. Client's vehicle and how the client fits in the vehicle
4. Adaptive driving equipment needs
5. In-traffic performance
6. Inspection and fitting of the vehicle with equipment installed

A driver rehabilitation therapist is an allied health professional, such as an occupational therapist, with advanced knowledge and skill in the specialized areas of driver evaluation, driver education, and driver rehabilitation for persons with disabilities. An occupational therapy **driver rehabilitation therapist** can develop an occupational profile and perform a formal clinical evaluation of a person's physical, visual, perceptual, cognitive, and psychological functioning as it relates to driving (Procedures for Practice 31-2).

Developing an Occupational Profile and Performance Skill Assessment for Driving

The occupational therapy driver rehabilitation therapist will first develop an occupational profile to understand the meaning and requirements of the occupation of driving for each client and detail the internal and external contextual factors that may influence independence in driving. Examples of the relationship of driving to the person's roles are (1) working as a mailman, (2) living in a rural area but working in a city (commuter), or (3) the grandparent who is responsible for picking up a grandchild after school. The person's driving habits and routines are also considered, such as what type of traffic environment he drives in and what time of day he drives.

The second step is a clinical assessment to determine any client factors that may hinder safe driving ability and then to complete an evaluation of overall performance skills as they relate to driving and operating a motor vehicle. The evaluation and testing procedures are similar to those used to determine readiness for any other BADL or IADL with an emphasis on specific skills related to driving and are described in the early chapters of this textbook. For example, evaluation of a client's strength and range of motion may determine that special adaptive equipment will be needed to compensate for deficits. A visual performance deficit (nystagmus) or a cognitive deficit (impulsivity) will suggest possible problems to be anticipated during the in-traffic assessment. Research indicated that the strongest independent predictors of crash-involved drivers was failure on the *Useful Field of Vision* test, which addresses several visual and cognitive processing domains, including visual sensory function, visual processing speed, and divided and selective attention (Sims et al., 1998). By understanding the client factors and specific deficits, the driver rehabilitation therapist can plan an evaluation road route that will challenge the known deficits during driving, thereby providing an accurate assessment of a person's capabilities and safety.

Vehicle Assessment

A driver rehabilitation therapist must evaluate the client's vehicle to assess its appropriateness. The client must be able to enter and exit the vehicle and store the wheelchair, scooter, or other orthotic device as needed (Fig. 31-24). The necessary adaptive equipment for driving must be compatible with the client's vehicle, or specific recommendations must be given regarding purchase of a more appropriate vehicle.

In past decades, the automobile industry produced many two-door cars from which disabled drivers could choose. The two-door cars allowed for easy loading of a folding-frame manual wheelchair behind the driver or passenger seat. Today few two-door cars exist that can accommodate loading the popular rigid-frame wheelchairs, but four-door cars, minivans, and trucks are now produced that allow easy loading of the rigid-frame wheelchair, either manually or electrically. Wheelchair-loading devices have particular vehicle and wheelchair requirements. The wheelchair measurements and weight must be taken to ensure that the loading device will accommodate the particular wheelchair or scooter. Likewise, the vehicle must be measured to determine that the particular vehicle model and make will accommodate not only the lifting device being recommended but also the wheelchair or scooter. It is a hand-in-glove process. The driver rehabilitation therapist evaluates the client, the wheelchair, and the vehicle for appropriateness, along with the client's ability to operate the loading device safely and efficiently.

A van can be set up for a person to drive from the wheelchair or to enable the person to make an independent transfer from the wheelchair to the driver's seat, as seen earlier in Figure 31-14. A van can be adapted with a device such as a wheelchair lift or a motorized ramp so that the person can ride the wheelchair into the vehicle. Structural modifications, such as a raised roof or lowered floor, are generally necessary to give the wheelchair user additional headroom, doorway clearance, and front windshield visibility. Full-size vans or minivans with structural modifications are very expensive (upward of $40,000.00, not including the cost of the driving equipment).

Equipment Assessment

After a clinical assessment is completed and the therapist understands the client factors, performance skills, and contextual factors, the equipment assessment can be completed. This step should be an objective, methodical approach to determine exactly what adaptive equipment the person requires for safe operation of the vehicle.

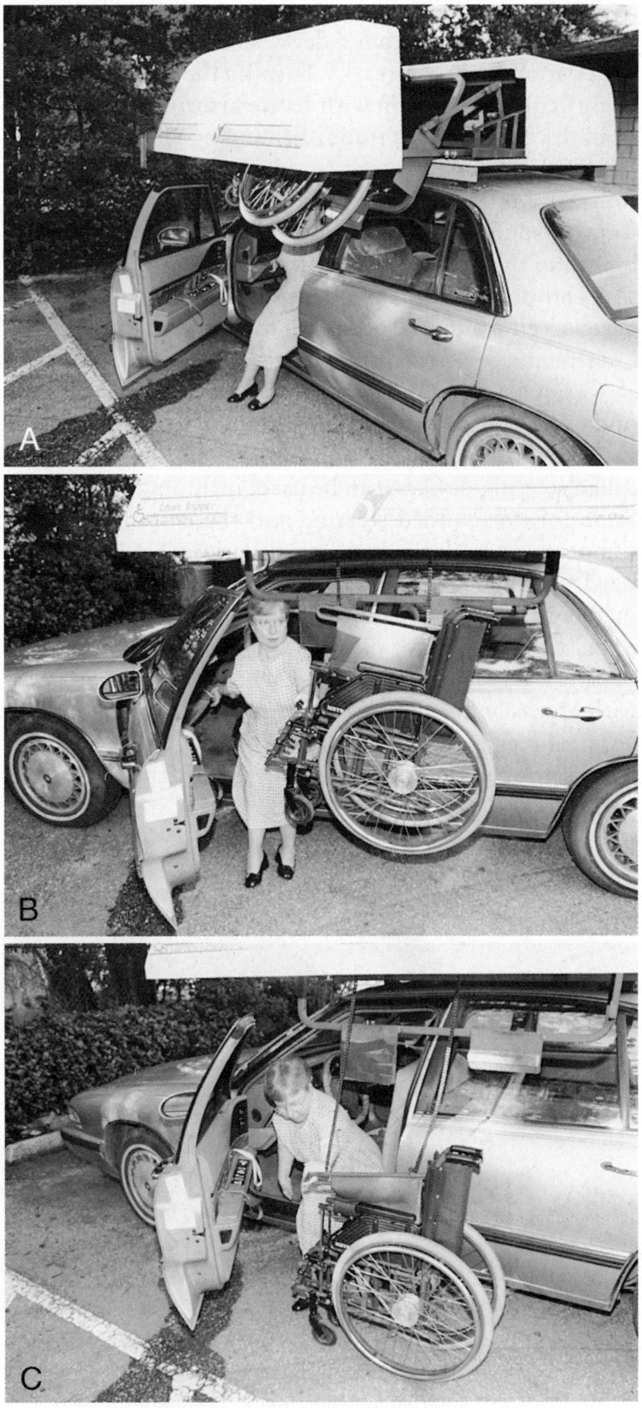

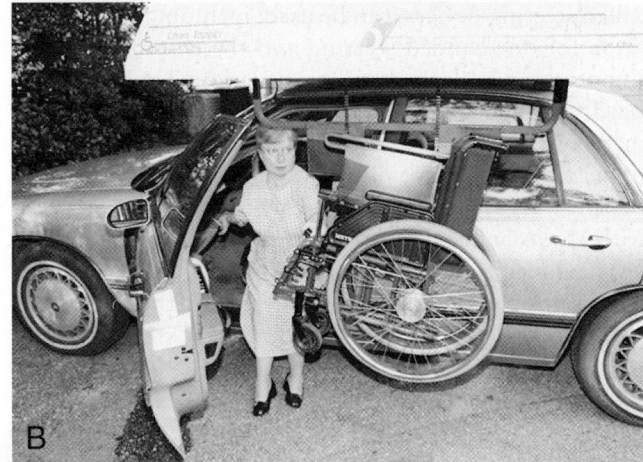

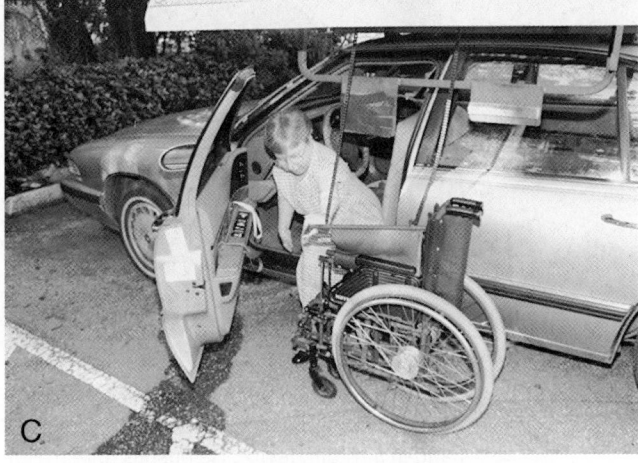

Figure 31-24 A woman with rheumatoid arthritis illustrates how she uses a Braun Chair Topper, a mechanical device, to unload her manual wheelchair.

Development of driving technology over the past 25 years has allowed persons with a variety of disabilities to drive. If there is funding available, a person with a severe physical disability can drive. Driving technology can cost as little as $85 for a steering device, $300 for a left-foot gas pedal, and $800 for simple mechanical hand controls, or as much as $100,000 for a modified van with a sensitive steering, gas, and brake system (Fig. 31-25).

Persons with physical deficits or mobility challenges may require special driving devices or aids to assist them with particular driving tasks. Turning the ignition key can be difficult for a person with severe arthritis. Turning the head to check for cars prior to changing lanes can be impossible for persons with fused necks without adaptations. Dynamic balance in the driver's seat may be difficult for a person with quadriplegia or ataxia. The driver rehabilitation therapist analyzes each driving task for the person and determines the client's needs and desires and what specific aids are necessary for safe driving (Monga, Ostermann, & Kerrigan, 1997).

Various add-on assistive devices for primary and secondary vehicle controls are shown in Figure 31-26. To assist with steering, add-on devices for the steering wheel, called steering devices, can be used, including the spinner knob for one-handed steering and the tri-pin device for the person who lacks hand grip. Various levels of sensitized steering in combination with varying steering wheel diameter and placement are available to compensate for upper extremity range of motion and strength deficits. A person with right hemiplegia can operate the gas pedal with an easily installed left-foot gas pedal. A person with left hemiplegia may benefit from a turn signal crossover to allow safe operation of the turn signal with the right hand. Persons of short stature can use pedal extensions that range in length from 1–10 inches, or a person with severe rheumatoid arthritis may require a key extension in order to turn the ignition key.

Electronic hand controls are available for a person with no use of the legs and limited range of motion and strength in the arms and hands. A handle on the control box moves 4–6 inches from full brake to full acceleration and operates with only 2 ounces of pressure. A person with muscular dystrophy or polio with proximal weakness but distal strength in the hands can use this control easily for gas and brake operation (Fig. 31-27). The driver rehabilitation therapist must consider the person's strength, range of motion, sensation, coordination, balance, and posture in determining which style of hand control is best for the individual. "Final determination of equipment needs should be confirmed in a moving assessment in an evaluation vehicle; however, the patient's own vehicle must be considered at some point" (Gillen & Burkhardt, 2004, p. 502).

In-Traffic Assessment

Following the pre-driving clinical assessment, an in-traffic assessment is necessary to make a final determination about a person's ability to drive. The person can be observed operating the vehicle and interacting in the traffic environment. An appropriate evaluation vehicle is used that is equipped with various adaptive equipment as well as dual controls for the instructor and other safety equipment. The purpose of the in-traffic assessment is to assess the person's driving knowledge, skills, and behaviors in the real driving environment on the road and in traffic. By knowing the deficits of the person, the driver rehabilitation therapist can plan a route to challenge them to determine whether the identified deficits interfere with safe driving. A structured

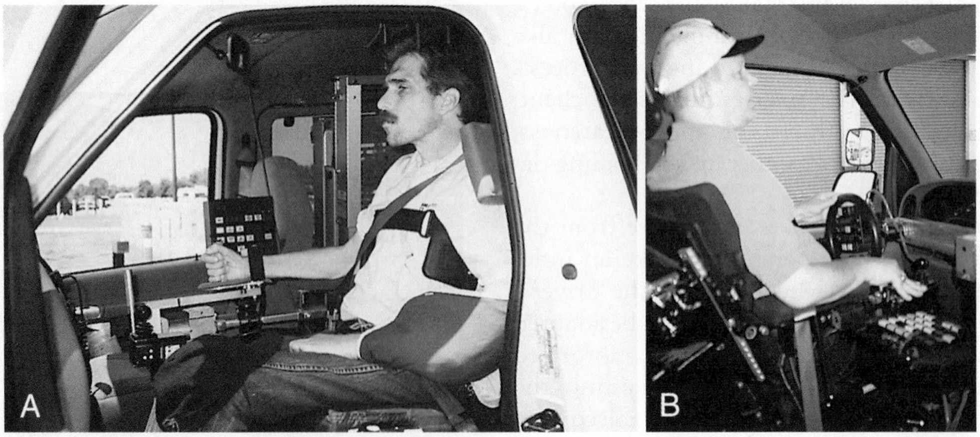

Figure 31-25 The Scott System allows many persons with polio, muscular dystrophy, C4–5 quadriplegia, and triplegia to drive independently. **A.** Person with C5 quadriplegia drives with the right hand in a tri-pin device. He pushes forward for gas and pulls back for braking, and supinates his forearm for turning right and pronates for turning left. **B.** One-handed steering with a small wheel by a person who uses his normal left extremity to push and pull the wheel for gas and brake; the wheel rotates 90° right or left for turning. (Courtesy of Driving Systems Inc., Van Nuys, CA.)

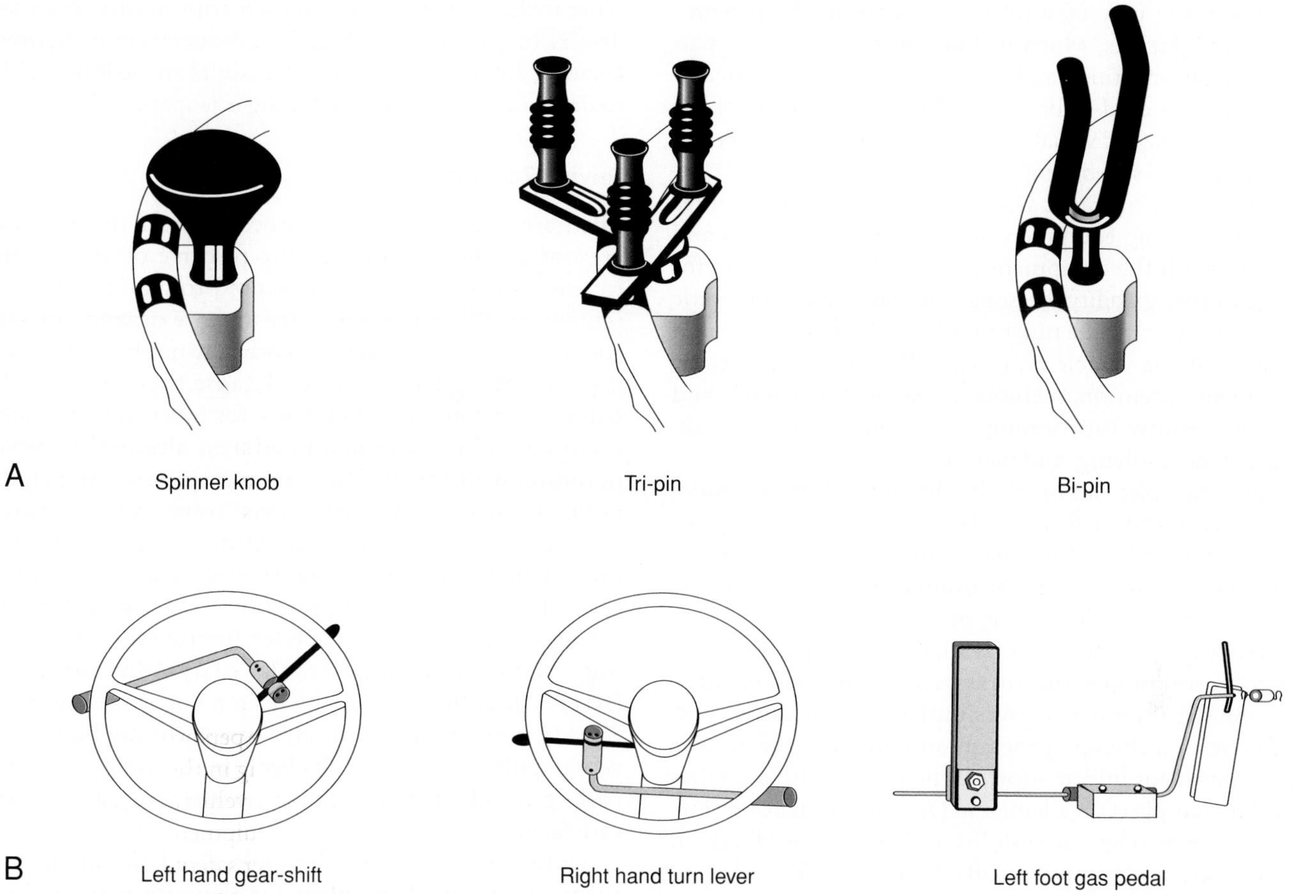

Figure 31-26 Various add-on assistive driving devices. **A.** Steering devices. **B.** Secondary control devices that cross over the functions of the gearshift (left), turn signal (middle), or gas pedal (right), which would be required by some persons after stroke.

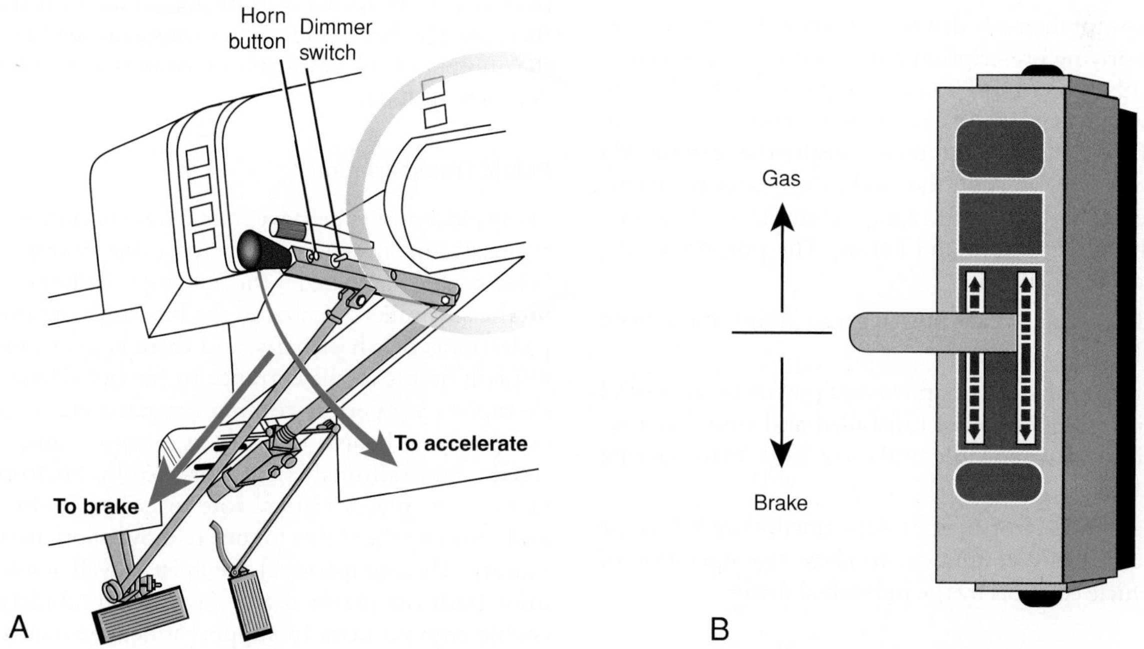

Figure 31-27 Mechanical hand controls or more expensive electromechanical hand controls aid in safe operation of gas and brake. **A.** Push right-angle mechanical hand controls. Requires scapular stabilization and 4− (good minus) strength of shoulder flexion, internal rotation, and elbow extension. **B.** Electroserver hand control requires 3 (fair) strength within a 4-inch range. Can be operated by weak fingers or shoulder flexion and extension.

driving route may take into consideration the person's contextual factors, which include his or her driving patterns, habits, routines, and roles. For example, a particular route may be used to bring out the known deficits of the client, such as left visual neglect, to evaluate whether the deficits permit safe driving.

During the in-traffic assessment, a driver who requires adaptive driving equipment may require instruction and practice with the equipment prior to being evaluated for overall driving ability. Persons who have had a traumatic brain injury or stroke must first be evaluated for physical control of the vehicle and, secondly, for reaction time, judgment, attention, memory, dynamic visual skills, and higher executive functioning such as quick decision making, problem solving, and planning.

The therapist can break the driving task into component parts for the new driver. The occupational therapist's knowledge and skill in task analysis and performance skills is very effective in the evaluation car whether the client is an experienced driver or a new driver.

Driving simulators are available but expensive, and their contribution to the full assessment of a person's driving abilities is limited. A few simulators are relatively cost effective to a therapy program and are designed to give more pertinent information on the person with a disability. An example is the Elemental Driving Simulator by Life Sciences, which has face validity and provides feedback on more visual and cognitive skills than other typical driving simulators (Gianutsos, 1997).

Final Steps

After a comprehensive driver evaluation has been completed, a driving prescription can be written that specifies the client's vehicle and adaptive equipment needs. The therapist can then advise the client or funding source on how to find a mobility equipment dealer that can modify the vehicle properly. After the modifications are complete, the driver rehabilitation therapist will meet the client for a final vehicle inspection and fitting. The purpose of the inspection and fitting is:

1. To determine if all prescription items have been installed
2. To determine if all adaptive equipment or structural modifications have been installed and completed according to applicable industry and manufacture standards
3. To determine proper fit or adjustments needed to the added adaptive equipment to allow safe operation of all vehicle controls by the individual driver

Community Mobility Alternatives

"Most adults, with or without disabilities, drive cars as their primary mode of transportation. People age 65 and older make more than 90% of their trips in cars, as either drivers or passengers" (American Association of Retired Persons, 2003, p. 87). When older adults are no longer able to drive, occupational functioning is jeopardized.

Driving Retirement

There are many persons seen by occupational therapy who are not candidates for learning to drive or are unable to drive for medical reasons or need to plan for driving retirement. When it is necessary to cease driving, the impact on lifestyle and independence may not be as difficult if pre-planning has occurred. Because these individuals still require community mobility for independent living, occupational therapy should address alternative transportation with clients. "Non-driving options can include public transportation such a fixed route rail, bus, paratransit, community transportation (e.g., community bus), demand-responsive transit (e.g., dial-a-ride), flex-route, Independent Transportation Networks, volunteer services, taxis, bicycles or tricycles, hitchhiking, and walking" (National Highway Traffic Safety Administration [NHTSA], 2006a, p. 10). In retirement states such as Florida, communities with golf cart paths are becoming very popular for older adults because the designated cart paths generally lead to shopping, social activity, and health care facilities.

Unfortunately, many older adults faced with driving retirement have made no plans for alternatives to driving. Some of those who have thought about alternatives expect to rely on friends and family for transportation rather than use other forms of transportation. Unfortunately, there are a higher number of persons who need a ride than the number who are available or willing to provide the ride (Yanochko, 2002).

Public Transportation

Many older adults perceive public transportation systems as unsafe, inconvenient, and inaccessible. Access to public buses can be hampered if the bus stops are not easy to get to, the sidewalks or paths to the bus stops are unsafe for pedestrians or wheelchairs, and there is poor lighting or difficult access to the entrance to the bus. Occupational therapists are perfect community partners to serve on city planning boards to assist in making transportation services more affordable and user-friendly. Environmental factors can play a critical role in either facilitating or undermining the ability for one to move about in the community. The occupational therapist is well suited to address both the personal and environmental factors that enable communities to support independence and safe transportation.

A person using a powered wheelchair who cannot drive a car generally needs a privately owned or public van or bus for transportation in the community. The van must be equipped with a wheelchair lift as well as a **wheelchair and occupant restraint system**, also called a WORS (Fig. 31-28). A proper WORS is a crash-tested passive or active restraint device that secures a wheelchair and the occupant separately and appropriately (Schneider, 1981). See information in Definition 31-2 for basic criteria for a proper wheelchair and occupant restraint system. As of 2000, wheelchair manufacturers must address the standards for restraining a wheelchair and the occupant in transit. The American National Standards Institute (ANSI) and the Rehabilitation Engineering Society of North America (RESNA) have contributed in an important way to the development of these standards (Bertocci, Hobson, & Digges, 2000).

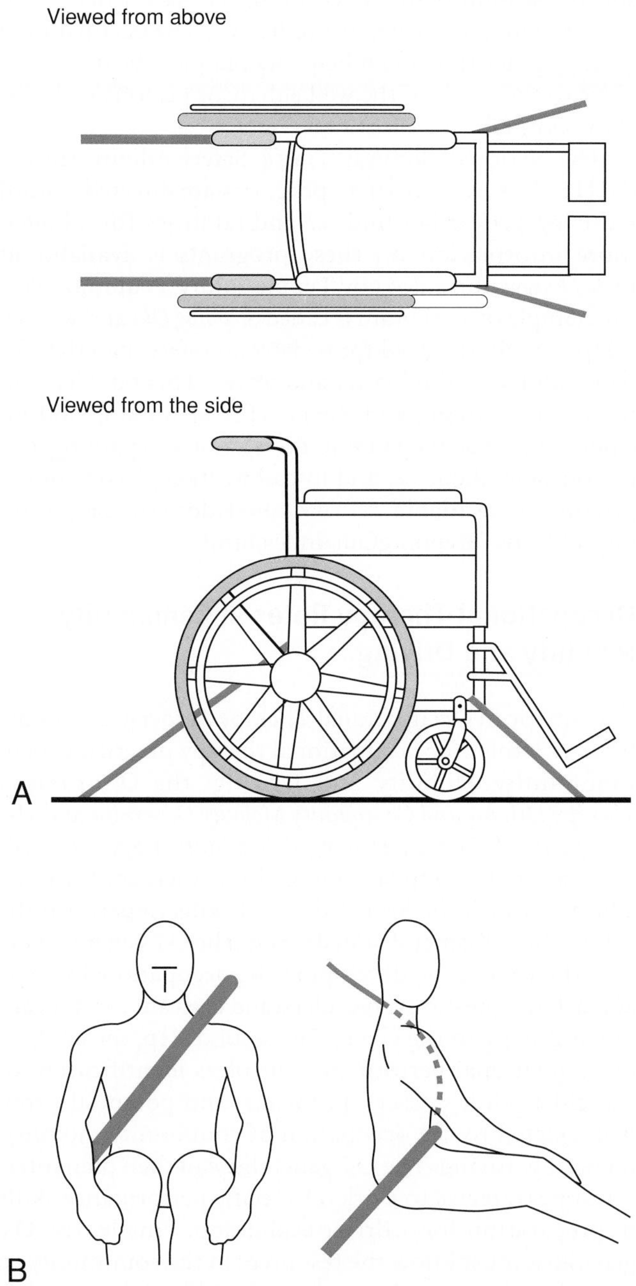

Figure 31-28 Wheelchair and occupant restraint system. **A.** Four points of attachment of tie-downs onto the wheelchair frame. **B.** An effective shoulder and lap belt restraint system requires proper belt angles. Incorrect belt placement can limit protection in a crash or load the occupant so as to cause injury. One end of the shoulder belt should be anchored higher than shoulder level. The lap belt should lie low across the bony structure of the pelvis.

DEFINITION 31-2

Basic Criteria for Proper Wheelchair Restraint

- There must be four points of attachment to the wheelchair.
- The attachment points must not be to any part of the wheelchair that is movable or removable, such as the armrests, footrests, or wheels.
- Proper strapping material and hardware must be used to withstand the forces generated by the wheelchair and the occupant in case of a collision.
- The occupant must be in a forward or rear-facing position, never a sideways or diagonal position.
- Occupant safety belts must be provided on the wheelchair.

Data from Bertocci, Hobson, & Digges, 2000; Schneider, 1981.

Performance Skill Requirements for Community Mobility Options

Alternative modes of transportation, whether it be driving a golf cart or scooter or using a public bus or a subway, require different performance skills. The abilities of the person may determine what options they are able to use. In addition, they must have the finances to pay for services if needed. For example, a bus passenger must be able to understand a bus schedule and strategize a route and timing as well as have the fare and physically offer the fare, get to a bus stop, and then climb on and off the bus. The passenger must then recognize where they need to get off the bus and appropriately notify the bus driver.

Each alternative mode of transportation has its own physical, visual processing, and cognitive skills required for safe utilization. The occupational therapy practitioner must include, in a comprehensive evaluation of a client, a community assessment for the use of alternative modes of transportation. Considering the person's contextual factors is very important so that the evaluation includes all aspects of the person's community. Then the occupational therapy intervention to enable community mobility should take place, if possible, near the person's home, on their chosen mode of transportation, and on the routes and paths that the person would be using.

Mobility as a Pedestrian

Walking should be encouraged as an alternate mode of transportation to motor vehicle travel. Walking is a form of transportation that also has the added benefit of being a healthy activity. Because walking is second nature to us, we forget that it is not only good exercise, but it also enables us to get where we need to go under our own steam, without having to rely on a vehicle. "Communities throughout the United States are mobilizing to promote walking and biking across the lifespan. Efforts include community design changes, health education, walking groups and media campaigns. . . .regular, moderate physical activity can extend the lifespan and prevent or slow the development of chronic disease such as heart disease and diabetes, as well as decrease the likelihood of falls, arthritis pain and depression" (NHTSA, 2006b, p. 1).

A United States Department of Transportation report on active aging describes strategic planning for creating active communities, from identifying audiences, to assessing barriers and opportunities for physical activity, to developing strategies for increasing the number of older adult walkers and cyclists. The catalogue of strategies includes public policy changes, improved community design, and information and education approaches. All reports are published by Partnership for Prevention in collaboration with the United States Department of Transportation, National Highway Traffic Safety Administration and are available at www.prevent.org/activeaging.htm.

Pedestrian Safety

In 2004, 4,641 pedestrians were killed in traffic crashes in the United States—a decrease of 15 percent from the 5,489 pedestrians killed in 1994. There were 68,000 pedestrians injured in traffic crashes in 2004. Most pedestrian fatalities in 2004 occurred in urban areas (72%), at non-intersection locations (79%), in normal weather conditions (89%), and at night (66%) (National Highway Traffic Safety Administration, 2004).

Accident rates for elderly pedestrians resemble those for elderly drivers; that is, the rate is higher than for any other age group. Elderly pedestrians are often hit in crosswalks or when crossing intersections and are generally hit when they have almost finished crossing. They are usually observing the law and not behaving dangerously. Many do not see the vehicle that hit them, and when they do see the vehicle, they usually believe that the driver has seen them and will avoid them. It follows that persons with walking impairments and those in wheelchairs may encounter the same dangers at intersections or crosswalks as the elderly do. Education about pedestrian safety could save lives. Education of community planners and city leaders could encourage changes in traffic signal intersections, pedestrian walkways, and pedestrian warnings. The occupational therapy practitioner can include this information when training a person to be mobile in the community via a wheelchair, cane, scooter, golf cart, or public bus. The occupational therapy practitioner can help city planners be more sensitive to the needs of the well elderly or persons with disabilities of all ages.

The National Highway Traffic Safety Administration (NHTSA) pedestrian safety programs are directed toward reducing pedestrian injuries and fatalities for all ages. More information on these programs is available at http://www.nhtsa.dot.gov/People/injury/Pedbimot/Ped. An example of a program is called *Stepping Out* and was developed to fill the need for pedestrian safety materials for older adults aged 65 years and above. This booklet promotes safe walking and the benefits of walking and includes tips for staying safe at intersections, in parking lots, in non-sidewalk areas, and in bad weather. A copy of the program is available at www.nhtsa.dot.gov/people/injury/olddrive/SteppingOut/index.html.

Occupational Therapy Roles in Community Mobility and Driving

The American Occupational Therapy Association has defined two roles for occupational therapy practitioners in Community Mobility and Driving: the *Occupational Therapy Driving and Community Mobility Generalist* and the *Occupational Therapy Driving Rehabilitation Specialist.* All occupational therapists emerge from their professional education with the knowledge and skills to perform the role of the OT generalist in driving. The OT generalist begins the process by developing the occupational profile and asking questions to understand the value and meaning of driving to the client. The second step, the analysis of occupational performance, involves identification of the older adult's assets, problems, and potential problems related to the occupation of community mobility, including driving. The OT generalist can then plan intervention strategies to work on specific performance skills in preparation for a driver evaluation. Finally, the OT generalist must know the resources in the community so a timely referral can be made to the OT specialist. A fair and objective assessment by a professional is very welcome by families of older drivers or of persons with acquired or congenital disabilities. The OT generalist must often steer the family toward the need for a driver evaluation and the resources of the OT specialist in driving and community mobility (Hunt & Pierce, 2005) (Resources 31-1).

CASE EXAMPLE

Mr. J.: Restoration of Mobility Following Stroke

Occupational Therapy Intervention Process	Clinical Reasoning Process	
	Objectives	**Examples of Therapist's Internal Dialogue**
Patient Information Mr. J. is a 67-year-old man with right hemiplegia and expressive aphasia from a left cerebral vascular accident (CVA). He was evaluated in an outpatient rehabilitation center, and the following problems were identified by the occupational therapist: 1. Client can roll over and sit up in bed but has difficulty moving his right leg off the bed in preparation for transferring and dressing. 2. Client cannot complete a stand-pivot transfer independently because he needs assistance coming to standing. 3. Client can propel his manual wheelchair with a one-arm drive on level surfaces but cannot negotiate a ramp or uneven terrain. 4. Client cannot perform bathroom activities at home because his bathroom is inaccessible to his wheelchair. 5. Client has not driven since the CVA but is very anxious to begin driving again. He is concerned about loading his wheelchair into a car by himself.	Appreciate the context	M J. is still young with a good medical history except for the CVA. Most importantly, he is motivated to improve his mobility skills so that he can be less dependent upon his wife. His home environment and spousal and family support will enable him to reach higher goals for mobility and independence.
	Develop intervention hypotheses	"Mr. J. has significant physical deficits that may be permanent, but with his young age and good health, I believe that his occupational performance could be enhanced greatly by improving his functional and community mobility skills."
	Select an intervention approach	"I will develop an intervention plan that emphasizes functional mobility first and community mobility needs second. I know that there are precursor mobility skills that are required in the areas of bed mobility, transfers, and wheelchair mobility, so I will need to address these performance skill areas first before I address the specific tasks that he is weak in such as handling his legs in bed or propelling his wheelchair outdoors. It will enhance my intervention if I talk with physical therapy to see if they can work on improving his leg strength and his ability to stand up independently. I will need to explain to the client and his family that we will address his driving ability as a long-term goal after we have accomplished the short-term goals in functional mobility. I will explain how the skills in functional mobility will prepare him for the driver evaluation when the time is appropriate. I will let the family know that I can research community transportation alternatives available in their community that he may be able to use in the meantime or in case it is found that he is not able to return to driving in the future."

Reflect on competence

"I am concerned that I do not know all of my responsibilities as an OT generalist in driving and community mobility. I need to research this area before I begin addressing the topic of driving and community mobility. I also need to find resources in my state for an OT specialist in driving and community mobility so I can talk intelligently about the specialist's services and purpose to the client and family."

Recommendations

The occupational therapist recommended two treatment sessions per week for 8 weeks. In collaboration with the client and his wife, the occupational therapist established the following long-term treatment goals: (1) Mr. J. will be independent in bed mobility and sitting on the edge of the bed; (2) Mr. J. will be able to perform a stand-pivot transfer independently; (3) Mr. J. will improve his ability to negotiate outdoor terrain and ramps with his manual wheelchair and be advised on motorized scooters for use in independent long-distance mobility in the community; (4) in collaboration with physical therapy, Mr. J. will be instructed in using his hemi-walker to walk into the bathroom and perform sink activities while standing; and (5) Mr. J. will be referred to an OT specialist in driving and community mobility once he is able to transfer in and out of his car.

Consider the patient's appraisal of performance

Consider what will occur in therapy, how often, and for how long

Ascertain the patient's endorsement of plan

"I do not believe that this client is aware of his potential for being more independent in functional mobility skills. Some of this may be related to his wife, who is unsure if he can drive again. I believe that he is motivated enough to be more independent and will have successful outcomes with an aggressive therapy program. I also believe that, when he sees that he can accomplish functional mobility goals and senses that his potential to drive again may be greater than he first thought, he will be highly motivated to work hard in occupational therapy. Mr. J. and his wife seem agreeable to the plan, and I hope that by including his wife that she will become more comfortable in letting him do more tasks for himself at home, which is very important to him."

Summary of Short-Term Goals and Progress

1. Mr. J. will be able to move his weak leg off the edge of a bed and come to a seated position with or without orthotic devices.

The therapist ascertained after a week of occupational therapy that Mr. J. could move his weak leg off the bed using his stronger left leg by putting his left foot under the weak right foot and then moving both feet over the edge of the bed. She determined, however, that he would require a device to use to pull against to come to a short-leg sitting position on the edge of the bed. In the second week, various techniques and assistive devices were demonstrated to him, and it was determined that a portable half bed rail worked best. By the fourth week, Mr. J. could come to a short-leg sitting position on the side of the bed independently. He was also shown how to use the bed rail to help him stand up and ready himself for a stand-pivot transfer.

2. Mr. J. will become independent in sink activities in the bathroom.

The first week of therapy revealed that the client's standing tolerance and balance were not sufficient to perform sink activities while standing even though he could walk short distances. In the second week, he was taught how to stand up from his wheelchair outside the bathroom door, walk into the bathroom using his hemi-walker and short leg brace, and sit on a tall-legged stool at the sink. The higher seat helped him come to standing when he pulled on the sink for assistance in standing up when ready to leave.

3. Mr. J. will be able to transfer into the passenger and driver side of his car independently.

By the third week, Mr. J. could handle his leg on and off the bed and could stand up independently. In the fourth week, Mr. J. was instructed in getting in and out of the passenger side of a car. After he could perform this transfer, he was taught how to transfer into the driver's side of the car, maneuvering his legs under the steering wheel.

Assess the patient's comprehension

Understand what he is doing

Compare actual to expected performance

Know the person

Appreciate the context

"Initially it was hard to motivate Mr. J. to work on bed mobility tasks, such as rolling over, coming to sitting, and moving his legs over the edge of the bed, because he had become used to his wife helping him in bed mobility. As she began to support him doing more on his own, I saw a big leap in his motivation. Once he could accomplish the first task of handling his legs, he was then very eager to move onto learning to stand up and transfer on his own. I could see his eyes light up every session as he accomplished another goal because he could see how it would all come together in the end and make him less dependent upon his wife. Even though he was unable to do some tasks completely on his own, he recognized quickly that there is much assistive technology out there that can benefit him."

"It has been very helpful for Mrs. J. to attend each of Mr. J.'s treatment sessions. As she has observed his weaknesses, she has been able to encourage him to complete his home therapy exercises and activities on days that he does not come to therapy. They have learned how to use the kitchen sink for support to let him work on standing tolerance 3–4 times a day. Mrs. J. has indicated that he will sometimes sit outside the bathroom and appear to long to just stand up and walk in. Mr. J. knows that they cannot afford to modify the bathroom doorway, so he understands that it is very important for him to have a good outcome with standing and this goal. He keeps asking me about a driving evaluation and is beginning to show some frustration in having to wait. Mrs. J. is very understanding of why this goal has been put off to later and has assured me that she will not let him drive before he is ready."

In the sixth week, he was referred to an OT specialist in driving and community mobility that I found in the next town. He was instructed by this specialist to use a left-foot gas pedal and a spinner knob for driving, and the adaptive equipment was installed in his own car. In collaboration with the OT driving specialist, we both decided that Mr. J. could not be independent in loading his wheelchair into his four-door sedan. He did not have the standing balance to use a wheelchair loader that is bumper or trunk mounted. He could, however, use a car topper that will electrically pick up, fold, and load his manual wheelchair into a box on the top of his car all while he sits in the driver seat. By the time of his discharge, he had received all necessary in-vehicle training by the OT driving specialist and was beginning to drive around his own community.

"Mr. J. is accomplishing his goals quickly. I see him working very hard because he can tell that a driver evaluation is getting closer to becoming to reality for him. Through my contact with the OT driving specialist, I was able to discover that Mr. J. can use an adaptive equipment rebate from General Motors to help him purchase some of his driving equipment since his car was bought new 6 months ago. This will enable him to afford to buy the car topper as well as the devices he requires for driving. I introduced Mr. J. to another client of mine who also drives with adaptive equipment and went to the same OT driving specialist. This was very encouraging to Mr. J., and he actually went to see some driving equipment in this gentleman's car. It was so great to see Mr. J. come into therapy after the first session of seeing the OT driving specialist. He was so excited and could finally see that he would be able to become much less dependent upon his family now. It was nice to hear him express his appreciation for my work, and he even admitted that he was glad I did not send him for a driving evaluation sooner."

Next Steps: Revised short-term goals (1 month):

1. Mr. J. will become independent in toilet transfers and tub transfers but will likely require some assistive technology such as elevated toilet seat, grab bars, and a tub bench.
2. Mr. J. will become independent in long-distance ambulation by using a motorized scooter but will require assistance for loading and unloading the scooter.
3. Mr. J. will be independent in driving himself to and from therapy.

Anticipate present and future patient concerns

Analyze patient's comprehension

Decide if the patient should continue or discontinue therapy and/or return in the future

"Mr. J. has made great progress over the past month. He does not seem as depressed as when I first saw him and is coming to therapy with more and more things that he would like to do. I have recommended that he obtain a referral for home health OT so that he can begin working in his own home environment. The home health OT can make sure he gets the right equipment in his bathroom and give him practice with his transfers in his own environment. He is totally agreeable to this plan. He is asking if he can drive now to and from his daughter's house, which is about 45 minutes away in another small town. I have referred him back to the OT driving specialist to address this issue with him. Mr. J. and I decided that he no longer needs outpatient OT but can be followed for his other goals by the OT consultant."

CLINICAL REASONING IN OCCUPATIONAL THERAPY PRACTICE

The Importance of a Client-Centered Approach

During the initial OT evaluation, Mr. J. appeared depressed and withdrawn. What observable signs did Mr. J. display during the evaluation from which the therapist might draw this conclusion? In what ways can the therapist investigate the cause of Mr. J.'s depression? What factors in the client's contextual environment could cause these depressed feelings?

Evidence Table 31-1
Best Evidence for Occupational Therapy Practice Regarding Occupational Therapy to Improve Mobility

Intervention	Description of Intervention Tested	Participants	Dosage	Type of Best Evidence and Level of Evidence	Benefit	Statistical Probability and Effect Size of Outcome	Reference
Targeted occupational therapy at home to increase outdoor mobility	Intervention: Assessment of barriers to outdoor mobility, set mobility goals with the client, and delivered interventions to meet the goals. Control: One OT session of advice, encouragement, and provision of leaflets describing local mobility services.	168 community-dwelling adults diagnosed with stroke within 36 months: 86 randomly assigned to the intervention group and 82 assigned to the control group.	Up to 7 occupational therapy interventions for up to 3 months. Mean dosage = 4.7 visits for a mean total of 230 minutes.	Randomized controlled trial. IA1a	Yes. The occupational therapy intervention that targeted specific mobility goals was successful in increasing outdoor mobility in both the short (4 months) and long term (10 months). Those with the worst self-reported outdoor mobility at the start of treatment benefited most.	Out of the house as much as you would like?: 65% for intervention; 35% for controls. How many journeys outdoors in last month?: 37 for intervention vs. 14 for controls; $p < 0.01$. *Nottingham Extended Activities of Daily Living Scale*: No significant difference. *Nottingham Leisure Questionnaire*: No significant difference. *General Health Questionnaire*: No significant difference. Effect sizes could not be calculated from data provided.	Logan et al., 2004

Transition from manual wheelchair to powered mobility device (PMD)	Prescribed (by a registered OT?) a PMD at point when no longer able to propel a manual wheelchair as primary mobility device.	Convenience sample of 8 community-living adults between ages 27 and 52 years, with static or progressive conditions, who had previously used a manual wheelchair before receiving a PMD between 6 and 24 months prior to the study (demarcation event).	Not applicable.	Retrospective study of behavior before and after the demarcation event of receiving a PMD (one group pre-/post-test design). IIIC2b	Yes. Results suggest that the transition to a PMD enhanced occupational performance, competence, adaptability, and self-esteem for persons with severe mobility impairments.	*Occupational Performance History Interview* (*OPHI*): significant improvement in role performance (Wilcoxon signed rank test, t $= 0, p = 0.001, r = 1.09$) after introduction of PMD. *Psychological Impact of Assistive Device Scale* (*PIADS*) (self-report): all participants rated adequacy, independence, quality of life, ability to adapt to ADL, and ability to take advantage of opportunities a score ≥ 2 (somewhat increased or better).	Buning, Angelo, & Schmeler, 2001

RESOURCE 31-1

Information and Professional Development in Driving and Community Mobility

Adaptive Mobility Services, Inc.
OT Professional Development Workshops
1000 Delaney Avenue
Orlando, FL 32806
Phone: (407) 426-8020
www.adaptivemobility.com

Association of Driver Rehabilitation Specialists (ADED)
711 S. Vienna
Ruston, LA 71270
Phone: (800) 290-2344
www.aded.net

American National Standards Institute
11 West 42nd Street, Floor 13
New York, NY 10036
Phone: (212) 642-4900
www.ansi.org

National Highway Traffic Safety Administration
Office of the Chief Counsel
400 7th Street, SW
Washington, DC 20590
Fax: (202) 336-3820
www.nhtsa.dot.gov/

Rehabilitation Engineering and Assistive Technology Society of North America (RESNA)
1700 North Moore Street, Suite 1540
Arlington, VA 22209-1903
Phone: (703) 524-6686
Fax: (703) 524-6630
E-mail: info@resna.org

Resources for Wheelchair Accessibility

AlumiRamp, Inc.
855 Chicago Road
Quincy, MI 49082
Phone: (800) 800-3864
www.alumiramp.com

Center for Accessible Housing
North Carolina State University
P.O. Box 8613
Raleigh, NC 27695-8613
Phone: (800) 647-6777
www.ncsu.edu/ncsu/design/cud

EZ-Access Ramps
1704 B Street NW, Suite 110
Auburn, WA 98001
Phone: (800) 451-1903
www.ezaccess.com

Driving Adaptive Equipment Manufacturers

Braun Corporation
1014 South Monticello
Winamac, IN 46996
Phone: (219) 946-6157
www.braunlift.com

Bruno Independent Living Aids
430 Armour Court
Oconomowoc, WI 53066
Phone: (800) 882-8183
www.bruno.com

Drivemaster Corporation
9 Spielman Road
Fairfield, NJ 07004
Phone: (201) 808-9709 or (800) 826-7368
www.drive-master.com

Driving Systems Incorporated
16139 Runnymede Street
Van Nuys, CA 91406
Phone: (818) 782-7693
www.drivingsystems.com

Electronic Mobility Controls, Inc.
6141 Crestmount Drive
Baton Rouge, LA 70809
Phone: (225) 927-5558
www.emc-digi.com

Q-Straint (w/c restraint)
5553 Ravenswood, Building 104
Ft. Lauderdale, FL 33312
Phone: (800) 987-9987
www.qstraint.com

SUMMARY REVIEW QUESTIONS

1. Define the two main areas of mobility for occupational therapy intervention and list three specific subareas under each main area of mobility.
2. Describe the hierarchy of intervention planning for mobility and identify two preparatory performance skills required for each area.
3. How can the principles of body mechanics be applied to training in transfer skills?
4. List the specific outdoor mobility skills that you should instruct a patient in who must now use a manual wheelchair.
5. List precursor abilities and skills that a patient with paraplegia must accomplish before learning to transfer into a wheelchair.
6. Describe the options available in teaching a patient how to negotiate a curb in a manual wheelchair.
7. Describe the different roles for evaluation and intervention planning for the OT generalist versus the OT driving and community mobility specialist.
8. List the performance skill factors to consider when determining whether your client or patient is appropriate to refer to an occupational therapy driver rehabilitation specialist for a driver evaluation.
9. For successful outcomes in mobility, identify specific areas of mobility intervention in which you will confer with an interdisciplinary team member and demonstrate your understanding of the interplay between the disciplines by defining each team member's responsibility for the areas you have identified.
10. Describe why planning for driving retirement is important and list the transportation alternatives that are available in some communities.

ACKNOWLEDGMENT

I thank Carol Blackburn, OTR/L, CDRS; Brenda Johnston, OTR; Daphne Cronin; Joan Bova; and Linda and Chuck Green for their assistance with the photography for this chapter.

References

American Association of Retired Persons [AARP]. (2003). *Beyond 50 2003: A report to the nation on independent living and disability*. Washington, DC: AARP.

American Medical Association [AMA]. (2003). *The physician's guide to assessing and counseling older drivers*. Available at www.ama-assn.org/go/olderdrivers.

American Occupational Therapy Association [AOTA]. (2002). Occupational therapy practice framework: Domain and process. *American Journal of Occupational Therapy, 56,* 609–639.

Americans with Disabilities Act [ADA]. (1990). *Public Law 101-336, 42 U.S.C. 12101*. Washington, DC: United States Department of Justice. Retrieved March 11, 2005 from http://www.usdoj.gov/crt/ada/adahom1.htm.

Bertocci, G. E., Hobson, D. A., & Digges, K. H. (2000). Development of a wheelchair occupant injury risk assessment method and its application in the investigation of wheelchair securement point influence on frontal crash safety. *IEEE Transactions of Rehabilitation Engineering, 8,* 126–139.

Buning, M. E., Angelo, J. A., & Schmeler, M. R. (2001). Occupational performance and the transition to powered mobility: A pilot study. *American Journal of Occupational Therapy, 55,* 339–344.

Carp, F. M. (1988). Significance of mobility for the well-being of the elderly. In *Transportation in an aging society: Improving mobility and safety for older persons* (Vol.1, pp. 1–20). Washington, DC: National Research Council Committee for the Study on Improving Mobility and Safety for Older Persons, Transportation Research Board.

Deusterhaus-Minor, M. A., & Deusterhaus-Minor, S. (1999). *Patient care skills* (4th ed.). Stanford, CT: Appleton & Lange.

Gianutsos, R. (1997). Driving and visual information processing in cognitively at-risk and older drivers. In M. Gentile (Ed.), *Functional visual behavior: A therapist's guide to evaluation and treatment options* (pp. 321–342). Bethesda, MD: American Occupational Therapy Association.

Gillen, G., & Burkhardt, A. (1998). *Stroke rehabilitation: A function-based approach*. St. Louis: Mosby, Inc.

Gillen, G., & Burkhardt, A. (2004). *Stroke rehabilitation: A function-based approach* (2nd ed.). St. Louis: Mosby, Inc.

Hunt, L., & Pierce, S. (2005). Driving and community mobility for older adults: Occupational therapy roles (online course). Bethesda, MD: American Occupational Therapy Association. Available at www.aota.org.

Kaplan, W. (1999). The occupation of driving: Legal and ethical issues. *American Occupational Therapy Association Physical Disabilities Special Interest Section Quarterly, 23,* 1–3.

Logan, P. A., Gladman, J. R. F., Avery, A., Walker, M. F., Dyas, J., & Groom, L. (2004). Randomised controlled trial of an occupational therapy intervention to increase outdoor mobility after stroke. *British Medical Journal, 10,* 1372–1375.

Monga, T., Ostermann, H., & Kerrigan, A. (1997). Driving: A clinical perspective on rehabilitation technology. In *Physical medicine and rehabilitation: State of the art reviews* (Vol. 11, pp. 69–92). Philadelphia: Hanley & Belfus.

National Highway Traffic Safety Administration (NHTSA) (2004). *Traffic safety facts*. Washington, DC: National Center for Statistics and Analysis. Retrieved November 3, 2006 from http://www.nrd.nhtsa.dot.gov/pdf/nrd-30/ncsa/TSF2004/809913.pdf

National Highway Traffic Safety Administration [NHTSA]. (2006a). Appendix 1: Literature review. Retrieved January 13, 2006 from http://www.nhtsa.dot.gov/people/injury/olddrive/OlderRoad/appendix.htm.

National Highway Traffic Safety Administration [NHTSA]. (2006b). Retrieved January 13, 2006 from http://www.nhtsa.dot.gov/people/injury/olddrive/FromTheField-ActiveAging/pages/FromtheField.

Nixon,V. (1985). *Spinal cord injury: A guide to functional outcomes in physical therapy management*. Gaithersburg, MD: Aspen.

Pierce, S. (1992). Driver's needs. *Team Rehab Report, 3,* 20–22, 38.

Pierce, S. (1993). Legal considerations for a driver rehabilitation program. *OT Practice, 16,* 1–4.

Pierce, S. (1996). A roadmap for driver rehabilitation. *OT Practice, 10,* 30–38.

Pierson, F. M. (1999). *Principles and techniques of patient care* (2nd ed.). Philadelphia: Saunders.

Schneider, L. W. (1981). Dynamic testing of restraint system and tie-downs for use with vehicle occupants seated in powered wheelchairs. UM-HSRI Report 81-18. Ann Arbor, MI: University of Michigan Transportation Research Institute.

Sims, R., Owsley, C., Allman, R., Ball, K., & Smoot, T. (1998). A preliminary assessment of the medical and functional factors associated with vehicle crashes by older adults. *Journal of the American Geriatrics Society, 46,* 556–561.

Wang, C. C., Kosinski, C. J., Schwartzberg, J. G., & Shanklin, A. V. (2003). *Physician's guide to assessing and counseling older drivers*. Washington, DC: National Highway Traffic Safety Administration.

Yanochko, P. (2002). *Traffic safety among older adults: Recommendations for California*. San Diego, CA: Center for Injury Prevention Policy and Practice, San Diego State University.

CHAPTER 32

Restoring Competence for Homemaker and Parent Roles

Susan E. Fasoli

LEARNING OBJECTIVES

After studying this chapter, the reader will be able to do the following:

1. State the principles of compensation and adaptation.
2. State the principles of work simplification.
3. Identify adapted methods and equipment that enable persons with varied physical challenges and diagnoses to regain competence in homemaking roles.
4. Identify adapted methods and equipment that enable persons with varied physical challenges and diagnoses to regain competence in parenting roles.
5. Describe and teach proper body mechanics for homemaking and parenting tasks and activities.

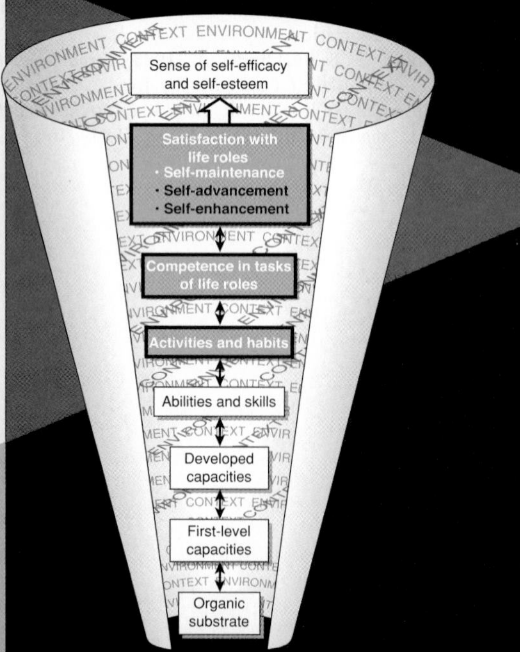

Restoring competence in homemaker and parenting roles following a disabling event can greatly enhance one's sense of efficacy and feelings of self-esteem. Therapists typically address impaired performance of these life roles after a client has regained independence in basic activities of daily living (e.g., self-care). Home management and parenting tasks, however, can be incorporated into the rehabilitation process at any time, depending on the individual's own priorities and needs.

Homemaking and parenting tasks may be used as both occupation-as-means and occupation-as-end, depending on the client's rehabilitation potential and desired goals. This chapter focuses on the use of occupation-as-end to restore a client's competence and participation in homemaker and parent roles. This treatment approach allows for addressing significant impairments in occupational performance skills (e.g., incoordination or visual impairments) via the principles for compensation and adaptation highlighted in Procedures for Practice 32-1.

Principles of work simplification and energy conservation can be taught to clients with physical impairments who lack sufficient endurance to accomplish daily life tasks. Work simplification and energy conservation principles are commonsense ideas to improve task efficiency and reduce energy expenditure during all occupational tasks and roles, including those related to homemaking and parenting (Procedures for Practice 32-1).

HOMEMAKER ROLES AND TASKS: TREATMENT PRINCIPLES AND METHODS

An important role of the occupational therapist is to learn what life roles and tasks are particularly meaningful to the client (i.e., to explore his/her occupational identity) and to allow him/her the opportunity to grieve for what is lost or

PROCEDURES FOR PRACTICE 32-1

Principles of Adaptation to Compensate for Functional Limitations

Principles for Compensation and Adaptation

- Limited ROM: Increase the person's reach via extended handles and organize needed items within a compact work space.
- Weakness and low endurance: Use lightweight and/or powered equipment and allow gravity to assist. Employ work simplification and energy conservation techniques.
- Chronic pain: Reinforce use of proper body mechanics and pacing during physical tasks.
- Unilateral loss of motor control and limb function: Use affected limb to stabilize objects when possible. Use adapted methods and/or assistive equipment to perform bilateral activities with one hand.
- Incoordination: Stabilize at proximal joints (e.g., elbow) to reduce degrees of freedom necessary for control. Use weighted objects to minimize distal incoordination.
- Visual impairments: Use senses of smell, touch, and hearing to substitute for low vision. Enhance performance of visual tasks by improving lighting, reducing glare, or increasing contrast.
- Cognitive limitations: Employ visual and auditory aids to enhance memory and organization. Plan steps prior to beginning task. Work in familiar environment (e.g., home kitchen) to enhance cognitive performance during homemaking tasks.

Principles of Work Simplification and Energy Conservation

- Limit the amount of work. When possible, avoid overfatigue by assigning heavy homemaking tasks (e.g., vacuuming, cleaning bathrooms) to family members or a housekeeper.
- Explore ways to reduce homemaking demands and expectations, such as using packaged mixes or frozen foods to decrease time and energy for meal preparation.
- Plan ahead. Schedule homemaking, child care tasks (e.g., changing bed linens, giving tub baths), and community outings (e.g., shopping, doctor visits) to distribute energy-demanding tasks throughout the week. Prioritize to complete important tasks before fatigue sets in.
- Use efficient methods. Organize work areas and store frequently used supplies in a convenient location. Avoid standing when it is possible to sit while doing the task (e.g., ironing). Slide objects across a counter or table rather than lift them. Identify needed items at the beginning of a task to avoid extra trips. Use a utility cart to transport items.
- Use correct equipment and techniques. Use assistive equipment (e.g., long-handled reachers) to decrease bending and stooping. Avoid prolonged holding by stabilizing items with non-skid mats. Adjust work height and use tools most appropriate for the job. When physical limitations are present, choose equipment that does not promote further deformity.
- Balance daily tasks with rest breaks. Clients should perform energy-demanding tasks early in the day, when they are most rested. Encourage self-pacing of tasks (don't rush!) to avoid fatigue. Frequent rest periods of 5–10 minutes can greatly enhance functional endurance during homemaking and parenting tasks.

changed (Unruh, 2004). Many factors, including psychosocial adjustment, cognitive or perceptual impairments, and physical limitations, can influence a client's ability to take part in homemaker roles and tasks.

Psychosocial Adjustment

When faced with the onset or progression of physical disability, a client and family may have a variety of psychological responses. These reactions may be characterized by lack of motivation and refusal to participate in therapy, expressed feelings of hopelessness or anger, and denial (American Occupational Therapy Association, 1997). For persons with chronic conditions, such as scleroderma or rheumatoid arthritis, the challenges encountered during household chores can strongly affect levels of life satisfaction and well-being (Sandqvist, Akesson, & Eklund, 2005). The family's expectations and reactions must also be considered when occupational therapists are setting intervention goals and establishing plans for treatment. These psychological reactions must be acknowledged and addressed by the occupational therapist if identified goals are to be achieved.

Barriers to Effectiveness

The occupational therapist must identify factors, in addition to psychosocial concerns, that can interfere with the effectiveness of intervention and inhibit performance during homemaking tasks. These factors include, but are not limited to, cognitive and perceptual impairments, poor vision, and environmental constraints including lack of family support.

Persons with cognitive impairments as a result of central nervous system disorders may have more difficulty learning compensatory techniques than persons with musculoskeletal or peripheral nervous system disorders. The client needs good memory, judgment, and problem-solving abilities to learn how an assistive device is used, when it is needed, and how it can safely enhance task performance (Moyers, 1999). Cognitive demands are increased when the adapted methods greatly alter the way the task is performed (e.g., ordering groceries online or learning to use a utility cart to transport items).

In the absence of intact cognitive abilities, clients may be able to learn new task methods, such as how to operate a microwave oven for meal preparation, if they can follow visual cues or instructions. The occupational therapist must ensure that the client can safely perform the task with the prescribed adaptations and meet unexpected challenges encountered during task performance.

Perceptual impairments, including poor figure-ground skills, poor spatial orientation, and visual neglect, can also interfere with one's ability to manage homemaking tasks independently. Limitations in perceptual processing can interfere with one's ability to find needed items in the cupboard, decrease safety of pouring hot coffee into a cup, and increase the likelihood of falls when vacuuming or sweeping floors. In addition, poor visual processing, such as loss of central vision or decreased contrast sensitivity, can inhibit safety during homemaking tasks. Environmental changes, such as increasing available lighting throughout the home and enhancing contrast (e.g., pouring coffee into a light-colored mug), can improve performance (Lampert & Lapolice, 1995).

Support of family or friends can be instrumental for carrying out recommended adaptations, reinforcing the use of assistive devices, and identifying additional concerns in need of intervention. When family assistance is not available, other support services (e.g., homemaker, companion) may be employed to ensure safety in homemaking tasks.

Preventing Decline in Homemaker Role and Tasks

Occupational therapists are often involved with preventing disability in persons who are at risk for developing impairments, activity limitations, and restrictions in the performance of life tasks and roles (Moyers, 1999). Prevention programs for elderly persons include exercise classes to reduce physical limitations in balance, range of motion, and strength, in addition to group activities that exercise cognitive abilities, such as judgment and problem solving (Jackson et al., 1998). Homemakers may be instructed in home safety tips directed toward reducing clutter, removing loose rugs, and arranging furniture to clear walkways and allow access to electrical plugs and windows. Environmental modifications, such as the installation of grab bars and railings, can significantly decrease the occurrence of falls (Plautz et al., 1996).

Occupational therapists can be instrumental in identifying hazards in the home and providing ideas that may enhance a person's safety and continued independence. Many limitations encountered by well elderly persons during homemaking tasks may be prevented or alleviated by relatively simple and inexpensive solutions.

Homemaking: Techniques and Therapeutic Aids

Competence in the role of homemaker can be attained in either of two ways, depending on the client's level of physical and cognitive ability: by managing and directing others to perform homemaking tasks or by direct participation.

Although persons with severe physical disabilities may not be able to perform many homemaking tasks without assistance, they can be effective home managers. For instance, individuals with high-level spinal cord injuries can independently manage household tasks by directing

RESOURCE 32-1

Books

Klinger, J. L. (1997). *Meal preparation and training: The health care professional's guide.* Thorofare, NJ: Slack.

Mayer, T. K. (2000). *One-handed in a two-handed world: Your personal guide to managing single handedly* (2nd ed.). Boston: Prince Gallison.

Organizations, Associations, and Services

The Internet offers a wealth of information concerning resources for specific disabilities. The following are some organizations that listed information specific to home management or parenting at the time of publication:

The Arthritis Foundation
Atlanta, GA
Phone: (800) 283-7800
www.arthritis.org

National Multiple Sclerosis Society
New York, NY
Phone: (800) FIGHT-MS or (800) 344-4867
www.nmss.org

American Heart Association
Dallas, TX 75231
Phone: (800) AHA-USA-1 or (800) 242-8721
www.americanheart.org

American Stroke Association
Dallas, TX 75231
Phone: (888) 4-STROKE or (888) 478-7653
www.strokeassociation.org

Through the Looking Glass (addresses the needs of parents with disabilities and parents of disabled children)
Berkeley, CA
Phone: (800) 644-2666
www.lookingglass.org

Computerized Information Services for Persons with Disabilities

ABLEDATA
Silver Springs, MD
Phone: (800) 227-0216.
www.abledata.com

Manufacturers and Distributors of Adaptive Devices

North Coast Medical
Morgan Hill, CA
Phone: (800) 821-9319
www.ncmedical.com

Sammons Preston Rolyan
Bolingbrook, IL
Phone: (800) 323-5547
www.sammonsprestonrolyan.com

family members or paid housekeepers, managing finances, and overseeing shopping. Computerized banking systems and shopping services are accessible to those with Internet access and are relatively easy to use. Occupational therapy at this level may focus on organizing how household tasks may be scheduled, instructing the client in computer use, or identifying service resources in the community. Homemaker services, home health aides, and Meals on Wheels may provide the support necessary for a person with limited abilities to remain at home.

Persons who can physically participate in homemaking tasks can benefit from a variety of interventions that maximize role performance. The following sections discuss equipment and adapted methods for homemaking.

Equipment Considerations

A number of factors contribute to the selection and use of assistive devices and adapted equipment for homemaking. Simple modifications in the way a task is performed sometimes eliminate the need for an assistive device, and this is the preferable solution. When equipment is recommended, a primary concern is that the assistive device satisfies the needs of the client and enables the person to accomplish tasks that are otherwise impossible or difficult (Axtell & Yasuda, 1993). The person must be comfortable with the idea of using an assistive device and satisfied with its appearance.

When making equipment recommendations, the occupational therapist must consider both the immediate and long-term needs of the client. Individuals with a progressive disease, such as rheumatoid arthritis or multiple sclerosis, benefit from equipment that can enhance current functional performance and provide for anticipated changes in physical status. In contrast, persons with nonprogressive conditions, such as acquired brain injury or spinal cord injury, often use fewer assistive devices as they regain physical abilities or learn alternate ways to accomplish their tasks without equipment.

Generally, assistive devices should be simple to use and maintain, as lightweight as possible, and dependable (Axtell & Yasuda, 1993). If a client has mild cognitive impairments that interfere with equipment use, family members may be taught ways to enhance carryover at home. Insurance providers generally do not pay for assistive devices and adapted equipment. For those who cannot afford to purchase such items, loaner equipment may be available from local organizations, including disability support groups and senior citizen centers.

Meal Preparation, Service, and Cleanup

Efficient work areas, adapted techniques, and assistive devices can greatly enhance a client's safety and participation in meal preparation tasks.

Kitchen Storage and Work Area

Kitchens should be organized so that frequently used items are within easy reach of the place they are most often used. On average, persons who use a wheelchair can reach to retrieve items between 15 inches (low reach) and 48 inches (high reach) from the floor. Those who are ambulatory but have difficulty bending generally can reach 30 inches (low reach) to 60 inches (high reach) from the floor, depending on the person's height (Anderson, 1981).

Pull-out shelves and turntables in cabinets can compensate for limited reach and maximize usable storage space. Pans, dishes, and so on may be stored vertically to alleviate the need to move unwanted items to obtain the one underneath. Pegboards with hooks can be attached to the back of closet doors to hold pots, pans, and utensils for easy access. Shelves attached to the inside of cabinet doors are handy for holding assorted wraps, canned goods, and cleaning supplies. Items that are seldom used should be removed to eliminate unnecessary clutter.

Safety and independence in the kitchen can be enhanced by the availability of clear and accessible workspaces. For persons in wheelchairs, work counters should be 28–34 inches from the floor and have a depth clearance of 24 inches underneath to allow room for wheelchair leg rests. A work area that is at least 30 inches wide is recommended to provide sufficient space for needed items during meal preparation (ADA-ABA, 2004).

Gathering and Transporting Items

An important role of the occupational therapist is to help the client solve problems about gathering and transporting items at home by using work simplification principles and proper body mechanics (Procedures for Practice 32-1 and 32-2). Long-handled reachers can be helpful but should be used primarily for retrieving lightweight unbreakable items.

The wide range of assistive devices for transporting items around the home includes cup holders and walker or wheelchair bags. Homemakers who use a wheelchair may benefit from using a lap tray that easily slides on and off the wheelchair arms (Fig. 32-1). A variety of wire baskets and trays that attach to a standard walker are available for purchase, but many of these devices accommodate only a few things at a time, such as a sandwich and covered beverage. Individuals who perform homemaking tasks either from a wheelchair or ambulatory level may prefer to use a wheeled utility cart because of its larger carrying capacity. The therapist can help clients learn to maneuver the cart efficiently. Homemakers who use an assistive device or adapted methods to transport hot foods and beverages must follow strict safety precautions to avoid burns.

When limited income inhibits a client's ability to purchase assistive aids, the creative therapist can work with the client to identify inexpensive workable alternatives. No-cost solutions, such as attaching a plastic grocery bag or used bike basket to a walker, can add to independence in transporting certain items.

Food Preparation

The use of assistive devices and adapted equipment can make food preparation easier and more enjoyable. Homemakers who have lost the use of one arm following stroke or fracture find an adapted cutting board extremely useful when peeling or cutting vegetables, fruit, or meat. A raised edge along one corner of the board can stabilize a slice of bread for spreading butter or jam (Fig. 32-2).

The occupational therapist helps clients with physical limitations to solve problems such as the safest way to open cereal boxes and juice cartons. Some persons can open packaged food with one-handed techniques, while others prefer to use adapted scissors with a looped handle

PROCEDURES FOR PRACTICE 32-2

Principles of Correct Body Mechanics

Principles of correct body mechanics that should be used during homemaking and parenting tasks (Melnik, 1994; Saunders, 1992) include:

- Keep the shoulders and hips parallel and facing the task. Do not twist the trunk when lifting.
- Maintain good balance by positioning the feet shoulder distance apart with one foot forward.
- When standing for long periods, reduce pressure on the lower back by placing one foot on a low stool and changing positions frequently.
- When sitting or standing, maintain a neutral position in the lower back by tilting the pelvis slightly forward to maintain the natural curve of the spine. Use this neutral back position when lifting as well.
- Use the strongest or largest muscles and joints when lifting (e.g., use legs rather than back, palms rather than fingers).
- Keep the back upright and bend at the hips and knees rather than bending forward at the waist when reaching for low items.
- Push before pulling and pull before lifting.
- While lifting or carrying, keep the object close to the body.
- Avoid rushing. Proper body mechanics are more effectively used when working at a comfortable pace.

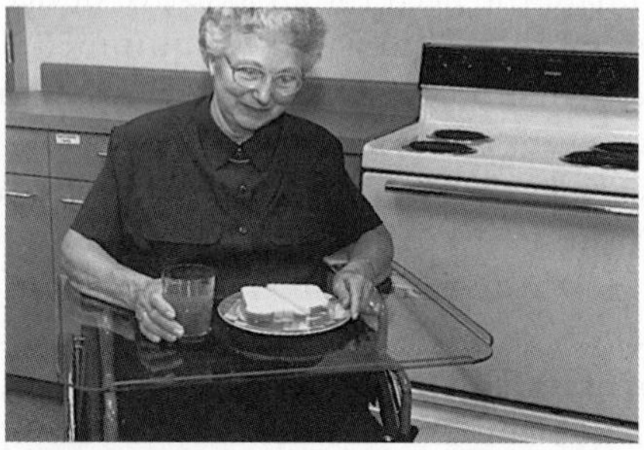

Figure 32-1 Woman eating her lunch on a clear acrylic wheelchair lap tray that allows her to observe her lower body. (Photo by Robert Littlefield.)

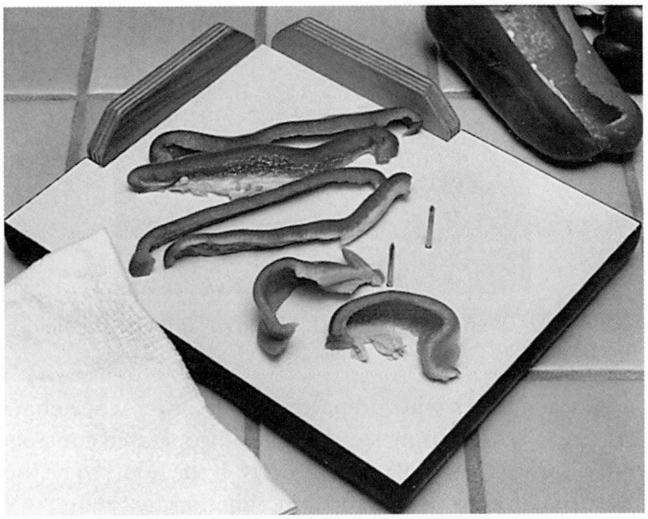

Figure 32-2 Spiked cutting board with corner guards. (Photo courtesy of North Coast Medical, Inc., Morgan Hill, CA.)

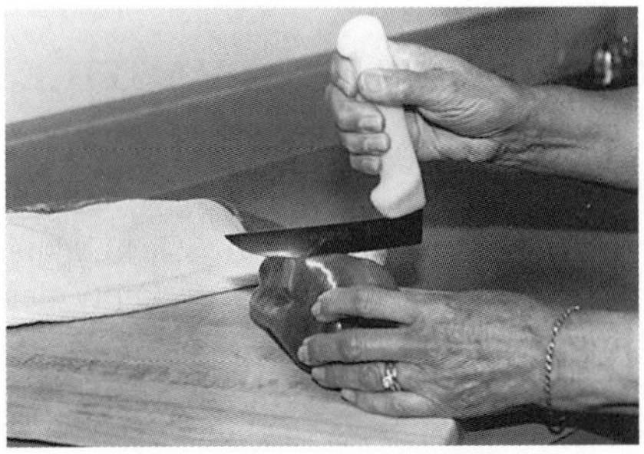

Figure 32-4 Ergonomic right-angled knife. (Photo by Robert Littlefield.)

(Fig. 32-3). Homemakers with weakness and impaired hand function may find it easier to open plastic milk jugs than cartons. Smaller containers are generally easier to manage than large ones. Non-slip mats or suction holders may be used under jars or bottles to hold them steady for opening with one hand and to reduce sliding or turning of bowls when mixing.

Knives, vegetable peelers, and other kitchen tools are available in many shapes and sizes. Clients with rheumatoid arthritis benefit from using utensils with ergonomically designed handles that require less hand strength and reduce ulnar drift (Fig. 32-4). Incoordination due to ataxia may be somewhat alleviated by the use of weighted utensils and tools. Freestanding or mounted jar openers can be helpful to persons with a variety of physical limitations. Homemakers can be taught adapted methods for cracking eggs (Fig. 32-5; Procedures for Practice 32-3).

Electric equipment, such as food processors, blenders, can openers, and electric knives, can conserve energy by reducing the physical demands and time needed for meal preparation. To be truly beneficial, this equipment must be easy to use and maintain and suited to the person's disability. For example, some one-handed cordless can openers are available only in right-handed models and therefore are not convenient for persons with significant right hemiparesis after stroke.

Homemakers with limited mobility or reach find a side-by-side refrigerator more accessible than other models. Loops of webbing or rope can be attached to the door handles to enable clients with limited hand function to pull the doors open. Heavy items should be stored on a shelf that is level with a lapboard or wheeled cart so they can be moved in and out with minimal lifting.

Cooking

Most persons with physical impairments find lightweight non-stick pots and pans to be the easiest to handle and maintain. Ergonomically designed cookware with easy-to-grip handles can be ideal for persons with limited distal strength (Fig. 32-6). The use of double-handled casserole dishes, pots, and pans can enable joint protection by evenly distributing the weight of the pan between both hands.

Ambulatory clients with back or lower extremity pain or limited endurance can save energy by sitting whenever possible while preparing meals. Individuals who prepare food in a wheelchair can use a mirror mounted at an angle over the stove to keep an eye on cooking foods. Persons with hemiparesis may use a suction cup holder to stabilize pot handles while stirring. Homemakers can conserve energy when straining vegetables or pasta by placing a french-fry basket in the pot before cooking or by using a slotted spoon. This practice eliminates the need to carry

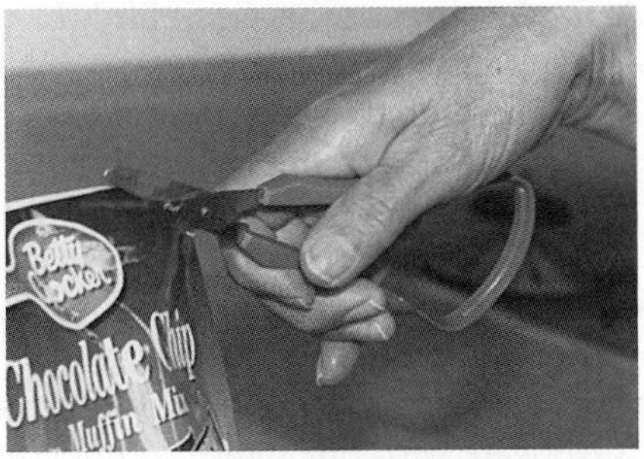

Figure 32-3 Looped scissors. (Photo by Robert Littlefield.)

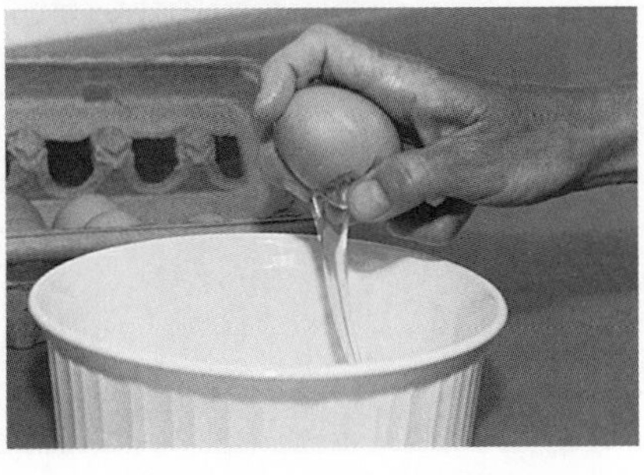

Figure 32-5 One-handed egg crack. (Photo by Robert Littlefield.)

PROCEDURES FOR PRACTICE 32-3

Methods for Breaking Eggs

Individuals with weak grasp can grossly hold the egg, throw it sharply into the bottom of an empty glass or metal bowl, where it will split in two, and then remove the shell.

Clients with functional use of only one hand may prefer to use the chef's method, as follows. Place the egg in the palm with one end held by the index and middle fingers and the other end held by the thumb to form a **"C"** around the egg. Sharply crack the egg on the side of a bowl, and then in one motion, pull the thumb down and the fingers up to pull the two halves apart (Fig. 32-5).

a hot pot to the sink to drain it. Those who can safely transport and drain hot foods at the sink can reduce the need for lifting and holding and enhance stability by resting the pot on the sink's edge when pouring. An adjustable strainer that clamps onto the top of a pot or pan can also be used.

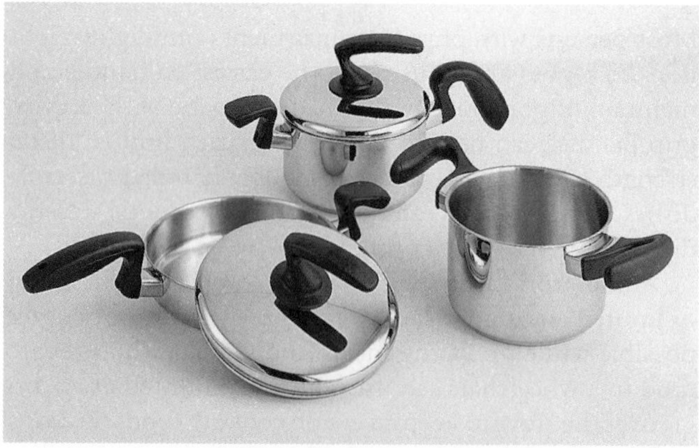

A

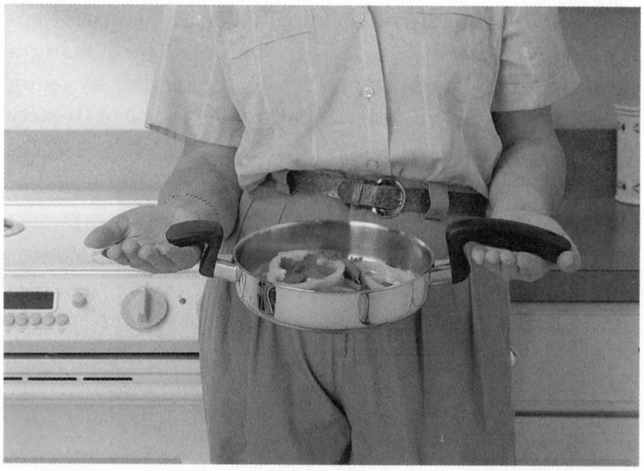

B

Figure 32-6 Ergonomic cookware with easy-grip handles. (Photo provided by Sammons Preston.)

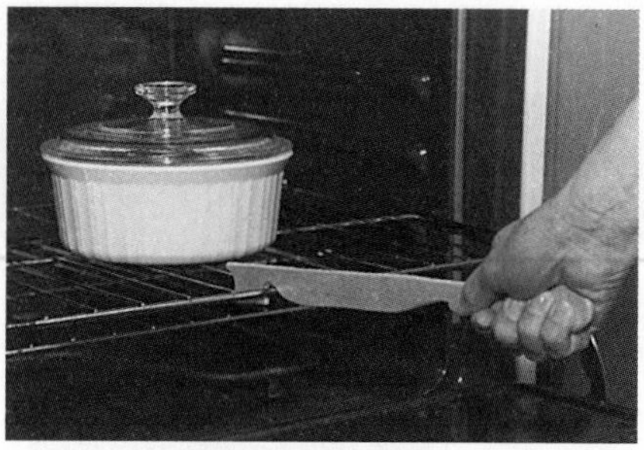

Figure 32-7 Oven push–pull stick. (Photo by Robert Littlefield.)

Homemakers who prepare meals from a wheelchair will find a self-cleaning stove with front-operated controls and a low wall oven (30–42 inches from the floor) to be the most practical to use and operate (Eberhardt, 1998).

Individuals with limited proximal arm strength or grasp should not remove hot items from a wall oven higher than waist level without supervision because of the potential for burns due to spilling or dropping. An oven push–pull stick may be used to manage oven racks or reposition hot dishes safely during baking (Fig. 32-7). If a client is planning to buy a new stove, the therapist may recommend a gas rather than electric range to reduce the risk of burns (Eberhardt, 1998) because the gas flames provide a visual cue that the burner is on.

Microwave ovens provide a cost-effective and safe alternative to conventional ovens and stoves. Elderly persons with arthritis, visual impairments, and limited endurance can be taught to use a microwave instead of a conventional stove to cook meals more easily and in less time (Kondo et al., 1997).

Dishwashing

Dishwashing can be made easier for individuals working in a wheelchair by placing a removable wooden rack in the bottom of a standard sink to reduce its depth to approximately 5 inches. The under-sink cabinet can be removed to allow persons in a wheelchair to face the sink head-on, with any exposed piping insulated to protect lower extremities from burns. A swing-away faucet with a single control lever can enhance the ability of a person with limited hand function to adjust water flow (Eberhardt, 1998). Installing this faucet beside rather than at the back of the sink further increases accessibility for persons in wheelchairs (Eberhardt, 1998).

Dishwashing in a double sink should be organized to allow the person to work from one direction to the other: dirty dishes, wash water, rinse water, and drying rack. Homemakers with hemiparesis may wash dishes with greater ease when the rinse water and dish rack are on their unaffected side. Suction bottlebrushes and scrub brushes can be attached to the sink to allow for cleaning glasses or silverware with one hand. A rubber mat at the bottom of the sink prevents plates from sliding when they are washed and reduces breakage. Persons with limited grasp may prefer to use a terry cloth mitt or sponge mitt when washing dishes.

Work simplification includes air drying versus towel drying dishes and reusing them directly from the dish rack or dishwasher. Use of an electric dishwasher aids energy conservation, particularly when little pre-rinsing of soiled dishes is required.

Whenever possible, the homemaker can eliminate unnecessary cleaning by using oven-to-table ware or by serving directly from the pot. Pans can be lined with foil to reduce washing after baking or broiling. It is recommended that individuals clean as they prepare the meal and soak hard to clean dishes while eating to reduce the amount of cleanup required when the meal is over.

Grocery Shopping

Persons with physical impairments or limited endurance can more easily participate in grocery shopping with a few task modifications or assistive devices. When transportation is readily available, individuals may find that frequent visits to the market are more manageable because they can purchase and carry smaller quantities of food items at one time. Shopping at a small local market, although sometimes more expensive, can be easier and less energy consuming than shopping at a superstore. Grocery shopping can become a social event when done with a friend. Shopping together may provide an additional advantage if the friend can assist with reaching items on high and low shelves or carrying the bags.

Planning

A well-organized shopping list is necessary to make the most efficient use of time and to conserve energy at the store. Individuals should keep the list in a convenient location at home, so that needed items can easily be added between shopping trips. Store maps, available at the customer service desk of many large grocery stores, can be used to organize the list. The homemaker or occupational therapist can arrange the items on the list (e.g., produce, dairy, meats) according to the store layout, aisle by aisle. Copies of this list can be used between store visits to record the items needed under each category.

The person should plan ahead and shop during off-peak hours, when the store is not crowded. Once at the store, a client can use the grocery list and signs above the aisles to find needed items.

Carts

Ambulatory persons with mild balance impairments can use a standard grocery cart when shopping; however, they should not use it for support when bending to reach items on low shelves. Individuals who use a wheelchair may find that adapted shopping carts that attach to the wheelchair are more convenient than a standard cart; although some have found that these attached carts interfere with their ability to reach items. When this is the case, homemakers who are independent with wheelchair mobility may prefer to leave a standard cart at the end of an aisle, gather needed items in a small lap basket, and transfer them into the cart before proceeding to the next aisle.

Large stores have motorized carts for shoppers with limited endurance and mobility. These carts are handy for getting around the store, but it may be necessary to call the store in advance to reserve one. The baskets on these carts are generally small, which may be problematic if the person is planning to purchase a large order. The client may need help to figure out the safest and most effective ways to obtain items from high or low shelves from a motorized cart.

Selecting and Retrieving Items

It is wise to shop for items that are easy to open and require little preparation. Persons with limited endurance can increase the ease of meal preparation by selecting frozen rather than fresh vegetables and skinless or boneless meats.

Individuals who have limited upper extremity range of motion or who use a wheelchair find it difficult or impossible to reach items on high shelves. A reacher can be used to retrieve lightweight unbreakable items, but assistance may be needed for heavier objects. Most stores provide an employee to assist with shopping if asked. Outgoing persons may prefer to ask people in the aisle for occasional help to increase opportunities for socialization.

Some individuals with traumatic brain injury or cerebrovascular accident have visual-perceptual problems that interfere with their ability to locate items (e.g., hemianopsia or impaired figure-ground skills). These persons can be taught to find objects more easily by scanning shelves in an organized manner, top to bottom and left to right. A person with severe visual impairments needs assistance to ensure safety and effectiveness while shopping.

Transporting Items Home

Generally, plastic grocery bags are easier to manage than paper. Foam tubing can be placed around the bag handles to reduce joint stress. At the checkout counter, the client should ask the clerk to keep grocery bags as light as possible and to bag refrigerated foods separately. Several half-filled bags are easier to manage than one or two full ones. Most stores provide assistance for transferring groceries into the car, but store workers should be instructed to place them within easy reach.

At home, a wheeled cart can be used to transport groceries into the house (Fig. 32-8). Persons with limited endurance can leave non-refrigerated items in the car until later, when the person has rested or a family member is available to bring them into the house.

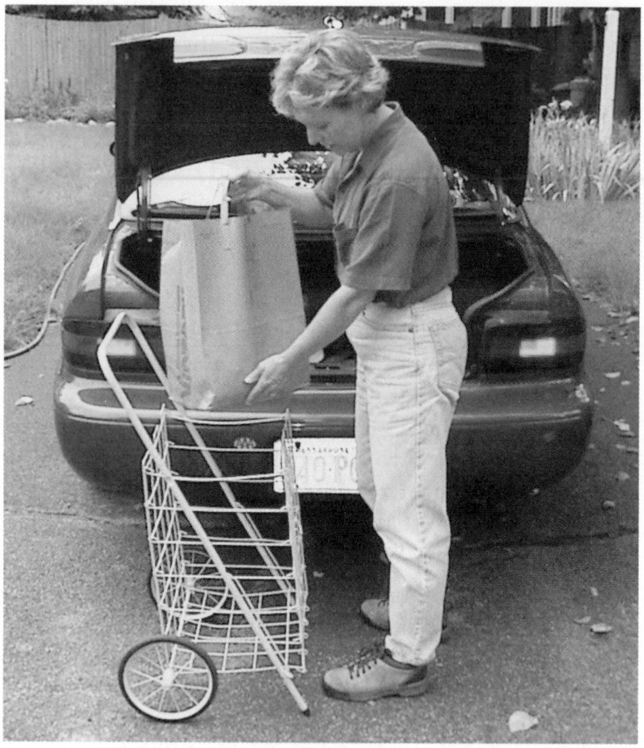

Figure 32-8 Using wheeled cart to conserve energy when transporting items.

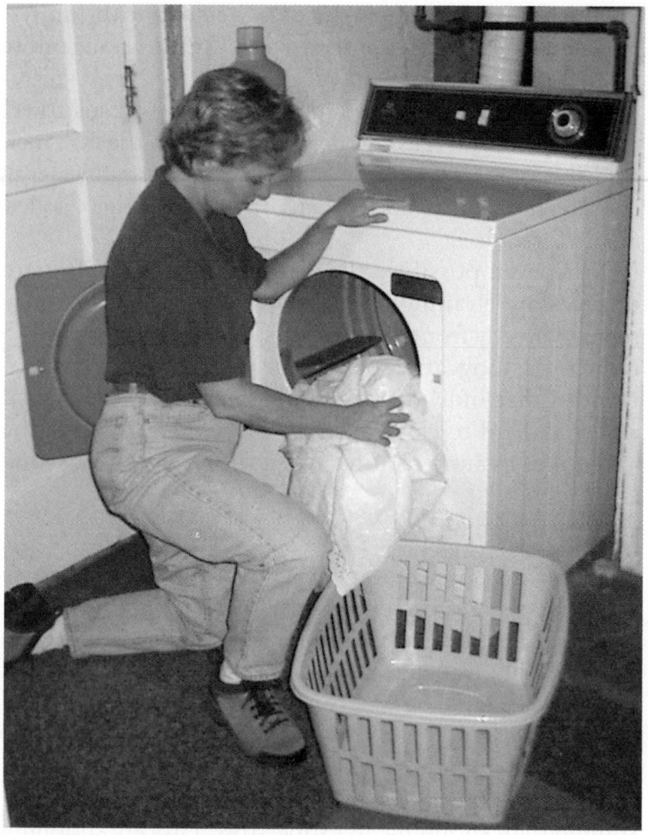

Figure 32-9 Kneeling to keep back straight when removing laundry from dryer.

Computerized Shopping

Clients with physical limitations and limited endurance may find computer shopping to be a wonderful, energy-efficient alternative to conventional shopping. Persons with Internet access find that grocery orders can be easily placed online. Deliveries are made directly to the home, eliminating transportation and accessibility issues that may arise at the grocery store. The occupational therapist can help the client identify which method of shopping is most practical based on the individual's priorities, physical limitations, knowledge of computer use, and financial situation.

Clothing Care

When a homemaker identifies clothing care as an important goal, the occupational therapist can help the person modify the way laundry tasks are performed. Even persons with severe physical impairments can engage in some aspect of clothing care (e.g., sitting at table to fold clothes).

In-Home Appliances Versus Self-Service Commercial Laundries

Although top-loading washers decrease the amount of bending required to load and unload clothing for persons who are ambulatory, they provide an additional challenge for persons in a wheelchair. Front-loading laundry machines are easier for seated individuals to access, but persons who are ambulatory may need training in body mechanics, particularly when loading or unloading wet clothes. For example, it is recommended that ambulatory clients with low back pain kneel on one knee, bending at the hips and knees and keeping the back upright, when loading or removing clothes from a front-loading machine (Fig. 32-9) (Saunders, 1992). Homemakers with limited hand function due to spinal cord injury or rheumatoid arthritis find it easier to use knob turners to set machine dials (Fig. 32-10).

Individuals who use a self-service commercial laundry for clothing care should bring needed coins and pre-measured packages of soap for each load. Many such laundries have rolling carts available for carrying wet clothes from washer to dryer. If possible, persons with physical impair-

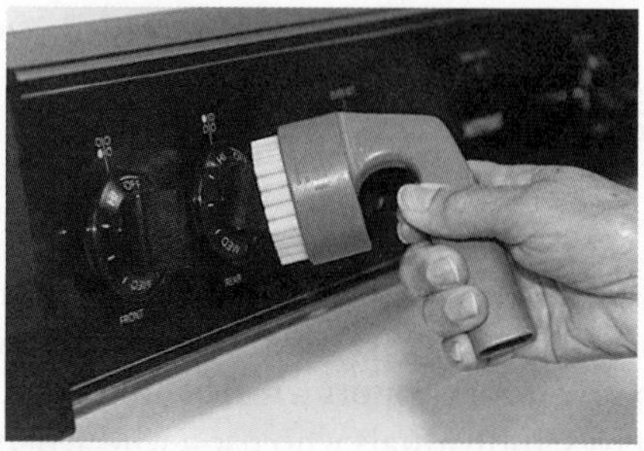

Figure 32-10 Knob turner. (Photo by Robert Littlefield.)

ments should choose a staffed laundry. These individuals can be called on for assistance if problems arise.

Collecting and Transporting Clothing

Ideally, the home laundry room should be on the same floor as the bedrooms to minimize the need to carry clothes up and down stairs. When this is not an option, family members can assist as needed to transport clothing to and from the laundry area.

Soiled clothing can be placed in a hamper lined with a plastic or cloth bag with handles. Seated individuals with good upper body strength can transport clothes to the washer by lifting the bag out of the hamper and either carrying it on their lap or hooking the drawstrings on the wheelchair handles. If the person is ambulatory but has difficulty bending, a clothes basket can be kept on a waist-high table or shelf to collect soiled laundry. A wheeled cart is handy for transporting clothes for persons at an ambulatory level.

Washing and Folding

Laundry detergents and bleaches should be kept within easy reach of the washing machine. Hand washing can be eliminated by laundering delicate clothing in a mesh laundry bag in the machine. Persons with visual impairments can fasten paired socks with pins when they are taken off so they don't have to be sorted when clean.

A person in a wheelchair can use a hand-held mirror and reacher to remove clothes from the bottom of a top-loading washer. Homemakers with very limited grasp due to spinal cord injury have found that stubborn items can be more easily removed from the washer tub after a wet towel or shirt is put back into the washer and the spin cycle is restarted. Movement of the wet towel inside the spinning washer can loosen clothes that are stuck to the tub.

Clothes can be folded while the person sits or stands at a table. An adjustable rod 42–60 inches high is convenient for hanging permanent-press items as they are removed from the dryer. Large items, like sheets and bath towels, can be reused immediately after cleaning so they don't have to be folded. Those who choose to fold sheets may find the task easier if they use the bed as a work surface.

Ironing

One challenging task for homemakers with physical impairments is to fold and unfold an ironing board. When possible, it is best to leave the ironing board set up in a convenient, out-of-the-way place. The board surface should be at waist level for persons who stand when ironing to reinforce good posture and body mechanics. Persons who iron while seated in a wheelchair will find a work surface of 28–34 inches high comfortable (ADA-ABA, 2004). A heat-resistant pad can be placed at the end of the ironing board to eliminate the need to stand the iron up while arranging clothes on the board.

When buying a new iron, individuals should select a lightweight model with an automatic shut-off switch. A cord holder can reduce effort and keep the iron cord from getting in the way. Permanent-press clothing requires less care than cotton or linen fabrics and thus reduces ironing needs. Persons who iron only occasionally may prefer to use a small tabletop ironing board if they have sufficient upper body strength to store and retrieve it from a closet easily.

Sewing

Homemakers may enjoy sewing as a hobby or may only make occasional alterations or repairs. Persons who have hemiparesis after a stroke can still sew with an electric machine by using the unaffected leg to operate foot or knee controls. Persons who do not have use of their lower extremities can place the foot pedal of an electric sewing machine on the table and use one hand or elbow to depress it. Sewing is generally most successful when there is an adequate workspace and adapted methods to stabilize materials when cutting or stitching.

Persons with limited use of an affected arm can hand sew by using an embroidery hoop attached to the edge of a table or counter with a C-clamp (Fig. 32-11). To minimize sewing needs, sticky iron-on tape or fabric glue can be

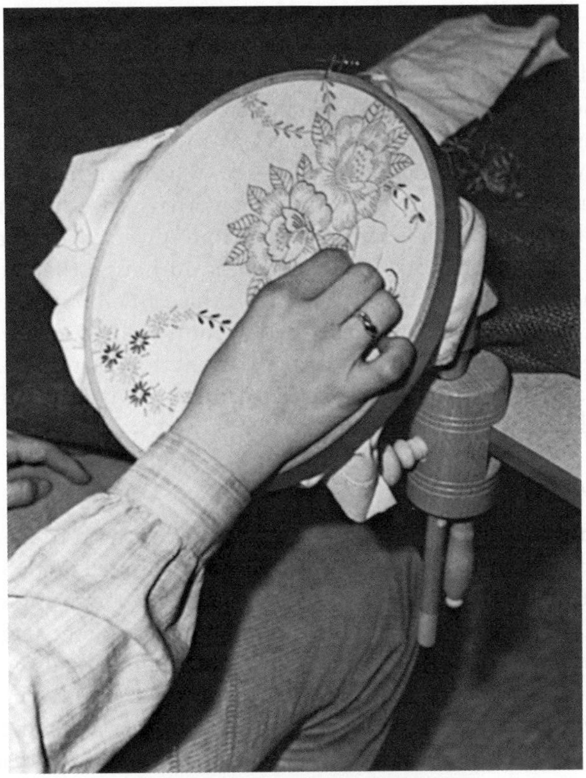

Figure 32-11 Embroidery adapted with use of a hoop that fastens to the table; requires only one hand.

used for hems and small repairs. Rotary cutters, instead of scissors, make cutting fabric easier.

Indoor Household Maintenance

The occupational therapist helps clients identify effective ways to do household maintenance tasks, such as bed making and floor care. Adapted techniques and assistive devices can help the client to safely perform necessary chores without assistance.

Bed Making

Bed making can be simplified by straightening the sheets and blankets as much as possible before rising in the morning. Homemakers with limited mobility or impaired upper extremity function find it easier to make the bed by completing one corner at a time, starting with the head of the bed. If the individual is working from a wheelchair, the bed should be positioned so that both sides are accessible. Persons with chronic back pain must adhere to proper body mechanics when making beds, being careful to eliminate excessive forward bending.

When changing the sheets, a person can reduce extra work by carefully pulling blankets and spreads toward the foot of the bed, trying not to dislodge them from under the mattress. In this way, the person will not have to expend unnecessary energy to find and reposition the top edge of the blankets or bedspread. Although the bottom sheet should be fitted, it should also be loose enough to be easily applied.

If the client or a friend is handy at sewing, several adaptations can be made to standard sheets to increase the ease of bed making. Fitted sheets can be adapted by opening the two fitted corners at the bottom end and sewing Velcro straps onto each side. When fastened, these straps securely hold the bottom corners together. Another adaptation is sewing the bottom edge of a top sheet to the bottom edge of a fitted sheet. Although this large sheet is more difficult to launder, this can eliminate the need to lift the mattress to tuck under the top sheet. Persons with limited upper body strength or hemiparesis may find lightweight blankets and spreads and satin pillowcases easier to manage.

Dusting

Physically challenged homemakers can dust hard-to-reach places with assistive devices. Persons with limited upper extremity reach because of orthopedic or neurological changes can use a long-handled duster that is lightweight and easily extended to reach high places. Individuals with good hand strength may prefer to hold a dust cloth with a long-handled reacher or use a vacuum cleaner attachment to clean hard-to-reach places. Persons who cannot afford assistive devices may find that a dust cloth secured to the end of a yardstick or dowel with a rubber band meets their needs. Clients with limited grasp or fine motor control may find that an adapted spray handle (see Fig. 30.7) attached to the furniture polish can and an old sock or duster mitten significantly enhance their independence in dusting.

Floor Care

Heavy homemaking tasks, such as floor care, are often the first activities that elderly persons or individuals with physical impairments find difficult because of the amount of strength and endurance required (Axtell & Yasuda, 1993). When the client's goal is independence in floor care, the occupational therapist must determine how this can be safely and efficiently accomplished.

Cleaning supplies can be conveniently stored and transported in a handled bin or canvas bag with a shoulder strap. When feasible, duplicate sets of equipment can be kept around the home to reduce the need to carry items. A number of lightweight, wet or dry floor cleaning tools are commercially available for quick cleanups. When a more thorough cleaning is needed, a dolly with large casters can reduce the physical demands of transporting heavy pails of water for mopping. Individuals should only partially fill cleaning pails to lessen their weight. A sponge mop with the squeeze lever on the handle minimizes bending and can be used with one hand. Individuals with limited hand function but adequate proximal arm strength can use a grasping cuff to help maintain a closed fist around mop or broom handles. Persons working from a wheelchair may find it best to start at the farthest corner and work backward out of the room. Furniture should be fitted with casters or Teflon slides if moved regularly.

Lightweight upright vacuums provide a good alternative to using heavier canister-style models because they work well and are easier to manage for both ambulatory and wheelchair-bound persons. A lightweight carpet sweeper is another good choice because it is maneuverable, is relatively inexpensive, and does not have to be plugged in to an electrical outlet. Although the carpet sweeper is easier to push, more repetitions are generally needed to clean the same area. Long-handled dustpans and brushes can ease cleanup because they eliminate the need for bending and stooping (Fig. 32-12). If the client has good hand function, cordless hand-held vacuum cleaners are handy for cleaning up small messes within easy reach.

Bathrooms

After a disabling event, a homemaker who cannot afford a housekeeper or does not have family members to assist may have to learn adapted ways to clean the bathroom. Cleaning needs can be reduced by rinsing the sink or tub immediately after use to wash away soap residue. Spray-on chemical products clean bathroom fixtures with little effort, substantially reducing physical demands. Toilet cleaning tablets can be dropped into the toilet tank to reduce the growth of bacteria between thorough cleanings.

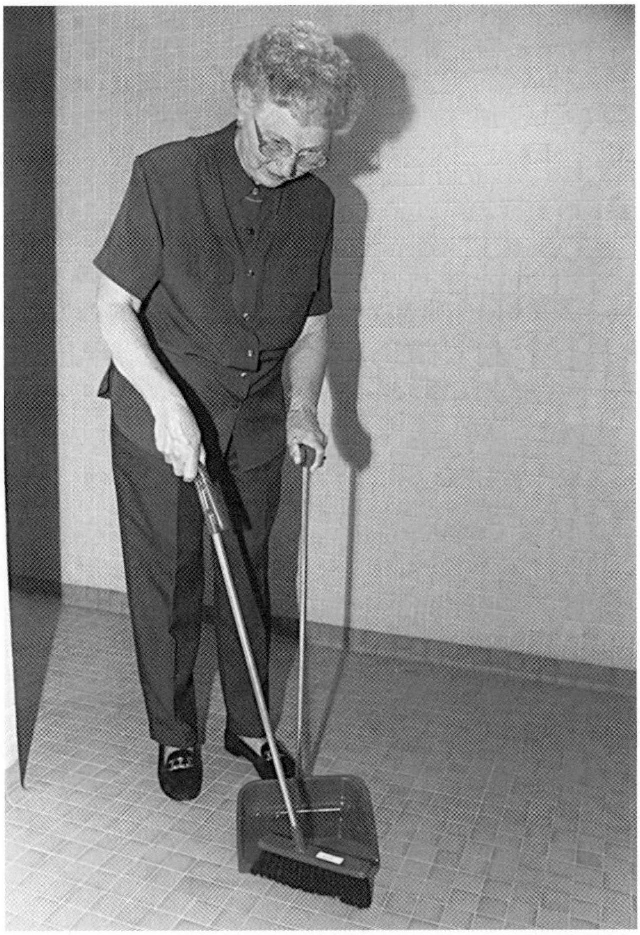

Figure 32-12 Use of a long-handled brush with dustpan. (Photo by Robert Littlefield.)

A long-handled mop with a small head is useful for cleaning inaccessible areas behind the toilet.

Many homemakers with physical impairments find that cleaning the bathtub is difficult or impossible. These suggestions may make it possible. Persons with limited endurance or balance concerns should sit to clean the tub. Cleaning sprays and foams can be easily applied and rinsed off from a seated position, particularly if a long-handled shower hose is used. A long-handled bathroom cleaner with a non-scratch scrubbing sponge can enable persons with limited reach to clean tubs and shower enclosures without assistance (Fig. 32-13). Replacing sliding doors with a plastic shower curtain can make the bathtub more accessible for bathing and cleaning. The plastic curtain can be laundered in the washing machine or inexpensively replaced when it becomes soiled.

Hard to Manage Tasks

No matter how creative the occupational therapist and client are, some household tasks may be impossible for persons with physical impairments. However, a large number of assistive devices are available to ease the physical requirements of previously difficult tasks. Electric outlet extensions can be plugged into existing baseboard outlets and secured to the wall to eliminate the need to bend when inserting or removing a plug. Devices that make it easier to replace hard to reach light bulbs are also available. The adaptive therapist is well able to analyze task demands and identify modifications or assistive devices that promote independence. When a client cannot accomplish household tasks despite adapted methods, the occupational therapist can initiate a referral to homemaker services.

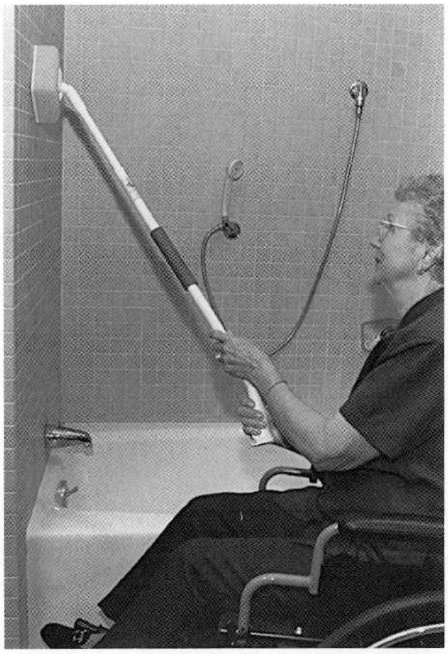

Figure 32-13 Cleaning bathroom tile using a long-handled cleaner. (Photo by Robert Littlefield.)

Outdoor Household Maintenance

When a client's goal is to do outdoor household maintenance, such as yard work or gardening, the occupational therapist can offer suggestions to increase safety and independence.

Yard Maintenance

Persons with mild physical impairments can return to some level of outdoor home maintenance if desired. Individuals with good endurance can mow with a self-propelled lawn mower and accomplish small projects, such as maintaining a patio area. To reduce the risk of back injury when mowing, individuals should avoid stopping and turning the mower. For this reason, a lawn with rounded rather than angled corners is easier to mow (Yeomans, 1992). Rechargeable battery-operated edgers are more convenient than models that must be connected to an electric cord when operated. Numerous ergonomically designed products have been developed to reduce injury during outdoor work. For example, bent-handled shovels reduce excessive back strain and forward bending by altering the fulcrum of movement (Fig. 32-14).

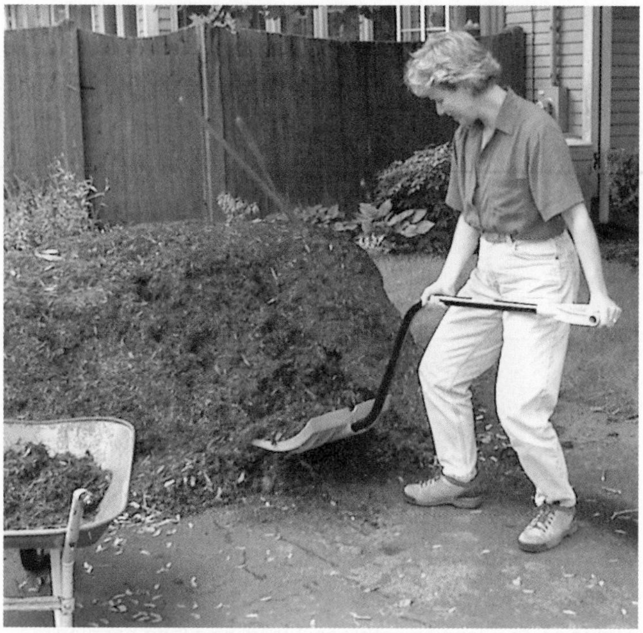

Figure 32-14 Protecting the back while shoveling by using an ergonomically designed shovel with bent handle and lifting with the legs, not the back.

Gardening

Homemakers who are physically challenged need not give up the joy of gardening. Tools can be adapted, flower and vegetable beds can be raised, and wider walkways or wheelways can be created to increase a person's access to the garden. Container gardening is also feasible for persons with limited mobility.

Gardeners with limited hand function can adapt ordinary hand tools with inexpensive foam pipe insulation, which is available at most building supply stores (Yeomans, 1992). This foam, pre-split for easy application, can significantly enhance the comfort of grasping and holding the tool. In a randomized study, Tebben and Thomas (2004) reported that a garden trowel labeled as "ergonomic" did not elicit better wrist positions during use when compared to an ordinary trowel. This reinforces the need to carefully assess whether "ergonomic" garden tools truly enhance body mechanics and positioning for a given client.

Individuals who garden from a wheelchair can increase their reach by using long-handled spades, shovels, and pruners. Persons with limited trunk mobility or balance may increase their safety by sitting on a garden stool and using long-handled tools. Gardeners who are fairly mobile can use a kneeling bench, with handles that assist them in getting up and down. Tools can be transported around the yard in apron pockets, a backpack, or a child's wagon, depending on the person's needs and available options. Tools with brightly colored handles are easy to see and therefore not likely to be lost in the garden (Yeomans, 1992).

Homemakers who return to gardening need to take care of themselves while caring for their flowers. Stretching exercises before gardening can reduce muscle stiffness and prevent injuries (Adil, 1994; Yeomans, 1992). Work simplification, energy conservation, and proper body mechanics are essential. Gardeners should keep themselves safe by using sun and insect protection, drinking plenty of fluids, and carrying a whistle around their neck in case they encounter unexpected problems when alone in the garden (Yeomans, 1992).

TASKS AND ACTIVITIES OF THE PARENTING ROLE: TREATMENT PRINCIPLES AND METHODS

The occupational therapist and client work closely to identify adapted methods and equipment that enhance participation and independence in parenting tasks. A holistic approach addresses parent and family needs within the home and community.

Psychosocial Adjustment

Parents whose physical limitations are due to an acute event, such as spinal cord injury or cerebrovascular accident, may initially lack a sense of competence, not only in their ability to care for themselves but also in their ability to care for their children. The occupational therapist must be sensitive to the client's psychosocial concerns. The impact of the client's impairments on family responsibilities and expectations must be considered when establishing a treatment plan. Restoration of parenting roles can be challenging for the client, the family, and the therapist.

Parents with diminished physical abilities following an acute event (e.g., spinal cord injury) are likely to have different intervention needs than parents with a chronic or progressive disease or disorder (e.g., rheumatoid arthritis or multiple sclerosis). Persons subjected to the acute onset of physical or cognitive impairments are confronted by sudden and sometimes drastic changes in the ways they can participate in important life roles and tasks. In contrast, individuals with progressive conditions and their families can gradually learn adapted ways to cope with changing abilities and levels of role participation over time.

During the evaluation, the occupational therapist should ask clients to identify which parenting tasks they highly value (e.g., play time, nursing, or bottle feeding) and which tasks are necessary for them to resume their parenting role. The client should then prioritize parenting goals in a way that addresses both valued and necessary tasks in a balanced way.

Barriers to Effectiveness

Barriers to a client's ability to return to parenting tasks and roles are similar to those for homemaker responsibilities. A client's child care needs within home and community environments must be identified and addressed. Factors such as the child's age, activity level, and obedience greatly influence the challenges encountered by the parent with physical impairments. The occupational therapist works to identify the barriers that interfere with a client's ability to accomplish important parenting tasks, devises adapted methods that reduce or remove these constraints, and assists the individual in regaining competence in his or her parenting role.

Child Care: Techniques and Therapeutic Aids

Caring for young children under the age of 4 years is physically demanding and can contribute to musculoskeletal pain, even in parents without physical disabilities (Sanders & Morse, 2005). Parents with rheumatoid arthritis, spinal cord injury, and stroke have reported that child care tasks that require lifting and carrying are the most challenging, followed by tasks that demand fine motor dexterity and/or grip strength (Joe, 1997; Ostensen & Rugelsjoen, 1992). A national survey of parents with physical disabilities revealed that parenting tasks such as traveling outside the home with a child, recreational activities, and chasing and retrieving children require the greatest assistance from others (Barker & Maralani, 1997). Funding for adapted parenting equipment and personal assistance services to help with child care is extremely limited. Therefore, the parent and therapist must work together to identify adapted methods and inexpensive solutions that best address parenting needs.

Equipment Considerations

The occupational therapist and client should initially explore whether simple adaptations to the way child care tasks are performed can enhance performance. When these simple solutions do not work, the client and therapist should evaluate whether commercially available child care equipment can feasibly meet the needs of the parent and child. If not, more creative solutions and adaptations must be devised.

The occupational therapist must consider the cost of the adapted equipment and whether it is acceptable to the client in terms of appearance and ease of use. In addition, the therapist must understand that the appropriateness of any equipment changes over time as the child grows and develops (DeMoss et al., 1995; Vensand et al., 2000).

Bathing

Parents need to be sure that all necessary equipment and clothes have been gathered and are within easy reach before they begin bathing their infant or young child. A terry cloth apron worn during bathing can protect clothing and dry the baby after the bath.

Persons who are ambulatory may find that bathing the infant in a portable plastic tub in or near the kitchen sink is a good option because the height of the sink or counter minimizes bending and the tub can be easily filled and drained at the sink. Parents who use wheelchairs, however, may find this arrangement inconvenient because it is too high for safely lifting the baby in and out of the tub. Persons in wheelchairs also find it difficult to bathe the infant if the baby tub is in a regular bathtub because it is too low (DeMoss et al., 1995; Vensand et al., 2000). An alternative is to secure the baby bathtub to a sturdy table or serving cart near a sink. A portable dishwasher hose can be connected to the sink faucet for filling the tub, and a separate hose can be used to drain the bath water (DeMoss et al., 1995; Vensand et al., 2000). It may be easier for the parent to use this arrangement to bathe the older infant until the child is mobile enough to help with getting in and out of a regular bathtub. This diminishes the parent's need to lift a wet, slippery child from a low tub.

Diapering and Dressing

Commercially available changing tables are usually inaccessible for persons who use a wheelchair because the wheelchair does not fit under the table for diapering or dressing the child. In addition, the surface may be too high for a seated parent to lift and transfer the baby safely, particularly as the infant grows (DeMoss et al., 1995; Vensand et al., 2000). The client and therapist should work together to determine the changing surface that most effectively and safely meets the individual's needs.

Safety straps should always be used to secure the active baby to prevent falls. These straps are particularly helpful when the parent needs extra time to manipulate diaper or clothing fasteners because of diminished fine motor control. A mobile attached to the changing table and assorted toys can keep the baby distracted during changing.

Although adapted fasteners for diapers and baby clothing can require initial assistance from family or friends, they can greatly enhance one's independence in child care during the day. For example, loops made of packing tape can be attached to disposable diaper tabs to reduce fine motor demands (DeMoss et al., 1995; Vensand et al., 2000). Wraps that hold either cloth or disposable diapers can be adapted by attaching metal key rings to small holes made in the Velcro tabs (DeMoss et al., 1995; Vensand et al., 2000). Small pieces of Velcro can also be sewn onto a variety of infant and baby clothes. Ideally, clothing should have full-length openings with closures that the parent can manage. When a zipper pull is used, zippers are easier to manipulate than snaps.

Feeding

Mothers with physical challenges may choose to nurse or bottle-feed their baby. After an initial adjustment period, breast-feeding can be easier than bottle-feeding because it eliminates formula preparation. If the mother is taking medications, it is important that she check with her physician before deciding to breast-feed to be sure that the medication will not harm the nursing infant. The mother should sit in a relaxed, comfortable position, using pillows to support the holding arm and baby while nursing. Pillows that are specifically designed to support the nursing infant are commercially available.

Some parents find bottle-feeding easier and more convenient with the older infant in a child seat, although others prefer to hold the child close to them when feeding (Fig. 32-15). Individuals with limited grasp may be able to hold a bottle and feed their infant after slipping their hand through a loop of webbing material attached to the bottle (DeMoss et al., 1995; Vensand et al., 2000). Lightweight plastic bottles with screw-on lids are recommended over glass bottles.

Older babies can be spoon-fed by a person with tetraplegia when the parent's wrist cock-up splint is adapted by attaching a Velcro loop to the palmar surface. The spoon is inserted into a utensil pocket made of Velcro hook and attached to the splint at the best angle for feeding (DeMoss et al., 1995; Vensand et al., 2000). An insulated baby dish can be used to keep food warm throughout the meal. Spoons should be rubber coated to protect the baby's gums and teeth if bumped while feeding.

Parents with impaired grasp and arm strength may not be able to attach or remove the tray on commercial high chairs (DeMoss et al., 1995; Vensand et al., 2000). In addition, it may be difficult for the parent to lift the child in and out of a standard high chair. Options to make high chairs more accessible for parents with physical limitations include altering the chair height, designing swing-away trays, and adding a climbing ladder to encourage the older infant to climb into the seat with supervision only (DeMoss et al., 1995; Vensand et al., 2000).

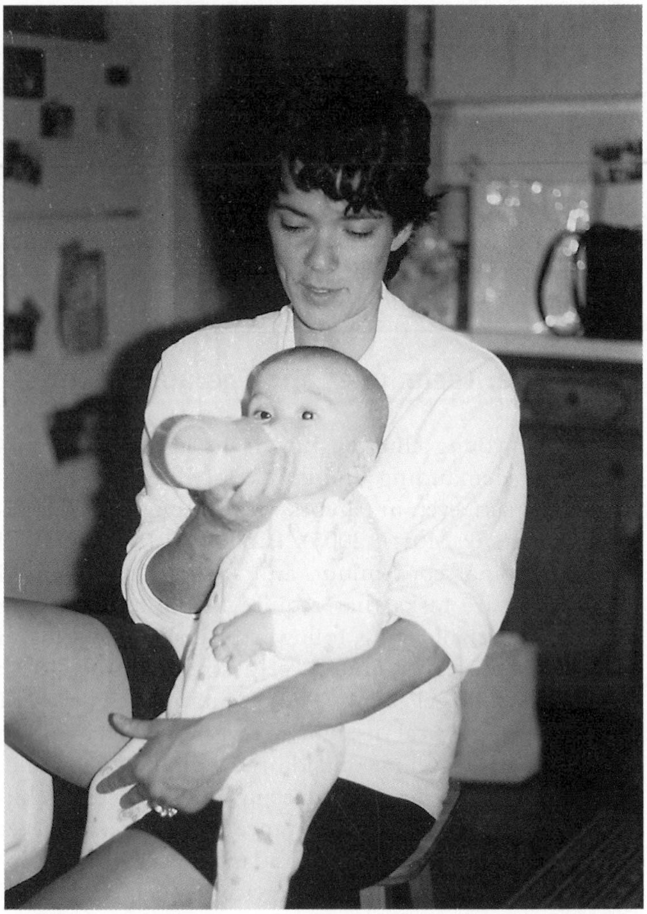

Figure 32-15 Alternative feeding position for mother with mild left hemiparesis following cerebrovascular accident.

Lifting and Carrying

Adapted equipment that provides alternative ways of carrying the infant or young child or reduces the need for multiple transfers can greatly enhance the parent's satisfaction and ability to care for the child. Parents with distal weakness and pain, as seen with rheumatoid arthritis, benefit from wearing wrist supports to reduce joint stress when lifting and carrying their child (Nordenskiold, Grimby, & Dahlin-Ivanhoff, 1998). Many clients prefer to practice lifting and carrying techniques with a weighted doll before trying to manage an active child.

A variety of cloth infant carriers and child front packs are available. Although these carriers allow the parent to transport a small child while leaving hands free, they may be contraindicated for persons with chronic back pain because the shoulders and back carry the weight of the child. Individuals who use wheelchairs may find child front packs handy for holding the infant while performing other homemaking tasks. Ease of use is important: adaptations may be needed to enable the parent with physical impairments to get the baby into and out of the infant carrier. The straps can be modified to reduce the parent's coordination needs (DeMoss et al., 1995; Vensand et al., 2000). Older babies with good neck and trunk control can safely ride on their parent's lap with only a safety belt attached to the wheelchair (Fig. 32-16).

Play

Parents with physical impairments may find that their ability to play with their young children is hindered because they cannot sit on the floor or bend to reach into standard playpens. Although infants can be entertained while they are sitting in a bouncy seat, older babies need a larger safe play area to develop gross motor skills. If cost is not an issue, a play care center, essentially a raised playpen that allows wheelchair access, can be built in the corner of a room (DeMoss et al., 1995; Vensand et al., 2000). If the center is equipped with swing-away doors, the parent can wheel up to the play center and easily reach into it to play with the

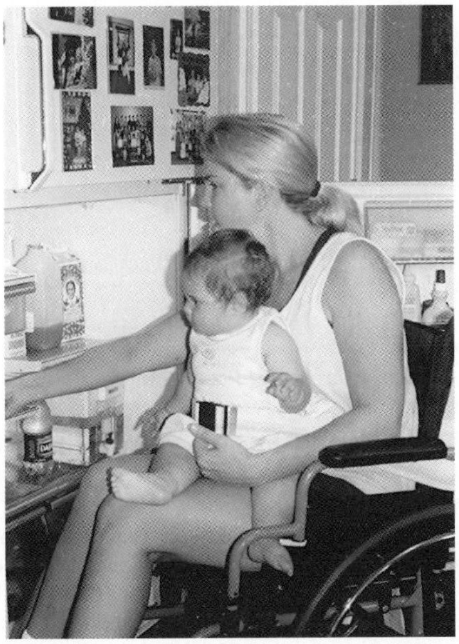

Figure 32-16 A mother confined to a wheelchair using a safety strap for an older baby while gathering items from the refrigerator.

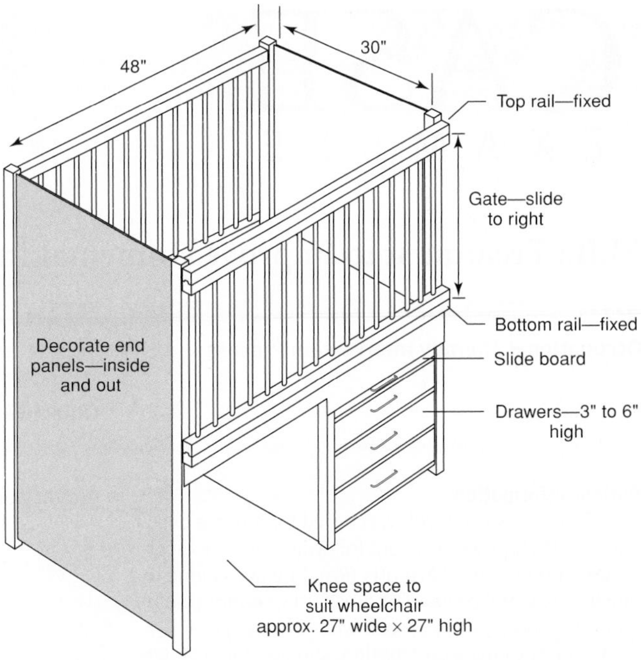

Figure 32-17 Crib with storage area, sliding gate side rails, and knee space to accommodate a wheelchair. (Designed by Lee Heintzman and Gordon Heintzman. Adapted from Dunn, V. M. [1978]. Tips on raising children from a wheelchair. *Accent on Living, 22,* 78–83.)

baby. This play area can also be used for the child's naps during the day, eliminating extra transfers in and out of the crib (DeMoss et al., 1995; Vensand et al., 2000). Walking toddlers and their parents may find that a child's table approximately 18 inches high is a convenient place to play while the parent is sitting in a wheelchair or standard chair.

Cribs

Standard cribs are inaccessible for parents who use wheelchairs, and they require ambulatory parents to bend forward when putting the baby in or out of bed. A standard drop-side crib can be adapted in several ways, depending on the parent's physical needs.

Persons who are ambulatory but have difficulty bending because of chronic back pain can raise the crib by inserting leg extenders or blocks of wood under the crib legs. The crib mattress can also be raised to the highest setting but should not remain in this position once the baby is old enough to sit or to climb over the crib rail.

Parents who use a wheelchair find it easier to transfer the baby in and out of the crib if the rail is adapted. One modification is cutting the rail in half to form two gates. These gates are attached with hinges to the head and foot of the crib. Center latches that are inaccessible to the child secure the gate when the baby is sleeping (DeMoss et al., 1995; Vensand et al., 2000). Another option is to adapt the crib rail so that it slides along a horizontal channel (DeMoss et al., 1995; Vensand et al., 2000; Dunn, 1978) (Fig. 32-17). Whatever crib design is used, the release mechanism for the crib rail must be child resistant yet manageable for the parent to manipulate with one hand or with limited coordination and dexterity.

EFFICACY AND OUTCOMES RESEARCH

Although the number of studies on occupational therapy outcomes continues to grow, there is a lack of evidence concerning specific effects on homemaking and parenting abilities. In fact, no effectiveness studies on occupational therapy and parenting skills of persons with physical disabilities were found. Generally, occupational therapy outcomes are based on more global measures of ADL or IADL, such as the *Functional Independence Measure (FIM)* or the *Nottingham Extended Activities of Daily Living Scale* (Granger et al., 1993; Nouri & Lincoln, 1987). The effects of OT intervention on homemaking, meal preparation, or household management abilities are often embedded within these broader IADL scales, making it challenging, if not impossible, to discern specific changes in task performance. Furthermore, descriptions of OT interventions tend to be vague, making it difficult to interpret research findings or compare evidence of treatment effects across studies (Wilkins et al., 2003).

Research is needed to examine the degree to which adapted methods and equipment (i.e., occupation-as-end) contribute to one's satisfaction and competence in homemaker and parenting roles after a disabling event. Empirical support for the cost effectiveness of adapted equipment and supportive services may lead to improved reimbursement from third-party payers.

CASE EXAMPLE

M.B.: Treatment to Improve Homemaking and Child Care Abilities

Occupational Therapy Intervention Process	Clinical Reasoning Processing: Objectives	Clinical Reasoning Processing: Examples of Therapist's Internal Dialogue
Patient Information M.B. is a 54-year-old widow referred for a home occupational therapy assessment following recent exacerbation of rheumatoid arthritis (RA). She lives alone in a ranch house and ordinarily cares for her 6-month-old granddaughter 3 days a week while her daughter works. Prior to her exacerbation, she was fairly active and able to manage all household and child care tasks independently with the exception of yard work. An avid gardener, she spent a good deal of time in her greenhouse prior to her exacerbation. She is able to use joint protection principles (e.g., avoiding positions of deformity, such as ulnar deviation) during functional tasks.	Appreciate the context	"M.B. is ordinarily a fairly active woman who has been caring for her 6-month-old granddaughter since she was a month old. She truly values the time she spends with the baby and is frustrated and somewhat depressed by her present limitations. Although her daughter has offered to find another child care provider while her mother recovers, this has been difficult to arrange in their small community. M.B.'s prior level of independence, combined with a strong desire to help her daughter and care for the infant, have motivated OT goals to optimize homemaking and child care abilities."
As a result of this exacerbation, she has decreased strength and dexterity in her hands and wrists, increased pain during activity, and a significant decrease in overall endurance. The occupational therapy evaluation identified the following problems: (1) moderately decreased ability to perform the household management tasks needed to maintain her independence at home, with fatigue after 30 minutes of activity; (2) moderate impairments in her ability to care for her granddaughter secondary to decreased strength and pain during resistive activities, such as opening baby food jars and attempting to lift the child; and (3) poor use of body mechanics and a tendency to rush through tasks when fatigued.	Develop intervention hypotheses	"I think that M.B.'s weakness, pain, and reduced endurance are the biggest barriers to her independence right now. Although she can tell me how to protect her joints during homemaking tasks, her pain and resulting fatigue are causing her not to use proper techniques. She tends to hurry through tasks so she can rest, and I'm concerned about her safety. I expect that, as her pain lessens, she'll do much better overall."
	Select an intervention approach	"I will develop an intervention plan that emphasizes compensation for deficits; this will help to protect her from injury long term. By engaging her in important home and child care tasks, we will use occupation-as-means to improve her physical abilities as well."
	Reflect on competence	"M.B. reminds me of a couple of other clients I've worked with in home care. It will be really important to involve her in problem solving of ways to best accomplish important tasks. This way she'll gain skills in handling unexpected situations outside of therapy."

Recommendations

The occupational therapist recommended three treatment sessions each week for 4 weeks. In collaboration with M.B. and her daughter, the therapist established the following long-term treatment goals: (1) M.B. will independently perform all indoor homemaking tasks, except floor care, with only occasional complaints of fatigue, using energy conservation and work simplification techniques; (2) M.B. will independently care for her granddaughter for 4-hour periods with only occasional complaints of pain, demonstrating appropriate use of assistive devices to protect joints during resistive activities; and (3) M.B. will use proper body mechanics when lifting and carrying her granddaughter and performing household tasks, such as meal preparation and laundry (see Home Program in Procedures for Practice 32-4).

Consider the patient's appraisal of performance

Consider what will occur in therapy, how often, and for how long

Ascertain the patient's endorsement of plan

"I think that OT in the home will be the most effective means of addressing M.B.'s current needs, especially because she is highly motivated to make changes that will optimize her home and child care abilities. Her house is pretty accessible, and I think small changes will really help improve her independence and safety. We should be able to accomplish a lot in the next 4 weeks."

PROCEDURES FOR PRACTICE 32-4

Home Program for Body Mechanics

M.B., please focus on using proper body mechanics during all of your daily tasks! Below are specific ideas for you to incorporate every day:

- Be sure to have a broad base of support when lifting your granddaughter. Keep feet shoulder distance apart, and place one foot forward of the other to help with balance.
- Face the task you're doing, and don't twist your trunk when lifting!
- When doing tasks around the house that take a while (like feeding your granddaughter or re-potting small plants) sit versus standing to conserve energy. Sit up straight, and think about keeping a neutral position in your lower back by tilting the pelvis slightly forward.
- When doing laundry, use your rolling basket to help transport clothes. When you do need to lift clothes, use your strongest muscles (legs vs. back) and bend at your hips and knees to avoid straining your back.
- Don't rush! It's best to take rests before you feel tired, and it's much easier to use good body mechanics when working at a comfortable pace!

Summary of Short-Term Goals and Progress

1. M.B. will independently and safely prepare a light meal for herself without complaints of fatigue, using work simplification and energy conservation principles after initial instruction.

The therapist and M.B. first reviewed work simplification principles in the context of preparing a hot beverage, taking the opportunity to organize work areas in the kitchen so frequently used items were easily accessible. They identified ways M.B. could conserve energy during meal preparation, such as by retrieving all items needed at one location (e.g., refrigerator) before moving on to the next and sitting when possible to prepare foods. After instruction in self-pacing, M.B. was more willing to take brief rests during meal preparation before fatigue or pain began to worsen. After practicing proper body mechanics, she was better able to obtain and carry items safely around the kitchen without increasing pain. In addition, use of a jar opener significantly reduced the discomfort in her hands. To reduce preparation time and effort, M.B. decided to use frozen rather than fresh vegetables until her endurance improved. M.B. found that these strategies greatly reduced her level of fatigue during meal preparation, and she began to apply these techniques to other tasks around the house.

Assess the patient's comprehension

"M.B. has cognitive strengths that I expect will help her to readily integrate new techniques with her current knowledge of joint protection."

Understand what he is doing

Compare actual to expected performance

"I was a bit concerned about her rushing through tasks when we first started therapy, but I think that was partly related to her desire to show us that she 'could do it.' I see that, as we gain rapport, she's becoming more comfortable with voicing her concerns about the long-term changes she is experiencing from her arthritis, and her fears about losing independence."

Know the person

Appreciate the context

"M.B. is lucky to have such a supportive daughter; she has helped to identify creative ways for her mother to manage the baby's care. I sense that she is concerned about her mother's chronic rheumatoid arthritis and the physical changes that M.B. is facing now. I wonder what their long-term plans will be regarding living arrangement, etc."

2. M.B. will safely and independently transfer her granddaughter from the infant seat to changing pad on the kitchen table with good body mechanics and safety and no complaints of discomfort.

M.B., her daughter, and the occupational therapist determined that the need for lifting and carrying the infant could be minimized by organizing essential child care materials, such as the infant seat, changing pad with straps, diapers, and toys, on one side of the oversized kitchen table and nearby hutch. M.B. found that bilateral wrist supports greatly reduced pain in her wrists when she lifted the baby.

Proper body mechanics were reinforced and practiced, such as standing close to the child with feet staggered and placed shoulder distance apart and using stronger muscles (legs rather than back) when lifting. M.B. progressed from requiring minimal assistance to lift and transfer the baby safely to performing the task independently. As she gained confidence in her abilities, her body mechanics improved and complaints of discomfort decreased.

Next Steps

Revised goals include the following: (1) M.B. will use work simplification techniques and proper body mechanics to do laundry independently; and (2) M.B. will safely and independently lift and transfer her granddaughter from a stroller to the infant seat with good body mechanics and will prepare and feed the child a warm meal without assistance.

Anticipate present and future patient concerns

Analyze patient's comprehension

Decide if the patient should continue or discontinue therapy and/or return in the future

"M.B. has been very responsive to therapy and has made great gains over the past couple of weeks. She is much more confident in her abilities, and her pain is being better managed through medication and the compensatory strategies she's learned to use. She's now ready to practice work simplification techniques during more physically challenging tasks. With a bit more therapy, she will be able to care for her granddaughter independently once again."

CLINICAL REASONING IN OCCUPATIONAL THERAPY PRACTICE

Effects of Arthritic Changes in the Wrists and Hands and Impaired Endurance During Gardening Tasks

Although M.B. was diagnosed with rheumatoid arthritis 15 years prior to this OT assessment, she managed homemaking and gardening tasks with little adapted equipment until this exacerbation. While M.B. worked in her greenhouse, the occupational therapist observed her bending from the waist to pick up a bag of potting soil and watering can from the floor. In addition, M.B. complained of wrist and hand pain and fatigue while standing at her work counter to transplant seedlings and plants into larger pots. She was very frustrated by the challenges she faced when trying to replant the flower boxes on her deck, a place she enjoyed with family and friends on warm summer days.

How could the therapist help M.B. solve problems and use compensatory strategies and adapted equipment to decrease pain and improve her safety while gardening? How might the therapist reinforce use of proper body mechanics? What work simplification and energy conservation techniques might be useful in addressing her joint protection and endurance needs?

SUMMARY REVIEW QUESTIONS

1. Describe how work simplification and energy conservation techniques can help persons with low endurance and shortness of breath due to chronic obstructive pulmonary disease with meal preparation and household maintenance tasks.
2. Identify at least three principles of correct body mechanics that a person with chronic back pain should use when doing laundry and transporting groceries from the store.
3. Describe how a homemaker who has pain and weakness in her hands and wrists due to rheumatoid arthritis can use adapted methods or assistive equipment when preparing brownies from a mix.
4. Using the principles of compensation and adaptation, what recommendations would you make to a client with limited upper extremity coordination and strength due to multiple sclerosis when gathering the items needed to prepare breakfast from a wheelchair?
5. Give two examples of adaptations that may assist a paraplegic parent with spinal cord injury at T4 (see Chapter 43) to lift and carry an 11-month-old infant from the crib to the changing area.
6. Describe how a mother with upper extremity weakness and limited hand function in her right arm after a stroke can use one-handed techniques and assistive equipment to prepare a bottle and feed her 5-month-old infant.
7. How would you recommend that a parent set up a baby bathtub and needed supplies to bathe a 2-month-old infant from a wheelchair?
8. Discuss proper body mechanics for a person with general pain related to fibromyalgia who is playing with a 10-month-old baby and putting the baby to bed.

ACKNOWLEDGMENT

Many thanks to Robert Littlefield, photographer, and to Sammons Preston Rolyan for the assistive devices pictured in this chapter. Special thanks to the individuals who shared their ideas about adapted techniques with me, based on their personal experience with physical challenges.

References

ADA and ABA Accessibility Guidelines for Buildings and Facilities. (2004). Retrieved March 10, 2006 from http://www.access-board.gov/ada-aba/final.htm.

Adil, J. R. (1994). *Accessible gardening for people with physical disabilities: A guide to methods, tools, and plants*. Bethesda, MD: Woodbine House.

American Occupational Therapy Association [AOTA]. (1997). The psychosocial core of occupational therapy. Position paper. *American Journal of Occupational Therapy, 51,* 868–869.

Anderson, H. (1981). *The disabled homemaker*. Springfield, IL: Charles C. Thomas.

Axtell, L. A., & Yasuda, Y. L. (1993). Assistive devices and home modifications in geriatric rehabilitation. *Clinics in Geriatric Medicine, 9,* 803–821.

Barker, L. T., & Maralani, V. (1997). *Challenges and strategies of disabled parents: Findings from a national survey of parents with disabilities: Final report*. Oakland, CA: Berkeley Planning Associates.

DeMoss, A., Rogers, A., Tuleja, C., & Kirshbaum, M. (1995). *Adaptive parenting equipment: Idea book I*. Berkeley, CA: Through the Looking Glass.

Dunn, V. M. (1978). Tips on raising children from a wheelchair. *Accent on Living, 22,* 78–83.

Eberhardt, K. (1998). Home modifications for persons with spinal cord injury. *OT Practice, 3,* 24–27.

Granger, C. V., Hamilton, B. B., Linacre, J. M., Heinemann, A. W., &

Wright, B. D. (1993). Performance profiles of the Functional Independence Measure. *American Journal of Physical Medicine and Rehabilitation, 72,* 84–89.
Jackson, J., Carlson, M., Mandel, D., Zemke, R., & Clark, F. (1998). Occupational lifestyle redesign: The well-elderly study occupational therapy program. *American Journal of Occupational Therapy, 52,* 326–336.
Joe, B. E. (1997). Small changes: Big differences. *OT Week, January 30,* 16–17.
Kondo, T., Mann, W. C., Tomita, M., & Ottenbacher, K. J. (1997). The use of microwave ovens by elderly persons with disabilities. *American Journal of Occupational Therapy, 51,* 739–747.
Lampert, J., & Lapolice, D. J. (1995). Functional considerations in evaluation and treatment of the client with low vision. *American Journal of Occupational Therapy, 49,* 885–890.
Melnik, M. (1994). *Understanding your back injury.* Rockville, MD: American Occupational Therapy Association.
Moyers, P. A. (1999). The guide to occupational therapy practice. *American Journal of Occupational Therapy, 53,* 247–322.
Nordenskiold, U., Grimby, G., & Dahlin-Ivanoff, S. (1998). Questionnaire to evaluate the effects of assistive devices and altered working methods in women with rheumatoid arthritis. *Clinical Rheumatology, 17,* 6–16.
Nouri, F. M., & Lincoln, N. B. (1987). An extended activities of daily living scale for stroke patients. *Clinical Rehabilitation, 1,* 301–305.
Ostensen, M., & Rugelsjoen, A. (1992). Problem areas of the rheumatic mother. *American Journal of Reproductive Immunology, 28,* 254–255.
Plautz, B., Beck, D. E., Selmar, C., & Radetsky, M. (1996). Modifying the environment: A community-based injury-reduction program for elderly residents. *American Journal of Preventive Medicine, 12 (Suppl. 4),* 33–38.
Sanders, M. J., & Morse, T. (2005). The ergonomics of caring for children: An exploratory study. *American Journal of Occupational Therapy, 59,* 285–295.
Sandqvist, G., Akesson, A., & Eklund, M. (2005). Daily occupations and well-being in women with limited cutaneous systemic sclerosis. *American Journal of Occupational Therapy, 59,* 390–397.
Saunders, H. D. (1992). *For your back.* Eden Prairie, MN: Viking.
Tebben, A. B., & Thomas, J. J. (2004). Trowels labeled ergonomic versus standard design: Preferences and effects on wrist range of motion during a gardening occupation. *American Journal of Occupational Therapy, 58,* 317–323.
Unruh, A. M. (2004). Reflections on: "So. . .what do you do?" Occupation and the construction of identity. *Canadian Journal of Occupational Therapy, 71,* 290–295.
Vensand, K., Rogers, J., Tuleja, C., & DeMoss, A. (2000). *Adaptive baby care equipment: Guidelines, prototypes & resources.* Berkeley, CA: Through the Looking Glass.
Wilkins, S., Jung, B., Wishart, L., Edwards, M., & Norton, S. G. (2003). The effectiveness of community-based occupational therapy education and functional training programs for older adults: A critical literature review. *Canadian Journal of Occupational Therapy, 70,* 214–225.
Yeomans, K. (1992). *The able gardener: Overcoming barriers of age and physical limitations.* Pownal, VT: Storey.

CHAPTER 33

Restoring Competence for the Worker Role

Valerie J. Rice and Stephen Luster

LEARNING OBJECTIVES

After studying this chapter, the reader will be able to do the following:

1. Understand and articulate the reasons people work.
2. Recognize and verbalize the unique role of occupational therapy in the return-to-work process.
3. Describe job analysis and how it is used in the return-to-work process, and identify other possible applications for the results of job analysis.
4. Describe functional capacity evaluations and considerations in selecting appropriate evaluations for clients.
5. Recognize how return-to-work evaluation tools can be used as treatment tools.

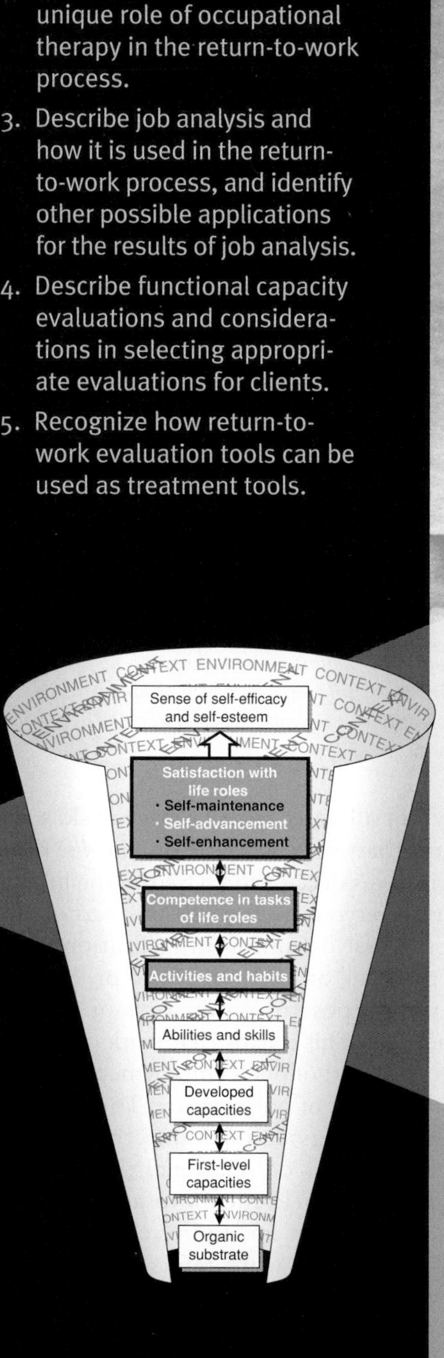

Glossary

Functional capacity evaluation (FCE)—Systematic process designed to assess a client's functional abilities. Functional abilities may include all physical and psychosocial abilities required in a work setting, such as musculoskeletal (strength, range of motion, etc.), cognitive, emotional, and communication abilities. The two performance categories include a general evaluation of physical abilities and an evaluation of job-specific capabilities.

Functional work assessment—Entire return-to-work evaluation process, including evaluations of (1) the individual client (occupational therapy and FCEs) and (2) the requirements of the job or potential jobs (job analysis).

Job analysis—Systematic evaluation of a job; a physical evaluation of the job site, observing workers performing their tasks, conducting a task analysis of the criterion tasks, measuring equipment and equipment placement, reviewing work-related documents such as job descriptions, and interviewing those who perform the job and their supervisors.

Task component testing, training—Functional capacity testing that identifies criterion tasks based on the most difficult, essential components of a job and develops specific evaluations or training programs based on those components. It is assumed that evaluating or training using task components critical to job success is a valid approach to determining work performance, as the content requirements of the job are used to develop the evaluation or training.

Work conditioning—Treatment program focused on functional requirements of a job or employment setting; incorporates basic physical conditioning such as restoration of flexibility, strength, coordination, and endurance. Work conditioning is conducted after completion of acute care and before work hardening.

Work hardening—Multidisciplinary structured, graded return-to-work treatment program that progressively introduces greater rehabilitation requirements on the client-worker to achieve full capability of the worker to meet the demands of a job. Work hardening includes all aspects required for the client to return to full function in employment, such as psychosocial, communication, physical, and vocational needs, and typically incorporates work simulation as part of the treatment process.

Work-related musculoskeletal disorder (WRMD)—Wide range of health problems arising from repeated stress to the body encountered in the workplace; may affect the musculoskeletal, nervous, and neurovascular systems and include the various occupationally induced cumulative trauma disorders, cumulative stress injuries, and repetitive motion disorders.

Two people meet for the first time at a social event. After introducing themselves, the inevitable question is asked: "What do you do?"

The focus of this chapter is on returning a worker who has been incapacitated in some way to the workforce. The intervention begins after an individual has been identified as being unable to meet the requirements of his or her job. Thus, the primary roles for the clinician are *evaluating* the individual's functional performance, strengths, and impairments as compared with the job requirements, *treating* the client, *matching* the client-worker with the job (enabling and integration process), and *reevaluation.* To understand the progression, it is first necessary to understand why people work, recognize how occupational therapists view work and their role in work rehabilitation, understand how the work role can be interrupted, and become acquainted with a few work-related assessments. An extensive explanation of the evaluation process is provided to enable a thorough understanding of the process and permit tailoring of the intervention to both the individual and the context in which the individual will work. With this knowledge, the occupational therapy process can be understood and implemented within the appropriate context.

WHAT IS WORK?

"He who complains against his work knoweth not life; work is an uplifting force by which all things may be moved. Repose is death, and work is life!" (Jastrzebowski, 1857, p. 1)

Although we may not all agree with Jastrzebowski's enthusiastic assertion that work is uplifting and *life itself,* there is some merit in his declaration. Used in the broadest sense of the term, everyone must work. It is part of life. Work, as seen in the first definition in Definition 33-1, consists of any physical or mental effort or activity directed toward the purposeful production or accomplishment of something. This means that work occurs in the home, in schools, as part of one's employment, during volunteer work, and as part of one's leisure. To work is *to do,* to accomplish. With this definition, returning the worker to work encompasses occupational therapy as a whole, as clinicians assist their clients to achieve their fullest capacity in all aspects of life. In this chapter, however, returning the worker to work refers to helping a client reenter the workforce, go to a place of employment

DEFINITION 33-1

Work-Related Definitions

Work (noun)

1. Physical or mental effort or activity directed toward the purposeful production or accomplishment of something: labor. 2. Employment: job [out of work]. 3. The means by which one earns one's livelihood. 4. a. Something that one is doing, making, or performing, esp. as part of one's occupation: a duty or task. b. The amount of effort required or done.

Work (verb)

1. To exert one's efforts for the purpose of doing or making something: labor. 2. To be employed. 3. To perform a function or act: operate.

Work (synonyms)

Business, employment, job, occupation. Core meaning: what one does to earn a living. Work, the most general of these terms, can refer to the mere fact of employment or to a specific activity.

Career

1. Chosen profession or occupation. 2. The general progression of one's life, especially in one's profession.

Job

1. An action that needs to be done: task. 2. An activity performed regularly for payment, especially a trade, occupation, or profession. 3. A specific piece of work to be done for a set fee. 4. A position in which one is employed.

Occupation

Any activity or task with which one occupies oneself, usually specifically the productive activity, service, trade, or craft for which one is regularly paid.

Vocation

A regular occupation or profession, especially one for which an individual is particularly suited or qualified.

or job (including volunteer positions), and/or develop a means to earn a livelihood.

MOTIVATIONS FOR WORK

Why would an individual want to reenter the labor force? Why do people work in the first place? For most people, work is an economic necessity. In earlier times, people traded their wares and their abilities to attain the goods they needed. Although this practice still exists in some small communities, most residents of industrialized countries have distinct employment and pay for their goods and services with money earned at their jobs.

Self-Creation and Self-Identity through Work

We work to finance lives, homes, families, education, and fun. However, especially in industrial societies, we do not have to work from dawn to dusk to earn a living, and we are also not required to enter jobs dictated by our birth or heritage. For the most part, we have choices. We can choose our line of work according to our own values. Occupations are key, not just to being a person, but to being a particular person and to creating and maintaining an identity (Christiansen, 1999; Unruh, 2004). The use of one's time during the day provides a sense of purpose and structure, as well as building an identity. We create ourselves through our actions. Although we may define ourselves daily through our work, we may also fulfill other needs. Our values and the meaning of our lives arise from (and are seen in) our work and how we spend our leisure, home, self-care, and family time.

Work can fulfill our primary motivations (needs), as defined by some of the great psychologists and psychiatrists of our time. Work can fulfill the need to find meaning in life as asserted by Frankl's (1984) logotherapy. Work can fulfill the need to find pleasure, on which Freudian psychology is based. Work can also fulfill the need for power or striving for superiority stressed by Adlerian psychology (Stein, 2002). The point is that work can answer a number of needs. For some, work meets multiple needs of financial achievement, a sense of accomplishment and competence, socialization and status within society, pleasure and gratification, a sense of meaning and purpose, self-respect, and an identity. For others, work answers a singular need, leaving them to meet other needs elsewhere in their lives.

Matching Personal Values with Work Requirements

If our work forces us to behave in ways that directly conflict with our view of ourselves, we feel discomfort and are motivated to change our line of work. This is because people try to maintain positive views of themselves and refute or avoid feedback that is negative or disagrees with their ideal self (Swann, 1987; Swann & Hill, 1982). As an example, Enid DuBois worked as a telephone solicitor for a newspaper. Often, the solicitors were told to tell the potential customers that a portion of their money would go to a particular cause to encourage people to subscribe. "After a while, I didn't care. Surely I could have fast-talked people. Just to continually lie to them. But it just wasn't in me. The disgust was growing in me every minute. I would pray and pray to hold on a little longer" (Terkel, 1974, pp. 94–97).

We have seen a change in the desires of the workforce. Besides emphasis on pay and security, workers value and expect their work to be psychologically meaningful. They expect to participate in decisions that affect their work lives (Hendrick, 1998). The current, better-educated workforce in industrialized nations seeks challenges, advancement, and a voice in their work lives.

Balance is particularly important to the younger generation entering today's workforce. Occupational balance refers to the integrating of one's work, home, and leisure activities (Backman, 2004). Other work-related values of younger persons in today's workforce include independence, autonomy, self-expression, recognition for their work, and continual learning (Chester, 2005). Younger workers need to feel valued and prefer work environments where they are mentored, treated with respect, and allowed to try some of their own ideas (even if they fail occasionally). More than past generations, they need to understand why things need to be done in a particular way, and they need to believe in and value the product, service, or mission they help to deliver (Chester, 2005). They value their social interactions at work, as well their own perception of the importance of the product created by their work (Polanyi & Tompa, 2004).

The importance of occupational involvement and the characteristics of work most valued differ according to one's culture (Hasan, 2004) and personal values. In fact, the importance of work within a single culture and perhaps within an individual can vary over time. For example, some researchers note that work alone is considered as a declining value, replaced by a high value of success in both personal and professional life (Deberdt, 2002). Similarly, people's values change over time, and their view of work can change accordingly. Thus, in rehabilitation, the therapist and the patient/client must explore the perceptions and values of the client, discover the client's occupational identity, and create an appropriate occupational balance intervention (Backman, 2004; Holmgren & Dahlin Ivanhoff, 2004).

INTERRUPTIONS IN THE ABILITY TO WORK

People's ability to work may be interrupted by changes in physical, psychosocial, or sociocultural status.

Physical Status

> Mr. L. worked in a collision repair shop. His brother was fond of saying that he "banged on cars" for a living. The job required him to stand and manually remove the dents from car fenders using specialized tools. He was physically strong because his job demanded it. He wasn't prepared for what happened after he broke his leg. It never seemed to heal correctly. He developed what they called reflex sympathetic dystrophy. The term didn't matter. All he knew was it hurt all the time and he couldn't stand or even sit for long periods. He received workers compensation and wondered if he'd ever work again (D. Rice, personal communication, 2000).

The direct result of injury or illness may be inability to resume work activities permanently or temporarily because the worker cannot fulfill the physical, cognitive, or emotional demands of the job. This mismatch between requirements and performance has been traditionally addressed by retraining the individual. The focus was on improving the deficits; thus the therapist worked to diminish individual shortfalls in strength, dexterity, coordination, range of motion, endurance, or memory. Whatever interrupted the client's ability to resume normal activities was addressed. More recently, the focus has broadened to include altering or redesigning the job to realign its requirements to the individual's residual abilities.*

Not all injuries or illnesses that disrupt the ability to work are the result of a sudden injury or illness. Non-traumatic injuries may also interfere with a person's ability to work. Non-traumatic injuries thought to be related to workplace demands include **work-related musculoskeletal disorders (WRMDs)**. These injuries are typically thought of as transient, although they can result in permanent disability. WRMDs include a wide range of health problems arising from repeated stress to the body encountered in the workplace. These health problems, which may affect the musculoskeletal, nervous, and neurovascular systems, include the various occupation-induced cumulative trauma disorders (CTDs), cumulative stress injuries, and repetitive motion disorders. Examples include damage to tendons and tendon sheaths and synovial lubrication of the tendon sheaths, bones, muscles, and nerves of the hands, wrists, elbows, shoulders, neck, back, and legs. Specific diagnoses include chronic back pain, carpal tunnel syndrome, de Quervain's disease, epicondylitis (tennis elbow), Raynaud's syndrome (white finger), synovitis, stenosing tenosynovitis crepitans (trigger finger), tendinitis, and tenosynovitis. (For a thorough review of WRMDs, see Kuorinka et al. [1995], Sanders [1997], Caryon, Smith, and Haims [1999], and Pransky et al. [1999].) Once again, the reason for not being able to return to work is the person's inability to fulfill the requirements of the job tasks, such as the administrative assistant with severe, chronic carpal tunnel symptoms who cannot use a keyboard without pain.

Traumatic injury, aging, or progressive disability may also alter self-perception and personal identity. When a person loses his or her sense of identity, life becomes less

* This same approach of designing the job or environment could enable older workers to continue working comfortably.

meaningful and can become meaningless (Debats, Drost, & Hansen, 1995; Moore, 1997; van Selm & Dittmann-Kohli, 1998), leading to depression so severe that it can interfere with a person's ability to carry out daily work. Thus, it is not always the initial injury that prevents a return to work; the resulting psychological adjustments can also interfere. Unless both the physical and psychological problems are addressed, the individual may not develop the skills needed to return to work.

Cognitive Status

People's cognitive abilities directly influence their ability to do a job and the type of job they can assume. For example, individuals who have had a brain injury (including mild to moderate traumatic brain injuries and strokes) can have difficulties with clear thinking, memory, concentration, decision making, and reasoning, as well as changes in their sensory processing and/or communication skills. After injury, they may suffer from depression, anxiety, or personality changes. All of these symptoms can interfere with their ability to return to work (National Institutes of Health [NIH], 2002).

Adults who have attention deficit disorder also experience thought and behavior patterns that differ from the "normal" population. These individuals are more likely to be fired and have difficulty keeping a job, yet 35% become self-employed (Barkley & Murphy, 1998 as cited in Adler and Cohen, 2002). A skilled therapist can help them recognize their strengths and the types of jobs or job structure that will take advantage of their skills and give them a good chance of success. For example, many adults with attention deficit hyperactivity disorder are innovative, energetic risk takers who can do well in jobs that permit multi-tasking, self-determination of scheduling, physical action, and out-sourcing of time-intensive detailed tasks.

Psychological and Behavioral Status

Psychosocial events may interrupt a person's ability to work, either temporarily or permanently. Divorce, severe illness, death of a family member, or change in job status sometimes triggers underlying psychopathology such as a mood or anxiety disorder. The disruption may be due not to underlying psychopathology but to the expression or manifestation of a normal reaction to a difficult situation.* Each individual reacts differently to life situations, and adaptation may come more quickly for some than for others. Examples of an individual's inability to meet work requirements include disruptions in the ability to concentrate and follow complex directions, react quickly to emergencies (psychomotor retardation), attend to detail, or handle the pressures and anxieties associated with the work environment. Although there is less information on individuals returning to work after a psychological disorder compared with after physical injuries/illnesses, this is no less a problem than is a physical injury. In fact, it may be more difficult to return to work because of the attitudes and lack of knowledge and empathy of employers and coworkers, in addition to fears and concerns of the workers themselves.

Depression is predicted to be one of the fastest-growing maladies of the 21st century and is often associated with physical injury or loss of work. Although treatment for depression and other psychological and emotional disturbances has vastly improved, there are definite implications for the individual's ability to work. Work seems to mitigate the rate of mental health deterioration, with employment status being more important for men than women (Llena-Nozal, Lindeboom, & Portrait, 2004).†

Sociocultural Status

Fewer than 10 years ago, millions of disabled Americans were guaranteed the ability to keep their government-funded health coverage when they accepted a paying job (Ross, 1999). This was offered because it is believed that many disabled individuals do not seek employment for fear of losing Medicare and Medicaid benefits. In fact, in this country and others, fewer than 1% of those who receive government disability ever leave that system (Ahlgren et al., 2005). In addition, many long-term sick-listed individuals (46%) move from vocational rehabilitation to permanent pensions rather than returning to work, with almost none of those receiving a temporary disability pension ever returning to work (Ahlgren et al., 2005). This law should remove some of the fear, and up to 550,000 disabled persons will receive rehabilitation and training in preparation for return to the workforce (Ross, 1999). The impact of this U.S. law is not yet known.

Aging and age discrimination may also prevent workers from continuing to work or from returning to work following physical or psychological problems or following a downsizing. This problem may become more evident as the proportion of workers aged 45–54 years increases, which will be followed in the next 10 years by a substantial increase in the proportion of workers 55 years of age and older (Yelin, 1999).

* This is also the basic explanation for a combat stress reaction, which is a normal reaction to an abnormal situation, such as a traumatic stressful event. When it interrupts a person's ability, it is often referred to as an acute stress disorder, which is typically short term. Post-traumatic stress disorder is longer term and has more impact on daily function over time (Lifelines, 2006).

† Although this chapter identifies some motivations for why people work, it is recognized that not all work exerts a positive influence on the worker. In fact, work-related stressors can contribute to psychological distress, occupational injury, or illness (Marchand, Demers, & Durand, 2005), thus influencing health, turnover, work attrition, and return to work. Certainly, therapists must ascertain whether these conditions exist for a client, an issue beyond the scope of this chapter.

WORK AND AGING

Society is challenged to consider three questions regarding older workers: (1) Can our nation "afford" older individuals who do not work? (2) Do older workers stand in the way of younger workers? (3) Are older workers less productive, slower, harder to supervise, less cognitively aware, and less physically able to do a job?

The workforce in 2012 will be more diverse and older, with a median expected age of 41.4 years and with 19% of workers aged 55 or older (Toosi, 2004). If all of these individuals did not work, there would be a severe shortage in multiple industries.

Yet barriers stand in the way of older individuals working. There is a concern about the safety of both the older worker and his colleagues among those hiring. A societal feeling of needing to "make room" for younger workers also exists. The attitude of retirement as a "public good" will have to change for older workers to get the jobs they seek. Perhaps it is happening, as there is a clear shift toward a longer work life in the United States (American Association of Retired Persons [AARP], 2006).

Who Are Our Older Workers and Why Do They Work?

The proportion of the population that works decreases with age (Tables 33-1 and 33-2). Not all older persons stop work as their own choice. Fifty-six percent of young retirees state that they were forced to retire, while 38% wanted to stop working (National Academy on an Aging Society, 2001). Those who work after age 60 tend to be male, educated, white, married, and in better health and better off monetarily than those who do not work (National Academy on an Aging Society, 2000). Older women who work feel more positive about growing older, report being in good physical health, and anticipate a better financial future than older women who are not working (National Center on Women and Aging, 2002).

Most older workers choose to work in order to remain active and productive, to do something fun, and for access to money and health care (AARP, 2006). Those who would like to work but cannot find a job report believing they lack necessary training or are experiencing age discrimination. Some of their fears may be founded as persons aged 55 and older are less likely to find a job than younger workers after displacement. Finding a job takes longer, wages are often lower when hired, and there are a number of age discrimination awards given by courts (Rix, 2005), even with U.S. anti-discrimination laws and European Union anti-discrimination directives on employment.

Three keys to successful aging are low probability of disease and disability, high mental and physical function, and active engagement with life (Rowe & Kahn, 1999). Active engagement with life includes having close personal relationships and pursuing activities that produce something of value (a product or service) (Rowe & Kahn, 1999). Thus, continuing to work (in the broad sense of the term) may lead to greater satisfaction with life and perhaps even a longer life of higher quality.

Paid Employment, Volunteer Work, and Occupation of Time

It is intuitive to expect that an individual's occupational identity and the meeting of his or her needs and values (mentioned earlier) can be met through paid employment, volunteer work, or meaningful activities that occupy their time. Insufficient literature exists, however, to clearly substantiate this claim. Instead, we surmise that portions of this may be true based on findings. For example, individuals with mental illness who engaged in paid (competitive)

Table 33-2. Older Persons Who Work

Age (years)	Percentage Who Work Full Time	Percentage Who Work Part Time
40–59	80	
51–59	76	
60–69	61	36
70+	28	72

Data from National Academy on an Aging Society (2000).

Table 33-1. The Aging U.S. Workforce

Age Group	Percentage of Work Force Expected in 2012	Percent Change		
		1982–1992	*1992–2002*	*2002–2012*
Youth (16–24 years old)	15	−12.2	3.7	9
Prime age worker (25–54 years old)	66	29.7	9.2	5.1
Older (55+ years old)	19.1	−0.2	34.4	49.3

Adapted from Toosi, 2004.

work reported being more satisfied with their daily occupations than those involved in seemingly meaningful work in a therapeutic setting and those with no regular daily activity, yet none of the three groups differed in terms of self-ratings of health and well-being (Eklund, Hansson, & Ahlqvist, 2004). Questions about life satisfaction were not included in the prior study, but satisfaction with life has been associated with working in asthmatics (Piirila et al., 2005), and people who are employed are more satisfied with their lives than those who are unemployed (this is true for the general population and those with schizophrenia or other forms of mental illness) (Priebe et al., 1998).

The switch from paid worker to volunteerism or other form of meaningful activity must be taken carefully because one does not automatically suffice for the other. Ibarra (2002) suggests that a change to another profession or career, attempting "bridge employment" in another area, or moving toward another occupation requires a person to "try on" the new identity through action and a "test-and-learn" model of change.

WORK AND OCCUPATIONAL THERAPY

Adolph Meyer advocated a "freer conception of work, a concept of free and pleasant and profitable occupation including recreation and any form of helpful enjoyment as the leading principle." He said the "whole of human organization has its shape in a kind of rhythm," and through structured use of time, people could achieve well-being (Meyer, 1922, pp. 1–2). By assisting the client to achieve a balanced lifestyle in work, play, rest, and sleep, early occupational therapists helped clients achieve a sense of homeostasis and health. Meyer broadly defined the term *occupation* as purposeful activity within the full spectrum of a person's life.

Occupational therapy is soundly based on the concept of returning the injured worker to work, as it was founded on the belief that merely eliminating the disease or providing immediate treatment for traumatic injury was insufficient for full recovery and ability to assume life roles. Instead, a client should be guided through a strengthening and training process, both physically and mentally, to prepare him or her to resume occupational status in society (Committee on Installations and Advice, 1928; Rice, 1999a). Therapists used "crafts" in their treatment. What were once called crafts are today considered jobs. The term *craft* included activities such as carpentry, metal work, and bookbinding, all of which were full-time vocations. Initially, a wide variety of crafts or jobs were used in occupational therapy clinics. Occupational therapists realized, however, that carefully chosen occupation-based activities resulted in a transfer of training to almost any occupation the recovered client chose to pursue. This is opposite the current trend of work hardening, which simulates specific job tasks that will be required of the client upon return to work. The latter certainly has greater face validity, but to date, no published outcome research clearly supports one approach as superior to the other.

Occupational Therapists' Unique Contributions

Occupational therapists, with their solid background in the full spectrum of human performance (physiological, biomechanical, psychosocial, and behavioral), are uniquely qualified to help clients return to work. A fundamental goal of occupational therapy is to facilitate the client's highest level of functional status in all occupations and all contexts of life, including physical, emotional, social, cognitive, and communicative dimensions. Occupational therapists recognize that successful return to work is likely to depend on adequate function in many aspects of life, not solely task performance at a work site. For example, occupational therapists use their knowledge of human performance and the human mind to determine whether the impediments to returning to work are physical, psychosocial, or both. Therapists also use their knowledge of human psychology to discern possible motivations for the client to achieve well-being.

With some clients, the urge toward competence is obvious, and they work quickly to master their environment (White, 1971). Therapists can motivate others by having them visualize what they want to be able to do or the type of person they want to be and by working with them to achieve their *possible selves* (Markus & Nurius, 1986). Those who value work or for whom we can find the motivational factors in work are most inclined to participate fully in rehabilitation. They are also the most likely to return to the workforce. Providing small successes along the way does much to encourage the process, but without work that has intrinsic value for the individual, the return to work is likely to be unsuccessful. The application of the full spectrum of human performance elucidates the unique contributions of occupational therapists in returning the injured worker to the workforce.

Burwash Model

One model depicting the knowledge and intervention necessary for occupational therapists to evaluate and intervene in work practices is that presented by Burwash (1999), which is shown in Figure 33-1 and further described in Table 33-3. Returning to work is seen as one of the triangles representing concerns of clients. To

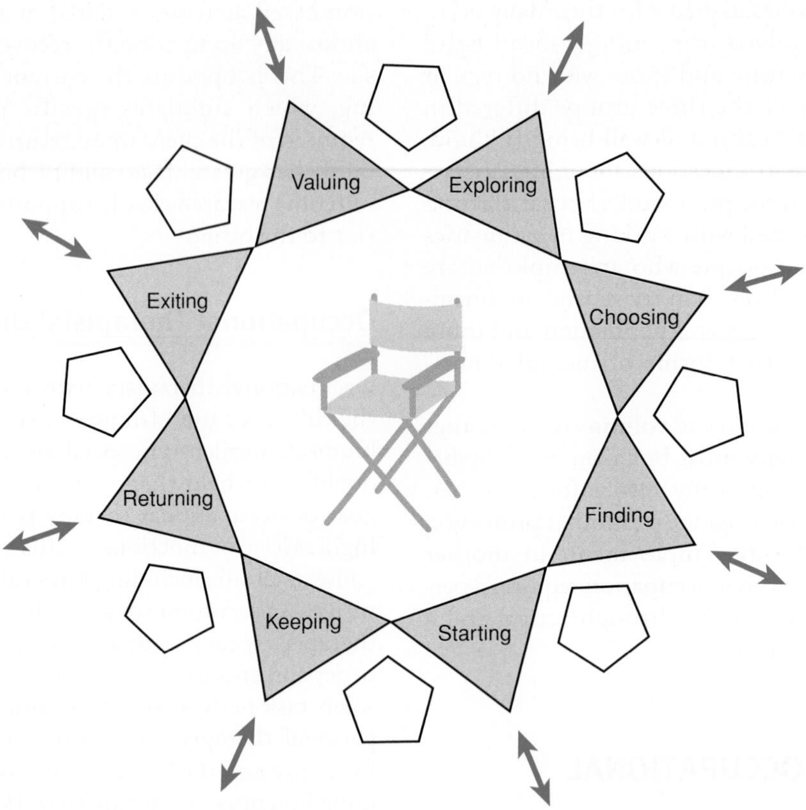

Figure 33-1 *Work Practice Model* (Burwash, 1999). The circular shape suggests many entry and exit points; intervention may progress in a linear fashion around the circle, or only one or two areas of concern may be addressed. The director's chair in the center is a reminder that focus is on the individual and his or her values, and the individual, rather than diagnosis or age, should be the director. The eight triangles represent concerns expressed by clients and are part of occupational therapy's professional heritage and within therapists' competencies. The pentagons suggest artists' palettes as a reminder that the intervention requires both art and science in dealing with productivity issues. The double-headed arrows represent environmental factors that influence and can be influenced by the client and therapist; they include social, cultural, and political factors, among others.

facilitate a return to work, however, the therapist may be involved in each of the eight areas. For example, the client may be leaving one line of work because of disease or disability and needs to reevaluate his or her values to explore and choose another career. While building the requisite physical and cognitive skills for the chosen job or career field, the client may also need to develop skills in searching for work along with the work habits needed to sustain a successful career.

The therapist must understand the client's value of work and self-perception as related to work (such as self-definition and self-esteem), so as to design the rehabilitation process and identify short-term goals and techniques to motivate the client. This client-centered approach to evaluation and treatment involves joint identification of goals and priorities by the therapist and the client (Law et al., 1994; Mattingly, 1991; Neistadt, 1995). For example, therapists can help clients ascertain whether they want their work to be a job rather than a career (see Definition 33-1) by examining where they fulfill their social, emotional, and achievement needs.

THE RETURN-TO-WORK PROCESS

Returning to work entails three main procedures: evaluation, intervention, and reevaluation.

Functional Work Assessments

Functional work assessments include evaluation of both the individual client and the work requirements the client will encounter. Individual evaluations incorporate the standard occupational therapy assessment, a delineation of the conditions preventing the client from returning to work, and a **functional capacity evaluation (FCE)**. The evaluation of the work requirements is often referred to as a **functional job analysis**, or simply job analysis.

Job Analysis

A job analysis is a systematic evaluation of the job that identifies its physical, cognitive, social, and psychological requirements. Conducting a job analysis entails going to

Table 33-3. Examples Using the *Burwash Model* (1999)

Model Segment	Client Concerns	Therapist Resources: Assessment Tools, Techniques, and Programs	Environmental Considerations
Valuing	"Why work?" "How does work fit into my life?" "What are my personal values and what types of work fit?" "Why am I not happy in this work?" "Is working worth it?"	Work Values Inventory, Life Roles Inventory, work values auction, spirituality of work questionnaire, Occupational Performance History Interview	Family and social group attitudes toward work; economic considerations for persons on disability pensions; religious beliefs about work; work and gender issues
Exploring	"I don't know what I'm physically capable of." "Are there any occupations that match my interests?" "What am I good at?"	Functional Capacity Evaluation, Self-Directed Search, work samples, computerized career exploration systems	Role definition of OT vs. other team members (career counselors, vocational rehabilitation counselor, teachers); family expectations
Keeping	"How is this health problem going to affect my work?" "I hurt so much after a day at work!" "I'm about to take stress leave; all of these changes are really getting to me." "I can't figure out how to get ahead at work; I'm really feeling stuck."	Ergonomic interventions, stress management and relaxation techniques, energy conservation and work simplification techniques, goal setting, injury prevention and health promotion programs, advocacy	Family and friends' expectations; public laws on disability and workplace ergonomic standards; employer, coworker, public attitudes toward persons with disabilities; client's support system; funding issues; job market; physical accessibility; access to transportation
Returning	"Will I be able to work again?" "How do I prevent reinjury?" "How do I deal with coworkers' comments about my illness?" "If I'm hurting at work, how do I cope with the pain?"	Work Environment Impact Scale, Worker Role Interview, graduated return-to-work programs, work hardening and chronic pain programs, assertiveness skills, Loma Linda Activity Sort, other resources in Exploring row above	Laws on injured workers and employers' responsibilities to them, job market, funding for retraining, family responsibilities, possible financial settlements, advice from lawyers and others, employer–employee relations

the job site, observing workers performing their tasks, measuring equipment and equipment placement, and interviewing those who perform the job and their supervisors. Some of the tools employed in the job analysis are video cameras, tape measures, scales, goniometers, stopwatches, dynamometers, still cameras, and strain gauges. The results of a job analysis can be used in several ways, as seen in Procedures for Practice 33-1.

Basic Components of Job Analysis

Components of any job analysis include the job title, basic description or objectives of the job, number of employees performing the job, the work and break schedule, a description of any rotation or enrichment program, and output requirements for the workers. A description of the environment should include temperature, available space,

PROCEDURES FOR PRACTICE 33-1

Ways to Use Job Analysis Data

- Develop FCE
- Match injured workers' capabilities to job task requirements
- Place workers on light duty
- Return previously injured workers to work
- Identify risk factors associated with work-related musculoskeletal disorders
- Develop pre-placement, post-job offer screenings
- Write job description (possibly using ADA terminology)
- Describe and advertise jobs

a list of fixed and movable equipment, personal protective equipment, and a sketch of the area. A sequential description of each task (essential function) and the component steps to complete it are also necessary. This should include measurements such as heights, weights, durations, distances, and so on.

Rationale for Conducting Job Analysis

The reason for conducting the job analysis dictates its questions and procedures. Purposes of conducting a job analysis include returning a person with a disability to work, identifying musculoskeletal risk factors, matching a rehabilitated or new worker with job demands, and developing assessments such as FCEs and pre-placement screening tests.

For example, if the results are to be used to return an individual classified as disabled according to the Americans with Disabilities Act (ADA) (Federal Register, 1991) to his or her work, the job must be described in terms of its essential functions (Definition 33-2). Therapists whose responsibilities include industrial rehabilitation and returning injured or disabled workers to the workforce or helping employers to advertise jobs should be well versed in Title I of the ADA. Several excellent book chapters for therapists are available (Bloswick et al., 1998; Isernhagen, 1995a; Kornblau, 1998a, 1998b), and therapists should also refer to the regulations and guides themselves (ADA Title I Regulations, 1991; Americans with Disabilities Act, 1990; Equal Employment Opportunity Commission, 1992).

DEFINITION 33-2

Essential Functions

Fundamental, Not Marginal, Job Duties

Some considerations in determining whether a function is essential include:

- Whether the position exists to perform that function
- The number of other employees available to perform the function or among whom the function can be distributed
- The degree of expertise required
- Whether past and/or present employees in the job have performed the function
- The time spent performing the function
- The consequences of not performing the function

Reasonable Accommodations

Modifications of the work environment include job restructuring and providing adaptive or adaptable equipment and similar modifications to enable equal opportunities for employment by individuals with disabilities.

If the reason for performing the job analysis is to identify risk factors that may predispose a person to musculoskeletal disorders, listing the essential functions is not compulsory. A job analysis primarily geared to injury prevention, such as work-related musculoskeletal disorders, should include descriptions of observed risk factors, such as repetitive motions, force, static postures, awkward postures, mechanical compressions, vibration, and the acceleration and velocity of dynamic motions, noted for each body part and quantified. For example, the duration of static hold using a pinch grip is noted in seconds. Literature on job analysis related to injury prevention can be found in several excellent sources (Alexander, 1999; Ellexson, 1997; Isernhagen, 1995b; Karwowski & Marras, 1999; Pulat & Alexander, 1992; Rice, 1998; Rogers, 1983, 1992; Sanders, 1997).

For matching workers' capabilities with the job requirements, placing workers on light duty, or returning previously injured workers to work, tasks (i.e., essential functions) are broken into their component steps and quantitatively described in enough detail to permit them to be matched with the worker's residual capabilities (Procedures for Practice 33-2). The therapist who only occasionally participates in returning injured workers to the workforce may prepare a unique job analysis for each client; those who work full time in industrial rehabilitation generally keep a file of job descriptions that lets them quickly determine whether a client can return by comparing the results of the FCE with the job description (Isernhagen, 1995b). One benefit of having occupational therapists involved in job analysis is the ability to combine these purposes for conducting job analysis and developing a comprehensive database for an industry's use.

Use of Job Analysis in Developing and Selecting a Functional Capacity Evaluation

A job analysis should be conducted *prior to development or selection of an FCE.* An FCE consists of two parts: a general evaluation of physical abilities and a job-specific evaluation. Before one can decide whether to use solely the general evaluation versus the job-specific evaluation, the therapist must know whether the client intends to return to a specific job or type of job. If so, the information from the job analysis can be used to develop one of two types of FCE using criterion-referenced tasks. The first uses task components, while the second uses work simulations (both discussed later in the chapter). In both cases, the initial information is gathered during the job analysis.

Predicting Work Performance

The results of job analysis can also be used to predict performance. A review of 21 research studies designed to predict work performance, found static, dynamic, and combined strength tests and simulations predicted job

pounds and a 50-pound toolbox. The criterion task includes the more difficult of the two tasks on the assumption that a worker who can accomplish the more difficult task is also competent for the lesser one. The criterion tasks, in the form of task components or work simulations, are used because they are believed to predict job performance. It is assumed that testing applicants on single aspects of job performance that are critical to job success is a valid approach to determining work performance, as the content requirements are used (Wigdor & Green, 1991). An example of the development of criterion-referenced tasks using both the task component and work simulation techniques can be seen in Procedures for Practice 33-3.

WORK SIMULATIONS

Work simulations differ from task components in that they replicate essential series of tasks required on a job. For example, a firefighter's task of removing a hose, attaching it to a nozzle, and holding the hose during spraying is one task simulation. The same task series analyzed according to its task components might include only two portions, lifting an item that weighs the same as the hose and pushing a sled whose weight equals the amount of hose pressure. Work simulations frequently involve multiple constructs, such as strength, balance, and agility, and they have more face validity.

Psychosocial Behaviors

Some evaluations include the individual's psychosocial behaviors as they apply to work habits and motivation; however, this is not consistently part of the process. This part of the FCE should describe the client's limitations in comprehension, recall, and ability to follow instructions. Other psychosocial issues, such as ability to handle work pressures, respond to supervision, and relate to coworkers or customers, should also be noted.

Many FCEs use an evaluation called the detection of sincerity of effort, which is said to be an indication of a client's motivation to perform optimally during an FCE. The belief is that a client who is not sincere may have a less successful recovery or prolonged recovery, overuse treatment, have increased costs of care, and receive unwarranted disability payments (Lechner, Bradbury, & Bradley, 1998). In their excellent review article, Lechner, Bradbury, and Bradley reviewed several sincerity-of-effort evaluation methods for reliability and validity. They also examined the concept of using the coefficient of variation in muscle performance tests, the correlation between musculoskeletal evaluations and FCEs. They concluded, "to date, none of the previously discussed methods for detecting sincerity of effort have been adequately studied for its use with clients with LBP" (low back pain). They further state that "therapists also are advised to avoid reporting test results as 'valid' or 'invalid' based on perceived levels of cooperation and to avoid using the terms 'symptom magnification' and 'exaggerated pain behavior' to describe client behavior" (Lechner, Bradbury, & Bradley, 1998, pp. 884–885).

Since alterations in mood and affect commonly coexist with and exacerbate physical problems, these issues should be included in the assessment. A brief screening tool can be used in conjunction with clinical observations to determine the influence of any psychosocial problems. The *Generalized Contentment Scale* is a quick 25-item paper and pencil measure of non-psychotic depression that is useful in determining the extent of mood alterations associated with loss of the work role (Hudson, 1982). If significant test results are obtained, assistance from psychological services may be indicated.

Selecting a Functional Capacity Evaluation

More than 55 FCEs are available, and selection of an appropriate one can be difficult. They differ in the physical and psychological factors they assess and the way the measures are administered. They also differ in the training required for competency in administration and interpretation. Some use a battery of tests that may or may not be based on a specific task analysis of the job in question. Such a battery may include strength, flexibility, and endurance tests. Others use actual simulations of the tasks required of the job. Few have undergone rigorous examination to determine whether the evaluation predicts actual job performance (Innes & Straker, 1999; Rice, 1999b). Although it may seem easy to select an FCE based on the availability of workshops and related products, the decision making process should be performed carefully. Some good review articles assist with selecting FCEs (Innes & Straker, 1999; King, Tuckwell, & Barrett, 1998) and pre-placement tests (Rice, 1999b). King, Tuckwell, and Barrett (1998) reviewed 10 FCEs for their years of availability, format, length of assessment and report, validity and reliability, availability of peer-reviewed published research, standardization of instruction, whether the FCE is norm or criterion referenced, and costs. Innes and Straker (1999) reviewed the test–retest, inter-rater, intra-test, and instrument precision reliability of 28 evaluations. Both articles contain charts that are well worth having as references for selection of evaluations. No single evaluation is likely to suffice in all cases for all clients. Therefore, clinicians should be familiar with various evaluations and select those most suitable for their setting and their clients.

Functional Work Assessments Conclusion

Knowledge of the two primary means of assessment in industrial rehabilitation, job analysis and functional capacity assessment, sets the stage for intervention. Individual clients' goals, work site design alterations, and bringing the capabilities of the worker closer into alignment with the demands of the job are all built on a well performed set of assessments. The practitioner must integrate into the intervention process the detail the assessments provide, and the results of the FCE should be used to indicate a client's potential to work. This information should be clearly communicated to the employer and to the client. The bottom line is this: The best "evaluation" is one that is holistic; it examines the work, the work environment, and the workers needs, interests, desires (motivations), behaviors (habits and lifestyle), and personal characteristics.

Intervention

Intervention that is specific for returning the individual to the workforce builds upon traditional occupational therapy intervention, taking it a few steps further into the daily work requirements of the client. Throughout intervention, the therapist should maintain communication with the client's work supervisor and iteratively determine the potential for work site modification to match the levels of performance being discovered during the evaluation. These modifications may continue throughout the process, permitting the client to return to a work setting much earlier and encouraging personal identification as a contributing, competent worker.

Work Conditioning

Work conditioning generally follows acute care and precedes **work hardening**. Like traditional occupational therapy intervention, work conditioning focuses on remediation of underlying physical or cognitive deficits to improve function. The difference between traditional rehabilitation and work conditioning is that the intervention is focused on functional requirements of a job or employment setting rather than on life skills required at home or for recreational activities. Restoration of flexibility, strength, coordination, and endurance may be addressed. Work conditioning should increase physical abilities, engineer successful performance, and provide realistic feedback regarding the client's capabilities (Fig. 33-2). The client's day may include a regimen of warm-up exercises tailored to the activities planned for the day, conditioning exercises based on job requirements, and job-related tasks using work samples that replicate essential task components of a job. A program may begin with sessions of an hour or two and progress as the client-worker's condition improves to 8 hours per day.

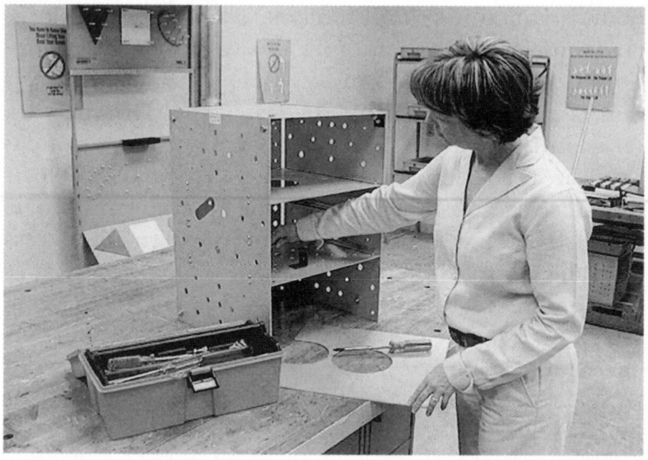

Figure 33-2 Work conditioning using a simulated work task. This is an initial simulation, as the requirements for bending and stooping have not yet been added.

Work Hardening

Work hardening is a multidisciplinary structured treatment designed to maximize a client's ability to return to employment. Work hardening includes all aspects required for the client to return to full employment function, such as psychosocial, communication, physical, and vocational needs. Although general physical abilities are addressed in work conditioning, work hardening is aimed more specifically at a particular job or classification of jobs, so it tends to use work simulation. Considerations added during work hardening include productivity (speed, accuracy, and efficiency), safety (ability to adhere to safety principles and use of safety equipment and algorithms), physical tolerances for specific tasks (endurance and ability to carry out the repetitive task requirements), organizational skills, and decision making. The key differences are the use of real or simulated work activities in a graded fashion, building to work over periods comparable with those in actual work settings; the full spectrum of work-related intervention; and the use of a multidisciplinary approach (Isernhagen, 1988). Disciplines included in a work hardening program can include occupational and physical therapy, psychology, vocational rehabilitation, social work, and social services. Other professionals who may participate full time or as needed include drug and alcohol counselors, nutritionists, and educators (special education or educational evaluators).

Work hardening environments should replicate the workplace as closely as possible. Sufficient space is needed for both traditional equipment for work conditioning and specialized equipment that may be brought from a job site. Also, the behaviors and interactions required of the clients should replicate a work setting, such as arriving and leaving on a set schedule, working with fixed breaks, having supervisors who give positive and negative feedback on performance, performance standards, and so on. Returning a client to a part-time or full-time light duty assignment during rehabilitation may help the client feel like part of the team. It may also assist employers by building their confidence in the process and by letting them observe first hand the capabilities of the client-worker.

All involved parties should be kept informed of the process. This includes employers, supervisors, insurance representatives, occupational health nurses, and the physician.

Reevaluation of the Client and Program Evaluation

Two types of intertwined evaluations should be conducted. Individual clients should be reevaluated, and the program as a whole should be evaluated. Monitoring clients' progress and annotating whether they have achieved functional goals should occur as in traditional occupational therapy during clinic-based treatment. Follow-up evaluations with the client and the client's supervisor are suggested so that, in case of a problem, the therapist can intervene before reinjury or exacerbation of the injury occurs. In addition, it is important to combine this information (having removed individual identifiers) with that of other clients to determine whether overall program goals are being met. It is important to know whether the program is meeting the needs of individual clients as well as those of the referral sources (employers). Tracking information such as the rate of successful return to work, the length of limited-duty time, and the subjective responses of past clients and their supervisors enables the therapist to improve the program. This information is important for showing the cost-benefit value of the services and should be available if reimbursement questions arise. The same information can be used in marketing strategies.

A CLINICAL IMPLEMENTATION OF THE RETURN-TO-WORK PROCESS

This chapter contains basic information about work-related assessment, intervention through work conditioning and work hardening, and reevaluation of both the individual and the program, along with background information on work motivation, interruption of work, and ways occupational therapists can intervene. Still, the application of this knowledge can be confusing without a framework. Therefore, this section describes a decision pathway and an example of an FCE (Fig. 33-3). The interventions identified in this decision pathway are closely aligned with the interventions articulated in the article "Occupational Therapy Practice Framework: Domain and Process" (American Occupational Therapy Association, 2002). These interventions are therapeutic use of self, education, consultation, and therapeutic use of occupations (occupation-based activity). These interventions are broad based, and it is probably beyond the scope of this chapter to present a meaningful discussion of their merits or limitations.

The return-to-work decision pathway shown in Figure 33-4 presents work rehabilitation processes in the larger context of injury, medical management, and acute rehabilitation. As cost containment is a paramount issue in any health care organization, the decision pathway encourages a logical process to return the client to the workforce in a time-efficient manner. As can be seen in Figure 33-4, the decision pathway begins with an interruption of the work process, includes medical and rehabilitative intervention, incorporates the return-to-work process of evaluation and intervention, and offers several junctures at which the client may return to work.

The FCE in Figure 33-3 is composed of measures that are routinely available in most clinical settings (Resource 33-1). Additional tests can be added as available and desired. The many available off-the-shelf FCEs all have some limitations as well as merits, and therapists should be broad minded in their selection of tools for the FCE. It may be most efficacious for therapists first to develop an understanding of the return-to-work evaluation and intervention process and then to develop a structured evaluation system composed of available components that are specific to individual patients and the specific environmental context to which they must return.

The first page of information seen on the FCE (Fig. 33-3) contains the evaluation of the findings, an explanation of the discrepancies between the job requirements and work performance, and recommendations. This arrangement seems to put the end (the results) at the beginning before permitting the reader to follow and understand the evaluative process. The format is designed so the "bottom line" is immediately available for the employer and/or client to read. Background information in the form of the evaluative process is then provided as substantiation of the findings.

Each section of the decision pathway and FCE is explained in the next section. Also refer to the Case Example, which further demonstrates the use of the FCE.

Medical Management and Acute Rehabilitation

The return-to-work process begins as soon as a patient enters the medical system for treatment. Medical management (Fig. 33-4) concerns the use of medical and surgical treatment to control and remedy acute medical problems that have interrupted the work role. Acute rehabilitation naturally follows medical management when medical problems and their treatments have caused physical debilitation, muscle weakness, impaired joint motion, decreased flexibility and/or coordination, or other limita-

Work Capacity Evaluation (Occupational Therapy Service)

Note:—Patient has been medically evaluated and cleared for Functional/Work Capacity Evaluation by ________________ MD

—Evaluation completed by ________________ OTR

Client Name ________________ Date ______

Assessment of Evaluation Findings

- ☐ Incomplete and/or invalid evaluation
  - ☐ Insufficient information to determine physical and/or work capacity
  - ☐ Client refused to participate or complete evaluation process
  - ☐ Client's symptoms prevented active participation in evaluation process
- ☐ Successful demonstration of work performance

Department of Labor Physical Demands of Work Level

Job Requirement	Client's Demonstrated Performance
☐ Less than Sedentary—Infrequent lifting <2 pounds, minimal walking, no carrying	☐
☐ Sedentary—Infrequent lifting of 10 pounds or less, no sustained walking or carrying	☐
☐ Sedentary-Light—Infrequent lifting of 15 pounds; frequent lifting of 10 pounds or less; intermittent, self-paced, no-load walking	☐
☐ Light—Infrequent lifting of 20 pounds; frequent lifting of 10 pound or less; no-grade, slow-speed, 10-pound load carry/walking	☐
☐ Light-Medium—Infrequent lifting of 35 pounds; frequent lifting of 20 pound or less; no-grade, slow-speed, 20-pound load carry/walking	☐
☐ Medium—Infrequent lifting of 50 pounds; frequent lifting of 25 pound or less; no-grade, slow-speed, 25-pound load carry/walking	☐
☐ Medium-Heavy—Infrequent lifting of 75 pounds; frequent lifting of 35 pound or less; no-grade, slow-speed, 35-pound load carry/walking	☐
☐ Heavy—Infrequent lifting of 100 pounds; frequent lifting of 50 pound or less; slow-speed, 50-pound load carry/walking	☐
☐ Very Heavy—Infrequent lifting in excess of 100 pounds; frequent lifting of 50 to 100 pounds; slow-speed, 50-pound load carry/walking	☐

Factors Explaining Discrepancies between Job Requirements and Work Performance

- ☐ Suboptimal voluntary effort in testing
- ☐ Discrepancies between diagnosis and symptoms presented
- ☐ Discrepancies between client's perception of ability & actual ability
- ☐ Limited physical abilities
  - ☐ Joint motion/flexibility
  - ☐ Strength
  - ☐ Physical endurance
  - ☐ Sensation
  - ☐ Hand dexterity
- ☐ Limited psychosocial abilities
  - ☐ Mood/affect
  - ☐ Cognition
  - ☐ Pain tolerance/behavior

Figure 33-3 Functional capacity evaluation (FCE).

(continued)

Recommendations

☐ Demonstrated work capacity matches job requirements

☐ Perform target job at full capacity

- ☐ Full time
- ☐ Part time _____ hr/day _____ days/week

☐ Demonstrated work capacity approximates job requirements and demonstrates client's potential to return to work.

☐ Perform target job with limits or light duty

"Safe" performance recommendations are calculated as maximum infrequent exertion/movement/lift (<1/hr in optimal position/conditions) calculated at 60% of measured maximum demonstration where applicable.

☐ Two-hand floor to thigh level lift	# ____________	
☐ Two-hand thigh to shoulder lift	# ____________	
☐ Two-hand shoulder to overhead lift	# ____________	
☐ Push (waist level)	# ____________	
☐ Pull (waist level)	# ____________	
☐ Overhead pull to shoulder level	# ____________	
☐ Sit	☐ Unlimited	☐ Limit to ____________
☐ Stand	☐ Unlimited	☐ Limit to ____________
☐ Walk	☐ Unlimited	☐ Limit to ____________
☐ Bend/stoop	☐ Unlimited	☐ Limit to ____________
☐ Reach overhead	☐ Unlimited	☐ Limit to ____________
☐ Precision tool use	☐ Unlimited	☐ Limit to ____________
☐ Hand/power tool use	☐ Unlimited	☐ Limit to ____________

☐ **Work Site Modification**

Ergonomic work site evaluation with recommendations for job pace/process or equipment modifications

☐ **Work Conditioning**

Structured, supervised work activity to physically and psychologically condition client for return to work

☐ **Retest Functional Capacity**

Following resolution of psychosocial and or physical issues

Background Information

Age ___ Sex ___ Hand Dominance ___

Current Employment ___ Full time ___ Part time ___ Days/week ___
Hrs/day ___ Full Duty ___ Light Duty ___ Not employed

Job Title ______________________________

Essential tasks of current or target job

Key physical and cognitive tasks required by job

Figure 33-3 (continued)

Background Information (*continued*)

Select the "Best Fit" rating of current job physical demands

- ☐ Less than Sedentary—Infrequent lifting <2 pounds, minimal walking, no carrying
- ☐ Sedentary—Infrequent lifting of 10 pounds or less, no sustained walking or carrying
- ☐ Sedentary-Light—Infrequent lifting of 15 pounds; frequent lifting of 10 pounds or less; intermittent, self-paced, no-load walking
- ☐ Light—Infrequent lifting of 20 pounds, frequent lifting of 10 pound or less, no grade slow speed 10-pound load carry/walking
- ☐ Light-Medium—Infrequent lifting of 35 pounds, frequent lifting of 20 pound or less; no-grade, slow-speed, 20-pounds load carry/walking
- ☐ Medium—Infrequent lifting of 50 pounds, frequent lifting of 25 pound or less, no grade, slow-speed, 25-pound load carry/walking
- ☐ Medium-Heavy—Infrequent lifting of 75 pounds; frequent lifting of 35 pound or less; no-grade, slow-speed, 35-pound load carry/walking
- ☐ Heavy—Infrequent lifting of 100 pounds, frequent lifting of 50 pound or less; slow-speed, 50-pound load carry/walking
- ☐ Very Heavy—Infrequent lifting in excess of 100 pounds, frequent lifting of 50 to 100 pounds; slow-speed, 50-pound load carry/walking

Medical Condition

Diagnosis related to work deficit ____________________

____

Concurrent medical conditions ____________________

____

Time off work ____________________

Surgery and medical treatment ____________________

____

Current Symptoms Relating to Work Situation

Symptom	Location	Intensity: Mild		Mod		Severe
Pain		•	•	•	•	•
Numbness		•	•	•	•	•
Weakness		•	•	•	•	•
Clumsiness		•	•	•	•	•
Fatigue		•	•	•	•	•
Anxiousness		•	•	•	•	•

Evaluation Data Demonstrated Work Capacity Using Selected Work Samples

Valpar Standardized Work Samples Rate quality of work performance (1 poor. . . to 5 excellent) during testing situation	Time in Seconds	MTM Rate
1 Small Tools 1 2 3 4 5 Follows instructions 1 2 3 4 5 Maintains physical stamina 1 2 3 4 5 Maintains motivation 1 2 3 4 5 Communicates 1 2 3 4 5 Shows self-confidence		

Figure 33-3 (continued)

Demonstrated Work Capacity Using Selected Work Samples (*continued*)

Valpar Standardized Work Samples Rate quality of work performance (1 poor. . . to 5 excellent) during testing situation	Time in Seconds	MTM Rate
4 Upper Extremity Range of Motion 1 2 3 4 5 Follows instructions 1 2 3 4 5 Maintains physical stamina 1 2 3 4 5 Maintains motivation 1 2 3 4 5 Communicates 1 2 3 4 5 Shows self-confidence		
9 Whole-Body Range of Motion and Endurance 1 2 3 4 5 Follows instructions 1 2 3 4 5 Maintains physical stamina 1 2 3 4 5 Maintains motivation 1 2 3 4 5 Communicates 1 2 3 4 5 Shows self-confidence		
15 Electrical Circuitry and Print Reading 1 2 3 4 5 Follows instructions 1 2 3 4 5 Maintains physical stamina 1 2 3 4 5 Maintains motivation 1 2 3 4 5 Communicates 1 2 3 4 5 Shows self-confidence		
19 Dynamic Physical capacity (Endurance test at PDC level set by BTE strength testing and actual job demand) PDC Test level _____ 1 2 3 4 5 Follows instructions 1 2 3 4 5 Maintains physical stamina 1 2 3 4 5 Maintains motivation 1 2 3 4 5 Communicates 1 2 3 4 5 Shows self-confidence	Number of completed tasks	

Perception of Ability to Perform Work
EPIC Hand Function (HFS) and Spinal Function Sorts (SFS)

	Sedentary		Light	
	HFS % of total	SFS % of total	HFS % of total	SFS % of total
Able				
Slightly Restricted				
Moderately Restricted				
Very Restricted				
Unable				
Don't Know				

Figure 33-3 (continued)

EPIC Hand Function (HFS) and Spinal Function Sorts (SFS) (*continued*)

	Medium HFS % of total	Medium SFS % of total	Heavy HFS % of total	Heavy SFS % of total
Able				
Slightly Restricted				
Moderately Restricted				
Very Restricted				
Unable				
Don't Know				

Client Description of Role Demands and Perceived Performance

	Required	Perform Well	Perform Poorly	Unable
Standing ≥50% of work day				
Sitting ≥50% of work day				
Frequent walking ≥30 min/hr				
Frequent/prolonged bending or stooping				
Occasional (1–2/day) max lift				
Circle "best fit" 100# 50# 20# 10#				
Frequent (1/hour) lift/carry				
Circle "best fit" 50# 20# 10# ,10#				
Frequent overhead reach ≥10 times/hr				
Frequent/prolonged computer use ≥45 min/hr				
Frequent/prolonged use of hand tools				
Frequent/prolonged use of vibrating power tools				
Frequent/prolonged use of precision instruments				
Analytical decision making				
Personnel supervision				

Abilities (Potential to Work) Work-Related Body Motion

	Right Normal	Right Impaired	Right Unable	Left Normal	Left Impaired	Left Unable
Raise arm over head						
Touch hand to back of neck						
Touch hand to middle of back						
Touch hand to opposite shoulder						
Elbow bend—palm up and down						
Wrist flex and extend						
Gross hand grasp and release						
Bend—stoop to touch floor						
Kneel (one knee) on floor						
Crawl (10 feet)						

Figure 33-3 (continued)

Abilities (Potential to Work) (*continued*)

Static Postures (time in minutes maintaining posture before onset of symptoms)

Sitting ____ Standing ____ Reaching above shoulder level ____________________

Hand Sensation

(Moving two-point discrimination at digit tips)

	Thumb	Index	Middle	Ring	Small
Right Hand					
Left Hand					

Hand Dexterity Jebsen-Taylor Hand Function Test
(Time in seconds) (Benchmark score = 2 SD below mean)

Item	Writing	Turning Cards	Pick Up Small Objects	Feeding	Placing Checkers	Stacking Light Cans	Stacking Heavy Cans
Raw score, Right hand							
Raw score, Left hand							
Male, Dom hand	19.2	5.8	7.9	8.2	4.7	3.8	4
Male, Non-dom hand	55.9	6.3	8	10.5	5	4.4	3.9
Female, Dom hand	15.9	7.1	7.1	8.9	4.5	4.1	4.2
Female, Non-dom hand	47.4	7	8	11.2	5.2	4.5	4.3

Static Isometric Strength BTE/Primus Work Simulator Testing

	Right			Left		
	In #	Percentile rank	CV	In #	Percentile rank	CV
Grip						
3 Jaw Pinch						
Wrist Extension						
Forearm Supination						
Elbow Flexion						
Shoulder Flexion						

	Pre-Test	Post-Test
Pulse		
Blood Pressure		

Dynamic Isotonic Lifting, Pushing, and Pulling (BTE/Primus Testing)

Perform to fatigue, initial onset of symptoms or evidence of deteriorating technique

	Tool	Weight Lifted/Pulled	Percentile Rank
Floor to Knuckle	191#		
Knuckle to Shoulder	191$		
Shoulder to Overhead	191+		
Push (Waist Level)	191@		
Pull (Waist Level)	191		
Overhead Pull	191%		

	Pre-Test	Post-Test
Pulse		
Blood Pressure		

Figure 33-3 (continued)

Physical Endurance

(Tuxworth Step Test) 5 min (25 steps/min rate) 16″ (40 cm) step

Formula = cumulative resting heart rates (HR)/body weight

HR 0.5 min—1 min ×2 ___ + HR 1.5 min—2 min ×2 ___ + HR 2.5 min—3 min ×2 ___

Body weight ___ Kg (1 Kg = 2.2 lb)

Mean = 5.40 SD = 1.145 Z score = ______

Cognitive/Behavioral

Generalized Contentment Scale ____________

(Range 25–125) Lower scores suggest greater life contentment

Decision-Making Test (record percentile ranking) ____________

Mini Mental Status Exam (MMSE) ____________

Range 0–30

Score <24 suggests need for detailed testing

Summary of Findings

Patient's description/perception of job requirements

Less than sedentary **Sedentary** **Sedentary-Light** **Light** **Light-Medium** **Medium** **Medium-Heavy** **Heavy** **Very Heavy**

Client's Perception of Performance Ability

Cognition/Behavior

Body Range of Motion

Static Standing and Sitting and Reaching Tolerance

Upper Body Strength, Lifting/Pushing/Pulling, and Consistency of Effort

Physical Endurance

Hand Sensation and Dexterity

Work Performance **Valpar Work Samples**		**Worker Qualification Profile** **Indicate level based on MTM percent rate of work**
Valpar 1	Small Tools (hand tool use in awkward and confined space)	Not tested Exceeds work standard Meets work standard Does not meet work standard (good potential to meet standard) Does not meet work standard (minimal potential to meet standard)
Valpar 4	Upper Extremity ROM in function (finger/hand dexterity in awkward and confined space)	Not tested Exceeds work standard Meets work standard Does not meet work standard (good potential to meet standard)

Figure 33-3 (continued)

Summary of Findings (*continued*)		
Valpar 9	Whole-Body ROM (hand function in combination with reaching and bending)	Not tested Exceeds work standard Meets work standard Does not meet work standard (good potential to meet standard) Does not meet work standard (minimal potential to meet standard)
Valpar 15	Electrical Circuitry and Print Reading (attention, memory, new learning, finger dexterity)	Not tested Exceeds work standard Meets work standard Does not meet work standard (good potential to meet standard) Does not meet work standard (minimal potential to meet standard)
Valpar 19	Dynamic Physical Capacity (manual materials handling)	Not tested Exceeds work standard Meets work standard Does not meet work standard (good potential to meet standard) Does not meet work standard (minimal potential to meet standard)

Figure 33-3 (continued)

tions. Acute rehabilitation for physical injuries can involve the use of physical agents, exercise, and education to restore abilities impaired by injury, illness, surgery, or enforced inactivity. Both medical management and acute rehabilitation entail evaluation, diagnosis, and procedures to remedy pathological conditions. At the end of each of these processes, a decision as to the potential for the client to return to work must be made. If the client is able and willing to return to work at these junctures, intervention is discontinued. Many clients with minimal residue of injury or illness and high internal motivation return to work without further intervention.

Work Rehabilitation

If medical management and acute rehabilitation do not result in a return-to-work status, efforts focus on the feasibility of returning the client to work. The method to determine return-to-work feasibility is the functional work assessment, which includes general medical information, a job analysis (if the job or type of job is known), an FCE, and an assessment of the client's perceptions of his or her abilities.

In addition to being evaluative, the functional work assessment forms the framework within which the therapist builds intervention strategies to bring about the return to work. The FCE used here can be carried out in seven steps.

Step 1: Pre-Evaluation Information

As indicated in Figure 33-3, information is recorded about the client's job, along with demographics and information regarding the client's medical condition and symptoms. Details about the job can be obtained though the client's self-report, a written job description, interviews with the employer, and/or an on-site job analysis.

Job Demands

The evaluator seeks to determine the specifics of the job in terms of physical, cognitive, and social demands. Careful review of the job description and interviews with client and supervisor allow the therapist to form a picture of the demands of the job. The therapist may also choose to conduct a job site analysis so that objective measurements and observations can further elucidate the demands. These job demands are key in setting up work samples later in the evaluation.

Medical History and Current Symptoms

In addition to a complete review of the medical record, the client is asked to describe his or her medical history, including medical treatment, surgery, rehabilitation, and time off work. Information about the client's current symptoms is gathered. The grid Current Symptoms Relating to Work Situation allows the client to describe symptoms and rate them on intensity. Clients are encouraged to state their desired resolutions to the current work/disability situation so

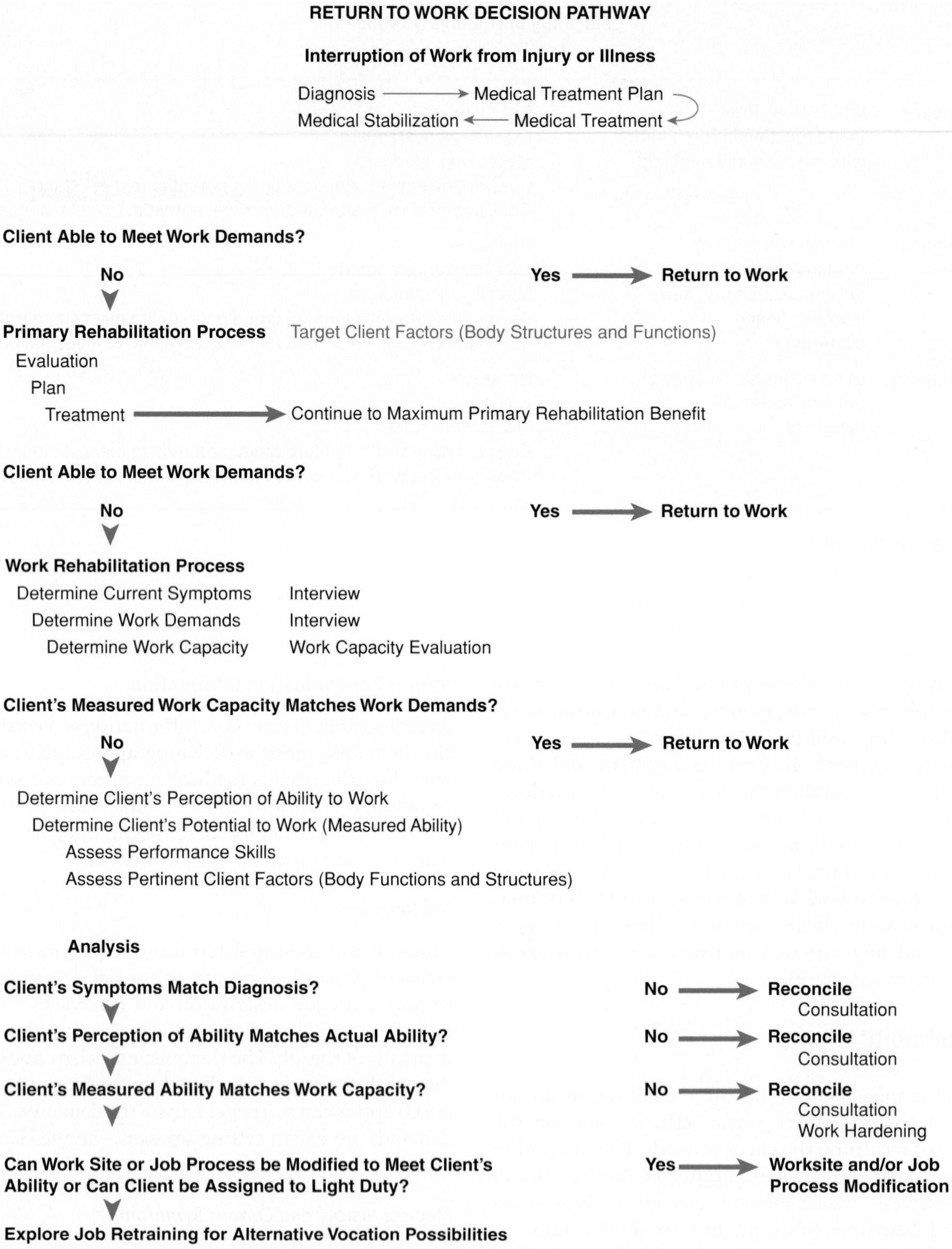
RETURN TO WORK DECISION PATHWAY
Interruption of Work from Injury or Illness
Diagnosis
Medical Treatment Plan
Medical Stabilization
Medical Treatment
Client Able to Meet Work Demands?
No
Yes
Return to Work
Primary Rehabilitation Process
Target Client Factors (Body Structures and Functions)
Evaluation
Plan
Treatment
Continue to Maximum Primary Rehabilitation Benefit
Client Able to Meet Work Demands?
No
Yes
Return to Work
Work Rehabilitation Process
Determine Current Symptoms
Interview
Determine Work Demands
Interview
Determine Work Capacity
Work Capacity Evaluation
Client's Measured Work Capacity Matches Work Demands?
No
Yes
Return to Work
Determine Client's Perception of Ability to Work
Determine Client's Potential to Work (Measured Ability)
Assess Performance Skills
Assess Pertinent Client Factors (Body Functions and Structures)
Analysis
Client's Symptoms Match Diagnosis?
No
Reconcile
Consultation
Client's Perception of Ability Matches Actual Ability?
No
Reconcile
Consultation
Client's Measured Ability Matches Work Capacity?
No
Reconcile
Consultation
Work Hardening
Can Work Site or Job Process be Modified to Meet Client's Ability or Can Client be Assigned to Light Duty?
Yes
Worksite and/or Job Process Modification
Explore Job Retraining for Alternative Vocation Possibilities

Figure 33-4 Return-to-work decision pathway.

RESOURCE 33-1

Work Evaluation Equipment Baltimore Therapeutic Equipment Co. 7455-L New Ridge Road Hanover, MD 21076 Phone: (410) 850-0333 www.bteco.com	**Valpar International Corporation** P.O. Box 5767 Tucson, AZ 85703 Phone: (800) 528-7070 www.valparint.com

as to enable the therapist and client to establish goals jointly. Even though the evaluation is in the early stages, at this point, there is usually sufficient information to initiate treatment that can coincide with the continuing evaluation.

The therapist should determine whether the cluster of symptoms presented by the client matches those usually associated with the diagnosis or disorder. Significant variances between diagnosis and expected symptoms can be a sign of a client being overwhelmed by the situation or an early indication of symptom magnification. At this point in the FCE, the process may change from evaluation to intervention. The therapist may now choose to use a consultation intervention in which the client is assisted in explaining the discrepancies between conflicting findings. Although a disconnect between diagnosis and symptoms may not be at the client's conscious level, it should be addressed at once. During this intervention, it is appropriate to provide the client with additional information about the medical condition and its usual presentation and course in rehabilitation. It is important during this consultation to allow the client a face-saving way out, such as the opportunity to restate or discuss symptoms. The purpose of the consultation process is to help the client to either clarify information or adjust behavior according to new information presented by the therapist. Alignment of symptoms may also help to delineate those who have a well-defined WRMD versus those who may have signs and symptoms of overuse that are not yet at a stage of clinical diagnosis. This process may also assist the client to accept and understand his or her symptoms.

Step 2: Work Performance Measurement

In accordance with the job demands identified in step 1, the therapist determines which of the available work performance measures best simulates the demands of the current or target job. Although testing of ability components can be fairly general and applied to many jobs and tasks, if the job to which the client will return is known, the evaluation should be tailored to it. Figure 33-3 has a reporting format for selected work performance measures, including the following:

- Valpar 1: Small tools; fine motor dexterity

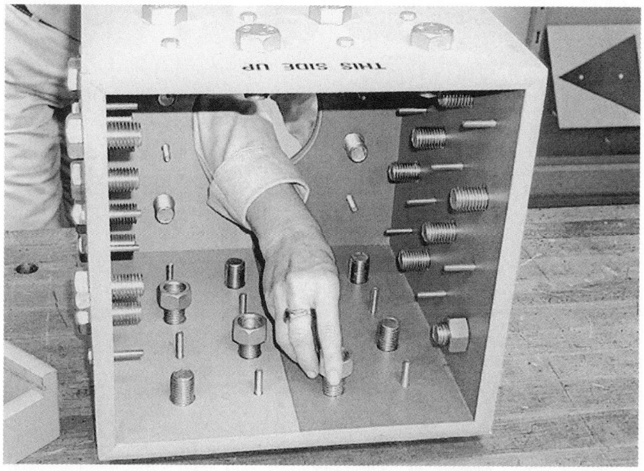

Figure 33-5 Valpar Work Sample 4. Upper extremity range-of-motion work sample.

- Valpar 4: Upper extremity range of motion; prolonged use of both hands in confined space with awkward angles (Fig. 33-5)
- Valpar 9: Whole-body range of motion; reaching, bending, and stooping while using hands
- Valpar 15: Electrical circuitry and print reading requiring attention, memory, new learning, and hand dexterity (Fig. 33-6)
- Valpar 19: Dynamic physical capacities; reaching, lifting, reading, decision making, and following directions (Fig. 33-7)

Methods Time Measurement (MTM) scoring criteria are used with all of these work performance measurements (Valpar International Corp., 1992). MTM compares work sample performance with an engineered standard that relates to competitive performance rather than to norma-

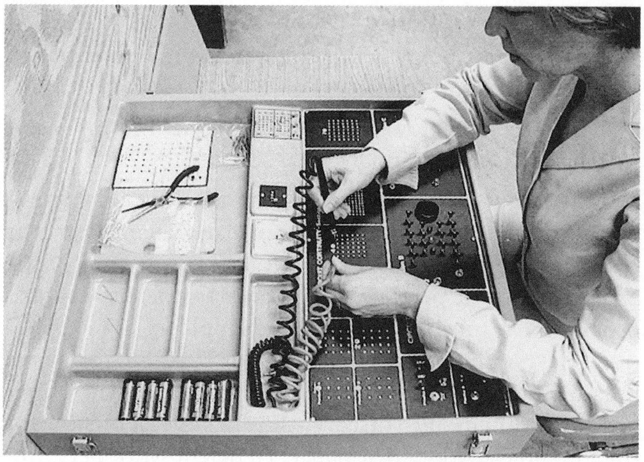

Figure 33-6 Valpar Work Sample 15. Electricity circuitry and print reading.

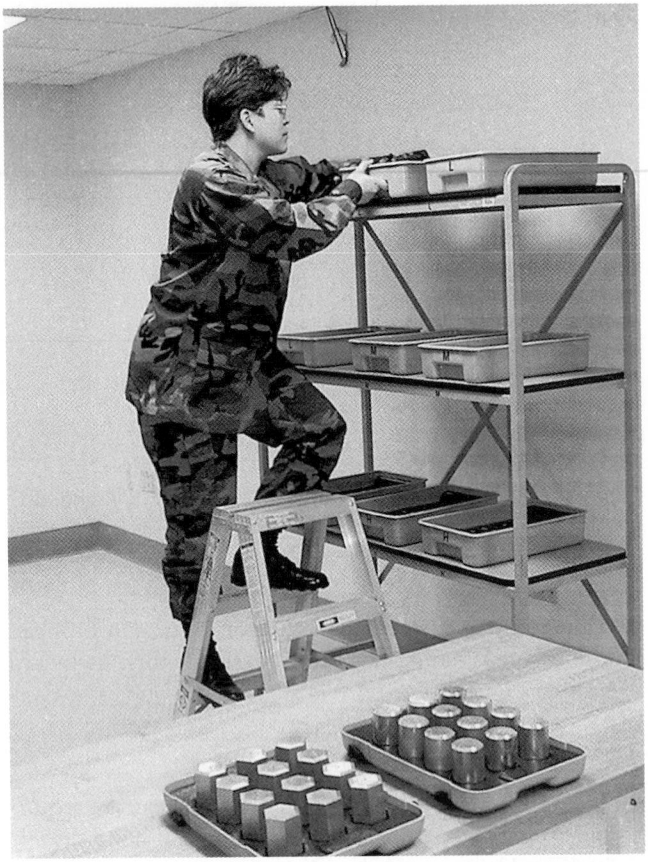

Figure 33-7 Valpar Work Sample 19. Work dynamic physical capacities.

tive data. The standards were developed by an engineering company and are designed to mimic the real pace of work rather than the burst activity common to testing. MTM grades performance in a percent rate of work from 0 to 150%. The percent rate of work is scaled against the following competitive work standards:

- Performance exceeding work standards
- Performance meeting work standards
- Performance below work standards with potential to meet standard
- Performance below work standard with minimal potential to reach standard

MTM can, at first, be confusing to clinicians accustomed to using only standard normative data, but it is essential for the therapist to understand it for proper analysis of work performance measurement data and to explain the results to the client and employer.

In the event that the client's work sample performance falls below competitive standards, steps 3 and 4 of the evaluation are used to discover the deficits responsible for the impaired work performance. Deficient work performance is generally the result of disconnects between job demands, internal motivation based on perception of ability, and/or performance and ability levels. If, however, demonstrated work performance on job-specific work samples meets the competitive standards, steps 3 and 4 can be omitted, and the therapist can proceed to data analysis and recommendations.

Step 3: Client's Perception of Ability to Work

Figure 33-3 shows two methods for gathering information regarding clients' perception of their abilities. The Employment Potential Improvement Corporation (EPIC) Hand Function Sort (HFS) and the Spinal Function Sort (SFS) (Fig. 33-8) are ratings of perceived capacity. These sorts require the client to view pictures of work situations (62 for the HFS and 50 for the SFC) and then sort them into four categories based on his or her perception of ability to perform the task within the situation. The categories include "able," "slightly restricted," "moderately restricted," and "unable."

The picture sort results can be analyzed in depth with the data compared with normative standards. The results can also be recorded in the format illustrated in Figure 33-3 as to the client's reported ability within each of the four physical demand characteristics categories of sedentary, light, medium, and heavy work. The second method of gaining the client's perception of ability is a self-rating of performance on a variety of common work tasks. Careful analysis of picture sort results and self-reports of ability give important information about the client's perception of his or her ability in relation to the diagnosis, presented symptoms, and the measures of ability that follow.

Step 4: Ability Measurement

Figure 33-3 incorporates tests and measures of ability, including body range of motion; static posture tolerance;

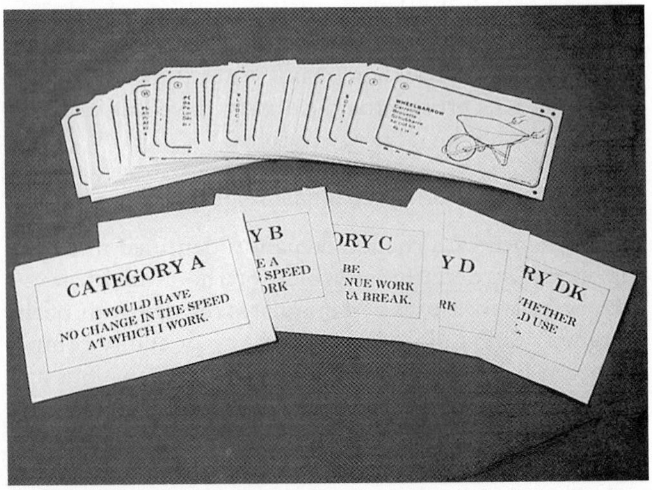

Figure 33-8 Patients sort cards based on their perceptions of ability to perform work tasks.

hand sensation and dexterity; extremity strength; lifting, pushing, and pulling strength; physical endurance; mood and affect; and cognitive problem solving. These are measures of performance skills and client factors that may affect an individual's capabilities at a number of jobs, rather than being tailored to any particular job or set of tasks. Examples include:

- Body range of motion, assessed by observing functional movements of the trunk and extremities to include reaching, touching hands to back of neck and middle of back, and bending or stooping toward the floor.
- Tolerance to the static postures of sitting and standing, observed and documented as the client performs other components of testing that require sitting or standing for extended periods.
- Physical strength, documented using both static strength and dynamic lift tests. A device such as the work simulator (Baltimore Therapeutic Equipment Co., 1999) can accomplish both static and dynamic lifting tests and allow comparison of strength between body sides and comparison against normative standards (Fig. 33-9).
- Physical endurance, using either a step test (Tuxworth & Shanawaz, 1977) or treadmill testing if available. *Before any strength or physical endurance testing, it is essential to ensure that the patient's medical record has been reviewed and the referring physician has given clearance for physical testing.*
- Hand dexterity and function, using any of a number of tests. The *Jebsen-Taylor Hand Function Test* is a standard in most clinical settings and can rapidly gather information on hand function using common objects rather than pegs or pins (Jebsen et al., 1969).

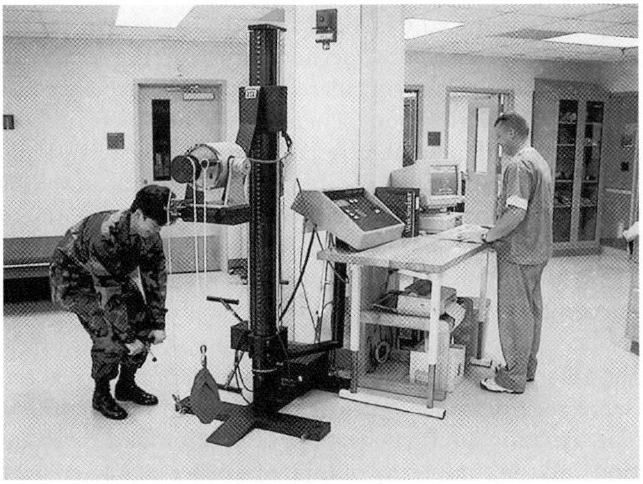

Figure 33-9 *BTE Work Simulator* used for dynamic strength testing.

- Mood and affect; alterations can exacerbate physical problems. This aspect of function should therefore be included in the assessment. A brief screening tool can be used in conjunction with clinical observations to determine any potential psychosocial problems. (See previous discussion of the *Generalized Contentment Scale.*) If significant findings are obtained, assistance from psychological services may be indicated.
- Cognition should be tested to determine whether difficulties with attention, memory, vision, reading skills, and problem solving are contributing to work deficits. The *Folstein Mini Mental Status Exam* (Folstein, Folstein, & McHugh, 1975) is a brief paper and pencil test that can give the clinician a quick look at the client's cognitive functioning. A score of less than 24 without obvious external confounding factors would strongly suggest the need for more formal cognitive testing before proceeding on in the evaluation. In addition, the *PSI Decision Making Test* is a 5-minute standardized paper-and-pencil test measuring attention, immediate memory, reading, and judgment (Ruch et al., 1981). Either or both of these tests can give the evaluator a general idea of cognitive function and help in determining whether further specialized testing is indicated.

Step 5: Summarize Test Data

The complexity of work demands and human behavior requires that therapists approach evaluation and intervention in a structured manner. If a structured approach is not used, there is a risk of being overwhelmed by the sheer amount of data or by the difficulties inherent in multifaceted behavioral interventions. To help manage information and use it as the basis for analysis, treatment, and recommendations, the sample FCE uses grids for summarizing and recording perception of ability, actual ability, and performance and work data. The evaluator summarizes observations from the tests and converts raw data to standard scores using either normative or MTM criteria. Completion of this section begins to paint a comprehensive picture of the patient's perceptions, abilities, and demonstrated performance in sample work situations. This information is the basis for the analysis in step 6.

Step 6: Analyze Findings

Under Assessment of Evaluation Findings, Figure 33-3 shows the variables to be considered in analyzing the results of test data. The first opinion relates to the quality of the FCE. Was this an incomplete or invalid evaluation, and if so, why did the therapist perceive it as such? The therapist annotates the client's demonstrated work performance to the job requirements on the Department of Labor Physical Demands of Work Level chart (United

States Employment Service Dictionary of Occupational Titles). If work performance in sample testing does not meet competitive standards of job requirements, the therapist explains the difference in terms of the client's abilities and/or motivation. In essence, this is a return-to-work equation involving several variables. The therapist must look for matches and disconnects in the data collected during the evaluation to present a meaningful analysis and recommendations.

1. The first match is between the diagnosis and symptoms. A given diagnosis usually results in a constellation of symptoms. The therapist must decide whether the symptoms match the diagnosis.
2. The next match is the agreement between the symptoms and the client's perception of his or her ability to work as expressed in the picture sort. An example of a disconnect is for the client to report hand paresthesias but not to indicate problems with precision tools on the card sort.
3. Next is assessment of the degree of agreement between the client's perception of ability to work and his or her demonstrated physical and cognitive abilities (potential to work). Examples of disconnects include the client who indicates inability to use heavy tools on the card sort but shows above-normal strength and endurance during physical testing.
4. The therapist compares the client's physical and cognitive abilities (potential to work) with actual work performance demonstrated during work simulations or task component testing to determine the level of agreement. Demonstrated physical and cognitive abilities should be close to those demonstrated during performance of work samples.

The analysis in this section is the basis for flowing the evaluation process seamlessly into treatment. Problems in incorrect perception can be addressed and reconciled through consultation and education about the pathophysiological aspects of the injury or disorder and expected course of recovery. Education in techniques such as joint protection, energy conservation, and body mechanics can increase the client's ability to deal with symptoms and limitations. Instruction in movement and stretching exercises can provide further skills for managing symptoms and limitations. Work conditioning can be initiated. Work conditioning using work samples can increase physical abilities, engineer successful performance, help the client to recognize his or her abilities, and assist the client to develop realistic goals.

Step 7: Recommendations

Figure 33-3 incorporates recommendation statements that can be supported from the information gathered in steps 1–4, summarized in step 5, and analyzed in step 6. The first section of recommendations concerns the client who can return to either full duty or limited or light duty. The referring physician may well use evaluation recommendations to determine the parameters of light duty, so it is important to base the definition of the limits of light duty on the results of test data and to include what the individual can do as well as what he or she cannot do. The recommendations section also addresses clients who are not ready to return to work but who may be brought to work standards with interventions such as education or work conditioning and hardening. Finally, for clients who do not appear to have the potential to return to target-level work or the pre-injury job, the practitioner may recommend pre-vocational testing and vocational exploration of jobs within the client's physical demand capability.

SPECIALIZED OCCUPATIONAL THERAPY PRACTICE

Return-to-work evaluation and therapeutic intervention are complicated yet fascinating and rewarding. Work-oriented therapy, also known as industrial therapy, pushes the envelope of professional practice by demanding the blending of expert skill in assessment and data gathering with clinical reasoning and behavioral treatment. Applying occupational therapy skills and knowledge to the process is equally challenging because of the necessity of using physical and biomechanical knowledge along with cognitive and psychosocial knowledge. One particular benefit of practicing in the return-to-work field is being able to see the results of therapeutic efforts beyond those seen when practicing exclusively within the confines of a clinic.

Although the core of occupational therapy practice can be used as a basis for work rehabilitation and following step-by-step procedures should greatly increase the probability of seamlessly moving clients through the return-to-work process, this is considered to be a practice area that requires specialization. Therapists who specialize in return-to-work rehabilitation must develop observational and communication skills that are clearly understood by the client worker, the supervisor, the insurance representative, and medical professionals. They must become comfortable in the work settings of their clients, just as they are comfortable in clinic settings.

Occupational therapists specializing in this area have the potential to contribute to the growth of empirical evidence regarding outcomes of work-related interventions. The dynamic interplay between evaluation and intervention and the complexity of injured worker characteristics, in part, explain the relatively weak body of evidence regarding return-to-work rehabilitation at present.

Therefore, there is no Evidence Table specific to the Case Example in this chapter.

Return-to-work rehabilitation programs that use a comprehensive multidisciplinary approach provide an improved service to clients, guiding clients through the medical and rehabilitation processes without abandoning them along the way to fend for themselves in their quest to return to meaningful employment. The needs of both client and employer are addressed, one by one, until the client is a client no more, having once again become a worker and a valued contributing member of the workforce and of society.

CASE EXAMPLE

Mr. B.: Return to Work After Hand Surgery

Occupational Therapy Intervention Process	Clinical Reasoning Process: Objectives	Clinical Reasoning Process: Examples of Therapists Internal Dialogue
Patient Information		
Mr. B. is a 37-year-old married civil service employee. He works as an audiovisual support assistant and has a 2-year history of right dominant hand radial wrist pain. Mr. B. was intermittently treated for stenosing tenosynovitis of the first dorsal wrist compartment (de Quervain's disease) during the previous year. Conservative treatment, including activity limitations, limiting wrist motion with a thermoplastic thumb spica-type splint, superficial heat and cold, deep heat using ultrasound, and trials of transcutaneous and percutaneous corticosteroid medication via phonophoresis, iontophoresis, and injection, did not relieve symptoms to a level allowing Mr. B. to work at full capacity. About 10 weeks prior to referral for FCE, Mr. B. underwent a surgical procedure to release the right first dorsal wrist compartment. The surgery and post-operative recovery period were unremarkable. By post-operative week 10, however, Mr. B. could not return to work because of continued pain in the radial wrist during job-specific tasks. His supervisor referred Mr. B. to occupational health services, and Mr. B. was subsequently referred to occupational therapy for FCE and recommendations for return to duty.	Appreciate the context	"I believe that Mr. B. has received a reasonable standard of treatment for the diagnosed condition. He has progressed through an expected treatment regimen with invasive (surgical) treatment initiated only when conservative had failed."
A review of Mr. B.'s medical record and results of an initial interview revealed that he was in reasonable health and, excluding de Quervain's tendonitis, was without significant pathological medical history. Mr. B. had not been working for a total of 10 weeks, including the post-operative phase of his treatment. He was now back to work and on unofficial light duty status administered by the good graces of his supervisor.		"Mr. B. seems to have a good working relationship with his supervisor as evidenced by the allowance of non-medically directed light duty."

Description of Assessment

Mr. B. gave the therapist a specific listing of job tasks that included infrequent lifting and carrying of 50-pound items and fairly frequent lifting of approximately 25-pound objects. As part of his additional duties, Mr. B. was required to lift with one hand and carry a flagpole base weighing 17 pounds. The lift and carry were usually done with the right wrist slightly flexed and in radial deviation. Aspects of Mr. B.'s job description were verified by review of his written job description, an interview with his supervisor, and on-site observation.

Mr. B. stated that any use of his right hand caused wrist pain. He could perform all basic and instrumental activities of daily living but could not perform his job except for answering the phone and doing paperwork. He stated that it had taken "the doctors" 2 years to figure out his problem and the surgery had not fixed it. When asked about his desired outcome, he replied that he needed either to be trained for another kind of job or receive disability for this work-related injury.

Based on his job demands, the OT decided to use the Valpar 1 (small tools), Valpar 9 (whole-body range of motion), and Valpar 19 (dynamic physical capacity) to sample Mr. B.'s actual work performance. Mr. B. performed at the MTM rate of 95% on the Valpar 1, 90% on the Valpar 9, and 78% on the Valpar 19. Work performance on the Valpar 1 and 9 met competitive work standards; performance on the Valpar 19 was below competitive work standards.

The OT gathered subjective and objective data about Mr. B.'s abilities to examine the possible causes of the discrepancy between his abilities and the test and job demands. The EPIC Hand Functions Sort and the Spinal Function Sort allowed Mr. B. to express his perceptions of his ability to perform common work and leisure tasks. Results of these two sorts revealed that he perceived he could perform 80.5% of the tasks at normal or subnormal rates and intensity (categories A, B, and C); 19.5% of the tasks were rated as unable to perform in his present condition. Many of the tasks in both categories that were reported as not performable did not fall into the work domains usually associated with hand and wrist pain.

Measurement of physical abilities revealed body range of motion, ability to maintain static postures, and hand sensation as within normal range. Three of the seven subtests on the Jebsen-Taylor Hand Function Test were significantly below the mean. Static isometric strength testing using the BTE Work Simulator indicated that the right arm was below the first percentile, while the left arm showed average strength ratings at the 60th percentile. Lifting, pushing, and pulling ability of both arms using the BTE dynamic lift tests was below the first percentile. The general contentment scale score was 62. Cognitive performance under time pressure (decision making test) was at the 45th percentile. Physical endurance using the step test was three standard deviations below the mean for age group.

Planning the evaluation	"My task is to try to discover the reason this medical condition continued to limit Mr. B.'s successful return to work despite successful surgical treatment and hand rehabilitation. I will need to consider his medical history in light of the job demands and try to determine his motivations regarding recovery and return to work. I will need to assess his ability to perform work tasks to see if he is actually "work ready." If he is not able to perform at job standards, then I will need to assess his physical, cognitive, and behavioral potentials to try to understand the 'why' of his work inability."
Interpret observations	"The severity level of Mr. B.'s symptoms does not seem to match the expected response to surgical treatment and recovery for de Quervain's disease. Mr. B.'s perception of his performance ability does not match the severity of his reported symptoms either but does match measurement of physical and cognitive abilities. Work sample performance was greater than I expected from the evaluation of his physical abilities. Finally, I don't think that the sample work performance fully met target job requirements."
	"In general, I am seeing mismatches between diagnosis and symptoms, symptoms and abilities, and abilities and performance. I believe that this fits a pattern of psychological overlay that limits the application of ability to work performance. Combined with this situation, there is a general physical debilitation from several months of inactivity. The duration of his symptoms and perceived slow postoperative recovery are no doubt influencing symptom intensity and may be limiting his willingness to exert full effort during ability testing. At this time, he does not appear ready or willing to return to full duty."
Develop intervention hypotheses Select an intervention approach	"At no time during the evaluation did Mr. B. appear to be exerting himself to the full extent of his ability, as would be evidenced in concentrated facial expression, sweating, or grimacing with effort. At no time did he express pain or appear to be in pain."

Recommendations The OT interpreted Mr. B.'s potential for return to work as moderate and recommended that Mr. B. participate in a work rehabilitation program. Skillful application of physical and psychosocial therapeutic interventions would be required to meet the long-term goal of return to full-time work. Mr. B.'s perceptions regarding his ability and performance would probably have to change to restore Mr. B.'s work role competency.	Consider the patient's appraisal of performance Consider what will occur in therapy, how often, and for how long Ascertain the patient's endorsement of plan	"Before we started treatment, I thought it would be important to review the results of the test data with Mr. B. and encourage him to explore and explain the variances in the data. Selective retesting (requested by Mr. B. and agreed upon by the therapist) allowed Mr. B. to clarify conflicts in data and demonstrate higher performance levels."
Summary of Short-Term Goals and Progress In 1 month, Mr. B. will be able to do the following: 1. Use principles of body mechanics, energy conservation, and work simplification to perform work simulations 2. Improve his endurance and work tolerance so that he can use his right hand and wrist during work activities 3. Problem solve with the therapist regarding necessary adaptations to work task and work area Here is a summary of Mr. B.'s formal work rehabilitation. The therapist provided several lessons on anatomy, pathophysiology, and wound healing, which related to Mr. B.'s surgical procedure. A focal point was that wound healing is a multiple-month process and that some pain during that process is normal.	Assess the patient's comprehension Understand what he is doing Compare actual to expected performance	"The plan and goals were devised in conjunction with Mr. B. so as to increase his compliance. The goals specifically avoided the psychosocial issues and focused on tangible items such as knowledge of the healing process, body mechanics, and increasing endurance. I wanted Mr. B. to have the opportunity to change his perceptions about his work ability by experiencing successful activity rather than psychological analysis."
Based on recommendations from the FCE, the referring physician assigned Mr. B. to an official light-duty status that specified physical demand limitations, with Mr. B. participating in work in accordance with FCE results. Mr. B. participated in daily 90-minute work conditioning treatment activities with emphasis on regaining physical endurance and progressive use of the right hand and wrist during work activities. A secondary purpose was to arrange for progressive successful work experiences, so Mr. B. would begin to habituate a positive work role. Mr. B. was provided training in body mechanics, energy conservation, and work simplification, especially as they related to his FCE results and the demands of his job. A formal work site and job analysis provided the work site supervisor with sufficient information to modify task and pace to match Mr. B.'s abilities. The occupational therapist fabricated an ergonomic tool adaptation to correct the identified injury-producing task. This modification corrected the extreme hand posture of radial deviation, allowing a more neutral posture. The device was adopted shopwide in Mr. B.'s work area.	Know the person Appreciate the context	"Analysis of the job tasks indicated that there were tasks that could cause a reoccurrence of wrist symptoms. I felt that it was important that Mr. B. know that the problem wasn't just related to his physical abilities but also to the job demands and that those job demands could be modified by changing the pace of work and by using adapted equipment."
Next Steps Following 1 month of work conditioning, Mr. B. completed a partial FCE. Testing with the Valpar work samples indicated ability to work at target job standards. Mr. B. subsequently returned to full duty.	Anticipate present and future patient concerns Analyze patient's comprehension Decide if the patient should continue or discontinue therapy and/or return in the future	"I am pleased as to how Mr. B. responded to intervention. We succeed in helping, in part, because at no time during the evaluation or intervention phases of Mr. B.'s participation in the return-to-work process was there any attempt to confront, catch, or expose his psychological issues. I was careful to remain neutral and request only that he try to explain the variances in the data. Mr. B. was always given "wiggle room" and face-saving avenues in all interactions. Over the course of the rehabilitation, the combination of education, non-judgmental interactions, and successful repetitive work experience encouraged Mr. B. to choose to alter his perceptions of ability and performance and regain work role competency."

CLINICAL REASONING IN OCCUPATIONAL THERAPY PRACTICE

Work Rehabilitation

Wrist pain was the dominant feature in Mr. B.'s inability to return to work. At the time of the evaluation, Mr. B. was 10 weeks post surgery from a right first dorsal wrist compartment release and still complaining of significant wrist pain with work-related activities. At that time, Mr. B.'s surgical wound was most probably at the end of the second stage of healing (proliferation) or early in the third stage (scar maturation). Conventional wisdom regarding soft tissue wound healing holds that the third and last phase may continue for 9 months or longer.

How should the therapist interpret Mr. B.'s emphasis on wrist pain? Is it real or enhanced? Should Mr. B. have been given a longer period of protection from work stressors following the surgery? What is a possible consequence of an extended recuperation period?

SUMMARY REVIEW QUESTIONS

1. List four reasons people work and explain how each might affect their ability to return to work.
2. List four reasons older persons choose to work, along with four methods of attracting older workers to continue working.
3. Describe the unique contributions of occupational therapy to the return-to-work process.
4. Describe how job analysis is used in both the evaluation and treatment phases of the return-to-work process.
5. Describe other potential uses for the results gained from a job analysis.
6. Compare and contrast the two types of performance evaluation suggested in a FCE.
7. Using the job of grocery store clerk and scanning, keying, and bagging as the essential tasks, write a brief description of a treatment program based on task components and a description of a treatment program based on work simulation.
8. Use the return-to-work decision pathway to develop an evaluation plan for a 42-year-old diabetic who has intermittent retinal bleeding (loss of sight) and who has recently lost his job as a computer systems analyst.

References

Adler, L. A., & Cohen, J. (2002). Adult ADHD: Recent advances in diagnosis and treatment. Retrieved December 2005 at www.medscape.com.

Ahlgren, A., Broman, L., Bergroth, A., & Ekholm, J. (2005). Disability pension despite vocational rehabilitation? A study from six social insurance offices of a county. *International Journal of Rehabilitation Research, 28,* 33–42.

Alexander, D. (Ed.). (1999). *Applied ergonomics case studies.* Atlanta: Engineering and Management.

American Association of Retired Persons [AARP]. (2006). The state of 50+ America 2006. Available at http://www.aarp.org/research/economy/trends/fifty_plus_2006.html

American Occupational Therapy Association [AOTA]. (2002). Occupational therapy practice framework: Domain and process. *American Journal of Occupational Therapy, 56,* 609–639.

Americans with Disabilities Act [ADA]. (1990). *Public Law 101-336, 42 U.S.C. 12101.* Washington, DC: United States Department of Justice. Retrieved March 11, 2005 from http://www.usdoj.gov/crt/ada/adahom1.htm.

Americans with Disabilities Act Title I Regulations (1991). 29 CFR '1630.01 et seq. and appendix.

Backman, C. L. (2004). Occupational balance: Exploring the relationships among daily occupations and their influence on well-being. *Canadian Journal of Occupational Therapy, 71,* 202–209.

Baltimore Therapeutic Equipment Co. (1999). *BTE Work Simulator operator's manual.* Hanover, MD: Baltimore Therapeutic Equipment Co.

Bloswick, D. S., Jefferies, D. C., Brakefield, S., & Dumas, M. (1998). Industrial setting case study: Ergonomics and Title I of the Americans with Disabilities Act. In V. Rice (Ed.), *Ergonomics in health care and rehabilitation* (pp. 307–334). Boston: Butterworth-Heinneman.

Burwash, S. C. (1999). A teaching model for work practice in occupational therapy. *Work, 12,* 133–137.

Calgary Fire Department (1999). http://content.calgary.ca/CCA/City+Hall/Business+Units/Calgary+Fire+Department/index.htm.

Carayon, P., Smith, M. J., & Haims, M. C. (1999). Work organization, job stress, and work-related musculoskeletal disorders. *Human Factors, 41,* 644–663.

Chester, E. (2005). *Getting them to give a damn: How to get your front line to care about the bottom line.* Chicago: Dearborn Trade Publishing, Kaplan.

Christiansen, C. H. (1999). Defining lives: Occupation as identity: An essay on competence, coherence, and the creation of meaning. 1999 Eleanor Clarke Slagle lecture. *American Journal of Occupational Therapy, 52,* 547–558.

Committee on Installations and Advice. (1928). Analysis of crafts. *Archives of Occupational Therapy, 6,* 417–421.

Crowe & Shannon Social Security Law Group (1997). The nuts and bolts of functional capacity evaluations. Available at http://www.croweshanahan.com/capacity2.html.

Debats, D. L., Drost, J., & Hansen, P. (1995). Experiences of meaning in life: A combined qualitative and quantitative approach. *British Journal of Psychology, 86,* 359–375.

Deberdt, J. P. (2002). Employment: A declining value. *La Presse Medicale, 31,* 488–490.

Eklund, M., Hansson, L., & Ahlqvist, C. (2004). The importance of work as compared to other forms of daily occupations for wellbeing and functioning among persons with long-term mental illness. *Community Mental Health Journal, 40,* 465–477.

Ellexson, M. (1997). Job analysis and work-site assessment. In M. Sanders (Ed.), *Management of cumulative trauma disorders* (pp. 195–213). Boston: Butterworth-Heinneman.

Equal Employment Opportunity Commission. (1992). *A technical assistance manual on the employment provisions (Title I) of the Americans with Disabilities Act.* Washington, DC: Equal Employment Opportunity Commission.

Federal Register (July 26, 1991). Part V: Equal Employment Opportunity Commission 29 CFR part 1630, *Equal Employment Opportunity for Individuals with Disabilities;* Final Rule.

Folstein, M. F., Folstein, S. E., & McHugh, P. R. (1975). Mini-Mental State: A practical method for grading the state of patients for the clinician. *Journal of Psychiatric Research, 12,* 189–198.

Frankl, V. (1984). *Man's search for meaning.* New York: Touchstone.

Gordon, C. C., Brandtwiller, B., Churchill, T., Clauser, C. E., McConville, J. T., Tebbetts, I., & Walker, R. A. (1989). *Anthropometric Survey of U.S. Army Personnel: Methods and Summary Statistics.* Natick/TR-89/044. Natick, MA: U.S. Army Natick R, D, and E Center.

Hasan, H. (2004). Meaning of work among a sample of Kuwaiti workers. *Psychology Report, 94,* 195–207.

Hendrick, H. (1998). Macroergonomics: A systems approach for dramatically improving occupational health, safety and productivity. In S. Kumar (Ed.), *Advances in occupational ergonomics and safety* (p. 26). Philadelphia: Taylor & Francis.

Holmgren, K., & Dahlin Ivanoff, S. (2004). Women on sickness absence-Views of possibilities on obstacles for returning to work. A focus group study. *Disability and Rehabilitation, 26,* 213–222.

Hudson, W. W. (1982). The Generalized Contentment Scale. In *The clinical measurement package.* Homewood, IL: Dorsey Press.

Ibarra, H. (2002). How to stay stuck in the wrong career. *Harvard Business Review, 80,* 132.

Innes, E. & Straker, L. (1999). Reliability of work-related assessments. *Work, 13,* 102–124.

Isernhagen, S. J. (1988). *Work Injury. Management and Prevention.* Rockville, MD: Aspen.

Isernhagen, S. J. (Ed.). (1995a). *The comprehensive guide to work injury management.* Gaithersburg, MD: Aspen.

Isernhagen, S. J. (1995b). Job analysis. In S. J. Isernhagen (Ed.), *The comprehensive guide to work injury management* (pp. 70–85). Gaithersburg, MD: Aspen.

Jastrzebowski, W. (1857). *An outline of ergonomics, or the science of work based upon the truths drawn from the science of nature.* Warsaw: Central Institute for Labor Protection, 1997; T. Baluk-Ulewiczowa (trans).

Jebsen, R. H., Taylor, N., Trotter, M. J., & Howard, L. A. (1969). An objective and standardized test of hand function. *Archives of Physical Medicine and Rehabilitation, 50,* 311.

Karwowski, W., & Marras, W. S. (Eds.). (1999). *The occupational ergonomics handbook.* New York: CRC.

King, P. M., Tuckwell, N., & Barrett, T. E. (1998). A critical review of functional capacity evaluations. *Physical Therapy, 78,* 852–866.

Kornblau, B. (1998). Health care ergonomics and the Americans with Disabilities Act: An introduction. In V. Rice (Ed.), *Ergonomics in health care and rehabilitation* (pp. 287–294). Boston: Butterworth-Heinneman.

Kornblau, B. (1998b). The Americans with Disabilities Act: Legal ramifications of ADA consultation. In V. Rice (Ed.), *Ergonomics in health care and rehabilitation* (pp. 295–306). Boston: Butterworth-Heinneman.

Kuorinka, I., Hagberg, M., Silverstein, B., Smith, M., Forcier, L., Perusse, M., Welb, R., & Hendrick, H. (Eds.). (1995). *Work related musculoskeletal disorders (WMSDs): A reference book for prevention.* Philadelphia: Taylor & Francis.

Law, M., Baptiste, S., Carswell, A., McColl, M. A., Polatajko, H., & Pollock, N. (1994). *Canadian Occupational Performance Measure* (2nd ed.). Toronto: Canadian Association of Occupational Therapists.

Lechner, D. E., Bradbury, S. F., & Bradley, L. A. (1998). Detecting sincerity of effort: A summary of methods and approaches. *Physical Therapy, 78,* 867–888.

Lifelines (retrieved 2006). Combat stress reactions: Normal responses to abnormal conditions. Available at http://www.lifelines.navy.mil/dav/lsnmedia/LSN/CombatStress/

Llena-Nozal, A., Lindeboom, M., & Portrait, F. (2004). The effect of work on mental health: Does occupation matter? *Health Economics, 13,* 1045–1062.

Marchand, A., Demers, A., & Durand, P. (2005). Does work really cause distress? The contribution of occupational structure and work organization to the experience of psychological distress. *Social Science and Medicine, 61,* 1–14.

Markus, H., & Nurius, P. S. (1986). Possible selves. *American Psychologist, 41,* 954–969.

Mattingly, C. (1991). The narrative nature of clinical reasoning. *American Journal of Occupational Therapy, 45,* 998–1005.

Meyer, A. (1922). The philosophy of occupational therapy. *Archives of Occupational Therapy, 1,* 1–10.

Moore, S. L. (1997). A phenomenological study of meaning in life in suicidal older adults. *Archives of Psychiatric Nursing, 11,* 29–36.

National Academy on an Aging Society. (2000). Who are young retirees and older workers? Data profiles: Young retirees and older workers, 1. Available at http://www.agingsociety.org/agingsociety/publications/young/index.html.

National Academy on an Aging Society. (2001). What benefits do young retirees and older workers receive? Data profiles: Young retirees and older workers, 6. Available at http://www.agingsociety.org/agingsociety/publications/young/index.html.

National Center on Women and Aging. (2002). 2002 National Poll: Women 50+. The Heller School for Social Policy and Management, Brandeil University. Executive Summary available at http://www.heller.brandeis.edu/national/research.htm#National_Poll.

National Institutes of Health [NIH]. (2002). Traumatic brain injury: Hope through research. Prepared by the Office of Communications and Public Liaison, National Institute of Neurological Disorders and Stroke, National Institutes of Health, Bethesda, MD. Available at http://www.ninds.nih.gov/disorders/tbi/detail_tbi.htm.

Neistadt, M. E. (1995). Methods of assessing clients' priorities: A survey of adult physical dysfunction settings. *American Journal of Occupational Therapy, 49,* 428–436.

Piirila, P. L., Keskinen, H. M., Luukkonen, R., Salo, S. P., Tuppurainen, M., & Nordman, H. (2005). Work, unemployment and life satisfaction among patients with diisocyanate induced asthma—A prospective study. *Journal of Occupational Health, 47,* 112–118.

Polanyi, M., and Tompa, E. (2004). Rethinking work-health models for the new global economy: A qualitative analysis of emerging dimensions of work. *Work, 23,* 3–18.

Pransky, G., Snyder, T., Dembe, A., & Himmelstein, J. (1999). Under-reporting of work-related disorders in the workplace: A case study and review of the literature. *Ergonomics, 42,* 171–182.

Priebe, S., Warner, R., Hubschmid, T., & Eckle, I. (1998). Employment, attitudes towards work and quality of life among people with schizophrenia in three countries. *Schizophrenia Bulletin, 24,* 469–477.

Pulat, B. M., & Alexander, D. C. (Eds.). (1992). *Industrial ergonomics: Case studies.* New York: McGraw-Hill.

Rice, V. (Ed.). (1998). *Ergonomics in health care and rehabilitation.* Boston: Butterworth-Heinemann.

Rice, V. J. (1999a). Ergonomics: An introduction. In K. Jacobs & C. Bettencourt (Eds.), *Ergonomics for therapists* (pp. 3–12). New York: Andover Press.

Rice, V. J. (1999b). Pre-placement strength screening. In W. Karwowski & W. Marras (Eds.), *The industrial ergonomics handbook* (pp. 1299–1319). Washington, DC: CRC Press.

Rix, S. E. (2005). Update on the older worker, 2004. AARP Public Policy Institute. Available at www.aarp.org.

Rogers, S. (Ed.). (1983). *Ergonomic design for people at work* (Vols. I and II). New York: Van Nostrand.

Rogers, S. (1992). A functional job analysis technique in ergonomics. In J. S. Moore & A. Garg (Eds.), *State of the art review* (Vol. 7, no. 4, pp. 679–711). Philadelphia: Hunley & Belfus.

Ross, S. (December 17, 1999). HistoryChannel.Com, Associated Press. 10:26 AM Eastern Standard Time.

Rowe, J. W., and Kahn, R. L. (1999). *Successful aging.* New York: Random House.

Ruch, W. W., Shub, S. M., Moinat, S. M., & Dye, D. A. (1981) *PSI Basic Skills Tests for Business, Industry and Goverment.* Glendale, CA: Psychological Services.

Sanders, M. (Ed.). (1997). *Management of cumulative trauma disorders.* Boston: Butterworth-Heinemann.

Stein, H. T. (2002). *The collected clinical works of Alfred Adler.* Bellingham, WA: Alfred Adler Institutes of San Francisco and Northwestern Washington.

Swann, W. B. (1987). Identity negotiation: Where two roads meet. *Journal of Personality and Social Psychology, 53,* 1038–1051.

Swann, W. B., & Hill, C. A. (1982). When our identities are mistaken: Reaffirming self-conceptions through social interaction. *Journal of Personality and Social Psychology, 43,* 59–66.

Terkel, S. (1974). *Working: People talk about what they do all day and how they feel about what they do.* New York: Pantheon.

Toosi, M. (2004). Labor force projections to 2012: The graying of the US workforce. *Monthly Labor Review, February,* 37–57.

Tuxworth, W., & Shanawaz, H. (1977). The design and evaluation of a step test for the rapid prediction of physical work capacity in an unsophisticated industrial work force. *Ergonomics, 20,* 181–191.

Unruh, A. M. (2004). Reflections on: "So. . .what do you do?" Occupation and the construction of identity. *Canadian Journal of Occupational Therapy, 71,* 290–295.

Valpar International Corp. (1992). *Valpar work sample administration manual* (pp. 2–3). Tucson, AZ: Valpar International Corp..

van Selm, M., & Dittmann-Kohli, F. (1998). Meaninglessness in the second half of life: The development of a construct. *International Journal of Aging and Human Development, 47,* 81–104.

White, R. W. (1971). The urge toward competence. *American Journal of Occupational Therapy, 25,* 271–274.

Wigdor, A. K., & Green, B. F. (1991). *Performance assessment for the workplace.* Washington, DC: National Academy.

Yelin, E. (1999). Measuring functional capacity of persons with disabilities in light of emerging demands in the workplace. In *Summary of a workshop: Measuring functional capacity and work requirements.* Washington, DC: Division of Health Care Services, Institute of Medicine and Committee on National Statistics, Commission on Behavioral and Social Sciences and Education, National Research Council.

Supplemental References

Barkley, R. A., & Murphy, K. R. (1998). *Attention-deficit hyperactivity disorder: A clinical workbook* (2nd ed.). New York: Guilford Publications Inc.

Kim, S., & Feldman, D. C. (2000). Working in retirement: The antecedents of bridge employment and its consequences for quality of life in retirement. *Academy of Management Journal, 43,* 1195–1210.

National Academy on an Aging Society (2001). Who are young retirees and older workers? Data profiles: Young retirees and older workers, 5. Available at http://www.agingsociety.org/agingsociety/publications/young/index.html.

CHAPTER 34

LEARNING OBJECTIVES

After studying this chapter, the reader will be able to do the following:

1. Define leisure in a conceptual and pragmatic fashion.
2. Evaluate the physiological and psychological benefits of engagement in active and quiet leisure.
3. Describe how leisure can be integrated into occupational therapy practice.
4. Identify various leisure assessments and describe how they are used.
5. Discuss barriers and challenges for clients and therapists engaging in leisure activities.

Restoring Competence in Leisure Pursuits

Carolyn Hanson

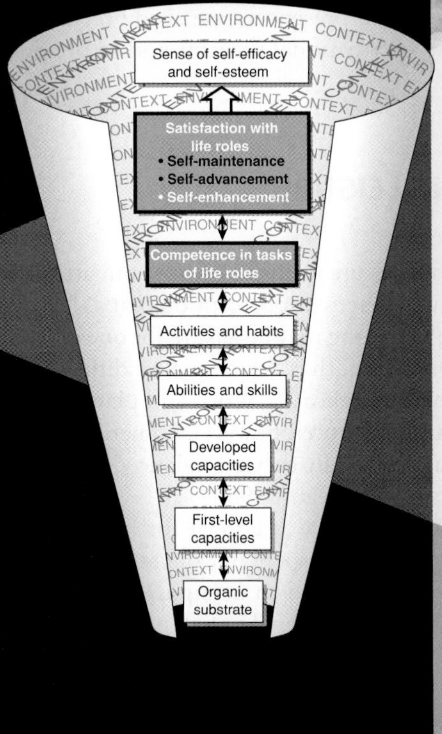

Glossary

Chat room—Internet site where people communicate with each other in real time during a certain period on specific topics.

Electronic mail (E-mail)—Correspondence with people via the computer; sending a letter electronically.

Free time—Time other than that spent in work or self-care activities.

Horticulture therapy—Gardening as a therapeutic intervention.

Leisure—Freely chosen activity that requires control and commitment. Active leisure involves mental and physical exertion (e.g., wheelchair sports), whereas quiet leisure involves activities, such as reading and crafts, that require less physical effort. Socialization entails contact with others via telecommunication, computer, and/or in person.

Internet surfing—Using the Internet to access information.

Occupational imbalance—Excessive time spent in one area, usually work, at the expense of another, usually leisure. May aggravate health and quality of life.

Recreation—Time that is not spent in work or self-care and may or may not result in observable activity; similar to free time.

Therapeutic recreation—Professional use of recreational activities as primary form of treatment with patients; sometimes called recreational therapy.

Therapeutic recreation specialist—Trained professional who uses recreational activities as a therapeutic intervention with patients.

Activities of daily living (ADL), work, and play/**leisure** are core aspects of occupational therapy intervention that promote self-efficacy and self-esteem. Although information concerning the use of play/leisure in occupational therapy is scarce compared to ADL and work, play/leisure is incorporated into key models that inform practice. In the Occupational Functioning Model, engagement in play/leisure is categorized as a self-enhancement role under the control of and chosen by the individual (Trombly, 2002). Participation in social roles (including that of leisure) is a key concept in the International Classification of Functioning, Disability and Health (Brachtesende, 2005), and the Occupational Therapy Practice Framework (American Occupational Therapy Association [AOTA], 2002) endorses participation in leisure activities as a legitimate goal in occupational therapy treatment.

Terms such as play, leisure, and recreation are often used interchangeably in conversation. Leisure can be viewed as the adult version of play, as many similarities are present. Also, leisure is viewed as a more encompassing concept than play or recreation and is the term most frequently used in the occupational therapy literature. **Recreation** is often used to describe how we occupy time that is not devoted to work or self-care. **Therapeutic recreation specialists**, professionals who are trained to use recreational activities to improve the quality of life for patients, have played a major role in developing leisure programs in medical settings. The profession of **therapeutic recreation (TR)** gained prominence and became more formalized after World War II, as recreational activities were used in the treatment of disabled war veterans. The history of TR is similar to the history of occupational therapy because our profession was launched after working with veterans from World War I. The distinguishing difference between the two professions is that treatment protocols for TR always use recreational activity as the primary form of treatment. Occupational therapists concentrate on the overall functioning of the individual, of which recreation is one component.

The purpose of this chapter is to review briefly the use of leisure with persons with disabilities; to highlight particular leisure assessments; to recommend the development of specific leisure programs and activities for adults with physical disabilities; to discuss barriers for both therapists and clients; to present a case study regarding the use of leisure in occupational therapy; and to provide leisure resources.

DEFINING LEISURE

A precise definition of leisure is elusive because our attitude toward a given activity shapes our perception of it as leisure or work. For example, sewing may be leisure for one person but considered work by another, which makes differentiation between the two complicated. Work and play are not always dichotomous experiences, however. Sometimes they become blended, and hopefully they are balanced, a central tenet of our profession (Primeau, 1996).

Balancing work and leisure is crucial for mental and physical health. Excessive time spent in work at the expense of leisure or vice versa may lead to **occupational imbalance** (Wilcock, 1998). Occupational imbalance may aggravate health and quality of life, resulting in injury or illness. Engagement in leisure activity is important to a balanced life and satisfaction with life. In fact, Kinney and Coyle

(1992) interviewed 790 adults with physical disabilities and found that leisure satisfaction was the most significant predictor of life satisfaction. To avoid occupational imbalance, leisure opportunities must be available and accessible to all people, including those with disabilities.

Recipients of occupational therapy services have a variety of leisure goals, which are shaped by the type of leisure preferred and the individual's cultural background. Here are some examples:

- Using **free time** in a meaningful way
- Developing or improving socialization skills
- Increasing physical components such as strength, range of motion, coordination, and endurance
- Facilitating emotional adjustment such as self-esteem, confidence, and relaxation
- Improving cognitive capacities such as maintaining attention and following instructions

Types of Leisure

Law et al. (1994) have partitioned leisure into three major categories: active leisure, which consists of recreational activities incorporating physical exertion such as wheelchair sports and travel; quiet leisure, which incorporates activities such as watching television, reading the newspaper, and crafts; and socialization, which consists of visiting and correspondence. Both quiet and active leisure activities appear to contribute to occupational balance, self-esteem, and wellness for persons with disabilities (Fig. 34-1).

Quiet Leisure

According to a British study surveying 54 OT fieldwork students in three practice settings, the most diverse and numerous activities used in treatment were from the leisure area as opposed to work or ADL areas. Using the *Canadian Occupational Performance Measure* (*COPM*) to categorize these leisure activities, the students reported that quiet recreational activities were prescribed more than twice as much as active leisure. Examples mentioned by the students included crafts and board games (Drew & Rugg, 2000). Generally, adults with physical disabilities tend to engage in quiet and passive activities (Law, 2002), such as needlecrafts like knitting, crochet, and embroidery.

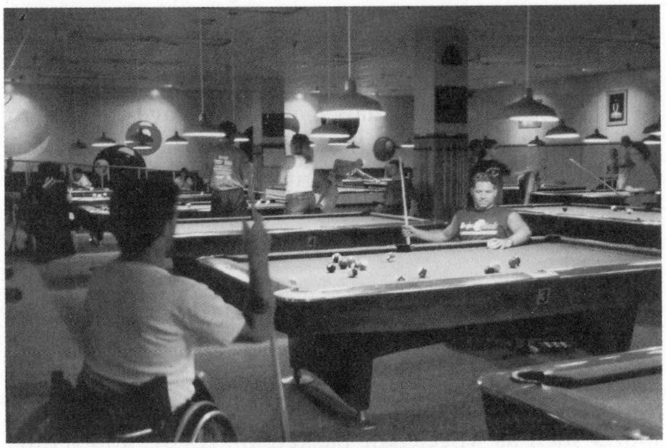

Figure 34-1 Recreational activity: billiards.

Another type of quiet leisure, **horticulture therapy** (HT), refers to gardening for therapeutic reasons. Occupational therapists have traditionally used HT to facilitate leisure and occupational skills in diverse populations. Gardening assists in enhancing the emotional well-being of patients by affirming life and establishing a sense of peace in addition to improving range of motion and endurance (Harnish, 2001). Raised flower boxes enable wheelchair users to employ gardening skills while improving functional, emotional, cognitive, and physical skills. Various tools are designed to allow people with arthritis and upper extremity weakness to garden (Resources 34-1).

Active Leisure

People with chronic musculoskeletal diseases may be afraid to engage in activities that require physical exertion and believe that their leisure options are limited to quiet activities. Occupational therapists may inadvertently contribute to this misperception. Therapists may not be introducing active leisure to clients because exercise recommendation guidelines have not been fully developed for people with physical disabilities. Sports for those with disabilities, however, have been connected to rehabilitation efforts since the 1940s when archery was used as therapy for paraplegic war veterans. Wheelchair sports have continued to expand in variety to encompass wheelchair basketball, tennis, and quad rugby as a few of the better established popular sports (Fig. 34-2).

EFFICACY AND OUTCOMES RESEARCH SPECIFIC TO LEISURE

Insufficient physical activity has been identified as the major factor in the deteriorating health of people with disabilities (Coyle & Santiago, 1995). Despite the increased growth of wheelchair sports, many people with disabilities lead sedentary lives. Research data on the activity patterns of those with disabilities are scarce since insufficient evidence is available to determine exactly what activity is best for an adult with a physical disability based on safety, effectiveness, and outcome measures. Utilizing the research on the able-bodied, we know that a properly designed physical activity program includes aerobic, flexibility, and strength components (Durstine et al., 2000). Exercise dosage (intensity, frequency, and duration of the physical activity) needs to be modified for persons with disabilities

RESOURCE 34-1

Organizations, Information, and Equipment for Leisure Pursuits

Sport Organizations

- Disabled Sports USA—Provides sports opportunities to people with disabilities. Listing of summer and winter sports and equipment for these sports; methods to contact existing chapters.
  http://www.dsusa.org
- Adaptive Sports Association—Offers snow skiing instruction and summer sports options to physically and cognitively disabled persons of all ages.
  http://www.frontier.net/~asa
- Mesa Association for the Disabled—Non-profit organization providing sports and recreational opportunities to people with disabilities. Other links to sports organizations.
  http://www.geocities.com/HotSprings/5896/
- National Wheelchair Basketball Association—Provides rules, team registration, divisions of wheelchair basketball, and listing of basketball camps. Additional links.
  www.nwba.org
- Paralyzed Veterans of America—Research and education, sports and recreation, resources for professionals, publications, and products. Includes Multiple Sclerosis Center of Excellence site.
  http://www.pva.org/
- National Disability Sports Alliance—Player classification for sports; information for those with cerebral palsy, traumatic brain injury, and stroke as well as programming for people with muscular dystrophy and multiple sclerosis.
  http://www.ndsaonline.org/
- Wheelchair Sports USA—Qualifying standards and rules for sports. Links to various organizations and sporting events.
  http://www.wsusa.org/

Specific Leisure Activities and Sports/Sport Magazines

- American Horticulture Therapy Association—Membership information, conferences and educational opportunities, publications and information packets, and other HT sites.
  www.ahta.org/
- Chicago Botanic Gardens—Information on plants and flowers in the Midwest. Hosts a horticultural therapy certificate program.
  www.chicagobotanic.org
- World travel options focusing on accessible services and transportation. Includes review of cruise ship accessibility. Excellent source of links to sports and other disability sources.
  http://www.accessable.com/; http://www.disabilitytravel.com/
- Quad rugby home page—History of the sport, rules, U.S. teams, and classification of players.
  http://www.quadrugby.com
- Sled hockey rules and regulations (using a sled instead of ice skates to play hockey).
  http://www.sledhockey.org/
- GatorSport Adult Exploration Camp—Camp designed for adults with physical disabilities. Resources and organizations for a variety of sports and leisure activities.
  http://www.gatorsport.net
- Active Living magazine—Feature articles on living with a disability, health and fitness, listing of amputee support groups, and a variety of links.
  www.activeliving-magazine.com
- New Mobility magazine—Health, fitness and recreation for people with disabilities.
  www.newmobility.com

Equipment

- Cycles for the physically challenged: hand cycles, tandem tricycles, tandem bicycles, seats, backrests, footrests, and accessories.
  http://www.haverich.com
- TRS—Prosthetic hands for sports and other leisure activities, such as photography and playing musical instruments. Highlights adult, children, and infant technology.
  http://www.oandp.com/trs
- KY Enterprises—Adaptive recreational equipment and controllers for video games for those with limited use of their hands.
  http://www.quadcontrol.com
- Adaptive recreation and sporting equipment for people with disabilities and the aged. Leisure activities range from crafts and gardening to motorcycling and sailing and skiing.
  http://www.achievableconcepts.com.au/; http://www.accesstr.com/; http://www.spokesnmotion.com (various programs as well as equipment offered); http://www.fhnbinc.org (Fishing has no boundaries-gear and programs for everyone)

to maintain a training effect that does not cause abnormal clinical symptoms/signs or injury. For example, it is recommended that adults with physical disabilities lower the intensity of the exercise but increase the duration and the frequency of the activity (Durstine et al., 2000). Progress would be slower when these parameters are altered.

Persons with Spinal Cord Injury

Researchers surveyed 160 persons with spinal cord injury (SCI) regarding their post-discharge activities (Hoffmann et al., 1995). On the basis of their activity level, respondents were placed in an active or an inactive group. Over a 1-year period, the active individuals spent, on average, 3.2 days in the hospital compared with 10.7 days for the inactive individuals. Inactive individuals were more than 2.5 times as likely to have pressure sores as the active ones. Results of this study underscore the cost-saving benefits of being physically active.

One hundred forty-three individuals with SCI from 18–55 years of age were surveyed regarding their engagement in physical activity before and after their injury (Wu & Williams, 2000). Individuals who participated in sports such as wheelchair basketball, rugby, and tennis were shown to have less depression, improved social

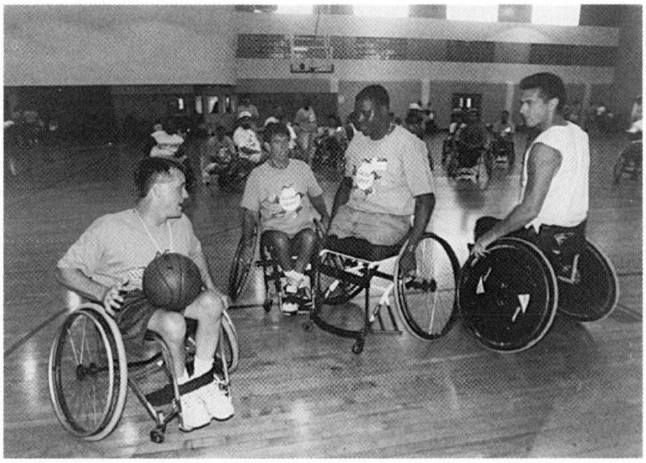

Figure 34-2 Active leisure: wheelchair basketball.

interaction, and less incidence of rehospitalization. The participants in this study reported that they engaged in sport because it was fun and provided a means to be fit and healthy and a means to interact with a variety of people. Peers with disabilities, as opposed to therapists, were invaluable in introducing newly injured people to wheelchair sports. Wu and Williams emphasized that therapists should take a more active role in educating clients about sports training and leisure activities (see the Case Example about K.J.).

Persons with Joint Replacements

Individuals with modern joint replacement can expect to have their joints last at least 10–15 years. This does not apply to people with hip and knee joint replacements who regularly jog or hike because this type of activity may endanger the integrity of the prosthetic components (Kuster, 2002). Since there are no prospective, randomized studies on physical activities post total joint replacement, the conservative opinions of orthopedic surgeons have guided current recommendations on suitable leisure activities. In general, speed, prior sport experience, and joint impact are factors when considering load or joint stress. High-impact activities requiring speed, such as football, soccer, and handball, are discouraged, whereas low-impact activities, such as swimming, cycling, and walking, are encouraged. Technically demanding sports (snow skiing, mountain biking) are not suggested for those individuals who have never engaged in these activities prior to their joint replacement. The rationale is that the learning curve for technical sports is too demanding on the replaced joints (Kuster, 2002).

Persons with Rheumatoid Arthritis

Minor and Lane (1996) noted that people with rheumatoid arthritis (RA) are prescribed rest and medication for their condition, which is appropriate for the acute condition but

CASE EXAMPLE

K.J.: Resuming Leisure Activities After Stroke

Occupational Therapy Intervention Process	Clinical Reasoning Process: Objectives	Clinical Reasoning Process: Examples of Therapist's Internal Dialogue
Patient Information K.J. is a 42-year-old woman who sustained a left cerebrovascular accident (CVA) resulting in right-sided paresis. She had good return of right upper extremity muscles but lacks coordination. Muscles of right lower extremity are spastic, and K.J. cannot safely ambulate, so she is learning to use a wheelchair. K.J. feels sad and helpless at times, although she is making steady gains in feeding, dressing, and transferring. Previous leisure interests include playing basketball and driving her sports car.	Appreciate the context	"K.J.'s past lifestyle was active, and she valued mobility. I will bring up leisure adaptations when she is receptive. I'll want to encourage gains in self-care activities and help her see how this success can transfer over into engaging in leisure pursuits. It will be important for me to listen to K.J.'s concerns and fears. I will provide examples of disabled athletes and information on wheelchair sports. Maybe I'll show a video of wheelchair athletes playing basketball."

Patient Information (cont'd)	Develop intervention hypotheses	"I will address attitudinal barriers regarding belief in self by structuring successful ADL sessions. A visit with a wheelchair basketball player may motivate K.J. to work harder and feel better about the rehab process. I will find a car with hand controls since this may also facilitate interest in driving again."
	Select an intervention approach	"I will strengthen K.J.'s upper extremities by having her engage in ADL tasks as well as using light weights and resistive bands. It makes sense to work on gross and fine motor coordination tasks. I will introduce adaptive equipment and sports chairs for wheelchair basketball and discuss driver training programs. I will remediate skills when possible (strength and coordination) and compensate when necessary (wheelchair for mobility and hand controls for driving)."
	Reflect on competence	"I will address ADL tasks and equipment, but I may need to refer K.J. to a wheelchair specialist to prescribe a custom chair. Local wheelchair sports camp (offering basketball and other sports) is available in the summer. I will provide contact info and web site addresses regarding sports chairs and the rules of wheelchair basketball. I will identify driver training programs in the area and refer her to a driving specialist."

Recommendations I will involve K.J. in treatment by making tasks relevant and meaningful. K.J. has begun to realize that basic ADL skills are needed to be able to leave the house. Leisure activities of playing basketball and driving a sports car may motivate her to make the most of her time in therapy. I will provide information on wheelchair basketball rules and sports chairs or refer to the Internet for specifics. I will contact an athlete with a disability (preferably a wheelchair basketball player) to demonstrate that K.J. can still be active even though she has had a stroke. This athlete (former patient) may most likely have a modified car or van if he is a wheelchair user. Having someone with a disability who is also an athlete will serve as an excellent role model for K.J., who is unsure about her abilities.	Consider the patient's appraisal of performance	"When K.J. can dress and groom independently (with or without devices), transfer safely from a variety of surfaces, and obtain and maneuver wheelchair efficiently for 30 minutes, she will be able to physically begin playing basketball with a local group of wheelchair players who practice weekly at the community college. I believe that playing basketball will motivate K.J. to gain strength.
	Consider what will occur in therapy, how often, and for how long	My therapy sessions will consist of grooming and dressing with adaptive equipment, increasing upper extremity strength by one muscle grade, increasing tolerance to activity, and practicing transfers from all surfaces and planes. I will expose K.J. to driving equipment and sports chairs. I'll conduct daily therapy sessions for 30 minutes for 2–3 weeks. I want to arrange for a wheelchair basketball athlete to visit K.J. (who may also have car controls on a modified vehicle).
	Ascertain the patient's endorsement of plan	Because K.J. is anxious to return to past activities, she is looking forward to meeting the wheelchair player and inspecting a car with hand controls. She is beginning to ask me for info on wheelchair basketball rules and specifics about team practices."

Summary of Short-Term Goals and Progress 1. Dresses and grooms self independently and uses assistive devices for lower extremity dressing (long-handled shoe horn, sock aid, elastic shoe laces). 2. Upper extremity strength has improved by one grade (from 3/5 to 4/5 on MMT). 3. Transfers from a variety of surfaces and planes. Able to perform car transfers and is practicing placing wheelchair in back of driver's seat independently. 4. Referred to a driving specialist. Appointment to be made when patient is ready. 5. Wheelchair athlete visited facility and played a one-on-one make-shift game with patient.	Assess the patient's comprehension	"I want K.J. to understand the importance of doing daily self-care activities to be independent as well as use muscles on a continuous basis. She told me that she feels better about herself now that she can do more and depend less on others."
	Understand what she is doing	"I have seen K.J. improve dramatically; she has been less tearful and more motivated to try activities. The visit with the disabled athlete really helped in introducing her to life in a new but satisfying way. She established an easy rapport with him and shared some of her frustrations and fears. K.J. told her family that she is excited about playing basketball again even though she's in a wheelchair."

Summary of Short-Term Goals and Progress (cont'd)	Compare actual to expected performance Know the person Appreciate the context	"K.J. has met and surpassed all my short-term goals. Although hesitant about using adaptive equipment, she has learned how to use devices well. I think that she'll continue to work on perfecting her turning skills in a wheelchair (for tight turns in basketball practices). I have noticed that K.J. has had a brighter affect since the visit with the wheelchair athlete. I think she finally realizes that she can still engage in her pre-stroke preferred leisure activities. I know that K.J.'s motivation has made a big difference in her therapy outcomes. K.J. enjoyed her active lifestyle before her stroke and thought that it was all over for her after the CVA. With encouragement and support from the wheelchair athlete and me, she was able to see that life would be slightly different but she could still engage in these favorite activities."
Next Steps 1. Prepare patient for discharge by providing specifics on driver training programs (in area in case identified specialist is not available), sports equipment, and stroke info. 2. Make sure that patient has all equipment (self-care, customized wheelchair) or knows about what equipment would be most beneficial to obtain (e.g., basketball chair). 3. Encourage patient to contact therapist if any problems or questions arise.	Anticipate present and future patient concerns Analyze patient's comprehension Decide if the patient should continue or discontinue therapy and/or return in the future	"I want to make sure K.J. understands how to manage paralysis as well as signs of stroke. I will review stroke risk factors and how to prevent stroke as well as review info on driver training programs." "I will ask K.J. to identify ways to minimize stroke. I will have her list strategies she will use at home to take care of daily tasks. Then I'll evaluate her competence in using assistive devices." "When K.J. is able to take care of all self-care skills and can use her wheelchair effectively, she is ready for discharge. I will make sure that she has all the necessary resources so that she can obtain info or items if she hasn't been issued them already."

CLINICAL REASONING IN OCCUPATIONAL THERAPY PRACTICE

Promotion of Leisure Exploration

Before her stroke, Ms. K.J. found meaning in her life through engagement in leisure activities. In what ways did providing her with experiences to reengage in interests motivate her to participate in her rehabilitation more fully?

harmful in the chronic state. People with RA often stop engaging in leisure and recreational activities. Unfortunately, inactivity produces the same symptoms as the rheumatoid disease process: muscle weakness, decreased flexibility, fatigue, incoordination, depression, and lowered pain threshold. People with RA who do engage in aerobic exercise may experience a significant reduction in swelling, which is attributed to increased synovial blood flow. Minor and Lane emphasized that vigorous activity is only supported in people with no joint inflammation; otherwise, joint damage may ensue.

Based on clinical experience, Minor and Lane (1996) made the following recommendations for people with chronic arthritic conditions and no active inflammation:

- Warm up prior to vigorous activity.
- Include range-of-motion movement in any physical activity program.
- Engage in low-impact activities.
- Reduce load on joints by swimming, biking, or rowing.
- Wear shoes with good support and use orthotics, if needed biomechanically.

- Avoid overstretching as well as running and climbing stairs (of all locomotor activity, stair climbing produces most stress on hip joints).

Elders

In the Northern Manhattan Stroke study of 1000 elders, those who engaged in physically active leisure were found to have a decreased incidence of ischemic stroke (Sacco et al., 1998). Researchers of this study stressed that physically active leisure be emphasized in stroke prevention campaigns. In addition to a variety of sports, physically active leisure, such as walking, armchair or wheelchair aerobics (exercising the upper extremities while seated), swimming, and weight training (using light weights or machines; using resistive bands), is ideal for increasing endurance and tone in elders. As elders constitute more of our population, it behooves us to create and promote leisure and socialization opportunities in assisted-living facilities and retirement homes.

T'ai Chi is available for elders in many communities. Known as a soft martial art, T'ai Chi involves moving the body slowly and smoothly through its range of motion. Over the past 5 years, there has been an exponential increase in randomized controlled trials on the effects of practicing T'ai Chi. In a meta-analysis performed by Klein and Adams (2004), 17 clinical trial studies were critically reviewed with all showing statistical significance in at least one outcome measure. Typical outcome measures included the positive effects T'ai Chi had on quality of life and physical function. In addition, T'ai Chi was credited in improving pain management and balance. Although T'ai Chi appears to improve balance, it has not been correlated in preventing the incidence of falls in elders. Evidence is available, however, that strength training in elders with chronic conditions reduces the incidence of falls as well as improves ADL independence (Durstine et al., 2000).

Potential Contributions from Occupational Therapy

Occupational therapists value and understand the power of occupation, thus we can facilitate role change in people with physical disabilities and encourage adaptation to a new lifestyle through engagement in leisure (Fig. 34-3). To facilitate role change, we must be knowledgeable about leisure activities appropriate for our patients, discuss leisure interests, and provide opportunities for exploration. Proactively, occupational therapists can create sports programs or provide physically active leisure opportunities for people with disabilities and inform patients about active, quiet, and socialization activities within their communities. Incorporating leisure activity into our assessment and treatment encourages the individual to take risks and be exposed to activities that they might not have attempted on their own.

ASSESSMENT TOOLS

Before recommending specific leisure activities or using leisure as an intervention, one should assess the patient's interest in leisure. The following are instruments that identify the types of activities that are meaningful to clients. Although this is not an exhaustive list of the leisure assessments available in the fields of occupational therapy and therapeutic recreation, the following sections present some of the better known instruments.

The Canadian Occupational Performance Measure

Designed by occupational therapists, the *Canadian Occupational Performance Measure* (*COPM*) detects self-perceived change in occupational performance over time (Law et al., 1994). The *COPM* contains three sections: self-care, productivity, and leisure. The leisure section is divided into quiet recreation, such as hobbies, crafts, and reading; active recreation, such as sports, outings, and travel; and socialization, such as visiting, phone calls, and correspondence. Individuals are requested to identify any problems in the three sections and to rate the importance of each activity on a scale of 1 to 10. Then five of the most important problems are identified, and individuals rate their performance and satisfaction with performance on these five problems (Table 34-1).

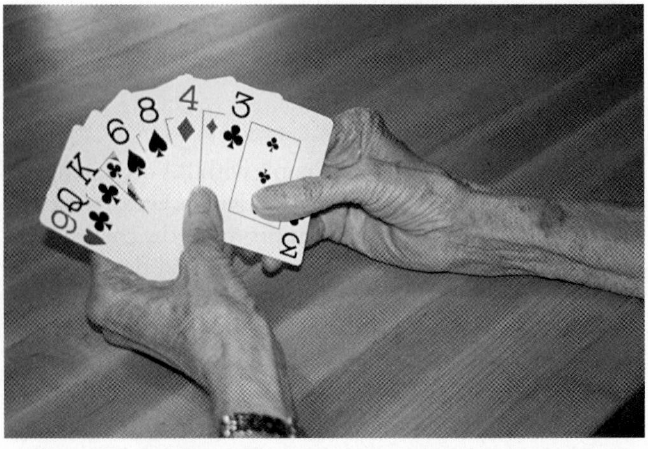

Figure 34-3 Large-print playing cards typify leisure adaptations available to elders. (Photo by Laurie Manuel.)

Table 34-1. Leisure Activity Chart

Activity Level	Paraplegia, Lower Extremity Amputation[a]	Tetraplegia[b]	Cerebrovascular Accident[c]	Traumatic Brain Injury[d]	Dementia[e]
Sedentary	Cards Board games Puzzles Painting, drawing Music listening Reading Computer activities Video games Needlecrafts Movies	Cards Board games Puzzles Painting, drawing Music listening Reading Computer activities Video games Movies	Cards Board games Puzzles Painting, drawing Music listening Mirror games Needlecrafts Computer activities Photo albums, scrapbooks Movies	Cards Board games Puzzles Painting, art, drawing Music listening Mirror games Needlecrafts Computer activities Photo albums, scrapbooks Movies	Matching games Sequencing games Sing alongs Show and tell
Mild	Archery Bowling Target shooting Billiards Flying Camping Fishing Photography Gardening Travel	Archery Target shooting Fishing Photography Gardening Travel	Paved nature walks Pet therapy Bowling Gardening	Paved nature walks Pet therapy Bowling Gardening	Putt putt Bowling Fishing Parties Gardening
Moderate	Sailing Swimming Weight training Horseback riding Scuba diving Golf Table tennis Dance	Sailing Swimming Weight training Creative movement, dance	Weight training Assisted swimming Creative movement, dance	Weight training Assisted swimming Creative movement, dance	Walking groups Creative movement, dance Weight training Swimming Table tennis
Vigorous	Wheelchair basketball Racing, track Tennis Softball Snow skiing Water skiing Rowing, kayaking Hand cycling Sled hockey	Quad rugby Racing Tennis	Stationary bicycle Rowing, kayaking Other activities depending on degree of paralysis or paresis	Stationary bicycle Rowing, kayaking Other activities depending on degree of paralysis or paresis	Speed walking, jogging Bicycling, tricycling Tennis Rowing

This table provides suggested activities for persons with disabilities. The appropriateness of any activity is greatly influenced by the individual's functional level. Specific adaptive equipment and special assistance may be required.

[a] Treatment should emphasize activities that reinforce functional independence and physical fitness.

[b] Specialized adaptive equipment is required for most activities. Functional independence is possible in many of these activities with proper planning and practice.

[c] Treatment should emphasize visual-perceptual and one-handed activities. Activities that improve range of motion and visual field on the impaired side are valuable.

[d] Activities should focus on cognitive challenges and games to strengthen fine and gross motor skills without complex rules or higher order thinking.

[e] Activities to improve socialization, cognitive orientation, and recollection are important.

Interest Checklists

Occupational therapists have developed and used many interest checklists. The *Nottingham Leisure Questionnaire*, developed in England for stroke patients, is a 38-item list of activities ranging from watching television to doing sporting activities (Drummond & Walker, 1994). A 5-point scale is used to describe frequency of doing the activity, ranging from regularly (every day) to never. In obtaining test–retest reliability scores, 21 subjects completed the same questionnaire on two occasions within a 2-week period. Using Cohen's kappa coefficient, it was discovered that reliability was excellent (0.75–1.00) and good (0.60–0.74) for 23 of the 38 items and fair (0.40–0.59) for another six items. Inter-rater reliability was tested using the ratings of two occupational therapists and showed excellent agreement on 40 items and good agreement on one item; the total was more than 38 items due to write-ins of other activities not specified in the questionnaire (Drummond & Walker, 1994).

The *Interest Checklist* (Matsutsuyu, 1967) consists of 80 items grouped into the following categories: ADL, manual skills, cultural-educational, physical sports, and social recreation. The rating given to each item ranges from no interest to casual interest to strong interest.

Kautzmann (1984) developed an interest checklist for persons with arthritis that uses similar categories as well as games, organizational activities, and entertainment. This instrument consists of 64 items rated according to their importance, ranging from none to high, and their relevance to the person with arthritis (importance of activity and whether a priority for further development) (Kautzmann, 1984).

Finally, the *Lin Interest Check List* (*LICL*), developed in 1991, contains 151 interests and activities within six categories: sports, physical activities, and nature; crafts; games; sociocultural and entertainment activities; community and education; and hobbies and miscellaneous. Level of interest, frequency, and history of participation are to be identified for each item. The *LICL* has high content validity and good test–retest reliability (Lin, 1991).

Occupational Therapy Assessment of Leisure Time

The *Occupational Therapy Assessment of Leisure Time* (*OTALT*) was based on a review of the leisure literature in occupational therapy and provides a frame of reference specifically for leisure (Soderback & Hammarlund, 1993). The purpose of the *OTALT* is to enable the client to use leisure time more effectively and to improve satisfaction with leisure activities. Using open-ended questions, the therapist interviews the client on the dimensional concepts of time, intrinsic motivation, and free choice of leisure activity; capability; structure of social and cultural environment; engagement in leisure activity; pleasure for pleasure's sake; goal self-fulfillment, goal diversion, recreation, and relaxation; leisure role; leisure behavior; and influence on his or her leisure role and leisure behavior. Although multiple questions are provided for each dimension, therapists are encouraged to structure the interview the best way they see fit.

Leisure Questionnaires from Therapeutic Recreation

Beard and Ragheb (1980) have developed four leisure questionnaires that are commonly used by therapeutic recreation specialists in medical settings. The *Leisure Satisfaction Measure* (*LSM*) contains 51 statements about how patients perceive their needs being met through leisure. The *Leisure Attitude Measurement* (*LAM*) contains 36 items that quantify the patient's attitude in 3 areas: cognitive, affective, and behavioral (Ragheb & Beard, 1982). The *Leisure Interest Measure* (*LIM*) identifies patients' interest in the following eight domains: physical, outdoor, mechanical, artistic, service, social, cultural, and reading (Beard & Ragheb, 1990). The *Leisure Motivation Scale* (*LMS*) contains 48 items regarding motivation to engage in leisure activities and reflects four areas: intellectual, social, competence-mastery, and stimulus avoidance (Beard & Ragheb, 1983). As a whole, reliability and validity are good for these measures because items and domains have been analyzed extensively according to the test manuals for the four aforementioned assessments.

Physical Activity Scale for Individuals with Physical Disabilities

A relatively new assessment is the *Physical Activity Scale for Individuals with Physical Disabilities* (*PASIPD*). *PASIPD* is recommended for use in studies of activity and health (Washburn et al., 2002). The brief scale consists of 13 items: six leisure time questions, six household questions, and one occupational activity question. Respondents indicate how many days and hours per session they engage in activity.

ARENAS FOR LEISURE INTERVENTION

Occupational therapists help clients resume pre-morbid leisure interests and explore new options. Table 34-1 describes leisure activities that persons with various diagnoses are typically able to perform. The discussion that follows highlights two other broad areas of leisure intervention: information technology and sports camps.

Information Technology

Computers can provide leisure outlets, such as accessing information on activities and organizations and developing intellectual and creative abilities. Computer activities such as communicating with people in **chat rooms**, using **electronic mail (E-mail)**, **Internet surfing**, and playing video games are popular and accessible. If there is interest, therapists ensure a proper match between the person and the hardware and software. A structured training program is recommended to allow experimentation with appropriate equipment before purchase. With the right match, the computer can provide educational and social opportunities. Although distinctly having many advantages, computers may encourage individuals to be sedentary, remaining indoors and in one position for extended periods. As with any activity, moderation is the key. Frequent breaks and repositioning are crucial.

Sports Camps

Camps have been developed to introduce sports and leisure activities to people with disabilities and to facilitate engagement in physically active leisure and to promote health (Hanson, 1998). Focus may be on one particular sport, such as with wheelchair tennis camp, or an introduction to a variety of sports. Some camps are specialized for individuals with particular diagnoses; others include anyone with a mental or physical disability. Due to the focused nature of the camp and the time invested (camps may last from several days to several weeks), participants have the chance to socialize and learn specific sport skills. In addition, camp participants often learn techniques and obtain tips from each other on daily living skills such as transferring and catheterization. Affiliation with others is a strong motivating factor in promoting leisure activities.

Occupational therapists realize the many benefits of directing a camp, which range from raising the awareness of the able-bodied to providing the disabled with opportunities to explore sport. Additional benefits may include training for students and staff who serve as camp volunteers. Volunteers assist in monitoring participants for heat exhaustion and any untoward effects of exercise (Safety Note 34-1) and assist with coaching. It is possible to conduct research in camps, such as collecting outcome data on clients who are active and inactive and their functional abilities and incidence of secondary medical complications. A wide range of research projects will ultimately enable us to promote wellness and sports opportunities for individuals with disabilities. It is not enough to give anecdotal accounts of our successful interventions with clients; we must back up our statements with research data.

SAFETY NOTE 34-1

Safety Considerations During Active Leisure

Spinal Cord Injury

Individuals with spinal cord injury (lesion at T6 and above) are at risk for autonomic dysreflexia, which is brought on by being overheated or having an obstructed fecal mass, a kink in a catheter tube, or pain. Symptoms and signs include hypertension, pounding headache, profuse sweating, flushing, pupil constriction, and nasal congestion. **This is a medical emergency.** Obtain medical help while removing restrictive binders or clothing, elevating head, checking leg bag for obstruction, and monitoring blood pressure (Hollar, 1995).

Monitoring during Active Leisure Pursuits

The new participant requires supervision from a therapist, with subsequent monitoring by the participant. Environmental conditions with extreme heat (outdoor wheelchair racing in Florida in July) or cold (snow skiing in Colorado) should be cautiously considered and consistently evaluated for potential ill effects. Terminate activity if safety is questionable.

- Monitor body temperature.
- Monitor sweating and color of skin.
- Observe for signs of fatigue.
- Check for incontinence.
- Encourage skin inspection.
- Encourage fluid intake.
- Recommend pressure relief.
- Evaluate positioning, cushioning, and strapping during activity.
- Consider special training for activity.

BARRIERS TO LEISURE ENGAGEMENT

A number of factors interfere with ensuring that persons with disabilities ultimately can engage in leisure activities that maintain a satisfactory occupational balance. Some factors stem from contemporary trends in occupational therapy; other interfering factors have to do with client access.

Barriers for Therapists

Occupational therapists often have limited time to work with clients and may feel they lack adequate knowledge about leisure activities and resources, but this is an important area for intervention. Asking about leisure interests and desires allows occupational therapists to provide exploratory experiences in a monitored and controlled setting and offer the "just right" challenge to their clients. Moreover, we can follow up by forging relationships with community and recreational centers to encourage continued participation upon discharge (Procedures for Practice 34-1).

Barriers for Clients

Access to recreational and leisure pursuits may be difficult for persons with disabilities. Personal, environmental, and societal factors may all limit leisure participation. Personal factors may include fatigue, pain, depression, comorbid illness, and medical condition. Activity safety and weather conditions may impact participation as well (Mallinson et al., 2005). Environmental barriers due to poorly designed parking lots and sidewalks without curb cuts may prevent access. A recreational facility may have outdated, inaccessible bathrooms. Transportation to a facility or center may also pose problems, as may the financial requirements for specialized equipment such as wheelchairs designed for specific sports and adapted sports equipment. It may be difficult to find coaches and other personnel who understand the needs of those with disabilities. Despite these possible barriers, it is vital that people with disabilities have support and encouragement from their family and friends to participate in leisure activities that interest them and are within their capabilities.

Attitudinal barriers in our society are often more disabling than personal and environmental barriers. Individuals with disabilities such as tetraplegia and bilateral upper or lower extremity amputations may not believe that they are capable of participating in a variety of activities because of the attitudes of others. Advances in technology and changes in attitudes have allowed people with spinal cord injury and neuromuscular diseases to water ski using a sit ski; people with hand amputations can wind surf using sport-specific prostheses; wheelchair users can rock climb with special equipment; fishermen can fish (Fig. 34-4); and individuals with lower extremity amputations can play tennis (Fig. 34-5). Self-defense classes have been formed for community dwellers with visual impairments (Fig. 34-6). Wheelchairs designed specifically for use on the beach have been developed in addition to numerous models for various sports. With developing technology, opportunities to engage in numerous activities are possible if there is interest and motivation on the part of the therapist and the individual (Fig. 34-7).

In conclusion, human occupation is commonly taken for granted, and its health benefits are not acknowledged (Wilcock, 1998). This is even more pronounced in leisure. Engagement in leisure promotes health and decreases medical costs. Efforts to provide leisure opportunities for adults with disabilities are gradually increasing as we shift from hospital- to community-based treatment. Our renewed interest in community-based intervention supports our efforts to encourage leisure exploration and develop leisure programs for *all* people. Occupational therapists can become more aware of existing leisure opportunities and integrate leisure activities into assessment and treatment. By forming partnerships to develop and promote leisure options in new areas for people with disabilities, we can improve quality of life.

PROCEDURES FOR PRACTICE 34-1

Strategies to Promote Leisure

- Elicit enthusiasm and support from health professionals through in-service education that links leisure, health, and quality of life.
- Elicit support from family and friends.
- Identify interest and enjoyment in activity via leisure assessments and interviewing techniques.
- Evaluate for special needs and assist in choosing an appropriate activity based on current abilities.
- Provide exposure to activity and establish a schedule to learn.
- Set basic goals for activity that can be mastered early, and establish more challenging goals with progress.
- Follow up to evaluate success and to make possible adjustments.
- Create opportunities to reinforce engaging in activity that may be external or internal (longer lasting effect).

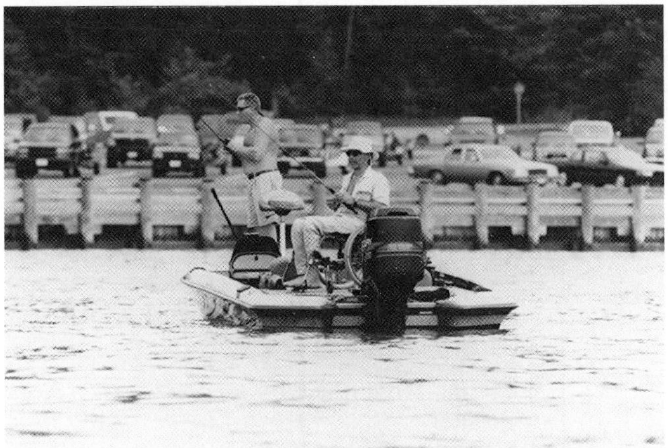

Figure 34-4 Technology to allow independent fishing from a wheelchair. (Photo by Gary Rudolph.)

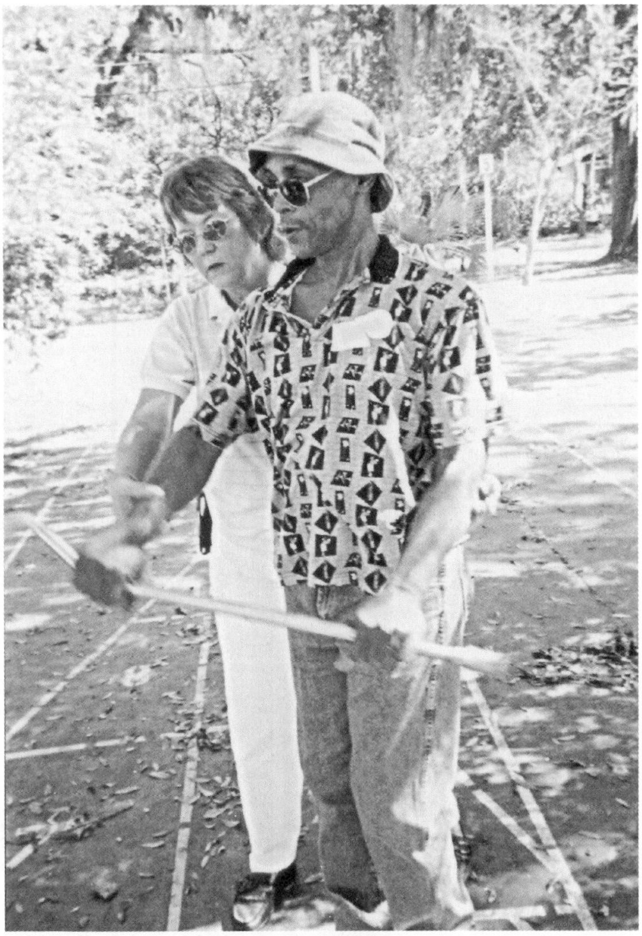

Figure 34-6 Self-defense training with the visually impaired.

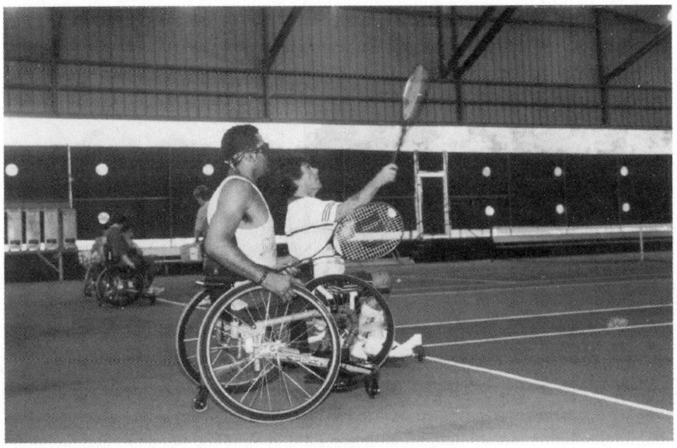

Figure 34-5 Active leisure: wheelchair tennis.

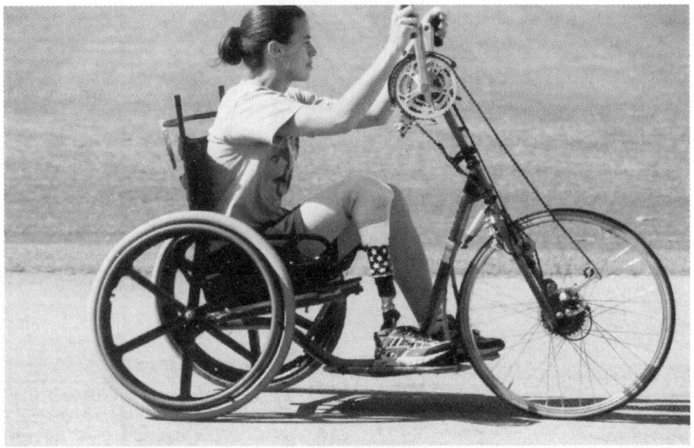

Figure 34-7 Independent or group activity: hand-crank three-wheeled bicycle.

Evidence Table 34-1

Intervention	Description of Intervention Tested	Participants	Dosage	Type of Best Evidence and Level of Evidence	Benefit	Statistical Probability and Effect Size of Outcome	Reference
Leisure rehab vs. IADL treatment	Leisure group: Sports and games, gardening, entertainment. IADL group: Mobility, transfer training, dressing, cooking, bathing.	309 stroke survivors.	Median number of sessions = 10 sessions; median duration of sessions = 55 minutes.	Randomized, controlled trial. 1A1a	No difference between leisure rehab group and IADL group on outcome measures of leisure participation or functional training.	N/A No statistically significant differences.	Logan et al., 2003
Leisure activity; in-home treatment	Leisure activity training vs. leisure discussion about effects of stroke.	40 stroke survivors; mean age = 69.6 years.	60-minute sessions once a week for 5 weeks.	Experimental and control group. IB1a	No. Leisure activities training group did not have significantly increased scores on *Katz Adjustment Index*. Low dose of therapy is ineffective.	No significant differences between groups on activity level and satisfaction with free-time activity.	Jongbloed & Morgan, 1991

SUMMARY REVIEW QUESTIONS

1. How would you define leisure to a patient?
2. What are the benefits of engaging in quiet leisure? Active leisure? Socialization?
3. How might leisure goals be different for someone with a stroke? Spinal cord injury? Lower extremity amputation?
4. Describe specific ways that occupational therapists can integrate leisure into evaluation and treatment.
5. What kinds of barriers limit leisure introduction and exploration? How would you remove those barriers in your own practice?
6. Describe the ways in which leisure activities enhance health and wellness for all people, including individuals with disabilities.
7. Discuss the advantages and disadvantages of the various types of leisure assessments described in this chapter.
8. What leisure activities would you recommend for people with no lower extremity use? No use of one side of the body? Overall general weakness?

ACKNOWLEDGMENT

We thank Pat Dasler for her case study contribution and Laurie Manuel and Gary Rudolph for the photographs.

References

American Occupational Therapy Association [AOTA]. (2002). Occupational therapy practice framework: Domain and process. *American Journal of Occupational Therapy, 56,* 609–639.

Beard, J. G., & Ragheb, M. G. (1980). Measuring leisure satisfaction. *Journal of Leisure Research, 12,* 20–33.

Beard, J. G., & Ragheb, M. G. (1983). Measuring leisure motivation. *Journal of Leisure Research, 15,* 219–228.

Beard, J. G., & Ragheb, M. G. (1990). Leisure Interest Measure. Paper presented at the meeting of the National Recreation and Park Association Symposium on Leisure Research, Phoenix, AZ.

Brachtesende, A. (2005). ICF: The universal translator. *OT Practice, 10,* 14–17.

Coyle, C. P., & Santiago, M. C. (1995). Aerobic exercise training and depressive symptomatology in adults with physical disabilities. *Archives of Physical Medicine and Rehabilitation, 76,* 647–652.

Drew, J., & Rugg, S. (2000). Activity use in occupational therapy: OT students' fieldwork experience. *British Journal of Occupational Therapy, 64,* 478–486.

Drummond, A., & Walker, M. (1994). The Nottingham Leisure Questionnaire for stroke patients. *British Journal of Occupational Therapy, 57,* 414–418.

Durstine, J. L., Painter, P., Franklin, B. A., Morgan, D., Pitetti, K. H., & Roberts, S.O. (2000). Physical activity for the chronically ill and disabled. *Sports Medicine, 30,* 207–219.

Hanson, C. S. (1998). A sports exploration camp for adults with disabilities. *OT Practice, 3,* 35–38.

Harnish, S. (2001). Gardening for life- adaptive techniques and tools. *OT Practice, 6,* 12–15.

Hoffmann, L., Williford, R., Mooney, B., Brown, C., & Davis, C. (1995). Leisure activities provide rehab potential. *Case Management Advisor, 6,* 71.

Hollar, L. D. (1995). Spinal cord injury. In C. A. Trombly (Ed.), *Occupational therapy for physical dysfunction* (4th ed., pp. 795–813). Baltimore: Williams & Wilkins.

Jungbloed, L., & Morgan, D. (1991). An investigation of involvement in leisure activities after stroke. *American Journal of Occupational Therapy, 45,* 420–427.

Kautzmann, L. (1984). Identifying leisure interests: A self-assessment approach for adults with arthritis. *Occupational Therapy in Health Care, 2,* 45–51.

Kinney, W. B., & Coyle, C. P. (1992). Predicting life satisfaction among adults with physical disabilities. *Archives of Physical Medicine and Rehabilitation, 73,* 863–869.

Klein, P. J., & Adams, W. D. (2004). Comprehensive therapeutic benefits of taiji: A critical review. *American Journal of Physical Medicine, 83,* 735–745.

Kuster, M. S. (2002). Exercise recommendations after total joint replacement. *Sports Medicine, 32,* 433–445.

Law, M. (2002). Participation in the occupations of everyday life. *American Journal of Occupational Therapy, 56,* 640–649.

Law, M., Polatajko, H., Pollock, N., McColl, M. A., Carswell, A., & Baptiste, S. (1994). Pilot testing of the Canadian Occupational Performance Measure: Clinical and measurement issues. *Canadian Journal of Occupational Therapy, 61,* 191–197.

Lin, S. (1991). Content validity and test-retest reliability of the Lin Interest Check List. Unpublished thesis. Richmond: Virginia Commonwealth University.

Logan, P. A., Gladman, J. R. F., Drummond, A. E. R., & Radford, K. A. (2003). A study of interventions and related outcomes in a randomized controlled trial of occupational therapy and leisure therapy for community stroke patients. *Clinical Rehabilitation, 17,* 249–255.

Mallinson, T., Waldinger, H., Semanik, P., Lyons, J., Feinglass, J., & Chang, R. W. (2005). Promoting physical activity in persons with arthritis. *OT Practice, 10,* 10–14.

Matsutsuyu, J. (1967). The Interest Checklist. *American Journal of Occupational Therapy, 11,* 170–181.

Minor, M. A., & Lane, N. E. (1996). Recreational exercise in arthritis. *Rheumatic Disease Clinics of North America, 22,* 563–577.

Primeau, L. A. (1996). Work and leisure: Transcending the dichotomy. *American Journal of Occupational Therapy, 50,* 569–577.

Ragheb, M. G., & Beard, J. G. (1982). Measuring leisure attitude. *Journal of Leisure Research, 14,* 155–167.

Sacco, R. L., Gan, R., Boden-Albala, B., Lin, I. F., Kargman, D. E, Hauser, W. A., Shea, S., & Paik, M. C. (1998). Leisure-time physical activity and ischemic stroke risk: The Northern Manhattan Stroke Study. *Stroke, 29,* 380–387.

Soderback, I., & Hammarlund, C. (1993). A leisure-time frame of reference based on a literature analysis. *Occupational Therapy in Health Care, 8,* 105–133.

Trombly, C. A. (2002). Conceptual foundations for practice. In C. A. Trombly & M. V. Radomski (Eds.), *Occupational therapy for physical dysfunction* (5th ed., pp. 1–15). Baltimore: Lippincott Williams & Wilkins.

Washburn, R. A., Zhu, W., McAuley, E., Frogley, M., & Figoni, S. F. (2002). The physical activity scale for individuals with physical disabilities: Development and evaluation. *Archives of Physical Medicine and Rehabilitation, 83,* 193–200.

Wilcock, A. A. (1998). Occupation for health. *British Journal of Occupational Therapy, 61,* 340–345.

Wu, S. K., & Williams, T. (2000). Factors influencing sport participation among athletes with spinal cord injury. *Medicine and Science in Sports and Exercise, 33,* 177–182.

CHAPTER 35

LEARNING OBJECTIVES

After studying this chapter, the reader will be able to do the following:

1. Integrate the psychosocial perspective in formulating a rehabilitation program.
2. Consider alternative practice models and value their application within the therapeutic relationship.
3. Place patients within life cycle and family contexts and recognize the implications of this placement for occupations and life roles.
4. Understand the impact of history and course of disability on psychosocial adaptation.
5. Appreciate existential issues raised by illness, injury, and disability; describe ways individuals construct meaning from these experiences.
6. Be alert for psychiatric complications and recognize indications for referral.

Optimizing Personal and Social Adaptation

Jo M. Solet

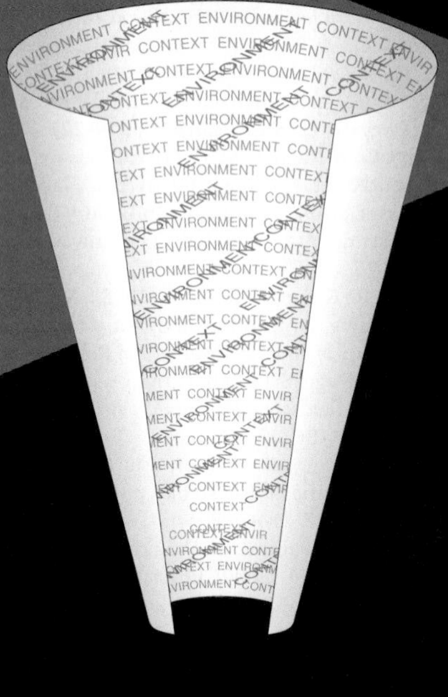

Glossary

Adaptation—Alteration or adjustment by which an individual or species improves its condition in relation to its situation or environment.

Attribution—Assigned cause or the process by which an individual assigns cause.

Continuity—The quality of persisting over time in an uninterrupted way.

Coping—Cognitive, emotional, and behavioral efforts individuals make to manage external and internal challenges that tax their ordinary resources.

Existential—Description of a perspective that emphasizes the human condition, including the felt necessity to create meaning in a universe that seems indifferent.

Pathography—Written personal story of illness or injury.

Post-Traumatic Stress Disorder (PTSD)—Lasting psychological response to witnessing or experiencing traumatic events, especially when helpless to prevent them.

Relaxation Response—Inborn human capacity to enter a special physiological state characterized by slowed brain waves, lowered heart and respiratory rates, and lowered blood pressure, which is believed to be health enhancing.

Retribution—That which is given or demanded as repayment or punishment for transgression; penance.

Termination—Period of closing a therapeutic relationship at the end of treatment.

"Man's origin is dust and his end is dust. He spends his life earning bread. He is a clay vessel, easily broken, like withering grass, a fading flower, a passing shadow, a fugitive cloud, a fleeting breeze, a scattering dust, a vanishing dream." —*Mazor for Rosh Hashanah and Yom Kippur: A Prayer Book for the Days of Awe* (1972)

The immediate change in physical functioning that an individual undergoes as a result of illness or injury is not alone a sufficient predictor of the capacity to benefit from treatment or of the future quality of life. Although the **adaptation** process may follow a general outline of stages, it is unique for each person and is influenced by the circumstances of onset and course, by the age and place in the life cycle, by the specific personality with characteristic ways of **coping** and finding meaning, and by the availability of family support. This chapter begins by introducing practice models and treatment structures that address the psychosocial perspective and then guides the reader through each of these life contexts, psychological, and social factors, which must be considered in individualizing occupational therapy treatment for physical disabilities (Procedures for Practice 35-1).

PRACTICE MODELS

Each practice model uses its own theoretical framework to interpret clinical observations, guide treatment planning, and promote recovery. Many occupational therapists use components of more than one of these models; they find this can lead to rich, empathic, creative treatment and fruitful participation with the treatment team.

Psychodynamic Model

The psychodynamic practice model, which had its origin in Freud's theories, emphasizes the relationship with the therapist as providing a safe, empathic, and consistent environment in which healing may take place (Rowe & MacIsaac, 1991). It considers patients' internal experiences; conscious and unconscious longings for wholeness, love, and protection; and conflicts about dependency and helplessness. Motivation is conceived as the critical element for successful rehabilitation. The psychodynamic model both values the symbolic nature of activities and mandates that they be selected for intrinsic meaning and relevance for the patient. It advises special care in the ending of treatment, known as **termination**.

Cognitive-Behavioral Model

The cognitive-behavioral practice model focuses therapeutic efforts on the development of patterns of thinking and specific behaviors (Burns, 1990). Therapists who use a cognitive-behavioral model are careful observers and recorders who look for patients' reactions to their environment and for interactions between their ways of thinking and ways of behaving. These therapists enhance motivation through planned rewarding of successive graded goals, called reinforcement; they shape thoughts and behaviors that indicate successful adaptation and

PROCEDURES FOR PRACTICE 35-1

Attending to Psychosocial Aspects of Physical Disabilities

In attending to the psychosocial aspects of physical disabilities, the occupational therapist works in partnership with patients to develop, reorganize, or restore occupational performance and life roles.

- The occupational therapist serves as a caring, consistent guide in patients' efforts to find meaning and as a resource for knowledge, skills, and competencies in personal, interpersonal, social, and vocational arenas.
- The occupational therapist, through both group and individual treatment, acknowledges and addresses patients' feelings, personal and social histories, and the contexts within which they live and work.
- The occupational therapist identifies strengths, assets, and possibilities with the goal of mobilizing patients' motivation and coping abilities and encouraging full participation in rehabilitation.
- The occupational therapist serves as an interface with patients' families.
- The occupational therapist directs the focus of the treatment team to the recognition and integration of the multiple dimensions of patients' life roles and relates the effect of altered capacities upon these life roles.

extinguish those that are maladaptive. For example, they reinforce treatment adherence and good self-care, such as wearing a splint or taking medication, and work to extinguish health-damaging habits, such as smoking, and socially isolating behaviors, such as aggressive outbursts. Skills for self-regulation, including the **relaxation response** and assertive communication, are also often components of cognitive-behavioral treatment (Basco, 1993).

Model of Human Occupation

Although the cognitive-behavioral and psychodynamic models are also applied by psychologists, social workers, and psychiatrists, the Model of Human Occupation (Kielhofner, 1992) evolved in the context of occupational therapy. This model focuses on engagement in purposeful activities and their central place in the experience of living. The client is recognized as "an occupational being for whom access and participation in meaningful and productive activities is central to health and well-being" (American Occupational Therapy Association [AOTA], 2002, p. 613). Human activities are defined as multidimensional physical, social, spiritual, and symbolic and as embedded within each individual's specific physical, psychological, and cultural contexts. Evaluation in this model considers strengths and difficulties in occupational behaviors that are necessary to the fulfillment of life roles such as worker, parent, or friend. Treatment seeks to develop, remediate, or enhance performance. Success in occupational performance is inherently organizing to the personality and is importantly related to feelings of mastery, competence, group acceptance, and sense of identity (AOTA, 1995a, 1995b).

Wellness Model

Research over the past decade confirms that we function as integrated organisms, with changes in one bodily system felt throughout. Separation of the mind from the body is increasingly understood to be an academic exercise rather than a true reflection of the functioning of the human organism. For example, mainstream medicine now recognizes important relationships between immune functioning and psychological health first proposed in the early 1980s (Ader, 1981). Psychological states such as depression (Denollet, 1998) and anxiety (Kubzansky et al., 1998) are now routinely assessed as risk factors for heart disease, not just as reactions to it. In addition, the growing preventive perspective in healthcare has begun to define the behaviors and habits related to sleep (Edinger & Erwin, 1992), nutrition (Buning, 1999), and exercise (Thoren et al., 1990) that, through multiple inter-connected channels, are likely to extend life and lead to greater physical and psychological well-being. Health behaviors may be difficult to address and psychological well-being may be difficult to achieve in the face of the stresses of physical disability; these often include pain and limited mobility, compromised social integration, and altered sleep and appetite. Specific health-promoting interventions support maintenance of function and reserve capacity of organ systems in those with chronic disabling conditions (Kemp, 2005; Stuifbergen et al., 2004). The occupational therapist works with other members of the clinical team to ensure that treatment addresses a foundation of these health-promoting behaviors that can be integrated into patient routines after discharge (Johnson, 1986).

PRACTICE STRUCTURES

Occupational therapists work with patients individually and in groups. Group participation is often an adjunct to or follow-up for individual treatment.

Individual Treatment

Individual treatment is framed by the therapeutic relationship, the alliance between a patient and therapist, which begins during the evaluation period. As the relationship develops, the occupational therapist learns not only about the physical capacities of the patient, such as strength and range of motion, but also about the type and degree of explanation the patient will find helpful during the course of treatment.

Patients who retain the capacity may wish to tell their story, describing to the occupational therapist how the illness or injury came to pass, their reactions to it, their losses, and their expectations of recovery. Listening attentively to patients' stories, even when their histories are available in some form in the charts, develops trust and tells patients that they are unique and their feelings and experiences are valued. Listening also supplies important information about interaction and communication ability, mood states such as depression or anxiety, ways of coping, and family and cultural contexts. All of these are critical to formulating social and psychological goals as part of intervention planning.

Group Treatment

Group treatment supplies a practice environment for patients' social participation, a therapeutic envelope or safe holding environment that is broader than that of individual treatment. Group treatment interrupts isolation and provides a context within which to identify and solve common problems (Ziegler, 1999). Groups may be organized to address goals related to specific disabilities, to promote mastery of skills, to practice leisure or creative activities, or to facilitate transitions. Although the primary focus of the group may not be to address psychological or social needs, treatment components influence patients' total well-being and provide a shared space for creating dignity, responsibility, meaning, and pleasure (Ziegler, 1999).

As groups evolve beyond parallel participation into interaction among members, patients support and learn from each other and begin to value themselves more highly. A group can also serve as a magnifying glass in which difficult behavior can be brought under the observation of others. When supportive confrontation is used to address and modify this behavior, it improves an individual's opportunities outside the treatment setting. When group discussions deepen, they provide for disclosure of grief and fears, for voicing **existential concerns**, for organizing personal narratives, and for engendering shared hopes (Alonso & Swiller, 1993; Weber, 1993). Occupational therapists include these social and psychological goals in all group planning, treatment, and documentation (Procedures for Practice 35-2).

PROCEDURES FOR PRACTICE 35-2

Planning Group Treatment

Choosing Goals for Group Participation

- Practicing social behaviors
- Following rules and recognizing group needs
- Identifying and solving common problems
- Learning specific skills and activities
- Accepting supportive confrontation and modifying behavior
- Disclosing feelings, existential concerns, and shared hopes
- Enhancing self-esteem through supporting others

Considerations for Choosing Group Members

- Cognitive and social capacities
- Readiness for broader interaction
- Congruence with other members
- Attention and memory
- Psychosis and dangerousness
- Communication ability
- Cultural background
- Energy limits

THE ADAPTATION PROCESS

The substantial variations in psychological and social adaptation to disability are related to the diability's onset and course, the patient's age and place in the life cycle, and individual differences in personality, ways of coping, and attributing meaning to experience.

Stage Theories

Viewing adaptation to disability as a natural course of stages such as shock, denial, anger, depression, and acceptance can be a useful way to conceptualize the psychological reorganization associated with an illness or injury (Miner, 1999). In reality, these stages may flow together and even be reexperienced as new challenges arise (Dewar & Lee, 2000). Clinicians may unconsciously protect themselves from recognizing the realities of living with a disability by assuming that all patients are passing through a natural series of stages that will eventually lead to a satisfying outcome; not all disabled individuals reach a stage of acceptance or well-being.

The four stages from acute injury through rehabilitation described by Morse and O'Brien (1995) constitute a template, summarized next, that may help therapists to recognize changing psychological states and anticipate the needs of their patients. The empirical study of traumatic injury and hospitalization upon which the stages are based demonstrates the special challenges of traumatic onset and offers illustrations of each stage using the language of patients' own recollections.

The first stage, "vigilance: becoming engulfed," encompasses the overwhelming physiological insult in which extraordinary cognitive efforts and heightened senses are recruited to preserve life. During this period immediately following traumatic injury, some patients in the study recalled detachment, a sense of being both observer and participant, as they began to direct the helpers who had arrived to care for them.

The second stage, "disruption: taking time out," begins when the individual relinquishes responsibility to caregivers or becomes unconscious. Patients remembered this part of their experience as a fog in which they were lost between nightmares and intolerable wakefulness. Patients in critical condition could not distinguish reality or focus beyond themselves. They were disoriented, heavily sedated, and not in control of their reactions. Patients at this stage sometimes perceived their caregivers as dangerous and the environment as hostile. Recognizing that during this stage many patients are afraid to be alone, the occupational therapist in the acute setting may facilitate the continuous presence of friends and family members, enlisting their help in orienting the patient.

The third stage, "enduring the self: confronting and regrouping," starts as the patient becomes more aware of his or her surroundings and begins to recognize the extent of the injuries. This is a time of focus on the present in which the conscious decision to carry on and rejoin the world must be made, even as growing awareness intensifies the psychological pain. Patients in the study described fear, panic over complete dependence, dread of painful treatments, and desperate efforts at control. During this stage, patients expressed shock at the loss of their former selves and began to anchor to staff and others for support and assistance. Some expressed an idealized view of their past selves as competent and attractive and their lives before the disablement as fully satisfying. Often they believed full recovery would occur in weeks or months, even with severe spinal cord injuries; the smallest gains were very important.

This is a time when the sensitivity of caregivers is critical for supporting hope. The occupational therapist is careful not to break the patient's denial prematurely because this defense serves as protection against psychologically overwhelming losses. The therapist should also avoid making promises about the expected degree of recovery, since it may later prove to be unattainable, compromising the therapeutic relationship and leaving the patient feeling cheated, angry, resentful, and depressed (Davidhizer, 1997). An early intervention for certain patients during this stage is training in diaphragmatic breathing to induce the relaxation response. Breathing may provide the first avenue for perceived self-control. In addition, the relaxation response is associated with reduced pain and anxiety (Kabat-Zinn, 1991).

The last stage, "striving to regain the self: merging the old and new reality," is the period of physical and psychological challenge in which active rehabilitation takes place. The goals of active rehabilitation include making sense of the event, getting to know the altered body, and accepting the consequences of the experience, including the possibility of continued dependency. This is the stage at which patients may begin to revise and reformulate expectations. The occupational therapy treatment plan integrates these psychological demands and addresses them in concert with activities of daily living, strengthening, endurance, mobility, and prevocational training. As preparation for the social situations that may be encountered after discharge from the protective rehabilitation environment, treatment anticipates and addresses fears of inadequacy and of rejection by others (Gardner, 1999). Participation in group treatment, including role playing specific situations, such as facing direct questions about the disability or about altered appearance, may be a component of this social preparation.

Onset and Course

The circumstances of onset and the course of the specific disability are important factors influencing the adaptation process.

Early Acquisition

When an individual is born with a disability such as spina bifida or has an injury in early childhood, the sense of self develops continuously with the disability, typically within the framework of the family and often with the support of therapy mandated through school programs. The challenge for the individual born with a disability or disabled in early childhood is to grow into each life stage encountering new developmental challenges—physical, psychological, and social. A disability that does not have major effects in childhood may later become significant as cognitive, emotional, and behavioral demands change and expectations for independence increase (King et al., 1993; Simkins, 1999). A significant proportion of individuals with early disabilities later develop new medical, functional, and support needs as they reach their forties and fifties (Kemp, 2005). Through a series of interviews with adults disabled as children, King et al. (2003) identified three pathways—belonging, doing, and understanding—through which challenges were met at these life "turning points." Successful adaptation came though social support, described as feeling "believed in," through determination and the conviction that challenges could be met, and through realization, by changing beliefs and expectations.

Degenerative Illness

When disability has a slow onset and course, as is the case with degenerative illnesses such as rheumatoid arthritis and multiple sclerosis, increasing disability is expected. Degenerative illnesses are not fully predictable; the course may be slow or rapid, complicating efforts to retain control over the life course. Each loss can feel like a reminder, a new insult. In multiple sclerosis, for example, there may be plateaus or even periods when symptoms remit but later recur (Mairs, 1996). Post-poliomyelitis syndrome (PPS) occurs in a different pattern. Seventy percent of individuals who had a primary polio infection years before, develop new symptoms, such as fatigue, pain, and atrophy, that require them to revisit struggles from their past (Jonsson, Moller, & Grimby, 1998; Kemp, 2005; Kemp & Krause, 1999). Some may stretch to the limits of their physical capacity in an effort to maintain occupations intrinsic to their life roles and to remain connected to valued peer groups. Ideally, as symptoms progress, processes of realization and reorganization bring with them adaptation and an acceptable compromise including altered patterns of daily occupations (Thoren-Jonsson, 2001). Maintenance of a hopeful attitude can be difficult when stabilization or recovery is not anticipated (Lynch, Kroencke, & Denney, 2001). The challenges of degenerative illness are to continually adapt to reorganized life roles, maintain internal resources, and evolve concrete supports in the face of impending decline (Boeije et al., 2002).

Traumatic Injury and Illness of Rapid Onset

Traumatic injuries, such as spinal cord injury, and disease processes with extremely rapid onset, such as Guillain-Barré syndrome, do not allow for psychological preparation. The dramatic nature of the onset may quickly exhaust the reserves of friends and family. Affected individuals may undergo not only an immediate change in ability to function but also a discontinuity in time and sense of self, a loss of personal identity, and a shift in confidence about the world as safe and just (Gardner, 1999; Morse & O'Brien, 1995). The individual is also at risk for development of post-traumatic stress disorder, characterized by hyperarousal and reexperience of the trauma (Herman, 1992). The occupational therapist considers each of these in evaluation and treatment planning.

Disability and the Life Cycle

The developmental tasks of each period of life are biologically, socially, and culturally determined, and they build upon those that have preceded them (Franz & White, 1985). Therefore, the point in a person's life at which he or she becomes disabled, together with the trajectory of the disability, help to determine what will be entailed in the long-term process of adaptation (Boeije et al., 2002). The occupational therapist must keep in mind the normal demands of patients' period of life and consider ways these demands may be met within the context of disability.

Adolescence

Currently, 90% of those born in the United States with a disability live to at least age 20 (Shultz & Liptak, 1998). Along with the usual challenges of young adulthood, including transition from school to work and from parents and family to the broader community, those disabled at birth or in childhood must negotiate the change from child to adult healthcare. This can include losing long-term supportive relationships and taking increased responsibility for care coordination and decision making (Shultz & Liptak, 1998). When adolescents or young adults who have already acquired some independence from their parents become disabled, they may find being thrown back into childhood dependence especially painful. Psychological distress in adult rehabilitation inpatients has been reported to be greatest among these younger patients, decreasing with age (Laatsch & Shahani, 1996).

The emphasis on peer acceptance, athletic ability, physical appearance, and emerging sexuality at this time of life puts the disabled young adult at special risk for rejection and social isolation; development of social competence is an especially important contributor to successful adaptation (King et al., 1993). In addition, as they reach the age that society presumes coincides with independence, young adults no longer qualify for the mandated instruction and therapy available through many public schools. Each year 300,000 of the disabled students who depart the secondary schools in the United States do not go on to live independently; rather, they watch from the sidelines as their peers move on without them (Betz, 1998). Research confirms the need for community-based transition services to support adolescents with disabilities in "building bridges" to the adult world (Stewart et al., 2001).

Adulthood

The developmental tasks of adulthood may include confirming career choice, finding a partner, and parenting children. When an adult at this point in the life cycle becomes disabled, plans and conceptions about the future, which may already have been the focus of substantial effort, require reorganizing. Adapting to disability occurring at this stage may require altering vocational course, finding different leisure activities, redesigning an intimate partnership, and rebalancing parenting roles, just when some sense of competence and direction has been won (Rena, Moshe, & Abraham, 1996).

Midlife

A disability that strikes in midlife may find the individual at the peak of his or her career mastery and earning capacity, sometimes with adolescent children or aging parents as dependents. Although a history of successful coping with multiple life roles may already exist, this may be a difficult time to accommodate change and reorganize responsibilities (Quigly, 1995). Available resources may be limited, especially when the disabled person is the head of the household. A person disabled at midlife may feel prematurely aged, deprived of the anticipated leisure activity of healthy retirement and the hard-earned relief that follows discharge of career and parenting duties. In addition, marriage or intimate partnership may be at risk, as some non-disabled partners choose to avoid additional demands or to seek a different mate.

Later Life

Disability in later life, even at a time when health decline may be anticipated, threatens the individual's ability to participate in the community in which he or she may have a long history and feel an important identification. Isolation is common. The elderly person may be realistically worried about losing his or her home or may already be institutionalized. He may be concerned about being a financial or care burden to an aging partner or to children who are stressed by their own responsibilities. Anticipated generative roles such as grandparent or mentor, with the opportunity to offer wisdom and nurturance, may be short-circuited. An elderly disabled person may already have lost his social cohort and main supporting relationships. When additional disability is imposed on an already frail system, accommodation can be extremely difficult. Interests and leisure activities developed over a lifetime may have to be abandoned and efforts made to find other satisfactions (Hasselkus, 1991). Furthermore, the devaluation of the elderly in our society, commonly combined with limited financial resources, can compromise care and undermine motivation (Kemp, 1993). The experience of overwhelming loss without hope for the future can lead to despair. Just as she does when working with younger patients, the occupational therapist models a problem-solving mindset with realistic expectations, reconciling capacities and marshalling patient strengths toward sense of fulfillment (Bontje et al., 2004). When remaining time before death is limited, some elderly people feel an urgent need to undertake a life review, drawing together the strands of meaning from their past. The occupational therapist recognizes the privilege of participating in this life review process.

Individual Differences

The occupational therapist will find it helpful to remember that patients come to treatment with formed personalities and ways of interacting with the world that may or may not have been healthy or effective even before the injury or illness. In addition, patients may regress during hospitalization when deprived of their usual occupations, relationships, and areas of control, which served as supports to their personal and cultural identities. Some must deal with lost bowel or bladder function or inability to walk, capacities that they developed as babies. Others may have brain damage, altering memory or the ability to make plans or follow directions. Some patients have been hospitalized following traumatizing events that compromise psychological functioning. Those hospitalized for medical problems are known to suffer more psychiatric illness than their healthy peers, especially depression (Joseph, 2005). Some patients seem easy to treat; others are recalcitrant, uncooperative, or resistant. Some become increasingly demanding, asking for special treatment, breaking rules, and exhausting all efforts (Main, 1957). Some appeal to the therapist's wish to rescue them; others, in their failure to improve, stir feelings of disappointment, shame, and helplessness in the therapist (Groves, 1978; Kahana & Bibring, 1964). It is some comfort for the new occupational therapist to recognize that these are all part of the normal experience of being a clinician. Collegial support and knowledgeable supervision help with the treatment of difficult patients and the management of the therapist's feelings.

Personality

Individual differences in personality, along with variations in cultural context and personal history, contribute to the uniqueness of responses to illness and injury. For example, it is often said about head injury that it is not just the injury but the head that matters. Serious stresses may intensify normal fears, longings, and relationship demands. Ongoing pain, with the attendant loss of sleep and degraded sense of mastery, can further alter functioning. Psychiatric illness and character problems can be exacerbated by threats to physical health and the integrity of the body (Zegans, 1991). Each individual must be treated as unique. The occupational therapist should be prepared to recognize and address distinctions among an array of personality styles (Kahana & Bibring, 1964) and ways of coping (Solet, 1991), some of which are summarized next.

Personality characteristics that have driven an individual's career choices and have helped define his or her relationships may be a mismatch for the requirements of hospitalization. Patients who are orderly, punctual, and conscientious may find that perceived loss of control distorts their self-esteem. They may react by becoming demanding, inflexible, and obstinate; if they become openly angry, they may feel ashamed and conscience stricken (Kahana & Bibring, 1964). A clinical approach that is congenial, efficient, predictable, and routine and that includes explanations as well as inclusion in decision-making is most reassuring for these individuals. The occupational therapist takes special care in pacing and grading challenges to provide for periods of control and success.

Patients who have a history of loss, helplessness, abuse, or abandonment may react to illness or injury with fears that no one will take care of them. They may make intense, urgent demands, seem over-dependent, easily disappointed, occasionally impulsive, and insatiable in their need for reassurance. Some, feeling unlovable, may expect abandonment and may withdraw rather than cling (Kahana & Bibring, 1964). A successful clinical approach for these individuals includes readiness to give care and to show concern along with limit setting that is consistent and not punitive. Good coordination between team members is especially important for these patients, who sometimes compare team members or complain about one team member to another.

Some individuals act guarded or suspicious when hospitalized (Kahana & Bibring, 1964). These characteristics may be an intensified part of their usual personality but may also arise from the disorientation and lost **continuity** accompanying illness or injury. Neurological and sensory changes can make relatively ordinary events difficult for patients to interpret; a right-hemisphere lesion or even the loss of eyeglasses or a hearing aid may have important ramifications. The occupational therapist is alert to the variety of conditions and diagnoses that may relate to such behavior. Wary, suspicious patients may need continual orienting and often benefit from the reassurance and company of friends or family. The occupational therapist uses language patients can understand to acknowledge their worries, answer questions, and address complaints without arguing or reinforcing false observations. Especially if suspiciousness evolves or becomes more elaborate, the occupational therapist seeks neurological or psychiatric consultation.

Patients may react to their helpless state by asserting their importance, being smug or grandiose, or demanding that only the most esteemed clinicians be involved in their care. When they are deprived of the surroundings, belongings, and roles from which they derive status and identity, patients need confirmation that these are recognized. The occupational therapist uses history taking as a time to begin offering this recognition and acknowledgment. Repeatedly feeling forced to confront their impairments can provoke some patients to make compensatory claims of superiority. The therapist resists the urge to put these difficult patients in their place because such expressions of entitlement are often a sign of deep vulnerability (Groves, 1978). The occupational therapist is hopeful and points out areas of strength and strategies for ongoing effort (Keith, 1999).

Some patients seem to reject caregivers' efforts to reduce their suffering. They may appear self-sacrificing, have a history of bad luck, or even seem to revel in their misery (Kahana & Bibring, 1965). When patients do not seem to wish to recover, their symptoms may be serving a hidden purpose, such as penance or atonement. The occupational therapist may have to refer a patient who appears excessively guilt ridden for psychotherapy. Alternatively, illness or injury sometimes returns isolated or lonely people to a caring social environment from which they do not wish to be separated by recovery. Treatment planning should recognize needs for social stimulation and companionship. In collaboration with the patient, the occupational therapist organizes in advance for appropriate social contact after discharge.

Ways of Coping

Coping can be defined broadly as the cognitive, emotional, and behavioral efforts individuals make to manage external and internal challenges that tax their ordinary resources. Coping includes what people think, feel, and do in response to stress. Ways of coping can be understood as organized between three sets of poles: seeking versus withdrawing from social connections; seeking versus avoiding information and control; and expressing or repressing emotional reactions. Coping efforts contribute to health because they help define capacity for perceiving and reporting symptoms, for decision making, for complying with treatment demands, and for accepting comforting and support, all of which affect physiological processes and the sense of well-being (Stone & Porter, 1995).

Although individuals may have characteristic ways of coping that align with their personalities, the demands of any particular situation, including the length of time the challenge has lasted, are also important in determining ways of coping. For example, the period before surgery that provides the opportunity for active coping by seeking information and making decisions is very different from the post-surgical period, in which little control can be exercised and detachment or distraction may be most useful. In parallel fashion, coping with an acute health crisis may draw on different coping capacities from a patient and family than those required by an ongoing disability. As coping requirements change or awareness increases, the patient and family may reappraise their situation, recognizing new possibilities and drawing on additional resources.

In the clinical setting, ways of coping are assessed by self-report questionnaires, clinical observation checklists, and interviewing (Lazarus & Folkman, 1984; Solet, 1991; Nochi, 2000). As part of evaluation, the occupational therapist asks the patient and family members about prior challenges or crises and the coping efforts that were made. Treatment then draws on successful coping such as securing arrangements for continued religious participation during hospitalization when this has proven to be an important source of strength in the past (Larson & Milano, 1995). Treatment may also include active teaching to enlarge the patient's universe of coping alternatives. Examples include keeping a journal to encourage emotional expression (Pennebaker, 1995); participating in a specialized group to enhance social connection (Weber, 1993); gaining companionship, comfort, or direct help from a pet or animal assistant (Gal, 1999); practicing the relaxation response to decrease perceived pain and anxiety (Kabat-Zinn, 1991); and learning assertive communication to feel more confident asking questions, identifying goals, and collaborating in treatment decisions.

No particular way of coping is in itself good or bad; it must suit the individual in his specific circumstances. For example, coping by wishful thinking, denial, and withdrawal may serve important protective purposes early after an injury, when recognition of the extent of losses could overwhelm the individual. Recognizing that successful adaptation can involve cycles of approach and avoidance, the occupational therapist is cautious about fracturing patients' protective ways of coping; she is aware of possible reactions including anxiety, shame, and resentment (Martz, 2004; Thoren-Jonsson, 2001). An avoidant coping strategy when it lasts over an extended period can prevent full participation in treatment and limit needed emotional expression, knowledge acquisition, and social reintegration. Lasting avoidance, denial, or withdrawal may indicate overwhelming fears, guilt, or self-loathing or signal cognitive impairments and is cause for seeking psychiatric or neurological consultation.

THE SEARCH FOR MEANING

Occupational therapists are confronted daily with illness and injury. We grapple with ways to continually affirm our profession and to make sense of the suffering we witness (Peloquin, 2002). Our patients, facing these same questions of meaning, look to us not just for help in physical recovery but for our vision to guide them in interpreting their experiences. Their confrontation with the fragile nature of life may bring their deepest longings to the surface; they wish for vanished loved ones, protection, belonging, vigor, significance, and relief.

Existential Questions

> "What is really important for a life to be worth living? What is it others will say about me when I die? What will my life say? Those are the kinds of questions my brain was filled with after the accident. It's no wonder I couldn't focus on details when the questions of life were asking to be answered." (Lowenstein, 1999)

Our patients ask us to recognize and acknowledge these questions and longings. They offer us the privilege of helping them to reclaim personal continuity and to create meaningful life narratives, which integrate their experiences of illness or injury with changing self-concepts (Boeije et al., 2002; Helfrich, Kielhofner, & Mattingly, 1994; Nochi, 2000). They challenge us to seek and reinforce their motivation to heal and to nurture their well-being at critical turning points and in the face of what for some will be lasting physical compromise (Brendel et al., 2001; King et al., 2003). They need us to join with them in celebrating the presence of interior life, personal connection, and the mystery of existence despite ambiguity, painful loss, and the final certainty of death (Fig. 35-1).

Attributions

Meaning and belief systems are fundamentally woven into the human mind and society. The way we make sense of experience not only describes but actually affects our reality (Kleinman, 1988; Peloquin, 2002). Most people with an illness, injury, or traumatic life event eventually ask "Why

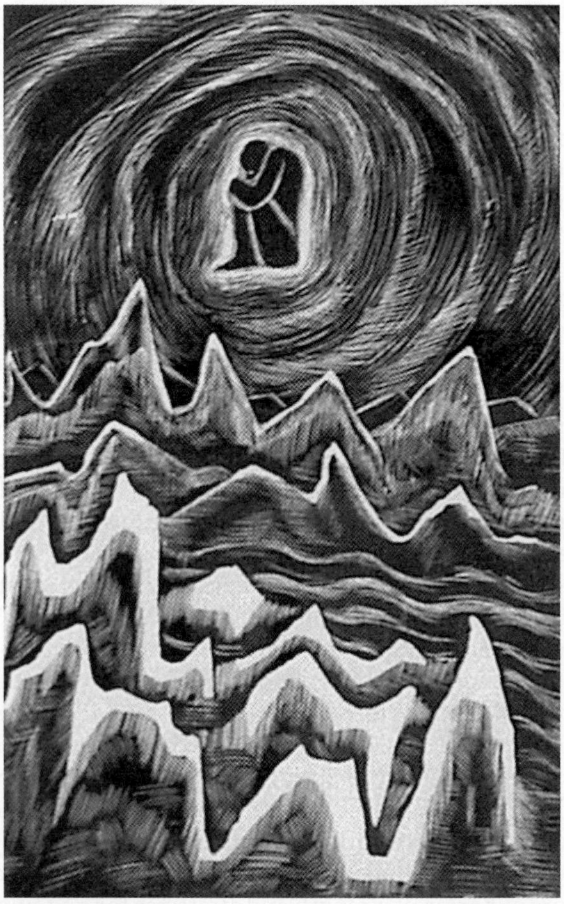

Figure 35-1 The Self in danger. (Pen and ink by Margaret Rusciano Tolksdorf, Pelham, NY.) See www.virtualeasel.com.

Table 35-1. Patient Attributions

Type of Attribution	Description of Individual and Situation	Quotation Showing Explanation for Illness or Injury
Retribution	Salesman drinking and driving, now a paraplegic following an accident	"I don't believe God could be persuaded to forgive me for killing a child in the accident."
Faith	Computer expert, mother, hit by an electronic garage door when dropping off her car for repair	"I have learned to live one level higher. Life requires a leap of faith when you no longer understand or validate in the same way. The intuitive comes to the forefront; before it stood behind."
Personal responsibility	Poet, mother, rode as a passenger on an icy day in a car she knew to be in poor repair	"I never thought about what I was doing then, but since my injury I think about that choice all the time."
Victimization	College student, former swim champ, attacked when skinny dipping by hoods offended by his exposure in front of their girlfriends	"I am afraid the possibilities for my future are diminished. It is so hard to see friends and younger sibs going through school, finishing, moving on with their lives. I am NOT an evil guy; what is this for? When this happened, I was sure I had died and gone to purgatory."
Acceptance	Biochemist hit by a bus crossing the street	"Is there any reason the owl eats the bunny and not the other way around? Injury and death are part of all nature. I am different now: I have lost my arrogance."
Chance	Engaged woman following an accident that disabled her and killed her boyfriend	"People like to take credit for the good things and blame others for the bad things, but really, an awful lot happens by chance. The important thing is to be ready for the good things—and I am ready."

me?" and try to make an **attribution** about or create an explanation for their experience. Clinical research has demonstrated the range and character of these attributions (Solet, 1991) (Table 35-1). Dangoor and Florian (1994) have established sense of coherence, a measure of ability to construct meaning from experience, as more important than actual degree of disability in contributing to well-being among chronically disabled women.

Retribution

Some individuals see their illness or injury as a punishment, penance, or **retribution**. As children we are taught that when we break rules, we will be punished; thus, it may be natural on some deep level to believe that a painful event indicates badness or unworthiness deserving punishment. In actuality, no realistic connection may be present between patients' behavior and their injuries, or they may be accurate in describing a connection, such as a history of drunk driving or unsafe sexual practices. In either case, attributions of retribution can render individuals immobilized by guilt and shame, unable to seek information or emotional support or to participate actively in their own recovery (Solet, 1991). They may require support to forgive themselves; some also need to focus on altering their dangerous behaviors. The opportunity to be heard and the reality of being accepted by the occupational therapist can help them begin to value themselves, feel worthy of treatment, and invest in the future.

Victimization

Again, either through a realistic analysis or based on deep feelings alone, some patients see themselves as victims. Especially when facts support the construction, such as in an assault or an accident from a faulty product, the occupational therapist validates the attribution and acknowledges the loss of trust that accompanies such an experience. The risk for patients who make attributions of victimization is that they may take on the role of victim more broadly as a lasting self-characterization. They may be unable, because of fear, anger, or sense of helplessness, to see the world as a place that is safe to rejoin. The occupational therapist helps by showing the realistic boundaries of these beliefs and by being a reliable and trustworthy caregiver.

Chance

Chance or luck is sometimes invoked by patients to explain illness or injury. Such an arbitrary universe as these patients perceive may be seen as dangerous and out of control, a form of impersonal victimization. Alternatively, an arbitrary universe may be benign and open to individual willingness to accept not just loss but opportunity. The occupational therapist encourages patients who endorse chance to see hopeful possibilities.

Faith

Many patients demonstrate faith that their experience of illness or injury will, in the end, have meaning and purpose. These attributions based on faith need not exist only within the context of formal religion to engender optimism and encourage adaptation (Benson, 1995). They may convey a deep conviction that there is a plan for the universe in which good will ultimately prevail, a plan beyond ordinary human understanding (Rankin, 1985). Attributions of faith may be especially poignant for those who are isolated and have few relationships because of their disability, allowing them to feel deeply valued beyond their difficult individual circumstances (Solet, 1991). Recent research points to the healing nature of deep self-disclosure such as may take place in prayer (Pennebaker, 1995). Occupational therapists are open to hearing about patients' spiritual lives and practices as elements of culture and daily life that can support healing.

Narratives and Metaphors

Patients want to tell their stories, and they need to be heard. The process of constructing and sharing a narrative of illness or injury organizes experience, shapes continuing perceptions, and breaks isolation. Through narrative, patients connect the present to the past, forming continuity in their lives and identities (Spencer et al., 1995; Boeije et al., 2002).

Increasingly patients are turning to the Internet, especially to disease- or disability-specific chat groups to exchange narratives of their experiences and to offer support and treatment information. Recent analyses of some of these virtual communities has shown the information offered can be surprisingly accurate and sophisticated, with patients helping each other and family members to be more aware of treatment possibilities and more ready to be active partners in decision making (Hoch & Ferguson, 2005). Occupational therapists may help patients identify virtual communities connected to reputable sources and may serve as translators and interpreters when relevant material is complicated.

Occupational therapists use specific structures to collaborate with patients in interpreting their lives, including life charts, assisted autobiographies, and occupational storytelling (Frank, 1996). Through attentive listening, occupational therapists not only validate patients' experiences but also enhance their own clinical reasoning, tailoring empathic language and treatment activities to match patients' individual needs and motivations (Kautzman, 1992).

A common characteristic of these narratives is the use of certain metaphors that connect individuals' experiences to universal themes of culture and help to place their suffering in meaningful contexts. Hawkins (1993) described five metaphors that frequently serve as frames for interpreting illness or injury; each can be understood as coordinating with role expectations for the therapist and with specific risks for patient adaptation (Solet, 1994).

Rebirth

The metaphor of rebirth is a central religious and mythological theme. Through it, illness, injury, and the closeness of death are seen as transformative and regenerative (Hawkins, 1993). It is common for patients to reevaluate their lives around their illness or injury and to describe a profound altering of values and priorities. The old self dies and a new and different self is born through suffering. The change brought about through this confrontation can be experienced like a religious conversion; wisdom and spiritual renewal can become the gift and compensation for suffering. Part of the role of the occupational therapist is to bear witness to these changes. Sometimes the illness is equated with a life of sinfulness: drugs, unsafe sex, smoking, bad diet, and aggressive treatment of others. The patient may wish the therapist to serve in a priest's role, to grant absolution and confirm worthiness for care. The risk to patients using this metaphor is its association with attributions of deserved punishment, described earlier. Patients may become passive in penance, feel undeserving of health, and be unable to mobilize for the rigors of treatment (Solet, 1991).

Battle

The metaphor of battle is very common and is the most congruent with the Western system of medical care (Hawkins, 1993); it is frequently used by clinicians and politicians. We hear often of "the war on cancer" and "the war on drugs." In this metaphor, the patient becomes the hero doing battle with a monstrous foe; the therapist is the ally in "fighting disease." The illness or disease is seen as exogenous, from the outside, and a crusade is launched to attack it. This metaphor combines aggression with social optimism and dignifies the active, courageous stance known colloquially as "fighting spirit" (Walker, 1999). Although some patients may relate easily to this aggressive position, others, by personality or beliefs, are a poor match and find the metaphor disturbing. Furthermore, the battle metaphor of attack on the invader may not be fully suitable for some illnesses. Cancer cells are, in fact, not an external threat, like plague or tuberculosis, but parts of the self turned unruly. Pain can also be difficult to conceptualize as an invading adversary with which to do battle, since it may be experienced as from within by the patient. In treating rheumatoid arthritis and other autoimmune diseases, the goal is quite the contrary: to help the patient's body to stop fighting itself.

Athlete

Somewhat related to the battle metaphor is that of the athlete. The patient deals with illness as a game or sport in which the central issues are courage, stamina, and endurance (Hawkins, 1993). The therapist is the coach; the patient is in training; new skills are learned through practice. This is particularly effective for individuals who have a history of sports participation or are sports fans. The risk to patients with this metaphor is in its implications regarding performance. There is an audience in sports; there is competition for who is best; there are rules and standards that must be followed, and trespass may lead to shame, as if the game were lost. The requirement to be courageous and strong throughout the ordeal so as not to lose or disappoint may prevent real communion with others over the reality of suffering and the inevitability of death. It may be helpful to emphasize that patients, caregivers, and family are all part of the team.

Journey

Illness as journey is a common metaphor found in narratives in which the patient travels to the kingdom of the sick, returning with the gift of wisdom. Susan Sontag (1988), writing about cancer, describes the disease as granting "a more onerous citizenship" (p. 3). Within this metaphor, the therapist serves as a guide, having accompanied others in this same land. The journey of illness or injury may be a rite of passage involving degradation, humiliation, and depersonalization (Hawkins, 1993). This metaphor fits especially well with the loss of vision (Hull, 1990) or with traumatic brain injury and the period of rehabilitation (Keith, 1999; Lowenstein, 1999). The individual leaves the world of ordinary sensations and consciousness and finds that expectations must be redefined; roles and relationships are changed, and activities that were once taken for granted must be relearned or abandoned (Pasciewicz, 1987). One risk to patients with the journey metaphor is that it can lead to a perception of exile; injury, illness, and disability can be isolating, sometimes permanently. In a real sense, withdrawal from society may be the result when the individual cannot cope with alterations in appearance, personality, mastery, or ability to communicate. Historically, exile has been forced when behavior or appearances ranged far from society's accepted norms or when the spread of infectious diseases threatened others, as with AIDS or leprosy. Group participation with other "travelers" may help limit isolation.

Nature

In contrast to the four metaphors described earlier, the New Age metaphor places faith in the healing powers of nature, especially the efficacy of positive emotions. This metaphor may be construed as a reaction to aspects of modern medical care, which has been faulted for defining the patient as the passive focus of technology, subject to external treatment forces, rather than as a vessel filled with self-healing resources. The therapist's role here is as caring partner. The disease or injury may be described as presenting an opportunity to alter values or to recognize and integrate hidden powers of the self. The risk to patients is the sense of bafflement, failure, and shame they may feel if conscientious efforts are not rewarded with health. This construction emphasizes the requirement to be "positive," and individuals may develop guilt about their own normal feelings of grief, fear, or anger, believing that they are hindering their own recovery. They may be deprived of legitimate ownership of authentic feelings. This metaphor works best when the occupational therapist demonstrates belief in the goodness of the full spectrum of human feelings and in the whole cycle of nature, which includes not only spring but also winter.

Pathography

Occupational therapists may prepare themselves to respond with empathy to their patients' narratives by exploring published accounts of illness or injury known as **pathographies** (see supplemental reading list). Authors have many motivations, including trying to find meaning in their own experiences, consolidating changed identities, breaking isolation, validating others, offering hope or counsel, exposing inhumane care, and giving specific information about treatment alternatives. Some pathographies are inspiring tales of recovery or of transcendence over pain or disability (Hull, 1990), even over imminent death (Bauby, 1997; Broyard, 1992). Some are offered by family members as a testimonial to a loved one or a journal of the shared ordeal (Wiltshire, 1994); others aim to elevate natural healing capacities and transform our health care system (Barasch, 1993). Numerous popular films also depict disabled characters and their struggles and ways of coping. Such films, even when their stories are fictional, help us understand views of disability in our culture. For some patients or their families, the occupational therapist selects readings or films as an educational component of treatment.

THE HEALING CONTEXT

Although health care policy-makers assume families will provide a healing context for their disabled members, very little formal structure is in place to support their efforts (Levine, 1999). As our population ages and as advances in medical technology extend lives, the burden on family members is expected to grow. Idealizing or romanticizing the position of disabled individuals and their families avoids confronting the real deprivations many suffer and camouflages important ethical questions regarding responsibility for the allocation of societal resources (Saetersdal, 1997).

Family Care Giving

In the United States, more than 25 million unpaid informal caregivers provide an estimated $196 billion worth of labor; the overwhelming majority of these caregivers are family members (Rolland, 1993). More than 400,000 children under 11 years old and more than 1 million U.S. adolescents provide care for an adult family member with a chronic illness (*Boston Globe*, 2005). Evidence as to stress on partners and family members suggests some carry a level of responsibility that can damage their own health and well-being.

Loss of disabled persons' income often places these families in financial jeopardy. Dangoor and Florian (1994) identify socioeconomic status as one of the criteria that are more important than actual degree of disability in contributing to adaptation among chronically disabled women. In 1997, one third of adults with disabilities lived in households with an annual income less than $15,000, compared with only 12% of the non-disabled; Americans with disabilities spent four times as much on medical care, services, and equipment as their non-disabled counterparts (Kilborn, 1999).

Family Reorganization and Identity

In the United States, 6% of adults, 15.5 million people, are unable to perform a major life activity. Half a million adults with developmental disabilities are living with parents over age 65. Families with a newly disabled member or a disabled member who is losing functional capacity through the common pattern of accelerated aging, experience grief, increased demands, and changes in routines, roles, structures, and expectations, often on top of increased financial burdens (Lynch, Kaplan, & Shema, 1997; Kemp, 2005). Additional stresses may exacerbate preexisting marital discord or substance abuse. Such problems are reflected in the divorce rate, which is higher than normal among couples when one spouse is disabled, with men leaving their wives more frequently than the reverse (Kilborn, 1999). Adaptation requires learning and concrete planning as well as transformation within the family unit parallel to that of the disabled person. Partners and families struggle to construct ways of coping with specific problems and ways to forge new identities among themselves and within their communities.

Engaging with Family Members

The occupational therapist, often working in concert with a nurse or social worker, may be the major preparatory interface with the formal health care system for a family planning to receive a disabled member at home. To initiate collaboration with the family, the occupational therapist assesses readiness and does not force premature instruction that could frighten, anger, or alienate the family (Levine, 1999). In all contacts with the family, the occupational therapist remains aware of and respects the rights and wishes of the patient with regard to privacy and confidentiality (Procedures for Practice 35-3).

Important differences between what occupational therapists and family members value as treatment and support are common (Humphrey, Gonzalez, & Taylor,

PROCEDURES FOR PRACTICE 35-3

Engaging with Family Members

Goals of Interaction with Patients' Families

- Seeking information about family medical and social history
- Offering specific information about disability and treatment
- Collaborating and fostering inclusion in decision making
- Validating feelings
- Acknowledging experiences
- Fostering hope and successful coping
- Guiding reconnection with patient
- Instructing in issues of patient care and safety, including home visits and use of assistive devices
- Facilitating use of community resources, including barrier-free opportunities and support groups

Considering the Family Context

Try to answer the following questions when assessing a patient's family context.

- Where is the patient in the life cycle, and what have been the patient's roles and responsibilities?
- How have the roles, responsibilities, and expectations of family members been altered?
- Is there lost income and/or added expense?
- What family problems may be exacerbated by this crisis?
- How has the family coped with crises in the past?
- How will the likely course of the disability affect the family?
- How is the family making sense of the experience? Do they have a specific cultural perspective or religious belief?
- To what communities do they belong that may be a source of help or strength?
- Do they need referral for family counseling?

1992). Hasselkus (1991, 1994) found that occupational therapists focused treatment planning on disabled individuals' level of independence; family members, however, were more likely to express concern that their returning member be safely cared for with a sense of maintained identity. Ongoing life satisfaction rather than level of self-care is becoming recognized as the most valuable measure of rehabilitation success and one that may be more congruent with patient and family needs and expectations (Levine, 1987).

If the patient is to be discharged home, the occupational therapist typically accompanies the patient on a pre-discharge visit to check for safety and to organize installation of assistive devices. This is a good time to facilitate social participation by helping the patient (and family) become aware of community resources and barrier-free opportunities. Community connection is especially important to those living independently with a disability. The occupational therapist also connects the patient and family with specific support and advocacy groups through which they may share problem-solving, feel a sense of camaraderie, and be empowered if they choose to work to improve the system for themselves and others.

Some patients are discharged to separate quarters or to institutional settings. Discharge of a family member to a long-term care facility involves wrenching decisions and can feel like abandonment, especially in families whose traditional culture and values include loyalty and strong bonds among members (Banks, 2003; Turner & Alston, 1994). This is true even when it seems clear to the clinical community that taking the individual home would seriously overtake the resources of the family. The occupational therapist acknowledges these feelings and helps organize ways to maintain family relationships even when the disabled member will not be living at home.

In certain cases, family stress may be extreme, communication difficult, and reactions overwhelming. Family members may disagree over what care is appropriate for individuals who are not legally competent to make decisions about their own care. This happened in the case of Terry Schiavo (Quill, 2005), in which national attention was drawn to the court battles between her husband and parents over whether this brain-damaged woman was responsive and whether her condition warranted continuing life-sustaining interventions.

In non-traditional family constructions and partnerships, additional stresses may result from lack of legal recognition of couple and parenting commitments with the associated rights to direct and oversee care and to health insurance coverage. Currently in the United States, only Massachusetts legally recognizes marriage between individuals of the same gender, with civil unions recognized in Vermont, New Hampshire, and Connecticut (October 1, 2005) and same-gender domestic partnership legal in California (www.glad.org; www.lamdalegal.org). The laws here are evolving, with issues of cross recognition and transportability of rights across states still to be further defined. The 1996 Federal Defense of Marriage Act prevents same-gender couples from receiving certain Federal protections and tax benefits afforded traditional couples. Gay marriage is legally recognized throughout Canada.

Although most people fail to prepare legally for sudden illness or disability, when decline can be anticipated, as with degenerative illness, individual wishes can be discussed, powers of attorney can be organized, and health care proxies completed. Some hospitals make a practice of making forms and information available (Dr. Andrea Patenaude, personal communication, Dana-Farber Cancer Center, Boston, MA). Social workers, psychologists, and attorneys specifically trained for assisting couples and families may serve a critical role in marshaling resources, modeling expression and compassion, and guiding direction. When an illness has been shown to have possible genetic links, additional questions arise, including whether other family members should undertake testing and what the implications might be for pregnancy. Specially trained genetic counselors can clarify the ethics and science, supporting informed decision making (Patenaude, 2005). The occupational therapist is alert to the possible necessity of specialized referrals (Procedures for Practice 35-3).

Partnership and Sexuality

The unique role of occupational therapists in addressing both activity and meaning places them in an ideal position to include sexual well-being among treatment goals. Sexual well-being correlates with adjustment and satisfaction in other areas of life and is an important component of the partnership bond (Woods, 1984). As one of the activities of daily living, sexual activity merits an accepting, problem-solving focus.

To acknowledge and accept the sexual identity of their patients, occupational therapists become aware of their own beliefs and values and suspend judgment when these values differ from those of their patients. Even when the primary sexual counseling is done by another team member, such as a nurse, occupational therapists are prepared to recognize intimate needs within different stages of the life cycle and sexual orientations. They are prepared to initiate discussion of sexual activity, including birth control and safe practices, without being seductive or eroding clinically appropriate boundaries. Embarrassment or a sense of undesirability may prevent patients from raising sexual concerns themselves. The occupational therapist acquires sufficient medical and psychological background related to disabilities and sexuality to anticipate patients' needs and questions and to organize appropriate referrals.

Desire, sexual responsiveness, sensory channels, and mobility may be altered by disability (Basson, 1998; Hulter & Lundberg, 1995). The occupational therapist explicitly helps the disabled person by encouraging him or her to reconceptualize sexuality and sexual activity more broadly and to explore new possibilities for sexual expression. When the disabled individual has a consistent sexual partner, the therapist may offer the opportunity to include him or her in teaching or treatment sessions. A satisfying sexual relationship is learned; it is based on more than simple instinct or appetite and does not have to be unplanned or spontaneous to be fulfilling (Woods, 1984). The disabled person and his or her sexual partner may learn to adapt to periods of fatigue, continence timing, or requirements for special positioning.

Fears may contribute to the disabled person's hesitancy about sexual activity. Fear of rejection may be based on altered appearance or on perceptions of the social acceptance of the needs and desires of disabled people. These fears can discourage efforts to establish or maintain relationships. In some cases, especially when this coincides with depression or social isolation, referral for psychotherapy can be valuable. Patients with certain diagnoses may have been warned about the danger of overexertion and may harbor fears about heart attacks or strokes. Some patients fear being injured by sexual activity or anticipate increases in their pain. Here a physician knowledgeable in sexual medicine can be a critical resource. Informed and sensitive medical management, sometimes including medications, can help disabled individuals successfully address problems and claim their sexual selves.

In some settings, disabled individuals are vulnerable to sexual exploitation or abuse, especially when cognitive or verbal limitations prevent them from reporting their experiences or serving as reliable witnesses in a court of law. A significant fear of parents of disabled young adults relates to their children's vulnerability in this regard (Hallum & Krumholtz, 1993). Occupational therapists who work with such patients are aware and alert to these possibilities and meet legal and ethical requirements for reporting concerns.

COMPLICATING FACTORS

Substance abuse, pain, depression, and post-traumatic stress disorder are common complications of illness and injury that hinder adaptation and mandate specific treatments.

Substance Abuse

Illicit drug use in our society is highest among those who are marginalized and culturally or economically disenfranchised (Li & Ford, 1998; Moore & Li, 1994), among whom are many disabled individuals. Social isolation, losses producing painful feeling states, and traumatic experiences related to injury confer special vulnerability and suggest reasons disabled individuals are at higher than normal risk for substance abuse. Consistent with this observation, disabled vocational rehabilitation clients were shown to have higher use of illicit drugs in all categories, including crack cocaine and heroin, than the general public (Moore & Li, 1998).

Alcohol and drug use have been implicated not just as reactions to but also as causative agents in disability, most notably in relation to auto accidents. Research evidence points to alcohol as having a role in a significant number of spinal cord injuries (Heinemann, Mamott, & Schnoll, 1990). Beyond health complications such as malnutrition and liver disease, which may affect all abusers, disabled abusers may be at increased risk for adverse drug interactions, falls due to balance or mobility impairments, and sores and gastrointestinal bleeding that may go undetected because of sensory losses (Heinemann, 1993; Yarkony, 1993).

In studying users' history of drug choice, Khantzian (1990), who posited a self-medication theory of substance abuse, found that many had experimented with various classes of drugs and settled on any that offered a particular type of needed relief. For example, individuals used stimulants to relieve depression and hyperactivity, opioids to mute psychologically disorganizing feelings such as rage and aggression, and alcohol to break emotional constriction and allow for release or connection. Primary motivations for substance abuse, he concluded, are difficulties in managing feelings, low self-esteem, lack of supporting relationships, and poor self-care, which are particularly common among individuals with abusive or traumatic histories or severely deprived circumstances. Other factors found to be associated with illicit drug use among those with disabilities include best friend's drug use and history of high risk-taking (Moore & Li, 1998).

Meyer (1999) studied not only the neurobiology of addiction but its sociology as well. He concluded that for some individuals, drug use becomes a "career." Drug seeking grows into a main source of activity and occupation, especially when no compelling or achievable alternative can be perceived. The addict's lifestyle then becomes a further barrier to other avenues of fulfillment.

As members of the treatment team, occupational therapists are alert to the possibility of substance abuse, prepared to make appropriate referrals, and able to participate in humane, respectful care (Procedures for Practice 35-4). Well-designed substance abuse treatment addresses appropriate stages of recovery; is sensitive to ethnic, cultural, and linguistic differences; and is responsive to patients' particular needs (Cambridge Health Alliance, 1995). Treatment addresses the factors that may have predisposed the individual

PROCEDURES FOR PRACTICE 35-4

Addressing Substance Abuse

Considering Substance Abuse

- Take an occupational history. Was the patient functioning in work or school? Was the patient maintaining relationships?
- Are any family members likely to be helpful in understanding the patient's history?
- Is there any evidence that substance abuse was a primary cause of the condition?
- Might the condition have provoked substance abuse?
- Are there predisposing factors such as depression, trauma, family history of substance abuse, or membership in a marginalized group?
- Does evidence support need for referral?

Treatment Goals for Substance Abuse

- Improve health habits and self-care.
- Develop skills in self-regulation and impulse control.
- Experience group participation; learn to communicate needs; learn to give and receive support.
- Prepare for constructive vocational role.
- Value a clean and sober identity.
- Connect with community resources to maintain change.

to substance abuse, not just the behavior itself. Suggested treatment goals for substance abuse are listed in Procedures for Practice 35-4.

Pain

Although pain is not a diagnosis in itself, it can accompany many illnesses, injuries, and disabilities including spinal cord injury, acquired amputation, cerebral palsy, multiple sclerosis, and post-polio syndrome (Ehde et al., 2003). Along with subjective assessment of independence and severity of disability, the existence of pain has been found to be directly related to well-being among those with severe motor impairments (Dudgeon et al., 2002). Dudgeon's subjects described their experiences of chronic pain as a "personal venture," as "mysterious" with "unclear causes and consequences" and with "little or dissatisfying communication" about it found to be possible. More than a simple sensation, pain is a perception that emerges at the intersection of body, mind, and culture. Pain is an ineffable private experience that each individual must learn to interpret, but it is also a universal phenomenon with broad influence on society at large. A major contributor to healthcare use and a significant reason for lost work days and disability benefits, pain also adds significantly to family and marital discord (Grunebaum, 1996). An estimated 50 million Americans are partially or fully disabled by pain, with arthritis, headaches, and back pain among the largest contributors (Mayday Fund, 1998).

The Personal Experience of Pain

The daily reality of the individual in pain often includes sleeping difficulties, problems concentrating, and decreased mobility, which can limit all areas of occupational performance including work, recreation, and sexual expression. Altered moods, especially agitation or lethargy with depression, are common among those who have had pain over an extended period, multiple assessments without diagnosis, or multiple treatments without relief. Grief over lost mastery and diminished life roles with feelings of rage, helplessness, victimization, and defectiveness can result, leading to social withdrawal. Prompt and preemptive treatment of pain is a strong priority, ideally before roles, relationships, and even identity become irretrievably eroded (Bridle, 1999; Carr & Goudas, 1999; Harris, Morley, & Barton, 2003).

Pain Treatment

A full pain treatment program includes pharmacological, educational, physical, and psychological components and is administered through a team of clinicians that includes an occupational therapist. Group and individual treatments are often combined. Education presents a mind–body pain model that both gives recognition to the stress and distress that accompany pain and supports the efficacy of several avenues of treatment (Solet, 1995). Recognition and validation are necessary elements because pain patients sometimes feel that no one understands or cares about the extent of their suffering (Main & Spanswick, 1991).

The mind–body model encourages patients to view their pain not as a simple response to tissue damage but as a complex experience that can be affected by many factors, such as positioning for activities, ways of thinking, and emotional reactions (Fields, 1997). Diary keeping (self-monitoring) provides information about which specific factors affect an individual's pain experience; this is vital for collaboration in treatment planning. Diary keeping also documents evidence of improvement, which bolsters patients' motivation and supports treatment adherence (see Clinical Reasoning box, Cognitions Associated with Pain).

The physical components of a pain treatment program can include instruction in body mechanics, and stretching, strengthening, aerobic exercise, pacing, massage, and acupuncture. The psychological components can include the relaxation response, biofeedback, cognitive therapy (modification of thought patterns), affect management

CLINICAL REASONING IN OCCUPATIONAL THERAPY PRACTICE

Cognitions Associated with Pain

Chronic pain is commonly associated with certain elements of self-narrative. As part of effective pain treatment, the individual must learn to become aware of and change thoughts or cognitions that are undermining function and self-esteem (Gallagher, 1997). The statements that follow might be uncovered through monitoring or in dialogue. Using Helplessness and Dependency as examples, write positive alternative statements for the other examples of Rumination and Retribution, Punishment in the spaces provided below.

Helplessness

- The pain prevents me from doing all the things I want to do.
- The pain makes me bad at everything I used to be good at.
- There is no point in trying.

Alternatives

- When I pace myself, I get things accomplished.
- It is harder to do some things, but I can still do many things well.

Dependency

- Everyone should take over for me because of the pain.
- I can't be expected to do anything when I feel like this.

Alternative

- Some things are harder to accomplish, but I can still do them. I will ask for help when I truly need it.

Rumination

- I have to attend to the pain every minute to be sure it is not getting worse.

Alternative ______________________________

____

Retribution, Punishment

- I must have done something to deserve this.

Alternative ______________________________

____

(control of emotional reactions), and training in assertive communication (Caudill, 1995; Gallagher, 1997). Each of these treatment components may contribute a degree of relief and help patients in managing their pain, even when complete relief is out of reach.

Depression

Theoretical debate and research over the etiology of depression continues, with exploration including reactions to loss, neurobiological mechanisms, and genetic predispositions. These explanations need not be mutually exclusive since the brain is the substrate for interpretation of personal experience. The frontal lobes, which mediate executive functions such as goal-directed activity, have been implicated in the neurobiological processes associated with depression (Powell & Miklowitz, 1994). Clinicians sometimes mistakenly assume that depression is simply a stage or normal reaction to a disabling illness or injury and that it will remit if left untreated. With periods of hospitalization so short in the current environment, those with lasting depression can be lost to follow-up.

Among medically ill older adults, major depression is experienced by an estimated 20%, and minor depression is experienced by an additional 20–30% (Koenig & George, 1998). Personal or family histories of depression constitute special risk factors following the onset of illness or injury. In some cases, depression is part of a larger picture that includes swings in energy level and emotions, called bipolar disorder or manic depression. Depression, whatever the cause or pattern, can undermine all areas of functioning and, when severe, is life-threatening. Presence of depression mandates referral for assessment, including for risk of suicide. As many as 15% of those who suffer from depression or bipolar disorder commit suicide each year; suicide is the ninth leading cause of death in the United States (Nemeroff, 1998).

Diagnosis and Treatment of Depression

Patients whose motivation to participate in treatment is sapped by significant or unrelenting depression not only lose a critical opportunity to reorganize life skills and identity in a protected setting but also fare poorly if depression remains untreated after discharge. Evidence supporting this relationship of mood to physical health is increasingly clear. Research demonstrates that depression is a risk factor for future heart disease (Denollet, 1998) and that depression increases the risk of dying after a heart attack or stroke (Nemeroff, 1998).

Making a diagnosis of depression in cases of ill, injured, or disabled patients can be complicated; symptoms customarily associated with depression, such as sleep or appetite change, can be directly related to the primary conditions for which some disabled patients are seeking care. In addition, actual brain damage may alter neurobiology.

Since occupational therapists often have a close and continuous relationship with their patients, their observations of behaviors, feelings, and ways of thinking contribute important information to diagnosis. The occupational therapist looks not only for somatic or bodily symptoms but also for cognitive and emotional signs of depression. These include indecisiveness, inability to concentrate, diminished interest or loss of pleasure in formerly enjoyable activities, feelings of worthlessness or excessive guilt, and recurrent thoughts of death or suicide (Nemeroff, 1998).

Patients with bipolar disorder commonly receive diagnostic attention during a depressive phase, and the full scope of their psychiatric illness is not always clear. As the implications for treatment are different, especially in terms of medications, it is important when considering depression also to look for any personal or family history of mania; symptoms include very high energy, sleeplessness, pressured speech, grandiose thinking, unbridled spending, and even delusions (Ghaemi & Sachs, 1999). Patients' lack of insight into and inability to report their own psychological state during manic periods is the rule.

The occupational therapist documents concerns about depression or mania in the medical record, including supporting observations, and brings this information to the attention of the treating physician or team to facilitate referral for psychiatric evaluation (Safety Note 35-1). Assessment for antidepressant and/or mood-stabilizing medications and psychotherapy is a high priority. Components of occupational therapy treatment for depression include restoring self-care and appetites, improving feelings of mastery through meaningful goal-directed activities, reframing self-defeating cognitions, and encouraging social integration.

SAFETY NOTE 35-1

Indications for Psychiatric Referral

- Inability or unwillingness to comply with treatment
- Substance abuse
- Uncontrolled pain
- Traumatic flashbacks or dissociation
- Depression with suicidal tendency
- Mania
- Hostility, agitation
- Paranoia, unwarranted fears
- Hearing voices, delusions
- Social isolation or withdrawal
- Extended denial
- Unresolved religious or existential crisis
- Overwhelming guilt
- Family upheaval

Post-Traumatic Stress Disorder

Individuals injured or disabled through war, natural disaster, accident, abuse, or violent crime are at special risk for the psychological symptom complex called **post-traumatic stress disorder (PTSD)**. Even those who have witnessed terror or extreme helplessness but are not themselves physically injured, which sometimes includes family members of the disabled person, may develop PTSD. Symptoms can include hyperarousal (vigilance), nervousness, fearfulness, nightmares, flashbacks (spontaneous re-experiencing), ruminations, and mental absence or dissociation (Herman, 1992). For some patients, the resulting disability may constitute life-long physical evidence of the traumatic experience, even serving as a proprioceptive cue or trigger for PTSD symptoms and continuing stress reactions. In addition, some disabilities, such as spinal cord injury, carry with them medical problems that can be life-threatening and serve as a further source of anxiety (Martz, 2004; Ville, 2001).

Individuals with symptoms of PTSD require immediate referral to be evaluated for specialized psychotherapy and medication. Coordination between caregivers is critical to a positive outcome for these patients, who need a safe, predictable environment in which they can make sense of their experiences. Listening to their narratives can be disturbing, so strong team support and supervision are important for all involved caregivers, including occupational therapists.

CASE EXAMPLE

Mr. D.: Adaptation Process after Stroke

I felt a Cleaving in my Mind-
As if my Brain had split-
I tried to match it-Seam by Seam-
But could not make them fit-
The thought behind, I strove to join
Unto the thought before-
But Sequence ravelled out of Sound-
Like Balls-upon a Floor-

Emily Dickinson (1830-1886)

Occupational Therapy Intervention Process	Clinical Reasoning Process	
	Objectives	**Examples of Therapist's Internal Dialogue**
Patient Information Mr. D. is a 53-year-old right-handed white man who suffered a severe right thalamic hemorrhage with rapid onset and steady improvement. His presenting problems at inpatient OT assessment included left hemiparesis; left homonymous hemianopsia; left neglect and anosognosia; disorientation to time and place; deficits in perception, attention, memory, and visuospatial processing; and complete dependence in activities of daily living. Mr. D. retained superior verbal ability, had an advanced education, strong family support, and adequate health insurance. He is a husband, father, and former university dean and public administrator and has been his family's primary breadwinner.	Appreciate the context	"Mr. D. was obviously in the prime of his career at the time of his stroke; it must have come as such a shock to him and his family. His vocational background suggests that he is used to being highly respected and in charge. He has been directing others, not accepting direction. I imagine that it will be particularly difficult for him to adjust to a dependent role of any duration. I will want to think of as many ways that he can be in control as possible and support his family in recognizing his needs in this regard." "With high school–aged children and a spouse who has not been working outside the home, financial pressures may add to the stress. I wonder if his wife may need to seek employment and may not be available as a caregiver for him when he returns home."
	Develop intervention hypotheses	"Mr. D.'s denial of the severity of his disability is a major obstacle to recognizing the need for and committing to OT treatment."
	Select an intervention approach	"I know it will be important that I show respect for his history of life roles by prioritizing OT goals related to intellectual and social skills and beginning with activities that emphasize compensation through his most preserved areas of function. This strategy should help increase his motivation and sense of personal continuity."
	Reflect on competence	"Mr. D.'s preserved verbal strengths will help in building our therapeutic alliance."
Recommendations Related to Personal and Social Adaptation The following goals were set for inpatient treatment (5 days/wk for 3 months) and outpatient follow-up: (1) foster therapeutic alliance; (2) identify/enlist motivating strategies; (3) consider past occupational roles and future adaptation; (4) encourage partnership in setting priorities for goals; (5) develop sense of mastery and control through specific skill development and relearning: reading, self-care, and mobility; and (6) guide the search for meaning.	Consider the patient's appraisal of performance Consider what will occur in therapy, how often, and for how long Ascertain the patient's endorsement of plan	"Trust will be critical in countering neurologically based denial. I must help him to believe there are good reasons for what I am asking of him. As his denial begins to break, the increased awareness of his losses will be painful; questions of meaning are likely to arise. I will try to help him find his own best way of making sense of his experiences. I will have to examine my own feelings about what has happened to him, a robust and gifted man at the height of his career." "I think that it is important to integrate safety and self-care goals into treatment if he is to return home without requiring a full-time aide. Continued dialogue will be needed to negotiate for attention to these goals and to address issues of physical dependency, which at present do not appear relevant to him."
Interventions Related to Personal and Social Adaptation Improve orientation to time and place. Solicit narrative of his experiences related to the stroke. Compensate for left visual field deficits and denial using cues from OT. Improve awareness/positioning and range of motion in left upper and lower extremities.	Assess the patient's comprehension Understand what he is doing	"I need to continually orient Mr. D. to his surrounding and circumstances and, later, to the OT role. Other staff and team members can be enlisted to help so that Mr. D. is getting a consistent message. Staff and team should be made aware of the effects of his neurological deficits on his reasoning and tendency to confabulate."

This case study follows the structure introduced in this chapter for integrating psychosocial components in treatment planning. The internal dialogue in the Case Example emphasizes these aspects as related to ongoing physical rehabilitation. The patient described, Mr. D., was in active inpatient rehabilitation for 3 months, followed by periodic home visits for outpatient treatment. Medical complications contributed to his unusually long length of stay. During the period following his stroke and after a second stroke until his death, he continued to correspond with this author, his occupational therapist. He expressed the wish that his experiences be used to help others. He often quoted the Emily Dickinson poem above. The accompanying series of drawings demonstrate his growing awareness during his inpatient stay (Fig. 35-2).

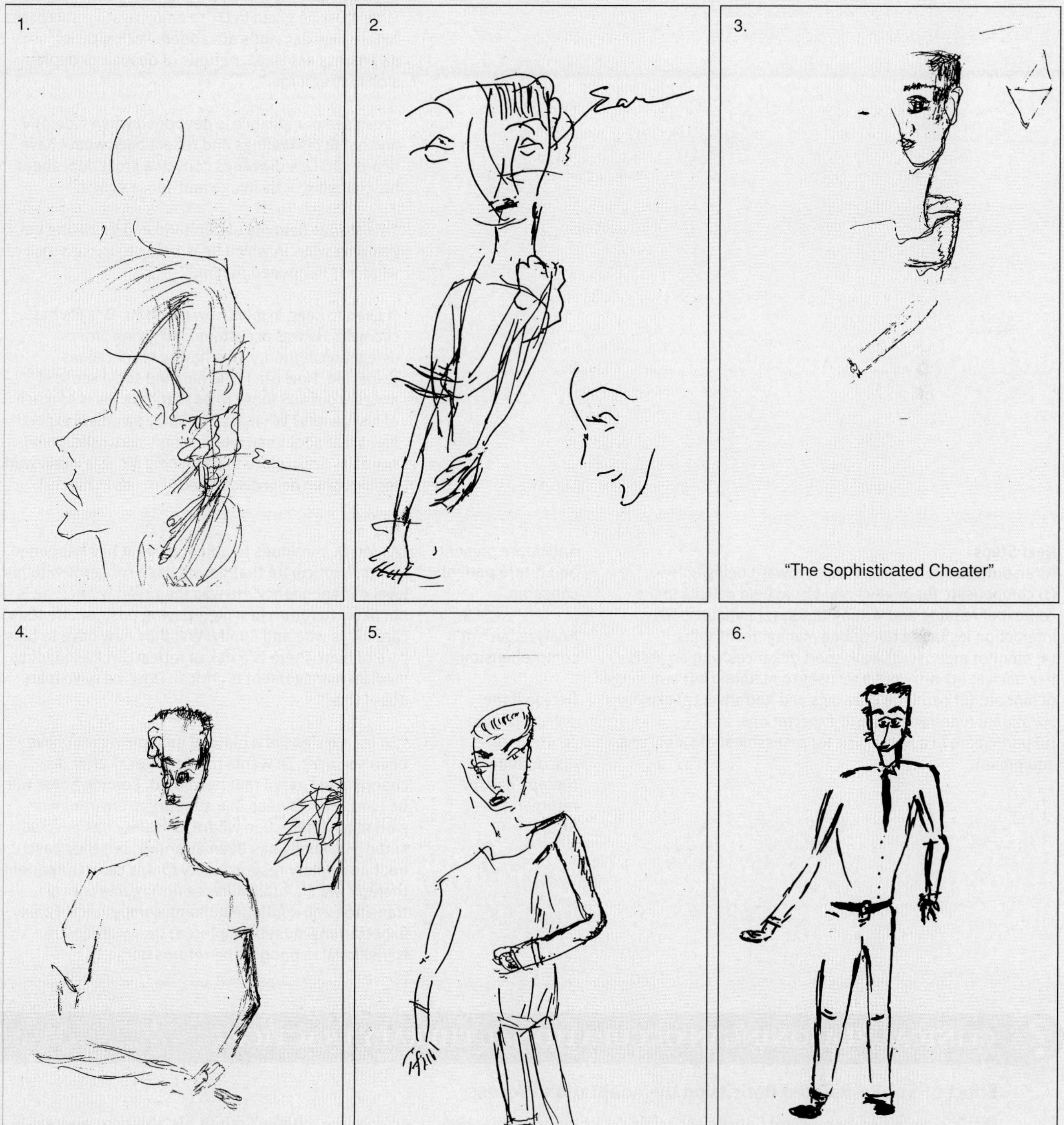

Figure 35-2 Six serial self-portraits drawn by Mr. D. during months 3, 4, and 5 after right-hemisphere stroke.

Maneuver the wheelchair for short distances. Practice supervised self-care. Attempt reading and writing. Facilitate personal continuity through narrative and drawings. Address existential questions. Open lines of communication with family.	Compare actual to expected performance Know the person	"Sometimes he sounds almost psychotic, but I appreciate that actually he is trying to make narrative sense of what he experiences through a limited field of vision and with a damaged perceptual framework normally supported by the right hemisphere."
	Appreciate the context	"With his denial breaking, I believe that it is crucial to avoid flooding Mr. D. with failures in these areas. Time must be given in OT to enjoy relative successes before new demands are added. With growing awareness of losses, periods of despair or depression may emerge." "I can see our alliance is deepened when I identify and name his feelings and reflect back what I have heard. Mr. D.'s drawings convey a great deal about his changing body image and sense of self." "His stories help me understand and guide the developing ways in which he is trying to make sense of what has happened to him." "I need to keep in mind how much Mr. D.'s life has changed. He was accustomed to giving orders, delegating authority, and having his decisions respected. How can I help him find some sense of mastery outside those roles that have been so much of his identity? What are his family members expecting? What additional relationships and institutional supports are in place that can help Mr. D.'s world work for him when he is discharged? Friends? Church?"
Next Steps As an outpatient, Mr. D. will work toward being able to: (1) compensate for neglect and visual field deficits in the context of reading and writing tasks; (2) initiate social interaction including telephone management skills; (3) monitor moods; (4) walk short distances with an assistive device; (5) carry out exercises to maintain left arm range of motion; (6) continue drawings and narrative; (7) explore vocational requirements and expectations; and (8) participate in a home visit for assessment of safety and equipment.	Anticipate present and future patient concerns Analyze patient's comprehension Decide if the patient should continue or discontinue therapy and/or return in the future	"As Mr. D. continues to adjust to what has happened to him, I anticipate that he will have concerns with his level of dependency. He was the bread winner; he is not likely to return to a high-paying position. He took care of his wife and family. Will they now have to take care of him? There is a risk of repeat stroke; ongoing medical management is critical. Does he have fears about this?" "So far, no signs of a plateau in improvement have been seen. Mr. D. wants to continue OT after discharge, and I agree that he should. Coming home will be hard. He has been in a supportive environment with much interaction where his safety has been assured. His family has been attentive, but they have not had primary responsibility for his care. Outpatient therapy will maintain alliance during this critical transition and continue building competence. Family expectations must be explored; they will require transitional support as he returns home."

? CLINICAL REASONING IN OCCUPATIONAL THERAPY PRACTICE

Effect of Stroke-Related Deficits on the Adaptation Process

Mr. D.'s cognitive-behavioral deficits associated with right-hemisphere brain damage initially limited his ability to appreciate his circumstances and adjust to his condition. He retained the ability, however, to verbalize his concerns and comprehend verbal input from others. How might the therapist's plans and goals specific to adaptation have changed if Mr. D. had impairments typically associated with left-hemisphere lesions (e.g., communication deficits)?

Evidence Table 35-1
Evidence for Occupational Therapy Practice That Incorporates Personal and Social Adaptation

Intervention	Description of Intervention Tested	Participants	Dosage	Type of Best Evidence and Level of Evidence	Benefit	Statistical Probability and Effect Size of Outcome	Reference
Client-centered, in-home ADL practice	In-home OT to achieve client-identified ADL or IADL goals plus routine services	138 stroke survivors (67 LCVA, 71 RCVA); mean age = 71 years.	30–45 minutes per visit for 10 visits over 6 weeks.	Randomized controlled study. IA2b (lacked control for difference in attention between treated and other group who received routine services only).	Yes. The treated group showed small improvement on *Nottingham Extended ADL Scale* and *Barthel Index* vs. other group.	*Nottingham*: $p = 0.02, r = 0.17$. *Barthel*: $p = 0.06$, $r = 0.13$.	Gilbertson et al., 2000
Task-specific practice of client-chosen BADL	Practice of specific tasks in a familiar context.	323 acute stroke survivors (147 LCVA, 156 RCVA); mean age, 72.5 years.	Ranged from 1–15 visits over a period of 6 weeks to 5 months.	Meta-analysis of 2 studies.	Yes. The treated groups improved in BADL as measured by the *Barthel Index*.	Mean weighted effect size was $r = 0.16$, equivalent to a 16% success rate over control treatment.	Trombly & Ma, 2002
Training neglect for enhancement of functional tasks	Tested association between neglect and function; study justifies therapeutic efforts at primary remediation of neglect.	40 right-handed adults with RCVA (19 with neglect, 21 without neglect).	Tested at 3 points: *LOTCA*, *FIM*, and *Rabideau Kitchen Evaluation*.	Longitudinal controlled study using consecutive admissions.	Neglect predicted lower performance on all areas of *LOTCA*/cognitive skills and *FIM*/daily functional tasks and longer hospitalization.	15.8% neglect group ADL independent vs. 81% non- neglect group; $\chi^2 = 4.27$; $p < 0.04$. Student's = 2.48, $p < 0.02$.	Katz et al., 2000

(continued)

Evidence Table 35-1
Evidence for Occupational Therapy Practice That Incorporates Personal and Social Adaptation (*continued*)

Intervention	Description of Intervention Tested	Participants	Dosage	Type of Best Evidence and Level of Evidence	Benefit	Statistical Probability and Effect Size of Outcome	Reference
Social support; family educational counseling; and leisure-focused therapy	Examined success of community reintegration efforts as reported in multiple studies.			Meta-analysis/literature review of 17 studies between 1970 and 2002: 4 on social support; 10 on family education; and 3 on leisure activities.	Social support: improves outcome. Family education: positive family impact. Leisure activities: no consensus.		Bhogal et al., 2003

Abbreviations: ADL, activities of daily living; IADL, instrumental activities of daily living; LCVA, left cerebrovascular accident; RCVA, right cerebrovascular accident; BADL, basic activities of daily living; LOTCA, Loewenstein Occupational Therapy Cognitive Assessment; FIM, Functional Independence Measure.

SUMMARY REVIEW QUESTIONS

1. Write a letter from the rehabilitation hospital to a close friend or family member describing your feelings and efforts to cope following a disabling accident.
2. Generate five short hypotheses through which to understand why a patient might seem unmotivated in treatment. Considering your hypotheses, what components would you expect interventions for pain and depression to have in common and why?
3. Present briefly the four stages from injury to rehabilitation as described by Morse and O'Brien. In what ways are stage theories helpful? What wrong assumptions can they produce?
4. What stresses might disabled patients' families or partners experience? What are three ways occupational therapists ease those stresses?
5. Explore an online chat room serving a virtual community of ill or disabled individuals. Give examples of support and information that you find being exchanged. What criteria would you use to evaluate the value of this chat room for its participants? In what ways might a chat room be like group treatment? In what ways might it be different?
6. Respond to this patient's question: "Why go on living with a severe disability?" What feelings or reactions in yourself over such a question would lead you to seek extra support or supervision?
7. List four indications that would cause you to seek psychiatric consultation or referral for the patient in Question 6.
8. View one or more of the films that portray a disabled person. What strategies for coping are depicted in the film(s)? What is demonstrated about the close relationships and occupations of disabled individuals? How might the film(s) influence the audience's understanding of living with a disability?

ACKNOWLEDGMENT

I would like to thank the patients who have been my teachers for the more than 30 years I have been an occupational therapist; Jenny Lee Olsen, Director of Library Services at Cambridge Health Alliance for her generous help and guidance in the literature search; Manu Thakral for thoughtful comments on the developing manuscript; and editors Mary Radomski and Catherine Trombly for their confidence in offering me the opportunity to contribute to this book.

References

Ader, R. (1981). *Psychoneuroimmunology*. Orlando, FL: Academic.

Alonso, A., & Swiller, H. (1993). *Group therapy in clinical practice*. Washington, DC: American Psychiatric Association.

American Occupational Therapy Association [AOTA]. (1995a). Position paper: Occupational performance: Occupational therapy's definition of function. *American Journal of Occupational Therapy, 49,* 1019–1020.

American Occupational Therapy Association [AOTA]. (1995b). Position paper: The psychosocial core of occupational therapy. *American Journal of Occupational Therapy, 49,* 1021–1022.

American Occupational Therapy Association [AOTA]. (2002). Occupational therapy practice framework: Domain and process. *American Journal of Occupational Therapy, 56,* 609–639.

Banks, M. E. (2003) Disability in the family: A life span perspective. *Cultural Diversity and Ethnic Minor Psychology, 9,* 367–384.

Barasch, I. B. (1993). *The healing path: A soul approach to illness*. New York: Putnam.

Basco, M. R. (1993). The cognitive behavior therapist's role in diabetes management. *Behavior Therapist, Summer,* 180–182.

Basson, R. (1998). Sexual health of women with disabilities. *Canadian Medical Association Journal, 159,* 359–362.

Bauby, J. (1997). *The diving bell and the butterfly*. New York: Random House.

Benson, H. (1995). Commentary: Religion, belief and healing. *Mind/Body Medicine, 1,* 158.

Betz, C. L. (1998). Adolescent transitions: A nursing concern. *Pediatric Nursing, 24,* 23–30.

Bhogal, S. K., Teasell, R. W., Foley, N. C., & Speechley, M. R. (2003). Community reintegration after stroke. *Topics in Stroke Rehabilitation, Summer,* 107–129.

Boeije, H. R., Duijnstee, M. S., Grypdonck, M. H., & Pool, A. (2002). Encountering the downward phase: Biographical work in people with multiple sclerosis living at home. *Social Science Medicine, 55,* 881–893.

Bontje, P., Kinebanian, A., Josephsson, S., & Tamuura, Y. (2004). Occupational adaptation: The experience of older persons with physical disabilities. *American Journal of Occupational Therapy, 58,* 140–149.

Boston Globe. (2005, December 26). Details of caregiver study. Health Science Section, C4.

Brendel, D. H., Florman, J., Roberts, S., & Solet, J. M. (2001). "In sleep I almost never grope": Blindness, neuropsychiatric deficits, and a chaotic upbringing. *Harvard Review of Psychiatry, 9,* 178–188.

Bridle, M. J. (1999). Are doing and being dimensions of holism? *American Journal of Occupational Therapy, 53,* 636–639.

Broyard, A. (1992). *Intoxicated by my illness*. New York: Fawcett Columbine.

Buning, M. E. (1999). Fitness for persons with disabilities: A call to action. *OT Practice, 8,* 27–32.

Burns, D. (1990). *The feeling good handbook*. New York: Plume.

Cambridge Health Alliance (1995). *Mental health and addictions*. Unpublished document.

Carr, D. B., & Goudas, L. C. (1999). Acute pain. *Lancet, 353,* 2051–2058.

Caudill, M. A. (1995). *Managing pain before it manages you*. New York: Guilford.

Dangoor, N., & Florian, V. (1994). Women with chronic physical disabilities: Correlates of their long-term psychosocial adaptation. *International Journal of Rehabilitation Research, 17,* 159–168.

Davidhizer, R. (1997). Disability does not have to be the grief that never ends: Helping patients adjust. *Rehabilitation Nursing, 22,* 32–35.

Denollet, J. (1998). Personality and coronary heart disease: The type-D scale-16. *Annals of Behavioral Medicine, 20,* 209–226.

Dewar, A. L., & Lee, E. A. (2000). Bearing illness and injury. *Western Journal of Nursing Research, 22,* 912–926.

Dickinson, E. (Franklin, R. W., Ed.) (1999). *The poems of Emily Dickinson*. Cambridge, MA: Belknap.

Dudgeon, B. J., Gerrard, B. C., Jensen, M. P., Rhodes, L. A., & Tyler, E. J. (2002). Physical disability and the experience of chronic pain. *Archives of Physical Medicine and Rehabilitation, 83,* 229–235.

Edinger, J. D., & Erwin, C. W. (1992). Common sleep disorders: Overview of diagnosis and treatment. *Clinical Reviews, November-December,* 60–88.

Ehde, D. M., Jensen, M. P., Engel, J. M., Turner, J. A., Hoffman, A. J., & Cardenas, D. D. (2003). Chronic pain secondary to disability: A review. *Clinical Journal of Pain, 19,* 3–17.

Fields, H. L. (1997). Brain systems for sensory modulation: Understanding the neurobiology of the therapeutic process. *Mind/Body Medicine, 2,* 201–206.

Frank, G. (1996). Life histories in occupational therapy clinical practice. *American Journal of Occupational Therapy, 50,* 251–264.

Franz, C. E., & White, K. M. (1985). Individuation and attachment in personality development: Extending Erikson's theory. *Journal of Personality, 53,* 224–256.

Gal, B. (1999). Veterinary update: Pets keep people healthy. *Veterinary Economics, Summer,* 3–4.

Gallagher, R. M. (1997). Behavioral and biobehavioral treatment in chronic pain: Perspectives on effectiveness. *Mind/Body Medicine, 2,* 176–186.

Gardner, D. (1999). The protective barrier in brain injury. *TBI Challenge, April/May,* 8–12.

Ghaemi, S. N., & Sachs, G. (1999, April 10). Practical psychiatric update: Improving assessment and treatment of the bipolar spectrum. *American Occupational Therapy Association Conference Proceedings,* Boston.

Gilbertson, L., Langhorne, P., Walker, A., Allen, A., & Murray, G. D. (2000). Domiciliary occupational therapy for patients with stroke discharged from hospital: randomised controlled trial. *British Medical Journal, 320,* 603–606.

Groves, J. E. (1978). Taking care of the hateful patient. *New England Journal of Medicine, 298,* 883–887.

Grunebaum, J. (1996). The importance for effective treatment of understanding the interpersonal context in which pain occurs. Unpublished manuscript.

Hallum, A., & Krumholtz, J. D. (1993). Parents caring for young adults with severe physical disabilities: Psychological issues. *Developmental Medicine and Child Neurology, 35,* 24–32.

Harris, S., Morley, S., & Barton, S. B. (2003). Role loss and adjustment in chronic pain. *Pain, 105,* 363–370.

Hasselkus, B. R. (1991). Ethical dilemmas in family caregiving for the elderly: Implications for occupational therapy. *American Journal of Occupational Therapy, 45,* 206–212.

Hasselkus, B. R. (1994). Working with family caregivers: A therapeutic alliance. In B. R. Bonder & M. B. Wagner (Eds.), *Functional performance in older adults* (pp. 339–351). Philadelphia: Davis.

Hawkins, A. H. (1993). *Reconstructing illness: Studies in pathography.* West Lafayette, IN: Purdue University.

Heinemann, A. W. (1993). *Substance abuse and physical disability* (pp. 93–106). New York: Hawor.

Heinemann, A. W, Mamott, B., & Schnoll, S. (1990). Substance abuse by persons with recent spinal cord injuries. *Rehabilitation Psychology, 35,* 217–228.

Helfrich, C., Kielhofner, G., & Mattingly, C. (1994). Volition as narrative: Understanding motivation in chronic illness. *American Journal of Occupational Therapy, 48,* 311–317.

Herman, J. L. (1992). *Trauma and recovery.* New York: Basic.

Hoch, D., & Ferguson, T. (2005). What I have learned from E-patients. *PLoS Medicine, 2,* e206.

Hull, J. (1990). *Touching the rock: An experience of blindness.* New York: Pantheon.

Hulter, B. M., & Lundberg, P. O. (1995). Sexual function in women with advanced multiple sclerosis. *Journal of Neurology, Neurosurgery, and Psychiatry, 59,* 83–86.

Humphrey, R., Gonzalez, S., & Taylor, E. (1992). Family involvement in practice: Issues and attitudes. *American Journal of Occupational Therapy, 47,* 587–593.

Johnson, J. (1986). Wellness and occupational therapy. *American Journal of Occupational Therapy, 40,* 753–758.

Jonsson, A. T., Moller, A., & Grimby, G. (1998). Managing occupations in everyday life to achieve adaptation. *American Journal of Occupational Therapy, 53,* 353–362.

Joseph, R. (2005). Integrated healthcare and disease management. Unpublished presentation. Cambridge, MA: Cambridge Health Alliance.

Kabat-Zinn, J. (1991). The power of breathing: Your unsuspected ally in the healing process. In *Full catastrophe living: The wisdom of your body and mind to face stress, pain, and illness* (pp. 47–58). New York: Delacorte.

Kahana, J. R., & Bibring, G. (1964). Personality types in medical management. In N. Zinberg (Ed.), *Psychiatry and medical practice in a general hospital* (pp. 108–123). New York: International Universities.

Katz, N., Hartman-Maieir, A., Ring, H., & Soroker, N. (2000). Relationship of cognitive performance and daily function of clients following right hemisphere stroke: Predictive and ecological validity of the LOTCA Battery. *Occupational Therapy Journal of Research, 20,* 3–16.

Kautzman, L. N. (1992). Linking patient and family stories to caregivers' use of clinical reasoning. *American Journal of Occupational Therapy, 47,* 169–173.

Keith, B. (1999). Psychological aspects of recovery from brain surgery. Unpublished manuscript.

Kemp, B. J. (2005). What the rehabilitation professional and consumer need to know. *Physical Medicine and Rehabilitation Clinics of North America, 16,* 1–18.

Kemp, B. J., & Krause, J. S. (1999). Depression and life satisfaction among people aging with post-polio syndrome. *Disability Rehabilitation, 21,* 241–249.

Kemp, J. K. (1993). Psychological care of the older rehabilitation patient. *Geriatric Rehabilitation, 9,* 841–857.

Keonig, H. G., & George, L. K. (1998). Depression and physical disability outcomes in depressed medically ill hospitalized older adults. *American Journal of Geriatric Psychiatry, 6,* 230–247.

Khantzian, E. J. (1990). Self-regulation and self-medication factors in alcoholism and the addictions. In M. Galanter (Ed.), *Recent developments in alcoholism* (Vol. 8, pp. 255–271). New York: Plenum.

Kielhofner, G. (1992). *Conceptual foundations of occupational therapy.* Philadelphia: Davis.

Kilborn, P. T. (1999, May 31). Disabled spouses increasingly face a life alone and a loss of income. *The New York Times,* A8.

King, G., Cathers, T., Brown, E., Specht, J. A., Willoughby, C., Polgar, J. M., MacKinnon, E., Smith, L. K., & Havens, L. (2003). Turning points and protective processes in the lives of people with chronic disabilities. *Qualitative Health Research, 13,* 184–206.

King, G. A., Shultz, I. Z., Steel, K., Gilpin, M., & Cathers, T. (1993). Self-evaluation and self-concept of adolescents with physical disabilities. *American Journal of Occupational Therapy, 47,* 132–140.

Kleinman, A. (1988). *The illness narratives: Suffering, healing, and the human condition.* New York: Basic.

Kubzansky, L. D., Kawachi, I., Weiss, S. T., & Sparrow, D. (1998). Anxiety and coronary heart disease: A synthesis of epidemiological, psychological, and experimental evidence. *Annals of Behavioral Medicine, 20,* 47–58.

Laatsch, L., & Shahani, B. T. (1996). The relationship between age, gender and psychological distress in rehabilitation inpatients. *Disability and Rehabilitation, 18,* 604–608.

Larson, D. B., & Milano, M. A. G. (1995). Are religion and spirituality clinically relevant in health care? *Mind/Body Medicine, 1,* 147–158.

Lazarus, R. S., & Folkman, S. (1984). *Stress, appraisal, and coping.* New York: Springer.

Levine, C. (1999). The loneliness of the long-term care giver. *New England Journal of Medicine, 340,* 1587–1590.

Levine, S. (1987). The changing terrains in medical sociology: Emergent concerns with the quality of life. *Journal of Health and Social Behavior, 28,* 1–6.

Li, L., & Ford, J. A. (1998). Illicit drug use by women with disabilities. *American Journal of Drug and Alcohol Abuse, 24,* 405–418.

Lowenstein, A. (1999). Alice's story: Notes from the rehabilitation center. Unpublished manuscript.

Lynch, J. W., Kaplan, G. A., & Shema, S. J. (1997). Cumulative impact of sustained economic hardship on the physical, cognitive, psychological and social functioning. *New England Journal of Medicine, 337,* 1889–1895.

Lynch, S. G., Kroencke, D. C., & Denney, D. R. (2001). The relationship between disability and depression in multiple sclerosis. *Multiple Sclerosis, 7,* 411-416.

Main, C. J., & Spanswick, C. C. (1991). Pain: Psychological and psychiatric factors. *British Medical Bulletin, 47,* 732-742.

Main, T. F. (1957). The ailment. *British Journal of Medical Psychology, 30,* 129-217.

Mairs, N. (1996). *Waist high in the world.* Boston: Beacon.

Martz, E. (2004). Do post-traumatic stress symptoms predict reactions of adaptation to disability after a sudden-onset spinal cord injury? *International Journal of Rehabilitation Research, 27,* 185-194.

Mayday Fund (1998). Facts and figures about pain in America. *Pain Link Resources.*

Mazor for Rosh Hashanah and Yom Kippur: A prayer book for the days of awe (1972). New York: Rabbinical Assembly.

Meyer, R. (1999). *Our models of addiction: Their promise and their problems.* Unpublished presentation, Psychiatry Grand Rounds, June 16, Cambridge Health Alliance.

Miner, L. (1999, March 25). The psychosocial impact of limb or digit amputation. *Occupational Therapy Week,* 10-11.

Moore, D., & Li, L. (1994). Substance abuse among applicants for vocational rehabilitation services. *Journal of Rehabilitation, 60,* 48-53.

Moore, D., & Li, L. (1998). Prevalence and risk factors of illicit drug use by people with disabilities. *American Journal on Addictions, 7,* 93-102.

Morse, J. M., & O'Brien, B. (1995). Preserving self: From victim, to patient, to disabled person. *Journal of Advanced Nursing, 21,* 88-896.

Nemeroff, C. B. (1998). The neurobiology of depression. *Scientific American, June,* 42-49.

Nochi, M. (2000). Reconstructing self-narratives in coping with traumatic brain injury. *Social Science and Medicine, 51,* 1795-1804.

Peloquin, S. M., (2002). Reclaiming the vision of reaching heart as well as hands. *American Journal of Occupational Therapy, 56,* 517-526.

Pasciewicz, P. V. (1987). The experience of a traumatic closed head-injury: A phenomenological study. Unpublished doctoral dissertation. Cincinnati, OH: The Union Institute (formerly Union for Experimenting Colleges and Universities).

Patenaude, A. F. (2005). *Genetic testing for cancer: Psychological approaches for helping patients and families.* Washington, DC: American Psychological Association.

Pennebaker, J. W. (1995). *Emotion, disclosure, and health.* Washington, DC: American Psychological Association.

Powell, K. B., & Miklowitz, D. J. (1994). Frontal lobe dysfunction in the affective disorders. *Clinical Psychology Review, 14,* 525-546.

Quigly, M. C. (1995). Impact of spinal cord injury on the life roles of women. *American Journal of Occupational Therapy, 49,* 780-786.

Quill, E. T. (2005). Terri Schiavo: A tragedy compounded. *New England Journal of Medicine, 325,* 1630-1633.

Rankin, W. (1985). A theologian's perspective on illness and the human spirit. *Linacre Quarterly, November,* 329-334.

Rena, F., Moshe, S., & Abraham, O. (1996). Couples' adjustment to one partner's disability: The relationship between sense of coherence and adjustment. *Social Science Medicine, 43,* 163-171.

Rolland, J. S. (1993). Mastering family challenges in serious illness and disability? In F. Walsh (Ed.), *Normal family processes* (2nd ed., pp. 444-473). New York: Guilford.

Rowe, C. E., & MacIsaac, D. S. (1991). *Empathic attunement: The technique of psychoanalytic self psychology.* Northvale, NJ: Jason Aronson.

Saetersdal, B. (1997). Forbidden suffering: The Pollyanna syndrome of the disabled and their families. *Family Process, 36,* 431-435.

Schultz, A. W., & Liptak, G. S. (1998). Helping adolescents who have disabilities negotiate transitions to adulthood. *Issues in Comprehensive Pediatric Nursing, 21,* 187-201.

Simkins, C. N. (1999). Pediatric brain injury may last a lifetime. *TBI Challenge, April/May,* 4-5.

Solet, J. M. (1991). *Coping and injury attribution in head-injured adults.* Unpublished doctoral dissertation. Boston: Boston University.

Solet, J. M. (1994). *Narratives: Empathic listening and therapist role expectations.* Unpublished Training Program Lectures. Cambridge, MA: Cambridge Health Alliance and Harvard Medical School.

Solet, J. M. (1995, August 17). Educating patients about pain. *Occupational Therapy Week,* 3-4.

Sontag, S. (1988). *Illness as metaphor and AIDS and its metaphors.* New York: Anchor.

Spencer, J., Young, M. E., Rintala, D., & Bates, S. (1995). Socialization to the culture of a rehabilitation hospital: An ethnographic study. *American Journal of Occupational Therapy, 49,* 53-62.

Stewart, D. A., Law, M. C., Rosenbaum, P., & Willms, D. G. (2001). A qualitative study of transition to adulthood for youth with physical disabilities. *Physical and Occupational Therapy Pediatrics, 21,* 3-21.

Stone, A. A., & Porter, M. A. (1995). Psychological coping: Its importance for treating medical problems. *Mind/Body Medicine, 1,* 46-54.

Stuifbergen, A. K., Harrison, T. C., Becker, H., Carter, P. (2004). Adaptation of a wellness program for women with chronic disabilities. *Journal of Holistic Nursing, 22,* 12-31.

Thoren, P., Floras, J. S., Hoffman, P., & Seals, D. R. (1990). Endorphins and exercise: Physiological mechanisms and clinical implications. *Medicine and Science in Sports and Exercise, 22,* 417-428.

Thoren-Jonsson, A. L. (2001). Coming to terms with the shift in one's capabilities: A study of adaptation to poliomyelitis sequelae. *Disability Rehabilitation, 23,* 341-351.

Trombley, C. A., & Ma, H. (2002). A synthesis of the effects of occupational therapy for persons with stroke, part l: Restoration of roles, tasks, and activities. *American Journal of Occupational Therapy, 56,* 250-259.

Turner, W. T., & Alston, R. J. (1994). The role of the family in psychosocial adaptation to physical disabilities for African Americans. *Journal of the National Medical Association, 86,* 915-921.

Ville, I., Ravaud, J. F., & Tetrafigap Group (2001). Subjective well-being and severe motor impairments: the Tetrafigap survey on the long-term outcome of tetraplegic spinal cord injured persons. *Social Science Medicine, 52,* 369-384.

Walker, L. G. (1999). Psychological intervention, host defenses, and survival. *Advances in Mind-Body Medicine, 15,* 273-281.

Weber, R. L. (1993). Group therapy training materials. Unpublished documents. Cambridge, MA: Cambridge Health Alliance and Harvard Medical School.

Wiltshire, S. F. (1994). *Seasons of grief and grace: A sister's story of AIDS.* Nashville: Vanderbilt University.

Woods, F. W. (1984). *Human sexuality in health and illness.* St. Louis: Mosby.

Yarkony, G. M. (1993). *Medical complications in rehabilitation.* New York: Hawor.

Zegans, L. (1991). The embodied self: Integration in health and illness. *Advances: Journal of the Institute for the Advancement of Health, 7,* 29-45.

Ziegler, R. G. (1999). Individual and group psychotherapy: Principles for an epilepsy practice. Unpublished manuscript. Boston: Seizure Unit, Children's Hospital.

Suggested References

Supplemental Readings

Barasch, I. B. (1993). *The healing path: A soul approach to illness.* New York: Putnam.

Bauby, J. (1997). *The diving bell and the butterfly.* New York: Random House.

Berti, A., Bottini, G., Gandola, M., Pia, L., Smania, N., Stracciari, A., Vallar, G., & Paulesu, E. (2005). Shared cortical anatomy for motor awareness and motor control. *Science, 309,* 488-491.

Broyard, A. (1992). *Intoxicated by my illness.* New York: Fawcett Columbine.

Hull, J. (1990). *Touching the rock: An experience of blindness.* New York: Pantheon.

Jamison, K. R. (1996). *An unquiet mind.* New York: Random House.

Luria, A. R. (1968). *The mind of a mnemonist.* Cambridge, MA: Harvard University.

Luria, A. R. (1972). *The man with a shattered world.* Cambridge, MA: Harvard University.

Ma, H., & Trombley, C. A. (2002). A synthesis of the effects of occupational therapy for persons with stroke, part 2: Remediation of impairments. *American Journal of Occupational Therapy, 56,* 260-274.

Mairs, N. (1996). *Waist high in the world.* Boston: Beacon.
Rogers, A. G. (1995). *A shining affliction.* New York: Viking.
Rosenberg, C. H., & Popelka, G. M. (2000) Post-stroke rehabilitation: A review of guidelines for patient management. *Geriatrics, 55,* 75–81.
Sacks, O. (1985). *The man who mistook his wife for a hat.* New York: Simon & Schuster.
Wakefield, D. (2005). *I remember running: The year I got everything I wanted and ALS.* New York: Marlowe.
Weber, R. J. (2000). *The created self: Reinventing body, persona, and spirit.* New York: Norton.
Wiltshire, S. F. (1994). *Seasons of grief and grace: A sister's story of AIDS.* Nashville: Vanderbilt University.

Suggested Films

A Beautiful Mind (2002)
Awakening (1990)
Born on the Fourth of July (1989)
Children of a Lesser God (2000)
Iris (2001)
My Left Foot (1989)
Memento (2000)
Murderball (2005)
Rainman (1988)
Ray (2004)
Regarding Henry (1996)
Scent of a Woman (1993)
The Best Years of Our Lives (194)
The Elephant Man (1989)

CHAPTER 36

Optimizing Access to Home, Community, and Work Environments

Dory B. Sabata, Shoshana Shamberg, and Michael Williams

LEARNING OBJECTIVES

After studying this chapter, the reader will be able to do the following:

1. Understand the historical background of civil rights for people with disabilities, the social model of disability, the independent living movement, and the establishment of the Americans with Disabilities Act.
2. Understand key events and policies that affect accessibility of home, work, and communities.
3. Describe four intervention techniques for maximizing access to participation at home, in the workplace, and in communities.
4. Recognize examples of products, design features, and other contextual factors that interact with a client's ability to perform occupations.
5. Explore intervention plans that reduce demands and facilitate access to home, workplace, and community.
6. Outline evidence-based best practices for reducing environmental demands and maximizing performance patterns.

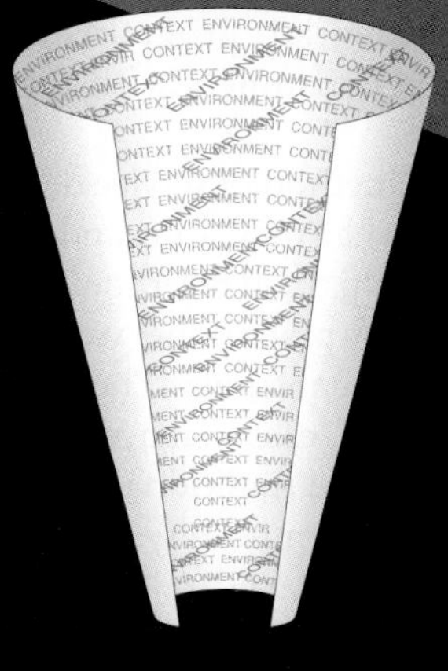

Glossary

Age in place—The concept that as people age, they can continue to live and participate within their own homes and communities of choice.

Assistive technology—Any item, piece of equipment, or product system, whether acquired commercially off the shelf, modified, or customized, that is used to increase, maintain, or improve functional capabilities of individuals with disabilities (Assistive Technology Act of 1998).

Electronic and information technology—Equipment or interconnected system or subsystem of equipment that is used in the creation, conversion, or duplication of data or information (Section 508 of the Rehabilitation Act).

Excess disability—Decreased ability to function beyond the functional impairment associated with a particular health condition.

Universal design—A design approach for creating products and spaces that addresses the need for access by all potential users.

Visitability—A movement started by Concrete Change that advocates that all homes have a no-step entrance, wide doorways, and access to a first floor bathroom for visitors.

Vocational rehabilitation—Therapeutic preparation for obtaining and participating in employment.

Workplace accommodation—Strategy to reduce barriers and maximize participation in employment for people with disabilities by changing the work environment, job task, or how the job is performed.

Occupational therapy intervention to optimize accessibility requires both knowledge of the process to implement changes in the physical environment and the product options available. This chapter highlights some of the historical events that have shaped this dimension of occupational therapy practice. Occupational therapists use four intervention strategies to optimize access to home, community, and work environments: universal design, environmental modifications, assistive technology, and task modification strategies. Application of strategies will be discussed for home, workplace, and community environments along with factors affecting the implementation of environmental modifications. Given the importance of evidence-based practice, some of the research that demonstrates efficacy for these types of interventions will be described in terms of client outcomes.

ACCESSIBILITY: AN HISTORICAL PERSPECTIVE OF ACCESS TO THE ENVIRONMENT FOR PEOPLE WITH DISABILITIES

Occupational therapists provide training and strategies to help people with disabilities to optimize participation in activities in a variety of contexts. One way this is accomplished is by promoting environments and attitudes that facilitate a person's right to decide how and where he or she will live, work, and socially participate. Political advocacy, legislation protecting civil rights, and changing demographics of the population are all influential in shaping current occupational therapy practices for optimizing environmental access.

Independent Living Movement

Services to increase quality of life for people with disabilities were established in accordance with the Comprehensive Rehabilitation Services Amendment of the Rehabilitation Act of 1973. This initiated the Independent Living Movement (ILM), which models itself on the Civil Rights Movement. The ILM stems from grassroot activists who promoted an alternative to the medical model perspective of disability. The ILM differs from the medical model in that it is consumer oriented and directed (American Occupational Therapy Association [AOTA], 1993).

Independent living is defined as control over one's life based on the choice of acceptable options that minimize physical and psychological reliance on others in making decisions and performing everyday activities (Frieden & Cole, 1985). With this movement and supporting legislation, Centers for Independent Living (CILs) were established to provide referral and direct services in housing, attendant care, transportation, recreation, housing, and social and vocational counseling. These centers are important because they provide a support system to consumers, often educating the family support network or compensating for the lack of one. CILs are unique community-based non-profit nonresidential programs that are substantially controlled by consumers with disabilities (Johnson, 1986).

With this client-centered method of service delivery, the client and caregivers define what they want and need, and the occupational therapists help them meet their goals. The role of the occupational therapy practitioner varies with the setting and/or the needs of the consumer. The practitioner may act as consultant, advocate, case manager, and, often, provider of both non-medical and traditional occupational therapy services in the home or community.

Legislation and Governmental Regulation of Accessibility

Over the past 50 years, a number of key legislative initiatives paved the way for fully ensuring that all citizens, including people with disabilities, have access to community, job, and residential environments. Federal legislation addressing accessibility issues began in 1954 with the Hill Burton Act (PL 83-565) to correct construction and design problems in federally funded hospitals. The Architectural Barriers Act of 1968 (PL 90-480) created the United States Architectural and Transportation Barriers Compliance Board (ATBCB), which was authorized to study architectural design and develop standards for the construction of accessible buildings. Their findings are reported in the Minimum Guidelines for Accessible Design (MGRAD). The Rehabilitation Act of 1973 (PL 93-112) expanded the powers of the ATBCB or Access Board, which was then authorized to enforce federal accessibility requirements in federally funded buildings, federally funded programs, subsidized and public housing, and transportation facilities. These standards, called the Uniform Federal Accessibility Standards (UFAS), are based on MGRAD and guidelines of the American National Standards Institute (ANSI).

The Fair Housing Amendments Act (FHAA) of 1988 established the Fair Housing Act Accessibility Guidelines (FHAAG) for multifamily housing of four units or more and civil rights housing protection for people with disabilities. The FHAA mandates accessibility compliance and civil rights protection in private housing. People with disabilities are provided equal access to housing and a mechanism for filing complaints when their civil rights are violated. According to this law, the resident cannot be denied the opportunity to modify the rented home to meet individual needs for accessibility. The cost of the modification, however, is the responsibility of the renter. The landlord may require that the work be done by an approved professional, and an escrow account may be established in which the tenant must place funds for returning the residence to its original state. Modifications that may be easily used by other tenants and do not change the nature of the residence are not required to be returned to the original state. Such modifications include widened doorways, levered handles, grab bar solid blocking, and the like. A ramp may have to be removed, cabinets under counters may have to be reinstalled, and the tub may have to be returned to the bathroom from which it was removed to create an accessible shower stall (Procedures for Practice 36-1).

In 1990, with Congressional approval of the Americans with Disabilities Act (ADA), 43 million Americans with disabilities were awarded civil rights protection by extension of equal rights protection established by the Civil Rights Act of 1964. The ADA is an attempt to correct the many loopholes of earlier legislation aimed at providing services and rights for people with disabilities and a method of enforcing specialized regulations through the courts. Part of the ADA stipulates that state and local accessibility regulations must be considered in the design or modification of public spaces including businesses, schools, parks and other recreational facilities, state and local government buildings, and public transportation. The ATBCB used both the Uniform Federal Accessibility Standards (UFAS) and FHAAG standards to create the Americans with Disabilities Act Accessibility Guidelines (ADAAG) (Table 36-1).

In addition to the federal policies and standards that affect the built environment, state and local governments also have established building codes and safety codes. These codes can affect the location, design, and layout of public and private spaces. Most building design is based on the functional abilities and physical stature of an average person. The ADAAG was developed to propose some specifications for designing more accessible public spaces. The ADAAG was based primarily on the needs of younger adults with disabilities, and today, these implemented environmental features are not designed to meet the needs of older adults (Sanford, 2001). Guidelines can serve as a starting point to creating accessible public places but should not be the only consideration.

PROCEDURES FOR PRACTICE 36-1

Guidelines, Standards, and Regulations of Accessible Design

Occupational therapists who work with contractors and designers familiarize themselves with the following standards, guidelines, and legislation that affect accessibility and the physical environment.

- American National Standards Institute (ANSI)
- Minimum Guidelines for Accessible Design (MGRAD)
- Section 504 of The Rehabilitation Act 1973
- Architectural and Transportation Barriers Compliance Board (ATBCB)
- Uniform Federal Accessibility Standards (UFAS)
- Fair Housing Amendments Act of 1988 (FHAA)
- The Fair Housing Act Accessibility Guidelines (FHAAG)
- Americans with Disabilities Act of 1990 (ADA)
- Americans with Disabilities Act Accessibility Guidelines (ADAAG)

AGING

In addition to trends related to governmental oversight of accessibility, changing demographics also influence occupational therapy intervention to optimize access to home,

Table 36-1. Sample of ADAAG Specifications[a]

Measure	Specification
Toilet height	17 in to 19 in
Grab bar diameter	1 1/4 in to 1 1/2 in
Space between wall and grab bar (see Fig. 36-6)	1 1/2 in
Length of grab bar behind the water close	36 in
Clear space for wheelchair for 180° turn (see Fig. 36-7)	60 in
Maximum high forward reach allowed	48 in
Minimum low forward reach	15 in
Minimum clear width of an accessible route	36 in
Curb ramp minimum width	36 in
Maximum slope of a ramp in new construction	1:12
Preferred ramp slopes (see Fig. 36-5)	Between 1:16 and 1:20
Minimum landing length	60 in
Minimum landing size if ramps change direction at landings	60 in × 60 in
Maximum threshold for exterior sliding doors	3/4 in
Maximum threshold for other doors	1/2 in

[a] This table does not include requirements for children's use, nor were these measurements and specifications intended for homes.

work, and community. Overall, the population is aging, and those with chronic disabilities are living longer. By 2020, an estimated 54 million people in the United States will be aged 65 and older (United States Census Bureau, 2004). Over one fifth of those aged 45–54 have a disability, and about 14% of these people are severely disabled. Numbers increase sharply for people aged 65–69, of whom nearly 45% have some type of disability and 30.7% have severe disabilities; for those aged 80 and older, the numbers are nearly 74% and 58%, respectively (McNeil, 2001). Even with increasing disability with increasing age, older adults are active members of communities. The majority of older adults continue to reside in a home rather than in institutions (Greenwald and Associates, Inc., 2003). Older adults are participating longer in the workplace as well (Toossi, 2004).

When environmental demands exceed a person's abilities, **excess disability** results, which greatly limits participation in activities at home, in the workplace, or in the community. The current housing stock is often not accessible, and it is not designed for people to **age in place**. Workplaces have not been designed with aging workers in mind either. Communities have experienced increasing urban sprawl, and zoning has often distanced housing from commercial services such as stores and social and medical services.

Aging in Place

Older adults indicate a strong preference to continue living in their own homes. Homes have not been designed for aging in place. Although older adults are increasingly recognizing the need for home modifications, often their homes still lack the needed accessibility features (Bayer & Harper, 2000).

Aging in the Workplace

The American Association of Retired Persons (Bayer & Harper, 2000) reports that 80% of boomers believe they will continue to work during retirement. From 2000 to 2015, the annual growth rate of people ages 55 and over in the U.S. labor force will be nearly four times that of the overall labor force (Toossi, 2004). The phenomenon of aging in the workplace will present many new challenges to accessibility. New skills will be required for older adults to engage in an ever-increasing technological environment. Computer technology and interfaces will need to be designed to adapt to changes in vision, hearing, sensation, motor skills, and cognition that may be experienced by aging workers.

Elder-Friendly Communities

The increasing number of aging adults need environments to be adapted, modified, and designed to meet the needs of increasing disability and age-related changes. Livable or elder-friendly communities that facilitate participation incorporate affordable, accessible housing, supportive service, and transportation options (Kochera, Straight, &

Guterbock, 2005). ADAAG was not designed with older adults in mind, and community environments will need to include alternative accessibility options beyond the ADAAG to maximize community participation for older adults.

ROLE OF OCCUPATIONAL THERAPY

Occupational therapists analyze the physical environment as it relates to human performance, determine specific functional and environmental problems, and negotiate intervention options in collaboration with the client and support network. The generalist practitioner understands that the environment can be changed to decrease demands or to maximize abilities to facilitate performance. Specialists in accessibility and environmental modifications understand the range of possibilities and are conversant in the language needed to communicate effectively with building professionals as well as with clients. Other specialist competencies have been identified by the American Occupational Therapy Association (AOTA) for the Specialty Certification in Environmental Modifications.

Decades of regulation to eliminate discriminatory practices have led to the Americans with Disabilities Act (ADA) of 1990. Occupational therapy practitioners who are knowledgeable about these changes in policies and demographics provide valuable consultation and information to help facilitate social participation and performance of occupations that are meaningful and purposeful. A client-centered approach to service delivery empowers the client to advocate for his or her own needs with knowledge and a wide array of resources.

OVERARCHING STRATEGIES TO OPTIMIZE HOME, WORK, AND COMMUNITY ACCESSIBILITY

Any effort to optimize accessibility is always informed by an understanding of how environmental changes fit into the broader context of a client's requirements and preferences. Environmental press theory and concepts related to meaning associated with personal space shed light on these issues (Resources 36-1).

Environmental Press Theory

A conceptual framework called the docility hypothesis or environmental press theory (Lawton & Nahemow, 1973) is often used to describe a "just-right fit" between the demands of the environment and the abilities of the person. Occupational performance is dependent on this person–environment fit. Occupational therapy practitioners understand the importance of occupations to their clients and can help to implement environmental interventions to promote safety and reduce activity demands.

Meaning Associated with a Person's Space

When entering the home, workplace, or even community of a client, occupational therapists recognize that the physical space is meaningful to the client. Some people may feel trapped or have negative feelings about their environment, while others find a particular environment nurturing and comforting (Marcus, 1995). Think about your own environments in which you perform occupations. For example, do you sit in a particular seat in class? One's choice may depend on where one's friends sit, the relationship with the instructor, being in the habit of sitting there, or a number of other reasons. Regardless of what the reasons are, meaning has been established with that place.

Objects can become symbolic of goals and affect the identity of the people who use them (Csikszentmihalyi & Rochberg-Halton, 1981). Occupational therapists recognize that removing objects can be interpreted as a loss to some clients. Some objects may not seem functional, but they do have meaning and purpose. When making changes to a particular environment, introducing new tools, or removing objects, be aware of their meaning to the client. The occupational therapy practitioner needs to be sensitive to the meaning of the context and recognize how that may affect compliance to recommended interventions.

Occupational therapists evaluate the occupational functioning of their clients in the physical context and make recommendations for changes to the environment to optimize accessibility. Practitioners, however, often become frustrated when clients do not follow recommendations. The Consumer Decision Model (Ohta & Ohta, 1997) proposes that people need to perceive a high threat and severe consequences to their current environment, as well as high efficacy and low cost to making changes to the environment. Often clients will not make changes until a crisis arises.

Intervention Strategies to Optimize Accessibility

Through activity analysis, occupational therapists can identify the barriers in technology and the environment that may contribute to further disabling a person with functional limitations. Regardless of whether

RESOURCE 36-1

Optimizing Access to Home, Community, and Work Environments

Training Programs and Designations in Housing Accessibility and Modification

- AOTA Continuing Education: http://www.aota.org/nonmembers/area3/index.asp
- Lifease, Inc., Margaret Christenson, MPH, OTR, FAOTA, phone: (800) 961-3273.
- RESNA Assistive Technology Practitioner (ATP) and Assistive Technology Supplier (ATS) Credentialing Program, RESNA, 1700 N. Moore Street, Suite 1540, Arlington, VA 22209-1903. (703) 524-6686 (V). (703) 524-6639 (TTY). (703) 524-6630 (TTY). http://www.resna.org
- National Association of Home Builders (NAHB) Certified Aging in Place Specialist (CAPS), 1201 15th Street, NW, Washington, DC 20005. Phone: (800) 368-5242. Fax: (202) 266-8400. http://www.nahb.org
- National Resource Center on Supportive Housing and Home Modification, University of Southern California, Andrus Gerontology Center, 3715 McClintock Avenue, Los Angeles, CA 90089-0191. Phone: (213) 740-1364. Fax: (213) 740-7069. http://www.homemods.org

Resources: Technical Assistance and Organizations

- ABLEDATA Phone: (800) 346-2742 www.abledata.com
- Abilities O.T. Services Inc. 3309 W. Strathmore Avenue, Baltimore, MD 21215-3718. Phone: (410) 358-7269. Fax: (410) 358-6454. E-mail: shoshamberg@yahoo.com
- Access Board (ATBCB) Phone: (800) 872-2253
- Adaptive Environments Center, Inc. (AEC) 347 Congress Street, Suite 301, Boston, MA 02210. Phone: (617) 695-1225. Fax: (617) 482-8099. http://www.adaptenv.org
- Accessible Space, Inc. (ASI) 2550 University Avenue, Suite 330 N., St. Paul, MN 55114. Phone: (800) 466-7722. Fax: (651) 645-0541. http://www.accessiblespace.org
- American Association of Homes and Services for the Aging (AAHSA) 901 E Street NW, Suite 500, Washington, DC 20004-2011. Phone: (202) 783-2242. Fax: (202) 783-2255. http://www.aahsa.org
- American Association of Retired People (AARP) 601 E Street NW, Washington, DC 20049. Phone: (202) 434-6120. http://www.aarp.org
- American National Standards Institute (ANSI) Phone: (212) 868-1220
- American Occupational Therapy Association (AOTA) 4720 Montgomery Avenue, P.O. Box 31220, Bethesda, MD 20814-1220. Phone: (800) SAY-AOTA. http://www.aota.org
- Association for Safe & Accessible Products (ASAP) 50 Washington St., Norwalk, CT 06854. Phone: (203) 857-0200.
- Center for Universal Design North Carolina State University, School of Design, Box 8613, Raleigh, NC 27695-8613. www.ncsu.edu/ncsu/design/cud
- Concrete Change 600 Dancing Fox Road, Decatur, GA 30032. Phone: (404) 378-7455. http://concretechange.home.mindspring.com/
- Consortium for Citizens with Disabilities (CCD) Housing Task Force http://www.c-c-d.org/tf-housing.htm
- Disability Rights Education Defense Fund Phone: (202) 986-0375
- Easter Seals 230 West Monroe Street, Suite 1800, Chicago, IL 60606. Phone: (800) 221-6827; (312) 726-6200; (312) 726-4258 (TTY). http://www.easter-seals.org/resources/easy.asp
- Future Home Foundation Inc. Att: Dave Ward, curator, 12900 Jarrettsville Pike, Phoenix, MD 21131. Phone: (410) 666-0086. E-mail: cdavidward@aol.com
- Habitat for Humanity International (HFHI) 1 Habitat Street, Americus, GA 31709-3498. Phone: (800) 422-4828 ([800] HABITAT); (912) 924-6935. http://www.habitat.org
- Independent Living Centers For a listing of local centers, call the national office at (314) 531-3055.
- IDEA Center for Inclusive Design and Environmental Access School of Architecture and Planning, State University of New York at Buffalo, Buffalo, NY 14214-3087. Phone: (716) 829-3485. Fax: (716) 829-3256. http://www.ap.buffalo.edu/;idea
- Industrial Design Society of America, IDSA-UD Special Interest Section 1141 Walker Road, Great Falls, VA 22066. Phone: (703) 759-0100. Fax: (703) 759-7679. http://www.idsa.org
- Lighthouse International http://www.lighthouse.org/
- National Association of Home Builders Research Center 400 Prince George's Center Boulevard, Upper Marlboro, MD 20774-8731. Phone: (301) 249-4000. Fax: (301) 249-0305. http://www.nahb.org
- National Association of the Remodeling Industry (NARI) 4900 Seminary Road, Suite 320, Alexandria, VA 22311. Phone: (800) 966-7601; (703) 575-1100. Fax: (703) 575-1121. http://www.nari.org
- National Home Modification Action Coalition (NHMAC) http://www.homemods.org
- National Kitchen & Bath Association (NKBA) 687 Willow Grove Street, Hackettstown, NJ 07840. Phone: (800) 367-6522; (800) 843-6522. Fax: (908) 852-1695. http://www.nkba.org
- Paralyzed Veterans of America (PVA) 801-18th Street NW, Washington, DC 20008. Phone: (800) 424-8200 (V); (800) 795-4327 (TTY). Fax: (202) 785-4452. http://www.pva.org
- Rebuilding Together 1536 Sixteenth Street. NW, Washington, DC 20036-1402. Phone: (800) 4-REHAB-9. Fax: (202) 483-9081. http://www.rebuildingtogether.org
- Remodeling Online http://www.remodeling.hw.net
- Siebert, C. (2005). Occupational therapy practice guidelines for home modifications. Bethesda, MD: American Occupational Therapy Association Press.

RESOURCE 36-1

- Technical Assistance Collaborative, Inc. One Center Plaza, Suite 310, Boston, MA 02108. Phone: (617) 742-5657. Fax: (617) 742-0509. www.tacinc.org
- TRACE Research and Development Center University of Wisconsin at Madison, 5901 Research Park Boulevard, Madison, WI 53719-1252. Phone: (608) 262-6966. www.trace.wisc.edu
- Universal Designers & Consultants, Inc. (UDC) 6 Grant Avenue, Takoma Park, MD 20912. Phone: (301) 270-2470 (V-TTY). Fax: (301) 270-8199. http://www.UniversalDesign.com
- U.S. Department of Housing and Urban Development (HUD). Phone: (800) 827-5005. www.hud.gov/fhe/fheo.html
- Volunteers for Medical Engineering Baltimore, MD. Phone: (410) 455-6395.

interventions are targeted at participation in the home, workplace, or community, the four strategies discussed in this section can be applied.

1. Universal design and other accessible design
2. Environmental modifications
3. Assistive technology
4. Task modification strategies

Universal Design and Other Accessible Design

Occupational therapists' understanding of occupational performance can offer valuable knowledge to an interdisciplinary team that implements universal design to help maximize occupational performance for all potential users. By understanding the needs of people with a variety of health conditions, occupational therapists can contribute to increasing accessibility of spaces and products that are used by many people (Definition 36-1; Procedures for Practice 36-2).

Products that are designed for use by everyone should use universal design principles. One example is the use of an automatic door opener. Automatic doors decrease the need for strength, motor skills, and cognitive skills. In addition to being useful to people with these types of functional limitations, automatic doors can be helpful to any worker who is carrying packages through the doorway. Figures 36-1, 36-2, and 36-3 illustrate some design features of both home and workplace that apply universal design to a bathroom, kitchen, and office space.

Environmental Modifications and Assistive Technology

Most environments have not been built with universal design features in mind, and therefore, environmental modifications are needed to increase accessibility. Environmental modifications are changes made to the current physical environment. Occupational therapy practitioners collaborate with the client and with other team members, such as design, construction, and other building professionals, to develop a plan for reducing environmental barriers.

A typical home bathroom does not contain the same features noted in the universal design bathroom (Fig. 36-1). Therefore, homes may need to be retrofitted to include them. For instance, someone who has a bathtub may need to replace it with a curbless shower to facilitate bathing in a wheelchair. Public Law 100-407 (1998) defines **assistive technology** as "any item, piece of equipment, or product system, whether acquired commercially off the shelf, modified, or customized, that is used to increase, maintain, or improve functional capabilities of individuals with disabilities." Assistive technology can be added to the environment.

Task Modification Strategies

Design features, modifications, and assistive technology are used to decrease environmental demands and to reduce barriers. Task modifications are changes in how or where a task is performed. Occupational therapists provide training to clients who need to learn how to do a task in a different way.

One way in which a task can be modified is by teaching a client to perform a task from a different position, such as seated rather than standing, or using a nondominant hand. Another type of task modification is performing a task in a different location (such as bathing in a shower rather than a tub or sleeping in the living room instead of the bedroom). Changing the time of day in which an activity is performed is another strategy used by people who fatigue and need to allocate their energy to their most important activities of the day. Objects in the environment can be grouped for a similar task, or the

DEFINITION 36-1

Types of Accessible Design

When providing consultation to designers, contractors, families, and patients, occupational therapists appreciate the breadth of access and functional performance strategies and aids that may be available to consumers. The following terms help to clarify the various ways that accessible environments can be created and labeled. This assists in communication with other professionals on the implementation team, especially the designers and building contractors.

- "**Universal design** is the design of products and environments to be usable by all people, to the greatest extent possible, without the need for adaptation or specialized design" (Mace, 1997). Environments created using the elements of universal design are accessible, adaptable, aesthetically pleasing (non-medical appearance), and often cost effective. Universal design is intended to eliminate barriers and the need for major structural modifications, and to provide features that can be used by people with a wide range of abilities and needs across the life span. This design approach minimizes the need for major costly structural modifications to accommodate a functional impairment or age-related decline (American Association for Retired People, 1996). Universal design features address the natural effects of aging, which may result in physical, sensory, and/or cognitive decline (ABLEDATA, 1995). Ideally, this type of design should address the general needs of people with a wide range of functional abilities and limitations.
- An accessible environment may be used, approached, and entered easily, especially by people with disabilities. It is not necessarily designed to address a specific functional limitation.
- An adaptable environment is one that is built or modified so that adaptation for individual and changing needs can be accomplished over time without major structural changes.
- Lifespan design incorporates accessible and adaptable features for use as occupants grow older to accommodate changes in functional ability (Shamberg, 1993).
- A barrier-free environment is built or altered to remove obstacles and maximize accessibility. It is usually designed to address the specific needs of individuals with functional limitations. An example of barrier-free design is a wide, flat entryway to accommodate wheelchairs. By modifying physical space, equipment, tasks, and behavior, a person can compensate for age-related changes or disability and maximize comfort, safety, and independence. Often the environment produces greater barriers to a person's functional performance than the actual disabling condition (Center for Universal Design, 1997).

PROCEDURES FOR PRACTICE 36-2

Principles of Universal Design

When designing a space or product to be used by all potential users, the following principles should be applied.

Equitable Use

The design is useful and marketable to people with diverse abilities.

Guidelines

- Provide the same means of use for all users: identical whenever possible; equivalent when not.
- Avoid segregating or stigmatizing any users.
- Provisions for privacy, security, and safety should be equally available to all users.
- Make the design appealing to all users.

Flexible in Use

The design accommodates a wide range of individual preferences and abilities.

Guidelines

- Provide choice in methods of use.
- Accommodate right- or left-handed access and use.
- Facilitate the user's accuracy and precision.
- Provide adaptability to the user's pace.

Simple and Intuitive

Use of the design is easy to understand, regardless of the user's experience, knowledge, language skills, or current concentration level.

Guidelines

- Eliminate unnecessary complexity.
- Be consistent with user expectations and intuition.
- Accommodate a wide range of literacy and language skills.
- Arrange information consistent with its importance.
- Provide effective prompting and feedback during and after task completion.

Perceptible Information

The design communicates necessary information effectively to the user, regardless of ambient conditions or the user's sensory abilities.

(continued)

PROCEDURES FOR PRACTICE 36-2 *(continued)*

Guidelines

- Use different modes (pictorial, verbal, tactile) for redundant presentation of essential information.
- Provide adequate contrast between essential information and its surroundings.
- Maximize "legibility" of essential information.
- Differentiate elements in ways that can be described (i.e., make it easy to give instructions or directions).
- Provide compatibility with a variety of techniques or devices used by people with sensory limitations.

Tolerance for Error

The design minimizes hazards and the adverse consequences of accidental or unintended actions.

Guidelines

- Arrange elements to minimize hazards and errors: most used elements should be most accessible; hazardous elements should be eliminated, isolated, or shielded.
- Provide warnings of hazards and errors.
- Provide fail-safe features.
- Discourage unconscious action in tasks that require vigilance.

Low Physical Effort

The design can be used efficiently and comfortably and with a minimum of fatigue.

Guidelines

- Allow user to maintain a neutral body position.
- Use reasonable operating forces.
- Minimize repetitive actions.
- Minimize sustained physical effort.

Size and Space for Approach and Use

Appropriate size and space is provided for approach, reach, manipulation, and use regardless of user's body size, posture, or mobility.

Guidelines

- Provide a clear line of sight to important elements for any seated or standing user.
- Make reach to all components comfortable for any seated or standing user.
- Accommodate variations in hand and grip size.
- Provide adequate space for the use of assistive devices or personal assistance.

© Copyright 1997 North Carolina State University, The Center for Universal Design.

The Center for Universal Design (1997). *The principles of universal design, version 2.0.* Raleigh, NC: North Carolina State University. Compiled by advocates of universal design, listed in alphabetical order: Bettye Rose Connell, Mike Jones, Ron Mace, Jim Mueller, Abir Mullick, Elaine Ostroff, Jon Sanford, Ed Steinfeld, Molly Story, and Gregg Vanderheiden

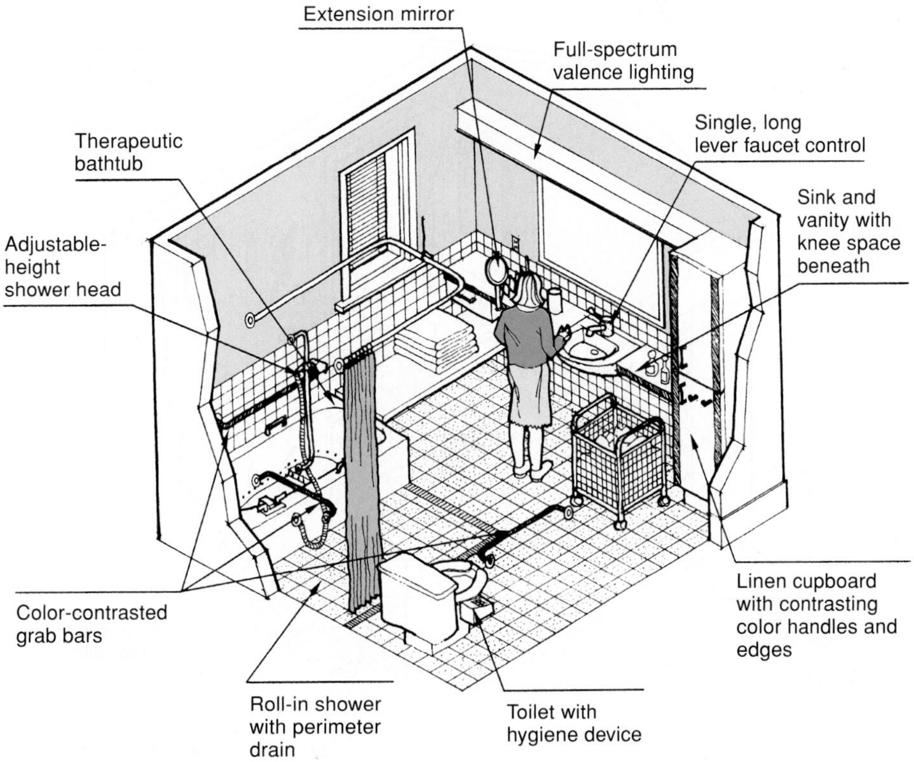

Figure 36-1 Example of universal-design bathroom. (Reprinted with permission from Canadian Mortgage Housing Corporation. [1992]. *Open house guidebook* [p. 10]. Ottawa, Ontario, Canada: Canadian Mortgage Housing Corporation Innovation Division.)

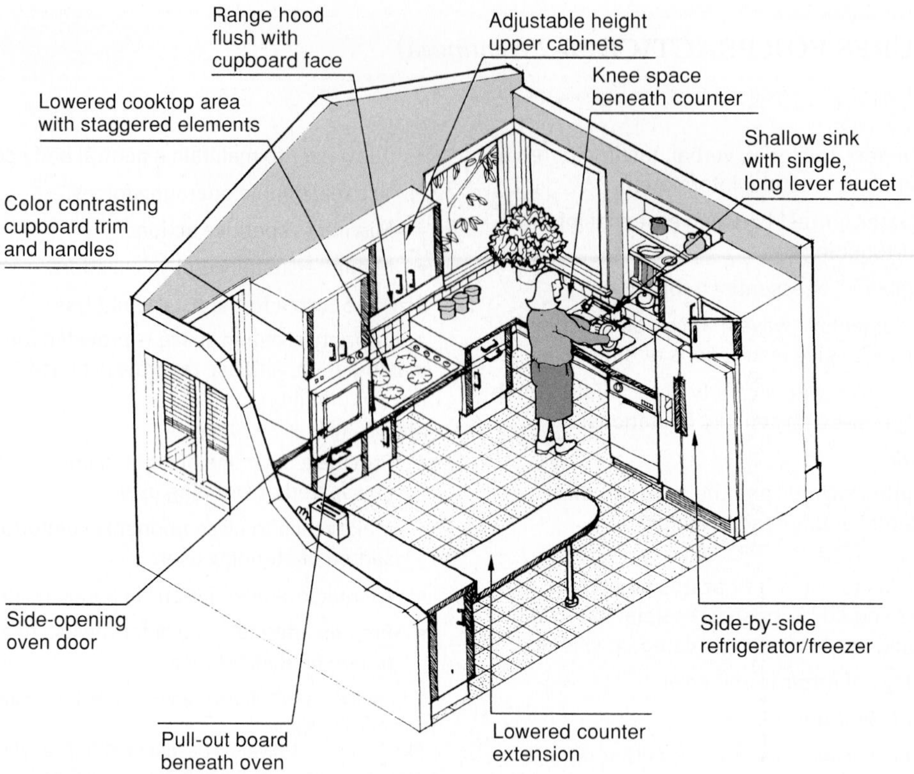

Figure 36-2 Example of universal-design kitchen. (Reprinted with permission from Canadian Mortgage Housing Corporation. [1992]. *Open house guidebook* [p. 14]. Ottawa, Ontario, Canada: Canadian Mortgage Housing Corporation Innovation Division.)

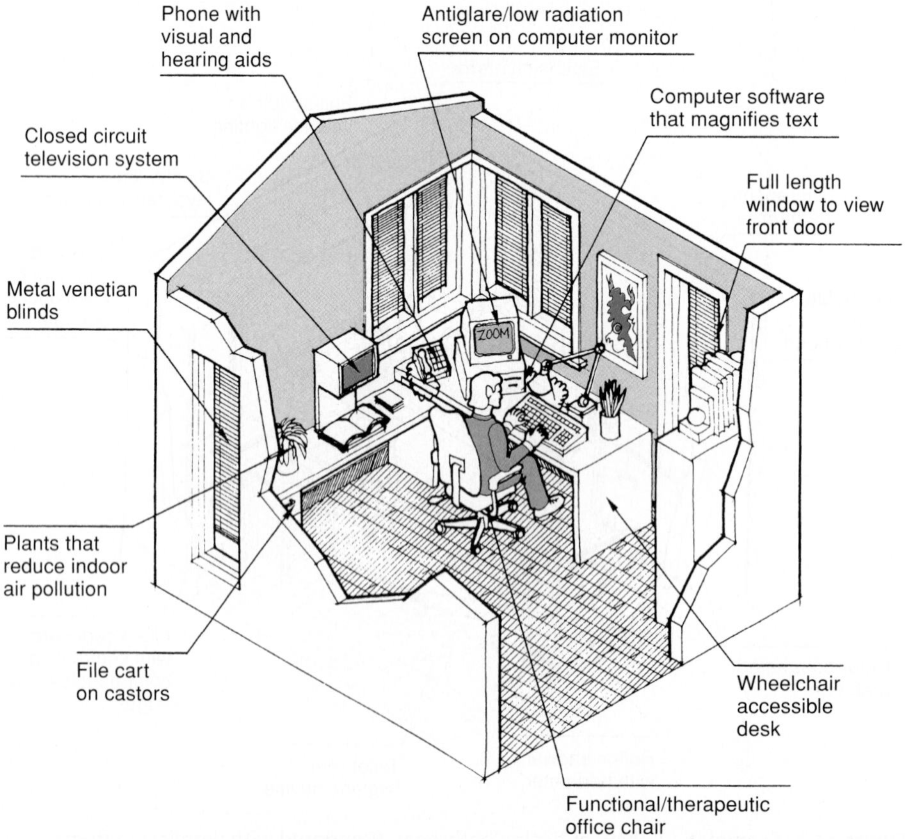

Figure 36-3 Example of universal-design office. (Reprinted with permission from Canadian Mortgage Housing Corporation. [1992]. *Open house guidebook* [p. 6]. Ottawa, Ontario, Canada: Canadian Mortgage Housing Corporation Innovation Division.)

PROCEDURES FOR PRACTICE 36-3

Therapeutic Intervention to Promote Safety and Independence: Principles of Work Simplification

- Use both hands to work with symmetrical motions when possible.
- Lay out work areas within normal reach. Work where the areas of both hands overlap and arrange supplies in a semicircle within easy reach. Plan storage within normal reaching ranges in the working area. Arrange storage at first point of use; have extras of the things you need at more than one work center, for example, measuring cups, spoons, knives, and so on. Create fixed workstations where there is a designated location for each job so that supplies and equipment can always be kept there ready for immediate use.
- Slide heavy objects rather than lifting and carrying. For example, slide pots from sink to range. Use a wheeled cart if counters are not contiguous.
- Avoid holding and grasping; instead, use utensils that rest firmly or suction cups or clamps, so both hands are free to work.
- Let gravity work for you by using a laundry chute, refuse chute, gravity-fed flour and sugar bins, or a pan below the level of a cutting board.
- Store small tools so that they are in the proper position to grasp and start working immediately. Store the eggbeater so its handle can be grasped in the left hand without shifting.
- Create efficient storage by using a pegboard on the wall with hooks for hanging, magnetic racks for knives and utensil storage, step shelves to maximize tight spaces with less reaching, and vertical storage racks.
- Have machine controls and switches within easy reach. Change the location and position of switches by using extension cords and minimize unplugging and plugging by using a multiplug outlet or extension cord with a single on-off switch.
- Whenever possible, sit to work in a comfortable chair and adjust the work surface or chair height for upright posture and forearm support. When you are seated, place feet flat on the floor or use a footrest. Use a chair with back support, especially in the lower back. Use a support cushion where needed, and slope the seat slightly to the back so that you do not slide forward. Ensure enough knee room to allow you to face the job to be done.
- Use the height appropriate for you, the worker, as well as the job. Jobs requiring hand activity need a higher work surface than those requiring arm motion or pressure. Since body proportions differ, use individualized measurements when possible. The arms and shoulders of a seated or standing person should be relaxed without raising hands above the level of elbows. A work surface a few inches lower than the elbows allows a person to work without hunching the shoulders and enables proper leverage for the work to be done.
- Create pleasant working conditions with a minimum of stress and strain. Natural lighting, halogen lighting, adequate ventilation, comfortable clothing, pleasing colors and music, windows looking onto natural settings, and organization of the environment facilitate this goal.

steps to completing an activity can be simplified (Procedures for Practice 36-3).

SPECIFIC INTERVENTIONS FOR ACCESS TO THE HOME ENVIRONMENT

When helping clients optimize access to their home environments, occupational therapists evaluate performance of activities of daily living (ADLs) and other activities that are currently performed in the home. Therapists assess the environment for hazards such as clutter, poor lighting, and broken steps. They also assess the person's behavior within the environment such as balance and strength when transferring, problem-solving skills in emergency situations, and sensory/perception such as for detecting temperature changes when cooking and bathing. (See Chapter 11 for a full discussion of assessing accessibility.)

The three most challenging areas of the home are the entrance, inside stairs, and the bathroom (Housing and Urban Development, 2001).

Entrance and Stairs

The front door may not be easily accessible by someone using a wheelchair or even a walker. Steps can provide a challenge when entering the home. For people who are ambulatory but unsteady, a solution may be adding secure handrails to support the body. Handrails may be a low-cost modification initially used to support an older person as they are trying to use the steps. People who use mobility devices (e.g., walkers and wheelchairs) may need more extensive modifications to the environment such as a ramp or lift.

Ramps are a lower cost option to creating a no-step entrance. The slope of a ramp needs to minimize the steepness without making too long of an entrance. Some alternatives for ramp configurations can be found in Figure 36-4. Often, there is a tradeoff between strength and endurance in relation to the slope of the ramp. Figure 36-5 demonstrates the rise to run ratio or ramp slope. When the entrance to a home is very steep or the yard space required to build a ramp is insufficient, lifts may be another alternative. An often aesthetically pleasing option is to use soil and ground covering to create a gradual sloping feature called an earth berm.

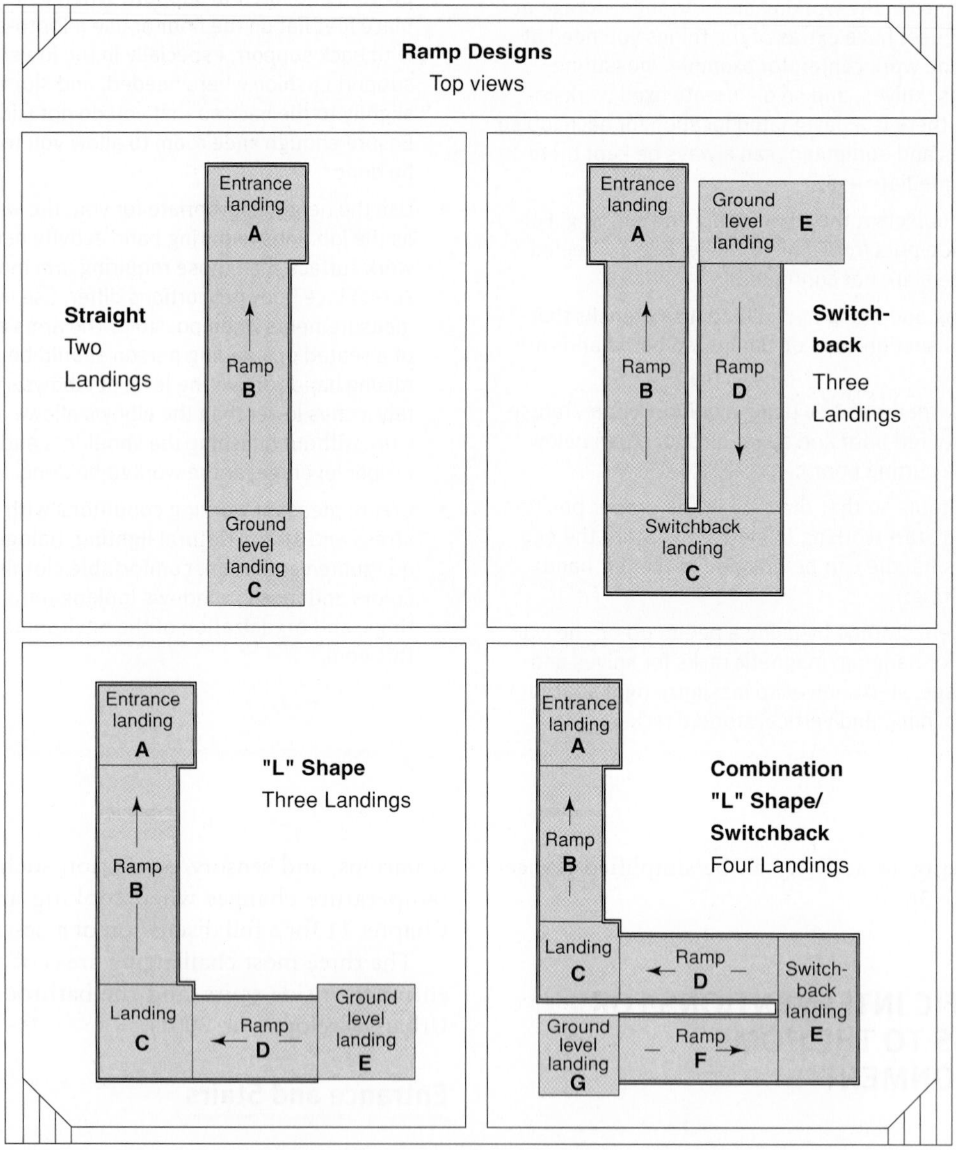

Figure 36-4 Typical ramp specifications. For an outdoor uncovered ramp, the ratio of height to length is 1:20 (for every inch of height, 20 inches of length). For a covered outdoor or indoor ramp, the ratio is typically 1:12. Landings are needed wherever the ramp changes direction and at 30-foot intervals on long ramps. The landing at the top of the ramp should be 5 × 5 feet for adequate maneuvering. The bottom of the ramp must have at least 5 feet of level area at the termination point. Recommended widths of ramps range from 36 to 48 inches with handrail grasping surface 30 to 34 inches high. (Reprinted from Henson J. [1988]. *Building a ramp* [p. 7]. Little Rock, AR: Arkansas Department of Human Services, Division of Rehabilitation Services.)

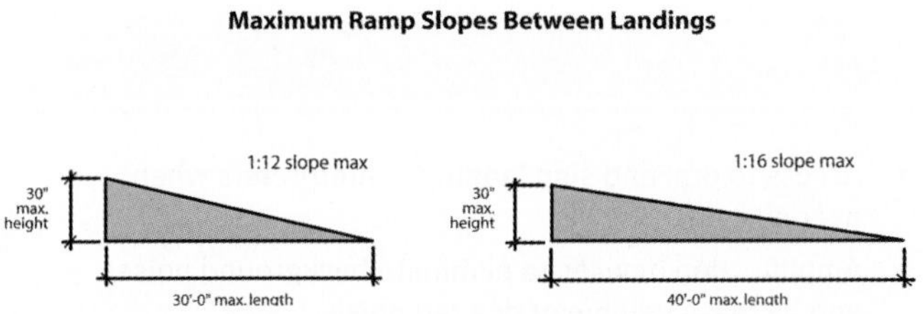

Figure 36-5 Sample ramp slope specifications.

Bathrooms

Bathing, grooming, and toileting are typically performed in the bathroom. When bathrooms are not accessible, people may perform these activities in other locations. Older adults may use a bedside commode to toilet in a bedroom or living room. People who cannot access their second-floor bathroom may sponge bathe in the kitchen sink. Figure 36-1 shows some features that offer different options for creating a more accessible bathroom.

INTERVENTIONS FOR ACCESS TO WORK ENVIRONMENT

Although the ADA does not apply to home modifications, Title I of the ADA ensures that workers with disabilities have access to accommodations that enable them to perform the tasks required for their job (see Chapter 33). Entering and exiting the workplace, moving around the workplace, and completing essential job tasks may be difficult if environmental barriers exist. Workplace accommodations can be used to reduce activity demands and therefore maximize occupational functioning at work. For example, heavy doors can be challenging to open. Guidelines indicate that doors should open with 5 pounds or less of pressure or with electronic controls. Other examples of common workplace accommodations include computer adaptations, such as voice input and output software, large-print screens, adapted keyboards, accessible workstations and bathrooms, adapted telephones, telecommunications display device (TDD) or text telephone, Braille and large print materials, sign language interpreter, and adapted controls on equipment (Fig. 36-3). In addition to accessing workstations, environmental barriers can also exist in accessing the restrooms and break rooms; this aspect of social participation is also the purview of the occupational therapist working to optimize access for clients.

As is clear from the previous discussion, occupational therapists can help clients optimize access to home and work in many ways. The interaction of the person's abilities and the environment is key in determining which interventions will best facilitate occupational performance. Procedures for Practice 36-4 details a wide array of modifications for various functional limitations.

INTERVENTIONS FOR ACCESS TO THE BROADER COMMUNITY

Homes and workplaces are part of communities. Schools, parks and recreational facilities, retail stores, and places for health and social services are also part of the community environment. These public spaces are subject to some of the established guidelines. Guidelines, such as the Fair Housing Act Accessibility Guidelines (FHAAG) and the Uniform Federal Accessibility Standards (UFAS), provide recommendations for design of architectural features, installation of equipment, and space planning, including height, width, type, and configuration of elements and fixtures (Architectural Transportation Barriers Compliance Board or Access Board, 1991). The FHAAG regulates the design of private multifamily housing, such as apartments. The ADAAG applies to public spaces, particularly the workplace and community. To further explain some of the specifications outlined in ADAAG, see Figure 36-6 for installing grab bars and Figure 36-7 for the turning radius for wheelchair users (Procedures for Practice 36-5).

Access to visiting one's neighbors is another issue around community accessibility. The concept of **visitability**, as discussed by Eleanor Smith of Concrete Change (Atlanta, Georgia), suggests that all home environments be designed so that people can visit one another. Visitability includes three basic features for access to homes, including a no-step entrance, wide doorways (32 inches) on the first floor of the home, and access to a first floor bathroom with an accessible toilet, sink, and light switch. For the most part, private homes are not required to be accessible. Recommendations can be made, however, to include basic features of access in the design of a home to meet future needs, eliminating the need for major and often costly modifications later (Concrete Change, 2001).

Access to the community goes far beyond just meeting set standards or adhering strictly to guidelines. Specialists who thoroughly understand the minimum accessibility features can advocate not only for implementation of these features, but also for exceeding them to further optimize accessibility.

FACTORS AFFECTING EFFECTIVENESS OF INTERVENTION STRATEGIES

The goal of environmental interventions is to improve accessibility to facilitate occupational functioning. To opti-

PROCEDURES FOR PRACTICE 36-4

Examples of Suggested Environmental Interventions for Specific Functional Limitations

The following are examples of environmental interventions for people with visual impairments:

- Adequate lighting with high lumens. Use non-glare lighting with sconces or shades. Halogen lighting is recommended for close work and task lighting in work areas for extra lighting when needed. Use switches that can provide adjustable light intensity for different tasks.
- Window treatments that allow for light filtering and adjustment and awnings on the outside of windows when direct sunlight is the most intense.
- Contrasting colors of surfaces to define objects and spaces, especially background and foreground, such as light switch covers contrasting with walls, chair seat contrasting with floor, wall contrasting with floor, countertops contrasting with sink, dark food on light-colored cutting board and the reverse, and step edges contrasting with step surface.
- Tactile indicators, raised letters, or voice output on controls and signs. Use large print with high contrast from the background. Vary textures to provide cues for directionality and dangerous situations.
- Elimination of busy and confusing patterns on such surfaces as rugs, upholstery, and wallpaper.
- Elimination of clutter and obstacles from access routes throughout the environment and removal of low-profile furniture or moving it against walls out of access routes.
- Visual aides such as closed-circuit television, magnifiers, large-print computer screens with high contrast, and talking devices.
- Illuminated switches for appliances and lights. Large knobs and handles that contrast in color and have a non-slip surface.
- Bathroom grab bar system that contrasts with the wall and that has a 1.5-inch diameter and a non-slip surface. Colored tape may be wrapped around the bar to create a pattern.

The following are common environmental interventions to address the needs of people with hearing impairments:

- Use of TDDs for telephone communication. Use of fax machine and telephone relay system.
- Handy access to paper and writing implement for communication.
- Vibrating or visual signal devices, such as alarm clocks, smoke alarms, telephones, doorbells, and baby monitors to place under pillow or bed when sleeping.
- Closed caption features on television and videos. Use of closed-loop or amplification devices for use in group settings or large spaces.
- Access to oral and sign language interpreters when needed.
- Amplification devices to eliminate background noises and increase volume of desired noise.
- Arrange furniture so people sit facing each other and ensure that there is adequate lighting so the person can use visual cues when conversing.

The following suggestions address the needs of people with mobility impairments:

- Ranch-style houses with at least one no-step entrance. The house should be on a flat lot with continuous sidewalks and street access from house to house and block to block. The house should be in an area with accessible public spaces like banks, shopping centers, library, post office, medical offices, parks, and recreation centers.
- Open, unobstructed spaces in each room with adequate turning radius for the wheelchair.
- Bathroom off the master bedroom with a wheel-in shower, transfer space on at least one side of the toilet, pull-down grab bars to use when needed.
- Open-bottom sink with counter space and a ground fault circuit interrupt (GFI) outlet within easy reach.
- Either a built-in transfer bench or portable one in the shower. Barrier-free shower doors or a shower curtain. Hand-held showerhead on an adjustable-height track.
- Wheelchair stair lift providing access to the finished basement.
- Patio or deck off the back door and master bedroom with access to a garden area.
- Environmental control system (ECU) to regulate the thermostat, lighting, television, stereo, and so on from one portable control unit.
- Wheelchair-accessible home office with computer station.
- Adjustable-height countertops, cabinets, and sinks.
- Wall oven and microwave at accessible heights.
- Stovetop with staggered burners and front or side controls.
- Angled mirror over the stove to show contents of pots for a seated person.
- Accessible switches for exhaust ventilation and fire extinguisher.
- Low-maintenance lawn covering and landscaping. Raised, vertical, or container beds for gardening from a wheelchair.
- Garbage can on wheels.
- Wheelchair-accessible table tennis, pool table, swimming pool with a lift.

PROCEDURES FOR PRACTICE 36-4 *(continued)*

The following recommendations address the needs of people with mild dementia living in their own homes:

- Environmental cues and assistive devices to address safety and memory deficits and communication deficits.
- Personal emergency response system with medication management. Training in use of devices and monitoring of ability to learn.
- Automatic medication management system that is set up weekly by a home care nurse.
- Burglar alarm and posted fire escape plan. Client instructed in emergency response and escape, with periodic reinforcement to ensure carryover of learning. Smoke alarms that are hard-wired with battery backup.
- Emergency lighting in case of power failure.
- Daily call to monitor self-care ability.
- Meals on Wheels and use of microwave with electric hot water pot. Electric range or microwave oven rather than gas stove. Step-by-step instructions for each appliance and any safety precautions on or next to the device. Ongoing monitoring for safety awareness and proper use.
- Pre-programmed telephone numbers used most for one-button speed calling.
- Well-organized environment to compensate for any problem-solving or memory deficits. Labeled cabinets or doors removed in the kitchen for viewing the cabinet contents.

mize client acceptance of accessibility recommendations, the occupational therapist tries to address client awareness of resources, funding issues, and interdisciplinary communication.

Awareness of Resources

Occupational therapy practitioners work with clients to make them aware of their options regarding ways in which environmental demands can be reduced. Clients can often identify the occupational areas that are difficult for them, but they may not realize that the environment presents barriers to their occupational functioning. People continue to believe that something is "wrong" with them rather than with their environment when they have difficulty performing their occupations. Occupational therapy practitioners identify the demands and barriers presented in the environment and help clients address these accessibility issues in treatment plans.

Additionally, when clients do identify the need for environmental interventions, they may not know who can make the modifications, where to go to get services, and how to pay for them (Bayer & Harper, 2000). Occupational therapy practitioners can help families identify needed home modifications and access services. Home modifications are often pieced together through a variety of service providers. Area Agencies on Aging and Centers for

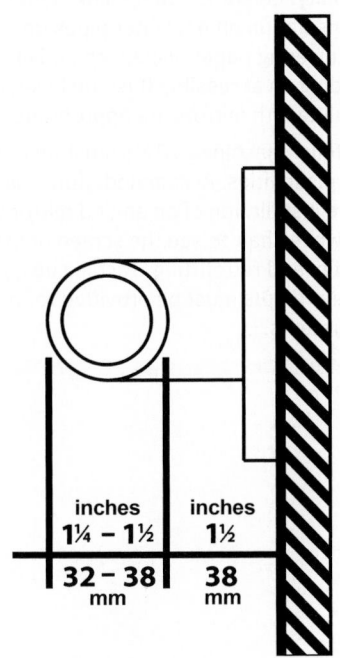

Figure 36-6 ADAAG specifications for placement of grab bars.

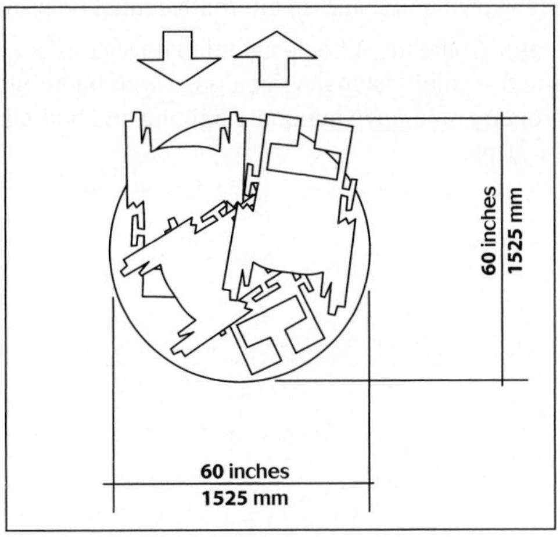

Figure 36-7 ADAAG specifications for wheelchair turning radius.

PROCEDURES FOR PRACTICE 36-5

Community Access: Accessible Design of Architectural Elements of Public Spaces and Multifamily Homes

The occupational therapy practitioner considers the following major elements of the environment when consulting about public spaces and multifamily homes, as specified in FHAAG and ADAAG:

- Accessible route. An accessible site must have a continuous unobstructed path connecting all elements and spaces of a building or facility, such as route from parking space to the entrance.
- Signage. ADAAG specifies the proportion, size, location, symbol usage, and level of contrast for character signage. Letters must contrast with background and must be raised and have Braille markings. Raised letters or numbers used to mark buildings, rooms, or offices must be placed on the right or left of the door 54–66 inches off ground or floor level.
- Parking spaces. Accessible parking spaces are required in every parking lot that services employees or visitors. The parking spaces must be convenient and marked for use for people with disabilities. Accessible spaces must have a minimum width of 12 feet, 5 feet of which serves as a drop-off zone and must be connected by an accessible route to an accessible entrance.
- Approaches. Paths must be a minimum of 36 inches wide. Pathways should be constructed of firm, smooth, non-slip continuous surfaces. Ramps must have handrails, curb guards, and non-slip surfaces. Landings must be provided at the base and top of each ramp. These landings must be no more than 30 feet apart.
- Doors and doorways. A doorway must have a clear opening of 36 inches (32 inches with door open) and must be operable by a single effort. Doorway entrances must be level at grade (0.5 inch or lower threshold). Fire doors are exempt from accessibility guidelines. Turnstile or revolving entrances are not accessible to those who use wheelchairs, and an alternative must be provided.
- Stairs. Stairs must be designed to have consistent tread and riser dimensions, be equipped with handrails, drain properly, and have adequate lighting and non-slip surfaces.
- Elevators. Elevators should be automatically operated and should have a cab door at least 32 inches wide, protective door and reopening devices, door and signal timing for hall calls, a door delay for cab calls, and an area large enough for wheelchair accessibility.
- Controls. Switches and controls for light, heat, ventilation, windows, curtains, fire alarms, and all similar controls must be placed within reach of people in wheelchairs, preferably approximately 42 inches off the floor.
- Warning signals. Warning signals must be both visual and audible in nature and located at appropriate accessible heights as designated by ADAAG. Fire or exit signage must be at least 7 feet from the floor.
- Lighting. Adequate non-glare lighting should be provided, and electrical outlets and rocker-style or pressure-sensitive switches must be located at accessible heights.
- Public telephones and water fountains. A public telephone must be placed so that the coin slot, dial, and headset are reachable from a wheelchair. Phones for people with hearing impairments should be labeled as such, with clear visual operating instructions. Coin slots should not be more than 54 inches off the floor. Similarly, water fountains should be fully accessible. The fountain should not be recessed. Its controls should be on the front of the unit. A wall-mounted unit should not be more than 36 inches off the floor. An accessible cup dispenser and a telephone amplification device are examples of reasonable accommodations.
- Bathrooms. Toilet stalls should have grab bars. Toilet partitions should be rearranged and widened to increase maneuverability. Clearance under sinks and counters is necessary. Insulation on hot water pipes under sinks is important. Lowering paper dispensers, raising toilet seats, providing an accessible flushing lever, and lower mirrors or full-length mirrors are appropriate.
- Automated teller machines. ATMs must be usable for people with disabilities. Accommodations may be as simple as the installation of an angled mirror to enable a person in a wheelchair to see the screen or may run to major redesign and retrofitting. Tactile cues, Braille, and/or voice prompts must be provided for people with visual impairments.

Independent Living are federally supported social service organizations that vary by location as to whether they offer home modification services. Rebuilding Together is a national non-profit provider of home modifications and home repair with local chapters across the country. The variability across geographic locations can be challenging in finding service providers who assist with creating accessible home environments.

Vocational rehabilitation services often assist with **workplace accommodations** for people with disabilities. Some workplaces have ergonomic consultants or departments that help create workplace environments that reduce the risk of injuries while optimizing work productivity. The needs of aging workers will be a new challenge for many workplaces to begin to address.

Accessibility of public spaces is somewhat regulated with regard to the ADA. Many buildings and spaces, however, were built prior to 1990 (when the ADA took effect). Older buildings continue to contain many accessibility barriers. New construction is subject to meeting ADAAG. Occupational therapists can serve not only as consultants to projects aimed at increasing community accessibility, but also as advocates raising awareness of the barriers to community participation.

Community coalitions, local building codes, and local services available can all affect community accessibility. Interested individuals and organizations may form local coalitions to promote changes in building codes or to better coordinate the delivery of services. Since the information age, virtual communities also exist through the Internet. Occupational therapy practitioners can assist with gaining access to **electronic and information technology** for people with disabilities. This can be achieved by understanding the various formats, software programs, and interfaces with the technology needed by people with disabilities.

Funding Issues

One of the major barriers to home, workplace, and community access is finding funding for the changes. Universal design is a relatively recent concept and is not yet a standard practice in the design of new building and construction of homes, workplaces, and communities. New construction with accessibility features costs less than retrofitting existing structures.

Funding must be pieced together from a variety of sources. Individuals pay out of pocket. Employers may assist with funding workplace accommodations. Some insurance companies may pay for home and/or workplace accommodations. Community organizations with grant funds may pay for services that improve community accessibility and home accessibility. Funding options vary greatly by location, organization, and reason for the intervention.

Communication and the Interdisciplinary Team

As in other areas of practice, occupational therapy practitioners work in collaboration with other professionals who have different perspectives and terminology. Building professionals, such as contractors, designers, architects, and building code officials, are not part of a typical health care team but can be part of the team providing environmental interventions to promote accessibility. Professionals of multidisciplinary teams need to develop a method of communication that promotes collaborative problem solving. Occupational therapy recommendations that address client's occupational functioning are made in collaboration with the contractor who understands structural and construction issues. As with any type of team, all members need to have a similar understanding of the goal to effectively achieve the desired outcome.

EFFICACY AND OUTCOMES

The desired outcomes when optimizing accessibility are to maximize occupational functioning and social participation. People with disabilities, older adults, caregivers, personal assistants, and potentially anyone who is part of a particular environment can all benefit from the outcomes of environmental interventions. As a person ages, changes with aging may be modulated by reducing participation in activities rather than in changing the environment. Unknowingly, by limiting activities, the older person may contribute to further declines in physical functioning. Research in the area of fall risk reduction has demonstrated that occupational therapy visits with home modification recommendations can be an effective approach to reducing fall risk among older adults with a history of falling (Cumming, Thomas, & Szonyi, 1999). Researchers also have found the use of home modifications and assistive technology to be a cost-effective alternative to institutional care (Mann et al., 1999).

Not only do people with disabilities benefit from environmental accessibility, but also all potential users of a particular space or setting benefit. In a study of people with dementia and their caregivers, the caregivers were better able to cope with difficult behaviors of the person with dementia following home-modification interventions (Gitlin et al, 2001).

Evidence Table 36-1
Best Evidence for Occupational Therapy Practice Regarding Home Modification Interventions

Intervention	Description of Intervention Tested	Participants	Dosage	Type of Best Evidence and Level of Evidence	Benefit	Statistical Probability and Effect Size of Outcome	Reference
Assistive technology (AT) and environmental interventions (EI) will result in greater ADL performance and reduced overall cost of health-related services	OT visit with recommendations, implementation of AT and EI.	Older adults in New York (N = 104; treatment, n = 52;- controls, n = 52).	For treatment group, mean AT devices received, n = 15; mean EI interventions, n = 1.44; mean visits from OT = 8.9; and mean visits from technician, n = 2.4.	Randomized, controlled study; level I evidence. IA2a	Significant difference in number of AT devices received. Significant difference in number of EIs received. Cost-effective alternative to long-term care.	AT devices: t = 6.57, $p < 0.001$, $r = 0.297$ EIs received: t = 4.1, $p < 0.001$, $r = 0.14$. Cost effectiveness compared with long-term care: d = 0.56, $r = 0.243$.	Mann et al., 1999
Home modifications for caregivers (CGs) of persons with dementia	Home visits by OT with educational strategies and home modifications to manage ADL and IADL dependency and difficult behaviors of persons with dementia.	Family CGs in Philadelphia area caring for family member with dementia: N = 171 (treatment,n = 93; controls, n = 78).	Five 90-minute home visits by OT.	Randomized, controlled study, stratified by race and gender; level I evidence. IA2a	Intervention group compared with controls reported: less decline in IADL performance of person with dementia; spousal CGs were less upset by behaviors of person with dementia; female CGs were able to better manage behaviors; and female and minority CGs showed improved management of functional dependency.	Decline in IADL performance: $p = 0.030$, t = 2.24, $r = 0.017$. Spousal CGs less upset by behaviors of person with dementia: $p = 0.049$, t = 1.97, $r = 0.15$. Female CGs better able to manage behaviors: $p = 0.037$, t = 1.97, $r = 0.16$.	Gitlin et al., 2001

						Improved management of functional dependency by female and minority CGs: $p = 0.049$, $r = 0.15$; and $p = 0.037$, $r = 0.16$, respectively.	
Home modification intervention to reduce falls in older adults	Standardized assessment of home hazards, recommendations, and supervised implementation by OT, follow-up visit.	530 community-dwelling older adults in Sydney, Australia, prior to being discharged from inpatient hospitalization. (controls, n = 266; intervention, n = 264); mean age = 77 years.	1-hour home visit, with additional visits as needed and follow-up.	Randomized, controlled study with block design; level I evidence. IA1b	Intervention group demonstrated a 19% reduction in falls compared with control group. Those with prior history of falls showed a 36% reduction in fall rates in the intervention group compared with controls.	Reduction in falls: $p = 0.05$, t = 1.96, $r = 0.15$. Reduction in falls in those with a prior history of falls: $p = 0.001$, t = 2.54, $r = 0.19$.	Cumming, Thomas, & Szonyi, 1999
Bathroom modifications to maximize self-care performance	OT recommendations for bathroom modifications	Pre-test, n = 34; post-test n = 20.	Two home visits from OT: initial evaluation and recommendations and follow-up reevaluation. Both visits included instruction on safe self-care.	Quasi-experimental study, one group pre and post measures; level III evidence.	From pre to post test, participants showed significant improvement in bathing, ADL performance, and transfers.	Bathing: t = 2.65, $p < 0.01$, $r = 0.269$. ADL performance: $t = 3.01$ $p < 0.01$, $r = .322$. Transfers: $t = 5.08$ $p < .000$, $r = .576$	Gitlin, Miller, & Boyce, 1999

CASE EXAMPLE

Mrs. P.: Implementing Environmental Interventions to Optimize Occupational Performance

Occupational Therapy Intervention Process	Clinical Reasoning Process	
	Objectives	**Examples of Therapist's Internal Dialogue**
Patient Information Mrs. P. is an 85-year-old woman who sustained a right-sided cerebrovascular accident (CVA) 2 months ago, resulting in left-sided hemiparesis. She was recently discharged from the rehabilitation center to an apartment that she has shared with her husband for more than 30 years. Mr. P. would like to hire an attendant to work a few hours a day to assist with Mrs. P.'s personal care and to help with the housekeeping, but financial constraints do not allow for this. Both Mr. P. and their daughter carry out most of the household tasks and have reported becoming increasingly frustrated and fatigued. They both say that they don't believe that they can leave Mrs. P. alone because of their concerns about her safety and independence. Prior to her stroke, Mrs. P. prided herself on her ability to care for her husband and her home. Mrs. P. has been referred to the community occupational therapist to address concerns about her independence and safety in her home environment.	Appreciate the context	(See related assessment chapter, Chapter 11, for description of the assessment process and patient's background.) "I know that Mrs. P. is returning home where she lives with her husband. She needs assistance with personal care and housekeeping. Her husband wants help but cannot financially afford to hire an assistant for his wife. Their daughter lives nearby and helps when she can. Her workplace does not like her to take off time during the day though. She needs to take her mother to doctor appointments and tries to schedule them around her lunchtime."
	Develop intervention hypotheses	"I anticipate that Mrs. P. will be able to safely engage in some self-care and housekeeping activities. I may be able to help her delay further decline or even delay institutionalization by implementing environmental interventions and helping her acquire assistive technology that promotes accessibility and optimizes her occupational performance."
	Select an intervention approach	"Since I am unsure of Mrs. P.'s readiness to change, I will apply the Consumer Decision Model and further assess her perceived threat and consequences of her situation and cost and efficacy of interventions. I will also approach the intervention plan by addressing components of the Person-Environment-Occupation Model and determine how to decrease demands in the home environment to increase occupational performance."
	Reflect on competence	"I have worked with several clients with unilateral hemiparesis resulting from a stroke who were discharged home. I am knowledgeable about various tools and databases (such as LifeEASE, ABLEDATA, and eCASPAR) and am confident that I will be able to offer some options of products that may be useful to the needs of my client. I will work with another therapist who is knowledgeable in other techniques for stroke recovery that focus more on remediation such as constraint-induced movement. I will also make referrals to social work for assistance with finding funding sources and locating caregiver support for the family members."

Recommendations

The occupational therapist recommended 3–5 visits to negotiate environmental modifications and assistive technology. In collaboration with Mrs. P., her husband, and her daughter, the occupational therapist established the following long-term treatment goals: (1) following bathroom modifications, Mrs. P. will safely complete bathing activities with minimal supervision and prompting; (2) after instruction on task modification, Mrs. P. will engage in light housekeeping tasks with minimal assistance from family; (3) Mrs. P. will complete dressing and grooming tasks with the use of assistive devices and verbal prompting; and (4) Mrs. P. will participate in activities at a senior center 2–3 times a week.

Consider the patient's appraisal of performance	"Mrs. P. lacks of awareness of safety risks. I suspect that she may have attention deficits or executive function disorder, and further assessment is needed. This might explain why she does not demonstrate any memory deficit but does seem to have difficulty with initiation and sequencing. She is aware of changes in her abilities to perform meaningful activities."
Consider what will occur in therapy, how often, and for how long	"Mrs. P. will have home modifications made to her bathroom including replacing the tub with a shower, placing non-skid strips on the shower floor, and installing grab bars. Here is how I plan to approach Mrs. P.'s other needs: provide Mrs. P. and her family members training on safety issues and how to protect and care for her paralyzed side, which is likely to be neglected; use task modification strategies to engage Mrs. P. in meaningful housekeeping tasks; provide visual and verbal cues to encourage visual scanning to the affected side and to avoid injury; and provide assistive devices to assist with dressing, grooming, and meal preparation activities."
Ascertain the patient's endorsement of plan	"Mrs. P. is motivated to engage in housekeeping tasks, which are important to her. She is agreeable to the plan and understands that her family will feel more secure if she follows through with the recommended safety features."

Summary of Short-Term Goals and Progress

1. Mrs. P. will complete dressing and grooming tasks daily with the use of assistive devices.
2. Mrs. P. will complete at least two IADLs with task modification strategies, assistive devices, and set-up from family.

The occupational therapist introduced task modification strategies and assistive devices that facilitate access to participation in self-care and household activities. The therapist recognized that Mrs. P. was motivated to contribute to her family and her household.

The occupational therapist recognized that Mrs. P. liked gadgets and that she was open to trying assistive devices that reduced physical barriers. The therapist assisted Mrs. P. and her family in selecting several assistive devices to increase ADL and IADL performance and then trained Mrs. P. to use them. Mrs. P.'s family reported that Mrs. P. was less dependent on them for self-care activities.

Assess the patient's comprehension Understand what he is doing	"I could see that Mrs. P. became frustrated with learning to use a button hook for dressing. We discussed other alternatives, and eventually, she preferred to have Velcro fasteners on her clothes to replace buttons."
Compare actual to expected performance	"Mrs. P. was able to use a spiked cutting board while seated at the kitchen table. Her family assisted with set-up, but otherwise, she was able to complete most meal preparation."
Know the person Appreciate the context	"I anticipated that Mrs. P. would improve her participation in activities with the strategies and devices. She was highly motivated. We did have to try some different strategies to get the expected outcome. An additional outcome was that her family caregivers felt less burdened."

Next Steps Revised short-term goals (1 month): Following bathroom modifications and training with assistive devices, Mrs. P. will complete bathing with minimal supervision 2 times per week.	Analyze patient's comprehension	"Mrs. P. does not want to be dependent on her husband to assist her with bathing. She is waiting for assistance from Rebuilding Together to provide a roll-in shower in place of her tub."
	Decide if the patient should continue or discontinue therapy and/or return in the future	"I am concerned about Mrs. P.'s visual left neglect. She doesn't seem to be aware of the deficit, and she is resistant to strategies for visual scanning to the left. Also, she has fallen a couple times in the past month. Her visual and sensory perception is impaired, and she has difficulty when getting up from a chair. I wonder if she is experiencing orthostatic hypotension, which is contributing to her fall risk. I have referred her to a physical therapist. Following her bathroom modifications, I will visit her again and provide training."

CLINICAL REASONING IN OCCUPATIONAL THERAPY PRACTICE

Interventions to Decrease Environmental Demands

The demands in Mrs. P.'s home environment did not match with her current abilities and resulted in decreased performance of meaningful self-care and housework activities. Describe at least two different intervention strategies used by the therapist to help Mrs. P. progress toward resuming self-care and homemaker roles.

SUMMARY REVIEW QUESTIONS

1. What historical events affect current practices and trends in accessibility of homes, workplaces, and communities? Why is knowledge of these important to the occupational therapy practitioner who consults on accessibility?
2. How do the evaluation results influence decisions about interventions used to optimize accessibility in the home, workplace, and community?
3. What are some of the design and product solutions that help to reduce activity demands within the home environment?
4. How can universal design principles be applied to the design of communities, homes, and workplaces to maximize occupational functioning and social participation?

References

ABLEDATA. (1995). Informed consumer guide to accessible housing. *Macro International, January, 1–11.*

American Association of Retired Persons [AARP]. (1996). *Housing Report, Summer/Fall, 4–7.*

American Occupational Therapy Association [AOTA]. (1993). Statement: The role of OT in the independent living movement. *American Journal of Occupational Therapy, 47,* 1112.

Architectural Transportation Barriers Compliance Board or Access Board. (1991). *UFAS retrofit manual.* Washington, DC: United States Access Board.

Bayer, A., & Harper, L. (2000). Fixing to stay: A national survey on housing and home modification issues research report. Washington DC: American Association of Retired Persons.

Canadian Mortgage Housing Corporation. (1992). *Maintaining seniors' independence: A guide to home adaptations.* Ottawa, Ontario, Canada: Project Open House.

Center for Universal Design. (1997). The principles of universal design. Retrieved November 20, 2006, from http://design.ncsu.edu/cud/about_ud/wdprinciples.htm

Concrete Change. (2001). Visit-ability: Inclusive home design. Retrieved October 3, 2005 from http://www.concretechange.org/.

Csikszentmihalyi, M., & Rochberg-Halton, E. (1981). *The meaning of things: Domestic symbols and the self.* New York: Cambridge University Press.

Cumming, R. G., Thomas, M., Szonyi, G., Salkeld, G., O'Neill, E., Westbury, C., & Frampton, G. (1999). Home visits by an occupational therapist for assessment and modification of environmental hazards: A randomized trial of falls prevention. *Journal of the American Geriatrics Society, 47,* 1397–1402.

Frieden, L., & Cole, J. A. (1985). Independence: The ultimate goal of rehabilitation for spinal cord-injured people. *American Journal of Occupational Therapy, 39,* 734–739.

Gitlin, L. N., Corcoran, M., Winter, L., Boyce, A., & Hauck, W. W. (2001). A randomized, controlled trial of a home environmental intervention: Effect on efficacy and upset in caregivers and on daily function of people with dementia. *The Gerontologist, 41,* 4–14.

Gitlin, L. N., Miller, K. S., & Boyce, A. (1999). Bathroom modifications for frail elderly renters: Outcomes of a community-based program. *Technology & Disability, 10*(3), 141–149.

Greenwald, M., & Associates Inc., (2003). *These four walls... Americans 45+ talk about home and community*. Washington DC: American Association of Retired Persons.

Housing and Urban Development [HUD]. (2001). Special Needs Housing and the HOME Program. HUD-2001-18-CPD, May 2001.

Johnson, W. G. (1986). The Rehabilitation Act and discrimination against handicapped workers. In M. Berkowitz and M. A. Hill (eds.), *Disability and the Labor Market* (pp. 241–261). Ithaca: Cornell University ILR Press.

Kochera, A., Straight, A., & Guterbock, T. (2005). Beyond 50.05: A report to the nation on livable communities: Creating environments for successful aging. Washington DC: American Association of Retired Persons.

Lawton, M. P., & Nahemow, L. (1973). Ecology and the aging process. In C. Eisdorfer & M. P. Lawton (Eds.), *Psychology of adult development and aging* (pp. 619–674). Washington, DC: American Psychological Association.

McNeil, J. (2001). Americans with disabilities: Household economic studies. Washington DC: United States Census Bureau.

Mace, R. (1997). What is universal design? Raleigh, NC: NC State University, Center for Universal Design. Retrieved on February 17, 2006 from http://design.ncsu.edu/cud/univ_design/ud.htm.

Mann, W. C., Ottenbacher, K. J., Fraas, L., Tomita, M., & Granger, C. V. (1999). Effectiveness of assistive technology and environmental interventions in maintaining independence and reducing home care costs for the frail elderly: A randomized controlled trial. *Archives of Family Medicine, 8,* 210–217.

Marcus, C. C. (1995). *House as a mirror of self: Exploring the deeper meaning of home*. Berkley, CA: Conari Press.

Ohta, R. J., & Ohta, B. M. (1997). The elderly consumer's decision to accept or reject home adaptations: Issues and perspectives. In S. Lanspery & J. Hyde (Eds.), *Staying put: Adapting the places instead of the people* (pp. 79–89). Amityville, NY: Baywood.

Public Law 100-407. (1998). Technology-Related Assistance for Individuals with Disabilities Act of 1998.

Sanford, J. (2001). Best practices in the design of toileting and bathing facilities for assisted transfers. Report for the U. S. Access Board. Retrieved November 20, 2006 from http://www.access-board.gov/research/Toilet-Bath/report.htm.

Shamberg, S. (1993). The accessibility consultant: A new role for occupational therapists under the ADA. *Occupational Therapy Practice, 4,* 14–23.

Siebert, C. (2005). Occupational therapy practice guidelines for home modifications. Bethesda, MD: American Occupational Therapy Association Press.

Toossi, M. (2004). Employment outlook: 2002–2012, Labor force projections to 2012: The graying of the US workforce. *Monthly Labor Review*. Retrieved August 6, 2005 from http://www.bls.gov/opub/mlr/2004/02/art3full.pdf.

United States Census Bureau. (2004). U.S. Interim projections by age, sex, race, and Hispanic origin. Retrieved on February 17, 2006 from http://www.census.gov/ipc/www/usinterimproj/.

CHAPTER 37

Preventing Occupational Dysfunction Secondary to Aging

Glenn Goodman and Bette R. Bonder

LEARNING OBJECTIVES

After studying this chapter, the reader will be able to do the following:

1. Describe normal age-related changes as they relate to areas of occupation, performance skills, performance patterns, and client factors (body functions and body structures).
2. Discuss activity patterns of older adults as related to activities of daily living, instrumental activities of daily living, education, work, play, leisure, and social participation.
3. Describe considerations in assessing the function of older adults.
4. Discuss interventions through which occupational therapists can facilitate function in older adults.
5. Describe the factors that make intervention following illness or injury for older adults different from that for younger adults.

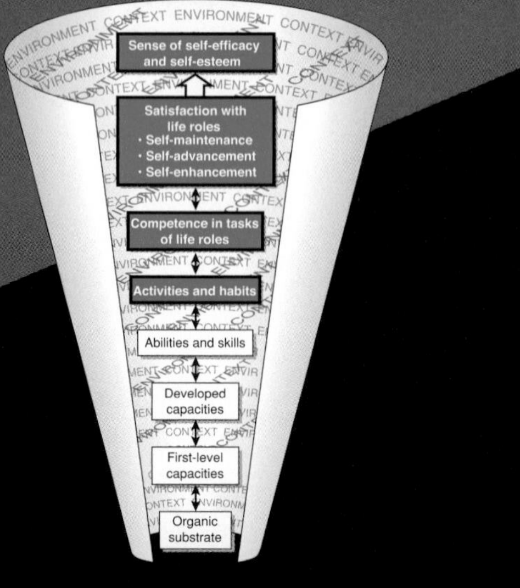

Glossary

Crystallized intelligence—Ability to use stored or previously learned information.

Dementia—Symptom caused by a number of conditions and characterized by loss of memory, language functions, ability to think abstractly, and ability to care for oneself.

Fluid intelligence—Ability to use new information.

Presbycusis—Age-related sensorineural hearing loss, especially for high-frequency sounds.

Presbyopia—Age-related vision change caused by loss of flexibility of the lens, which leads to poor near vision.

Productivity—Activities that make an economic contribution to society, including but not limited to paid employment, volunteer work, child care, and homemaking.

From 1950 to 2000, the total resident population of the United States increased from 150 million to 281 million, representing an average annual growth rate of 1% (Administration on Aging, 2004; Federal Interagency Forum on Aging Related Statistics [FIFARS], 2004). During the same period, the population 65 years of age and over grew almost twice as rapidly and increased from 12 to 35 million people. The population 75 years of age and over grew almost three times as quickly as the total population, increasing from 4 to 17 million people. Projections indicate that the rate of population growth during the next 50 years will be somewhat slower for all age groups and older age groups will continue to grow more than twice as rapidly as the total population. From 2000 to 2050, it is anticipated that the percentage of the population 65 years and over will increase substantially. Between 2000 and 2050, the percentage of the population 65 to 74 years of age will increase from 7% to 9%, and the population 75 years and over will increase from 6% to 12%. By 2040, the population 75 years and over will exceed the population 65 to 74 years of age. The aging of the population has important consequences for the health care system (Administration on Aging, 2004; FIFARS, 2004). As the older fraction of the population increases, more services will be required for the treatment and management of chronic and acute health conditions. Providing health care services needed by Americans of all ages will be a major challenge in the 21st century (Administration on Aging, 2004, p. 21).

These figures have considerable import for health care providers, particularly occupational therapists, who are concerned with assisting individuals to maintain or regain ability to perform valued daily activities. Enhancing functional performance of older adults can have economic, social, and personal benefits for these individuals, their families, and society as a whole.

The emphasis in this chapter is on the normal aging process. Older adults are, of course, subject to all of the illnesses and injuries that affect younger people, as well as some that are far more likely to occur in older individuals, such as cerebrovascular accidents, dementing illnesses, and cancer. Other chapters in this volume address mechanisms by which therapists can provide effective intervention for these conditions. When illness or injury occurs, however, the therapist must put the consequences in the context of the individual's life stage, which makes understanding normal aging essential. Special considerations in intervening with older adults are also discussed in this chapter.

NORMAL AGING

Changes that accompany normal aging occur in every sphere, both internal to the individual, including the cognitive-neuromuscular substrate, first-level capacities, and developed capacities, and external to the individual, as in social situations and responses to the physical environment. It is essential to remember, however, the wide range of variation among individuals. All of us know individuals who, at age 55, have stooped shoulders, shuffling gait, and poor vision and hearing and whose favorite activity is napping. We also know individuals who, at age 80, have a vigorous stride and engage in activities that would exhaust many a younger person. The existence of a physical change does not necessarily lead to a commensurate decrement in function. This section considers typical cognitive-neuromuscular, first-level, and developmental changes that accompany normal aging. These changes occur to varying degrees among older adults, with varying effects on performance.

COGNITIVE-NEUROMUSCULAR SUBSTRATE

Without question, genetic factors influence the aging process (Jones, Bland, & Quinn, 2003). Perhaps most important from the perspective of aging is the contribution of genetics to predisposition to illness and disability, including type II diabetes, some cancers, and high blood pressure (Jones, Bland, & Quinn, 2003). The interaction of genetic predisposition with personal behaviors and environmental circumstances leads to expression of genetic tendencies. Thus it may be possible to reduce risk of most genetic disorders by half or more through modification of behaviors (Rowe & Kahn, 1998). For example, exercise can reduce risk of high blood pressure and heart disease even in individuals with a strong genetic risk (Kell, Bell, & Quinney, 2001).

FIRST-LEVEL CAPACITIES

This section summarizes age-related changes in the following systems and capacities that allow for reflex-based responses: sensory, neuromuscular, cardiovascular, and cognitive. These first-level capacities are client factors as described in the Occupational Therapy Practice Framework (American Occupational Therapy Association [AOTA], 2002).

Sensory Changes

Some sensory changes normally occur with aging; others result from disease processes common among older adults (Hooper, 2001). One role of the occupational therapist is to evaluate the level of dysfunction caused by change in client factors such as sensation and process skills that allow individuals to interpret sensory input. Therapists then can determine strategies to compensate for problems that interfere with abilities, activities, tasks, and life roles in performance areas of occupation.

Changes typically occur in all sensory spheres, including vision, hearing, gustation, olfaction, touch, and vestibular sensation. Changes in multiple sensory channels require careful intervention to optimize function. Furthermore, decrements may occur at the level of reception or of interpretation or integration, that is, either peripherally or centrally in the nervous system (Bottomly & Lewis, 2003). Sensory loss can severely impair the older person's ability to communicate with other humans; the psychosocial consequences can be devastating (Heine & Browning, 2002).

Vision

In 2002, 18% of non-institutionalized people 65 years of age and older were visually impaired, which is defined as full or partial blindness or other trouble seeing. The prevalence of visual impairment increases with age, from 14% of people 65 to 74 years of age to 33% of people 85 years of age and over. Cataracts, glaucoma, and macular degeneration are primary causes of visual impairment among the older population (FIFARS, 2004).

Deterioration of near vision, called **presbyopia**, begins to affect most people when they are about age 40 (Boyce, 2003). The lens loses its elasticity and becomes less able to focus because of weakness in the ciliary body (Lewis, 2003) Presbyopia is easily accommodated through the use of a well-known assistive device: eyeglasses.

Another common change is development of degenerative opacities (cataracts) of the lenses, which lead to decreased sensitivity to colors, increased sensitivity to glare, and diminished acuity (Boyce, 2003).

Several diseases, including diabetic retinopathy and retinitis pigmentosa, can affect the retina at any age. The effects of these diseases, both of which may lead to total blindness, are most pronounced in the elderly population because both are progressive degenerative diseases (Boyce, 2003). Macular degeneration, a disorder causing loss of central vision as the macula deteriorates, is most common among older individuals. Most older individuals with macular degeneration retain sufficient peripheral vision to assist in mobility but not enough for activities such as reading or watching television (Boyce, 2003).

Musculature that controls eye movement tends to lose strength and tone (Tideiksaar, 2002). Tear secretion may be reduced and degenerative changes may occur in the sclera, pupil, and iris (Bottomly & Lewis, 2003). Such changes can result in excessive dryness, loss of light/dark accommodation, and poor night vision. Finally, decreased color vision and changes in the vitreous body that affect retinal function occur with aging (Bottomly & Lewis, 2003).

Hearing

Approximately 47% of men and 30% of women over 65 years old have severe hearing loss, especially for high frequencies (FIFARS, 2004). Conductive hearing loss may be the result of problems in the external or middle ear, such as wax buildup, Eustachian tube blockage, or stiffness of the ossicles and membranes (Lewis, 2003). Age-related sensorineural hearing loss, known as **presbycusis**, results from dysfunction of the sensory hair cells of the cochlea, neural connections from the cochlea to the cerebral cortex and brainstem, or vascular changes in the auditory system (Lewis, 2003). Functional consequences of these changes include difficulty hearing high-frequency sounds, distinguishing consonants during conversation, and filtering background noise during conversation, and challenges to balance due to inner ear changes (Tideiksaar, 2002).

Taste and Smell

Thresholds for taste and smell increase with age (Rawson, 2003). This has several functional implications. First, the ability to appreciate food flavor is closely related to olfaction (Lewis, 2003). Inability to detect aromas may cause food to seem tasteless, possibly resulting in secondary nutritional disorders. Safety may become a concern, as individuals may not be able to detect harmful odors such as natural gas, spoiled food, or smoke (Aldwin & Gilmer, 2003). Smoking or environmental exposures may exacerbate age-related changes in taste and olfaction (Bottomly & Lewis, 2003).

Tactile Changes

Tactile changes can occur due to normal aging, but there is more evidence to suggest tactile changes occur more frequently due to pathological conditions of the skin and nervous system (Aldwin & Gilmer, 2003; Bottomly & Lewis, 2003; Ebersole & Hess, 1998). Changes in the number and sensitivity of touch and pressure receptors have been reported, but studies showing definitive loss of pain and temperature sense are not yet conclusive (Aldwin & Gilmer, 2004; Ebersole & Hess, 1998; Lewis, 2003).

Proprioceptive and Kinesthetic Changes

Documentation of changes in proprioception or kinesthesia that are purely related to aging is scant. Some studies, however, have reported a decline in lower extremity proprioception among elderly patients that was not found when the upper extremities were tested (Bottomly & Lewis, 2003). Changes in proprioception secondary to loss of vision, peripheral vascular disease, arthritis, cardiovascular disorders, stroke, disorders of the inner ear, and diabetes have also been reported (Bottomly & Lewis, 2003; Ebersole & Hess, 1998).

Vestibular Function

Vestibular changes are particularly significant because of the importance of falls as a health risk for older adults. Approximately 33% of older adults fall each year (Balogun & Katz, 2002), and 15% of these individuals are subjected to serious health consequences, such as broken hips (Tideiksaar, 2002). The mortality rate following hip fracture approaches 50% (Kell, Bell, & Quinney, 2001).

Older adults have more postural sway than younger adults (Waddington & Adams, 2004), a condition that is exacerbated when vision is impaired. Vestibular righting response diminishes with age, which can lead to problems in maintaining balance. Age-related changes in static balance, dynamic balance, and gait appear to increase the probability of falls (Aldwin & Gilmer, 2003; Bottomly & Lewis, 2003; Ebersole & Hess, 1998, Lewis, 2003; Tideiksaar, 2002).

Central Nervous System

With age, the cerebrum atrophies (Bottomly & Lewis, 2003; Ebersol & Hess, 1998), and cerebrospinal fluid space increases. Neurons are lost or atrophy, particularly in the precentral gyrus, postcentral gyrus, superior temporal gyrus, and Purkinje cells of the cerebellum (Bottomly & Lewis, 2003). The number of synapses falls, and neurotransmitter systems change. In addition, plaques, fibrillary tangles, and other cellular abnormalities have been found in the brains of functionally normal older adults (Lewis, 2003). Responses to stimuli as measured by electroencephalogram also slow down. Neurotransmission can be impaired by aging, leading to behavioral abnormalities (Strong, 1998).

Peripheral Nervous System

Among the changes in the peripheral nervous system seen in aging are loss of both myelinated and unmyelinated nerve fibers, axonal atrophy, and nerve conduction velocity (Verdu et al., 2000). Some sources, however, indicate that the manifestations of nervous system deterioration (reduced sensibility, coordination, cognitive abilities, and reaction time) observed with aging do not correspond to the relatively small physical changes seen at the cellular level (Bottomly & Lewis, 2003). In addition, variation between individuals makes functional and structural generalizations problematic.

Musculoskeletal System

The musculoskeletal system is affected by the aging process. The effects of normal change can have consequences for mobility and function. The following sections describe the normal aging process as it affects muscles and bone, as well as the impact of various diseases on the musculoskeletal system.

Muscles

The number and size of muscle fibers decrease with age (Kell, Bell, & Quinney, 2001). Increase in fatty and connective tissue, decreased strength, and loss of type II fast-twitch anaerobic muscle fibers that are responsible for phasic movement have been reported, as have decreases in muscle flexibility and endurance.

Joints

Joint function declines steadily after age 20. Ligaments and tendons become less resilient and more prone to injury (Bottomly & Lewis, 2003). The quantity and viscosity of synovial fluid decrease with aging. Cartilage becomes opaque, with an increase in cracks and fraying

(Bottomly & Lewis, 2003). The effects of weight bearing and stress on joints and the effects of diseases, such as the various kinds of arthritis, make the rate and nature of cartilage deterioration highly variable. Once cartilage is destroyed or damaged, it does not regenerate. This has special significance to the elderly, who must rely on prevention or corrective surgery to manage the potentially disabling effects of loss of cartilage (Bottomly & Lewis, 2003; Lewis, 2003).

Bones

The progressive loss of bone mineral content with aging results in loss of bone mass and density. The rate of these changes is affected by diet, exercise, and gender (Kell, Bell, & Quinney, 2001). Osteoporosis has been studied extensively. Women after age 39 have a rate of bone loss double that of men. Post-menopausal women are affected most. By age 65, at least 50% of women have developed some form of osteoporosis. The rate of degeneration slows by age 70 (Lewis, 2003).

Effect of Disease on the Musculoskeletal System

Arthritis, osteoporosis, connective tissue diseases, orthopedic injuries from falls and trauma, and repetitive motion disorders are most prevalent in elderly individuals (Tideiksaar, 2001). Almost 50% of men and women have some form of arthritis by age 65 (FIFARS, 2004). In 1996, hip fractures alone were responsible for more than 300,000 hospitalizations among people 65 years of age and older, of whom 80% were women. Among people 85 years of age and older, 90% of women and 54% of men had measurably reduced hipbone density.

Cardiovascular Changes

The cardiovascular system loses efficiency with age, which is the result of changes in the frequency and regularity of the conduction system (Dean, 2001), a reduction in pacemaker cells (Bottomly & Lewis, 2003), alterations in blood pressure (Newman, 1995), changes in the elasticity, length, and thickness of the arteries (Bottomly & Lewis, 2003), a decrease in heart rate and stroke volume (Dean, 2001), and a general thickening of specific heart tissues, such as the atria and valves (Bottomly & Lewis, 2003).

Aging affects every component of the cardiopulmonary system (Dean, 2001; Kell, Bell, & Quinney, 2001). Elastic tissues decrease and fibrous tissues increase. This especially affects the medium and small airways constructed of smooth muscle. The joints of the chest wall stiffen, the muscles of the diaphragm flatten, and the chest wall becomes more barrel shaped and less compliant (Dean, 2001). Approximately 50% of individuals over age 65 have blood pressure greater than 140/90 (Ebersole & Hess, 1998).

New research suggests that the effects of aging on the cardiovascular system once thought to be irreversible and consistent are highly variable among individuals (Chodzko-Zajko, 2001) and cultures (Ebersole & Hess, 1998) and reversible with exercise and dietary and behavioral changes (Blair et al., 1996; Chodzko-Zajko, 2001).

Cognitive Changes

As it is difficult to differentiate between first-level and developed capacities in cognition, the following discussion combines these two aspects of age-related changes. Age-related changes occur in some aspects of intelligence, problem solving, abstract reasoning, memory, memory processing, and attention. In all of these functions, changes are most noticeable after age 70, although gradual decline occurs when individuals reach the age of 30 (Anstey & Low, 2004).

As measured by the *Wechsler Adult Intelligence Scale*, intelligence quotient decreases with advancing age, largely the result of decreases in the performance rather than verbal subscales (Riley, 2001). Performance subscales may depend on **fluid intelligence** (the ability to use new information), whereas verbal subscales may use **crystallized intelligence** (recall of stored memories) (Anstey & Low, 2004). In particular, flexibility in reasoning tasks seems to decline (Riley, 2001), although older adults show wide individual variation in these cognitive tasks. Problem-solving skills also seem to become less efficient (Anstey & Low, 2004).

To remember, one must attend to the matter to be recalled and be able to receive information through sensory channels. The information must be processed (interpreted) and stored. Initial storage may be relatively short term. Overall, well older adults do not have memory loss in processing and short-term storage of information, although some have difficulty encoding large amounts of information at once (Anstey & Low, 2004).

Decrements in long-term memory and encoding are noticeable (Anstey & Low, 2004). Older adults have more trouble recalling information than do younger ones, although retrieval difficulty is not as noticeable for recognition. For example, on seeing a name, an older person may remember the face and personality of an acquaintance but, on seeing the person, have difficulty retrieving the name. This difficulty is much less pronounced when the information has practical significance. Remote or very long-term memory appears not to decline. This finding, however, is more anecdotal than data based and must be viewed with caution (Riley, 2001).

Another common phenomenon is increased difficulty with word finding, accompanied by subtle deficits in short-term memory, such as difficulty remembering names or where one put an object. Dubbed mild cognitive impairment, this irritating but not disabling condition seems to begin in late middle age (Royall et al., 2005). In most instances, the individual remembers the information later. For some individuals, memory training has helped minimize associated functional decrements (Riley, 2001).

One challenge in examining cognitive change in older adults is the clear association between sensory decline and cognition (Valentin et al., 2005). Visual or hearing deficits may reduce the individual's ability to respond accurately to questions or to follow instructions, creating the illusion of greater cognitive problems than may actually be present.

CASE EXAMPLE #1

Mrs. P.: Optimizing Occupational Function Despite Limitations Associated with Aging

Occupational Therapy Intervention Process	Clinical Reasoning Process: Objectives	Clinical Reasoning Process: Examples of Therapist's Internal Dialogue
Patient Information Mrs. P. is a 73-year-old woman who lives alone in a ranch-style house in a small town. Her grown daughter visits about four times a year; her son visits once a year. Mrs. P. was divorced 12 years ago and never remarried. Mrs. P. worked as a nurse for more than 20 years at a large university hospital. Now she works 2 days a week at a nursing home three blocks from her house, where she reviews charts for quality assurance. Mrs. P. has always enjoyed work and feels that the staff are close friends. Other than her income from the job, Mrs. P.'s only source of funds is Social Security. Throughout her adult life, Mrs. P. has been in a sorority consisting of about a dozen women who have been friends since they were young women. They live nearby. For many years, she was a member of a women's group that raised funds for the ballet in the nearby city. When she is at home, Mrs. P. enjoys working on a dollhouse that she built. Mrs. P. has a long history of health problems. She survived breast cancer when she was in her 40s, and 3 years ago, she had surgery to remove a cancerous tumor from her colon. She has high blood pressure, which is controlled with medication. She also has a significant hearing loss that is gradually worsening.	Appreciate the context	"Mrs. P. strikes me as a very independent woman, someone who is used to calling the shots. I will want to be very careful to respect that in her throughout this process." "Clearly, Mrs. P. has a strong social network. It impresses me that she has maintained strong connections with both her friends from work and her sorority sisters. I wonder if she would consider allowing these life-long friends to help her out now."
Reason for Referral to Occupational Therapy Recently Mrs. P.'s sorority sisters noted changes in her social behavior (missing meetings, not answering her phone, refusing social invitations) and contacted her son with their concerns. He urged his mother to make an appointment with her family physician, her primary care provider for the past 30 years. During the visit, the physician discovered that her high blood pressure has worsened, as has her hearing. She also reported being very tired and having difficulty managing around the house. The physician ordered a series of medical tests and asked a home health agency to send an occupational therapist to evaluate the home and Mrs. P.'s function. He assured her that her son agreed to pay for this evaluation.		"It's important for me to get a sense of how Mrs. P. is functioning in her own environment, and I am pleased that a home visit was ordered. She will likely be the most comfortable here, and I'll be able to get a clearer sense of what the barriers are to her occupational functioning."

Results of Occupational Therapy Assessment Mrs. P. agreed to a home visit by the occupational therapist. The therapist decided to evaluate Mrs. P.'s home and her performance of basic self-care and instrumental activities of daily living. The therapist used the *Check It Out Check-List* (Pynoos & Cohen, 1990), the *Interest Checklist*, and the *Self Assessment of Occupational Functioning*. She also asked Mrs. P. to give her a tour of the house and to describe problems encountered in daily tasks.		"I decided to use these instruments because they will help identify areas of occupation that are most important to Mrs. P as we collaborate to develop an intervention plan, and they apply a theoretical model of practice—the Model of Human Occupation."
	Develop intervention hypotheses	"I have a number of core hypotheses as I approach this consultation: (1) return to work is feasible and valued by employer and client; (2) consultation with physical therapy, physician, audiology, and social work is feasible; (3) client's reasons for social withdrawal need further assessment; (4) client continues to have interests in current occupations; and (5) client may be interested in alternative occupations to replace current work and leisure activities if these are not feasible."
	Select an intervention approach	"Consultative, adaptive, collaborative, client-centered, and rehabilitative approaches could all possibly be implemented."
	Reflect on competence	"I have knowledge and skills that I believe can help Mrs. P. Occupational therapy has strengths in energy conservation, adaptation of work and home for safety, meaningful occupations, and social skills. Physical therapy, audiology, physician, and social work could provide assistance with hearing, hypertension, financial, and social problems."
Recommendations 1. Develop an intervention plan in consultation with client, family, employer, and sorority sisters if appropriate. 2. Recommend consultation with physical therapy, social work, physician, and audiology. 3. Prioritize goals with interventions that are financially and functionally feasible in consultation with all stakeholders.	Consider the patient's appraisal of performance Consider what will occur in therapy, how often, and for how long	"Mrs. P. seems to want help to improve her functioning, but I do feel that I am somewhat limited as to how much I can do for her in just one session. I will want to make sure that I am addressing her priorities and, if she is interested, am willing to work with her to explore availability of alternative resources to fund care."
	Ascertain the patient's endorsement of plan	"I find myself wondering about whether or not other stakeholders are invested in the client over the long term? What are they willing and able to provide in support?"
Problem List and Solutions The therapist and Mrs. P. discussed these concerns and worked jointly toward identifying potential solutions. Since the therapist was asked to do an evaluation, not to provide long-term intervention, she must provide Mrs. P. with sufficient information to address her concerns.	Assess the patient's comprehension	"Mrs. P. was very forthright about her concerns and could readily agree with some of my observations about the potential safety hazards related to all of her clutter. I can't tell whether her reluctance to get rid of things reflected difficulty with decision

Problem List and Solutions (cont'd)

Home safety

Mrs. P. acknowledged that the house was cluttered with old papers, knickknacks, and clothes. She was reluctant to throw anything away but agreed to have her daughter store some of the items for her. Mrs. P. also indicated that she had no funds to replace the worn carpet, although both agree that worn spots and loose edges contribute to falls. She and the therapist identified several possible sources of funds and discussed the possibility of taking the carpet up entirely.

Physical deconditioning

Mrs. P. indicated that she had much less energy than she used to and quickly becomes short of breath when walking around the house. She agreed to begin a gradual plan of physical activity, starting with a stroll around the block each day.

Social isolation

Mrs. P.'s hearing loss was quite noticeable. The therapist encouraged her to see an audiologist to have her hearing evaluated. Mrs. P. expressed concern about paying for a hearing aid but agreed to ask her son for help.

Mrs. P. indicated that her friends were all in poor health and "no fun" anymore. She also said she was worried about falling at work. She was unwilling to discuss any alternatives for maintaining ties with her friends but agreed that she could discuss her concerns about work with her supervisor.

Understand what she is doing	making or, perhaps, her overall fatigue and deconditioning."
Compare actual to expected performance	"Mrs. P. is remarkably insightful. She realizes that falling at home or at work could have serious health consequences, but she may be self-limiting her activities more than is necessary. She seemed very receptive to my suggestions regarding how she could
Know the person	safely increase her activity level."
Appreciate the context	

Next Steps

1. Client will consult with physician to address hypertension and fatigue.
2. Client will consult with physical therapy to address lack of endurance.
3. Client will consult with audiologist to address hearing loss.
4. Client will return to work.
5. Client will employ methods of energy conservation to work,
   self-care, and home maintenance tasks and will report ability to complete these tasks with fewer incidence and severity of fatigue symptoms.
6. Client will address safety hazards in the home, such as clutter and unsafe flooring, by removing these dangerous barriers.
7. Client will engage in activities with sorority sisters twice a week.

Mrs. P. and her occupational therapist developed a time line for Mrs. P. to call her doctor, her daughter, her son, and her boss, and Mrs. P. and her therapist agreed that the therapist will make a follow-up call to check on her progress in 2 weeks. On follow-up, the therapist learned that Mrs. P. had accomplished a great deal. Mrs. P.'s physician determined that she had pernicious anemia and instituted monthly injections of vitamin B12. Mrs. P. reported that she already felt more energetic.

Mrs. P. started walking around her yard twice a day. Her daughter came to visit and helped her organize the house. Her son sent a check for a new hearing aid. Mrs. P. had not yet talked with her boss and was worried about doing it. She and the therapist practiced the conversation to provide Mrs. P. with a strategy. A week later, Mrs. P. called the therapist to tell her she was back at work.

Anticipate present and future patient concerns	"I wonder if the employer is satisfied with Mrs. P.'s work performance. Is Mrs. P. enjoying her work? "
Analyze patient's comprehension	"I should ask Mrs. P. about her interactions with the sorority sisters and her family. Are there more frequent interactions? What is the quality of those interactions?"
	"Is Mrs. P. falling at home or at work and, if so, how frequently? How could I best evaluate for this? How about incidence of shortness of breath? I should consider these factors before deciding to discontinue intervention. Is the client able to manage daily activities including work without a worsening of hypertension or fatigue?"
	"If I am only able to intervene in one session, how could I most effectively address these complex issues using consultation, advocacy, and ethical/professional behavior? Can communication with the physician, the family, and other professionals involved address this concern adequately?"

Analysis of Reasoning

The therapist's initial task was to gather the information needed to clearly identify the problem. As the therapist secured information, it became evident that both Mrs. P. and her family needed to be consulted. Goals were identified based on their input. In this case, the occupational therapist provided an assessment and recommendations but left implementation of the plan to this capable client and family.

Decide if the patient should continue or discontinue therapy and/or return in the future

CLINICAL REASONING IN OCCUPATIONAL THERAPY PRACTICE

Intervention to Prevent Performance Decrements

The occupational therapist focused on screening and prevention in this consultative intervention. How might the therapist's assessment and intervention approaches have been different if Mrs. P.'s function had deteriorated to the extent that she was placed in a long-term care facility?

A Special Note about Dementia

Dementing illnesses are extremely common among older adults. **Dementia**, which is characterized by forgetfulness, difficulty finding words, and other cognitive loss, is not a normal condition of aging. Rather, it is a symptom of any of several disease processes (Corcoran, 2001). Some, such as depression, sensory deprivation syndrome, malnutrition, and drug toxicity, are reversible; others are not. Alzheimer's disease, the most common form of dementia, is a progressive disorder that eventually leads to total disability and death.

It is beyond the scope of this chapter to deal with the methods for intervening with individuals with dementing disorders. A few suggested intervention strategies are included in Procedures for Practice 37-1 and in Chapter 29 of this book. Health care professionals should be familiar with the early symptoms of cognitive disorder, such as difficulty finding words, forgetfulness about everyday events and procedures, and lack of recollection of familiar individuals. When noted, these symptoms should be carefully evaluated by a geriatrician, a physician trained to work with older individuals. Reversible causes may be treated relatively easily. If the individual has an irreversible dementing illness, a variety of management strategies can help informal and formal caregivers to cope with resulting problems. This enhances quality of life for both the ill person and the caregivers. One excellent source of information about management is *The 36-Hour Day: A Family Guide to Caring for Persons with Alzheimer Disease, Related Dementing Illnesses, and Memory Loss in Later Life* (Mace, Rabins, & McHugh, 1999).

DEVELOPED CAPACITIES: CHANGES IN VOLUNTARY RESPONSES

Changes in organic substrates and first-level capacities may impair such voluntary responses as rising from a chair and gait speed (Fiatarone et al., 1990). Weakness in ankle dorsiflexion and knee extension has been correlated with falls in older individuals (Tideiksaar, 2001).

PROCEDURES FOR PRACTICE 37-1

Strategies for Working with Individuals with Dementia

- Place items used frequently in visible locations.
- Use simple, one-step instructions.
- Maintain habitual activities as much as possible; simplify as needed.
- Obtain a bracelet identifying the person as memory impaired in case of wandering.
- Encourage physical activity during the day to improve nighttime sleep.
- Provide activities that stimulate memory (for example, baking or music that the person used to enjoy).
- Avoid excessively crowded or unfamiliar surroundings that might lead to catastrophic reactions.
- Contact the local Alzheimer's association for resource lists and support groups.

Loss of dexterity and coordination with aging is well-documented (Desrosiers et al., 1995). Scores on the *Jebsen Hand Function Test* (Jebsen et al., 1969), the *Nine-Hole Peg Test* (Mathiowetz, Weber et al., 1985), and the *Box and Block Test of Manual Dexterity* (Mathiowetz, Volland et al., 1985) all decline with age. The result can be increased difficulty in activities requiring such skill.

ABILITIES AND SKILLS: PHYSICAL CAPACITY

The following changes in physical capacity typify skills and abilities that are affected by normal aging: postural alignment, sway, and instability with postural changes (Tideiksaar, 2001); gross motor coordination (Bottomly & Lewis, 2003); fine motor coordination and dexterity (Desrosiers et al., 1995); strength and endurance (Bottomly & Lewis, 2003); walking speed, step length, and step height (Bottomly & Lewis, 2003; Tideiksaar, 2001); and reaction time (Bottomly & Lewis, 2003).

ACTIVITIES AND HABITS

Activities and habits are prominently discussed in the Practice Framework (AOTA, 2002). The category labeled performance patterns considers habits, routines, and roles. As with physiological change, activity patterns are highly individual (Bonder & Martin, 2000). In fact, older adults have great freedom of choice in our culture. Some older

CASE EXAMPLE # 2

Mrs. S.: Optimizing Occupational Function for a Senior in a Nursing Home Setting

Occupational Therapy Intervention Process	Clinical Reasoning Process: Objectives	Clinical Reasoning Process: Examples of Therapist's Internal Dialogue
Patient Information Mrs. S., an 80-year-old nursing home resident, has five children. Four of them live within 50 miles. Mrs. S. worked as the personal secretary for the provost of a small college for 20 years. She had a variety of interests, including reading, cooking, and baking; participating in church and local theater; and gardening. Mrs. S. faced a number of challenges in her life, including the early death of her father, the Great Depression, her husband's absence for 3 years of service in World War II, raising a child with schizophrenia, the early and sudden death of her husband (she was 51 when he died), and adjusting to a move from her home to an apartment and now to a nursing home. Mrs. S.'s medical history is fairly typical for a person her age. She developed osteoarthritis in both knees, resulting in several microscopic surgeries and two total knee replacements. She was hospitalized for a brief bout of depression secondary to menopause. She has presbyopia with resulting losses of both near and far vision that are well corrected with eyeglasses. She has severe hearing loss in both ears that is partially corrected with hearing aids. Mrs. S. also had a series of strokes that began when she was 70. The strokes left her with mild spasticity, about 50% of proximal upper extremity active range of motion, and only a	Appreciate the context	"I should focus on past and current occupations and performance in areas of occupation. I want to take note of the current status of body functions and structures and how these may influence performance in the areas of occupation. It's important that I identify performance patterns, habits, and routines and try to make sense of all that relative to the cultural, spiritual, physical, social, personal, temporal, and virtual contexts of Mrs. S.'s past and current environment. For example, I wonder how possible changes in these factors have influenced her occupations and what areas of occupation may be compromised by these changes."

Patient Information (cont'd)

mass grasp in her left hand. She had full use of lower extremities except for a loss of about 15° of right active knee flexion and mild spasticity and weakness in the left lower extremity. She lost approximately 25% of the visual field on the left side to hemianopsia but can accommodate for this by turning her head. Mrs. S. also had mild dysarthria and dysphagia. She dribbled urine because of changes in bladder function and weak sphincter musculature. She wore a small protective pad and took medication to control this. She was hospitalized a year ago for an attempted suicide and major depression as a result of the breaking of her knee replacement and difficulty adjusting to the idea of another major surgery. She received psychiatric services and a long rehabilitation stay after she agreed to have the knee replacement. Her recovery from the knee replacement was very good except for her complaint of chronic pain in the knee that has not responded to medication.

Prior to the failure of her first knee replacement, Mrs. S. was totally independent in all basic activities of daily living. After her knee replacement and rehabilitation stay, a trial in her assisted-living facility became problematic because of her declining ability to walk and transfer to the bathroom and inability to do her own personal care. She and her family decided that Mrs. S. should be admitted to a nursing home, where she would receive closer supervision and assistance for her personal care.

Reason for Referral to Occupational Therapy

The nursing home staff was concerned about Mrs. S.'s safety and social withdrawal. Mrs. S. was still using a wheeled walker but found placing her left hand on the walker handle difficult. She was able to move from her bed to the bathroom independently but had several recent falls. She dressed independently if her clothes were placed on a chair beside her bed. However, she displayed poor judgment in activities such as bending too far over the edge of the bed and dangerously reaching for things she dropped on the floor. She also tripped over things while walking. She used a wheelchair on outings with her family and with the activities program at the nursing home. Mrs. S. rarely smiled, and nursing staff reported difficulty getting her to participate in group activities or outings, even though she was physically able to do so. Her family was supportive. Her oldest daughter had power of attorney and durable medical power of attorney. Mrs. S. paid privately for nursing home care and had funds remaining to cover about 2 more months of care. She was willing to pay privately for brief occupational therapy intervention.

"Are there standardized or non-standardized assessments that could be used to address functional mobility, ADL, depression?"

Results of Occupational Therapy Assessment

After reviewing the medical records, the occupational therapist evaluated Mrs. S.'s life roles, tasks, activities, skills, abilities, and developed capacities. Mrs. S. was interviewed along with her oldest daughter and primary nurse. Some of the critical questions raised during the interviews were:

What safety issues are you most concerned about?
What is your level of satisfaction with life right now? What do you think could be done to improve it?
What things do you like to do right now? What things irritate you?
If you could change five things around here to make things better for yourself, what would you change?
What worries you most? What makes you happiest?
Do you have any goals to improve yourself, your environment, or your living situation?

Results of Occupational Therapy Assessment (cont'd)	Develop intervention hypotheses	"I have a number of core hypotheses as I approach intervention planning: (1) the client is motivated to improve; (2) the caregivers are motivated to collaborate on the established goals; (3) the family is supportive and motivated to assist in achieving the goals; (4) direct intervention as well as consultation and collaboration are necessary to achieve the goals; (5) the client has the potential to achieve the goals; (6) the other stakeholders have the resources to collaborate in accomplishing the agreed upon goals; and (7) it is financially possible to consult other professionals such as physical therapy, urology, orthopedic surgery, pain management specialist, audiology, and social work."
	Select an intervention approach	"Rehabilitative, client-centered, consultative, adaptive, and collaborative approaches may all apply to this client."
	Reflect on competence	"Skills from other professionals will be needed to address many of the issues. OT has strengths in the areas of safety, urinary incontinence, meaningful occupations, functional mobility, ADLs, and psychosocial issues."
Recommendations 1. Interview client, family, caregivers, and nurses to identify problems that are of highest priority for each stakeholder. 2. Further assess safety and performance of ADLs. 3. Recommend consultation with physical therapy, social work, audiology, psychiatry, and urology. 4. Develop a plan of care in consultation with all stakeholders.	Consider the patient's appraisal of performance Consider what will occur in therapy, how often, and for how long Ascertain the patient's endorsement of plan	"I need to address issues that are most important to the client, the family, and the caregivers. I wonder if there is consensus among all stakeholders about these issues and their relative importance. I will need to consider what can be done in the way of consultation, direct OT intervention, and collaboration with others considering the client's strengths and weaknesses, the motivation of all stakeholders, and the context. Who will be responsible for goal achievement using which model of team intervention?"
Summary of Short-Term Goals and Progress The interviews and evaluation revealed the following problems: 1. Mrs. S. tends to get upset and take things into her own hands when she has to wait for assistance. This results in unsafe or dangerous behavior and activities. 2. Mrs. S. gets depressed and does not feel like socializing with others, especially residents with problems similar to hers or worse. 3. Mrs. S. needs some meaningful activities to replace the wide variety of activities that formerly gave her pleasure. 4. Mrs. S. needs some modifications to her environment to increase safety and orientation to reality and current events. 5. Mrs. S. is easily embarrassed and has difficulty asking for personal assistance, especially with urination and personal hygiene. 6. Mrs. S. would like more interaction and visits from her family.	Assess the patient's comprehension Understand what she is doing Compare actual to expected performance Know the person Appreciate the context	"How can I and the team best monitor falls, frequency of urinary incontinence, quality and quantity of participation in mandatory or optional leisure activities, and the list of positive and negative feelings?" "What can be done to assess motivation of client, staff, and family in monitoring follow-through with recommendations, and do I need to adjust instructions and goals depending upon progress or lack of progress achieved?" "I should consider standardized assessments of depression, occupational function, cognition/judgment, and ADL function."

Occupational Therapy Goals

The following goals were agreed upon by Mrs. S., her family, and the nursing staff:

1. Mrs. S. will request and wait for assistance or supervision for trips to the bathroom or will use a female urinal at bedside.
2. Mrs. S. will call for assistance should she drop any item on the floor that is not within easy reach of her long-handled reacher. Otherwise, she will continue to dress herself independently with setup at bed or chair level.
3. Mrs. S. will attend at least two outings per week with family or with the nursing home activities program. She will provide constructive criticism to the staff as to how the activity could be improved.
4. Mrs. S. will learn to propel her wheelchair so that she can safely navigate throughout the building without falling. She will be supervised for walks to the bathroom or in the hall.
5. Mrs. S. will choose and successfully complete three leisure activities within a month using adaptive equipment or techniques recommended by the occupational therapist.
6. Mrs. S. will complete a list of things that she is unhappy with as well as a list of things she is grateful for and review them with her daughter at least once a week to encourage her to express her feelings appropriately.

Next Steps The occupational therapist decided to see Mrs. S. once or twice a week for a month to achieve these goals. Mrs. S. agreed to pay for the therapy because she did not qualify for skilled services under Medicare regulations. **Direct Intervention** 1. Instruction in safety for mobility within her room; 2. Adjustment of call signal button and chairs and removal of throw rugs and other barriers to safe mobility in the room; 3. Provision of long-handled reachers and instruction in use of them; 4. A session to assess safety issues during dressing and hygiene activities; 5. Suggestions for adaptive equipment for playing cards, reading, and plant care; 6. A daily calendar and structured time to read the paper or watch the news on television for current events; 7. A meeting with Mrs. S. and her family at the end of the month to review progress on goals and to make decisions about continuance of therapy or discharge. The occupational therapist suggested referrals to physical therapy for a program to maintain or enhance mobility and physical conditioning, speech pathology to review issues related to dysphagia and dysarthria, and social work to help Mrs. S. and her family apply for Medicaid or other support, as financial concerns were becoming an issue. The therapist consulted the nursing and activities staff and provided written copies of suggestions for the staff to facilitate accomplishment of the therapy goals. Suggestions were also made to Mrs. S. and her family to explore a visit to a chronic pain specialist for the knee pain and to a urologist for follow-up on bladder control issues.	Anticipate present and future patient concerns Analyze patient's comprehension Decide if the patient should continue or discontinue therapy and/or return in the future	"Are the goals being met? Why or why not? Did the other consultants contribute to the interventions and what were the outcomes? How are the client, caregivers, and family responding? What barriers could be further addressed to address the problems and goals more effectively? Is additional support needed to ensure safety? Has the client reached maximum potential to achieve the goals based upon progress notes and consultation with all stakeholders? What progress can be documented? Do all stakeholders agree that further therapy would be beneficial in reaching particular goals?"

CLINICAL REASONING IN OCCUPATIONAL THERAPY PRACTICE

Intervention Despite Age-Related Deterioration

What strategies did the therapist use to collaborate with patient, family, and nursing home staff? What else could be done to ensure that stakeholders maintain their contribution to Mrs. S.'s function long after the occupational therapy intervention is complete?

adults engage in many activities; others focus on one or two. For example, some older adults report activities that are related primarily to family, while others may be active in volunteer work, several hobbies, social relationships, and care of their personal needs.

The importance of habits must be emphasized. Evidence shows that when a familiar task is undertaken in a familiar environment, the effect of aging on performance is reduced (Rogers, Holm, & Stone, 1997). Where such habits can be followed closely, task performance is improved.

Most older adults accommodate to age-related changes well by modifying routines or finding and accepting assistance. This is especially true when the activity is one for which it is socially acceptable to receive help. Help with driving, cooking, or managing finances is often acceptable. Some older adults are determined to do for themselves, while others are accepting, even relieved, when they can rely on others to take care of them.

Driving

Older drivers have higher rates of fatal crashes, based on miles driven, than any other group except very young drivers, according to the Insurance Institute for Highway Safety (IIHS). The high death rate is due in large part to their greater physical frailty. They are less likely to survive after an injury than a younger person. By 2030, people age 65 and older are expected to represent 25% of the driving population and 25% of fatal crash involvements, IIHS says. According to the National Highway Traffic Safety Administration (NHTSA), there were 19.9 million licensed drivers age 70 and older in the United States in 2002 (latest data available), or 10% of all licensed drivers (Insurance Information Institute, 2004).

Model driving evaluation and rehabilitation programs for the older driver include measuring driver potential before on-road evaluation (visual, cognitive, auditory, motor, neuropsychological, and psychosocial factors; driver/vehicle fit; reaction time; and driver simulation); measuring and improving driver performance with on-road testing and intervention; proper documentation of fitness to drive; environmental and ergonomic factors impacting drivers, passengers, and pedestrians; and communication with all of the stakeholders in making a decision about the safe performance of an older driver (College of Health Professionals, University of Florida, n.d.; Pellertino, 2006).

Self-Care

A significant issue for older adults has to do with level of independence in self-care (Hayase et al., 2004). If personal ability is compromised, the issue is availability and acceptance of assistance. Most older adults show decline in ADL performance over time (Hayase et al., 2004). Among the deficits that are commonly seen are complex actions such as cutting toenails. Heavy housework, such as mopping floors and washing windows, is difficult for many individuals and may be hired out or done by family members. In addition, most elders spend more time on self-care activities than they did when younger (Christiansen & Hammecker, 2001). Issues of time can be significant when self-care consumes such a significant proportion of the day that other desired activities cannot be pursued.

Substantial disability in self-care is most likely to be perceived when there is a sudden change due to illness or change in social circumstances rather than the gradual ones that affect most well elders. If the change is loss related, emotional reactions that typically accompany loss must be addressed. Changes perceived as positive, however, such as a move to a long-desired retirement location, can also cause unanticipated emotional difficulties.

Urinary Incontinence

Urinary incontinence affects more than 13 million Americans. Up to 35% of community-dwelling people over age 60 experience incontinence; two thirds of these are women (Neumann, 2002). Ability to bathe and urinary and bowel incontinence are issues that can influence life-altering decisions for elders. Those who are unable to bathe or who are incontinent are most likely to be placed in institutional settings, which is an event that most elders wish to avoid. Interventions for urinary/ bowel incontinence include surgery, medications, and behavioral treatment. Occupational therapists provide behavioral interventions that may include regular scheduling of toileting, pelvic muscle reeducation (Kegel exercises), biofeedback, bladder training, urge inhibition, bowel management, and dietary and fluid modifications (Burgio et al., 2002; Neumann, 2002).

Work

Emerging patterns in work and retirement reflect increasing diversity in the older population (Sterns, Laier, & Dorsett, 2001). For example, some older adults are creating a trend to earlier retirement followed by a second career in a different area, a return to part-time work, or a move to volunteer work.

Physiological changes seen in normal aging do not typically interfere with work abilities (Sterns, Laier, & Dorsett, 2001). Elders require somewhat different kinds of in-service training to maintain or expand competency, requiring slightly more time than younger adults to learn new skills. They respond best to learning that is based on practical examples. If these special needs are accommodated, however, they are as capable of maintaining their skills as younger people.

Substantial evidence exists that voluntary retirement is not viewed as a negative event (Bambrick & Bonder, 2005). When retirement is involuntary, however, either as a result of a personal situation such as failing health or external events such as layoffs, individuals are likely to be dissatisfied with retirement.

Retirement often does not mean the cessation of productive activity (Bambrick & Bonder, 2005; Herzog & House, 1991). Herzog and House note that individuals who engage in volunteer work, child care, other service for family members, or other forms of unpaid service report that these have value both to them and to others. Bambrick and Bonder found that older adults describe several major themes in their perceptions of work, including (1) contribution to self-concept, (2) giving back to the community, and (3) staying engaged.

At present, work as undertaken by older adults is receiving considerable attention for several reasons. Some of these reasons relate to demographics and public policy (Bergstrom & Holmes, 2004), some relate to the preferences of older adults (Altschuler, 2004; Bambrick & Bonder, 2005), and others are related to the age-related changes that affect ability to work (Bosma et al., 2003).

With regard to demographic and policy issues, several factors emerge in current discussion of older workers (Bergstrom & Holmes, 2004). As previously noted, the population of older adults in the United States is becoming a larger proportion of the population as a whole. This means fewer young adult workers, those individuals historically viewed as the productive members of society. The so-called dependency ratio is changing such that, within a decade or so, there will be only two adult workers for every adult over 65. This has implications for public programs, such as Social Security, that depend on worker contributions to support retirees (Bergstrom & Holmes, 2004). At the same time, historical discrimination against older workers is being addressed through policy initiatives like the Age Discrimination in Employment Act and the Americans with Disabilities Act. Changing demographics require fundamental reconsideration of policies designed to either encourage or discourage elders' choices about paid employment.

At the same time, many older adults are making choices that differ from those of previous generations. Although there is a trend toward earlier retirement compared with previous generations, there is also a trend toward continued paid employment, albeit in new work circumstances (Altschuler, 2004; Bambrick & Bonder, 2005). Elders describe multiple reasons for wanting to continue to work, including issues of independence, sense of self-worth, and a wish to continue to contribute to society.

Considerable evidence shows that elders remain capable of work far beyond the traditional retirement age of 65 (Sterns, Laier, & Dorsett, 2001). Due to changes in cognition and physical status, older adults may require modest modifications in training and in work tasks; given these accommodations, however, they can continue to be productive and valuable workers far into later life. Elders in the workplace benefit from training that is practical and from repetition of new information. With regard to the content of work tasks, there is some speculation that cognitively challenging work delays deterioration of cognitive function (Bosma et al., 2003) and that remaining at work can reduce incidence of depression (Tian et al., 2004). Decreases in physical capacity require adjustment in the physical demands of work tasks (Savinainen, Nygard, & Ilmarinen, 2004) (Fig. 37-1).

Leisure

Leisure is extremely important to older adults (Bundy, 2001). It provides a sense of identity for individuals who are no longer working. It appears to delay onset of some disabling conditions, and it is linked to life satisfaction. Furthermore, it offers opportunities for expression of important personal meanings (Bonder & Martin, 1998). For older adults, the line between leisure and work may be indistinct, with activities providing both a sense of usefulness to others and satisfaction of personal need for engagement and challenge (Bambrick & Bonder, 2005) (Fig. 37-2).

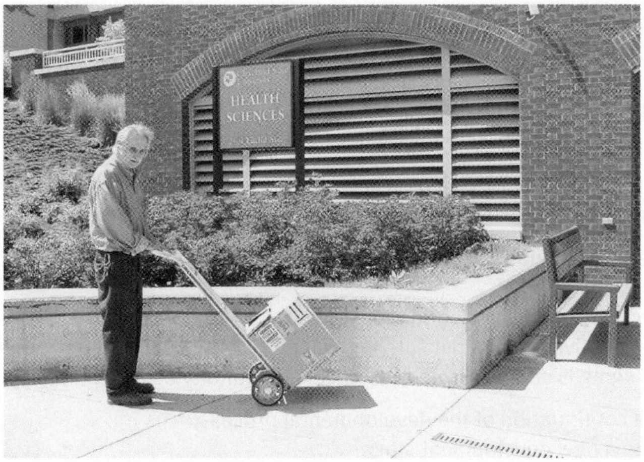

Figure 37-1 The gentleman pictured is still on the job, despite the physical demands of his work in delivering supplies around his organization.

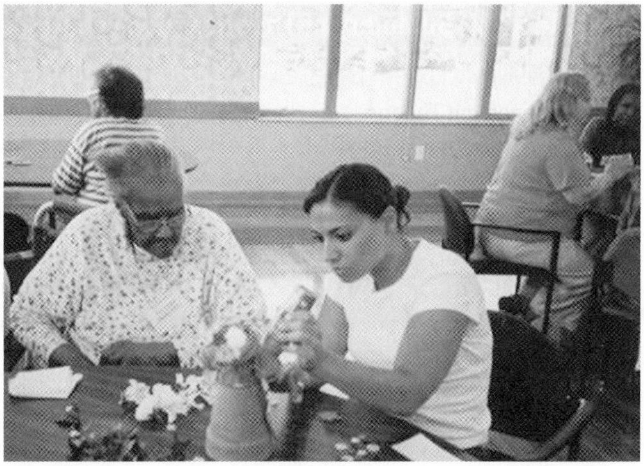

Figure 37-2 Even elders with substantial impairments derive great satisfaction from meaningful leisure activities.

The general belief, consistent with activity theory, is that maintaining a high level of activity is positive (Rosenfeld, 1997). This theory, however, has been challenged by some who believe that an important component of later life is reflection and life review (Ekerdt, 1986; Rowles, 1991).

TASKS AND LIFE ROLES

Elders also have greater personal choice in determining their tasks and life roles than do younger individuals. Although some individuals must continue to work to support themselves, most have the option of retiring from paid employment. Those who have children typically have finished rearing them. Since living in certain school districts is no longer an issue, some elders opt to sell their home and move to an apartment or to new community.

Satisfaction of Emerging Personal Needs and Meanings

In recent years, researchers have made increasing attempts to understand the occupations of older adults (Bambrick & Bonder, 2005; Bonder & Martin, 1998; Bonder & Martin, 2000; Rudman, Cook, & Polatajko, 1997). In particular, researchers are interested in knowing what is important to elders and how their occupations contribute to quality of life (Johansson, 2003).

Physical health is not, in and of itself, sufficient to ensure good quality of life (Johansson, 2003). Occupational therapists theorize that individuals are most satisfied with their lives when they engage in a variety of occupations that balance self-care, work, and leisure (Kielhofner, 1995). Research suggests that this is true for older adults as well as younger individuals (Rowe & Kahn, 1998).

Elimination or Alteration of Roles

Clearly, although elders often make choices about self-enhancement roles, far less choice is involved in the elimination of tasks associated with changes in social roles. Death of a spouse, siblings, or friends dramatically shifts occupational tasks. Many elders find that they must modify their roles to accommodate them. As an example, one woman who had made her living as a weaver found that she could no longer sit at a large floor loom. She chose to weave at a small table loom or use finger looms (Bonder, 2001a). The salient issue seems to be the ability to find outlets for expression of personal meaning (Bonder & Martin, 2000).

Additional Roles

Elders not only lose or choose to end previous roles; they also add roles. An elder who stops paid employment becomes a retiree and may become a volunteer. A parent whose children are grown may become a grandparent. A notable rite of passage in the United States is the receipt of the letter at age 50 that indicates one is eligible for membership in the AARP; individuals electing to join add this role, too.

New chosen roles can enhance life satisfaction. In some instances, even roles that are not chosen may be satisfying. For example, some elders become not only grandparents but surrogate parents for their grandchildren. As many

Table 37-1. Summary of Theories of Psychological Processes of Older Adults

Theorists	Constructs
Disengagement Theory (Cummings & Henry, 1961)	1. Elderly withdraw from activity 2. Elderly disengage emotionally from people and events
Activity Theory (Havighurst, 1963; Longino & Kart, 1982)	1. Elderly strive to maintain activity 1. High levels of activity correlate with well-being
Continuity Theory (Atchley, 1989)	1. Elderly attempt to continue activities that were always important to them 2. Elderly perceive activities as continuous 3. Elderly adapt activity to compensate for change 4. Successful aging is characterized by degree of continuity achieved
Lifespan Theories (Erikson, 1963; Levinson, 1986; Neugarten, 1975)	1. Old age is a continuation of the developmental process, representing a new development stage 2. Tasks specific to the stage can be identified 3. Successful aging results from accomplishing tasks
Person-Environment-Occupation (Christiansen & Baum, 1997)	1. Successful occupational engagement results from an interaction of the person, the environment, and the occupation 2. Intervention can occur in any of these three elements to enhance performance

Based on Table 3-1 in Bonder, B. R. (2001). The psychosocial meaning of occupation. In B. R. Bonder & M. Wagner (Eds.), *Functional performance in older adults* (p. 46). Philadelphia: F.A. Davis Co. Reprinted with permission.

as 10% of elders are custodial grandparents (Fuller-Thompson, Minkler, & Driver, 1997). Although this may be perceived by some as a burden, many grandparents express great satisfaction with this role.

COMPETENCE AND SELF-ESTEEM: PSYCHOSOCIAL CHANGES

Psychosocial status may well be a more significant predictor of occupational function than any other factor. Highly motivated, enthusiastic individuals tend to fare well, often despite what appear to be substantial physical limitations. Practitioners must attend to situations in which the individual, following an injury or illness, becomes depressed, loses motivation, and becomes increasingly disabled.

Changes in psychosocial status must be separated into those that are psychological and those that are social. For a well older adult, the former relate to developmental tasks of later life. The latter relate to external factors, including major life changes such as retirement and the loss of social contacts through moves, retirement, or death of peers.

A number of theorists have attempted to identify the normal psychological processes that accompany aging. Among the theories are disengagement, activity, continuity, and life span models. The principal characteristics of these theories are noted in Table 37-1. Although each theory has appeal, each also has limitations in explaining the psychological functioning of older individuals, and all remain to be carefully tested.

Social changes are also less than clear. It is well established that older individuals have significant losses of social contacts (Bye, Llewellyn, & Christi, 2001). It is less clear, however, whether or how individuals compensate for those losses. For example, loss of a spouse is devastating for most older individuals (Bye, Llewellyn, & Christi, 2001). Some individuals compensate for the loss within a year or so, while others never recover.

IMPEDIMENTS TO OCCUPATIONAL FUNCTION

We review two categories of barriers to occupational function: disease and environmental factors.

Impact of Disease

Almost all older adults eventually fall ill or have an injury that may call for secondary or tertiary preventive interventions, that is, minimizing consequences early in treatment or enhancing rehabilitation once severe disability has occurred. The following special characteristics of older adults must be considered in planning intervention.

Differential Severity of Condition

Some conditions that are relatively innocuous in younger individuals can have severe consequences for older individuals (Rowe & Kahn, 1998). One example is influenza, which is unpleasant for younger adults but may be lethal for older ones. On the other hand, cancers that may be terminal in younger adults are often quite slow growing in older individuals, leading to much less severe outcomes.

Multiple Health Problems

Otherwise well older adults are likely to have two or three chronic health problems (Administration on Aging, 2004), each of which may require a different intervention. A common example is a client who has both rheumatoid arthritis and osteoporosis. Although moderately strenuous weight-bearing exercise may be the treatment of choice to prevent bone loss, such activity may exacerbate the arthritis.

Duration of Recuperation

Older adults generally recuperate more slowly than younger ones. Even if the eventual outcome is every bit as good, it is likely to take the older individual longer to arrive at that point. Treatment often ends too soon for older individuals.

Consequences of Dysfunction

Most elders prefer to live independently or "age in place" (Rowe & Kahn, 1998). It is their wish to remain in the living situation to which they have grown accustomed. Illness and dysfunction, however, can lead to a decision to institutionalize. Functional abilities are central to such decisions. In particular, bathing and toileting abilities influence family decisions. For this reason, occupational therapists often find that elders want to emphasize these abilities in treatment.

Environmental Factors

As with all clients, environmental factors, both physical and social, can have a profound influence on function. Issues described in Chapters 10 and 11 of this text should be carefully considered during interaction with elderly clients, since changes to the personal, social, cultural, and environmental context can greatly facilitate personal abilities.

FACILITATORS OF OCCUPATIONAL FUNCTION

Clinicians consider each patient's age as they plan assessment and treatment to optimize occupational function.

Evaluation

Careful evaluation is vital to successful intervention focused on supporting functional performance of older adults. Perhaps most attention has been given to assessment of self-care (Wilkins, Law, & Letts, 2001). In assessing older adults, however, it is important to be cognizant of the goals of the individual (Canadian Association of Occupational Therapists, 2002). Assessment should begin with identification of the individual's goals and proceed to determination of factors that support or impede those goals. The Practice Framework (AOTA, 2002) recommends completing an occupational profile and an analysis of occupational performance. The two combined provide information about what the individual needs and wants to do and what factors limit ability to accomplish those tasks.

Several instruments may be helpful in determining those goals. The *Canadian Occupational Performance Measure* (Law et al., 2005) involves interview of the client and joint identification of goals for therapy. These goals then become the measures of outcome. Other instruments that may be helpful include the *Role Change Assessment* (Jackoway, Rogers, & Snow, 1987) and *Interest Checklist* (Matsutsuyu, 1963).

Legislation, particularly the Omnibus Budget Reconciliation Act (OBRA) (Glantz & Richman, 1991), requires that people in nursing homes have an environmental assessment, but such assessment should be done in community settings as well. A number of good environmental assessment instruments are available (Mann, 2001; Tiedeksaar, 2001) (see Chapter 11).

Instruments are also being developed to assess driving ability (Pellerito, 2006) because transportation is an important concern in accomplishing occupations. In addition, it is important to evaluate risk for falls (Nandy, 2004) because falls are common among older adults, have a high risk of significant injury, and can, therefore, significantly affect occupation. It is important to evaluate both the physical and the social environment to understand fully the individual's situation.

Therapists must be aware that some assessment is mandated by third-party payers. For example, the U.S. government has implemented a minimum data set (MDS) (Health Care Financing Administration, 1999) for residents of nursing homes, and the Outcomes Assessment Information (OASIS) for home health. Furthermore, accreditation bodies, such as the Joint Commission on

Accreditation of Healthcare Organizations (1999), require that a patient's age be considered in both assessment and treatment planning.

Intervention

An important role for occupational therapists working with older adults is prevention or remediation of functional disability (AOTA, 2002). Intervention may include prevention, screening, environmental modifications, modification or substitution of activities, educational interventions, and acceptance of individual needs and wishes by health care providers.

Prevention

The wellness movement (Gallup, 1999) is based on the principle of maximizing both health and performance. Activities such as stress management, exercise to increase physical fitness, maintenance of adequate nutrition, safe driving habits, avoidance of alcohol and drugs, cessation of smoking, and activities to increase safety are associated with this model (Bonder, 2001b). In prevention programs, occupational therapists work with other health care providers to maximize the individual's physical and functional well-being. The occupational therapist may emphasize activities that encourage socialization and physical fitness, modification of the environment to reduce the possibility of accidents, and identification of roles and activities that are satisfying to the individual. Such interventions have demonstrated benefit (Clark et al., 1997).

One particularly important issue with regard to prevention is falls. Older adults are particularly prone to falls (Lach, 2005; Tideiksaar, 2002). As many as one third of elders fall in a given year, and of these, as many as half sustain serious injuries such as hip fracture. These injuries are associated with high mortality rates, making falls a serious concern for older adults. In addition, because they are aware of the potential for falls, many older adults have considerable fear of falling (Lach, 2005). While fear of falling is particularly prominent among individuals who have a previous history of falling, it is also common among elders who have not fallen. Some older adults significantly curtail their activities because of this fear; thus, their accomplishment of desired occupations suffers even in the absence of a physical injury.

Falls are multifactorial in nature. Among the contributing factors are: changes in sensation necessary to avoid falls (Tideiksaar, 2002), changes in musculoskeletal and vestibular function that compromise balance and gait (Nitz & Choy, 2004; Waddington & Adams, 2004), and environmental hazards such as wet or uneven surfaces (Hantula, Bragger, & Rajala, 2001). Risk factors shared both by falls and fear of falling include stroke, Parkinson's disease, comorbidity, and White race (Friedman et al., 2002).

Similarly, recent research on fall prevention suggests that the most effective strategies are multifactorial (Chang et al., 2004). Recommended interventions fall into three main categories: education (Deery, Day, & Fildes, 2000), environmental modification such as improved lighting and removal of objects posing trip hazards (Boyce, 2003; Tideiksaar, 2001), and interventions to modify client factors and performance skills. These last interventions include such approaches as balance training (Nitz & Choy, 2004; Waddington & Adams, 2004) and t'ai chi (Verhagen et al., 2004).

Outcomes of these strategies suggest that modest reductions in risk for falls can be achieved (Kempton et al., 2000; Vassallo et al., 2004). Some evidence has shown that environmental modifications are less successful than modifications in individual capacities and knowledge, although the data are not sufficiently compelling to eliminate the possibility that environmental modifications can be helpful (Gill, 1999).

Screening

During the course of prevention activities, occupational therapists should be alert to potential problems (Wilkins, Law, & Letts, 2001). If individuals who are nutritionally compromised or who have recently had a life-changing loss receive early intervention, disability may be minimized or avoided. For example, if a client becomes unable to drive because of increasing visual impairment, the therapist may acquaint him or her with community transit services or help make contact with friends and relatives who can provide occasional transportation. Such an intervention helps reduce the likelihood of social isolation, which can lead to depression and perhaps to significant disability.

Environmental Modifications

If it is not feasible to increase the individual's performance ability, another highly effective intervention is to reduce some demands through alteration of the environment (Procedures for Practice 37-2).

Technological Aids to Function

Numerous technological assists can maximize function (Procedures for Practice 37-3). Some are simple, such as an alarm on the doorknob to warn family members that a person is wandering away or automatic off switches

PROCEDURES FOR PRACTICE 37-2

Environmental Modifications for Elderly Individuals

Cognitive Problems

- Reduce clutter.
- Label drawers and cabinets by their contents; for individuals who have dementia or other serious cognitive deficits, pictures may be easier to understand than words.
- Use color, texture, and lighting changes to provide location cues, such as changes from carpet to tile signaling the move from dining area to hallway.
- Use timers as reminders for specific functions.
- Put safety off switches on stoves and furnaces.

Visual Problems

- Use high-tone colors and low-gloss finishes to improve visual acuity and depth perception (Tideiksaar, 2001).
- Incorporate devices to increase magnification or enlarge print, contrasting colors, and dependence on other sensory systems such as touch.
- Maintain a consistent environment to allow the visually impaired individual to function more effectively.
- Write with felt-tipped pens and in bold print to help improve visibility (Mann, 2001).
- Access optometrists, ophthalmologists, and staff at sight centers or the Society for the Blind for helpful input.
- Provide high-intensity, low-glare light; avoid fluorescent lights; and put glare-reducing screens over televisions and windows (Tideiksaar, 2001).
- Teach compensatory techniques to individuals who have reduced peripheral vision or who have only peripheral vision (Lewis, 2003).

Hearing and Communication Problems

- Refer for a thorough evaluation from a speech pathologist, audiologist, or otolaryngologist.
- Speak slowly and clearly and use a deep voice with someone who has high-frequency loss; do not shout.
- Make sure the individual can see you when you speak (Hooper, 2001).
- Write messages if necessary.
- Select activities for which verbal interaction may not be essential, such as bowling, swimming, checkers, and walks.
- Check that hearing aids are fitted and used properly and that batteries are fresh; remember that these aids do not restore normal hearing and may not help everyone with hearing impairment.
- Use visual cues, such as flashing lights, to get the client's attention.

Neuromuscular, Motor, or Mobility Problems

- Make sure the environment is free of hazards such as slippery floors, poorly marked stairs, and architectural barriers.
- Adjust the height of chairs, beds, dressers, clothes, and toilet seats, and provide a bath chair if needed; ensure that grab bars are within easy reach.
- Provide task-oriented treatment in the individual's environment; numerous repetitions enhance learning, and simulated activities may not be easily transferred to real situations.
- In institutional settings, keep in mind OBRA regulations that mandate reduced use of restraints. Careful evaluation of seating can eliminate the need for restraints; for example, a chair that is higher in front than in back can make it more difficult to rise, and well-fitted chairs can enhance balance.

Self-Care: Toileting and Continence Problems

- Make sure that the bathroom is physically accessible. Add grab bars and non-skid mats.
- Mark the bathroom clearly. Use large, clear words, pictures, and color coding if necessary.
- Reduce liquid intake prior to bedtime.
- Institute regular reminders to use the bathroom.
- Use behavior modification techniques to assist elders to notice full bladders.

on stoves to reduce fire hazard. Others, such as the computer-operated Smart House, are highly sophisticated and expensive.

There are limits to the application of technology with older clients. Some clients may resist learning to use the new technologies. Devices can break down and may be expensive to repair. Acquiring the devices may be expensive and not covered by insurance. It is difficult to keep up with advances, and sometimes, a new and better device appears on the market as soon as a client has purchased an expensive piece of equipment. Many older adults, however, enjoy technological devices, quickly learn to use them, and with them gain considerable independence (Mann, 2001).

Modification and Substitution of Activity

Activity analysis, a cornerstone of occupational therapy, can be particularly helpful in assisting older clients. The

PROCEDURES FOR PRACTICE 37-3

Assistive Technology for Problems Associated with Aging

- Telephones with amplifiers, large-print numbers, one-touch dialing, and memory features; cordless, cellular, or digital phones; external speakers
- Screen magnification, print enhancements, and voice synthesizers for computer screen reading
- Assistive listening devices, telecommunication devices (TDDs), or computer software/hardware to facilitate communication via Internet (e.g., chat rooms and instant messaging), closed captioning for television; devices to convert auditory output to flashing lights for smoke detectors, telephones, and doorbells
- Life call systems that provide a link with emergency services
- Advances in technology for mobility, such as wheelchair seating systems, power carts that are easy to disassemble, lightweight wheelchairs, wheeled walkers with brakes and built-in seating systems, and adaptive controls for cars

PROCEDURES FOR PRACTICE 37-4

Promoting Activity Choice for Intervention with Elders

- Link older adults with activities that express important personal meanings, especially connectedness with others, spirituality, service to others, and self-expression (Bonder & Martin, 2000).
- Recognize the vast individual variability in selection of activities that express personal meanings. One individual may choose to express spirituality through attendance at church, another through meditation.
- Find out what specific self-care activities are perceived as vital to elders who are concerned about remaining in their homes.
- Remember that older adults persist for longer periods with activities that are purposeful (Nelson, 1988).
- Employ reminiscence as a means to establish and maintain connections with others.
- Use activity inventories to stimulate an older client to think about what he or she values.
- Adapt the activity or help the client identify an activity that meets similar needs when preferred activities become too difficult for a client. To do so, ascertain what component of the activity is meaningful. For example, if he or she likes to cook because it is a way to socialize, substituting an activity that is not social will not be satisfying.

process involves matching present skills, interests, and motivation with activities that are stimulating, challenging, enjoyable, goal directed, and purposeful. Some specific suggestions are presented in Procedures for Practice 37-4.

In conclusion, intervention with older adults requires understanding of the normal developmental processes that affect performance as well as the special life circumstances of older adults. To be most effective, intervention must address all spheres of function. The special factors that alter intervention with older adults must be taken into account. With older adults, the goal of good quality of life as measured by satisfying activities is in reach in many situations. Thoughtful intervention by occupational therapists can ensure it.

SUMMARY REVIEW QUESTIONS

1. In a well elderly individual, what are the most typical changes in sensation? How can they affect function?
2. How do normal neuromuscular changes that accompany aging affect mobility? How can these changes ultimately affect occupational function?
3. What are some key differences in the cognitive complaints of adults with age-associated memory impairment versus Alzheimer's disease? Describe ways the therapeutic response to these complaints may differ.
4. In general, what effect does retirement have on an older individual who has planned for the event?
5. What is the first step an occupational therapist should take in assessing the status of an older individual?
6. What factors are important in selecting substitute activities for an older adult?
7. In deciding about technological interventions, what factors must be considered to ensure acceptance of the device?
8. What factors complicate intervention with an older adult who falls ill or is injured?

Evidence Table 37-1 Best Evidence for Occupational Therapy Practice for Older Adults

Intervention	Description of Intervention Tested	Participants	Dosage	Type of Best Evidence and Level of Evidence	Benefit	Statistical Probability and Effect Size of Outcome	Reference
Reactivating occupational therapy (OT)	A technique used to improve engagement in activity cognitively.	44 participants, with slight to moderate dementia, each randomly assigned to one of two treatment groups (age 65–95 years).	2 hours per week (in addition to traditional OT).	Randomized, control study. IA1b	Yes. After 12 and 24 weeks, subjects who received reactivating O.T. plus functional rehabilitation had signifcantly better scores in cognitive performance, psychosocial functioning, and subjective well-being compared to those receiving functional rehabilitation only.	$p < 0.01$	Bach et al., 1995
3R Program	Reminiscence, Reality orientation, and Remotivation used in small-group therapy sessions.	30 participants; 15 in the control group and 15 in the treatment group.	8 weeks, 1 session per week.	Quasi-experimental study. IIB2b	Yes. Improvement in mental state noted.	$p < 0.001$	Koh et al., 1994
Leisure activities after a stroke	Leisure activities.	40 participants, 20 in control group and 20 in treatment group; mean age = 69.6 years.	5 weekly visits.	Randomized, control study. IB1a	No. None found.		Jongbloed & Morgan, 1991
Occupational therapy for community-residing elders	Studied preventive occupational therapy intervention.	361 culturally diverse older adults living independently in the community (age 60 years and older).	1 hour per week for 9 months.	Randomized controlled study (3 groups: OT, activity, and no intervention). IA1a	Yes. OT intervention produced superior outcomes on health, functional status, pain, and physical and social functioning.	$p < 0.05$ or better (depending on outcome variable).	Clark et al., 1997

continued

Evidence Table 37-1 Best Evidence for Occupational Therapy Practice for Older Adults(*continued*)

Intervention	Description of Intervention Tested	Participants	Dosage	Type of Best Evidence and Level of Evidence	Benefit	Statistical Probability and Effect Size of Outcome	Reference
Follow-up of health promotion for independent-living elders	Reevaluation of participants in health promotion OT after 6 months (see Clark et al., 1997).	285 of original 361 participants.	No treatment; follow-up assessment only		Yes. Outcomes were sustained on many measures over the 6-month period.	$p < 0.05$ or better (depending on outcome variable)	Clark et al., 2001
OT interventions	Meta-analysis of various OT interventions.	Review of 15 studies about OT with older adults.		Meta-analysis	Yes. OT helps with physical outcomes and daily living and psychosocial outcomes.	$p < 0.001$; effect size of 0.51.	Carlson et al., 1996

References

Administration on Aging. (2004). Statistics: A profile of older Americans: 2004. Retrieved June 3, 2005, from http://www.aoa.dhhs.gov/prof/Statistics/profile/2004/15_pf.asp.

Aldwin, C. M., & Gilmer, D. F. (2003). *Health, illness, and optimal aging: Biological and psychosocial perspectives*. Thousand Oaks, CA: Sage Publications.

Altschuler, J. (2004). Beyond money and survival: The meaning of paid work among older women. *International Journal of Aging and Human Development, 58,* 223–239.

American Occupational Therapy Association [AOTA]. (2002). Occupational Therapy Practice Framework: Domain and process. *American Journal of Occupational Therapy, 56,* 609–639.

Anstey, K. J., & Low, L. (2004). Normal cognitive changes in aging. *Australian Family Physician, 33,* 783–787.

Atchley, R. C. (1989). Continuity theory of normal aging. *Gerontologist, 29,* 183–190.

Bach, D., Bach, M., Bohmer, F., & Grilc, B. (1995). Reactivating occupational therapy: A method to improve cognitive performance in older adulthood. *Age and Aging, 24,* 222–226.

Balogun, J. A., & Katz, J. S. (2002). Physiological changes and functional limitations associated with aging: A critical literature review. *Fizyoterapi Rehabilitasyon, 13,* 37–59.

Bambrick, P., & Bonder, B. (2005). Older adults' perception of work. *Work: A Journal of Prevention, Assessment, and Rehabilitation, 24,* 77–84.

Bergstrom, M. J., & Holmes, M. E. (2004). Organizational communication and aging: Age-related processes in organizations. In J. Nussbaum (Ed.), *Handbook of communication and aging research* (2nd ed., pp. 305–327). Mahwah, NJ: Lawrence Erlbaum Associates.

Blair, S. N., Kampert, J. B., Kohl, H. W. 3rd, Barlow, C. E., Macera, C. A., Paffenbarger, R. S. Jr., & Gibbons, L. W. (1996). Influences of cardiorespiratory fitness and other precursors on cardiovascular disease and all-cause mortality in men and women. *Journal of the American Medical Association, 276,* 205–210.

Bonder, B. R. (2001a). Culture and occupation: A comparison of weaving in two traditions. *Canadian Journal of Occupational Therapy, 68,* 310–319.

Bonder, B. R. (2001b). The psychosocial meaning of activity. In B. R. Bonder & M. B. Wagner (Eds.), *Functional performance in older adults* (2nd ed., pp. 42–58). Philadelphia: Davis.

Bonder, B. R., & Martin, L. (1998). Meaning of activity for older women. Unpublished paper presented at the American Occupational Therapy Association Annual Conference, Indianapolis, IN.

Bonder, B. R., & Martin, L. (2000). Personal meanings of occupation for women in later life. *Women and Aging, 12,* 177–193.

Bosma, H., van Boxtel, M. P. J., Ponds, R. W. H. M., Houx, P. J. H., & Jolles, J. (2003). Education and age-related cognitive decline: The contribution of mental workload. *Educational Gerontology, 29,* 165–173.

Bottomly, J. M., & Lewis, C. B. (2003). *Geriatric rehabilitation: A clinical approach*. Upper Saddle River, NJ: Prentice Hall.

Boyce, P. R. (2003). Lighting for the elderly. *Technology and Disability, 15,* 165–180.

Bundy, A. (2001). Leisure. In B. R. Bonder & M. B. Wagner (Eds.), *Functional performance in older adults* (2nd ed.). Philadelphia: Davis.

Burgio, K., Goode, P., Locher, J., Umlauf, M., Roth, D., Richter, H., Varner, R. E., & Lloyd, L. K. (2002). Behavioral training with and without biofeedback in the treatment of urge incontinence in older women: A randomized controlled trial. *Journal of the American Medical Association, 288,* 2293–2299.

Bye, R. A., Llewellyn, G. M., & Christi, K. E. (2001). The end of life. In B. R. Bonder & M. B. Wagner (Eds.), *Functional performance in older adults* (2nd ed., pp. 500–519). Philadelphia: Davis.

Canadian Association of Occupational Therapists. (2002). *Enabling occupation: An occupational therapy perspective* (revised ed.). Ottawa, Ontario, Canada: Canadian Association of Occupational Therapists.

Carlson, M., Fanchiang, S. P., Zemke, R., & Clark, F. (1996). A meta-analysis of the effectiveness of occupational therapy for older persons. *American Journal of Occupational Therapy, 50,* 89–98.

Chang, J. T., Morton, S. C., Rubenstein, L. Z., Mojica, W. A., Maglione, M., Suttorp, M. J., Roth, E. A., & Shekelle, P. G. (2004). Interventions for the prevention of falls in older adults: Systematic review and meta-analysis of randomised clinical trials. *British Medical Journal, 328,* 680.

Chodzko-Zajko, W. (2001). Biological theories of aging: Implications for functional performance. In B. Bonder & M. Wagner (Eds.), *Functional performance in older adults* (2nd ed., pp. 28–41). Philadelphia: Davis.

Christiansen, C., & Baum, C. (1997) Person-environment occupational performance: A conceptual model for practice. In C. Christiansen & C. Baum (Eds.), *Occupational therapy: Enabling function and well-being* (2nd ed.). Thorofare, NJ: Slack Inc.

Christiansen, C., & Hammecker, C. (2001). Activities of older adults: Self-care. In B. R. Bonder & M. B. Wagner (Eds.), *Functional performance in older adults* (2nd ed., pp. 155–178). Philadelphia: Davis.

Clark, F., Azen, S. P., Carlson, M., Mandel, D., La Bree, L., Hay, J., Zemke, R., Jackson, J., & Lipson, L., (2001). Embedding health-promoting changes into the daily lives of independent-living older adults: Long-term follow-up of occupational therapy intervention. *Journal of Gerontology: Series B: Psychological Sciences and Social Sciences, 56,* P60–P63.

Clark, F., Azen, S. P., Zemke, R., Jackson, J., Carlson, M., Mandel, D., Hay, J., Josephson, K., Cherry, B., Hessel, C., Palmer, J., & Lipson, L. (1997). Occupational therapy for independent-living older adults: A randomized controlled trial. *Journal of the American Medical Association, 278,* 1321–1326.

College of Health Professionals, University of Florida. (n.d.) National older driver research and training center web site. Retrieved July 23, 2005 from http://driving.phhp.ufl.edu/.

Corcoran, M. A. (2001). Dementia. In B. R. Bonder & M. B. Wagner (Eds.), *Functional performance in older adults* (2nd ed., pp. 287–304). Philadelphia: Davis.

Cummings, E. M., & Henry, W. E. (1961). *Growing old: The process of disengagement*. New York: Basic.

Dean, E. (2001). Cardiopulmonary development. In B. R. Bonder & M. B. Wagner (Eds.), *Functional performance in older adults* (2nd ed., pp. 86–120). Philadelphia: Davis.

Deery, H. A., Day, L. M., & Fildes, B. N. (2000). An impact evaluation of a falls prevention program among older people. *Accident Analysis and Prevention, 32,* 427–433.

Desrosiers, J., Hebert, R., Bravo, G., & Dutil, E. (1995). Upper extremity performance test for the elderly (TEMPA): Normative data and correlates with sensorimotor parameters. *Archives of Physical Medicine and Rehabilitation, 76,* 1125–1129.

Ebersole, P., & Hess, P. (1998). *Toward healthy aging: Human needs and nursing response* (5th ed.). St. Louis: Mosby.

Ekerdt, D. J. (1986). The busy ethic: Moral continuity between work and retirement. *Gerontologist, 26,* 239–244.

Erikson, E. (1963). *Childhood and society*. New York: Norton Publications.

Federal Interagency Forum on Aging-Related Statistics. (2004). *Older Americans 2004: Key indicators of well-being*. Washington, DC: United States Government Printing Office.

Fiatarone, M., Marks, E., Ryan, N., Merideth, C., Lipsitz, L., & Evans, W. (1990). High intensity strength training in nonagenarians. *Journal of the American Medical Association, 263,* 3029–3034.

Friedman, S. M., Munoz, B., West, S. K., Rubin, G. S., & Fried, L. P. (2002). Falls and fear of falling: Which comes first? A longitudinal prediction model suggests strategies for primary and secondary prevention. *Journal of the American Geriatrics Society, 50,* 1329–1335.

Fuller-Thompson, E., Minkler, M., & Driver, D. (1997). A profile of grandparents raising grandchildren in the United States. *Gerontologist, 37,* 406–411.

Gallup, J. W. (1999). *Wellness centers: A guide for the design professional*. New York: Wiley.

Gill, T. M. (1999). Prevention falls: To modify the environment or the individual? *Journal of the American Geriatrics Society, 47,* 1471–1472.

Glantz, C., & Richman, N. (1991). *Occupational therapy: A vital link to implementation of OBRA*. Rockville, MD: American Occupational Therapy Association.

Hantula, D. A., Bragger, J. L. D., & Rajala, A. K. (2001). Slips and falls in stores and malls: Implications for community-based injury prevention. *Journal of Prevention and Intervention in the Community, 22,* 67–79.

Havighurst, R. J. (1963). Successful aging. In R. H. Williams, C. Tibbitts, & W. Donahue (Eds.), *Processes of aging* (Vol. 1, pp. 299–320). New York: Atherton.

Hayase, D., Mosenteen, D., Thimmaiah, D., Zemke, S., Atler, K., & Fisher, A. G. (2004). Age-related changes in activities of daily living ability. *Australian Occupational Therapy Journal, 51,* 192–198.

Health Care Financing Administration. (1999). MDS 2.0 information site. Retrieved on July 14, 2005 from http://www.cms.hhs.gov/quality/mds20/.

Heine, C., & Browning, C. J. (2002). Communication and psychosocial consequences of sensory loss in older adults: Overview and rehabilitation directions. *Disability and Rehabilitation, 24,* 763–773.

Herzog, A. R., & House, J. S. (1991). Productive activities and aging well. *Generations, Winter,* 49–54.

Hooper, C. R. (2001). Sensory and sensory integrative development. In B. R. Bonder & M. Wagner (Eds.), *Functional performance in older adults* (2nd ed., pp. 121–137). Philadelphia: Davis.

Insurance Information Institute. (2004). *Older drivers.* Retrieved July 23, 2005 from http://www.iii.org/media/hottopics/insurance/older-drivers/

Jackoway, I. S., Rogers, J. C., & Snow, T. L. (1987). The Role Change Assessment: An interview tool for evaluating older adults. *Occupational Therapy in Mental Health, 7,* 17–37.

Jebsen, R., Taylor, N., Trieschmann, R., Trotter, M., & Howard, L. (1969). An objective and standardized test of hand function. *Archives of Physical Medicine and Rehabilitation, 50,* 311–319.

Johansson, C. (2003). Rising with the fall: Addressing quality of life in physical frailty. *Topics in Geriatric Rehabilitation, 19,* 239–248.

Joint Commission on Accreditation of Healthcare Organizations. (1999). *Comprehensive accreditation manual for hospitals.* Oakbrook Terrace, IL: Joint Commission on Accreditation of Healthcare Organizations.

Jones, D. S., Bland, J. S., & Quinn, S. (2003). Health aging and the origins of illness: Improving the expression of genetic potential. *Integrative Medicine: A Clinician's Journal, 2,* 16–25.

Jongbloed, L., & Morgan, D. (1991). An investigation of involvement in leisure activities after a stroke. *American Journal of Occupational Therapy, 45,* 420–427.

Kell, R. T., Bell, G., & Quinney, A. (2001). Musculoskeletal fitness, health outcomes, and quality of life. *Sports Medicine, 31,* 863–873.

Kempton, A., van Beurden, E., Sladden, T., Garner, E., & Beard, J. (2000). Older people can stay on their feet: Final results of a community-based falls prevention programme. *Health Promotion International, 15,* 27–33.

Kielhofner, G. (1995). *A model of human occupation: Theory and application.* Baltimore: Williams & Wilkins.

Koh, K., Ray, R., Lee, J., Nair, A., Ho, T., & Ang, P. (1994). Dementia in elderly patients: Can the 3R mental stimulation programme improve mental status? *Age and Aging, 23,* 195–199.

Lach, H. W. (2005). Incidence and risk factors for developing fear of falling in older adults. *Public Health Nursing, 22,* 45–52.

Law, M., Baptiste, S., Carswell, A., McColl, M. A., Polatajko, H., & Pollock, N. (2005). *Canadian Occupational Performance Measure* (4th ed.). Ottawa, Ontario, Canada: Canadian Occupational Therapy Association.

Levinson, D. J. (1986). A conception of adult development. *American Psychologist, 49,* 3–13.

Lewis, S. C. (2003). *Elder care in occupational therapy* (2nd ed.). Thorofare, NJ: Slack Inc.

Longino, C. F., & Kart, C. S. (1982). Explicating activity theory: A formal replication. *Journal of Gerontology, 37,* 713–722.

Mace, N. L., Rabins, P. V., & McHugh, P. R. (1999). *The 36-hour day: A family guide to caring for persons with Alzheimer disease, related dementing illnesses, and memory loss in later life* (3rd ed.). Baltimore: Johns Hopkins University.

Mann, W. C. (2001). Technology. In B. Bonder & M. Wagner (Eds.), *Functional performance in older adults* (2nd ed., pp. 429–447). Philadelphia: Davis.

Mathiowetz, V., Volland, G., Kashman, N., & Weber K. (1985). Adult norms for the Box and Block Test of manual dexterity. *American Journal of Occupational Therapy, 39,* 386–391.

Mathiowetz, V., Weber, K., Kashman, N., & Volland G. (1985). Adult norms for the Nine Hole Peg Test of finger dexterity. *Occupational Therapy Journal of Research, 5,* 24–38.

Matsutsuyu, J. (1963). The Interest Checklist. *American Journal of Occupational Therapy, 32,* 628–630.

Nandy, S. (2004). Development and preliminary examination of the predictive validity of the Falls Risk Assessment Tool for use in primary care. *Journal of Public Health, 26,* 138–143.

Nelson, D. (1988). Occupation: Form and performance. *American Journal of Occupational Therapy, 42,* 633–638.

Neugarten, B. L. (1975). *Middle age and aging.* Chicago: University of Chicago.

Nuemann, B. (2002). Using behavior treatment for urinary incontinence. *Occupational Therapy Practice, 7,* 10–15.

Newman, L. (1995). *Maintaining function in older adults.* Newton, MA: Butterworth Heinemann.

Nitz, J. C., & Choy, N. L. (2004). The relationship between ankle dorsiflexion range, falls, and activity level in women aged 40–80 years. *New Zealand Journal of Physiotherapy, 32,* 121–125.

Pellerito, J. M. (2006). *Driver rehabilitation and community mobility.* St. Louis: Mosby.

Pynoos, J., & Cohen, E. (1990). *Home safety guide for older people: check it out, fix it up.* Washington, DC: Serif.

Rawson, N. E. (2003). Age related changes in perception of flavor and aroma. *Generations, 27,* 20–26.

Riley, K. (2001). Cognitive development in later life. In B. R. Bonder & M. Wagner (Eds.), *Functional performance in older adults* (2nd ed., pp. 139–152). Philadelphia: Davis.

Rogers, J. C., Holm, M., & Stone, R. (1997). Evaluation of daily living tasks: The home care advantage. *American Journal of Occupational Therapy, 51,* 410–422.

Rosenfeld, M. (1997). *Motivational strategies in geriatric rehabilitation.* Bethesda, MD: American Occupational Therapy Foundation.

Rowe, J. W., & Kahn, R. L. (1998). *Successful aging.* New York: Pantheon.

Rowles, G. D. (1991). Beyond performance: Being in place as a component of occupational therapy. *American Journal of Occupational Therapy, 45,* 265–271.

Royall, D. R., Palmer, R., Chiodo, L. K., & Polk, M. J. (2005). Executive control mediates memory's association with change in instrumental activities of daily living: The Freedom House study. *Journal of the American Geriatrics Society, 53,* 11–17.

Rudman, D. L., Cook, J. V., & Polatajko, H. (1997). Understanding the potential of occupation: A qualitative exploration of seniors' perspectives on activity. *American Journal of Occupational Therapy, 51,* 640–650.

Savinainen, M., Nygard, C., & Ilmarinen, J. (2004). A 16-year follow-up study of physical capacity in relation to perceived workload among ageing employees. *Ergonomics, 47,* 1087–1102.

Sterns, H., Laier, M. P., & Dorsett, J. G. (2001). Work and retirement. In B. R. Bonder & M. Wagner (Eds.), *Functional performance in older adults* (2nd ed., pp. 179–195). Philadelphia: Davis.

Strong, R. (September). Neurochemical changes in the aging human brain: Implications for behavioral impairment and neurodegenerative disease. *Geriatrics, 53,* S9–S12.

Tian, H., Sturm, R., Pincus, H. A., & Tanielian, T. L. (2004). Depression and leaving employment among older adult Americans. *Psychiatric Services, 55,* 10.

Tideiksaar, R. (2001). Falls. In B. R. Bonder & M. Wagner (Eds.), *Functional performance of older adults* (2nd ed., pp. 267–286). Philadelphia: Davis.

Tideiksaar, R. (2002). Sensory impairment and fall risk. *Generations, 26,* 22–27.

Valentin, S. A., van Boxtel, M. P., van Hooren, S. A., Bosma, H., Beckers, H. J., Ponds, R. W., & Jolles, J. (2005). Change in sensory functioning predicts change in cognitive functioning: Results from a 6-year follow-up in the Maastricht aging study. *Journal of the American Geriatrics Society, 53,* 374–380.

Vassallo, M., Vignaraja, R., Sharma, J. C., Hallam, H., Binns, K., Briggs, R., Ross, I., & Allen, S. (2004). The effect of changing practice on fall prevention in a rehabilitative hospital: The Hospital Injury Prevention Study. *Journal of the American Geriatrics Society, 52,* 335–339.

Verdu, E., Ceballos, D., Vilches, J. J., & Navarro, X. (2000). Influence of aging on peripheral nerve function and regeneration. *Journal of the Peripheral Nervous System, 5,* 191–208.

Verhagen, A., Immink, M., van der Meulen, A., & Biema-Zeinstra, S. M. (2004). The efficacy of Tai Chi Chuan in older adults: A systematic review. *Family Practice, 21,* 107–113.

Waddington, G. S., & Adams, R. D. (2004). The effect of a 5-week wobble-board exercise intervention on ability to discriminate different degrees of ankle inversion, barefoot and wearing shoes. A study in healthy elderly. *Journal of the American Geriatrics Society, 52,* 573–576.

Wilkins, S., Law, M., & Letts, L. (2001). Assessment of functional performance. In B. R. Bonder & M. B. Wagner (Eds.), *Functional performance in older adults* (2nd ed.). Philadelphia: Davis.

Supplemental References

Baron, K., & Curtin, C. (1990). A manual for use with the Self-Assessment of Occupational Functioning. Unpublished manuscript. Department of Occupational Therapy, University of Illinois, Chicago, IL.

Pollack, N. (1993). Client-centered assessment. *American Journal of Occupational Therapy, 47,* 298–301.

Rapkin, B. D., & Fischer, K. (1992). Framing the construct of life satisfaction in term of older adults' personal goals. *Psychology and Aging, 7,* 138–149.

SECTION VI: Treatment to Promote Occupational Function for Selected Diagnostic Categories

CHAPTER 38

Stroke

Anne M. Woodson

LEARNING OBJECTIVES

After studying this chapter, the reader will be able to do the following:

1. Define stroke, or cerebrovascular accident, and briefly describe the causes, incidence, and impairments and disabilities that can result from stroke.
2. Describe the continuum of care for individuals recovering from stroke, including the interdisciplinary team, the various settings for care, and the phases of recovery and intervention.
3. Describe methods for evaluating occupational performance and component abilities and capacities of patients recovering from stroke.
4. Suggest goals and methods for treatment to improve the occupational performance and component abilities and capacities of patients recovering from stroke.
5. Analyze the effectiveness of occupational therapy intervention in improving a patient's quality of life and adjustment to life with stroke.

Glossary

Aphasia—Language disorder caused by brain damage that affects production and/or comprehension of written or spoken language.

Apraxia—Impairment of motor planning or organized, controlled movement not explained by motor or sensory impairment.

Backward chaining—Process of breaking a task into steps and guiding or assisting learner through all but the last step, which learner performs independently. Preceding steps of task are added until learner can perform entire sequence independently.

Hemiparesis—Weakness or partial paralysis on one side of the body caused by brain damage.

Hemiplegia—Paralysis on one side of the body caused by brain damage.

Hemorrhage—Bleeding resulting from the rupture of a blood vessel.

Homonymous hemianopsia—Visual field deficit caused by brain damage in which patient cannot perceive half of visual field of each eye.

Ischemia—Loss of blood flow through a vessel resulting in an insufficient supply of blood and oxygen to surrounding tissues, as when a blood clot blocks a cerebral artery.

Learned non-use—Phenomenon observed in patients with hemiparesis in which patient avoids functional use of involved arm after failed attempts to use it and successful attempts to use uninvolved arm.

Postural adaptation—Ability of body to maintain balance automatically and remain upright during alterations in position and challenges to stability.

Shoulder subluxation—Incomplete dislocation of humerus out of glenohumeral joint caused by weakness, stretch, or abnormal tone in the scapulohumeral and/or scapular muscles.

Unilateral neglect—Disturbance in the ability to notice, orient, or respond to stimuli in space on side of body opposite site of brain damage.

Stroke, or cerebrovascular accident (CVA), describes a variety of disorders characterized by the sudden onset of neurological deficits caused by vascular injury to the brain. Vascular damage in the brain disrupts blood flow, limits oxygen supply to surrounding cells, and leads to brain tissue death or infarction. The mechanism, location, and extent of the lesion determine the symptoms and prognosis for the patient. This chapter focuses on patients with stroke, but non-vascular brain trauma or disease, such as gunshot wounds or tumors, may manifest many of the same neurological deficits and may be treated similarly.

CAUSATION

Strokes are usually classified by the mechanism and location of the vascular damage. The two broad causes are **ischemia** and **hemorrhage**. Ischemic strokes result from a blockage of a cerebral vessel and can further be categorized as caused by thrombosis or embolism. Thrombosis is the stenosis or occlusion of a vessel, usually as a result of atherosclerosis. This occlusion is typically a gradual process, often with preceding warning signs, such as transient ischemic attack (TIA). An embolism is dislodged platelets, cholesterol, or other material that travels in the bloodstream and blocks a vessel. Ischemic strokes are the most common type, representing roughly 80% of strokes (Brandstater, 2005).

Hemorrhagic strokes result from a rupture of a cerebral blood vessel. In such strokes, blood is released outside of the vascular space, cutting off pathways and leading to pressure injuries to brain tissue. Hemorrhages, which are either intracerebral (bleeding into the brain itself) or subarachnoid (bleeding into an area surrounding the brain), may be caused by hypertension, arteriovenous malformation, or aneurysm (Bartels, 2004). Hemorrhagic strokes are less common (an estimated 20% of strokes), but they result in a higher mortality rate than ischemic strokes (American Heart Association, 2005).

Location of Involvement

Most lesions are either anterior circulation strokes, which present signs and symptoms of hemispheric dysfunction, or posterior circulation strokes, which display signs and symptoms of brainstem involvement (Aminoff, Greenberg, & Simon, 2005). Another distinction related to location of CVA is whether the lesion results from large-vessel or small-vessel disease. Thrombosis occurs most often in the large cerebral blood vessels. Small-vessel, or lacunar, strokes are very small infarctions that occur only where small arterioles branch off the larger vessels in deeper portions of the brain, such as the basal ganglia, internal capsule, thalamus, and pons. Lacunar strokes can produce distinctive syndromes and have a good prognosis for recovery (Brandstater, 2005).

CASE EXAMPLE #1

Mrs. H.: Right Cerebrovascular Accident

Occupational Therapy Process	Clinical Reasoning Process: Objectives	Clinical Reasoning Process: Examples of Therapist's Internal Dialogue
Patient Information Mrs. H. is an 82-year-old widow who lived alone independent in ADL and IADL except for community transportation. She was found unresponsive at home by a neighbor and diagnosed with a large right middle cerebral artery infarction. During her acute hospital stay, an occupational therapist evaluated Mrs. H. and reported inconsistent levels of awareness, no spontaneous movement on the left side, and signs of left hemianopsia and spatial neglect. Treatment consisted of involving the patient in simple self-care tasks and initiating a bed positioning and mobility program in conjunction with nursing and physical therapy to prevent secondary complications. Ten days post stroke, Mrs. H. was able to sit in a wheelchair for 1-hour periods, follow one-step commands consistently, and perform simple grooming and bed mobility tasks with minimal assistance. She was transferred to an inpatient rehabilitation unit for more intensive treatment. At the time of discharge from acute care, Mrs. H. was incontinent of bowel and bladder and had a small area of skin breakdown over her coccyx. The social worker reported that Mrs. H. had led a sedentary life and enjoyed going to church, visiting with neighbors and family, reading her Bible, and watching television. Staff reported her verbal skills, comprehension, and memory to be good, although Mrs. H. expressed frustration at her continued hospitalization and stated that she expected a full recovery and return home. Mrs. H.'s family consisted of four adult grandchildren and their families, who were unable to change their work or living situations to care full time for Mrs. H. The family was supportive and hopeful that Mrs. H. could return home with a hired care provider, although they were willing to consider skilled nursing home placement if Mrs. H. did not gain sufficient functioning to return home.	Understand the patient's diagnosis or condition Know the person	"The large size of Mrs. H.'s lesion, persistent altered levels of consciousness, initial severe ADL dependence and motor deficits, visuospatial deficits, and incontinence all predict poor functional outcomes and lengthy recovery period. In her favor, Mrs. H. was able to live alone at home and has no significant prior medical history." "Mrs. H. seems to have limited knowledge and understanding of the nature of her stroke and resulting impairments. She appears to be someone with limited experience living in a dependent role. Because she had not been a physically active person, she may fatigue easily during an intense rehabilitation program. It would not be difficult for her, however, to resume valued roles and activities from a wheelchair level, especially with supportive friends and family. The fact that her thinking skills appear intact will help Mrs. H. achieve her rehabilitation goals, but her visual-perceptual impairments will hinder learning new techniques."
Reason for Referral to Occupational Therapy Mrs. H. was referred to occupational therapy to increase self-care independence, increase awareness of left visual spatial field, recommend proper management of the left arm, and assist in determination of optimum discharge plans. She will also be seen daily by physical therapy and periodically by speech-language pathology, social work, psychology, and therapeutic recreation.	Appreciate the context Develop provisional hypotheses	"I will coordinate my services closely with other disciplines to avoid patient fatigue and develop consistent strategies. I will involve family in therapy early because it seems likely that Mrs. H. will need moderate to maximum skilled care upon discharge."

Assessment Process and Results

The rehabilitation team completed the *Functional Independence Measure* (*FIM*) (Keith et al., 1987) for Mrs. H. as part of the standard care process for the unit. Mrs. H. scored a 28 (out of a possible 91) on the *FIM* motor score, and 30 (out of a possible 35) on the cognitive score. In areas assessed by OT, Mrs. H. required minimal (25%) assistance with eating, grooming, and upper body dressing; maximum (75%) assistance with bed bathing and toilet transfers; and total (more than 75%) assistance for lower body dressing, toileting, and tub transfers. During interview/observation of leisure skills, Mrs. H. described difficulty reading ("I think I need new glasses") and watching TV ("The picture isn't very good"). Mrs. H. was observed consistently keeping her head turned to the right and having difficulty finding or concentrating on people or objects in her left visual field.

OT assessment of component abilities and capacities revealed impaired sensation in the left arm; inconsistent minimal movement in left pectorals, internal rotators, and biceps only; and mild shoulder pain with movement above shoulder level. In addition, a screen of visual field function found significant loss of left peripheral field perception.

The speech-language pathologist reported swallowing difficulties and recommended a pureed diet with no thin liquids. Physical therapy described Mrs. H. as requiring maximum (75%) assistance to perform a scooting transfer and unable to sit unsupported, stand, or propel a wheelchair.

Consider evaluation approach and methods

"From the PT assessment, I learned of Mrs. H.'s postural control deficits. It was important to observe her performance in self-care rather than rely on self-report because she seems to have limited insight into her disabilities.

Interpret observations

Although observation of ADL gave me information about her visual field and inattention problems, I will consider more in-depth testing of her visual function, perhaps portions of the *Brain Injury Vision Assessment Battery for Adults* (Warren, 1996), because of her desire to resume reading."

"I can observe that Mrs. H.'s limited ability in lower extremity dressing, bathing, and transfers are due to her poor sitting balance and lack of mobility. Her difficulties with upper extremity dressing, grooming, and feeding are a result of decreased attention to left visual space and left side of body. Her left side somatosensory and motor deficits and her lack of awareness of her visual problems add to her left inattention."

Occupational Therapy Problem List

- Loss of independence in basic ADL
- Loss of independence in IADL and leisure activities
- At risk for injury or complications in left arm because of lack of voluntary movement, decreased sensation, and visual-spatial neglect
- Limited insight into impairments and disabilities resulting from stroke and the predicted course of recovery

Synthesize results

"Mrs. H.'s stroke has severely reduced her ability to live independently in her home, although returning home is her discharge goal. Her degree of hemiparesis, postural instability, and neglect, along with her lack of awareness, increases her risk for secondary complications."

Occupational Therapy Goal List

Patient will be able to do the following:

- Perform feeding, grooming, and upper body dressing with supervision and minimal cueing
- Perform lower body dressing, toilet transfers, and bathing on a tub bench with moderate (50%) assistance
- Independently operate television by remote control and tape recorder for books on tape
- Maintain sitting balance on the side of bed for at least 2 minutes while engaged in upper body activity
- Properly position left arm during change of position in bed and while seated in wheelchair
- Independently perform stretching and range-of-motion activities for left hand, wrist, forearm, and elbow; perform stretching and range-of-motion activities for shoulder with moderate assistance

Develop intervention hypotheses

"I do not think Mrs. H. will be able to return to independent living, but improving basic capacities (balance, visual attention) would allow her to succeed in simple meaningful activities. Education will assist with continuity of care in a new setting and allow the patient and family to feel they can contribute to the recovery process."

Select an intervention approach

"Occupational therapy intervention will include restoration, compensation, and prevention approaches."

Occupational Therapy Goal List (cont'd) Patient's family will be able to do the following: • Demonstrate proper techniques for positioning • Assist with self-care • Assist with left arm mobility • Encourage attention to left visual field	Consider what will occur in therapy, how often, and for how long	"I predict that Mrs. H. will progress slowly in therapy but will benefit from multidisciplinary treatment. She will need at least 2 weeks of inpatient rehabilitation. She will be seen daily in OT, twice a day for shorter periods (30 minutes) to allow rest between sessions."
Intervention The treatment program during Mrs. H.'s 2-week inpatient rehabilitation stay consisted of (1) an activity program emphasizing basic and instrumental ADL training to address sitting balance, transitional movements, management of left upper extremity, and attention to and scanning of the left visual field and (2) patient and family education regarding the consequences and course of recovery of stroke, safety awareness and prevention of secondary impairments, and compensatory techniques and adaptations to promote functional independence. At discharge, Mrs. H. was able to feed herself, perform simple grooming activities, and use her television and tape recorder with setup and supervision. Status in all other ADL remained unchanged. Sitting balance remained poor, and left spatial neglect remained pronounced. Mrs. H. required maximum assistance with protection and mobilization of her left arm. Mrs. H.'s family attended family training sessions prior to discharge and was provided with written instructions of material covered in training.	Assess the patient's comprehension Understand what she is doing Compare actual to expected performance Know the person Appreciate the context	"Mrs. H. had difficulty learning new techniques for familiar activities, so she required repeated practice and reinforcement from nursing and other disciplines. Because Mrs. H. could not recognize or monitor her visual or balance impairments, interventions to improve these capacities had to rely more on external rather than internal adjustments. Mrs. H. was always pleasant and cooperative and continued to feel that soon she would get better and go home. It was disappointing that she did not gain more independence, but I feel the family understands the impact of Mrs. H.'s stroke and the probability of a lengthy recovery period."
Next Steps Mrs. H. was transferred to a skilled nursing facility, where she will continue occupational and physical therapy. Copies of all therapy documentation were forwarded to the center and information was shared through phone calls. During a conference prior to discharge, the family was informed of possible future settings for continuing care for Mrs. H, and provided with a list of home health agencies, outpatient services, and provider services.	Anticipate present and future patient concerns Analyze patient's comprehension Decide if the patient should continue or discontinue therapy and/or return in the future	"I felt it was important to talk directly to the therapists at the skilled nursing facility to discuss Mrs. H.'s unique problems. It has been less than a month since the onset of her stroke, which is too soon to determine the extent of her recovery. I have emphasized to the patient and family that transfer from the rehabilitation unit does not mean her recovery is over, but it is merely moving to a different stage. I have tried to give the patient and family as much information as possible to help them recognize signs of progress or regression so that they can be advocates to ensure that Mrs. H. receives the proper type of therapy at the proper time."

CLINICAL REASONING IN OCCUPATIONAL THERAPY PRACTICE

Role of Family and Caregiver in Continuing Therapeutic Goals

One of the problems interfering with Mrs. H.'s progress in inpatient rehabilitation was her left visual field deficit and unilateral neglect. How would this problem affect Mrs. H.'s awareness of and involvement in her new environment at a skilled nursing facility? How would this problem affect her performance of self-care tasks and valued leisure activities? How would the therapist explain this problem to the patient and family? What instruction could the therapist give family members so that they could help Mrs. H. learn to compensate for her visual-perceptual deficits? What adaptations could they make in Mrs. H.'s environment?

CASE EXAMPLE # 2

Mr. G.: Left Cerebrovascular Accident

Occupational Therapy Process	Clinical Reasoning Process	
	Objectives	**Examples of Internal Dialogue**
Patient Information Mr. G. is a 38-year-old man with a history of hypertension who had abrupt onset of right-sided weakness and loss of speech. He was hospitalized quickly and diagnosed with a left subarachnoid hemorrhage. He spent 9 days in acute care and 2 weeks on an inpatient rehabilitation unit before being discharged home to live with his wife and two children aged 10 and 12. During his hospitalization, Mr. G. made rapid progress and regained most of his speech and movement on the right side. Upon discharge, Mr. G. could perform self-care tasks, simple meal preparation, and household walking using a straight cane with supervision and increased amount of time. He had mild apraxia resulting in delays initiating and sequencing multistep tasks. He had decreased control of his right arm, particularly when he tried to raise it above shoulder level or attempted fine motor activities. Before his stroke, Mr. G. worked in the parts department of an automobile dealership. His job included inventory, ordering, stocking, and pickup and delivery of parts. His wife was a teacher who was home for the summer but planned to return to work when school started in 2 months.	Understand the patient's diagnosis or condition Know the person	"Mr. G.'s rapid recovery and young age predict good functional recovery. He should continue to gain independence in basic self-care, but persisting problems with higher level right arm and leg function, with higher level communication skills, and with skilled motor planning may interfere with his participation in desired life roles." "Mr. G. was quite successful in achieving inpatient rehabilitation goals and will probably expect similar rapid progress after he returns home. He and his wife will be anxious for him to gain higher levels of function within 2 months. The early months after discharge home can be stressful and frustrating as patients encounter difficulty resuming previous roles."
Reason for Referral to Occupational Therapy Mr. G. was referred to outpatient occupational therapy to continue progress in ADL and IADL independence and to assist with resuming community roles. He was also referred for outpatient physical therapy to work on improving balance and upgrading gait and for speech therapy to improve word retrieval and higher level reading and math skills.	Appreciate the context Develop provisional hypotheses	"Home is the best place for Mr. G. to practice and refine his ADL/IADL skills. As he gains confidence at home and competence in performance skills, he will look more to resuming community roles, especially his worker/provider role."
Assessment Process and Results Mr. G.'s goals for occupational therapy were to function safely alone at home after his wife returned to work, to regain normal function of his right dominant arm, and to return to work as soon as possible. Initial outpatient assessments included the *Stroke Impact Scale* (Duncan et al., 1999), which allowed Mr. G. to rate how various impairments and disabilities caused by his stroke affected his quality of life.	Consider evaluation approach and methods Interpret observations	"I like using the *Stroke Impact Scale* and *Functional Test for the Hemiplegic/Hemiparetic Upper Extremity* because they are specific to stroke and help patients focus on functional results and appreciate that their problems are typical. These assessments are both useful for tracking progress over a long period of time." "Mr. G is at a stage where he is beginning to experience and realize the effects of his stroke on his

Assessment Process and Results (cont'd) Responses to this scale and further interview revealed that Mr. G. is concerned about the continuing difficulty in using his right arm; worries about being a burden on his family and returning to work; feels foolish and inadequate because of frequent mistakes in speech, reading, writing, and math; admits that he is very slow with his daily care routine and household tasks and depends on his wife for help more than he would like; and feels unable to participate in most previous leisure or social activities. A home assessment was completed to observe Mr. G. perform his morning bathing/dressing/grooming tasks and to assess safety risks. He took almost 2 hours to complete these tasks, needed occasional physical assistance for balance, needed occasional verbal cueing for sequencing, and had difficulty with fine motor tasks such as buttoning. The *Functional Test for the Hemiplegic/Paretic Upper Extremity* (Wilson, Baker, & Craddock, 1984a, 1984b) was administered to determine level of functional use of his right arm (see Fig. 38-3).		unique life roles. He shows good insight into his problems, and that will help him achieve or adapt his goals. His ADL deficits are due to a combination of dynamic balance problems, delays in initiation, and decreased coordination of his right arm. He is able to use his right arm effectively as a stabilizing assist and for simple grasp and release, but he has difficulty with activities involving moving the arm above shoulder level or right-hand fine motor prehension or manipulation."
Occupational Therapy Problem List • Requires supervision and extended time to complete bathing, grooming, and dressing • Requires supervision and/or increased time to perform home IADL tasks (writing checks, preparing meals) • Unable to perform tasks required for job, including using computer, lifting boxes up to 50 pounds, and driving • Unable to resume leisure activities, including bowling and coaching son's baseball team • Difficulty using right arm for activities above shoulder level • Unable to use right hand for fine motor prehension or manipulation tasks • Depressed, anxious over loss of independence and role functioning and financial uncertainties	Synthesize results	"Mr. G. has shown good functional recovery in a short period of time and is working hard to readapt to his home environment. However, his deficits in higher level occupational and component skills hinder his role competence."
Occupational Therapy Goal List • Perform morning self-care independently in 45 minutes or less • Assume partial meal preparation and laundry tasks to help wife • Use right arm to comb hair and to place and retrieve objects on shelf at eye level • Use right hand to tie shoelaces, manipulate coins, sign name, and perform simple computer functions • Participate in gross motor recreational activities with children (swimming, table tennis) • Perform job simulation activities for 2 hours without rest break • Complete pre-driving evaluation • Be able to use community transportation independently	Develop intervention hypotheses	"I think Mr. G. will gain independence in basic ADL and limited IADL. I think he will make substantial progress in resuming valued roles, but this may take a long time, and he may need to accept modified roles."
	Select an intervention approach	"Occupational therapy intervention will primarily be restorative, with compensation/adaptation intervention used as needed."
	Consider what will occur in therapy, how often, and for how long	"Because Mr. G. has a time goal (his wife's return to work), I will see him 3 times a week for 1 month, and then 2 times a week for a month."

Intervention Treatment consisted of the following: (1) Task-specific training in ADL, IADL, and job activities. Activities were adapted, graded, and expanded as Mr. G. gained competency. (2) Repetitive task-oriented program to improve motor planning, postural adaptation, and right arm strength and control. This program was designed to be carried over to home. (3) Education concerning safety issues, home and activity adaptations, social supports, and available community resources. His wife and children attended therapy sessions at least once a week and provided valuable suggestions and encouragement for carryover of therapy in the home. All goals were achieved at the end of 2 months. He scored significant improvements on both the *Functional Test for the Hemiplegic/Paretic Upper Extremity* and the *Stroke Impact Scale*. Mr. G was able to demonstrate independence with written home programs addressing component skills and was able to verbalize appropriate safety precautions.	Assess the patient's comprehension Understand what he is doing Compare actual to expected performance Know the person Appreciate the context	"Mr. G. was highly motivated for therapy and was relieved to see incremental improvements. He had problems that seemed to respond best to familiar, meaningful, repetitive treatment activities. Treatment was designed to provide structure to substitute for his loss of employment, to allow him to resume alternative roles at home, and to allow him to explore the feasibility of returning to his previous job."
Next Steps Mr. G. was scheduled for follow-up visits with his neurologist in the outpatient stroke clinic every 3 months for a year post stroke, which allowed OT a chance to contact him and monitor his progress. He was referred for behind-the-wheel driving assessment and training. He initiated application procedures for his state's vocational rehabilitation financial aid and training services. He and his wife were given the names of counseling resources to help them deal with the stresses of his continued recovery.	Anticipate present and future patient concerns Analyze patient's comprehension Decide if the patient should continue or discontinue therapy and/or return in the future	"I anticipate that Mr. G. will continue to gain competence in component skills and occupational functioning but that his rate of recovery will slow down. I am glad I will have a chance to check with him periodically to alter his home program if necessary and to determine if he will benefit from additional therapy. Depending on the results of vocational screening, he may decide to pursue different employment that might require specific job training. Both he and his wife seem to understand that depression is a common complication of stroke."

CLINICAL REASONING IN OCCUPATIONAL THERAPY PRACTICE

Use of ADL and IADL to Improve Component Impairments: Occupation-As-Means

Although he showed rapid recovery, Mr. G. was unable to resume occupational roles after returning home because of residual impairments. How would training in meal preparation and laundry activities help to lessen Mr. G.'s particular impairments? How could these activities be graded to increase active shoulder range of motion? Improve hand dexterity? Upgrade balance requirements? What compensatory strategies could Mr. G. use to improve initiation and sequencing of kitchen and laundry tasks? What safety techniques should he employ?

INCIDENCE

Stroke is the third leading cause of death in the United States and a leading cause of chronic disability among adults. Of the estimated 700,000 persons who have first or recurrent CVAs in the United States each year, approximately two thirds survive, bringing the number of stroke survivors in the U.S. population at any one time to over two and a half million (American Heart Association, 2005). Stroke is the most common diagnostic category among patients seen by occupational therapists (Rijken & Dekker, 1998). The projected aging of the U.S. population is expected to raise the incidence of stroke because about two thirds of all strokes occur in those over age 65 (Aminoff, Greenberg, & Simon, 2005).

MEDICAL MANAGEMENT

Acute stroke care focuses on determining the cause and site of the stroke, preventing progression of the lesion, reducing cerebral edema, preventing secondary medical complications, and treating acute neurological symptoms (Bartels, 2004). Advances in the use of technology and pharmaceuticals have transformed acute stroke care from mainly supportive to possible prevention and intervention. Improved techniques of diagnosis, including computed tomography (CT) and magnetic resonance imaging (MRI), can distinguish ischemic from hemorrhagic lesions and define their location, size, and vascular territory (Caplan, 2002).

In acute ischemic stroke, treatment concerns include restoration of blood flow and limitation of neuronal damage. Anti-platelet and anti-coagulation drugs, such as aspirin and heparin, are frequently used to improve flow through occluded vessels and prevent further clotting or thrombosis. Newer pharmacological treatments include thrombolytic drugs, such as tissue plasminogen activator (t-PA), that can open occluded cerebral vessels and immediately restore circulation (Bartels, 2004). Their use is limited, however, by the associated increased risk of hemorrhage and the fact that they must be administered within 3–6 hours after stroke onset. As the effectiveness of various medical treatments has not been established, only a small percentage of patients with ischemic stroke are treated with thrombolytic drugs (Caplan, 2002). With hemorrhagic stroke, acute treatment includes control of intracranial pressure, prevention of rebleeding, maintenance of cerebral perfusion, and control of vasospasm (Bartels, 2004).

RECOVERY FROM STROKE

The degree and time course of recovery from stroke vary with the nature and severity of the initial injury (Dobkin, 2005). Early initial improvement or spontaneous recovery occurs because pathologic processes in the brain resolve and neurotransmission resumes near and remote from an infarct or hemorrhage (Dobkin, 2005). Later, ongoing improvement occurs with structural and functional reorganization within the brain, or neuroplasticity. Neuroplasticity includes greater excitability and recruitment of intact neurons in both hemispheres of the brain as a response to stimulation, participation, training, and experience (Dobkin, 2005). Langton Hewer (1990) described a model of stroke recovery that includes both intrinsic and adaptive recovery. Intrinsic recovery refers to the remediation of neurological impairments, such as return of movement to a paralyzed limb. Adaptive recovery entails regaining the ability to perform meaningful activities, tasks, and roles without full restoration of neurological function, such as using the unaffected hand for dressing or walking with a cane or walker. Most patients gain some degree of both intrinsic (neurological) and adaptive (functional) recovery (Langton Hewer, 1990). Rehabilitation, including occupational therapy, is designed to promote maximum possible functional recovery from stroke.

Neurological Impairments and Recovery

Each survivor of a CVA has a unique combination of deficits determined by the location and severity of the lesion. Definition 38-1 lists the most commonly encountered neurological impairments following stroke and describes the possible effect of each on occupational functioning. The most typical manifestation of CVA is **hemiparesis** or **hemiplegia**, ranging from mild weakness to complete paralysis on the side of the body opposite the site of the CVA. As much as 88% of patients with acute stroke have hemiparesis (Foulkes et al., 1988), although the rate of physical impairment usually decreases after the first 3–6 months post stroke (Dobkin, 2005).

Certain impairments are associated with lesions in a particular hemisphere. For example, left CVA may cause right hemiparesis, aphasia or other communication deficits, and/or apraxia or motor planning deficits. Right CVA may result in left hemiparesis, visual field deficits or spatial neglect, poor insight and judgment, and/or impulsive behavior (Brodie, Holm, & Tomlin, 1994).

Many patients do not regain full movement or function of the upper extremity. Studies found that 69% of patients admitted to a rehabilitation unit following CVA had initial mild to severe upper extremity dysfunction, but only 14% experienced complete motor recovery, and 30% regained partial motor recovery in the arm (Nakayama et al., 1994). Historically, motor recovery in the patient with hemiparesis is described as progressing from proximal to distal movement and from mass, patterned, undifferentiated movement to selective, coordinated movement (Brunnstrom, 1970; Fugl-Meyer et al., 1975). Therapists now rarely see such a distinct progression of motor recovery in patients, perhaps because improved medical treatments limit brain damage or because of arbitrarily shortened time frames for rehabilitation services (see Definition 38-1).

Functional Recovery

Much attention is given to the functional outcomes of patients surviving stroke. Although residual neurological deficits can lead to permanent impairments, disabilities, and handicaps, impairments alone do not predict levels of disability or occupational functioning (Kelly-Hayes et al., 1998). Important aspects of functional recovery include the amount of assistance required to carryout daily living tasks and whether a stroke survivor can resume function at home. Studies indicate that independence in

DEFINITION 38-1

de·fin·i·tion

Neurological Impairments Following Stroke

Hemiplegia, hemiparesis	Impaired postural adaptation, bilateral integration Impaired mobility Decreased independence in any or all ADL, IADL
Hemianopsia, other visual deficits	Decreased awareness of environment; decreased ability to adapt to environment Impaired ability to read, write, navigate during mobility, recognize people and places, drive; can affect all ADL, IADL
Aphasia	Impaired speech and comprehension of verbal or written language; inability to communicate, read, or comprehend signs or directions Decreased social, community involvement; isolation
Dysarthria	Slurred speech, difficulty with oral motor functions such as eating, altered facial expressions
Somatosensory deficits	Increased risk of injury to insensitive areas Impairment of coordinated, dexterous movement
Incontinence	Loss of independence in toileting Increased risk of skin breakdown Decreased social, community involvement
Dysphagia	At risk for aspiration Impaired ability to eat or drink by mouth
Apraxia	Decreased independence in any motor activity (ADL, speech, mobility), decreased ability to learn new tasks or skills
Cognitive deficits	Decreased independence in ADL, IADL; decreased ability to learn new techniques; decreased social interactions
Depression	Decreased motivation, participation in activity; decreased social interaction

activities of daily living (ADL) improves with time after an acute stroke. A large prospective community-based study (Jorgensen et al., 1995) using the *Barthel Index* of ADL scores (Mahoney & Barthel, 1965) found that, after completing inpatient rehabilitation, 64% of patients with acute stroke were discharged to their homes and 15% were discharged to nursing homes. After completing rehabilitation, 28% of stroke survivors were considered moderately to severely disabled in self-care, 26% were mildly disabled in self-care, and 46% were independent in self-care.

Few studies have addressed the recovery of instrumental activities of daily living (IADL), such as home management, vocational, leisure, or community skills. Most persons surviving stroke report decreased levels of activity, socialization, and overall quality of life, with only an estimated 25% returning to the level of everyday participation of community-matched persons who have not had a stroke (Lai et al., 2002).

Factors Influencing Recovery

Research in stroke outcomes has sought to identify characteristics and indicators that predict survival rate, degree of disability, and functional status. No simple predictors have been identified from numerous prospective studies. Patients with similar impairments after stroke may achieve wide ranges in outcomes: individuals with mild neurological impairments may end up with serious disabilities or handicaps, while other individuals with severe residual stroke impairments achieve satisfactory functional recovery (Kelly-Hayes et al., 1998).

The type, size, and site of the brain lesion, of course, influence the extent and course of recovery. Advanced age and the presence and severity of co-existing disease, such as diabetes, heart disease, and peripheral vascular disease, can impede optimal functional recovery. The effect of age may partly be related to more frequent co-impairments, such as arthritis or dementia, in the elderly. Many elderly patients with poor outcomes following a stroke had reduced function prior to the stroke (Brandstater, 2005).

Other factors associated with poor functional outcomes include severe initial motor deficits, poor sitting balance, dependence in basic ADL, prior stroke, persistent bowel and urinary incontinence, severe visuospatial deficits, severe cognitive impairments, depression, severe aphasia, altered level of consciousness, and poor social supports (e.g., living alone). Factors that may predict good quality of life after stroke include family support, independence in basic ADL, and access to continued services (Brandstater, 2005).

Time Frame for Recovery

It has traditionally been reported that recovery of function following stroke occurs most rapidly during the first 1–3 months, but slower improvement can continue for up to a year (Wade, 1992). Policy makers tend to regard stroke as an acute disorder following a circumscribed recovery course rather than as a chronic, changing condition. Plateaus in recovery often reflect the insensitivity of measurement scales to incremental improvements rather than a patient's reduced potential for learning new tasks or gaining skill (Dobkin, 2005). Multiple studies have shown that patients more than 1 year post stroke can exhibit substantial motor and functional improvement after participation in novel rehabilitation protocols (Page, Gater, & Bach-y-Rita, 2004). Individual stroke survivors who have successfully resumed life roles or taken on new ones report the process of recovery as continuing years after onset of stroke, with gains reported both in component skills and occupational performance (Buscherhof, 1998; Matola, 2001).

SPECTRUM OF CARE

Since the brain damage resulting from stroke has the potential to affect any aspect of an individual's health and functioning, a wide array of disciplines are involved in caring for survivors of stroke. A patient recovering from stroke may receive care in multiple settings as he or she progresses from onset through a rehabilitation program to a return to the community. Coordination of services and ongoing communication among patients, families, and care providers at each step of rehabilitation is mandatory for optimum outcomes.

Interdisciplinary Team

Ideally, members of the stroke rehabilitation team include the patient, the patient's family, the primary physician (internal medicine, family medicine, or geriatrics), a neurologist or physical medicine specialist (physiatrist), rehabilitation nurse, occupational therapist, physical therapist, social worker, speech-language pathologist, clinical psychologist, therapeutic recreation specialist, and dietitian. Team members vary with the patient's needs and available resources. Frequent communication in the form of clear documentation, team meetings, and individual exchanges among members is vital for effective and efficient teamwork.

Settings for Care

Occupational therapists treat patients recovering from stroke in a variety of settings, including acute-care hospitals, skilled nursing facilities, inpatient rehabilitation centers, outpatient clinics, and home care settings. A study of 1991 Medicare claims for rehabilitation services found that 73% of patients who survived stroke received services in one or more of these settings, with 17% treated in inpatient rehabilitation programs, 23% admitted to nursing facilities, and 40% receiving either home health or outpatient services (Gresham et al., 1995). To facilitate a patient's transition from one setting of care to another, occupational therapists should be familiar with facilities and available services in the patient's area and communicate pertinent information to the next setting, particularly the patient's goals of resuming life roles.

ASSESSMENT

Numerous evaluations exist to identify stroke impairments and disability. To help in the selection and ordering of assessment tools, therapists are guided by models of practice and evidence-based practice guidelines. Occupational function is the focus of occupational therapy; thus, assessment of a patient post stroke begins with determination of roles, tasks, and activities important to that individual. From this context, the occupational therapist assesses the individual's competence in performing these valued roles, tasks, and activities. Where disabilities are discovered, further evaluation identifies specific impairments in abilities and capacities and residual abilities that can lead to restoration of function.

In response to growing demands for standards of quality health care, the U.S. Department of Health and Human Services' Agency for Health Care Policy and Research (now the Agency for Healthcare Research and Quality) published the *Post-stroke Rehabilitation Clinical Practice Guideline* (Gresham et al., 1995). Concerning assessment, this guideline recommends that practitioners "use well-validated standardized measures" throughout acute care and rehabilitation to achieve consistency of treatment decisions, facilitate team communication, and monitor progress for each survivor (Gresham et al., 1995, p. 7). Often, multiple assessment instruments must be used because of the wide variation in individual stroke manifestations and the patient's changing needs over the course of recovery. The guideline recommends specific assessments based on the instrument's validity, reliability, sensitivity to change, and practicality.

Therapists should be familiar with commonly used standardized stroke deficit scales because they are frequently used as an interdisciplinary summary of baseline function and as indicators of recovery or treatment outcomes. The *National Institute of Health Stroke Scale* (Brott et al., 1989) is a brief, well-validated tool that can be administered by physicians, nurses, or therapists. Items scored include consciousness, vision, extraocular movements, facial palsy, limb strength, ataxia, sensation, speech, and language. The *American Heart Association Stroke Outcome Classification* (Kelly-Hayes et al., 1998) was devised to summarize the neurological impairments, disabilities, and handicaps that occur post stroke. This classification formula records the number of neurological domains affected (motor, sensory, visual, language, cognitive, affective), the severity of these impairments, and the functional (ADL) performance rating resulting from these impairments. Such a classification system can be used to assess recovery, determine response to various treatments, and track long-term effects of stroke on survivors.

Assessment of Occupational Performance

The patient's ability to perform the self-care, recreational, and vocational tasks that he or she hopes to continue is evaluated by observation rather than report because there can be a difference between what a patient can do and actually does. Evaluation to determine a patient's level of occupational functioning is administered early to predict answers to the following questions (Wade, 1992): (1) Where will the patient live, and what physical adaptations will be necessary? (2) How much and what type of assistance will the patient need? (3) What roles will the patient be able to fulfill, and how will he or she spend his or her time?

A patient's ADL performance in a structured clinical setting may not indicate performance at home. For example, patients who can put on and remove clothing during therapy sessions may not be able to find and retrieve their clothes in a cluttered closet, select clothing appropriate for the weather, or initiate the dressing routine without prompting (Campbell et al., 1991). Conversely, a patient may be unable to master simple meal preparation in the unfamiliar environment of a clinic kitchen but may readapt easily to this task upon return home. A home evaluation can help determine what resources and means a patient has to achieve independence in tasks as well as assessing safety and accessibility (see Chapter 11).

Self-Care

Methods for assessing self-care, or basic ADL, and examples of evaluation tools are discussed in Chapter 4. Measures of disability in ADL recommended by the *Post-Stroke Rehabilitation Clinical Practice Guideline* (Gresham et al., 1995) are the *Barthel Index* (Mahoney & Barthel, 1965) and the *Functional Independence Measure* (Keith et al., 1987). These interdisciplinary measures are well known and widely used in stroke research. Their use can strengthen the team approach to stroke, with occupational therapists typically completing the self-care portions of these assessments and practitioners of other disciplines completing portions pertaining to bowel and bladder control, mobility, communication, cognition, and social interaction. These functional scales tend to have ceiling effects and are limited in their ability to measure higher levels of function or quality of life (Lai et al., 2002).

Instrumental Activities of Daily Living

A patient's goals and probable discharge situation may direct a therapist to evaluate more complex areas of occupational performance. Measures of IADL recommended by the *Post-Stroke Rehabilitation Clinical Practice Guideline* include the *Frenchay Activities Index* (Holbrook & Skilbeck, 1983) and the *Philadelphia Geriatric Center Instrumental Activities of Daily Living Scale* (Lawton, 1988). The *Frenchay Activities Index* is a self-report tool developed specifically for patients with stroke that compares how frequently a patient engaged in activities, such as washing clothes, going on social outings, and gardening, prior to a stroke with frequency of participation in the same activities afterward. The stated purposes of this evaluation are to record changes in patterns of activity after stroke and to reflect quality of life rather than to measure performance in survival skills. The *IADL Scale*, on the other hand, is an observed measure that ranks quality of performance of activities such as using a telephone, managing medications, and handling finances. The *Stroke Impact Scale* (Duncan et al., 1999) was developed to be a more comprehensive measure of outcomes for stroke survivors (Lai et al., 2002). The scale is a self-report interviewer-administered measure with questions pertaining to higher-level functions of affected limbs, memory and thinking, mood and emotions, communication skills, home and community mobility, typical daily activities, and participation in meaningful life roles. Items included in this scale were derived from feedback of stroke patients and their caregivers who identified the persistent consequences of stroke that interfered the most with quality of life.

When appropriate, potential for driving and return to work may be evaluated by an occupational therapist or other specialist trained in these areas. A patient's ability to resume driving and/or vocational tasks is discussed later in this chapter; see also Chapters 31 and 33.

Assessment of Component Abilities and Capacities

Observation of a patient's ADL performance suggests to the therapist probable deficits in components of independent functioning, which can be measured directly by administration of selected tests. Areas to be evaluated include postural adaptation, specific components of upper extremity function, and motor learning ability.

Postural Adaptation

Postural adaptation, or postural control, refers to the individual's ongoing ability to remain upright against gravity for stability and during changes in body position (Bobath, 1990; Warren, 1990). The recognition and treatment of deficits in postural adaptation constitute an important aspect of therapy for stroke patients because so many daily living tasks (e.g., putting on socks, getting in and out of a bathtub, housework, and participating in sports) depend on this skill. Evaluation and treatment limited to a patient securely supported in bed or in a wheelchair fail to address most usual daily tasks that require dealing with gravity. A person with hemiplegia typically has decreased trunk control, poor bilateral integration, and impaired automatic postural control. As a result, the patient must devote considerably more effort to remaining upright, with decreased ability to focus on purposeful tasks (Warren, 1991). When engaging in a challenging activity, the hemiplegic patient often resorts to a developmentally lower level compensatory strategy to help maintain stability, such as using upper extremities to help with standing balance (Warren, 1990).

Postural adaptation capacities such as balance can best be observed during the performance of meaningful functional activities, although the *Berg Balance Scale* (Berg et al., 1989) has been listed as a recommended tool in the *Post-Stroke Rehabilitation Clinical Practice Guideline*. Determining status of a patient's trunk control after stroke is an important starting point for assessing component capacities or skills because poor trunk control can lead to dysfunctional limb control, increased risk of falls, contracture and deformity, diminished sitting and standing endurance, decreased visual feedback and swallowing effectiveness secondary to head and neck malalignment, and impaired ability to interact with the environment (Gillen, 2004a). A patient's posture and balance, both static and dynamic, can be observed and noted while the patient is seated and standing and during self-care tasks such as dressing, transfers, and bathing. Definition 38-2 compares functional seated posture with the dysfunctional positioning typically observed in patients recovering from stroke.

Upper Extremity Function

Occupational therapists are the clinicians most often involved with the evaluation and treatment of motor deficits in the hemiplegic or hemiparetic upper extremity. Evaluation of the involved upper extremity should address sensation; the mechanical and physiological deterrents to movement; the presence and degree of active or voluntary movement; the quality of this movement, including strength, endurance, and coordination; and the extent of function resulting from movement.

Somatosensory Assessment

During evaluations of sensory deficits in the stroke patient, it is important to remember that sensation is a component of function and not a focus for treatment except as it relates to the ability to perform usual daily living tasks. When somatosensory disturbances are present, they usually accompany motor impairment in the same anatomic distribution (Brandstater, 2005).

Most tests of sensation require attention, recognition, and response to multiple stimuli; therefore, sensory testing is difficult in patients with aphasia, confusion, and other cognitive deficits. It is often necessary to determine the patient's level of comprehension and communication, including yes/no reliability. An expressively aphasic patient can nod, gesture, point to written or pictured cues, or select a stimulus object from an array of objects. When testing with standard procedures is not possible, information may still be gained from observing a patient's reactions to the testing. The presence of gross protective sensation (flinching when pricked with a sharp pin) can be documented even if discriminatory perception cannot be determined.

Patients who have had mild CVAs and who have intact primary sensory awareness may need to be tested for more subtle discriminatory problems using the two-point discrimination test (Callahan, 1995) or the *Moberg Pick-up Test* (Dellon, 1981). Such testing is indicated when motor return is good but hand dexterity remains impaired. Chapter 7 provides details of sensory assessment.

Mechanical and Physiological Components

Factors that can interfere with movement and function of the hemiplegic upper extremity include limitations in passive range of motion, joint malalignment, abnormal muscle tone, and pain. Interview and medical records can help determine whether these conditions resulted from the stroke or were present prior to onset. Passive movement restrictions in the joints and soft tissues of the extremity may result from an individual's anatomy and lifestyle or from pre-morbid conditions such as arthritis or injury. Limitations may result more directly from the stroke, with sudden and prolonged immobilization of joints due to weakness or spasticity in muscles. Persistent stereotyped positioning of joints without counteracting movement results in the shortening and eventual contracture of muscles, tendons, and ligaments. In the shoulder, adhesions, tendinitis, and bursitis are common

DEFINITION 38-2

de·fin·i·tion

Common Impairments in Sitting Posture Seen After Stroke

Body Part	Normal Sitting Posture Ready for Function	Abnormal Sitting Posture Typical of Stroke
Head, neck	Neutral	Forward Flexed to weak side Rotated away from weak side
Shoulders	Symmetrical height Aligned over pelvis	Uneven height Involved shoulder retracted
Spine, trunk	Straight from posterior view Appropriate lateral curves Lateral trunk muscle lengths equal bilaterally	Curved from posterior view Thoracic kyphosis Shortened lateral trunk muscles on one side, elongation on opposite side
Arms	Not used to maintain static upright posture Relaxed	Use of stronger arm to maintain upright posture Increased or decreased muscle tone in involved arm
Pelvis	Symmetrical weight bearing through both ischial tuberosities Neutral to slight anterior pelvic tilt Neutral rotation	Asymmetrical weight bearing Posterior pelvic tilt One hip retracted forward
Legs	Hips at 90° flexion Knees aligned with hips; hips in neutral adduction or abduction and internal or external rotation Feet under knees Feet flat on floor, able to bear weight	Hips in more extension Hips adducted so that knees touch or involved hip externally rotated so that knees wide apart Feet in front of knees Feet not flat on floor, unable to bear weight

complications of hemiparesis, and all can result in limited range of motion (Andersen, 1985). Edema secondary to reduced circulation and loss of muscle action can further limit passive joint motion, particularly in the hand. Goniometric measurement of passive range of motion is usually not indicated unless treatment is specifically aimed at increasing passive motion, such as when trying to eliminate an elbow flexion contracture. More useful in assessing patients with stroke is a comparison of the involved to the uninvolved arm to determine probable baseline joint motion.

Shoulder subluxation, or malalignment of the glenohumeral joint, occurs in 30–50% of stroke patients. This condition is probably caused by the weight of the arm pulling down the humerus when the supraspinatus and deltoid muscles are weak and by weakness of scapular muscles that allows the glenoid cavity to rotate downward (Brandstater, 2005). Shoulder subluxation can be identified by palpation: the patient's arm hangs freely with trunk stabilized while the examiner palpates the subacromial space for the separation between the acromion and the head of the humerus. The distance separating the two is measured in finger widths, that is, the number of fingers that can be inserted in the space (Bohannon & Andrews, 1990).

The role of subluxation in the painful shoulder is controversial; other processes that may cause pain in the hemiplegic shoulder include spasticity and/or contracture, impingement, soft tissue trauma, rotator cuff tears, glenohumeral capsulitis, bicipital tendonitis, complex regional pain syndrome, and traction neuropathy (Walsh, 2001). Most patients with shoulder pain will have varying combinations of these disorders (Brandstater, 2005; Walsh, 2001).

Abnormal muscle tone is a common component of movement deficits in hemiplegia but is also associated with range-of-motion limitations and pain. Definitions of states of increased and decreased muscle tone and methods for evaluating muscle tone are found in Chapter 6. See Chapter 5 for descriptions of pain evaluation.

Voluntary Movement

Determining the amount and quality of voluntary movement a patient can produce is one of the first steps in assessing movement potential (Warren, 1991). The patterns of motion available are different for each stroke patient. Movement can change dramatically or subtly with time; hence, it requires careful reassessment throughout recovery. Factors to consider when evaluating motor control of the involved upper extremity include:

- Can the patient perform reflexive but not voluntary movement? Example: Patient demonstrates active elbow extension in the involved arm when balance is disturbed (equilibrium reaction) or flexes the hemiparetic elbow while yawning (associated reaction) but cannot perform these movements on request.
- Do proximal segments (neck, trunk, shoulder, hip) stabilize as needed to provide firm support for movement of the distal parts? Example: A patient cannot keep his balance when attempting arm movement and can raise his hemiparetic arm only with pronounced lateral bending of the trunk and excessive elevation of the shoulder girdle.
- Can voluntary movement be performed unassisted against gravity, or is assistance required in the form of positioning, support, or facilitation? Example: A patient can bring her hand to her mouth only by flexing her elbow in a horizontal plane with gravity eliminated.
- Can voluntary movement be performed in an isolated fashion or only in a synergistic pattern? Example: A patient can reach for an object on a table only with a pattern of shoulder abduction, elbow flexion, and trunk flexion, rather than with the more efficient pattern of shoulder flexion and elbow extension.
- Can reciprocal movement (the ability to perform agonist/antagonist motion in succession in an individual joint) be performed with practical speed and precision? Examples: A patient cannot produce a smooth pattern of elbow extension-flexion-extension needed to grasp a glass, take a drink, and set it back on the table but can perform both movements separately. A patient cannot perform the rapid alternating movements necessary to brush teeth.

One of the major movement difficulties following stroke is attaining the capacity and ability to isolate and control single muscle actions and combine them in a pattern appropriate for the task at hand. In motor patterns typical in hemiplegia, movement initiated in one joint results in automatic contraction of other muscles linked in synergy with that movement. This results in limited, stereotyped movement patterns rather than adaptive, selective motions. Typical stereotyped patterns are described as flexor or extensor synergy patterns according to the motion at the elbow (Brunnstrom, 1970) (see Chapter 25). There is considerable variation in synergistic patterning, and other causes of abnormal stereotyped patterns include compensatory movements, unnecessary movement, muscle tension resulting from exertion or stress, and movement in response to gravity (e.g., pronation).

Several methods for evaluating voluntary movement post stroke are described in Chapters 6 and 22 to 25. Valid and reliable evaluation tools recommended by the *Post-Stroke Rehabilitation Clinical Practice Guidelines* include the *Fugl-Meyer Assessment of Motor Function* (Fugl-Meyer et al., 1975) (Chapter 25) and the *Motor Assessment Scale* (Carr et al., 1985) (Chapters 6 and 23).

Strength and Endurance

Muscle weakness ranging from slightly less than normal strength to total inability to activate muscles has been recognized as a limiting factor in the rehabilitation of patients with hemiplegia (Andrews & Bohannon, 2000). The measurement of muscle strength to monitor recovery after stroke has been controversial because of the debate regarding the influence of muscle weakness versus spasticity (Teixeira-Salmela et al., 1999) and the theory that applied resistance increases spasticity (Bobath, 1990). Clinical studies, however, suggest that strengthening of hemiplegic upper extremity musculature is appropriate for many patients (Kluding & Billinger, 2005). The motor assessment evaluations mentioned in this chapter and techniques described in Chapter 5 are recommended to establish baseline levels of muscle strength.

Reduced endurance, seen as a decrease in the ability to sustain movement or activity for practical amounts of time, is an important limiting factor in the motor performance of stroke patients because it affects the patient's ability to participate fully in rehabilitation (deGroot, Phillips, & Eskes, 2003) (Research Note 38-1). Decreased endurance can be the result of physical and/or mental fatigue caused by the exertion required to move weakened limbs or the result of comorbid cardiac or respiratory conditions (see Chapter 5).

Functional Performance

Assessing functional use of a hemiparetic arm post stroke is problematic because, although occupational performance evaluations identify deficits in ADL and IADL, they do not accurately reflect a patient's ability to use the affected arm for tasks. As observed in a population-based study, recovery of function in more than half of patients with significant upper extremity paresis was achieved only with compensatory use of the unaffected arm (Nakayama et al., 1994). Similarly, physical component skill evaluations may predict a patient's potential

RESEARCH NOTE 38-1

Fatigue After Stroke: Ingles, J. L., Eskes, G. A., & Phillips, S. J. (1999). Fatigue after stroke. *Archives of Physical Medicine and Rehabilitation, 80*, 173–178.

Abstract

The objective was to determine the frequency and outcome of fatigue, its effect on functioning, and its relationship to depression in patients 3 to 13 months post stroke. Participants included 88 individuals from a pool of consecutive patients previously admitted to an acute stroke service who were willing and able to complete the self-report questionnaires and 56 elderly control subjects living independently in the community. The main outcome measures were the *Fatigue Impact Scale*, a self-report measure of the presence and severity of fatigue and its effect on cognitive, physical, and psychosocial functions, and the *Geriatric Depression Scale*. Results showed that the frequency of self-reported fatigue was greater in the stroke group (68%) than in the control group (36%; $p < 0.001$) and was not related to time post stroke, stroke severity, or lesion location. Among the stroke group, 40% reported that fatigue was either their worst or one of their worst symptoms. Patients attributed more functional limitations to fatigue than did control subjects with fatigue. Although fatigue was accompanied by depressed mood in a substantial number of subjects in the stroke group (29%), an even greater number (39%) reported fatigue without feelings of depression. The authors concluded that, although fatigue was independent of depression, the effect of fatigue on functional abilities was strongly influenced by depression.

Implications for Practice

- Fatigue is expected to be a problem soon after stroke but is not always considered a deterrent to functional capacity or occupational therapy treatment several months post stroke. Therapists should recognize the long-term effect of fatigue symptoms when planning therapy in community or home programs.
- Training in energy conservation and work simplification techniques, including pacing and balancing of rest with activity, is appropriate for patients with stroke.
- The use of objective measures of functional and physical performance and standardized measures of fatigue and depression can help patients and families understand the effect of fatigue on function and recommend treatments to lessen that effect.

for functional use of a hemiparetic arm but are not measures of occupational performance. Many tests are described in the literature as useful for evaluating function of the involved upper extremity. Okkema and Culler (1998) reviewed 13 evaluations that include functional or task-oriented items and concluded that few of these tests are actually functional; that is, few use relevant real-life activities. Most of these tests can be categorized as task-oriented evaluations, with portions or simulations of familiar activities.

One difficulty in measuring function after stroke results from the normal differences in performance ability between dominant and non-dominant arms (Bornstein, 1986). Eating with utensils, combing hair, and writing, for example, are normally performed by the dominant arm; testing the ability of a hemiparetic non-dominant arm to perform these tasks is not relevant or useful to a patient. The arm has a wide range of functions, and any single test assesses only a portion of the actual possible functions (Wade, 1989). Therapists must choose tests that seem best suited for the individual patient.

One functional test developed specifically for use with stroke patients is the *Action Research Arm Test* (Lyle, 1981). This test is divided into four categories (grasp, grip, pinch, and gross movement) and has 19 items that are graded on a 4-point scale. This test can be quickly administered, was found to have high validity and reliability, and correlates well with the *Fugl-Meyer Assessment of Motor Function* (DeWeerdt & Harrison, 1985). However, the test requires specific handmade and difficult to obtain materials, and items tested are simulations rather than true occupational tasks.

The *Frenchay Arm Test* was developed as a battery of functional tasks used to study recovery after stroke (DeSouza, Langton Hewer, & Miller, 1980). The most recent abbreviated version includes five tasks (Heller et al., 1987) requiring use of the affected arm (Fig. 38-1). The test takes little time to administer, and materials are easy to assemble. Validity and reliability were established, but this test has relatively low sensitivity for patients on the low and high ends of the performance scale (Okkema & Culler, 1998).

A standardized test developed by occupational therapists specifically to evaluate patients' ability to use the hemiplegic upper extremity for purposeful tasks is the *Functional Test for the Hemiplegic/Paretic Upper Extremity* (Wilson, Baker, & Craddock, 1984a, 1984b). This test consists of 17 tasks divided into seven functional levels that range from absence of voluntary movement to selective and coordinated movement (Figs. 38-2 and 38-3). The tasks follow a pattern of increasing difficulty and complexity and reflect Brunnstrom's hierarchy of motor recovery in hemiplegia. This test was found to have inter-rater reliability and validity, and scores showed a strong correlation to scores on the *Fugl-Meyer Assessment of Motor Function* (Filiatrault et al., 1991). The *Functional Test for the Hemiplegic/Paretic Upper Extremity* is dominance neutral in that most items are activities normally performed by either arm or bilaterally. Disadvantages of this test are that it does not provide specific information about why a patient has failed a task (Wilson, Baker, & Craddock, 1984a) and it uses pass/fail

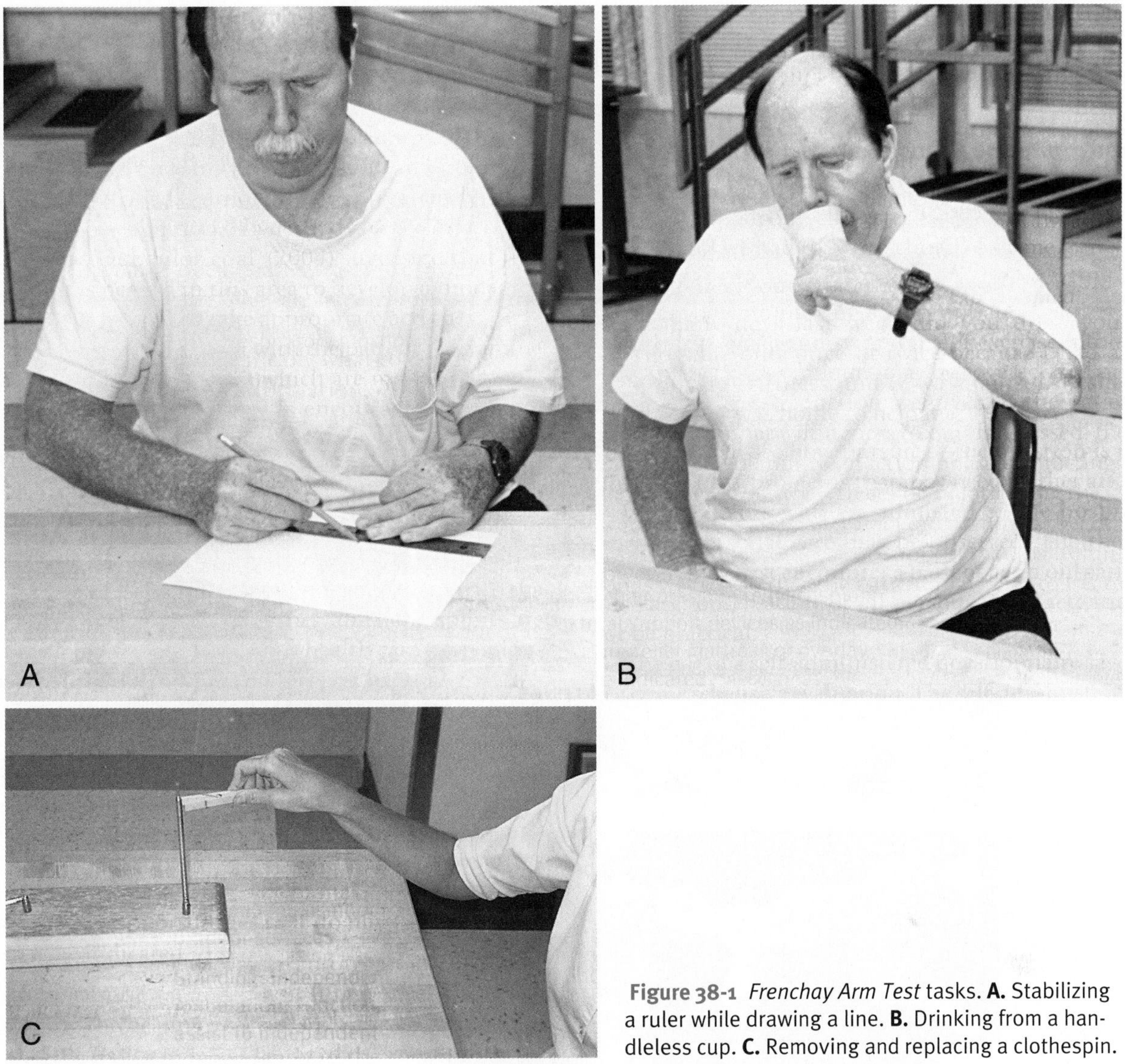

Figure 38-1 *Frenchay Arm Test* tasks. **A.** Stabilizing a ruler while drawing a line. **B.** Drinking from a handleless cup. **C.** Removing and replacing a clothespin.

scoring rather than an ordinal scale, making it difficult to use for documenting partial progress.

Motor Learning Ability

Motor learning ability refers to a patient's ability to learn and organize movement for adaptation to the environment (Warren, 1991). The motor learning model of rehabilitation states that regaining the ability to perform purposeful tasks entails setting a recognizable goal, practicing, and receiving feedback (Carr & Shepherd, 1987). In this context, therapists should assess factors that can affect a patient's ability to learn or relearn, including visual function, speech and language disorders, motor planning ability, cognitive disorders, and psychosocial adjustments. Although discussed as separate categories, these factors operate as parts of an integrated system. It is often difficult to discern or separate, for example, cognitive functioning from visual-perceptual or speech-language skills. Does a patient fail to respond to a request to brush his teeth because he can't locate the toothbrush in his visual field, because he has forgotten how to sequence this task, because he cannot understand the verbal request, or because he is not motivated to perform grooming tasks? These classifications are meant to assist the therapist in recognizing the components of learning impairments that follow stroke.

Visual Function

The visual system is a complex of almost all parts of the central and peripheral nervous system; therefore, any type or degree of brain damage is expected to have some effect on the function of the visual system (Warren, 1999). Chapter 8 describes assessments of vision and visual perception.

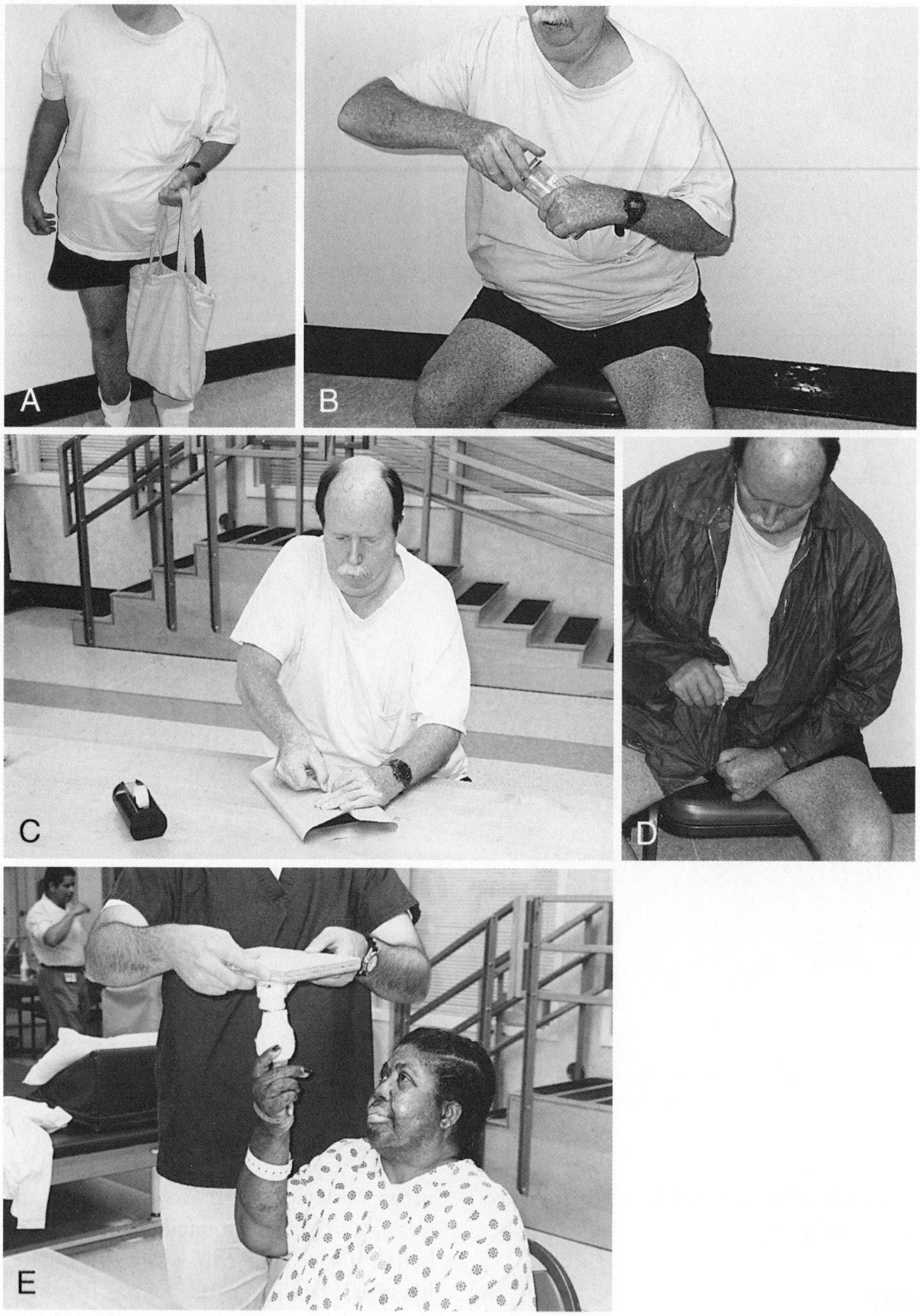

Figure 38-2 *Functional Test for the Hemiplegic/Paretic Upper Extremity*, sample tasks. **A.** Holding a pouch with a 1-pound weight. **B.** Stabilizing a jar while removing lid. **C.** Stabilizing a package while wrapping. **D.** Hooking and zipping a zipper. **E.** Putting in light bulb.

The most common visual disturbance associated with stroke is **homonymous hemianopsia**. Hemianopsia is a visual field defect affecting half of the visual field. Homonymous means the deficit involves both eyes. A patient with left homonymous hemianopsia has decreased or absent vision in the nasal field of the right eye and the temporal field of the left eye. Deficits in visual attention in stroke patients are hemi-inattention and hemineglect, or **unilateral neglect**. Unilateral neglect is a failure to notice, orient, or respond to stimuli on one side of visual space (Heilman & Valenstein, 1979). Patients can have hemianopsia without neglect or hemi-inattention without a visual field deficit, but neglect, the most severe form of decreased visual attention, usually indicates a visual field deficit in addition to hemi-inattention (Warren, 1999). Neglect is almost always associated with right parietal lobe damage (Shinsha & Ishigami, 1999) and is highly predictive of poor functional recovery (Cherney et al., 2001).

FUNCTIONAL TEST FOR THE HEMIPLEGIC/PARETIC UPPER EXTREMITY

Patient Name E.G. (L CVA)

LEVEL	TASK	DATE: 6-17-06 EXAMINER: AMW GRADE	TIME	DATE: 7-13-06 EXAMINER: AMW GRADE	TIME	DATE: 8-12-06 EXAMINER: AMW GRADE	TIME
1	Patient is unable to complete higher level tasks						
2	A. Associated reaction	(NA)		(NA)		(NA)	
	B. Hand into lap	+	2 sec	+	2 sec	+	2 sec
3	C. Arm clearance during shirt tuck	+	5 sec	+	5 sec	+	3 sec
	D. Hold a pouch	+	15 sec	+	15 sec	+	15 sec
	E. Stabilize a pillow	+	25 sec	+	14 sec	+	8 sec
4	F. Stabilize a jar	+	12 sec	+	8 sec	+	5 sec
	G. Stabilize a package	+	75 sec	+	66 sec	+	40 sec
	H. Wringing a rag	+	32 sec	+	15 sec	+	10 sec
5	I. Hold a pan lid	+	20 sec	+	20 sec	+	19 sec
	J. Hook and zip a zipper	+	55 sec	+	22 sec	+	15 sec
	K. Fold a sheet	–	>3 min	+	90 sec	+	50 sec
6	L. Blocks and box	+	35 sec	+	20 sec	+	18 sec
	M. Box on shelf	–	helped w/ L. hand	+	15 sec	+	7 sec
	N. Coin in coin gauge	–	unable to pick up dime	–	dropped dime	+	15 sec
7	O. Cat's cradle			–		+	45 sec
	P. Light bulb			–		+	30 sec (difficult)
	Q. Remove rubber band					+	15 sec

Figure 38-3 *Functional Test for the Hemiplegic/Paretic Upper Extremity*. Copyright 1980 by the Occupational Therapy Department, Rancho Los Amigos Hospital, Downey, California. Reprinted with permission. See Wilson, Baker, and Craddock (1984a, 1984b) for a description of the items.

Because visual deficits are disabling to the degree that they prevent completion of necessary ADL, observation of the patient's functional performance provides the most valuable information concerning the visual system (Warren, 1993, 1999). Patients with significant field deficits or unilateral neglect may display behaviors such as not noticing food only on the left side of the tray, shaving only the right side of the face, or bumping into walls or furniture on the left while walking.

Speech and Language

Disturbances in the ability to communicate or to comprehend verbal or written information can significantly affect the ability to resume or relearn usual activities. **Aphasia** is an acquired language disorder that can cause impairment in listening, speaking, reading, writing, arithmetic, or using appropriate gestures (Cherney, 1995). Stroke is the leading cause of aphasia, with damage to the left cerebral hemisphere the usual origin. A simplified clinical classification of aphasia recognizes fluent and non-fluent aphasias based on the patient's ability to produce speech (Goodglass, 1993). In the fluent aphasias, patients can easily produce spontaneous speech, but auditory comprehension and understanding of language is limited. The most common type of fluent aphasia is Wernicke's aphasia, or receptive aphasia, characterized by the smooth articulation of speech but marked by incorrect word or sound substitutions and the inability to name objects, repeat phrases, or follow commands. Reading and writing impairments are also common to this disorder (Sarno, 1994). Non-fluent aphasia is speech output that is difficult to produce and is characterized by slow, awkward articulation with limited vocabulary and grammar usage in the presence of relatively well-preserved auditory comprehension. An example is Broca's aphasia or expressive aphasia, in which the patient can follow commands but cannot name objects, repeat phrases, or convey ideas. Patients with non-fluent aphasia may be able to sing familiar songs or speak in other automatic ways, such as praying or swearing. Patients with non-fluent aphasia may also have agraphia, or the inability to express themselves in writing (Sarno, 1994).

Dysarthria is a speech disorder characterized by slurred speech, poor articulation, drooling, or decreased facial expression caused by weakness or incoordination of facial and oral musculature. Oral apraxia is another communication problem in which the patient has difficulty initiating and sequencing the movements necessary to produce speech. In these disorders, the patient can understand and express symbolic language (Sarno, 1994).

The speech-language pathologist evaluates functions and dysfunctions of speech and speech musculature. The occupational therapist needs to confer with the speech-language pathologist to learn the results of a patient's communication evaluation, support the patient's language goals, and request suggestions for the most effective communication strategies (Sarno, 1994).

Motor Planning

Motor planning deficits, or **apraxia**, are deficits of skilled, organized, purposeful movement sequences that cannot be explained by motor or sensory impairments. These deficits are best identified during performance of daily living tasks. Clinical manifestations of motor planning difficulties include the following (Warren, 1991):

- Failure to orient the head or body correctly to a task, such as a patient attempting a toilet transfer who tries to sit on the toilet before correctly positioning the body in front of it.
- Failure to orient the hand properly to objects and/or poor tool use, such as a patient who has to be reminded of the correct way to hold a pen when writing with the uninvolved hand.
- Difficulty initiating or carrying out a sequence of movements, such as a patient with nearly normal motor performance who cannot put on a shirt without step-by-step verbal and physical cueing.
- Movements characterized by hesitations and perseveration, such as a patient who, after brushing his teeth, is handed a razor and asked to shave. After a delay, the patient brings the razor to his mouth and tries to brush his teeth with it.
- Movements that can be performed only in context or in the presence of a familiar object or situation, such as a patient who does not follow a command to move hand to mouth unless given something to eat or drink.

These deficits are most pronounced during learning sessions, such as when training in wheelchair propulsion or one-handed buttoning, and in activities with multiple steps, such as making a sandwich.

Cognition

Disorders in higher brain functions, including problems with attention, orientation, concentration, memory, reasoning, judgment, or problem solving, are common after stroke (Gresham et al., 1995). Patients with cognitive dysfunction may not achieve rehabilitation goals due to difficulty learning new techniques for performing tasks and decreased safety awareness. Cognitive impairment can be assessed during evaluation and treatment of occupational performance by focusing on the adaptive abilities of planning, judgment, problem solving, and initiation. Chapter 9 describes specific assessment techniques. Mental status screening tests recommended by the *Post-Stroke Rehabilitation Clinical Practice Guideline* are the *Mini-Mental State Examination* (Folstein, Folstein, & McHugh, 1975) and the *Neurobehavioral Cognitive Status Examination* (Kiernan et al., 1987). Therapists must be careful to differentiate between cognitive deficits and communication difficulties common to stroke (Gresham et al., 1995).

Psychosocial Aspects

Adjustment to disability is a critical component of rehabilitation, although effective measures of adjustment have not been described (Morris, 1998). Most patients have natural emotional reactions to their stroke, including denial, anxiety, anger, and depression (Gresham et al., 1995). Depression is the most frequently reported reaction, affecting 25–40% of patients within the first year after a stroke (Eriksson et al., 2004). Depression tends to develop over time and is more likely to be seen as rehabilitation proceeds than during the acute period post stroke (Gresham et al., 1995). Depression in stroke is both a physiological result of biochemical changes in the brain and a reaction to the personal losses of patients who realize, with time, that they will not fully recover (Eriksson et al., 2004).

Denial, an adaptive emotional mechanism employed to cope with depression or anxiety, is seen when the survivor of a stroke is unable or unwilling to acknowledge the short- and long-term consequences of stroke (Remer-Osborn, 1998). It presents a challenge for the rehabilitation team because the patient may deny the need for treatment, set unreasonable personal goals, and fail to accommodate to the condition in the expectation of complete recovery (Versluys, 1995).

Emotional lability is an emotional response, such as laughing or crying, that is disproportionate to the emotional stimulus (Remer-Osborn, 1998). A patient may cry whenever seeing a family member or when asked about a valued activity.

Emotional reactions, compounded by cognitive, perceptual, and language impairments, may lead to behavioral outcomes including frustration, anger, impatience, irritability, overdependence, insensitivity to others, and rigid thinking (Versluys, 1995). These responses can further result in impaired personal interactions, inability to perform social and leisure activities or roles, and eventual isolation. Patients 3 months or more post stroke have reported decreased socialization and quality of life despite improved physical functioning (Lai et al., 2002). Evaluation of the patient's and family's adjustments to the stroke, to rehabilitation, and to the prospect of living with the aftermath of the stroke can be done through interview and observation and by sharing information with other members of the rehabilitation team.

TREATMENT

A careful interpretation of evaluation results helps determine a patient's assets and deficits in areas of occupational functioning. Possible goals for patients recovering from stroke include the following:

- The patient will gain competence in valued and necessary basic ADL and IADL in order to perform at the highest level of independence possible in the desired post-discharge setting.
- The patient will improve postural control in order to perform daily living tasks requiring balance and changes in body position.
- The patient will gain increased somatosensory perception and/or will employ compensatory strategies in order to perform ADL safely.
- The patient and/or caregiver will demonstrate appropriate management techniques for the hemiparetic upper extremity to prevent pain and other secondary mechanical or physiological movement restrictions.
- The patient will gain the necessary strength, endurance, and control of movement of the involved upper extremity in order to use the involved upper extremity spontaneously during the performance of ADL.
- The patient will gain visual function or will employ compensatory strategies in order to resume previously performed ADL safely.
- The patient will improve motor planning ability in order to relearn old methods or learn new methods of performing ADL.
- The patient and/or caregiver will demonstrate appropriate strategies for improving or compensating for cognitive deficits during the performance of ADL.
- The patient and/or caregiver will be able to verbalize the reality and impact of emotional reactions to stroke and identify coping strategies or resources to help adjust to living with a stroke.
- The caregiver will demonstrate appropriate methods and problem-solving strategies for assisting the patient with ADL and with home activities to improve component skills.
- The patient will gain competence in tasks and activities necessary to resume valued roles or to assume new meaningful roles in the community.

Safety of the patient is a concern during and after treatment (Safety Note 38-1). In this chapter, the description of occupational therapy for stroke patients is divided into three stages: the acute phase, the rehabilitation phase, and reentry to the community. For most patients, progression of recovery and provision of services are not this clear cut. For a variety of reasons, many patients do not have access to the full spectrum of services with smooth continuity of care. Any treatment described, therefore, may apply to any or all other stages for a particular patient and should be viewed as part of a continuum of care adapted to meet changing needs over time (Sabari, 1998). Specific recommendations from the *Post-Stroke Rehabilitation Clinical Prac-*

SAFETY NOTE 38-1

Precautions with Stroke Patients

- In the acute period after stroke, ascertain the patient's medical status and stability daily before treatment. Know the symptoms of progressing or recurrent stroke.
- Determine whether cardiac or respiratory precautions apply for a particular patient and monitor accordingly, watching for signs of cardiac distress and blood pressure changes, including dizziness, breathing difficulties, chest pain, excessive fatigue, and altered heart rate or rhythm.
- Guard against falls by providing appropriate supervision and assistance during transfers and other transitional movements.
- To avoid shoulder injury or pain, never pull or lift a patient by or under the weak arm during transfers or other transitional movements.
- Use appropriate precautions in the presence of insensitive skin, particularly if a patient also has visual field deficits and/or unilateral neglect.
- Ascertain a patient's ability to swallow and follow recommended management techniques during feeding.
- Provide appropriate supervision for patients who demonstrate impulsive behavior and/or poor safety awareness.
- Teach the patient, family members, and other health care workers about safety concerns for an individual patient.

tice Guideline are included and indicated by **colored print.** These recommendations are backed by research evidence and/or expert opinion.

Acute Phase

Stroke rehabilitation begins "as soon as the diagnosis of stroke is established and life-threatening problems are under control" (Gresham et al., 1995, p. 53). Length of stay in acute hospital beds is typically just long enough for necessary diagnostic tests, for initiation of appropriate medical treatment, and for making decisions and arrangements for the next phase of rehabilitation. Patients who have just had a stroke may need to be seen bedside because of precautions, monitoring, and varying levels of consciousness. During this phase, the patient must adjust to the sudden, unexpected shift from usual life roles to the role of patient.

Early Mobilization and Return to Self-Care

The patient with acute stroke should be mobilized as soon after admission as is medically feasible. The patient should be encouraged to perform self-care as soon as medically feasible and, if necessary, should be offered compensatory training to overcome disabilities. The early introduction of basic ADL, such as rolling in bed, sitting on the side of the bed, transferring to a wheelchair or commode, self-feeding, grooming, and dressing, helps the patient reestablish some control over the environment and begin to improve occupational functioning and component abilities and capacities (Gresham et al., 1995). Even at this early stage, the occupational therapist's assessment of a patient can help determine the most appropriate setting for rehabilitation and discharge. **Discharge planning should begin at the time of admission. Goals are to determine the need for rehabilitation, arrange the best possible living environment, and ensure continuity of care after discharge.** The occupational therapist in an acute-care setting should take an active role in rehabilitation triage, basing recommendations on the patient's identified deficits and abilities (Radomski, 1995).

Lowering Risk for Secondary Complications

As part of the stroke care team, the occupational therapist should practice methods to prevent or lessen complications resulting from stroke.

Skin Care

It is estimated that up to 21% of patients with stroke develop pressure sores (Langhorne et al., 2000). Those who are comatose, malnourished, obese, or incontinent or who have severe paralysis or muscle spasticity are at greatest risk. The occupational therapist helps patients maintain skin integrity by doing the following:

- Using proper transfer and mobility techniques to avoid undue skin friction
- Recommending appropriate positioning for bed and sitting and participating in scheduled position changes as needed
- Assisting with wheelchair and seating selection and adaptation
- Teaching patient and caregiver precautions to avoid injury to insensitive skin and involved side of body
- Watching for signs of skin pressure or breakdown on a patient (bruising, redness, blisters, abrasions, ulceration), especially over bony areas, and alerting nursing or medical staff as appropriate

Maintaining Soft Tissue Length

Contractures, or shortening of skin, tendons, ligaments, muscles, and/or joint capsules, may result from the immobilization following stroke. Risk factors include muscle paralysis, spasticity, and imbalance between agonist and antagonist muscle groups. Contractures restrict movement, may be painful, and may limit functional recovery

(Gresham et al., 1995). The appropriate management is therefore a preventive program of proper positioning and soft tissue and joint mobilization. Suggested bed positioning for patients with stroke, based on a literature review (Carr & Kenney, 1992), is summarized in Procedures for Practice 38-1. However, bed positioning, like any treatment, must be adapted to meet the individual needs of the patient. Care must be taken to protect the weak upper extremity during treatment because handling, positioning, and transferring can exert great stress on the vulnerable shoulder early after stroke (Walsh, 2001). Specific techniques for supporting the hemiparetic shoulder are discussed later in this chapter. Resting hand splints are often applied to prevent soft tissue shortening, but their use has not been found to significantly prevent or reverse contracture of wrist and finger flexor muscles (Lannin et al., 2003).

Controlled and frequent movement of body parts is the preferred method to prevent contractures. When a patient cannot use the involved side to engage in meaningful activities, therapists should initiate supervised active or active-assistive movement activities. When active movement is not possible, therapists should see that immobile body parts go through passive range of motion at least once daily. If performing passive range of motion on the involved arm, ensure proper scapulohumeral rhythm by relaxing and mobilizing the scapula before elevation of the arm and by manually assisting upward rotation of the scapula (Bobath, 1990). The humerus should be externally rotated during abduction to prevent impingement of the supraspinatus between the greater tubercle of the humerus and the acromion process. Whenever possible, a patient should attend closely to passive movement as a first step in relearning motion (Carr & Shepherd, 1987). A study using positron emission tomography (PET) on early post-stroke patients who had no active movement showed that passive elbow movements elicited some of the same brain activation patterns as active movement in more recovered patients (Nelles et al., 1999).

PROCEDURES FOR PRACTICE 38-1

Recommended Bed Positioning for Patients With Hemiplegia

Supine Positioning

- Head and neck slightly flexed
- Trunk straight and aligned
- Involved upper extremity supported behind scapula and humerus with a small pillow or towel, shoulder protracted and slightly flexed and abducted with external rotation, elbow extended or slightly flexed, forearm neutral or supinated, wrist neutral with hand open
- Involved lower limb with hip forward on pillow, nothing against soles of feet

Lying on the Unaffected Side

- Head and neck neutral and symmetrical
- Trunk aligned
- Involved upper extremity protracted with arm forward on pillows, elbow extended or slightly flexed, forearm and wrist neutral, and hand open
- Involved lower extremity with hip and knee forward, flexed, and supported on pillows

Lying on the Affected Side

- Head and neck neutral and symmetrical
- Trunk aligned
- Involved upper extremity protracted forward and externally rotated with elbow extended or slightly flexed, forearm supinated, wrist neutral, and hand open
- Involved lower extremity with knee flexed
- Uninvolved lower extremity with knee flexed and supported on pillows

Information from Carr & Kenney (1992).

Fall Prevention

For patients hospitalized with stroke, falls are the most common cause of injury (Gresham et al., 1995). Factors that increase the risk of falls include advanced age, confusion, impulsive behavior, mobility deficits, poor balance or coordination, visual impairments, and communication deficits that interfere with a patient's ability to request assistance in a timely manner. Treatment that helps to prevent falls includes detecting and removing environmental hazards, optimizing motor control, recommending appropriate adaptive devices, and teaching safety measures to the patient and family.

Patient and Family Education

Early in recovery, support for patients who have had strokes and their families may best be provided in the form of education to promote a realistic understanding of the consequences of stroke and the purposes and methods of various treatments (Gresham et al., 1995). All aspects of occupational therapy assessment and treatment for survivors of stroke should be considered opportunities for education: to engage cooperation and participation in the identification of meaningful treatment goals, to highlight residual abilities as well as disabilities, and to promote carryover of treatment gains. As the period after stroke is stressful, emotional, and tiring for both the patient and family, education sessions provided during the acute phase should be brief, simple, and reinforced as needed with repetition or appropriate learning aids (see Chapter 14).

Rehabilitation Phase

Part of discharge planning during the acute phase of stroke is screening for rehabilitation services. Rehabilitation choices depend on a patient's condition, the social support system, and the resources available in a community. To qualify for further treatment in a rehabilitation program, a patient must be medically stable, have at least one functional disability, have sufficient endurance to sit supported for at least an hour, and be able to learn and to participate actively in therapy (Gresham et al., 1995). Patients who meet these criteria are referred for inpatient rehabilitation programs, for multidisciplinary rehabilitation services at a skilled nursing facility, or for treatment by one or more disciplines in home care or in an outpatient clinic. Patients who do not meet these criteria should continue to receive appropriate medical or support services at home, in a skilled nursing facility, or in a chronic care facility; they may be reassessed later for rehabilitation services.

During this phase of recovery, the patient and family are focused on getting better and are usually more concerned with recovering lost function than on adapting to a life of chronic disability (Sabari, 1998). Successful occupational therapy intervention coordinates a patient's striving for restoration of function with the potential for compensation and alternative occupational roles.

Treatment to Improve Performance of Occupational Tasks

The occupational therapist's primary goal in stroke rehabilitation is to improve independence in daily living tasks and hence the patient's quality of life. **Patients with persistent, non-remediable functional deficits should be taught compensatory methods for performing important tasks and activities, using the affected limb when possible and, when not, the unaffected limb.** Many consider that early ADL training focusing on compensatory techniques results in faster success and is therefore more cost effective and more satisfying to the patient, who again feels competent (Nakayama et al., 1994). Others contend that, when ADL training focuses entirely on one-handed techniques, the patient fails to relearn bilateral movements and, instead, develops unilateral habits (Bobath, 1990; Roberts et al., 2005). Skilled occupational therapy intervention combines both compensatory and remedial treatment strategies and attempts to reduce both disabilities and impairments by engaging the patient in meaningful activities. Putting on a front-buttoning shirt, for example, besides helping a patient gain independence in the task of dressing, addresses the following component abilities, capacities, and conditions:

- Joint and soft tissue integrity (self-stretching or relaxation techniques for involved arm in preparation for dressing, positioning of arm on a surface to prevent stretching of weak shoulder structures)
- Voluntary movement and function of involved upper extremity (abducting shoulder to put on a sleeve, extending elbow to push the hand through the sleeve, pinching one side of the shirt to stabilize while buttoning)
- Somatosensory perception (the texture of the shirt, the position of the affected arm)
- Postural adaptations (anterior pelvic tilt, trunk rotation, weight shifting)
- Visual-perceptual skills (finding the shirt in the visual field, distinguishing top from bottom, finding the sleeve opening)
- Cognitive skills and emotional reactions (sequencing, attention span, frustration tolerance, motivation)

ADL training with stroke patients begins with simple tasks and gradually increases in difficulty as a patient gains competency (Gresham et al., 1995). Several studies discerned a hierarchy of achievement of self-care skills. Results of one study showed that bathing, dressing, and climbing stairs were the activities for which stroke survivors most often required assistance, with 32% of patients needing help with bathing, 25.5% needing help with dressing, and 32% requiring assistance with stairs 12 months post stroke (Carod-Artal et al., 2002). Aspects of dressing that are particularly difficult for stroke patients are putting a sock and shoe on the affected foot, lacing shoes, and pulling up trousers or pants (Walker & Lincoln, 1990). A study that investigated the relationship between dressing abilities and cognitive, perceptual, and physical deficits found that, in general, lower extremity dressing correlates more with motor performance and upper extremity dressing correlates more with cognitive or perceptual performance (Walker & Lincoln, 1991). **Adaptive devices should be used only if other methods of performing the task are not available or cannot be learned. The device should have proven reliability and safety, and the patient and/or caregiver should be thoroughly trained in its proper use.**

As the patient progresses, occupational performance tasks other than basic self-care may have to be addressed. IADL tasks such as homemaking, home management, and community mobility involve greater interaction with the physical and social environment and require higher level problem-solving and social skills than basic ADL tasks (Carod-Artal et al., 2002). Avocational interests, including adapted methods of continuing familiar hobbies, are an important area of treatment. Many stroke survivors are faced with increases in leisure time because of inability to go back to work; however, a reduction in social and leisure participation has been found to be a common occurrence after stroke (Lai et al., 2002). Chapter 30 discusses specific techniques for regaining independence in ADL/IADL for those with loss of the use of one side of the body.

Treatment to Improve Component Abilities and Capacities

Performance component goals are based on the impairments associated with an individual's stroke and are directly linked to occupational performance goals. The goals and modalities used to address these component deficits must be purposeful and meaningful from the patient's point of view (Trombly, 1995). Thus, a floor game may be used to improve sitting balance needed to don socks, or resistive grasp activities may be taught to strengthen muscles needed to squeeze a tube of toothpaste. Treatments for stroke deficits are described individually in the following sections, but most patients in rehabilitation programs have multiple interacting problems necessitating efficient, integrated treatment plans that address several deficit areas at once (Warren, 1991).

Postural Adaptation

The ability to make automatic postural adjustments, including trunk control and the maintenance of balance, is a prerequisite for successful performance of occupational tasks. Part of the occupational therapist's role in training a patient in ADL independence post stroke is in teaching the patient the safest, most effective and efficient "ready" position for engaging in activities (see Definition 38-2) and strategies for adapting to changes in body position. Various techniques can be used to accomplish these goals as long as the therapist has a clear understanding of each patient's particular strengths and weaknesses regarding stability and mobility. Treatment to improve postural control for the performance of daily living activities is aimed at reestablishing the prerequisites for mature postural adaptation, including the following abilities (Warren, 1990):

1. To produce full range of movement in the trunk and extremities.
2. To differentiate body parts from one another, such as rotating the shoulders independently of the hips.
3. To stop and hold movement at midrange to stabilize against gravity.
4. To increase and decrease postural tone in body segments automatically and appropriately to support movement and/or stability.
5. To move both sides of the body symmetrically.

The incorporation of transitional movement patterns (i.e., strategies to change body positions, such as from supine to side-lying or seated to standing) and the use of strategically placed activities allow patients to practice effective postural adjustment while focusing on the task at hand (Warren, 1990).

A particularly challenging impairment of postural control is pusher behavior. Pusher behavior is clinically defined to describe hemiplegic patients who actively push away from their non-paralyzed side with their stronger limbs and resist attempts to make them more upright (Davies, 2000). It is observed in approximately 5% of stroke patients, usually in the most involved patients, and negatively affects functional recovery (Pedersen et al., 1996). A pilot study by Perennou et al. (2002) concluded that pusher behavior does not result from disrupted processing of vestibular information but from a higher order disruption in the processing of somesthetic information from the left side of the body, possibly an extinction or neglect phenomenon. Because patients with pusher behavior resist hands-on attempts to correct their alignment, therapists should select treatment that manipulates the environment (reaching for objects to encourage weight shift to the strong side) and provides external cues ("bring your right shoulder toward the wall") (Gillen, 2004a) (see Definition 38-2).

Upper Extremity Function

Bilateral use of the upper extremities is crucial to efficient and effective occupational performance. Patients recovering from stroke usually place a high priority on regaining function in the involved arm. The occupational therapist must determine which deficits most affect a patient's upper extremity performance and plan realistic multilevel, task-oriented treatment to restore function or promote adaptation to the loss of function.

Somatosensory Deficits

Treatment for sensory dysfunction of stroke patients has not been systematically developed, although therapists attempt remediation as well as compensation for these deficits (Trombly, 1989). Remedial treatment entails a sequence of presentation of a tactile stimulus, response by the patient, exact feedback, and practice (Weinberg et al., 1979). Compensatory treatment entails substituting intact senses for those lost or dysfunctional. Therapists must determine the appropriateness of either type of treatment for individual patients. For example, sensory retraining is unrealistic for patients with minimal voluntary movement, visual field neglect, or poor cognitive skills.

Yekutiel and Guttman (1993) conducted a controlled trial in which 20 hemiplegic patients 2 or more years post stroke received systematic sensory training for the hemiplegic hand for 6 weeks. Their sensory reeducation program included exploring with each patient the nature and extent of sensory loss, selecting sensory tasks of interest to the patient that promoted learning, and encouraging constant use of vision and the uninvolved hand to teach tactics of perception. At the end of the training period, the treatment group showed significant gains in all sensory tests, whereas the control group showed no changes.

Treatment to restore tactile awareness and teach compensation for sensory loss is discussed in Chapter 27. One method of providing repetitive stimulation is to encourage the patient to use the involved hand in ADL as soon as possible. The use of different textures (e.g., foam, terry cloth, Velcro) on weight-bearing surfaces or on the holding surfaces of commonly used utensils, such as cups, forks, and pens, can increase sensory input to the affected hand (Eggers, 1984).

Mechanical and Physiological Components of Movement

Techniques for maintaining soft tissue length and avoiding pain in the involved upper extremity initiated during the acute phase of stroke recovery should be continued and adapted in response to changes in the patient's movement or muscle tone. As the patient in a rehabilitation program gains in mobility, measures should be taken to protect weak upper extremity structures from stretching or injury due to the effects of gravity and improper movement. Procedures for Practice 38-2 summarizes handling techniques for an affected upper extremity.

Treatment of problems related to the hemiplegic shoulder centers on prevention and management of symptoms and underlying causes. The use of a sling as a prevention or treatment for subluxation of the hemiplegic shoulder is not supported by empirical research (Gresham et al., 1995; Turner-Stokes & Jackson, 2002). Reasons for using slings are to reduce the subluxation of the glenohumeral joint, provide support for the arm, protect against trauma, and prevent or reduce pain. Carr and Shepherd (1987) found that radiographs of hemiplegic shoulders in slings revealed no significant reduction of subluxation. Bobath (1990) maintained that flexor spasticity in the upper extremity is reinforced with the use of a sling. Pain control is a valid reason for use of a positioning device; however, the relation between subluxation and shoulder pain is unclear. Several studies have found no association between shoulder pain and subluxation after stroke (Bohannon & Andrews, 1990; Turner-Stokes & Jackson, 2002), including one that found a low correlation between shoulder pain after stroke and subluxation, age, and arm motor function but a high correlation between shoulder pain and limited passive shoulder external rotation (Zorowitz et al., 1996). These studies support a general recommendation that the hemiplegic arm should be appropriately supported but that shoulder supports should not be issued uniformly to all patients with shoulder subluxation. If considering a sling, therapists should address the following questions (Andersen, 1985; Ridgway & Byrne, 1999). A positive response to the following questions might indicate a sling:

- Does pain or edema increase when the arm hangs down?
- Is the patient's balance during standing, walking, or transfers improved by the use of a sling?
- Is the patient unable to attend to and protect the arm during movement?
- Can the patient or caretaker independently put on and take off a sling correctly?

A positive response to the following questions might contraindicate a sling:

- Would the sling prevent or hinder active movement or function in the arm?
- Would a sufficiently supportive sling impair circulation or cause excessive pressure on the neck?
- Would the sling put the patient at risk for contracture as a result of immobilization?
- Would a sling decrease sensory input and promote unilateral disregard?

Alternative positioning methods and devices for shoulder support include taping of the shoulder and scapula (Ridgway & Byrne, 1999), wheelchair lapboards and armrest troughs, use of a table while seated or standing, putting the hand in a pocket or under a belt, and using an over-the-shoulder bag while standing (Gillen, 2004b) (Fig. 38-4). Functional electrical stimulation has been used to prevent or improve shoulder subluxation, decrease pain, and improve range of motion. Studies evaluating the effectiveness of this treatment showed benefits during treatment but reduction of gains after treatment was discontinued (Walsh, 2001). Any patient with shoulder pain that persists and consistently interferes with function or progress in therapy should be referred to specialists best qualified to diagnose and treat specific shoulder problems.

Along with protection, patients learning to manage their involved arm should know techniques of active, active-assistive, or passive movement designed to maintain range of motion, stretch tight tissues, or relax hypertonicity. The combination of positioning for comfort and muscle imbalances brought on by spasticity and weakness can lead to the development of stereotyped non-functional positioning for the hemiplegic upper extremity with

PROCEDURES FOR PRACTICE 38-2

Proper Handling of the Hemiparetic Upper Extremity

- Teach the patient as early as possible to be responsible for the positioning of the arm during transfers, bed mobility, and other activities involving change of position.
- Use gait belts or draw sheets, rather than the affected arm, to assist the patient in moving his or her body.
- Avoid shoulder range of motion beyond 90° of flexion and abduction unless there is upward rotation of the scapula and external rotation of the humerus (Gresham et al., 1995).
- Avoid overhead pulley exercises, as they appear to increase the frequency of pain in the shoulder because neither scapular nor humeral rotation occurs, and the force may be excessive (Kumar et al., 1990).

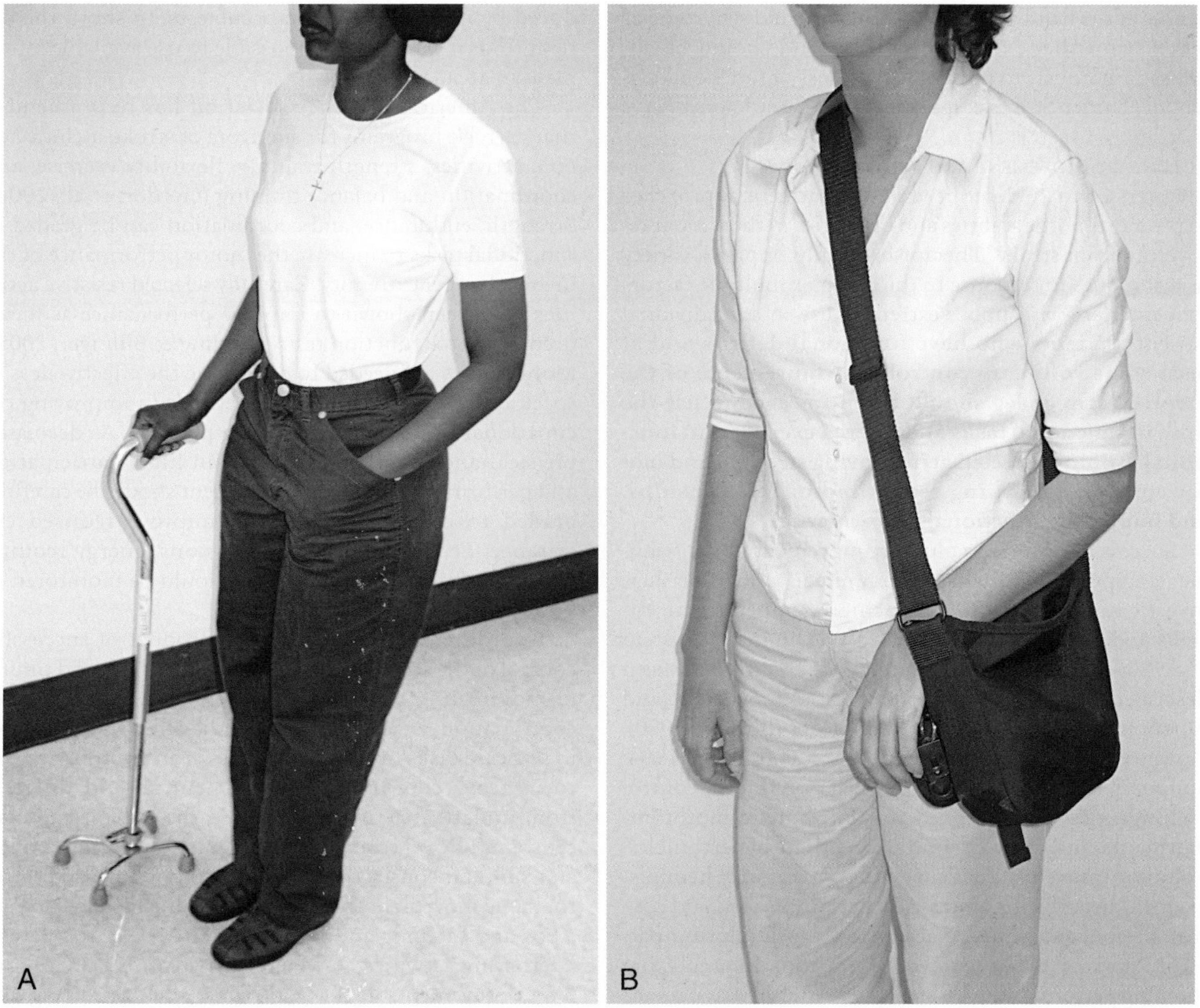

Figure 38-4 Alternative methods for supporting the hemiplegic arm while standing. **A.** Hand in pocket. **B.** Use of shoulder bag.

shoulder retraction, adduction, and internal rotation; elbow flexion; forearm pronation; and wrist and finger flexion. Therapists should emphasize frequent changes of position to prevent contractures and pain.

Even in the absence of motor recovery, normal movement is an important model for movement reeducation (Van Dyck, 1999). Passive and assisted active movement can be incorporated into activities, with the patient experiencing and concentrating on movement in a functional context. Methods of teaching self-managed range of motion entail bilateral activities such as having the patient clasp his or her hands while leaning forward to reach for the floor or pushing both hands forward with arms supported on a table (Eggers, 1984). Advantages of these activities are that they can easily be given a functional context, such as picking up objects off the floor or dusting a table, and the patient can monitor his or her own pain threshold and is therefore not apprehensive about movement of the arm (Andersen, 1985). Nelson et al. (1996), in a study of persons with hemiplegia, found that using a simple dice game to achieve bilaterally assisted forearm supination brought better results (more range of motion, more repetitions) than use of a rote exercise routine (Evidence Table 38-1). Self-management of range of motion should be closely supervised and may not be appropriate for patients who have decreased awareness of the involved side, who move too quickly, who do not respect pain, or who lack a mobile scapula.

Hand edema is a frequent complication of hemiplegia. Edema control techniques include elevation of the hand, retrograde massage, and use of pressure gloves. Patients with minimal voluntary movement should avoid allowing the hand and arm to hang down for long periods. Prolonged hand edema can lead to limited passive movement, pain, and soft tissue contractures. Edema combined with severe pain, hypersensitivity, and vasomotor disturbances of the hand are signs of shoulder-hand syndrome or reflex sympathetic dystrophy (RSD) and should be addressed vigorously to prevent further loss of functional potential (Turner-Stokes & Jackson, 2002) (see Chapter 42).

Voluntary Movement and Function

Chapters 21 to 26 describe various treatment approaches to promote motor abilities and capacities in the patient recovering from stroke. Therapists usually employ a variety of techniques in response to the complex multiple factors that interfere with upper extremity use in an individual patient. **Patients who have functional deficits and at least some voluntary control over movements of the involved arm or leg should be encouraged to use the limb in functional tasks and offered exercise and functional training directed at improving strength and motor control, relearning sensorimotor relationships, and improving functional performance.**

Success in restoring voluntary movement in the hemiplegic upper extremity has been limited, perhaps because investigation of factors enhancing or impeding motor skills and processes following stroke is limited (Winstein et al., 2004). Spasticity, for example, has traditionally been described as a major barrier to normal movement and function in the patient with hemiplegia (Bobath, 1990). However, clinical studies (Fellows & Thilmann, 1994; Sommerfeld et al., 2004) suggest that poor motor control with weakness is more likely to contribute to motor impairments and activity limitations than hypertonicity. Voluntary movement deficits in the patient with hemiplegia include problems of muscle force production and control, of abnormal muscle activation and inhibition patterns, and of synergistic organization. In analyzing reaching performance, Wu et al. (1998) found that persons with stroke produced movements that were less efficient, less direct, less smooth, and slower than movements produced by neurologically intact subjects. In short, the patient finds it difficult or impossible to use available movement in an adaptive way.

The American Heart Association has recommended that exercise programs for survivors of stroke include aerobic activities, strength training, flexibility exercise, and coordination and balance training (Gordon et al., 2004). Strength, endurance, and coordination can be graded in functional tasks to increase the motor performance of the involved upper extremity. Carefully selected resistive activities have been shown to improve performance as measured by motor function tests (Kluding & Billinger, 2005). More studies are needed to determine the effectiveness of specific clinical strengthening methods in improving occupational performance of stroke patients. As decreased physical and mental endurance can limit participation and performance in therapy, treatment should be carefully graded to compensate for and improve reduced endurance. Length of treatment sessions, energy requirements, and need for rest periods should be monitored to meet patients' needs.

Coordinated movement is the product of successful control of the strength, range, speed, direction, and timing of movement. As almost all purposeful activity requires coordination, encouraging use of the affected extremities in self-care tasks or leisure activities is an appropriate way to improve coordination. Treatment should progress from unilateral activities, in which the patient can concentrate fully on control of the hemiparetic arm, to bilateral simultaneous activities, in which both arms perform the same movement together (such as lifting and carrying a box and catching and throwing a large ball), to bilateral alternating activities, in which the two arms perform different movements at the same time (such as sorting and assembling nuts and bolts). Grading fine motor activities entails progressing from gross to precise manipulation

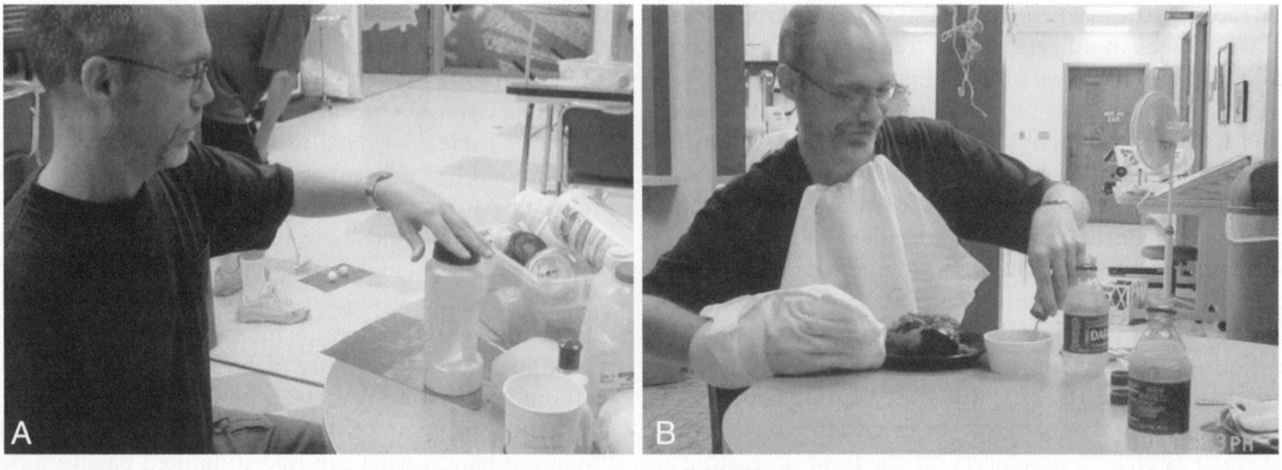

Figure 38-5 Constraint-induced movement therapy. **A.** Applying and removing jar lids. **B.** Eating a meal with involved upper extremity while non-involved hand is restrained.

tasks and attempting more difficult patterns of grasp and pinch. Because hand and arm control for patients with hemiplegia becomes more difficult as the arm moves away from the body, the placement of activities should be varied. Writing is a highly coordinated task that is frequently a goal for stroke patients who need at least to be able to sign documents. Training in writing may be necessary if a patient plans to use the hemiparetic hand or the uninvolved non-dominant hand.

Task-Specific and Task-Oriented Interventions

In light of the range and complexity of possible motor impairments and the myriad of treatment strategies available, the occupational therapist should design treatment to fit the patient's level and interests and to guide and extend combinations of muscle action into meaningful tasks (Carr & Shepherd, 1987). There is growing evidence that intervention strategies providing context-relevant, meaningful engagement in activities are more beneficial for skill acquisition than rote exercise or passive modalities (Winstein et al., 2004). Task-specific training is aimed at improving component skills of selected tasks, such as using hand muscles to practice gripping a fork. An example of task-oriented training is a patient simulating a useful or familiar activity such as using a spoon to transfer dried beans from one container to another. Occupational engagement, such as a patient using a hemiparetic arm to eat a meal at home, involves the greatest degree of patient self-choice, motivation, and meaning (American Occupational Therapy Association, 2002), although therapists must judge adaptations necessary to allow patients to succeed. Trombly and Wu (1999) found that providing a meaningful object within a functional context during treatment (e.g., reaching for food on a plate) leads to improved performance over exercise or reaching for a neutral target. Similarly, Fasoli et al. (2002) found that, during functional reaching tasks, internally focused instructions (e.g., "straighten your elbow") resulted in slower, less forceful reach than externally focused instructions (e.g., "think about the size, shape, and weight of the object") in samples of adults with and without CVA.

Therapists should review the wide range of possible functions of the upper extremity to select activities patients can succeed in. In normal function, the hand performs as a prehensile tool, and the arm places the hand in a wide variety of different and precise positions (Savinelli et al., 1978). Bard, Hirschberg, and Tolleson (1964) proposed a classification of function of the upper extremity, including (1) non-manipulatory activities, (2) prehension and manipulation, and (3) skilled individual finger movements, such as typing. Non-manipulatory activities, such as weighting down a checkbook while writing, can be incorporated into functional activities by patients who have limited movement or no voluntary hand movement.

Constraint-Induced Movement Therapy

It is important to promote functional use of the involved upper extremity early and consistently because patients tend to have difficulty translating limited upper extremity movement into functional use. They often report that their arm is "dead" or "useless" despite sufficient arm movement for simple activities. Movement may return spontaneously, but it appears that function or purposeful use of the arm is enhanced with therapeutic intervention and practice (Blanton & Wolf, 1999). Based on studies involving both animal and human subjects, Taub et al. (1993) described a phenomenon of **learned non-use**: the person with hemiparesis notices negative consequences of efforts to use the affected limb that are reinforced by successful compensatory use of the unaffected limb (Blanton & Wolf, 1999). The intervention termed forced use, or constraint-induced movement therapy (CIMT), was developed to counteract the effects of learned non-use (Fig. 38-5). In a comparative clinical study, Taub et al. (1993) restrained the unaffected upper extremity of chronic stroke patients (at least 1 year post onset) in a sling during waking hours for 2 weeks. This group also participated in sessions of intensive practice of functional tasks with the impaired arm. A comparison group was given activities designed to encourage use of the impaired arm but without practice and without restraint of the unimpaired arm. The restraint subjects showed greater improvement on measurements of motor function than the control group and showed carryover of this function to life tasks and maintenance of gains during a 2-year follow-up period. Dromerick, Edwards, and Hahn (2000) found that CIMT could be implemented during acute rehabilitation (1–2 weeks after stroke) with resulting improvement in involved arm function at the end of 14 days of treatment. This study suggests that preventing or minimizing learned non-use with early intervention is preferable to extinguishing learned behaviors.

Although CIMT is described as providing "the most promising evidence that motor recovery can be facilitated (after stroke)" (Duncan, 1997, p. 3), it is difficult to implement in standard clinical practice. CIMT emphasizes massed practice by combining daily 6-hour training sessions for the paretic arm with restraint of the uninvolved arm in a sling or mitt during 90% of waking hours for a duration of 2–6 weeks (Page et al., 2004). Patients included in CIMT studies had to meet minimal voluntary movement requirements including the ability to initiate 20° or more of wrist extension and 10° or more of finger extension. As a result, benefits from this treatment are limited to those with less severe motor involvement, or approximately 20–25% of patients with chronic stroke (Blanton & Wolf, 1999). Other problems limiting the application of CIMT techniques include poor compliance with patient restraint schedules, concerns over safety and limitations on independence caused by the restrictive device, lack of facility resources to provide intensive training sessions, and concerns about reimbursement (Page et al., 2004).

Recent research involving CIMT has deviated from the original research protocol by varying target populations, altering inclusion criteria, and modifying intensity and duration of treatment (Roberts et al., 2005). Ploughman and Corbett (2004) studied the effects of restraining patients' uninvolved arm without extensive shaping therapy. Roberts et al. (2005) monitored patient performance and satisfaction after 2 weeks of CIMT in the home environment incorporating meaningful daily activities chosen by the patient. Page et al. (2004) describes a modified CIMT for outpatients that combines involving the affected arm in functional tasks during structured 30-minute sessions 3 times a week with restraint of the unaffected arm every weekday for 5 hours. All studies reported improved motor function using standardized measurements, supporting the observation that techniques that induce a patient to use an affected limb should be considered therapeutically effective (Taub, Uswatte, & Pidikiti, 1999).

Motor Learning Ability

As occupational therapists mainly teach skills, they must address the learning process to help patients improve occupational performance. Learning to dress, for example, entails performing the task effectively and efficiently in a variety of circumstances or contexts (Carr & Shepherd, 1987). Therapists can best assist patients with stroke by helping them develop their own problem-solving techniques and strategies to deal with their environment.

Visual Dysfunction

Chapter 28 describes treatment for patients with visual deficits. In general, therapists can employ either of two basic approaches for patients with visual problems following stroke, determined by the extent of visual impairment and a patient's intact capabilities (Warren, 1999). With an active approach, the goal of therapy is to improve a patient's visual perceptual processing, either by improving component skills, such as visual scanning ability, or by training in compensatory skills, such as turning the head to the left. With a passive approach, treatment emphasis is on altering the patient's environment to improve occupational performance, such as positioning all food in the right visual field before a meal.

There is limited research to support the effectiveness of visual training procedures used with patients following stroke (Ma & Trombly, 2002). Results of one study (Weinberg et al., 1977), however, suggest that visual-perceptual deficits following stroke must be confronted and patients must be taught to recognize their deficits for treatment to be effective. Sharing results of objective evaluations with the patient and family, giving feedback on the effects of visual deficits on functional performance, and teaching patients to recognize and correct errors in performance have been suggested as techniques for increasing a patient's awareness of his or her deficits (Warren, 1993).

Studies of the effects of visual training skills on unilateral neglect (Cherney, Halper, & Papachronis, 2003) and visual-perceptual deficits (Edmans, Webster, & Lincoln, 2000) indicate that treatment involving forced awareness of neglected space, task-specific practice, and use of consistent strategies to accomplish functional activities improve cognitive-perceptual abilities after stroke. To ensure transfer of training, Toglia (1991) recommended a multicontext approach of practicing strategies in multiple environments with varied tasks and component demands. Therapists, for example, can provide a stronger learning event by reinforcing a visual searching task (finding all the forks in a dishwasher bin) with touching and moving the targets (picking up the forks and putting them in the correct space in a drawer). Training must be specific to the individual's deficits and goals for occupational functioning. A patient with hemianopsia and unilateral visual neglect who is unsafe with wheelchair propulsion and is not interested in reading or writing as a leisure activity will benefit more from specific environmental scanning activities in a wheelchair (obstacle courses, grocery shopping) than from paper and pencil or computer activities.

Speech and Language Disorders

Occupational therapists should work closely with speech-language pathologists to contribute to a patient's improvement in speech and language functioning. Therapists can promote proper posture as an assist to respiration and eye contact important to speech. Therapy sessions also provide a social context supportive of communication (Sarno, 1994). Whenever possible, therapists should incorporate speech and language goals into their treatment sessions, such as requiring verbal responses (counting repetitions of an activity or naming objects used) or addressing functional reading and writing tasks (reading signs and recipes, writing checks). Occupational therapists can assist in selecting and adapting a non-verbal form of communication for a patient, such as writing, drawing, use of a communication board, and gestures. Suggestions for working with patients with aphasia and their families include the following (American Heart Association, 1994):

- Avoid unnecessary noise: turn off television, find a quiet space.

- Do not speak to the patient or request speech when he or she is engaged in a physical activity.
- Allow enough time for the patient to respond; do not rush or force communication; do not switch topics quickly.
- Never assume that the person with aphasia can't understand what's being said; never allow others to ignore the person with aphasia.
- Speak slowly and clearly using simple, concise language; do not speak loudly unless hearing is impaired; do not talk down as if to a child.
- Use demonstration, visual cues, and gestures as needed to help with comprehension.

Motor Planning Deficits

Motor planning deficits, or apraxia, are serious learning disorders and among the most difficult to rehabilitate. The emphasis of treatment is on teaching compensatory skills rather than on remediation due to the complexity of these impairments (Warren, 1991), with goals of competent performance of desired habitual or novel activities (Gresham et al., 1995). Suggestions for treatment include manually guided movement, repetitive graded use of objects and contexts to evoke more automatic responses, explaining clearly the components of a task, **backward chaining**, and practicing activities as closely as possible to the patient's usual context or routine (Gresham et al., 1995). Language can facilitate movement planning; it assists in the sequencing of actions required for a task, helps focus concentration and identify mistakes, and reduces perseveration (Warren, 1991). Therapists can have patients verbalize step by step what they have done and are going to do, for example, "I have taken the cap off the toothpaste. Now I will pick up my toothbrush and put toothpaste on it."

Cognitive Deficits

Treatment to optimize cognitive abilities is discussed in Chapter 29. As in other areas of dysfunction, treatment for cognitive problems after stroke can include retraining of specific component skills, teaching compensation techniques or substitution of intact abilities, and/or adaptation of the environment (Gresham et al., 1995). Examples include using prompts or cues to shape desired behavior; providing feedback on performance with suggestions and strategies for improvement; providing visual aids, such as memory logs, checklists, maps, or diagrams for deficits of memory, sequencing, or organization; and simplifying the environment and grading tasks for patients with attention deficits. Caregivers must be educated regarding recommended adaptations, safety precautions, and the need for supervision.

Psychosocial Adjustment

Patients and families usually need assistance in making healthy emotional adjustments after stroke. It may be unreasonable to expect compliance to treatment instructions when patients and their families are coping poorly with the losses associated with stroke (Evans et al., 1992). Patients typically employ hope and determination to cope with hospitalization, the hard work of rehabilitation, and changes in body image but many cling to the belief that they will be "normal" again (Sabari, 1998). Therapists should reinforce the efforts of the rehabilitation team and encourage patients and families to talk about their reactions to stroke and their comprehension of its progression and prognosis. In light of the shortening time frames for rehabilitation, therapists should make sure patients and families understand that recovery from stroke does not end with discharge from a hospital or rehabilitation program. Therapists should also help patients and families to realize that the ultimate goal of rehabilitation is not complete recovery from physical and intellectual impairments but the ability to resume valued life roles.

Therapists should recognize the signs and symptoms of depression and inform appropriate team members if treatment has not been initiated. For the patient with emotional lability, both patient and family need to be reassured that lability is a symptom of the stroke and that control will improve with time (Carr & Shepherd, 1987). The therapist can instruct the patient in techniques such as deep breathing or redirecting attention to help him modify his behavior (Carr & Shepherd, 1987). Group activities, social interactions, and community outings are important methods for allowing a patient to practice roles from before the stroke and to realize that the patient role is a temporary transition to getting on with life despite residual impairments.

Transition to the Community

"For many stroke survivors and their families, the real work of recovery begins after formal rehabilitation. One of the most important tasks of a rehabilitation program is to help those involved to prepare for this stage of recovery." (Gresham et al., 1995, p. 143)

Discharge Planning

Discharge planning takes place throughout the rehabilitation phase. Successful planning allows the patient and family to feel comfortable with the decisions made for discharge, feel capable of maintaining gains and continuing progress without the intense level of support provided by rehabilitation specialists, and feel able to monitor for changes requiring adjustments or further intervention.

Occupational therapists assist in identifying the most appropriate discharge setting; training the patient, family, and caregiver in essential skills; and arranging for continuity of care with community services. Factors determining discharge setting include patient's and family's preferences, level of patient's disabilities, level of caregiver's support, and safety and accessibility of the home (Gresham et al., 1995). Often a patient with a fairly high level of physical functioning cannot return home because there is no caregiver or the residence is unsafe or inaccessible, whereas a more disabled patient can return home because a healthy spouse is willing to assume the role of caregiver and the residence is safe and accessible. Therapists perform a major role by participating with patients and families in home visits and safety assessments and recommending necessary home alterations or adaptive equipment.

Patient, Family, and Caregiver Education

Ideally, every treatment session is an opportunity to teach the patient, family, or caregiver techniques and problem-solving strategies for use after rehabilitation. Although learning styles vary, patients and their families are best served by a combination of demonstration, experiential sessions, and written instructions. Repetition is important, and caregivers should demonstrate, rather than simply verbalize, their ability to assist the patient safely and independently. At the time of discharge from a rehabilitation program, patients and their families are often overwhelmed with information from several disciplines that they must try to assimilate. After formal therapy sessions have ended, many patients and caregivers report good intentions of following home programs as prescribed but admit that the routine of daily activity leaves little time or energy for carrying out therapeutic recommendations at home. The most effective home programs therefore are those that incorporate treatment for component limitations into self-care and leisure routines (Van Dyck, 1999), for example: "Before bathing or dressing, briefly perform the following stretching movements to get the best posture and arm movement for these tasks." This is more likely to be complied with than: "Perform the following exercises, 10 repetitions each, at least twice a day." Home programs should, of course, be individualized and should remind the patient of skills already mastered, of skills the patient can reasonably expect to gain, and of possible problems common to stroke. Patients and families should be well informed of sources for information or assistance as new capabilities or problems evolve. Fall prevention is a necessary component of the home program and should encourage greater independence in mobility while identifying and reducing the risks of falls (Gresham et al., 1995).

Resuming Valued Roles and Tasks

Although most individuals who have had stroke improve in basic functional abilities such as walking and self-care, most have limitations in physical and social role functioning (Lai et al., 2002). Sabari (1998) refers to the third phase of stroke recovery as that of reestablishing social roles and suggests that this is the critical phase in defining one's quality of life. Occupational therapists should facilitate this adaptive process by helping patients set and achieve reasonable goals for task performance so as to assume adapted or new roles.

Work

For patients who expect to resume working, prevocational or vocational evaluation and appropriate work readiness training should be encouraged (see Chapter 33). A literature review (Teasell, McRae, & Finestone, 2000) examining return to work among working-age stroke patients found that between 17% and 51% of the patients were able to return to work. The wide variability seen in return to work is explained by differences in stroke severity and differences in defining work. A smaller percentage of patients were able to resume full-time competitive employment, and a greater percentage returned to part-time or home-based work. A majority of those returning to work acknowledged that their jobs required modifications (Teasell, McRae, & Finestone, 2000). Those able to return to work reported significantly higher levels of subjective life satisfaction (Vestling, Tufvesson, & Iwarsson, 2003). The factors generally found to predict likelihood of returning to work included independence in self-care, ability to walk, younger age, high educational and occupational levels, stable marital status, and preserved language and cognitive capacities (McMahon & Crown, 1998; Vestling, Tufvesson, & Iwarsson, 2003).

Leisure and Recreation

Throughout rehabilitation, **valued leisure activities should be identified, encouraged, and enabled.** Effective therapy incorporates leisure interests into treatment so that the patient recovering from stroke can begin to analyze the effects of impairments on valued activities and anticipate strategies for return to these activities. A study of 40 individuals discharged from rehabilitation programs post stroke found that individuals with a large variety of interests were more likely to resume at least one leisure activity than those with limited leisure interests (Jongbloed & Morgan, 1991). Other factors influencing leisure participation include family and social support, transportation or financial barriers, attitudes toward altered leisure performance, and amount of free time available (Jongbloed & Morgan, 1991). Many patients following stroke report decreased time and energy for leisure pursuits because of the increased demands of self-care. Many do not accept performance of a valued activity at a lower standard; for example, a patient with hemiparesis may give up golf rather than play at a reduced level of performance. Many patients, particularly those who were working at the time of their stroke, do not have established leisure roles or do not admit to any leisure interests. Methods to promote leisure and recreation after stroke include finding ways to overcome physical barriers in the home or community in order to adapt a valued activity; introduction of new leisure activities suitable for a patient's abilities; and education and advocacy regarding available community resources (Gresham et al., 1995).

Sexuality

Surveys of patients and their spouses show that typical effects of stroke on sexuality include decreased libido, impaired erectile functioning in men, decreased vaginal lubrication in women, and decreased frequency of sexual activity (Korpelaineu, Nieminen, & Myllyla, 1999). Causes may be physiological (decreased motor, sensory, or cognitive functioning; dependency in ADL; decreased endurance; incontinence; co-existing disease; or side effects of medications) or psychosocial (poor self-image, depression, role changes, impaired communication ability, fear of impotence, or fear of recurring stroke) (Farman & Friedman, 2004; Gresham et al., 1995; Korpelaineu, Nieminen, & Myllyla, 1999).

To assist with sexual expression, all therapists can impart the message that patients are permitted to have concerns and seek information about sexual problems after stroke. Therapists should reassure their clients that these problems are common and that sexual activity after stroke is not contraindicated (Farman & Friedman, 2004; Gresham et al., 1995). Other possible interventions include providing or referring to resources to increase the patient's knowledge, encouraging open communication between partners, suggesting adaptations such as changes in positioning or timing, and referring to a qualified specialist (Farman & Friedman, 2004; Gresham et al., 1995).

Driving

Nearly all adults in the United States drive (Warren, 1999), so the ability to resume driving is a high priority for most individuals with brain damage and is seen as a way to continue community independence and avoid isolation (Gresham et al., 1995). Improved survival rates and longevity after stroke increase the need for health professionals to make recommendations regarding a patient's ability to drive (Korner-Bitensky et al., 2000). Due to its complexity and danger, driving after stroke is usually not addressed until a patient has returned home and gained a satisfactory level of independence with self-care and short-distance mobility. It has been reported that only 30% of those who drove before stroke are able to resume driving, and 87% of those who drove before stroke did not receive any form of driving evaluation (Fisk, Owsley, & Pulley, 1997). Although it is not known with certainty which deficits necessitate the use of adaptive driving aids or render a stroke survivor unfit to drive, perceptual and cognitive deficits are recognized as having a serious effect on driving safety (Korner-Bitensky et al., 2000). Hemiparesis alone does not appear to prevent a return to driving because vehicles or techniques can be adapted to compensate for most motor deficits seen post stroke. There are no standard evaluation procedures for determining the ability of cerebrally injured patients to return to driving, but consistent practices include: (1) a pre-driving evaluation battery to test for visual scanning, visual attention, higher level visual-cognitive skills, distractibility, mental slowness, problem solving, and ability to follow directions; (2) a driving simulator evaluation; and (3) a road test, both on a protected course and in traffic (Galski, Ehle, & Williams, 1997; Korner-Bitensky et al., 1998). Studies have failed to establish the accuracy of various components of pre-driving assessment in predicting on-road driving performance, although road tests appear to have the highest correlation (Akinwuntan et al., 2002).

Few studies have substantiated the effectiveness of rehabilitation to improve driving-related deficits (Klavora et al., 1995). Current practices include in-car driver retraining, driving simulator training, and attempts to remediate underlying impairments. Klavora et al. found significant improvement in behind-the-wheel driving assessments in post-stroke subjects who trained with Dynavision, which is an apparatus "designed to train visual scanning, peripheral visual awareness, visual attention, and visual-motor reaction time across a broad, active visual field" (Klavora et al., 1995, p. 535). Therapists must remember that the decision to allow a person who has had a stroke to resume driving rests with the state licensing bureau (Gresham et al., 1995) (see Chapter 31).

Community Support and Resources

Methods to reintegrate the patient into the community (e.g., transportation options, dealing with architectural barriers, assistance from family or friends, access to senior citizen centers) should be addressed throughout rehabilitation because failure to resume pre-morbid community activities has been significantly correlated with isolation and depression in stroke patients (Logan, Dyas, & Gladman, 2004). Successful reintegration into the community, according to individuals who have had strokes, can take years rather than months (Buscherhof, 1998; Matola,

2001), continuing after a patient has regular contact with rehabilitation specialists. **Acute-care hospitals and rehabilitation facilities should maintain up-to-date inventories of community resources; provide this information to stroke survivors, their families, and their caregivers; and offer assistance in obtaining needed services.** In general, supports for patients and their families include educational, instrumental, and emotional supports (Gresham et al., 1995). Educational resources are available through organizations (Resources 38-1) that offer direct audiotaped, videotaped, printed, and/or online information specific to stroke. Instrumental supports are physical assistance programs such as personal provider services, Meals on Wheels, and volunteer groups who can build wheelchair ramps. Emotional support can come from family, friends, mental health professionals, and other survivors of stroke.

Support for long-term caregivers is especially important because caregivers appear to be at substantial risk for burnout, depression, isolation, and general health problems (Gresham et al., 1995; Han & Haley, 1999). Therapists can encourage and suggest sources for respite care, support groups, or counseling. Many communities, unfortunately, are limited in resources for the patient and family. Therapists can be advocates and consultants for the development of community programs; this can range from referring patients and families to others in the community living with stroke, to organizing a stroke club, to identifying opportunities for volunteer jobs for patients.

RESOURCE 38-1

National Stroke Association
9707 East Easter Lane
Englewood, CO 80112
Phone: (303) 649-9299; (800) STROKES ([800] 787-6537)
www.stroke.org

American Stroke Association (division of American Heart Association)
7272 Greenville Avenue
Dallas, TX 75231
Phone: (888) 4STROKE ([888] 478-7653)
www.strokeassociation.org
www.americanheart.org

Internet Stroke Center
Washington University School of Medicine, Department of Neurology
660 South Euclid, Box 8111
St. Louis, MO 63110
Phone: (314) 362-3458
www.strokecenter.org

Stroke Support Groups—obtain listings of local stroke clubs from above web sites or organizations.

National Aphasia Association
P.O. Box 1887, Murray Hill Station
New York, NY 10156-0611
Phone: (800) 922-4622
www.aphasia.org

Post-Discharge Monitoring

Because of the varying rates of recovery and adjustment after stroke and the trends toward earlier discharges from acute centers and rehabilitation programs, occupational therapists should facilitate provision of services along a smooth continuum. **The stroke survivor's progress should be evaluated within 1 month after return to a community residence and at regular intervals during at least the first year, consistent with the person's condition and the preferences of the stroke survivor and family.** The 12 months after stroke is considered a high-risk time crucial to the redevelopment of satisfactory life roles (Gresham et al., 1995; Sardin, Cifu, & Noll, 1994).

Managed health care programs tend to focus resources on the most acute patients and on those showing the greatest response to therapy. As patients become more chronic and/or fail to progress in therapy (commonly termed recovery plateau), they are frequently terminated from rehabilitation services (Page, Gater, & Bach-y-Rita, 2004). Studies have shown, however, that patients with chronic CVA (greater than 1 year post stroke) can exhibit substantial motor and functional improvement with novel rehabilitation protocols requiring repetitive, task-specific practice (Page, Gater, & Bach-y-Rita, 2004; Page et al., 2004). Rather than indicating a permanent diminished capacity for improvement, plateaus may represent patient adaptations to an unvaried treatment regimen (Page, Gater, & Bach-y-Rita, 2004).

Radomski (1995) recommends greater emphasis on outpatient programming to enhance quality of life and health care effectiveness. Occupational performance and component abilities should be assessed during follow-up visits to determine whether a patient is maintaining the functional level achieved during rehabilitation or is progressing or regressing from this level. A period at home often provides patients the opportunity to experience and acknowledge their strengths and weaknesses and focuses their interest on improving specific skills needed to reintegrate into the home and community. Long-term survivors of stroke report the value of timely interventions over an extended period as they slowly regained confidence in a new self and resumed meaningful life roles (Buscherhof, 1998; Matola, 2001).

EFFECTIVENESS OF TREATMENT

In compiling the *Post-Stroke Rehabilitation Clinical Practice Guideline*, a panel of experts and consultants concluded after an extensive review of the literature that "few well-controlled clinical studies document benefits from rehabilitation" (Gresham et al., 1995, p. 11). Difficulties in determining effectiveness of treatment for the stroke population include differentiating benefits of rehabilitation from spontaneous neurological recovery after stroke (Gresham et al., 1995); the heterogeneous nature of the population of stroke survivors with their diverse causes and impairments; and the ethical and practical problems inherent in assigning patients to control groups.

Recent emphasis on evidence-based practice has resulted in greater efforts to use empirical research findings to guide treatment decisions.

Studies analyzing the effects of stroke rehabilitation in general suggest that patients benefit from early intervention, that favorable ADL and neuromuscular outcomes are associated with higher intensities of rehabilitation, and that improvements in impairments do not automatically lead to improvements in ADL (Kwakkel et al., 1997; Ottenbacher & Jannell, 1993). Although treatment effects for rehabilitation were small, they were significantly practical in that small improvements in independent functioning can make the difference between discharge to home and institutionalization.

Duncan (1997) reviewed clinical trials and summarized evidence for interventions to improve motor control after stroke. The trials compared various therapeutic approaches, such as traditional biomechanical and rehabilitative therapy versus neurodevelopmental or proprioceptive neuromuscular facilitation treatment. Based on this review of research, remediation programs appear to improve motor control in patients with some initial voluntary movement. There were no statistically significant differences among treatment groups receiving various types of sensorimotor treatment as measured for motor or functional outcomes and no evidence that reduction of motor impairment carries over to functional performance.

Steultjens et al. (2003) conducted a systematic review of available literature to determine whether OT interventions improve outcome for stroke patients. Their meta-analysis of 32 studies looked at the effects of six specific OT intervention categories on primary outcome measures of basic ADL (BADL) and IADL and on secondary process measures of arm and hand function, muscle tone, and cognitive functions. The reviewers established small but significant effect sizes favoring OT effectiveness on BADL and IADL. They concluded that evidence establishing efficacy of training of cognitive functions, of advice and instruction regarding assistive devices, and of providing splints is lacking. No study was available to determine effectiveness of family or caregiver training.

Trombly and Ma (2002) reviewed 36 studies for level of evidence to support OT treatment for the restoration of roles, tasks, and activities and for the remediation of psychosocial, cognitive-perceptual, and sensorimotor impairments. Acknowledging the limitations of this small body of research and the lack of replication, the authors summarize evidence for OT practice for stroke patients as follows (see Evidence Table 38-1 for best evidence):

- To improve performance of BADL and IADL and role participation, provide opportunities for practice of client-chosen activities in a familiar context and provide necessary adaptations and training in the use of the adaptations.
- To improve cognitive abilities and capacities, use homemaking or other occupational tasks and activities rather than paper-and-pencil tasks.
- To improve function in those patients with unilateral neglect, provide training that involves moving into neglected space for goal accomplishment.
- To improve visual-perceptual abilities, use functional (task-specific) training and consistent strategies of compensation.
- To increase participation and endurance, use goal-directed and meaningful activities, such as games.
- To increase voluntary movement and coordination, practice with goal-directed and meaningful objects, preferably using bilateral simultaneous movement, rather than rote exercise.
- To improve motor performance, teach the patient to imagine functional use of the affected limb.
- To promote voluntary movement after discharge, provide a written and illustrated home program of movement exercises and activities.

The authors also concluded that two treatments, splinting to reduce spasticity and exercise to recruit motor units in the prime mover to improve movement were not supported by evidence. The effects of OT on reducing depression after stroke has not been studied enough to warrant recommendation (Trombly & Ma, 2002; Ma & Trombly, 2002).

In conclusion, more research is needed to determine evidence-based OT interventions for stroke patients. Limitations in determining OT effectiveness include the variability of treatment approaches among OT practitioners and settings (Steultjens et al., 2003) and the team approach to patient treatment, which makes it difficult to isolate OT effects from those of other disciplines (Trombly & Ma, 2002). Current studies additionally provide no information regarding the effectiveness of OT programs in reducing the need for and relative costs of health care services for stroke patients (Landi & Bernabei, 2003). Future research must focus on verifying findings of existing studies, determining which treatments are effective for desired outcomes, which patients will most benefit from these services, and what are the appropriate times, settings, and intensities of treatment.

Evidence Table 38-1 Best Evidence for Occupational Therapy Practice Regarding Stroke

Intervention	Description of Intervention Tested	Participants	Dosage	Type of Best Evidence and Level of Evidence	Benefit	Statistical Probability and Effect Size of Outcome	Reference
Task-specific practice of client-chosen BADL or IADL	Practice of specific tasks in a familiar context	323 acute stroke survivors (147 with left cerebrovascular accident [LCVA], 156 with right cerebrovascular accident [RCVA]). Mean age = 72.5 years.	Ranged from 1 to 15 visits over a period of 6 weeks to 5 months.	Meta-analysis of 2 studies.	Yes. The treated groups improved in BADL as measured by *Barthel Index*, and improved in IADL as measured by *Nottingham EADL Scale*.	Mean weighted effect size was $r = 0.16$, equivalent to a 16% success rate over control treatment.	Trombly & Ma, 2002
Use of cueing strategies to improve scanning function in unilateral neglect	Practice of scanning tasks with visual or motor cues.	13 acute stroke survivors (0 with LCVA, 13 with RCVA). Mean age = 57.5 years.	21 trials/day for 4 consecutive days.	Randomized controlled study. IC1b	Yes. Bias Index of Line Bisection improved in all cued conditions compared with controls (strongest effect with motor cueing).	Mean effect size was $r = 0.87$.	Lin et al., 1996

continued

Practice of goal-directed tasks to increase voluntary active range of motion	Experimental group: use of exercise apparatus and game to increase forearm supination. Control: use of same apparatus without game.	30 acute stroke survivors (11 with LCVA, 15 with RCVA, 4 with other). Mean age = 68.4 years.	2 sets of 10 trials for each condition; different days.	Randomized controlled study. IC2c	Yes. Mean gain of 13.4° more supination (handle rotation) in experimental group.	$r = 0.42$	Nelson et al., 1996
Use of goal-directed object-present activity to enhance quality of movement	Practice of reaching movement with object present or to accomplish functional goal versus reaching without object or without functional goal.	28 chronic stroke survivors (17 with LCVA, 9 with RCVA, 2 with other). Mean age = 63.4 years.	10 trials/condition within 1 day.	Meta-analysis of 2 studies.	Yes. Better organization of reaching movement for functional goal as described by kinematic variables for speed, smoothness, strategy used, and force.	Combined effect size: $r = 0.62$.	Ma & Trombly, 2002
Use of written and illustrated home exercise program to improve coordinated movement	Experimental group: home therapy by individualized written and illustrated program of upper extremity exercises. Control Group: no treatment.	22 acute stroke survivors (13 with LCVA, 9 with RCVA). Mean age = 58 years.	3–4 visits for an average of 9 weeks; patients practiced home program 2–3 times a day.	Comparison of 2 treatment groups without randomization. IIC2b	Yes. Experimental group showed improved performance in Upper Extremity Reaching Subtest of *Southern Motor Group's Motor Assessment* and in *Timed 10-Hole Peg Test*.	$r = 0.30$ (for reaching subtest); $r = 0.50$ (for *Timed 10-Hole Peg Test*).	Turton & Fraser, 1990

SUMMARY REVIEW QUESTIONS

1. Name the two main categories of stroke and the subtypes and causes of each.
2. Name six neurological deficits that can result from stroke and describe how each may interfere with dressing.
3. What is the difference between neurological recovery and functional recovery after stroke? How might occupational therapy facilitate both types of recovery in a patient?
4. Name five settings where occupational therapists work with patients recovering from stroke and describe characteristics of a patient who might be treated in each setting.
5. Define postural adaptation and name three ways impairments in this area affect occupational performance. Describe treatment methods to improve postural control.
6. What mechanical and physiological components of movement should be evaluated in the hemiplegic upper extremity? What methods can be used to prevent development of a painful shoulder?
7. What variables should be considered during evaluation for voluntary movement in the hemiplegic upper extremity?
8. What factors can affect a stroke patient's ability to learn and organize movement? Describe how deficits in each of these areas affect self-care.
9. Select a treatment activity for a patient recovering from stroke and describe how this activity can both increase ADL independence (reduce disability) and improve component abilities and capacities (reduce impairment).
10. Describe methods to assist a post-stroke patient resume self-enhancement and self-advancement roles after discharge from rehabilitation services.

References

Akinwuntan, A. E., Feys, H., DeWeerdt, W., Pauwels, J., Baten, G., & Strypstein, E. (2002). Determinants of driving after stroke. *Archives of Physical Medicine and Rehabilitation, 83,* 334–341.

American Heart Association. (1994). *Caring for the person with aphasia.* Brochure. Dallas: American Heart Association.

American Heart Association. (2005). *Heart disease and stroke statistics –2005 update.* Dallas: American Heart Association.

American Occupational Therapy Association [AOTA]. (2002). Occupational Therapy Practice Framework: Domain and process. *American Journal of Occupational Therapy, 56,* 609–639.

Aminoff, M. J., Greenberg, D. A., & Simon, R. P. (2005). *Clinical neurology* (6th ed.). New York: Lange Medical Books/McGraw-Hill.

Andersen, L. T. (1985). Shoulder pain in hemiplegia. *American Journal of Occupational Therapy, 9,* 11–19.

Andrews, A. W., & Bohannon, R. W. (2000). Distribution of muscle strength impairments following stroke. *Clinical Rehabilitation, 14,* 79–87.

Bard, G., Hirschberg, G. G., & Tolleson, G. C. B. (1964). Functional testing of the hemiplegic arm. *Journal of the American Physical Therapy Association, 44,* 1081–1086.

Bartels, M. N. (2004). Pathophysiology and medical management of stroke. In G. Gillen & A. Burkhardt (Eds.), *Stroke rehabilitation: A function-based approach* (2nd ed., pp. 1–30). St. Louis: Mosby.

Berg, K., Wood-Dauphinee, S., Williams, J. I., & Gayton, D. (1989). Measuring balance in the elderly: Preliminary development of an instrument. *Physiotherapy Canada, 41,* 304–311.

Blanton, S., & Wolf, S. L. (1999). An application of upper-extremity constraint-induced movement therapy in a patient with subacute stroke. *Physical Therapy, 79,* 847–853.

Bobath, B. (1990). *Adult hemiplegia: Evaluation and treatment* (3rd ed.). London: Heinemann Medical.

Bohannon, R. W., & Andrews, A. W. (1990). Shoulder subluxation and pain in stroke patients. *American Journal of Occupational Therapy, 44,* 506–509.

Bornstein, R. A. (1986). Normative data on intermanual differences on three tests of motor performance. *Journal of Clinical and Experimental Neuropsychology, 8,* 12–20.

Brandstater, M. E. (2005). Stroke rehabilitation. In J. A. De Lisa et al. (Eds.), *Physical medicine and rehabilitation principles and practice* (4th ed., pp. 1655–1676). Philadelphia: Lippincott Williams & Wilkins.

Brodie, J., Holm, M. B., & Tomlin, G. S. (1994). Cerebrovascular accident: Relationship of demographic, diagnostic and occupational therapy antecedents to rehabilitation outcomes. *American Journal of Occupational Therapy, 48,* 906–913.

Brott, T., Adams, H. P., Olinger, C. P., Marler, J. R., Barsan, W. G., Biller, J., Spilker, J., Holleran, R., Eberle, R., Hertzberg, V., Rorick, M., Moomaw, C. J., & Walker, M. (1989). Measurements of acute cerebral infarction: A clinical examination scale. *Stroke, 20,* 864–870.

Brunnstrom, S. (1970). *Movement therapy in hemiplegia.* New York: Harper & Row.

Buscherhof, J. R. (1998). From abled to disabled: A life transition. *Topics in Stroke Rehabilitation, 5,* 19–29.

Callahan, A. (1995). Sensibility assessment: Prerequisites and techniques for nerve lesions. In J. M. Hunter, E. J. Mackin, & A. D. Callahan (Eds.), *Rehabilitation of the hand: Surgery and therapy* (4th ed., pp. 129–152). St. Louis: Mosby.

Campbell, A., Brown, A., Scheldroth, C., Hastings, A., Ford-Booker, P., Lewis-Jack, O., Adams, C., Gadling, A., Ellis, R., Wood, D., Dennis, G., Adeshoye, A., Weir, R., & Coffey, G. (1991). The relationship between neuropsychological measures and self-care skills in patients with cerebrovascular lesions. *Journal of the National Medical Association, 83,* 321–324.

Caplan, L. R. (2002). Treatment of patients with stroke. *Archives of Neurology, 59,* 703–707.

Carod-Artal, F. J., Gonzales-Gutierrez, J. L., Herrero, J. A. E., Horan, T., and deSeijas, E. V. (2002). Functional recovery and instrumental activities of daily living: Follow-up 1-year after treatment in a stroke unit. *Brain Injury, 16,* 207–216.

Carr, E. K., & Kenney, F. D. (1992). Positioning of the stroke patient: A review of the literature. *International Journal of Nursing Studies, 29,* 355–369.

Carr, J. H., & Shepherd, R. B. (1987). *A motor relearning programme for stroke* (2nd ed.). Rockville, MD: Aspen.

Carr, J. H., Shepherd, R. B., Nordholm, L., & Lynne, D. (1985). Investigation of a new motor assessment scale for stroke patients. *Physical Therapy, 65,* 175–180.

Cherney, L. R. (1995). Management approaches for aphasia [Foreword, special issue]. *Topics in Stroke Rehabilitation, 2,* vi.

Cherney, L. R., Halper, A. S., Kwasnica, C. M., Harvey, R. L., & Zang, M. (2001). Recovery of functional status after right hemisphere stroke: Relationship with unilateral neglect. *Archives of Physical Medicine and Rehabilitation, 82,* 322–328.

Cherney, L. R., Halper, A. S., & Papachronis, D. (2003). Two approaches to treating unilateral neglect after right hemisphere stroke: A preliminary investigation. *Topics in Stroke Rehabilitation, 9,* 22–33.

Davies, P. M. (2000). *Steps to follow: A guide to the treatment of adult hemiplegia* (2nd ed.). Berlin: Springer-Verlag.

deGroot, M. H., Phillips, S. J., & Eskes, G. A. (2003). Fatigue associated with stroke and other neurologic conditions: Implications for stroke rehabilitation. *Archives of Physical Medicine and Rehabilitation, 84,* 1714–1720.

Dellon, A. (1981). *Evaluation of sensibility and re-education of sensation in the hand.* Baltimore: Williams & Wilkins.

DeSouza, L. H., Langton Hewer, R. L., & Miller S. (1980). Assessment of recovery of arm control in hemiplegic stroke patients. I: Arm function tests. *International Rehabilitation Medicine, 2,* 3–9.

DeWeerdt, W. J. G., & Harrison, M. A. (1985). Measuring recovery of arm-hand function in stroke patients: A comparison of the Brunnstrom-Fugl-Meyer Test and the Action Research Arm Test. *Physiotherapy Canada, 37,* 65–70.

Dobkin, B. H. (2005). Rehabilitation after stroke. *New England Journal of Medicine, 352,* 1677–1684.

Dromerick, A. W., Edwards, D. F., & Hahn, M. (2000). Does the application of constraint-induced movement therapy during acute rehabilitation reduce arm impairment after ischemic stroke? *Stroke, 31,* 2984–2988.

Duncan, P. W. (1997). Synthesis of intervention trials to improve motor recovery following stroke. *Topics in Stroke Rehabilitation, 3,* 1–20.

Duncan, P. W., Wallace, D., Lai, S. M., Johnson, D., Embretson, S., & Laster, L. (1999). The Stroke Impact Scale Version 2.0: Evaluation of reliability, validity, and sensitivity to change. *Stroke, 30,* 2131–2140.

Edmans, J. A., Webster, J., & Lincoln, N. B. (2000). A comparison of two approaches in the treatment of perceptual problems after stroke. *Clinical Rehabilitation, 14,* 230–243.

Eggers, O. (1984). *Occupational therapy in the treatment of adult hemiplegia.* London: Heinemann Medical.

Eriksson, M., Asplund, M. D., Glader, E. L., Norrving, B., Stegmayr, B., Terent, A., Asberg, K. H., & Wester, P. O. (2004). Self-reported depression and use of antidepressants after stroke: A national survey. *Stroke, 35,* 936–941.

Evans, R. L., Hendricks, R. D., Haselkorn, J. K., Bishop, D. S., & Baldwin, D. (1992). The family's role in stroke rehabilitation. *American Journal of Physical Medicine and Rehabilitation, 71,* 135–139.

Farman, J., & Friedman, J. D. (2004). Sexual function and intimacy. In G. Gillen & A. Burkhardt (Eds.), *Stroke rehabilitation: A function-based approach* (2nd ed., pp. 533–549). St. Louis: Mosby.

Fasoli, S. E., Trombly, C. A., Tickle-Degnen, L., & Verfaellie, M. H. (2002). Effect of instructions on functional reach in persons with and without cerebrovascular accident. *American Journal of Occupational Therapy, 56,* 380–390.

Fellows, S. J., & Thilmann, A. F. (1994). Voluntary movement at the elbow in spastic hemiparesis. *Annals of Neurology, 36,* 397–407.

Filiatrault, J., Arsenault, A. B., Dutil, E., & Bourbonnais, D. (1991). Motor function and activities of daily living assessments: A study of three tests for persons with hemiplegia. *American Journal of Occupational Therapy, 45,* 806–810.

Fisk, F. D., Owsley, C., & Pulley, L. V. (1997). Driving after stroke: Driving exposure, advice and evaluations. *Archives of Physical Medicine and Rehabilitation, 78,* 1338–1345.

Folstein, M. F., Folstein, S. E., & McHugh, P. R. (1975). Mini-mental State: A practical method for grading the cognitive state of patients for the clinician. *Journal of Psychiatric Research, 12,* 189–198.

Foulkes, M. A., Wolf, P. A., Price, T. R., Mohr, J. P., & Hier, D. B. (1988). The stroke data bank: Design, methods, and baseline characteristics. *Stroke, 19,* 547–554.

Fugl-Meyer, A. R., Jaasko, L., Leyman, I., Olsson, S., & Steglind, S. (1975). The post-stroke hemiplegic patient: I. A method for evaluation of physical performance. *Scandinavian Journal of Rehabilitation Medicine, 7,* 13–31.

Galski, T., Ehle, H. T., & Williams, J. B. (1997). Off-road driving evaluations for persons with cerebral injury: A factor analytic study of predriver and simulator testing. *American Journal of Occupational Therapy, 46,* 324–332.

Gillen, G. (2004a). Trunk control: A prerequisite for functional independence. In G. Gillen & A. Burkhardt (Eds.), *Stroke rehabilitation: A function-based approach* (2nd ed., pp. 119–144). St. Louis: Mosby.

Gillen, G. (2004b). Upper extremity function and management. In G. Gillen & A. Burkhardt (Eds.), *Stroke rehabilitation: A function-based approach* (2nd ed., pp. 172–218). St. Louis: Mosby.

Goodglass, H. (1993). *Understanding aphasia.* San Diego: Academic Press, Inc.

Gordon, N. F., Gulanick, M., Costa, F., Fletcher, G., Franklin, B. A., Roth, E. J., & Shephard, T. (2004). AHA Statement: Physical activity and exercise recommendations for stroke survivors. *Circulation, 109,* 2031–2041.

Gresham, G. E., Duncan, P. E., Stason, W. B., Adams, H. P., Adelman, A. M., Alexander, D. N., Bishop, D. S., Diller, L., Donaldson, N. E., Granger, C. V., Holland, A. L., Kelly-Hayes, M., McDowell, F. H., Myers, L., Phipps, M. A., Roth, E. J., Siebens, H. C., Tarvin, G. A., & Trombly, C. A. (1995). *Post-stroke rehabilitation. Clinical Practice Guideline 16.* (AHCPR Publication 95-0662). Rockville, MD: United States Agency for Health Care Policy and Research.

Han, B., & Haley, W. E. (1999). Family caregiving for patients with stroke: Review and analysis. *Stroke, 30,* 1478-1485.

Heilman, K., & Valenstein, E. (1979). Mechanisms underlying hemispatial neglect. *Annals of Neurology, 5,* 166–170.

Heller, A., Wade, D. T., Wood, V. A., Sunderland, A., Langton Hewer, R., & Ward, E. (1987). Arm function after stroke: Measurement and recovery over the first three months. *Journal of Neurology, Neurosurgery and Psychiatry, 50,* 714–719.

Holbrook, M., & Skilbeck, C. E. (1983). An activities index for use with stroke patients. *Age and Ageing, 12,* 166–170.

Jongbloed, L., & Morgan, D. (1991). An investigation of involvement in leisure activities after a stroke. *American Journal of Occupational Therapy, 45,* 420–427.

Jorgensen, H. S., Nakayama, H., Raaschou, H. O., Vive-Larsen, J., Stoier, M., & Olsen, T. S. (1995). Outcome and time course of recovery in stroke: Part I. Outcome. Copenhagen Stroke Study. *Archives of Physical Medicine and Rehabilitation, 76,* 399–405.

Keith, R. A., Granger, C. V., Hamilton, B. B., & Sherwin, F. S. (1987). The Functional Independence Measure: A new tool for rehabilitation. In M. G. Eisenberg & R. C. Grzesiak (Eds.), *Advances in clinical rehabilitation* (Vol. 2, pp. 6–18). New York: Springer.

Kelly-Hayes, M., Robertson, J. T., Broderick, J. P., Duncan, P. W., Hershey, L. A., Roth, E. J., Thies, W. H., & Trombly, C. A. (1998). The American Heart Association Stroke Outcome Classification. *Stroke, 29,* 1274–1280.

Kiernan, R. J., Mueller, J., Langston, J. W., & Van Dyke, C. (1987). The Neurobehavioral Cognitive Status Examination: A brief but differentiated approach to cognitive assessment. *Annals of Internal Medicine, 107,* 481–485.

Klavora, P., Gaskovski, P., Martin, K., Forsyth, R. D., Heslegrave, R. J., Young, M., & Quinn, R. P. (1995). The effects of Dynavision rehabilitation on behind-the-wheel driving ability and selected psychomotor abilities of persons after stroke. *American Journal of Occupational Therapy, 49,* 534–542.

Kluding, P. & Billinger, S. A. (2005). Exercise-induced changes of the upper extremity in chronic stroke. *Topics in Stroke Rehabilitation, 12,* 58–69.

Korner-Bitensky, N. A., Mazer, B. L., Safer, S., Gelinas, I., Meyer, M. B., Morrison, C., Tritch, L., Roulke, M. A., & White, M. (2000). Visual testing for readiness to drive after stroke: A multicenter study. *American Journal of Physical Medicine and Rehabilitation, 79,* 253–259.

Korner-Bitensky, N. A., Safer, S., Gelinas, I., & Mazer, B. L. (1998). Evaluating driving potential in persons with stroke: A survey of occupational therapy practices. *American Journal of Occupational Therapy, 52,* 916–919.

Korpelaineu, J. T., Nieminen, P., & Myllyla, V. V. (1999). Sexual functioning among stroke patients and their spouses. *Stroke, 30,* 715–719.

Kumar, R., Metter, E. J., Mehta, A. J., & Chew, T. (1990). Shoulder pain in hemiplegia: The role of exercise. *American Journal of Physical Medicine and Rehabilitation, 69,* 205–208.

Kwakkel, G., Wagenaar, R. C., Koelmen, T. W., Lankhorst, G. J., & Koetsier, J. C. (1997). Effects of intensity of rehabilitation after stroke: A research synthesis. *Stroke, 28,* 1550–1556.

Lai, S.-M., Studenski, S., Duncan, P. W., & Perera, S. (2002). Persisting consequences of stroke measured by the Stroke Impact Scale. *Stroke, 33,* 1840–1844.

Landi, F., & Bernabei, R. (2003). Occupational therapy for stroke patients: When, where and how? *Stroke, 34,* 686–687.

Langhorne, P., Stott, D. J., Robertson, L., MacDonald, J., Jones, L., McAlpine, C., Dick, F., Taylor, G. S., & Murray, G. (2000). Medical complications after stroke: A multicenter study. *Stroke, 31,* 1223–1229.

Langton Hewer, R. (1990). Rehabilitation after stroke. *Quarterly Journal of Medicine, 76,* 659–674.

Lannin, N. A., Horsley, S. A., Herbert, R., & McCluskey, A. (2003). Splinting the hand in the functional position after brain impairment: A randomized, controlled trial. *Archives of Physical Medicine and Rehabilitation, 84,* 297–302.

Lawton, M. P. (1988). Instrumental activities of daily living (IADL) scale: Original observer-rated version. *Psychopharmacology Bulletin, 24,* 785–787.

Lin, K.-C., Cermak, S. A., Kinsbourne, M., & Trombly, C. A. (1996). Effects of left-sided movements on line bisection in unilateral neglect. *Journal of the International Neuropsychological Society, 2,* 404–411.

Logan, P. A., Dyas, J., & Gladman, J. R. F. (2004). Using an interview study of transport use by people who have had a stroke to inform rehabilitation. *Clinical Rehabilitation, 18,* 703–708.

Lyle, R. C. (1981). A performance test for assessment of upper limb function in physical rehabilitation treatment and research. *International Journal of Rehabilitation Research, 4,* 483–492.

Ma, H., & Trombly, C. A. (2002). A synthesis of the effects of occupational therapy for persons with stroke, Part II: Remediation of impairments. *American Journal of Occupational Therapy, 56,* 260–274.

Mahoney, F. I., & Barthel, D. W. (1965). Functional evaluation: The Barthel Index. *Maryland State Medical Journal, 14,* 61–65.

Matola, T. (2001). Stroke: A bird's eye view. *Topics in Stroke Rehabilitation, 7,* 61–63.

McMahon, R., & Crown, D. S. (1998). Return to work factors following a stroke. *Topics in Stroke Rehabilitation, 5,* 54–60.

Morris, J. (1998). The role of psychology in stroke rehabilitation. *Topics in Stroke Rehabilitation, 5,* 1–10.

Nakayama, H., Jorgenson, H. S., Raaschou, H. O., & Olsen, T. (1994). Compensation in recovery of upper extremity function after stroke: The Copenhagen study. *Archives of Physical Medicine and Rehabilitation, 75,* 852–857.

Nelles, G., Spiekermann, G., Jueptner, M., Leonhardt, G., Muller, S., Gerhard, H., & Diener, C. (1999). Reorganization of sensory and motor systems in hemiplegic stroke patients: A positron emission tomography study. *Stroke, 30,* 1510–1516.

Nelson, D. L., Konosky, K., Fleharty, K., Webb, R., Newer, K., Hazboun, V. P., Fontane, C., & Licht, B. C. (1996). The effects of an occupationally embedded exercise on bilaterally assisted supination in persons with hemiplegia. *American Journal of Occupational Therapy, 50,* 639–646.

Okkema, K., & Culler, K. (1998). Functional evaluation of upper extremity use following stroke: A literature review. *Topics in Stroke Rehabilitation, 4,* 54–75.

Ottenbacher, K. J., & Jannell, S. (1993). The results of clinical trials in stroke rehabilitation research. *Archives of Neurology, 50,* 37–44.

Page, S. J., Gater, D. R., and Bach-y-Rita, P. (2004). Reconsidering the motor recovery plateau in stroke rehabilitation. *Archives of Physical Medicine and Rehabilitation, 85,* 1377–1381.

Page, S. J., Sisto, S., Levine, P., & McGrath, R. E. (2004). Efficacy of modified constraint-induced movement therapy in chronic stroke: A single-blinded randomized controlled trial. *Archives of Physical Medicine and Rehabilitation, 85,* 14–18.

Pedersen, P. M., Wandel, A., Jorgensen, H. S., Nakayama, H., Raaschou, H. O., & Olsen, T. S. (1996). Ipsilateral pushing in stroke: Incidence, relation to neuropsychological symptoms, and impact on rehabilitation. The Copenhagen Stroke Study. *Archives of Physical Medicine and Rehabilitation, 77,* 25–28.

Perennou, D. A., Amblard, B., Laassel, E. M., Benaim, C., Herisson, C., & Pelissier, J. (2002). Understanding the pusher behavior of some stroke patients with spatial deficits: A pilot study. *Archives of Physical Medicine and Rehabilitation, 83,* 570–575.

Ploughman, M., & Corbett, D. (2004). Can force-used therapy be clinically applied after stroke? An exploratory randomized controlled trial. *Archives of Physical Medicine and Rehabilitation, 85,* 1417–1423.

Radomski, M. V. (1995). There is more to life than putting on your pants. *American Journal of Occupational Therapy, 49,* 487–490.

Remer-Osborn, J. (1998). Psychological, behavioral, and environmental influences on post-stroke recovery. *Topics in Stroke Rehabilitation, 5,* 45–53.

Ridgway, E. M., & Byrne, D. P. (1999). To sling or not to sling? *OT Practice, 4,* 38–42.

Rijken, P. M., & Dekker, J. (1998) Clinical experience of rehabilitation therapists with chronic diseases: A quantitative approach. *Clinical Rehabilitation, 12,* 143–150.

Roberts, P. S., Vegher, J. A., Gilewski, M., Bender, A., & Riggs, R. V. (2005). Client-centered occupational therapy using constraint-induced therapy. *Journal of Stroke and Cerebrovascular Diseases, 14,* 115–121.

Sabari, J. S. (1998). Occupational therapy after stroke: Are we providing the right services at the right time? *American Journal of Occupational Therapy, 52,* 299–302.

Sardin, K. J., Cifu, D. X., & Noll, S. F. (1994). Stroke rehabilitation: 4. Psychologic and social implications. *Archives of Physical Medicine and Rehabilitation, 75,* S-52–S-55.

Sarno, M. T. (1994). Neurogenic disorders of speech and language. In S. B. O'Sullivan & T. J. Schmitz (Eds.), *Physical rehabilitation: Assessment and treatment* (3rd ed., pp. 633–653). Philadelphia: Davis.

Savinelli, R., Timm, M., Montgomery, J., & Wilson, D. J. (1978). Therapy evaluation and management of patients with hemiplegia. *Clinical Orthopaedics and Related Research, 131,* 15–29.

Shinsha, N., & Ishigami, S. (1999). Rehabilitation approach to patients with unilateral spatial neglect. *Topics in Stroke Rehabilitation, 6,* 1–14.

Sommerfeld, D. K., Eek, E. U., Svensson, A.-K., Holmqvist, L. W., & vonArbin, M. H. (2004). Spasticity after stroke: Its occurrence and association with motor impairments and activity limitations. *Stroke, 35,* 134–139.

Steultjens, E. M. J., Dekker, J., Bouter, L.-M., van de Nes, J. C. M., Cup, E. H. C., & van den Ende, C. H. M. (2003). Occupational therapy for stroke patients: A systematic review. *Stroke, 34,* 676–687.

Taub, E., Miller, N. E., Novack, T. A., Cook, E. W. III, Fleming, W. C., Nepomuceno, C. S., Connell, J. S., & Crago, J. E. (1993). Technique to improve chronic motor deficit after stroke. *Archives of Physical Medicine and Rehabilitation, 74,* 347–354.

Taub, E., Uswatte, G., & Pidikiti, R. (1999). Constraint-induced movement therapy: A new family of techniques with broad application to physical rehabilitation—Clinical review. *Journal of Rehabilitation Research and Development, 36,* 237–251.

Teasell, R. W., McRae, M. P., & Finestone, H. M. (2000). Social issues in the rehabilitation of younger stroke patients. *Archives of Physical Medicine and Rehabilitation, 81,* 205–209.

Teixeira-Salmela, L. F., Olney S. J., Nadeau, S., & Brouwer, B. (1999). Muscle strengthening and physical conditioning to reduce impairment and disability in chronic stroke survivors. *Archives of Physical Medicine and Rehabilitation, 80,* 1211–1218.

Toglia, J. P. (1991). Generalization of treatment: A multicontext approach to cognitive perceptual impairment in adults with brain injury. *American Journal of Occupational Therapy, 45,* 505–516.

Trombly, C. A. (1989). Stroke. In C. A. Trombly (Ed.), *Occupational therapy for physical dysfunction* (3rd ed., pp. 454–471). Baltimore: Williams & Wilkins.

Trombly, C. A. (1995). Occupation: Purposefulness and meaningfulness as therapeutic mechanisms. *American Journal of Occupational Therapy, 49,* 960–972.

Trombly, C. A., & Ma, H. (2002). A synthesis of the effects of occupational therapy for persons with stroke, Part I: Restoration of roles, tasks, and activities. *American Journal of Occupational Therapy, 56,* 250–259.

Trombly, C. A., & Wu, C.-Y. (1999). Effect of rehabilitation tasks on organization of movement after stroke. *American Journal of Occupational Therapy, 53,* 333–344.

Turner-Stokes, L., & Jackson, D. (2002). Shoulder pain after stroke: A review of the evidence base to inform the development of an integrated care pathway. *Clinical Rehabilitation, 16,* 276–298.

Turton, A., & Fraser, C. (1990). The use of home therapy programmes for improving recovery of the upper limb following stroke. *British Journal of Occupational Therapy, 53,* 457–462.

Van Dyck, W. R. (1999). Integrating treatment of the hemiplegic shoulder with self-care. *OT Practice, 4,* 32–37.

Versluys, H. P. (1995). Facilitating psychosocial adjustment to disability. In C. A. Trombly (Ed.), *Occupational therapy for physical dysfunction* (4th ed., pp. 377–389). Baltimore: Williams & Wilkins.

Vestling, M., Tufvesson, B., & Iwarsson, S. (2003). Indicators for return to work after stroke and the importance of work for subjective well-being and life satisfaction. *Journal of Rehabilitation Medicine, 35,* 127–131.

Wade, D. T. (1989). Measuring arm impairment and disability after stroke. *International Disability Studies, 11,* 89–92.

Wade, D. T. (1992). Stroke: Rehabilitation and long term care. *Lancet, 339,* 791–793.

Walker, M. F., & Lincoln, N. B. (1990). Reacquisition of dressing skills after stroke. *International Disability Studies, 12,* 41–43.

Walker, M. F., & Lincoln, N. B. (1991). Factors influencing dressing performance after stroke. *Journal of Neurology, Neurosurgery and Psychiatry, 54,* 699–701.

Walsh, K. (2001). Management of shoulder pain in patients with stroke. *Postgraduate Medical Journal, 77,* 645–649.

Warren, M. (1990). A developmental treatment approach for adults with postural dysfunction. *Occupational Therapy Practice, 1,* 53–62.

Warren, M. (1991). Strategies for sensory and neuromotor remediation. In C. Christensen, & C. Baum (Eds.), *Occupational therapy: Overcoming human performance deficits* (pp. 632–662). Thorofare, NJ: Slack.

Warren, M. (1993). A hierarchical model for evaluation and treatment of visual perceptual dysfunction in adult acquired brain injury: Part 2. *American Journal of Occupational Therapy, 47,* 55–66.

Warren, M. (1996). *Brain Injury Vision Assessment Battery for Adults.* Birmingham, AL: visABILITIES Rehabilitation.

Warren, M. (1999). *Evaluation and treatment of visual perceptual dysfunction in adult brain injury, part I* (continuing education handbook). Birmingham, AL: visABILITIES Rehabilitation.

Weinberg, J., Diller, L., Gordon, W. A., Gerstmann, L. J., Leiberman, A., Lakin, P., Hodges, G., & Ezrachi, O. (1977). Visual scanning training effect on reading-related tasks in acquired right brain damage. *Archives of Physical Medicine and Rehabilitation, 58,* 479–486.

Weinberg, J., Diller, L., Gordon, W. A., Gerstmann, L. J., Leiberman, A., Lakin, P., Hodges, G., & Ezrachi, O. (1979). Training sensory awareness and spatial organization in people with right brain damage. *Archives of Physical Medicine and Rehabilitation, 60,* 491–496.

Wilson, D. J., Baker, L. L., & Craddock, J. A. (1984a). Functional test for the hemiparetic upper extremity. *American Journal of Occupational Therapy, 38,* 159–164.

Wilson, D. J., Baker, L. L., & Craddock, J. A. (1984b). Protocol: Functional test for the hemiplegic/paretic upper extremity. Unpublished manuscript. County Rehabilitation Center, Rancho Los Amigos, Occupational Therapy Department, Downey, CA

Winstein, C. J., Rose, D. K., Tan, S. M., Lewthwaite, R., Chui, H. C., & Azen, S. P. (2004). A randomized controlled comparison of upper-extremity rehabilitation strategies in acute stroke: A pilot study of immediate and long-term outcomes. *Archives of Physical Medicine and Rehabilitation, 85,* 620–628.

Wu, C.-Y., Trombly, C. A., Lin, K., & Tickle-Degnen, L. (1998). Effects of object affordances on reaching performance in persons with and without cerebrovascular accident. *American Journal of Occupational Therapy, 52,* 447–456.

Yekutiel, M., & Guttman, E. A. (1993). A controlled trial of the retraining of the sensory function of the hand in stroke patients. *Journal of Neurology, Neurosurgery and Psychiatry, 56,* 241–244.

Zorowitz, R. D., Hughes, M. B., Idank, D., Ikai, T., & Johnston, M. V. (1996). Shoulder pain and subluxation after stroke: Correlation or coincidence? *American Journal of Occupational Therapy, 50,* 194–201.

CHAPTER 39

Traumatic Brain Injury

Mary Vining Radomski

LEARNING OBJECTIVES

After studying this chapter, the reader will be able to do the following:

1. Describe the similarities and differences in the typical course of recovery for persons with severe, moderate, and mild traumatic brain injury.
2. Select appropriate assessment tools and strategies for persons with traumatic brain injury during acute medical management and inpatient and post-acute rehabilitation.
3. Apply information from related chapters of this text to the treatment of motor, cognitive, behavioral, and emotional aspects of traumatic brain injury.
4. Analyze how needs of family members change during recovery and adaptation and determine how to meet their needs in occupational therapy.
5. Anticipate possible roles for occupational therapists in addressing long-term needs of survivors of traumatic brain injury.

Glossary

Agitation—Subtype of delirium that is unique to survivors of TBI in altered states of consciousness in which there are excesses in behavior that include some combination of aggression, disinhibition, restlessness, and confusion.

Anterograde amnesia—Inability or impaired ability to remember events beginning with the onset of a condition (Lezak, 1995).

Diffuse axonal injury—Axonal damage (torn axons, shearing of axon clusters, and reactive swelling of strained and damaged axons) resulting from acceleration or deceleration and contracting waveform movements of the brain matter and accompanying fast rotational propulsion of the brain in the skull (Lezak, 1995).

Hematoma—Masses of blood confined to an organ or space that is caused by a broken blood vessel (Scott & Dow, 1995).

Mild brain injury—Trauma-induced physiological disruption of brain function as manifested by at least one of the following: any period of loss of consciousness, any loss of memory for events immediately before or after the accident, any alteration in mental state at the time of the accident, focal neurological deficit that may or may not be transient (American Congress of Rehabilitation Medicine, 1995a).

Post-traumatic amnesia—Inability to remember day to day events after brain injury. The time elapsed from injury to recovery of continuous memory is one indicator of severity of brain damage.

Traumatic brain injury (TBI)—Insult to the brain, not degenerative or congenital, that is caused by an external physical force. This insult may produce a diminished or altered state of consciousness and resultant impairment of cognitive, behavioral, emotional, or physical functioning (Brain Injury Association, 2000).

People who have had a **traumatic brain injury (TBI)** often undergo changes in their ability to carry out valued roles, tasks, and activities. In fact, moderate to severe brain injury affects virtually every area of life for the survivor and his or her family (Pagulayan et al., 2006). These individuals are often young adults at the time of injury, thus, changes in capacities and abilities may affect their occupational functioning for months, years, or decades. The complex interaction of factors associated with impairment and context require a multidisciplinary approach to treatment. Therefore, occupational therapists who work with patients with TBI must appreciate the contributions and expertise of other team members as they offer the patient all that is unique to occupational therapy.

To enable the reader to appreciate the effect of TBI on society, this chapter begins with a discussion of its incidence and causes. Next, mechanisms of injury are explained. A review of the typical clinical course of recovery from severe TBI emphasizes how occupational therapy contributes to remediation of impairments and adaptation to deficits throughout the continuum of care. The unique needs of persons with **mild brain injury** are also highlighted, but it is hoped that readers can determine appropriate evaluation and treatment approaches for persons with moderate TBI based on descriptions of the two extremes of severity of injury. Since brain injury rehabilitation requires an integration of many aspects of occupational therapy evaluation and treatment, the reader will frequently be referred to other chapters of this text.

INCIDENCE, PREVALENCE, AND CAUSATION

The Brain Injury Association (BIA) (2000) defines traumatic brain injury (TBI) as an insult to the brain, not degenerative or congenital, that is caused by an external physical force. This insult may produce a diminished or altered state of consciousness and hence impairment of cognitive, behavioral, emotional, or physical functioning. Rates of TBI-related hospitalization have declined by approximately 50% since 1980 because of successes in prevention and a shift in treatment of relatively mild cases from inpatient to outpatient settings (Thurman et al., 1999). The BIA, however, estimates that 5.3 million Americans are living with disabilities resulting from TBI. Each year, approximately 1.4 million people in the United States sustain a TBI, and an estimated 80,000–90,000 each year have onset of disabilities resulting from TBI (Langlois, Rutland-Brown, & Thomas, 2004). Beyond the sheer numbers of persons with TBI, demographic characteristics of this population have many implications for society and rehabilitation. After children ages 0–4 years, adolescents and young adults have the highest incidence of TBI in the United States (1995–2001 data), followed by people over age 75 years (Langlois, Rutland-Brown, & Thomas, 2004). Adults aged 75 years and older have the highest rate of TBI-related hospitalization and death (Langlois, Rutland-Brown, & Thomas, 2004). Regardless of age, men have more TBIs than women (Langlois, Rutland-Brown, &

Thomas, 2004). Age of onset appears to be related to cause of TBI (Elovic & Antoinette, 1996).

Falls are the leading cause of TBI, but motor vehicle accidents result in the greatest numbers of TBI-related hospitalizations (Langlois, Rutland-Brown, & Thomas, 2004). Motor vehicle accidents that result in TBI cause the highest rates of hospitalization and death and are the leading cause of TBI for persons aged 15–19 years (Langlois, Rutland-Brown, & Thomas, 2004). Falls result in the greatest number of TBI-related ED visits and are the leading cause of TBI among the elderly (Langlois, Rutland-Brown, & Thomas, 2004). Interpersonal violence ranks third, although in some urban areas, the percentage of TBIs caused by violence may exceed that caused by falls or motor vehicle accidents (Elovic & Antoinette, 1996; Harrison-Felix et al., 1996). Alcohol use is a contributing factor to accidents resulting in TBI, with estimates that approximately 50% of people who sustain TBI were intoxicated at the time of injury (Agency for Health Care Policy and Research, 1999). Pre-injury alcohol use has implications for outcome, treatment, and long-term adjustment to TBI. Patients who were intoxicated when injured reportedly have a longer hospitalization, longer duration of **agitation**, and lower cognitive status at discharge than those who were not intoxicated (Kelly et al., 1997; Sparadeo & Gill, 1989). Furthermore, a history of TBI increases a person's risk of TBI. The BIA estimates that after one TBI, the risk of a second is three times normal, and after a second TBI, the risk of a third injury is eight times normal.

Finally, it is important to appreciate the incidence of TBI based on severity. TBI is characterized as mild, moderate, or severe (Definition 39-1). Most people who sustain a TBI have a relatively mild injury (at least 75% of all TBIs in the United States [National Center for Injury Prevention and Control, 2003]), although trauma centers appear to have a much higher proportion of patients with severe injuries (Harrison-Felix et al., 1996).

DEFINITION 39-1

Defining Severity of TBI

Severe—Loss of consciousness longer than 6 hours; initial *Glasgow Coma Scale* score of 8 or less (O'Dell & Riggs, 1996).
Moderate—Initial *Glasgow Coma Scale* score of 9 to 12 (Hall & Johnston, 1994); **post-traumatic amnesia** of 1 to 24 hours (Bond, 1990).
Mild—Trauma-induced physiological disruption of brain function as manifested by at least one of the following: any period of loss of consciousness, any loss of memory for events immediately before or after the accident, any alteration in mental state at the time of the accident, focal neurological deficit that may or may not be transient (American Congress of Rehabilitation Medicine, 1995a), and initial *Glasgow Coma Scale* score of 13 to 15 (Hall & Johnston, 1994).

MECHANISMS OF INJURY AND CLINICAL IMPLICATIONS

A TBI is usually caused by a dynamic loading or impact to the head from direct blows or from sudden movements produced by blows to other body parts. This loading can result in any combination of compression, expansion, acceleration, deceleration, and rotation of the brain inside the skull (Bakay & Glasauer, 1980). The type of damage is directly related to the nature and severity of the injury (Katz, 1992).

Diffuse Versus Focal Injuries

Brain injuries may be diffuse, focal, or both. Motor vehicle accidents and falls produce acceleration, deceleration, and rotation of the brain inside the skull. The brainstem is more stable than the cerebrum, which rotates around the brainstem during impact. The rotation places a stretch or shear force on the long axons that transmit information throughout the brain and brainstem (Leech & Shuman, 1982). These injuries, termed **diffuse axonal injuries**, are likely to result in coma because of the damage to the axons in the midbrain reticular activating system (Duff, 2001).

Coma caused by diffuse axonal injuries may quickly reverse if the axonal damage was mild or may continue as a vegetative state if axons were ruptured. Recovery from coma progresses to a period of confusion with impaired attention and **anterograde amnesia**. When confusion clears, any cognitive impairments become more evident. Impairments may include diminished mental processing speed and efficiency and difficulty with divided-attention tasks, which require the patient to respond simultaneously to two sources of information. There is a reduced capacity for higher level cognitive functions, including abstract reasoning, planning, and problem solving. Typical behavioral outcomes range from impulsivity, irritability, and exaggerated pre-morbid traits to apathy and poor initiative (Katz, 1992). Diffuse injuries often include damage to the brainstem and cerebellar pathways, resulting in ataxia, diplopia, and dysarthria (Trexler & Zappala, 1988).

Focal lesions include contusions, lacerations of the brain, and intracranial hematomas (Duff, 2001). Although focal lesions can occur anywhere beneath the impact, they are usually seen at the anterior poles and inferior surfaces of the frontal and temporal lobes. They occur when the brain hits the skull and scrapes over the irregular bony structures at these locations (Katz, 1992). The occipital and parietal lobes, which have smooth surfaces, are less likely to incur damage. The folds of the dural membranes, especially the falx cerebri and the tentorium, can also cause damage to the brainstem, the medial aspect of the occipital lobe, and the superior surface of the cerebellum (Bakay & Glasauer, 1980).

Focal lesions to the prefrontal and anterior temporal areas interrupt connections to subcortical limbic structures and affect modulation of memory, emotion, and drive (Katz, 1992). Damage to the orbitofrontal areas results in impulsivity that is greater than with diffuse damage, but there are no motor impairments of the extremities or of speech (Trexler & Zappala, 1988). Damage to the frontolateral cortex results in hemiparesis, impulsivity, and attentional impairments. There is decreased accuracy and decreased mental flexibility, which affects the quality of performance (Trexler & Zappala, 1988).

Cranial Nerve Damage Associated with TBI

Cranial nerves can be torn, stretched, or contused. The olfactory nerve (I) is often abraded or torn when the frontal lobes scrape across the orbital surface of the skull (Leech & Shuman, 1982). The optic nerve (II) may be damaged directly, or vision can be compromised by injury to the eye, the optic tracts, or the visual cortex (Brandstater et al., 1991). Cranial nerves III, IV, and VI, which control eye movements, are all vulnerable to injury (Brandstater et al., 1991; Leech & Shuman, 1982). The oculomotor nerve (III) is stretched when edema, bleeding, or a tumor expands the contents of the skull, causing the uncus of the temporal lobe to herniate into the foramen magnum and compress the brainstem (Leech & Shuman, 1982). The abducens nerve (VI) is very long and consequently vulnerable to injury. The facial and vestibulocochlear nerves (VII and VIII, respectively) may be damaged if the temporal bone is fractured at the base of the skull (Brandstater et al., 1991; Leech & Shuman, 1982). Cranial nerves V and IX to XII are rarely damaged (Leech & Shuman, 1982).

Fractures Associated with TBI

The skull may fracture from the force of the blow in the area of or at a distance from the actual impact site. The patient with a brain injury from a motor vehicle accident or a fall may have other systemic trauma, such as fractures of the extremities, shoulder girdle, pelvis, or face; cervical fractures with possible spinal cord injury; abdominal trauma; and pneumothorax or other chest cavity trauma.

Secondary Effects of TBI

Secondary effects of the TBI can occur immediately or develop within hours or days (Jennett & Teasdale, 1981). Trauma can abolish or disrupt autoregulation of cerebral blood flow, the blood–brain barrier, and vasomotor functions, resulting in disordered cerebral energy metabolism, intracranial hypotension, cerebral vasospasm, and increases in intracranial pressure (ICP) and cerebral edema (Duff, 2001; Jennett & Teasdale, 1981). Other secondary effects of brain trauma include intracranial hemorrhage, ischemic brain damage, uncal herniation resulting in brainstem compression, general systemic reactions to the neural impairment, electrolyte abnormalities, altered respiratory regulation, intracranial infection, and abnormal autonomic nervous system responses (Lillehei & Hoff, 1985). Usually by the time the patient is stabilized and occupational therapy is ordered, the secondary effects of brain trauma are present, influencing the patient's ability to respond to therapy.

FOUR PHASES OF LIFE FOR THE SURVIVOR OF TBI

Based on their review of the literature, authors of the Agency for Health Care Policy and Research evidence report on the effectiveness of rehabilitation for persons with TBI described four phases of life for the adult survivor of moderate to severe TBI: pre-injury, medical treatment, rehabilitation, and survivorship (Fig. 39-1) (Chestnut et al., 1999). While management of TBI is typically a multidisciplinary enterprise, the following description of each phase is based on a typical recovery from severe TBI with emphasis on occupational therapy evaluation and treatment. Note how the role of occupational therapy changes with each phase, increasingly and uniquely focusing on occupational functioning the further the patient progresses in recovery.

Pre-Injury Phase

> "In Chris's first 17 years she became used to being called 'outstanding.' She usually was one of the top students in every honors class. . . . Chris was a fairly good organist and gymnast too. In her first 17 years, outstanding was normal. Outstanding was easy." (Rain, 2000, p. 6)

Occupational therapists always appreciate the person as distinct from his or her condition, impairment, or disability. People who sustain a TBI bring their personal, social, and cultural backgrounds to recovery (see Chapter

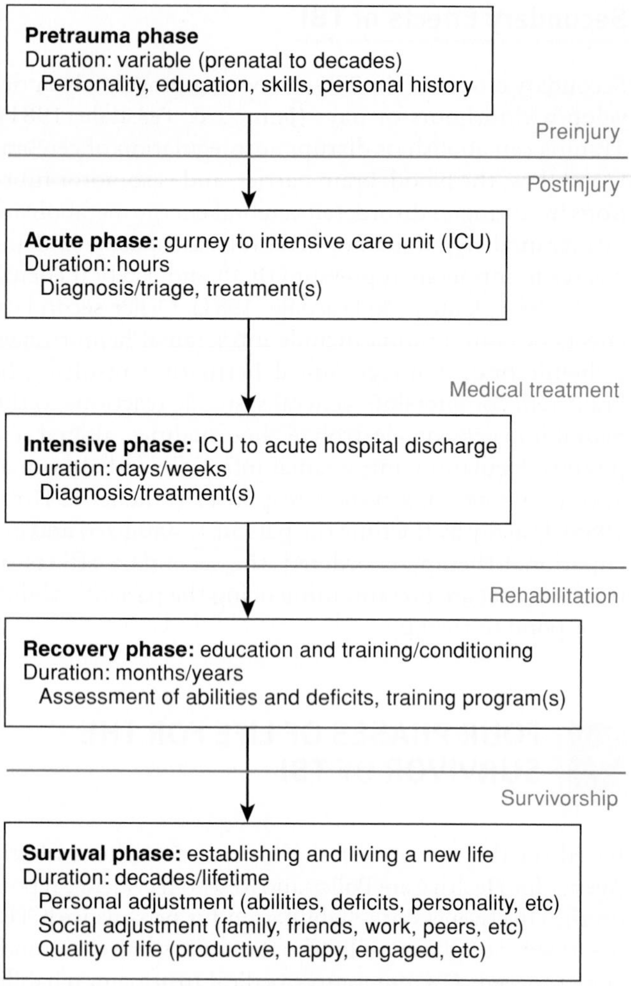

Figure 39-1 Four phases of life of the TBI survivor. (Reprinted with permission from Chestnut, R. M., Carney, N., Maynard, H., Mann, N. C., Patterson, P., & Helfand, M. [1999]. Summary report: Evidence for the effectiveness of rehabilitation for persons with traumatic brain injury. *Journal of Head Trauma Rehabilitation, 14,* 176–188.)

10). Chestnut et al. (1999) suggested that, while standard treatments are appropriate for the acute medical treatment phase of TBI, consideration of individual differences becomes increasingly important as patients progress through recovery and adaptation.

Rosenthal and Bond (1990) summarized the importance of understanding pre-morbid factors that may affect the patient's recovery. They reported that researchers have noted a high frequency of pre-injury learning disabilities and behavior disorders in persons with TBI. They suggested finding out about the patient's pre-morbid cognitive strengths and weaknesses through school records or family interviews and investigating any pre-existing neurological conditions, such as previous TBI, epilepsy, dementia, or stroke. Eames, Haffey, and Cope (1990) further recommended asking family members how the patient previously reacted to frustration so as to recognize and avoid stress-provoking situations.

Medical Treatment of TBI

> "As I gradually regain consciousness in the hospital, I imagine I am having a nightmare. . . . As I open my eyes and stare around the room at the monitors and plugs and dripping IV bottles, I hope this nightmare will end quickly." (Rain, 2000, p. 6)

The primary goals of this phase of recovery center on survival, achieving medical stability, and preventing or minimizing the secondary effects of TBI.

Emergency Medical Treatment

Paramedics are typically the first medical specialists to respond to the needs of a person with severe TBI. Once they have ensured an adequate airway and stabilized blood pressure, they usually immobilize the patient on a rigid backboard with the neck in a rigid cervical spine collar (Marion, 1996). As most secondary brain injury occurs during the first few hours of TBI, vital signs are checked frequently en route to the trauma center, and any deterioration is addressed immediately (Marion, 1996).

Once in the emergency department, the medical team continues to ensure protection of the airway and adequacy of breathing and blood pressure (Marion, 1996). The medical team performs a general assessment of injuries and neurological status, often using the *Glasgow Coma Scale* (*GCS*) (Teasdale & Jennett, 1974). The *GCS* provides an objective assessment of moderate to severe TBI using a 15-point system to test motor, eye-opening, and verbal capabilities (Table 39-1) (Teasdale & Jennett, 1974), although in some cases, alcohol or other drug intoxication or sedation prevents an accurate neurological assessment in the emergency department (Marion, 1996).

Computed tomography (CT) of the head is usually obtained within 30 minutes after the patient arrives in the emergency department; it is the most reliable test for determining the presence of intracranial hematomas (Marion, 1996). **Hematoma**, a mass of blood confined to an organ or space and caused by a broken blood vessel (Scott & Dow, 1995) must be evacuated as soon as possible to optimize chances for survival and recovery (Marion, 1996).

Intensive Medical Management

After appropriate evaluation and treatment for life-threatening injuries, the patient is taken to the intensive care unit (ICU). Medical treatment aims to optimize cerebral perfusion and brain tissue oxygenation, minimize brain swelling, and maintain all other physiological variables within the normal range (Marion, 1996). The length of stay in the ICU

Table 39-1. Glasgow Coma Scale

Eye opening (*E*)	Spontaneous	4
	To speech	3
	To pain	2
	Nil	1
Best motor response (*M*)	Obeys	6
	Localizes	5
	Withdraws	4
	Abnormal flexion	3
	Extensor response	2
	Nil	1
Verbal response (*V*)	Oriented	5
	Confused conversation	4
	Inappropriate words	3
	Incomprehensible sounds	2
	Nil	1

Coma score = (E + M + V) = 3 to 15.

Reprinted with permission from Jennett, B., & Teasdale, G. (1981). *Management of head injuries* (p. 78). Philadelphia: F. A. Davis Company.

is primarily determined by the ability to manage the patient's brain swelling, which usually subsides within 4–5 days (Marion, 1996). A physiatrist is typically consulted on the day the patient is admitted to the ICU, and he or she follows the patient throughout the hospital stay and often through reentry to the community. The physiatrist orders rehabilitation services for the coma patient that may begin in the ICU, including occupational therapy. Rehabilitation for patients with alterations in consciousness, as described in this overview, may also occur in medical, rehabilitation, or subacute units or in long-term care facilities.

Patients with Severe Alterations in Consciousness

A person with TBI may exhibit any of a number of altered states of consciousness, depending on the severity of the injury (Talbot & Whitaker, 1994). Various terms are used to describe the continuum from complete consciousness to complete absence of consciousness (Definition 39-2). Patients with severe TBI begin in coma, which is a time-limited state (Duff, 2001). Some patients gradually or abruptly recover consciousness directly from coma, while others shift over 2–4 weeks into the vegetative state (Duff, 2001). Vegetative patients may still recover consciousness, but they do so gradually, spending long periods in a minimally conscious state in which there is verifiable evidence of conscious processing (Phipps et al., 1997). Giacino and Kalmar (1997) suggested that the distinction between vegetative state and minimally conscious state is important in terms of diagnosis and prognosis. Patients diagnosed with minimally conscious state at admission to rehabilitation attained significantly more favorable outcomes 1–12 months after injury than did those in the vegetative state. The ability to sustain visual pursuit eye movement seems to be one of the first signs of the transition out of vegetative state (Giacino & Kalmar, 1997) and is an early indicator of possible readiness for rehabilitation (Ansell, 1993).

DEFINITION 39-2

Definitions of Severe Alterations of Consciousness (American Congress of Rehabilitation Medicine, 1995b)

Coma

Coma denotes unarousability with absence of sleep-wake cycles on electroencephalogram (EEG) and loss of capacity for environmental interaction. Neurobehavioral criteria for this diagnosis include:

1. Patient's eyes do not open either spontaneously or to external stimulation.
2. Patient does not follow commands.
3. Patient does not mouth or speak recognizable words.
4. The patient does not demonstrate intentional movement (may show reflexive movement such as posturing, withdrawal from pain, or involuntary smiling).
5. Patient cannot sustain visual pursuits through a 45° arc in any direction when the eyes are held open manually.
6. These criteria cannot be attributed to use of paralytic agents.

Vegetative State

Vegetative state indicates complete loss of ability to interact with the environment despite the capacity for spontaneous or stimulus-induced arousal. This state always follows an initial period of coma after TBI and is further characterized by behavioral responses that consist of reflexive reactions only. Sleep-wake cycles may be present on EEG. Neurobehavioral criteria for this diagnosis include:

- Patient opens his or her eyes spontaneously or after stimulation.
- Criteria 2 to 6 under coma are met.

Minimally Responsive State

Minimally responsive state describes patients who are no longer comatose or vegetative but who are severely disabled. Patients in this state have the capacity for environmental interaction evidenced through observation or testing. Meaningful responses are inconsistent and depend on external stimulation. Patients in this category are sometimes referred to as slow to recover (Ansell, 1993). The neurobehavioral criterion for this diagnosis includes:

- Patient demonstrates a meaningful behavioral response after a specific command, question, or environmental prompt.

Assessment

Diagnosis of specific alterations in consciousness and prognostic decisions must be reserved for physicians and other professionals with experience in neurological assessment of patients with impaired consciousness (American Congress of Rehabilitation Medicine, 1995b). The rehabilitation team, however, including occupational therapists, uses a number of objective assessments to monitor changes in function and response to pharmacological, environmental, and behavioral interventions and for early detection of neuromedical complications (O'Dell & Riggs, 1996).

Rancho Los Amigos Levels of Cognitive Functioning Scale

The *Rancho Los Amigos Levels of Cognitive Function Scale* uses behavioral observations to categorize a patient's level of cognitive function (Table 39-2) (Hagen, Malkmus, & Durham, 1979; Hagen, 1998). It helps clinicians to communicate about a patient's level of cognitive function among themselves and with families and to develop appropriate rehabilitation strategies. The first three levels of the *Rancho Los Amigos Levels of Cognitive Functioning Scale* describe the response to stimulation and the environment of patients emerging from coma.

Behavior-Based Assessment Instruments

In addition to the *GCS*, the instruments described in Table 39-3 are all brief assessments that occupational therapists and other rehabilitation team members can use at bedside to evaluate patients with severe alterations in consciousness.

Use of Single-Subject Experimental Methodology

As many scales do not adequately operationalize or define stimuli and target behaviors, DiPasquale and Whyte (1996) proposed that clinicians use single-subject experimental methodology as a means of answering individualized questions about responsiveness. They described how these methods were used to determine whether or not a patient with a brain injury was able to follow a verbal command to squeeze her hand. The protocol began with the therapist performing passive range of motion to the patient's right hand, placing the patient's hand in hers, and then waiting 1 minute. There were three conditions: correct command ("Squeeze my hand"); incorrect command ("Tie your shoes"); and observation period (equal duration but no command given). Six trials were performed in random order in which the command was given and then the therapist waited for 5 seconds to observe the patient's response. If the patient did not respond in 5 seconds, the command was given again. If again, there was no response in 5 seconds, the trial was recorded as no response. The results of assessment using this approach cast doubts on family reports of volitional hand squeezing and helped inform team/family planning. They describe a similar methodology to assess vision in minimally responsive patients (Whyte & DiPasquale, 1995) (see Chapter 8).

Prognosis and Outcome

Early prediction of outcome presumably helps direct expensive medical treatment or rehabilitation to patients who have the best chance for survival with fewer residual impairments and enables the family to make informed, realistic decisions on immediate and long-term care (Davis &

Table 39-2. Rancho Los Amigos Levels of Cognitive Functioning

Level	Description
I	No response: unresponsive to stimuli
II	Generalized response: non-specific, inconsistent, and non-purposeful reaction to stimuli
III	Localized response: response directly related to type of stimulus but still inconsistent or delayed
IV	Confused, agitated: response heightened, severely confused, may be aggressive
V	Confused-inappropriate: some response to simple commands, but confusion with more complex commands; high level of distractibility
VI	Confused-appropriate: response more goal directed but cues necessary
VII	Automatic-appropriate: response robotlike, judgment and problem solving lacking
VIII	Purposeful-appropriate (*with standby assistance*): response adequate *to familiar tasks*, subtle impairments *require standby assistance with acknowledging other people's needs and perspectives, modifying plans*
IX	*Purposeful-appropriate (with standby assistance on request): responds effectively to familiar situations but generally needs cues to anticipate problems and adjust performance; low frustration tolerance possible*
X	*Purposeful and appropriate (modified independent): responds adequately to multiple tasks but may need more time or periodic breaks; independently employs cognitive compensatory strategies and adjusts tasks as needed*

Rancho levels I to VIII are widely used in brain injury rehabilitation. The addition of levels IX and X in 1998 (revisions italicized) describe higher level cognitive, behavioral, and emotional barriers to optimal functioning (Hagen, Malkmus, & Durham, 1979; Hagen, 1998).

Table 39-3. Behavior-Based Assessment Tools for Altered States of Consciousness

Coma/Near Coma Scale[a] (Rappaport et al., 1992)	Measures small clinical changes in patients with severe TBI and non-traumatic brain injuries who function at levels characteristic of near-vegetative or vegetative states; consists of 8 parameters, each with a specified number of stimuli and trials. Based on the numerical scoring system, patient falls into 1 of 5 categories: no coma, near coma, moderate coma, marked coma, extreme coma.
Western Neuro Sensory Stimulation Profile (Ansell & Keenan, 1989)	Assesses cognitive function in severely impaired adults (Rancho levels II–IV) and monitors change in non-comatose patients who are slow to recover. Battery consists of 32 items related to arousal, attention, response to stimuli, and expressive communication and results in a profile of 6 subscales that summarize individual patterns of responses.
Coma Recovery Scale (Giacino et al., 1991)	Detects subtle changes in neurobehavioral status; predicts outcome in acute rehabilitation patients with severe alterations in consciousness (Rancho levels I–IV); consists of 35 items in 6 areas: auditory, visual, motor, oromotor-verbal, communication, and arousal. Responses are criterion referenced: specific stimuli are administered to elicit specific responses.
Disability Rating Scale[a] (Rappaport et al., 1982)	Single instrument to provide quantitative information on recovery from severe TBI from coma to community; consists of 8 items in 4 categories: arousal and awareness; cognitive ability to handle self-care functions; physical dependence upon others; and psychosocial adaptability for work, housework, or school. Scoring takes 30 seconds (if clinician is very familiar with both tool and patient) to 15 minutes (Center for Outcome Measurement in Brain Injury [COMBI], 2006). Scale is thought to be relatively insensitive in detecting problems and progress for persons with mild TBI (COMBI, 2006).
Agitated Behavior Scale[a] (Corrigan, 1989)	Allows objective measurement of agitation, particularly as a serial assessment to evaluate effectiveness of interventions to reduce agitation (COMBI, 2006); consists of 14 items; total score reflects overall agitation, with subscales specific to disinhibition, aggression, and lability.

[a] Available online at http://www.tbims.org/combi.

Cunningham, 1984; Jennett & Teasdale, 1981). Many researchers have attempted to assess the predictive power of age, clinical observations (such as the *GCS*, pupillary reactions, and eye movements), data from CT, surgical lesion, length of post-traumatic amnesia (i.e., the length of time after the accident before the return of continuous memory), brainstem dysfunction, evoked potentials, increased ICP, or a combination of these factors (Braakman et al., 1980; Bricolo, Turazzi, & Feriotti, 1980; Karnaze, Weiner, & Marshall, 1985; Salcman, Schepp, & Ducker, 1981). Even with sophisticated clinical and radiological techniques, however, during the first days after injury, it is not possible to predict outcome with sufficient accuracy to guide early treatment or justify withholding treatment (Marion, 1996). Repeated observations of neurological recovery over weeks or months remain the best means to predict complete or nearly complete recovery (Marion, 1996).

As mentioned previously, the *GCS* is often used to predict outcome. An initial score of 8 or below that is maintained for 6 hours post injury predicts a mortality rate of 50% or survival with moderate to severe disabilities. Choi et al. (1988) found that a low motor score on the *GCS*, a fixed and dilated pupil, and age greater than 60 years strongly predicted death or severe disability and that the combination of factors had more predictive accuracy than any one of them used independently. The length of post-traumatic amnesia is another frequently used predictor of outcome. Post-traumatic amnesia is a loss of memory of day-to-day events after an injury. Post-traumatic amnesia lasting less than 1 hour indicates mild injury; 1–24 hours indicates moderate injury; 1–7 days indicates severe injury; and more than 7 days indicates very severe injury (Bond, 1990).

Outcome scales have been developed to allow physicians to correlate "final" recovery levels to early treatment and prognostic indicators. The *Glasgow Outcome Scale* (*GOS*) is widely used. Its categories are death, vegetative state, severe disability (conscious but dependent), moderate disability (independent but disabled), and good recovery (able to participate in normal social life and return to work), with 90% accurate assessment of prognosis possible 6 months post injury (Jennett & Teasdale, 1981; Satz et al., 1998). The *GOS* does assess some aspects of mental and physical function in assigning outcome categories (Jennett et al., 1981). Some researchers consider that more detailed neuropsychological and/or social factors should be considered in determining outcome (Hall, Cope, & Rappaport, 1985). When these factors are added, more residual disability is identified than by the *GOS*, and improvements in levels of disability are identified more accurately (Hall, Cope, & Rappaport, 1985). Addition of these factors also allows assessment of continued subtle recovery to be made beyond 6 or 12 months post injury (Hall, Cope, & Rappaport, 1985; Najenson et al., 1974).

The therapist is not required to predict but should consider the predictive factors listed herein when deciding on treatment goals or length of rehabilitation efforts. Cognition, personality, and motivation, all of which may substantially affect quality of survival (Jennett et al., 1981), are also to be considered in determining treatment goals. Outcome predictions are based on groups of patients, not on individuals, who may have family and character strengths that allow them to recover more completely than anticipated.

Intervention for Patients with Severe Alterations in Consciousness

Rehabilitation for patients with severe alterations in consciousness aims to foster alertness and behavioral responsiveness (Giacino et al., 1997) and to prevent complications associated with prolonged immobilization (Mysiw, Fugate, & Clinchot, 1996). Early intervention is believed to result in shorter rehabilitation stays and higher Rancho levels at discharge (Lippert-Grüner, Wedekind, & Klug, 2003). With contradictory evidence regarding its effectiveness, however, sensory stimulation remains particularly controversial (Giacino et al., 1997). Giacino et al. (1997) recommended that, at a minimum, patients with alterations in consciousness receive intervention that includes range-of-motion exercise, positioning protocols, and tone alteration methods. They suggested that the additional provision of sensory stimulation trials be considered on a case-by-case basis, appreciating that it is often difficult to distinguish between brain recovery and an intervention effect (Davis & Gimenez, 2003). Finally, reducing possible agitation (Eames, Haffey, & Cope, 1990) and supporting and educating overwhelmed family members are critical aspects of rehabilitation at this phase (Phipps et al., 1997).

For patients with alterations in consciousness, members of the rehabilitation team often have similar roles and responsibilities. For example, both occupational and physical therapists often perform range-of-motion exercises and collaborate to optimize positioning. All team members, including family, follow a consistent sensory stimulation protocol to enhance the reliability and interpretability of observations. For patients at this phase of recovery, intervention typically addresses first-level and developed capacities to lay the foundation for later focus on activities, tasks, and roles (Procedures for Practice 39-1). Because of the medical acuity of many of these patients, occupational therapists attend to the safety precautions summarized in Safety Note 39-1.

PROCEDURES FOR PRACTICE 39-1

Goal Setting for and with Persons with TBI

Occupational therapy treatment goals address changing aspects of occupational functioning as patients with severe TBI progress through recovery and adaptation. Here are some examples based on Chestnut et al.'s (1999) phases of recovery and adaptation.

Medical Treatment Phase (treatment focuses on first-level and developed capacities)

- In 3 weeks, the patient will make localized responses in less than 15 seconds after the presentation of tactile, olfactory, auditory, or visual stimuli at least 75% of the time to lay the foundation for using a communication board.
- In 3 weeks, the patient will demonstrate improvement in upper extremity range of motion, gaining at least 10% in shoulders and elbows, to facilitate ease and thoroughness with caregiver-provided hygiene activities.

Rehabilitation Phase (treatment primarily focuses on abilities and skills, activities and habits, and task competency)

- In 2 weeks, the patient will be able to follow a checklist to carry out personal hygiene tasks with no more than occasional specific cues.
- In 2 weeks, the patient will independently locate and follow a daily schedule in his planner.
- In 2 weeks, the patient will independently follow written and pictorial instructions to carry out his upper extremity range of motion exercises.

Survivor Phase (treatment primarily focuses on habits, competency in tasks, and satisfaction with life roles)

- In 4 weeks, the client will use compensatory cognitive strategies to structure his children's afternoon activities.
- In 4 weeks, the client will use an alarm cueing device to improve his completion of time-specific tasks at work.

POSITIONING

Occupational therapists collaborate with other members of the rehabilitation team to optimize positioning to normalize muscle tone and ultimately affect motor performance (Rinehart, 1990). Some typical abnormal positions seen in patients with severe traumatic brain injuries include abnormally forward head, protracted and forward-tipped scapulae with or without elevation, posterior pelvic tilt with unilateral retraction and/or elevation, severe trunk tightness with lack of trunk dissociation from neck and head, hip flexor and adductor tightness, and foot plantar flexion and inversion.

The patient's position must be reevaluated frequently. Assistive positioning supports are used intermittently and removed as the patient's neuromuscular status improves. The nursing staff and the patient's family must be made aware of the desired bed and wheelchair positioning and

SAFETY NOTE 39-1

Safety Precautions for Treating Patients in Altered States of Consciousness

The patient with a severe TBI may be referred for occupational therapy before he or she is completely medically stable. Precautions may be numerous because of systemic injuries, secondary effects of the brain injury itself, disturbance of basic body regulatory systems, and the life support equipment used to treat the patient; such precautions must be heeded by the therapist. Typical precautions are described here; other precautions may also be necessary and should be ascertained from the nurse, physician, or patient's chart before the evaluation begins.

- A major concern with acute brain trauma is control of intracranial pressure (ICP). Sustained increased ICP can be fatal (Jennett & Teasdale, 1981). The patient with an ICP monitor can be readily checked during treatment sessions. The therapist must closely observe patients not on a monitor for pupil changes; decreased neurological responses; abnormal brainstem reflexes; flaccidity; behavioral changes; vomiting; and changes in pulse rate, blood pressure, and respiration rate. Fluids may be restricted, or the patient's head may be positioned in neutral at 30° of elevation in an attempt to regulate ICP (Turner, 1985). Turning the patient's head to one side may obstruct the internal jugular vein and result in a sudden increase of ICP (Boortz-Marx, 1985). The neck should be neither flexed nor extended but kept in neutral for maximum venous drainage and decreased ICP. The presence of a family member, gentle touching, quiet talking, and stroking the face have been found to decrease ICP in adults (Mitchell, 1986). Side-lying with the head of the bed elevated is the most desirable position. Side-lying avoids the increased extensor tone promoted in supine. Prone lying is contraindicated with increased ICP, and supported sitting at 90° is used as soon as tolerated to help breathing, to provide symmetrical body alignment, and to increase awareness of surroundings (Palmer & Wyness, 1988).
- Early post-traumatic epilepsy occurs in 5% of patients with brain injuries, and late-onset epilepsy affects 20% of those with prolonged unconsciousness, depressed skull fracture, or intracranial hematoma (Jennett & Teasdale, 1981; Schaffer, Kranzler, & Siqueira, 1985). To reduce the chance of a seizure during treatment, begin tactile stimulation and range of motion slowly to assess the patient's physiological response. Monitor the heart rate, blood pressure, and facial color and any autonomic changes, such as sudden perspiration or increased restlessness. As the therapist becomes more familiar with the patient's responses, he or she gradually increases intensity of stimulation. Use seizure precautions: avoid rapid, repetitive stimuli, such as vibration, flickering lights, and an oscillating fan. If a seizure does occur, ensure that the airway is open, position the patient on his or her side to prevent aspiration of stomach contents, and summon medical assistance (Greenberg, Aminoff, & Simon, 1993). The patient's limbs should not be restrained during a seizure.
- If the patient has had a craniotomy for evacuation of a hematoma, the bone flap may be left off, and the brain may be covered only by scalp to allow the brain to expand. Direct pressure to this site must be avoided.
- The patient may have a tear in the dura and cerebrospinal fluid leak. In this case, the patient initially is treated with head elevation, antibiotics, and precautions against nose blowing (Jennett & Teasdale, 1981; Schaffer, Kranzler, & Siqueira, 1985).
- If the patient has other systemic trauma, such as fractures or chest cavity trauma, appropriate precautions must be taken when he or she is stimulated or moved. Care must also be taken to avoid disturbing intravenous lines, tracheostomy, nasogastric tube, endotracheal or respirator tubes, and traction for extremity fractures. If the patient has a nasogastric tube, caution must be taken that the patient's head remains above the level of his or her stomach to avoid regurgitation and aspiration (Miller, Pentland, & Berrol, 1990).

of the wearing schedule for any splints. To reduce abnormal tone and to reduce or prevent contractures, the positioning must continue throughout the day and night.

Bed

Side-lying or semiprone, if permitted, with good body alignment is preferable to supine if the patient has abnormal posture (Carr & Shepherd, 1980; Farber, 1982). Lying supine triggers an extensor response. In side-lying, the head, resting on a small pillow, should be in neutral alignment with the trunk; the bottom upper extremity should be in scapular protraction and humeral external rotation; the top upper extremity should be in scapular protraction, slight shoulder flexion, and resting on a pillow to avoid horizontal adduction; the bottom elbow should be flexed; the top elbow should be extended; wrists should be in extension; and cones should be placed in the hands to decrease spasticity and maintain thumb web spaces. A pillow between the knees decreases hip internal rotation and adduction. The lower leg also may need pillow support to align it with the thigh. The hip and knee are flexed only slightly. Elongation of the lower side of the trunk between the shoulder and pelvis is desirable. A side-lying trunk position may have to be maintained by a pillow or sandbag behind the back and shoulder. Footboards should be avoided because they elicit extensor thrust. Splints or special shoes (Farber, 1982) that are cut to avoid pressure to the ball of the foot but still maintain ankle flexion to 90° and reduce foot drop are used to avoid stimulating an extensor thrust.

If the patient must be supine, a small pillow under the head is used, with small rolled pillows under that pillow to keep the head in midline if the patient cannot do so. Furthermore, small pillows are placed under the scapulae to protract them, shoulders are positioned in slight abduction and external rotation, elbows are extended, and cones or finger spreaders position the fingers (Charness, 1986). If the pelvis is retracted on one side, a small folded towel is placed behind it, and that leg is positioned in neutral rotation. Some knee flexion should be encouraged by a small towel roll placed under the distal thigh just above the knee. Keep in mind that experts recommend a semirecumbent bed positioning (with head-of-bed angle maintained at 45°) to minimize risk of aspiration and pneumonia for patients on mechanical ventilators (Helman et al., 2003).

Wheelchair

Early and correct upright positioning in a wheelchair helps to facilitate arousal by stimulating the visual and vestibular systems, inhibiting abnormal tone, providing normal proprioceptive input, and reducing the likelihood and/or extent of contractures and complications from prolonged bed rest. The pelvis must be positioned correctly before other areas can be addressed. The pelvis should be in a neutral position or have a slight anterior tilt and should be symmetrical, without one side retracted or elevated. Weight bearing equally through both buttocks is essential to improvement of tone. Solid seat and back inserts are necessary, as the typical wheelchair seat and back sag and facilitate posterior pelvic tilt, unequal weight bearing through the hips, and hip internal rotation and adduction. If necessary, a small, flat lumbar roll is placed above the pelvis and below the scapula to facilitate anterior pelvic tilt. If the pelvis is retracted on one side, wedged back pieces may be helpful for positioning. If unequal weight bearing with habitual elongation of one side of the trunk is occurring, an insert under the habitual weight-bearing buttock may be helpful. The back of the chair may be reclined 10–15° to position the trunk and head more appropriately. Hip flexion of 90° can be achieved by a wedge cushion with the high end at the distal thigh. The seat belt should come from the corners of the seat at a 45° angle and fasten over the lower pelvis and hip area to help maintain the anterior pelvic tilt and equal weight bearing through the buttocks. The patient may need firm pads on the outer aspect of the thighs to reduce excessive abduction or a knee abductor to decrease excessive adduction. If the seat belt cannot keep the patient from scooting forward in the chair, a removable padded bar may have to be placed close to the pelvis and femurs.

The trunk, positioned next, should be symmetrical and in midline, with shoulders over pelvis in sagittal, frontal, and horizontal planes. Lateral trunk supports can be used to decrease lateral trunk flexion. Experimentation with the positioning is essential because trunk control varies among patients. The therapist must not provide too much trunk support, only enough to facilitate the patient's normal movement and control. With a solid seat and back, the patient may not require additional trunk support.

A harness, shoulder straps, or a chest strap may be necessary to prevent forward trunk flexion. These should not fasten directly on top of the shoulders but should extend a little higher before going through the seat back to fasten. An additional seat belt can also be placed horizontally across the anterior superior iliac crests to provide backward pressure (Charness, 1986).

Knees and ankles are flexed to 90°, heels are slightly behind the knees in sitting, feet are in neutral pronation-supination and inversion-eversion. The footplate should be large enough to support the whole foot. Ankle straps are avoided because they encourage plantar flexion in some patients; a foot wedge, heel loops, an insert behind the foot, special shoes, toe guards, or a combination of these may be helpful in decreasing abnormal tone and in achieving weight bearing on the heel.

The ideal upper extremity position is neutral scapular elevation or depression with the scapulae in slight protraction, slight shoulder external rotation, and slight flexion and abduction. Elbows are in comfortable flexion, and the forearm is in pronation. The wrists are in neutral flexion-extension and neutral ulnar-radial deviation; the fingers are relaxed; and the thumb is radially abducted. Excessive scapular retraction may require contouring of the seat back or reclining the seat unit by about 10°. Positioning of shoulder straps, chest straps, and/or lateral trunk supports may help to obtain adequate shoulder position.

A lapboard positioned at the proper height to allow good upper extremity weight bearing is helpful. The lapboard should not be pushed against the patient's abdomen but placed far enough away so the patient can flex forward slightly at the hips. There should be a cutout so that the lapboard fits around the patient, and the lapboard should be large enough to accommodate the whole arm. A V-shaped piece of dense foam can be positioned behind the patient's elbow to decrease elbow flexion and retraction of the arm off the back of the lapboard. The lapboard may also have a contoured surface for the hands. Hand fixation is avoided because it usually causes the patient to pull back against the fixation.

Ideally the head should be in midline, with cervical elongation and the chin tucked in slightly. It is important that positioning eliminate chin jutting and neck hyperextension. The position of the patient's shoulders and upper trunk influences head position. A customized head support may be required (Farber, 1982). Pressure directly to the occipital area elicits increased extensor tone of the head and trunk. Therefore, the pressure to right the head is applied up from the occipital process to each side of midline and around the forehead with a backward and downward pressure. Such a head support has to be fastened to a headrest, which is recessed so that the patient's head cannot push or rest against it. Lateral head supports may be necessary to position the patient's head adequately. See Chapter 18 for further discussion of wheelchair selection and positioning.

Passive Range of Motion

Passive range of motion (PROM) can be difficult when muscle tone is increased. Inhibitory movements opposite the abnormal tone are performed slowly, holding the stretch until muscles relax. Sudden stretch and inappropriate stimulation and handling should be avoided. Scapular mobility should be addressed before upper extremity PROM to free the scapula and facilitate normal scapular and humeral movement during the rest of PROM (Palmer & Wyness, 1988). PROM within the limits of pain and positioning helps to minimize contractures from heterotopic ossification (Citta-Pietrolungo, Alexander, & Steg, 1992). See Chapter 21 for a complete discussion of exercise to improve range of motion.

Splinting and Casting

The goals of splinting and casting are to decrease abnormal tone and increase the patient's functional movement. The patient's quality of movement is constantly reassessed to determine continued necessity of the splints or the need for modifications. Splints should be very carefully monitored when used with severely spastic or posturing patients, as they can aggravate abnormal tone and rapidly create pressure areas.

With severe spasticity in elbow, wrist, knee, ankle, or foot, plaster or fiberglass serial casting may be indicated (Mortenson & Eng, 2003; Pohl et al., 2002). Serial cylinder casting provides neutral warmth and more even skin pressure and allows for less movement than splints (Fig. 39-2). Casts are usually left on for 1–7 days before being replaced by a new one. Pohl et al. (2002) found that shorter cast-change intervals (1–4 days) provided improvements in range of motion that were comparable to longer intervals (5–7 days) but with fewer complications. Dropout casts, which leave a portion of the limb free to relax out of a tightly contracted position; bivalve casts, which are split in two, with moleskin protecting the edges so they can be removed during therapy and nursing procedures; and weight-bearing inhibitory casts, which are fabricated to approximate the ideal weight-bearing posture of the foot or hand, can also be used (Carr & Shepherd, 1980). Hill (1994) found casting more effective than traditional treatment of PROM, stretching, and splinting in reducing contractures in a group of 15 head-injured patients. The effect of casting on spasticity was variable, and Hill recommended further study. Decisions to use serial casting are informed by the patient's cognitive level. If the patient has

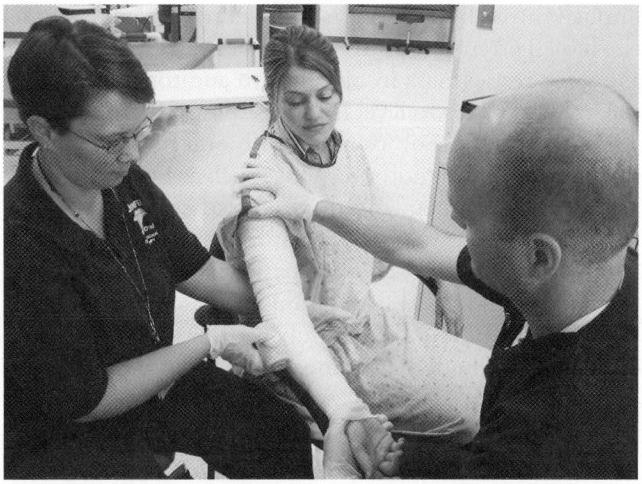

Figure 39-2 Occupational therapists fabricate a series of casts to help patients with brain injury improve range of motion and decrease spasticity. Casts are relatively inexpensive (as compared to splints), and can be replaced with new ones as the patient gains range of motion.

severe agitation, casts may pose safety problems (O'Dell, Bell, & Sandel, 1998). Casting is contraindicated with uncontrolled hypertension, major open wounds, unhealed fracture, impaired circulation, acute inflammation, and recent episode of autonomic dysreflexia, or if professionals need access to the extremity for lines or vitals (Stoeckmann, 2001). Rinehart (1990) recommended against casting more than one joint if the patient is confused or easily agitated or has short-term memory problems.

Sensory Stimulation

The goals of a sensory stimulation program are to promote arousal, appropriate patterns of movement, and interaction with the environment (Rinehart, 1990) by enhancing recovery processes such as neuroplasticity (Davis & Gimenez, 2003). Sensory stimulation programs are individualized to the patient's physical and cognitive functioning, but they always include multiple periods of observation and careful data collection (Mysiw, Fugate, & Clinchot, 1996). Clinicians use consistent protocols to standardize the administration of stimuli and data sheets to record observations regarding rate of response and changes in respiration, pulse, blood pressure, head movements, eye opening, eye movements, eye fixations, mimic responses, aimed and non-aimed motor reactions, and articulations (Lippert-Grüner & Terhaag, 2000). Responses are measured at the beginning and end of every session and as each sense is stimulated. Clinicians monitor observation records in the hopes of seeing patterns of increasingly specific responses to stimuli, signifying improved responsiveness.

Each stimulus is provided with a desired motor response in mind. The response is verbally requested and/or implied through the therapist's handling. Patients at Rancho level II often demonstrate non-specific responses, such as motor restlessness in response to auditory stimuli. As the patient moves to level III, the responses become more stimulus specific. For example, with oral motor stimulation, one expects a motor response such as lip closure.

Tactile, vestibular, olfactory, kinesthetic, proprioceptive, auditory, and visual stimuli are used. Gustatory stimulation may be used if the patient's oral motor status permits. Pleasant and unpleasant and familiar and unfamiliar stimuli are used; stimuli with emotional significance to the patient may be most likely to elicit a response. Trials of organized stimulation periods of 15–30 minutes each are scheduled throughout the day (for up to 90 minutes total). These sessions must be spaced to allow for rest and nursing care. The patient's response to stimulation may be quite slow because central nervous system processing is slowed or prevented by the damage. The therapist should wait for a response to the stimulation and, if necessary, repeat the stimulus. Procedures for Practice 39-2 describes how to administer various types of stimuli.

Management of Agitation

Once patients begin localizing stimuli, they may become quite agitated and restless (Scott & Dow, 1995). Post-traumatic agitation is reported to occur in the acute setting in 33–50% of patients with TBI (Sandel, Bell, & Michaud, 1998) and may last for days or weeks (Malkmus,

PROCEDURES FOR PRACTICE 39-2

Multisensory Stimulation

Stimuli are presented in a consistent and meaningful manner, typically one sensory modality at a time. The patient is told what the therapist is doing and often given an instruction specific to a desired response. Minimize competing visual and auditory stimuli by turning off the television, closing the door, or pulling the drape. Give simple, clear verbal feedback on every response elicited such as, "Good. You are turning your head toward my voice." Here are examples of how various types of stimuli are presented.

- Tactile stimulation focuses on the qualities of touch, pressure, and temperature (Lippert-Grüner & Terhaag, 2000). For example, rub patient's skin with items of various texture or temperature and use a firm or moving touch on the patient's limbs with verbal cues to orient the patient to his or her body. Performing passive range of motion provides both tactile and kinesthetic stimulation. Bathing and dressing are excellent sources of varied input, especially if verbal orientation to body parts being washed or moved is included.
- Provide gentle kinesthetic, proprioceptive, vestibular stimuli by changing body position (from supine to sitting, sitting to side-lying), by head and neck movements, rolling, tilting the bed to sitting, side-to-side or antero-posterior movement of the patient in bed or on a mat, or rocking. Gelling et al. (2003) recommend standing coma and minimally conscious patients (using electric standing frames or tilt tables) as the optimal means of enhancing arousal and awareness of the environment. **Kinesthetic, proprioceptive, vestibular stimulation may be contraindicated, however, in patients with a tracheostomy, elevated ICP, or seizures and therapists must seek physician approval and orders before providing intervention of this nature. The patient's reaction must be closely monitored during and after all stimulation, with careful attention to desired ranges of heart rate, ICP, and blood pressure.**
- Stimulate the olfactory sense with noxious or pleasant odors, such as spices, almond, vanilla, banana, lemon, perfume, coffee, or other smells familiar to the patient. This stimulation may be most effective when it is done before the patient is fed. The therapist must offer an effective concentration of the odor. Saturated cotton balls or a sniff bottle are held close to but not touching the patient's nose for 2–5 seconds (Farber, 1982). This cranial nerve is sometimes injured in TBI, so olfactory stimulation may not elicit a response (Jennett & Teasdale, 1981). **Avoid odors with fumes, such as ammonia and artificial vanilla, because they irritate cranial nerve V.** A tracheostomy or nasogastric tube eliminates or reduces the air passing through the nostrils and hence reduces the effectiveness of olfactory stimuli.
- Auditory stimulation consists of tapes of favorite music or familiar voices, bells, loud alerting noises such as clapping hands, direct conversation to the patient, verbal commands, explanations, and feedback. The therapist uses clear, firm speech, often presenting information to the patient regarding his or her circumstances and whereabouts. During therapy sessions, radios, televisions, and other noises should be eliminated as much as possible so that voice commands for motor responses or the selected auditory stimuli are the most prevalent auditory input.
- Provide visual stimulation to elicit attention, focus, and visual tracking with brightly colored objects, a mobile over the bed, mirrors, colored lights, a flashlight in a darkened room, or pictures of family and friends of the patient. Move brightly colored objects in front of the eyes, if they are open. Have the family label the pictures to assist in orienting the patient to them. Environmental changes from the bed to the therapy room or from indoors to outdoors are important sources of visual stimulation.

Booth, & Kodimer, 1980). Agitation is a subtype of delirium in the coma-emerging patient that is associated with frontotemporal injury, disorientation, comorbid medical complications, and/or use of anticonvulsant medication (Kim, 2002). Agitation causes excesses of behavior that include some combination of aggression, akathisia (motor restlessness or a sense of inner restlessness [Ivanhoe & Bontke, 1996]), disinhibition, and emotional lability (Center for Outcome Measurement in Brain Injury, 2006; Sandel, Bell, & Michaud, 1998).

Behavioral disorders associated with TBI have distinct causes and characteristics at various points of recovery (Eames, Haffey, & Cope, 1990). Eames, Haffey, and Cope suggested that efforts to manage behavior be preceded by a contextual assessment in which clinicians attempt to determine what factors are contributing to the problem. Clinicians examine the following variables:

- Personal context—extent and location of brain damage, state of bodily dysfunction, including pain, and pre-morbid factors such as intellect, personality traits, and coping style
- Social context—persons present during maladaptive behavior; reinforcers
- Physical context—properties of the environment in which problematic behavior occurs

During the period of medical instability, patients may exhibit agitation that stems from post-traumatic confusion and inability to process information (Eames, Haffey, & Cope, 1990). Patients may demonstrate apparently non-goal-directed body movements, such as thrashing; goal-directed behaviors, such as trying to remove life-sustaining tubes or get out of bed; screaming, moaning, or bizarre verbalizations; and disinhibited behavior, such as uncontrolled laughter or inappropriate sexual behavior (Eames, Haffey, & Cope, 1990). The primary aim of behavior management at this phase is to ensure the continuation of medically necessary treatment and to do as little as possible to impede the natural course of recovery (Eames, Haffey, & Cope, 1990). Procedures for Practice 39-3 has specific suggestions regarding management of agitation during occupational therapy sessions.

PROCEDURES FOR PRACTICE 39-3

Managing Agitation: Rancho Level IV

During this stage of recovery, occupational therapists primarily seek to decrease the patient's agitation by attempting to normalize the environment and employing appropriate physical management methods that allow the patient to move and release energy without jeopardizing safety (Eames, Haffey, & Cope, 1990; Kim, 2002). Remember that the patient is not accountable for the agitation, hostility, or aggressiveness. He or she is responding to internal confusion, not specifically to you as a person or professional. At the same time, you must structure your interactions to protect the patient and yourself.

Strategies to Normalize the Environment

- Minimize the influence of confusion by asking family members to bring in familiar objects (photographs or belongings) and position them so they are visible to the patient (Eames, Haffey, & Cope, 1990).
- Work in a quiet environment with minimal distracters that may further alarm or confuse the patient.
- Attempt to provide orientation information and maintain a predictable daily structure and routine to reduce confusion.
- Normalize interactions by introducing yourself at each session, telling the patient where he or she is and what you are going to do (Eames, Haffey, & Cope, 1990). Extend the same courtesies, even to comatose patients, that you would to patients without cognitive impairments (Eames, Haffey, & Cope, 1990).

Strategies for Physical Management

- Use equipment and devices that maximize freedom of movement along with safety. Mittens without separations for the thumb may keep patients from resisting care or from pulling out tubes. A floor bed (a mattress on the floor that is surrounded by portable walls lined with therapy mats) allows the patient to move freely in bed without risk of falling. Extensions to the wheelchair so that it can neither tip over backward nor fit through doorways also allow for safe mobility (Eames, Haffey, & Cope, 1990).
- Engage the patient in gross motor activities such as face washing, catching a ball, hitting a balloon, and putting on simple clothing, if he or she is able. Physical activity, walking, or even being wheeled in the wheelchair may help decrease agitation (Baggerly, 1986).
- Be prepared to change activity at the first sign that the patient is becoming restless or agitated. Consider moving to another environment or offering a drink or snack if the patient has normal oral motor activity. Avoid responding to obscenities or bizarre verbalizations; simply view them as cues to distract the patient with another activity.
- Exude calm, confidence, and acceptance; the patient needs you to provide consistency and predictability that counters his or her confusion.

Family Support and Education

TBI has almost as many implications for family members as it does for the patient. After a loved one undergoes a severe TBI, family members are typically relieved that the patient has survived but have little experience to help them understand the situation or what lies ahead (Phipps et al., 1997). Television portrayals of people who abruptly "wake" from coma with no apparent deficits may lead families to expect full recovery, and they may have difficulty processing information that is inconsistent with that hope (Phipps et al., 1997).

To truly collaborate with family members and provide right-timed education, clinicians try to learn about patient and family background. Clinicians are advised to employ interpersonal communication skills such as the use of reframing statements or clarifying questions to inquire about such matters as family structure, family routines and activities, and experiences with service providers (Sohlberg et al., 2001).

Many families relish the opportunity to contribute to their loved one's recovery. They support the therapist's efforts to position the patient and learn to perform PROM exercises. Family members also make important contributions to the sensory stimulation program by providing information about the patient's preferences, typical manner of responding, and background. They may also receive instruction so they can perform the sensory stimulation protocol and collect data on responses. Families often see a level of responsiveness that is not verifiable by staff, and early in recovery, they tend to interpret unresponsiveness in ways other than as a reflection of cognitive status, such as deafness, lack of interest, or laziness (Phipps et al., 1997). Since the patient's level of responsiveness often drives decisions about what services are appropriate, how long they will be provided, and whether the patient is making progress, tension between the overwhelmed family and rehabilitation team is fairly common (Phipps et al., 1997). By providing the family with clear and concise information that matches their most immediate concerns, therapists can help families begin to understand what has happened in ways that neither inflame expectations nor squelch hope.

Holland and Shigaki (1998) proposed a three-phase model for educating families and caretakers of persons with TBI. They suggested that families benefit from information that is relevant to the patient's stage of recovery and their own stage of adjustment. They recommended that, during the first phase (ICU through acute hospitalization), family education should focus on providing basic orientation to help the family decipher what is unfolding and to clarify terms and procedures associated with trauma care and TBI. Family members also need help to understand the disordered and occasionally bizarre behavior associated with agitation and to appreciate it as a natural part of recovery (Eames, Haffey, & Cope, 1990). Finally, conversations and instructions have to be repeated frequently, as the family is under considerable stress and flux (Livingston, 1990). (See Holland and Shigaki's excellent bibliography of phase-specific materials available for families, some of which are in Spanish, as well as Resources 39-1 for materials that could be used in family education.)

RESOURCE 39-1

Traumatic Brain Injury
American Occupational Therapy Association
Brain Injury Evidence Briefs and Structured Abstracts
www.aota.org (members only)

Brain Injury Association (BIA)
Provides information on brain injury, including resources for survivors, families, professionals, and on state BIA associations.
http://www.biausa.org

Among the excellent resources on this site is the "The Road to Rehabilitation" series, which are articles written for laypersons on an array of relevant topics that can be downloaded for free.
http://www.biausa.org/Pages/road_to_rehab.html

Center for Outcomes Measurement in Brain Injury (COMBI)
Assessment tools used in brain injury rehabilitation
http://www.tbims.org/combi

Family Caregiver Alliance
Provides resources for caregivers of individuals with chronic conditions including TBI
http://caregiver.org

MossRehab Resource Net
Provides consumer resources for persons with TBI
http://www.mossresourcenet.org/tbires.htm

National Institute of Neurological Disorders and Stroke.
Traumatic brain injury: Hope through research. Bethesda, MD: National Institutes of Health; 2002 Feb., NIH Publication No.: 02–158.
http://www.ninds.nih.gov/disorders/tbi/detail_tbi.htm

National Resource Center for Traumatic Brain Injury
The mission of this Federally funded center is to provide practical, relevant information about products to professionals, persons with brain injury, and family members.
http://www.neuro.pmr.vcu.edu/

Traumatic Brain Injury.com
Offers brief educational videos on TBI that can be viewed via the website on a personal computer
http://www.traumaticbraininjury.com

Traumatic Brain Injury Model Systems
Seventeen centers funded by the National Institute on Disability and Rehabilitation Research, National Institute of Health
http://www.tbindc.org

Rehabilitation

> "My occupational therapist (OT) has promised to take me to the hospital chapel to play the organ. My mom brought my organ books to the hospital. . . . Now I can show the therapists that I don't need their exercises . . .[and] don't belong here in the hospital." (Rain, 2000, p. 6)

Rehabilitation occurs in inpatient, outpatient, and residential settings for weeks, months, or years, although not continuously, until goals are achieved and/or the patient no longer appears to benefit from intervention. In general, the primary goals of inpatient rehabilitation are medical stability, reduction of physical impairments, and acquisition of basic self-care skills. Post-acute rehabilitation emphasizes reducing the obstacles of community integration posed by cognitive and behavioral impairments (Malec et al., 2000). Decreases in lengths of stay, however, often due to expiration of funding, results in many patients being discharged from inpatient rehabilitation settings without realizing their potential to recover capacities and basic skills (Yody & Strauss, 1999). Therefore, post-acute rehabilitation increasingly addresses medical needs, fundamental capacities, and basic skill acquisition before or instead of community reentry (Yody & Strauss, 1999).

Inpatient Rehabilitation

Patients can fully participate in intensive inpatient rehabilitation when they demonstrate stimulus-specific responses and when post-traumatic confusion and agitation either resolve or do not present a barrier to participation in intensive therapies, such as Rancho levels V and VI. At level V, patients are still disoriented and confused but increasingly goal directed (Heinemann et al., 1990) and capable of teaching–learning interactions (Abreu & Toglia, 1987). They cannot process information at a normal rate or produce an appropriate response to all environmental situations. A patient at this level may require maximum assistance for independent living skills, exhibit significant neuromuscular impairments, need maximum cueing for orientation, display severe memory impairment, possibly show confused verbal and mental processes, and have little carryover of new learning. As patients progress to Rancho level VI, they remain inconsistently oriented but begin to be aware of appropriate responses to staff and family and demonstrate carryover for relearned, familiar tasks (Hagen, 1998).

The value and effectiveness of inpatient rehabilitation are generally recognized by providers, consumers, and payers. Najenson et al. (1974) studied the outcome of 169 patients with severe brain injury who underwent a program using postural reflexes, self-care tasks, locomotor tasks, and communication training. The statistics showed that 84% of the patients were independent in daily living skills at discharge. The authors found recovery continuing up to 3 years after injury and stressed the need for continued follow-up of these patients after discharge from a rehabilitation hospital. Gerstenbrand (1972) described a rehabilitation program beginning in the acute stage after trauma that included use of reflexes to influence muscle tone and more active mobilization and socialization techniques later. He briefly stated the results for 170 patients in terms of being back at work and concluded that rehabilitation at full intensity was essential. Cope and Hall (1982) studied two groups of patients with severe brain injuries and compared the time required for rehabilitation and the outcome. The first group was admitted for rehabilitation less than 35 days post injury, and the second group was admitted more than 35 days post injury. The researchers concluded that those admitted later required twice as much rehabilitation as those admitted early, despite similar severity of initial injury. Outcome 2 years post injury, however, was not significantly different between groups. Finally, Heinemann et al. (1990) demonstrated that persons with moderate to severe TBI who received inpatient rehabilitation improved in self-care and mobility skills and maintained those gains at follow-up.

Assessment: Inpatient Rehabilitation

Patients with TBI who are in rehabilitation can participate in formal assessment. Occupational therapists often begin by screening vision, visual perception, and cognition. Chapters 8 and 9 detail numerous assessment tools and methods appropriate for persons at this phase of recovery from TBI, such as the *Galveston Orientation and Amnesia Test* (Levin, O'Donnell, & Grossman, 1979), *Loewenstein Occupational Therapy Cognitive Assessment* (Katz et al., 1989), and the *Patient Competency Rating Scale* (Prigatano et al., 1986). Clinicians must determine the extent to which patients can scan, attend, follow, and retain instructions to interpret performance on other traditional assessments, including upper extremity strength and function and activities of daily living. A number of tools developed specifically to assess patients with TBI are used in a variety of rehabilitation disciplines, including occupational therapy (Table 39-4). Others are detailed at www.tbims.org/combi.

Treatment: Inpatient Rehabilitation

Occupational therapy during inpatient rehabilitation is aimed at optimizing motor, visual-perceptual, and cognitive capacities and abilities; restoring competence in fundamental self-maintenance tasks; contributing to the patient's continuing behavioral and emotional adaptation; and supporting the patient's family as they prepare for discharge.

Optimizing Motor Capacities and Abilities

Therapists initially help patients optimize their motor capacities and abilities by engaging them in gross motor

Table 39-4. Assessment and Outcomes Tools for TBI Patients in Rehabilitation

Instrument	Brief Description
Supervision Rating Scale (SRS)[a] (Boake, 1996)	Measures level of supervision patient receives from caregivers. Based on interviews with patient and caregiver (such as nurse or family member), clinician rates on 13-point ordinal scale reflecting intensity and duration of supervision needed for safety. Ratings automatically sort patient into one of five levels of supervision: independent, overnight supervision, part-time supervision, full-time indirect supervision, or full-time direct supervision.
Functional Assessment Measure[a] (Hall, 1997)	12-item addition to *FIM*; relates to community functioning (i.e., car transfers, employability, adjustment to limitations, swallowing). Makes *FIM* more sensitive to the problems of persons with TBI.
Neurobehavioral Rating Scale (Levin et al., 1987)	27-item clinical rating scale measures common cognitive, behavioral, and emotional disturbances associated with TBI; used to track neurobehavioral recovery, measure behavioral change in response to intervention.
Mayo-Portland Adaptability Inventory[a] (Malec & Thompson, 1994)	Designed for interdisciplinary post-acute rehabilitation; covers broad range of observable attributes, such as physical function (including pain and mobility), cognitive capacity, emotional status, social behavior, self-care, work, and driving status. Based on team consensus, patient's status on 30 items is rated on a 4-category scale: no impairment; impairment on clinical examination but does not interfere with everyday function; impairment does interfere with everyday function; or complete or nearly complete loss of function.
Community Integration Questionnaire[a] (Willer, Ottenbacher, & Coud, 1994)	15-item instrument to assess home integration, social integration, productivity (employment, volunteer work, school); can be completed by self-report with assistance from family member.

[a] Available online at http://www.tbims.org/combi. *FIM, Functional Independence Measure.*

activities that they can perform almost automatically, such as playing catch or hitting a punching bag (Fig. 39-3). Such activities minimize the demands on weakened cognitive capacities, such as attention, concentration, and memory for instructions. Intervention increasingly focuses on refining motor capacities and abilities as the patient's motor and cognitive recovery progress. Patients perform traditional exercise regimens as well as exercise and activity delivered by virtual reality to improve strength and balance (Holden, 2005; Thorton et al., 2005) (Fig. 39-4). Occupational therapists use approaches that best match therapy goals and the patient's abilities, many of which are detailed in Chapters 21 to 27.

Optimizing Visual-Perceptual Capacities and Abilities

TBI frequently results in visual-perceptual disturbances that impair occupational function (Bouska & Gallaway, 1991). With TBI, the visual field loss is often in the superior fields; loss of acuity relates to loss of contrast sensitivity; and the oculomotor system is frequently impaired, with poor fixation, deviation of the eyes resulting in diplopia, and difficulty in visual scanning (Scott & Dow, 1995). Limitations in complex visual processing become evident during perceptual evaluation (Warren, 1993). Chapter 8 details specific assessments applicable to patients with TBI. As Quintana recommends in Chapter 28, intervention for primary visual deficits emphasizes environmental adaptation, compensatory techniques, assistive devices, and patient and family education. It is important to identify possible visual impairments as early as possible so that appropriate patients are referred for ophthalmology assessments and therapists can make an effort to circumvent the influence of visual impairments on performance. The efficacy of perceptual remediation is controversial. Based on her review of research on remedial perceptual retraining, Neistadt (1994a) was pessimistic about its appropriateness for TBI patients: "Far and very far transfer from remedial to functional tasks will not occur for clients with diffuse brain injuries and severe cognitive deficits, in either early or late stages of recovery, even with a variety of training tasks and up to 6 weeks of training" (p. 232).

Optimizing Cognitive Capacities and Abilities

Chapter 29 presents four general strategies for optimizing cognitive capacities and abilities: remediating the deficit, changing the physical or social context, acquiring behavioral routines, and learning compensatory cognitive strategies; all are appropriate for persons with TBI. Inpatients with TBI are typically in a period of relatively rapid improvement, so therapists provide cognitive remediation activities and exercises to challenge and stimulate primary cognitive domains (orientation, attention, memory) in the hope that natural recovery will be enhanced and accelerated. Card or board games, puzzles, and paper and pencil tasks, such as word recognition or letter or number cancellation drills, may be used. Computer programs can

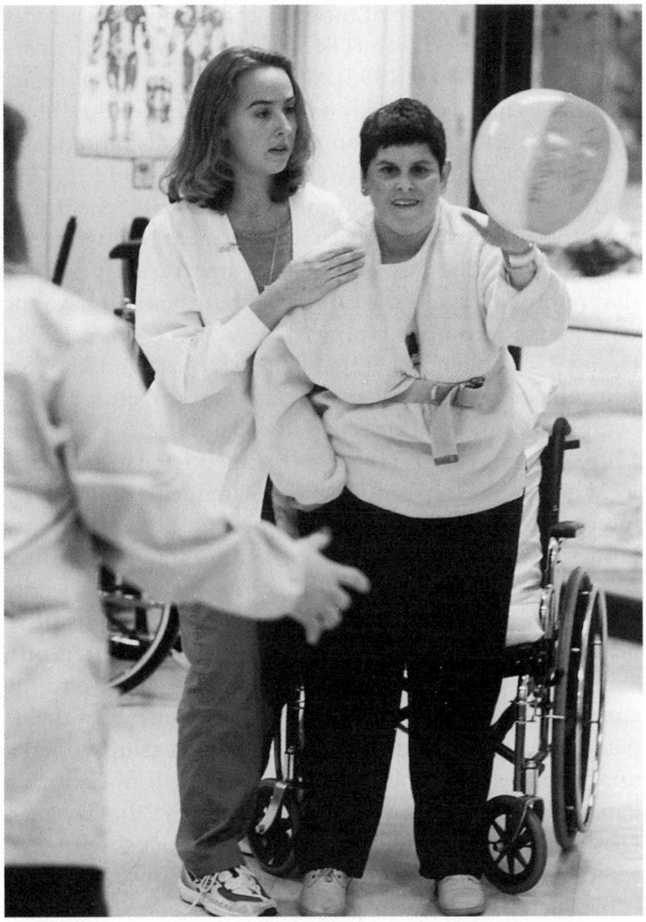

Figure 39-3 Early efforts to optimize motor function focus on eliciting automatic movement. Occupational and physical therapy co-treatment sessions are common.

help retrain the patient's ability to focus attention, increase visual scanning, improve reaction time, improve visual-motor coordination, improve simple problem-solving skills, and increase frustration tolerance. Patients may participate in group treatment, such as an orientation group in which they rehearse and reinforce awareness of date, place, and circumstances.

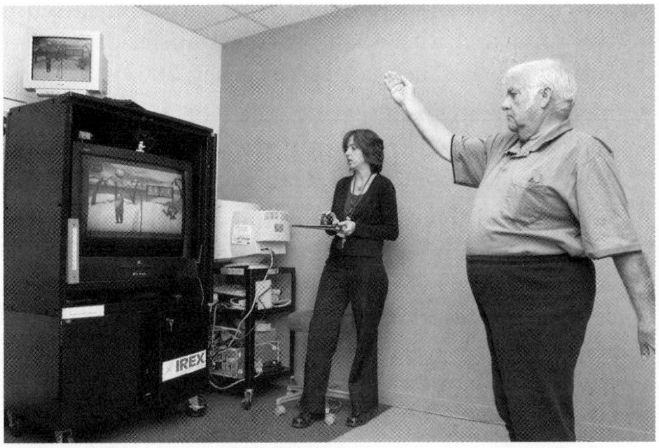

Figure 39-4 Virtual reality allows patients with brain injury to practice skills while participating in interesting and motivating activities that might otherwise be unsafe or unavailable to them.

The effectiveness of cognitive remediation has been questioned (Carney et al., 1999; Salazar et al., 2000), and other methods of optimizing cognitive capacities and abilities should also be employed. For example, Cicerone et al. (2000, 2005) suggest that evidence supports strategy training for attention deficits but not sole reliance on repeated exposure to and practice of computer-based tasks devoid of clinician involvement. Occupational therapists often use a dynamic investigative approach (Toglia, 1989) in which cognitive retraining activities become opportunities for assessing performance under a variety of circumstances. Careful activity analysis and logging of observations and environmental variables informs discharge recommendations to families regarding the circumstances in which their loved one is best able to function. Such information is invaluable to families as they assume day-to-day responsibility for structuring the patient's time and activities.

Occupational therapists also use the physical context to optimize patients' cognitive capacities and abilities during this phase of recovery. Specialized brain injury units typically incorporate signage and physical landmarks that enhance orientation and technology, such as monitoring systems, that allow the patient to move even though he or she may be confused and disoriented. Occupational therapists also strategically place familiar pictures and objects, calendars, and clocks in the patient's room to optimize orientation.

Patients in this phase of recovery rarely appreciate the significance and implications of cognitive impairments and therefore are usually not ready to learn to use compensatory cognitive strategies that require initiation and insight. Occupational therapists, however, often assemble a simple memory log and help patients use it to follow a schedule, reconstruct previous activities and instructions, and remember names of staff.

Restoring Competence in Basic Self-Maintenance Tasks

As previously mentioned, inpatient rehabilitation usually focuses on helping patients reacquire basic self-care skills, such as bathing, dressing, hygiene, and eating. In general, a given self-care task is simplified until the patient is consistently successful in performing it, and then the complexity is gradually increased while the externally provided structure is gradually decreased. Environmental distractions are kept to a minimum. The therapist structures the task, gathers the items to be used, and sequences the task by providing the patient with the appropriate item and instructions, one step at a time. For example, in dressing, the therapist first hands the patient his undershorts and then gives simple verbal instructions and physical assistance as necessary to have the patient put the shorts over his legs and pull them up. The therapist does not present the patient's tee shirt until the shorts are on. Initially, the therapist selects solid colors with minimal fastenings to decrease perceptual confusion. The therapist may also choose to limit the task by having the patient do only one or two steps of the entire task (e.g., put on tee shirt only) if the patient has very low endurance, low frustration tolerance, or limited motor skills. Selection of the position of the patient (i.e., dressing in bed, sitting in the wheelchair, or sitting on the edge of the bed) and the method of dressing is based on the patient's neuromuscular function. Gradually, as the patient becomes more successful in dressing, the therapist decreases verbal and physical cueing, using checklists and/or graded cues (see Chapter 29). Bathing, hygiene training, feeding, and wheelchair transfer training are structured in the same fashion. Occupational therapists can help set the stage for establishing consistent and automatic self-care routines at home by outlining the sequence of steps in which the patient is most successful.

During inpatient rehabilitation, occupational therapists assess the patient's ability to handle other self-maintenance tasks, such as preparing a sandwich, counting and handling money, and using the telephone (Fig. 39-5). Again, a dynamic investigative approach is employed to determine under what circumstances the patient can safely and competently carry out these activities.

Contributing to Behavioral and Emotional Adaptation

Behavioral sequelae may intermittently influence the patient's ability to participate in therapy at this stage. Brain damage itself may cause psychosocial changes, such as irritability, aggressiveness, or apathy (Prigatano, 1992). As the patient becomes more alert, his or her awareness of the situation may increase irritability, uncooperativeness, or mood fluctuations. Patients who lack awareness of deficits may also become frustrated with staff and family who limit their activities. Furthermore, patients who repeatedly fail on a variety of tasks may become depressed or anxious (Prigatano, 1992). It is important for occupational therapists to appreciate the state of internal chaos and vulnerability of many patients with TBI at this phase of recovery (Groswasser & Stern, 1998). Without the anchor of intact memory to make connections between experiences, "life is downgraded to a collection of unrelated, disjointed, and sporadic episodes" (Groswasser & Stern, 1998, p. 73). Rather than force confrontation of deficits, therapists avoid placing patients in situations that are fraught with frustration and failure and instead structure experiences that reinforce patients' confidence that they still have the potential to accomplish things (Groswasser & Stern, 1998). Doing so establishes therapeutic trust, the foundation for later phases of recovery, when patients are better able to compare pre-morbid and current capabilities. See Chapter 15 for guidelines to establish a therapeutic relationship.

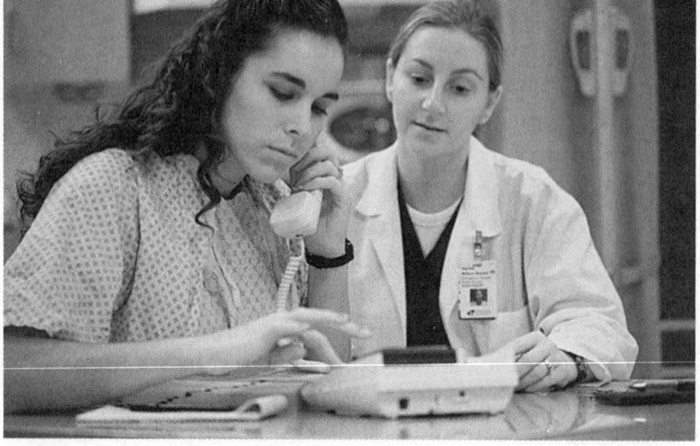

Figure 39-5 Occupational therapists often simulate real-life activities, such as using the telephone book and gathering information over the telephone.

When behavioral sequelae associated with brain injury interfere with progress and the potential for community reintegration, the rehabilitation team establishes an interdisciplinary plan to minimize or eliminate socially unacceptable behavior and promote prosocial, adaptive behavior. Eames, Haffey, and Cope (1990) pointed out, "Since the primary aim of rehabilitation is a return to the community, simple containment or toleration of disordered behavior within the rehabilitation setting is inadequate because the community at large will not adopt a lenient attitude toward such behavior" (p. 420). Ylvisaker, Jacobs, and Feeney (2003) recommend focusing on antecedents associated with positive behavior and less on consequences related to problems. The following are examples of strategies that contribute to patients' ability to learn effective behaviors during inpatient rehabilitation and beyond:

- Redesign or normalize the environment (Ylvisaker, Jacobs, & Feeney, 2003). For example, if noise and distractions seem to contribute to a patient's irritability and aggressiveness, provide treatment and care in areas that are calm and quiet.
- Capitalize on the superiority of procedural over declarative memory by helping patients learn context-sensitive routines rather than broader transfer-dependent strategies (Ylvisaker, Jacobs, & Feeney, 2003).
- Identify positive competing behavior, and as a team, consistently and frequently reward all instances of adaptive behavior (Eames, Haffey, & Cope, 1990).
- Withhold all rewards that maintain maladaptive behavior. Use time-outs in a calm, mechanical manner that does not reward the patient with increased social contact (Eames, Haffey, & Cope, 1990).
- Address cognitive impairments that may be contributing to maladaptive behavior.
- Help the patient to learn new skills and to experience success to reduce frustration-induced maladaptive behavior.

Supporting the Patient's Family

Patients' families continue to require information and support to understand the recovery and rehabilitation process and to inform their decision making and discharge planning. Holland and Shigaki (1998) recommended that the rehabilitation team provide the family with information about the following topics: (1) the full spectrum of possible TBI outcomes to enhance realistic expectations; (2) the effects of TBI on family systems and possible alterations in family dynamics post discharge; (3) the benefits, challenges, and responsibilities of caretaking and supervision post discharge; and (4) resources available for post-acute rehabilitation. Furthermore, by attending occupational therapy treatment sessions, family members encourage their loved one while learning about the patient's strengths and weakness and techniques for helping him or her optimize performance. Participation in inpatient rehabilitation also helps families to frame gains and improvements as continuations of a new start and to minimize expectations of an abrupt recovery to the "same person" the patient was before the injury (Phipps et al., 1997).

Post-Acute Rehabilitation

Malec and Basford (1996) described the array of post-acute rehabilitation programs in the literature and possibly available to clients with TBI. (The transition to references to the "client" rather than "patient" signifies the increasingly collaborative therapeutic relationship between therapist and TBI survivor during post-acute rehabilitation and survivor phases.) Occupational therapists are typically involved in all of these options, including the following:

- Home-based therapy provides a single discipline or interdisciplinary intervention for clients who are either unable to get to clinic-based services or who require context-specific training within the home environment.
- Residential neurobehavioral programs provide intensive treatment for clients with severe behavioral disturbances.
- Residential community reintegration programs provide integrated cognitive, emotional, behavioral, physical, and vocational rehabilitation to clients who cannot participate in outpatient programs because of severe cognitive and behavioral impairments or lack of availability of outpatient options.
- Comprehensive (holistic) day treatment programs provide integrated, multidisciplinary rehabilitation that emphasizes self-awareness, social skills, and cognitive compensation as precursors to return to work.
- Outpatient community reentry programs provide specific rehabilitation therapies as well as vocational services.

In their review article comparing outcomes of post-acute brain injury rehabilitation with natural recovery after TBI, Malec and Basford (1996) concluded, "Although generally uncontrolled, the studies reviewed document benefits for many individuals with brain injury, including increased independence and a rate of return to independent work or training that exceeds 50% and may reach 60% to 80% for intensive comprehensive (holistic) day treatment programs" (p. 198). Post-acute rehabilitation typically is not a continuous sequence of rehabilitation services but, more often, a time-limited, goal-specific series of rehabilitation episodes.

In general, the aim of post-acute rehabilitation is to prepare the client to reenter the community, although some programs also offer specialized tracks or pathways that focus on prerequisite physical, behavioral, cognitive, or self-care skills (Abreu et al., 1996). Compensation is emphasized; rarely do these programs focus on deficit remediation. While the occupational therapist's roles and responsibilities vary with the type and even location of the program, this section of the chapter reviews areas that are typically addressed. This section also discusses mild brain injury, as these survivors rarely receive inpatient rehabilitation services.

Occupational Therapy Assessment: Post-Acute Rehabilitation

Occupational therapists continue to use many of the instruments and methods described earlier in this chapter (see Table 39-4) and text. As clients have more real-world experiences and their self-awareness continues to improve, tools like the *Canadian Occupational Performance Measure* (*COPM*) (Law et al., 1994) become important for identifying treatment goals that are important to the client. Trombly, Radomski, and Davis (1998) used the *COPM* to select treatment goals with 16 adults with TBI who were in outpatient occupational therapy and to measure treatment outcome. This instrument, however, is not useful for clients with significant problems with insight and self-awareness because these individuals are unlikely to view themselves as having problems that can be addressed in therapy (E. S. Davis, personal communication, September 7, 1998). In the aforementioned study, for some clients, progress was marked by self-rated decreases in performance scores at discharge, reflecting improved accuracy of self-appraisal (E. S. Davis, personal communication, September 7, 1998).

Treatment: Post-Acute Rehabilitation

After discharge from acute rehabilitation, many clients require occupational therapy treatment aimed at teaching them to compensate for residual cognitive and visual-perceptual impairments so that they may resume self-maintenance, self-advancement, and self-enhancement roles.

Optimizing Cognitive Capacities and Abilities

In post-acute rehabilitation, clients (usually in Rancho level VII or VIII) may continue to demonstrate specific impairments in short- and long-term memory, reasoning, conceptualization, comprehension, abstract thinking, information-processing speed, organization of information, simplification of problems, judgment, and problem solving (Dikmen, Reitan, & Temkin, 1983; Gianutsos, 1980). They may display decreased attention during attempts to store information, inability to determine the salient or relevant details of what they hear or read, decreased ability to structure or associate incoming information appropriately, and decreased cognitive flexibility (Scherzer, 1986). Especially if the client also has decreased self-awareness, these impairments will affect his or her ability to make coherent decisions and plan for the future.

Occupational therapists continue to help clients and their families to change the physical and social context to optimize occupational functioning. This may include decreasing stimulus arousal properties and increasing important visual cues at the home and work site to optimize cognitive function. Home and work site visits allow therapists to identify opportunities for these modifications. Also, because clients in post-acute rehabilitation have a more stable living situation than they did as inpatients, their occupational therapists can capitalize on consistency of clients' environments and daily activities to help them create routines and habits that minimize the demands of information processing with frequently performed tasks. Occupational therapists also use a variety of activities and exercises, such as computer games, worksheets, crafts and projects, and simulated work tasks, to help clients improve their awareness of strengths and weaknesses. As clients appreciate the significance of residual cognitive impairments and implications for resumption of roles, occupational therapists teach them to use compensatory cognitive strategies, such as day planners, alarm cueing devices, and problem-solving schemata, in the context of personally relevant real-world tasks (see Chapter 29).

Optimizing Visual-Perceptual Capacities and Abilities

Similarly, occupational therapists continue to help clients make changes in environment and strategy to circumvent the influence of visual-perceptual impairments. For example, Williams (1995) described occupational therapy intervention for problems with reading and writing of a woman who was more than 12 months post TBI. A comprehensive low-vision evaluation performed by an ophthalmologist and occupational therapist revealed adequate central visual acuity, slightly reduced contrast sensitivity, an inferior visual field cut in both eyes, and a dense scotoma bordering the fovea in both eyes. Intervention, which consisted of changes in lighting for reading and writing, oculomotor exercises, and strategy training, ultimately allowed her to resume these valued activities.

Restoring Competence in Self-Maintenance Roles

Clients who have not achieved independence in basic self-care and homemaking tasks continue to work toward those goals in post-acute rehabilitation. Giles et al. (1997) used behavioral training to help TBI clients in a transitional living center develop independence in dressing and washing skills in a relatively short period (11–37 days) of treatment. Even clients with proficient self-care skills benefit from treatment that links individual skills to automatic routines (see Chapter 29). Based on performance on the *Rabideau Kitchen Evaluation-Revised* (Neistadt, 1992), Neistadt (1994b) used a meal preparation protocol to help outpatients with TBI learn to prepare a hot beverage and snack. After three 30-minute sessions per week for 6 weeks, participants made gains reflecting improvements in independence and decreased their performance times. Intervention specific to self-care and homemaking always involves input from family and/or caregivers and measures to ensure transfer of newly acquired skills to the client's living environment.

When client and family are satisfied with the client's ability to perform physical daily living skills and homemaking tasks, such as cleaning, meal preparation, and laundry, occupational therapy addresses community and necessary survival skills. Many clients rely on occupational therapy to help them relearn to manage money, write checks, go shopping, use the bank and post office, move in crowds, handle architectural barriers, and use public transportation, the telephone, the newspaper, and the phone book. To do so, clinicians again adapt the environment, help clients acquire behavioral routines, and teach clients to use compensatory strategies.

The therapist must carefully assess the amount of supervision and structuring necessary because of impaired judgment and problem-solving ability. The client's ability to bend over and get something from a lower cupboard, climb on an escalator, cross the street safely, organize time adequately, manage finances, and interact with others in a functional manner factor into occupational therapy recommendations regarding the need for continuing assistance or supervision.

Almost as soon as they are discharged from the hospital, many survivors of TBI inquire about their readiness to drive. The client's residual physical, cognitive, perceptual, and visual dysfunction must be thoroughly assessed to determine his or her ability to drive safely. The client's psychosocial status, including self-control, impulse control, and frustration tolerance, must be also carefully considered. A complete history of the medical status, current medications, and driving record is also taken. Simulated driving on a computer is helpful if available. A car can be adapted to compensate for some physical problems (see Chapter 31), and the client can be trained to compensate for visual field neglect (Scott & Dow, 1995). No compensation, however, can be made for slowed reaction to emergencies, lack of judgment or problem-solving ability, spatial or directional confusion on the road, impairment in depth perception, or decreased endurance (Jones, Giddens, & Croft, 1983). Following evaluation, if the client appears suitable for driving, an on-the-road test covering all driving situations is performed in a dual-control car or the patient's own car, with the assistance of an adaptive driving instructor (Jones, Giddens, & Croft, 1983). The therapist performing a driving evaluation should be familiar with the department of motor vehicle regulations applicable in that state.

Restoring Competence in Self-Enhancement and Self-Advancement Roles

Occupational therapy plays an important role on the post-acute rehabilitation team by helping the client resume previous leisure activities or determine new leisure outlets that are more in line with current abilities. Since lack of initiative and cognitive inflexibility may hinder independence in play and leisure skills, occupational therapists teach clients to use planning and structuring strategies to ensure an optimal balance in their activities.

Many survivors of TBI have to change not only what they do for fun but also with whom they do it. Few friendships withstand the cognitive, behavioral, and emotional upheaval that comes with TBI. Occupational therapy intervention may focus on helping the client initiate new social contacts, participate in support groups, and reestablish the social skills necessary for maintaining and building a social network. Social skills retraining following severe head injury develops skill in social behaviors and facilitates successful social interactions. In general, behavioral learning methods are the most effective for training severely brain-injured individuals to overcome social skill impairments (Giles & Clark-Wilson, 1993). Treatment typically entails instruction and modeling of the social skill, practicing the skill with feedback, and shaping the skill until it is used correctly (Boake, 1991). For example, Yuen (1997) reported how positive talk training (learning to give compliments) in occupational therapy helped a man who was 20 years post TBI to engage in social interactions that were not riddled with what had become his usual style of negative, sarcastic comments. Gutman (1999) described use of a set of guidelines for occupational therapy to help adult men with TBI to achieve greater satisfaction with male social roles.

Once clients reestablish their competence in self-maintenance roles, they are ready to explore return to work. Post-acute occupational therapy facilitates that process with pre-vocational programs that focus on work behaviors and habits, such as punctuality, thoroughness, response to feedback, and ability to take and use notes. Occupational therapists may also link clients with appropriate volunteer jobs where they can employ newly learned compensatory cognitive strategies and build their endurance and work tolerance.

Contributing to Behavioral and Emotional Adaptation

As clients attempt to resume familiar activities, they cannot escape the awareness that they have changed in some manner (Groswasser & Stern, 1998). Emotional and behavioral difficulties can be attributed to pre-morbid personality and coping style, cognitive consequences of TBI, and/or grief associated with injury-related losses (Hanks et al., 1999). These emotional and behavioral changes may include social or sexual disinhibition, low tolerance for frustration or stress, reduced insight or judgment, labile affect, irritability, impulsivity, and depression (Jorge et al., 1993). In the extreme, the patient may experience psychiatric disorders such as paranoia, phobias, confusion, or delusional ideation (Ashman et al., 2004; Benton, 1979). Regardless of the specific goals of therapy, occupational therapists support and guide clients with TBI as the clients confront and address impairments and inefficiencies that interfere with performance. Clinicians maintain dual roles as reassuring companion and objective observer by providing sensitive and timely feedback regarding behaviors that could otherwise result in rejection and social isolation in the community. As depression negatively influences psychosocial functioning after TBI (Hibbard et al., 2004; Ownsworth & Fleming, 2005), occupational therapists also respond to indicators that clients may be in need of psychological or psychiatric intervention and make referrals as needed (see Chapters 10 and 35).

Supporting the Client's Family

In most cases, the client's family ultimately provides long-term assistance and support for the survivor, and the family's stresses apparently do not decrease over time as do the stresses related to other traumatic injuries (Muir, Rosenthal, & Diehl, 1990). As time passes and the client moves through the rehabilitation continuum, the implications of the injury become clearer, and many families feel losses as "partial death" (Muir, Rosenthal, & Diehl, 1990, p. 436). The person they knew, loved, and depended on to fulfill their expectations is "dead," and long-established roles within the family have changed. Since the course of recovery is unknown (filled with hope, euphoria, and despair), family members undergo mourning that is intense, disorganized, and prolonged (Muir, Rosenthal, & Diehl, 1990).

Many roles within a marriage change when a spouse has a TBI, including roles as provider and parent. Less discussed are changes in sexual roles because of primary and/or secondary sexual dysfunctions (Griffith, Cole, & Cole, 1990). Primary sexual dysfunctions result directly from the brain injury and resultant neural or endocrine disorders influencing sexual interest, activity, responses, and fertility (Griffith, Cole, & Cole, 1990). For example, sexual activities may be altered or inhibited by any of a number of motor or sensory disorders, such as hypertonicity or apraxia (Griffith, Cole, & Cole, 1990). Secondary sexual dysfunctions and disturbances of psychosocial abilities or sexual responses because of cognitive impairments and psychological reactions range from hypersexuality syndromes to total apathy and inactivity (Griffith, Cole, & Cole, 1990). Partners with TBI may exhibit disinhibited behaviors that are inappropriately provocative or seductive or break unwritten rules regarding personal space and touching (Gronwall, Wrightson, & Waddell, 1998). Forgetfulness regarding aspects of personal hygiene further add to the distance and even engender repulsion between previously affectionate partners. Occupational therapists can help clients and their partners resume satisfying sexual roles, first by being willing to discuss matters of intimacy and sexuality. Couples may be referred for medical assessment of primary sexual dysfunctions and counseling for some aspects of secondary sexual dysfunctions. Inappropriate social and sexual behaviors should be addressed in a deliberate and consistent manner by the rehabilitation team.

Finally, occupational therapists continue to support families by providing education (Research Note 39-1). Holland and Shigaki (1998) recommended emphasis on the following topics in family education at this phase of recovery and adaptation: (1) the protracted nature of TBI recovery, (2) the experience of recovery from the patient's perspective, (3) adjustment to and possible management of behavioral and personality changes, (4) sexuality issues, (5) community resources, and (6) home adaptation.

Mild Brain Injury

It is estimated that, each year, more than 1.1 million people in the United States experience a mild brain injury (National Center for Injury Prevention and Control, 2003). Mild brain injury has been defined as a traumatically induced physiological disruption of brain function as manifested by at least one of the following: any period of loss of consciousness, any loss of memory of events immediately before or after the accident, any alteration in mental state at the time of the accident, and focal neurological deficits that may or may not be transient (American Congress of Rehabilitation Medicine [ACRM], 1995a). Symptoms of mild brain injury may include nausea, dizziness, headache, blurred vision, cognitive deficits, and behavioral changes (ACRM, 1995a). Most people with a mild brain injury return to normal functioning within 1–3 months (Ruff, Camenzuli, & Mueller, 1996), although approximately 10% of patients continue to have problems a year after injury (Ruff, Camenzuli, & Mueller, 1996).

Experts disagree about the persistence and cause of cognitive problems after mild TBI (Dikmen, Machamer, & Temkin, 2001). Some link cognitive inefficiencies to acute stress disorder (Bryant et al., 2003), while others attribute disability to brain damage (deKruijk, Twijnstra, & Leffers, 2001). Montgomery (1995) described a multifactor explanation for disability after mild TBI. He suggested that personal factors (perfectionism or tendency toward negative

RESEARCH NOTE 39-1

Abstract: Wells, R., Dywan, J., & Dumas, J. (2005). Life satisfaction and distress in family caregivers as related to specific behavioural changes after traumatic brain injury. *Brain Injury*, 19, 1105–1115.

The purpose of this study was to determine the extent to which TBI-related behavioral sequelae, coping strategies, and life circumstances predicted caregiver satisfaction. TBI-related neurobehavioral changes, caregiver coping strategies, satisfaction with caregiver role, and overall life satisfaction were examined using multivariate regression analyses. Seventy-two pairs (survivor with TBI and family caregiver) completed questionnaire packets. Family members had an average of 10 years in the caregiving role. Survivors with TBI completed a self-report version of the *Brock Adaptive Functioning Questionnaire* (*BAFQ*) (ratings of neurobehavioral functioning). Caregivers completed the *Caregiving Questionnaire, Symptoms Checklist, Satisfaction with Life Questionnaire,* and *Methods of Coping Inventory* and also a version of the BAFQ to capture their appraisal of their loved one's neurobehavioral functioning.

Overall, caregivers in this study expressed more positive than negative feelings about their caregiving role. The nature of their loved ones' neurobehavioral deficits and coping strategies employed appeared to affect caregiver outcomes. Engaging the support of family appeared to be the most effective way to avoid depression and anxiety. While poor impulse control on behalf of the survivor was associated with caregiver anger and irritability, lack of empathy on behalf of the survivor was identified as most detrimental to the caregiver's life satisfaction.

Implications for Practice

- Because family caregivers assume long-term responsibility for survivors of severe traumatic brain injury, their coping and satisfaction are of importance to occupational therapists.
- As social support appears to be linked to caregiver coping and satisfaction, occupational therapists encourage family caregivers to avail themselves of friends' and family assistance as well as to participate in local brain injury support groups.
- It is critical that family caregivers understand the neurobehavioral consequences of traumatic brain injury, especially the possibility that cognitive dysfunction may contribute to problems with empathy. As family members understand that the survivor with TBI may be cognitively unable to appreciate or even recognize their sacrifices and efforts, they may adjust expectations and seek affirmation and support from other sources.
- Occupational therapists assure family members that, despite the challenges involved, many long-term caregivers report positive feelings about their caregiving roles.

thinking) interact with transient sequelae of mild brain injury, such as headache and mental inefficiency, that lead to short-term decrements in performance. Premature resumption of normal activities places an undue load on information-processing capacities that leads to errors and slowness of performance. Over time, the individual begins to make misattributions of causation and starts questioning his or her fundamental competence and even sanity (Montgomery, 1995). These individuals profit from outpatient rehabilitation services that address residual physical symptoms, provide information and support, and teach them to use cognitive compensatory strategies that decrease the demands on working memory. By normalizing and explaining cognitive inefficiencies, helping reestablish routines, and teaching use of memory backups such as day planners, occupational therapists can play a pivotal role in helping these clients resume pre-morbid tasks and roles.

Clinicians need to appreciate that persons with mild brain injury who find their way to rehabilitation professionals represent a fraction of the cases with mild TBI and that cognitive problems may be observed for a variety of reasons that have nothing to do with brain injury (artifacts from testing, pre-existing conditions, litigation, emotional problems) (Dikmen, Machamer, & Temkin, 2001). Given the disagreement regarding the mechanism underlying cognitive problems after mild TBI, it is not surprising that there is little consensus about the best intervention. At present, there is little in the literature to guide occupational therapists looking for an evidence-based approach to intervention. Existing studies do not specifically mention occupational therapy intervention, which is why there is no evidence table to accompany the mild brain injury case example in this chapter.

Survivorship

> "I have been living with multiple effects of a severe TBI for 23 years. . . . Many of these years were spent in lonely isolation, wondering when the nightmare would end. . . . Now, I am focusing my energy on reaching out as well as within to live this life." (Rain, 2000, p. 6)

The medical treatment and rehabilitation phases of life for the survivor are relatively brief compared to the years, even decades, during which he or she will continue to live with the consequences of TBI. Most survivors ultimately achieve independence in self-care skills and recover motor function (Olver, Ponsford, & Curran, 1996), but cognitive, behavioral, and emotional problems are long-term barriers to good quality of life (Klonoff, Snow, & Costa, 1986; Koskinen, 1998). Olver, Ponsford, and Curran (1996) compared outcome after TBI 2 years and 5 years post injury for Australian survivors of moderate to severe injury. Survivors improved in terms of independence in self-maintenance tasks but had more complaints about cognitive, behavioral, and emotional issues at 5 years post injury than at 2 years post injury. More than 60% of their subjects 5 years post injury complained of memory problems, fatigue, and irritability; more than 50% reported that they had lost friends and had become more socially isolated. Koskinen (1998) described a similar pattern in her follow-up study of Finnish survivors of severe TBI 10 years post injury. Subjects indicated that the most unsatisfying aspects of their lives were contacts with friends, sexuality, and leisure activities. Neurobehavioral and emotional consequences of TBI had significant effects on both the quality of life of survivors and level of strain felt by family caregivers.

Olver, Ponsford, and Curran (1996) reported that fewer survivors were working 5 years post injury than 2 years post injury (50% of the sample was employed at 2 years; 40% was employed at 5 years), which is of particular concern, since employment appears to be linked to quality of life after TBI (O'Neill et al., 1998). O'Neill et al. found that being employed part or full time contributed to survivors' sense of well-being, social integration, and pursuit of meaningful home activities. In fact, individuals who worked part time had fewer unmet needs, were better integrated socially, and more often engaged in home activities than full-time workers, presumably because of more discretionary time and energy.

These long-term and often unmet needs underscore the importance of intermittent long-term rehabilitation services and community resources for persons with TBI. Unfortunately, most rehabilitation services remain medically oriented, focusing heavily, often exclusively, on intervention for physical impairments. Koskinen (1998) reported that survivors with physical deficits received rehabilitation services over a 10-year period, but physically functioning individuals with cognitive, behavioral, or emotional problems had no possibilities for rehabilitation of any kind. Unfortunately, depression represents a barrier to psychosocial functioning for years after TBI (Hibbard et al., 2004).

The contrast between need and service availability is particularly disturbing to occupational therapists who have the education and skills to make a difference in the lives of survivors of TBI. For example, Nelson and Lenhart (1996) described a case in which weekly outpatient occupational therapy sessions over 5 months helped a woman who was 5 years post TBI to improve her ability to handle school, household, and social responsibilities. Trombly, Radomski, and Davis (1998) and Trombly et al. (2002) found that adults with TBI met self-identified goals in outpatient occupational therapy, many of whom were more than 2 years post injury.

The survivorship phase of life for persons with TBI presents opportunities for clinicians to employ all that is truly unique to occupational therapy, synthesizing the totality of our education, philosophy, and values to enhance occupational functioning in society. Readers are challenged to consider the following ways to poise themselves for action:

- Recommend that a life care plan be prepared for survivors of moderate to severe TBI (Sherer, Madison, & Hannay, 2000). Based on expert diagnosis and prognosis, a life care plan delineates the services and items required for the current and long-term care of the survivor as well as the costs of these services (Sherer, Madison, & Hannay, 2000). The life care plan can be used clinically to plan appropriate long-term care, including intermittent follow-up, and for forensic purposes, such as determination of an appropriate settlement that will provide for the lifetime needs of the injured person (Sherer, Madison, & Hannay, 2000). In fact, occupational therapists have the background to be credentialed to prepare life care plans for the disabled.
- Promote to possible referral sources what you as an occupational therapist are able to do to enhance community integration and quality of life for persons with TBI. Join your local brain injury association; connect with your state's vocational rehabilitation division; familiarize yourself with key personnel supporting disabled students at local colleges and universities. Showcase your contribution to clients' occupational function in your documentation. Access resources that will allow you to maintain your expertise (Resources 39-1).
- Establish the kind of therapeutic relationship with clients that will make them want to return to you for help. Respecting the client's readiness for treatment means sometimes not intervening but making sure that he or she knows that your door is open in the future.
- Make sure that the discharge from outpatient occupational therapy incorporates plans for follow-up and clear information regarding possible circumstances in the future when further occupational therapy services may be helpful. Provide information to the survivor and his or her family regarding mechanisms to reinstate services. Remember that the nature of TBI interferes with survivors' ability to advocate for themselves (e.g., lack of initiation, impaired memory), and so you must build in opportunities to discern and respond to their needs.

CASE EXAMPLE #1

K.R.: Occupational Therapy During Acute and Rehabilitation Phases of Recovery from Severe TBI

Occupational Therapy Intervention Process	Clinical Reasoning Process: Objectives	Clinical Reasoning Process: Examples of Therapist's Internal Dialogue
Patient Information K.R. is a 20-year-old college student who sustained a TBI in a motor vehicle accident. Prior to the accident, K.R. was a physics major described by family as dependable and hard-working, with a 3.8 grade point average during his first 2 years of college.	Understand the patient's diagnosis or condition	"K.R.'s recent medical history suggests that he had a severe brain injury and will likely require occupational therapy services and other rehabilitation services throughout the continuum of care (acute medical, inpatient, outpatient, follow-up)."
Examination in the emergency department revealed a laceration over his forehead and right pneumothorax. His blood alcohol level was 0.226 (more than twice the legal limit). He had an initial *Glasgow Coma Scale* score of 3. Intracranial pressure was elevated. He sustained facial fractures and an undisplaced right suprapubic ramus fracture. Serial computed tomography demonstrated diffuse axonal injury, edema, and right posterior temporoparietal intraparenchymal hemorrhage. Within the first week of the TBI, a tracheostomy and feeding tube were inserted, and shortly	Know the person	"From what his parents tell me, K.R. sounds like a really hard-working guy. Apparently, in addition to his course work, K.R. worked 16 hours a week as a dishwasher in his dormitory. It sounds like K.R. tends to be quiet and soft-spoken but enjoys the company of a small circle of friends. I found out that his leisure interests include golf, cross-country skiing, and playing piano. It was really worth the time it took to talk with K.R.'s parents. I can tell that I will like working with them, and the information they provided me with will

thereafter, K.R. underwent open reduction and internal fixation of the right zygomatic maxillary complex fracture.

Occupational and physical therapy were initiated 10 days post injury, with orders for range of motion, positioning, and assessment of response to sensory stimuli. At the time he was first seen in occupational therapy just before his transfer from ICU to the medical unit, his passive range of motion (PROM) was within normal limits for all extremities; muscle tone was unremarkable. K.R. did not speak or follow commands consistently. He was frequently observed to thrash around, primarily moving his left side, and at times, his movement appeared purposeful (pulling at tubes, seeming to scratch his right leg with his left foot). He appeared to track objects with his left eye inconsistently. His initial total score on the *Western Neuro Sensory Stimulation Profile* was 23, and he was believed to be functioning at a Rancho level II to III (increasingly responsive to specific stimuli).

help me as I try to make therapy interesting and engaging for K.R."

Reason for Referral to Occupational Therapy

After less than a week on the medical step-down unit, K.R. was transferred to the inpatient brain injury rehabilitation unit and was again referred to occupational therapy and to physical therapy, speech-language pathology, and neuropsychology (he was 3 weeks post injury). He was referred to occupational therapy to assess responsiveness to stimuli, positioning, neuromuscular reeducation, and ADL training as appropriate. Consistent with his acute hospitalization, a family member (typically his mother) was present at most therapy sessions.

Appreciate the context

"The transfer from the medical unit to the rehabilitation unit represents a significant change in K.R.'s care. There is much more stimulation on the rehabilitation unit, and the overall emphasis of care changes from one of medical survival to recovery and adaptation."

Develop provisional hypotheses

"I anticipate that, by putting in place formal interventions and observational protocols, we will be able to maximize K.R.'s responsiveness to stimuli and ultimately his ability to benefit from rehabilitation. It will be important to involve his family for their sake as much as for his."

Assessment Process and Results

- *Western Neuro Sensory Stimulation Profile* was readministered, and K.R. obtained scores ranging from 54–80, with notable improvements in auditory comprehension, visual tracking, object manipulation, and arousal and attention.
- During assessment, K.R. sustained eye contact less than 25% of the time and was awake for approximately 15 minutes of each session. He horizontally tracked across midline with both eyes approximately 50% of the time and tracked vertically in one direction somewhat less. He generally followed gross motor commands approximately 25% of the time.
- Minimal formal assessment of K.R.'s right upper extremity function was performed, but he was observed to not use or move it. His range of motion appeared to within normal limits for both upper extremities.
- During assessment, it was evident that K.R. could not contribute to any aspect of ADL.

Consider evaluation approach and methods

"I need to primarily rely on observational methods during assessment and carefully document what I am seeing so that I will be able to detect changes in responsiveness and function."

Interpret observations

"I am finding that my assessment sessions really blur with treatment; it seems I am doing both at all times. I am encouraged that K.R. is demonstrating more specificity in his overall responses. While his speech is not intelligible, he seems to be making more frequent verbalizations. Since he came to the rehab unit, I am noticing that he can participate for longer periods of time, and that is encouraging as well."

Occupational Therapy Problem List

- Decreased arousal and attention
- Decreased and inconsistent visual tracking
- Inability to follow commands consistently
- Decreased right upper extremity function
- Dependence in activities of daily living (ADL)

Synthesize results

"K.R.'s overall responsiveness appears to be steadily improving based on records of his status on the acute medical unit. I am going to try to use my interventions related to ADL and upper extremity function as vehicles to improve arousal and attention."

Initial Occupational Therapy Goal List

Because it was difficult to predict the patient's rate of recovery or response to therapy, the team set goals for 2-week intervals, with the understanding that the patient's length of stay on the rehabilitation unit would be dictated by his apparent ability to profit from intervention. Meanwhile, the patient's family was exploring possible discharge options to home for continued home-based services or to a subacute rehabilitation facility.

K.R. will stay awake for two 20-minute sessions per day, demonstrating sensory-specific responses to visual and auditory stimuli at least 50% of the time.

K.R. will respond to one-step commands at least 50% of the time, such as during light hygiene activities.

K.R. will safely sit upright during occupational therapy sessions with proper wheelchair positioning.

K.R.'s parents will be able to perform systematic sensory stimulation and track responses on a data collection form.

Develop intervention hypotheses	"My underlying assumption is that, as we provide that 'just-right' amount of stimulation and structure, K.R. will become increasingly aroused and attentive, which is necessary for him to be truly engaged in the rehabilitation process."
Select an intervention approach	"At this point, my primary approach to intervention is remedial."
Consider what will occur in therapy, how often, and for howlong	"K.R. is at the beginning of what will likely be a long course of rehabilitation, and it is impossible to come up with firm projections as to how long that process might be. Based on my experience, I expect that it may be a matter of a couple of weeks before K.R. can consistently follow instructions and truly participate in therapy. I will be seeing him at least three times per day throughout his inpatient rehabilitation stay, which could be 3 to 4 weeks. I am always reluctant to talk about specifics at this point, especially to family members, because it really is hard to project the outcome with any certainty."

Intervention

K.R. was seen three times daily, twice in the therapy clinic, with sessions lasting 10–30 minutes as tolerated. He participated in daily light hygiene activities in which, for example, he was instructed to turn on the faucet and was handed a wet washcloth and asked to wash his face. Nursing, occupational therapy, and family collaborated to ensure that K.R. was fully dressed each morning. As recommended by the therapist, K.R.'s parents brought in pictures of friends and family and posted them in his room. PROM for the right upper extremity was incorporated into his sensory stimulation program, and efforts were made to elicit automatic upper extremity movement by, for example, challenging K.R. to catch or hit a balloon. He made steady gains in all areas, so that within 3 weeks of his admission to rehabilitation, he followed one-step commands approximately 70% of the time and participated in morning hygiene activities for 20-minute intervals with ongoing verbal and tactile cues. He was able to feed himself with the utensil in his right hand once the therapist scooped food. K.R. started speaking in short phrases approximately 6 weeks after onset and progressed rapidly to whole sentences, indicating, for example, when he had to go to the bathroom. As K.R.'s cognitive recovery progressed, the occupational therapist helped him to become more independent in dressing, grooming, and his upper extremity exercise program and to increase his orientation and attention span. He was able to use a memory log (with entries recorded by others) to answer questions about his daily activities.

Assess the patient's comprehension Understand what he is doing Compare actual to expected performance	"At the time of his transfer to the rehabilitation unit and referral to occupational therapy, K.R's cognitive status posed the primary barrier to his functioning, specifically his low levels of arousal and attention. Motor and ADL activities are means by which I can try to promote arousal, tracking, responsiveness, and K.R.'s ability to follow commands. I can begin to provide more of a learning-based intervention when K.R. begins to show within-session carryover."
Know the person Appreciate the context	"I am beginning to see glimpses of K.R.'s personality and so are his family members. Even though he is disoriented and quite unaware of his circumstances, he can be easily engaged in therapy tasks, especially if he views them as competitive."

At the time of discharge, K.R. needed supervision with grooming and upper extremity dressing and moderate assistance with lower extremity dressing and bathing. K.R.'s mother was taught methods to assist him at home. He was able to walk with a quad cane and moderate assistance; he needed contact guard assistance with standing balance. At discharge, he was oriented to person, place, and time, scoring in the normal range on the *Galveston Orientation and Amnesia Test*, and demonstrated at least some degree of session-to-session carryover. The therapist recommended 24-hour supervision because of continued impairments in memory, problem solving, and judgment. He was discharged to his parents' home 2 months post TBI with plans to return for daily therapy in the day hospital program (supervised all-day multidisciplinary therapies with return home each evening).

"K.R. was discharged home before he was fully competent in self-maintenance because his parents were able to provide assistance and supervision and because intensive outpatient services were available."

Next Steps

The occupational therapy intervention plan during K.R.'s 3 weeks in the day hospital focused on use of a memory aid and reestablishing competence in instrumental ADL, including light meal preparation, laundry, checkbook management, and bill paying. His living situation contributed to motivation and improved insight more than the insulated experience of the rehabilitation unit. When he no longer required all-day supervision, he was discharged from the day hospital but continued outpatient occupational therapy three times a week.

Anticipate present and future patient concerns

Analyze patient's comprehension

Decide if the patient should continue or discontinue therapy and/or return in the future

"I feel good about the fact that we can offer K.R. and his family comprehensive and long-term rehabilitation services. They will need us off and on as they face new milestones over the next year such as driving, return to independent living, and return to school and work. His parents have joined a support group and are working closely with our staff to carry over what he is working on in therapy."

CLINICAL REASONING IN OCCUPATIONAL THERAPY PRACTICE

Occupational Therapy Intervention in the Survivor Phase of Recovery

K.R. had a neuropsychological evaluation a year after he sustained the TBI. Results suggested that, despite his considerable neurological and behavioral recovery, K.R. demonstrated general cerebral dysfunction that affected his information-processing speed, expressive abilities, abstraction, higher level reasoning, planning, organization, and memory. K.R.'s pre-morbid attributes, such as above-average intelligence and diligence, appeared to contribute to his recovery, and K.R. had plans to reenter college within 2 months of testing. The neuropsychologist advised against this plan, suggesting that K.R. allow himself more time to recover and that he further develop compensatory cognitive strategies to optimize the likelihood for successful return to school. The neuropsychologist further recommended that K.R. establish connections with a counseling psychologist, anticipating a point when K.R.'s expectations to fully resume his career track might clash with his post-injury capabilities. K.R. felt that the neuropsychologist was unduly pessimistic, but with the encouragement of his parents, he agreed to participate in occupational therapy and at least meet with the counseling psychologist.

Assuming that K.R. has not been actively involved in occupational therapy for the past 6 months, what assessment tools and methods would you use to guide your treatment plan? What aspects of occupational functioning do you anticipate having to address in treatment?

CASE EXAMPLE # 2

Dr. N.: Occupational Therapy after Mild Brain Injury

Occupational Therapy Intervention Process	Clinical Reasoning Process	
	Objectives	**Examples of Therapist's Internal Dialogue**
Patient Information Dr. N. is a 29-year-old single woman who sustained a mild TBI when she fell off her bicycle; she was not wearing a helmet. She reports that she did not lose consciousness, and her *Glasgow Coma Scale (GCS)* score in the emergency department was 13. She was hospitalized for 2 days with a small epidural hematoma over the right occipital region and significant headaches. Dr. N. returned to work 2 days after her hospital discharge despite continued headaches and balance and memory problems. Dr. N. has a degree in biochemistry and works as a postdoctoral fellow at a university. Her parents and four siblings reside in another state, and she lives with her significant other of 4 years. Dr. N. participated in neuropsychological assessment approximately 6 months post injury because cognitive inefficiencies continued to interfere with her function, especially at work. Findings suggested mild impairment for recent verbal and non-verbal memory and subtle impairment for executive abilities. These cognitive changes contributed to decreased efficiency at work (slowness in problem solving, needing to reread professional literature, frequent note taking). Furthermore, Dr. N. was anxious and depressed. She reported difficulty falling asleep despite overwhelming fatigue. She worried about whether or not she had completed intended tasks, checking and double-checking herself throughout the day. She described herself as easily frustrated, lacking confidence, and overdependent on her significant other. She continued to have headaches approximately 4 days a week. The neuropsychologist expected Dr. N. to maintain her job successfully and pursue pre-morbid career goals with assistance in adjusting self-expectations and information-processing habits.	Understand the patient's diagnosis or condition Know the person	"Given her GCS score and the fact that she did not lose consciousness, I can assume that her TBI was not severe and that she has a good prognosis for a full recovery." "My guess is that Dr. N. is used to pushing herself, as evidenced by a rather speedy return to work after her hospitalization. Clearly, Dr. N. is a bright woman and has high expectations of herself. The cognitive inefficiencies since her injury must be frightening and confusing for her. I am glad that she appears to have social support."
Reason for Referral to Occupational Therapy Dr. N. was referred to occupational therapy for assistance in developing compensatory cognitive strategies and behavioral routines that would improve her efficiency at home and work. She was also referred to a psychologist for support and biofeedback to help her manage her headaches.	Appreciate the context Develop provisional hypotheses	"Dr. N. was referred to an outpatient brain injury clinic that specializes in serving people with mild brain injury. The staff knows to avoid overemphasizing concerns about permanent cognitive impairment and encourage clients to reinterpret symptoms as short term and manageable."

Assessment Process and Results • Interview and self-report questionnaire related to client's problems, inefficiencies, and concerns and learn about how Dr. N. manages information at present • Interview regarding "typical day" • Observations of response to orally-presented homework and follow-through	Consider evaluation approach and methods	"Because I have reviewed the results of Dr. N.'s neuropsychological evaluation, it is not necessary or appropriate to assess cognition in occupational therapy. In fact, repeated assessment of similar domains might be detrimental, potentially overemphasizing cognitive inefficiencies that will likely be short term. Instead, I will try to find out about performance patterns and daily functioning."
	Interpret observations	"When I asked her to bring photographs to her next session, Dr. N. wrote a note to herself on 1 of approximately 8 'sticky notes' that were affixed to her wallet. She seems comfortable with note taking, but I'm guessing that her notes do little to supplant her memory as she likely doesn't find them when she needs them."
Occupational Therapy Problem List • Misattributions and misperceptions regarding personal competence • Inadequate use of external information-processing strategies • Disruption of personal routines, especially surrounding bedtime	Synthesize results	"Dr. N. did not link distracters, such as headache and fatigue, to episodes of memory failure and absent-mindedness or understand the implications of a limited working memory. I noticed that Dr. N. started writing lots of notes to herself but did not store or refer to them in a systematic manner; she worked off a mental plan each day but could not set priorities among multiple tasks. I am concerned about so much sleep in the early evening followed by more active household tasks. It's no wonder she is having difficulty with sleep."
Initial Occupational Therapy Goal List The anticipated length of treatment was four to six sessions. Dr. N. will independently employ compensatory cognitive strategies to increase her effectiveness and efficiency with work and personal tasks. Dr. N. will make changes in her daily routine that contribute to improved balance among work, leisure, and rest.	Develop intervention hypotheses	"There seem to be many contributions to Dr. N.'s problems right now, including the after-effects of mild brain injury, anxiety associated with misattributions related to the problems she's experiencing, and a rather limited repertoire of external information-processing strategies. Interventions in occupational therapy will focus on helping her make correct attributions related to performance problems and broadening her repertoire of information-processing strategies."
	Select an intervention approach	"I will use an education-consultative approach, teaching her about information processing and helping her refine her information management strategies."
	Consider what will occur in therapy, how often, and for how long	"I think that she will need a relatively short duration of occupational therapy. I recommend that she come to therapy once per week for a few weeks, which will allow her to try out the strategies that we discuss, and we can work together to refine them accordingly."

Intervention Dr. N. participated in five treatment sessions over 3 months, attending weekly sessions for 3 weeks and two follow-up sessions over 6 weeks. As cognitive inefficiencies were reframed as partly consequences of a working memory overload related to stress and the distraction of physical symptoms, Dr. N. eagerly explored methods to decrease the demands on internal information processing. She purchased a day planner and, with input from the therapist, established daily and weekly planning routines. Daily and weekly plans helped her set priorities among tasks and allocate time for leisure. She experimented with establishing routines for certain aspects of her "typical" day, scheduling breaks and allocating tasks with low cognitive demands to periods when her energy tended to be low. Her after-work routine changed as well: she set the timer to take a 20- to 30-minute nap followed by a 30-minute walk. She also established a bedtime wind-down routine that ultimately decreased the amount of time she needed to fall asleep.	Assess the patient's comprehension Understand what she is doing Compare actual to expected performance Know the person Appreciate the context	"Dr. N. had relatively mild or subtle impairments that changed her cognitive capacity. Similar to many bright individuals, Dr. N. had never thought about her own thinking strategies and did not have a broad repertoire of techniques or habits of mind that she could default to. Furthermore, in her attempts to understand changes resulting from her injury and their implications, Dr. N. failed to appreciate the cumulative effect that subtle impairments, stress, reliance on pre-morbid cognitive strategies, and distractions associated with pain exerted on her information processing. She was relieved to learn that she was not 'losing it' and quickly engaged in problem solving with me regarding possible changes in strategies and routines that would buoy her everyday performance. Her relatively brief involvement in treatment shows the benefit of holistic occupational therapy services in dramatically improving an individual's occupational functioning and quality of life."
Next Steps Discharge from occupational therapy.	Anticipate present and future patient concerns Analyze patient's comprehension Decide if the patient should continue or discontinue therapy and/or return in the future	"I do not expect that Dr. N. will need further therapy and anticipate that, as her headaches and fatigue abate, her overall functioning will improve. She seems to now make correct attributions related to cognitive inefficiencies and has a good sense of when to employ compensatory strategies to lighten her load."

CLINICAL REASONING IN OCCUPATIONAL THERAPY PRACTICE

Implications of Severity of TBI on Treatment Planning

Because Dr. N.'s cognitive impairments were relatively mild, she was aware of cognitive changes and able to learn information-processing principles and independently apply them in novel situations. Explain how the treatment plan would likely change if Dr. N. had sustained a moderate or severe TBI. How might Dr. N.'s cognitive profile be different? What would be the implications in terms of therapist's role, treatment methods, length of treatment, and outcome expectations?

Evidence Table 39-1
Best Evidence for Interventions Used in Occupational Therapy after Severe Brain Injury

Intervention	Description of Intervention Tested	Participants	Dosage	Type of Best Evidence and Level of Evidence	Benefit	Statistical Probability	Reference
Multisensory stimulation[a]	Experimental group received multisensory stimulation protocol (auditory, tactile, olfactory, gustatory, visual, kinesthetic, proprioceptive, vestibular) that was administered by family members; controls did not receive this intervention.	Total of 24 patients (ages 17–42 years) who were 2–12 days post severe brain injury and who had a *Glasgow Coma Scale* (*GCS*) score less than 8 (n = 12 in experimental group; n = 12 matched controls).	Multisensory stimulation provided to experimental group for approximately 1 hour, 1–2 times per day for duration of coma. (Coma was said to have ended when patient was observed to obey commands and make purposeful movements.)	Quasi-experiment, cohort study; 12 patients in each of the 2 conditions. II C 3 c	Total duration of coma was significantly less for experimental group than control group. Experimental group showed signs of greater responsiveness (based on weekly averages of *GCS*), but researchers did not test the significance of these differences.	$p < 0.05$; $r = 0.5830$	Mitchell et al., 1990

(continued)

Evidence Table 39-1
Best Evidence for Interventions Used in Occupational Therapy after Severe Brain Injury *(continued)*

Intervention	Description of Intervention Tested	Participants	Dosage	Type of Best Evidence and Level of Evidence	Benefit	Statistical Probability	Reference
Multisensory Stimulation[a]	Same as above.	31 patients (ages 6–75 years) who were in coma or persistent vegetative state 2 weeks after severe brain injury received multisensory stimulation; outcomes compared with historical reference group from the literature with similar characteristics (n = 135).	Multisensory stimulation provided to experimental group up to 8 hours per day, 7 days per week, until the participant was accepted for conventional rehabilitation therapy.	Case-control study with 31 patients in experimental group. II B 3 c	No significant differences in either time taken to follow a simple command or in *Glasgow Outcome Scale* 10–12 months post injury.	N/A	Pierce et al., 1990
Self-care skills training	Subjects received a washing and dressing protocol that involved behavioral methods (behavioral observation, task analysis, consistent practice, faded cueing).	4 patients living in a residential setting (3 sustained a TBI; 1 had brain injury after cerebral bleed) who were at least 7 months post injury and who had severe physical and cognitive impairments.	Daily ADL retraining with fading physical assistance and cueing.	4 single-subject studies. IV C 2 b	3 of 4 subjects achieved independence in washing and dressing (in 20, 37, and 11 days, respectively); 1 of 4 did not.	No formal statistical tests reported.	Giles et al., 1997

[a]Note how two studies with similar levels of evidence come to different conclusions regarding effectiveness.

SUMMARY REVIEW QUESTIONS

1. What are some treatment planning implications related to age of onset of TBI? Describe the relevance of the cause of injury, developmental stage, and possible comorbidities.
2. In what ways do occupational therapists use information regarding mechanisms of injury of each patient in the clinical reasoning process? For example, how is the clinical presentation of a diffuse brain injury different from that of a focal brain injury? How can the therapist obtain information about the mechanisms of injury for a given patient?
3. Describe specific ways a patient's pre-injury characteristics and background may affect rehabilitation and outcome.
4. Summarize terms used to describe patients in altered states of consciousness and why distinctions between these states are important to the occupational therapist.
5. Analyze the similarities and differences between providing sensory stimulation and managing agitation for a minimally responsive patient.
6. What are some of the frequently cited predictors of prognosis and rehabilitation outcome after TBI? What are the occupational therapy implications of these predictors in planning treatment for patients in terms of goals, length of treatment, and role or needs of the family?
7. Describe the adjustment and adaptation process of the patient with TBI as compared to that of the family. Detail what support and education patients and family members need from occupational therapy during each phase of recovery and adaptation.
8. How might the treatment approach used to optimize cognitive capacities and abilities for an inpatient be different from the treatment approach used in post-acute rehabilitation or if the patient returns for services years later?
9. Compare Montgomery's multifactor explanation for disability after mild TBI with your own explanation of disability after severe TBI.

References

Abreu, B. C., Seale, G., Podlesack, J., & Hartley, L. (1996). Development of paths of postacute brain injury rehabilitation: Lessons learned. *American Journal of Occupational Therapy, 50,* 417–427.

Abreu, B. C., & Toglia, J. P. (1987). Cognitive rehabilitation: A model for occupational therapy. *American Journal of Occupational Therapy, 41,* 439–448.

Agency for Health Care Policy and Research. (1999). Rehabilitation for traumatic brain injury. AHCPR publication 99-E006. Rockville, MD: United States Public Health Service.

American Congress of Rehabilitation Medicine. (1995a). Definition of mild traumatic brain injury. *Journal of Head Trauma Rehabilitation, 8,* 86–87.

American Congress of Rehabilitation Medicine. (1995b). Recommendations for use of uniform nomenclature pertinent to patients with severe alterations in consciousness. *Archives of Physical Medicine and Rehabilitation, 76,* 205–209.

Ansell, B. J. (1993). Slow-to-recover patients: Improvement to rehabilitation readiness. *Journal of Head Trauma Rehabilitation, 8,* 88–98.

Ansell, B. J., & Keenan, J. E. (1989). The Western Neuro Sensory Stimulation Profile: A tool for assessing slow to recover head injured patients. *Archives of Physical Medicine and Rehabilitation, 70,* 104–108.

Ashman, T. A., Spielman, L. A., Hibbard, M. R., Silver, J. M., Chandna, T., & Gordon, W. A. (2004). Psychiatric challenges in the first 6 years after traumatic brain injury: Cross-sequential analyses of Axis I disorders. *Archives of Physical Medicine and Rehabilitation, 85,* S36–S42.

Baggerly, J. (1986). Rehabilitation of the adult with head trauma. *Nursing Clinics of North America, 21,* 577–587.

Bakay, L., & Glasauer, F. E. (1980). *Head injuries.* Boston: Little, Brown.

Benton, A. (1979). Behavioral consequences of closed head injury. In G. L. Odom (Ed.), *Central nervous system trauma research status report* (pp. 220–231). Bethesda, MD: National Institute of Neurological and Communicative Disorders and Stroke.

Boake, C. (1991). Social skills training following head injury. In J. S. Kreutzer & P. H. Wehman (Eds.), *Cognitive rehabilitation for persons with traumatic brain injury* (pp. 181–189). Baltimore: Paul H. Brookes.

Boake, C. (1996). Supervision rating scale: A measure of functional outcome from brain injury. *Archives of Physical Medicine and Rehabilitation, 77,* 765–772.

Bond, M. R. (1990). Standardized methods of assessing and predicting outcome. In M. Rosenthal, E. R. Griffith, M. R. Bond, & J. D. Miller (Eds.), *Rehabilitation of the adult and child with traumatic brain injury* (2nd ed., pp. 59–76). Philadelphia: Davis.

Boortz-Marx, R. (1985). Factors affecting intracranial pressure: A descriptive study. *Journal of Neurosurgical Nursing, 17,* 89–94.

Bouska, M. J., & Gallaway, M. (1991). Primary visual deficits in adults with brain damage: Management in occupational therapy. *Occupational Therapy Practice, 3,* 1–11.

Braakman, R., Gelpke, G. J., Habbema, J. D. F., Maas, A. I. R., & Minderhoud, J. M. (1980). Systematic selection of prognostic features in patients with severe head injury. *Neurosurgery, 6,* 362–370.

Brain Injury Association. (2000). The costs and causes of traumatic brain injury. http://www.fha.state.md.us/cphs/sa/html/tbi_cost.html.

Brandstater, M. E., Bontke, C. F., Cobble, N. D., & Horn, L. J. (1991). Rehabilitation in brain disorders: 4. Specific disorders. *Archives of Physical Medicine and Rehabilitation, 72,* S332–S340.

Bricolo, A., Turazzi, S., & Feriotti, G. (1980). Prolonged posttraumatic unconsciousness: Therapeutic assets and liabilities. *Journal of Neurosurgery, 52,* 625–634.

Bryant, R. A., Moulds, M., Guthrie, R., & Nixon, R. D. V. (2003). Treating acute stress disorder following mild traumatic brain injury. *American Journal of Psychiatry, 160,* 585–587.

Carney, N., Chestnut, R. M., Maynard, H., Mann, N. C., Patterson, P., & Helfand, M. (1999). Effect of cognitive rehabilitation on outcomes for persons with traumatic brain injury: A systematic review. *Journal of Head Trauma Rehabilitation, 14,* 277–307.

Carr, J. H., & Shepherd, R. B. (1980). *Physiotherapy in disorders of the brain.* London: Heinemann Medical.

Center for Outcome Measurement in Brain Injury. (2006). *List of scales.* http://www.tbims.org/combi/

Charness, A. L. (1986). *Stroke/head injury: A guide to functional outcomes in physical therapy management* (Rehabilitation Institute of Chicago Series). Rockville, MD: Aspen.

Chestnut, R. M., Carney, N., Maynard, H., Mann, N. C., Patterson, P., & Helfand, M. (1999). Summary report: Evidence for the effectiveness of rehabilitation for persons with traumatic brain injury. *Journal of Head Trauma Rehabilitation, 14,* 176–188.

Choi, S. C., Narayan, R. K., Anderson, R. L., & Ward, J. D. (1988). Enhanced specificity of prognosis in severe head injury. *Journal of Neurosurgery, 69,* 381–385.

Cicerone, K. D., Dahlberg, C., Kalmar, K., Langenbahn, D. M., Malec, J. F., Bergquist, T. F., Felicetti, T., Giacino, J. T., Preston Harley, J., Harrington, D. E., Herzog, J., Kneipp, S., Laatsch, L., & Morse, P. A. (2000). Evidence-based cognitive rehabilitation: Recommendations for clinical practice. *Archives of Physical Medicine and Rehabilitation, 81,* 1596–1615.

Cicerone, K. D., Dahlberg, C., Malec, J. F., Langenbahn, D. M., Felicetti, T., Kneipp, S., Ellmo, W., Kalmar, K., Giacino, J. T., Harley, J. P., Laatsch, L., Morse, P. A., & Catanese, J. (2005). Evidence-based cognitive rehabilitation: Updated review of the literature from 1998 through 2002. *Archives of Physical Medicine and Rehabilitation, 86,* 1681–1692.

Citta-Pietrolungo, T. J., Alexander, M. A., & Steg, N. L. (1992). Early detection of heterotopic ossification in young patients with traumatic brain injury. *Archives of Physical Medicine and Rehabilitation, 73,* 258–262.

Cope, D. N., & Hall, K. (1982). Head injury rehabilitation: Benefit of early intervention. *Archives of Physical Medicine and Rehabilitation, 63,* 433–437.

Corrigan, J. D. (1989). Development of a scale for assessment of agitation following traumatic brain injury. *Journal of Clinical and Experimental Neuropsychology, 11,* 261–277.

Davis, A. E., & Gimenez, A. (2003). Cognitive-behavioral recovery in comatose patients following auditory sensory stimulation. *Journal of Neuroscience Nursing, 35,* 202–214.

Davis, R. A., & Cunningham, P. S. (1984). Prognostic factors in severe head injury. *Surgery, Gynecology and Obstetrics, 159,* 597–604.

DeKruijk, J. R., Twijnstra, A., & Leffers, P. (2001). Diagnostic criteria and differential diagnosis of mild traumatic brain injury. *Brain Injury, 15,* 99–106.

Dikmen, S., Machamer, J., & Temkin, N. (2001). Mild head injury: Facts and artifacts. *Journal of Clinical and Experimental Neuropsychology, 23,* 729–738.

Dikmen, S., Reitan, R. M., & Temkin, N. R. (1983). Neuropsychological recovery in head injury. *Archives of Neurology, 40,* 333–338.

DiPasquale, M. C., & Whyte, J. (1996). Use of quantitative data in treatment planning for minimally conscious patients. *Journal of Head Trauma Rehabilitation, 11,* 9–17.

Duff, D. (2001). Review article: Altered states of consciousness, theories of recovery, and assessment following a severe traumatic brain injury. *Axon, 23,* 18–23.

Eames, P., Haffey, W. J., & Cope, D. N. (1990). Treatment of behavioral disorders. In M. Rosenthal, E. R. Griffith, M. R. Bond, & J. D. Miller (Eds.), *Rehabilitation of the adult and child with traumatic brain injury* (pp. 410–432). Philadelphia: Davis.

Elovic, E., & Antoinette, T. (1996). Epidemiology and primary prevention of traumatic brain injury. In L. J. Horn & N. D. Zasler (Eds.), *Medical rehabilitation of traumatic brain injury* (pp. 1–28). Philadelphia: Hanley & Belfus.

Farber, S. D. (1982). *Neurorehabilitation: A multisensory approach.* Philadelphia: Saunders.

Gelling, L., Shiel, A., Elliott, L., Owen, A., Wilson, B., Menon, D., & Pickard, J. (2004). Commentary on Oh H. and Seo W. (2003) Sensory stimulation programme to improve recovery in comatose patients. *Journal of Clinical Nursing, 12,* 394–404.

Gerstenbrand, F. (1972). The course of restitution of brain injury in the early and late stages and the rehabilitative measures. *Scandinavian Journal of Rehabilitation Medicine, 4,* 85–89.

Giacino, J. T., & Kalmar, K. (1997). The vegetative and minimally conscious states: A comparison of clinical features and functional outcome. *Journal of Head Trauma Rehabilitation, 12,* 36–51.

Giacino, J. T., Kezmarksy, M. A., DeLuca, J., & Cicerone, K. (1991). Monitoring rate of recovery to predict outcome in minimally responsive patients. *Archives of Physical Medicine and Rehabilitation, 72,* 897–901.

Giacino, J. T., Zasler, N. D., Katz, D. I., Kelly, J. P., Rosenberg, J. H., & Filley, C. M. (1997). Development of practice guidelines for assessment and management of the vegetative and minimally conscious states. *Journal of Head Trauma Rehabilitation, 12,* 79–89.

Gianutsos, R. (1980). What is cognitive rehabilitation? *Journal of Rehabilitation, 46,* 36–40.

Giles, G. M., & Clark-Wilson, J. (1993). *Brain injury rehabilitation: A neurofunctional approach.* San Diego: Singular.

Giles, G. M., Ridley, J. E., Dill, A., & Frye, S. (1997). A consecutive series of adults with brain injury treated with a washing and dressing retraining program. *American Journal of Occupational Therapy, 51,* 256–266.

Greenberg, D. A., Aminoff, M. J., & Simon, R. P. (1993). *Clinical neurology* (2nd ed.). East Norwalk, CT: Appleton & Lange.

Griffith, E. R., Cole, S., & Cole, T. M. (1990). Sexuality and sexual dysfunction. In M. Rosenthal, E. R. Griffith, M. R. Bond, & J. D. Miller (Eds.), *Rehabilitation of the adult and child with traumatic brain injury* (pp. 206–224). Philadelphia: Davis.

Gronwall, D., Wrightson, P., & Waddell, P. (1998). *Head injury: The facts* (2nd ed.). New York: Oxford University.

Groswasser, Z., & Stern, M. J. (1998). A psychodynamic model of behavior after central nervous system damage. *Journal of Head Trauma Rehabilitation, 13,* 69–79.

Gutman, S. A. (1999). Alleviating gender role strain in adult men with traumatic brain injury: An evaluation of a set of guidelines for occupational therapy. *American Journal of Occupational Therapy, 53,* 101–110.

Hagen, C. (1998). *Rancho Levels of Cognitive Functioning: The revised levels* (3rd ed.). Downey, CA: Rancho Los Amigos Medical Center.

Hagen, C., Malkmus, D., & Durham, P. (1979). *Levels of cognitive functioning, rehabilitation of the brain-injured adult: Comprehensive physical management.* Downey, CA: Professional Staff Association of Rancho Los Amigos Hospital.

Hall, K. M. (1997). The Functional Assessment Measure. *Journal of Rehabilitation Outcomes Measurement, 1,* 63–65.

Hall, K., Cope, D. N., & Rappaport, M. (1985). Glasgow outcome scale and disability rating scale: Comparative usefulness in following recovery in traumatic head injury. *Archives of Physical Medicine and Rehabilitation, 66,* 35–37.

Hall, K. M., & Johnston, M. V. (1994). Part II: Measurement tools for a nationwide data system. *Archives of Physical Medicine and Rehabilitation, 75,* SC-10–SC-18.

Hanks, R. A., Temkin, N., Machamer, J., & Dikmen, S. S. (1999). Emotional and behavioral adjustment after traumatic brain injury. *Archives of Physical Medicine and Rehabilitation, 80,* 991–997.

Harrison-Felix, C., Newton, C. N., Hall, K. M., & Kreutzer, J. S. (1996). Descriptive findings from the Traumatic Brain Injury Model Systems National Data Base. *Journal of Head Trauma Rehabilitation, 11,* 1–14.

Helman, D. L., Sherner, J. H., Fitzpatrick, T. M., Callender, M. E., & Shorr, A. F. (2003). Effect of standardized orders and provider education on head-of-bed positioning in mechanically ventilated patients. *Critical Care Medicine, 31,* 2285–2290.

Heinemann, A. W., Saghal, V., Cichowski, K., Ginsburg, K., Tuel, S. M., & Betts, H. B. (1990). Functional outcome following traumatic brain injury rehabilitation. *Journal of Neurological Rehabilitation, 4,* 27–37.

Hibbard, M. R., Ashman, R. A., Spielman, L. A., Chun, D., Charatz, H. J., & Seton, M. (2004). Relationship between depression and psychosocial functioning after traumatic brain injury. *Archives of Physical Medicine and Rehabilitation, 85,* S43–S53.

Hill, J. (1994). The effects of casting on upper extremity motor disorders after brain injury. *American Journal of Occupational Therapy, 48,* 219–224.

Holden, M.K. (2005). Virtual environments for motor rehabilitation: A review. *CyberPsychology and Behavior, 8,* 187–211.

Holland, D., & Shigaki, C. L. (1998). Educating families and caretakers of traumatically brain injured patients in the new health care environment: A three phase model and bibliography. *Brain Injury, 12,* 993–1009.

Ivanhoe, C. B., & Bontke, C. F. (1996). Movement disorders after traumatic brain injury. In L. J. Horn & N. D. Zasler (Eds.), *Medical rehabilitation of traumatic brain injury* (pp. 395–410). Philadelphia: Hanley & Belfus.

Jennett, B., Snoek, J., Bond, M. R., & Brooks, N. (1981). Disability after severe head injury: Observations on the use of the Glasgow Outcome Scale. *Journal of Neurology, Neurosurgery, and Psychiatry, 44,* 285–293.

Jennett, B., & Teasdale, G. (1981). *Management of head injuries.* Philadelphia: Davis.

Jones, R., Giddens, H., & Croft, D. (1983). Assessment and training of brain-damaged drivers. *American Journal of Occupational Therapy, 37,* 754–760.

Jorge, R. E., Robinson, R. G., Arndt, S. V., Starkstein, S. E., Forrester, A. W., & Geisler, F. (1993). Depression following traumatic brain injury: A 1 year longitudinal study. *Journal of Affective Disorders, 27,* 233–243.

Karnaze, D. S., Weiner, J. M., & Marshall, L. F. (1985). Auditory evoked potentials in coma after closed head injury: A clinical-neurophysiological coma scale for predicting outcome. *Neurology, 35,* 1122–1126.

Katz, D. I. (1992). Neuropathology and neurobehavioral recovery from closed head injury. *Journal of Head Trauma Rehabilitation, 1,* 1–15.

Katz, N., Itzkovich, M., Averbuch, S., & Elazar, B. (1989). Loewenstein Occupational Therapy Cognitive Assessment (LOTCA) battery for brain-injured patients: Reliability and validity. *American Journal of Occupational Therapy, 43,* 184–192.

Kelly, M. P., Johnson, C. T., Knoller, N., Drubach, D. A., & Winslow, M. M. (1997). Substance abuse, traumatic brain injury and neuropsychological outcome. *Brain Injury, 11,* 391–402.

Kim, E. (2002). Agitation, aggression, and disinhibition syndromes after traumatic brain injury. *NeuroRehabilitation, 17,* 297–310.

Klonoff, P. S., Snow, W. G., & Costa, L. D. (1986). Quality of life in patients 2 to 4 years after closed head injury. *Neurosurgery, 19,* 735–743.

Koskinen, S. (1998). Quality of life 10 years after a very severe traumatic brain injury (TBI): The perspective of the injured and the closest relative. *Brain Injury, 12,* 631–648.

Langlois, J. A., Rutland-Brown, W., & Thomas, K. E. (2004). *Traumatic brain injury in the United States: Emergency department visits, hospitalization, and deaths.* Atlanta, GA: Centers for Disease Control and Prevention, National Center for Injury Prevention and Control.

Law, M., Baptiste, S., McColl, M. A., Carswell, A., Polatajko, H., & Pollock, N. (1994). *Canadian Occupational Performance Measure.* Toronto, Ontario, Canada: Canadian Association of Occupational Therapists.

Leech, R. W., & Shuman, R. M. (1982). *Neuropathology: A summary for students.* New York: Harper & Row.

Levin, H. S., High, W. M., Goethe, K. E., Sisson, R. A., Overall, J. E., Rhoades, H. M., Eisenberg, H. M., Kalisky, A., & Gary, H. E. (1987). The Neurobehavioral Rating Scale: Assessment of the behavioral sequelae of head injury by the clinician. *Journal of Neurology, Neurosurgery, and Psychiatry, 50,* 183–193.

Levin, H. S., O'Donnell, V. M., & Grossman, R. G. (1979). The Galveston Orientation and Amnesia Test. *Journal of Nervous and Mental Disease, 167,* 675–684.

Lezak, M. D. (1995). *Neuropsychological assessment* (3rd ed.). New York: Oxford University.

Lillehei, K. O., & Hoff, J. T. (1985). Advances in the management of closed head injury. *Annals of Emergency Medicine, 14,* 789–795.

Lippert-Grüner, M., & Terhaag, D., (2000). Multimodal early onset stimulation in rehabilitation after brain injury. *Brain Injury, 14,* 585–594.

Lippert-Grüner, M., Wedekind, C., & Klug, N. (2003). Outcome of prolonged coma following severe traumatic brain injury. *Brain Injury, 17,* 49–54.

Livingston, M. G. (1990). Effect on the family system. In M. Rosenthal, E. R. Griffith, M. R. Bond, & J. D. Miller (Eds.), *Rehabilitation of the adult and child with traumatic brain injury* (pp. 225–235). Philadelphia: F. A. Davis Company.

Malec, J. F., & Basford, J. S. (1996). Postacute brain injury rehabilitation. *Archives of Physical Medicine and Rehabilitation, 77,* 198–207.

Malec, J. F., Moessner, A. M., Kragness, M., & Lezak, M. D. (2000). Refining a measure of brain injury sequelae to predict postacute rehabilitation outcome: Rating scale analysis of the Mayo-Portland Adaptability Inventory. *Journal of Head Trauma Rehabilitation, 15,* 670–682.

Malec, J. F., & Thompson, J. M. (1994). Relationship of the Mayo-Portland Adaptability Inventory to functional outcome and cognitive performance measures. *Journal of Head Trauma Rehabilitation, 9,* 1–15.

Malkmus, D., Booth, B. J., & Kodimer, C. (1980). *Rehabilitation of the head injured adult: Comprehensive cognitive management.* Downey, CA: Professional Staff Association of Rancho Los Amigos Hospital.

Marion, D. W. (1996). Pathophysiology and initial neurosurgical care: Future directions. In L. J. Horn & N. D. Zasler (Eds.), *Medical rehabilitation of traumatic brain injury* (pp. 29–52). Philadelphia: Hanley & Belfus.

Miller, J. D., Pentland, B., & Berrol, S. (1990). Early evaluation and management. In M. Rosenthal, E. R. Griffith, M. R. Bond, & J. D. Miller (Eds.), *Rehabilitation of the adult and child with traumatic brain injury* (2nd ed., pp. 21–51). Philadelphia: F. A. Davis.

Mitchell, P. H. (1986). Intracranial hypertension: Influence of nursing care activities. *Nursing Clinics of North America, 21,* 563–576.

Mitchell, S., Bradley, V. A., Welch, J. L., & Britton, P. G. (1990). Coma arousal procedures: A therapeutic intervention in the treatment of head injury. *Brain Injury, 4,* 273–279.

Montgomery, G. K. (1995). A multi-factor account of disability after brain injury: Implications for neuropsychological counseling. *Brain Injury, 9,* 453–469.

Mortenson, P. A., & Eng, J. J. (2003). The use of casts in the management of joint mobility and hypertonia following brain injury in adults: A systematic review. *Physical Therapy, 83,* 648–658.

Muir, C. A., Rosenthal, M., & Diehl, L. N. (1990). Methods of family intervention. In M. Rosenthal, E. R. Griffith, M. R. Bond, & J. D. Miller (Eds.), *Rehabilitation of the adult and child with traumatic brain injury* (2nd ed., pp. 433–448). Philadelphia: Davis.

Mysiw, W. J., Fugate, L. P., & Clinchot, D. M., (1996). Assessment, early rehabilitation intervention, and tertiary prevention. In L. J. Horn & N. D. Zasler (Eds.), *Medical rehabilitation of traumatic brain injury* (pp. 53–76). Philadelphia: Hanley & Belfus, Inc.

Najenson, T., Mendelson, L., Schechter, I., David, C., Mintz, N., & Grosswasser, Z. (1974). Rehabilitation after severe head injury. *Scandinavian Journal of Rehabilitation Medicine, 6,* 5–14.

National Center for Injury Prevention and Control. (2003). *Report to Congress on mild traumatic brain injury in the United States: Steps to prevent a serious public health problem.* Atlanta, GA: Centers for Disease Control and Prevention.

Neistadt, M. E. (1992). The Rabideau Kitchen Evaluation-Revised: An assessment of meal preparation skill. *Occupational Therapy Journal of Research, 12,* 242–253.

Neistadt, M. E. (1994a). Perceptual retraining for adults with diffuse brain injury. *American Journal of Occupational Therapy, 48,* 225–233.

Neistadt, M. E. (1994b). A meal preparation treatment protocol for adults with brain injury. *American Journal of Occupational Therapy, 48,* 431–438.

Nelson, D. L., & Lenhart, D. A. (1996). Resumption of outpatient occupational therapy for a young woman five years after traumatic brain injury. *American Journal of Occupational Therapy, 50,* 223–228.

O'Dell, M. W., Bell, K. R., & Sandel, M. E. (1998). Brain injury rehabilitation. 2. Medical rehabilitation of brain injury. *Archives of Physical Medicine and Rehabilitation, 79,* S-10–S-15.

O'Dell, M. W., & Riggs, R. V. (1996). Management of the minimally responsive patient. In L. J. Horn & N. D. Zasler (Eds.), *Medical rehabilitation of traumatic brain injury* (pp. 103–131). Philadelphia: Hanley & Belfus.

Olver, J. H., Ponsford, J. L., & Curran, C. A. (1996). Outcome following traumatic brain injury: A comparison between 2 and 5 years after injury. *Brain Injury, 10,* 841–848.

O'Neill, J., Hibbard, M. R., Brown, M., Jaffe, M., Sliwinski, M., Vandergroot, D., & Weiss, M. J. (1998). Quality of life and community integration after traumatic brain injury. *Journal of Head Injury Rehabilitation, 13,* 68–79.

Ownsworth, T., & Fleming, J. (2005). The relative importance of metacognitive skills, emotional status, and executive function in psychosocial adjustment following acquired brain injury. *Journal of Head Trauma Rehabilitation, 20,* 315–332.

Pagulayan, K., Temkin, N. R., Machamer, J., & Dikmen, S. S. (2006). A longitudinal study of health-related quality of life after traumatic brain injury. *Archives of Physical Medicine and Rehabilitation, 87,* 611–618.

Palmer, M., & Wyness, M. A. (1988). Positioning and handling: Important considerations in the care of the severely head-injured patient. *Journal of Neuroscience Nursing, 20,* 42–50.

Phipps, E. J., DiPasquale, M., Blitz, C. L., & Whyte, J. (1997). Interpreting responsiveness in persons with severe traumatic brain injury: Beliefs in families and quantitative evaluations. *Journal of Head Trauma Rehabilitation, 12,* 52–69.

Pierce, J. P., Lyle, D. M., Quine, S., Evans, N. J., Morris, J., & Fearnside, M. R. (1990). The effectiveness of coma arousal intervention. *Brain Injury, 4,* 191–197.

Pohl, M., Rückriem, S., Mehrholz, J., Ritschel, C., Strick, H., & Pause, M.R. (2002). Effectiveness of serial casting in patients with severe cerebral spasticity: A comparison study. *Archives of Physical Medicine and Rehabilitation, 83,* 784–790.

Prigatano, G. P. (1992). Personality disturbances associated with traumatic brain injury. *Journal of Consulting and Clinical Psychology, 60,* 360–368.

Prigatano, G. P., Fordyce, D. J., Zeiner, H. K., Rouche, J. R., Pepping, M., & Wood, B. C. (1986). *Neuropsychological rehabilitation after brain injury.* Baltimore, MD: John Hopkins University Press.

Rain, K. (2000). Survivor's voice. *TBI Challenge!, 4,* 6.

Rappaport, M., Dougherty, A. M., Devon, L, & Kelting, B. A. (1992). Evaluation of coma and vegetative states. *Archives of Physical Medicine and Rehabilitation, 73,* 628–634.

Rappaport, M., Hall, K. M., Hopkins, K., Belleza, & Cope, N. A. (1982). Disability Rating Scale for severe head trauma: Coma to community. *Archives of Physical Medicine and Rehabilitation, 63,* 118–123.

Rinehart, M. A. (1990). Strategies for improving motor performance. In M. Rosenthal, E. R. Griffith, M. R. Bond, & J. D. Miller (Eds.), *Rehabilitation of the adult and child with traumatic brain injury* (2nd ed., pp. 331–350). Philadelphia: F. A. Davis Company.

Rosenthal, M., & Bond, M. R. (1990). Behavioral and psychiatric sequelae. In M. Rosenthal, E. R. Griffith, M. R. Bond, & J. D. Miller (Eds.), *Rehabilitation of the adult and child with traumatic brain injury* (pp. 179–192). Philadelphia: F. A. Davis Company.

Ruff, R. M., Camenzuli, L., & Mueller, J. (1996). Miserable minority: Emotional factors that influence the outcome of mild traumatic brain injury. *Brain Injury, 10,* 551–565.

Salazar, A. M., Warden, D. L., Schwab, K., Spector, J., Braverman, S., Walter, J., Cole, R., Rosner, M. M., Martin, E. M., Ecklund, J., & Ellenbogen, R. G. (2000). Cognitive rehabilitation for traumatic brain injury: A randomized trial. *Journal of the American Medical Association, 283,* 3075–3081.

Salcman, M., Schepp, R. S., & Ducker, T. B. (1981). Calculated recovery rates in severe head trauma. *Neurosurgery, 8,* 301–308.

Sandel, M. E., Bell, K. R., & Michaud, L. J. (1998). Brain injury rehabilitation: 1. Traumatic brain injury: Prevention, pathophysiology, and outcome prediction. *Archives of Physical Medicine and Rehabilitation, 79,* S-3–S-9.

Satz, P., Zaucha, K., Forney, D. L., McCleary, C., Asarnow, R. F., Light, R., Levin, H., Kelly, D., Bergsneider, M., Hovda, D., Martin, N., Caron, M. J., Namerow, N., & Becker, D. (1998). Neuropsychological, psychosocial and vocational correlates of the Glasgow Coma Scale at 6 months post-injury: A study of moderate to severe traumatic brain injury patients. *Brain Injury, 12,* 555–567.

Schaffer, L., Kranzler, L. I., & Siqueira, E. B. (1985). Aspects of evaluation and treatment of head injury. *Neurology Clinics, 3,* 259–273.

Scherzer, B. P. (1986). Rehabilitation following severe head trauma: Results of a three-year program. *Archives of Physical Medicine and Rehabilitation, 67,* 366–374.

Scott, A. D., & Dow, P. W. (1995). Traumatic brain injury. In C. A. Trombly (Ed.), *Occupational therapy for physical dysfunction* (4th ed., pp. 705–733). Baltimore: Williams & Wilkins.

Sherer, M., Madison, C. F., & Hannay, H. J. (2000). A review of outcome after moderate to severe closed head injury with an introduction to life care planning. *Journal of Head Trauma Rehabilitation, 15,* 767–782.

Sohlberg, M. M., McLaughlin, K. A., Todis, B., Larsen, J., & Glang, A. (2001). What does it take to collaborate with families affected by brain injury: A preliminary model. *Journal of Head Trauma Rehabilitation, 16,* 498–511.

Sparadeo, F. R., & Gill, D. (1989). Focus on clinical research: Effects of prior alcohol use on head injury recovery. *Journal of Head Trauma Rehabilitation, 4,* 75–82.

Stoeckmann, T. (2001). Casting for the person with spasticity. *Topics in Stroke Rehabilitation, 8,* 27–35.

Talbot, L. R., & Whitaker, H. A. (1994). Brain-injured persons in an altered state of consciousness: Measures and intervention strategies. *Brain Injury, 8,* 689–699.

Teasdale, G., & Jennett, B. (1974). Assessment of coma and impaired consciousness: A practical scale. *Lancet, 2,* 81–84.

Thorton, M., Marshall, S., McComas, J., Finestone, H., McCormick, A., & Sveistrup, H. (2005). Benefits of activity and virtual reality based balance exercise programmes for adults with traumatic brain injury: Perceptions of participants and their caregivers. *Brain Injury, 19,* 989–1000.

Thurman, D. J., Alverson, C., Dunn, K. A., Guerrero, J., & Sniezek, J. E. (1999). Traumatic brain injury in the United States: A public health perspective. *Journal of Head Trauma Rehabilitation, 14,* 602–615.

Toglia, J. P. (1989). Approaches to cognitive assessment of the brain-injured adult. *Occupational Therapy Practice, 1,* 36–55.

Trexler, L. E., & Zappala, G. (1988). Neuropathological determinants of acquired attention disorders in traumatic brain injury. *Brain and Cognition, 8,* 291–302.

Trombly, C. A., Radomski, M. V., & Davis, E. S. (1998). Achievement of self-identified goals by adults with traumatic brain injury: Phase I. *American Journal of Occupational Therapy, 52,* 810–818.

Trombly, C. A., Radomski, M. V., Trexel, C., & Burnett-Smith, S. E. (2002). Occupational therapy and achievement of self-identified goals by adults with acquired brain injury: Phase II. *American Journal of Occupational Therapy, 56,* 489–498.

Turner, M. S. (1985). Pediatric head injury. *Indiana Medicine, 78,* 194–197.

Warren, M. (1993). A hierarchical model for evaluation and treatment of visual perceptual dysfunction in adult acquired brain injury: Part 1. *American Journal of Occupational Therapy, 47,* 42–54.

Wells, R., Dywan, J., & Dumas, J. (2005). Life satisfaction and distress in family caregivers as related to specific behavioural changes after traumatic brain injury. *Brain Injury, 19,* 1105–1115.

Whyte, J., & DiPasquale, M. C. (1995). Assessment of vision and visual attention in minimally responsive brain injured patients. *Archives of Physical Medicine and Rehabilitation, 76,* 804–810.

Willer, B., Ottenbacher, K. J., & Coud, M. L. (1994). The Community Integration Questionnaire. *American Journal of Physical Medicine and Rehabilitation, 73,* 103–111.

Williams, T. A. (1995). Low vision rehabilitation for a patient with a traumatic brain injury. *American Journal of Occupational Therapy, 49,* 923–926.

Ylvisaker, M., Jacobs, H. E., & Feeney, T. (2003). Positive supports for people who experience behavioral and cognitive disability after brain injury. *Journal of Head Trauma Rehabilitation, 18,* 7–32.

Yody, B. B., & Strauss, D. (1999). The effect of decreasing length of stay on long-term TBI patient outcomes. *Journal of Rehabilitation Outcomes Measurement, 3,* 42–50.

Yuen, H. K. (1997). Positive talk training in an adult with traumatic brain injury. *American Journal of Occupational Therapy, 51,* 780–783.

LEARNING OBJECTIVES

After studying this chapter, the reader will be able to do the following:

1. Describe four neurodegenerative diseases, including their courses and their symptoms.
2. By completing the occupational therapy evaluation, select appropriate assessment and evaluation tools for clients with neurodegenerative diseases based on individual clients' characteristics and requirements.
3. Determine appropriate interventions for clients with neurodegenerative disease based on their individual characteristics and requirements.
4. Select appropriate equipment for home, work, and community to help a client with neurodegenerative disease maintain independent function at the highest possible level.

CHAPTER 40

Neurodegenerative Diseases

Susan J. Forwell, Lois F. Copperman, and Lucinda Hugos

Glossary

Akinesia—Impaired ability to initiate voluntary and spontaneous motor responses, such as the interruption of performance in movement when attention is distracted (e.g., freezing in Parkinson's disease).

Axonal transection—Separation of an axon from its postsynaptic neuron, permanently interrupting action potential propagation.

Bradykinesia—Slowness or poverty of body movement.

Cogwheel rigidity—Series of catches in the resistance during passive motion.

Fasciculations—Rapid, flickering twitching movements of a part of a muscle occurring irregularly in time and location.

Festinating gait—Marked by very small rapid steps and occurs in persons with Parkinson's disease when the posture of the head and trunk involuntarily lean forward ahead of the feet, moving the center of gravity (COG) forward. Rather than taking a large step to correct the imbalance, several hurried small steps increasing gait velocity occurs, resulting in running or "chasing" one's COG, which remains in front of the feet.

Myelin—Lipid-rich insulating material covering nerve fibers that speeds conduction of impulses.

Rigidity—Hypertonicity of agonist and antagonist muscles that offers a consistent, uniform resistance to passive movement.

Neurodegenerative diseases are generally chronic and potentially progressive and frequently require coping with existing disability and the threat of future loses. The underlying pathologies of these diseases are described in this chapter and are shown to have mechanisms that attack the peripheral nervous system (PNS) and central nervous system (CNS), resulting in impairments and limitations that affect all aspects of life. Although the underlying diseases are not curable, research and medical advances have led to treatments that alter the progressive course of many neurodegenerative diseases and allow people to live longer, more productive lives.

This chapter begins with an overview of occupational therapy for persons with neurodegenerative diseases. Broad considerations related to evaluation, goal setting, and intervention are reviewed, followed by detailed discussions of multiple sclerosis (MS) and Parkinson's disease (PD), amyotrophic lateral sclerosis (ALS), and Guillain-Barré syndrome (GBS).

OCCUPATIONAL THERAPY FOR NEURODEGENERATIVE DISEASES

Occupational therapy frequently begins at diagnosis and continues throughout the continuum of comprehensive care; it may take place in inpatient acute care, inpatient rehabilitation, outpatient, in-home, or long-term care settings. Inpatient acute treatment usually follows a relapse or deterioration in the disease and/or a crisis and is generally short and limited to stabilizing symptoms with medical interventions. Inpatient rehabilitation may last 1 to several weeks, with daily therapy sessions geared to develop new strategies to deal with changed symptoms and to identify and obtain equipment. Outpatient therapy is usually weekly, with 1-hour individual sessions to demonstrate strategies to maximize independence, instruct in home programs, minimize the effects of symptoms on daily activities, and identify and obtain needed equipment. Occupational therapy in long-term care facilities may be similar to inpatient rehabilitation for people adjusting to changing symptoms or developing palliative care plans for patients whose neurodegenerative disease has progressed to the point they cannot be cared for at home.

Neurodegenerative diseases affect most aspects of life and commonly individuals in their young and middle adult years. It is imperative occupational therapy focus on activities and occupations that are most relevant, valued, and important to the individual and significant other(s). Evaluative screens help the therapist to determine the client's most relevant activities and to target these specific areas during assessment. For example, an individual may set a high priority on continuing employment and be willing to delegate home and self-care tasks. Assessment and intervention for this person would focus on maximizing independence in activities necessary for work and setting up the support systems needed for home functions. Occupational therapists must also keep an eye on their own coping and objectivity, especially when treating clients whose disease course portends increasing disability or death.

Occupational Therapy Evaluation

Occupational Profile

The occupational therapy evaluation begins with an interview that gathers information about the client's relevant history of disease, valued roles and occupations, and screens for specific concerns or problems. This interview must be sensitive to the client's changing function and fear of the unknown as well as illuminate problem areas that may not be spontaneously discussed such as fatigue, depression, sexual function, and cognitive concerns that impact their occupations and social network. With this information, an occupational profile assists to direct further assessment.

Occupational Analysis

Based on the occupational profile, the occupational therapist will select assessments and measurement tools that will provide in-depth information on occupational areas of concern. For persons with neurodegenerative disease, the content of these measures may be limited to a few or cover a broad spectrum of occupational performance areas (such as ADLs, IADLs, and work) or symptoms (such as sensation, spasticity, weakness, memory, and fatigue).

Occupational Therapy Intervention Process

Goal Setting

The primary goals of intervention are to reduce the effects of disability resulting from disease impairments and to maintain or promote independence and quality of life; that is, safe, functional, and comfortable participation in chosen tasks and roles. Goal setting is a collaborative process that includes the client, occupational therapist, and as appropriate, family and other significant persons. The unplanned and profound impact of neurodegenerative disease frequently makes realistic goal setting complex, and requires sensitivity, flexibility, and negotiation skills of the occupational therapist. The therapist frequently helps the client modify behaviors and assumptions of a lifetime while assisting the person and significant others to move toward realistic new goals. Treatment goals should be in sync with the client's priorities and grounded in evidence-based research. Given the progressive nature of many neurodegenerative diseases, regular reassessment and reordering of goals and priorities may be necessary.

Intervention Implementation

Due to the complexity of disability, intervening in one area may affect several other factors, such as fatigue, pain, and weakness. Interventions are varied and frequently involve significant others, especially as the disease progresses. The following is an overview of ways occupational therapy optimizes performance in key occupational roles for persons with neurodegenerative diseases.

Self-Maintenance Roles

In basic and instrumental ADL, the occupational therapist assists the client to attain safety, maintain independence in priority activities, use specialized equipment, and participate using energy-conserving methods. Treatment strategies include the following:

- Priority setting
- Education in areas such as the disease process affecting motor or cognitive changes
- Environmental modifications at home and work to promote safety and independence
- Exercise to prevent loss of range of motion and strength needed to dress
- Behavior modification such as use of energy conservation and time management techniques
- Identifying and obtaining equipment to compensate for weakness or other symptoms
- Balancing independence with assistance from others

Self-Advancement Roles

The onset of neurodegenerative diseases affects employment in or outside of the home. Contrary to popular expectations, however, many individuals can and should continue to work rather than claim disability. Medical treatments affecting disease progression and legislation mean that modification of employment is frequently more appropriate than an immediate disability claim. Continued employment has implications for financial independence, health care choices, socialization, identity, and self-esteem. Occupational therapists critically review job expectations and, as required, make modifications to the environment, recommend behavioral changes, prescribe equipment, identify resources, and make recommendations to the individual or the employer. Nonprofit groups such as the National Multiple Sclerosis Society (NMSS) provide resources and are excellent sources of information for both patients and therapists (Resources 40-1).

Self-Enhancement Roles

Maintaining leisure pursuits may be a high priority for individuals with neurodegenerative diseases but are often the first roles to be abandoned. Modifying activities and proper equipment often enable the individual to continue to carry out these important meaningful occupations.

Members and Roles of Rehabilitation Team

Depending on the type and severity of functional limitations, involvement of the rehabilitation team may vary, although it is essential in maintaining the highest level of function and quality of life (Martin & Weiler, 2003). When cognitive problems interfere with everyday occupations, psychologists, speech therapists, and occupational thera-

RESOURCE 40-1

Neurodegenerative Diseases

Amyotrophic Lateral Sclerosis

ALS Association
21021 Ventura Boulevard,
Suite 321
Woodland Hills, CA 91364-2206

Muscular Dystrophy Association, ALS Division
3300 East Sunrise Drive
Tucson, AZ 85718-3208
Phone: (602) 529-2000
Publications include *ALS: Maintaining Mobility, Meals,* and others.

Cleveland Clinic ALS Center
ALS Coordinator, Department of Neurology
9500 Euclid Avenue
Cleveland, OH 44195
Publication: *ALS Care Manual.*

Guillain-Barré Syndrome

Guillain-Barré Syndrome Foundation International
P.O. Box 262
Wynnewood, PA 19096
Phone: (610) 667-0131
www.gbsfi.com

Guillain-Barré Syndrome Support Group
Eastgate, Sleaford
Lincolnshire, NG34 7EB
United Kingdom
+44 1529 304615
www.gbs.org.uk

Multiple Sclerosis

National Multiple Sclerosis Society (NMSS)
733 Third Avenue
New York, NY 10017
Phone: (800) FIGHT-MS.
www.nmss.org
Local chapters provide "Fatigue: Take Control!" video-based series for fatigue management.

Multiple Sclerosis Association of America (MSAA)
National Headquarters
706 Haddonfield Road
Cherry Hill, NJ 08002
Phone: (800) 532-7667
www.msaa.com

Consortium of Multiple Sclerosis Centers (CMSC)
c/o Gimbel MS Center, Holy Name Hospital
718 Teaneck Road
Teaneck, NJ 07666
Phone: (201) 837-0727

Cooling Vests

Coolsport (20% discount for people with MS)
1880 West Carson Street
Torrence, CA 40501
Phone: (310) 618-1590
www.coolsport.net

MicroClimate Cooling Systems, Inc.
968 East Saginaw Road
Sanford, MI 48657
Phone: (800) 642-9077
www.microclimate.com

Parkinson's Disease

Parkinson's Disease Update Newsletter
Phone: (800) 947-6658

Parkinson Foundation of Canada
National Office, 4211 Yonge Street, Suite 316
Toronto, Ontario, M2P 2A9
Canada
Phone: (800) 565-3000
www.parkinson.ca

American Parkinson Disease Association, Inc.
1250 Hylan Boulevard,
Suite 4B
Staten Island, NY 10305
Phone: (800) 223-2732
www.apdaparkinson.org

National Parkinson Foundation, Inc.
Bob Hope Research Center,
1501 N.W. 9th Avenue
Miami, FL 33136-1494
Phone: (800) 327-4545
www.parkinson.org

Michael J. Fox Foundation for Parkinson's Research
P.O. Box 2010
Grand Rapids, MN 55745
www.michaeljfox.org

Miscellaneous

National Organization of Rare Disorders (NORD)
55 Kenosia Avenue, P.O. Box 1968
Danbury, CT 06813-1968
Phone: (203) 744-0100
www.rarediseases.org

Paralyzed Veterans of America (PVA)
801 Eighteenth Street NW
Washington, DC 20006
Phone: (800) 424-8200
www.pva.org

Clearinghouse on Disability Information
U.S. Department of Education,
202-205-8241
www.ed.gov/about/offices/list/osers/codi.html

pists are often consulted (Brown & Kraft, 2005). Neuropsychologists may be called upon to conduct in-depth cognitive assessments, make recommendations, and engage in intervention. In addition to cognitive issues, the speech therapist may be involved when dysarthria is present or expressive communication is labored. In the presence of dysphagia, an occupational therapist, speech therapist, and/or dietician commonly form the intervention team. Social work services assist when there is a shift in financial or care needs to advise on and make application to appropriate programs and counsel individuals and significant others to better cope with role change and demands. Physical changes as a result of weakness, spasticity, sensory problems, pain, and decreased endurance and range of motion necessitate the services of physical and occupational therapy to enhance mobility, upper extremity function, and overall conditioning to reduce falling and to provide guidance for appropriate exercise programs. Occupational therapy services are used when individuals are having difficulty caring for themselves or their immediate environment or engaging in work and/or familiar leisure occupations.

SPECIFIC NEURODEGENERATIVE DISEASES

The following sections present four specific neurodegenerative diseases: multiple sclerosis (MS), Parkinson's disease (PD), amyotrophic lateral sclerosis (ALS), and Guillain-Barré syndrome (GBS). The first section discusses MS and provides detailed insights into the clinical reasoning that is involved in occupational therapy treatment and evaluation that may be applicable across conditions. For example, a client with ALS who has fatigue may benefit from the energy conservation techniques mentioned in the section on MS. As such, issues that occur across neurodegenerative diseases are not elaborated upon in subsequent sections. Each neurological disorder, however, has its own underlying pathology, peculiarities, and prognosis. Understanding these issues helps the therapist develop appropriate intervention plans.

Multiple Sclerosis

MS is the most commonly diagnosed neurological disease that can cause disability in young adults (Stolp-Smith et al., 1997). An estimated 400,000 people in the United States have MS (NMSS, 2006). MS causes severe disability in some people, but many continue to lead active, productive lives and are not severely disabled (Rodriguez et al., 1994; Stolp-Smith et al., 1997). Therapists may have a skewed perspective because it is the relatively severely disabled people who are typically referred for therapy. Unfortunately, by the time a person requires wheeled mobility, a tremendous window of opportunity has passed for interventions such as upgrading ambulation skills, fatigue management, and employment modifications. Therefore, therapists should work to alert physicians and other referral sources to the need for early intervention with persons with MS.

The cause of MS remains unknown. The present theory is an environmental trigger initiates the autoimmune response in people with genetic susceptibility (Trapp et al., 1998). The *multiple* in multiple sclerosis refers to both time and location. The *sclerosis* refers to the hardened or sclerotic plaques that are the scar tissue resulting from autoimmune attacks on the CNS (axons and **myelin** covering).

Axonal transection is considered as significant as demyelination in MS damage (McGavern et al., 2000; Trapp et al., 1998). At least temporarily, demyelinated axons may remyelinate and provide conduction of nerve impulses. Transected axons are permanently destroyed and lose all potential for conduction. At autopsy, Trapp et al. (1998) found as many as 11,236 ± 2,775 transected axons in a cubic millimeter of active lesions in subjects with definite MS compared to 0.7 ± 0.7 in white matter of subjects without brain disease. Evidence has also been seen of continued disease activity even during periods that are clinically quiet (Trapp et al., 1998). The demyelination and axonal damage occur in the presence of inflammation, which may explain the rapid improvement often seen in treatment of relapses with corticosteroid anti-inflammatory agents.

Diagnosing MS

Individuals who are diagnosed with MS are typically between the ages of 15 and 50 years, although children are increasingly being diagnosed (Krupp & Macallister, 2005). Peak age of onset is 20 to 30 years. Women are two to three times as likely to get MS as men. Caucasians of northern European descent have the greatest risk of developing MS (Bourdette, 1997). The incidence of MS increases with distance from the equator, both north and south, similar to the pattern of European settlement (Frankel, 1990; Kurland, 1952). The individual risk is related to where a person spends the first 15 years of life (Alter, 1978; Frankel, 1990) and is about 1:1,000 in the United States (NMSS, 2006).

The diagnosis of MS is based on findings of the history, neurological examination, and overall clinical picture. Additional tests, such as analysis of cerebrospinal fluid and magnetic resonance imaging, are used only to prove the clinical signs and not solely as the basis of the diagnosis. Objective demonstration of two or more white matter lesions in discrete parts of the CNS is necessary to make the diagnosis (Poser et al., 1983). Episodes of CNS dysfunction must be reported or demonstrated over time, or there must be ongoing progression over 6 months with no other explanation of these problems.

Signs of MS include weakness, hyperreflexia, positive Babinski sign, dysmetria, nystagmus, and impaired vibratory or position sensation. The *Expanded Disability Status Scale* (*EDSS*) (Kurtzke, 1983) and the *MS Functional Composite* (*MSFC*) (Fischer et al., 2001) are the most commonly used impairment rating instruments in both clinical and research settings. The presence of several signs and symptoms may result in profound limitations such as unemployment and loss of independence.

The Course of MS

The course of MS is typically categorized into four types: relapsing-remitting, secondary progressive, primary progressive, and progressive-relapsing. The relapsing-remitting course of MS produces clearly defined relapses of acute worsening of neurological function followed by partial or complete improvement and then stable periods of remission between attacks. The most common course of MS at the time of diagnosis, relapsing-remitting MS often becomes secondary progressive MS with time (NMSS, 2006; Trapp et al., 1998). People with secondary progressive MS start with a relapsing-remitting course of up to 10–15 years following diagnosis. The secondary progressive diagnosis is typically made when there is continued neurological deterioration. People with primary progressive MS have continuously declining neurological function from onset (Lublin & Reingold, 1996; NMSS, 2006). The fourth course of MS is progressive-relapsing, which differs from relapsing-remitting MS because disease progression continues through the periods between relapses.

Two other terms occasionally used to refer to MS disease course are benign and malignant (Lublin & Reingold, 1996). People with benign MS are fully functional 15 years after the disease onset. People with malignant MS have rapid progression leading to significant disability or death in a short period.

Disease-Modifying Medications for MS

Four immune-modulating medications approved for use in the United States (NMSS, 2006) have been shown to have positive effects on slowing the disease progression: interferon-beta-1a (Avonex); interferon-beta-1b (Betaseron); glatiramer acetate (Copaxone), and interferon-beta-1a (Rebif). A fifth medication, utilized primarily when the other four drugs no longer seem effective, is mitoxantrone (Novantrone). Medications are also used for the treatment of MS signs and symptoms, such as Amantadine and Provigil for fatigue, baclofen for spasticity, numerous antidepressants for depression, gabapentin for pain, and ditripan for selected urinary problems.

Clients commonly discuss with therapists and ask their opinion on the value of medications. This is true particularly of MS disease-modifying medications because they are not designed to improve the patient's condition or reverse disability but rather slow disease progression. Clients often wonder whether it is worth taking the medications when they are not seeing improvement. The therapist's responsibility is to understand and reinforce the importance of continuing to take appropriate medications.

With the increased stability of the disease course that results from these medications, patients may realize greater benefits from rehabilitation intervention, such that they live fuller lives, remain employed, and participate in high-priority occupations longer. The costs of these medications may make maintaining employment-related prescription coverage a very desirable outcome of therapy.

Potential Emotional, Social, and Economic Consequences

A disease that primarily strikes young adults has substantial economic and employment consequences. Between the ages of 20 and 40, people typically are entering the labor market, establishing themselves in their careers, and forming families. MS, with its common symptoms of fatigue, weakness, difficulties with prolonged standing or walking, and cognitive problems, can impede productivity both at work and at home. Studies conducted prior to the development of disease-modifying medications revealed that more than 70% of individuals with MS were out of the labor force 10–15 years after initial diagnosis (Kalb, 1996). The influence of disease-modifying drugs (data is being collected to look at the effect), however, together with employment disability legislation such as the Americans with Disabilities Act, has resulted in opportunities for people to maintain productive paid employment for longer periods. Persons with MS who leave the labor market are likely to have greater social isolation and psychological distress, lower incomes, and more limited access to health insurance than if they remain employed (Kalb, 1996).

Symptoms Typically Addressed in Occupational Therapy

A number of symptoms associated with MS may include weakness, sensory changes, balance disturbance, visual changes, bowel and bladder disturbance, cognitive changes, dysarthria and dysphagia, dizziness or vertigo, pain, ataxic gait, tremor, sexual dysfunction, depression, spasticity, and fatigue. The most common and pervasive symptom is fatigue (Freal, Kraft, & Coryell, 1984; Paralyzed Veterans of America [PVA], 1998). A few of these symptoms are described here as they present in MS to provide examples for the implications for occupational therapy services.

Fatigue

Fatigue, one of the most common MS symptoms, affects approximately 60–80% of people with MS (PVA, 1998). Fatigue is a significant contributor to disability and a primary reason people with MS are referred to occupational therapy. People with MS often report that their symptoms tend to worsen when they tire. Fatigue can vary from slight to severe, worsening in the afternoon, and may be related to increased core body temperature (Fig. 40-1). Therapists must be alerted to the types and potential sources of fatigue associated with MS (Definition 40-1) (PVA, 1998). With the types of fatigue identified, the therapist can then target treatments appropriately (Forwell, 2007).

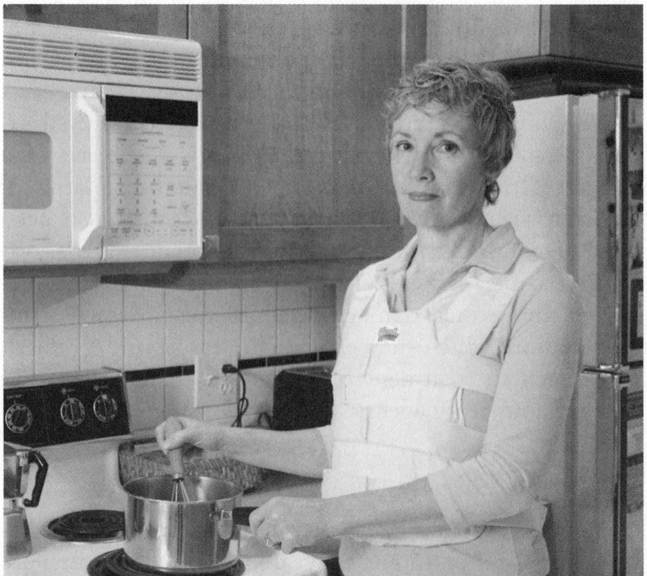

Figure 40-1 Woman in cooling vest cooking at the stove.

DEFINITION 40-1

Types of Fatigue in MS

- Primary MS fatigue— Fatigue directly due to MS disease process. Causation is poorly understood.
- Fatigue due to poor sleep—Sleep problems are often related to muscle spasms, depression, or urinary problems.
- Fatigue due to depression.
- Nerve fiber or motor fatigue—Fatigue probably related to inefficient nerve conduction.
- Fatigue due to impairments, such as weakness and spasticity.
- Fatigue secondary to medication side effects or infections.

Weakness

Weakness is another common symptom resulting in referral to therapy. Weakness may occur in all parts of the body. One of the most common initial complaints is weakness in the foot dorsiflexors resulting in stumbling or falling, especially on uneven surfaces.

Cognition

Approximately 40–60% of people with MS have cognitive problems that vary considerably in severity (Beatty et al., 1995; Rao et al., 1991). In an electronic survey conducted by the Rocky Mountain MS Center in 2003, 73% of respondents reported some cognitive difficulty; of these, 44% had not discussed the subject with a health provider. Cognitive problems are seen at all stages of the disease and are not directly correlated with motor impairments (Maurelli et al., 1992). Studies have found correlations between cognitive impairments and the extent of brain damage on weighted magnetic resonance brain scans (Foong, Rozewicz, & Quaghebeur, 1997; Rovari et al., 1998).

Common cognitive problems of people with MS include word retrieval difficulties; slowed speed of information processing and difficulties learning new material; and problems with attention, concentration, memory, and executive functions, such as diminished judgment, difficulty with abstract reasoning, and reduced verbal fluency organization (NMSS, 1998). People with MS may have other perceptual-cognitive problems, such as visual-spatial impairments that might be evidenced by a tendency to get lost or a history of motor vehicle accidents.

Cognitive problems are likely to vary during the day, increasing in the afternoon or when the client has performed tasks requiring sustained mental concentration (Krupp & Lekins, 2000). The cognitive problems of MS are frequently subtle. Both individuals and their families may be unaware that cognitive problems are related to the disease and are not personality or psychological issues. There is no "MS personality," but executive function problems, such as reduced insight and inflexible thinking, may be mistaken for personality changes.

Many areas of cognition may remain intact, and screens such as the *Mini-Mental State Exam* are unlikely to detect such problems (Beatty & Goodkin, 1990). Consequently, it has been necessary to complete a lengthy neuropsychological evaluation. More recently, however, a group of experts came to consensus on a 90-minute, 6-measure neuropsychological battery designed specifically for MS called the *Minimal Assessment of Cognitive Function in MS* (*MACFIMS*) (Benedict et al., 2002). Baselining individual cognitive performance using appropriate cognitive tests is encouraged for documentation of future change and possible future employment disability claim. Identification of cognitive impairments, information about their effects on function, and the development of individualized compensation strategies may reduce the impact of the problems.

No medications have been proven effective in treating cognitive problems. Intervention, however, that includes group therapy, stress management, computer-assisted retraining, and cognitive-behavioral therapy, has been shown to have positive effects on cognitive function (Brown & Kraft, 2005).

Pain

Pain is estimated to be a problem for 40–60% of people with MS (Moulin, Foley, & Ebers, 1988). Pain directly due to the neurological lesions is considered primary to MS and is usually treated with medications. Pain that is secondary to MS and is often a result of poor posture, positioning, or spasticity is often relieved by therapy.

Spasticity

Spasticity in MS is usually greater in the lower extremities than in the upper extremities. Therapists should be familiar with the standard medications for spasticity, such as baclofen and tizanidine, and their side effect of drowsiness, which may increase fatigue (PVA, 2003). The intrathecal baclofen pump may help to improve function for people with moderate to severe spasticity.

Tremor and Ataxia

Intention tremor occurs during motor performance and is the most common tremor seen in MS. It is one of the most difficult problems to manage (NMSS, 2006). As an activity progresses, the tremor increases such that the tremor is at its worst at the end of range or when the activity is at its target or goal, a point when the greatest control and precision is required. Intention tremor occurs in the upper extremity and is evidenced primarily in the fingers, hand,

and wrist. Intention tremor may also occur in the lower extremities, torso, and neck (NMSS, 2006).

Ataxia presents in the trunk and lower extremities where postural responses tend to occur before upper extremity movements. As such, the proximal segments are too early to counteract the destabilizing effects of the upper extremity. The functional challenges of ataxia are further magnified because of the multiple joints involved in the ataxic movement.

Dysphagia

Swallowing problems in MS are receiving increased attention because research that did not use videofluoroscopy (VF) suggested that 34–43% of individuals studied experienced dysphagia, although only half of these patients reported swallowing difficulties (Calcagno et al., 2002; Thomas & Wiles, 1999). When VF was used, most asymptomatic persons with MS were shown to have abnormalities (Weiser et al., 2002). These studies indicated that risk factors for dysphagia were severity of disease and cerebellar or brainstem involvement. This suggests that occupational therapists should routinely screen for choking, aspiration, and swallowing difficulties.

Adjusting to MS

Although only a small percentage of people with MS are severely disabled, the diagnosis is often devastating. The continual need to adjust to changing symptoms and varying impairments and the fear of and uncertainty about the disease process affect self-esteem, relationships, sexuality, physical activities, vocational goals, and recreational interests. From questions about pregnancy to cognitive changes influencing competence or safety, MS subtly or not so subtly affects every role and relationship. The variability of the disease and the hidden nature of many of the symptoms, such as cognitive changes and fatigue, often make it difficult and uncomfortable to explain to friends, coworkers, and family members.

Each person's reaction to MS events varies and has implications for adjustment. Research has shown that emotion-focused coping techniques were used more often by those experiencing an MS relapse, whereas problem solving and using one's social network were used by persons with MS in remission (Pakenham, 1999). This is supported by evidence that emotional involvement was a marginal indicator of new MS lesions as shown on MRI (Mohr et al., 2002). It has also been demonstrated in a 1-year follow-up study that a greater use of problem-solving strategies to cope was an indicator of better psychological adjustment (Warren, Warren, & Cockerill, 1991).

Initially, people are typically quite preoccupied with their diagnosis because it represents a major new and unknown threat that suddenly challenges former assumptions about the future. As time passes, particularly if the individuals with MS return to full function, they frequently ignore the diagnosis and pay little attention to MS issues. As long as the inattention does not result in adverse decisions, this may be a healthy attitude. The occupational therapist helps clients process the implications of changes and identifies modifications to minimize their effects. Information about new symptoms may be all a person needs to make a successful adjustment.

Occupational Therapy Evaluation

During the evaluation process of a person with MS, there are unique features that must be understood and incorporated from the individual's history with MS and from his or her life experience. The occupational therapist can then select evaluation tools and methods appropriate for the person with MS.

Occupational Profile

The occupational therapy assessment begins with an interview about the person's goals for therapy and a brief history of symptoms and treatment since diagnosis. This gives the therapist an idea of the course of the disease and the person's past coping style. Throughout the interview, the therapist actively listens for hints of cognitive difficulties. The therapist should always remember that many people with MS who appear symptom free may have significant hidden impairments. Brief questions regarding dizziness, thinking problems, dropping things, numbness and tingling, manual dexterity, prolonged walking and standing, employment, home physical and social environment, leisure interests, bladder problems, ADL, IADL, fatigue, sleeping pattern, equipment, muscle cramping, pain, fine motor activities, falling and balance problems, and stiffness can provide clues to the specific assessments that are likely to be relevant to the person's problems. If possible, particularly if cognitive problems are present, a family member or significant other should be encouraged to attend the evaluation if the client consents. The therapist can best probe for symptoms if the client completes selected survey instruments, such as the *Pain Severity Scale* (PVA, 1998), and lists his or her medications prior to the interview.

Analysis of Occupational Performance: Tools and Methods

The initial interview and history give the therapist a quick indication of what evaluation tools and methods to use. Upper extremity range-of-motion and manual muscle tests, manual dexterity, and dynamometer evaluations are routine unless clearly inappropriate. An evaluation tool being used in MS drug studies that measures short-distance walking, hand function, and cognition is the *MS Functional Composite* (*MSFC*) measure, which includes a timed 25-ft walk, the *Nine-Hole Peg Test*, and the *Paced Auditory Serial Addition Test* (*PASAT*) (Fischer et al., 2001).

Therapists select a variety of other standardized evaluation tools and methods based on the client's history and priorities, including:

- Fatigue assessment, such as *Modified Fatigue Impact Scale* and a qualitative assessment (PVA, 1998)
- The *6-Minute Walk Test* to assess endurance and fatigue (Pankoff et al., 2000)
- Sleep history, questionnaire, or diary (PVA, 1998)
- Cognitive screening such as the *MACFIMS* (Benedict et al., 2002)
- Vision evaluation
- Depression instruments such as the *Beck Depression Inventory*-18 (BDI-18) (Mohr et al., 1997)
- Gait, bed mobility, and/or transfer assessment such as the mobility section of the *Functional Independence Measure* (*FIM*)
- ADL, IADL, and dysphagia assessments
- Manual dexterity and coordination tests, such as the *Nine-Hole Peg Test* or *Purdue Pegboard*
- Sensory testing, including *Semmes-Weinstein Monofilaments* and proprioception
- Spasticity assessment using the *Modified Ashworth Scale*
- Tremor and ataxia assessments
- Trigger point evaluation for head, neck, and shoulder muscles
- Vestibular evaluation

Administering such measures, however, requires the therapist to accurately interpret findings in the context of the client's situation. For example, therapists must attempt to differentiate among various types of fatigue by considering results of several assessments. A high score on a depression index, for example, may indicate that depression is contributing to the patient's report of fatigue, while slow times on the *6-Minute Walk Test* may also suggest a nerve fiber or motor fatigue component. Alternatively, information from a sleep questionnaire may provide evidence that disturbed sleep due to urinary frequency is a source of daytime fatigue. It is common for persons with MS to have several different sources of fatigue (Forwell et al., 2007), and multiple health care professionals may be involved in treating them. Finally, if the person reports repeated falling or safety issues, a home visit may also be appropriate.

Occupational Therapy Intervention Process

Goal Setting

Clients' priorities and interests are the cornerstone of goal setting and treatment planning. Frequently, however, both they and the referring provider mistakenly believe they have to live with problems as a result of MS that, in fact, are treatable through therapy. The collaborative process of goal setting assists to achieve realistic and satisfying outcomes.

Intervention Plan

Following the evaluation and a full discussion of the findings, the occupational therapist discusses the various types of interventions that may help the person manage the identified problems. Due to the progressive nature of the disease, occupational therapy is generally compensatory, teaching the client techniques to manage the symptoms and compensate for disability resulting from impairments rather than alleviating them.

The intervention plan must also take into account the unique issues of individuals with MS. For example, Finlayson (2004) suggests that, for older adults with MS, the occupational therapist must ensure they feel a sense of control over their future, work with families affected by the MS, and advocate for enhanced community support options.

Intervention Implementation

Increasingly, evidence is demonstrating the benefits of occupational therapy intervention for clients with MS. In a meta-analysis of occupational therapy intervention for MS, a positive effect on MS symptoms emerged (Baker & Tickle-Degnen, 2001). Although the level of evidence was not strong and research design flaws were noted, the body of literature is growing to support evidence-based practice.

Due to the interaction of multiple symptoms, intervention usually addresses the relevant occupations where problems present. Isolated treatment of symptoms is unlikely to be very effective, and concurrent occupational and physical therapy is often indicated. For example, physical therapists may treat fatigue by obtaining gait equipment, promoting aerobic exercises, and educating on the difference between energy expenditure during functional activities and exercise routines to increase endurance, while the occupational therapist instructs the client in energy conservation, identifies adaptive equipment, and helps the client modify home and work tasks. Taken together, these changes may significantly reduce fatigue. Occupational therapy intervention typically involves one or more of the following: instruction in activity strategies and energy conservation; establishing an appropriate exercise program; addressing pain and spasticity; implementing cognitive compensations; and identifying equipment, environmental, and employment modifications.

Activity Strategies and Energy Conservation

If a client complains of fatigue, the occupational therapist should suspect multiple types of fatigue and direct interventions appropriately. Fatigue treatment begins as the therapist provides written and oral explanations of each relevant underlying type of fatigue in an easily understood fashion. Guidelines for the treatment of fatigue are available (PVA, 1998). At the beginning of intervention, the client typically fills out a detailed activity diary and makes a list of individual goals and priorities (PVA, 1998). The occupational therapist and client use the diary as a starting point to identify and develop activity modifications to reduce fatigue through a systematic analysis of daily work, home, and leisure activities in all environments relevant to the individual.

Most energy conservation strategies are designed to enable persons with MS to use their limited energy on useful, meaningful activities that are important to them. This approach allows the client to exercise choice and control in everyday occupations. Research has demonstrated the effectiveness of occupational therapist-led group intervention for people with MS in energy conservation strategies (Mathiowetz, Matuska, & Murphy, 2001; Mathiowetz et al., 2005; Vanage, Gilbertson, & Mathiowetz, 2003). In addition, throughout the United States, chapters of the NMSS offer a 6-week video course called *Fatigue: Take Control!* developed by Copperman and Hugos (NMSS, 2003). Preliminary studies of course effectiveness have demonstrated positive outcomes (Campbell, 2006). The course provides both information and treatment on MS fatigue and is useful for therapists and people with MS.

Essentially, the therapist helps the client analyze activities, understand rest-activity ratios, incorporate energy conservation strategies and exercise routine, and identify modifications and equipment to help the individual perform valued tasks and activities. Recommended changes may include the following:

- Decrease prolonged standing and walking by modifying tasks and using powered mobility devices for distances.
- Alternate periods of activity with intervals of rest, such as walking, sitting, and then walking again.
- Teach the client about the relationship between increased body temperature and increased fatigue, a phenomenon probably due to a decrease in the efficiency of nerve conduction in a demyelinated CNS.
- Identify modifications to help maintain cooler body temperature, such as layering clothing, purchasing an air conditioner, eliminating hot showers, sitting when showering, using a cooling vest (Figs. 40-1 and 40-2) when walking or active, and not using down comforters when sleeping.
- Shift important activities to the morning.
- Use appropriate equipment, such as a hinged ankle–foot orthosis, to compensate for weakness and reduce the energy required to walk.
- Obtain seating systems for trunk support in wheelchairs and properly fit ergonomic chairs with armrests and possibly headrests for computer and work activities.

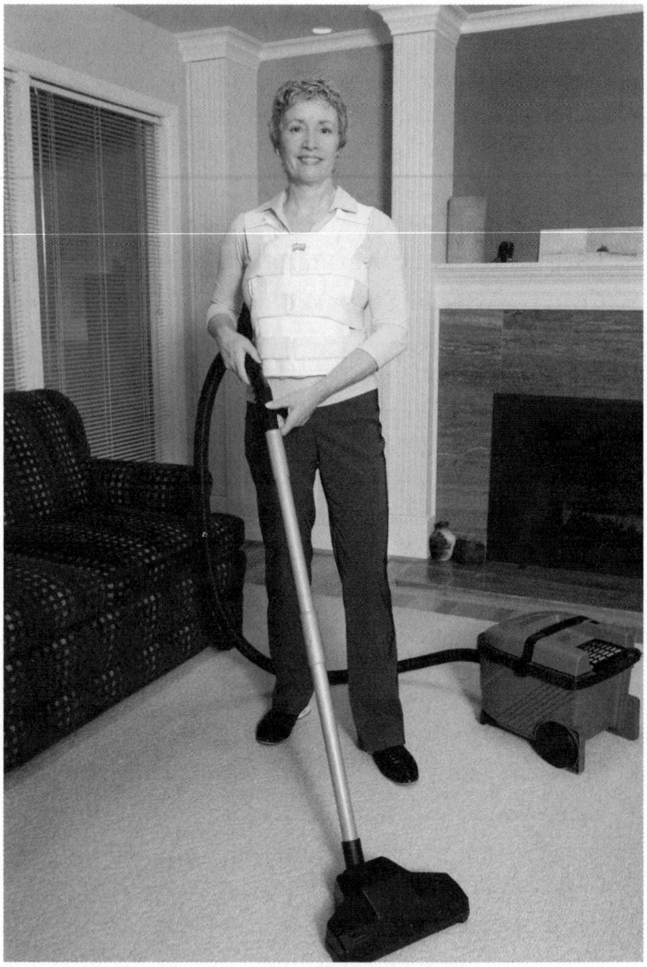

Figure 40-2 Woman in cooling vest vacuuming.

Written recommendations and summaries should always be provided at the end of the 2- to 4-hour sessions usually necessary to treat fatigue. Clients should also be encouraged to return to occupational therapy if changes in their symptoms result in problems in their function. Follow-up is recommended in 2–3 months.

Equipment, Behavioral, and Environmental Modifications

Generally, equipment, environmental, and behavioral modifications help patients compensate for weakness, spasticity, tremor, fatigue, ataxia, and cognitive problems. Environmental modifications may help in areas as diverse as providing access to mobility equipment, maintaining independence in ADL, and decreasing the distance to the bathroom. Many standard pieces of adaptive equipment are helpful. Computers and voice-activated software and memory aids may help decrease limitations due to weakness or tremor. Powered wheeled mobility devices, such as scooters or electric wheelchairs, are frequently effective in limiting fatigue and aiding functional limitations related to weakness and spasticity. Powered mobility devices that are capable of adaptation later, such as adding a tilt feature to an electric wheelchair, accommodate to changing status. Because of fatigue, self-propelling manual wheelchairs are often not indicated. When appropriate, the therapist identifies needed equipment and helps the client arrange equipment trials. Home and/or work visits may be necessary to identify environmental modifications.

Behavioral changes, such as switching an exercise program from lunch to after work and incorporating a lunchtime nap, frequently improve an individual's ability to perform productively. Changing behavior to use the elevator, for instance, might be combined with obtaining a scooter for distance walking and widening the doorways. The combination of the right equipment, behavior changes, and environmental modifications depend upon the individual's needs, resources, and personal preferences. Scheduled follow-ups are recommended to determine the need for new or further modifications as changes occur.

Exercise Programs

Occupational therapists teach clients to monitor the effects of any MS exercise program on both fatigue and their ability to perform high-priority activities to achieve the right activity balance. Two common MS symptoms, fatigue and spasticity, often decrease with regular exercise. Fatigue may be reduced by a structured aerobic program (Petajan et al., 1996; PVA, 1998), and spasticity may be managed with a stretching program done independently or by a caregiver. People with MS who have limited energy must carefully consider the optimal time of day to exercise and the most effective exercises because exercise often reduces the ability to perform activities immediately following the exercise for minutes to hours. Occupational therapists may help the client integrate exercise into his or her routine and to identify the best timing for the exercise regimen.

An aerobic home program will vary based on several considerations. For example, for an employed individual with limited time and leg weakness, a home stationary biking program for 25 minutes three or four times a week may be best. Alternatively, a water exercise program at the recreation center may be beneficial because the buoyancy helps reduce the effects of weakness. Of note, aquatic programs for people with MS should occur in cool pools due to heat sensitivity. Stretching programs for persons with MS generally emphasize relatively few repetitions and holds of 30–60 seconds. Finally, a strengthening program is indicated after a motivated client has successfully maintained a stretching and aerobic exercise program. The neurological weakness in MS cannot be reversed by strengthening, but deconditioning weakness may be reduced.

In general, MS exercise regimens are most likely to be successful if they start slowly and gradually increase in time, repetitions, and/or intensity. A realistic exercise program performed regularly is more desirable than an ideal program that is never followed. Good illustrations and written instructions should accompany every home program.

Spasticity Interventions

The appropriate intervention for spasticity depends on the severity and the extent to which it interferes with function. In addition to stretching exercises, adapted dressing techniques may prove helpful, such as using a stool to maintain hip flexion to decrease extensor spasm and/or using dressing sticks to compensate for inability to reach the feet. A standing home program may also be employed, using a standing frame for 30–60 minutes per day. Other interventions include resting splints and posture and positioning techniques, such as bringing the hips into 90° or more of flexion to decrease extensor tone in the lower extremities (PVA, 2003). Should a baclofen pump be indicated, the therapist may be involved in assessment prior to pump implantation and should reevaluate following implantation.

Cognitive Compensation

Occupational therapy for cognitive problems helps clients compensate for deficits and inefficiencies. Careful attention to timing of cognitive problems, fatigue levels, nature of the problem, and the environment in which problems occur helps the therapist develop individualized compensations. For example, treating fatigue with energy conservation techniques and mobility equipment often improves self-reported cognitive performance. Performance is also optimized as clients schedule cognitively demanding tasks for periods during the day when they typically feel their best, in minimally distracting environments. For example, tasks requiring higher levels of cognitive function should generally be performed in the morning if possible. Employment responsibilities and requirements should be scheduled to reduce the influence of the problems on job performance.

Education of both the client and his or her significant others regarding the problems is often beneficial. As families and others become aware that these problems are due to disease and not personality, the pressures on the individual can be eased, and modifications can be undertaken. Caution should be exercised in the disclosure of specific cognitive problems to employers, with careful consideration given to individual employment circumstances. Examples of modifications to facilitate cognitive functions include:

- Changing the environment to reduce distractions and interruptions and promote organization
- Teaching problem-solving techniques and reinforcing use of social network to assist with decision making, while showing the disadvantages of emotion-focused strategies

- Using a memory aid, such as a day planner or personal data appliance (PDA)
- Providing simple step-by-step written home and/or work directions
- Changing the difficult cognitive tasks to the morning
- Doing one activity at a time
- Incorporating assistive technology to improve function in high-order IADL, such as money management and bill payment
- Increasing the time allotted for an activity
- Delegating difficult tasks to others
- Using repetition in the learning process
- Assessing driving safety and recommending appropriate interventions

Pain Intervention

For pain related to weakness or spasticity, interventions such as posture training, ergonomic seating, stretching, and focal heat modalities on muscle trigger points may be effective. An ergonomic workstation should be used to minimize pain and fatigue in the employment environment.

Tremor and Ataxia Intervention

The hallmark of occupational therapy intervention for tremor and ataxia is proximal stabilization or support, modified approach to occupations, and adapted equipment and orthoses. Proximal stabilization includes supporting the trunk and larger joints of the upper and lower extremities. For example, for meals, lean one's torso against the table and have arms resting on the table (Gillen, 2000); because the position is sitting, the lower extremity is supported, the trunk is stabilized by leaning against the table, and the shoulder and elbows are supported. A modified approach may be the use of hand-over-hand for writing or dialing a cell phone. If one hand is unaffected by tremor, consider retraining the unaffected hand as tolerated. Orthoses might include a cervical collar to reduce the travel of the head and neck or wrist splints to minimize travel and number of joints in motion in the presence of tremor (NMSS, 2006).

Employment Modifications

The problems described in the preceding sections may affect the performance of individuals with MS at work. Many people with MS apply for disability benefits prematurely because they fear problems that may occur later or do not know about possible modifications. With the advent of medications that slow disease progression, interventions can frequently help individuals continue productive employment for many years. Job modifications may include:

- Changing the times at which tasks are performed
- Limiting prolonged walking and standing by using conference calls, increasing e-mail consultation, using powered mobility devices, and changing to an office near the bathroom
- Alterations in workstations, such as ergonomic chair with armrests, headsets, and mouse and keyboard trays
- Modifying work hours
- Working completely or partly at home
- Using voice-activated software and other technology
- Setting up a place where one can rest periodically

Parkinson's Disease

Parkinson's disease (PD) is a progressive, variable condition. It is most common in later adult years, with the mean age of onset 55–60 years. The incidence of PD is 1%, or 1,000 per 100,000 persons (Stern, 1993). Generally, PD is gradual at onset, and symptoms may take years to develop (Baker & Graham, 2004). PD is typically defined by the three cardinal signs of tremor, **rigidity**, and **bradykinesia**. Postural instability is often added to this list (Conley & Kirchner, 1999). Tremor, commonly the first complaint, is a resting tremor that increases with stress and may present as pill-rolling (Gelb, Olliver, & Gilman, 1999; Uitti, 1998). Rigidity is not a diagnostic feature of PD because it tends to occur at a more advanced stage (Conley & Kirchner, 1999; Gelb, Olliver, & Gilman, 1999). Bradykinesia causes a lack of facial expression, or "mask face," and affects walking, involvement in activities, and eye blink (Conley & Kirchner, 1999). Postural instability begins with reduced arm swing, head and trunk leaning forward, and shorter strides that progress to a shuffling gait. Lack of postural reflexes often results in increasing falls and **akinesia**, or episodes of "freezing" that reduce or eliminate spontaneous initiation of gait and impede turning and crossing thresholds (Conley & Kirchner, 1999; Gelb et al., 1999; Hass et al., 2005; Ward & Robertson, 2004).

Other symptoms of PD, particularly in the middle to later stages, include swallowing changes, **festinating gait**, autonomic deficits, psychiatric complications (particularly depression), and dementia (Conley & Kirchner, 1999; Gelb et al., 1999; Giladi et al., 2001; Phillip, 1999). When festinating gait is coupled with "freezing" of gait, 37% of those with PD report an increased occurrence of falls (Giladi et al., 2001). For swallowing problems, research has shown that overall disease severity is not related because a high percentage of those in early stages have difficulties with delayed swallow reflex, residues of food materials, and abnormal tongue control that may result in nutritional problems (Colcher & Stern, 1999; Fuh et al., 1997).

Dementia related to PD occurs in 15–20% of individuals and tends to occur in those who are older at the time of diagnosis and who have a long history of the disease and depression (Aarsland et al., 1996). The areas of cognitive function that seem to be most affected are motor planning, abstract reasoning, concentration, organizing, and sequencing (Monza et al., 1998; Ward & Robertson, 2004). It has also been shown that persons with PD rely on external cues, feedback, and repetition when learning new tasks (Ward & Robertson, 2004).

The cause of PD is thought to stem from both hereditary and environmental factors. Hereditary factors have been linked to a chromosome 4 mutation in 5–10% of cases, although the contribution of this mutation to PD is uncertain (Conley & Kirchner, 1999; Muenter, Forno, & Hornykiewicz, 1998). Environmental factors implicated in PD include exposure to well water and pesticides and living on a farm (Conley & Kirchner, 1999; Marder et al., 1998).

The pathogenesis of PD is related to the loss of dopaminergic neurons of the substantia nigra that provide input to the corpus striatum and, in part, modulate the thalamus and its connections to the motor cortex (Conley & Kirchner, 1999; Ward & Robertson, 2004). There is also suggestion that further biochemical anomalies in the basal ganglia are present (Conley & Kirchner, 1999).

DEFINITION 40-2

Stages of Parkinson's Disease

Hoehn & Yahr (1967)

Stage 1: Unilateral symptoms, no or minimal functional implications, usually a resting tremor.
Stage 2: Midline or bilateral symptom involvement, no balance difficulty, mild problems with trunk mobility and postural reflexes.
Stage 3: Postural instability, mild to moderate functional disability.
Stage 4: Postural instability increasing, though able to walk; functional disability increases, interfering with ADL; decreased manipulation and dexterity.
Stage 5: Confined to wheelchair or bed.

Bradley (1996)

Early: Not disabling: monosymptomatic; responds well to medication; may remain at this level for years.
Non-fluctuating: Some disability; levodopa added to medication regimen; 80% of function is restored.
Fluctuating: Function limited; side effects to levodopa; difficult-to-control symptoms, postural instability, and gait disturbance become debilitating.

Diagnosing PD

In autopsy studies, PD has been shown to be misdiagnosed in 25% of cases (Calne, 1995). In part, the difficulty is a result of the lack of definitive biological markers. Clinical imaging techniques (positron emission tomography) remain experimental (Conley & Kirchner, 1999). At present, diagnosis is based on clinical evidence using clinical diagnostic criteria.

The Course of PD

PD has been described as having either five stages (Hoehn & Yahr, 1967) or three stages (Bradley, 1996) (Definition 40-2). These stages are broadly described by presence of symptoms, functional implications, and response to medications.

Potential Emotional, Social, and Economic Consequences

In the initial stages of PD, the degree of physical disability is minimal. The emotional burden and social consequences, however, can be marked. Resting tremor, rarely resulting in motor disability, is a frequent source of psychological distress, with many individuals reporting feeling embarrassed or self-conscious (Uitti, 1998). In later stages, Peto, Jenkinson, and Fitzpatrick (1995) found that tremor and rigidity were highly correlated with distress and reduced quality of life. Another study found that the highest predictors of poor quality of life for persons with PD were depression, sleep disorders, and increasing dependence (Karlson et al., 1999). Major depression or depressive symptoms have been found in 45% of those with PD, suggesting that early identification and intervention are crucial (Karlson et al., 1999). Self-esteem is challenged when the person with PD is unable to perform previous roles or mundane tasks, such as feeding or dressing oneself (Gillen, 2000). Persons with PD report that fatigue, pain, and social isolation contribute to distress and compromised quality of life (Friedman & Friedman, 1993; Karlson et al., 1999).

The economic implications of PD are frequently related to the cost of medications, wheeled mobility, accessibility modifications, self-care and safety equipment, and in-home support. If the individual is employed, increasing limitations may require employment modifications and early application for disability benefits accompanied by loss of income. PD-related dementia may decrease the ability of the person to manage finances. An elderly caregiver is also likely to require caregiver assistance and/or respite care, which is a further financial consideration. Finally, if required, placement in a long-term care facility is costly.

The social consequences of PD are striking. In the early stages, for example, handwriting may be somewhat shaky and micrographic, which reduces legibility (Conley & Kirchner, 1999; Gillen, 2000; Uitti, 1998). In the intermediate and later stages, the voice softens and becomes monotone. Reduced facial expression and minimal hand gesturing also contribute to decreased communication with others (Tickle-Degnen, 2006; Uitti, 1998). The person with PD may have waning interest in social and/or previously enjoyed leisure activities. PD challenges ability to cope and alters relationships and roles in families with increasing dependence. Both the individual and family members may have feelings of guilt, despair, and anger as care giving increases and falls to a spouse or adult child (Baker & Graham, 2004).

Occupational Therapy Evaluation

In the early stages of PD, occupational therapy is rarely indicated unless there are functional limitations or psychological issues. At this stage, it is recommended that interests and roles are maintained within and outside of the home including employment, social activities, and driving (Baker & Graham, 2004). Occupational therapy is most often required in the intermediate and later stages of the disease (Hoehn and Yahr [1967] stages 3 to 5). Evaluation should include a brief history and, in the intermediate stages, identify occupational performance problems related to reduced mobility, safety issues, swallowing, fine motor incoordination and dexterity, slowed movements, **cogwheel rigidity**, and depressed affect. Another area of evaluation concerns occupations that have been eliminated or where reduced time is spent (Gillen, 2000). Some examples of individual impairments and limitations in activities that may be included in screening are:

- Difficulties with coordination and manipulation in home, community, and work activities (writing, manipulating utensils/tools, and managing clothes fasteners)
- Difficulties with safe mobility, such as walking on even and uneven surfaces, stair climbing, driving, and moving from sit to stand, that limit home, community, and work tasks
- Bradykinesia, postural instability, and rigidity that limit chosen occupations
- Difficulties with ADL and IADL due to bradykinesia, rigidity, and cognitive function
- Difficulties with swallowing or other meal time problems that prolong eating and reduce intake
- Fatigue and cognitive problems that affect activities and competence
- Sexual activity limitations related to bradykinesia, rigidity, fatigue, depression, anxiety, and psychosocial problems
- Sleep disturbances

Occupational Therapy Intervention Process

Goal Setting

When setting goals with the client with PD and significant others, the occupational therapist must be mindful of and balance activity energy demands with motivation and frustration as well as caregiver time in the context of the dependence-interdependence-independence continuum (Gillen, 2000). Participation of others in this process is frequently crucial to the viability and success of interventions.

Intervention Implementation

Interventions vary with the individual's and significant other's priorities and resources, stage of the disease, occupational difficulties identified through the evaluation, and activities in which they participate. In addition to the client, many of the procedures described in Procedures for Practice 40-1 should also be suggested to significant others to incorporate at home and in other relevant environments. Occupational therapy intervention for persons with PD has been evaluated in numerous studies showing an overall effectiveness of occupational therapy and other rehabilitation therapeutic interventions (Murphy & Tickle-Degnen, 2001).

Amyotrophic Lateral Sclerosis

Amyotrophic lateral sclerosis (ALS), popularly known as Lou Gehrig's disease, is a late-onset fatal neurodegenerative disease of upper motor neurons (UMN) and lower motor neurons (LMN). The prevalence of ALS is 5 to 8 cases per 100,000, and it occurs more often in men (Mitsumoto, Chad, & Pioro, 1998). No special test is available to establish the diagnosis and the cause is unknown. Initial symptoms vary widely and diagnosis is a careful, multistep system of exclusion.

The average age at onset is 58 years, although adults as young as 20 have been diagnosed. Age-specific incidence and mortality rates in sporadic ALS increase until the eighth decade, with a peak between 55 and 75 years of age. Age at onset and the pattern of symptom development is useful for determining an individual's prognosis, with a younger onset of upper motor neuron origin having a somewhat better prognosis. It has also been shown that baseline scores on the *Short Form-36* are significant predictors of health status over time (Norquist et al., 2003). Generally the prognosis for individual patients is best left to neurologists with expertise in ALS.

In ALS, voluntary muscle control is affected, and early manifestations indicating UMN or LMN disease vary with the site of the initial disease process. UMN damage results in general weakness, spasticity, and hyperreflexia. LMN involvement results in weakness or muscle atrophy of the extremities, cervical extensor weakness, **fasciculations**, muscle cramps, and loss of reflexes. Speech, swallowing, and breathing may be affected by damage to the bulbar nerves. Early bulbar involvement and/or advanced age at time of diagnosis tend to indicate a quicker course of the disease (Mitsumoto et al., 1998). Speech impairment is common (Ball et al., 2004a). Generally people with ALS develop both UMN and LMN symptoms as the disease

PROCEDURES FOR PRACTICE 40-1

Occupational Therapy for PD

Interventions Related to Decreasing Isolation and Communication Problems

- Education about timing important activities to synchronize with medication regimen so that participation can occur when medications are at the height of effectiveness
- Modification of leisure activities to encourage participation and decrease isolation
- Information on support and advocacy groups
- Caregiver training for modifying communication and social activities
- Writing modifications, including enlarged felt-tip pen and writing when rested
- Communication aids, including speed dial, large-key telephones, dictating devices, and remote control systems for lights, television, and other frequently used devices
- Providing home exercise program to maintain facial movement and expression

Interventions Related to Safety

- Instruction in sit-to-stand techniques and bed mobility
- Instruction to manage "freezing" while walking, includes avoiding crowds, narrow spaces, and room corners; reduce distractions such as not carrying items while walking; reduce clutter in pathway; doing one activity at a time; not hurrying to answer the phone; focusing when changing directions; rhythmic beat or counting to maintain momentum
- Demonstration of equipment to increase independence and safety, such as a raised toilet seat, toilet grab bars, shower bench, sink chair, soap on a rope
- Prescribing walking aids (walker for festinating gait)
- If required, a wheelchair having a proper seating system, cushion, and adjusted foot/leg rests and arm rests that is appropriate for transporting within the community
- Good, uniform lighting, particularly in narrow spaces and at doorways
- Providing home and group exercises to maintain mobility, coordination, posture, and tolerance and reduce effects of festinating gait, bradykinesia, and postural instability
- Home assessment and modifications that might include alterations to the bathroom (e.g., non-skid surfaces, bath bench/chair) and flooring (e.g., eliminating throw rugs), horizontal strips on carpet where "freezing" episodes occur, and reducing furniture congestion (Gillen, 2000)

Interventions to Maintain Independence and Participation

- Modifying eating routine to include small portions, reduced distractions, more frequent meals that allow adequate time, and adapted equipment as required, such as non-slip surfaces for plates, built-up handles, and lids on cups
- Instruction in using adult absorbent underwear if necessary
- Demonstrating voice and facial exercise programs
- Advising on modifying sexual routine, such as to occur after resting and urination
- Instruction of energy effectiveness strategies in home, leisure, and work activities
- Modifications to reduce or eliminate the need for fine motor control, such as clothing with minimal fasteners or velcro closures
- To reduce impact of cognitive and perceptual limitations, use visual cues, rhythmic music, and a non-distracting environment; speak slowly and clearly; use simple instruction; provide one new concept at a time; and practice with repetition (Ward & Robertson, 2004)
- Home assessment

CLINICAL REASONING IN OCCUPATIONAL THERAPY PRACTICE

Justifying a Home Assessment for a Client with Parkinson's Disease (PD)

An occupational therapist considers it essential to complete a home assessment for someone with PD who lives alone and is falling and losing weight. Why does the therapist consider it necessary, and how could it be justified to a third-party payer?

progresses. Cognition may be affected, although this is relatively rare, whereas eye function, bowel and bladder control, and sensation are spared.

No known cure or effective pharmacological treatment is available for ALS, although riluzole (Rilutek), an antiglutamate agent, is the only Food and Drug Administration–approved medication for the treatment of ALS. Other medications can assist in the management of symptoms such as fasiculations, spasticity, anxiety, insomnia, and excessive saliva but do not affect the progression of the disease. Tracheotomies, gastrostomies, and assisted ventilation are used to ease problems with eating and breathing (Mitsumoto et al., 1998). Due to the progressive nature of ALS and vast array of symptoms and potential interventions, a multidisciplinary health care team approach improves the quality of life for individuals with ALS (Van der Berg et al., 2005).

The Course of ALS

Six stages of ALS are recognized and described according to clinical features (Table 40-1). The median duration of life after diagnosis ranges from 23 to 52 months, but a significant proportion of patients survive 5 years or more (Mitsumoto et al., 1998). Focal weakness of the arm, leg, or bulbar area is a common initial symptom (Mitsumoto et al., 1998). Atrophy may begin in the hands, with wasting of the thenar and hypothenar eminences, as well as in the shoulder musculature. Finger extension is usually affected earlier than grip strength because of dorsal and palmar interossei wasting. Walking and bed mobility are affected, and falling is common with lower extremity weakness. Upper and lower extremity weakness makes transfers and getting up from the floor after a fall increasingly difficult. Speech and swallowing problems may arise early in the disease course.

Potential Emotional, Social, and Economic Consequences

ALS is a devastating disease for individuals and their families. Its relatively fast progression, frequently involving early loss of upper extremity function and possibly speech and swallowing, means that the disease quickly affects quality of life and the ability to perform ADL, IADL, and employment tasks. It has been shown that those with ALS, as compared to normal controls, have more depression, external locus of control, and feelings of hopelessness (McDonald et al., 1994) and that this is not related to physical function or sociodemographic factors (Plahuta et al., 2002; Robbins et al., 2001).

People with ALS and their families have little time to make psychological adjustment to the diagnosis and its implications before having to deal with their loved one's increasing disability. The acceptance by family members of the ALS diagnosis may affect willingness to be involved in planning, incorporating changes necessary to maximize the independence of the person with ALS, and making informed choices for intervention (Ball et al., 2004a).

People frequently withdraw from employment soon after the diagnosis and may also have to confront economic problems due to loss of income and possibly health insurance issues. Since the age group most commonly affected is often employed and actively involved in family and community activities, the abrupt change in status is devastating.

Occupational Therapy Evaluation

The specifics of the occupational therapy assessments should be based on clearly defined levels of function (see Table 40-1) and the individual's needs and priorities. Early interventions should target the individual's symptoms as these affect their occupations. As ALS progresses, interventions not only focus on individual function, but also on the physical environment and social network. This is supported by Neudert, Wasner, and Borasio (2004), who showed that the quality of life of a person with ALS with a supportive family and social network remains stable over time despite reduced health status.

Table 40-1. Rehabilitation of Patients with ALS at Various Stages

Stage	Characteristic Clinical Features	Activities to Maintain Motor Function	Equipment
I	Ambulatory, no problems with ADL, mild weakness	Normal activities, moderate exercise in unaffected muscles, active range-of-motion (ROM) exercise	None
II	Ambulatory, moderate weakness in certain muscles	Modification in living; modest exercise; active, assisted ROM exercise	Assistive devices
III	Ambulatory, severe weakness in certain muscles	Active life; active, assisted, passive ROM exercise; joint pain management	Assistive devices, adaptive devices, home equipment
IV	Wheelchair-confined, almost independent, severe weakness in legs	Passive ROM exercise, modest exercise in uninvolved muscles	Assistive devices, adaptive devices, wheelchair, home equipment
V	Wheelchair confined; dependent; pronounced weakness in legs, severe weakness in arms	Passive ROM exercise, pain management, decubitus prevention	Adaptive devices, home equipment, wheelchair
VI	Bedridden, no ADL, maximal assistance required	Passive ROM exercise, pain management, prevention of decubitus ulcers and venous thrombosis	Adaptive devices, home equipment

Information from Sinaki, M. (1980). Rehabilitation. In D. W. Mulder (Ed.), *The diagnosis and treatment of amyotrophic lateral sclerosis* (pp. 169–193). Boston: Houghton Mifflin. Reprinted with Permission from Mitsumoto, H., Chad, D., & Pioro, E. (1998). *Amyotrophic lateral sclerosis. Contemporary neurology series.* Philadelphia: Davis.

To assist with the occupational therapy evaluation process, a number of measures are suggested such as the *ALS Functional Rating Scale* (Mitsumoto, Chad, & Pioro, 1998). To determine ongoing functional ability, ADL and IADL assessments should be included in all evaluations. Functional limitations may be due to reduced upper extremity ability, and thus the *Purdue Pegboard* or other timed upper extremity function tests and standard range-of-motion and manual muscle testing are useful measures. Limitations may be due to fatigue, which has been shown to affect physical quality of life (Lou et al., 2003) and can be assessed with the *Multidimensional Fatigue Inventory*. As oral communication and swallowing function declines (Higo et al., 2004), assessment and intervention is required to ensure ongoing nutritional needs are met and social participation is maintained. As the disease is progressive, reevaluations should be done at repeated visits.

Occupational Therapy Intervention Process

Goal Setting

The progressive nature of the disease necessitates that rehabilitation in ALS be compensatory, focusing on adapting to disability and preventing secondary complications. Goals center on keeping the person as active and independent as possible for as long as possible. Here are some examples of occupational therapy goals for a client with ALS in the early stages:

- Optimize strength and range of motion using home exercise programs (Drory et al., 2001).
- Maintain function in ADL and IADL through use of assistive or adaptive devices.
- Decrease pain and fatigue in the neck and extremities through use of splints and orthotics.
- Employ joint protection, pain management, energy conservation, and work simplification techniques.

As motor function declines, mobility and self-care become increasingly difficult. Home evaluations and/or in-home therapy are important in the later stages of the disease, and intervention goals largely focus on enabling the caregiver to assist the client safely and effectively. The occupational therapist helps the caregiver–client team to do the following:

- Optimize safety, assess positioning, perform safe transfers, and maintain skin integrity
- Employ augmentative communication equipment (Ball et al., 2004a)
- Assess and manage dysphagia (Higo et al., 2004)
- Optimize social participation (Ball et al., 2004b)
- Identify and obtain equipment, such as a hospital bed, to allow continued mobility
- Employ environmental modification

Throughout the stages of the disease, the therapist remains sensitive to the client's, family's, and caregiver's needs and stresses as the demands of care giving perpetually change. Physical demands, financial concerns, and transformation of the home into a hospital-like setting produce enormous strain on the client and the caregivers (Mitsumoto et al., 1998). Open discussions and close collaboration with clients, caregivers, and the ALS team help to address and plan for the client's changing needs.

Intervention Implementation

When treating clients with ALS, therapists must be aware of the client's level of gadget tolerance, financial resources, and social and cultural context. Special considerations for exercise, equipment, assistive technology, and dysphasia management for this diagnostic group are briefly reviewed.

Exercise

Active and passive range-of-motion, strengthening, endurance, stretching, and home breathing exercise programs are all appropriate at various stages of the disease. Research indicates that they are effective for minimizing secondary complications (Mitsumoto et al., 1998). Attention to overexertion, potential secondary problems, muscle spasms, and careful monitoring of fatigue are important to a successful exercise program. A client may initially be able to perform an independent home stretching program, but as the disease progresses, the program may become too fatiguing or difficult. At that time, the caregiver may be asked to learn how to perform the program.

Equipment and Assistive Technology

A variety of assistive and adaptive equipment may help the client achieve the highest possible level of independence at the various stages of ALS (see Table 40-1). Assistive equipment such as a neck collar or universal cuff may be helpful. Mobility equipment or aids, depending on level of function, may include a foot-drop splint, cane, and/or walker. In a study by Trail et al. (2001), 57% of a moderately disabled group used a mobility device in addition to a wheelchair. The occupational therapist's role is to inform clients and caregivers about potentially helpful adaptive equipment at the various stages of ALS.

As the disease progresses, home assessment and client caregiver consultation inform selection of a wheelchair. Since independent walking becomes difficult in a rapidly progressing disease such as ALS, ordering the wheelchair may need to be expedited. Desirable features for a manual wheelchair are lightweight frame, small turning radius, high reclining back, and supports for head, trunk, and extremities (Trail et al., 2001). As ALS progresses, ideally a power wheelchair has adaptable controls; maneuverability;

the ability to add tilt or recline features; supports head, trunk, and extremities; and enables the client to access the community (Trail et al., 2001). Transporting the wheelchair in a vehicle should be considered when making purchase decisions as well as ramps or elevators required to access home and public spaces.

If the social network is prepared to adapt to the use of such technology, environment controls are extremely useful as the disease progresses. This technology, for example, includes hands-free operation of phone, lighting, call alert systems, door (un)locking systems, computers, TV, radio, and other equipment and devices.

Dysphasia

Swallowing difficulties present at various stages, particularly when bulbar involvement is apparent. Interventions may include, but are not limited to, reducing distractions during mealtime (limit conversation and other activities), altering food consistency (i.e., thicken liquids), teaching manual techniques to swallow, and ensuring adequate time for meals. Early introduction of an alternate route of nutrition may be indicated if nutrition and weight maintenance become issues.

Guillain-Barré Syndrome

Guillain-Barré syndrome (GBS) is an inflammatory disease resulting in axonal demyelination of peripheral nerves (Dematteis, 1996; Meythaler, DeVivo, & Braswell, 1997). Characteristics of GBS include a quickly progressing, symmetrical ascending paralysis starting with the feet; pain, particularly in the legs; absence of deep tendon reflexes; mild sensory loss in glove-and-stocking distributions; cranial nerve dysfunction with possible facial palsy; an autonomic nervous system response of postural hypertension and tachycardia; respiratory muscle paralysis; and pain, fatigue, and urinary dysfunction (Gregory, Gregory, & Podd, 2005; Hughes & Rees, 1997; Meythaler et al., 1997). Severity of symptoms varies from so mild that medical attention is unlikely to severe disease that may cause death reportedly in 1–10% of cases (Hughes & Rees, 1997; Carroll et al., 2003; Khan, 2004).

The cause of GBS is unclear. Its distribution is known to be worldwide, with an incidence of 1.3 to 2 per 100,000 (Hughes & Rees, 1997). Men are slightly more commonly affected than women, and GBS most often occurs in adults 20–24 years and 70–74 years of age (Hughes & Rees, 1997; Jiang et al., 1997). No evidence supports hereditary susceptibility or vaccinations as causes of GBS, although there are reports concerning previous viral infections (Hughes & Rees, 1997). Enteritis precedes GBS in 41% of cases, and respiratory tract infections and HIV or AIDS may also precede it (Hughes & Rees, 1997; Jiang et al., 1997; Carroll et al., 2003).

Diagnosing GBS

Diagnosis of GBS entails a detailed history of symptoms and a complete physical and neurological examination that includes nerve conduction velocity tests and cerebral spinal fluid analysis (Hughes & Rees, 1997; Muscular Dystrophy Association of Canada, 1997). The medical interventions for GBS attempt to lessen the severity and hasten recovery but do not cure the disease (Muscular Dystrophy Association of Canada, 1997). Treatments for GBS include intravenous immunoglobulin, plasma exchange otherwise known as plasmapheresis, and steroids (Rees et al., 1998).

The Course of GBS

GBS has three phases. In more than 95% of people with GBS, the onset, or acute inflammatory phase, manifests as an acute weakness in at least two limbs that progresses and reaches its maximum in 2–4 weeks with increasing symptoms (Hughes & Rees, 1997; Dematteis, 1996). Mechanical ventilation is required for 20–30% of individuals with GBS (Dematteis, 1996). This is followed by the plateau phase when the greatest disability is present, as are many symptoms described earlier. During this phase, which may last for a few days or weeks, there is no significant change. Finally, the progressive period of recovery, when remyelination and axonal regeneration occur, may last for up to 2 years, although the average length of this phase is 12 weeks (Jiang et al., 1997; Meythaler, DeVivo, & Braswell, 1997). The recovery generally starts at the head and neck and proceeds distally (Karavatas, 2005). The degree of recovery varies, with complete return of function in approximately 50% of patients, whereas 35% experience some residual weakness that may not resolve. The remaining 15% of patients experience more significant permanent disability (Dematteis, 1996). In a study by Parry (2000), fatigue was the most common residual problem for 93% of patients. Gregory, Gregory, and Podd (2005) suggest that subtle cognitive deficits may be present as limitations in executive functions, short-term memory, and decision making.

Potential Emotional, Social, and Economic Consequences

Emotional and psychological reactions are a response to the rapid onset of symptoms and the degree of disability. Shock, despair, fear, and anger may be consuming (Dematteis, 1996). At the height of the acute phase of the disease, should the individual be unable to speak or move, fear of the unknown and frustration are often overwhelming (Muscular Dystrophy Association of Canada, 1997). As recovery progresses and improvement is slow, the psychological adjustment, impatience, and frustration associated with residual disability may be daunting.

For young adults, the impact of GBS can have educational, employment, and/or economic implications. This age group is launching careers and may have debt with only small savings. For those who develop GBS in later years, particularly in retirement, the economic effect may be less. Should the recovery phase last several months, the burden on family, colleagues, and/or friends who may be required to absorb the roles previously held by the person with GBS may be profound. A New Zealand survey describes the marked psychosocial impact of GBS and the need for professional intervention (Gregory et al., 2005).

Occupational Therapy Evaluation

Referral to occupational therapy is common when the course of GBS is moderate to severe. Approximately 40% of all GBS patients require rehabilitation services (Meythaler et al., 1997).

Screening and assessment during the plateau phase typically occur in intensive care, when the individual is undergoing extensive medical procedures such as plasma exchange or intravenous immunoglobulin. During this period, occupational therapists evaluate communication, control of the environment as appropriate, comfort, and level of anxiety.

During the recovery phase, occupational therapists evaluate mobility, self-care, communication, leisure, and reintegration into the workplace as appropriate. During this phase, OT services can be provided in an inpatient rehabilitation facility, through an outpatient program, and/or at home or work (Karavatas, 2005).

Occupational Therapy Intervention Process

Goal Setting

As the natural course of GBS is improvement, patients and caregivers tend to be optimistic about recovery. The long-term goal is full recovery, so that the individual performs at the same level as prior to the onset of GBS with or without modification.

Intervention Implementation

Modifications during the plateau phase should be considered temporary. Examples of interventions include:

- Developing communication tools, such as sign or picture board
- Ensuring access to the nurse call button, TV, and lights by remote control, as appropriate
- Modifying the telephone for hands-free use
- Modifying lying and sitting positions for optimal function and comfort
- Positioning for trunk, head, and upper extremity stability
- Teaching about GBS and strategies to reduce anxiety

Recovery-phase interventions are oriented to the resumption of activities and roles. Examples of occupational therapy interventions include:

- Providing activities and dynamic splints to maintain range of motion, particularly of wrists, fingers, and ankle (hinged drop-foot orthosis)
- Instructing in safe mobility and independent transfers
- Training in modified self-care techniques and adapting other daily activities
- Adapting modes of communication according to the person's priorities
- Encouraging access to the community
- Modifying and encouraging reengagement in routine activities, as appropriate
- Adapting equipment and modifying behavior in home, leisure, and work activities
- Instructing in energy conservation and fatigue management strategies
- Modifying employment roles, tasks, and environment, as indicated
- Fine motor program to enhance strength, coordination, and sensation
- Home assessment and modifications, as appropriate, to facilitate return to home

EVIDENCE-BASED RESEARCH ON OCCUPATIONAL THERAPY FOR NEURODEGENERATIVE DISEASES

Although expert consensus (PVA, 1998) may agree that occupational therapy is effective in treating neurodegenerative diseases, little empirical evidence confirms these views. Consequently, occupational therapy described here is based on commonly held assumptions about treatment and not on well-designed randomized controlled trials establishing its effectiveness. Even in the randomized controlled trials that have been published, occupational therapy is frequently not studied alone but is one of several interventions with other rehabilitation therapies (Aisen, 1999; Baker & Tickle-Degnen, 2001; Solari et al., 1999), typically in an inpatient rehabilitation setting (Freeman et al., 1997). Most occupational therapy for persons with these diseases takes place in outpatient, home health, or long-term care facilities, and consequently, the generalizability of these team-based inpatient studies is questionable. The study by Mathiowetz et al. (2005) of the effectiveness of outpatient group occupational therapy in energy conservation strategies in MS is a notable exception. It remains useful, however, to refer to a meta-analysis in which 10 of 15 studies demonstrated the positive effect of occupational therapy intervention on the capabilities and abilities of clients and 9 of 15 studies showed favorable outcomes in activities and tasks (Murphy & Tickle-Degnen, 2001). This analysis also showed that 63% of those with PD who received therapy improved as compared to 37% who did not receive therapy.

Problems, however, with existing research are the lack of attention to placebo groups, small sample size, selection bias, poor internal validity, and lack of control for medications. At a time when evidence-based outcomes are increasingly required for reimbursement, occupational therapists must carry out well-designed research studies of interventions and publish findings in peer-reviewed journals to support the effectiveness of interventions in achieving positive outcomes.

CASE EXAMPLE

Mrs. K: Multiple Sclerosis

Occupational Therapy Process	Clinical Reasoning Process: Objectives	Clinical Reasoning Process: Examples of Therapist's Internal Dialogue
Patient Information Ms. K., a 37-year-old woman diagnosed with relapsing-remitting multiple sclerosis (MS) 2 years prior to her first visit to occupational therapy, had recently submitted her resignation to her employer of 15 years. Upset by having to quit her administrative job, she reported the following problems: (1) severe fatigue, which had increased in the past year and resulted in her inability to do her normal household tasks, perform her ADL, and work without becoming exhausted; (2) a marked increase in lower extremity weakness, with decreased ability to perform tasks requiring prolonged walking or standing; (3) a feeling of heaviness and stiffness in upper and lower extremities; (4) decreased manual dexterity; (5) frequent falling; (6) daily headaches; (7) dizziness; (8) bladder problems; (9) vision problems; (10) disturbed sleep; and (11) increased attention and memory problems. Her adaptive equipment at the time of her initial therapy visit included a manual wheelchair and a quad cane. She had quit driving. Her husband was very supportive and had recently stopped adoption proceedings because of her MS changes. Medications included a bladder medication and a MS disease-modifying drug.	Understand the patient's diagnosis and context of OT services Know the person	"This is not a new diagnosis for Ms. K., though it is her first interaction with occupational therapy because she may not have needed services in the past." "I will want to get to know how long Ms. K. has experienced her current problems and how she has tried to address them before her resignation from work. It appears that she has made some rather significant and life-altering decisions about her future. In my experience, some patients respond to the relapse of MS symptoms by fearing the worst, not really understanding MS and all the potential treatment options. Getting a sense of 'where she is at' will be my priority."
Reason for Referral to Occupational Therapy Fatigue management and work evaluation.	Appreciate the context Develop provisional hypotheses	"Ms. K. is not working and is having difficulty at home. Since her husband is supportive, he will likely help to make any changes I suggest in therapy. She is probably using inadequate fatigue management strategies."

Assessment Process and Results

The occupational therapy evaluation showed the following areas of concern: decreased strength bilaterally in the lower extremities and her dominant upper extremity; increased tone bilaterally in the lower extremities; decreased sensation and manual dexterity in the dominant upper extremity; high levels of dizziness with head movement; head, neck, and shoulder muscle trigger points; and marked fatigue. Ms. K., determined not to give in to the disease, had made no adaptations to reduce energy expenditure in daily activities. She was scheduled to have a neuropsychological assessment to identify her current baseline function and problem areas. Her equipment was self-selected and inappropriate for her problems. She was not taking any medications to manage spasticity or fatigue. Her seating at home and work was not supportive. Ms. K. purposefully climbed the stairs in the morning and had a desk distant from the bathroom to get exercise, since she had no exercise program.

Consider evaluation approach and methods

"I think I will start with an interview to get to know Ms. K., her past coping strategies, and her primary concerns. Depending on that information and what I already know from the client information, I will use some specific assessments such as the *Modified Fatigue Impact Scale, Modified Ashworth Scale,* and the *Functional Independence Measure.*"

Interpret observations

"I'm thinking that fatigue underlies most of her occupational performance problems and that weakness and spasticity are adding to this. It also seems that her current equipment and environmental setup are not helping her. I am also very concerned about what (I think) is a premature resignation from her work and withdrawal from driving."

Occupational Therapy Problem List

1. Use of inappropriate equipment
2. Minimal understanding and use of fatigue management strategies
3. Has recently resigned from work without knowledge of options
4. Is not involved in a home exercise program
5. Has stopped driving without investigating options

Synthesize results

"Her occupational performance problems are due to inadequate information and modifications related to fatigue, equipment, ergonomic layout, and exercise routine."

Occupational Therapy Goal List

In collaboration with Ms. K., the following goals were established:

- Identify and obtain appropriate power mobility equipment
- Incorporate at least six energy-saving strategies into her day
- Withdraw resignation notice from employer
- Make changes in work area by obtaining a headset and ergonomic chair and move her desk closer to the bathroom
- Submit a request to her employer for power automatic door openers on bathroom
- Apply to vocational rehabilitation and work with therapist and vendor to install hand controls on her vehicle
- Demonstrate that she can independently perform head, neck, and shoulder stretching exercises

Develop intervention hypotheses

"I will sequence the intervention by focusing on what is most important to Ms. K. I hypothesize that education on energy effectiveness strategies will improve success in performing daily tasks and assessment and alteration of the work environment while appropriate equipment will make it possible for her to return to work. I advocate the use of hand controls to return Ms. K. to independent driving."

Select an intervention approach

"I think the compensatory and educational approach will be most useful."

Consider what will occur in therapy, how often, and for how long

"I recommend one outpatient treatment session a week for 6 weeks. We will work closely with the physical therapist who will attend to pain, gait, and exercise interventions."

Intervention

The occupational therapy intervention included: (1) instruction in and adoption of energy conservation techniques at home, at work, and in community (Mathiowetz, Matuska, & Murphy, 2001; Mathiowetz et al., 2005); (2) identifying and obtaining powered mobility equipment (Mathiowetz and Matuska, 1998); (3) decreasing daily headaches with head, neck, and shoulder stretching and focal heat; (4) identifying and obtaining equipment to decrease energy consumption at home and work (Mathiowetz et al., 2005; PVA, 1998); (5) with

Assess the patient's comprehension

Understand what she is doing

Compare actual to expected performance

"Ms. K. was motivated to participate in therapy sessions, particularly because there was a potential to return to work. From my experience, I realize the success of therapy depends on her ability (and her husband's) to incorporate suggested techniques, access and use equipment appropriately, and implement ergonomic changes into her daily life."

"When we started talking about fatigue, Ms. K. realized she was fighting the fatigue rather than managing it. At first, it was tough to incorporate the sug-

therapist assistance, identifying and obtaining ergonomic seating and workstation to decrease pain and energy consumption; (6) increasing independence in driving with hand controls; (7) continuing full- or part-time employment; (8) instruction in vestibular and strengthening home exercise program (Petajan et al., 1996); and (9) identifying and obtaining equipment and modifications to decrease cognitive problems at home and work.	Know the person Appreciate the context	gestions like taking rests, but Ms. K. immediately began to reduce long walks in favor of a short home exercise program." "While she didn't want a lot of equipment, Ms. K. was interested in getting appropriate items if it meant she could continue to do her usual activities at home and work." "Because both her husband and employer were supportive, modifications at home and work could be accommodated."
Next Steps Following the therapy evaluation, Ms. K. withdrew her resignation at her job and began making modifications in her work. She was also planning to resume driving with the appropriate hand control modifications.	Anticipate present and future patient concerns Analyze patient's comprehension Decide if the patient should continue or discontinue therapy and/or return in the future	"I will follow-up with Ms. K. when she has returned to work to assist with any concerns related to the ergonomic changes and to help problem solve difficult job situations. I think this is important so that she has a positive experience upon her return and does not begin to have reservations." "After that, I will follow-up at the annual visit or earlier if there is a change in her function."

CLINICAL REASONING IN OCCUPATIONAL THERAPY PRACTICE

Work and Managing Symptoms of MS

In accordance with the outpatient occupational therapy evaluation and goals, Ms. K.'s therapist suggested that Ms. K. withdraw her resignation to her employer until she had tried to manage her MS symptoms. What factors influenced this advice, and why would the therapist make this recommendation?

Evidence Table 40-1
Best Evidence for Occupational Therapy Practice Regarding Intervention Related to Multiple Sclerosis (MS)

Intervention	Description of Intervention Tested	Participants	Dosage	Type of Best Evidence and Level of Evidence	Benefit	Statistical Probability and Effect Size of Outcome	Reference
Efficacy and effectiveness of an energy conservation course on fatigue, quality of life (QOL), and self-efficacy for persons with MS	Community-based energy conservation course included but was not limited to importance of rest through the day, effective communication, proper body mechanics, and modification of environment.	N = 169 persons with MS; 140 women, 29 men; mean age = 48 years.	Energy conservation course for 2 hours a week for 6 weeks.	Level 1 randomized control trial with a crossover design.	The energy conservation course significantly reduced the impact of the fatigue, improved vitality, and increased self-efficacy for performing energy conservation strategies.	Results were established at $p < 0.05$. Moderate to large effect sizes were established for the fatigue subscales (0.52–0.74) and for 3 of the *Short Form-36* subscales (0.53–0.99).	Mathiowetz et al., 2005
Rehabilitation program for individuals with MS	Self-care activities using compensatory strategies, equipment, and conditioning were evaluated on admission, at discharge, and 6 weeks post discharge.	N = 30 adults with MS; 27 women, 3 men; mean age = 45 years. Rating of less than 5 on at least 1 item on the *Research Institute of Chicago Functional Assessment Scale.*	5–7 days of intensive occupational and physical therapy.	Level 4 case series before and after repeated measures.	Improved in tub/shower transfers, toileting, feeding, grooming, and upper and lower extremity dressing; 100% had high or very high satisfaction with OT services.	Results were established at $p < 0.05$ or better.	Mathiowetz and Matuska, 1998

(continued)

Evidence Table 40-1 (*continued*)

Intervention	Description of Intervention Tested	Participants	Dosage	Type of Best Evidence and Level of Evidence	Benefit	Statistical Probability and Effect Size of Outcome	Reference
Efficacy of an energy conservation course on fatigue impact, self-efficacy, and QOL for persons with MS	Experimental intervention group received energy conservation course by trained OTs that addressed importance of rest, effective communication, proper body mechanics, and ergonomic principles. Control intervention group: support group involving discussion of MS topics.	N = 54 persons with MS; 36 women, 18 men; mean age = 50 years; 83% reported fatigue as a primary symptom; 11% reported taking medications for fatigue.	6 weeks, 2 hours a week of control intervention followed by 6 weeks, 2 hours a week of experimental intervention.	Level 3, repeated measures with control and experimental interventions.	Efficacy for the energy conservation course was demonstrated because participants had less fatigue impact, increased self-efficacy, and improved QOL.	Results were established at $p < 0.05$ or better. Moderate to large effect sizes were established for the fatigue subscales (0.53–0.66), self-efficacy (0.52), and 3 of the *Short Form-36* subscales (0.49–0.78).	Mathiowetz, Matuska, & Murphy, 2001
Aerobic exercise program and its effects on fatigue, mood, and daily tasks	Treatment group (n = 21) participated in combined arm and leg ergometry. Control group (n = 25) did not alter usual activities for 15 weeks.	N = 46; 31 females, 15 males; mean age = 40 years; *Expanded Disability Status Scale* score of less than 6.	40 minutes three times a week for 15 weeks.	Level 1; randomized control trial.	The treatment group showed significant improvement in aerobic capacity, physical work capacity, upper and lower extremity strength, ambulation, and self-care. Depression, anger, and fatigue were significantly reduced at 10 weeks.	Results were established at $p < 0.05$.	Petajan et al., 1996

SUMMARY REVIEW QUESTIONS

1. What are the various courses of MS?
2. What symptoms of MS may require occupational therapy intervention?
3. What are the main modifications that a therapist might recommend for a woman with severe MS fatigue who is working full time and has two young children?
4. How can an occupational therapist help a person with neurodegenerative disease stay employed?
5. What factors and symptoms should a therapist consider when ordering wheeled mobility for a patient with neurodegenerative disease?
6. What environmental modifications may be necessary in PD?
7. List the items you would check and primary modifications you might recommend during a home safety visit for a person with a neurodegenerative disease.
8. Why is it important to include the significant others when developing interventions?
9. Plan an outpatient therapy session to treat a person with PD who has akinesia, bradykinesia, and rigidity and who is falling regularly.

References

Aarsland, D., Tandberg, E., Larsen, J. P., & Cummings, J. L. (1996). Frequency of dementia in Parkinson disease. *Archive of Neurology, 53,* 538–542.

Aisen, M. L. (1999). Justifying neurorehabilitation: A few steps forward. *Neurology, 52,* 8–10.

Alter, M. (1978). Migration and risk of multiple sclerosis. *Neurology, 28,* 1089.

Baker, M.G. & Graham, L. (2004). The journey: Parkinson's disease. *British Medical Journal*, 329, 611–614.

Baker, N. A., & Tickle-Degnan, L. (2001). The effectiveness of physical, psychological and function interventions in treating clients with multiple sclerosis: A meta-analysis. *American Journal of Occupational Therapy, 55,* 385–392.

Ball, L.J., Beukelman, D.R. & Pattee, G.L. (2004a). Acceptance of augmentative and alternative communication technology by persons with amyotrophic lateral sclerosis. *Augmentative and Alternative Communication*, 20(2), 113–122.

Ball, L.J., Beukelman, D.R. & Pattee, G.L. (2004b). Communication effectiveness of individuals with amyotrophic lateral sclerosis. *Journal of Communicative Disorders*, 37, 197–215.

Beatty, W. W., & Goodkin, D. E. (1990). Screening for cognitive impairment in multiple sclerosis: An evaluation of the Mini-Mental State Examination. *Archives Neurology, 47,* 297–301.

Beatty, W. W., Paul, R. H., Wilbanks, S. L., Hames, K. A., Blanco, C. R., & Goodkin, D. E. (1995). Identifying multiple sclerosis patients with mild or global cognitive impairment using the Screening Examination for Cognitive Impairment (SEFCI). *Neurology, 45,* 718–723.

Benedict, R. H.., Fischer, J. S., Archibald, C. J., Arnett, C. A., Beatty, W. W., Bobholz, J., Chelune, G. J., Fisk, J. D., Langdon, D. W., Caruos, L., Foley, F., LaRocca, N. G., Vowels, L., Weinstein, A., DeLuca, J., Rao, S. M., & Munschauer, F. (2002). Minimal neuropsychological assessment of multiple sclerosis patient: A consensus approach. *Clinical Neuropsychology, 16,* 381–397.

Bourdette, D. (1997). Multiple sclerosis. In R. E. Rakel (Ed.), *Current therapy* (pp. 937–946). Philadelphia: Saunders.

Bradley, W. E. (1996). *Neurology in clinical practice* (2nd ed.). Boston: Butterworth- Heinemann.

Brown, T. R., & Kraft, G. H. (2005). Exercise and rehabilitation for individuals with multiple sclerosis. *Physical Medicine and Rehabilitation Clinics of North America, 16,* 513–555.

Calcagno, P., Ruoppolo, G., Grasso, M. G., De Vincentiis, M., & Paolucci, S. (2002). Dysphagia in multiple sclerosis: Prevalence and prognostic factors. *Acta Neurological Scandinavia, 105,* 40–43.

Calne, D. B. (1995). Diagnosis and treatment of Parkinson's disease. *Hospital Practice, 30,* 83–86, 89.

Campbell, G. (2006). Pilot study of Fatigue: Take control! in a veteran's cohort. Poster presentation at Consortium of MS Centers Annual Meeting, Scottsdale, AZ.

Carroll, A., McDonnell, G. & Barnes, M. (2003). A review of the management of Guillian-Barre syndrome in a regional neurological rehabilitation unit. *International Journal of Rehabilitation Research*, 26, 297–302.

Colcher, R.A. & Stern, M.B. (1999). Therapeutics in the neurorehabilitation of Parkinson's disease. *Neurorehabilitation and Neural Repair, 13,* 205–218.

Conley, C. C., & Kirchner, J. T. (1999). Parkinson's disease: The shaking palsy. *Post Graduate Medicine, 109,* 39–52.

Dematteis, J. A. (1996). Guillain-Barré syndrome: A team approach to diagnosis and treatment. *American Family Physician, 54,* 197–200.

Drory, V.E., Gotsman, E., Reznick, J.G., Mosek, A. & Korczyn, A.D. (2001). The value of nuscle exercise in patients with amyotrophic lateral sclerosis. *Journal of Neurological Sciences*, *191*, 133–137.

Finlayson, M. (2004). Concerns about the future among older adults with multiple sclerosis. *American Journal of Occupational Therapy, 58,* 54–63.

Fischer, J. S., Jak, A. J., Kniker, J. E., Rudick, R. A., & Cutter, G. (2001). *Multiple Sclerosis Functional Composite (MSFC): Administration and scoring manual.* New York: National Multiple Sclerosis Society.

Foong, J., Rozewicz, L., & Quaghebeur, G. (1997). Executive functions in multiple sclerosis: The role of frontal lobe pathology. *Brain, 20,* 15–26.

Forwell, S. J. (2007). Clinical approach to identification and evaluation of fatigue. *International Journal of Multiple Sclerosis Care.*

Forwell, S. J., Brunham, S., Tremlett, H., Morrison, W., & Oger, J. (2007). Differentiating primary and non-primary fatigue in MS. *International Journal on MS Care.*

Frankel, D. I. (1990). Multiple sclerosis. In D. A. Umphred (Ed.), *Neurological rehabilitation* (2nd ed., pp. 531–549). St. Louis: Mosby.

Freal, J. E., Kraft, G., & Coryell, J. (1984). Symptomatic fatigue in multiple sclerosis. *Archives of Physical Medicine and Rehabilitation, 65,* 135–138.

Freeman, J. A., Langdon, D. W., Hobart, J. S., & Thompson, A. J. (1997). Health-related quality of life in people with multiple sclerosis undergoing inpatient rehabilitation. *Journal of Neurologic Rehabilitation, 10,* 17–20.

Friedman, J., & Friedman, H. (1993). Fatigue in Parkinson's disease. *Neurology, 43,* 2016–2018.

Fuh, J.-L., Lee, R.-C., Wang, S.-J., Lin, C.-H., Wang, P.-N., Chiang, J.-H., & Liu, H.-C. (1997). Swallowing difficulty in Parkinson's disease. *Clinical Neurology and Neurosurgery, 99,* 106–112.

Gelb, D. J., Olliver, E., & Gilman, S. (1999). Diagnostic criteria for Parkinson disease. *Archive of Neurology, 56,* 33–39.

Giladi, N., Shabtai, H. Rozenberg, E., & Shabtai, E. (2001). Gait festination in Parkinson's disease. *Parkinsonism and Related Disorders, 7,* 135–138.

Gillen, G. (2000). Improving activities of daily living performance in an adult with ataxia. *American Journal of Occupational Therapy, 54,* 89–96.

Gregory, M. A., Gregory, R. J., & Podd, J. V. (2005). Understanding Guillain-Barré syndrome and central nervous system involvement. *Rehabilitation Nursing, 30,* 207–212.

Hass, E.J., Waddell, D.E., Fleming, R.P., Juncos, J.L. & Gregor, R.J. (2005). Gait initiation and dynamic balance control in Parkinson's disease. *Archives of Physical Medicine and Rehabilitation, 86,* 2172–2176.

Higo, R., Tayama, N., & Nito, T. (2004). Longitudinal analysis of progression of dysphagia in amyotrophic lateral sclerosis. *Auris Nasus Larynx, 31,* 247–254.

Hoehn, M. M., & Yahr, M. D. (1967). Parkinsonism: Onset, progression and mortality. *Neurology, 17,* 427–442.

Hughes, R. A. C., & Rees, J. (1997). Clinical and epidemiologic features of Guillain-Barré syndrome. *Journal of Infectious Diseases, 176 (Suppl. 2),* S92–S98.

Jiang, G. X., Chang, Q., Ehmst, A., Link, H., & de Pedro-Cuesta, J. (1997). Guillain-Barré syndrome in Stockholm County, 1973–1991. *European Journal of Epidemiology, 13,* 25–32.

Kalb, R. C. (1996). *Multiple sclerosis: The questions you have–The answers you need.* New York: Demos.

Karavatas, S. G. (2005). The role of neurodevelopmental sequencing in the physical therapy management of a geriatric patient with Guillain-Barré syndrome. *Topics in Geriatric Rehabilitation, 21,* 133–135.

Karlson, K. H., Larsen, J. P., Tandberg, E., & Maeland, J. G. (1999). Influences of clinical and demographic variables in quality of life in patients with Parkinson's disease. *Journal of Neurology, Neuropsychiatry and Psychiatry, 66,* 431–435.

Khan, F. (2004). Rehabilitation in Guillain-Barré syndrome. *Australian Family Physician, 33,* 1013–1017.

Krupp, L. B., & Lekins, L. E. (2000). Fatigue and declines in cognitive functioning in multiple sclerosis. *Neurology, 55,* 934–939.

Krupp, L. B., & Macallister, W. S. (2005). Treatment of pediatric multiple sclerosis. *Current Treatment Options in Neurology, 7,* 191–199.

Kurland, L. T. (1952). The frequency and geographic distribution of multiple sclerosis as indicated by mortality statistics and morbidity surveys in the United States and Canada. *American Journal of Hygiene, 55,* 457.

Kurtzke, J. F. (1983). Rating neurologic impairment in multiple sclerosis: An Expanded Disability Status Scale (EDSS). *Neurology, 33,* 1444–1452.

Lou, J-S., Reeves, A., Benice, T., & Sexton, G. (2003). Fatigue and depression are associated with poor quality of life in amyotrophic lateral sclerosis. *Neurology, 60,* 122–123.

Lublin, F. D., & Reingold, S. C. (1996). Defining the clinical course of multiple sclerosis: Results of an international survey. *Neurology, 46,* 907–911.

Marder, K., Logroscino, G., Alfaro, B., Mejia, H., Halim, A., Louis, E., Cote, L., & Mayeux, R. (1998). Environmental risk factors for Parkinson's disease in an urban multiethnic community. *Neurology, 50,* 279–281.

Martin, W. R., & Wieler, M. (2003). Treatment of Parkinson's disease. *Canadian Journal of Neurological Science, 30 (Suppl. 1),* S27–S33.

Mathiowetz, V., Finlayson, M. L., Matuska, K. M. Chen, H. Y., & Luo, P. (2005). Randomized controlled trial of an energy conservation course for persons with multiple sclerosis. *Multiple Sclerosis, 11,* 592–601.

Mathiowetz, V., & Matuska, K. M. (1998). Effectiveness of inpatient rehabilitation on self-care activities of individuals with multiple sclerosis. *Neurorehabilitation, 11,* 141–151.

Mathiowetz, V., Matuska, K. M., & Murphy, M. E. (2001). The effects of an energy conservation course for persons with multiple sclerosis. *Archives of Physical Medicine and Rehabilitation, 82,* 449–456.

Maurelli, M., Marchioni, E., Cerretano, R., Basone, D., Bergamaschi, R., Citterio, A., Martelli, A., Sibilla, L., & Savoldi, F. (1992). Neuropsychological assessments in MS: Clinical, neurophysiological and neuroradiological relationships. *Acta Neurologica Scandinavica, 86,* 124–128.

McDonald, E. R., Wiedenfeld, S. A., Hiller, A., Carpenter, C. L., & Walter, R. A. (1994). Survival in amyotrophic lateral sclerosis: The role of psychological factors. *Archives of Neurology, 51,* 17–23.

McGavern, D. B., Murray, P. D., Rivera-Quinones, C., Schmelzer, J. D., Low, P. A., Rodrigues, M. (2000). Axonal loss results in spinal cord atrophy, electrophysiological abnormalities and neurological deficits following demyelination in a chronic inflammatory model of multiple sclerosis. *Brain, 123,* 519–531.

Meythaler, J. M., DeVivo, M. J., & Braswell, W. C. (1997). Rehabilitation outcomes of patients who have developed Guillain-Barré syndrome. *American Journal of Physical Medicine and Rehabilitation, 76,* 411–419.

Mitsumoto, H., Chad, D., & Pioro, E. (1998). *Amyotrophic lateral sclerosis. Contemporary neurology series.* Philadelphia: Davis.

Mohr, D. C., Goodkin, D. E., Likosky, W., Beutler, L., Gatto, N., & Langan, M. K. (1997). Identification of the Beck Depression Inventory items related to multiple sclerosis. *Journal of Behavioural Medicine, 20,* 407–414.

Mohr, D. C., Goodkin, D. E., Nelson, S., Cox, D., & Weiner, M. (2002). Moderating effects of coping on the relationship between stress and the development of the new brain lesions in multiple sclerosis. *Psychosomatic Medicine, 64,* 803–809.

Monza, D., Soliveri, P., Radice, D., Fetoni, V., Testa, D., Caffarra, P., Caraceni, T., & Girotti, F. (1998). Cognitive dysfunction and impaired organization of complex motility in degenerative parkinsonian syndromes. *Archive of Neurology, 55,* 372–378.

Moulin, D. E., Foley, K. M., & Ebers, G. C. (1988). Pain syndromes in multiple sclerosis. *Neurology, 38,* 1830–1834.

Muenter, M. D., Forno, L. S., & Hornykiewicz, O. (1998). Hereditary form of parkinsonism: Dementia. *Annals of Neurology, 43,* 768–781.

Murphy, S., & Tickle-Degnen, L. (2001). The effectiveness of occupational therapy-related treatments for persons with Parkinson's disease: A meta-analytic review. *The American Journal of Occupational Therapy, 55,* 385–392.

Muscular Dystrophy Association of Canada. (1997). *Guillain-Barré syndrome.* InfoSMDAC. Toronto, Ontario, Canada: Muscular Dystrophy Association of Canada.

National Multiple Sclerosis Society [NMSS]. (1998). Clinical Bulletin: Disease Management Consensus Statement, New York. *Neurology, 77,* 231–249.

National Multiple Sclerosis Society [NMSS] (2003). *Fatigue: Take Control! Video based series and workbook.* New York: NMSS.

National Multiple Sclerosis Society [NMSS]. (2006). About MS. Retrieved on April 16, 2006 from http://www.nationalmssociety.org.

Neudert, C., Wasner, M., & Borasio, G. D. (2004). Individual quality of life is not correlated with health-related quality of life or physical function in patients with amyotrophic lateral sclerosis. *Journal of Palliative Medicine, 7,* 551–557.

Norquist, J.M., Jenkinson, C., Fitzpatrick, R., Swash, M. & the ALS-HPS Steering Group. (2003). Factors which predict physical and mental health status in patients with amyotrophic lateral sclerosis over time. *ALS and Other Motor Neuron Disorders, 4,* 112–117.

Pakenham, K. I. (1999). Adjustment to multiple sclerosis: Application of stress and coping model. *Health Psychology, 18,* 383–392.

Pankoff, B., Overend, T., Lucy, D., & White, K. (2000). Validity and responsiveness of the 6 minute walk test for people with fibromyalgia. *Journal of Rheumatology, 27,* 2666–2670.

Paralyzed Veterans of America [PVA]: Multiple Sclerosis Council for Clinical Practice Guidelines. (1998). *Fatigue and multiple sclerosis: Clinical Practice Guidelines.* Washington, DC: Paralyzed Veterans of America.

Paralyzed Veterans of America [PVA]: Multiple Sclerosis Council for Clinical Practice Guidelines. (2003). *Spasticity management in multiple sclerosis: Clinical Practice Guidelines.* Washington, DC: Paralyzed Veterans of America.

Parry, G. J. (2000), Residual effects following Guillain-Barré. Retrieved from http://www.angelfire.com/home/gbs/residual.html.

Petajan, J. H., Gappmaier, E., White, A. T., Spencer, M. K., Mino, L., & Hicks, R. W. (1996). Impact of aerobic training on fitness and quality of life in multiple sclerosis. *Annals of Neurology, 39,* 432–441.

Peto, V., Jenkinson, C., & Fitzpatrick, R. (1995). The development of validation of a short measure of functioning and well being for individuals with Parkinson's disease. *Quality of Life Research, 4,* 241–248.

Plahuta, J.M., McCulloch, B.J. Kasarskis, E.J., Ross, M.A., Walter, R.A., & McDonald, E.R. (2002). Amyotrophic lateral sclerosis and hopelessness: psychosocial factors. *Social Science and Medicine, 55,* 2131–2140.

Poser, C. M., Paty, D., Scheinberg, L., McDonald, W., Davis, F., Ebers, G., Johnson, K., Sibley, W., Silberberg, D., & Tourtellotte, W. (1983).

New diagnostic criteria for multiple sclerosis: Guidelines for research protocols. *Annals of Neurology, 13,* 227–231.

Rao, S. M., Leo, G. J., Bernardin, L., & Unverszagt, F. (1991). Cognitive dysfunction in multiple sclerosis. *Neurology, 41,* 685–696.

Rees, J. H., Thompson, R. D., Smeeton, N. C., & Hughes, R. A. (1998). Epidemiological study of Guillain-Barré syndrome in south east England. *Journal of Neurology, Neurosurgery and Psychiatry, 64,* 74–77.

Robbins, R.A., Simmons, Z. Bremer, B.A., Walsh, S.M., & Fischer, S. (2001). Quality of life in ALS is maintained as physical function declines. *Neurology, 56,* 442–444.

Rodriguez, M., Siva, A., Ward, J., Stolp-Smith, K., O'Brien, P., & Kurland, L. (1994). Impairment, disability, and handicap in multiple sclerosis: A population-based study in Olmsted County, Minnesota. *Neurology, 44,* 28–33.

Rovari, N. M., Filippi, M., Falautano, M., Minicucci, L., Rocca, V., Marinelli, V., & Comi, G. (1998). Relation between MR abnormalities and patterns of cognitive impairment in multiple sclerosis. *Neurology, 50,* 1604–1608.

Ruggieri, R. M., Palermo, R., Vitello G., Gennus, M., Settipani, N., & Piccoli, F. (2003). Cognitive impairment in patients suffering from relapsing-remitting multiple sclerosis with EDSS < or = 3.5. *Acta Neurologica Scandinavica, 108,* 323–326.

Solari, A., Filippini, G., Gasco, P., Colla, L., Salmnaggi, A., La Mantia, L., Farinotti, M., Eoli, M., & Mendozzi, L. (1999). Physical rehabilitation has a positive effect on disability in multiple sclerosis patients. *Neurology, 52,* 57–62.

Stern, M. B. (1993). Parkinson's disease: Early diagnosis and management. *Journal of Family Practice, 36,* 439–446.

Stolp-Smith, K. A., Carter, J. L., Rohe, D. E., & Knowland, D. P. (1997). Management of impairment, disability and handicap due to multiple sclerosis. *Mayo Clinic Proceedings, 72,* 1184–1196.

Thomas, F. J., & Wiles, C. M. (1999). Dysphagia and nutritional status in multiple sclerosis. *Journal of Neurology, 246,* 677–682.

Tickle-Degnen, L. (2006). Wilma West Lectureship, USC Occupational Science Symposium. March 3, 2006, University of Southern California, Los Angeles, CA.

Trail, M., Nelson, N., Van, J.N., Appel, S.A., & Lai, E.C. (2001). Wheelchair use by patients with amyotrophic lateral sclerosis: A survey of user characteristics and selection preferences. *Archives of Physical Medicine and Rehabilitation, 82,* 98–102.

Trapp, B. D., Peterson, J., Ransohoff, R. M., Rudick, R., Mork, S., & Bo, L. (1998). Axonal transection in the lesions of multiple sclerosis. *New England Journal of Medicine, 338,* 278–285.

Uitti, R. J. (1998). Tremor: How to determine if the patient has Parkinson's disease. *Geriatrics, 53,* 30–36.

Vanage, S. M., Gilbertson, K. K., & Mathiowetz, V. (2003). Effects of an energy conservation course on fatigue impact for persons with progressive multiple sclerosis. *American Journal of Occupational Therapy, 57,* 315–323.

Van den Berg, J.P., Kalmijn, S., Lindeman, E., Veldink, J.H., de Visser, M., Van er Graaff, M.M., Wokk, J.H.J., & Van der Berg, L.H. (2005). Multidisciplinary ALS care improves quality of life in patients with ALS. *Neurology,* 65, 1264–1267.

Ward, C. D., & Robertson, D. (2004). Rehabilitation in Parkinson's disease. *Reviews in Clinical Gerontology, 13,* 223–239.

Warren, S., Warren, K. G., & Cockerill, R. (1991). Emotional stress and coping in multiple sclerosis exacerbations. *Journal of Psychosomatic Research, 35,* 37–47.

Weiser, W., Wetzel, S. G., Kappos, L., Hoshi, M. M., Witte, U., Radue, E. W., & Steinbrich, W. (2002). Swallowing abnormalities in multiple sclerosis: Correlation between videofluoroscopy and subjective symptoms. *European Radiology, 12,* 789–792.

CHAPTER 41

Orthopaedic Conditions

Colleen Maher and Jane Bear-Lehman

LEARNING OBJECTIVES

After studying this chapter, the reader will be able to do the following:

1. Identify the role of the occupational therapist in assessing and planning treatment for persons with occupational dysfunction secondary to injuries or diseases affecting the musculoskeletal system.
2. Select appropriate assessments and plan treatment according to the stages of recovery following a musculoskeletal injury or disease of the upper extremity.
3. Describe how to accomplish daily life tasks without causing adverse sequelae following fracture or surgery to the hip.
4. State the principles of body mechanics and describe how to apply them to activities and tasks of daily life.
5. Describe the phases of fracture management of the upper extremity and how to optimize occupational functioning at each stage.

Glossary

Clinical union—Evidence of bony callus on radiographic examination, although the fracture line is still apparent (Salter, 1999).

Codman's pendulum exercises—Exercises prescribed for most shoulder surgeries in early recovery. The standing or sitting patient bends over at the hips so that the trunk is parallel to the floor. The arm assumes a position away from the body and perpendicular to the floor, either with or without a sling. In this gravity-assisted position, the patient moves the arm passively or actively, depending on the surgical protocol, forward into humeral flexion and backward into humeral extension; across and away from the body for shoulder abduction and adduction; and then in a circle for circumduction (Salter, 1999).

Collar-and-cuff sling—Commercially available sling that supports the upper extremity in an adducted and internally rotated position against the abdomen.

Controlled range of motion—Active or passive movement within a predetermined safe arc. Often the allowed movement begins in the middle of the range and is gradually upgraded toward the full arc as healing occurs. A splint can be used to set the boundaries or block unwanted movement.

Deep pressure tissue massage—Firm manual pressure applied to the skin for about 5 seconds to blanch the underlying scar. This massage is initiated once sutures are removed. On a closed wound, lanolin or vitamin E can be used. Massage begins at the perimeter and gradually works toward and then over the surgical scar site.

Occupation-specific training—Occupation-as-means using the equipment and in the context specific to one's occupation (e.g., patient who enjoys golfing practices golf swings using golf clubs and ball, under supervision of the occupational therapist). Same as task-specific training.

Shoulder immobilizer—Used if strict immobilization is required. Adjustable elastic band that fits around the waist with two straps that position and secure the arm in internal rotation.

Skateboard—Wooden or plastic board with four ball-bearing wheels (one at each corner) that support the skateboard and reduce friction when the patient attempts to move the upper extremity. The forearm rests on the skateboard, and the patient moves it to active range of motion in gravity-lessened plane.

Theraband—Exercise bands that come in various levels of resistance (denoted by different colors) used to improve strength.

Trendelenburg gait—Gait pattern that results from a weakened gluteus medius muscle. The patient lurches toward the injured side to place the center of gravity over the hip. It is characterized by dropping of the pelvis on the unaffected side at heel strike of the affected foot.

Volkmann's ischemia—Increased compartment pressure in one anatomic area of the extremity as a result of a fracture or crush injury. In the upper extremity, it is most common in the forearm. Closure of the small vessels results in increased pressure. The patient will experience severe pain, especially with passive stretching. Pressure greater than 30 mm Hg is considered a surgical emergency in which a fasciotomy would be performed (Bednar & Light, 2003).

Wall climbing, finger walking, palm gliding—Exercise to develop shoulder flexion. The patient faces the wall, places the injured shoulder's hand on the wall, and either finger walks or glides the palm toward the ceiling and then the floor. For shoulder and scapular abduction, the patient turns parallel to the wall and abducts the shoulder to place the fingers or palm on the wall for finger walking or palm gliding. Commercially available finger climbers can be mounted on the wall or used on a tabletop with set increments for the finger walk; some climbers can be adjusted to different angles to allow for varying degrees of movement.

Orthopaedic conditions include injuries, diseases, and deformities of bones, joints, and their related structures: muscles, tendons, ligaments, and nerves. These conditions can be caused by traumatic events, such as motor vehicle, recreational, or work-related accidents; by cumulative trauma; or by congenital anomaly. The rising incidence rate of musculoskeletal injuries is attributed to an increase in "individual participation in high-speed travel by land, sea, and air, complex industry, and competitive and recreational sports" (Salter, 1999, p. 417). Furthermore, more individuals are reaching old age, and as they age, the incidence of injuries from falls increases.

This chapter provides an overview of the occupational therapy assessments and treatments used with adult patients who have orthopaedic or musculoskeletal conditions. Specifically, it reviews upper extremity and hip fractures and their sequelae, hip surgery for trauma and disease, shoulder injuries and their effects on function, and pain with a focus on low back pain.

PURPOSE AND ROLE OF OCCUPATIONAL THERAPY IN ORTHOPAEDICS

The aim of occupational therapy in orthopaedic rehabilitation is to help the patient achieve maximal function of body and limb to restore occupational functioning. In the acute stage of recovery, the therapist's role is to help relieve pain, decrease swelling and inflammation, assist in wound care, maintain joint or limb alignment, and restore function at the injury site. The therapist teaches the patient to safely perform tasks and activities while protecting the injury site for healing. As healing progresses to **clinical union** and then to consolidation, the occupational therapist retrains the patient in activities of daily living (ADL) and other occupational tasks.

For individuals who have a chronic joint disease, such as osteoarthritis, or cumulative trauma, such as low back pain, the occupational therapist's role depends on the stage of recovery and the directives of the treatment team. The occupational therapist may directly help relieve pain, realign structures, or reduce the stress on soft tissue. Or the occupational therapist may work closely with the physical therapist to relate the functional program to treatment offered in physical therapy to heal the wound. As the acute episode of pain calms, the occupational therapist focuses on an individually tailored education program to help the patient physically and psychologically make the required lifestyle changes to reach and sustain optimal occupational functioning.

OCCUPATIONAL THERAPY EVALUATION IN ORTHOPAEDICS

Evaluation is an ongoing process that is carefully coordinated with the stage of recovery. The therapist selects assessments that will provide sufficient information to plan and to direct treatment but will not threaten the injured or inflamed structure during healing. The therapist chooses assessments that correspond to the level of bone healing, the chosen method of reduction and stabilization, and the plan for movement during healing or the acute inflammatory episode. The therapist assesses participation in life roles, areas of occupations, performance skills and performance patterns, and impairments of capacities and abilities.

Participation in Life Roles

Although resumption of life roles may not be possible at the start of the aftercare program, life roles regulate the choices made during treatment planning and serve as the end point for treatment planning. In addition to noting the activities and tasks the patient can and cannot accomplish, using the assessment tools described in Chapter 5, the therapist observes whether the patient is magnifying the injury or appears to be adopting a sick role.

Impairments of Abilities and Capacities

Physical impairments are directly measured by various assessment instruments. See Chapter 5 for assessment of pain, edema, range of motion (ROM), strength, and endurance. The surgeon's protocol may stipulate no movement or no force at or near the fracture site, or it may require **controlled range of motion** beginning immediately or within the first 3–4 weeks after stabilization (Fig. 41-1). If the surgeon's protocol requires complete rest of the injured bone or joint, ROM measurements are deferred until movement is permissible. If the patient is on

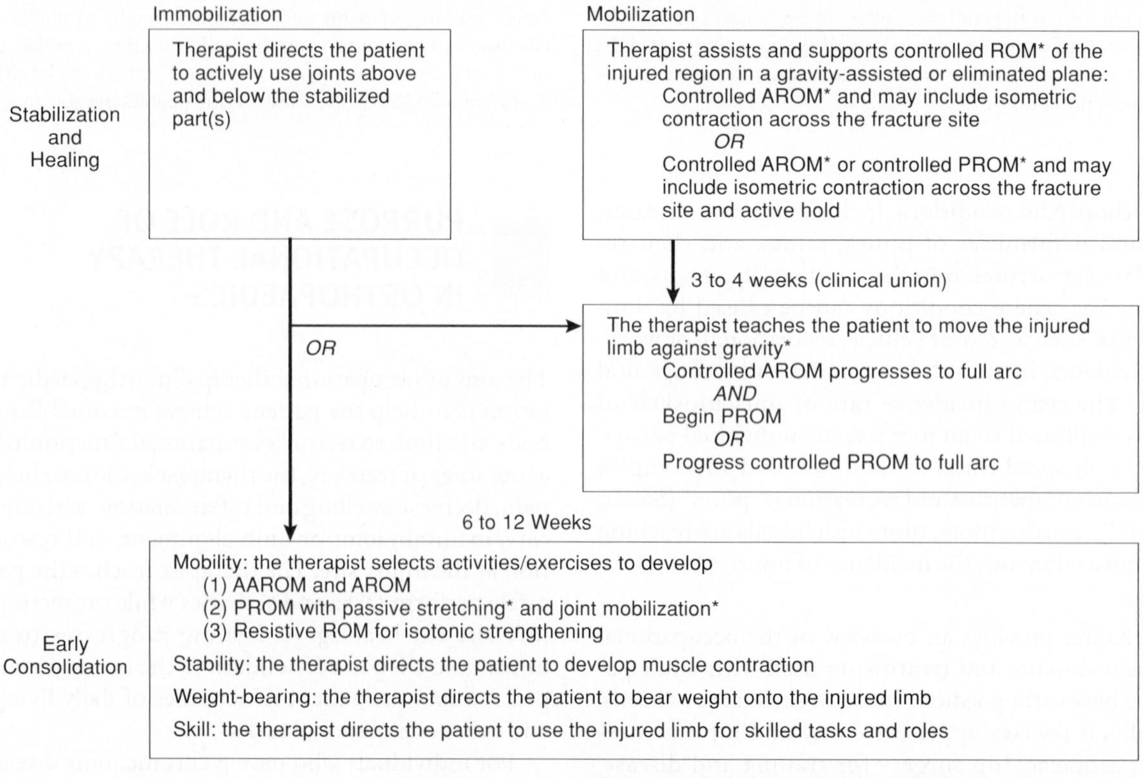

Figure 41-1 Guidelines for therapeutic intervention during fracture healing and consolidation.

a specific program, such as controlled range of motion, the therapist measures the joint, adhering to the precautionary boundaries, and does not allow the patient to exceed the limits of the directive. The adjacent joints are measured, and a treatment program is designed for any adjacent joint that demonstrates less than normal function. Detailed strength testing with applied resistance is deferred until there is bony consolidation or the acute inflammation has calmed. Due to the force required, grip and pinch testing are usually deferred for 2–4 weeks following cast removal in forearm fractures. Assessing strength after a fracture should only be performed when ordered by the orthopaedist. The occupational therapist not only focuses on direct measure of the injured and adjacent anatomical regions but also closely observes the patient's total body response in terms of postural changes, pain responses, and psychological reactions.

OCCUPATIONAL THERAPY TREATMENT IN ORTHOPAEDICS

The most important treatment goal is the restoration of occupational functioning. To achieve this, the patient needs to be directed from the start of recovery to move and to use all joints that are not affected by the injury or the disease. For patients who have an upper limb fracture or a short-term inflammation, the therapist may recommend temporary use of the uninjured hand alone to perform some ADL, assisted by adaptations such as pump bottles for toothpaste and shampoo, a button hook, or a rocker knife. Other ADLs may require the temporary assistance of another person so as not to disturb the healing region. When the patient is medically ready, the occupational therapist, through careful activity analysis, ascertains how the patient can safely resume tasks that correspond with the achieved recovery status to reintegrate the injured or inflamed limb into activity safely. Attention is directed toward redeveloping the function of the injured limb to resume its capacity in mobility, stability, weight bearing, and ultimately skill (see Fig. 41-1). When a condition is chronic, such as status post total hip replacement or low back pain, the therapist recommends alternative methods, adaptive equipment, or environmental modification for safe task completion.

Acute Trauma: Fractures

As long as orthopaedic surgeons have been treating fractures, there has been a controversy between the "movers" and the "resters." The surgeons prescribing rest as a fracture treatment keep their patients immobilized in traction, plaster, or fiberglass for long periods after stabilization. For many surgeons, however, the goal in fracture treatment is to mobilize the injured structures as quickly as is compatible with healing and return the patient to work and leisure activities (Salter, 1999).

The goal of fracture treatment is to achieve a precise and effective stabilization for optimal recovery and resolution of function. Closed fractures that are relatively undisplaced and stable may be managed by protection alone, without reduction or immobilization. Fractures that are undisplaced but unstable do not need reduction but do require positioning and immobilization in a cast or a fracture brace. Surgical reduction is performed to reduce open fractures and those closed fractures where the bone fragments cannot be approximated accurately by closed manual reduction alone. The bone fragments are brought into a closer anatomical alignment during surgical reduction and are stabilized by insertion of an internal fixation device, such as a nail, pin, screw, rod, compression plate, or an external fixator. Surgical repair also can include prosthetic devices that are implanted to restore joint motion (Smith et al., 2003).

Fracture healing, when the part is immobilized by a cast, splint, or fracture brace (Figs. 41-2 and 41-3), is accomplished through the formation of immature woven bone or external callus. The woven bone then consolidates and remodels so that the fracture is repaired with lamellar bone (Smith et al., 2003). When internal fixation provides complete bone immobilization, external callus does not form, and direct healing occurs. When external callus forms first, more healing time is required. Fracture healing has a general timetable that is confirmed routinely by physical exam

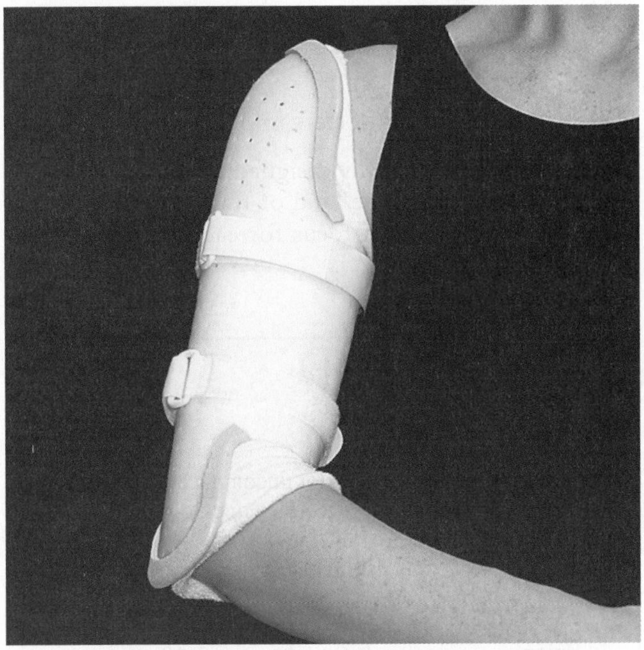

Figure 41-2 Thermoplastic humeral fracture brace to support the length of the humerus during healing. (Courtesy of Smith & Nephew, Inc., Germantown, WI.)

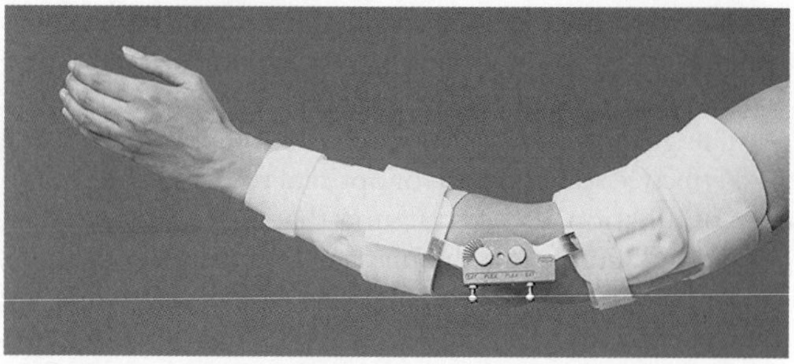

Figure 41-3 Upper extremity fracture brace with adjustable hinge joint designed to position the elbow statically in flexion or extension, block undesirable motion, and allow some free elbow motion. (Courtesy of Smith & Nephew, Inc., Germantown, WI.)

and x-rays to reveal the healing status before advancing the rehabilitation program (Definition 41-1). Restoring bone to its optimal function is evident when consolidation or complete fracture repair has occurred when the callus is ossified, the fracture site is no longer tender and painful, and there is no movement when the fractured bone is manipulated (Krop, 2002; Smith et al., 2003).

Rehabilitation begins as soon as the plaster cast dries or within a day or two after reduction. The timing, amount, and kind of activity depend on the place and kind of fracture, the method of fracture reduction selected by the orthopaedic surgeon, and, in some instances, the age of the patient. Clinical experience has shown that early specific use of the injured limb during healing diminishes or eliminates the need for treatment after immobilization (Salter, 1999). Early movement prevents the unwanted side effects of immobilization: stiff joints, disuse atrophy, and muscle weakness.

Evaluation Process in Aftercare for Fractures

The evaluation is carefully designed and adjusted to the stage of recovery and the kind of fracture. This chapter presents the specialized focus for each fracture by the stage of recovery: immobilization and early mobilization or early consolidation.

Immobilization or Early Mobilization (Zero–6 weeks)

The therapist identifies the tasks and activities for which the patient needs to learn an adaptation or obtain assistance during the temporary period of restricted movement so that the fracture site remains undisturbed. Measurements of ROM and circumference for swelling are conducted on adjacent joints. Assessment of ROM of the injured joints depends on the type of protection and stabilization used and the orthopaedic surgeon's protocol for aftercare, as discussed earlier. Patients with secure internal fixation of bone fragments may begin gentle ROM of the involved joints before the consolidation phase. This usually occurs at 2 weeks post-op under the close supervision of the surgeon.

Early Consolidation (6–8 weeks)

The therapist determines whether and to what extent the patient can safely reintegrate the injured limb into occupational tasks. The therapist continually assesses the patient's ability to use the injured limb for functional tasks to correspond with clinical progress. The therapist initially measures active ROM (AROM) of the involved joints with the exception of shoulder fractures, which are measured for AA/PROM (active assisted, passive range of motion). Edema and sensibility should be assessed. A 10-cm visual analog scale should be used to assess the patient's pain level. Grip and pinch measurements are not taken until the surgeon orders strengthening. Observe the patient for signs of infection: redness, heat, swelling, pain, loss of function, or changes in circulation. To do so, look at the limb's skin color: purple, dusky, or white coloration indicates alterations in circulation, as does a skin surface that is too warm or too cold to the touch. ***Immediately report abnormal findings to the surgeon.***

Treatment Process in Aftercare for Fractures

Intervention strategies for addressing orthopaedic injuries are based on the stage of recovery and the orthopaedic treatment protocol. The therapist selects and applies intervention strategies that are consistent with the orthopaedic surgeon's immobilization or mobilization plan, the restrictions or precautions, and goals.

Immobilization or Early Mobilization

Early mobilization treatment programs have specific and focused protocols indicating the timing, type, and quantity of desired movement (see Fig. 41-1). Advancement of the therapeutic program is determined for each patient based on the stability of the fracture and radiographic signs of fracture healing (Brotzman et al., 2003). The

DEFINITION 41-1

Fracture Healing

The estimate of healing time for uncomplicated fractures in tubular bones, according to Apley and Solomon (1994), is as follows:

	Upper Limb	Lower Limb
Callus visible	2–3 weeks	2–3 weeks
Union	4–6 weeks	8–12 weeks
Consolidation	6–8 weeks	12–16 weeks

cautiously controlled movement usually begins in a gravity-assisted or gravity-eliminated plane. The movement may be active assistive range of motion (AAROM) or AROM restricted to midrange and gradually upgraded to full ROM. Under careful guidance and manual handling, isometric contraction of the muscles whose bellies extend across the fracture site is encouraged to facilitate circulation and bone healing. Some protocols require controlled PROM, often followed by an active hold pattern. That is, the therapist passively moves the injured part through the prescribed arc, and then the patient isometrically holds the achieved position briefly.

The therapist may have to fit the patient with a sling, shoulder immobilizer, splint, or fracture brace during healing either to add protective support or to begin early controlled movement. To add to a patient's comfort during stabilization in an external fixator, the therapist may recommend and fabricate a supportive static splint. Thermoplastic splinting alone is often used to achieve relative immobilization for fractures of the metacarpals and phalanges (see Chapters 16 and 42). Following the initial treatment of closed reduction of fractures in the shaft of long bones, the surgeon may prescribe a functional fracture brace as popularized by Sarmiento and shown in Figures 41-2 and 41-3 (Sarmiento, 2000). The lightweight thermoplastic fracture brace allows for motion above and below the fracture site and minimizes detrimental effects of prolonged immobilization. The metal hinge controls the amount of movement available. The patient is closely monitored for circulation, biomechanical alignment, and desired (controlled) movement. The therapist adjusts the shell to facilitate comfort, to respond to changes such as a reduction of limb volume, and to adjust the amount of movement the splint permits.

Early Consolidation

Therapy usually begins with focused, active use of the limb. Active therapy consists of activities and tasks to remediate the use of the muscles in the injured region. The therapist directs the patient in a graduated program to resolve the presenting impairments and to reintegrate the limb into normal and customary use for functional tasks and role performance. If secondary changes are noted in the adjacent body parts or if there is a change in body posture, therapy is also directed to resolving those impairments.

Should edema persist even with elevation and active muscle contraction, additional methods, such as compression gloves or sleeves, contrast baths and retrograde massage, or manual lymph drainage, are applied. To ameliorate stiffness and pain, the therapist may introduce modalities such as paraffin, fluidotherapy, or heat packs before or with exercise or activity (see Chapter 20). If stiffness prevails and the fracture is stable, joint mobilization and passive stretching are performed to facilitate the arthrokinetic accessory movements to increase the passive movement potential. Dynamic splinting, static progressive splinting, or the use of continuous passive motion may also increase passive mobility over time. Adherent or hypertrophic scar formation after open reduction or soft tissue repair can also limit movement, increase pain, and alter sensation. To prevent this, the therapist teaches the patient **deep pressure tissue massage** and applies continuous pressure to the scar with an agent such as silastic gel to facilitate scar remodeling (see Chapter 45).

FRACTURES

The care of fractures challenges both the surgeon and the occupational therapist to help the patient ultimately reincorporate the injured limb into functional performance tasks. To initiate the care of a patient who sustained a fracture, the therapist must understand the anatomy and biomechanics of the extremity and select intervention strategies that are consistent with the physiological process of fracture repair.

Shoulder Fractures

The shoulder complex is composed of the glenohumeral joint, scapulothoracic joint, sternoclavicular joint, and acromioclavicular joint. The shoulder complex provides a wide range of movements for hand placement but also provides the important functions of stabilization for hand use, lifting and pushing, reaching, and weight bearing (Greene & Roberts, 2005). The shoulder is considered the most challenging portion of the body to rehabilitate. After traumatic, degenerative, or surgical shoulder lesions, the therapy goals are delicately balanced to relieve pain, to restore movement and muscle strength, and to allow for callus formation and the approximation of the bony fragments in the injured region.

Immobilization of the shoulder results in stiffness and pain; therefore, non-operative and post-operative therapy programs call for a specific regimen of PROM, AAROM, or AROM within a controlled, guarded range. Shoulder fractures are closely monitored by radiographs as initial controlled PROM and AAROM begin. There is controversy with regard to PROM. Some argue that passive motion is contraindicated, particularly in the elderly (Goldstein, 1999). Others say that passive movement is safe if the provided range corresponds to the surgeon's prescribed limitations. Emphasis is on the patient resuming non-resistive functional activities and using the injured limb as soon as movement is allowed.

Since immobilization quickly results in stiffness, active shoulder motion begins as soon as the acute pain diminishes in stable shoulder fractures. Unstable shoulder fractures usually require surgical intervention for fixation. The protocols are based on the classification of fracture, the type of surgical procedure, and age and activity level of the patient, and they often follow the guidelines as originally described by Neer (1990). Some post-operative protocols start isometrics for external rotation and shoulder abduction across the repair site immediately to facilitate stability. Assisted isotonic shoulder motions follow about 3–4 weeks later, once the shoulder fragments are approximated as confirmed by radiograph (Kelley & Clark, 1995). If shoulder stability is achieved with internal fixation, AROM or pain-free AAROM exercises may begin as early as 7–10 days after surgery (Kelley & Clark, 1995).

During the first 6–8 weeks, isometric exercises, a stimulant for fracture healing and callus formation, are performed along with **wall climbing**, non-resistive therapeutic activities, and **Codman's pendulum exercises**. Codman's exercises are performed with the patient bending over so that the injured upper limb is perpendicular to the floor. In this gravity-assisted plane, the patient does clockwise and counterclockwise circular movements and flexion, extension, abduction, and adduction. ***Codman's exercises may be contraindicated if the upper extremity is edematous.***

Barring complications, when clinical union is achieved at approximately 6 weeks, progressive shoulder exercises for flexion, extension, abduction, and internal and external rotation are started (Kelley & Clark, 1995). Passive stretching, joint mobilization, and resistive exercises begin once there is established clinical union, the inflammation has decreased, and there is no fear of disrupting the fracture (Kelley & Clark, 1995).

Humeral head fractures that are unstable and significantly displaced are often medically treated with humeral head replacement, known as hemiarthroplasty. A total shoulder arthroplasty is often considered for patients with severe arthritis in combination with a proximal humerus fracture (Keenan & Waters, 2003). Therapy for total prosthetic joint replacement of the shoulder varies with the design of the prosthesis and the surgical procedure. The rehabilitation program begins within the first 2–3 days after surgery. The exercises should not cause any pain. The key to a satisfactory functional result is early achievement of shoulder forward flexion and external rotation in the plane of the scapula. Some protocols require the use of continuous passive motion for forward shoulder flexion immediately following surgery (Salter, 1999).

Codman's pendulum exercises, passive shoulder elevation done lying supine with the opposite hand assisting the affected limb, and use of an exercise wand to perform passive external rotation are introduced during the first 2–3 days after surgery (Tan, Leggin, & Williams, 2002). The patient is instructed to perform the exercises 4–6 times daily. Since the subscapularis tendon and the rotator cuff are violated during the surgery, some surgeons introduce external rotation slowly in the first 4 weeks; others incorporate passive external rotation on the second post-operative day. The preferred position for passive external rotation exercise is with the humerus adducted. For the first 4–5 weeks of rehabilitation, external rotation is often limited to what was obtained at the time of wound closure or the operative ROM value for external rotation (Kelley & Clark, 1995; Tan, Leggin, & Williams, 2002). During this phase, the patient is instructed to begin non-resistive occupational tasks, such as brushing teeth and self-feeding.

One to 2 weeks post-operatively, the patient is instructed to add passive internal rotation, extension, and horizontal adduction. The patient can progress to isometric strengthening of the rotator cuff at 4–6 weeks. If the subscapularis was detached during surgery, the surgeon may restrict strengthening of this muscle at this time. At 6 weeks, with medical advisement, the program is upgraded to include active resistive exercise and activities to strengthen the rotator cuff muscles and the three parts of the deltoid muscle (Tan, Leggin, & Williams, 2002). Theraband exercises, free weights, and occupational tasks that emphasize abduction and rotational movements are initiated. Weight bearing on the injured arm is not allowed for at least 6 months.

Management of humeral shaft or humeral neck fractures is divided into three phases. Phase I includes positioning, Codman's pendulum exercises, and passive assistive exercises. Fractures of the humeral shaft and humeral neck both respond well to early passive movement and positioning. Codman's pendulum exercises and passive assistive movement of the shoulder are performed several times a day to prevent stiffness. The occupational therapist may make a fracture brace conforming to the length of the humerus to provide the initial support after a humeral shaft fracture (see Fig. 41-2). The therapist must be careful to flare and roll the edges of the shell to prevent compromise to circulation and nerve impingement while allowing available movement. In the case of humeral shaft fracture, there is a risk of radial nerve damage due to the location of the injury relative to the course of the radial nerve. Radial nerve injury is characterized by the inability to extend the elbow, wrist, and digits. Other complications that are not uncommon with humeral shaft fractures are delayed union and non-union. These complications may occur as a result of an injury to the nutrient artery located at midshaft when the humerus is fractured (Macklin et al., 2002). A bone stimulator may be used to facilitate bone healing.

For phase II, the therapist encourages active assisted concentric and eccentric exercise, progressing to lightly resistive exercises. These patterns often begin with the patient supine and progress to seated, in which position the weight of the extremity is first supported by the therapist or a **skateboard**.

Phase III addresses both stretching and strengthening. As healing permits, the patient can combine shoulder forward flexion with abduction with or without external rotation (Basti et al., 1994). Use of the injured extremity in occupation-as-end is encouraged.

Elbow Fractures

Elbow motion gives the individual the capacity to position the hand in space close to or far from the body for manipulation of objects and to function as a stabilizer for strength activities (Davila, 2002). These movements are accomplished by two degrees of freedom: flexion and extension at the ulnohumeral and radiohumeral joints and pronation and supination at the proximal radioulnar joint. Supracondylar fractures of the humerus are the most common and the most serious elbow fracture (Salter, 1999). These fractures are associated with a high incidence of malunion and have a risk of **Volkmann's ischemia**, a compartment syndrome of the forearm. Ischemia, considered an urgent medical matter, can be caused by edema within a fascia-surrounded compartment or by acute elbow flexion that compresses an artery against bone. ***Signs of ischemia include pale, bluish skin color; absence of forearm radial pulse; and decreased hand sensation accompanied by severe pain. Report these signs immediately.*** Immediate action is important because the peripheral nerves can withstand only 2–4 hours of ischemia, although they do have some potential to regenerate. The muscle can withstand up to 6 hours of ischemia, but it cannot regenerate (Salter, 1999). Prolonged occlusion allows for the progression to a contracture as the necrotic muscle becomes dense, shortened, fibrous scar tissue.

The uncomplicated supracondylar fracture may be treated with immobilization in a removable plaster cast or thermoplastic splint following open reduction. The elbow is held in 90–100° of flexion, and the arm may be supported in a **collar-and-cuff sling** (Salter, 1999). After the first week, the splint is removed daily for gentle, non-resistive active movement in a gravity-eliminated position. Therapy for elbow fractures emphasizes active, not passive, movement and flexion rather than extension to minimize the risk of ischemia and excessive bone formation (heterotopic ossification) (Salter, 1999). Many patients achieve close to full movement after 6–12 months without specific treatment; some, however, do not achieve complete elbow extension even with therapy (Davila, 2002).

Complex elbow fractures are often treated with open reduction and well-secured fixation. Active motion begins 3–5 days after surgery. Similar to the supracondylar fracture, the elbow fracture is splinted in flexion rather than extension; flexion has a greater functional importance. If a contracture occurs, the hand can be raised to the face for eating and hygiene (Davila, 2002). In the elderly, elbow fractures are often treated with a collar-and-cuff sling alone, and active movement begins early to prevent stiffness and pain. A functional arc of motion for daily activities can be regained, but full ROM is not always achieved.

Radial head fractures can be treated with closed reduction or, depending on the severity, may require radial head excision. Radial head fractures seldom require more than a sling for immobilization. Active pronation and supination exercises are encouraged early. Emphasis should be placed on regaining active supination. Full supination is more difficult and painful than pronation (Davila, 2002). Supination and pronation exercises should be performed seated or standing, with the shoulder adducted to the side and elbow flexed to 90°. Exercises should be performed 6 times daily, with a minimum of 2 sets of 10 repetitions. Exercises should be pain free. Continuous passive motion (CPM), dynamic supination splint, and static progressive splinting can be used to further encourage forearm rotation. See Chapter 42 for wrist and hand fractures.

ROTATOR CUFF PATHOLOGIES

The shoulder complex is the foundation of all upper extremity movements. The rotator cuff musculature plays an integral part in the function and control of the shoulder complex. The supraspinatus performs shoulder elevation, the infraspinatus and teres minor perform external rotation, and the subscapularis performs internal rotation. Besides the actions they produce, the rotator cuff musculature functions as a force couple to control the head of the humerus on the glenoid fossa. Its anatomical location at the subacromial space, between the coracoacromial arch and the head of the humerus, makes the rotator cuff extremely vulnerable to compression. The supraspinatus also has an area of hypovascularity known as the critical zone. This zone is where the supraspinatus tendon inserts on the greater tuberosity of the humerus. Due to its anatomical location and area of hypovascularity, the supraspinatus is the most commonly impinged rotator cuff tendon. Patients with rotator cuff pathology are often faced with the inability to perform the most personal self-care tasks. Activities such as toileting, hair care, and hooking a bra are all dependent on a normally functioning rotator cuff.

Shoulder Impingement Syndrome

Shoulder impingement syndrome is a compression of the structures found in the subacromial space. Structures found in the subacromial space (superior to inferior) include the subacromial bursa, supraspinatus, joint capsule, and long head of the biceps. Shoulder impingement syndrome is most commonly caused by repetitive or sustained elevation of the shoulder above 90°. If shoulder impingement syndrome goes untreated, it can result in a rotator cuff tear. Charles Neer developed a classification system to better understand the progression of shoulder impingement syndrome. Stage I is described as edema, inflammation, and hemorrhage. In this stage the bursa and/or the tendons become irritated and inflamed. The symptoms can be reversed with occupational therapy intervention. The focus should be on activity modification. In stage II, the bursa and tendons become thick and fibrotic. At this stage, a person can be treated conservatively; however, recovery may take longer. In stage III, a person may present with bone spurs and partial or full thickness tears (Neer, 1990). A small tear is less than 1 cm, a medium tear is 3 cm, a large tear is less than 5 cm, and a massive tear is greater than 5 cm (Post, Silver, & Singh, 1983).

Rotator Cuff Tendonitis and Bicipital Tendonitis

A person may have rotator cuff tendonitis and or bicipital tendonitis but not shoulder impingement syndrome. The chief complaint of tendonitis is pain during humeral movement above 90°. In most cases, the patient is independent with activities of daily living; however, the patient will experience pain while performing these tasks. Common causes are repetitive overhead use, curved or hooked acromion, weakness of shoulder or scapula musculature, and capsular tightness. Tendonitis can be treated conservatively with pain modalities, activity modification, strengthening exercises, and **occupation-specific training**.

Bursitis

Shoulder bursitis is inflammation of the subacromial bursa. Bursitis can be differentiated from rotator cuff tendonitis if the patient has pain during passive shoulder elevation and is pain free during AROM and muscle testing of the rotator cuff. It is rarely the major source of pain and usually coexists with shoulder impingement syndrome (Malone, Richmond, & Frick, 1995). See the section on shoulder impingement for causes.

Calcific Tendonitis

Calcific tendonitis results from calcium deposits laid down at the insertion of the tendon on the bone. In the shoulder, calcific tendonitis most commonly occurs in the supraspinatus and infraspinatus tendons. The cause is unknown. This type of tendonitis usually heals on its own by spontaneous reabsorption. Reabsorption of the calcium can take several months. During this time, the person may experience significant pain. Physical agent modalities, pain-free ROM, and activity modification are used to address the pain.

Rotator Cuff Tear

Tears of the rotator cuff can be partial or full thickness. See the section on shoulder impingement syndrome for description of size of tear. Causes include trauma, progression of impingement syndrome, and degenerative changes of the tendon. Patients with rotator cuff tears will present with difficulty performing activities above shoulder level and will often compensate by hiking the shoulder using the upper trapezius muscle. Rotational movements, such as reaching the small of the back to tuck a shirt in or remove a wallet from a back pocket, can also be limited. Rotator cuff tears can significantly limit a person's occupational functioning. Rotator cuff tears are diagnosed using magnetic resonance imaging (MRI) and magnetic resonance arthrography (MRA) (Toyoda et al., 2005). Some partial tears can be treated conservatively with activity modification and strengthening of scapula and rotator cuff muscles. Surgical options for those patients who don't benefit from conservative treatment include arthroscopic, mini-open, and open repairs. Post-operative therapy focuses on regaining full ROM, scapula and rotator cuff strengthening, practicing activities of daily living, and occupational tasks.

Evaluation (of the non-surgical patient)

The evaluation should begin with a thorough history. Discuss the mechanism of injury. Was it a sudden onset or gradual onset? If it was a gradual onset, try to determine what activity or sustained posture led to the rotator cuff problem. Also discuss the patient's level of pain (scale of 0–10). Is the pain localized or referred? What activities or occupations cause pain? Can the patient sleep on the involved side? The therapist should also observe the patient's posture and symmetry of the scapula at rest and during upward rotation. The physical assessments can then begin with asking the patient to perform various functional movements such as reaching the small of the back, reaching the opposite axilla, and touching the top of the head. See Chapter 5 for assessment of AROM and PROM and manual muscle testing of the shoulder. Active cervical ROM and sensory testing the C4 to T1 dermatomes (see Chapter 7) should be performed to eliminate the possibility of cervical involvement. Palpation of the rotator cuff tendons will assess tenderness and swelling. Special tests should be administered to determine all the involved structures. Special tests for rotator cuff pathology include the Neer impingement sign, Hawkins test, empty can test, drop arm test, and biceps speed's test (Procedures for Practice 41-1). Activities of daily living should be assessed by

PROCEDURES FOR PRACTICE 41-1

Special Tests for Rotator Cuff Injuries

1. *Neer Impingement Sign:* Forced forward flexion with the shoulder internally rotated. If the patient expresses pain, the sign is positive, indicating compression and/or inflammation of the supraspinatus and/or long head of the biceps (Fig. 41-4).
2. *Hawkins test:* Shoulder and elbow are flexed to 90° followed by forced internal rotation. If the patient expresses pain (Fig. 41-5), the test is positive, indicating compression and/or inflammation of the supraspinatus and long head of the biceps.
3. *Empty can test:* Shoulder elevation to 45° and internal rotation (thumb facing down). Therapist applies resistance to abduction (downward force) (Fig. 41-6). Positive sign is weakness or pain. This test indicates a tear of the supraspinatus tendon. Repeat the same test at 90°. If pain is only experienced at 90° position, suspect bursitis.
4. *Drop arm test:* Patient's arm is positioned in 90° of abduction. The patient slowly lowers his or her arm to the side. The test is positive if the patient drops the arm to the side, indicating a supraspinatus tear (Fig. 41-7).
5. *Biceps speed's test:* Shoulder flexed to 90°, forearm supinated, and elbow extended. Resistance is applied to flexion (downward force using a long lever arm). Positive sign is pain over bicipital groove (Fig. 41-8).

observing the patient using the involved extremity during activities that are within low range (waist level), mid range (shoulder level), and high range (above shoulder level). The therapist should note any compensating or expressions of pain while performing the activities. Numerous shoulder questionnaires can also be administered to address pain,

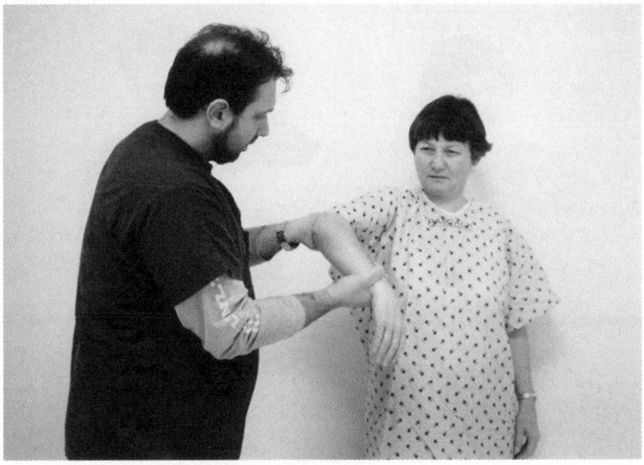

Figure 41-5 Hawkins test.

function, and activity. Examples of these questionnaires include *The Disabilities of the Arm, Shoulder and Hand* (*The DASH*) (Hudak, Amadio, & Bombardier, 1996) and the *Western Ontario Rotator Cuff Index* (Kirkley, Alvarez, & Griffin, 2003).

Evaluation (of the post-surgical patient)

The evaluation for the post-surgical patient will be guided by the surgeon. Request for occupational therapy services can begin as early as 24 hours after surgery. Assessments of pain, PROM, and activity adaptation are the usual orders post-operatively. Depending on the type of repair, AROM can be assessed at 4–6 weeks, and strengthening can be tested at 8 weeks.

Treatment (of the non-surgical patient)

Conservative treatment should begin with educating the patient on activity modification. The patient should be instructed to avoid above shoulder level activities

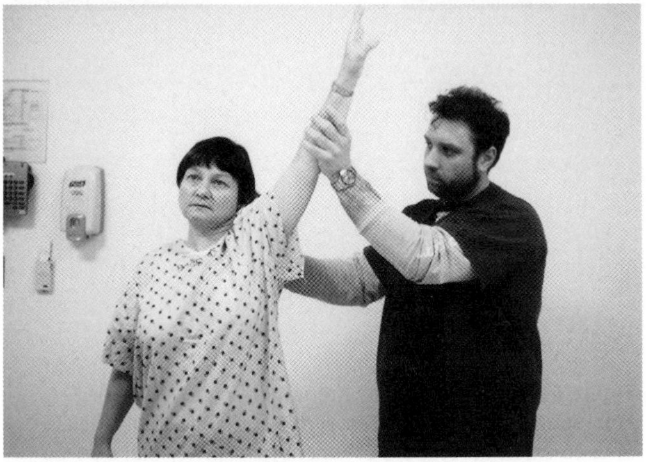

Figure 41-4 Neer Impingement Sign.

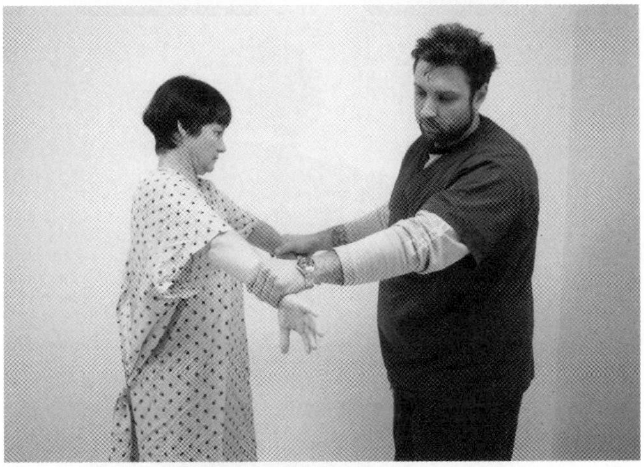

Figure 41-6 Empty can test.

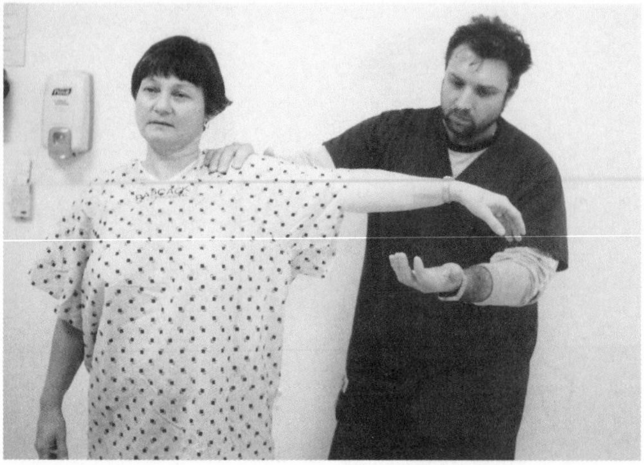

Figure 41-7 Drop arm test.

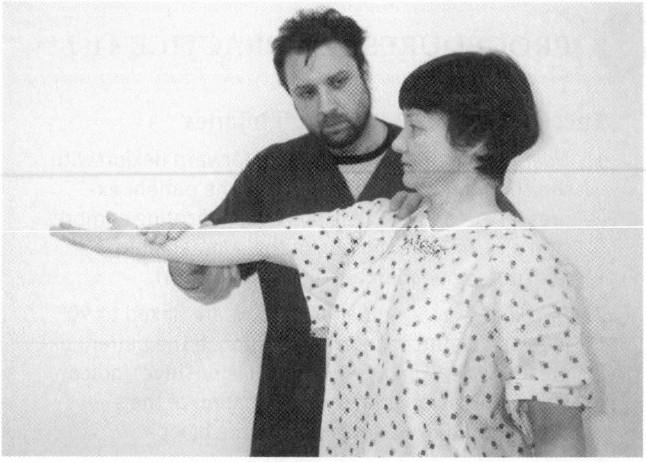

Figure 41-8 Biceps speed's test.

until pain subsides. Sleeping postures should also be addressed. The patient should avoid sleeping with the arm above shoulder level or in an adducted and internally rotated position. Combined adduction and internal rotation for a long period of time can further compromise the blood supply of the supraspinatus tendon. Exercise should focus on pain-free ROM. Begin with PROM. As pain decreases, progress to AROM. Strengthening should include isometric and isotonic exercises for the rotator cuff and scapula musculature. Also improve ROM and strengthen through functional activities such as dressing (Fig. 41-9, A–C). Investigate what

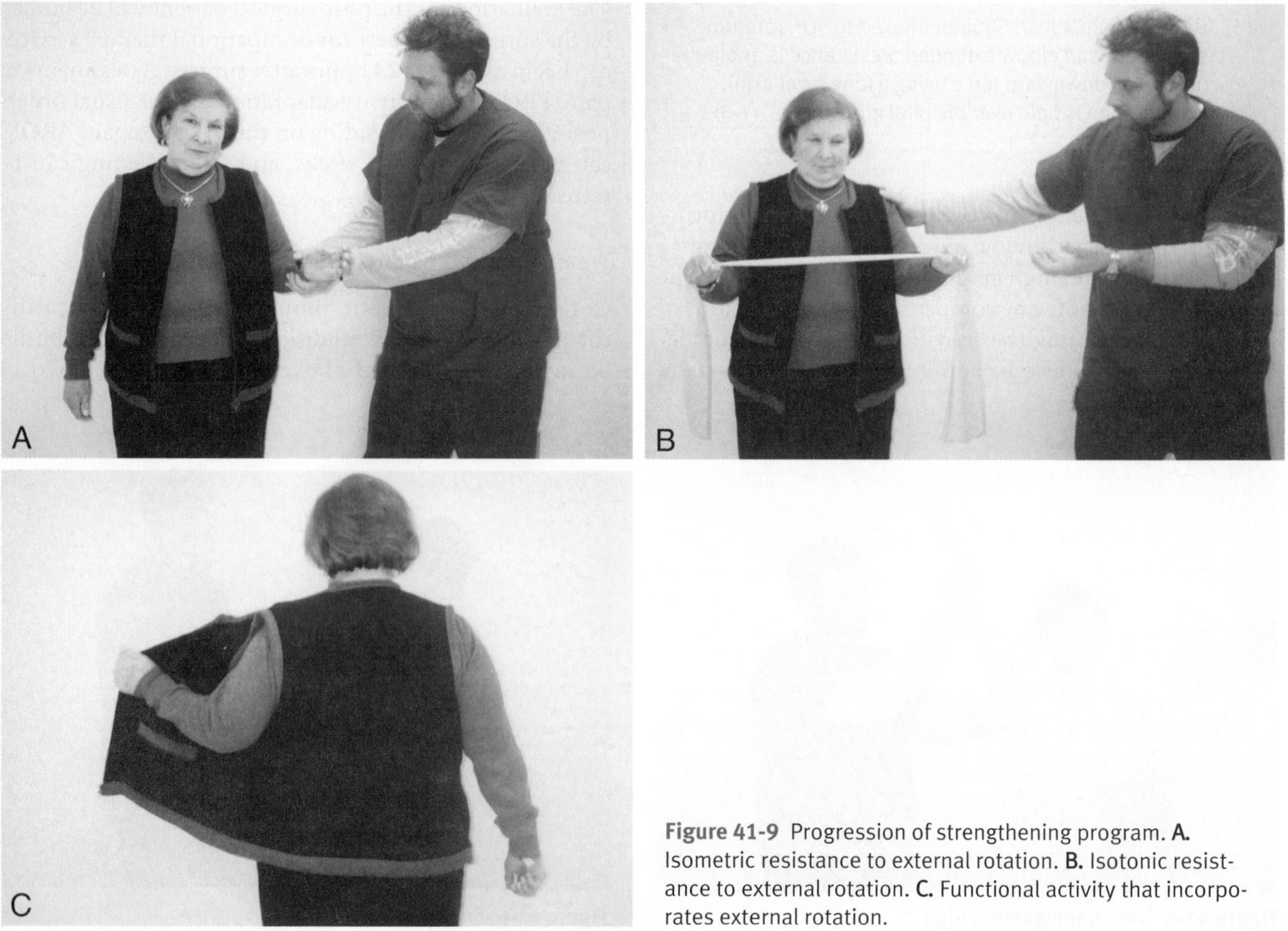

Figure 41-9 Progression of strengthening program. **A.** Isometric resistance to external rotation. **B.** Isotonic resistance to external rotation. **C.** Functional activity that incorporates external rotation.

occupations are most important to the patient and have him or her bring in the necessary equipment such as a golf club or tennis racquet. The long-term goal is to return the patient to unrestricted, pain-free occupational functioning.

Treatment (of the post-surgical patient)

Immediately following rotator cuff repair, the patient will begin with PROM/AAROM for the next 4–6 weeks. The movements emphasized should include pain-free Codman's pendulum exercises, passive shoulder elevation, and internal/external rotation in the adducted or slightly abducted position. An ice pack should be used before, during, and after exercise to decrease pain and swelling. The patient should be instructed to perform these exercises at home using the uninvolved arm to supply the power. Internal and external rotation is performed with the patient supine and the shoulder adducted to the side and elbow flexed to 90°. A cane or stick is held in both hands, while the uninvolved arm supplies the power to move the involved extremity toward the stomach (internal rotation) and away from the stomach (external rotation). Pulleys are only used if requested by the surgeon because repetitive shoulder elevation may irritate the repair. During this time, the patient should be instructed in one-handed techniques to perform activities of daily living. The involved shoulder should not be used for any activity at this time, unless indicated by the surgeon. In between exercise sessions, the shoulder is often protected in a **shoulder immobilizer**. At 4–6 weeks the patient progresses to AROM. Begin in gravity-lessened positions and progress to against-gravity movements. Shoulder extension and internal rotation to the small of the back are added. Encourage the patient to achieve functional ROM. Engage the patient in light activities of daily living. Avoid compensatory movements such as hiking the scapula or lateral bending of the trunk. When performing against-gravity activities of daily living, progress from waist level to above shoulder level activities. Strengthening can be initiated at 6 weeks to prepare the patient for functional activities. Initially the strengthening program begins with isometric exercises for the rotator cuff and scapula stabilization exercises.

Eight weeks after surgery, the patient progresses to isotonic exercises using **Theraband** and free weights. Activities of daily living above shoulder level should be emphasized, including cooking and laundry. At 12 weeks, the patient can begin resistive occupational tasks. Again, the long-term goal is to return the patient to normal pain-free occupational functioning. These treatment protocols are only guidelines. Communication with the surgeon should be ongoing throughout the patient's rehabilitation.

HIP FRACTURES

Intertrochanteric hip fractures are very common in adults over 50 years of age and are more common in women than in men (Altizer, 2005). These fractures occur in bone that is markedly weakened by osteoporosis (Salter, 1999). Many of these patients have comorbidities, including congestive heart failure, coronary artery disease, hypertension, chronic obstructive pulmonary disease, or diabetes, that affect the duration and potential of the rehabilitation program (Altizer, 2005).

Hip fractures are treated with closed reduction and immobilization in plaster or open reduction with internal fixation using pins, nails, screws and plate, or rods (Keenan & Waters, 2003). Partial joint replacement is the treatment for some fractures of the neck and head of the femur. In partial joint replacement, the femoral head and neck are replaced by a prosthesis composed of a metal head and stem. After excision of the femoral head, the stem of the prosthesis is inserted distally into the medullary canal of the femur so that its head articulates with the normal acetabulum. If destructive changes have taken place in both the femur and the acetabulum, a total hip arthroplasty is necessary (Keenan & Walters, 2003).

Occupational Therapy Following a Hip Fracture and Surgery

The restrictions for weight bearing and hip movement on the operated leg are directly related to the severity and location of the fracture, the surgical approach, the ability of the fixation device or prosthesis to withstand stress, the integrity of the bone, the weight of the patient, and the patient's cognitive status (Goldstein, 1999; Smith et al., 2003). The physical therapist teaches the patient to use a walker or crutches, depending on percentage of body weight allowed on the operated limb (Definition 41-2). The occupational therapist teaches the patient to complete ADL safely, corresponding to the medical orders and the physical therapy progression for post-operative weight bearing. For some patients, pre-existing factors or the risk of dislodging the new hip joint may necessitate the assistance of another person for lower extremity dressing and for bathing.

The rate of progression of weight bearing and mobility is individually tailored for the patient by the rate of fracture healing and the patient's response (Goldstein, 1999). Close communication among the rehabilitation team is imperative to provide the patient with the best quality of care and consistency in learning how to function after surgery. Essential to the planned discharge following a hospital stay of less than a week for most is the therapist's

DEFINITION 41-2

Progression of Weight Bearing After Hip Surgery (Goldstein, 1999)

Weight-Bearing Status	Percentage of Body Weight on Operated Limb	Ambulatory Device
Non-weight bearing	0	Walker or crutches
Touchdown weight bearing	10–15	Walker or crutches
Partial weight bearing	30	Walker or crutches
50% weight bearing	50	Cane
Full weight bearing	75–100	Cane or no device

evaluation of the patient's ability to perform basic and instrumental ADL safely and independently and the need for adapted equipment and/or assistance of others (Bargar, Bauer, & Borner, 1998).

It is best to teach the patient who is restricted to non-weight bearing or touchdown weight bearing to sit to perform ADL to conserve energy and increase safety. Once the patient can do partial weight bearing, he or she can safely stand while grooming. For some, this may be as early as the first week, and for others, it may be as late as the third or fourth week (Goldstein, 1999). For at least 6 weeks, and for some patients longer, movement is restricted. As these restrictions preclude bending over or bringing the foot closer to the hands, adaptations (Procedures for Practice 41-2) are required to resolve problems in bathing, dressing, functional mobility, and home management.

The patient must be reminded that the operated hip is not to be flexed actively or passively or the leg adducted beyond the midline (Safety Note 41-1). Long-handled dressing and grooming devices are provided, and the therapist teaches the patient to bathe and dress the operated side using these devices to avoid bending over (flexion) or crossing the operated leg (adduction). For bathing, if permitted, some patients shower standing and require a grab assist bar and non-skid bath mat in the tub area for safety. Others prefer to sit to conserve energy or feel secure, and they require a bath bench. The bath bench must be high enough so the hip does not flex more than 80–90°. These patients also require a non-skid bath mat and grab assist rail. Procedures for Practice 41-3 describes the procedure to get into and out of a bathtub after hip surgery.

To reduce hip flexion during sitting and rising, the patient is instructed to use a raised toilet seat, bed, and chair. Bed and chair heights are raised by putting wooden blocks under the legs. To increase mattress and chair cushion

PROCEDURES FOR PRACTICE 41-2

Adaptations for ADL After Hip Replacement Surgery

Problem	Adaptation
Bathe feet	Long-handled bath sponge
Get in and out of tub	Non-skid bath mat; grab bar; tub bench
Don, doff shoes	Extended-handled shoe horn; elastic laces
Don, doff socks	Sock aide
Don pants	Reacher or dressing stick
Transfer to and from toilet, tub, and bed	Raised toilet seat, increased height of chair and bed
Sit in and rise from a chair	Wedge cushion with thick end of the wedge at the back of the chair
Open and close cabinets	Relocate frequently used items to eliminate the need to bend; use a reacher

SAFETY NOTE 41-1

Movement Restrictions After Hip Surgery

- No hip flexion beyond 90°
- No hip rotation (avoid internal rotation for posterolateral approach and external rotation for anterolateral approach)
- No crossing the operated leg over the unoperated leg
- No adduction of the operated leg

PROCEDURES FOR PRACTICE 41-3

Transferring Into and Out of a Bathtub After Hip Surgery

To Get into the Bathtub

1. Stand with feet parallel to the tub with the operated leg next to the bathtub.
2. Shift body weight to unoperated leg.
3. Hold onto a grab assist rail for support.
4. Position the operated leg into hip extension and knee flexion; then abduct the hip to allow the leg to go over the edge of the bathtub.
5. Extend the knee on the operated side once the leg is over the tub edge.
6. Place the foot on the non-skid bath mat inside the tub.
7. When balance is secure, transfer the body weight to the operated leg.
8. Lift the unoperated leg over the edge of the tub and place the foot on the bath mat.

To Get out of the Bathtub

1. Position self so feet are parallel to the side of the tub and the operated leg leads (goes out of the tub first).
2. Use the same procedure as for getting into the tub.

firmness and prevent passive hip flexion, plywood is inserted between the mattress and box spring or between the chair cushion and its frame. The patient is encouraged to sit in a reclined position enhanced by a wedge cushion or a small rolled pillow or towel at the junction of the chair's seat and back, as originally described by McKee (1975).

The patient who must sit in a regular-height chair is taught to stand up without over flexing the operated hip. In a chair with armrests, the patient scoots to the front edge of the seat, keeping the operated hip extended, and uses the armrests to push straight up without bending the trunk forward. In a chair without armrests, the patient moves to the side of the chair so that the operated thigh is over the edge with the foot placed at the midline of the chair. This places the operated hip in extension, puts the foot close to the center of gravity, and enables the person to gain momentum to stand without excessive hip flexion. With this technique, the unoperated hip, knee, and ankle are in position for weight bearing.

By 6 weeks, almost all patients walk with a cane, and some walk unassisted; most can return to driving a car, swimming, and work (Goldstein, 1999). Physical restrictions against bending to put on shoes or socks, sleeping on the operated side, and using a regular-height toilet seat are often lifted 8–12 weeks after surgery.

CHRONIC CONDITIONS

Some orthopaedic conditions are chronic. One is progressive hip pain from degenerative disease. When that pain interferes with activities and tasks of daily life despite medication, rest, reduction in lower extremity loading by the use of a cane, walker, or crutches, and physical therapy, hip surgery is indicated (Salter, 1999). After hip replacement surgery, therapists teach the patient to move the operated leg within the ordered weight-bearing and movement restrictions. Another chronic condition seen by therapists who practice in orthopaedics is low back pain. Medical costs for low back pain range between $20–50 billion annually (Hu et al., 2003). This section discusses occupational therapy both after hip replacement surgery and to relieve low back pain to enable occupational performance.

Occupational Therapy After Elective Hip Surgery Resulting from Disease

A number of surgical procedures are used for reduction of hip pain. They include osteotomy; arthrodesis, or hip fusion; hip resurfacing; and partial or total hip arthroplasty. To select the procedure, the orthopaedic surgeon considers not only the patient's age and physical status but also his or her occupational requirements and lifestyle.

Osteotomy is a procedure to correct the alignment of the femur to relieve weight bearing on the hip joint. When the osteotomy is done, compression plates stabilize the bone, and the patient can begin early post-operative mobilization with passive movement. Only partial weight bearing on the operated leg using crutches is allowed for 6 months, until the bone is healed. Osteotomies are not the treatment of choice for treating hip pain as a result of arthritis (Namba, Skinner, & Gupta, 2003).

Hip joint arthrodesis fuses the acetabulum with the femoral head at about 25–30° of flexion and in neutral abduction and rotation. Arthrodesis is considered for patients under age 60 years who are in good physical condition and who have only one painful hip. A candidate is a person who is not a candidate for a prosthetic hip implant because of heavy physical demands at work or recreational pursuits that are beyond the tolerances of an implant. This is also considered a salvage procedure for those whose prosthetic hip implant has failed. The patient is mobilized a week after the hip fusion and is allowed gradual weight bearing up to full weight in 2 months. Some patients do use a cane for a long time after surgery. The patient requires long-handled devices to assist with reaching the feet during bathing and dressing because of early post-operative flexion restrictions (Dalseth & Lippincott, 1991). In 6 months, when complete healing is established, the patient may be able to put on a sock and shoe when seated by flexing the knee to the side of the chair and reaching behind, using touch without visual guidance. The arthrodesis does leave the patient with a residual disability, but the hip is strong, stable, and pain free, and the patient has adequate endurance for standing at work and participating in active sports, such as walking, hiking, sailing, and horseback riding (Kostuik, 1991).

A total hip arthroplasty (THA) surgically replaces the entire hip joint destroyed by disease or trauma. The main benefit of hip replacement is to resolve arthritic pain. Joint replacement surgery can also restore the length of the limb and its alignment, which has the potential to improve ROM and function (Drake, Ace, & Maale, 2002). This surgery replaces the arthritic acetabular cup with a metal cup and polyethylene plastic liner. The femoral head is replaced with a femoral head implant and stem component. Other typical joint-bearing surface materials include plastic and ceramic balls and sockets. The surgical approach to perform the THA varies among surgeons. The most common is the posterolateral approach (Youm et al., 2005). With this approach, there is no disruption to the gluteus medius and minimus muscles, and therefore, hip abduction is not compromised. The risk of the posterolateral approach is posterior dislocation. To avoid dislocation, immediately following surgery the patient is placed in an abduction pillow. Some surgeons also opt to place the ipsilateral knee in a knee immobilizer to further decrease the risk of dislocation. The patient is instructed to avoid hip flexion beyond 90°, adduction, and internal rotation. The second most common approach is the anterolateral approach (Youm et al., 2005). Although this approach decreases the risk for posterior dislocation and does not require an abduction pillow, the surgery requires division of the gluteus medius and minimus muscles and could disrupt the superior gluteal nerve, which leads to hip abductor weakness (Bertin & Rottinger, 2004). This weakness can result in a limp. The patient is instructed to avoid flexion beyond 90°, adduction, and external rotation.

Another decision the surgeon must make when performing a THA is what type of implant fixation he or she will use. The choices are cemented, cementless, or hybrid prostheses (Namba, Skinner, & Gupta, 2003). The cemented total replacement usually requires 4–6 weeks of weight bearing to tolerance (WBTT) using a standard or rolling walker, and then the patient progresses to straight cane. The cementless prosthesis, which depends on ingrowth of porous bone for stability, requires 6–12 weeks of partial weight bearing before a cane is used. Some surgeons may initially order non-weight bearing. In the case of the hybrid prosthesis, in which the femoral portion is cemented and the acetabulum is uncemented, 4–6 weeks of partial weight bearing precedes introduction of a cane (Youm et al., 2005).

Pre-operative education should be the first phase of occupational therapy for the patient receiving a THA. Hip precautions, demonstration of long-handled equipment, and medically necessary durable medical equipment should be presented. Pre-operative education has been linked to reducing anxiety (Spalding, 2003). The first 2 months after total hip arthroplasty is critical for protection and function of the new hip joint. The post-surgical program is designed to allow for healing of the trochanter and soft tissues and for development of a capsule around the joint for future stability. ***Until soft tissue is healed, hip flexion beyond 90°, hip adduction, and hip rotation (internal rotation for posterolateral approach and external rotation for anterolateral approach) are avoided.*** The extremes of these movements during the first 2 months can dislocate the prosthesis. If dislocation occurs, the hip must be treated with closed reduction or be surgically realigned. The patient may be placed in a hip spica cast or knee immobilizer, delaying rehabilitation (Best, 2005). To protect the prosthesis, the occupational therapist instructs the patient in adaptive procedures and in methods to modify the environment to allow for safe performance of ADL and homemaking (Definition 41-2). The techniques used to help the patient following a total hip arthroplasty parallel those described earlier under hip fracture surgery: hip flexion and adduction are discouraged, and weight-bearing guidelines are carefully adhered to. Rehabilitation starts as early as the third day after surgery.

For at least 3 weeks and, for some patients, up to 8 weeks after surgery, the operated hip is positioned in extension and abduction. A splint or a foam abduction wedge is used with the patient lying down or sitting to encourage hip abduction. Once the patient achieves 55° of hip flexion in physical therapy, the patient can sit reclined on a raised chair using a rolled pillow or wedge cushion between the seat and the back of the chair and a foam abduction wedge between the legs. The patient learns to transfer from supine to standing without flexing the operated hip beyond 90° by keeping the knees apart (hips abducted) and sliding out of a raised bed to take weight on the unoperated leg. Some patients use an overhead trapeze bar to assist this transfer. The patient also needs to practice transferring from a variety of surfaces such as high chair (Fig. 41-10, A–C), tub bench, raised toilet seat, and a car seat.

The patient with a cemented or hybrid total hip prosthesis usually begins partial weight bearing with a walker or crutches immediately after surgery. In some instances, these patients can withstand full weight bearing within the first 3 days; however, many orthopaedic surgeons wait 3 weeks before ordering full weight bearing (Goldstein, 1999). The ADL program, which can be taught with the patient standing, uses the bathing and lower extremity dressing techniques described for fractures (Procedures for Practice 41-2 and Safety Note 41-1). The patient with a cementless total hip arthroplasty is usually touchdown weight bearing for the initial recovery phase and is conservatively progressed to partial weight bearing (Goldstein, 1999). This necessitates learning ADL from the seated position (Fig. 41-11). Once

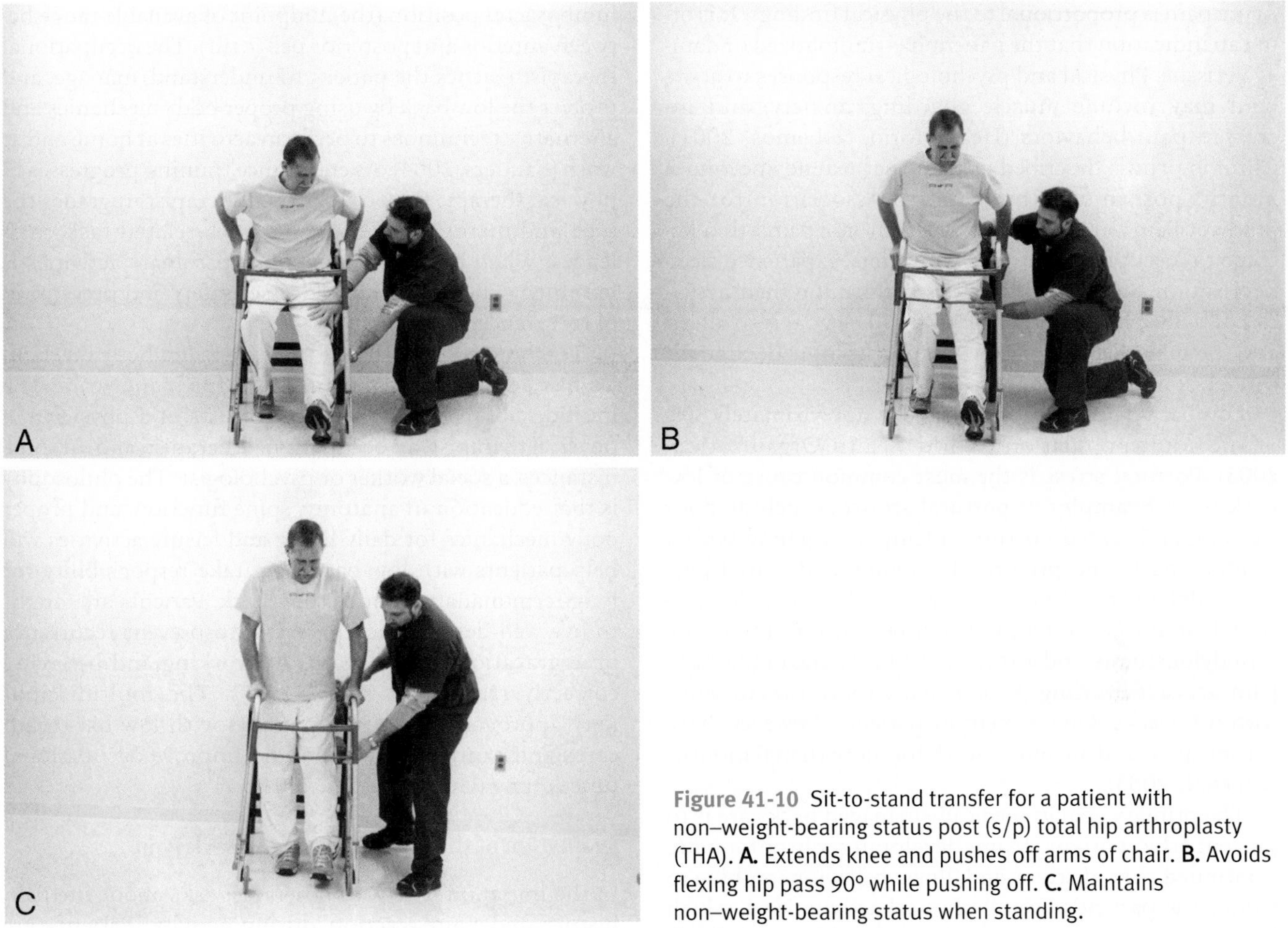

Figure 41-10 Sit-to-stand transfer for a patient with non–weight-bearing status post (s/p) total hip arthroplasty (THA). **A.** Extends knee and pushes off arms of chair. **B.** Avoids flexing hip pass 90° while pushing off. **C.** Maintains non–weight-bearing status when standing.

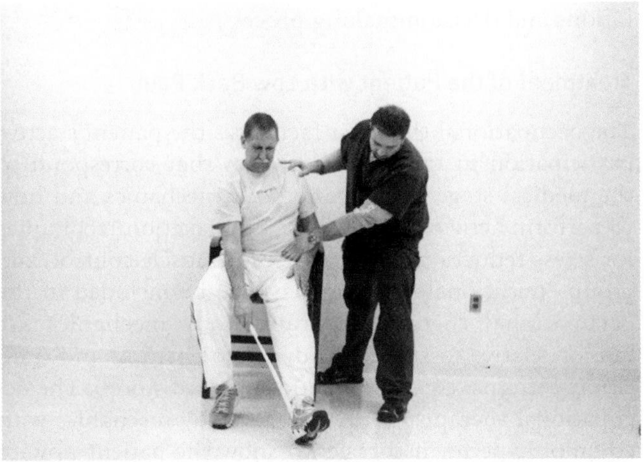

Figure 41-11 Removing shoe status post total hip arthroplasty (THA). Approach medial aspect of shoe with long-handled shoe horn to prevent internal rotation.

50% weight bearing is ordered, the ADL program is upgraded to allow for standing with a cane. The cane is used until the **Trendelenburg gait** disappears.

Usually, after a total hip arthroplasty, patients do not receive outpatient therapy following inpatient rehabilitation, although many may receive home care occupational and physical therapy for safety assessment and/or treatment. Between the second and third month after surgery, patients usually resume all routine daily activities, with the restrictions listed in Safety Note 41-1 still applicable. For some, this restriction may persist for a long time, even for life. Mayo Clinic has recommended the following low-impact sport activities permissible at >12 weeks after surgery: golf, swimming, cycling, bowling, sailing, and scuba diving (Healy, Iorio, & Lemos, 2001). Tennis, skiing, and jogging are discouraged.

Low Back Pain

"Pain is an unpleasant sensory and emotional experience associated with actual or potential tissue damage" (International Association for the Study of Pain, 2004).

Acute pain is proportional to the physical findings. It is often an indication that the patient has traumatized or damaged tissue. Physical and psychological responses to acute pain may include muscle guarding, anxiety, and increased pain behaviors (Healy, Iorio, & Lemos, 2001). Chronic pain is described as pain that extends beyond 3 months post injury (International Association for the Study of Pain, 2004). Patients with chronic pain often become preoccupied with their symptoms, experience sleep deprivation, and have difficulties performing their activities of daily living (Cieza et al., 2004). The goal is to alleviate the pain early to prevent psychological changes (Andersson, 1992).

Low back pain has been reported by approximately 80% of the adult population (World Health Organization, 2003). Postural stress is the most common cause of low back pain. Examples of postural stressors include poor sleeping and seated postures, lifting or reaching with a rounded back, and prolonged standing and seated postures (McKenzie, 2005). Other causes of back pain include spinal stenosis, vertebral fracture, tumor, infection, spondylolisthesis, and arthritis. Most episodes of low back pain are self-limiting; 90% of patients return to work within 6 weeks. One percent of patients, however, have chronic pain and are out of work for more than 6 months (Hu et al., 2003).

The primary goal in medically managed back care is to prevent the patient from developing chronic pain. Continued pain, distress, and illness behavior combine to reduce the patient's overall physical activity level, which leads to disuse syndrome, deconditioning (Waddell, 1992), and occupational dysfunction. If pain is not alleviated, the objective findings over time may have little or no association to a nociceptive stimulus. Chronic pain and disability become increasingly associated with emotional distress, depression, disease conviction (convince self and others that the disease exists), failure to cope, catastrophizing (feelings of total misfortune), and adaptation to chronic invalidism. This situation becomes self-sustaining and is often resistant to traditional medical management alone (Waddell, 1992).

The primary focus when treating patients with acute or chronic low back pain is to return them back to work and to resume their daily activities as quickly as possible. All efforts should be made to prevent the development of chronic pain syndrome by adopting practices used in sports medicine treatment to calm the pain and relax the muscles. Bed rest is replaced with early application of physical therapy, a flexibility program, and active involvement in a graduated program of occupation-as-end. Studies have shown that exercise can significantly reduce sick leave in patients with low back pain (Kool, 2004). As physical therapy helps the patient develop dynamic control of the lumbar spine through flexibility training, stretching, and ROM exercises, the occupational therapist directs the patient in performance of activities in a neutral lumbosacral position (the midpoint of available range between anterior and posterior pelvic tilt). The occupational therapist teaches the patient to understand, manage, and protect the low back by using proper body mechanics and alternative techniques to perform activities at home and at work (Sanders, 2004). As endurance training progresses in physical therapy, the occupational therapist upgrades the type and quantity of ADL and work-related task challenges. When return to usual and customary activities is imminent, the treatment addresses safety and prevention of recurrence.

Teaching patients about their back and body mechanics has been part of rehabilitation for many years. The multidisciplinary team usually consists of a physician, a physical therapist, an occupational therapist, and, in some instances, a social worker or psychologist. The philosophy is that education in anatomy, spine function, and proper body mechanics for daily living and leisure activities will help patients with low back pain take responsibility for long-term management of their back. Patients are taught to live well despite back pain and to prevent recurrence or aggravation of symptoms by working and behaving correctly (Kumar & Konz, 1997). The multidisciplinary approach to treating patients with low back pain can significantly reduce pain and improve occupational functioning (Guzman et al., 2001).

Evaluation of the Patient with Low Back Pain

In the initial interview, the therapist asks about the pain history and pain reaction during activity. Patients are asked to describe their pain in relation to location, intensity (using a 0–10 pain scale), quality (is pain sharp, throbbing, burning, etc.), and duration. Inquiry into occupational function determines the person's extent of accommodation and methods for task completion. Observation of actual or simulated performance of tasks may be indicated to reveal the patient's functional limitations and decision-making process.

Treatment of the Patient with Low Back Pain

The occupational therapist facilitates the patient's active participation in tasks and activities that correspond to the medical stage by teaching body mechanics and how to perform activities safely. Use of relaxation techniques for stress reduction, biofeedback for muscle control, and group educational sessions may also be included in the occupational therapy program. Body mechanics are taught relative to static and dynamic postures and transition patterns (e.g., sit to stand, stand to stoop). The occupational therapist demonstrates body mechanics with commonly performed tasks to show the patient how to apply the principles to everyday tasks. Emphasis is on both cognitive and motor learning to develop the patient's understanding and ability to self-regulate motor activity safely. Therapeutic activity, including

PROCEDURE FOR PRACTICE 41-4

Principles of Body Mechanics (Fig. 41-12, A–C)

The patient is taught to do the following:

- Incorporate a pelvic tilt during static sitting or standing to unload the facet joints, aid in pelvic awareness, and decrease muscular tension in the low back.
- Position the body close to and facing the task. This aids in balance by getting the objects as close to the center of gravity as possible. Objects held away from the body require increased force of all muscles to lift or hold them. Getting closer also helps to avoid twisting or bending the spine.
- Avoid twisting. Twisting causes stress on the ligaments and small muscles of the spine. Instead, turn the body by stepping with both legs to face the activity.
- Use the hip flexors and extensors to lower and raise the body. These are large muscles with leverage and power to handle heavy loads. The joints and muscles of the spine are much smaller, with less leverage and power.
- Avoid prolonged repetitive activity or static positions. Take microbreaks and walk briefly or stretch every hour.
- Balance activity with rest to facilitate endurance and safety. Incorporate rest periods into the course of a particular activity or alternate between two work patterns that challenge different muscle groups.
- Use a wide base of support. Stability while lifting is increased when the feet are at least hip distance apart. One foot slightly in front of the other provides additional support.
- Keep the back in proper alignment, ear over shoulder, shoulder over hips, and hips over knees and feet to maintain the natural curves of the back. Practice in front of a mirror.
- Test a load before lifting to decide whether the lift should be modified. Describe how to modify the lift: get help, split the load into more than one lift, or put the object on wheels.
- Stay physically fit. Strong muscles and flexible joints are the best defense against injury or recurrence of an injury.

games, crafts, ADLs, and work tasks, are selected for practice. Through feedback, the therapist guides the patient's performance during the activities and encourages development of self-regulation.

Body Mechanics

Good body mechanics entails practices to reduce the load or stresses on the spine in various positions or when moving objects. Compression and twisting of the spine are avoided, as are attempts to exert force in positions that poorly support the spine (Procedures for Practice 41-4). Suggestions for application of principles of body mechanics in various postures are as follows:

- While standing, for example to cook or wash dishes in the kitchen or to brush teeth at the bathroom sink, the patient places one foot on the shelf under the sink

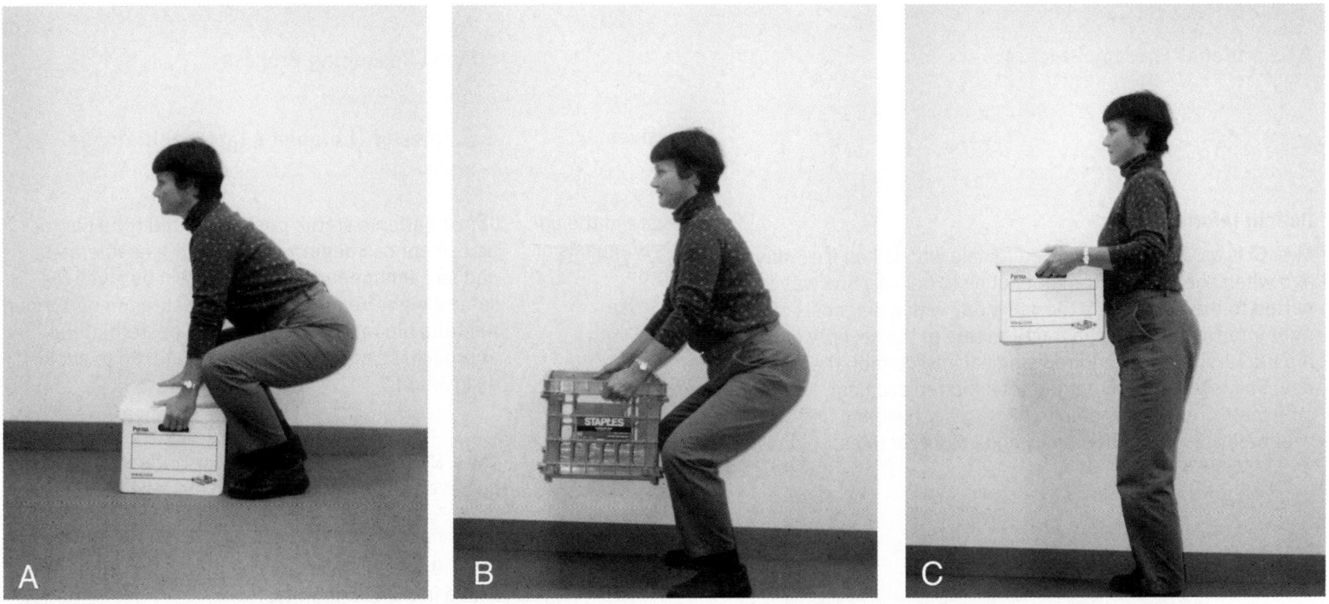

Figure 41-12 Lift using proper body mechanics. **A.** Move close to object being lifted. **B.** Lift with legs and maintain lumbar curve. **C.** Maintain lumbar curve throughout lifting activity.

or on a low stool to achieve posterior pelvic tilt. This technique is used whenever prolonged standing is a requirement.

- To sit, the patient lowers the body by flexing the knees and hips without bending the spine. To do so, the patient places the hands on the chair's armrest, both to guide the descent and to provide support through the transition. A raised seat is recommended because it requires less muscle power, which reduces pain and stress on the back. A slightly reclined sitting posture is preferred for prolonged sitting. When seated to work at a table, the patient avoids bending over the work by moving the chair close to the work and raising or inclining the work surface as needed.
- For tasks that ordinarily require excessive reaching and bending of the spine, such as sweeping, vacuuming, or raking, the patient is taught to move the body close to the task, that is, to walk with the broom or rake rather than reaching with it.
- For lifting objects from the floor, the choice of position depends on the size and weight of the object. To pick up a lightweight object, such as a newspaper, the patient faces the newspaper and lowers both knees in a semisquat (or a ballet position of plié) toward the floor while keeping the back straight and maintaining posterior pelvic tilt. When lifting a large or heavy object or a small child, the patient adds more central support by lowering one knee to the floor (half-kneeling) so that the body is close to and facing the object. The goal is to bring and keep the weighted mass as close to the body's center of gravity as possible. A small child is encouraged to climb up into the lap. Once the object or child is grasped securely, the knee on the floor helps push the body up, and then both legs extend to lift the weight. The patient should be instructed to lift to an intermediate height, such as a chair, if possible, rest briefly, and then lift to carry.
- The patient is taught to carry light, well-balanced loads of laundry, groceries, and parcels close to the body. Infants are best transported in a front or back baby carrier or a stroller. Through practice sessions, the patient learns his or her safe load tolerances over given distances and time. It is important that practice employ common items, such as half a gallon of milk, which weighs 4 pounds, or a gallon of bottled water, which weighs 8 pounds.

CASE EXAMPLE

Mrs. B.: Total Hip Replacement

Occupational Therapy Process	Clinical Reasoning Process	
	Objectives	**Examples of Therapist's Internal Dialogue**
Patient Information Mrs. B. is a 72-year-old married female who fell on ice 3 days ago when she walked from her house to her car. She was admitted to the hospital on the same day with a diagnosis of a right intertrochanteric hip fracture. Due to the severity of the hip fracture, Mrs. B. required surgical intervention the same day. She received a cemented total hip replacement. Mrs. B. anticipates returning home to be with her husband and eventually resuming her family and volunteer roles.	Understand the patient's diagnosis or condition	"Most patients status post cemented total hip replacement can begin weight bearing as tolerated, and so I am hopeful that Mrs. B. will be given the same weight-bearing orders. The surgeon performed the total hip replacement using a posterolateral approach, so precautions must be taken to avoid dislocation."
	Know the person	"Mrs. B. has a history of osteoarthritis in both hips; however, she has been able to manage the pain with Advil." "Mrs. B. obviously values her home life and being active in the community."

Reason for Referral to Occupational Therapy Mrs. B. was referred to occupational therapy (OT) for the duration of her acute-care post-operative hospital stay, approximately 5 days, to learn how to move safely while adhering to hip precautions, to practice transferring, and to begin to resume personal activities of daily living. She was also referred to physical therapy.	Appreciate the context Develop provisional hypotheses	"Mrs. B. will have to follow the hospital's total hip replacement critical pathway, which allows a 5-day stay. I am glad she was referred to physical therapy, as we will be able to coordinate our services as well as co-treat during some of our sessions. I anticipate at the end of her 5 day stay that Mrs. B. will have improved occupational functioning by understanding hip precautions and practicing with long-handled equipment. The co-treatments with physical therapy will help to improve her confidence and ability to transfer."
Assessment Process and Results • The evaluation began with an interview concerning the patient's home environment. Mrs. B. reports that she lives with her husband in a one-story ranch-style home. There are four steps to enter her home. The bathroom has a combined tub and shower. • Bed mobility and transfers were assessed. Mrs. B. required minimal assistance for bed mobility and contact guard (CG) with verbal cues for tub and toilet transfer (using standard walker). • Self-care: Dressing: hip precautions were reviewed and use of long-handled adaptive equipment was demonstrated prior to the assessment. Mrs. B. was independent with upper body dressing but required moderate assistance for lower body dressing. Mrs. B. required constant verbal cueing on hip precautions during dressing assessment. Bathing: Mrs. B. is (I) sponge bathing (bedside) her upper body and requires moderate assistance bathing her lower body (with aide of long-handled sponge). • Upper extremity ROM: AROM is within functional limits (WFLs) throughout both upper extremities. • Manual Muscle Test (MMT): 4/5 muscle strength throughout both upper extremities. • Pain (scale 0–10): Mrs. B. reported a 7/10 for her right hip. Mrs. B. reports her pain is constant and interferes with her sleep and any movements she has been requested to do by nursing.	Consider evaluation approach and methods Interpret observations	"Due to the orthopaedic nature of Mrs. B.'s injuries, a biomechanical approach that focused on her impaired occupational functioning was used to assess her impaired abilities and capabilities." "Pain was reported throughout the entire evaluation, which I was concerned might interfere with her progress. I contacted the patient's surgeon, and pain medications will be increased and administered to coordinate with occupational and physical therapy treatment sessions. ROM and muscle strength of both upper extremities were assessed to determine their ability to assist with transfers. Her major limitations are with her ADLs and mobility activities."
Occupational Therapy Problem List • Pain that interferes with sleep and movement • Impaired ADL status • Unsafe transfers and mobility due total hip replacement (THR) • THR restrictions	Synthesize results	"Mrs. B. has the typical problems one faces following a THR."
Occupational Therapy Goal List 1. Mrs. B. will have a pain level of 3/10 during all self-care activities. 2. Mrs. B. will be able to transfer to and from a chair, bed, tub bench, and toilet while adhering to the hip precautions. 3. Mrs. B. will demonstrate how to use long-handled equipment to independently perform functional tasks in the kitchen, bedroom, and bathroom while adhering to hip precautions.	Develop intervention hypotheses Select an intervention approach Consider what will occur in therapy, how often, and for how long	"I feel Mrs. B. will have improved occupational functioning by learning total hip replacement precautions. The structured daily therapy will also build her confidence for performing mobility and transfer tasks." "The occupational therapy intervention will use a combined compensatory approach and biomechanical approach." "Following the critical pathway, Mrs. B. will have five individualized treatments from occupational during her inpatient stay. An additional 3 co-treatments with physical therapy will be added to address mobility and transfers."

Intervention Mrs. B. participated in 8 treatments over a 5-day inpatient stay. Her pain medication was coordinated with OT visits. Both the occupational therapist and physical therapist taught Mrs. B. postures and movements that would be safe for her operated hip during transfers, sitting, standing, lying in bed, and bending and reaching during ADLs and IADLs. Transfers were performed using a standard walker. She practiced with long-handled equipment while adhering to hip precautions. Tasks or components of tasks that she could not complete satisfactorily were identified. Mr. B. attended all of the OT sessions with his wife, and he agreed to assist his wife with those activities identified as being difficult for Mrs. B. The therapist taught Mrs. B. energy conservation techniques to be used during ADLs and IADLs. Mrs. B. was given a written and illustrated brochure concerning restrictions related to ADL. The therapist determined that Mrs. B.'s husband, with the assistance of a home health aide, could provide the necessary care for ADL and IADL that she could not manage because of hip precautions. Therefore, the recommendation was to discharge her home rather than to a skilled nursing facility.	Assess the patient's comprehension Understand what she is doing Compare actual to expected performance Know the person Appreciate the context	"Mrs. B. made significant improvement in her occupational functioning with intensive therapy that used a team approach and family support."
Next Steps Discharge to home with assistance of home health aide. Recommend home care OT.	Anticipate present and future patient concerns Analyze patient's comprehension Decide if the patient should continue or discontinue therapy and/or return in the future	"Mrs. B. is a highly motivated individual who will benefit from home care occupational therapy to further maximize her occupational functioning. She understands the importance of her home program as well as continuing with structured supervised occupational therapy. I feel confident that, in 6 months, Mrs. B. will be successfully participating in those occupational roles that she identified as valuable in her life (wife, homemaker, and volunteer)."

CLINICAL REASONING IN OCCUPATIONAL THERAPY PRACTICE

Effects of Surgical Approach on ADLs

During her inpatient stay, Mrs. B. required multiple verbal cues to avoid flexing beyond 90°. Mr. B. informed you that he ordered an over-the-toilet commode for when Mrs. B. is discharged home. What adjustments can be made on the commode to ensure she does not flex beyond 90° or dislocate? Would you recommend the same adjustments for Mrs. B. if she had an anterolateral approach?

Evidence Table 41-1
Best Evidence for Occupational Therapy Practice Regarding Pain Management

Intervention	Description of Intervention Tested	Participants	Dosage	Type of Best Evidence and Level of Evidence	Benefit	Statistical Probability and Effect Size of Outcome	Reference
Multidisciplinary Pain Management Program	The program included physical, psychological, activity-based, and social interaction–based training and education. The team consisted of occupational therapist, psychologist, physician, physiotherapist, and social worker. Group-oriented program (8–9 patients per group) but with individually tailored treatment for each patient.	188 patients with pain diagnoses (fibromyalgia, low back, whiplash, and myalgia). Males: 42; females: 146. Mean age = 41 years. Mean pain duration was 7.6 years for females and 5.8 years for males.	5–7 hours each session, once a week for 5 weeks.	One group, repeated-measures design. IIIA2a	Yes. There was significant improvement in occupational performance and performance satisfaction as measured by the *Canadian Occupational Performance Measure* (*COPM*); 30–37% of patients increased 2 or more points on the *COPM*; 44–56% increased more than 1 point in performance and satisfaction.	$p < 0.001$; insufficient data to allow calculation of the effect sizes.	Persson, Rivano-Fischer, & Eklund, 2004

Evidence Table 41-2
Best Evidence for Occupational Therapy Practice Regarding Regarding Hip Fracture

Intervention	Description of Intervention Tested	Participants	Dosage	Type of Best Evidence and Level of Evidence	Benefit	Statistical Probability and Effect Size of Outcome	Reference
Early Post-Operative Individualized Occupational Therapy (OT)	OT group: individual daily ADL and IADL training, including the use of technical aids. Control group (conventional care).	100 eligible patients aged ≥65 years with independent residence. Did not use walking or technical aids prior to hospitalization.	After the 3rd to 4th post-operative day, the OT group received 45–60 minutes of individualized training (including technical aids) each weekday morning for 3–33 days. The control group received conventional care from the nursing staff for 3–23 days. All patients received instruction in walking with mobility aids.	Randomized controlled trial. IB1b	Yes. OT sped up the ability of patients to perform ADL, enhancing probability of discharge home. At discharge, the OT group had significantly better ability to dress, to take care of personal hygiene, to toilet, and to bathe independently compared with the control group. No other factors (e.g., age, sex, type of fracture, etc.) explained the outcome. After 2 months, all patients had regained their ADL and IADL abilities.	*Klein-Bell ADL Scale* subtests: Dressing: $F_{(2,91)} = 79$, $p = 0.0001$, $r = 0.31$. Toileting: $F_{(2,90)} = 5.97$, $p = 0.02$, $r = 0.20$. Bathing/hygiene: $F_{(2,91)} = 17$, $p = 0.0001$, $r = 0.31$. Mobility: $F_{(2,91)} = 2.20$, $p = 0.1$, $r = 0.13$. 52% of the OT group (only group evaluated) needed technical aids and adaptation of their homes. Preventative changes (remove loose rugs, etc.) were needed in 90% of the homes.	Hagsten, Svensson, & Gardulf, 2004

SUMMARY REVIEW QUESTIONS

1. What are the unwanted side effects of immobilization of any fracture?
2. How would you direct your patient to prevent adverse side effects of prolonged immobilization?
3. What is a major treatment goal for any patient with an upper extremity fracture?
4. Why is passive motion not used in the treatment of fractures of the elbow?
5. What are the guiding principles for advancing a patient in the aftercare therapy program following orthopaedic surgery?
6. What is clinical union, and why is it significant in terms of the therapy program?
7. Why are isometric contractions across the fracture site encouraged?
8. Describe the type of exercise performed at 6, 8, and 12 weeks post-op rotator cuff repair.
9. What is the occupational therapist's role for the patient who underwent hip replacement surgery after a fractured hip?
10. After a hip fracture or total hip joint arthroplasty, the therapist directs the patient to perform occupational performance tasks safely. What specific tasks may threaten the integrity of the surgical procedure? Why?
11. List precautions that must be taught to a patient with a total hip arthroplasty (posterolateral and anterolateral approaches).
12. Describe how lower extremity dressing should be taught to a patient with low back pain, using all applicable body mechanic principles. Do the same for the tasks of sweeping the floor and working at a computer.

References

Altizer, L. (2005). Hip fractures. *Orthopaedic Nursing, 24,* 283–292.

Andersson, G. B. F. (1992). Concept and development of back schools. In M. V. Jayson (Ed.), *The lumbar spine and back pain* (4th ed., pp. 409–415). New York: Churchill Livingstone.

Apley, A. G., & Solomon, L. (1994). *Concise system of orthopaedics and fractures* (2nd ed.). London: Butterworth Heinemann.

Bargar, W. L., Bauer, A., & Borner, M. (1998). Primary and revision total hip replacement using the Robodoc system. *Clinical Orthopaedics and Related Research, 354,* 82–91.

Basti, J. J., Dionysian, E., Sherman, P. W., & Bigliani, L. U. (1994). Management of proximal humeral fractures. *Journal of Hand Therapy, 7,* 111–121.

Bednar, M. S., & Light, T. R. (2003). Hand surgery. In H. B. Skinner (Ed.), *Current diagnosis and treatment in orthopedics* (3rd ed., pp. 559–558). New York: Lange Medical Books/McGraw-Hill.

Bertin, K. C., & Rottinger, H. (2004). Anterolateral mini-incision replacement surgery: A modified Watson-Jones approach. *Clinical Orthopedic Related Research, 429,* 248–255.

Best, J. T. (2005). Revision total hip and total knee arthroplasty. *Orthopaedic Nursing, 24,* 174–179.

Brotzman, S. B., & Wilk, K. E. (2003). Clinical orthopaedic rehabilitation (2nd ed.) Philadelphia: Mosby.

Cieza A., Stucki, G., Weigl, M., Kullmann, L., Stoll, T., Kamen, L., Kostanjsek, N., & Walsh, N. (2004). ICF core sets for chronic widespread pain. *Journal of Rehabilitation Medicine, 44,* 63–68.

Dalseth, T., & Lippincott, C. (1991). Postoperative rehabilitation. In H. C. Amstutz (Ed.), *Hip arthroplasty* (pp. 379–390). New York: Churchill Livingstone.

Davila, S. A. (2002). Therapist's management of fractures and dislocations of the elbow. In E. J. Mackin, A. D. Callahan, T. M. Skirven, L. H. Schneider, A. L. Osterman, & J. M. Hunter (Eds.), *Rehabilitation of the hand and upper extremity* (5th ed., pp. 1230–1244). St. Louis: Mosby.

Drake, C., Ace, M., & Maale, G. E. (2002). Revision total hip arthroplasty. *AORN Journal, 76,* 414–428.

Goldstein, T. S. (1999). *Geriatric orthopaedics: Rehabilitative management of common problems* (2nd ed.). Gaithersburg, MD: Aspen.

Greene, D. P., & Roberts, S.L. (2005). *Kinesiology: Movement in the context of activity* (2nd ed.). St. Louis: Elsevier Mosby.

Guzman, J., Esmail, R., Karjalainen, K., Malmivaara, A., Irvin, E., & Bombardier, C. (2001). Multidisciplinary rehabilitation for chronic low back pain: Systematic review. *Journal of British Medicine, 322,* 1511–1516.

Hagsten, B., Svensson, O., & Gardulf, A. (2004). Early individualized postoperative occupational therapy training in 100 patients improves ADL after hip fracture: A randomized trial. *Acta orthopedica Scandinavica, 75* (2), 177–183.

Healy, W. L., Iorio, R., & Lemos, M. (2001). Athletic activity after joint replacement. *American Journal of Sports Medicine, 29,* 377–388.

Hu, S. S., Tribu, C. B., Tay, B. K., & Carlson, G. D. (2003). Disorders, diseases, and injuries of the spine. In H. B. Skinner (Ed.), *Current diagnosis and treatment in orthopedics* (3rd ed., pp. 228–231). New York: Lange Medical Books/McGraw-Hill.

Hudak, P. L., Amadio, P. C., & Bombardier C. (1996). Development of an upper extremity outcome measure: The DASH (disabilities of the arm shoulder and hand). *American Journal of Industrial Medicine, 29,* 602–608.

International Association for the Study of Pain [IASP]. (2004). IASP pain terminology. Retrieved January 12, 2005 from http://www.iasp-pain.org/terms-p.html.

Keenan, M. E., & Waters, R. L. (2003). Rehabilitation. In H. B. Skinner (Ed.), *Current diagnosis and treatment in orthopedics* (3rd ed., pp. 691–69). New York: Lange Medical Books/McGraw-Hill.

Kelley, M. J., & Clark, W. A. (1995). *Orthopedic therapy of the shoulder.* Philadelphia: Lippincott.

Kirkley A., Alvarez, C., & Griffin, S. (2003). The development and evaluation of a disease-specific quality-of-life questionnaire for disorders of the rotator cuff: The Western Ontario Rotator Cuff Index. *Clinical Journal of Sports Medicine, 13,* 84–92.

Kool, J., Bie, R. D., Oesch, P., Knusel, O., Brandt, P. V. D., & Bachmann, S. (2004) Exercise reduces sick leave in patients with non-acute non-specific low back pain: A meta analysis. *Journal of Rehabilitation Medicine,* 36, 49–62.

Kostuik, J. P. (1991). Arthrodesis of the hip. In H. C. Amstutz (Ed.), *Hip arthroplasty* (pp. 929–940). New York: Churchill Livingstone.

Krop, P. N. (2002). Fractures: General principles of surgical management. In E. J. Mackin, A. D. Callahan, T. M. Skirven, L. H. Schneider, A. L. Osterman, & J. M. Hunter (Eds.), *Rehabilitation of the hand and upper extremity* (5th ed., pp. 377–378). St. Louis: Mosby.

Kumar, S., & Konz, S. (1997). Workplace adaptation for the low back region. In M. Nordin, G. J. Andersson, & M. H. Pope (Eds.), *Musculoskeletal disorders in the workplace* (pp. 316–328). St. Louis: Mosby.

Mackin, E. J., Callahan, A. D., Skierven, T. M., Schneider, L. H., Osterman, A. L., & Hunter, J. M. (Eds.), *Rehabilitation of the hand and upper extremity* (5th ed.). St Louis: Mosby.

Malone, T. R., Richmond, G. W., & Frick, J. L. (1995). Shoulder pathology. In M. J. Kelley & W. A. Clark (Eds.), *Orthopedic therapy of the shoulder* (pp. 104–119). Philadelphia: J.B. Lippincott Company.

McKee, J. I. (1975). Foam wedges aid sitting posture of patients with total hip replacement. *Physical Therapy, 55,* 767.

McKenkie, R. (2005). *Treat your own back* (7th ed.). New Zealand: Spinal Publication.

Namba, R. S., Skinner, H. B., & Gupta, R. (2003). Adult reconstructive surgery. In H. B. Skinner (Ed.), *Current diagnosis and treatment in orthopedics* (3rd ed., pp. 388–390). New York: Lange Medical Books/McGraw-Hill.

Neer, C. S., II (1990). *Shoulder reconstruction.* Philadelphia: Saunders.

Persson, E., Rivano-Fischer, M., & Eklund, M. (2004). Evaluation of changes in occupational performance among patients in a pain management program. *Journal of Rehabilitation Medicine, 36,* 85–91.

Post, M., Silver, R., & Singh, M. (1983). Rotator cuff tear: Diagnosis and treatment. *Clinical Orthopedic, 173,* 78.

Salter, R. B. (1999). *Textbook of disorders and injuries of the musculoskeletal system* (3rd ed.). Baltimore: Williams & Wilkins.

Sanders, M. J. (2004). Ergonomics of child care. In M. J. Sanders (Ed.), *Ergonomics and the management of musculoskeletal disorders* (2nd ed., pp. 410–417). St. Louis: Butterworth & Heinemann.

Sarmiento, A. (2000). Functional bracing for the treatment of fractures of the humerus diaphysis. *American Journal of Bone and Joint Surgery, 82,* 478.

Smith, W. R., Shank, J. R., Skinner, H. B., Diao, E., & Lowenberg, D. W. (2003). Musculoskeletal trauma. In H. B. Skinner (Ed.), *Current diagnosis and treatment in orthopedics* (3rd ed., pp. 76–154). New York: Lange Medical Books/McGraw-Hill.

Spalding, N. J. (2003). Reducing anxiety by pre-operative education: Make the future familiar. *Occupational Therapy International, 11,* 278–293.

Tan, V., Leggin, B. G., & Williams, G. R. (2002). Surgical and postoperative management of the rheumatoid shoulder. In E. J. Mackin, A. D. Callahan, T. M. Skirven, L. H. Schneider, A. L. Osterman, & J. M. Hunter (Eds.), *Rehabilitation of the hand and upper extremity* (5th ed., pp. 1608–1623). St. Louis: Mosby

Toyoda, H., Ito, Y., Tomo, H., Nakao, Y., Koike, T., & Takaoka, K. (2005). Evaluation of rotator cuff tears with magnetic resonance arthrography. *Clinical Orthopaedics and Related Research, 439,* 109–115.

Waddell, G. (1992). Understanding the patient with a backache. In M. V. Jayson (Ed.), *The lumbar spine and back pain* (4th ed., pp. 469–485). New York: Churchill Livingstone.

World Health Organization. (2003). WHO Technical Report Series. The burden of musculoskeletal conditions at the start of the new millennium. Geneva: World Health Organization.

Youm, T., Mauer, S. G., & Stuchin, S. A. (2005). Postoperative management after total hip and knee arthroplasty. *The Journal of Arthroplasty, 20,* 322–324.

Supplemental References

Brophy, R. H., Beauvais, R. L., Jones, E. C., Cordasco, F. A., & Marx, R. G. (2005). Measurement of shoulder activity level. *Clinical Orthopaedics and Related Research, 439,* 101–108.

Cameron, H., & Brotzman, B. (2003).The arthritic lower extremity. In S. B. Brotzman & K. E. Wilk (Eds.), *Clinical orthopaedic rehabilitation* (2nd ed., pp. 441–457). Philadelphia: Mosby.

LEARNING OBJECTIVES

After studying this chapter, the reader will be able to do the following:

1. State principles and general precautions of hand therapy evaluation and intervention.
2. Select splint positions that minimize, prevent, or correct hand deformity.
3. Describe clinical features of common hand impairments.
4. Recognize and foster favorable tissue responses to hand therapy interventions.
5. Promote pain-free occupational functioning of persons with hand impairment.

CHAPTER 42

Hand Impairments

Cynthia Cooper

Glossary

Anti-deformity position, intrinsic-plus position—Position of digital MP flexion and IP extension that maintains the length of the collateral ligaments and volar plate.

Buddy straps—Straps between an injured and an adjacent digit to protect or to promote movement.

Carpal tunnel syndrome—Nerve entrapment involving compression of the median nerve at the wrist causing sensory symptoms typically involving the thumb, index, and long finger and radial half of the ring finger.

Cervical screening—Proximal screening assessment of neck and shoulder to identify causes of or contributors to distal symptoms.

Claw deformity—Position of MP hyperextension and PIP flexion associated with muscle imbalance in ulnar-innervated structures.

Complex regional pain syndrome (CRPS)—Previously called reflex sympathetic dystrophy. CRPS is characterized by pain that is disproportionate to the injury, along with swelling, stiffness, and discoloration. Sudomotor (sweating) changes are often seen.

Contracture—Lack of passive motion due to tissue shortening.

Counterforce strap—Support or strap used over flexor or extensor muscle wads to support muscles and prevent maximum muscle contraction, decreasing load on the tendon. Often used to reduce symptoms of lateral or medial epicondylitis.

Cubital tunnel syndrome—Nerve entrapment involving compression of the ulnar nerve at the elbow between the medial epicondyle and olecranon. Sensory symptoms affect the small finger and ulnar half of the ring finger. Motor symptoms affect the FCU, FDP of the ring and small fingers, AP, and interossei.

de Quervain's disease—Tenosynovitis involving the abductor pollicis longus and EPB tendons at the first dorsal compartment.

Extensor lag—Inability to extend a joint actively while passively being able to.

Hard end feel—Unyielding quality of joint motion at end range passively. Indicates an established joint restriction.

Kirschner wires—Fixation devices used alone or in conjunction with other forms of fixation to treat unstable fractures of the hand.

Neuroma—Disorganized mass of nerve fibers that can occur following nerve injury. Significant nerve pain with associated hypersensitivity is elicited by tapping over the neuroma.

Oscillations—Rhythmic movements that may be helpful to reduce guarding and pain.

Place-and-hold exercises—Passive motion used gently to achieve a position, with the patient then actively sustaining or holding that position.

Soft end feel—Spongy quality of joint motion at end range passively. Indicates favorable potential for tissue remodeling.

Tenolysis—Surgical procedure to release tendon adhesions that restrict movement.

Hand problems, which may be cosmetic or functional or both, are hard to hide. Hands function exquisitely to gesture and express, touch and care, dress and feed (Tubiana, Thomine, & Mackin, 1996). Impairment can be devastating. The purposes of this chapter are to introduce readers to the elements of hand therapy, to highlight the breadth of material that hand therapy encompasses, and to identify resources for further study.

The complex arrangement of the hand, with its intimate anatomy and multiarticulate structures, is unforgiving of stiffness, scar, or edema. Injury at one site can lead to stiffness of other parts of the hand. To test this for yourself, passively hold your ring finger in extension and then try to make a fist. This example, called the quadregia effect, demonstrates the interconnectedness of digits, whereby limited movement of one digit may cause restricted motion in uninjured digits (Burkhalter, 1995). For this and other reasons, hand therapists must look at more than the isolated site of injury and must continually reexamine the patient's performance in the areas of occupation.

Hand therapy originated during World War II. Devastating upper extremity injuries of that era and of subsequent wars prompted a team approach to medical care (Hunter, 1986). Today, members of the rehabilitation team in hand therapy can include physicians and physician assistants, nurses, occupational therapists and occupational therapy assistants, physical therapists and physical therapy assistants, and aides or technicians. Workers' compensation representatives or case managers representing payers may also be involved.

Certified hand therapists are occupational therapists or physical therapists with advanced clinical skills who have passed the examination for certification in hand therapy. A minimum of 5 years of clinical experience and other criteria are prerequisites to taking the examination. It is advisable to establish a strong generalist background in occupational therapy before specializing in hand therapy.

RESOURCE 42-1

Brochures
American Society for Surgery of the Hand; phone: (303) 771-9236.

Consumer Guides and Books
Arthritis Foundation; phone: (800) 283-7800; www.arthritis.org

- *Arthritis of the Basilar Joint of the Thumb*
- *Carpal Tunnel Syndrome*
- *Dupuytren's Disease*
- *Trigger Finger/Trigger Thumb*
- *Osteoarthritis*
- *Carpal Tunnel Syndrome*
- *Using Your Joints Wisely*

American Occupational Therapy Association (AOTA) phone: (301) 652-2682; http://www.aota.org

- Dellon, A. L. (1997). *Somatosensory testing and rehabilitation.* Bethesda, MD: AOTA.
- Lee, K., & Marcus, S. (1990). *Home rehabilitation exercises: Hand.* Rockville, MD: AOTA.
- Melvin, J. L. (1995). *Rheumatoid arthritis: Caring for your hands.* Bethesda, MD: AOTA.

Minnesota Hand Rehabilitation, Inc.;
phone: (612) 646-4263

- Reiner, M. (2004). *The illustrated hand.* St. Paul: Minnesota Hand Rehabilitation.

CD ROM
Primal Pictures Ltd.; phone: +44-171-494-4300

McGroutier, D. A., & Colditz, J. (1998). *Interactive hand therapy.* London: Primal Pictures.

Tests
Physiopro, 805 rue Longpre, Sherbrooke, Quebec, Canada J1G 5B8
TEMPA.

Hand therapy differs from other occupational therapy specializations, such as pediatrics or gerontology, because it merges occupational therapy and physical therapy, and it has its own professional organizations. Although most hand therapists are occupational therapists, actual clinical practice may often look more like physical therapy than occupational therapy. Occupational therapy hand therapists should embrace an occupational therapy identity by grounding intervention in core concepts of our profession. To this end, hand therapists should not become so focused on specific anatomical structures that they overlook the person attached to the hand. They should treat the hand and should also address performance skills and performance patterns of the occupational human whose hand it is.

PSYCHOSOCIAL FACTORS AFFECTING THERAPEUTIC OUTCOMES

Why do some people with minor hand injuries wind up with large disabilities and others with devastating injuries have only small disabilities? Adaptive responses to hand impairment are influenced by body image as well as individual functional needs and contextual elements. The personal or symbolic meaning of the hand, self-esteem, family and friend support systems, and coping strategies all influence outcome (Grunert et al., 1991). Whenever possible, encourage patients to participate in their care. Introduce yourself, maintain eye contact, listen well, use non-medical terminology and instructional diagrams, and encourage some amiable conversation as appropriate (Moskowitz, 1996). It can be helpful to touch patients' hands supportively and to make positive remarks (see Chapter 15).

Motivation is the most important variable favorably influencing recovery (Chin et al., 1999). Realistic expectations and appropriate communication that emphasizes education are also important (Bryan & Kohnke, 1997; Moskowitz, 1996). Psychological symptoms related to hand trauma resolve best when intervention occurs early (Grunert et al., 1991).

HAND THERAPY CONCEPTS

The following concepts are keys to clinical reasoning for all diagnoses of hand impairment. Intervention should not be determined by diagnosis per se. Rather, hand therapy relies on an understanding of anatomy and physiology, wound healing, biomechanics, tissue tolerances, psychosocial issues, and probable outcomes. Given the infinite variations among people, no two intervention plans should be the same.

Tissue Healing

Tissue heals in phases as follows: inflammation, fibroplasia, and maturation or remodeling. The inflammation phase lasts several days. It includes vasoconstriction followed by vasodilation, with white blood cell migration to promote phagocytic removal of foreign bodies and dead tissue. Depending on the diagnosis, immobilization to provide rest is often advised during the inflammation phase (Smith & Price, 2002).

The fibroplasia phase starts at approximately day 4 and continues for 2–6 weeks. In this phase, fibroblasts synthesize scar tissue. The wound's tensile strength increases gradually with the increase in collagen fibers. At this time, active range of motion (AROM) and splints may be appropriate to protect healing tissues and promote balance in the hand (Fess & McCollum, 1998).

The maturation, or remodeling, phase may last for years, but tissue is usually more responsive early rather than late in this period. The remodeling phase reflects the changing architecture and improved organization of collagen fibers, and the associated increased tensile strength. Gentle resistive activity may be appropriate during maturation, but it may also generate inflammatory responses, which should be avoided. Gentle application of corrective dynamic or static splinting may also be appropriate (Fess, 1993). Tolerance of tissues to controlled stress requires monitoring throughout all phases of intervention.

As tissue continues to heal, the wound contracts, and the scar shrinks. Collagen continues to remodel, as it is constantly doing in uninjured tissue (Smith & Price, 2002).

Anti-Deformity Positioning

Upper extremity injury and disuse are associated with predictable deforming hand positions. Edema, which typically accompanies injury, creates tension on extrinsic extensor structures. This leads to a zigzag collapse with a resulting deformity position of flexed wrist, hyperextended metaphalangeals (MPs), flexed proximal interphalangeals (PIPs) and distal interphalangeals (DIPs), and adducted thumb (Pettengill, 2002).

Hand joints are anatomically destined to stiffen in predictable positions. Specifically, the MP joint is prone to stiffen in extension. This is because the protruding or cam shape of the metacarpal head causes the collateral ligament to be slack in MP extension and taut in MP flexion. Conversely, the interphalangeal (IP) joints are prone to become stiff in flexion because the volar plate folds on itself (Tubiana, Thomine, & Mackin, 1996).

When prolonged or constant immobilization is necessary and range of motion (ROM) is at risk, it is usually best to splint the patient's hand in the **anti-deformity position**, also called the intrinsic-plus position (Fig. 42-1). This position places the wrist in neutral or extension, the MPs in flexion, the IPs in extension, and the thumb in abduction and opposition. The anti-deformity position allows the collateral ligaments at the MP joints and the volar plate at the IP joints to maintain their length, which counteracts the forces that promote zigzag collapse. Certain diagnoses, such as flexor or extensor tendon repair, are not compatible with anti-deformity positioning. The physician can assist in this determination.

RESEARCH NOTE 42-1

Zhao, C., Amadio, P. C., Tanaka, T., Yang, C., Ettema, A. M., Zobitz, M. E., & An, K. N. (2005). Short-term assessment of optimal timing for postoperative rehabilitation after flexor digitorum profundus tendon repair in a canine model. *Journal of Hand Therapy, 18,* 322–329.

Abstract

The purpose of this study was to compare the short-term outcome following flexor tendon repair for postoperative rehabilitation commencing on day 1 (a common clinical choice) versus day 5 (the day on which, with postoperative immobilization, the initial gliding resistance is least in this model) in an in vivo canine model. Work of flexion (WOF) and tendon strength were evaluated following tendon laceration and repair in 24 dogs sacrificed 10 days postoperatively. Starting postoperative mobilization at day 5 resulted in no tendon ruptures compared with tendon ruptures in four of the dogs (33%) in the group subjected to mobilization starting at day 1. Although no statistically significant difference was found in WOF between groups at day 10, there was a trend toward lower resistance favoring the day 5 start group, and the statistical power to detect a difference in WOF was diminished by the ruptures in the day 1 group. We conclude that starting rehabilitation on day 5, when initial gliding resistance is lower, may have an advantage over earlier starting times, when surgical edema and other factors increase the initial force requirements to initiate tendon gliding. We plan further studies to evaluate the longer-term benefits of this rehabilitation program.

Implications for Practice

- Initial gliding resistance is lower on post-operative day 5 than on post-operative day 1 due to the effects of surgical edema and other factors.
- This study validates previous studies and confirms that post-operative mobilization of flexor tendons is safer to initiate on day 5 instead of day 1.

The Myth of No Pain, No Gain

Regarding tissue tolerances, the myth of no pain, no gain must be dispelled in hand therapy. A better mindset would be no pain, more gain. Well-intentioned therapists and overzealous family members of patients have too often caused irreversible damage by applying passive range-of-motion (PROM) forces beyond the tissues' tolerances (Fess, 1993). Pain induced by therapy can also cause

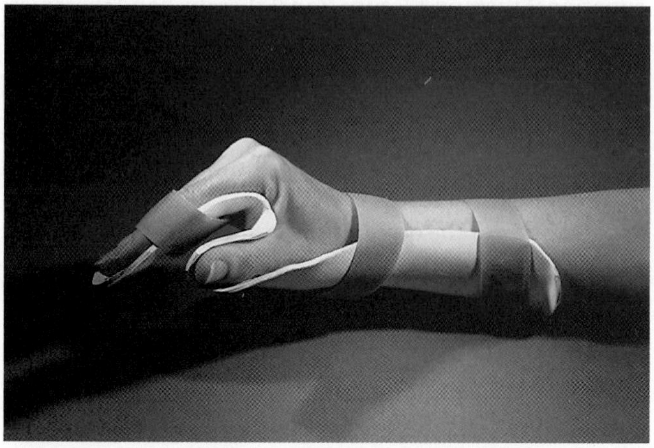

Figure 42-1 Anti-deformity or intrinsic-plus position: Wrist in neutral or extension; MPs in flexion; IPs in extension; and thumb in abduction and opposition.

complex regional pain syndrome (CRPS), which is discussed later.

People with upper extremity problems often arrive at therapy prepared for painful intervention. Some patients do not tell the therapist when intervention hurts. It is essential to educate patients about this. In addition, watch the patient's body language and face for signs of pain. Wincing and withdrawing the upper extremity are obvious signals. Proximal guarding is another revealing response. Change the intervention accordingly, and if necessary, try a hands-off approach wherein the therapist coaches and instructs while the patient self-treats.

Passive Range of Motion Can Be Injurious

PROM can be injurious to the delicate tissues of the hand. Specifically, PROM can disturb healing tissues and incite further inflammatory reactions, resulting in increased scar production. PROM can damage articular structures and can even trigger CRPS (Fess, 1993). Tissue's timeline for remodeling is maximized by non-inflaming intervention and is cut short by intervention that is inflaming or provoking. For all of these reasons, if PROM is clinically appropriate, be sure it is done gently and in a pain-free manner. The potential for harm may be compounded if PROM is performed following external application of heat. Instead, low-load, long-duration splinting is a safer and more effective method for remodeling tissue and increasing PROM (Fess & McCollum, 1998).

Judicious Use of Heat

External application of heat, such as a hot pack, is a popular way to prepare tissues for stretching. Unfortunately, the clinical concerns of externally applied heat have received less attention than they deserve. Heat increases edema, which acts like glue. Heat may degrade collagen and contribute to microscopic tears (Miles, Burjanadze, & Bailey, 1995). Heat may also incur a rebound effect, with stiffening following its use. ***Do not use heat on patients who have edema or whose limb appears inflamed.*** Overall, it is safer to use aerobic exercise to warm up the tissues of people with hand impairments. If external application of heat is used, elevate the upper extremity, be gentle with exercise, and promote active movement in conjunction with the heat. Continue to monitor for immediate and subsequent signs of inflammation.

Isolated Exercise, Purposeful Activity, and Therapeutic Occupation

Technically, it is necessary to treat hand impairments with a structure-specific approach to isolate and care for the discrete components that are involved. It may seem easiest to accomplish this type of exacting intervention in the form of isolated exercise. Traditional valuing of the appearance of highly technical clinical environments, medical model indoctrination, busy schedules, and financial or material constraints may contribute to the perpetuation of hand therapy identifying itself within an environment that looks like an exercise gymnasium. Although some hand therapists do incorporate purposeful activity into intervention, more support is needed for an alternative approach to hand therapy that leads with concepts of therapeutic occupation (Cooper & Evarts, 1998). One way to achieve this is to integrate patient-directed goals and activities of daily living (ADLs) into hand therapy intervention planning and implementation. Whenever possible, encourage upper extremity use in ordinary daily activities as appropriate to the diagnosis. Explore the capabilities in the clinic and then teach patients to do so at home. For example, folding socks and underwear can be upgraded to folding heavy towels and jeans, which require greater strength and endurance.

Occupation elicits adaptive responses that do not occur with exercise alone. Compared to isolated exercise, purposeful activity or occupation promotes more coordination and better movement quality (Nelson & Peterson, 1989). An example of isolated hand therapy exercise to increase grip strength is gross grasp with therapy putty or exercise grippers. An example of purposeful activity to increase strength would be putting away groceries, starting with light items and progressing to heavier objects.

Occupation-as-means instills occupational therapy's heritage in what might otherwise be a less function-oriented context (Trombly, 1995). The examples cited earlier become therapeutic occupation with the use of activity that is meaningful to the particular person to accomplish the therapeutic goal. If the patient enjoys baking, then rolling dough with a rolling pin would be a therapeutic occupation to promote grip function.

EVALUATION

History

History taking as part of the occupational profile offers an excellent opportunity to establish therapeutic rapport (Bryan & Kohnke, 1997). Review medical reports, including radiographs, when possible; learn hand dominance, age, occupation, and avocational interests (Aulicino, 2002). Assess deficits in the areas of occupation by asking what the patient cannot do that he or she wants to do, needs to do, or is expected to do. Also, discuss the case with the physician.

For trauma, learn the date of injury, dates of any surgery, where and how injury occurred, mechanism of injury, posture of the hand when it was injured, and any previous intervention. For non-traumatic problems, learn the date of onset, whether the symptoms are worsening, sequence of onset of symptoms, functional effects, and what worsens and/or lessens the symptoms (Aulicino, 2002).

Pain

Pain may be acute or chronic. Acute pain has a sudden and recent onset, usually has a limited course with an identifiable cause, and can last a few minutes to 6 months. Acute pain serves a physiological purpose, signaling the need to protect tissue from further damage. Chronic pain lasts months or years longer than expected and may not serve a physiological purpose (Maurer & Jezek, 1992). Myofascial pain, which may be chronic or acute, stems from local irritation in fascia, muscle, tendon, or ligament. It has specific reproducible pain patterns and associated autonomic symptoms (Travell & Simons, 1983). Evaluation of pain may include a graphic representation of pain, in which the patient marks painful areas on a drawing of the human body; analog pain rating scales (see Chapter 5); joint or muscle palpation to identify areas of local pain or qualitative changes in soft tissue; and trigger point sensitivity (Maurer & Jezek, 1992).

Physical Examination

It is helpful to observe the positioning and use of the patient's upper extremity in the waiting area before the meeting. On examination, look at the entire unclothed upper extremity for posture, guarding and gesturing, atrophy, and edema (Aulicino, 2002). Since distal symptoms are often caused by proximal problems, it is important to perform a **cervical screening**, which is a proximal screening assessment of the neck and shoulder, to identify additional areas requiring intervention. For more detail on cervical screening, see Cyriax (1982).

Wounds

Always follow universal precautions (Chapter 49). Evaluate wound size in terms of length, width, and depth. Wound drainage (exudate) is bloody (sanguinous), serous (clear or yellow), purulent (pus), or deep or dark red (hematoma). Wound odor is absent or foul (Baldwin, Weber, & Simon, 1992).

The three-color concept (red, yellow, or black) dictates wound care. Wounds can be one of or a combination of these three colors. A red wound is healing, uninfected, and composed of revascularization and granulation tissue. A yellow wound has an exudate that requires cleansing and debridement. A black wound is necrotic and requires debridement. The goal of wound care is to convert yellow and black wounds to red wounds (Evans & McAuliffe, 2002).

Scar Assessment

Observe scar location, length, width, and height. Hypertrophic scars stay confined to the area of the original wound and usually resolve within a year. Keloids proliferate outside the area of the original wound and do not usually become smaller or less pigmented with time. Note any scar tethering or adherence of skin and tendon causing restricted movement. Any wound or scar crossing a joint may form a **contracture**, which restricts passive motion. Immature scar has a red or purplish color imparted by its vascularity. It blanches to touch. Mature scar is flatter and softer. It has neutral color and does not blanch to touch (Baldwin, Weber, & Simon, 1992).

Vascular Assessment

Cyanosis, erythema, pallor, gangrene, or grayish color indicates vascular compromise. To test digital capillary refill, apply pressure to the fingernail or distal pad of the involved digit. Color should return within 2 seconds of release of pressure. Compare the refill time to that of uninvolved digits (de Herder, 1992).

Edema

Circumferential measurement is quick to perform and provides a good alternative when it is not possible to use a volumeter (Fess, 2002a). Be consistent with measuring tape placement and tension. Volumetric measurement is contraindicated over open wounds, percutaneous pinning such as Kirschner wires, plaster casts, or vasomotor instability (Fess, 1993). See Chapter 5 for volumetric measurement procedures.

Range of Motion

In hand therapy, ROM is measured as AROM, PROM, or torque range of motion (TROM), which is a more consistent and objective type of PROM in which the therapist documents the amount of force applied externally to achieve maximal PROM (Breger-Lee, Bell-Krotoski, & Brandsma, 1990). At a minimum, both AROM and PROM should be evaluated and compared to the uninjured extremity (Adams, Topoozian, & Greene, 1992) (see Chapter 5). Facilities usually have their own guidelines for measuring ROM. As expected, consistency of retesting is important.

Total active motion or total passive motion measures the sum of composite digital flexion and extension. This measurement is used in some studies. Normal total active motion and total passive motion are 270° (Fess, 2002a) (Procedures for Practice 42-1).

PROCEDURES FOR PRACTICE 42-1

Total Active Motion and Total Passive Motion

- Add the measurements for flexion of the MP, PIP, and DIP joints.
- Subtract the combined deficits in extension for those joints.

Grip and Pinch

When properly calibrated, the Jamar dynamometer is one of the best instruments to assess grip strength because of its reliability, face validity, and accuracy (see Chapter 5). Hand therapy authorities recommend comparing scores to those of the contralateral extremity rather than using norms (Fess, 2002a). Goals for grip and pinch strength depend on occupational factors and dominance. There may be approximately 10–15% difference in strength between dominant and non-dominant hands, with dominant hands usually being stronger. Interpretation of maximal effort with grip testing exceeds the scope of this chapter. However, grip testing at all five notch settings of the dynamometer typically reveals a bell-shaped curve when consistent effort is used. For more on this subject, see Smith et al. (1989). It is routine to measure three pinch patterns: lateral, three-jaw chuck, and tip. As with grip, compare pinch scores to those of the contralateral extremity.

No linear relationship exists between improvement in grip and pinch strength and improvement in function. Rice, Leonard, and Carter (1998) noted that even debilitated, deformed hands could be surprisingly functional. These authors found only weak relationships between grip and pinch strength and the forces required to open six containers used commonly in the home. Thus, grip and pinch testing are not substitutes for ADL assessment with contextual relevance (Rice, Leonard, & Carter, 1998). To promote occupational functioning of people with hand impairments, it is far better to have intervention and goals reflect personally meaningful ADLs than grip or pinch strength measures.

Manual Muscle Testing

Manual muscle testing is particularly useful for monitoring progress following peripheral nerve lesions (see Chapter 5). Facilities usually have their preferred method of grading, which may be numerical or descriptive (Shultis-Kiernan, 1992).

Sensibility

Inspect the patient's hand for dryness, moistness, and calluses (see Chapter 7). Blisters may be an alert to injurious hand use due to sensory loss. "Wear marks" illustrate where and how the hand is used and which parts of the hand avoid use, indicating sensory impairment (Callahan, 2002).

Hand therapy does not yet have one tool that evaluates the hand's functional sensibility (Moberg, 1991). The *Semmes-Weinstein Monofilament Test* and the *Two-Point Discrimination* (*2PD*) test are most commonly used in hand therapy. The *Semmes-Weinstein Monofilament Test* assesses pressure threshold, and the *2PD* assesses density of receptors. The *Moberg Pickup Test* (see Chapter 7) is a functional test appropriate for use on patients with median or median and ulnar nerve lesions.

Dexterity and Hand Function

No one evaluation covers all features of hand function (Jarus & Poremba, 1993). Standard terminology regarding hand function is lacking, and there is limited evidence that the assessment of hand function indicates the patient's actual performance in ADL (Desrosiers et al., 1993; Lynch & Bridle, 1989). Thus, hand function tests should not substitute for assessments of ADL or other areas of occupation. Hand function tests, however, can be helpful measures of improvement of performance skills.

For dexterity tests to be reliable, therapists must administer them using the standard procedures from the original articles or test manuals, and they must decide whether a specific test is valid for the intended use (Mathiowetz & Bass Haugen, 1995; Rider & Linden, 1988). The tests described in this section all require further validation study.

Minnesota Rate of Manipulation Test

The *Minnesota Rate of Manipulation Test* (1969) addresses manual or gross motor dexterity. It assesses the speed and accuracy of repetitive reaching, picking up, manipulating, and placing disks the size of double checkers. It has a 3-foot-long frame with four horizontal rows of openings in which the 60 disks are placed. Five subtests comprise the test: placing, turning, displacing, one-hand turning and placing, and two-hand turning and placing. The patient performs the test while standing. Each subtest starts with a practice trial and is tested three to five times. The score is the total time for the subtest trials. This test has been standardized with adaptations for use with patients who are visually impaired (Mathiowetz & Bass Haugen, 1995).

Test–retest reliability ranges from 0.87 to 0.95 for two-trial administration. Percentile tables are available, with norms based on young adults (n = 11,000) and on older unemployed adults (n = 3,000). Procedures for Practice 42-2 presents recommendations for interpretation of a particular patient's score using normative data from a percentile table.

PROCEDURES FOR PRACTICE 42-2

Interpretation of a Score Using Normative Data From a Percentile Table (Mathiowetz & Bass Haugen, 1995)

- Administer the test according to standard procedures.
- Compare the patient's score with the most appropriate percentile table (e.g., worker category, sex, age).
- A patient scoring at the 20th percentile performed better than 20% and worse than 80% of the normative sample.
- A score at 2.3 percentile or higher is usually interpreted to be normal or within normal limits.
- A score falling between 2.3 and 0.1 percentile is interpreted to be a mild deficit.
- A score below 0.1 percentile is interpreted to be a moderate to severe deficit.

Interpretation of a Score Using Normative Data From a Mean and Standard Deviation Table (Mathiowetz et al., 1985a)

- Administer the test according to the standard procedures.
- Compare the right-hand score with the right-hand normative data appropriate to the age and sex of the patient.

For example, if a 23-year-old man transported 66 blocks within 1 minute with his right hand, his score of 66 would be compared with the mean of 88.2 and the standard deviation (SD) of 8.8 (Table 42-1). Using the formula below, it is found that he scored 2.5 SD below the mean relative to his age group and gender.

- Use this formula to determine the SD above or below the mean for a specific patient's score:[a]

Client's score − mean ÷ SD = SD ± mean

Example:

$$66 - 88.2 = -22.2$$
$$-22.2 \div 8.8 = -2.5 \text{ SD}^{a}$$

[a]In tests such as the *Box and Block Test*, for which a high score indicates a better performance, a negative score means below the mean. In tests such as the *Nine-Hole Peg Test*, for which a high score indicates a poor performance, a negative score means above the mean (better than average performance). Thus the therapist can document objectively that the patient's right-hand performance on the *Box and Block Test* of manual dexterity was 2.5 SD below the mean. To determine the statistical meaning of the patient's score, the therapist must assume that the *Box and Block Test* scores are normally distributed. In a standard normal distribution table, 97.7% of the sample scores are greater than 2 SD below the mean; 2.2% are between 2 and 3 SD below the mean; and 0.1% are more than 3 SD below the mean. By convention, a score that falls 2 SD below the mean or higher is usually interpreted to be normal or within normal limits. A score falling between 2 and 3 SD below the mean is interpreted to show a mild deficit. A score more than 3 SD below the mean is interpreted to show moderate to severe deficit. Thus the example patient would be considered to have a mild deficit in manual dexterity relative to the normative data.

Table 42-1. Average Performance of 628 Normal Subjects on the Box and Block Test[a]

	Males		Females			Males		Females	
Age (Years)	*Mean*	*SD*	*Mean*	*SD*	Age (Years)	*Mean*	*SD*	*Mean*	*SD*
20–24					50–54				
Right hand	88.2	8.8	88.0	8.3	Right hand	79.0	9.7	77.7	10.7
Left hand	86.4	8.5	83.4	7.9	Left hand	77.0	9.2	74.3	9.9
25–29					55–59				
Right hand	85.0	7.5	86.0	7.4	Right hand	75.2	11.9	74.7	8.9
Left hand	84.1	7.1	80.9	6.4	Left hand	73.8	10.5	73.6	7.8
30–34					60–64				
Right hand	81.9	9.0	85.2	7.4	Right hand	71.3	8.8	76.1	6.9
Left hand	81.3	8.1	80.2	5.6	Left hand	70.5	8.1	73.6	6.4
35–39					65–69				
Right hand	81.9	9.5	84.8	6.1	Right hand	68.4	7.1	72.0	6.2
Left hand	79.8	9.7	83.5	6.1	Left hand	67.4	7.8	71.3	7.7
40–44					70–74				
Right hand	83.0	8.1	81.1	8.2	Right hand	66.3	9.2	68.6	7.0
Left hand	80.0	8.8	79.7	8.8	Left hand	64.3	9.8	68.3	7.0
45–49					75+				
Right hand	76.9	9.2	82.1	7.5	Right hand	63.0	7.1	65.0	7.1
Left hand	75.8	7.8	78.3	7.6	Left hand	61.3	8.4	63.6	7.4

[a]Values are number of cubes transferred in 1 minute. Mathiowetz et al., 1985a.

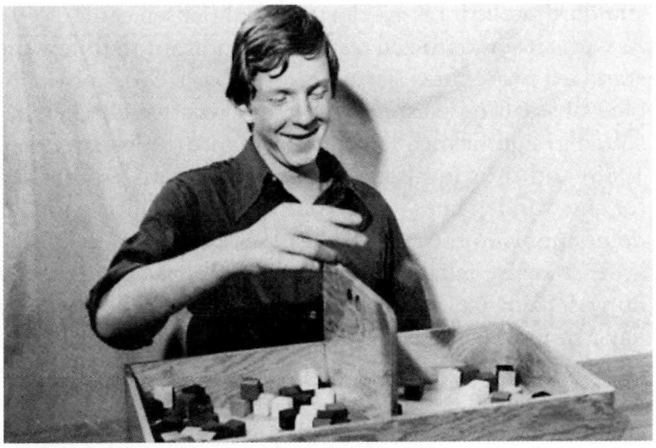

Figure 42-2 *Box and Block Test* of manual dexterity.

Box and Block Test

The *Box and Block Test* measures gross manual dexterity. It was developed to test people with severe problems affecting coordination (Fig. 42-2). This test must be constructed according to specific dimensions and published specifications (Mathiowetz et al., 1985a). The subject transfers 1-inch blocks from one side of the box to the other. The score is the number of blocks transferred in 1 minute for each hand. Procedures for Practice 42-3 presents procedures for administration of the test (Mathiowetz et al., 1985a).

Test–retest reliability of the *Box and Block Test*, established at a 6-month interval, was high (r = 0.94 for left hands and r = 0.98 for right hands) (Cromwell, 1976). Inter-rater reliability reflected strong correlations (r = 1.00 for right hand and r = 0.999 for left hand) (Mathiowetz et al., 1985a). Concurrent validity (r = 0.91) was established with the placing subtest of the *Minnesota Rate of Manipulation Test* (Cromwell, 1976).

The *Box and Block Test* is preferred to the *Minnesota Rate of Manipulation Test* because the normative data for the *Box and Block Test* have a broader range, the patient is allowed to sit while being tested, and it is time limited (Mathiowetz & Bass Haugen, 1995) (Procedures for Practice 42-3).

Purdue Pegboard Test

The *Purdue Pegboard Test* of finger dexterity (Tiffin, 1968) assesses picking up, manipulating, and placing little pegs into holes with speed and accuracy. It tests finger or fine motor dexterity (Mathiowetz et al., 1986). It has a wooden board with two rows of tiny holes plus reservoirs for holding pins, collars, and washers. The four subtests are per-

PROCEDURES FOR PRACTICE 42-3

Administration Procedures for the *Box and Block Test* (Mathiowetz et al., 1985a)

- Place the test box lengthwise along the edge of a standard-height table (Fig. 42-2).
- The 150 cubes are in the compartment of the test box to the dominant side of the patient.
- Sit facing the patient to monitor the blocks being transported.
- Give these instructions: "*I want to see how quickly you can pick up one block at a time with your right [left] hand [the therapist points to the dominant hand]. Carry the block to the other side of the box and drop it. Make sure your fingertips cross the partition. Watch me while I show you how.*"
- Transport three cubes over the partition in the same direction the patient is to move them.

  After the demonstration, say, "*If you pick up two blocks at a time, they will count as one. If you drop one on the floor or table after you have carried it across, it will still be counted, so do not waste time picking it up. If you toss the blocks without your fingertips crossing the partition, they will not be counted. Before you start, you will have a chance to practice for 15 seconds. Do you have any questions? Place your hands on the sides of the box. When it is time to start, I will say 'Ready' and then 'Go.'*"
- Start the stopwatch at the word *go*. After 15 seconds, say "*Stop.*"
- If the patient makes mistakes during the practice period, correct them before beginning the actual testing.
- On completion of the practice period, return the transported cubes to the compartment.
- Mix the cubes to ensure random distribution, and then say, "*This will be the actual test. The instructions are the same. Work as quickly as you can. Ready; go. [After 1 minute:] Stop.*"
- Count the blocks transported across the partition. This is the patient's score for the dominant hand.
- If the patient transports two or more blocks at the same time, subtract the number of extra blocks from the total.
- After counting, return the blocks to the original compartment and mix randomly.
- Turn the test around so that the blocks are on the non-dominant side.
- Administer the test to the non-dominant hand using the same procedures as for the dominant hand, including the 15-second practice.

formed with the subject seated. To begin, there is a brief practice. The subtests for preferred, non-preferred, and both hands require the patient to place the pins in the holes as quickly as possible, with the score being the number of pins placed in 30 seconds. The subtest for assembly requires the patient to insert a pin and then put a washer, collar, and another washer on the pin, with the score being the number of pieces assembled in 1 minute (Mathiowetz & Bass Haugen, 1995). The *Purdue Pegboard Test* manual provides normative data using percentile tables for adults and different categories of jobs and for children 5–15 years of age by age and sex.

One-trial administration of the *Purdue Pegboard Test* produced test–retest reliability of 0.60 to 0.79. Three-trial administration test–retest reliability ranged from 0.82 to 0.91 (Mathiowetz et al., 1986). Administering three trials for the four subtests took more time (20 minutes instead of 10) but provided better reliability. Gallus (1999) reported high test–retest reliability ($r = 0.85$–0.96) and no practice effects based on individuals with multiple sclerosis. A limitation of the *Purdue Pegboard Test* is that it was developed to select industrial employees. The validity of its use in identifying a need for occupational therapy should be evaluated (Mathiowetz, 1993).

Nine-Hole Peg Test

The *Nine-Hole Peg Test* measures finger dexterity among patients with physical disabilities. This test is sold commercially, or it can be constructed according to published details (Mathiowetz et al., 1985a). Test administration is brief, involving the time it takes to place nine pegs in holes in a 5-inch square board and then remove them. The *Nine-Hole Peg Test* had high inter-rater reliability ($r = 0.97$ for right hand and $r = 0.99$ for left hand). Test-retest reliability was moderate: ($r = 0.69$ for right hand and $r = 0.43$ for left hand) (Mathiowetz et al., 1985b). Concerns exist about the transferability of these norms to data collected with commercial versions of the test that use different materials (Davis et al., 1997).

The *Purdue Pegboard Test* is preferred to the *Nine-Hole Peg Test* in the measurement of finger dexterity. Of the two, the *Purdue Pegboard Test* has better test–retest reliability; it is time limited; it is for both unilateral and bilateral assessment; and its normative data reflect a broader age range (Mathiowetz & Bass Haugen, 1995).

Jebsen Test of Hand Function

The *Jebsen Test of Hand Function* assesses hand function in terms of simulated ADL (Jebsen et al., 1969). It can be administered quickly (Jarus & Poremba, 1993). The test's seven timed subtests consisting of writing a sentence, simulated page turning, picking up small common objects, stacking checkers, simulated eating, moving empty cans, and moving heavy cans. Construction specifications and standard procedures are documented (Jebsen et al., 1969). As with all standardized tests, it is important to follow the standard procedures (Jarus & Poremba, 1993). For example, substituting plastic checkers for wooden checkers resulted in significantly lower performance (Rider & Linden, 1988) and thus invalidated the use of norms established for the wooden checkers. In addition, reliability statistics do not apply to the adapted test (Fess, 1993).

Test–retest reliability of the *Jebsen Hand Function Test* ranged from 0.60 to 0.99, based on 26 patients whose hand impairments had leveled off. No significant practice effect was demonstrated between two sessions with these patients (Jebsen et al., 1969). Although the researchers reported data on reliability of the *Jebsen Hand Function Test*, their data represented patient groups, not normal subjects (Mathiowetz et al., 1985b). Stern confirmed the test–retest reliability with 20 normal subjects, but she also found a significant practice effect for writing and simulated feeding subtests between the first and third sessions (Stern, 1992).

The *Jebsen Hand Function Test* does discriminate between subjects with and without different physical disabilities (Jebsen et al., 1969; Spaulding et al., 1988). A moderate correlation ($r = 0.64$) between the *Jebsen Hand Function Test* and the *Klein–Bell ADL Scale* suggests that the Jebsen test may have some usefulness in predicting functional ability, but it would not be an appropriate substitute for an ADL evaluation (Lynch & Bridle, 1989). Norms for adults aged 20–94 years (n = 300) are published (Jebsen et al., 1969).

The *Jebsen Hand Function Test* has several limitations. One is that it does not really address the proximal upper extremity (Desrosiers et al., 1993). In addition, it measures speed, not quality, of hand function (Jarus & Poremba, 1993; Spaulding et al., 1988). In addition, some of its subtests are not representative of ordinary daily activity. Mathiowetz (1993) questioned its content validity when he found that the page turning and feeding subtests do not actually duplicate those tasks in daily life. He also questioned why writing is evaluated as a timed test and why the non-dominant hand is tested in handwriting.

TEMPA

TEMPA is an acronym from the French for *Upper Extremity Performance Test for the Elderly* (Desrosiers et al., 1993). It consists of nine tasks, five bilateral and four unilateral, reflecting daily activity. Each task is measured by the three subscores of speed, functional rating, and task analysis. The nine tasks are pick up and move a jar, open a jar and take a spoonful of coffee, pour water from a pitcher into a glass, unlock a lock, take the top off a pillbox, write on an envelope and affix a postage stamp, put a scarf around one's neck, shuffle and deal cards, use coins, and pick up and move small objects. Instructions are in the manual. The test takes about 15–20 minutes for an unimpaired elderly subject and about 30–40 minutes for an impaired elderly subject (Desrosiers et al., 1993). Advantages of the *TEMPA* are clinical utility, especially with hand patients over 60 years of age; provision of both quantitative and qualitative data; simulation of ADL; test applicability; test availability; and acceptability to patients (Rudman & Hannah, 1998). A possible disadvantage of this test is its cost of approximately $500. Questions have surfaced concerning the quality control in production of the test (Humiston, 2000).

TEMPA norms were established on adults 60 years of age or older (n = 360) by 10-year age groups and by gender. Inter-rater reliability of the *TEMPA* ranged from 0.96 to 1.00. Test–retest reliability ranged from 0.77 to 1.00. Concurrent validity with the *Action Research Arm* test was 0.90 to 0.95, and with the *Box and Block Test*, it was 0.73 to 0.78 (Desrosiers et al., 1994). Some support for construct validity was demonstrated by correlating the *TEMPA* with basic personal care ($r = 0.68$) (Desrosiers et al., 1993).

CLINICAL REASONING AND INTERVENTION

Questions to Ask

Close communication with the patient's physician is always advisable. Choosing which questions to ask depends on the diagnosis and structures involved. General categories of questions may include the physician's expectations for functional recovery; tendon status, such as fraying or vascular compromise; whether the patient is medically cleared for AROM only or AROM and/or PROM; and whether the patient is medically cleared for low-load, long-duration dynamic splinting.

ADL and Occupational Role Implications

The functional use of the upper extremity and the patient's ability to perform in the areas of occupation are what really matter. Hand therapists must be careful not to become so focused on the technical aspects of the patient's injury that they overlook the patient's function, personal goals, and life needs. In some circumstances, it may actually be better for patients to accept a stiff finger and get on with life using compensatory techniques than to interrupt the flow of their lives for therapy (Merritt, 1998). This may be true if gains are exceedingly slow, if function is not dramatically compromised, or if there are other priorities, such as ill family members, for example.

Goal Setting

Express hand therapy goals or projected outcomes in terms that reflect the patient's occupational functioning. Ultimately, the number of degrees achieved in ROM is less important than whether the patient can open a door, get dressed, or return to work. One way to integrate concrete and functional outcomes is to measure the movement needed to accomplish an appropriate patient-specific functional task and incorporate that measurement into the stated goal. For example, if a patient wants to be able to splash water on his or her face but lacks forearm supination to do so, have the patient perform the activity with the opposite upper extremity. Measure the supination needed to perform the task. In this instance, the goal could be stated as "sufficient forearm supination (60°) for ability to wash the face" (C. Skotak, personal communication, 1999).

Quality of Movement

Poor quality of movement (called dys-coordinate cocontraction) may result from cocontraction of antagonist muscles. The cause may be habit, fear of pain, guarding, or excessive effort. Poor quality of movement looks awkward and unpleasant. It is important to identify dys-coordinate cocontraction early and to work on retraining a smooth, comfortable, effective quality of motion. Pain-free activity or pain-free occupation is the best way to promote good quality of motion. **Oscillations** are rhythmic therapeutic movements that may be helpful, but they must be pain free. Imagery, such as pretending to move the extremity through water or gelatin, may also help (Cooper, Liskin, & Moorhead, 1999). Biofeedback may aid in muscle reeducation as well.

What Structures Are Restricted, and Does PROM Exceed AROM?

Hand therapists strive to be structure specific in identifying and treating upper extremity limitations. It is not adequate to identify a general problem, such as decreased ROM. Rather, it is important to understand and treat the specific structures causing the restriction. Limited PROM may be due to pericapsular structures, such as adhered or shortened ligaments, or actual joint limitations, such as mechanical block or adhesions. PROM that exceeds AROM may be due to disruption of the musculotendinous unit, adhesions restricting excursion of the tendon (Fess, 1993), or weakness. When PROM exceeds AROM, promote active movement and function of the restricted structures with differential tendon gliding exercises, blocking exercises, place-and-hold exercises, and functional splints (discussed later). When PROM equals AROM, discern whether the restriction is joint or musculotendinous or both (see section on joint versus musculotendinous tightness), and promote both passive and active flexibility.

Joint Versus Musculotendinous Tightness

With joint tightness, the PROM of the particular joint *does not change* with repositioning of the joints proximal and/or distal to it. With musculotendinous tightness, the PROM of the particular joint *does vary* with repositioning of joints crossed by that multiarticulate structure (Colditz, 2002b). Treat joint tightness with dynamic splinting, static progressive splinting, or serial casting, followed by AROM. Treat musculotendinous tightness the same as extrinsic tightness (discussed later).

Lag Versus Contracture

A lag is a limitation of active motion in a joint that has passive motion available. A joint contracture is a passive limitation of the joint. A patient with a PIP **extensor lag** cannot actively extend the PIP joint even though passive extension is available. A patient with a PIP joint flexion contracture lacks passive extension of that joint.

Treat lags by facilitating motion of the restricted structure with scar management, blocking exercises in mechanically advantageous positions, place-and-hold exercises, static splinting to promote normal length of the involved structure, and functional splints. Treat contractures the same as for joint tightness (discussed later).

An advantageous position to test or treat extensor lag at the PIP level is to maintain MP flexion while trying to extend actively at the PIP. An advantageous position to test or treat extensor lag at the DIP level is to maintain MP and PIP flexion while trying to extend actively at the DIP. This is contraindicated if the diagnosis is acute mallet finger (see section on extensor tendon injury).

Intrinsic Versus Extrinsic Tightness

Compare the PROM of digital PIP and DIP flexion with the MP joint flexed and again with the MP joint extended. With extrinsic tightness, there is less PIP and DIP passive flexion with the MP joint flexed. With intrinsic tightness, there is less PIP and DIP passive flexion with the MP joint extended (Colditz, 2002b).

Treat intrinsic tightness with functional splinting with MPs hyperextended and IPs free. In other words, promote IP flexion with MPs hyperextended. Treat extrinsic extensor tightness with MPs flexed and IPs free, and promote composite digital flexion. Use blocking exercises with an advantageous proximal position (discussed later). Try dynamic or static progressive splinting.

Tightness of Extrinsic Extensors or Extrinsic Flexors

With extrinsic extensor tightness, there is less passive composite digital flexion available with the wrist in flexion than with the wrist in extension. In contrast, with extrinsic flexor tightness, there is less passive composite digital extension available with the wrist in extension than with the wrist in flexion (Colditz, 2002b). Treat extrinsic flexor or extensor tightness with place-and-hold exercises, static splinting comfortably at end range (especially useful at night), dynamic or static progressive splinting during the day, and functional splinting.

BASIC INTERVENTIONS

Edema Control

Elevation, active exercise, contrast baths, and compression have been the mainstays of edema control. Treatment of upper extremity edema has also historically included retrograde massage, string wrapping, compressive garments, and modalities such as an intermittent pressure pump. Compression garments should not be too tight.

Research has challenged hand therapists recently to reexamine the anatomical and physiological bases of our treatment of edema. This inquiry has resulted in a new approach to the treatment of upper extremity edema, called manual edema mobilization (Artzberger, 2002), a technique for stimulating the lymphatic system to remove the excess large plasma proteins that cause sustained edema leading to fibrotic tissue and stiffness. This hands-on technique, which must be learned in workshops that last 2 days or longer, can lead to dramatic and effective results. The approach used in manual edema mobilization is very different from and, in some ways, opposite to traditional retrograde massage techniques. Furthermore, manual edema mobilization raises questions about whether retrograde massage is sometimes more damaging than helpful. Manual edema mobilization is a wonderful example of the groundbreaking changes in hand therapy, based on scholarly questioning and research, that keep the profession interesting.

Scar Management

Compression (e.g., Isotoner gloves, Tubigrip, or Coban wrap) and desensitization are traditionally used to promote scar softening and maturation. Silicone gel applied over the scar (Baum & Busuito, 1998) helps promote scar maturation, presumably through neutral warmth. Other inserted materials such as padding, otoform, or elastomer can also be used. Application of micropore tape over incision scars has been suggested more recently.

Although friction massage has typically been advocated for scar softening, legitimate questions have been raised as to whether this more aggressive technique may in fact cause inflammation, resulting in deposition of even more scar tissue. Manual edema mobilization may be a more effective alternative. Research is needed in this area.

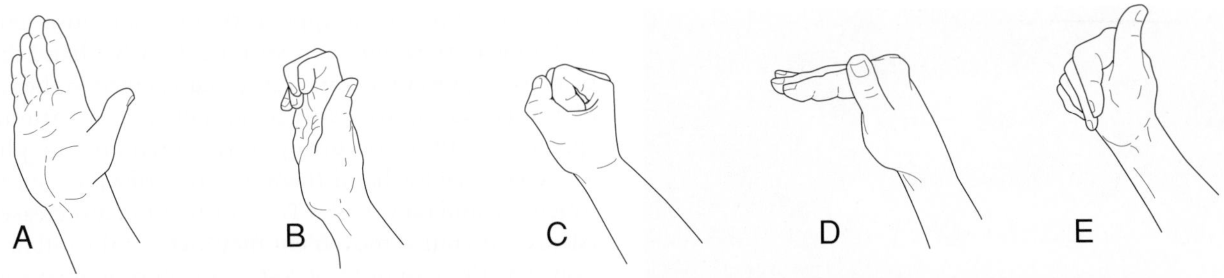

Figure 42-3 Differential flexor tendon gliding exercises. The five positions: **A.** Straight. **B.** Hook. **C.** Fist. **D.** Tabletop. **E.** Straight fist. (Adapted with permission from Rozmaryn, L. M., Dovelle, S., Rothman, E. R., Gorman, K., Olvey, K. M., & Bartko, J. J. [1998]. Nerve and tendon gliding exercises and the conservative management of carpal tunnel syndrome. *Journal of Hand Therapy, 11,* 171–179.)

Differential Digital Tendon Gliding Exercises

Tendon gliding exercises maximize total gliding and differential gliding of digital flexor tendons at the wrist (Fig. 42-3) (Rozmaryn et al., 1998; Pettengill & van Strien, 2002). Since tendon gliding exercises promote digital and joint motions, they are a mainstay of most home exercise programs.

Blocking Exercises

Various blocking tools and splints are available commercially or can be made easily with scraps of splinting materials (Fig. 42-4) (Skirven & Trope, 1994). Digital cylinders blocking the IPs help to isolate and exercise MP flexion and extension. A blocking splint with the MPs extended promotes intrinsic stretch as well as IP flexion. A blocking splint with the MPs flexed promotes extrinsic extensor stretch and recovery of composite fisting. A PIP cylindrical block encourages DIP isolated flexion and flexor digitorum profundus (FDP) excursion at the DIP. A DIP cap facilitates PIP flexion and flexor tendon excursion at the PIP.

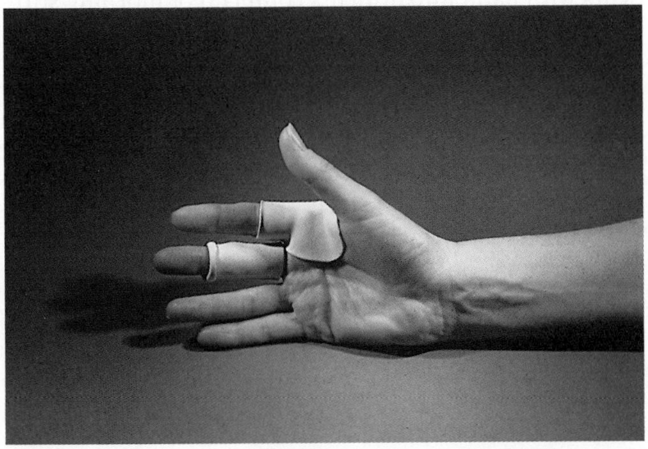

Figure 42-4 Blocking splints. MP splint blocks MP motion, promoting PIP and DIP motion. Digital splint blocks PIP motion, promoting MP and/or DIP motion.

Instruct patients who do blocking exercises to exercise comfortably into the end range to remodel the tissue. Teach them to do the exercises frequently and slowly, holding at the comfortable end range for 3–5 seconds (Schneider & Feldscher, 2002).

Place-and-Hold Exercises

Place-and-hold exercises are effective for achieving increased ROM when PROM exceeds AROM. To perform them, use comfortable PROM to position the hand (e.g., composite fisting). Then release the assisting hand while the patient tries to sustain the position in a pain-free way (Collins, 1993; Pettengill & van Strien, 2002). Place-and-hold exercises can be effective in combination with blocking exercises.

End Feel and Splinting

If there is a **soft end feel** (a favorable spongy quality at end range indicative of potential to remodel), it is reasonable to try low-load, long-duration dynamic splinting for a medically cleared patient. Dynamic splint forces must be prolonged and gentle for tissue to remodel. Forceful splinting is contraindicated because it causes pain and injury, hence inflammation and scarring (Brand, 2002; Fess, 2002b). Follow dynamic splint use with activity that challenges and incorporates the limited motion. For a firmer or **hard end feel** (an unyielding quality at end range), try increasing the time in the splint and decreasing the force. If there is a hard end feel, dynamic splinting may not be effective, and serial casting or static progressive splinting may be more useful.

Splints

Functional splints can be used in ordinary daily activity to promote mobility of restricted structures. For example, if

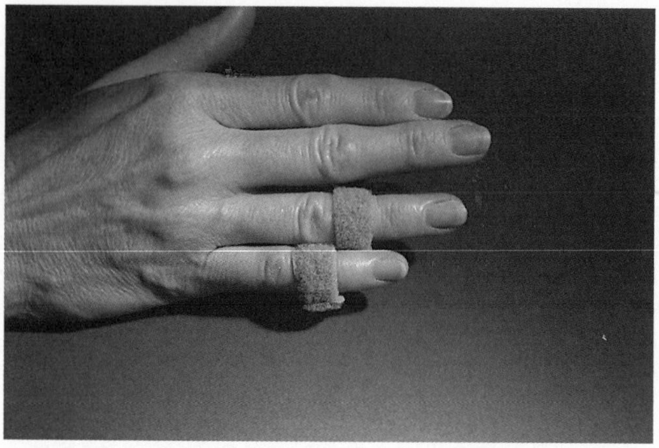

Figure 42-5 Offset buddy straps. Inter-digital strap accommodates different phalangeal lengths of adjacent digits. Used to allow one digit to assist the next in achieving motion and for protection.

the index finger PIP joint lacks flexion and the MP joint moves normally, try a hand-based index finger MP blocking splint, used off and on through the day. When the splint is in use, the patient achieves PIP flexion exercise while performing normal grasping activities.

Buddy straps allow one digit to assist a neighboring digit to achieve greater motion. The offset buddy strap (Fig. 42-5) accommodates different phalangeal lengths of adjacent digits (Jensen & Rayan, 1996). Buddy straps are also useful to retrain keyboard users who habitually maintain the small finger MP in hyperextension or repetitively hyperabduct the small finger when keyboarding.

A dorsal MP flexion blocking splint promotes composite flexion incorporating MP flexion and is particularly helpful when there is extrinsic extensor tightness. If the patient has difficulty incorporating MP flexion into composite fisting and, instead, extends the MPs while flexing the IPs, a dorsal hood maintaining MP flexion promotes recovery of composite fist incorporating MP flexion. (See Chapters 16 and 17 for further splinting guidelines.)

COMMON DIAGNOSES

Hand therapists 15 years ago treated more hand trauma than cumulative trauma, and surgical cases constituted most of the caseload. Nowadays, many hand therapists see a substantially greater number of patients with a soft tissue diagnosis, such as tendinitis or cumulative trauma disorders.

Stiff Hand

Any upper extremity injury can result in the serious and sometimes irreversible problem of a stiff hand. Even an injury in the proximal upper extremity can cause serious stiffening of the digits. The stiff hand is what hand therapists try to prevent. Edema is the main culprit in the series of events leading to a stiff hand. Edema is a natural response to trauma, occurring in the inflammatory phase. The challenge for hand therapy is to strike a balance between rest and movement. Too much rest may increase the edema. Too much movement may increase the inflammation. The right amount of rest in an appropriate position reduces inflammation and promotes healing. Proximal motion plus well-tolerated hand and wrist exercise and functional use, particularly while elevated, help to reduce edema and restore motion.

Encourage the patient to achieve gentle full arcs of available motion with functional use or exercise instead of performing quick or incomplete arcs of motion that are less effective. Make exercises relevant to occupational functioning or at least goal oriented whenever possible (e.g., grasping and releasing items). If the patient's hand is painful or more swollen after use or exercise, it is imperative to decrease temporarily the amount of exercise being performed (Colditz, 2002b).

Avoid aggressive PROM. It is okay to coax tissues to lengthen within their available comfortable range, but always respect the feeling of tissue resistance, and do not exceed it. Gentle passive motion, if indicated, should be accompanied by joint traction to promote gliding of the joint surfaces. Sustained holding of a position is much more effective than fast jerky stretches, which frequently add to the inflammation (Colditz, 2002b).

During the acute inflammatory stage, static splinting is usually most appropriate. After the inflammation has subsided and while the joint displays a soft end feel, dynamic splinting is productive. Inflamed tissue is not as flexible as uninflamed tissue (Brand, 2002). Watch closely for signs of inflammation and return to static splinting as indicated. Later, if there is a hard end feel, serial static or static progressive splinting will most likely be needed. Many patients with hand impairments complain of morning stiffness. Night splinting, which can be very helpful for this problem, also corrects tissue tightness that limits daytime use of the hand (Colditz, 2002b).

Tendinitis/Tendinosis

The pain associated with tendinitis/tendinosis can be severe and can seriously impact performance in all areas of occupation. Symptoms include pain with AROM, with resistance, and with passive stretch of the involved structures. Tendons are made up of connective tissues that are not well vascularized. Tendinitis has been treated historically as if it is an inflammatory phenomenon. Recent histological evidence has shown that the pathology of tendinitis includes alterations in tissue with disorganized and degenerated collagen and atypical vascular granulation tissue. These findings are described as angiofibroblastic hyperplasia or angiofibroblastic tendinosis. It is now believed by authorities that the patients who are diagnosed with tendinitis actually have tendinosis. Since the pathology is not primarily inflammatory, treatment approaches now emphasize interventions that restore nourishment to collagen (Ashe, McCauley, & Khan, 2004; Nirschl, 1992). The question of use of modalities with this diagnosis remains intriguing. Most authorities report that modalities are effective in reducing pain, normalizing the vascular status of the involved tissue, and quieting inflammation if it exists.

Debate is ongoing over the cause of musculoskeletal problems; whether such problems are work related remains controversial (Terrono & Millender, 1996). Tendons are vulnerable because they are relatively avascular. Cell damage may become chronic (Pitner, 1990). Biomechanical deficits include muscular weakness, inflexibility, and scar tissue. Early treatment of an acute traumatic case typically has a better prognosis than after the injury has become chronic.

Evaluation

An overaggressive evaluation that provokes pain can set the treatment timetable back significantly and undermine the trust of and rapport with the patient. Start the evaluation with a cervical screening to look for proximal causes of distal symptoms. Compare both extremities. Assess for pain that may be local or diffuse, swelling, sensory changes, and loss of function. Tendinitis typically is accompanied by pain with AROM, with resistance, and with passive stretch of the involved structures. Compare subjective and objective findings, but remember that symptoms are often elusive and may occur dynamically or intermittently. Patients who seem angry or hostile may understandably be depressed over their loss of function.

It is essential to identify the activity causing the pain. Occupational therapists possess unique skills for ergonomic-related analysis of occupational performance and activity modification. It is best to observe the actual activity. If this is not possible, simulate the activity. Ergonomic risk factors for tendinitis include forceful, rapid, repetitive movements. A movement is considered repetitive if it is performed more than once every 30 seconds or for more than half the total work time. Additional risk factors include a history of soft-tissue problems, pressure and shear forces, stress and muscle tension, and hypermobility (Idler, 1997; Keller, Corbett, & Nichols, 1998).

Intervention

Treat the acute phase with ice, compression, elevation of the involved structures, and rest if needed to manage pain. Anti-inflammatory physical agent modalities may be useful at this time (see Chapter 20), but remember that this diagnosis is no longer thought to be primarily inflammatory. Splinting is individualized to the patient's and physician's preferences. Splinting may be most beneficial and least problematic at night. Although some physicians advocate immobilization for weeks (Idler, 1997), there are also clinical compromises associated with disuse from immobilization (Bulthaup, Cipriani, & Thomas, 1999; Skirven & Trope, 1994). Soft supports may be very helpful. In weighing the advantages and disadvantages of splint use, consult closely with the referring physician, try to avoid pain, and monitor the clinical responses. Active pain-free motion is the best way to begin revascularizing the involved tissues.

After the inflammation subsides, upgrade intervention to restore normal function through gradual mobilization balanced with rest. Most importantly, pain must be avoided. Instruct in tendon gliding exercises in a pain-free range appropriate to the particular structures involved. Progress from isometric exercises with gentle contractions of involved structures to isotonic exercises (Johnson, 1993). Gradually introduce low-load, high-repetition strengthening in short arcs of motion. Then increase the arc of motion and modify proximal positions to be more challenging if appropriate for work simulation. Instruct in gentle flexibility exercises in a pain-free range. It is often difficult for patients to learn to perform slow and pain-free passive stretch. Aerobic exercises and proximal conditioning are essential (Pitner, 1990).

Prevent reinjury through education (Furth, Holm, & James, 1994). Simulation and biofeedback (see Chapter 20) can promote biomechanically efficient upper extremity use. Teach the patient to avoid reaching and gripping with an extended elbow or a flexed or deviated wrist. First, solve the easily recognizable issues, such as obviously poor posture or trunk twisting with reaching and lifting. Instruct in pacing to avoid fatigue that leads to re-inflammation. Unsupported upper extremity use is taxing, as are non-symmetrical upper extremity use, non-frontal trunk or upper extremity alignment, and unilateral upper extremity work. Many people with distal symptoms recover well by focusing intervention on posture, conditioning, and proximal strengthening. Using hand-held tools with ergonomic design can be helpful (Johnson, 1993). Even a small ergonomic adjustment, such as learning to lift bilaterally with proper body mechanics or making use of a telephone headset instead of laterally flexing the neck and elevating the shoulder to hold the receiver, can often lead to dramatic improvement.

Lateral Epicondylitis, or Tennis Elbow

Lateral epicondylitis involves the extrinsic extensors at their origin. The extensor carpi radialis brevis is most commonly involved. Pain is at the lateral epicondyle and extensor wad (the proximal portion of the extensor muscles) (Wuori et al., 1998). This diagnosis is differentiated clinically from radial tunnel syndrome, in which tenderness occurs more distally over the radial tuberosity. Test for radial tunnel syndrome with the middle finger test (positive if there is pain secondary to resisting the middle finger proximal phalanx while the patient maintains elbow extension, neutral wrist, and MP extension) or by percussing distally to proximally over the superficial radial nerve. This percussion test is positive if it elicits paresthesias (Skirven & Trope, 1994; Terrono & Millender, 1996).

Exercises should include proximal conditioning and scapular stabilizing. Use built-up handles. If using a splint, support the wrist in extension, especially at night. Splinted wrist position recommendations range from neutral to about 30°. Also try a **counterforce strap**, which is a strap placed over the extensor wad to prevent full muscle contraction and to reduce the load on the tendon during the day with activity (Skirven & Trope, 1994; Wuori et al., 1998). ***Avoid applying the counterforce strap too tightly, as this can cause radial tunnel syndrome.***

Medial Epicondylitis, or Golfer's Elbow

Medial epicondylitis involves the extrinsic flexors at their origin (Johnson, 1993). The flexor carpi radialis (FCR) is most commonly involved. Pain is at the medial epicondyle and flexor wad (the proximal portion of the flexor muscles) and worsens with resisted flexion and pronation. Exercise should promote proximal conditioning. Avoid activity that requires force at end ranges. Provide built-up handles. If using a splint, maintain the wrist in neutral, and try a counterforce strap over the flexor wad.

De Quervain's Disease

De Quervain's disease is tendinitis involving the abductor pollicis longus (APL) and extensor pollicis brevis (EPB) tendons at the first dorsal compartment. It is the most common upper extremity tenosynovitis. Finkelstein's test is positive if there is exquisite pain with passive wrist ulnar deviation while flexing the thumb (Fig. 42-6) (Mooney, 1998). This diagnosis occurs frequently among golfers, knitters, racquet sports players, mail sorters, and filing clerks (Verdon, 1996). Thumb posture in sustained hyperabduction at the computer space bar may also be provoking (Pascarelli & Kella, 1993). Differential diagnosis is for carpometacarpal (CMC) arthritis, scaphoid fracture, intersection syndrome, and FCR tendinitis (Stern, 1990).

Teach patients to avoid wrist deviation, especially in conjunction with pinching. Provide built-up handles. If splinting, use a forearm-based thumb spica, leaving the IP free. Watch for irritation from the radial splint edge along the first dorsal compartment (Skirven & Trope, 1994).

Intersection Syndrome

Intersection syndrome presents as pain, swelling, and crepitus of the APL and EPB muscle bellies approximately 4 cm proximal to the wrist, where they intersect with the wrist extensor tendons (extensor carpi radialis brevis and extensor carpi radialis longus). This diagnosis is associated with repetitive wrist motion and occurs in weight lifters, rowers, and canoers (Servi, 1997). Differential diagnosis is for de Quervain's disease (Stern, 1990), and both diagnoses can occur concomitantly. Teach patients to avoid painful or resisted wrist extension and forceful grip. Splinting is the same as for de Quervain's disease.

Extensor Pollicis Longus Tendinitis

Also called drummer boy palsy, tendinitis of the extensor pollicis longus (EPL) reveals pain and swelling at Lister's tubercle (a dorsal prominence at the distal radius around which the EPL passes). It is less common than other forms of tendinitis, but if left untreated, it can lead to tendon rupture. EPL tendinitis is associated with activities requiring repetitive use of the thumb and wrist, as seen in drummers. Rupture of the EPL may occur in persons with rheumatoid arthritis or Colles' fracture (Verdon, 1996).

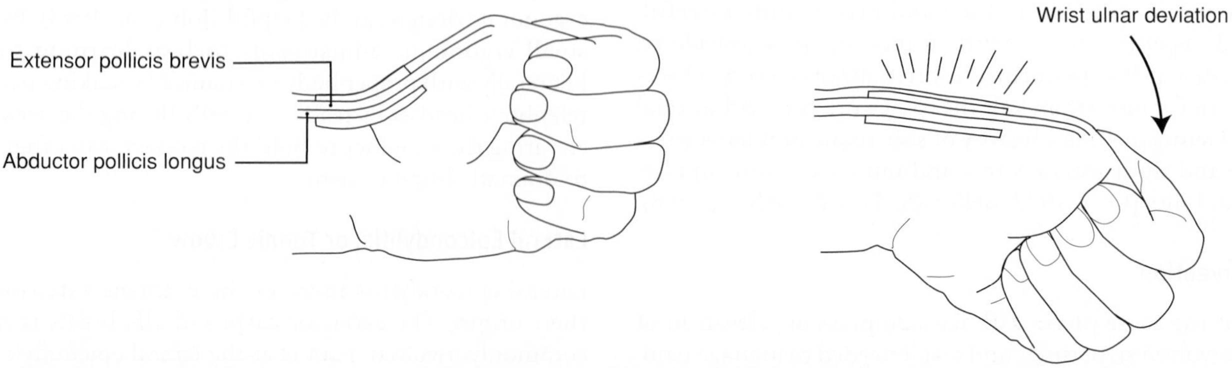

Figure 42-6 Finkelstein's test for de Quervain's disease. (Adapted with permission from American Society for Surgery of the Hand. [1990]. *The hand: Examination and diagnosis* [3rd ed.]. New York: Churchill Livingstone.)

Help patients to identify and eliminate provocative activities. Enlarge the girth of utensils. The splinting choice is a forearm-based thumb spica that includes the IP.

Extensor Carpi Ulnaris Tendinitis

Tenosynovitis of the extensor carpi ulnaris (ECU) occurs fairly frequently. It causes pain and swelling distal to the ulnar head and is associated with repetitive ulnar deviation motions. Subluxation of the ECU tendon elicits a painful snap with forearm supination and wrist ulnar deviation. Differential diagnosis includes instability of the distal radioulnar joint (Stern, 1990) and ulnocarpal abutment or tears of the triangular fibrocartilage complex.

Teach patients to avoid ulnar deviation with activities. Splinting consists of a forearm-based ulnar gutter or a wrist cock-up splint.

Flexor Carpi Radialis Tendinitis

With tendinitis of the FCR, pain is over the FCR tendon just proximal to the wrist flexor creases. Differential diagnosis is for a volar ganglion (Stern, 1990) or arthritis of the scaphotrapeziotrapezoid joint. Splinting consists of a wrist cock-up in neutral or a position of comfort.

Flexor Carpi Ulnaris Tendinitis

Flexor carpi ulnaris (FCU) tendinitis is more common than FCR tendinitis. It causes pain along the volar-ulnar side of the wrist. Inflammation occurs where the FCU inserts at the pisiform. Differential diagnosis is pisiform fracture and pisotriquetral arthritis (Verdon, 1996) or triangular fibrocartilage complex injury. Teach patients to avoid wrist flexion with ulnar deviation. Splinting consists of a forearm-based ulnar gutter. For comfort, pad the ulnar head if it is prominent, so the splint does not rub or irritate it.

Flexor Tenosynovitis, or Trigger Finger

Trigger finger is also called stenosing tenosynovitis of the digital flexor. The usual cause is stenosis at the A-1 pulley, which is part of the fibro-osseous tunnel that prevents bow-stringing of the digital flexors (Culp & Taras, 2002). Tenderness is over the A-1 pulley of the digital flexor (Fig. 42-7) along with pain with resisted grip and painful catching or locking of the finger in composite flexion (Lee, Nasser-Sharif, & Zelouf, 2002).

The origin of this impairment can be inflammatory or not. It has been strongly associated with diabetes and rheumatoid arthritis (Lee, Nasser-Sharif, & Zelouf, 2002). Medical management often consists of a mixture of steroid and local anesthetic injected into the flexor sheath. The injection may be repeated a few times. Therapy consists of splinting the MP in neutral to prevent composite digital flexion (preventing triggering), while promoting tendon gliding, and place-and-hold fisting that avoids triggering. Built-up handles, padded gloves, and pacing strategies are helpful. Instruct the patient to avoid triggering, as this re-inflames the tissue. See the classic article by Evans, Hunter, and Burkhalter (1988). If symptoms persist, the surgeon may surgically release the A-1 pulley.

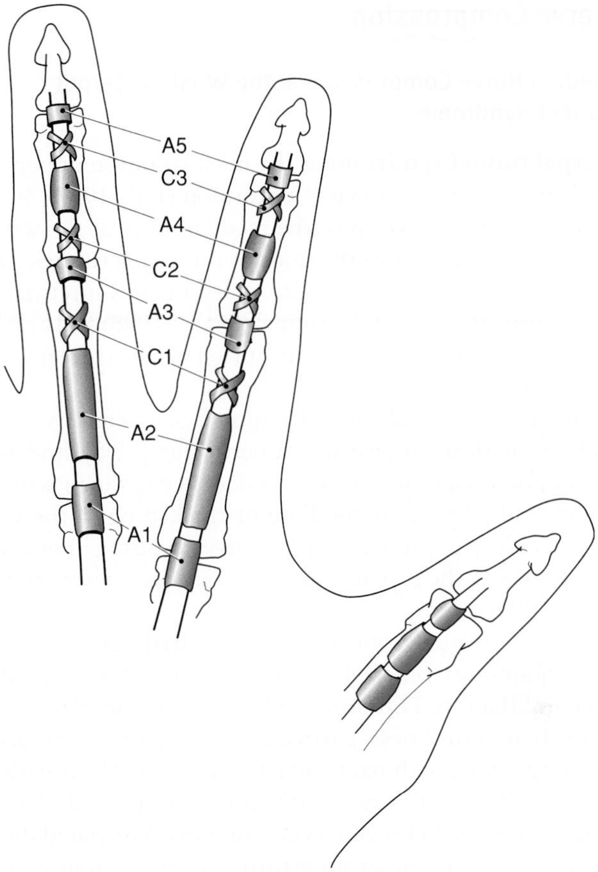

Figure 42-7 Pulley system. (Adapted with permission from Reiner, M. [1991]. *The illustrated hand.* St. Paul: Minnesota Hand Rehabilitation.)

Nerve Injury

When injury or disease occurs to a neural structure in the upper extremity, there is a high likelihood that multiple areas of neural pathology will develop. This phenomenon is known as the double or multiple crush syndrome (Posner, 1998). Remembering this concept lessens the possibility of missing relevant clinical findings.

The various mechanisms of nerve injury include acute or chronic compression, stretch ischemia, electrical shock, radiation, injection, and laceration (Smith, 2002). Compression and laceration, impairments that are commonly seen by hand therapists, are described next.

Nerve Compression

Median Nerve Compression at the Wrist, or Carpal Tunnel Syndrome

Carpal tunnel syndrome is the most common upper extremity nerve entrapment (Concannon et al., 1997). It results from compression of the median nerve at the wrist. The carpal bones form the floor of the carpal tunnel. The transverse carpal ligament, also called the flexor retinaculum, forms the roof of the tunnel (Szabo, 1998) and acts as a pulley for the flexor tendons during gripping (Netscher et al., 1998).

Inside the carpal canal are nine flexor tendons (four FDP, four flexor digitorum superficialis [FDS], and the flexor pollicis longus) and the median nerve, which is most superficial (Fig. 42-8). Swelling or thickening of the tendons can lead to pressure on the nerve, resulting in sensory symptoms in the distribution of the median nerve (Hayes et al., 2002).

Carpal tunnel syndrome occurs with greatest frequency among women 40–60 years of age and is frequently bilateral (Lam & Thurston, 1998). Typical complaints include hand numbness, particularly at night or when driving a car, along with pain and paresthesias in the distribution of the median nerve (thumb through radial ring finger pads), and clumsiness or weakness. Associated diagnoses include rheumatoid arthritis, Colles' fracture, diabetes, deconditioning (Mooney, 1998), obesity (Lam & Thurston, 1998), and thyroid disease (Szabo, 1998). Transient carpal tunnel syndrome is fairly common in pregnancy (Stolp-Smith, Pascoe, & Ogburn, 1998). Carpal tunnel syndrome may be associated with repetitive use (Keir, Bach, & Rempel, 1998) or flexor tenosynovitis (Donaldson et al., 1998) caused by increased friction between the tendons and nerve (Mooney, 1998). For these people, focus intervention on resolving the tendinitis.

Evaluation

Perform a cervical screening, and evaluate posture, ROM, grip and pinch, and manual muscle testing looking for independent excursion of FDP and FDS. Also do Tinel's, Phalen's, *Semmes-Weinstein Monofilament*, and two-point discrimination tests (Sailer, 1996). Tapping at the volar wrist elicits Tinel's sign, which is a sensation of tingling or electric shock if the median nerve is compromised. Phalen's test provokes sensory symptoms in the median nerve distribution if positive, created by maintaining the wrist in flexion for 60 seconds (Tubiana, Thomine, & Mackin, 1996). Phalen's test should be done with extended elbows to avoid confusing these findings with a positive elbow flexion test (see section on cubital tunnel syndrome). Advanced cases of carpal tunnel syndrome reveal thenar atrophy of the abductor pollicis brevis, which can be functionally debilitating (Aulicino, 2002; Concannon et al., 1997).

Intervention

Conservative medical management may include steroid injection (Terrono & Millender, 1996). Conservative therapy for carpal tunnel syndrome includes night splinting with the wrist in neutral because this position minimizes pressure in the carpal tunnel; exercises for median nerve gliding at the wrist (Fig. 42-9); differential flexor tendon gliding exercises (Fig. 42-3); aerobic exercise; proximal conditioning; ergonomic modification; and postural training (Donaldson et al., 1998; Rozmaryn et al., 1998). Teach patients to avoid extremes of forearm

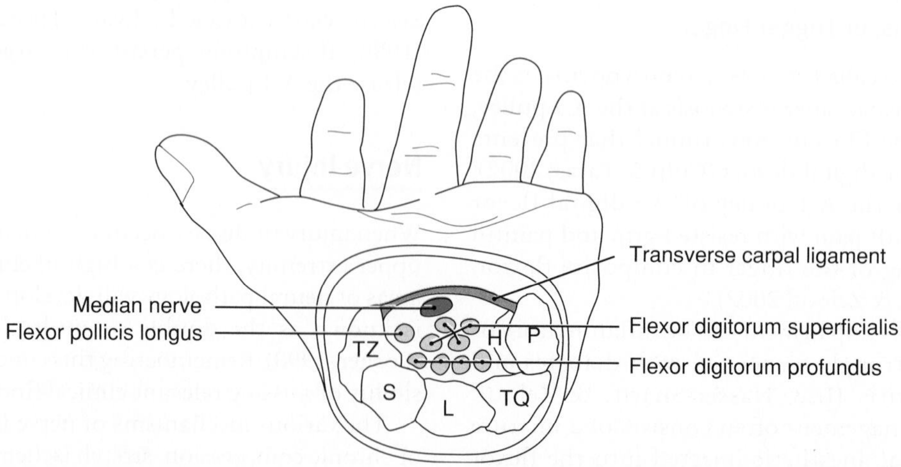

Figure 42-8 Carpal tunnel cross-section. TZ, trapezium; S, scaphoid; L, lunate; TQ, triquetrum; P, pisiform; H, hook of Hamate. (Adapted with permission from Reiner, M. [1991]. *The illustrated hand.* St. Paul: Minnesota Hand Rehabilitation.)

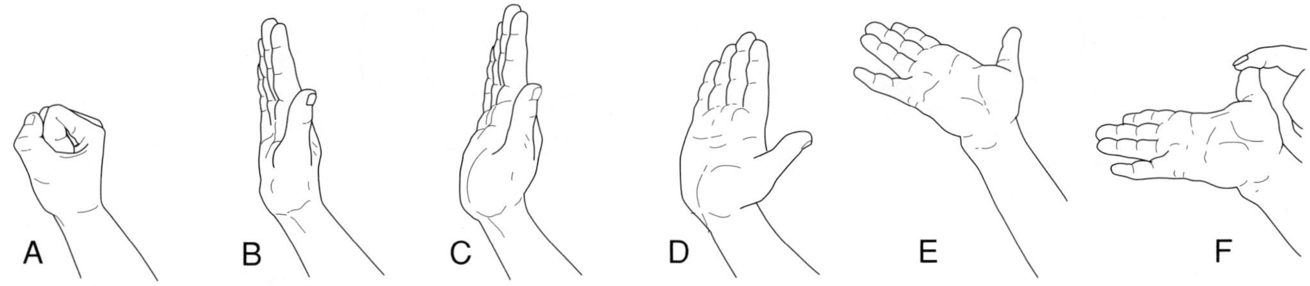

Figure 42-9 Median nerve gliding exercises at the wrist. Positions: **A.** Neutral wrist with finger and thumb flexion. **B.** Fingers and thumb extended. **C.** Wrist and fingers extended with thumb in neutral; **D.** Thumb extended. **E.** Forearm supinated. **F.** Thumb gently stretched into extension. (Adapted with permission from Rozmaryn, L. M., Dovelle, S., Rothman, E. R., Gorman, K., Olvey, K. M., & Bartko, J. J. [1998]. Nerve and tendon gliding exercises and the conservative management of carpal tunnel syndrome. *Journal of Hand Therapy, 11,* 171–179.)

rotation or of wrist motions and to avoid sustained pinch or forceful grip. Provide padded gloves and built-up handles (Sailer, 1996). Thick padded steering wheel covers are helpful.

Surgical intervention consists of decompression of the carpal tunnel by division of the transverse carpal ligament (Hayes et al., 2002). Carpal tunnel release is one of the 10 most frequent surgeries performed in the United States (Rozmaryn et al., 1998). Post-operative therapy, when necessary, consists of edema control, scar management, desensitization as needed, nerve and tendon gliding exercises (Skirven & Trope, 1994), and eventual strengthening. Many therapists postpone strengthening exercises until at least 6 weeks following carpal tunnel release to avoid inflammation. Patients with new and mild symptoms tend to recover best (Aulisa et al., 1998).

Ulnar Nerve Compression at the Elbow, or Cubital Tunnel Syndrome

Cubital tunnel syndrome is the second most common upper extremity nerve entrapment and is the most commonly compressed site of the ulnar nerve, at its location between the medial epicondyle and the olecranon (Posner, 1998). Typical complaints include proximal and medial forearm pain that is aching or sharp; decreased sensation of the dorsal and palmar surfaces of the small finger and the ulnar half of the ring finger; and weakness of interossei, adductor pollicis, flexor carpi ulnaris, and flexor digitorum profundus of the ring and small fingers. Clawing may be more evident if the FDP is not involved because the long flexors are unopposed. Wartenberg's sign, the inability to adduct the small finger, and Froment's sign, in which effort at lateral pinch elicits thumb IP flexion due to weakness of the adductor pollicis, may be seen. Grip and pinch strength are decreased, and patients complain of dropping things (Khoo, Carmichael, & Spinner, 1996). Symptoms are worse when the elbow is flexed repeatedly or is kept in flexion because this position dramatically reduces the volume of the cubital tunnel (Bozentka, 1998). Understandably, symptoms may increase at night if the person sleeps with the elbow flexed (Blackmore, 2002).

Cubital tunnel syndrome may result from trauma, such as a blow to the elbow or fracture or dislocation of the supracondylar or medial epicondylar area, or it may be due to chronic mild pressure on the elbow. Associated diagnoses include osteoarthritis, rheumatoid arthritis, diabetes, and Hansen's disease (Osterman & Davis, 1996).

Evaluation

Tapping over the cubital tunnel elicits a positive Tinel's sign. However, Tinel's sign may also be positive in 20% of normal people (Khoo, Carmichael, & Spinner, 1996). The elbow flexion test is positive if passively flexing the elbow and holding it flexed for 60 seconds produces sensory symptoms (Tetro & Pichora, 1996). Keep the wrist neutral while performing the elbow flexion test so as not to confound the findings with Phalen's test. Look for digital clawing and for muscle atrophy in the first web space, hypothenar eminence, and medial forearm. Perform grip and pinch testing and manual muscle testing as appropriate, and test sensation (Osterman & Davis, 1996).

Intervention

Conservative therapy for cubital tunnel syndrome includes edema control; splinting or padding the elbow; and positioning guidelines to avoid leaning on the elbow, to avoid elbow flexed postures, and to avoid elbow-intensive activity (Khoo, Carmichael, & Spinner, 1996). Elbow splinting helps prevent sleeping with the elbow flexed. Types of splints include elbow pads or soft splints, pillows, and anterior or posterior thermoplastic splints. The splinted elbow position for sleeping is usually about 30° of flexion. Additional therapy includes proximal conditioning, postural and ergonomic training, and ulnar nerve gliding exercises (Fig. 42-10).

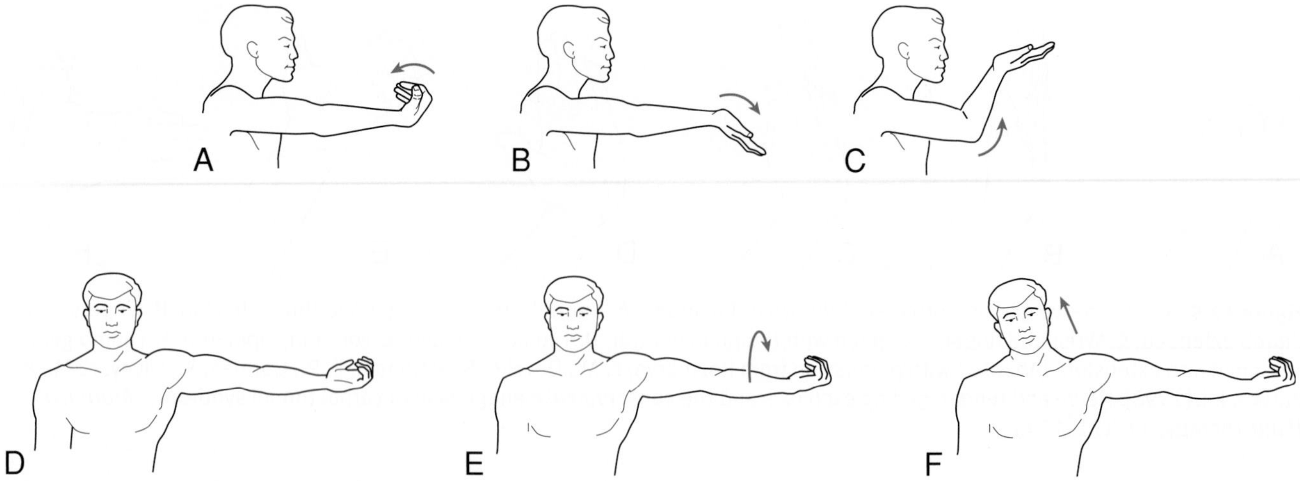

Figure 42-10 Ulnar nerve gliding exercises. **A.** Extend the arm with elbow straight and wrist and fingers flexed. **B.** Extend the wrist and fingers. **C.** Flex the elbow. **D.** Abduct the shoulder with wrist and fingers flexed. **E.** Externally rotate the shoulder. **F.** Laterally flex the neck. (Adapted with permission from Byron, P. M. [1995]. Upper extremity nerve gliding programs used at the Philadelphia Hand Center. In J. M. Hunter, E. J. Mackin, & A. D. Callahan [Eds.], *Rehabilitation of the hand: Surgery and therapy* [4th ed., p. 954]. St. Louis: Mosby.)

Radial Nerve Compression, or Posterior Interosseous Nerve Syndrome

Posterior interosseous nerve syndrome is purely motor. It presents two clinical pictures. In one, paralysis affects all muscles innervated by the posterior interosseous nerve, with inability to extend the MP joints of thumb, index, long, ring, or small fingers. Wrist extension occurs only radially because of paralysis of extensor digitorum and ECU. In the other presentation of this syndrome, the person cannot extend the MP joint of one or more digits. Paralysis may spread to other digits if it is not treated on a timely basis (Spinner, 1995).

A common site of entrapment of the posterior interosseous nerve is at the supinator muscle, where it pierces the two heads of this muscle. Other causes include soft tissue tumors, rheumatoid arthritis with synovial proliferation, and radial head fractures or dislocations (Spinner, 1995). Therapy focuses on maintaining PROM and splinting to prevent deformity and promote function.

Nerve Laceration

Nerve lacerations are categorized as complete or partial. Stretching and contusion injuries can occur along with the laceration. Nerve reconstruction is termed primary if within 48 hours, early secondary if within 6 weeks, and late secondary after 3 months. The advantages associated with primary repair are that nerve stump retraction is limited and electrical stimulation can be used to identify distal fascicles (Smith, 2002).

A **neuroma**, a disorganized mass of nerve fibers, can follow nerve injury. Significant nerve pain is elicited by tapping over the neuroma, with hypersensitivity limiting functional use of the hand. Desensitization techniques are helpful, along with padding over the painful area to promote functional use (Smith, 2002).

Following nerve injury, therapy promotes functional performance in the areas of occupation with ADL training and adaptive equipment and assists in prevention of deformity with splinting and appropriate PROM. Hand therapy provides valuable education to patients about their diagnosis and general recovery sequence and teaches protective guidelines to compensate for sensory loss. Hand therapy monitors changes in sensory and motor function and helps prevent joint contractures and imbalance by reevaluating ROM, sensation, and muscle status. Splint modifications are based on clinical changes over time.

Low Median Nerve Lesion

Median nerve laceration at the wrist results in low median nerve palsy, with denervation of the opponens pollicis (OP) and abductor pollicis brevis of the thumb and of the lumbricals to the index and long fingers. Clawing of the index and long fingers does not usually occur because the interossei remain ulnarly innervated. Loss of sensation of the radial side of the hand is present. With the absence of thumb abduction and opposition, the thumb rests in adduction, where it may become contracted (Fig. 42-11). Fabricate a hand-based thumb abduction splint to maintain balance, to substitute for lost thumb opposition, and to prevent overstretching of denervated muscles (Colditz, 2002a).

Median nerve laceration creates serious functional loss of manipulation and sensibility of the thumb, index, and

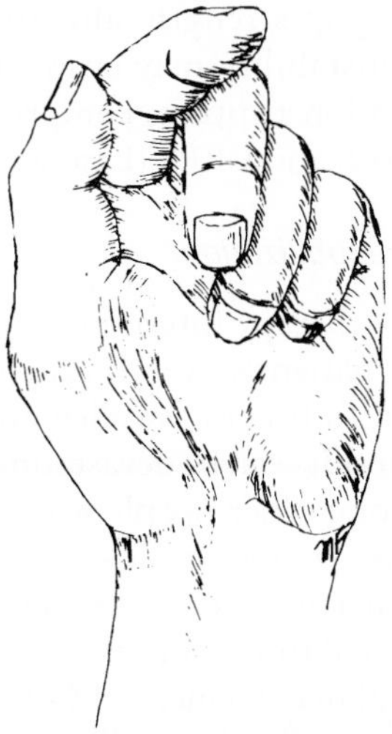

Figure 42-11 Thenar wasting (atrophy of thumb) due to median nerve problem. (From Snell, R. S. [2003]. *Clinical anatomy* [7th ed.]. Baltimore: Lippincott Williams & Wilkins.)

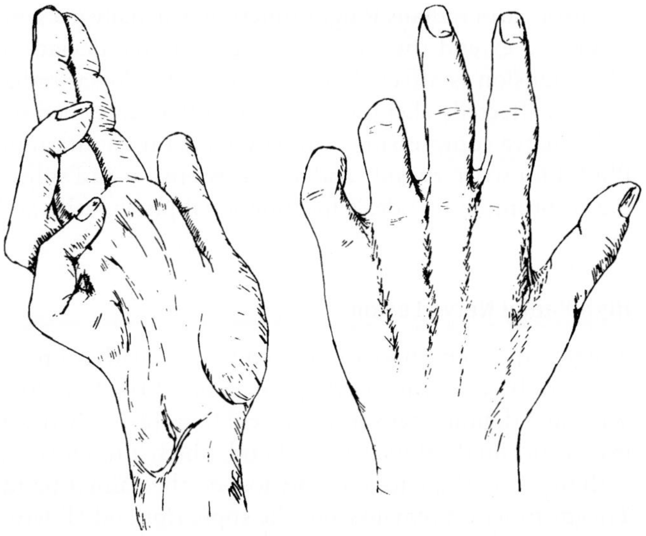

Figure 42-12 Clawing of digits seen with ulnar nerve problems. (From Snell, R. S. [2003]. *Clinical anatomy* [7th ed.]. Baltimore: Lippincott Williams & Wilkins.)

long fingers. Motor recovery usually occurs before sensory recovery. Be sure to teach compensatory strategies to avoid reinjury while sensibility is impaired (Colditz, 2002a). Instruct the patient to perform PROM to maintain joint mobility. Fabricate splints to sustain thumb abduction and digital MP flexion with IP extension to promote functional hand use and to counteract the deforming forces of the injury.

High Median Nerve Lesion

Injury near or at the elbow is called a high median nerve injury. Along with the motor loss identified earlier, there is denervation of FDP to index and long fingers, FDS to all digits, pronator teres, and pronator quadratus. The median nerve is considered the most important sensory nerve, and its loss severely compromises hand function. In therapy, prepare patients for probable tendon transfers by preventing deformity with splinting and by maintaining PROM of pronation, of digital MPs in flexion, of digital IPs in extension, and of thumb CMC abduction (Colditz, 2002a). Visual cues, adaptive devices, and modified handles may help compensate for the functional loss.

Low Ulnar Nerve Lesion

Laceration of the ulnar nerve at the wrist level is called a low ulnar lesion. This injury results in loss of most of the hand intrinsics. Denervation of the adductor digiti minimi, flexor digiti minimi, and opponens digiti minimi results in flattening of the hand with loss of the ulnar transverse metacarpal arch; denervation of thumb adductor pollicis (AP) and deep head of flexor pollicis brevis results in loss of thumb adduction and MP support; denervation of dorsal and volar interossei results in loss of digital abduction or adduction; and denervation of lumbricals to the ring and small fingers results in extrinsic imbalance. The ring and small fingers present a **claw deformity**, a position of MP hyperextension and PIP flexion associated with muscle imbalance in ulnar-innervated structures (Fig. 42-12). Fine manipulation skills are compromised (Colditz, 2002a). Sensory loss involves the ulnar digits.

Splinting for ulnar nerve palsy aims to prevent overstretching of the denervated ring and small finger intrinsics. An MP blocking splint that maintains slight MP flexion and prevents MP extension is recommended (Colditz, 2002a) (see Chapter 16). Teach patients to compensate for sensory loss and to maintain passive range of the MPs in flexion and the IPs in extension. It is very important to prevent PIP flexion contractures. Built-up handles in conjunction with the MP blocking splint may be helpful.

High Ulnar Nerve Lesion

A high ulnar nerve lesion is often identified with trauma at or proximal to the elbow. There is involvement of the muscles listed earlier and denervation of FDP of ring and small fingers and of FCU. Ring and small finger clawing is less apparent with the high lesion but becomes noticeable as the FDP are reinnervated and are unopposed by the still-absent intrinsics. Splinting and treatment are the same as for a low ulnar nerve lesion. If the FDP is absent, teach the patient to maintain full PROM of the IPs of the ring and small fingers to prevent contractures (Colditz, 2002a).

Low Radial Nerve Lesion

Low radial nerve injury of the deep motor branch is called posterior interosseous palsy. Presentations vary (see section on radial nerve compression), but brachioradialis and extensor carpi radialis longus function is usually present. Efforts to extend the wrist yield strong radial deviation. MP extension is affected. Sensation on the dorsal radial hand is affected. Therapy is similar to that described for radial nerve compression, with emphasis on maintaining PROM for wrist, thumb, and digital extension and splinting to promote tenodesis for functional pinch, grip, and release.

High Radial Nerve Lesion

A high radial nerve injury is seen commonly with humeral fractures because this nerve spirals around the humerus. Wrist and digital extensors are absent (Fig. 42-13). Sensory loss occurs on the dorsal-radial hand, which interferes less with function than does sensory loss on the palmar hand. Triceps function remains, but the supinator and all wrist and finger extensors lose function. Tenodesis is lost (Colditz, 2002a).

Splinting restores tenodesis and may be useful for many months during the wait for reinnervation, which occurs at approximately 1 inch per month. Various static and dynamic splints are available; the dynamic splints are most useful functionally. Many patients make good use of both types of splints. Compliance tends to be good because of the functional value of these splints. It is important to maintain joint suppleness while awaiting reinnervation or reconstructive surgery (Colditz, 2002a).

Fractures

Distal Radius Fracture

Distal radius fractures are among the most common upper extremity fractures (Laseter, 2002). Hand therapists frequently treat patients with this diagnosis. Distal radius fractures should not be confused with fractures of the carpal bones. The main complication associated with distal radius fracture is traumatic arthritis due to poor articular congruency (Leibovic, 1999). Decreased wrist ROM, decreased grip strength, alteration of the carpal alignment, and instability may ensue. Other complications include tendon rupture, compression of the median or ulnar nerve, and CRPS (Laseter, 2002).

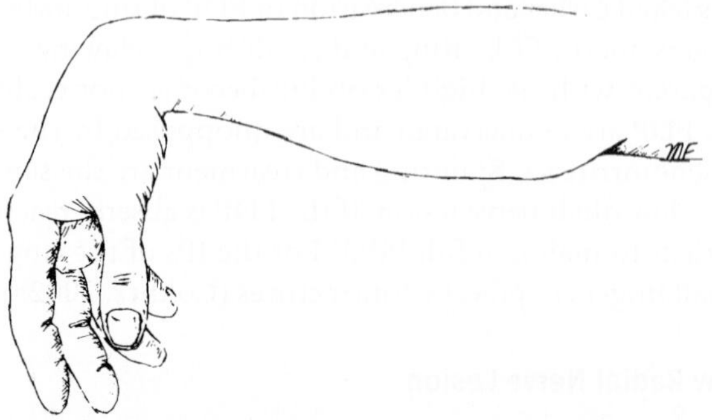

Figure 42-13 Wrist drop due to radial nerve problem. (From Snell, R. S. [2003]. *Clinical anatomy* [7th ed.]. Baltimore: Lippincott Williams & Wilkins.)

Therapy During Immobilization

Appropriate early therapy intervention can make a huge difference in the patient's overall functional recovery. If digits are allowed to become swollen and stiff, the long-term functional results can be devastating. These fractures are common among older people with osteoporosis and balance problems. Temporary loss of independence following fracture can trigger an irreversible downward spiral in their occupational functioning.

Typical medical management of Colles' fracture is cast immobilization, usually above elbow with the elbow in 90° of flexion to prevent forearm rotation during the first 3 weeks. When the patient is put in a short arm cast and the elbow is freed, begin elbow AROM for flexion and extension, but avoid resisted elbow motion so as not to stress the fracture healing. Do not perform elbow PROM without medical clearance, and be very gentle. Biceps tightness commonly follows elbow immobilization.

Certain fractures require an external fixator and/or internal fixation. Some physicians delay the referral of patients to therapy, but postponing the initiation of therapy can result in significant problems with edema and decreased ROM. It is a good idea to communicate with referring physicians and encourage routine early therapy referral for this diagnosis.

While the patient is in an external fixator, provide pin site care as the physician prescribes using sterile technique and universal precautions (Bryan & Kohnke, 1997). Teach the patient digital ROM and tendon gliding exercises, and instruct in precautions related to cast wearing. It is critical to monitor for cast tightness because this can cause CRPS. Call the physician if the cast is too tight. Discourage the use of slings because they promote unnecessary proximal stiffness, guarded posture, and disuse (Collins, 1993).

Insidious onset of shoulder restrictions is problematic and best avoided. Physicians most assuredly appreciate therapists' input regarding early signs of this problem. To prevent a frozen shoulder, proximal ROM is a high treatment priority (Skirven & Trope, 1994). Instruct in shoulder flexion, abduction, internal rotation, and external rotation (Collins, 1993). Perform as thorough a physical assessment as tolerated and as cast constraints permit. This may have to be done in phases. Early identification of guarding, excessive pain, or autonomic signs can alert the team to the possibility of CRPS.

Following distal radius fracture, the recovery of function depends on restoration of motion and strength and on maximizing the length-tension relationship of the digital flexors and extensors (Collins, 1993). Edema can contribute to decreased ROM at uncasted areas. Patients are often surprised that uninjured and uncasted areas can stiffen.

The goals of early therapy during immobilization are to normalize edema and to achieve as nearly normal AROM of uncasted areas as possible (Collins, 1993). During this period, intrinsic tightness, extrinsic tightness, and digital joint tightness may occur (Skirven & Trope, 1994). The chance of tendon adherence is increased following open reduction and its accompanying incisional scar. Various blocking splints may be used with functional activity and exercise to resolve joint or musculotendinous tightness (Fig. 42-4). Differential tendon gliding exercises are extremely important. Frequent exercise throughout the day is better than a few long sessions. It is generally advised to perform exercises every hour or two, perhaps 5–10 repetitions each, maintaining the end position comfortably for 3–5 seconds. Incorporate exercises into occupation, including ADL, as much as possible (Bryan & Kohnke, 1997).

If extrinsic musculotendinous tightness persists, it may be appropriate to add night static progressive splinting or low-load, long-duration dynamic splinting in conjunction with exercise to normalize extrinsic length (Collins, 1993). Consult the physician before making this determination.

Therapy After Cast or Fixator Is Removed

When fracture immobilization is discontinued, physicians often recommend a custom-fabricated volar wrist splint. This is protective and can be corrective to help restore functional wrist motion (usually extension). This temporary support is particularly helpful if the patient maintains habitual wrist flexion because this "doggy paw" posture leads to development of the undesirable deformity position of MP extension, PIP flexion, and thumb adduction and extension discussed earlier (Skirven & Trope, 1994).

Following removal of the cast or external fixator, there is usually measurable limitation in ROM, with patients reporting awkwardness and decreased function (Byl, Kohlhase, & Engel, 1999). Consult the physician for medical clearance and guidelines for forearm and wrist ROM. ***Do not initiate PROM of the wrist without medical clearance because this may be injurious.*** Teach the patient to wean off the protective splint according to the physician's guidelines, which are individualized. Edema control continues to be the highest priority until it is resolved. AROM and ADL can help correct the edema.

At any time, but especially in this early stage, overzealous therapy is harmful. Patients and families who think they should be aggressive in their home programs need education and reinforcement to avoid overdoing it. Use written material and illustrations to teach them how to observe tissue responses and monitor inflammation (Colditz, 2002b). Temperature elevation over the joints of digits may indicate that intervention is eliciting an inflammatory reaction and should be adjusted accordingly (Fess, 1993).

It is extremely important to retrain the wrist extensors to function independently of the extensor digitorum (Laseter & Carter, 1996). Have the patient practice wrist extension with available composite digital flexion, being especially sure the MPs are flexed. Then have the patient flex the wrist with digits relaxed but extended to isolate the wrist flexors. As substitution patterns are hard to overcome, early training of biomechanically efficient movement is best. Progressive grasp-and-release activities reinforce this tenodesis training. It is also important to retrain the extensor digitorum to function independently of the intrinsics. Have the patient extend the MPs with the IPs slightly flexed to isolate the extensor digitorum.

Gradually upgrade therapy with increasingly challenging motions, combined motions, and activities aiming to restore joint suppleness and musculotendinous lengths. Dexterity activities, such as cat's cradle, and games, such as pick-up sticks, promote spontaneous functional movements. Sorting drawers and folding small items of clothing are good home activities. Initiate graded functional strengthening with medical clearance, usually after good motion has been achieved. Again, it is easy to be too aggressive with these patients. Upgrade carefully, monitor patient and tissue responses, and adjust the intervention accordingly.

Scaphoid Fracture

Some 60% of carpal fractures affect the scaphoid (also called the navicular) bone. The mechanism of injury is usually a fall on the outstretched hand (called FOOSH). Associated ligamentous injury may also be present. Tenderness in the anatomical snuffbox, a depression at the base of the thumb between the EPL and EPB tendons, where snuff used to be placed, is a classic finding. Scaphoid fracture may be difficult to confirm radiographically initially and may not become apparent until 3 weeks following injury due to resorption at the fracture site. Once fracture is confirmed, the thumb is usually included in the cast, with the IP joint free.

Proximal scaphoid fractures may be at risk for developing avascular necrosis because of the pattern of vascular supply. Casting time may be long for this reason. Hand therapy principles are the same as for distal radius fracture (Dell & Dell, 2002).

Non-Articular Hand Fracture

Fracture occurs more often in the hand than any other area, and more than 50% of hand fractures occur at work. Motor vehicle accidents, household injuries, and recreational accidents also account for many of these injuries (Meyer & Wilson, 1995) (Fig. 42-14).

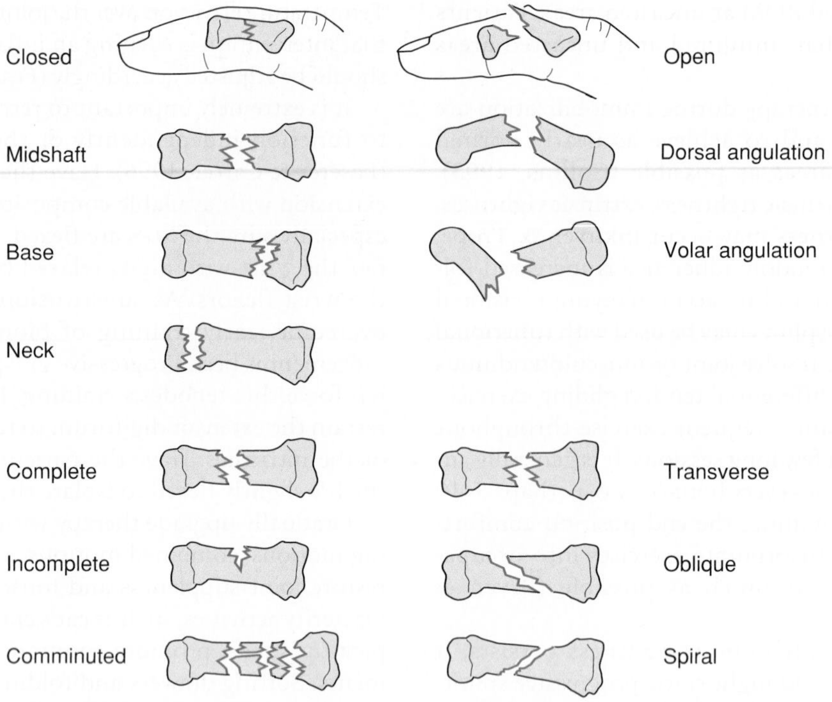

Figure 42-14 Fracture terminology. (Adapted with permission from American Society for Surgery of the Hand. [1990]. *The hand: Examination and diagnosis* [3rd ed.]. New York: Churchill Livingstone.)

Distal Phalanx Fracture

Distal phalanx digital fractures typically result from a crushing injury and occur most often in the thumb and middle finger. Tuft fractures occur at the distal tip. They are extremely painful, in part because there is often a subungual (i.e., beneath the nail) hematoma (Meyer & Wilson, 1995). Following a distal phalanx fracture, hypersensitivity, pain, and decreased ROM of the DIP joint may occur (Skirven & Trope, 1994). Monitor closely for signs of DIP extensor lag or the inability to extend the DIP joint actively despite full available passive extension (Meyer & Wilson, 1995).

Middle Phalanx Fracture

At the middle phalanx, fractures angulate according to their relation to the FDS insertion. Medical management and early positioning guidelines vary among caregivers. Following middle phalanx fractures, decreased PIP and DIP ROM are common problems. Fractures at this site may require long immobilization time for healing, with resulting stiffness. When the patient is medically cleared for therapy, isolated FDS exercises are very important. Here, too, PIP joint flexion contractures are serious complications that can occur in as little as 2 weeks of immobilization in flexion. Consult with the physician for therapy guidelines based on fracture stability and healing (Russell, 1999).

Proximal Phalanx Fracture

At the proximal phalanx, fractures tend to angulate with a palmar apex. This deforming force is due to the action of the intrinsic muscles on the proximal fragment (Purdy & Wilson, 2002). With proximal phalanx fractures, a hand-based splint in intrinsic-plus (anti-deformity) position is useful at night. A digit-based extension splint provides support and protection in the day except during exercise. Again, the physician provides therapy guidelines based on fracture stability and healing. PIP joint flexion contractures are the most likely and difficult complication. Watch for these, and catch them early. Better yet, avoid them with appropriate splinting and structure-specific exercise. PIP extensor lag and flexor tendon adherence at the fracture site are other serious problems (Purdy & Wilson, 2002).

Metacarpal Fracture

Unless there is associated trauma, metacarpal fractures at the base are frequently stable. Metacarpal fractures at the shaft may be transverse, oblique, or spiral. Metacarpal fractures at the neck are common, occurring most often in the small finger. They may result in muscle imbalance between the intrinsics and extrinsics (Purdy & Wilson, 2002).

With metacarpal fractures, dorsal hand edema is a frequent complication that can contribute to MP joint dorsal capsular tightness. If there is associated soft tissue injury, intrinsic contracture or extensor digitorum adherence may occur (Skirven & Trope, 1994). Appropriate early therapy and preventive edema control are important (Purdy & Wilson, 2002).

Unstable fractures require fixation to achieve stability and allow early ROM. **Kirschner wires**, a common form of fixation used for hand fractures, may be used alone or in conjunction with additional fixation. Other forms of internal fixation include tension band wires, lag screws, plates, and mini external fixators (Leibovic, 1999). Functional recovery relates to anatomical restoration. To maximize functional outcomes, the ideal situation allows for early motion. Preventing stiffness of uninvolved digits is a high priority that can itself be challenging. Prolonged immobilization is associated with edema and pain. Persistent edema results in joint and tendon scar and adhesions; atrophy occurs, as well as osteoporosis (Meyer & Wilson, 1995).

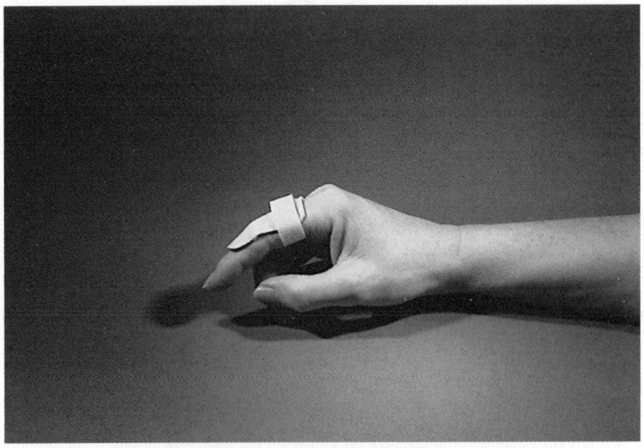

Figure 42-15 Dorsal PIP extension–blocking splint. Protective digit-based splint maintains slight PIP flexion. Used to prevent full extension to protect volar plate injury.

Collateral Ligament Injury

PIP Joint Sprain

PIP joint sprains often result from sports involving balls. Their severity, which may be underappreciated, is described as grade I through grade III. In grade I, the ligament remains intact, but there is diffuse individual fiber disruption. In grade II, there is complete disruption of one of the joint capsule's major retaining ligaments. In grade III, there is complete disruption of one collateral ligament in addition to injury to dorsal and/or volar capsular structures. Pain, decreased ROM, and risk of flexion contracture are the most common problems associated with grade I and II injuries. Joint instability may occur with grade III injuries (Campbell & Wilson, 2002).

Therapy focuses on edema control, joint protection, and ROM. Buddy straps are helpful to protect or to promote movement. They may be offset to improve fit (Fig. 42-5) (Jensen & Rayan, 1996). Splinting is both protective and corrective. A dorsal extension blocking splint is often ordered early on for volar plate injuries associated with dorsal PIP joint dislocation (Fig. 42-15) (Lairmore & Engber, 1998). Persistent thickening about the joint commonly occurs, interfering with recovery of ROM.

Skier's Thumb

Disruption of the ulnar collateral ligament of the thumb MP joint occurs with acute radial deviation. This diagnosis, which may entail avulsion of bone fragment at the ligamentous insertion, is often seen among people who fall while skiing (Lairmore & Engber, 1998). Injury to the radial collateral ligament of the thumb MP occurs only one tenth as often (Campbell & Wilson, 2002). Following surgical repair, the wrist and thumb are casted. When therapy begins, IP ROM is the priority because full MP flexion may not be achieved, especially among older patients. Avoid resistive exercise until medically cleared. Then begin with lateral pinch but avoid tip pinch until further medical clearance, which may not be for 12 weeks, as tip pinch is strenuous on the injured structures. Use a hand-based spica splint for protection. Scar hypersensitivity due to the underlying radial sensory nerve is common.

Flexor Tendon Injury

Surgical repair of flexor tendon injury is a complex undertaking performed by specialists in the field. Like the surgery, hand therapy for these patients is a complicated and specialized area. Therapy can be time consuming, and it entails substantial education of the patient, with subtle but significant changes in splinting and exercise at every session to promote function while protecting fragile repaired structures. Multiple structures are often involved, and there are many precautions and contraindications that vary according to the details of the patient's surgery and the surgeon's specifications and preferences. It is essential to maintain close communication with the patient's surgeon. A therapist experienced in the treatment of these patients should closely supervise their care.

Five anatomical zones describe flexor tendon injury to the index, long, ring, and small digits (Fig. 42-16). Zone I is from the insertion of the FDS to the insertion of the FDP. Zone II is the area where the FDS and FDP both lie within the flexor sheath, from the A-1 pulley to the FDS insertion. This region has memorably been dubbed "no man's land" to reflect the technical challenge and historically poor prognosis for repair in this area (Wang & Gupta, 1996). Zone III describes the area from the distal edge of the carpal tunnel to the A-1 pulley of the flexor

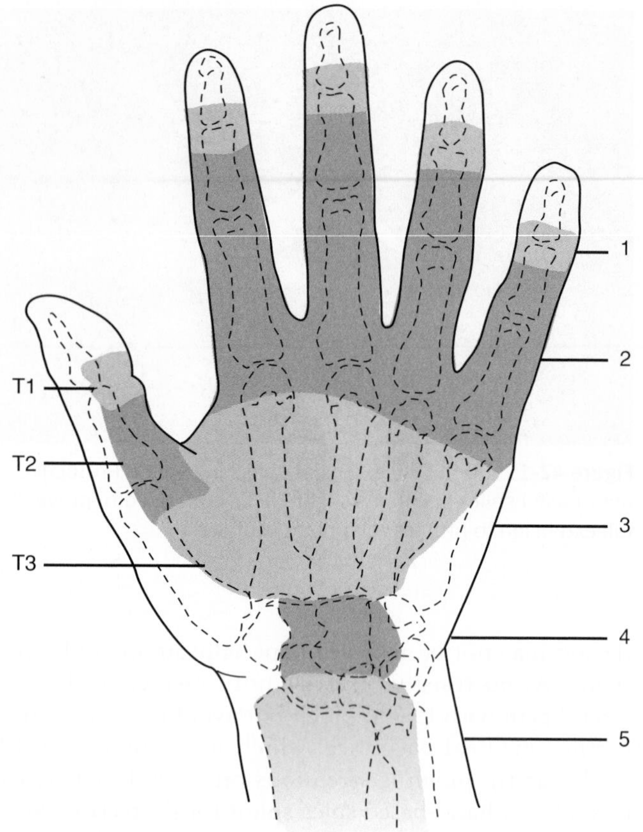

Figure 42-16 Flexor tendon zones. (Adapted with permission from Kleinert, H. H., Schepel, S., & Gill, T. [1981]. Flexor tendon injuries. *Surgical Clinics of North America, 61,* 267–286. Stewart, K. M., & van Strien, G. [1995]. Postoperative management of flexor tendon injuries. In J. M. Hunter, E. J. Mackin, & A. D. Callahan [Eds.], *Rehabilitation of the hand: Surgery and therapy* [4th ed., pp. 433–462]. St. Louis: Mosby.)

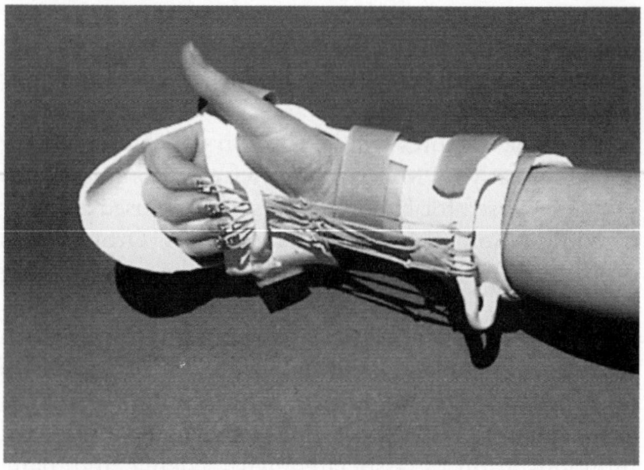

Figure 42-17 Modified Kleinert splint. Dorsal splint maintains the wrist in 30° of flexion, MPs in 70° of flexion, and IPs in extension. Rubber band attachments provide passive digital flexion.

sheath, including the lumbrical muscles. Zone IV is where the flexor tendons lie under the transverse carpal ligament in the carpal tunnel. Injuries in this zone may include the median and ulnar nerves. Zone V is the area from the forearm flexor musculotendinous junction to the border of the transverse carpal ligament (Culp & Taras, 2002).

Physicians usually indicate specific postoperative positioning guidelines to protect repaired structures following flexor tendon repair. The goals are twofold and contradictory: to minimize adhesion formation and to prevent gap or attenuation of the repaired tendon (Silva et al., 1998). These dual goals highlight the complexity of therapy associated with this diagnosis. Various protocols exist for controlled mobilization, using a dorsal splint with the wrist in about 30° of flexion, MP joints in about 70° of flexion, and IP joints ideally in full extension (Wang & Gupta, 1996). The involved IP joints may have to be in some flexion if a digital nerve has been repaired. The Duran protocol entails passive digital flexion and extension within the protective splint to achieve 3–5 mm of differential digital tendon excursion. With this protocol, gentle active motion begins with medical clearance about 4 or 5 weeks after surgery (Culp & Taras, 2002).

The passive flexion–active extension protocol, also called the Kleinert protocol, uses rubber band attachments to the fingernails to provide passive digital flexion within the protective dorsal splint (Fig. 42-17). The patient performs gentle active digital extension and the rubber band provides passive digital flexion within the confines of the protective splint. Exercises are gradually increased to 10 repetitions comfortably every waking hour. At night, the digits may be strapped carefully and comfortably to the dorsal hood of the splint to counteract the tendency to develop PIP or DIP flexion contractures (Wang & Gupta, 1996).

The Chow protocol uses a combination of the Duran and Kleinert techniques. With advances in suture techniques, some caregivers are advocating early active motion protocols (Winters et al., 1998).

When the physician gives medical clearance to discontinue the dorsal protective splint, begin a graded program to promote functional movement. Edema control and scar management remain high clinical priorities. Assess closely and determine tissue-specific limitations that guide the therapy program. Tendon gliding exercises and place-and-hold exercises are typical early techniques. Corrective splinting is useful, along with ADL, graded activity, and upgraded exercise as appropriate.

Staged Flexor Tendon Reconstruction

Staged flexor tendon reconstruction is a complex two-part procedure. It is highly advisable to have an experienced hand therapist supervise the treatment. Staged

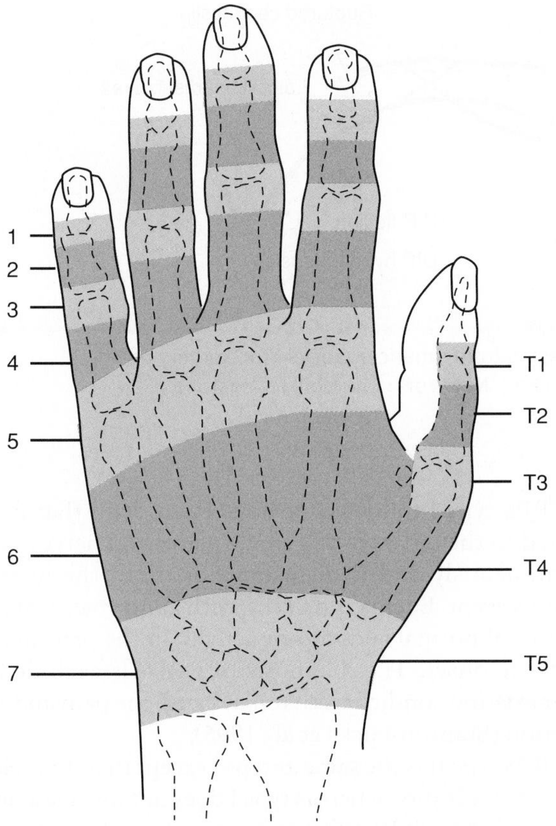

Figure 42-18 Extensor tendon zones. (Adapted with permission from Kleinert, H. H., Schepel, S., & Gill, T. [1981]. Flexor tendon injuries. *Surgical Clinics of North America, 61,* 267–286; Evans, R. B. [1995]. An update on extensor tendon management. In J. M. Hunter, E. J. Mackin, & A. D. Callahan [Eds.], *Rehabilitation of the hand: Surgery and therapy* [4th ed., pp. 565–606]. St. Louis: Mosby.)

flexor tendon surgery is chosen when there is significant scarring of the tendon yet potential for eventual function. It may be used in cases of flexor tendon rupture or when primary repair is not possible, such as with a complex injury involving bone and multiple tissues. In the first stage, a tendon implant replaces the scarred tendon; capsular contractures are released; and pulleys are reconstructed. The implant, which may be active or passive, stimulates formation of a new biological sheath. In the second stage, after about 3 months, a tendon graft replaces the implant (Hunter & Mackin, 2002).

Extensor Tendon Injury

Therapy of extensor tendon injuries is complicated and requires supervision by experienced hand therapists. Various protocols are available for immobilization, controlled passive motion, or active short arc of motion following extensor tendon repair (Evans, 2002).

Seven zones describe the digital extensors for the index, long, ring, and small fingers, and five zones describe the thumb extensors (Fig. 42-18). Injury in zones I and II leads to a mallet deformity (Evans, 2002), which follows disruption of the terminal extensor tendon and manifests itself as DIP extensor lag (Fig. 42-19). Depending on the nature of the problem, in non-operative cases, therapy may include continuous splinting of the DIP in extension for 6–8 weeks as determined by the physician while the tendon heals. It is essential to maintain normal PIP ROM during immobilization at the DIP. When initiating ROM of the DIP after the terminal tendon has healed, watch closely for recurrence of DIP extensor lag and resume splinting as needed to recover DIP extension (Evans, 2002). Some physicians recommend continuation of night splinting when DIP AROM is begun.

Extensor injuries in zones III and IV lead to a boutonniere deformity, an imbalanced digital position of PIP flexion and DIP hyperextension (Fig. 42-20). The deformity is due to volar displacement of the lateral bands secondary to involvement of the central slip (Evans, 2002) . In non-operative cases, splint the PIP in full extension for 6 weeks, and promote DIP active and passive flexion to prevent stiffness of the oblique retinacular ligament. In operative cases, follow the physician's guidelines, which may vary in timing and technique of mobilization and splinting. When the patient is medically cleared to begin PIP active exercises, watch closely for PIP extensor lag, and modify therapy and splinting accordingly (Crosby & Wehbe, 1996).

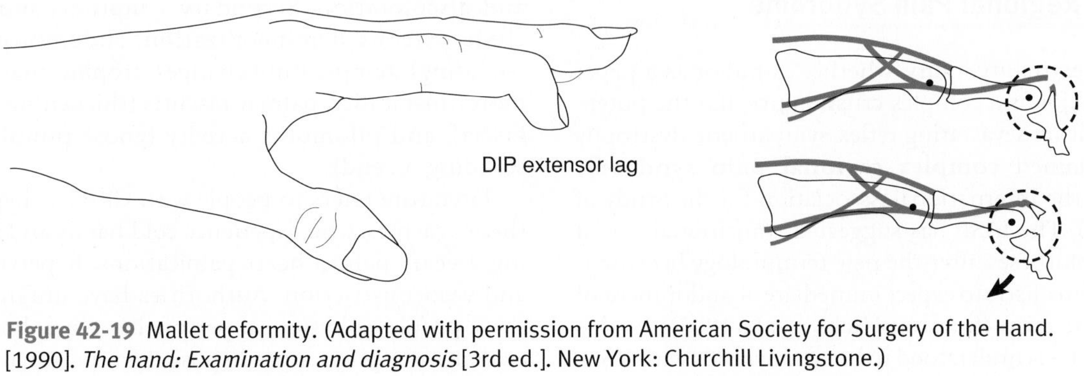

Figure 42-19 Mallet deformity. (Adapted with permission from American Society for Surgery of the Hand. [1990]. *The hand: Examination and diagnosis* [3rd ed.]. New York: Churchill Livingstone.)

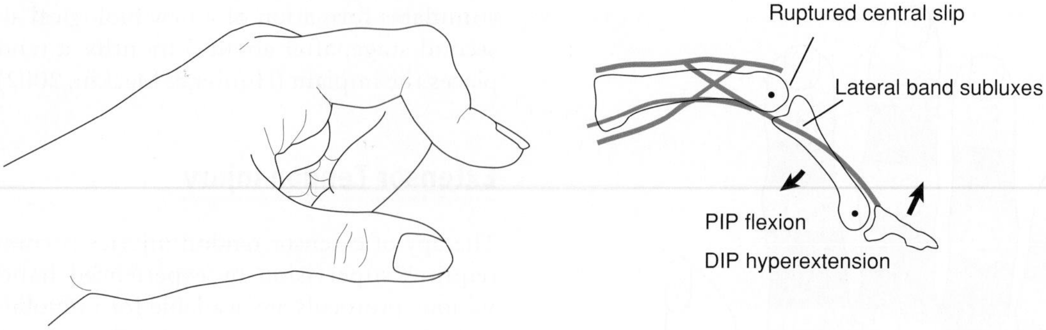

Figure 42-20 Boutonniere deformity. (Adapted with permission from American Society for Surgery of the Hand. [1990]. *The hand: Examination and diagnosis* [3rd ed.]. New York: Churchill Livingstone.)

Injury in zones V and VI may be treated by immobilization or by controlled early motion (Evans, 2002). Specific positioning and motion guidelines vary from surgeon to surgeon and are modified according to each patient's tissue responses. Multiple complex splints may be needed to achieve a program that balances rest and motion appropriately.

Injury in zone VII is likely to result in restrictions due to development of adhesions (Evans, 2002). Communicate closely with the surgeon for specific positioning and motion guidelines.

Tenolysis

Tenolysis is a surgical procedure to release tendon adhesions that restrict movement. Physicians do not usually perform this procedure until injured tissues have matured and PROM is maximized, as demonstrated by a plateau in progress during therapy. Therapy following tenolysis may begin as early as a few hours after surgery. The first few days following surgery are considered crucial. The physician's referral should include information on the integrity of the tendon and expected ROM goals based on intraoperative findings (Schneider & Feldscher, 2002). First priorities are edema control and ROM; observe and respect these fragile tissues' tolerances.

Complex Regional Pain Syndrome

Any upper extremity injury, whether as minor as a paper cut or as major as a complex crush injury, has the potential to result in devastating reflex sympathetic dystrophy (RSD), renamed **complex regional pain syndrome (CRPS)** by the International Association for the Study of Pain (IASP). The IASP has suggested transitional use of RSD in parentheses after the new terminology because it would be unrealistic to expect immediate abandonment of this familiar term (Stanton-Hicks et al., 1995). In this chapter, CRPS is understood to be synonymous with RSD.

CRPS type I follows a noxious event. Pain that is not limited to the territory of a single peripheral nerve occurs spontaneously and is disproportionate to the inciting noxious event. Edema is present, with abnormality of skin color or abnormal sudomotor activity in the painful area since the onset. The diagnosis of CRPS is excluded by other existing conditions that may cause the pain and dysfunction (Stanton-Hicks et al., 1995).

CRPS type II is the same as type I except that it develops after a nerve injury, whereas type I does not involve a nerve injury. CRPS type III refers to a group not otherwise specified and includes patients who do not fulfill the criteria for types I or II (Stanton-Hicks et al., 1995).

Pain that is disproportionate to the injury is the hallmark of CRPS. Constant attention to the patient's pain level and autonomic responses can lead to early medical management, if not prevention, of this challenging problem. The earlier this problem is diagnosed, the more successfully it may resolve (Walsh & Muntzer, 2002).

Over the years, many terms have been used to describe CRPS, including causalgia, Sudeck's atrophy, and shoulder-hand syndrome. Although clinical presentation is variable, traditional hand therapy literature identifies five clinical types as minor causalgia, minor traumatic dystrophy, shoulder-hand syndrome, major traumatic dystrophy, and major causalgia (Koman, Smith, & Smith, 2002).

Historically, the four cardinal symptoms and signs of CRPS have been identified as pain, swelling, stiffness, and discoloration. Secondary symptoms and signs include osseous demineralization, sudomotor changes (sweating), temperature changes, trophic changes, vasomotor instability, palmar fasciitis (thickening of palmar fascia), and pilomotor activity (goose pimples or hair standing on end).

Literature refers to people with CRPS as hypersympathetic reactors, who experience cold hands and feet, fainting, sweaty palms, heart palpitations, hyperventilation, and vasoconstriction. Authorities have unfairly labeled these people as hysterical personality types, but no good evidence supports a predispositional personality profile for this diagnosis. A lot of methodologically bad evidence, however, unfortunately stigmatizes those with the diagnosis and biases caregivers (Lynch, 1992).

Elegant animal studies have shown that self-protection through immobilization, intended to avoid pain, is itself a risk factor for the diagnosis of CRPS. People with CRPS must learn to use the extremity in ways that are pain free and biomechanically efficient. Normalizing sensory input also helps interrupt the vicious cycle of pain and stiffness (Byl & Melnick, 1997).

Therapy for CRPS

The most important therapy guideline is no PROM or painful intervention. The first thing is to control the pain. This includes management through medications, sympathetic blocks such as stellate ganglion blocks, and modalities such as transcutaneous electrical nerve stimulation (TENS) as appropriate. Close communication with medical experts specializing in pain management is ideal.

Provide vasomotor challenge through stress loading (described later), temperature biofeedback, and posture changes during activity. Hardy and Hardy (1997) recommend resetting the sensory thresholds through contrast, vibration, and desensitization (see Chapter 27). Water aerobics and functional activities are excellent ways to provide active movement incorporating reciprocal motion. Use stress loading routinely with patients who are at risk for CRPS. Stress loading is proposed to change sympathetic efferent activity. Although the physiological mechanisms of stress loading are not known (Carlson & Watson, 1988), it is popular among hand therapists for treating active CRPS, not the sequelae.

The two components of stress loading are "scrubbing the floor" (performed literally on all fours if possible), in brief sessions, 3 times per day initially, and carrying a weighted briefcase, done with the extremity in extension. The weight should be light and tolerable. Be sure it is not too heavy. Scrubbing and carrying achieve compressive loading and distraction of the upper extremity. If actual scrubbing cannot be tolerated, substitute comfortable weight-bearing exercises.

The frequency and duration of scrub and carry are upgraded as tolerated. If wrist ROM limitations or injury precautions do not allow the patient to assume the scrub position, positions may be adapted to accomplish comfortable weight bearing (see Chapter 24). Also instruct the patient to perform frequent pain-free proximal AROM bilaterally.

Avoid PROM or other therapy until the pain and swelling begin to subside, and then monitor responses closely. Incorporate traditional hand therapy, including splinting and other non-aggravating modalities, with edema control, joint ROM, differential tendon gliding, restoration of musculotendinous lengths, strengthening, desensitization, physical agents including transcutaneous electrical nerve stimulation and ultrasound as appropriate, and functional activity within tolerance. Manual edema mobilization is effective with this diagnosis.

Perhaps with CRPS more than other diagnoses, patient-directed therapy is essential. It is better to perform gentle, pain-free active exercises frequently for short periods than fewer and longer sessions. Light massage and active exercise help to interrupt the pain cycle. Make the exercise program bilateral and include reciprocal upper extremity motions (Byl & Melnick, 1997). Allow the progress to be as slow as necessary to prevent worsening of symptoms. This diagnosis can be overwhelming and discouraging. Provide the patient with appropriate encouragement and reassurances that progress can be made over time.

CRPS typifies the difficult clinical problems that hand therapists are trying to avert or avoid. Intervention programs that are progressing well can be suddenly and unexpectedly derailed by this disorder. For this reason, it is advisable to approach all hand therapy patients supportively and with a very careful eye, regardless of their diagnosis. Early identification of CRPS is a key to resolving it.

Osteoarthritis

Idiopathic osteoarthritis (OA) is the most common type of OA. In the upper extremity, it often affects the DIP and PIP joints. Osteophytes at the DIP are called Heberden's nodes, and osteophytes at the PIP are called Bouchard's nodes. For painful DIP nodes, small cylindrical splints or light Coban wrap may promote function while decreasing pain (Melvin, 1989).

Hand therapy for osteoarthritis focuses on alleviating symptoms through education in principles of joint protection, protective and supportive splinting, and provision of adaptive devices for ADL. For osteoarthritis of the thumb CMC, a hand-based thumb spica splint (Fig. 42-21) is often extremely helpful (Swigart et al., 1999). Some

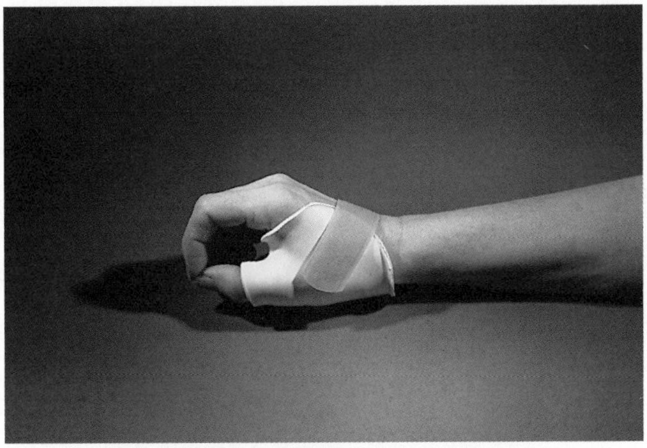

Figure 42-21 Hand-based thumb spica splint. Used to provide pain relief and promote functional pinch.

therapists prefer to use a forearm-based spica splint, particularly when there is pantrapezial involvement rather than just CMC joint involvement (Melvin, 2002, 1989).

Thumb CMC arthroplasty is a common post-operative diagnosis seen by hand therapists. Surgical techniques and timelines for therapy vary among physicians. Patients are often sent to therapy a few weeks after surgery for fabrication of a static forearm-based thumb spica splint with the IP free. The physician indicates appropriate guidelines for AROM according to the particular surgical procedures performed. Post-operative therapy goals are to promote pain-free stability and function. ADL modification and joint protection remain a priority.

Rheumatoid Arthritis

Unlike osteoarthritis, rheumatoid arthritis (RA) is a systemic disease that primarily affects the synovium. Its debilitation and crippling effects can be severely disabling. Rheumatoid arthritis presents as inflammation of synovial membranes of joints and of tendon sheaths, with redness, swelling, pain, and heat in the areas of involvement (Melvin, 1989).

Digital involvement at the DIP is less common than at the PIP. If DIP involvement does occur, a mallet finger may result. Involvement at the PIP may result in swan-neck or boutonniere deformities. (See section on extensor tendons for clinical management of mallet and boutonniere deformities.) A swan-neck deformity presents as MP flexion, PIP hyperextension, and DIP flexion (Fig. 42-22). Fabricate a digital dorsal splint in slight PIP flexion to minimize deforming forces and enhance FDS function. At the level of the MP joints, deformity usually manifests as MP ulnar drift and palmar subluxation (Melvin, 1989). Thumb deformities include boutonniere (primary thumb MP involvement) and swan-neck (primary CMC involvement) deformities. The thumb may also demonstrate stiff, unstable, and painful joints at the levels of the IP, MP, or CMC. Rheumatoid arthritis often affects the wrist. This is significant because the wrist is anatomically critical to proper hand function. Wrist involvement is compounded by concomitant hand deformity. Synovitis at the wrist can lead to flexor or extensor tendon ruptures (Melvin, 1989).

In evaluating patients with rheumatoid arthritis, observe deformities and abnormal posture, any atrophy, and skin condition. Identify crepitus of joint or tendon, palpable nodules, tendon integrity, and joint stability. Ask about morning stiffness, fatigue, and pain. The appearance of the deformity (cosmesis) is also relevant (Biese, 2002).

The goals of upper extremity splinting for rheumatoid arthritis include reducing inflammation, supporting weak tissues, and minimizing deforming forces. Splinting also provides functional assistance. Splinting is used especially in the acute stage, when inflamed structures are at risk for further damage. Forearm-based resting splints may support the wrist and entire hand, the wrist and MPs, or only the wrist.

Determine splint design according to the pathomechanics of the disease. Involved MP joints are at risk for volar subluxation. Therefore, splint the wrist in neutral or slight extension, the MP joints in available extension, and the PIP joints in slight flexion (Biese, 2002). Radial deviation of the wrist encourages ulnar drift of the digits at the MP joints because of the zigzag deformity. A splint to correct MP ulnar drift often improves the biomechanics of hand use. Talk with the patient to identify individual preferences and needs in terms of ADL and joint protection. Adapt the straps and practice with patients to be sure they can open and close them. For some people who require bilateral splints, it may be easier to use one at a time on alternate nights.

CONCLUSION

Wilson (1998) states, "The hand is not merely a metaphor or an icon for humanness, but often the real-life focal point—the lever or the launching pad—of a successful and genuinely fulfilling life" (Wilson, 1998, p. 14). Occupational therapy can be the launching pad for people with hand impairments to reestablish fulfilling lives.

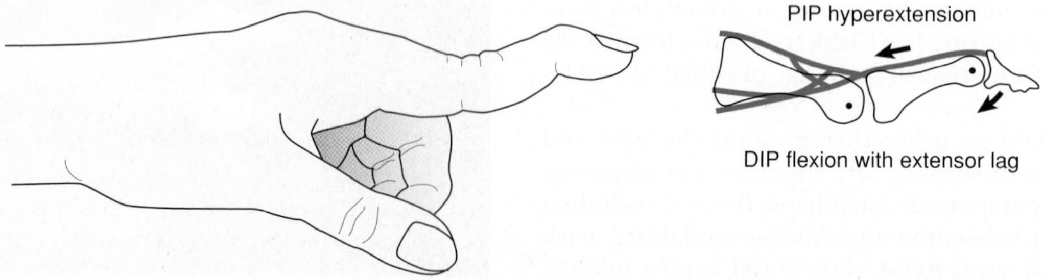

Figure 42-22 Swan-neck deformity. (Adapted with permission from American Society for Surgery of the Hand. [1990]. *The hand: Examination and diagnosis* [3rd ed.]. New York: Churchill Livingstone.)

CASE EXAMPLE

P. L.: Hand Impairments

Occupational Therapy Process	Clinical Reasoning Process: Objectives	Clinical Reasoning Process: Examples of Therapist's Internal Dialogue
Patient Information P.L. is a 49-year-old athletic computer software manager with dominant right hand. She is single and lives alone. P.L. fell on an outstretched hand while on vacation out of state, sustaining a comminuted displaced right distal radius fracture. She was initially treated with closed reduction and a long-arm cast. Ten days later, after returning home, she underwent open reduction internal fixation of the right distal radius with percutaneous pins, synthetic bone graft material, and application of an external fixator. Family members came to stay with her to assist with self-care and ADL needs. At the time of her injury, she was looking forward to a kayaking vacation.	Understand the patient's diagnosis or condition Know the person	"P.L. sustained a significant injury to her dominant upper extremity (UE) requiring fixation and bone grafting. The amount of immobilization time required for healing (6 weeks) could potentially lead to significant stiffness of multiple structures." "P.L. is an independent and active woman who hopes to go on a kayaking trip in a few months. She is not used to depending on others for self-care or other assistance. She likes living alone, driving her sports car, and going on business trips, and right now these aspects of her life are disrupted."
Reason for Referral to Occupational Therapy P.L. was referred to outpatient hand therapy the day after surgery to maximize her functional abilities while her dominant hand was immobilized and to promote wound and fracture healing, edema control, and mobility of non-immobilized structures.	Appreciate the context Develop provisional hypotheses	"P.L.'s family is with her initially to help her function while relying on her non-dominant UE for use. Although she prefers living alone, it is good that she has some help initially. Her desire to perform her occupational roles will help her recover more quickly."
Assessment Process and Results P.L. had severe pain (9/10), significant edema, and increased autonomic signs including vasomotor instability and guarded positioning of the right UE. She had extremely limited ROM of the digits of her right hand and was also hesitant to actively move her shoulder or elbow.	Consider evaluation approach and methods Interpret observations	"I do not want to impose pain with my evaluation, so I will measure only AROM in a gentle fashion. I will provide encouragement and explain how autonomic responses can be normalized with pain-free motion, elevation, and edema control." "P.L. is at risk for CRPS and for significant stiffness of joints and tendons. Managing the edema is a high priority in order to normalize all tissue responses."
Occupational Therapy Problem List • Disruption of independent living and job performance • Interruption of frequent job-related travel • Inability to sleep or to perform self-care or home activities due to pain, edema, and decreased ROM • Risk of developing CRPS with degradation of functional and clinical status as evidenced by increased autonomic signs	Synthesize results	"P.L. has multiple severe problems that could lead to permanent stiffness and loss of function. Despite this, she is a highly motivated successful professional and she is eager to recover."

Occupational Therapy Goal List

1. Normalize autonomic signs and ameliorate pain interfering with function and sleep
2. Promote spontaneous pain-free use of the right upper extremity in daily activity
3. Achieve independent self-care and homemaking and resume job-related travel and engagement in athletic activity

Develop intervention hypotheses	"I believe that a gradual and gentle upgrade of exercises to promote healing and recover flexibility will be far more effective than overstressing her delicate healing tissues."
Select an intervention approach	"Occupational therapy will focus on promoting healing and restoring normal joint motions and musculotendinous lengths in order to recover UE function."
Consider what will occur in therapy, how often, and for how long	"P.L. will need upgrades to her home program weekly. Splints will need to be revised, as well as exercises and instructions/practice in using her right UE for self-care and non-resistive home tasks."

Intervention

P.L. began a home program of education about the expected clinical course and recovery; pin site care; edema control; and shoulder, elbow, and digital ROM in pain-free ranges. Emphasis was on shoulder active exercise and upper extremity elevation. A week after surgery, P.L.'s autonomic signs were resolving. Her digits remained edematous, and AROM was still limited throughout the upper extremity except for her shoulder, which was functional.

At 2 weeks after surgery, digital AROM and PROM were slowly improving but still limited (Fig. 42-23, A & B). P.L.'s home program was upgraded to include edema control, functional grip and release activities, blocking exercises with thermoplastic supports, place-and-hold exercises, night composite digital extension static splinting, and day dynamic digital composite extension splinting. Differential digital flexor tendon gliding was restricted by adherence at the volar distal forearm incisional site, which was still healing. She had extrinsic extensor tightness, extrinsic flexor tightness, and intrinsic tightness. Fortunately, P.L. was not developing PIP flexion contractures. She had been relying on her non-dominant left hand for handwriting and all self-care. She returned to work soon after surgery and was once again traveling frequently on business.

At 3 weeks after surgery, when incisional sites were healed, manual edema mobilization began, and all functional activities, splints, and exercises were upgraded in a pain-free fashion. Silicone gel was applied to incision sites at night for scar management. P.L. continued to make slow but measurable progress. Her physician reported good radiographic alignment.

At 6 weeks after surgery, P.L.'s fixator was removed. Her physician reported good reduction and stability of the distal radioulnar joint. She was severely limited in forearm pronation and supination and in wrist AROM and PROM. She was instructed in pain-free forearm and wrist AROM. A thermoplastic volar wrist splint was fabricated for support and to correct limited wrist extension. P.L. began to resume use of her right upper extremity for handwriting intermittently and for home activities as tolerated. Although she was very compliant with her home program, her progress was slow. She had become quite adept at using her left hand for dexterity tasks.

Assess the patient's comprehension Understand what she is doing Compare actual to expected performance	"I can tell that P.L. understands her instructions because she demonstrates her activities well. She is exploring what new abilities she has with her right hand and is trying to use it as much as possible in a pain-free way. She demonstrates accurate placement of her splints and describes effective choices in using them. Her follow-through at home is exactly as I hoped it would be. And she understands when to rest her hand so that she does not develop new signs of swelling or pain."

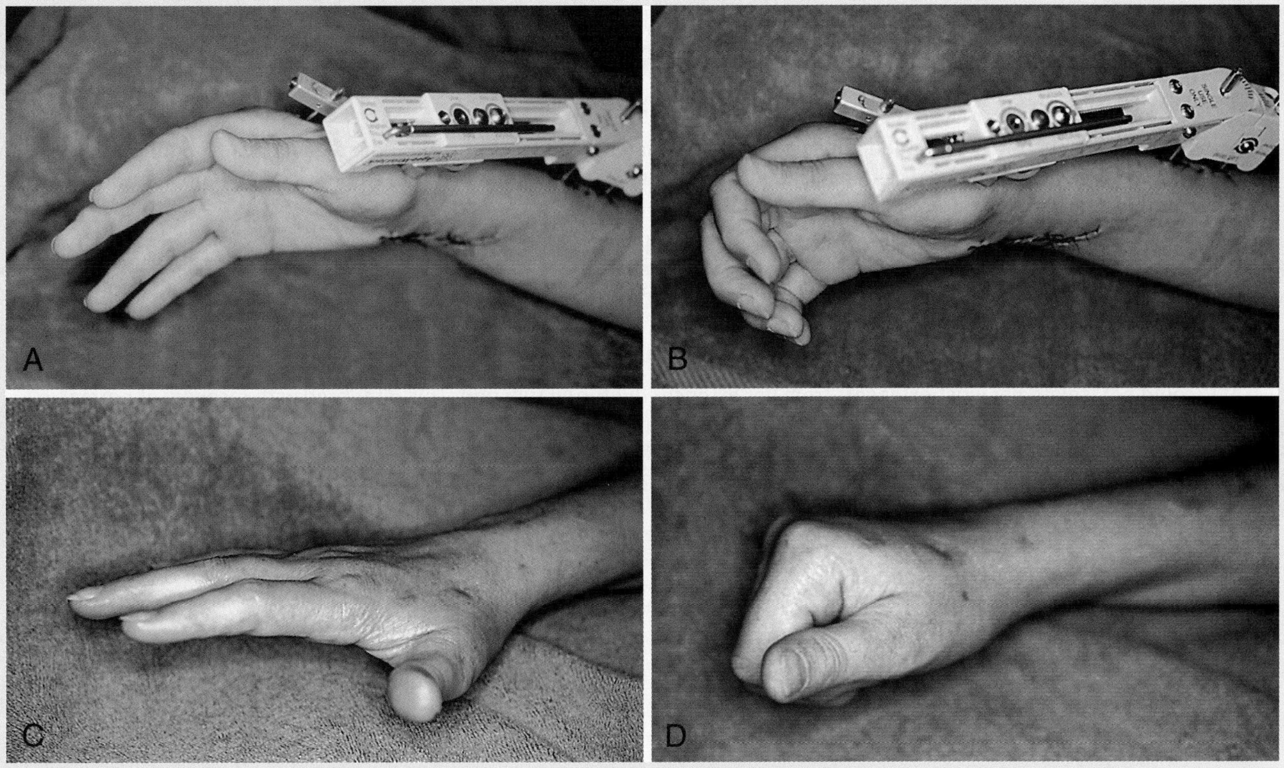

Figure 42-23 At 2 weeks post surgery, P.L.'s active digital extension (**A**) and flexion (**B**); at 10 weeks post surgery, P.L.'s active digital extension (**C**) and flexion (**D**).

Intervention (cont'd)

At 10 weeks after surgery, P.L. began to demonstrate dramatic gains in suppleness (Fig 42-23, C & D). She was significantly improved in digital edema and in all ROM. Elbow extension was normal. Forearm supination and pronation were better, with AROM being equal to PROM. Isolated wrist extension was improved. Digital composite fisting and FDP and FDS differential tendon gliding were nearly normal, and tightness of the extrinsic flexors was almost fully resolved. P.L. was using her right hand for all handwriting and grooming and for driving her sports car. She was eager to begin simulating kayaking, as she had kept her plans for a kayaking vacation. P.L. said that her dynamic splints and night static composite extension splints were helpful to her, so these were modified and upgraded. Strengthening exercises were gradually and cautiously upgraded as well.

Next Steps

Discharge from occupational therapy with home activities and splints

Anticipate present and future patient concerns

"P.L. was able to go on her kayaking trip and enjoyed it. She still exercises and knows that it is important not to overdo it. She has learned how to keep her tissues flexible and has gained good strength as well."

Analyze patient's comprehension

Decide if the patient should continue or discontinue therapy and/or return in the future

CLINICAL REASONING IN HAND THERAPY PRACTICE

Effects of CRPS on Functional Use of the Involved Extremity

Initially, P.L. demonstrated a guarded upper extremity position associated with autonomic signs. How might upper extremity posturing influence pain, edema, and ROM? What should the home program emphasize to promote autonomic normalization?

Effects of Edema on Upper Extremity Pain, ROM, and Function

Persistent edema of P.L.'s hand worsened her pain, stiffness, and function. What treatment techniques are helpful in resolving upper extremity edema?

Effects of Substitution Patterns on Wrist and Hand Function

P.L. could not isolate her wrist extensors from her extensor digitorum function. This interfered with recovery of normal grasp and release patterns. What clinical problems contribute to the inability to isolate wrist extensors? What functional exercises would help retrain isolated wrist extension with simultaneous grip (i.e., normal tenodesis patterns)? What choice of splint or splints might help recover these motions?

Evidence Table 42-1
Best Evidence for Occupational Therapy Practice Regarding Treatment of Hand Impairments

Intervention	Description of Intervention Tested	Participants	Dosage	Type of Best Evidence and Level of Evidence	Benefit	Statistical Probability and Effect Size of Outcome	Reference
Exercise to improve elbow extension	Active elbow flexion and extension with elbow extension prolonged with and without resistance.	10 subjects with elbow motion deficits of at least 30° after injury (mean age = 52 years, 6 women and 4 men, 9 right-hand dominant, 7 subjects with injury to dominant side) and 10 controls with unrestricted elbow range of motion and no history of elbow injury (mean age = 31 years, 9 women and 1 man, 9 right-hand dominant).	Two 9-second trials of alternating elbow flexion and extension on verbal command; also passive elbow extension with forearm unweighted and with a 3-lb cuff weight.	Non-randomized, two-group design. IIC2b And non-randomized, one-group, two-condition design. IIIC2b	No. Adding weight to a forearm in an effort to gain elbow extension resulted in increased activity of elbow flexors and may be contraindicated for those patients whose stiff elbow has the active component of muscle contraction in addition to the passive restrictions such as capsular tightness.	During active elbow flexion and extension, all elbow flexor muscles of stiff elbow group showed statistically significantly greater ($p < 0.05$) EMG activity compared with the control group. During prolonged extension, there was a significant ($p < 0.05$) increase of activity of the 3 flexor muscles of the stiff elbow group when weight was added. Effect sizes could not be calculated from the data provided.	Page, Backus, & Lenhoff, 2003

(continued)

Evidence Table 42-1 (*continued*)

Intervention	Description of Intervention Tested	Participants	Dosage	Type of Best Evidence and Level of Evidence	Benefit	Statistical Probability and Effect Size of Outcome	Reference
Corrective splinting for flexion contracture	Dynamic (Capener) finger extension splints were compared to belly gutter static splints to improve flexion contracture, hand strength, and hand function.	24 patients with rheumatoid arthritis and digital PIP/DIP flexion contractures randomized to group. Group 1: dynamic splints. Group 2: static splints. 22 women and 2 men; mean age = 37.08 years; all right-hand dominant; all had diagnosis of rheumatoid arthritis with finger flexion contractures <45°.	Group 1 used dynamic splint 4 times a day for variable duration with minimum of 6 hours daily for 6 weeks. Group 2 used static splint at rest for at least 6 hours daily for 6 weeks.	Matched pairs experimental design. IC1a	Yes. All subjects improved significantly. Severity of flexion contractures decreased, while strength and hand function increased. Both types of splints were effective.	Significant improvement in extension ROM of both groups ($t_{23} = 13.84, p < 0.0005, r = .94$); grip strength ($t_{23} = -3.61, p = 0.001, r = 0.60$); pinch strength ($t_{23} = 3.45, p = 0.002, r = 0.58$); hand function (Jebsen) ($t_{23} = 5.21, p < 0.0005, r = 0.73$). There was no significant difference in these outcome variables between types of splints.	Li-Tsang, Hung, & Mak, 2002

SUMMARY REVIEW QUESTIONS

1. Why should painful treatment be avoided? What signs are indicative of overaggressive intervention?
2. Name the phases of tissue healing and approximate timelines.
3. Define joint versus musculotendinous tightness, intrinsic versus extrinsic tightness, and tightness of extrinsic extensors versus extrinsic flexors.
4. Describe the anti-deformity position of the wrist and hand and explain why it is used.
5. What function is lost with a low radial nerve injury? What kind of splinting is appropriate, and why?
6. What distribution of sensation is usually impaired with carpal tunnel syndrome? What musculature might be atrophied in an advanced case? What night splint position is best for carpal tunnel syndrome, and why?
7. Describe complex regional pain syndrome and discuss intervention priorities for this diagnosis.
8. What symptoms are associated with a trigger finger?
9. Name four self-care or home activities that are safe and therapeutic for a person in a short arm cast with a healing distal radius fracture.

ACKNOWLEDGMENT

Heartfelt thanks to John L. Evarts, BS, for the photography and for his valuable ideas, contribution to content, and ongoing technical and emotional support. I also thank Cecelia M. Skotak, OTR, CHT; Virgil Mathiowetz, PhD, OTR; Michelle Pressman, MS, OTR; and Kevin Renfree, MD, for their input to a previous version of this chapter. I also acknowledge Michelle Pressman Abrams, MS, OTR, for her assistance in applying Occupational Therapy Practice Framework (OTPF) terminology to this revision.

References

Adams, L. S., Topoozian, E., & Greene, L. W. (1992). Range of motion. In J. S. Casanova (Ed.), *Clinical assessment recommendations* (2 ed., pp. 55–70). Chicago: American Society of Hand Therapists.

Artzberger, S. (2002). Manual edema mobilization: Treatment for edema in the subacute hand. In E. J. Mackin, A. D. Callahan, T. M. Skirven, L. H. Schneider, & A. L. Osterman (Eds.), *Rehabilitation of the hand and upper extremity* (5th ed., pp. 899–913). St. Louis: Mosby.

Ashe, M. C., McCauley, T., & Khan, K. M. (2004). Tendinopathies in the upper extremity: A paradigm shift. *Journal of Hand Therapy, 17,* 329–334.

Aulicino, P. L. (2002). Clinical examination of the hand. In E. J. Mackin, A. D. Callahan, T. M. Skirven, L. H. Schneider, & A. L. Osterman (Eds.), *Rehabilitation of the hand and upper extremity* (5th ed., pp. 120–142). St. Louis: Mosby.

Aulisa, L., Tamburrelli, F., Padua, R., Romanini, E., Lo Monaco, M., & Padua, L. (1998). Carpal tunnel syndrome: Indication for surgical treatment based on electrophysiologic study. *Journal of Hand Surgery, 23A,* 687–691.

Baldwin, J. E., Weber, L. J., & Simon, C. L. (1992). Wound/scar assessment. In J. S. Casanova (Ed.), *Clinical assessment recommendations* (2nd ed., pp. 21–28). Chicago: American Society of Hand Therapists.

Baum, T. M., & Busuito, M. J. (1998). Use of a glycerin-based gel sheeting in scar management. *Advances in Wound Care, 11,* 40–43.

Biese, J. (2002). Therapist's evaluation and conservative management of rheumatoid arthritis in the hand and wrist. In E. J. Mackin, A. D. Callahan, T. M. Skirven, L. H. Schneider, & A. L. Osterman (Eds.), *Rehabilitation of the hand and upper extremity* (5th ed., pp. 1569–1582). St. Louis: Mosby.

Blackmore, S. M. (2002). Therapist's management of ulnar nerve neuropathy at the elbow. In E. J. Mackin, A. D. Callahan, T. M. Skirven, L. H. Schneider, & A. L. Osterman (Eds.), *Rehabilitation of the hand and upper extremity* (5th ed., pp. 679–689). St. Louis: Mosby.

Bozentka, D. J. (1998). Cubital tunnel syndrome pathophysiology. *Clinical Orthopaedics and Related Research, 351,* 90–99.

Brand, P. W. (2002). The forces of dynamic splinting: Ten questions before applying a dynamic splint to the hand. In E. J. Mackin, A. D. Callahan, T. M. Skirven, L. H. Schneider, & A. L. Osterman (Eds.), *Rehabilitation of the hand and upper extremity* (5th ed., pp. 1811–1817). St. Louis: Mosby.

Breger-Lee, D., Bell-Krotoski, J., & Brandsma, J. W. (1990). Torque range of motion in the hand clinic. *Journal of Hand Therapy, 3,* 7–13.

Bryan, B. K., & Kohnke, E. N. (1997). Therapy after skeletal fixation in the hand and wrist. *Hand Clinics, 13,* 761–776.

Bulthaup, S., Cipriani, D. J., & Thomas, J. J. (1999). An electromyography study of wrist extension orthoses and upper-extremity function. *American Journal of Occupational Therapy, 53,* 434–440.

Burkhalter, W. E. (1995). Mutilating injuries of the hand. In J. M. Hunter, E. J. Mackin, & A. D. Callahan (Eds.), *Rehabilitation of the hand: Surgery and therapy* (4th ed., pp. 1037–1056). St. Louis: Mosby.

Byl, N. N., Kohlhase, W., & Engel, G. (1999). Functional limitation immediately after cast immobilization and closed reduction of distal radius fractures: Preliminary report. *Journal of Hand Therapy, 12,* 201–211.

Byl, N. N., & Melnick, M. (1997). The neural consequences of repetition: Clinical implications of a learning hypothesis. *Journal of Hand Therapy, 10,* 160–174.

Callahan, A. D. (2002). Sensibility assessment for nerve lesions-in-continuity and nerve lacerations. In E. J. Mackin, A. D. Callahan, T. M. Skirven, L. H. Schneider, & A. L. Osterman (Eds.), *Rehabilitation of the hand and upper extremity* (5th ed., pp. 214–239). St. Louis: Mosby.

Campbell, P. J., & Wilson, R. L. (2002). Management of joint injuries and intraarticular fractures. In E. J. Mackin, A. D. Callahan, T. M. Skirven, L. H. Schneider, & A. L. Osterman (Eds.), *Rehabilitation of the hand and upper extremity* (5th ed., pp. 396–411). St. Louis: Mosby.

Carlson, L. K., & Watson, H. K. (1988). Treatment of reflex sympathetic dystrophy using the stress-loading program. *Journal of Hand Therapy, 1,* 149–154.

Chin, K. R., Lonner, J. H., Jupiter, B. S., & Jupiter, J. B. (1999). The surgeon as a hand patient: The clinical and psychological impact of hand and wrist fractures. *Journal of Hand Surgery, 24A,* 59–63.

Colditz, J. C. (2002a). Splinting the hand with a peripheral nerve injury. In E. J. Mackin, A. D. Callahan, T. M. Skirven, L. H. Schneider, & A. L. Osterman (Eds.), *Rehabilitation of the hand and upper extremity* (5th ed., pp. 622–634). St. Louis: Mosby.

Colditz, J. C. (2002b). Therapist's management of the stiff hand. In E. J. Mackin, N. Callinan, T. M. Skirven, L. H. Schneider, & A. L. Osterman (Eds.), *Rehabilitation of the hand and upper extremity* (5th ed., pp. 1021–1049). St. Louis: Mosby.

Collins, D. C. (1993). Management and rehabilitation of distal radius fractures. *Orthopedic Clinics of North America, 24,* 365–378.

Concannon, M. J., Gainor, B., Petroski, G. F., & Puckett, C. L. (1997). The predictive value of electrodiagnostic studies in carpal tunnel syndrome. *Plastic and Reconstructive Surgery, 100,* 1452–1458.

Cooper, C., & Evarts, J. L. (1998). Beyond the routine: Placing therapeutic occupation at the center of upper-extremity rehabilitation. *OT Practice, 3,* 18–22.

Cooper, C., Liskin, J., & Moorhead, J. F. (1999). Dyscoordinate contraction: Impaired quality of movement in patients with hand disorders. *OT Practice, 4,* 40–45.

Cromwell, F. S. (1976). *Occupational therapist's manual for basic skill assessment: Primary prevocational evaluation.* Altadena, CA: Fair Oaks Printing.

Crosby, C. A., & Wehbe, M. A. (1996). Early motion after extensor tendon surgery. *Hand Clinics, 12,* 57–64.

Culp, R. W., & Taras, J. S. (2002). Primary care of flexor tendon injuries. In E. J. Mackin, A. D. Callahan, T. M. Skirven, L. H. Schneider, & A. L. Osterman (Eds.), *Rehabilitation of the hand and upper extremity* (5th ed., pp. 415–430). St. Louis: Mosby.

Cyriax, J. (1982). *Textbook of orthopaedic medicine* (Vol. 1, 8th ed.). London: Bailliere Tindall.

Davis, J., Fenlon, P., Proctor, T., & Watson, W. J. (1997). The Nine Hole Peg Test: A comparison study. Unpublished Master's thesis. Kirksville College of Osteopathic Medicine, Kirksville, MO.

de Herder, E. F. (1992). Vascular assessment. In J. S. Casanova (Ed.), *Clinical assessment recommendations* (2nd ed., pp. 29–39). Chicago: American Society of Hand Therapists.

Dell, P. C., & Dell, R. B. (2002). Management of carpal fractures and dislocations. In E. J. Mackin, A. D. Callahan, T. M. Skirven, L. H. Schneider, & A. L. Osterman (Eds.), *Rehabilitation of the hand and upper extremity* (5th ed., pp. 1171–1184). St. Louis: Mosby.

Desrosiers, J., Hebert, R., Dutil, E., & Bravo, G. (1993). Development and reliability of an upper extremity function test for the elderly: The TEMPA. *Canadian Journal of Occupational Therapy, 60,* 9–16.

Desrosiers, J., Hebert, R., Dutil, E., Bravo, G., & Mercier, L. (1994). Validity of the TEMPA: A measurement instrument for upper extremity performance. *Occupational Therapy Journal of Research, 14,* 267–281.

Donaldson, C. C., Nelson, D. V., Skubick, D. L., & Clasby, R. G. (1998). Potential contributions of neck muscle dysfunctions to initiation and maintenance of carpal tunnel syndrome. *Applied Psychophysiology and Biofeedback, 23,* 59–72.

Evans, R. B. (2002). Clinical management of extensor tendon injuries. In E. J. Mackin, A. D. Callahan, T. M. Skirven, L. H. Schneider, & A. L. Osterman (Eds.), *Rehabilitation of the hand and upper extremity* (5th ed., pp. 542–579). St. Louis: Mosby.

Evans, R. B., Hunter, J. M., & Burkhalter, W. E. (1988). Conservative management of the trigger finger: A new approach. *Journal of Hand Therapy, 1,* 59–68.

Evans, R. B., & McAuliffe, J. A. (2002). Wound classification and management. In E. J. Mackin, A. D. Callahan, T. M. Skirven, L. H. Schneider, & A. L. Osterman (Eds.), *Rehabilitation of the hand and upper extremity* (5th ed., pp. 311–330). St. Louis: Mosby.

Fess, E. E. (1993). Hand rehabilitation. In H. L. Hopkins & H. D. Smith (Eds.), *Willard and Spackman's occupational therapy* (8th ed., pp. 674–690). Philadelphia: J.B. Lippincott Co.

Fess, E. E. (2002a). Documentation: Essential elements of an upper extremity assessment battery. In E. J. Mackin, A. D. Callahan, T. M. Skirven, L. H. Schneider, & A. L. Osterman (Eds.), *Rehabilitation of the hand and upper extremity* (5th ed., pp. 263–284). St. Louis: Mosby.

Fess, E. E. (2002b). Principles and methods of splinting for mobilization of joints. In E. J. Mackin, A. D. Callahan, T. M. Skirven, L. H. Schneider, & A. L. Osterman (Eds.), *Rehabilitation of the hand and upper extremity* (5th ed., pp. 1818–1827). St. Louis: Mosby.

Fess, E. E., & McCollum, M. (1998). The influence of splinting on healing tissues. *Journal of Hand Therapy, 11,* 157–161.

Furth, H. J., Holm, M. B., & James, A. (1994). Reinjury prevention follow-through for clients with cumulative trauma disorders. *American Journal of Occupational Therapy, 48,* 890–898.

Gallus, J. M. (1999). Test-retest reliability of the Purdue Pegboard for individuals with multiple sclerosis. Unpublished Master's thesis. University of Minnesota, St. Paul, MN.

Grunert, B. K., Matloub, H. S., Sanger, J. R., Yousif, N. J., & Hettermann, S. (1991). Effects of litigation on maintenance of psychological symptoms after severe hand injury. *Journal of Hand Surgery, 16A,* 1031–1034.

Hardy, M. A., & Hardy, S. G. P. (1997). Reflex sympathetic dystrophy: The clinician's perspective. *Journal of Hand Therapy, 10,* 137–150.

Hayes, E. P., Carney, K., Wolf, J., Smith, J. M., & Akelman, E. (2002). Carpal tunnel syndrome. In E. J. Mackin, A. D. Callahan, T. M. Skirven, L. H. Schneider, & A. L. Osterman (Eds.), *Rehabilitation of the hand and upper extremity* (5th ed., pp. 643–659). St. Louis: Mosby.

Humiston, L. (2000). Upper Extremity Performance Test for the Elderly (TEMPA): Normative data for ages 20-29. Unpublished Master's thesis. University of Minnesota, St. Paul, MN.

Hunter, J. M. (1986). Philosophy of hand rehabilitation. *Hand Clinics, 2,* 5–24.

Hunter, J. M., & Mackin, E. J. (2002). Staged flexor tendon reconstruction. In E. J. Mackin, A. D. Callahan, T. M. Skirven, L. H. Schneider, & A. L. Osterman (Eds.), *Rehabilitation of the hand and upper extremity* (5th ed., pp. 469–497). St. Louis: Mosby.

Idler, R. S. (1997). Helping the patient who has wrist or hand tenosynovitis. *Journal of Musculoskeletal Medicine, 14,* 21–35.

Jarus, T., & Poremba, R. (1993). Hand function evaluation: A factor analysis study. *American Journal of Occupational Therapy, 47,* 439–443.

Jebsen, R. H., Taylor, N., Trieschmann, R. B., Trotter, M. J., & Howard, L. A. (1969). An objective and standardized test of hand function. *Archives of Physical Medicine and Rehabilitation, 50,* 311–319.

Jensen, C., & Rayan, G. (1996). Buddy strapping of mismatched fingers: The offset buddy strap. *Journal of Hand Surgery, 21,* 317–318.

Johnson, S. L. (1993). Therapy of the occupationally injured hand and upper extremity. *Hand Clinics, 9,* 2889–2898.

Keir, P. J., Bach, J. M., & Rempel, D. M. (1998). Fingertip loading and carpal tunnel pressure: Differences between a pinching and a pressing task. *Journal of Orthopedic Research, 16,* 112–115.

Keller, K., Corbett, J., & Nichols, D. (1998). Repetitive strain injury in computer keyboard users: Pathomechanics and treatment principles in individual and group intervention. *Journal of Hand Therapy, 11,* 9–26.

Khoo, D., Carmichael, S. W., & Spinner, R. J. (1996). Ulnar nerve anatomy and compression. *Orthopedic Clinics of North America, 27,* 317–337.

Koman, L. A., Smith, B. P., & Smith, T. L. (2002). Reflex sympathetic dystrophy (complex regional pain syndromes-types 1 and 2). In E. J. Mackin, A. D. Callahan, T. M. Skirven, L. H. Schneider, & A. L. Osterman (Eds.), *Rehabilitation of the hand and upper extremity* (5th ed., pp. 1695–1706). St. Louis: Mosby.

Lairmore, J. R., & Engber, W. D. (1998). Serious, often subtle, finger injuries: Avoiding diagnosis and treatment pitfalls. *The Physician and Sportsmedicine, 26,* 57–69.

Lam, N., & Thurston, A. (1998). Association of obesity, gender, age and occupation with carpal tunnel syndrome. *Australian and New Zealand Journal of Surgery, 68,* 190–193.

Laseter, G. F. (2002). Therapist's management of distal radius fractures. In E. J. Mackin, A. D. Callahan, T. M. Skirven, L. H. Schneider, & A. L. Osterman (Eds.), *Rehabilitation of the hand and upper extremity* (5th ed., pp. 1136–1155). St. Louis: Mosby.

Laseter, G. F., & Carter, P. R. (1996). Management of distal radius fractures. *Journal of Hand Therapy, 9,* 114–128.

Lee, M. P., Nasser-Sharif, S., & Zelouf, D. S. (2002). Surgeon's and therapist's management of tendonopathies in the hand and wrist. In E. J. Mackin, A. D. Callahan, T. M. Skirven, L. H. Schneider, & A. L. Osterman (Eds.), *Rehabilitation of the hand and upper extremity* (5th ed., pp. 931–953). St. Louis: Mosby.

Leibovic, S. J. (1999). Bone and joint injury in the hand: Surgeon's perspective. *Journal of Hand Therapy, 12,* 111–120.

Li-Tsang, C. W. P., Hung, L. K., & Mak, A. F. T. (2002). The effect of corrective splinting on flexion contracture of rheumatoid fingers. *Journal of Hand Therapy, 15,* 185–191.

Lynch, K. B., & Bridle, M. J. (1989). Validity of the Jebsen-Taylor Hand Function Test in predicting activities of daily living. *Occupational Therapy Journal of Research, 9,* 316–318.

Lynch, M. E. (1992). Psychological aspects of reflex sympathetic dystrophy: A review of the adult and paediatric literature. *Pain, 49,* 337–347.

Mathiowetz, V. (1993). Role of physical performance component evaluations in occupational therapy functional assessment. *American Journal of Occupational Therapy, 47,* 225–230.

Mathiowetz, V., & Bass Haugen, J. B. (1995). Evaluation of motor behavior: Traditional and contemporary views. In C. A. Trombly (Ed.), *Occupational therapy for physical dysfunction* (pp. 157–185). Baltimore: Williams & Wilkins.

Mathiowetz, V., Rogers, S. L., Dowe-Keval, M., Donahoe, L., & Rennells, C. (1986). The Purdue Pegboard: Norms for 14- to 19-year-olds. *American Journal of Occupational Therapy, 40,* 174–179.

Mathiowetz, V., Volland, G., Kashman, N., & Weber, K. (1985a). Adult norms for the Box and Block Test of manual dexterity. *American Journal of Occupational Therapy, 39,* 386–391.

Mathiowetz, V., Weber, K., Kashman, N., & Volland, G. (1985b). Adult norms for the Nine Hole Peg Test of finger dexterity. *Occupational Therapy Journal of Research, 5,* 24–38.

Maurer, G. L., & Jezek, S. M. (1992). Pain assessment. In J. S. Casanova (Ed.), *Clinical assessment recommendations* (2nd ed., pp. 95–108). Chicago: American Society of Hand Therapists.

Melvin, J. L. (1989). *Rheumatic disease in the adult and child: Occupational therapy and rehabilitation* (3rd ed.). Philadelphia: F.A. Davis Co.

Melvin, J. L. (2002). Therapist's management of osteoarthritis in the hand. In E. J. Mackin, A. D. Callahan, T. M. Skirven, L. H. Schneider, & A. L. Osterman (Eds.), *Rehabilitation of the hand and upper extremity* (5th ed., pp. 1646–1663). St. Louis: Mosby.

Merritt, W. H. (1998). Written on behalf of the stiff finger. *Journal of Hand Therapy, 11,* 74–79.

Meyer, F. N., & Wilson, R. L. (1995). Management of nonarticular fractures of the hand. In J. M. Hunter, E. J. Mackin, & A. D. Callahan (Eds.), *Rehabilitation of the hand: Surgery and therapy* (4th ed., pp. 377–394). St. Louis: Mosby.

Miles, C. A., Burjanadze, T. V., & Bailey, A. J. (1995). The kinetics of the thermal denaturation of collagen in unrestrained rat tail tendon determined by differential scanning calorimetry. *Journal of Molecular Biology, 245,* 437–446.

Moberg, E. (1991). The unsolved problem: How to test the functional value of hand sensibility. *Journal of Hand Therapy, 4,* 105–110.

Mooney, V. (1998). Overuse syndromes of the upper extremity: Rational and effective treatment. *Journal of Musculoskeletal Medicine, 15,* 11–18.

Moskowitz, L. (1996). Psychological management of postsurgical pain and patient adherence. *Hand Clinics, 12,* 129–137.

Nelson, D. L., & Peterson, C. (1989). Enhancing therapeutic exercise through purposeful activity: A theoretical analysis. *Topics in Geriatric Rehabilitation, 4,* 12–22.

Netscher, D., Steadman, A. K., Thornby, J., & Cohen, B. J. (1998). Temporal changes in grip and pinch strength after open carpal tunnel release and the effect of ligament reconstruction. *Journal of Hand Surgery, 23A,* 48–54.

Nirschl, R. P. (1992). Elbow tendinosis/tennis elbow. *Clinics in Sports Medicine, 11,* 851–870.

Osterman, A. L., & Davis, C. A. (1996). Subcutaneous transposition of the ulnar nerve for treatment of cubital tunnel syndrome. *Hand Clinics, 12,* 421–433.

Page, C., Backus, S. I., & Lenhoff, M. W. (2003). Electromyographic activity in stiff and normal elbows during elbow flexion and extension. *Journal of Hand Therapy, 16,* 5–11.

Pascarelli, E. F., & Kella, J. J. (1993). Soft-tissue injuries related to use of the computer keyboard. *Journal of Occupational Medicine, 35,* 522–532.

Pettengill, K. M. S. (2002). Therapist's management of the complex injury. In E. J. Mackin, A. D. Callahan, T. M. Skirven, L. H. Schneider, & A. L. Osterman (Eds.), *Rehabilitation of the hand and upper extremity* (5th ed., pp. 1411–1427). St. Louis: Mosby.

Pettengill, K. M. S., & van Strien, G. (2002). Postoperative management of flexor tendon injuries. In E. J. Mackin, A. D. Callahan, T. M. Skirven, L. H. Schneider, & A. L. Osterman (Eds.), *Rehabilitation of the hand and upper extremity* (5th ed., pp. 431–456). St. Louis: Mosby.

Pitner, M. A. (1990). Pathophysiology of overuse injuries in the hand and wrist. *Hand Clinics, 6,* 355–364.

Posner, M. A. (1998). Compressive ulnar neuropathies at the elbow: II. Treatment. *Journal of the American Academy of Orthopedic Surgeons, 6,* 289–297.

Purdy, B. A., & Wilson, R. L. (2002). Management of nonarticular fractures of the hand. In E. J. Mackin, A. D. Callahan, T. Skirven, L. H. Schneider, & A. L. Osterman (Eds.), *Rehabilitation of the hand and upper extremity* (5th ed., pp. 382–395). St. Louis: Mosby.

Rice, M. S., Leonard, C., & Carter, M. (1998). Grip strengths and required forces in accessing everyday containers in a normal population. *American Journal of Occupational Therapy, 52,* 621–626.

Rider, B., & Linden, C. (1988). Comparison of standardized and nonstandardized administration of the Jebsen Hand Function Test. *Journal of Hand Therapy, 1,* 121–123.

Rozmaryn, L. M., Dovelle, S., Rothman, E. R., Gorman, K., Olvey, K. M., & Bartko, J. J. (1998). Nerve and tendon gliding exercises and the conservative management of carpal tunnel syndrome. *Journal of Hand Therapy, 11,* 171–179.

Rudman, D., & Hannah, S. (1998). An instrument evaluation framework: Description and application to assessments of hand function. *Journal of Hand Therapy, 11,* 266–277.

Russell, C. R. (1999). Bone and joint injury in the hand: Therapist's commentary. *Journal of Hand Therapy, 12,* 121–122.

Sailer, S. M. (1996). The role of splinting and rehabilitation in the treatment of carpal and cubital tunnel syndromes. *Hand Clinics, 12,* 223–241.

Schneider, L. H., & Feldscher, S. B. (2002). Tenolysis: Dynamic approach to surgery and therapy. In E. J. Mackin, A. D. Callahan, T. M. Skirven, L. H. Schneider, & A. L. Osterman (Eds.), *Rehabilitation of the hand and upper extremity* (5th ed., pp. 457–468). St. Louis: Mosby.

Servi, J. T. (1997). Wrist pain from overuse. *The Physician and Sportsmedicine, 25,* 41–44.

Shultis-Kiernan, L. (1992). Manual muscle testing. In J. S. Casanova (Ed.), *Clinical assessment recommendations* (2nd ed., pp. 47–53). Chicago: American Society of Hand Therapists.

Silva, M. J., Hollstien, S. B., Fayazi, A. H., Adler, P., Gelberman, R. H., & Boyer, M. I. (1998). The effects of multiple-strand suture techniques on the tensile properties of repair of the flexor digitorum profundus tendon to bone. *Journal of Bone and Joint Surgery, 80A,* 1507–1514.

Skirven, T., & Trope, J. (1994). Complications of immobilization. *Hand Clinics, 10,* 53–61.

Smith, G. A., Nelson, R. C., Sadoff, S. J., & Sadoff, A. M. (1989). Assessing sincerity of effort in maximal grip strength tests. *Archives of Physical Medicine and Rehabilitation, 68,* 73–80.

Smith, K. L. (2002). Nerve response to injury and repair. In E. J. Mackin, A. D. Callahan, T. M. Skirven, L. H. Schneider, & A. L. Osterman (Eds.), *Rehabilitation of the hand and upper extremity* (5th ed., pp. 583–598). St. Louis: Mosby.

Smith, K. L., & Price, J. L. (2002). Care of the hand wound. In E. J. Mackin, A. D. Callahan, T. M. Skirven, L. H. Schneider, & A. L. Osterman (Eds.), *Rehabilitation of the hand and upper extremity* (5th ed., pp. 331–343). St. Louis: Mosby.

Spaulding, S. J., McPherson, J. J., Strachota, E., Kuphal, M., & Ramponi, M. (1988). Jebsen Hand Function Test: Performance of the uninvolved hand in hemiplegia and of right-handed, right and left hemiplegic persons. *Archives of Physical Medicine and Rehabilitation, 69,* 419–422.

Spinner, M. (1995). Nerve lesions in continuity. In J. M. Hunter, E. J. Mackin, & A. D. Callahan (Eds.), *Rehabilitation of the hand: Surgery and therapy* (4th ed., pp. 627–634). St. Louis: Mosby.

Stanton-Hicks, M., Janig, W., Hassenbusch, S., Haddox, J. D., Boas, R., & Wilson, P. (1995). Reflex sympathetic dystrophy: Changing concepts and taxonomy. *Pain, 63,* 127–133.

Stern, E. B. (1992). Stability of the Jebsen-Taylor Hand Function Test across three test sessions. *American Journal of Occupational Therapy, 46,* 647–649.

Stern, P. J. (1990). Tendinitis, overuse syndromes, and tendon injuries. *Hand Clinics, 6,* 467–476.

Stolp-Smith, K. A., Pascoe, M. K., & Ogburn, P. L. (1998). Carpal tunnel syndrome in pregnancy: Frequency, severity, and prognosis. *Archives of Physical Medicine and Rehabilitation, 79,* 1285–1287.

Swigart, C. R., Eaton, R. G., Glickel, S. Z., & Johnson, C. (1999). Splinting in the treatment of arthritis of the first carpometacarpal joint. *Journal of Hand Surgery, 24A,* 86–91.

Szabo, R. M. (1998). Acute carpal tunnel syndrome. *Hand Clinics, 14,* 419–429.

Terrono, A. L., & Millender, L. H. (1996). Management of work-related upper-extremity nerve entrapments. *Orthopedic Clinics of North America, 27,* 783–793.

Tetro, A. M., & Pichora, D. R. (1996). Cubital tunnel syndrome and the painful upper extremity. *Hand Clinics, 12,* 665–677.

The Minnesota Rate of Manipulation Tests: Examiner's Manual (1969). Minnesota: Circle Pines.

Tiffin, J. (1968). *Purdue Pegboard: Examiner manual.* Chicago: Science Research Associates.

Travell, J. G., & Simons, D. (1983). *Myofascial pain and dysfunction: The trigger point manual.* Baltimore: Williams & Wilkins.

Trombly, C. A. (1995). Occupation: Purposefulness and meaningfulness as therapeutic mechanisms. 1995 Eleanor Clarke Slagle Lecture. *American Journal of Occupational Therapy, 49,* 960–972.

Tubiana, R., Thomine, J.-M., & Mackin, E. J. (1996). *Examination of the hand and wrist* (2nd ed.). London: Martin Dunitz.

Verdon, M. E. (1996). Overuse syndromes of the hand and wrist. *Primary Care, 23,* 305–319.

Walsh, M. T., & Muntzer, E. (2002). Therapist's management of complex regional pain syndrome (reflex sympathetic dystrophy). In E. J. Mackin, A. D. Callahan, T. M. Skirven, L. H. Schneider, & A. L. Osterman (Eds.), *Rehabilitation of the hand and upper extremity* (5th ed., pp. 1707–1724). St. Louis: Mosby.

Wang, A. W., & Gupta, A. (1996). Early motion after flexor tendon surgery. *Hand Clinics, 12,* 43–55.

Wilson, F. R. (1998). *The hand: How its use shapes the brain, language, and human culture.* New York: Pantheon Books.

Winters, S. C., Gelberman, R. H., Woo, S. L. Y., Chan, S. S., Grewal, R., & Seiler, J. G. (1998). The effects of multiple-strand suture methods on the strength and excursion of repaired intrasynovial flexor tendons: A biomechanical study in dogs. *Journal of Hand Surgery, 23A,* 97–104.

Wuori, J., Overend, T. J., Kramer, J. F., & MacDermid, J. (1998). Strength and pain measures associated with lateral epicondylitis bracing. *Archives of Physical Medicine and Rehabilitation, 79,* 832–837.

Zhao, C., Amadio, P. C., Tanaka, T., Yang, C., Ettema, A. M., Zobitz, M. E., & An, K. N. (2005). Short-term assessment of optimal timing for postoperative rehabilitation after flexor digitorum profundus tendon repair in a canine model. *Journal of Hand Therapy, 18,* 322–329.

LEARNING OBJECTIVES

After studying this chapter, the reader will be able to do the following:

1. Define key terms and concepts central to spinal cord injury and its care.
2. Value the physical, psychosocial, and occupational challenges associated with spinal cord injury.
3. Describe the tests and procedures appropriate for occupational therapy assessment.
4. List the roles and priorities of the occupational therapist in each of the treatment phases.
5. Recognize functional expectations of patients with various levels of injury.

CHAPTER 43

Spinal Cord Injury

Michal S. Atkins

Glossary

Dermatome—"The area of the skin innervated by the sensory axons within each segmental nerve (root)" (ASIA, 2000, p. 5).

Complete injury—"Absence of sensory and motor function in the lowest sacral segment" (ASIA, 2000 p. 7).

Incomplete injury—"Partial preservation of sensory and /or motor function below the neurological level and including the lowest sacral segment" (ASIA, 2000 p. 7).

Paraplegia—Loss or impairment in motor and/or sensory function in the thoracic, lumbar, or sacral segments of the cord resulting in impairment in the trunk, legs, and pelvic organs and sparing of the arms (ASIA, 2000).

Tenodesis grasp—Passive opening of the fingers when the wrist is flexed and closing of the fingers when the wrist is extended (Wilson et al., 1984).

Tetraplegia—Loss or impairment in motor and/or sensory function in the cervical segments of the spinal cord resulting in functional impairment in the arms, trunk, legs, and pelvic organs (ASIA, 2000).

A spinal cord injury (SCI) is a devastating event that disrupts every facet of life. Diminished physical capacities, inability to get around and carry out daily routines, and feelings of confusion and despair are coupled with loss of gainful employment and questions about the ability to return home. The occupational therapist may share this burden. With such devastating losses, where does the therapist begin? How do we help patients rebuild a sense of efficacy and self-esteem? How do we set priorities for our treatment interventions?

This chapter provides beginning answers to these questions. It outlines occupational therapy evaluations, goal setting, and treatments used with persons with SCI and introduces epidemiological data, definitions, and classifications of injuries. Next, it discusses the course after injury, followed by occupational therapy evaluations and interventions. A case study of a person who was recently injured is presented. Research data, resources, and suggested readings are listed to assist the therapist in exploring SCI beyond the material outlined in this chapter.

EPIDEMIOLOGY

Spinal cord injury is relatively rare, afflicting approximately 11,000 people a year in the United States. The numbers of people with SCI alive today in the United States is estimated to be in the range of 225,000 to 288,000 (National Spinal Cord Injury Statistical Center [NSCISC], 2005). Most SCIs occur in young males. A ratio of four injured males per female persists over the past decades. The average age at injury is 37.8 years, and 52.6% of injuries occurred between the ages of 16 to 30 years (NSCISC, 2006).

The National Spinal Cord Injury Statistical Center (NSCISC), a federally funded organization established in 1973, collects SCI epidemiological data in the United States. The causes of SCI as tracked by NSCISC since 2000 are as follows: approximately 47%, motor vehicle accidents; 23%, falls or hit by object; 14%, violence; and 10%, sports injuries. Other causes, such as non-traumatic SCI, account for the remaining 7% (NSCISC, 2006). Non-traumatic SCI is caused by spinal stenosis, tumors, ischemia, infection, and myelitis (McKinley, Seel, & Hardman, 1999). In large metropolitan areas in the United States, violence, specifically gun violence, accounts for a greater percentage of SCIs (Nobunaga, Go, & Karunas, 1999). In other countries, violence accounts for only a small fraction of injuries.

In the United States, ethnic distribution of injured persons includes 62.9% whites, 22% African Americans, 12.6% Hispanics, and 2.5% from all other ethnic groups (NSCISC, 2006). This distribution shows greater representation of minority groups than the ethnic distribution of the U.S. population. NSCISC also notes a trend in the rise of injuries to minority groups (Jackson et al., 2004; NSCISC, 2005).

Most persons with SCI (59.3%) have completed high school, and 59.6% were employed at onset. Generally, the level of education of injured individuals is somewhat lower and the unemployment rate higher than in the general population. Considering the young age of onset, it is not surprising that most persons are single when the injury occurred (Stover et al., 1995).

The clinical implications of the SCI epidemiological data have great relevance to the work of occupational therapists. Therapists must appreciate that the patients' ethnic, gender, socioeconomic, and educational backgrounds may differ from their own (see Chapters 10 and 11). Additionally, given the typical age and sex of patients with SCI, sexual, bowel, and bladder management issues must be addressed with great sensitivity, and therapists must become comfortable with their role in these matters (Trieschmann, 1988).

COURSE AFTER SPINAL CORD INJURY

Spinal cord injury causes a disruption in the motor and sensory pathways at the site of the lesion (Fig. 43-1). Since the nerve roots are segmental, a thorough evaluation of motor and sensory function can identify the level of lesion (Fig. 43-2). For example, if the spinal cord is completely severed at the level of the sixth cervical nerve root, motor and sensory information below that level no longer can travel to and from the brain. This results in paralysis of muscular activity and absence of sensation below the level of injury (Hollar, 1995).

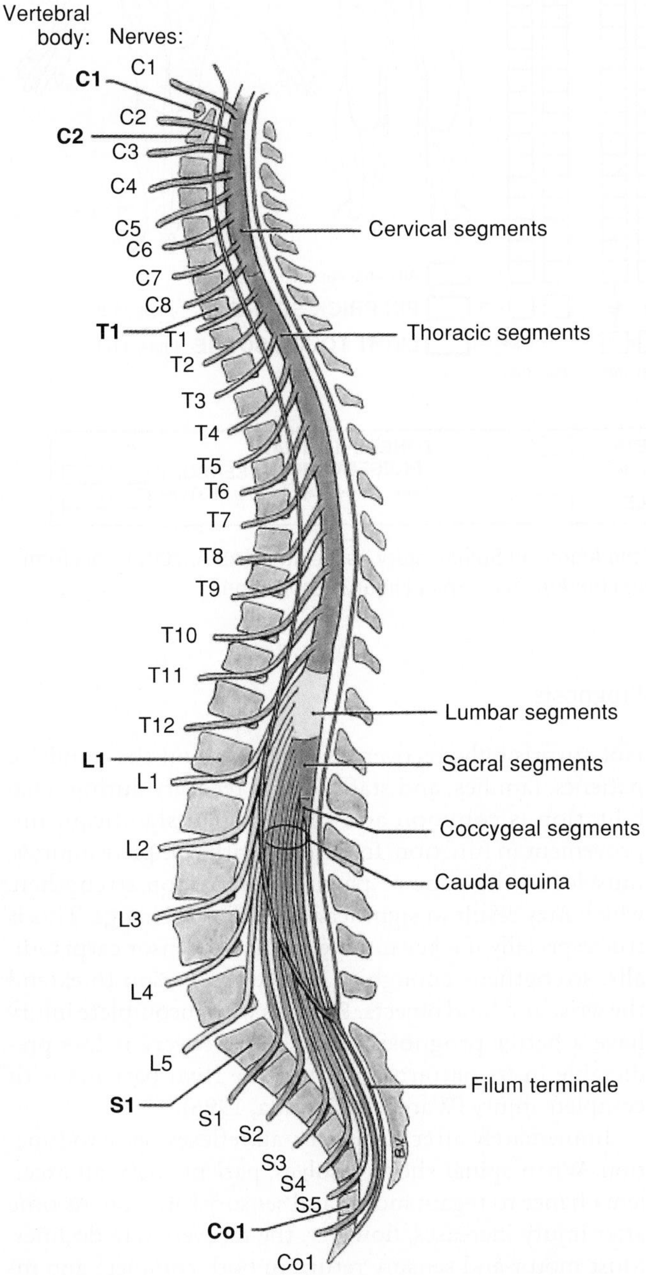

Figure 43-1 Spinal cord and spinal nerves in relation to the vertebrae. (From Agur A. M. R. [1991]. *Grant's atlas of anatomy* [9th ed.]. Baltimore: Williams & Wilkins.)

Immediately after the injury, a period of spinal shock occurs, characterized by areflexia at and below the level of injury. Spinal shock may last hours, days, or weeks. As soon as spinal shock subsides, reflexes below the level of injury return and become hyperactive. At the level of injury, areflexia may remain as the reflex arc is interrupted.

Neurological Classification of SCI

To understand the typical course of recovery from SCI, occupational therapists must be familiar with commonly used terms that describe SCI impairment and know how levels of impairment relate to prognosis.

Definitions

Tetraplegia results in functional impairment in the arms, trunk, legs, and pelvic organs. The term tetraplegia, which has replaced quadriplegia, is defined as an impairment in motor and/or sensory function in the cervical segments of the spinal cord (American Spinal Injury Association [ASIA], 2000). It is caused by damage to neural elements within the vertebral canal, and the term is not used to describe injuries to peripheral nerves. **Paraplegia** refers to motor and sensory impairment at the thoracic, lumbar, or sacral segments of the cord. Likewise, it refers only to damage to the neural elements inside the vertebral canal. Paraplegia results in sparing of arm function and, depending on the level of the lesion, impairment in the trunk, legs, and pelvic organs. The terms paraparesis and quadriparesis, which were used in the past to describe incomplete injuries, should no longer be used (ASIA, 2000).

The neurological level is diagnosed by the physician according to the motor and sensory level. The motor level is determined by testing 10 key muscles on each side of the body, and the sensory level is determined by testing sensation of 28 key points on each side of the body (Fig. 43-2). The **neurological** level is the lowest level at which key muscles grade 3 or above out of 5 on manual muscle testing (MMT), and sensation is intact for this level's **dermatome**. Also, the level above must have normal strength and sensation. For example, a person is diagnosed as having C6 tetraplegia when radial wrist extensors test 3 out of 5 and sensation is intact for the C6 dermatome. Furthermore, all motor and sensory status above the C6 level is intact. Skeletal level refers to the level of greatest vertebral damage (ASIA, 2000).

Functional level, a term used by occupational and physical therapists, refers to the lowest segment at which strength of key muscles is graded 3+ or above out of 5 on MMT and sensation is intact. Key muscles are those that significantly change functional outcomes (Occupational

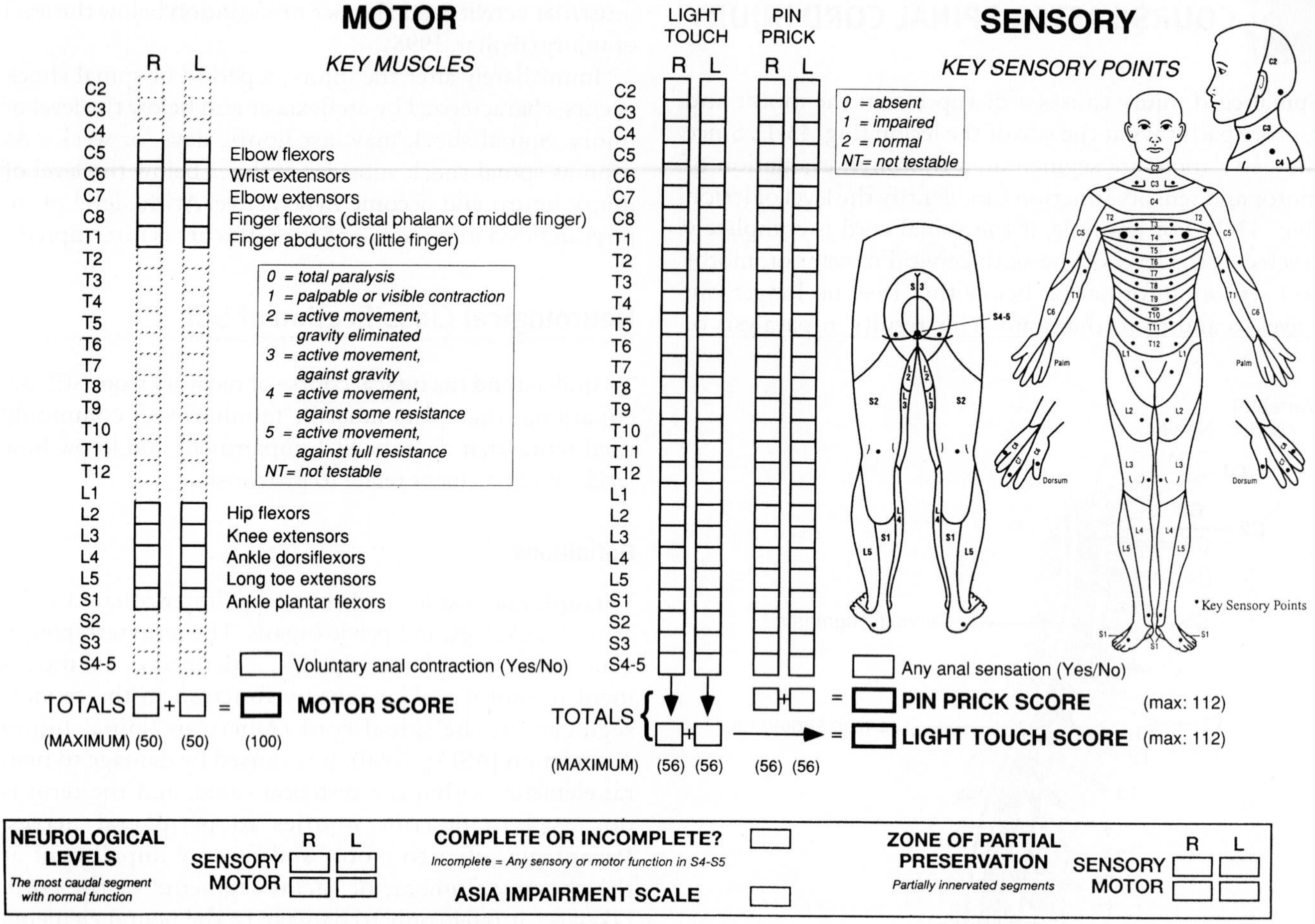

Figure 43-2 Standard neurological classification of SCI. (Courtesy of the American Spinal Injury Association [ASIA, 2000]. This form may be copied freely but should not be altered without permission from the American Spinal Injury Association.)

Therapy Department, 1990). The ASIA muscle list for the physician's motor examination (Fig. 43-2) includes only some of the muscles considered important to determine a functional level.

Two other terms commonly used with people with spinal injuries are complete and incomplete injuries (Definition 43-1). **Complete injury** consists of absence of sensory or motor function in the lowest sacral segments (S4-S5) (ASIA, 2000). The term **incomplete injury** should be used only when there is partial preservation of sensory and/or motor function below the neurological level and including the sacral segment (ASIA, 2000). The physician tests innervation at the lowest sacral segment, including anal sensation and sphincter contraction.

The term **zone of partial preservation** is used for patients with complete injuries who have partial innervation in dermatomes below the neurological level (ASIA, 2000). A patient may have a C5 neurological level complete injury, although radial wrist extensors innervated by C6 are functional (zone of partial preservation). Finally, some specific cord lesions cause a common pattern of clinical findings (see Definition 43-1).

Prognosis

Not surprisingly, recovery is very much on the minds of patients, families, and staff. Neural recovery during rehabilitation is common and can result in significant improvement in function. In patients with complete injuries, muscles in the zone of partial preservation strengthen, which may result in significant functional change. This is true especially if a key muscle, such as extensor carpi radialis, strengthens enough to enable the person to extend the wrist and hold objects. Patients with incomplete injury have a better prognosis, and their recovery is less predictable in its pattern and outcome than patients with complete injury (Waters & Yoshida, 1996).

Immediately after the injury, all reflexes cease to function. When spinal shock resolves, patients have an excellent chance to regain motor and sensory function. As time after injury increases, however, the recovery rate declines. Most motor and sensory return in both complete and incomplete injuries occurs in the first 6 months post onset; the rate of recovery is minimal after a year (Waters & Yoshida, 1996; Kirshblum et al., 2004).

DEFINITION 43-1

ASIA Scale and Clinical Syndromes

ASIA Impairment Scale

The following scale is used in grading the degree of impairment:

A = Complete—No sensory or motor function is preserved in the sacral segments S4-S5.
B = Incomplete—Sensory but not motor function is preserved below the neurological level and includes the sacral segments S4-S5.
C = Incomplete—Motor function is preserved below the neurological level, and more than half of key muscles below the neurological level have a muscle grade less than 3.
D = Incomplete—Motor function is preserved below the neurological level, and at least half of key muscles below the neurological level have a muscle grade greater than or equal to 3.
E = Normal—Motor and sensory functions are normal.

Note: To receive a grade of C or D, a person must have sensory or motor function in the sacral segments S4-S5. In addition, the individual must have either (1) voluntary anal sphincter contraction or (2) sparing of motor function more than three levels below the motor level.

Clinical Syndromes

Central Cord Syndrome—Incomplete injury most common to the cervical region in which the center part of the cord is damaged. This lesion results in greater weakness in the upper limbs than in the lower limbs, with sacral sparing (ASIA, 2000).
Brown-Sequard Syndrome—Half of the cord is damaged, causing ipsilateral proprioceptive and motor loss and contralateral loss of pain and temperature sensation (ASIA, 2000).
Anterior Cord Syndrome—Lesion with variable motor and sensory loss and preservation of proprioception (ASIA, 2000).
Conus Medullaris Syndrome—Lesions to the sacral cord and lumbar nerve roots within the spinal canal; commonly results in areflexic bladder, bowel, and lower limbs (ASIA, 2000).
Cauda Equina Syndrome—Lower motor neuron injury to the lumbosacral nerve roots within the spinal canal; results in areflexic bladder, bowel, and lower limbs (ASIA, 2000).

ASIA Impairment Scale reprinted with permission from the American Spinal Injury Association. (2000). *International standards for neurological classification of spinal cord injury.* Chicago: American Spinal Injury Association.

As patients and significant others hope for complete recovery, it is important that the therapist maintain hope while planning a realistic course of treatment. Research data can assist the clinician in predicting recovery and outcomes. One such source is the booklet *Recovery Following Spinal Cord Injury: A Clinician's Handbook* (Waters et al., 1995), although the therapist should be cautious about sharing this information with patients when they are most vulnerable.

Long-term survival of people with SCI has improved dramatically over the past 50 years. However, their life expectancy remains somewhat less than for the able-bodied population (NSCISC, 2006).

Impairments and Their Therapeutic Implications

Paralysis is the most common result of SCI. This injury is accompanied by a variety of frequent complications. The therapist must be aware of these impairments to provide a safe therapeutic environment and educate patients in understanding how to live a safe and healthy life.

Respiration

Many patients with SCI have compromised breathing. This is true especially for individuals with cervical injuries. Respiratory complications, specifically pneumonia, have been identified as the leading cause of death in the first year of life after SCI. In lesions above C4, damage to the phrenic nerve results in partial or complete paralysis of the diaphragm. These patients require ventilatory support (Fig. 43-3). Lower cervical and thoracic spine injuries can result in paralysis of other breathing muscles, such as the intercostals, abdominals, or latissimus dorsi (Kendall, McCreary, & Provance, 1993). Thus, patients with such injuries also have impaired respiration.

Use of proper techniques and infection control standards are important for respiratory care. Under the direction of the physician, the physical and respiratory therapists and the health care team work to achieve adequate bronchial hygiene and to facilitate good breathing at rest and during activities. Good communication with the team allows the occupational therapist to support breathing goals.

Autonomic Dysreflexia

Autonomic dysreflexia, a sudden dangerous increase in blood pressure, is a possibly life-threatening complication associated with lesions at the T6 level or above (Safety Note 43-1). It is brought on by an unopposed sympathetic

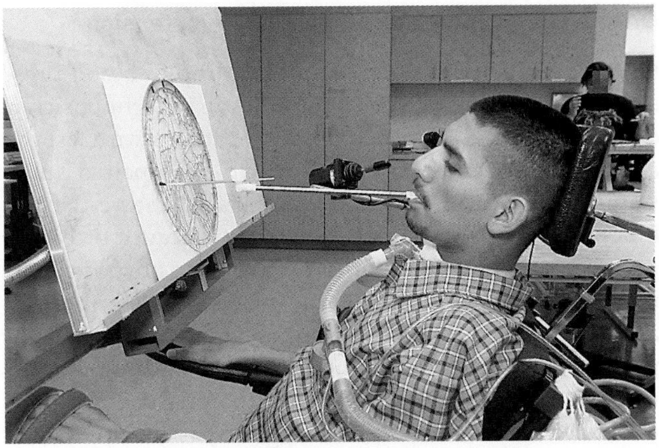

Figure 43-3 A person with C2 complete tetraplegia, ventilator dependent, using a mouthstick.

SAFETY NOTE 43-1

Safety Concerns for Patients with SCI

Autonomic Dysreflexia

Individuals with injuries at the T6 level or above may develop dangerously high blood pressure in response to a noxious stimulus. This condition is brought about by unopposed hyperactivity of the autonomic nervous system. If not promptly treated, autonomic dysreflexia may result in a stroke or sudden death. An increase of 20 mm Hg or more in systolic blood pressure is a sign that must be attended to. A pounding headache is the most common symptom. Other signs and symptoms include heavy sweating, flushed skin, goose bumps, blurry vision, a stuffy nose, anxiety, difficulty breathing, and chest tightness (Consortium for Spinal Cord Medicine, 1997a).

Take the following steps:

1. Ask the person to stop any ongoing activity, as it may further increase blood pressure.
2. Check blood pressure. If high:
3. Have the person sit up with head elevated to avoid excessive blood pressure to the brain.
4. Loosen clothing, abdominal binder, and any other constrictive devices.
5. Check the urinary catheter for kinks or folds and straighten any.
6. Continue to monitor blood pressure and seek medical assistance, which may include bladder irrigation, manual fecal evacuation, and medications.

Orthostatic or Postural Hypotension

In contrast to autonomic dysreflexia, in orthostatic hypotension, blood pressure drops to dangerously low levels in response to assuming an upright position. If it is not treated immediately, the person may lose consciousness. Symptoms of orthostatic hypotension include light-headedness, pallor, and visual changes. To resolve the problem:

1. Check blood pressure.
2. If the person is in bed, lower the head of the bed.
3. If the person is in a wheelchair, lift his or her legs and observe for signs of relief. If symptoms persist, recline the wheelchair to place the head at or below the level of the heart.
4. If symptoms persist, put the patient to bed.
5. Continue to monitor blood pressure and seek medical assistance. Do not leave the patient unattended until a nurse or a physician is present.

Principles for treatment of autonomic dysreflexia are derived from Consortium for Spinal Cord Medicine (1997a) and Zejdlik (1991). Principles for treatment of postural hypotension are derived from Zejdlik (1991).

response to noxious stimuli. Some of the more common causes of autonomic dysreflexia are distended bladder, urinary tract or other infection, bladder or kidney stones, fecal impaction, pressure ulcers, ingrown toenails, invasive procedures such as urinary catheterization or enema, and pain. The main symptoms are hypertension and a pounding headache (Consortium for Spinal Cord Medicine, 1997a).

Orthostatic Hypotension, or Postural Hypotension

Orthostatic hypotension is a sudden drop in blood pressure occurring when a person assumes an upright position (Safety Note 43-1). Most common in patients with lesions at the T6 level and above, it is caused by impaired autonomic regulation. A decrease occurs in the returning blood supply to the heart, commonly because of blood pooling in the lower extremities. Orthostatic hypotension is aggravated by a prolonged stay in bed. When the patient attempts to sit up, the blood rushes down to the legs. The patient may complain of light headedness or dizziness and may faint on moving from reclined to upright. The therapist must use caution when sitting the patient up by having the patient move slowly and in stages and letting the blood pressure adjust to the change. Elevating the head of the bed, using a tilt table, or using a reclining wheelchair can accomplish this. To control this problem further, patients benefit from wearing abdominal binders and elastic stockings (Zejdlik, 1991).

Pressure Ulcers and Pressure Relief

Pressure ulcers are a common problem for people with SCI. Most patients do not have the sensory feedback that periodically cues them to shift position in their bed or wheelchair. The constant pressure caused by maintaining a static position without shifting weight can lead to skin breakdown. All patients must be placed on a weight-shifting pressure-relief schedule.

Although most pressure relief efforts are aimed at the buttocks, many other parts of the body are vulnerable in patients with higher lesions. All insensate areas must be inspected daily. For high tetraplegic patients, these areas may also include the spine of the scapula and the back of the head.

The pressure relief program is successful only if patients with SCI incorporate this practice in their daily routines following hospitalization (Wolfe, Potter, & Sequeira, 2004). They must become responsible for carrying out pressure relief procedures themselves or for asking assistance in doing so. Educational materials, such as The Consortium for Spinal Cord Medicine Clinical Practice Guidelines, *Consumer Guides—Pressure Ulcers: What You Should Know* (2002), are helpful supplements for further reinforcing the program. No exact optimal interval of pressure relief standards is defined at this time; however, there is general agreement that, in bed, patients must change their position every 2 hours and, in a wheelchair, they must relieve pressure on their buttocks every hour for 1 minute (Buss, Halfens, & Abu-Saad, 2002).

Any client interaction must be viewed as an opportunity for a "teachable moment" (Wolfe, Potter, & Sequeira, 2004). Examples of our roles in pressure ulcer prevention include:

- Training in motor skills, such as checking the skin in bed and in the wheelchair.
- Establishing routines, such as inspecting and wiping any wetness in vulnerable areas.
- Assessing environmental and contextual factors, such as helping select high-protein, healthy foods when going to the market (Clark et al., 2006; Ryan, 2003).

Bowel and Bladder Function and Management

Bowel and bladder function is controlled in the S2-5 spinal segments. Therefore, all persons with complete lesions at and above the S2-5 levels lose their ability to void and defecate voluntarily. With the presence of intact reflex activity but with a lack of cortical voluntary control, patients void and defecate reflexively. Incomplete injuries and disruption at the S2-5 levels, as seen in conus medullaris and cauda equina, may present with a mixed sensory and/or motor picture. For example, a person may feel the urge but may lack the ability to void and defecate voluntarily. The goal of a sound bowel and bladder program is to allow the person to develop an elimination routine that supports health, reduces potential complications, and allows the freedom to engage in life roles without disruption (Consortium for Spinal Cord Injury, 1998b).

Following a thorough medical examination that includes studies of the structure and function of the digestive and urinary tracts, a physician establishes a safe elimination program. Most programs involve behavioral and pharmacological interventions (Pires, 2002). Surgery is also an option that is typically offered months or years post injury to further ease elimination and reduce problems.

Nurses are the primary trainers of bowel and bladder routines, and occupational therapists have a vital role in supporting the acquisition of these new skills and habits. A typical bowel program for a person with paraplegia includes taking oral medications to allow for optimal feces consistency and establishing a daily routine of transferring to the toilet, managing clothing, inserting a suppository, and, after waiting for some time, inserting a finger to the anus (called digital stimulation), which causes reflexive defecation. The occupational therapist may assist in facilitating skill acquisition in a person with poor vision and/or cognitive deficits. A magnifying mirror and a lamp may be placed on the floor to help the person see and further break down the activity to better reinforce each step. Persons with low tetraplegia have added challenges in becoming independent in bowel care. They may achieve independence or assist in managing their bowel care only after much practice. To compensate for poor trunk control, individuals perform the bowel program on a commode; to compensate for finger paralysis, they require a tool called the dill stick to stimulate the anal reflex to defecate (Fig. 43-4); and to compensate for lack of sensation in the anus and/or parts of the hand, they require a mirror. For safe task performance, occupational therapists may practice commode mobility and dill stick insertion focusing on effective visual compensation. When patients become skillful at bowel evacuation practices, they decrease the risk of complications. Most individuals, after discharge, opt to carry out their bowel program in the morning every other day and can complete the procedure within 45 minutes (Kirshblum et al., 1998).

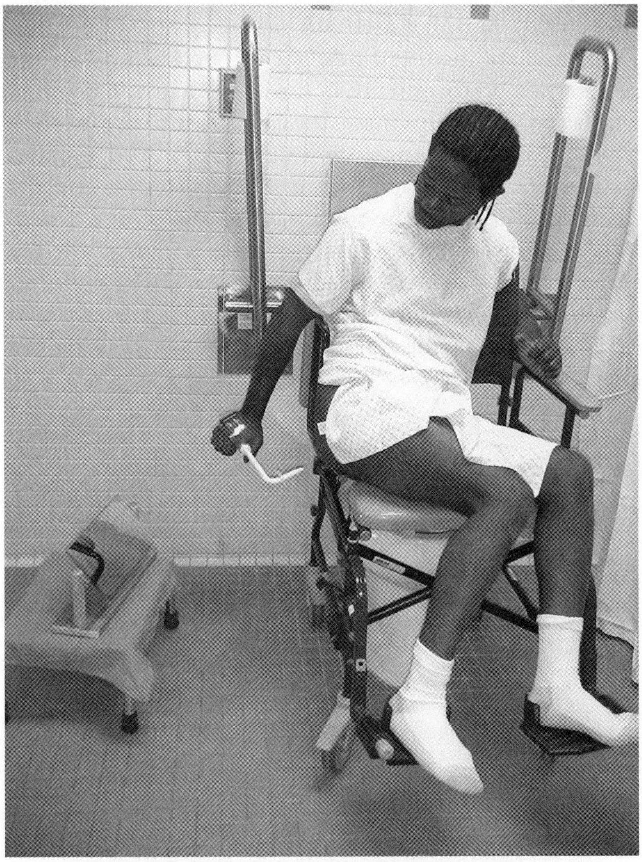

Figure 43-4 A simulation of a bowel program for a person with low-level tetraplegia (ASIA A). The person is hooking his left arm under the handle for stability. He is using a dill stick to stimulate reflexic evacuation and a mirror to compensate for his lack of sensation in the anal area.

As with the bowel program, the goal of the bladder program is to achieve a simple routine with minimal risk of complications. Recurring urinary tract infection is a frequent complication and the most frequent cause of rehospitalization after spinal cord injury (Cardenas et al., 2004). To avoid complications, patients must empty their bladder routinely.

An indwelling catheter, which is a catheter that stays in the urethra and is changed only periodically, is commonly inserted soon after the person is admitted to the acute care hospital. Although some patients stay with the indwelling catheter, an effort is made to find other ways to empty the bladder (Yarkony & Chen, 1996).

Common bladder practices include use of either intermittent catheterization or reflex voiding. Intermittent catheterization (IC) involves the manual insertion of a catheter into the bladder (Fig. 43-5) at fixed intervals of approximately 4–6 hours. Reflex voiding refers to the spontaneous micturition when the bladder is full. This voiding method requires that males use a condom catheter and a leg bag and that females use a diaper (Pires, 2002). As with the bowel program, the bladder programs of persons with tetraplegia need more intervention, and the occupational therapist must become thoroughly familiar with individual techniques. Interventions may include finding a way to keep down the pants when performing IC in the wheelchair and training with a tool that helps insert the catheter into the urethra. Urinary management is more challenging to females than to males. Women have a shorter urethra and the opening is between the folds of the labia, so it is much harder for women to insert a catheter. In addition, women often need to wear diapers because their shorter urethra is more prone to leakage, and there are currently no acceptable female external collection devices that can keep the skin dry.

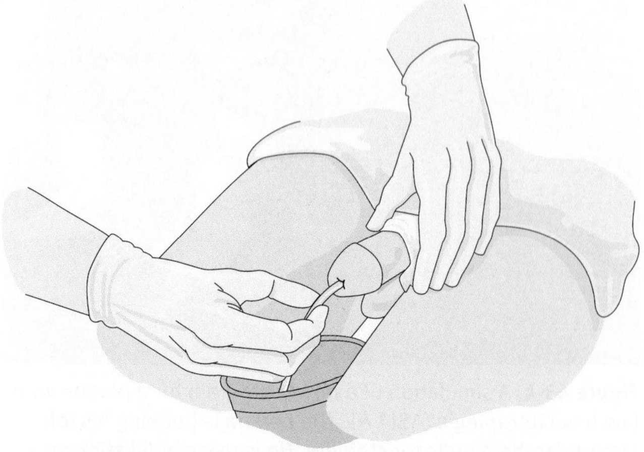

Figure 43-5 Catheterization: Inserting a catheter into the bladder and waiting for urine to flow.

To best meet the person's environmental and contextual demands, the occupational therapist must think and practice beyond the hospital or clinic when helping patients rehearse and refine bowel and bladder routines. As patients rebuild new routines and habits, the therapist helps identify and imbed these new functional skills in real-life scenarios such as emptying a full leg bag at a party, changing clothes when an accident happens in a mall, and performing intermittent catheterization while attending school.

Sexual Function

The need for emotional and physical intimacy does not diminish after SCI, and questions about intimacy, sexuality, fertility, and reproduction must be answered by a team of sensitive and knowledgeable professionals. SCI affects both sexual intercourse and reproduction. Usually, male patients with complete injuries are unable to have psychogenic (voluntary) erections and ejaculations. They can, however, have reflex erections that may be controlled by stimulation, such as pulling the pubic hairs (Ducharme & Gill, 1997). Patients with complete injuries at S2-5 lose bowel, bladder, and genital reflexes and have a complete loss of erection. As with physical performance, male fertility is decreased after SCI. Advances in technology, however, provide ways for male patients to sustain an erection and improve the chances of fathering children (Ducharme & Gill, 1997).

Although sexual and reproductive functioning is less affected in women, sex, fertility, and menopause are still issues of concern. Some consequences related to these issues are dysreflexia and bladder incontinence during intercourse and complications of pregnancy and delivery (Jackson & Wadley, 1999).

For both men and women, other psychological, social, and physical issues add to the difficulty in resuming satisfying sexual roles. Problems with mobility, dependency, and societal role expectations are some of the issues the person with SCI must face. Knowledgeable members of the team must address sexual issues with patients. Individual counseling, often by a psychologist, takes place after a thorough evaluation by a physician. The following four areas are typically addressed: sexual satisfaction, sexual function, fertility, and desirability. Patients learn that, despite their injury, they can continue to be desirable and have an active sex life (Ducharme & Gill, 1997).

The occupational therapist addresses many issues that relate to sexuality. Therefore, therapists must develop the necessary expertise and comfort level to deal with this sensitive and important subject. Some examples for the therapist's involvement may be helping people groom themselves to improve their appearance and to feel more attractive, creating a cozy environment that allows for intimacy, and finding equipment to compensate for lack of hand function.

Temperature Regulation

Many people with SCI cannot regulate body temperature, which can lead to hypothermia or heat stroke (Zejdlik, 1991). Due to decreased sensation, patients may become severely sunburned or frostbitten. Education in the importance of neutral temperatures and the prevention of skin exposure to sun and severe temperatures is an important part of the occupational therapy program (Hill, 1986).

Pain

Acute and chronic pain (duration of more than half a year) is common after SCI. Approximately 65% of individuals with SCI report having chronic pain, and persons with tetraplegia report having more pain than persons with paraplegia (Siddall & Loeser, 2001). Considering the violent nature of most injuries, it is not surprising that most patients have pain at onset and that pain persists for a long time. Although many types of pain are present, they are most commonly classified as follows:

- Mechanical pain: Local soft tissue pain associated with the injury. Mechanical pain, common in the shoulder of the person with tetraplegia, may be caused by direct trauma, muscle imbalance, and overuse of weak muscles. It is the most common pain in people with SCI (Siddall et al., 2003).
- Radicular pain (also called segmental root pain): Pain that often follows the segmental distribution of the nerve.
- Neuropathic pain (also called deafferentation or central pain). Pain that originates in the spinal cord and is thought to be the result of misdirected neural sprouting after the injury.

For many people with SCI, pain contributes to activity limitations, lack of participation, and depression. Available treatments include prescription and non-prescription medications, physical agent modalities, medical procedures such as nerve blocks, and psychotherapy (Widerstrom-Noga & Turk, 2003). The occupational therapist's contribution to pain management includes a thorough evaluation and a myriad of interventions. Although treatment goals are often directed toward reducing impairments, our main contribution is in changing habits and roles and facilitating engagement in meaningful activities and full participation. This approach is especially valuable because most persons continue to live with some pain throughout their lives and new pains arise with aging.

Fatigue

Physiological, psychological, and environmental factors all contribute to patients' fatigue. Persistent pain, antispasmodic medications, and prolonged bed rest are physical factors that can make the patient feel tired or sleepy. These factors are often compounded by restless nights interrupted by hospital routines, such as repositioning patients in bed and waking them for checking vital signs and administering medications. Occupational therapists must be aware of these constraints and observe and listen to the patient. They must find the optimal waking hours for activities and report nighttime sleep disturbances, any changes of behavior that medication may cause, and other factors.

Spasticity and Spasms

An injury to the spinal cord often results in an increase in transmission within the synaptic stretch reflex. This results in spasticity. Spasticity develops into clonic or tonic spasms triggered by sensory stimuli such as sudden touch, infection, or other irritation. Management of spasticity is important in maximizing a patient's functional independence. Severe spasticity may hinder function; for example, the hypertonicity of the hip and knee adductors can make donning pants difficult. The most common way to decrease spasticity is to use a muscle relaxant, such as baclofen. An intrathecal pump, motor point, or nerve blocks may be used in severe cases. Spasticity can lead to contractures, so routine positioning in bed (Fig. 43-6) and in the wheelchair and range of motion are essential; patient and family must participate in these measures for continuity of care (see Chapter 21).

Deep Vein Thrombosis

Deep vein thrombosis is the formation of a blood clot, most often in a lower extremity or the abdomen or pelvic area. A clot may develop further and dislodge from the venous wall, forming an embolus. This condition poses a threat to the patient because the embolus may travel and occlude pulmonary circulation (Consortium for Spinal Cord Medicine, 1997b). The therapist helps prevent this condition by observing any asymmetry in the lower extremities in color, size, and/or temperature. When deep vein thrombosis is identified, the patient must have complete bed rest and anti-coagulants to prevent embolus (Consortium for Spinal Cord Medicine, 1997b). This is a good time to inform the patient and family about the symptoms, prevention, and care of deep vein thrombosis.

Heterotopic Ossification

Heterotopic ossification, which is pathological bone formation in joints, has been recorded in 15–53% of SCI patients (van Kuijk, Geurts, & van Kuppevelt, 2002). It is a condition in which connective tissue calcifies around the joint. Heterotopic ossification usually appears 1–4 months after injury. The symptoms are a warm, swollen extremity, fever, and/or range-of-motion limitations.

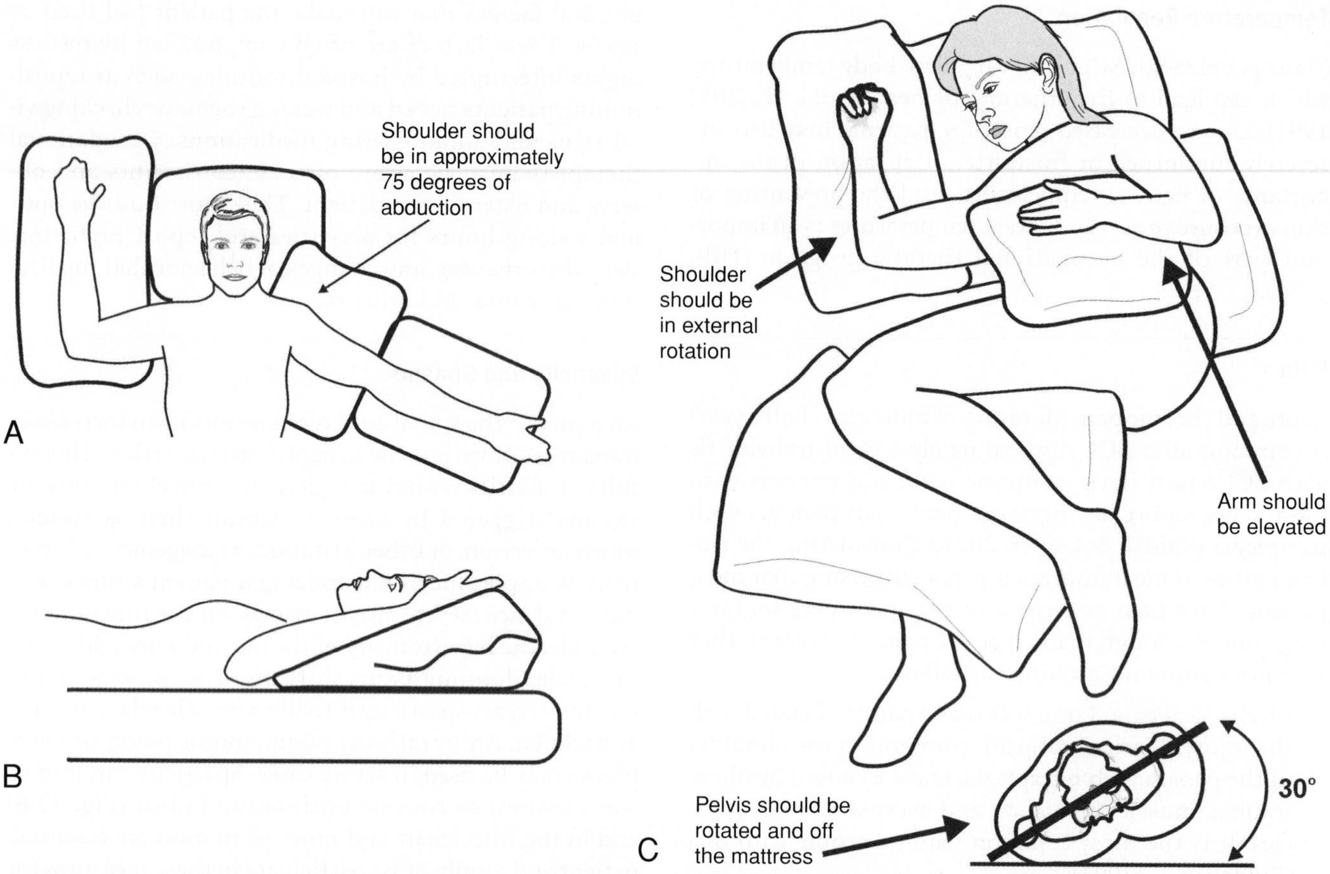
Shoulder should be in approximately 75 degrees of abduction
A
B
Shoulder should be in external rotation
Arm should be elevated
30°
Pelvis should be rotated and off the mattress
C

Figure 43-6 Positioning in bed. **A.** Alternate the arm in shoulder abduction and external rotation. **B.** Side view of **A**, showing placement of foam wedge. **C.** During side-lying, keep the upper back flat on the bed to protect the weighted shoulder. (Printed with permission from Rancho Los Amigos National Rehabilitation Center, Downey, CA.)

Most often seen in the hip and shoulder joints, heterotopic ossification can result in joint contractures. Positioning in bed and in the wheelchair (see Fig. 43-6) and daily range of motion prevent or control heterotopic ossification. As the first indication of heterotopic ossification most typically is range-of-motion limitation, the occupational therapist must use each range-of-motion session to monitor joint ranges, especially in patients with spastic muscles (Garland, 1991).

Psychosocial Adaptation

As mentioned earlier, SCI dramatically disrupts life (see Chaper 35). What coping mechanisms are enlisted to enable the individual to adjust to these dramatic life challenges? Despite inconclusive and conflicting research, many authors agree that reactions to SCI may include periods of shock, anxiety, denial, depression, internalized and externalized anger, adjustment, and acknowledgment. These coping behaviors may be enlisted in a different order, and some may be skipped (Livneh & Antonak, 1997).

Depression

Although it is not universal, many patients have varying degrees of depression, sadness, or grief (Consortium for Spinal Cord Medicine, 1998a). Logically, we associate depression with the grieving time right after the injury; depression, however, may persist long after the injury. Fuhrer et al. (1993) estimated that, after SCI, up to 25% of men and 47% of women have symptoms of depression. Depressive symptoms are also associated with lack of social and occupational involvement. Injured individuals who show more symptoms of depression participate less in worker, volunteer, and student roles. Interestingly, level of injury does not appear to be associated with depressive symptoms. Individuals with a high cervical lesion are not necessarily more commonly or intensely depressed than individuals with paraplegia (Fuhrer et al., 1993).

To understand the complexity of the psychosocial adjustment to SCI, we must also examine the reactions of the patient's family and significant others. The family and significant others may also go through these psychological reactions. Concurrently, they may have to reassess their future commitment to the injured person. A mother, for example, may grieve and be sad while having to decide whether to take her fully dependent son home after a turbulent adolescence.

SCI, independent of its severity, is an emotionally traumatic and overwhelming event. Therefore, in every encounter with the patient, we must ask ourselves: Is the person ready to hear this information? Is this "chunk" of information too much for the person? Often, the patient may answer these questions directly, but at times, the therapist may need to collect cues from facial expressions and/or from body language if patients have arm and trunk movement (Potter et al., 2004; Wolfe, Potter, & Sequeira, 2004).

Occupational therapists and other health care professionals must also examine their emotional reactions and the influence of these emotions on the patient and therapeutic process. For example, sometimes upon interviewing a newly injured person, I become especially sad as I strongly identify with something in the patient's life narrative (e.g., the struggles of a mother with two young children). I am reminded of my projection, as the patient may be perfectly accepting and cheerful. Furthermore, studies show that health care professionals may overestimate the degree of patients' distress and depression. Patients' descriptions of their own depression are often milder than perceived by the health care professional (Cushman & Dijkers, 1990).

As occupational therapists, we contribute to psychosocial adaptation after SCI by incorporating the following considerations into evaluation and treatment.

- Set aside all preconceived biases about who the patient is and how he or she should feel or behave. Instead, concentrate on learning to know patients, their unique life contexts, and their individual reactions to their trauma.
- Provide psychological support. At times when the patient is overwhelmed with sadness, it is okay just to be present and available to the person. It is okay to stop an activity, find a quiet environment, possibly outside, and listen, affirm, and educate.
- Select activities with a just-right challenge. After weeks of being dependent, patients find hope by being able to feed themselves or turn on a CD player independently.
- When providing information, don't overwhelm the person with too much detail. Find the opportunity for a "teachable moment" for a particular "chunk" of information and be sensitive of patients' signs to help you determine how to proceed and when to stop (Potter et al., 2004; Wolfe, Potter, & Sequeira, 2004).
- Accept patients' emotional states without judging them (Hammell, 1995). Lack of evidence of depression or anger does not necessarily mean that individuals are coping poorly with their injury. They may be using ways of coping that are not the textbook ones. Remember that there is no requirement to mourn to learn to accept and live with the injury (Cushman & Dijkers, 1990).
- Create opportunities for peer education and support. Peers with SCI are often very effective in reaching patients and in making them feel less isolated and more optimistic. Individuals with similar levels of injury can truly understand the pain that comes with SCI and may help the therapeutic process.

ASSESSMENT: GETTING TO KNOW THE PERSON

Prior to the assessment, the occupational therapist checks the medical chart for medical clearance to begin the evaluation. The patient often has other trauma, such as lacerations of internal organs, closed head injury, and fractures. Special care is taken to review records and communicate with the physician to ensure the safety of the patient. The initial evaluation is often difficult, as the newly injured patient may be sedated, in pain, and/or confused. Furthermore, this assessment may be interrupted by numerous medical procedures and may be restricted by medical and spinal precautions. Therefore, the occupational therapist must be flexible in choosing appropriate evaluation time, in gathering bits of information in interrupted sessions, and in choosing the right tool for the moment when the patient is available. In essence, the evaluation process should not be limited to set scheduled intervals, and the therapist must view each encounter with the patient as part of an ongoing assessment. Information should be also collected from significant others and other team members. Thus, at the end of the assessment period, the therapist assembles all fragments of information into a full, initial evaluation. Treatment begins while the evaluation is in progress. This prevents further complications, such as range-of-motion limitations and edema. The therapist may also address patients' immediate needs, for example making them more comfortable in bed, which further establishes rapport and trust.

Often various members of the interdisciplinary team repeat parts of the evaluation. A positive trend toward an interdisciplinary team evaluation in which a few members of the team evaluate the patient together brings organized information gathering to the process that is not redundant. Assessment in occupational therapy after SCI includes all levels of occupational functioning.

Occupational Profile

The goals of the initial evaluation include beginning to establish rapport and trust, teaching patients about their potential, and learning about who they are and what is important to them. From the first encounter, the therapist also begins to educate the patient and to plan discharge. This is true especially today, when hospital stays have been cut to a bare minimum. In the acute phase and shortly after the injury, patients may be quite limited in their knowledge of the nature of their injury, prognosis for recovery, and potential for function. It is important not to overwhelm the patient with more than can be absorbed at that moment. The therapist must always leave room for hope without deceiving the patient.

To gather deeper understanding of patients' roles, activities, and the meaning behind the activities, use open-ended questions. Charting a typical day's schedule prior to injury allows for creative questioning and enables the therapist to sketch a person's habits, routines, and other activities.

The *Canadian Occupational Performance Measure* (*COPM*) is an excellent tool for working with the SCI population. It focuses on finding out patients' occupational goals and their priorities (Donnelly et al., 2004) (see Chapters 4 and 10). If patients are not psychologically ready to formulate goals that are important to discharge, first goals may be directed toward their attaining more control over their immediate environment.

Evaluation of Performance Skills

Spinal stability must be established prior to any physical contact with the patient. The occupational therapist must clarify with the primary physician how much movement and load are allowed without jeopardizing spinal integrity.

The physical assessment includes upper extremity range of motion, strength, muscle tone, and sensation (see Chapters 6 and 7). The therapist also observes the patient's endurance, trunk balance, fatigability, and pain. *The Manual Muscle Test* is most widely used to measure strength. This test is useful in determining the functional level of the person. The appearance of the upper extremities can reveal signs of reflex sympathetic dystrophy, which is an upper limb disease marked by severe pain and swelling. Such findings are vital for prevention of further deformity by immediately initiating an aggressive treatment regimen.

Hand and Wrist of the Patient with Tetraplegia

Evaluation of the hands and wrists is both physical and functional. Most therapists observe hand use while the person is performing activities such as picking up coins or pieces of a game or eating. Most hand motor function tests are not specific to tetraplegia, and although they prove somewhat useful in determining abilities and capacities, many are old and require much time to administer. Some such tests are the *Sollerman Hand Function Test* (Sollerman & Ejeskar, 1995) and the *Jebsen Test of Hand Function* (Jebsen et al., 1969). New hand tests have been developed to specifically assess hand function before and after hand reconstruction surgeries. Some such tests are the *Standardized Object Test* (*SOT*) and the *VadenBerge Hand and Arm Function Test* (van Tuijl, Janssen-Ptten, & Seelen, 2002). New tetraplegia hand-specific functional assessments are needed. The *Tetraplegia Hand Activity Questionnaire* (*THAQ*) (Land at el., 2004) may prove useful but has yet to be tested. Pinch and grip strength are measured by dynamometers when hand muscles are functioning (van Tuijl, Janssen-Potten, & Seelen, 2002). To measure weak pinch and grip, more sensitive instruments than the standard dynamometer and pinch meter are used. Finally, using the client-centered approach of *The Canadian Occupational Performance Measure*, clinicians find out what is most relevant to the person. By asking the person to list functions they want and need to perform with their hands and examining their performance in these areas, the therapist can concentrate on those functional components most relevant to the person.

Evaluation of Performance in Areas of Occupation

Selection of appropriate functional evaluations is determined by level of injury and stage of recovery. Occupational therapists rely on observations and standardized and nonstandardized assessments to evaluate basic and instrumental activities of daily living (ADL), leisure, school, vocational interests, and aptitudes (see Chapter 4).

Activities of Daily Living and Instrumental Activities of Daily Living

Often full ADL evaluation is postponed because of medical and spinal restrictions, and predictions regarding length of stay and functional outcomes are rendered without complete data. The *Functional Independence Measure* (*FIM*) (see Chapter 4) is widely used to assess function; however, some instruments are designed specifically for the patient with SCI, such as the *Quadriplegia Index of Function* (Gersham et al., 1986) and the *Modified Barthel Index* (Yarkony et al., 1987). A relatively new and promising instrument dedicated to the person with spinal cord injury in *The Catz-Itzkovich Spinal Cord Independence Measure* (*Catz-Itzkovich SCIM*) (Catz, Itzkovich, Ring, et al., 2001). This functional instrument measures self-care, respiration, sphincter management, and mobility (Catz, Itzkovich, Steinberg, et al., 2001).

Leisure

Persons with SCI have high unemployment rates and much free time (Schoherr et al., 2005; Yerxa & Locker, 1990). Finding past relevant and meaningful leisure activities is of great importance for improving quality of life (see Chapters 4 and 34). Leisure assessments may include the *COPM* and interest inventories. Most SCIs occur to young men, thus, it is not surprising that sports are meaningful to many patients. Assessing the potential for engaging in sports following the injury may include activities such as an outing to a game and/or being introduced to a wheelchair sports program.

School and Vocation

A full vocational evaluation is rarely performed during acute rehabilitation because patients are focused on more immediate challenges. Many have lost the physical ability to engage in prior occupations. Vocational exploration begins with defining patients' abilities and interests. Observation of factors such as hand function and work habits contribute information for the prevocational team and department of vocational rehabilitation.

Home and Community

The home visit is an invaluable assessment tool for the person with SCI, and the earlier it is performed, the better. This visit allows the therapist to assess home accessibility and safety and to evaluate the capacity of patients and their families to problem solve (Atkins, 1989). Assessing transportation issues is important, as persons with SCI must often find new ways to get around. This evaluation may involve taking a bus for the first time or referring the patient to special disabled driving services (see Chapters 31 and 36).

SETTING GOALS: ORDERING PRIORITIES FOR MEANINGFUL AND RELEVANT ACTIVITIES

Setting treatment goals in the acute phase may seem overwhelmingly difficult for both patient and therapist. Complications seem to hinder progress, and patients are often confused, fearful, and uncertain about their impairments and abilities. Answers to the following questions help patient and therapist set priorities, establish short-term goals, and start treatment while evaluation is still in progress:

- What must be done to prevent further deformities and complications?
- What activity is important to the patient to engage in right now?

The development of short-term goals stems from the therapist's ability to perform an activity analysis. Short-term goals may address functional performance areas and tasks, underlying problems, or the component skills necessary to perform an ADL. For example, a person with C4 tetraplegia who wants to use a mouthstick for word processing on the computer must first tolerate sitting upright in the wheelchair for significant periods. Increasing tolerance for sitting upright is an appropriate short-term goal for achieving the independence of mouthstick computer use.

Functional Expectations

Expected functional outcome charts predict the degree of functional independence for a particular level of injury. One such chart was published in a 1999 document, *Outcomes Following Traumatic Spinal Cord Injury: Clinical Practice Guidelines for Health Care Professionals* (Consortium for Spinal Cord Medicine, 1999). The consortium is administered and financed by the Paralyzed Veterans of America. This document is presented here in part. It includes an evidence-based expected functional outcome chart (see Appendix). Not surprisingly, when the patient and therapist agree on the task and the expected functional outcome, the outcome of those predictions are most successful. In a 2000 study, Schonherr et al. (2000) explored the relationship between the expected predictions and their outcomes. The researchers also identified the effect of patient versus rehabilitation team predictive agreement and lack of agreement on outcomes. They found that prognosis on self-care and mobility was clearer with paraplegia than with tetraplegia and that predicting mobility and function of persons with incomplete injuries was less accurate and more complex (Schonherr et al., 2000).

Age-Specific Considerations

Although every patient has unique considerations in treatment planning, this chapter highlights the unique needs of adolescents and older adults.

Adolescence and Young Adulthood

The adolescent with SCI must deal with complicating normal developmental factors coupled with new impairments and disabilities (Smith et al., 1996). Psychological adaptation to the injury may be especially difficult for adolescents, as the injury comes in the midst of development of adult self-image, identity, and independence. The therapist is challenged to maintain a delicate balance between the sometimes competing needs to support patients and families and to encourage the young person to be self-reliant. Warning the family about avoiding overindulgence can lead to more engaged and assertive participation by the patient (Smith et al., 1996). At times, when the adolescent exhibits brooding or defiant behaviors that are harmful to progress, a strict behavioral program becomes necessary to draw the adolescent into positive participation (Massagli &

RESEARCH NOTE 43-1

Abstract: Donnelly, C., Eng, J. J., Hall, J., Alford, L., Giachino, R., Norton, K. & Kerr, D. S. (2004). Client-centered assessment and the identification of meaningful treatment goals for individuals with spinal cord injury. *Spinal Cord, 42,* 302–307.

In this retrospective study, Canadian researchers examined the rehabilitation records of 41 individuals with SCI. The researchers reviewed and compared the *Canadian Occupational Performance Measure* (*COPM*) and individuals' *Functional Independent Measure* (*FIM*) scores. Their objectives included finding patients' identified goals, self-perceived performance, and satisfaction in the areas of self-care, productivity, and leisure. They also examined the relationship between subjects' *COPM* and *FIM* outcome scores. Results: The most frequent goals listed by subjects were in the areas of self-care (79%). Of those goals, the most frequently mentioned ones were functional mobility, dressing, grooming, and feeding. Goals relating to productivity were listed by 12% of participants followed by leisure (9%). The researchers found fair relationship between specific *COPM* performance and satisfaction scores and *FIM* motor change scores. These data suggest that individuals perceived positive changes in their performance (subjectively measured by the *COPM*) as their function increased (as objectively measured by the *FIM*).

Implications for Practice

Finding meaningful treatment goals for each individual is the key to a successful outcome of the rehabilitation process. It serves to engage the patient in the rehabilitation process and directs the therapist and, often, the rest of the team in choosing relevant performance areas. This is especially important with shortened length of stay, as the list of potential areas for intervention can be overwhelmingly long, yet not necessarily relevant to an individual patient.

The most frequently identified patient goals in descending order were functional mobility, dressing, grooming, and feeding. These goals reflect the wish of many patients to gain independence in managing their own body first. Many patients shift their focus to productivity, leisure, and social activities at a later time.

The *FIM* is a widely used measurement scale for documenting the severity of disability, team performance goals, and outcomes of rehabilitation. If patient-identified goals are similar to the prescribed *FIM* items as described by this study, the rehabilitation process will be both predictable and smooth. The *FIM* is limited, however, in the case of people with high tetraplegia (C1-4 ASIA A) who remain fully dependent on others and also for those patients who are interested in achieving individual goals not included in the *FIM* list. Unlike the *FIM*, the *COPM* requires patients to identify their goals and to prioritize them. This assessment is client-centered and closely reflects occupational therapy values, and thus has been gaining in popularity since its introduction in 1998. Since the *FIM* is most widely used in rehabilitation hospitals in the United States and accepted by third-party payers in charting interventions and lengths of stay, it becomes our challenge to honor and advocate for patient goals even when they are not part of the *FIM* list.

Jaffe, 1990). Along with establishing independence, primary goals for the adolescent must include the following:

- Reentering the student role—Goals may include meeting with school personnel and visiting the school with the patient (Massagli & Jaffe, 1990).
- Sexual roles—Adolescents must be assured that individuals with SCI can remain sexually active (Massagli & Jaffe, 1990).
- Driver role—Initial evaluation and referral may be carried out in the acute rehabilitation phase and may be continued in the transition and adaptation phases. Driving, if possible, may provide the adolescent with a valuable sense of empowerment, independence, and increased motivation.
- At times, it is hard to remember that adolescents are minors and that all fundamental decisions must be made with parental participation and consent. The parents must be supported and must be part of the team, helping the patient make appropriate choices. Parents must also participate in educational sessions to ensure consistency in treatment, for example, with pressure relief.

The Older Adult

Having SCI and being elderly may be considered a dual diagnosis. The physiological process of aging can make rehabilitation from SCI particularly difficult, and older patients tend to have more medical complications (Scivoletto et al., 2003). Most geriatric SCIs are attributed to falls that result in lesions at the cervical level (DeVivo & Stover, 1995). The central cord syndrome is common among the elderly SCI population.

The geriatric patient may require downgrading of expected functional outcomes, given physical and/or cognitive limitations. Some important factors are decreases in muscle strength, endurance, energy, and physical fitness (McColl et al., 2003); joint degeneration; bone decalcification; skin integrity; cognition; vision; and emotional changes. Older patients may require more assistance in activities of daily living, and hence, the focus of rehabilitation may be helping them identify resources in the community and teaching them to direct their care effectively (Scivoletto et al., 2003).

Aging with Spinal Cord Injury

Long-term survival rates of patients with SCI have improved dramatically in the past few decades, and many people with SCI live for decades after injury (DeVivo, Krause, & Lammertse, 1999). Along with normal aging issues, some unique problems arise in this population. Using the upper limbs for mobility (pushing a wheelchair, transferring), overuse of weak muscles, and muscle imbalance may cause chronic shoulder pain and less often, elbow and wrist pain (Consortium for Spinal Cord Medicine, 2005; Curtis et al., 1999). Other body changes may include skin changes with increasing susceptibility to pressure ulcers, decreased bone density, susceptibility to fractures, impaired cardiovascular fitness, and renal and bowel complications. Additional problems include depression, an increase in functional dependence, and decreased mobility (Liem et al., 2004; Whiteneck et al., 1993).

The occupational therapist, using knowledge of energy conservation, joint protection, and activity analysis, must communicate with and educate the patient in restructuring activities to accommodate the new condition. An aging patient, once independent in all self-maintenance skills, may need help in the morning to conserve energy for work. A grandmother who wants to interact with her toddler grandson may have to train him to climb onto her lap rather than picking him up.

INTERVENTION

The occupational therapist treats individuals with SCI at various settings and at various times. Throughout this treatment continuum of acute care, acute rehabilitation, transition, and adaptation, most treatment principles remain the same. The focus of care changes, however, as the patient's internal processes and external environment change.

Acute Recovery: Focus on Support and Prevention

Immediately after injury, most patients are admitted into an intensive care unit, where the focus is on preservation of life and stabilizing fluids, electrolytes, and cardiopulmonary and other vital functions. The patient is immobilized in traction and waiting to hear whether surgery is required to stabilize the spine. For prevention of pressure ulcers, the patient is put in a rotating bed (Yarkoni & Chen, 1996). In the intensive care unit, medical and surgical procedures take precedence over therapy. The therapist must be flexible, often seeing the patient for brief periods throughout the day. One or two 15-minute sessions per day are often helpful to the patient, who may be in pain, fatigue easily, and become confused or overwhelmed by this fast-paced environment of electronic devices and medical procedures. The occupational therapist's initial contact should be within 24 hours of admission. Treatment begins as the initial evaluation is in progress, allowing the therapist to begin to gain a full picture of the patient (Hammell, 1995). In addition to ongoing patient and family support and education, the goals of therapy in the acute recovery phase include:

1. Provide some environmental controls to help the patient get some control.
2. Maintain normal upper limb joint range of motion and prevent deformities (Yarkoni & Chen, 1996).

To prevent range-of-motion limitations, therapists use positioning techniques and assist with range-of-motion exercises. In bed, most persons with tetraplegia tend to lie with their arms adducted close to their body, internally rotated, and with elbows flexed (Consortium for Spinal Cord Medicine, 2005). Therefore, movement in joints particularly susceptible to contractures must be monitored daily (van Kuijk, Geurts, & van Kuppevelt, 2002). These are scapular rotation, shoulder scaption (the functional motion between abduction and flexion), shoulder external rotation, elbow extension, and forearm pronation. Hands are fitted with resting hand splints. Upper limbs are placed in either some abduction or external rotation (see Fig. 43-6, A and B). Alternating arms between these positions puts all vulnerable joints in stretch. It is important to note, however, that although the goal is to preserve range of motion, one must consider the comfort of patients and allow them a good night sleep.

Range of motion to the hand of the tetraplegic patient is performed in a special way to facilitate **tenodesis grasp**: passive opening of the fingers when the wrist is flexed and closing of the fingers when the wrist is extended (Fig. 43-7) (Wilson et al., 1984). The patient, family, and others are taught how to perform range-of-motion exercises to facilitate tenodesis. Again, range-of-motion exercises must be augmented with proper positioning in bed and in the wheelchair.

Acute Rehabilitation: Focus on Support, Education, and Meaningful Activities

In the 1970s, the mean length of stay in acute SCI rehabilitation was 144.8 days. By the late 1990s, mean length of

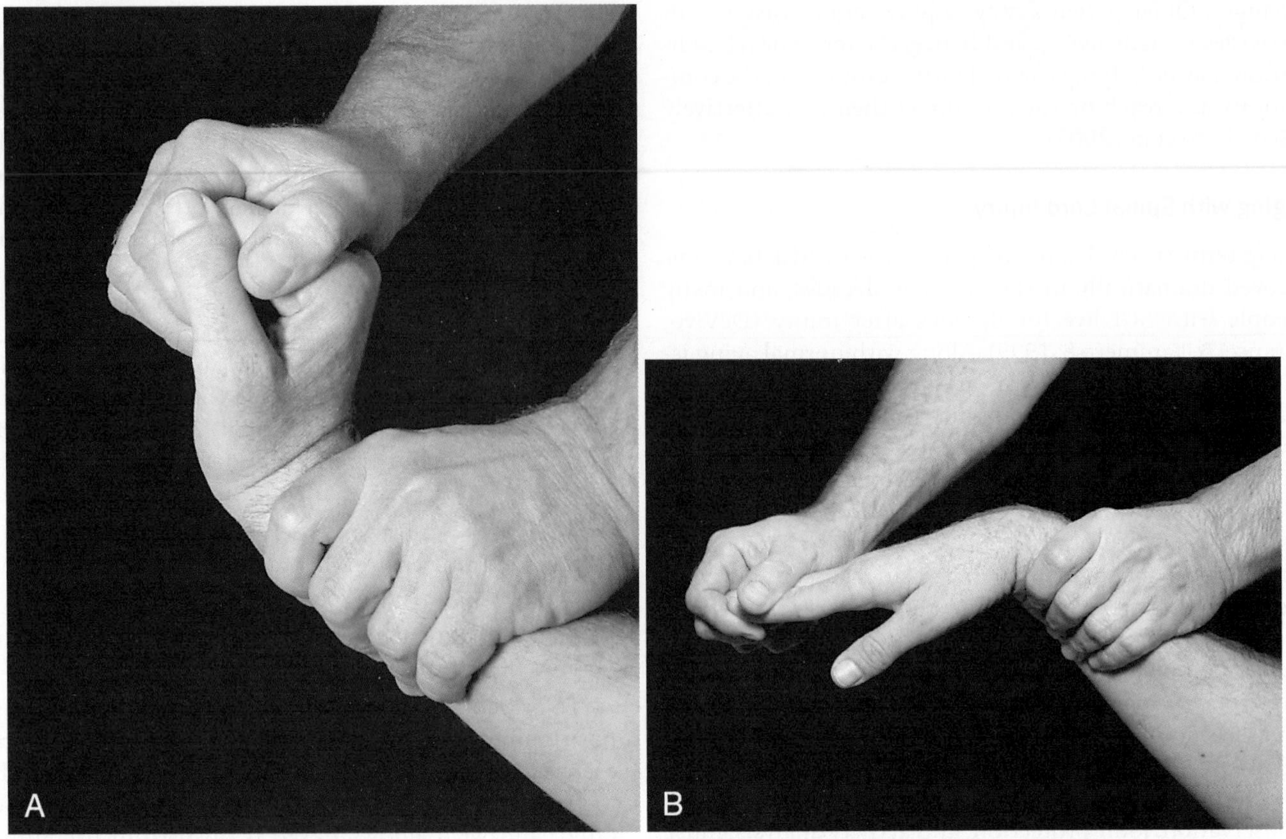

Figure 43-7 Ranging to facilitate tenodesis grasp. **A.** When the wrist is extended, the fingers are flexed. **B.** When the wrist is flexed, the fingers are extended.

stay had decreased to 44 days and to 39 days by 2006 (NSCISC, 2006). To make matters worse, at present, insufficient health care money is being allocated for outpatient services, and patients' needs are being only partially met (Zigler et al., 1998). Consequently, therapists are often frustrated, trying to accomplish too much in too little time. It helps to conceptualize rehabilitation as a lifelong endeavor, with acute rehabilitation being only the beginning phase. Shortened hospital stays serve as a catalyst for making tough decisions about what is most important to accomplish during inpatient stay.

During acute rehabilitation, occupational therapy continues to focus on providing education and support to patients and helping them begin to explore meaningful activities that restore a sense of efficacy and self-esteem. Treatments must always be structured with these overriding goals in mind. This chapter offers basic information. For specific detailed interventions, consult the reference list.

Educating Patients and Family

Each encounter with patients and families must be viewed as an educational opportunity. The style, quantity, and direction of each session must be carefully considered (Hammell, 1995; Wolfe, Potter, & Sequeira, 2004). While patients are learning to put on a shoe, for example, the therapist may ask if they have checked skin integrity and, by so doing, draw attention to the importance of skin inspection. This discussion may also inform the patient about preferable shoe styles and sizes, pedal edema, and deep vein thrombosis. These "teachable moments" arise often and help imbed details in newly learned skills and routines (Wolfe, Potter, & Sequeira, 2004). Nurses, the only team members who see the patient throughout the day, are pivotal in enforcing a daily routine. The therapist must communicate with them daily to ensure a coherent and consistent program.

Education is often enhanced by learning and problem solving with a peer or in a group (Hammell, 1995; Wolfe, Potter, & Sequeira, 2004). Group learning is widely used in SCI centers, to inform and invite group dialogue on topics such as home modifications, accessibility rights, attendant management, assertiveness, travel, and driving. Experiential group activities, such as going to a restaurant, are recommended for building emotional and social alliances with peers while learning from each other's successes and failures. Educational materials and videos are available through groups such as the Paralyzed Veterans of America and the Spinal Cord Injury Association (Resource 43-1). Participation in self-initiated learning, such as surfing the Internet, empowers the patient. On the

RESOURCE 43-1

Paralyzed Veterans of America (PVA)
801 Eighteenth Street, NW
Washington, DC 2006
Phone: (800) 424-8200; (202) 872-1300
www.pva.org
This organization offers many resources for consumers and for clinicians. Consortium for Spinal Cord Medicine publications of clinical practice guidelines available to clinicians and consumers (see reference list for individual guidelines). Guides for people with SCI. Booklets cover topics such as depression, autonomic dysreflexia, and bowel management.

Hammond, M. C., & Burns, S. C. (2000). *Yes, you can! A guide to self-care for persons with spinal cord injury* (3rd ed.). Washington, DC: Paralyzed Veterans of America.

Monthly Magazines

Paraplegia News and Sports 'n Spokes

Other Spinal Cord Injury Organizations

American Paralysis Association and the Christopher Reeve Paralysis Foundation (CRPF)
500 Morris Avenue
Springfield, NJ 07081
Phone: (800) 225-0292; Hotline: (800) 526-3456
www.apacure.com and www.ChristopherReeve.org

National Spinal Cord Injury Association (NSCIA)
6701 Democracy Boulevard, Suite 300-9
Bethesda, MD 20817
Phone: (800) 962-9629
www.spinalcord.org

Resources and Data

The Spinal Cord Injury Statistical Center (NSCISC) and the Spinal Cord Injury Information Network National Spinal Cord Injury Statistical Center
1717 6th Avenue South, Room 544
Birmingham, AL 35233-7330
Phone: (205) 934-3320
Fax: (205) 934-2709
http://main.uab.edu/show.asp?durki=10766 or www.spinalcord.uab.edu

Christopher & Dana Reeve Paralysis Resource Center
636 Morris Turnpike, Suite 3A
Short Hills, NJ 07078
www.paralysis.org

Other Publications

New Mobility
www.newmobility.com

Paralinks
www.paralinks.net

Internet, many SCI consumer web sites offer tips, personal stories, and chat rooms, which can provide a lively forum for communication, self-expression, and information. Family education must result in competence in range of motion, positioning, pressure relief, assistance in ADL, and use of equipment. Home and weekend passes provide an excellent opportunity to develop and refine skills.

Self-Efficacy and Self-Management Skills

Patients' medical and psychological status, as well as being in a hospital environment, invite passivity and submission to hospital routines and to professional staff recommendations of care. The therapist and the rest of the health care team must encourage patients in taking an active role in managing their care, in evaluating behaviors, and self-reflecting about failures and successes (Lorig, 2003; Radomski, 2000). In addition, our challenge as therapists is to recruit, educate, and empower our patients to be problem solvers. By so doing, we encourage active participation, generalization of information, and the transfer of learning to the discharge environment (Radomski, 1998; Wolfe, Potter, & Sequeira, 2004). When planning an outing, ask the group to prepare a list of items to be checked to ensure a safe, successful outing. Upon return to the hospital, encourage discussion of the outing to reflect on ways future outings can be improved. Practical issues like restaurant accessibility to wheelchairs and self-catheterization in public bathrooms may arise. This discussion is also a good time to reflect on performance accomplishments during the outing and to share failures and success experiences in a supportive environment.

Focusing on the Discharge Context: Objects, Locations, Activities, and People Central to the Patient

An early home visit can save many hours of therapy as the therapist obtains a visual image of the patient's discharge environment (Atkins, 1989). Engaging the patient in visualizing post-discharge activities at home helps make treatment relevant. For a bath evaluation, for example, the therapist must look for a setting that resembles the patient's home as closely as possible.

Balancing Self-Maintenance Skills and Meaningful Activities

In acute rehabilitation, most patients are relearning skills that they mastered in childhood, such as eating and dressing independently. This training is an important part of our job. For many patients, however, this training is frustrating, time consuming, tiring, and a constant reminder of their impairments and disabilities. The therapist has the difficult task of helping the patient see when relearning skills is valuable and when the skill should be accomplished by an attendant, either for now or permanently. The ultimate goal of rehabilitation is no longer viewed as the attainment of maximal functional independence. Rather, it is the attainment of optimal desired functional independence. Functional expectations charts (see Appendix 43-1 at the end of this chapter) help us understand the range of expectations for a given level of injury considering only the motor and sensory status of the patient. These charts do not answer such questions as these: Why should the patient dress for half an hour when his wife can dress him in 5 minutes? Will it still take that long after adequate training? What will the patient do when his wife is away? Such discussions encourage patients and families to explore the range and consequences of their choices. The novice therapist will find books such as *Spinal Cord Injury: A Guide to Functional Outcomes in Occupational*

Therapy (Hill, 1986) and *Physical Management for the Quadriplegic Patient* (Ford & Duckworth, 1987) especially valuable because they contain photographs that demonstrate various skills, their sequencing, and the use of assistive devices.

Choosing Equipment

Initially, when pain, spinal precautions, and orthoses, such as a body jacket, may stand in the way of accomplishing goals, assistive devices may be handy facilitators. When obstacles diminish, some equipment, such as a dressing stick, can be eliminated. Only essential equipment should be sent home with the patient, since much of it is costly and it may further complicate the person's life. Also, a universal device should be favored over multiple assistive devices (Clark, Waters, & Baumgarten, 1997).

Most persons with SCI require lifetime use of wheelchairs for their mobility. Choosing the optimal wheel chair requires great expertise and has important implications for ease of mobility, accessibility, and participation (see Chapter 18). The therapist and the patient must consider many factors in weighing the advantages and disadvantages of specific chairs (Consortium for Spinal Cord Medicine, 2005). For example, if a young adult with a functional level of C6 is returning to college following a rehabilitation stay and would like to use an attractive looking manual wheelchair to look and feel less disabled, questions about the layout of campus, the terrain, and distances between classes must first be answered prior to recommending the optimal wheelchair. The person's endurance, posture, and transportation are factors that must all be weighed in selecting either a manual wheelchair or a power wheelchair.

Patients and families should be involved also in the purchase of any other major equipment, such as commode, other bathroom equipment, or a bed.

Special Treatment Considerations Based on Level of Injury

The level of injury dictates the degree of motor, sensory, and autonomic nervous system impairments. Consequently, treatment considerations and outcomes vary greatly with each level. Most evidence-based data, as in the following discussion of the levels of SCI, describe individuals with complete injuries, as the clinical picture is similar from person to person. Outcome of incomplete injuries cannot be easily predicted or generalized because impairment varies greatly between individuals.

The Patient with High Tetraplegia: C1 to C4

Patients with complete C1-3 require an external breathing device because their diaphragm is either paralyzed or only partially innervated (C3). Most persons with C4 tetraplegia require assistance with ventilation during acute care, but as the diaphragm strengthens, they are able to breathe independently. The most common device for assisted breathing is the ventilator, a pneumatic electric machine that forces room air into the lungs. Expiration is passive. This device is attached via plastic tubes directly to a hole in the trachea (see Fig. 43-3).

People with complete high tetraplegia are paralyzed from the neck down. These patients require a highly specialized team to stabilize them medically and to prevent further complications, such as respiratory infections and pressure sores. The occupational therapist who works with this population must be comfortable with nursing procedures. These tasks include suctioning (removing secretions from the trachea), manually ventilating the patient with a manual resuscitator (Ambu-bag), and proficiently managing a ventilator (Nead & Hughes, 1997). The rehabilitation team must also be well coordinated, providing the patient and family with care while preparing them for discharge. Patients with high lesions have a myriad of issues to deal with in many domains of their life. It may be surprising to realize that, despite seemingly insurmountable obstacles to success, many patients with such lesions live healthy and meaningful lives (Whiteneck et al., 1989).

Some additional roles the therapist may have in treating persons with high cervical injury include teaching them to direct their own care; helping them select specialized and sophisticated equipment (see Chapter 19) for life support, mobility, and ADL; and training them in the use of mouth sticks, which are rigid long rods held in the mouth that allow the patient to perform activities such as turning pages, drawing, typing, painting, and playing board games (see Fig. 43-3) (Adler, 1989; Hammell, 1995).

The Patient with Lower Cervical Injuries: C5 to C8

As in the acute recovery phase, physical intervention includes positioning in bed and in the wheelchair (see Fig. 43-6), splinting the upper extremities, daily upper extremity range of motion, and strengthening. Strengthening, an important goal in this phase, can be performed by using weights, pulley systems, skateboards, suspension slings, mobile arm supports (discussed later), and modalities such as biofeedback and neuromuscular electrical stimulation (Sadowsky, 2001; Trombly, 1989) (see Chapters 20–22). See Procedures for Practice 43-1 for resources to inform intervention to improve hand function.

Patients with C5 Tetraplegia

Initially, the deltoids and biceps, key muscles for this level of injury, are weak, so upper limbs require support to function. The mobile arm support, also called a ball-bearing feeder, is a mechanical device attached to the wheelchair. This shoulder and elbow support carries the weight of the arm and reduces friction in motion (Wilson

PROCEDURES FOR PRACTICE 43-1

Intervention to Improve Hand Function for Persons with Tetraplegia

The following references offer practical information about helping patients improve their grasp.

Education and Training in Compensatory Hand Grips (Curtin, 1999)

- Analyses of hand grips of 30 individuals with C6, C7, or C8 tetraplegia
- Provides helpful criteria and vocabulary for understanding the function and compensatory techniques of the tetraplegic hand
- Provides analyses of pre-grip preparation and grasping techniques for which there are excellent drawings included

Regimen of Hand Splinting Principles Designed to Promote Tenodesis Hand Function (Harvey, 1996)

- Analysis of muscle adaptation explains kinesiological mechanism of hand tenodesis.
- This explanation aids the therapist in deciding on a sound splinting regimen to promote tenodesis hand function.

et al., 1984). The mobile arm support can assist the patient in driving the wheelchair, feeding, hygiene and grooming, and carrying out tabletop activities, such as writing and cooking (Atkins, Clark, & Waters, 2003). If and when the strength of the deltoids and biceps is 3+/5 or greater and endurance is good, patients can engage in activities without mobile arm supports (Zigler et al., 1998).

Patients with C5 complete tetraplegia need a way to grasp and hold objects, since their wrists and hands are paralyzed. First, the wrist must be stabilized with a splint or orthosis. Next, a device is attached to the hand to enable the person to perform activities. The universal cuff is a simple, inexpensive utensil holder that rests around the palm (Fig. 43-8). Other U- or C-shaped clamps can be attached to objects such a telephone receiver or a shaver. Some splints, devices, and orthoses accommodate the wrist and the hand as a unit. One is the Ratchet wrist-hand orthosis, which is made of metal and manually controlled. To maximize functional gain with this orthosis, the patient must be carefully trained.

Most patients with C5 tetraplegia can master tabletop activities. They lack trunk control and muscles below the shoulder, however, so they are mostly dependent in dressing and bathing (see Appendix 34-1) (Consortium for Spinal Cord Medicine, 1999). With adequate emotional and financial resources, persons with C5 tetraplegia engage in meaningful, productive activities. Case in point: Mr. L. is a financial consultant who lives on his own and has part-time attendants. He lives a busy life full of business trips and leisure activities with friends. He attributes his success to much planning and good organizational skills.

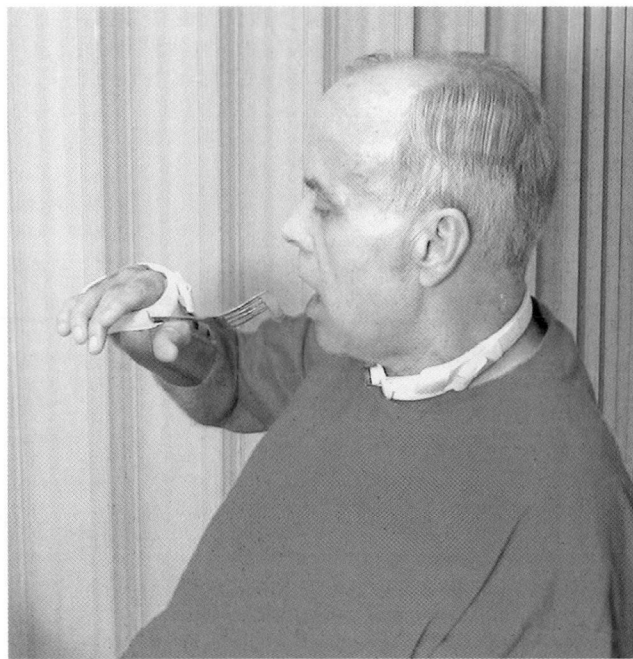

Figure 43-8 A person with C5 tetraplegia using a universal cuff.

Patients with C6 and C7 Tetraplegia

Patients with C6 and C7 tetraplegia may attain significantly higher levels of independence than the C5 patient. The addition of radial wrist extensors allows patients to close their fingers with a tenodesis grasp. This is a critical functional enhancement because, with it, light objects may be picked up, held, and manipulated. The wrist-driven wrist-hand orthosis, or the flexor hinge splint and tenodesis splint, is a metal device that transfers power from the extended wrist to the radial fingers, allowing a stronger pinch (Fig. 43-9) (Atkins, Clark, & Waters, 2003; Consortium for Spinal Cord Medicine, 1999).

More fully innervated proximal scapular and shoulder muscles, such as the rotator cuff, deltoids, and biceps, allow for an increase in upper limb strength and endurance. Patients can also roll in bed, and their arms can cross the midline more forcefully, with the addition of the clavicular pectoralis muscle. The ability to use the triceps, the key muscle for C7 tetraplegia, allows the patient to reach for objects above head level, such as items on a store shelf; transfer with greater ease; and push a manual wheelchair.

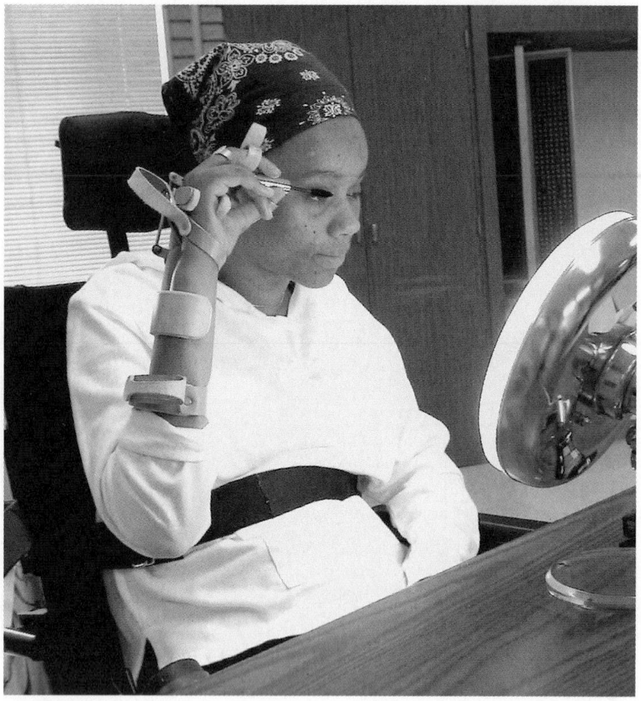

Figure 43-9 A person with C6 complete tetraplegia using the wrist-driven wrist–hand orthosis.

Patients with C8 Tetraplegia

Hand function is significantly improved with the addition of extrinsic finger muscles and thumb flexors. Hand dexterity and strength are limited by the absence of intrinsic finger and thumb muscles. A person with complete C8 tetraplegia grasps objects with the metacarpophalangeal joints in extension and the proximal interphalangeal and distal interphalangeal joints in flexion. This is called a claw hand or intrinsic minus hand (Formal & Smith, 1996).

Surgical Options for the Upper Extremities

Restoring hand function is the top priority of many individuals with tetraplegia (Moberg, 1978, Snoek et al., 2004). To improve hand function, persons with C5, C6, C7, or C8 injuries may have surgical options. These options do not provide for a normal hand but aim to restore pinch, grasp, and reach. Tendon transfer surgeries are recommended only after full spontaneous motor and sensory recovery has occurred and no earlier than a year after injury because most of these procedures permanently alter the musculoskeletal structures (Waters et al., 1996).

Upper limb reconstructive surgeries, although not frequently performed, are available for increasing motion and function of the upper extremities (Bryden et al., 2004). These surgeries may shorten or change the direction of pull of tendons of passive (paralyzed) muscles to provide a mechanical advantage to the thumb or fingers. Other common procedures may entail tendon transfers of functioning muscles. Typically, a proximal functional muscle with strength of 4/5 or above is attached to a tendon of a distal paralyzed muscle. Following the surgery, the patient learns to contract a proximal muscle to move a distal joint (Waters et al., 1996). An example of a hand tendon transfer surgery is the brachioradialis to flexor pollicis longus. This surgery restores lateral pinch by attaching the tendon of a strong (4/5 muscle or above) brachioradialis to a paralyzed flexor pollicis longus. To pinch an object, the patient flexes the elbow while the forearm is in pronation. To improve the stability of the thumb, the interphalangeal joint is fused.

The pre-operative and post-operative evaluation, education, wound care, and muscle reeducation must be carried out by an experienced therapist. Additionally, consistent communication with the operating physician is vital for favorable outcomes. Overall, patients who have gone through reconstructive surgeries perceive their surgeries positively and as improving their function and appearance (Bryden et al., 2004).

A select number of centers worldwide offer a relatively new and complex procedure for achieving hand function. A hand grasp neuroprosthesis, a permanently implanted electrical stimulation system, allows the person with C5-6 injury to open and close the hand by moving the opposite shoulder. This electrical device is composed of eight electrodes implanted into various muscles; electrode leads; transmitter; and a shoulder sensor. An external controller box on the wheelchair controls the device remotely with no connecting wires. Often the neuroprosthesis surgery is either combined with or follows other hand surgeries that allow for optimal use of the device (Kilgore et al., 1997).

The Patient with Paraplegia

Most people with complete or incomplete paraplegia are independent in self-maintenance, self-enhancement, and self-advancement roles, although they require assistance with heavy housekeeping and physically demanding vocational pursuits (Consortium for Spinal Cord Medicine, 1999). Paraplegics with injuries at T10 and below may attain skills more easily and rapidly than patients with higher injuries. Good trunk control enables a person with low paraplegia to bend down and from side to side without fear of falling forward. Skills performed while upright (e.g., bowel management, lower body dressing, undressing, and bathing) require the patient with a higher injury to secure the trunk by supporting the body with one arm while performing the activity with the other to prevent falls (Zigler et al., 1998).

Typically, patients with paraplegia have fewer medical complications than those with tetraplegia, and self-maintenance skills are learned quickly. Thus, the therapist and patient may shift the focus to self-enhancement and self-advancement roles. Community outings are encouraged as soon as possible to facilitate early integration and participation (Zigler et al., 1998) (Fig. 43-10).

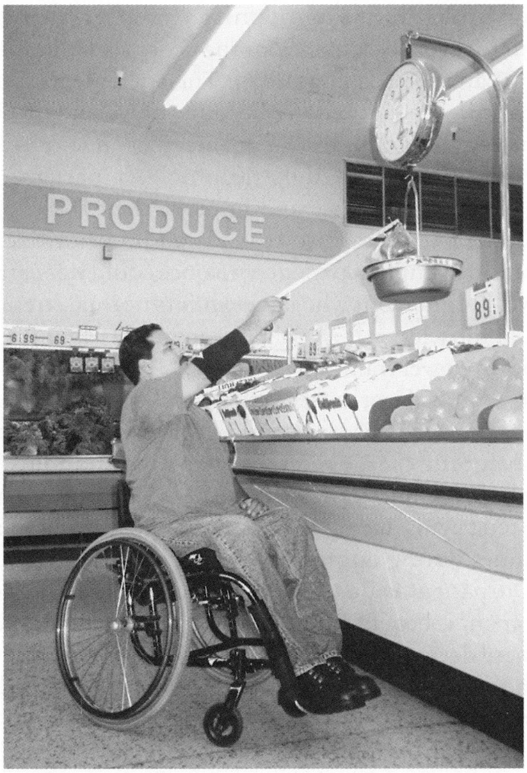

Figure 43-10 A person with paraplegia using a reacher to retrieve hard-to-reach items on a shopping outing.

The Ambulatory Patient: Incomplete Paraplegia and Tetraplegia

Typically when we think of spinal cord injuries, we picture a person using a wheelchair. Yet many individuals with incomplete SCI are able to walk (Fig. 43-11). Data shows that there has been an increase in incomplete injuries in the United States in recent decades (Jackson et al., 2004). This positive trend brings with it some unique challenges to the patient and occupational therapist.

For expedient and relevant treatment planning, the occupational therapist must clearly understand ambulation goals soon after admission. Early discussion with the physical therapist helps clarify goals and enables the occupational therapist to outline a treatment course that takes walking into consideration. Answers to the following questions guide treatment planning:

1. Will upper extremity aids be needed to assist in walking (e.g., a forearm trough walker)? If so, how will the patient carry objects if both hands are occupied?
2. What lower extremity braces are needed? Will the patient require assistance in donning and doffing the braces?
3. Is the goal walking short distances only? Will the patient need a wheelchair for mobility in the community?

Not surprisingly, ambulatory patients with tetraplegia pose the greatest challenge with their often weak upper extremities. In the wheelchair, equipment such as lapboards, armrests, and mobile arm supports support weak arms and allow for function. When upper limb proximal muscles are weak, hand function becomes difficult or impossible, since the patient lacks a mechanism for bringing the hand to the mouth or face. Various devices are available, which enable the person to both lift and support the arm. A solution for supporting the arm depends on the pattern of upper extremity muscle strength (e.g., a table vs. a chair-mounted mobile arm support). Frequently, however, these devices are less than optimal.

Concomitant Brain Injury and Cognitive Deficits

Much attention is given to the visible paralysis of the injured patient, while less visible traumatic brain injury may be overlooked and unattended to (Zejdlik, 1991). If we think about the velocity of the body at the time of impact in injuries such as motor vehicle accidents and falls, it becomes apparent that head injuries are common. The percentage of patients who suffer concomitant injuries to the brain and spinal cord may be as high as 40–50% (Davidoff, Roth, & Richards, 1992). These injuries may be diffuse or focal and mild or severe (Zejdlik, 1991). Since Chapter 39 is solely devoted to traumatic brain injury, the discussion here is limited to elements that are unique to the dual diagnosis.

The occupational therapist must be vigilant for clues of brain injury in the first encounters with the patient. A period of unconsciousness and post-traumatic amnesia raises a red flag. Therapists should ask patients directly whether they have trouble remembering events or sense any changes in their thinking. Patients may lack insight, however. Often, the family is an excellent source of information as they usually know the pre-morbid cognitive

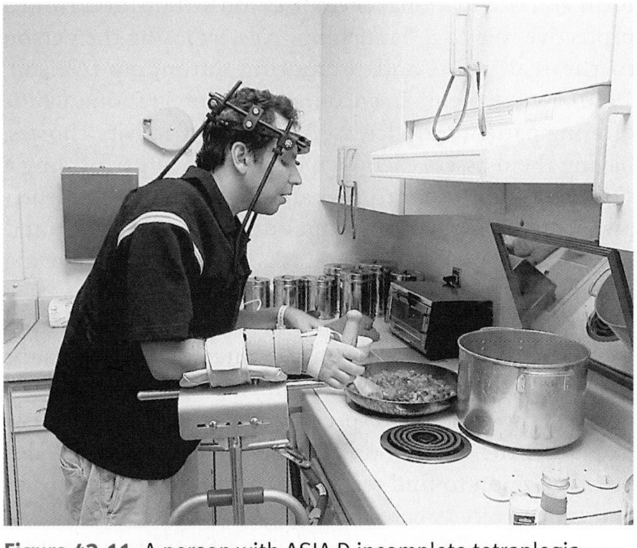

Figure 43-11 A person with ASIA D incomplete tetraplegia cooking while using an arm trough walker. The 8- to 10-pound Halo vest interferes with balance and limits vision.

status of the patient. The evaluation of the patient is made more challenging with factors such as fatigue, medication side effects, pain, depression, sleep deprivation, and sensory deprivation (Davidoff, Roth, & Richards, 1992). A formal screening can determine whether consultation with a communication specialist is indicated. It is common in many hospitals to request such consultations automatically if the patient had any period of unconsciousness or post-traumatic amnesia.

Cognitive deficits in the SCI population may not be limited to those incurred as a result of the injury. Factors such as previous head injuries, learning disabilities, and a history of alcohol and drug abuse are often present, and they affect the patient's cognitive functioning (Davidoff, Roth, & Richards, 1992). Although the effects of a mild brain injury associated with SCI may diminish over time, the prognosis for recovering from a preexisting cognitive deficit is poor (Davidoff, Roth, & Richards, 1992).

Transitions: Restoring Roles at Home and in the Community

A growing body of literature challenges the old concepts of traditional rehabilitation services in its success at helping smooth the transition from hospital to home. A quicker, more effective transition is essential as acute rehabilitation lengths of stay continue to decrease (NSCISC, 2006). Along with impairment reduction and increased physical independence, the rehabilitation team must engage in moving the person toward a life of managing disability, maintaining general health, preventing complications, and managing social, occupational, and financial environments that are often difficult and complex (Kendall, Ungerer, & Dorsett, 2003; Potter et al., 2004).

As time passes in acute rehabilitation, the health care team and occupational therapists must transition from a protective role to a "launching" role, exposing the person to the real world and promoting autonomy (Nelson, 1990). Key elements in encouraging reintegration include offering patients an increased number of activity choices, having them assess their own confidence in performing a skill, requiring them to prepare for the activity on their own (call in preparation for an outing or search the internet, for example), and when tasks are completed, having patients reflect on their successes and failures.

If therapists conclude that the rehabilitation program is too short for achieving optimal outcomes, they must be prepared to articulate and document the need for longer hospitalization. This is especially true if the short stay may jeopardize the safety of the patient. The therapist may also be called upon to find resources that allow the patient to continue to receive care and engage in occupations following discharge. Often the patient is referred to an outpatient clinic to continue treatment. Most patients continue to gain strength during the first year after their injury and after their discharge from the acute rehabilitation facility (Waters & Yoshida, 1996). This increase in strength may allow the patient to become more independent. Outpatient programs teach patients to use new movement and offer intensive ADL training. As patients gain strength and endurance and improve their balance, they should be encouraged to reassess and reprioritize their goals. For example, a patient who once could not carry out a bowel program but who later exhibits normal strength in manual muscle testing of the triceps and latissimus dorsi can begin bowel training.

Customized orthoses, such as the wrist-driven wrist-hand orthosis, are commonly given to the patient soon before discharge because production and adjustment of orthoses require much time. Therefore, orthotic training often begins during the last days of hospitalization and continues during outpatient visits to ensure good fit and use. Outpatient evaluation and training in the use of other equipment is beneficial because the patient and family can use these devices at home immediately.

The outpatient occupational therapist should begin and/or continue working on goals and skills that move the patient toward greater community integration (e.g., driving and vocational evaluation and training). The outpatient education of family members and attendants must continue to assure continuity and progress.

With the help of the social worker, liaison nurse, or case manager, the therapist can minimize barriers to receiving therapy after discharge. A frequent barrier is lack of transportation. If patients cannot leave home, an agency such as the Visiting Nurses Association may provide occupational therapy services at home for a limited time.

Other transitional services, such as support groups and transitional living centers, must be identified. Independent living centers are federally funded programs designed to promote reintegration. They are located in most large cities in the United States and provide resources and access to financial, vocational, rehabilitative, and community-based programs (Forchheimer & Tate, 2004).

To further ease clients' transition from hospital to home, models are continuing to emerge and evolve that reflect third-party payers' growing awareness of the benefits of less costly alternatives to hospitalization, preventing complications, enhancing health and quality of life, and supporting the goal of full participation. Examples for such models include:

- Clients living for days to months in a transitional residence with family members and /or attendants. Clients and their families are encouraged to seek health care providers' help only when they cannot solve problems independently. Such residential programs are often housed either at or near the acute rehabilitation center.

- Following discharge, clients receiving the assistance of a federal or state transitional services team, which may include a case manager, an occupational therapist, a physical therapist, a vocational counselor, and others. They may assist in finding accessible housing, implementing home modifications, and finding monetary benefits.

Adaptation: Focus on Facilitation Toward Full Participation

The path from being a dependent patient to becoming a person with a sense of efficacy and self-esteem is long and individual. The occupational therapist must encourage persons with SCI to develop competencies and satisfaction in life roles (Trombly, 1995). Although some laws (e.g., Americans with Disabilities Act) aim to encourage individuals with SCI to participate fully in all societal roles, many barriers continue to hinder full participation. The unemployment rate of individuals with SCI is significantly higher than in the general population, and income is lower (Krause et al., 1999; Mead et al., 2004).

Yerxa and Locker (1990) studied the pattern of engagement in daily occupations and quality of life among people with SCI. They found that people with SCI had much more free time than their nondisabled counterparts. Other studies show that life satisfaction was not related to the level of injury but to social integration, access to the environment, and occupation (Richards et al., 1999; Schonherr et al., 2005). These studies heighten the importance of looking beyond treating impairments and analyzing the daily activities of each individual, revealing meanings of these activities, and promoting them.

Occupational therapy literature emphasizes the role of the occupational therapist in helping individuals with SCI analyze their daily life, find solutions to simplify daily routines, and engage in experiential creative problem solving in the community (Hammell, 1995). This occupational therapy role has yet to be fully practiced because models for independent living are few, and only a few of these models employ occupational therapists. To fill this role, we must seek work in group homes and governmental agencies and rely less on traditional hospital-based employment. We must also engage in shaping public policy (Baum, 2000; Hammell, 2004).

The World Health Organization's (WHO) development of *The International Classification of Functioning, Disability and Health* (WHO, 2001) reflects a growing global recognition of the importance of viewing people with disabilities in a more holistic way, as healthy, functional, human beings engaged in social, vocational, and avocational pursuits. This model, therefore, parallels occupational therapy values and beliefs more closely than previous disease-oriented models (Brachtesende, 2005; Hemmingsson & Jonsson, 2005).

As occupational therapists, we have the opportunity and obligation to educate consumers, the public, and policy makers to help enable people with SCI to live a full, meaningful life by facilitating full participation in their desired life roles.

CASE EXAMPLE

Able: Spinal Cord Injury

Occupational Therapy Process	Clinical Reasoning Process: Objectives	Clinical Reasoning Process: Examples of Therapist's Internal Dialogue
Patient Information Able is a 19-year-old man with C6 ASIA A (complete) tetraplegia resulting from an ocean diving accident 3 months ago. Able is a sophomore at a community college. He came to the United States from Samoa to attend college on a football scholarship. Able is single and lives with fellow students	Understand the patient's diagnosis or condition	"If Able has a functional level of C6 he may be able to achieve independence in many areas. Unfortunately, because he has an ASIA A (complete) injury, his muscle and sensory return will most likely be only in the Zone of Partial Preservation (ZPP)."

in a rented house near campus. He has a large and supportive family in Samoa. After his injury, Able's mother, aunt, and two of his sisters came to be with him for a month. Able is fluent in English. He was hoping to stay in California and resume his studies. He did not have a discharge destination. Following his injury, Able was sent to a trauma center, where he underwent posterior fusion surgery to stabilize C4 to C7 vertebrae and was placed in a Philadelphia collar, a rigid collar that limits neck motion. Following surgery, Able was prescribed spine restrictions in order to protect the surgical site. Precautions allowed Able to perform shoulder bilateral/symmetrical activities with minimal resistance (no greater than 3+/5) and unilateral, active only activities with no resistance. During the post-operative hospital stay, Able was on a rotating bed to prevent pressure sores. The occupational therapist performed daily upper limb range-of-motion exercises. She established a shoulder-positioning program and fitted Able with prefabricated resting hand splints. In conversations with the patient and his family, the therapist began to explain rehabilitation. The occupational therapist documented that the family was engaged and supportive and that the patient appeared passive and quiet. Able was transferred to a rehabilitation center 3 weeks post injury.	Know the person	"Able is passive and quiet and seems quite depressed. Knowing that the best predictor of future behaviors and disposition is pre-morbid personality and behaviors, I am very hopeful that he soon will feel better, as he sees his renewed abilities. It is excellent that he has such a supportive, loving family; however, we will most likely request that they limit their visits somewhat, in order to enable Able to see that he can manage without them, to allow him to become more active in his rehabilitation, and to encourage him to begin directing his own care. Prompt identification of discharge destination and potential caregivers is crucial for goal setting. Therefore, the social worker must address these important issues as soon as possible."
Reason for Referral to Occupational Therapy Able was referred to occupational therapy to address limitation in self-maintenance, self-advancement, and self-enhancement roles.	Appreciate the context Develop provisional hypotheses	"Able's past accomplishments and tough school/sports schedule required him to be disciplined and structure his time efficiently. I think this will help him in the acute rehabilitation setting, a place that requires hard work. More importantly, his past level of engagement is an indicator that he will be able to continue a life full of participation in meaningful occupations."
Assessment Process and Results **Occupational profile:** Interviews included establishing rapport; in-depth interviews about Able's typical day, interests, routines, habits and roles; and administering of the *Canadian Occupational Performance Measure*. Initially, because of Able's withdrawn mood, the therapist secured Able's permission and interviewed his family about his life and about family goals. **Findings:** Able was clear about wanting to stay in California and resume his studies. His family was going to go back to Samoa in a few weeks. He and his family described his busy schedule. Football occupied most of his non-study time. For fun, he "hung out" with his roommates, some of whom where also from Samoa. Information from the social worker indicated no clear discharge destination and no knowledge of who will assist Able with his care. **Physical evaluation:** Included measuring both upper extremities (BUE) passive range of motion, tone, sensation (pain, light touch, proprioception and object identification), and *Manual Muscle Test* (*MMT*). Observations of reach and hand use included activities such as picking up a coin or a tissue and pushing a button.	Consider evaluation approach and methods	"Two casual contacts were made, establishing rapport with Able and his family and meeting Able's immediate needs. These included making Able more comfortable in bed and assessing his ability to press buttons (nurse call light, phone use, bed and TV controls)."

Results of *MMT*:

Scapulae and shoulder muscles: 3+ or above/5 throughout.
Elbows: 4/5 flexion; 0/5 extension.
Forearms: 4/5 supination; 2−/5 pronation.
Wrist: Radial wrist extensors: Right 3+/5; left 3/5; bilateral ulnar wrist extension and flexion 0/5
Fingers and thumbs: 0/5
Sensory level: C2-6 dermatomes intact; impaired C7 and absent below (see Fig. 43-2).
Tone throughout both upper limbs: Within normal limits.
Hand use: Drags objects to edge of table; picks up objects with the two hands

"I hope that Able's roommates and friends will help and support him when his family is no longer here. When he will indicate that he wants his friends around, we will encourage them to visit and be involved in his therapy."

"Able had a large repertoire of occupations prior to his injury. He has excellent potential for resuming his studies. I need to further explore his engagement with football and, as he gains skills and feels more self-confident and competent, explore with him the range of options of engaging in sports. For example, either being a spectator and/or acquainting him to wheelchair sports."

Summary of upper limb findings: Right hand dominant. Symmetry in strength with right arm slightly stronger than left. Shoulder strength 3+/5 and above. Deficits in reaching away from body and in pronation. Fair tenodesis action bilaterally; beginning effective hand compensatory techniques for picking up and manipulating objects.

Activities of daily living: Able was given a universal cuff in the acute hospital, and he is able to feed himself with a spoon and a fork and to brush his teeth. He needs assistance with set up for these activities (*Functional Independent Measure*-5). He is dependent with all other self-maintenance skills.

Interpret observations

"Initial spinal precautions limit full resistive exercises to neck, scapulae, and shoulders and allow only for minimal resistance, symmetrical exercises. This will be achieved with routine activities such as washing the face. A full strengthening program can be carried out to elbows and wrists. Left wrist will also benefit from neuromuscular electrical stimulation (NMES) to radial wrist extensors."

"Able is beginning to compensate for his finger paralysis. He has learned to drag objects to edge of table and to hold objects with two hands to compensate for weak grip. Further education and experiential training will help him with other compensatory techniques such as weaving objects through his fingers and using extreme ranges."

Occupational Therapy Problem List

- Decreased performance skills: Moderate depression, lack of engagement with the rehabilitation team, excessive dependency on family.
- Decreased performance skills: Upper limbs' weakness, sensory deficit, decreased endurance and control.
- Limitations in all occupational areas including ADL, IADL, education, work, leisure, and social participation.
- Decreased knowledge of spinal cord injury management, resources, and of directing own care.

Synthesize results

"The problem list is overwhelming as Able's disability is devastating, affecting physical capacities and all his occupational roles. I have to remind myself that tackling this long list will sort itself out daily, as we reassess Able's engagement in the program, his progress, and his evolving list of priorities."

Occupational Therapy Goal List

Initially Able had difficulty coming up with goals, as he appeared overwhelmed with his paralysis and was not able to determine what he would be able to physically do. With the help of his therapist, the team, and his family, his short-term goals included feeding, brushing his teeth, shaving, dressing, writing, and using the phone and the computer.

After approximately 5 weeks, with renewed hope, Able expressed interest in resuming his studies.

Toward discharge, goals included visiting a transitional living center, visiting Able's college, going to his college football game, and becoming independent in self-catheterization.

Develop intervention hypotheses

"Feeding, brushing teeth, and writing and using the computer are skills that will be easy for Able to develop. This will improve his self-confidence and feelings of competence. Able will have a harder time dressing his lower body. The reality of the amount of energy and time it takes to complete this task right now may help Able sort out his priorities as to what an attendant will do for him and what he will do himself."

Select an intervention approach

"The occupational therapy intervention approach will focus on compensatory or adaptive approach."

Other goals included: Increase upper limb strength and endurance and improve hand function (tenodesis hand). Learn routine spinal cord injury (SCI) precautions for skin care, pressure relief, bowel and bladder care, and autonomic nervous system functioning. Learn to direct own care. Learn SCI resources in the community. Choose cushion and wheelchair.	Consider what will occur in therapy, how often, and for how long	"I must remember that the interventions in acute care are only the beginning of a long process of rehabilitation toward participation. In acute rehabilitation Able will be seen for 2 to 3 hours a day, 6 days a week for 8 weeks. As a discharge destination emerges, we will help find the appropriate OT program to continue his care."
Intervention **First 3 weeks:** ADL training including feeding, brushing teeth, and grooming using a universal cuff. Evaluation for the use of right wrist-driven wrist–hand orthosis with clinic trial equipment. Ordering, checking fit, and training in orthosis use. Exploration and training in writing, computer skills, and telephone use. Hand use in routine activities, such as compensatory techniques in swiping a card, handling money, and opening pill bottles. Individual, short educational sessions focused on specific interventions, such as how to use the hand and how to best maximize hand function. Wrist strengthening program through exercises, activities, and NMES. Selecting and trying different wheelchairs. **Weeks 4 through 6:** Spinal precautions were lifted, allowing Able to move his neck and shoulders freely and engage in a full strengthening program. Able was referred to a progressive resistive exercise physical therapy group. Training in upper body dressing and beginning of lower body dressing. Expanded on student role activities such as using a tape recorder and handling books and papers. Education: Individual and group. Group experiential training in topics such as taking public transportation, assertiveness training, and directing care. Individual: Daily self range-of-motion exercises. Training in hand use with and without the orthosis through activities with peers (for example, board games). At 5 weeks, Able identified a new goal of wanting to attend his team's football game at his school. Ordering of cushion and permanent wheelchair.	Assess the patient's comprehension	"Able's pre-morbid self-discipline and high level of occupational engagement were, indeed, reliable predictors of his ability to engage in therapy despite his depression. In the first few weeks, he talked little, and although not fully engaged, he went along with the program as if "going through the motions" of therapy. As he gained some independence, he became more animated. He enjoyed working with the computer because he realized that going back to school would be possible. It was wonderful to get to know Able as his warm and engaging personality began to emerge when his depression lifted. He began initiating ideas, solved problems easily, and seemed interested in newly introduced equipment. He also became more outgoing and started socializing with other patients. Able's family needed to return to Samoa 5 weeks into his rehabilitation stay. The shift from family to friends' support happened naturally as all his acquaintances understood his need for support. This transition also helped facilitate his community reentry and thinking about football and school. Able and his friends began preparing for his attendance at the college football game. Able had to plan by calling and asking for his friends' assistance before and during the game. "Because Able decided to stay in California with no family around, team meetings involved finding alternatives for further care because all felt that Able would not be ready to live alone post discharge. Able liked the idea of an interim discharge to a transitional living facility. This would enable him to acquire more skills and to attain greater self-efficacy prior to returning to school and to independent living."
Weeks 7 through 8: Able trained in doing intermittent self-catheterization with a wrist-wrist-driven hand–orthosis.	Understand what he is doing	
Able, his friend and the occupational therapist planned and attended the team's football game.	Compare actual to expected performance	
Able and his therapist contacted his college, met with the Disabled Student Counselor and toured the college to assess its accessibility.	Know the person	
Prior to his discharge Able traveled with the social worker and occupational therapist and toured the discharge Transitional Living Center.	Appreciate the context	

Next Steps Post discharge, Able was accepted to a Transitional Living Center (TLC). This facility offered continued rehabilitation services at reduced intensity and cost. Able continued to receive occupational therapy, for the purpose of resuming his studies and for facilitating training of an attendant. After approximately 1 year, Able rented an apartment with a flat mate he met at the TLC and resumed college.	Anticipate present and future patient concerns Analyze patient's comprehension Decide if the patient should continue or discontinue therapy and/or return in the future	"Able wanted to maintain contact with his rehabilitation team. It was wonderful to chat with him over the phone and hear about his progress. He missed his family but had close supportive friends. Despite his severe disability, Able resumed a meaningful life, fully participating in social and vocational pursuits." "I hope that he will continue to be vigilant with his preventative care, taking meticulous care of his skin, bladder, and bowel in order to maintain his good health."

CLINICAL REASONING IN OCCUPATIONAL THERAPY PRACTICE 43-1

Effects of Depression and Lack of Involvement on Rehabilitation

In interviews and observations in acute care and acute rehabilitation, Able's therapists noted that the patient appeared depressed and uninvolved in his care. What could the therapist do to facilitate greater involvement and participation by the patient? What bodily and environmental factors might exaggerate these problems? What bodily and environmental factors might improve these problems?

CLINICAL REASONING IN OCCUPATIONAL THERAPY PRACTICE 43-2

Bladder Management for a Person with C6 Tetraplegia

Near the time of his discharge from the rehabilitation center, Able expressed interest in taking care of his bladder. Will he be able to carry it out independently? What steps will you take in training him in his bladder care?

Evidence Table 43-1
Best Evidence for Interventions Used in Occupational Therapy after Spinal Cord Injury

Intervention	Description of Intervention Tested	Participants	Dosage	Type of Best Evidence and Level of Evidence	Benefit	Statistical Probability	Reference
Intervention to improve upper extremity strength and tenodesis grasp	Comparison of 4 treatment groups: conventional, electrical stimulation, biofeedback, and combined electrical stimulation and biofeedback.	Persons with tetraplegia who were receiving inpatient rehabilitation services.	Intervention 1 time per day, 5 days per week for 5–6 weeks.	IC3a (random assignment; small treatment groups [10–13 per group]; attrition; no controls who did not receive treatment)	No treatment group was superior to the others. Analysis of data pooled from all groups shows statistically significant pre–post treatment differences.	N/A	Kohlmeyer et al., 1996
Self-care skills training	Occupational therapy and physical therapy provided during inpatient rehabilitation.	Persons with tetraplegia from traumatic or non-traumatic spinal cord injury who were receiving inpatient rehabilitation (55 individuals at admission; 45 at discharge).	Not specified.	IIIB3c (1 group, pre–post only, attrition of subjects)	Yes. Statistically significant improvement in self-care and motor skills (based on *Functional Independence Measure* scores).	Paired t score = 10.3; $p < 0.0005$; $r = 0.84$.	Lysack et al., 2001

Appendix 43-1
*Expected Functional Outcomes**

USING EXPECTED FUNCTIONAL OUTCOMES CHARTS

Outcome-based practice guidelines can provide estimates of the effect of rehabilitation on functional status or activity restrictions. In the Expected Functional Outcomes charts that follow, the Consortium for Spinal Cord Medicine has put forth its best description, based on outcome studies and expert consensus, of outcomes of people with motor complete spinal cord injury (SCI) 1 year after injury. These outcome guidelines are presented with the full recognition that outcomes are not fully under the influence or control of health care providers. Differences in patient characteristics; the course of medical events; psychological, social, and environmental supports; and cognitive abilities have strong influences on outcomes.

These outcome-based guidelines can be used to establish goals, provide information for quality improvement, and compare performance across facilities with similar populations. When used appropriately, outcome-based practice guidelines provide a benchmark for comparing programs and services while improving both the processes and outcomes of care that have an enduring impact on long-term functioning in the community. Disability outcome measures are generally focused on the degree to which a person can independently complete an important function or activity of daily living (ADL). This definition of disability is consistent with the World Health Organization (WHO) model of disablement in which disability is measured at the level of the person interacting with the environment during daily routines. In the completion of daily tasks, adaptive equipment becomes a crucial adjunct to the independence of the person with SCI.

The following charts present expectations of functional performance of SCI at 1 year post injury for each of eight levels of injury (C1-3, C4, C5, C6, C7-8, T1-9, T10-L1, and L2-S5). The outcomes reflect a level of independence that can be expected of a person with motor complete SCI, given optimal circumstances.

The categories presented reflect expected functional outcomes in the areas of mobility, activities of daily living, instrumental activities of daily living, and communication skills. The guidelines are based on consensus of clinical experts, available literature on functional outcomes, and data compiled from the Uniform Data System (UDS) and the National Spinal Cord Injury Statistical Center (NSCISC). Within the functional outcomes for people with SCI listed in the tables that follow, the panel has identified a series of essential daily functions and activities, expected levels of functioning, and the equipment and attendant care likely to be needed to support the predicted level of independence at 1 year post injury. These outcome areas include:

- **Respiratory, bowel, and bladder function.** The neurological effects of spinal injury may result in deficits in the ability of the individual to perform basic bodily functions. Respiratory function includes ability to breathe with or without mechanical assistance and to adequately clear secretions. Bowel and bladder function includes the ability to manage elimination, maintain perineal hygiene, and adjust clothing before and after elimination. Adapted or facilitated methods of managing these bodily functions may be required to attain expected functional outcomes.
- **Bed mobility, bed/wheelchair transfers, wheelchair propulsion, and positioning/pressure relief.** The neurological effects of SCI may result in deficits in the ability of the individual to perform the activities required for mobility, locomotion, and safety. Adapted or facilitated methods of managing these activities may be required to attain expected functional outcomes.
- **Standing and ambulation.** Spinal cord injury may result in deficits in the ability to stand for exercise or psychological benefit or to ambulate for functional activities. Adapted or facilitated methods of management may be required to attain expected functional outcomes in standing and ambulation.
- **Eating, grooming, dressing, and bathing.** The neurological effects of SCI may result in deficits in the ability of the individual to perform these activities of daily living. Adapted or facilitated methods of managing these activities of daily living may be required to attain expected functional outcomes.
- **Communication (keyboard use, handwriting, and telephone use).** The neurological effects of SCI may result in deficits in the ability of the individual to communicate. Adapted or facilitated methods of communication may be required to attain expected functional outcomes.
- **Transportation (driving, attendant-operated vehicle, and public transportation).** Transportation activities are critical for individuals with SCI to become maximally independent in the community.

* Reprinted with permission from the Paralyzed Veterans of America (PVA). Consortium for Spinal Cord Medicine (1999). *Outcome following traumatic spinal cord injury: Clinical practice guidelines for health care professionals.* Washington, DC: Paralyzed Veterans of America.

Adaptations may be required to facilitate the individual in meeting the expected functional outcomes.

- **Homemaking (meal planning and preparation and home management).** Adapted or facilitated methods of managing homemaking skills may be required to attain expected functional outcomes. Individuals with complete SCI at any level will require some level of assistance with homemaking activities. The hours of assistance with homemaking activities are presented in the tables.

- **Assistance required.** The Expected Functional Outcomes charts include the number of hours that may be required from a caregiver to assist with personal care and homemaking activities in the house. Personal care includes hands-on delivery of all aspects of self-care and mobility, as well as safety interventions. Homemaking assistance is also included in the recommendation for hours of assistance and includes activities previously presented. The number of hours presented in both the panel recommendations and the self-reported *Craig Handicap Assessment and Reporting Technique* (*CHART*) (Whiteneck et al., 1992) data is representative of skilled and unskilled and paid and unpaid hours of assistance. The 24-hour-a-day requirement noted for the C1-3 and C4 levels includes the expected need for unpaid attendant care to provide safety monitoring.

  Adequate assistance is required to ensure that the individual with SCI can achieve the outcomes set forth in the Expected Functional Outcomes charts. The hours of assistance recommended by the panel do not reflect changes in assistance required over time as reported by long-term survivors of SCI (Gerhart et al., 1993), and they also do not take into account the wide range of individual variables mentioned throughout this document that may affect the number of hours assistance is required. The *Functional Independence Measure* (*FIM*) estimates are widely variable in several categories. One does not know whether the representative individuals with SCI in the individual categories attained the expected functional outcomes for their specific level of injury or whether there were mitigating circumstances such as age, obesity, or concomitant injuries that would account for variability in assistance reported. An individualized assessment of needs is required in all cases.

- **Equipment requirements.** Minimum recommendations for durable medical equipment and adaptive devices are identified in each of the functional categories. Most commonly used equipment is listed, with the understanding that variations exist among SCI rehabilitation programs and that use of such equipment may be necessary to achieve the identified functional outcomes. Additional equipment and devices that are not critical for the majority of individuals at a specific level of injury may be required for some individuals. The equipment descriptions are generic to provide for variances in program philosophy and financial resources. Rapid changes and advances in equipment and technology will be made and therefore must be considered.

  Health care professionals should keep in mind that the recommendations set forth in Appendix 43-1 are not intended to be prescriptive, but rather to serve as a guideline. The importance of individual functional assessment of people with SCI prior to making equipment recommendations cannot be overemphasized. All durable medical equipment and adaptive devices must be thoroughly assessed and tested to determine medical necessity to prevent medical complications (e.g., postural deviations, skin breakdown, or pain) and to foster optimal functional performance. Environmental control units and telephone modifications may be needed for safety and maximal independence, and each person must be individually evaluated for the need for this equipment. Disposable medical product recommendations are not included in this document.

- ***FIM***. Evidence for the specific levels of independence provided in Appendix 43-1 relies both on expert consensus and data from the *FIM* in large-scale, prospective, and longitudinal research conducted by NSCISC. *FIM* is the most widely used disability measure in rehabilitation medicine, although it may not incorporate all of the characteristics of disability in individuals recovering from SCI, it captures many basic disability areas. *FIM* consists of 13 motor and 5 cognitive items that are individually scored from 1 to 7. A score of 1 indicates complete dependence, and a score of 7 indicates complete independence. The sum of the 13 *FIM* motor score items can range from 13, indicating complete dependence for all items, to 91, indicating complete independence for all items. *FIM* is a measure usually completed by health care professionals. Different observers, including the patient, family members, and caregivers, can contribute information to the ratings. Each of these reporters may represent a different type of potential bias. It should also be noted that, although the sample sizes of *FIM* data for certain neurological level groups are quite small, the consistency of the data adds confidence to the interpretation. Other pertinent data regarding functional independence must be factored into outcome analyses, including medical information, patient factors, social participation, quality of life, and environmental factors and supports. In Appendix 43-1, *FIM* data, when available, are reported in three areas. First, the expected *FIM* outcomes are documented based on expert clinical consensus. The second number reported is the median *FIM* score, as compiled by NSCISC. The interquartile range for NSCISC *FIM* data is the third set of numbers. In total, the *FIM* data represent 1-year post-injury *FIM* assessment of 405 survivors with complete SCI. Sample size for *FIM* and Assistance Data is provided for each level of injury. Different outcome expectations should clearly apply to different patient subgroups and populations. Some populations are likely to be significantly older than the referenced one. Functional abilities may be limited by advancing age (Penrod, Hedge, & Ditunno, 1990; Yarkony et al., 1988).

- **Home modifications.** To provide the best opportunity for individuals with SCI to achieve the identified functional outcomes, a safe and architecturally accessible environment is necessary. An accessible environment must take into consideration, but not be limited to, entrance and egress, mobility in the home, and adequate setup to perform personal care and homemaking tasks.

Appendix 43-1. Expected Functional Outcomes Level C1-3

Functionally relevant muscles innervated: Sternocleidomastoid; cervical paraspinal; neck accessories
Movement possible: Neck flexion, extension, rotation
Patterns of weakness: Total paralysis of trunk, upper extremities, lower extremities; dependent on ventilator

FIM/Assistance Data: Exp = Expected FIM Score / **Med** = NSCISC Median / **IR** = NSCISC Interquartile Range
NSCISC Sample Size: FIM=15 / Assist=12

	Expected Functional Outcomes	Equipment	FIM/Assistance Data		
			Exp	*Med*	*IR*
Respiratory	• Ventilator dependent • Inability to clear secretions	• 2 ventilators (bedside, portable) • Suction equipment or other suction management device • Generator or battery backup			
Bowel	Total assist	Padded reclining shower—commode chair (if roll-in shower available)	1	1	1
Bladder	Total assist		1	1	1
Bed mobility	Total assist	Full electric hospital bed with Trendelenburg feature and side rails			
Bed, wheelchair transfers	Total assist	• Transfer board • Power or mechanical lift with sling	1	1	1
Pressure relief, positioning	Total assist; may be independent with equipment	• Power recline and/or tilt wheelchair • Wheelchair pressure relief cushion • Postular support and head control devices as indicated independent with equipment • Hand splints may be indicated • Specialty bed or pressure relief mattress may be indicated			
Eating	Total assist		1	1	1
Dressing	Total assist		1	1	1
Grooming	Total assist		1	1	1
Bathing	Total assist	• Hand-held shower • Shampoo tray • Padded reclining shower—commode chair (if roll-in shower available)	1	1	1

Appendix 43-1. Expected Functional Outcomes *(continued)*
Level C1-3

	Expected Functional Outcomes	Equipment	FIM/Assistance Data Exp	Med	IR
Wheelchair propulsion	Manual: Total assist Power: Independent with equipment	• Power recline and/or tilt wheelchair with head, chin, or breath control and manual recliner • Vent tray	6	1	1–6
Standing, ambulation	Standing: Total assist; Ambulation: Not indicated				
Communication	Total assist to independent, depending on workstation setup and equipment availability	• Mouth stick, high-tech computer access, environmental control unit • Adaptive devices everywhere as indicated			
Transportation	Total assist	Attendant-operated van (e.g., lift, tie-downs) or accessible public transportation			
Homemaking	Total assist				
Assist required	• 24-hour attendant care to include homemaking • Able to instruct in all aspects of care		24*	24*	12–24*

*Hours per day

Level C4

Functionally relevant muscles innervated: Upper trapezius; diaphragm; cervical paraspinal muscles
Movement possible: Neck flexion, extension, rotation; scapular elevation; inspiration
Patterns of weakness: Paralysis of trunk, upper extremities, lower extremities; inability to cough, endurance and respiratory reserve low secondary to paralysis of intercostals

FIM/Assistance Data: Exp = Expected FIM Score / **Med** = NSCISC Median / **IR** = NSCISC Interquartile Range
NSCISC Sample Size: FIM=28 / Assist=12

	Expected Functional Outcomes	Equipment	FIM/Assistance Data Exp	Med	IR
Respiratory	May be able to breathe without a ventilator	If not ventilator free, see C1-3 for equipment requirements			
Bowel	Total assist	Reclining shower—commode chair (if roll-in shower available)	1	1	1
Bladder	Total assist		1	1	1
Bed mobility	Total assist	Full electric hospital bed with Trendelenburg feature and side rails			
Bed, wheelchair transfers	Total assist	• Transfer board • Power or mechanical lift with sling	1	1	1

Appendix 43-1. Expected Functional Outcomes *(continued)*
Level C4

	Expected Functional Outcomes	Equipment	FIM/Assistance Data *Exp*	*Med*	*IR*
Pressure relief, positioning	Total assist; may be independent with equipment	• Power recline and/or tilt wheelchair • Wheelchair pressure relief cushion • Postural support and head control devices as indicated • Hand splints may be indicated • Specialty bed or pressure relief mattress may be indicated			
Eating	Total assist		1	1	1
Dressing	Total assist		1	1	1
Grooming	Total assist		1	1	1
Bathing	Total assist	• Shampoo tray • Hand-held shower • Padded reclining shower—commode chair (if roll-in shower available)	1	1	1
Wheelchair propulsion	Power: independent Manual: Total assist	• Power recline and/or tilt wheelchair with head, chin, or breath control and manual recliner • Vent tray	6	1	1–6
Standing, ambulation	Standing: Total assist Ambulation: Not usually indicated	• Tilt table • Hydraulic standing table			
Communication	Total assist to independent, depending on workstation setup and equipment availability	Mouth stick, high-tech computer access, environmental control unit			
Transportation	Total assist	Attendant-operated van (e.g., lift, tie-downs) or accessible public transportation			
Homemaking	Total assist				
Assist required	• 24-hour care to include homemaking • Able to instruct in all aspects of care		24*	24*	16–24*

*Hours per day.

Appendix 43-1. Expected Functional Outcomes *(continued)*
Level C5

Functionally relevant muscles innervated: Deltoid, biceps, brachialis, brachioradialis, rhomboids, serratus anterior (partially innervated)
Movement possible: Shoulder flexion, abduction, and extension; elbow flexion and supination; scapular adduction and abduction
Patterns of weakness: Absence of elbow extension, pronation, all wrist and hand movement; total paralysis of trunk and lower extremities
FIM/Assistance Data: Exp = Expected FIM Score / **Med** = NSCISC Median / **IR** = NSCISC Interquartile Range
NSCISC Sample Size: FIM=41 / Assist=35

	Expected Functional Outcomes	Equipment	FIM/Assistance Data		
			Exp	*Med*	*IR*
Respiratory	Low endurance and vital capacity secondary to paralysis of intercostals; may require assist to clear secretions				
Bowel	Total assist	Padded shower, commode chair or padded transfer tub bench with commode cutout	1	1	1
Bladder	Total assist	Adaptive devices may be indicated (electric leg bag emptier)	1	1	1
Bed mobility	Some assist	• Full electric hospital bed with Trendelenburg feature with patient's control • Side rails			
Bed, wheelchair transfers	Total assist	• Transfer board • Power or mechanical lift	1	1	1
Pressure relief, positioning	Independent with equipment	• Power recline and/or tilt wheelchair • Wheelchair pressure relief cushion • Hand splints • Specialty bed or pressure relief mattress may be indicated • Postural support devices			
Eating	Total assist for setup, then independent eating with equipment	• Long opponens splint • Adaptive devices as indicated	5	5	25–55
Dressing	Lower extremity: Total assist Upper extremity: Some assist	• Long opponens splint • Adaptive devices as indicated	1	1	1–4
Grooming	Some to total assist	• Long opponens splints • Adaptive devices as indicated	1–3	1	1–5
Bathing	Total assist	• Padded tub transfer bench or shower—commode chair • Hand-held shower	1	1	1–3
Wheelchair propulsion	Power: Independent Manual: Independent to some assist indoors on uncarpeted, level surface; some to total assist outdoors	Power: Power recline and/or tilt with arm drive control Manual: Lightweight rigid or folding frame with hand rim modifications	6	6	5–6
Standing ambulation	Total assist	Hydraulic standing frame			

Appendix 43-1. Expected Functional Outcomes *(continued)*
Level C5

	Expected Functional Outcomes	Equipment	FIM/Assistance Data Exp	Med	IR
Communication	Independent to some assist after setup with equipment	• Long opponens splint • Adaptive devices as needed for page turning, writing, button pushing			
Transportation	Independent with highly specialized equipment; some assist with accessible public transportation; total assist for attendant-operated vehicle	Highly specialized modified van with lift			
Homemaking	Total assist				
Assist required	• Personal care: 10 hours/day • Home care: 6 hours/day • Able to instruct in all aspects of care		16*	23*	10–24*

*Hours per day.

Level C6

Functionally relevant muscles innervated: Clavicular pectoralis; supinator; extensor carpi radialis longus and brevis; serratus anterior; latissimus dorsi
Movement possible: Scapular protraction; some horizontal adduction, forearm supination, radial wrist extension
Patterns of weakness: Absence of wrist flexion, elbow extension, hand movement; total paralysis of trunk and lower extremities

FIM/Assistance Data: Exp = Expected FIM Score / **Med** = NSCISC Median / **IR** = NSCISC Interquartile Range
NSCISC Sample Size: FIM=43 / Assist=35

	Expected Functional Outcomes	Equipment	FIM/Assistance Data Exp	Med	IR
Respiratory	Low endurance and vital capacity secondary to paralysis of intercostals; may require assist to clear secretions				
Bowel	Some to total assist	• Padded tub bench with commode cutout or padded shower—commode chair • Other adaptive devices as indicated	1–2	1	1
Bladder	Some to total assist with equipment; may be independent with leg bag emptying	Adaptive devices as indicated	1–2	1	1
Bed mobility	Some assist	• Full electric hospital bed • Side rails • Full to king standard bed may be indicated			
Bed, wheelchair transfers	Level: Some assist to independent Uneven: Some to total assist	• Transfer board • Mechanical lift	3	1	1–3

Appendix 43-1. Expected Functional Outcomes *(continued)*
Level C6

	Expected Functional Outcomes	Equipment	FIM/Assistance Data		
			Exp	*Med*	*IR*
Pressure relief, positioning	Independent with equipment and/or adapted techniques	• Power recline wheelchair • Wheelchair pressure relief cushion • Postural support devices • Pressure relief mattress or overlay may be indicated			
Eating	Independent with or without equipment except cutting, which is total assist	Adaptive devices as indicated (e.g., U-cuff, tenodesis splint, adapted utensils, plate guard)	5–6	5	4–6
Dressing	Independent upper extremity; some to total assist for lower extremities	Adaptive devices as indicated (e.g., button hook; loops on zippers, pants, socks; Velcro on shoes)	1–3	2	1–5
Grooming	Some assist to independent with equipment	Adaptive devices as indicated (e.g., U-cuff, adapted handles)	3–6	4	2–6
Bathing	Upper body: Independent Lower body: Some to total assist	• Padded tub transfer bench or shower—commode chair • Adaptive devices as needed • Hand-held shower	1–3	1	1–3
Wheelchair propulsion Standing, ambulation	Power: Independent with standard arm drive on all surfaces Manual: Independent indoors; some to total assist outdoors Standing: Total assist Ambulation: Not indicated	Manual: Lightweight rigid or folding frame with modified rims Power: May require power recline or standard upright power wheelchair Hydraulic standing frame	6	6	4–6
Communication	Independent with or without equipment	Adaptive devices as indicated (e.g., tenodesis splint; writing splint for keyboard use, button pushing, page turning, object manipulation)			
Transportation	Independent driving from wheelchair	• Modified van with lift • Sensitized hand controls • Tie-downs			
Homemaking	Some assist with light meal preparation; total assist for all other homemaking	Adaptive devices as indicated			
Assist required	• Personal care: 6 hours/day • Home care: 4 hours/day		10*	17*	8–24*

*Hours per day.

Appendix 43-1. Expected Functional Outcomes *(continued)*
Level C7-8

Functionally relevant muscles innervated: Latissimus dorsi; sternal pectoralis; triceps; pronator quadratus; extensor carpi ulnaris; flexor carpi radialis; flexor digitorum profundus and superficialis; extensor communis; pronator/flexor/extensor/abductor pollicis; lumbricals [partially innervated]
Movement possible: Elbow extension; ulnar/wrist extension; wrist flexion; finger flexion and extension; thumb flexion/extension/abduction
Patterns of weakness: Paralysis of trunk and lower extremities; limited grasp release and dexterity secondary to partial paralysis intrinsic muscles of the hand

FIM/Assistance Data: Exp = Expected FIM Score / **Med** = NSCISC Median / **IR** = NSCISC Interquartile Range
NSCISC Sample Size: FIM=43 / Assist=35

	Expected Functional Outcomes	Equipment	FIM/Assistance Data *Exp*	*Med*	*IR*
Respiratory	Low endurance and vital capacity secondary to paralysis of intercostals; may require assist to clear secretions				
Bowel	Some to total assist	• Padded tub bench with commode cutout or shower—commode chair • Adaptive devices as needed	1–4	1	1–4
Bladder	Independent to some assist	Adaptive devices as indicated	2–6	3	1–6
Bed mobility	Independent to some assist	Full electric hospital bed or full to king standard bed			
Bed, wheelchair transfers	Level: Independent Uneven: Independent to some assist	With or without transfer board	3–7	4	2–6
Pressure relief, positioning	Independent	• Wheelchair pressure relief cushion • Postural support devices as indicated • Pressure relief mattress or overlay may be indicated			
Eating	Independent	Adaptive devices as indicated	6–7	6	5–7
Dressing	Independent upper extremities; independent to some assist lower extremities	Adaptive devices as indicated	4–7	6	4–7
Grooming	Independent	Adaptive devices as indicated	6–7	6	4–7
Bathing	Upper body: Independent Lower extremity: Some assist to independent	• Padded transfer tub bench or shower—commode chair • Hand-held shower • Adaptive devices as needed	3–6	4	2–6
Wheelchair propulsion	Manual: Independent all indoor surfaces and level outdoor terrain; some assist with uneven terrain	Manual: Rigid or folding lightweight or folding wheelchair with modified rims	6	6	6
Standing, ambulation	Standing: Independent to some assist Ambulation: Not indicated	Hydraulic or standard standing frame			
Communication	Independent	Adaptive devices as indicated			
Transportation	Independent car if independent with transfer, wheelchair loading and unloading; independent driving modified van from captain's seat.	• Modified vehicle • Transfer board			
Homemaking	Independent light meal preparation and homemaking; some to total assist for complex meal prep and heavy housecleaning	Adaptive devices as indicated			
Assist required	• Personal care: 6 hours/day • Home care: 2 hours/day		8*	12*	2–24*

*Hours per day.

Appendix 43-1. Expected Functional Outcomes *(continued)*
Level T1-9

Functionally relevant muscles innervated: Intrinsics of the hand including thumbs; internal and external intercostals; erector spinae; lumbricals; flexor/extensor/abductor pollicis
Movement possible: Upper extremities fully intact; limited upper trunk stability. Endurance increased secondary to innervation of intercostals
Patterns of weakness: Lower trunk paralysis, Total paralysis lower extremities

FIM/Assistance Data: Exp = Expected FIM Score / **Med** = NSCISC Median / **IR** = NSCISC Interquartile Range
NSCISC Sample Size: FIM=144 / Assist=122

	Expected Functional Outcomes	Equipment	FIM/Assistance Data		
			Exp	*Med*	*IR*
Respiratory	Compromised vital capacity and endurance				
Bowel	Independent	Elevated padded toilet seat or padded tub bench with commode cutout	6–7	6	4–6
Bladder	Independent		6	6	5–6
Bed mobility	Independent	Full to king standard bed			
Bed, wheelchair transfers	Independent	May or may not require transfer board	6–7	6	6–7
Pressure relief, positioning	Independent	• Wheelchair pressure relief cushion • Postural support devices as indicated • Pressure relief mattress or overlay may be indicated			
Eating	Independent		7	7	7
Dressing	Independent		7	7	7
Grooming	Independent		7	7	7
Bathing	Independent	• Padded tub transfer bench or shower—commode chair • Hand-held shower	6–7	6	5–7
Wheelchair propulsion	Independent	Manual rigid or folding lightweight wheelchair	6	6	6
Standing, ambulation	Standing: Independent Ambulation: Typically not functional	Standing frame			
Communication	Independent				
Transportation	Independent in car, including loading and unloading wheelchair	Hand controls			
Homemaking	Independent with complex meal prep and light housecleaning; total to some assist with heavy housekeeping				
Assist required	Homemaking: 3 hours/day		2*	3*	0–15*

*Hours per day.

Appendix 43-1. Expected Functional Outcomes *(continued)*
Level T10-L1

Functionally relevant muscles innervated: Fully intact intercostals; external obliques; rectus abdominis
Movement possible: Good trunk stability
Patterns of weakness: Paralysis of lower extremities

FIM/Assistance Data: Exp = Expected FIM Score / **Med** = NSCISC Median / **IR** = NSCISC Interquartile Range
NSCISC Sample Size: FIM=71 / Assist=57

	Expected Functional Outcomes	Equipment	FIM/Assistance Data		
			Exp	*Med*	*IR*
Respiratory	Intact respiratory function				
Bowel	Independent	Padded standard or raised padded toilet seat	6–7	6	6
Bladder	Independent		6	6	6
Bed mobility	Independent	Full to king standard bed			
Bed, wheelchair transfers	Independent		7	7	6–7
Pressure relief, positioning	Independent	• Wheelchair pressure relief cushion • Postural support devices as indicated • Pressure relief mattress or overlay may be indicated			
Eating	Independent		7	7	7
Dressing	Independent		7	7	7
Grooming	Independent		7	7	7
Bathing	Independent	• Padded transfer tub bench • Hand-held shower	6–7	6	6–7
Wheelchair propulsion	Independent all indoor and outdoor surfaces	Manual rigid or folding lightweight wheelchair	6	6	6
Standing, ambulation	Standing: Independent Ambulation: Functional, some assist to independent	• Standing frame • Forearm crutches or walker • Knee, ankle, foot orthosis (KAFO)			
Communication	Independent				
Transportation	Independent in car, including loading and unloading wheelchair	Hand controls			
Homemaking	Independent with complex meal prep and light housecleaning; some assist with heavy housekeeping				
Assist required	Homemaking: 2 hours/day		2*	2*	0–8*

*Hours per day.

Appendix 43-1. Expected Functional Outcomes *(continued)*
Level L2-S5

Functionally relevant muscles innervated: Fully intact abdominals and all other trunk muscles; depending on level, some degree of hip flexors, extensors, abductors, adductors; knee flexors, extensors; ankle dorsiflexors, plantar flexors.
Movement possible: Good trunk stability. Partial to full control lower extremities.
Patterns of weakness: Partial paralysis lower extremities, hips, knees, ankle, foot

FIM/Assistance Data: Exp = Expected FIM Score / **Med** = NSCISC Median / **IR** = NSCISC Interquartile Range
NSCISC Sample Size: FIM=20 / Assist=16

	Expected Functional Outcomes	Equipment	FIM/Assistance Data *Exp*	*Med*	*IR*
Respiratory	Intact function				
Bowel	Independent	Padded toilet seat	6–7	6	6–7
Bladder	Independent		6	6	6–7
Bed mobility	Independent				
Bed/wheelchair transfers	Independent	Full to king standard bed	7	7	7
Pressure relief/ positioning	Independent	• Wheelchair pressure-relief cushion • Postural support device as indicated			
Eating	Independent		7	7	7
Dressing	Independent		7	7	7
Grooming	Independent		7	7	7
Bathing	Independent	• Padded tub bench • Handheld shower	7	7	6–7
Wheelchair propulsion	Independent on all indoor and outdoor surfaces	Manual rigid or folding lightweight wheelchair	6	6	6
Standing/ ambulation	Standing: Independent Ambulation: Functional, independent to some assist	• Standing frame • Knee-ankle-foot orthosis or ankle-foot orthosis • Forearm crutches or cane as indicated			
Communication	Independent				
Transportation	Independent in car, Including loading and unloading wheelchair	Hand controls			
Homemaking	Independent complex cooking and light housekeeping; some assist with heavy housekeeping				
Assist required	Homemaking: 0–1 hour/day		0–1*	0*	0–2*

*Hours per day.

SUMMARY REVIEW QUESTIONS

1. List three key epidemiological factors of the SCI population and describe how these factors influence evaluation and treatment.
2. List three precautions the therapist must consider in planning for an outing with a patient with C5 injury.
3. What is a tenodesis grasp? Why is it important, and how can the occupational therapist facilitate it?
4. List five parts of the initial occupational therapy evaluation of a patient with SCI.
5. Describe a typical feeding setup for person with C5 tetraplegia.
6. What are the functional expectations for the patient with a C7 injury?
7. You read in the medical chart that a patient lost consciousness at the time of injury. How do you modify your evaluation? Describe how concomitant brain injury may alter your treatment goals and interventions.
8. What are the roles of the occupational therapist in the transition phase?

ACKNOWLEDGMENT

I thank the patients and staff at Rancho Los Amigos National Rehabilitation Center, who have inspired and taught me so much over the years. I also thank my husband, Richard Atkins, for his assistance in editing this chapter. Last, I thank the photographer, the late Paul Weinreich.

References

Adler, C. (1989). Equipment considerations. In G. Whiteneck, D. P. Lammertse, M. Scott, & R. Mentor (Eds.), *The management of high quadriplegia* (pp. 207–231). New York: Demos.

American Spinal Injury Association [ASIA]. (2000). *International standards for neurological classification of spinal injury patients*. Chicago: American Spinal Injury Association.

Atkins, M. S. (1989). A descriptive study: The occupational therapy predischarge home visit program for spinal cord injured adults. Unpublished Master's thesis. University of Southern California, Los Angeles, CA.

Atkins, M. S., Clark, D., & Waters, R. (2003). Upper limb orthoses. In V. W. Lin (Ed.), *Spinal cord medicine: Principles and practice* (pp. 663–674). New York: Demos.

Baum, C. (2000). Occupation-based practice: Reinventing ourselves for the new millennium. *OT Practice, 1,* 12–15.

Brachtesende, A. (2005). ICF the universal translator. *OT Practice*. The American Occupational Therapy Association.

Bryden, A. M., Wuolle, K. S., Murray, P. K., & Peckham, P. H. (2004). Perceived outcomes and utilization of upper extremity surgical reconstruction in individuals with tetraplegia at model spinal cord injury systems. *Spinal Cord, 42,* 169–176.

Buss, I. C., Halfens, R. J. G., & Abu-Saad, H. H. (2002). The most effective time interval for repositioning subjects at risk of pressure sore development: A literature review. *Rehabilitation Nursing, 27,* 59–66.

Cardenas, D. D., Hoffman, J. M., Kirshblum, S., & McKinley, W. (2004). Etiology and incidence of rehospitalization after traumatic spinal cord injury: A multicenter analysis. *Archives of Physical Medicine and Rehabilitation, 85,* 1757–1763.

Catz, A., Itzkovich, M., Ring, H., Agranov, E., & Tamir, A. (2001). The spinal cord independence measure (SCIM): Sensitivity to functional changes in subgroups of spinal cord lesion patients. *Spinal Cord, 39,* 97–100.

Catz, A., Itzkovich, M., Steinberg, F., Philo, O., Ring, H., Ronen, J., Spasser, R., Gepstein, R., & Tamir, A. (2001). The Catz-Itzkovich SCIM: A revised version of the Spinal Cord Independence Measure. *Disability and Rehabilitation, 23,* 263–268.

Clark, F. A., Jackson, J. M., Scott, M. D., Carlson, M. E., Atkins, M. S., Uhles-Tanaka, & Rubayi, S. (2006). Data-based models of how pressure ulcers develop in daily-living contexts of adults with spinal cord injury. *Archives of Physical Medicine & Rehabilitation, 87,* 1516–1525.

Clark, D. R., Waters, R. L., & Baumgarten, J. M. (1997). Upper limb orthoses for the spinal cord injured patients. In B. Goldberg & J. D. Hsu (Eds.), *Atlas of orthoses and assistive devices* (3rd ed., pp. 291–303). St. Louis: Mosby.

Consortium for Spinal Cord Medicine. (1997a). *Acute management of autonomic dysreflexia: Adults with spinal cord injury presenting to health care facilities*. Washington, DC: Paralyzed Veterans of America.

Consortium for Spinal Cord Medicine. (1997b). *Prevention of thromboembolism in spinal cord injury: Clinical practice guidelines*. Washington, DC: Paralyzed Veterans of America.

Consortium for Spinal Cord Medicine. (1998a). *Depression following spinal cord injury: A Clinical practice guideline*. Washington, DC: Paralyzed Veterans of America.

Consortium for Spinal Cord Medicine. (1998b). *Neurogenic bowel management in adults with spinal cord injury: Clinical practice guidelines*. Washington, DC: Paralyzed Veterans of America.

Consortium for Spinal Cord Medicine. (1999). *Outcome following traumatic spinal cord injury: Clinical practice guidelines for health care professionals*. Washington, DC: Paralyzed Veterans of America.

Consortium for Spinal Cord Medicine. (2002). *Consumer Guideline. Pressure ulcers: what you should know*. Washington, DC: Paralyzed Veterans of America.

Consortium for Spinal Cord Medicine. (2005). *Preservation of upper limb function following spinal cord injury: A clinical practice guidelines for healthcare professionals*. Washington, DC: Paralyzed Veterans of America.

Curtin, M. (1999). An analysis of tetraplegic hand grips. *British Journal of Occupational Therapy, 62,* 444–450.

Curtis, K. A., Tyner, T. M., Zachary, L., Lentell, G., Brink, D., Didyk, T., Gean, K., Hall, J., Hooper, M., Klos, J., Lesina, S., & Pacillas, B. (1999). Effect of a standard exercise protocol on shoulder pain in long-term wheelchair users. *Spinal Cord, 37,* 421–429.

Cushman, L .A., & Dijkers, M. (1990). Depressed mood in spinal cord injured patients: Staff perceptions and patient realities. *Archives of Physical Medicine and Rehabilitation, 71,* 191–196.

Davidoff, G. N., Roth, E. J., & Richards, J. S. (1992). Cognitive deficits in spinal cord injury: Epidemiology and outcome. *Archives of Physical Medicine and Rehabilitation, 73,* 275–284.

DeVivo, M. J., Krause, J. S., & Lammertse, D. P. (1999). Recent trends in mortality and causes of death among persons with spinal cord injury. *Archives of Physical Medicine and Rehabilitation, 80,* 1411–1419.

DeVivo, M. J., Stover, S. L. (1995). Long-term survival and causes of death (pp. 289–316). In S. L. Stover, Whiteneck, G. G., & DeLisa, J. A., *Spinal cord injury: Clinical outcomes from the model systems*. Gaithersbury, MD: Aspen.

Donnelly, C., Eng, J. J., Hall, J., Alford, L., Giachino, R., Norton, K., & Kerr, D. S. (2004). Client-centered assessment and the identification of meaningful treatment goals for individuals with spinal cord injury. *Spinal Cord, 42,* 302–307.

Ducharme, S. H., & Gill, K. M. (1997). *Sexuality after spinal cord injury*. Baltimore: Paul H. Brookes.

Forchheimer, M., & Tate, D. G. (2004). Enhancing community re-integration following spinal cord injury. *NeuroRehabilitation, 19,* 103–113.

Ford, J. R., & Duckworth, B. (1987). *Physical management for the quadriplegic patient* (2nd ed.). Philadelphia: Davis.

Formal, C., & Smith, J. (1996). Upper extremity function in spinal cord injury. *Topics in Spinal Cord Injury Rehabilitation, 1,* 1–13.

Fuhrer, M. R., Rintala, D. H., Hart, K. A., Clearman, R., & Young, M. E. (1993). Depressive symptomatology in persons with spinal cord injury who reside in a community. *Archives of Physical Medicine and Rehabilitation, 74,* 255–260.

Garland, D. E. (1991). A clinical perspective on common forms of acquired heterotopic ossification. *Clinical Orthopaedics and Related Research, 242,* 169–176.

Gerhart, K. A., Bergstrom, E., Charlifue, S. W., Menter, R. R., & Whiteneck, G. G. (1993). Long-term spinal cord injury: Functional changes over time. *Archives of Physical Medicine and Rehabilitation, 74,* 1030–1034.

Gersham, G. E., Labi, M. I., Dittmar, S. S., Hicks, J. T., Joyce, S. Z., & Phillips Stehlik, M. A. (1986). The Quadriplegia Index of Function (QIF): Sensitivity and reliability demonstrated in a study of thirty quadriplegic patients. *Paraplegia, 24,* 38–44.

Hammell, K. W. (1995). *Spinal cord injury rehabilitation.* Suffolk, United Kingdom: Chapman & Hall.

Hammell, K. W. (2004). Exploring quality of life following high spinal cord injury: A review and critiques. *Spinal Cord, 42,* 491–502.

Harvey, L. (1996). Principles of conservative management of a non-orthotic tenodesis grip in tetraplegics. *Journal of Hand Therapy, 9,* 238–242.

Hemmingsson, H., & Jonsson, H. (2005). The issue is: An occupational perspective on the concept of participation in the international classification of functioning, disability and health: Some critical remarks. *American Journal of Occupational Therapy, 59,* 569–576.

Hill, J. (1986). Spinal cord injury: A guide to functional outcomes in occupational therapy. Rockville, MD: Aspen.

Hollar, L. D. (1995). Spinal cord injury. In C. A. Trombly (ed.), *Occupational therapy for physical dysfunction* (4th ed., 795–813). Baltimore, MD: Williams & Wilkins.

Jackson, A. B., Dijkers, M., DeVivo, M. J., & Poczatek, R. B. (2004). A demographic profile of new traumatic spinal cord injuries: Change and stability over 30 years. *Archives of Physical Medicine and Rehabilitation, 85,* 1740–1748.

Jackson, A. B., & Wadley, V. (1999). A multicenter study of women's self-reported reproductive health after spinal cord injury. *Archives of Physical Medicine and Rehabilitation, 80,* 1420–1428.

Jebsen, R., Taylor, N., Trieschmann, R., Trotter, M., & Howard, L. (1969). An objective and standarized test of hand function. *Archives of Physical Medicine and Rehabilitation, 50,* 311–319.

Kendall, F. P., McCreary, E. K., & Provance, P. G. (1993). *Muscles: Testing and function* (4th ed.). Baltimore: Williams & Wilkins.

Kendall, M. B., Ungerer, G., & Dorsett, P. (2003). Bridging the gap: Transitional rehabilitation sercies for people with spinal cord injury. *Disability and Rehabilitation, 25,* 1008–1015.

Kilgore, K. L., Peckham, P. H., Keith, M. W., Thrope, G. B., Woulle, K. S., Bryden, A. M., & Hart, R. L. (1997). An implanted upper-extremity neuroprosthesis. *Journal of Bone and Joint Surgery, 79-A,* 533–541.

Kirshblum, S. C., Gulati, M., O'Conner, K. C., & Voorman, S. J. (1998). Bowel care practices in chronic spinal cord injury patients. *Archives of Physical Medicine and Rehabilitation, 79,* 20–23.

Kirshblum, S., Millis, S., McKinley, W., & Tulsky, D. (2004). Late neurologic recovery after traumatic spinal cord injury. *Archives of Physical Medicine and Rehabilitation, 85,* 1811–1817.

Kohlmeyer, K. M, Hill, J. P., Yarkony, G. M., & Jaeger, R. J. (1996). Electrical stimulation and biofeedback effect on recovery of tenodesis grasp: A controlled study. *Archives of Physical Medicine & Rehabilitation, 77,* 702–706.

Krause, J. S., Kenman, D., DeVivo, M. J., Maynard, F., Coker, J., Roach, M. J., & Ducharme, S. (1999). Employment after spinal cord injury: An analysis of cases from the Model Spinal Cord Injury Systems. *Archives of Physical Medicine and Rehabilitation, 80,* 1492–1500.

Land, N. E., Odding, E., Duivenvoorden, H. J., Bergen, M. P., & Stam H. J. (2004). Tetraplegia Hand Activity Questionnaire (THAQ): The development, assessment of arm-hand function-related activities in tetraplegic patients with a spinal cord injury. *Spinal Cord, 42,* 294–301.

Liem, N. R., McColl, M. A., King, W., & Smith, K. M. (2004). Aging with a spinal cord injury: Factors associated with the need for more help with activities of daily living. *Archives of Physical Medicine and Rehabilitation, 85,* 1567–1577.

Livneh, H., & Antonak, R. F. (1997). Psychosocial adaptation to chronic illness and disability. Gaithersburg, MD: Aspen.

Lorig, K. L. (2003). Self-management education, more that a nice extra. *Medical Care, 41,* 699–701.

Lysack, C. L., Zafonte, C. A., Neufeld, S. W., & Dijkers, M. (2001). Self-care independence after spinal cord injury: Patient and therapist expectations and real life performance. *Journal of Spinal Cord Medicine, 24,* 257–265.

Massagli, T. L., & Jaffe, K. M. (1990). Pediatric spinal cord injury: Treatment and outcome. *Pediatrician, 17,* 244–254.

McColl, M. A., Arnold, R., Charlifue, S., Glass, C., Savic, G., & Frankel, H. (2003). Aging, spinal cord injury, and quality of life: Structural relationships. *Archives of Physical Medicine and Rehabilitation, 84,* 1137–1144.

McKinley, W. O., Seel, R. T., & Hardman, J. T. (1999). Nontraumatic spinal cord injury: Incidence, epidemiology, and functional outcome. *Archives of Physical Medicine and Rehabilitation, 80,* 619–623.

Mead, M. A., Lewis, A., Jackson M. N., & Hess, D. (2004). Race, employment, and spinal cord injury. *Archives of Physical Medicine and Rehabilitation, 85,* 1782–1792.

Moberg, E. (1978). *The upper limb in tetraplegia.* Stuttgart: Thieme.

National Spinal Cord Injury Statistical Center. (2005). *Annual report for the model spinal cord injury care systems.* Birmingham: University of Alabama.

National Spinal Cord Injury Statistical Center. (2006). *Spinal cord injury: Facts and figures at a glance.* Birmingham: University of Alabama.

Nead, C., & Hughes, M. B. (1997). Patients with spinal cord injuries who are ventilator dependent: The practitioner's role. *Physical Disabilities: Special Interest Section Quarterly, 20,* 4. Bethesda, MD: American Occupational Therapy Association.

Nelson, A. L., (1990). Patients' perspectives on a spinal cord injury unit. *SCI Nursing, 7,* 44–63.

Nobunaga, A. I., Go, B. K., & Karunas, R. B. (1999). Recent demographic and injury trends in people served by the Model Spinal Cord Injury Systems. *Archives of Physical Medicine and Rehabilitation, 80,* 1372–1382.

Occupational Therapy Department. (1990). *Functional goals for patients with quadriplegia.* Unpublished form. Rancho Los Amigos National Rehabilitation Center, Downey, CA.

Penrod, L. E., Hegde, S. K., & Ditunno, J. F. Jr. (1990). Age effect on prognosis for functional recovery in acute traumatic central cord syndrome (CCS). *Archives of Physical Medicine and Rehabilitation, 71,* 963–968.

Pires, M. (2002). Bladder elimination and continence. In S. P. Hoeman (Ed.), *Rehabilitation nursing: Process, application and outcomes* (3rd ed.). Philadelphia: Mosby.

Potter, P. J., Wolfe, D. L., Burkell, J. A., & Hayes. (2004). Challenges in educating individuals with SCI to reduce secondary conditions. *Topics in Spinal Cord Injury Rehabilitation, 10,* 30–40.

Radomski, M. V. (1998). Problem-solving deficits: Using a multidimensional definition to select a treatment approach. *Physical Disabilities Special Interest Section Quarterly, 21,* 1. Bethesda, MD: American Occupational Therapy Association.

Radomski, M. V. (2000). Self-efficacy: Improving occupational therapy outcomes by helping patients say "I can". *Physical Disabilities Special Interest Section Quarterly, 23,* 1–3. Bethesda, MD: American Occupational Therapy Association.

Richards, J. S., Bombardier, C. H., Take, D., Dijkers, M., Gordon, W., Shewchuk, R., & DeVivi, M. J. (1999). Access to the environment and life satisfaction after spinal cord injury. *Archives of Physical Medicine and Rehabilitation, 80,* 1501–1506.

Ryan, J. M. (2003). The role of occupational therapy in the prevention of pressure ulcers. *Home and Community Health Special Interest Section Quarterly, 10,* 1-3. Bethesda, MD: American Occupational Therapy Association.

Sadowsky, C. L. (2001). Electrical stimulation and spinal cord injury. *NeuroRehabilitation, 16,* 165–169.

Schonherr, M. C., Groothoff, J. W., Mulder, G. A., & Eisma, W. H. (2000). Prediction of functional outcome after spinal cord injury: A task for the rehabilitation team and the patient. *Spinal Cord, 38,* 185–191.

Schonherr, M. C., Groothoff, J. W., Mulder, G. A., & Eisma, W. H. (2005). Participation and satisfaction after spinal cord injury: Results of a vocational and leisure outcome study. *Spinal Cord, 43,* 241–248.

Scivoletto, G., Morganti, B., Ditunno, P., Ditunno, J. F., & Molinari, M. (2003). Effects on age spinal cord lesion patients' rehabilitation. *Spinal Cord, 41,* 457–464.

Siddall, P. J., & Loeser, J. D. (2001). Pain following spinal cord injury. *Spinal Cord, 39,* 63–73.

Siddall, P. J., McClelland, J. M., Rutkowski, S. B., & Cousins, M. J. (2003). A longitudinal study of the prevalence and characteristics of pain in the first 5 years following spinal cord injury. *Pain, 103,* 249–257.

Smith, Q. W., Frieden, L., Nelson, M. R., & Tilbor, A. G., (1996). Transition to adulthood for young people with spinal cord injury. In R. R. Benz & M. J. Mulcahey (Eds.), *The child with a spinal cord injury* (pp. 601–612). Rosemont, IL: American Academy of Orthopedic Surgeons.

Snoek, G. J., Ijzerman, M. J., Hermens, H. J., Maxwell, D., & Biering-Sorensen, F. (2004). Survey of the needs of patients with spinal cord injury: Impact and priority for improvement in hand function in tetraplegics. *Spinal Cord, 42,* 526–532.

Sollerman, C., & Ejeskar, A. (1995). Sollerman Hand Function Test: A standardized method and its use in tetraplegia patients. *Scandinavian Journal of Plastic Reconstructive Surgery and Hand Surgery, 29,* 167–176.

Stover, S. L., Whiteneck, G. G., & DeLisa, J. A. (1995). *Spinal cord injury: Clinical outcomes from the model systems.* Gaithersburg, MD: Aspen.

Trieschmann, R. B., Ed. (1988). *Spinal cord injuries: Psychological, social and vocational rehabilitation* (2nd ed.). New York: Demos.

Trombly, C. A., Ed. (1989). *Occupational therapy for physical dysfunction* (3rd ed.). Baltimore: Williams & Wilkins.

Trombly, C. A. (1995). Theoretical foundations for practice. In C. A. Trombly (ed.), *Occupational therapy for physical dysfunction* (4th ed., pp. 15-20). Baltimore: Williams & Wilkins.

van Kuijk, A. A., Geurts, A. C. H., & van Kuppevelt, H. J. (2002). Neurogenic heterotopic ossification in spinal cord injury. *Spinal Injury, 40,* 313–326.

van Tuijl, J. H., Janssen-Potten, Y. J. M., & Seelen, H. A. M. (2002). Evaluation of upper extremity motor function tests in tetraplegics. *Spinal Cord, 40,* 51–64.

Waters, R. L., Adkins, R. H., Yakura, J. S., & Sie, I. (1995). *Recovery following spinal cord injury: A clinician's handbook.* Downey, CA: Los Amigos Research and Educational Institute.

Waters, R. L., Sie, I. H., Gellman, H., & Tognella, M. (1996). Functional hand surgery following tetraplegia. *Archives of Physical Medicine and Rehabilitation, 77,* 86–94.

Waters, R. L., & Yoshida, G. M. (1996). Prognosis of spinal cord injuries. In A. M. Levine (Ed.), *Orthopedic knowledge update: Trauma* (pp. 303–310). Rosemont, IL: American Academy of Orthopedic Surgeons.

Whiteneck, G. G., Charlifue, S. W., Gerhart, K. A., Lammertse, D. P., Manely, S., Menter, R. R., & Seedroff, K. R., Eds. (1993). *Aging with spinal cord injury.* New York: Demos.

Whiteneck, G. G., Charlifue, S. W., Gerhart, K. A., Overholser, J. D., & Richardson, G. N. (1992). Quantifying handicap: A new measure of long-term rehabilitation outcomes. *Archives of Physical Medicine and Rehabilitation, 73,* 519–526.

Whiteneck, G. G., Lammertse, D. P., Manley, S., & Mentor, R., Eds. (1989). *The management of high quadriplegia.* New York: Demos.

Widerstrom-Noga, E. G., & Turk, D. C. (2003). Types and effectiveness of treatments used by people with chronic pain associated with spinal cord injuries: Influence of pain and psychosocial characteristics. *Spinal Cord, 41,* 600–609.

Wolfe, D. L., Potter, P. J., & Sequeira, K. A. J. (2004). Overcoming challenges: The role of rehabilitation in educating individuals with SCI to reduce secondary conditions. *Topics in Spinal Cord Injury Rehabilitation, 10,* 41–50.

World Health Organization. (2001). *International classification of functioning, disability and health.* Geneva, Switzerland: World Health Organization.

Wilson, D. J., McKenzie, M. W., Barber, L. M., & Watson, K. L. (1984). *Spinal cord injury: A treatment guide for occupational therapists* (2nd ed.). Thorofare, NJ: Slack.

Yarkony, G. M., Roth, E. J., Heinemann, A. W., & Lovell, L. L. (1988). Spinal cord injury rehabilitation outcomes: The impact of age. *Journal of Clinical Epidemiology, 41,* 173–177.

Yarkony, G. M., Roth, E. J., Heinemann, A. W., Wu, Y. C., Katz, R. T., & Lovell, L. (1987). Benefits of rehabilitation for traumatic spinal cord injury: Multivariate analysis in 711 patients. *Archives of Neurology, 44,* 93–96.

Yarkony, G. M., & Chen, D. (1996). Rehabilitation of patients with spinal cord injuries. In R. L. Braddom (Ed.), *Physical medicine and rehabilitation.* Philadelphia: Saunders.

Yerxa, E. J., & Locker, S. B. (1990). Quality of time use by adults with spinal cord injuries. *American Journal of Occupational Therapy, 44,* 318–326.

Zejdlik, C. P. (1991). *Management of spinal cord injury* (2nd ed.). Boston: Jones & Bartlett.

Zigler, J. E., Atkins, M. S., Resnik, C. D., & Thompson, L. (1998). Rehabilitation. In A. Levine, F. Eismont, S. Garfin, & J. E. Zigler (Eds.), *Spine trauma* (pp. 585–606). New York: Saunders.

Suggested Reading

American Spinal Injury Association. (2000). *International standards for neurological classification of spinal injury patients.* Chicago: American Spinal Injury Association.

Consortium for Spinal Cord Medicine. (1999). *Outcome following traumatic spinal cord injury: Clinical Practice guidelines for health care professionals.* Washington, DC: Paralyzed Veterans of America.

Ford, J. R., & Duckworth, B. (1987). *Physical management for the quadriplegic patient* (2nd ed.). Philadelphia: Davis.

Hammell, K. W. (1995). *Spinal cord injury rehabilitation.* London: Chapman & Hall.

Hill, J. (1986). *Spinal cord injury: A guide to functional outcomes in occupational therapy.* Rockville, MD: Aspen.

Maynard, F. M., Bracken, M. B., Creasey, G., Ditunno, J. F., Donovan, W. H., Ducker, T. B., Graber, S. L., Marino, R. J., Stover, S. L., Tator, C. H., Waters, R. L., Wilberger, J. E., & Young, W. (1997). International standards for neurological and functional classification of spinal cord injury. *Spinal Cord, 35,* 266–274.

Reeve, C. (1998). *Still me.* New York: Ballantine.

Trieshmann, R. B., Ed. (1988). *Spinal cord injuries: Psychological, social and vocational rehabilitation* (2nd ed.). New York: Demos.

Zejdlik, C. P. (1991). *Management of spinal cord injury* (2nd ed.). Boston: Jones & Bartlett.

CHAPTER 44

Rheumatoid Arthritis, Osteoarthritis, and Fibromyalgia

Y. Lynn Yasuda

CHAPTER OBJECTIVES

After studying this chapter, the reader will be able to do the following:

1. Describe key features of rheumatoid arthritis, osteoarthritis, and fibromyalgia.
2. Identify clinical sequelae that interfere with meeting occupational functioning goals.
3. Select assessments to optimize occupational functioning for patients with rheumatoid arthritis, osteoarthritis, and fibromyalgia.
4. Describe interventions to enable patients to meet their occupational functioning goals.
5. Identify preventive interventions to enable prolonged continuance of desired occupational goals.

Glossary

Allodynia—Pain in response to a normally non-painful stimulus.

Crepitus—Grating, crunching, or cracking sound or sensation during joint or tendon motion.

Daily activity log—Recording of experiences or impressions by patients as they occur.

Energy conservation—Breaking up physically active periods with rest periods, resulting in increased amount of physical activity (Cordery & Rocchi, 1998).

Hyperalgesia—Increased response to painful stimuli.

Joint protection—Methods to reduce external stress applied to impaired joints.

Lag—Difference of active ROM subtracted from passive ROM, measured in degrees.

Morning stiffness—Subjective complaint of local or general lack of easy mobility of the joints upon arising. This is a nonspecific indication of inflammation in RA; duration is directly proportional to the severity of the inflammatory process. Complaints vary from none to many hours. Patients with OA may also complain of morning stiffness, but it tends to be milder and brief.

Rheumatoid nodules—Firm, usually painless lumps of variable size found in patients with RA. They can be found over areas that are subject to mechanical trauma (e.g., elbows, heels, and hands) and on finger flexor and extensor tendons.

Although more than 100 rheumatic diseases have been identified, this chapter focuses on rheumatoid arthritis (RA) and osteoarthritis (OA) because they are the most common rheumatic diseases encountered in an occupational therapy clinic. Both can be disabling, and both require intervention to allow optimal occupational functioning. Other rheumatic diseases may have some symptoms similar to RA or OA, and the principles used to manage these two diseases can be used when encountering others. Each rheumatic disease has unique manifestations, however, and occupational therapists must address these as well. This chapter also briefly discusses fibromyalgia (FM). FM is a complex syndrome that commonly has multidimensional physical and psychological characteristics. The best treatment results appear to occur when a multidisciplinary approach is used to manage the various features of the condition (Goldenberg, Burckhardt, & Crofford, 2004).

RHEUMATOID ARTHRITIS

Rheumatoid arthritis (RA) is a systemic, inflammatory disease that affects joints and can affect the major organs of the body, including eye, skin, lungs, heart, gastrointestinal system, kidneys, nervous system, or blood. Common symptoms are symmetric polyarticular pain and swelling during the inflammatory stage, **morning stiffness** (usually lasting more than 2 hours), malaise, and fatigue. Remissions and exacerbations are common with the course of disease, ranging from self-limiting disease to severe chronic disease. Estimates of prevalence range from 0.3–1% of the adult population, with RA occurring 2.5 times more often in women and commonly being seen in women aged 40 to 50 years (Gornisiewicz & Moreland, 2001; Goronzy & Weyand, 2001).

The etiology of RA remains unknown and is likely multifactorial, including genetic factors and exposure to unknown environmental factors. The joints most often involved are the wrists, PIP, MCP, elbows, metatarsophalangeal, and temporomandibular joints, although other joints can be involved as well (Gornisiewicz & Moreland, 2001).

OSTEOARTHRITIS

Osteoarthritis (OA), the etiology of which is still unknown, is currently thought to be a group of disorders in which biomedical, biochemical, and genetic factors play a role (Lozada & Altman, 2001). Commonly, a gradual loss of articular cartilage can be seen, combined with thickening of the subchondral bone, bony outgrowths at joint margins, and mild, chronic nonspecific synovial inflammation (Hochberg, 2001). Excessive biomechanical loading, which may occur after trauma to a joint or to normal cartilage or bone or both, can lead to cartilage loss. Repetitive impact loading to specific joints, such as seen in selected vocations and avocations, can lead to joint problems. Joints most commonly involved are the knees, hips, interphalangeal joints, the first CMC joint, and the spine, although other joints can be involved. Common symptoms are joint tenderness, sometimes accompanied by crepitus, limitation of movement, pain after use that is relieved by rest, and progression of pain at rest and at night. Morning stiffness in the involved joint generally lasts less than 30 minutes (Lozada & Altman, 2001). One third of people aged 65 years and older have knee OA. Before the age of 50, men are more likely than women to have OA, but after age 50, OA is more prevalent in women. Diagnosis is based on the history, physical examination, and radiographic features of joint space narrowing, sclerosis of bone, marginal osteophytes, and bony remodeling (Hochberg, 2001).

Assessment (RA and OA)

In response to a request for services, the occupational therapist reviews the chart, observes and interviews the patient concerning occupational functioning, and may use screening tests to determine whether referral for occupational therapy is indicated. A patient who risks decline in occupational functioning because of pain, fatigue, loss of strength, endurance, or joint range of motion (ROM); change in environment, including social support; or loss of coping skills or whose function may be improved can benefit from occupational therapy (Backman, 1998; Feinberg & Trombly, 1995).

Assessment begins with obtaining an occupational profile through interviewing to find out the occupational history of the client's typical day. This occupational history interview can yield information in several areas. For example, it can give information about the balance of rest and activity, the meaning and importance of various occupations, the environmental and social supports and/or barriers to performance, and the effect of client factors on performance, adjustment to disability, and a sense of self-efficacy. It also allows the therapist to learn the patient's perspective on occupational functioning in relation to the severity of the physical impairment.

From the occupational profile, the occupational therapist obtains information about the patient's important occupations and beginning information about impairment and context issues that affect the performance of these occupations. This will facilitate occupation goal setting by the patient through an instrument such as the *Canadian Occupational Performance Measure* (*COPM*) to determine areas of occupational functioning that are important to the person and that are at risk or are compromised (Backman, 1998; Law et al., 1994). As initial patient-identified goals are recognized, all subsequent aspects of assessment are related to finding out whether more detailed occupational functioning deficits or impairment issues exist. Occupational functioning and performance context assessments may include specific ADL evaluations and environmental analyses, including social support and architectural issues, to determine the influence of the environment on the patient's ability to function (Backman, 1998). Common assessments of impairments of abilities and capacities may include but are not limited to ROM evaluation, strength testing, and evaluation of hand deformities, pain, fatigue, and psychosocial status. Sensory evaluation should be done if systemic involvement has led the patient to make complaints that indicate polyneuropathies or nerve compression.

Psychosocial Factors to Consider before Goal Setting

To identify the patient's goals, the therapist must recognize the patient's response to the impairment issues that the disease has imposed. This helps establish the treatment plan. For example, a person who recognizes that the diagnosis is accurate and who understands and accepts the consequences of the disease process may design goals that can be met immediately, such as finding appropriate adapted equipment to continue working. Another person may not accept the diagnosis and, therefore, deny that any issues are present, believe that normalcy will soon return, and feel that dependency on others is appropriate.

If patients are situationally depressed or angry at having the condition, the therapist may be entreated to try harder to reduce the impairment, or the patient may look for questionable alternative interventions. Clear and attainable objectives established with the patient at this time may be significant in helping the patient to continue to engage in meaningful occupations. Meeting treatment objectives successfully, even in small increments, is important with these patients.

Dubouloz et al. (2004) were concerned that patients with RA have difficulty using the help-seeking strategies recommended in occupational therapy, such as using social support or pacing, which often carry associated meaning perspectives (i.e., personal beliefs, values, feelings, and knowledge) that have been identified as barriers to change. It has been suggested that these barriers can be overcome through a process of transformation of meaning perspectives. Following their study to determine meaning perspectives of women with RA, they concluded that clinicians could encourage patient self-reflection during interventions to guide the discovery of meaning perspectives and meaning perspective transformation of importance to individual clients. For example, if the therapist asks what does the illness mean to her/him and the patient responds, "This illness has made me give up almost all of my social relations," then this illness meaning perspective provides a beginning understanding of what impact the illness has had on occupational balance. This type of discussion could eventually lead to a transformative meaning perspective, in which the patient integrates the occupational therapy intervention (for example, "this illness has led me to pace my activities, so I can once again have lunch with friends, although not as frequently") as a result of a new recognition of a desired change in occupational balance. Dubouloz et al. (2004) suggested that further research is needed in this area to develop a model for therapists (and others) to take appropriate action.

The therapist should work with the patient to examine all activities and to determine which are most important to the individual. The patient is encouraged to decide which activities can be eliminated or performed differently. The skill of the therapist in helping patients recognize the value of assistive devices or alternative ways of performance is often needed to enable lifestyle redesign because some devices or alternative ways of performance connote a sense of disability that is not congruent with the person's body image. Crutches, canes, and hand splints are prime examples. People, even some health care professionals, find it difficult to use these devices because they denote a negative body image despite their advantages of prolonging walking and functional hand use. Alternatives, which may include change of vocation, also may require significant counseling to enable the patient to recognize the advantages to the change. For example, if the patient's job requires much stooping and lifting and no alternatives are available for this at work, vocational counseling to examine other job opportunities that do not stress involved joints may be indicated.

Personal Care and Instrumental ADLs

Survival skills to live independently in the community include personal care skills and instrumental activities of daily living (IADLs) skills. Patients may not always identify these skills as their most important occupational performance goals because they presume that someone will be there to do these tasks for them. It is not always possible to obtain assistance, however, and it may, in fact, be inconvenient to find help. Therefore, many patients can be helped to choose accomplishment of these tasks as part of their goals. Backman (1998) described ADL and IADL instruments for occupational therapists working with patients who have rheumatic disease. Observation of skills is important to assess how the person accomplishes tasks. Are joint protection methods used? Is the person aggravating impaired joints while doing these tasks? Are **energy conservation** techniques used? Is adapted equipment used? It is important to ask the person how often these tasks are performed and when assistance is sought. Although the patient may answer questions about personal care in an idealized manner during an interview, it is up to the therapist to aim for accuracy in obtaining the information. For example, consider the following scenario:

"Do you dress yourself?" "Yes."

"Did you dress yourself this morning before arriving to the clinic?" "No, because we were in a hurry to get here."

"Did you dress yourself yesterday?" "No, because it was late and we had to get to church on time."

"Did you dress yourself in the past week?" "Yes."

"How many days last week did you dress yourself?" "Possibly only once or twice because I had a lot of morning stiffness and it was painful. Besides, my daughter was home to help me."

The reader can see how pursuit of the question is important to identify problems that may need further attention.

With patients who are admitted to the hospital, all morning personal care may be observed. The therapist, however, may first encounter a patient as an outpatient. In this case, observation of all personal care activities may not be practical.

The use of a self-administered questionnaire saves time in a comprehensive evaluation. The self-administered *Evaluation of Daily Activity Questionnaire* (Nordenskiold, Grimby, & Dahlin-Ivanoff, 1998) has been tested with women with RA in Sweden. This 102-item checklist asks the respondent to indicate degree of difficulty of various tasks. The therapist can use a scoring procedure to note changes as function improves with the use of assistive devices.

For patients who work, a number of interviews and observational tools exist that are not specific to arthritis (Backman, 1998). These instruments can be used, but the evaluator must pay special attention to joint and systemic problems unique to these diseases as this assessment is done. The person may be able to do tasks, but repetition and effort during a test may not pose the problems that are seen when translated to an 8-hour workday. Another method to look at IADL skills when evaluation time is limited is to simulate key areas that may be problematic. For example, if patients say they cannot reach and place items in cupboards above the counters in the kitchen, having the person lift an item of similar weight to a cupboard in the occupational therapy clinic may provide clues as to whether the problem lies in grip strength, shoulder ROM, pain, or weakness.

An area of ADL that is sometimes overlooked is sexual expression. This area can be problematic for the person with arthritis because of pain, discomfort, fatigue, limited ROM, and other physical limiting factors. It can be awkward for patients to bring up this topic as part of ADL. The therapist must be sensitive to patients' cultural background in pursuing this aspect of ADL, but this topic should be brought up to allow the patient to discuss problems in this area (Majerovitz & Revenson, 1994). If the sexual expression problems are related to psychological areas unrelated to the disease, a referral to a psychologist may be indicated. In interviewing patients for problems with sexual expression, the approach is similar to that for other aspects of ADL: ask whether the problem is inability to perform activities, impairment of an ability area, or due to contextual or environmental factors. Depending on which factors are problems, provide intervention appropriately.

Range of Motion

Observation and measurement of upper extremity active ROM from an upright position gives the examiner useful information about functional ROM that the patient has for use in occupational functioning (see Chapter 5). Pain is often a reason for limited active ROM in arthritis, but limited ROM also can be from weakness, contractures, or joint derangement. Radiographs that show osteophytes, erosions, joint narrowing, and other skeletal problems rule out strengthening for the purpose of increasing active ROM. It is important to limit measurement to those areas of concern.

Strength

Testing of muscle groups or motion in areas of involvement with the patient in an upright posture provides information about function (see Chapter 5). For example, the patient who actively flexes the shoulder to 60° and takes moderate resistance without pain is likely to be able to lift a light plate to place it on a low shelf above the counter. Testing resistance to joint motions also enables the examiner to record whether pain limits the amount of resistance taken by the joint. It is important to use principles of joint protection in applying resistance to joints at the end of active ROM, to observe the patient's face for an indication of pain, and to stop immediately. Otherwise, the patient may have more pain than usual after leaving the testing session.

Strength in the hand can be measured with grasp meters and pinch meters (see Chapter 5). The Jamar dynamometer is a common instrument that is used to measure grasp. Although the metal of the dynamometer is bothersome to some patients because of deformities and pain, it is still useful, as most objects used in everyday life are inflexible. If, however, a patient has grasp strength less than 5 pounds, the Jamar dynamometer does not provide accurate measures of differences in strength as a result of intervention. In this case, other tools, such as an adapted sphygmomanometer (Melvin, 1998) or the *Grippit* (Nordenskiold & Grimby, 1993) show small increments of change brought about by intervention. Standard pinch meters can be used with patients, although the standard method of measurement, advocated by Mathiowetz et al. (1985), cannot always be used with patients with RA because of significant thumb and finger deformities and, therefore, the norms would not apply. Even though the norms cannot be used for comparison, it can be useful to describe how the pinch was achieved, for example, "the thumb pad is pressed against the index finger proximal phalanx, secondary to limited thumb abduction." Although this may be accompanied by ulnar deviation by the second MCP, this is useful for actively holding a small object. These compensatory mechanisms used by patients with severe deformity must be thoroughly evaluated, especially when surgery to improve hand function is considered. Some patients with severe RA have pinch strength greater than the available gross grasp strength.

Hand Assessment

Among the various hand assessments, Backman and Mackie (1995) and van Lankveld, Graff, and van't Pad Bosch (1999) developed instruments specifically for this population. Others that were not designed for this population can be useful for some purposes (Backman, 1998). Standardized hand assessments are useful as a baseline measure if an intervention is intended to show change in hand function or to assist in decision making for elective hand surgeries.

Endurance

In arthritis, especially RA, the ability to sustain functional motion can be limited by fatigue, weakness, or pain. Self-assessment measures of ability to sustain functional performance are useful for determining how fatigue interferes with meaningful occupations. If the patient has to rest all day because the previous day's activity caused fatigue or increased pain, activities of a prolonged, sustained nature must be curtailed to enable participation in occupations of highest choice. This is discussed further under fatigue management.

Pain

Pain can be evaluated during joint examination and/or during performance of occupations. At times, specific knowledge of pain location, severity, and time of day is useful, especially if intervention is to alter any of the parameters of pain. The *Visual Analog Scale* for pain has been found to be a simple and reliable tool to measure pain (Huskisson, 1974) (see Chapter 5).

Hand and Wrist Deformities

It is useful to record hand and wrist deformities to determine the best course of action for intervention to allow occupational performance. For each joint of the wrist and hand, the following problems should be palpated and recorded: (1) swelling, heat, and/or redness (cardinal signs of inflammation); (2) pain; (3) subluxation or dislocation;

(4) **crepitus**; (5) tendon rupture; and (6) **rheumatoid nodules**.

In OA, common hand deformities include spurs at the dorsolateral and medial margins of the DIP joints of the fingers, which generally develop slowly and are called Heberden's nodes. Heberden's nodes can cause volar and lateral deviation of the distal phalanx. Heberden's nodes are 10 times as prevalent in women as in men. A similar enlargement at the PIP joints of the fingers is called Bouchard's nodes. When the first CMC joint is involved, tenderness and pain at the base of the metacarpal and a squared appearance of the hand are present, which is evidence of subluxation at this joint (Brandt & Slemenda, 1993). Precision and power pinches are most at risk when the first CMC is significantly involved. In a review of 99 patients with hand OA, more than half had functional loss. Nearly half of the 99 had a concomitant history of OA of the knee (Altman et al., 1990). McFarlane et al. (1990) found, in following 32 patients with hand osteoarthritis from entry to a year later, that osteophytes, particularly when fast growing, produced pain. The slower the change in size, the less likely it is that the joint was seriously compromised.

The deformities that can be found in RA are complex. The following description of common deformities and how they develop will enable the therapist to apply appropriate interventions, such as hand splints, joint protection techniques, and/or patient education programs that dispel myths and increase the patient's understanding of causation of deformity.

Deformities of the Wrist

It is estimated that 95% of persons with persistent RA develop bilateral wrist joint involvement (Wilson, 1986). Three pathological processes that can produce deformity are cartilage degradation often seen early in RA, synovitis with erosion, and ligamentous laxity. Cartilage degradation may cause bony erosion and may lead to ruptured tendons, especially the extensor tendons of the ulnar fingers or the flexor pollicis longus (Shapiro, 1996). Even without erosion, synovial expansion can lead to volar subluxation of the proximal carpal row, which has been noted in 80% of RA wrists. The new positioning of all of the carpals can elicit pain. If intercarpal pressure increases during gripping motions, pain increases concomitantly, leading to a desire to reduce grip strength to reduce pain (Shapiro, 1996). Both cartilage loss and synovitis can lead to lax ligaments and further carpal derangement with wrist instability, which can lead to a radial shift of the carpus on the radius (Taliesnik, 1989). Even if the synovial destruction stops prior to significant deformity, fibrous ankylosis of some wrist joint surfaces may occur. Synovial erosion that proliferates and causes massive joint destruction, including any combination of tendon ruptures and joint derangement, can produce a floppy wrist (Shapiro, 1996).

Deformities of the Metacarpophalangeal Joints

Although ulnar drift of the MCP joints is uncommon in the early stages of RA, Wilson (1986) reports that 45% of patients whose disease has persisted longer than 5 years demonstrate this deformity. Ulnar drift is a combination of deviation of the phalanx from the metacarpal head and a lateral shift of the phalanx upon the metacarpal (Wilson, 1986) (Fig. 44-1). Wilson suggests that the following are contributors to this deformity:

1. Synovitis within the MCP joint stretching the radial collateral ligaments, which are weaker than their ulnar counterparts.
2. When the synovitis subsides, the extensor tendons migrate ulnarly, eventually ending up in the valleys between the metacarpal heads.
3. As the fingers flex, the flexors pull the digits ulnarly unopposed by the weakened radial collateral ligaments.
4. Contractures of the intrinsic muscles caused by a reflex protective muscle spasm secondary to the synovitis contribute MCP volar subluxation. This disrupts the balance of the volar plate, sagittal bands, transverse metacarpal ligament, and collateral ligament.
5. When wrist synovitis causes radial deviation of the wrist, the dynamics of the finger flexor tendons change as they cross the MCP, providing an ulnar force.

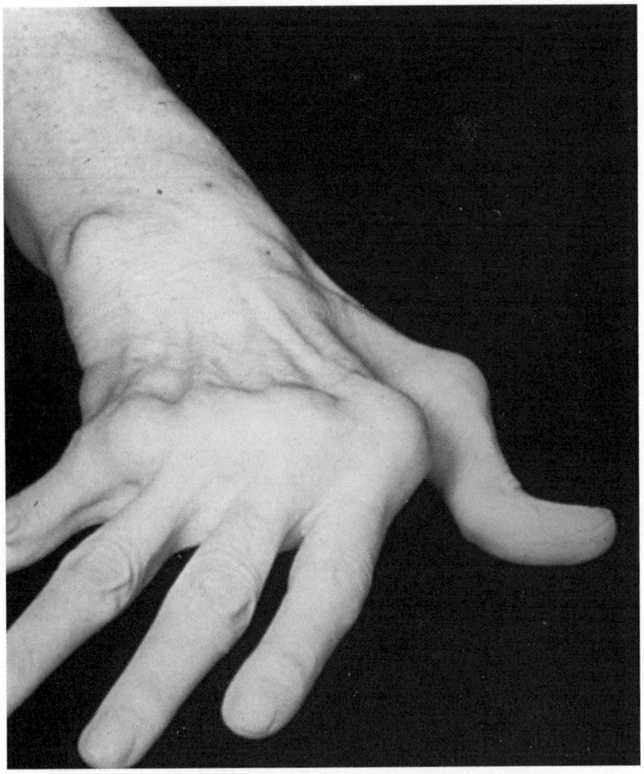

Figure 44-1 MCP ulnar deviation and subluxation. (Reprinted from the ARHP Arthritis Teaching Slide Collection. Used with permission of the American College of Rheumatology.)

6. MCP joint cartilage loss and bony erosion lead to volar subluxation, pulling the finger flexors ulnarly during flexion.
7. Flexor tenosynovitis can also lead to volar subluxation of the MCP joint.

The MCP collateral ligaments normally tighten on MCP flexion. Thus, abnormal laxity of the radial collateral ligament at the MCP joint can be evaluated by placing each of the patient's MCP joints in full passive flexion. Each digit is then pushed toward the ulna. In a normal hand, the digit has little or no movement laterally. If the radial collateral ligament is stretched, the finger can be easily displaced ulnarly.

When and if the MCP joints become fixed in flexion because of disease, the midpalmar crease may become moist and macerated from lack of exposure to air. This can be accompanied by a foul odor as it becomes difficult for the person to clean the hand; therefore, patient, therapist, and physician must be attentive in preventing this deformity.

Deformities of the Interphalangeal Joints

Swan-neck and boutonniere deformities are the most common finger deformities (Rizio & Belsky, 1996) (Figs. 44-2 and 44-3). Prolonged synovitis of the PIP joint can spread proximally under the central extensor slip, which becomes attenuated, and between the extensor and intrinsic tendons. When the central slip and lateral bands stretch, they migrate volarly, and a boutonniere deformity is produced (Rizio & Belsky, 1996; Wilson 1986). Nalebuff (1984) has described three stages of the boutonniere deformity. Stage I exhibits only a slight extensor **lag**, and a slight loss of DIP flexion occurs. A 40° PIP flexion deformity is considered stage II. In stage III, the PIP joint has a fixed flexion deformity.

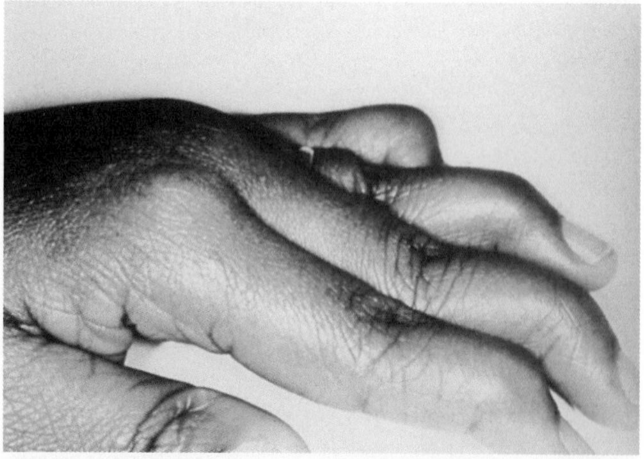

Figure 44-2 Swan-neck deformity: PIP hyperextension with DIP flexion. (Reprinted from the ARHP Arthritis Teaching Slide Collection. Used with permission of the American College of Rheumatology.)

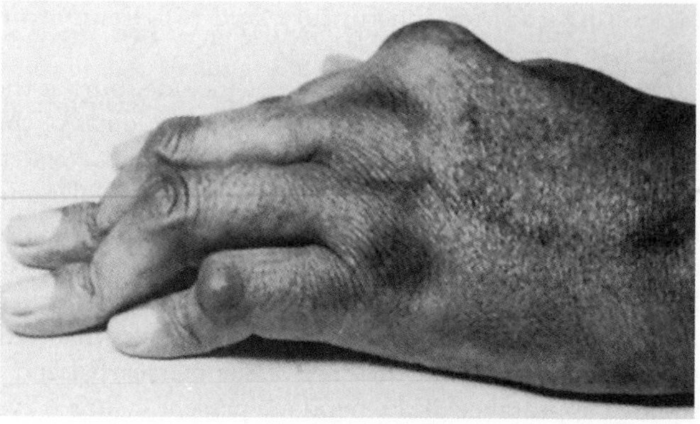

Figure 44-3 Boutonniere deformity: PIP flexion with DIP hyperextension. (Reprinted with permission from Feinberg, J. R. [1992]. Effect of the arthritis health professional on compliance with use of resting hand splints by patients with rheumatoid arthritis. *Arthritis Care and Research, 5,* 17–23.)

If the initiating PIP synovitis is anterolateral, it can stretch the transverse retinacular ligament, allowing the lateral band to migrate dorsally, resulting in a PIP joint hyperextension, or swan-neck deformity. Lateral bands in this position prevent the normal volar and lateral shift that allows PIP flexion. With progression of the synovitis, joint erosion and, finally, destruction occur with fibrous articular adhesions or bony ankylosis (Wilson, 1986). The swan-neck deformity can also be caused by the destructive effect of the synovitis beginning at any one of the three digital joints (Rizio & Belsky, 1996). The disturbance in function in patients with a swan-neck deformity is directly caused by the loss of flexibility of the PIP joint (Rizio & Belsky, 1996). Four types of swan-neck deformities have been described (Wilson, 1986). Type I deformity is characterized by full flexibility of the PIP joint. Patients complain of transient locking and trouble initiating PIP flexion. Type II deformity exhibits a flexible PIP when the MCP is flexed, but when the MCP is extended, there is limited PIP flexion. When there is significant loss of PIP motion, the deformity is designated type III. In type IV, there is intra-articular destruction and limited motion.

Deformities of the Thumb

Nalebuff's (1984) description of four types of common thumb deformities provides a shorthand for complex problems. Type I, or boutonniere deformity, is the most common and is characterized by MCP joint flexion and IP joint hyperextension (Fig. 44-4). This usually occurs when synovitis of the MCP joint stretches the extensor mechanism, including the dorsal capsule, extensor pollicis brevis tendon, and extensor hood. This results in MP flexion; volar subluxation of that joint may occur also. The stretching of the extensor pollicis brevis tendon allows it to displace ulnarly and volarly. Type II begins at the carpometacarpal (CMC) joint and results in MCP flexion and

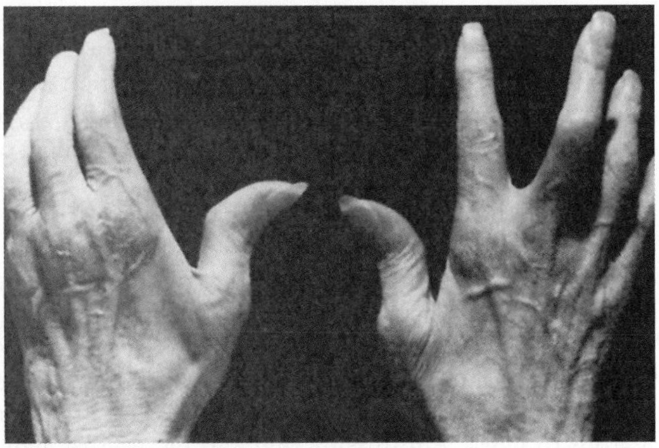

Figure 44-4 Nalebuff type I thumb deformity. (Reprinted from the ARHP Arthritis Teaching Slide Collection. Used with permission of the American College of Rheumatology.)

adduction and IP hyperextension. This type is not common. Type III, or swan-neck deformity, is common; it is characterized by MCP joint hyperextension and adduction and IP joint flexion. The origin of this deformity is synovitis at the CMC joint (Stein & Terrono, 1996).

Three other types of thumb deformity have been recognized and classified (Stein & Terrono, 1996). The most common of these is type IV, gamekeeper's deformity. This is characterized by MCP adduction and lateral instability of the MCP joint and is the result of attenuation of the ulnar collateral ligament. As the proximal phalanx deviates radially at the MCP joint, the first MCP assumes an adducted position, and the web space contracts. Type V consists of MCP hyperextension and IP flexion. The first metacarpal is not always adducted, and the CMC joint is usually not involved. Initiating cause is instability or attenuation of the volar plate at the MCP joint. Type VI consists of marked skeletal collapse and loss of bone substance called arthritis mutilans; the thumb becomes quite short and typically is unstable, with skin that appears to be redundant in relation to the underlying skeleton. It is ordinarily associated with similar deformities in the other digits.

Intervention (RA and OA)

Intervention addresses the problems identified by evaluation and is guided by the manifestation of the disease, the patient's adjustment to disease progression, and the patient-identified limitations in occupational functioning. The understanding of the altered biomechanical forces on joints, the systemic aspects and progression of rheumatoid arthritis, and the patient's level of engagement in meaningful occupation drive the occupational therapy intervention. Intervention in RA varies as the disease progresses from the acute (characterized by synovial inflammation and proliferation and systemic symptoms such as fever and pain) to the subacute, non-inflammatory phase and then to the chronic stage, in which the disease is burned out, but deformities are created or remain. In all stages, fatigue and exacerbation of pain are avoided. The occupational functioning goals identified by patients may be impaired by any of the following:

- Limited knowledge of the disease and its progression
- Limited knowledge and skill to modify activities at home or in the community to protect joints and conserve energy
- Limited ability to manage a full day, balancing between rest and activity
- Joint limitations and deformities
- Limited strength
- Limited knowledge of use of splints
- Limited knowledge on how to adapt or modify the environment
- Limited sense of self-efficacy to redesign lifestyle

The key intervention in OA is patient education concerning unloading and protecting involved joints and strengthening the muscles around joints. Other interventions include modification of the environment, prescription of assistive devices, splinting, and lifestyle redesign.

Patient and Family Education

With RA, all interventions require teaching the patient and family about the disease, its symptoms, and how prolonged synovitis can lead to irreversible joint destruction. Physicians and nurses explain how medications work. Occupational therapists must reinforce the importance of following medication guidelines and the reasons for it. Patients must understand that joint deformities cannot be prevented if the disease progresses unchecked without anti-inflammatory or disease-modifying medications. Although not all cases can be controlled easily or well with medications, the large number of choices allows the opportunity to try a variety until the appropriate compound and dose are discovered. Those who do not respond early to the medication can feel discouraged. The occupational therapist teaches adaptation to the disease progression. Besides helping the patient and family to understand the disease, the occupational therapist must instill hope that the use of adaptation and modifications as needed throughout the course of the disease can permit continued meaningful occupational functioning.

With OA, the goal of education is to enable the patient to control long-term management of OA. Understanding how OA affects joints and understanding OA-related **joint protection** principles and their application to daily living are key areas for education.

Joint Protection and Fatigue Management

With RA, the occupational therapist uses joint protection techniques to reduce pain and deformity. The goals of joint protection are to reduce loading to vulnerable joints, develop strategies to help preserve the present integrity of joint structures, relieve joint pain during activities, and reduce local inflammation (Cordery & Rocchi, 1998). The principles of joint protection described by Cordery and recently revised by Cordery and Rocchi (Procedures for Practice 44-1) require the therapist to apply teaching-learning techniques that will lead to these behavioral changes.

Joint protection principles are appropriate to OA, although the rationale varies from that of RA, since OA is limited to selective joint involvement without systemic effect. Joint protection guidelines for OA include the following: avoid pain in activities, maintain joint ROM and increase muscle strength and fitness, reduce excessive forces on involved joints, avoid staying in one position for long periods, and balance activity and rest (Cordery & Rocchi, 1998).

Respect Pain

The pain-sensitive structures in the joint are the fibrous capsule, ligaments, fat pads, and periosteum. Pain during the inflammatory process of RA is common. Pain can also be elicited when attenuated ligaments and deranged joint spaces are aggravated through use that lengthens the ligaments further or resistive motion that compresses the joint spaces (Shapiro, 1996). When pain is present at rest during the inflammatory process, reducing activity level to prevent increasing pain and to promote reduction of inflammation is indicated. In the chronic phase, the aggravating postures or precipitating activities are avoided, or adaptations are devised.

In OA, joint pain produced by engagement in activities is a useful symptom that may indicate stress to joints by use that exceeds the limits of comfort to the involved joint. Examples of this include prolonged kneeling and squatting, both of which can aggravate knee symptoms. Kneeling and squatting can usually be avoided by relocating items from low surfaces to higher levels and sitting on a stool to work. Equipment that can be used to avoid kneeling and squatting includes such items as long-handled dustpan and reachers. To avoid lifting heavy loads, when the spine and lower extremities are painful, usual equipment can be replaced by lighter versions made of materials such as aluminum, plastic, or nylon canvas. Examples of this are nylon canvas suitcases and briefcases. A rolling cart and luggage roller can be used. Postures that aggravate back symptoms when the spine is involved, such as prolonged leaning over a desk, can be modified by use of an upright reading rack. Leaning over a railing to pick up an infant from a crib can be avoided by adapting the railing to open to mattress level and sitting to transfer the infant to one's lap or an elevated stroller (see Chapter 32). Raising the height and firmness of chairs, toilet seats, beds, and other furniture avoids knee or hip pain during arising. Lateral supports or armrests may also be used to assist with rising from the seated position. To avoid pain when the thumb CMC is affected, the person can use jar openers, electric can openers, electric scissors, and lightweight or large-handled utensils to prevent undue stresses to this joint (Cordery & Rocchi, 1998; Stein & Terrono, 1996).

PROCEDURES FOR PRACTICE 44-1

Principles of Joint Protection

- Respect pain as a signal to stop the activity.
- Maintain muscle strength and joint ROM.
- Use each joint in its most stable anatomical and functional plane.
- Avoid positions of deformity and forces in their direction.
- Use the largest, strongest joints available for the job.
- Ensure correct patterns of movement.
- Avoid staying in one position for long periods.
- Avoid starting an activity that cannot be stopped immediately if it proves to be beyond capability.
- Balance rest and activity.
- Reduce the force.

From Cordery, J., & Rocchi, M. (1998). Joint protection and fatigue management. In J. Melvin & G. Jensen (Eds.), *Rheumatologic rehabilitation series, vol. 1: Assessment and management* (pp. 279–321). Bethesda, MD: American Occupational Therapy Association. Reprinted with permission.

Maintain Muscle Strength and Joint ROM

Balanced strength around unstable joints can reduce further injury to the capsule, ligaments, and cartilage. Joint protection during therapeutic exercise includes ensuring that muscle pull does not accentuate deformity. Joint position and ROM are critical for optimum functioning of muscles. Limited range at one joint, such as the shoulder, requires exaggerated motions at distal joints to accomplish a task.

In the presence of acute joint inflammation with RA, when range can become limited, joint protection includes use of gentle, pain-free ROM exercise. Attempts to go beyond this range can raise intra-articular pressure and aggravate existing pain.

In OA, maintaining daily activities within the limitations of the patient's pain prevents disuse atrophy. Strengthening around an unstable joint can increase stability and reduce pain. Bony enlargement around the

CMC joint of the thumb can inhibit motion. When this occurs, a bony block can prevent attempts to increase ROM and lead to further pain; therefore, attempts to increase ROM are avoided.

Use Each Joint in Its Most Stable Anatomical and/or Functional Plane

The most stable anatomical and/or functional plane is one in which muscle, not ligament, provides resistance to the motion (Cordery & Rocchi, 1998). For example, in a type I thumb deformity with flexible hyperextension of the IP joint, pinch with IP flexion against the pad of the thumb provides increased stability.

Avoid Positions of Deformity and Forces in Their Direction

Avoid external loads and internal forces that facilitate deformity when the degree of disease puts them at risk (Cordery & Rocchi, 1998). Turning resistive round doorknobs in an ulnar direction when the finger MCP joints are subluxed volarly and ulnarly is an example of force to be avoided by use of a lever door opener.

Use the Strongest Joints Available for the Job

Use of stronger, larger joints can handle greater forces. Examples of this principle include lifting objects from the floor by using the hips and knees instead of bending at the spine; pushing or pulling objects rather than carrying them; and using a belted waist pack rather than holding the purse with hook grasp (Fig. 44-5, A & B).

Ensure Correct Patterns of Movement

Incorrect patterns may be the result of pain, tenosynovitis, deformity, muscle imbalance, or habit (Cordery & Rocchi, 1998). For example, to raise the arm, the shoulder hikes (scapular elevation and upward rotation) as substitution for painful glenohumeral flexion. Using the glenohumeral joint within pain limits keeps this joint mobile. Another example is to push up when arising from a chair by using the flat surface of the palm rather than the dorsum of the fingers to prevent deforming forces toward MCP flexion.

Avoid Staying in One Position for Long Periods

This advice has been recommended for workers in general, as prolonged static postures can lead to muscle fatigue. When fatigued muscles cannot provide stability around a joint, the load transfers to the underlying joint capsule and ligaments that may already be stretched secondary to disease (Cordery & Rocchi, 1998). People with OA are prone to "gelling" or stiffness and discomfort that follow periods of inactivity. If, in addition, the activity requires static hold of involved joints over a long time, the muscles surrounding that joint tire and are less effective in supporting the joint (Cordery & Rocchi, 1998). Change of position or taking breaks and performing active ROM during activities that are normally prolonged, such as use of the computer, is recommended to prevent muscle fatigue and soreness and subsequent poor patterns of use. This principle is difficult to follow, as patients, like every-

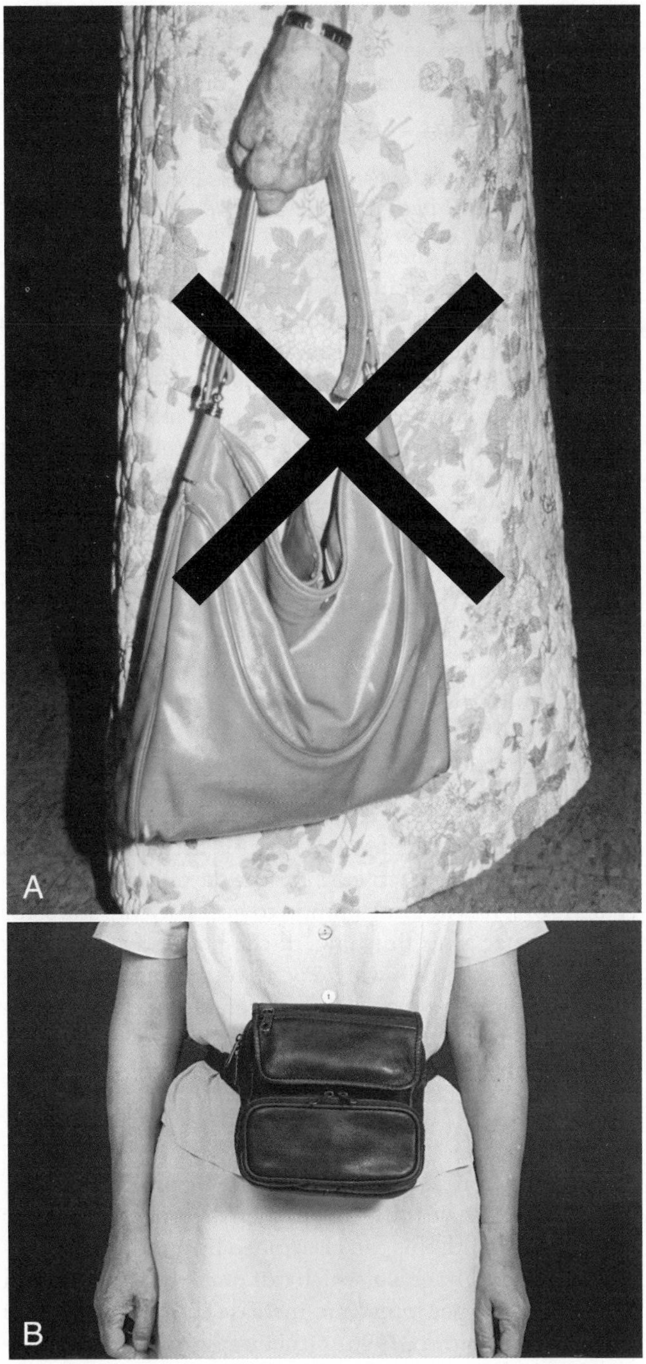

Figure 44-5 How to distribute a load over a larger area and use the largest joint available for a task. **A.** Problem: Patient carries her handbag using the small joints of the hand. **B.** Solution: Patient uses a belted waist pack. (Courtesy of the Collection of Rancho Los Amigos National Rehabilitation Center, Downey, CA.)

one else, want to complete tasks. Performing active ROM to affected joints every 15–20 minutes may minimize stiffness and facilitate muscle function (Brandt & Slemenda, 1993).

Avoid Starting an Activity that Cannot Be Stopped Immediately if It Proves to Be Beyond the Person's Ability

This principle requires planning and is not always easy, especially for an unfamiliar task. Fatigued muscles surrounding affected joints can lead to poor patterns of use and increased pain when timely rest is impossible. This principle has been well applied in newer designs of compact walkers that have seats and trays to make them convenient to use shopping, in the community, or in the kitchen. These walkers have enabled many who engage in community activities to sit when desired, rather than searching for and perhaps not finding a sitting surface. Another example of application of this principle is having patients identify midway locations, such as a chair on the porch that is located between the car and the kitchen. The patient can sit on this chair if unable to ambulate the complete distance to the target location.

Balance Rest and Activity

People with RA generally need more rest than others. Individuals must plan balance between activity and rest to accomplish priority activities for the day and week (Furst et al., 1987). It is not uncommon to hear patients state, for example, that after finishing all the housecleaning, they stayed in bed the following day. Determining and implementing appropriate balance between rest and activity requires self-monitoring, the value of which is further described in the section on Fatigue Management.

Reduce the Force

Strong effort or resistive motions can be problematic for involved joints, leading to further destruction and/or pain. In the hand, this can be avoided by building up handles to avoid tight grasp, which can put excessive stress on problematic finger joints and increase compressive forces at the wrist (Shapiro, 1996). Other ways to reduce resistive motions are the use of assistive devices, such as lightweight cooking utensils and jar openers that use the power of the upper arm rather than involved hand and wrist joints.

Work simplification methods also reduce stress on joints. Rather than carrying objects back and forth in the kitchen repeatedly, placing them all on a rolling cart to push them across the room at one time reduces the force on small hand joints. Resistive activities that push unstable MCP joints toward the ulna should be avoided (Fig. 44-6). If, however, a patient's favored leisure activity has been a hobby such as knitting and if satisfactory substitute activities cannot be found, the therapist must assess how the patient can knit without use of undue force. Suggestions include building up the needles and using large doweling for needles, taking frequent rest breaks, searching for loose-weave patterns, and other solutions that patients may suggest.

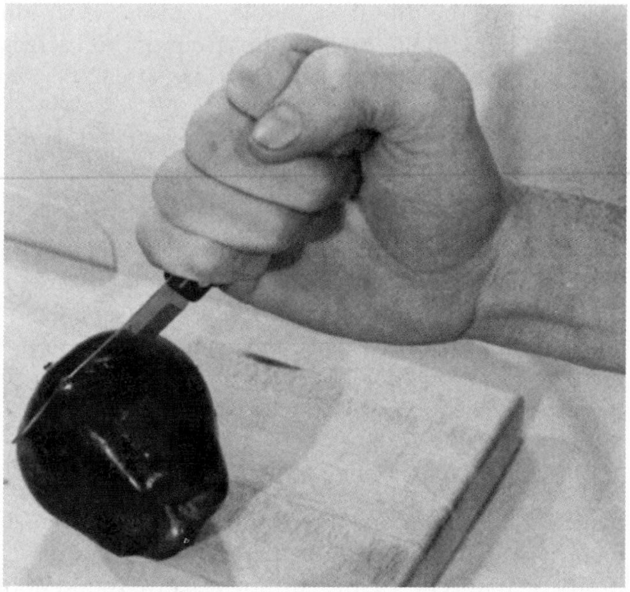

Figure 44-6 Avoidance of ulnar deviation forces: cutting an apple using a dagger grip on the knife to push the fingers radially.

In OA, the cartilage is too thin to protect against repetitive use of force, which produces destructive effects on cartilage. Patients' understanding of joint physiology and the role of the proprioceptors can help them to understand which daily occupations use excessive force, such as the effect of carrying heavy loads up and down stairs. This understanding lets the patient recognize the need to use alternative methods to accomplish the task; for example, in this case, to have others carry the load down the stairs or carry small amounts of load in a backpack and use the handrail to reduce the impact load to involved knee joints.

Fatigue Management

Fatigue has been described as the enduring subjective sensation of generalized tiredness or exhaustion (Belza, 1995). Contributors to fatigue are multidimensional and include physiologic, behavioral, and environmental factors (Belza, 2001). To control the effects of fatigue on everyday activities, the therapist teaches the patient to analyze daily activities to determine activities that increase pain and fatigue (Cordery & Rocchi, 1998). Gerber et al. (1987) found that rest breaks during the day can support a full day of activity. This was shown in a study of a 6-week course of energy conservation and joint protection training for patients with RA in which participants were taught to take periodic short rest periods during prolonged activities. As a result, 50% of these persons increased the amount of time they were active, compared with 11% of the control subjects (Gerber et al., 1987). In the 6-week course, the patients used worksheets to determine what may and may not be changed in their daily schedules to self-assess realistic changes. Additional activities provided in the workbook for the course continued this self-analysis to enable patients to plan their fatigue management. *Managing Your Fatigue*, a useful brochure published by the Arthritis Foundation, can accompany patient education programs on this topic.

Although fatigue that accompanies systemic disease in RA does not exist in OA, continued use of affected joints, along with other joints, can increase the discomfort level in these joints. Self-monitoring by recognizing onset of pain and discomfort with a routine daily schedule should be used to determine when activity should be stopped to rest the joints. By recording length of time in a task that is followed by moderate to severe pain and/or fatigue, patients can reduce the time in the task to decrease pain and/or fatigue. Cordery and Rocchi (1998) advocate rest periods shorter than 30 minutes several times a day between tasks.

Maintain Joint Mobility

Patients with RA commonly have limited ROM because of inflammation, joint destruction, weakness, reflex inhibition from pain, or limited use. The cause of the limitation directs the intervention.

During acute joint inflammation, joint motion should be maintained with at least one complete ROM exercise daily. The brochure *Exercise and Your Arthritis* by the Arthritis Foundation (Resources 44-1) is an example of information that patients can follow. It is important not to overstretch inflamed tissues in RA, as tensile strength can be reduced by as much as 50%, leading to tears (Minor, 1996). Active and active assistive ROM are commonly used during this period. If the patient's effort against gravity leads to discomfort or there is lag in the joint (most notable in the shoulder), passive ROM may be used to ensure that contractures do not occur during this period. It is imperative to pay attention to

RESOURCE 44-1

Patient and Professional Education

Arthritis Foundation—www.arthritis.org
A national resource with branches in every state. Patient education brochures can be obtained free or downloaded and printed. Examples of brochures are: *Golf and Arthritis, Managing Your Pain, Managing Your Activities, Protect Your Joints, Living with Osteoarthritis, Living with Rheumatoid Arthritis,* and *Living with Fibromyalgia.* Local offices can be found from the national website. Local offices may sponsor community programs, such as PACE (People with Arthritis Can Exercise) and aquatic exercise classes, as well as self-help courses and education and support groups. A magazine for the lay public, *Arthritis Today,* provides education as well as resources, such as travel agencies accommodating people with disability. Professional materials may also be found at the website.

MedlinePlus—www.medlineplus.gov
This website is co-sponsored by the U.S. National Library of Medicine and the National Institutes of Health. It provides health information for the lay public on over 700 topics on conditions, disease, and wellness. Information on fibromyalgia, rheumatoid arthritis, and osteoarthritis can be found here.

Fibromyalgia Network—www.fmnetnews.com
Publishes quarterly the *Fibromyalgia Network Health Journal,* which has current information for patients. Also has free patient-education brochures and information on the website.

National Fibromyalgia Association—www.fmaware.org
Provides free patient-education brochures and publishes a lay health journal 3 times/year, *Fibromyalgia AWARE.* On the medical advisory board are well-respected health professionals who focus on treatment and/or research for this condition.

The Oregon Fibromyalgia Foundation (OFF)—www.myalgia.com
This organization was founded in 1995 by Robert Bennett, MD, and Sharon Clark, PhD, and their colleagues from a well-known fibromyalgia center at the Oregon Health & Science University. The website provides a comprehensive synopsis of the research from medical journals, useful books in publication, as well as more basic lay information on many aspects of fibromyalgia.

Information About or for Purchase of Assistive Devices

ABLEDATA
www.abledata.com

Sammons Preston
www.sammonspreston.com

North Coast Medical
www.blvd.com/northcoast/

Maddak, Inc.
http://service.maddak.com

AliMed Catalogs
www.alimed.com/

Supplemental Reading

Foltz-Gray, D. (2005). *Alternative treatments for arthritis.* Atlanta: Arthritis Foundation.
This paperback book provides information on alternative treatments for arthritis. Each treatment is described, along with common uses, scientific evidence, side effects and interactions, safety concerns, dose, and ways to find a practitioner.

the patient's response if outside assistance is given because stoicism and the desire to not lose range may prevent the patient from reacting to pain overtly. Gentle active ROM in the evening can reduce morning stiffness (Minor, 1996), although some have found that the best time for performing this activity is in the morning after they take anti-inflammatory medication.

When joint inflammation has subsided, increasing ROM with gentle, controlled stretching can regain all or some of the loss that occurred during the inflammatory stage. General guidelines for ROM exercises for patients with RA include the following (Coppard, Gale, & Jensen, 1998; Minor, 1996):

- Exercise daily when stiffness and pain are the least.
- Take a warm shower or apply heat and/or cold before or after exercise.
- Perform gentle ROM exercise in the evening to reduce morning stiffness and in the morning to limber up prior to arising.
- Modify exercise (decrease frequency or adapt movement) to avoid increasing joint pain either during or after the exercise. Pain following exercise is a guide to reduce the number of repetitions.
- Use self-assistive techniques, such as wand exercises, to perform gentle stretching.
- Reduce number of repetitions when the joint is actively inflamed.

Strengthening

Patients with chronic RA are at risk for the ill effects of inactivity, including muscle atrophy and decreased exercise capacity, endurance, and cardiovascular fitness, resulting in a deconditioned state (Komatireddy et al., 1997). Research suggests that exercise may not be as detrimental as previously believed.

Isometric exercise is often used prior to or in conjunction with dynamic resistive and aerobic exercise programs. Initially, isometric exercise may be indicated to improve muscle tone, static endurance, and strength and to prepare joints for more vigorous activity (Minor, 1996). Isometric contractions performed at 70% of the maximal voluntary contraction, held for 6 seconds, and repeated 5–10 times daily can increase strength significantly (Minor, 1996). Minor recommends that while performing isometric exercise: (1) maintain the contraction for no more than 6 seconds, (2) avoid maximal effort, (3) exhale during the contraction and inhale during a similar period of relaxation, and (4) avoid contracting more than two muscle groups at a time. Dynamic exercise can improve both strength and endurance (Minor, 1996). Protect unstable or inflamed joints from damage during resistance exercises and perform within pain-free range. Start with 8–10 antigravity repetitions without pain before adding resistance. Reduce intensity, frequency, or ROM if joint swelling or pain occurs (Minor, 1996).

Splinting

In the treatment of OA, the use of a hand splint can be useful to stabilize an unstable first CMC joint in palmar abduction and thus balance forces on an unstable joint. Weiss et al. (2000) concluded that wearing a thumb CMC splint provided pain relief. Additionally, for those with early OA, which is defined as subluxation of MC base and osteophyte less than 2 mm, the amount of subluxation was reduced when wearing the splint. In the treatment of RA, hand splints have been used for a variety of purposes (Falconer, 1990). The effectiveness of splints for all of these purposes has not been extensively documented, although some studies have addressed pain reduction, grip strength, and comfort of a variety of orthoses (Kjeken, Moller, & Kvien, 1995; Stern et al., 1996; Ter Schegget & Knipping, 2000; Tijhuis et al., 1998). The following are some reasons splinting has been found useful with people with RA.

Reduce Inflammation

During the inflammatory process, joint rest by means of immobilization has been found to reduce joint inflammation, as was shown in an early study (that apparently has not been replicated more recently) when the ring size was significantly reduced in a small sample of persons with RA who were treated by immobilization versus those not immobilized (Partridge & Duthie, 1963). It is very common for resting hand splints to be prescribed during the inflammatory period. Some patients state that, when they awaken in the morning, the hand is more comfortable, having rested in a comfortable position during the night. The joints that are covered by a splint should be determined by the location of the inflammation. For example, if only the wrist is involved, a wrist splint is indicated. If the whole hand and wrist are involved, the orthosis should include all joints. The occupations of the patient may require fitting two orthoses for the inflamed hand. A night resting splint that covers all joints may be alternated with a shorter orthosis that allows the fingers to be free to perform pain-free non-resistive activities during the day.

Provide Support and Reduce Pain to Unstable Joints during Function

During the post-inflammatory stage, if unstable or subluxed joints or other joint deformities occur, the external support of an orthosis can enhance stability or prevent joint motion. Stability is provided only to joints posing problems. Feinberg and Brandt (1984) found that, when splinting relieved pain, adherence to splint wearing was good. Feinberg (1992) also found that patient education enhanced patient adherence to wearing of splints.

Prevent Undesirable Motion during Occupational Performance

A key example of this is to prevent hyperextension of the finger PIP joints (swan-neck deformity) through the use of a three-point splint that allows flexion but prevents hyperextension. Another example is to use an orthosis in the early stage of the Nalebuff type I deformity of the thumb, hyperextension of the IP joint. Although patients can be taught to remember to flex the IP joint when using a pinch motion, an orthosis that limits hyperextension can be a passive reminder to prevent further hyperextension and stretch to collateral ligaments. A practice that is controversial is immobilizing the finger PIP joint into extension when an early boutonniere deformity is seen. Some positive results have been seen in controlling the deformity for a limited time (Palchik et al., 1990).

Increase ROM or Prevent Deformity

Dynamic splinting, using an orthosis with finger extension outriggers, has been commonly used after finger MCP Silastic implant arthroplasty. This use of dynamic orthoses has been proposed for other purposes, such as to reduce contractures secondary to the disease, but little evidence supports this outcome or the use of dynamic splinting to prevent deformity.

Position Joints for Occupational Performance

An example of positioning joints for occupational performance is the use of the MCP ulnar deviation orthosis (Fig. 44-7, A & B) to permit continued use of the IP joints of the hand, when, if unsplinted, pain would be induced at the MCP joint with activity. Information regarding types of splints and use of custom versus prefabricated orthoses is discussed in Chapters 16 and 17.

Modify Environment

Ways to modify the environment to maintain the ability to participate in occupations of choice include changing the physical environment, recommending use of assistive devices, and assisting the patient to recognize and choose work or leisure environments that accommodate the disability. Examples of each of these are given for a variety of problems. The reader should be able to recognize readily what joint problems these modifications accommodate. The adaptations generally can be done with equipment from a local hardware store.

Change the Physical Environment

The patient and therapist must think about modifying all environments important to the patient's occupational

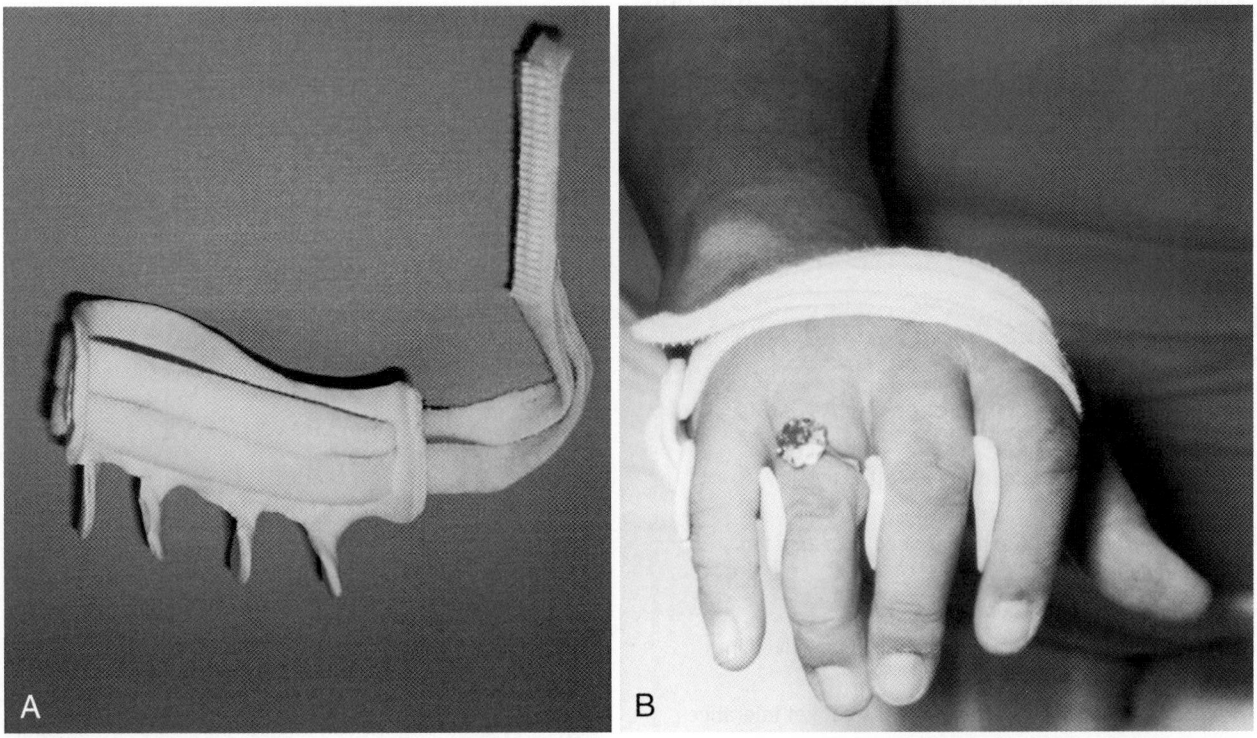

Figure 44-7 Splint to control ulnar deviation of the MCP joints during hand use. **A.** Ulnar deviation correction splint. **B.** Splint in place on the patient's hand. (Courtesy of the Collection of Rancho Los Amigos National Rehabilitation Center, Downey, CA.)

functioning, especially home and work. The following are some examples (Axtell & Yasuda, 1993).

Home:

- Remove doors of cabinets or attach loops to door handles.
- Lower the height of above-counter cupboards.
- Replace shelves in low cupboards with swivel or pull-out shelves.
- Replace standard oven with a microwave oven on a surface that accommodates available reach.
- Replace doorknobs with lever handles.
- Replace faucet handles with long lever handles.
- Use remote control devices to automate on/off switching of commonly used electrical devices, such as light switches.
- Lower closet rods if reach is limited.

Work:

- Organize workstation so that shelves are within reach and the table and chairs are at ergonomically correct heights.
- Attach forearm and wrist supports to computer areas.
- Use hands-free speaker phone.

Recommend Assistive Devices

Many assistive devices are available to the public. These devices can assist the person with RA or OA to limit stresses to joints. It is useful to teach patients joint protection principles so they can search independently for the products that produce the least amount of stress to joints. Criteria to consider when helping patients choose devices are found in Procedures for Practice 44-2. Excellent resources are available for special devices made for people with joint problems when common everyday products do not accommodate the problems (Procedures for Practice 44-3 and Resources 44-1). Generally, selection of these products requires professional advice and an opportunity to try the device to ensure that it will serve the purpose desired by the patient. Therefore, it is important for the

PROCEDURES FOR PRACTICE 44-2

Criteria to Consider When Choosing Assistive Devices

- Lightweight, durable, compact, attractive in appearance
- Multipurpose use to prevent need to search for multiple devices
- Simplicity of operation
- Reduce stress to all multilinked joints involved in operating the device
- Suitable for the individual patient's gadget tolerance
- In accord with the self-image of the user

PROCEDURES FOR PRACTICE 44-3

Commercially Available Common Assistive Devices

- **Self-care**—Buttonhook, dressing stick (various lengths can be used for dressing as well as reach for distant items), sock cone, reacher, long-handled sponge, extended handle for managing toilet paper, long-handled comb, electric toothbrush, pump toothpaste dispensers.
- **Meal preparation**—Rolling cart, knob turner for stove, built-up handles on cooking utensils, knives with right-angled handles (Fig. 44-8), electric can opener, jar opener, spring-lever scissors, cutting board with spikes to stabilize food, electric chopper, high kitchen stool, high stool on roller such as EZ Stand Mobile Stool (Fig. 44-9).
- **Home maintenance**—Long-handled dustpan, bucket on rollers, reachers to pull items out of areas and from floor.
- **Work and school**—Luggage cart, rolling cart, backpack, fanny pack, computer forearm-wrist rest, adapted key holder, built-up handle for writing implements, telephone headset, adapted hand tools, electric stapler and pencil sharpener, car door opener (Fig. 44-10A).
- **Leisure**—Adapted gardening tools, rolling stool for gardening, card holder, reading rack, embroidery hoop holder, rolling golf cart, knob turner (Fig. 44-10B).

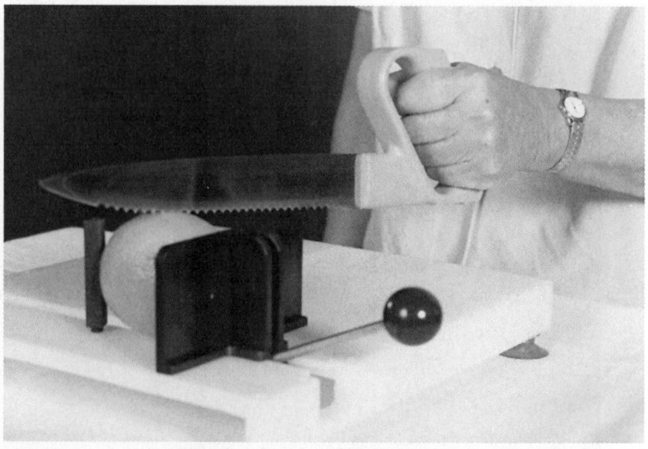

Figure 44-8 Cutting with an angled knife on a cutting board with vegetable spike. (Courtesy of Paul Weinreich, Rancho Los Amigos National Rehabilitation Center, Downey, CA.)

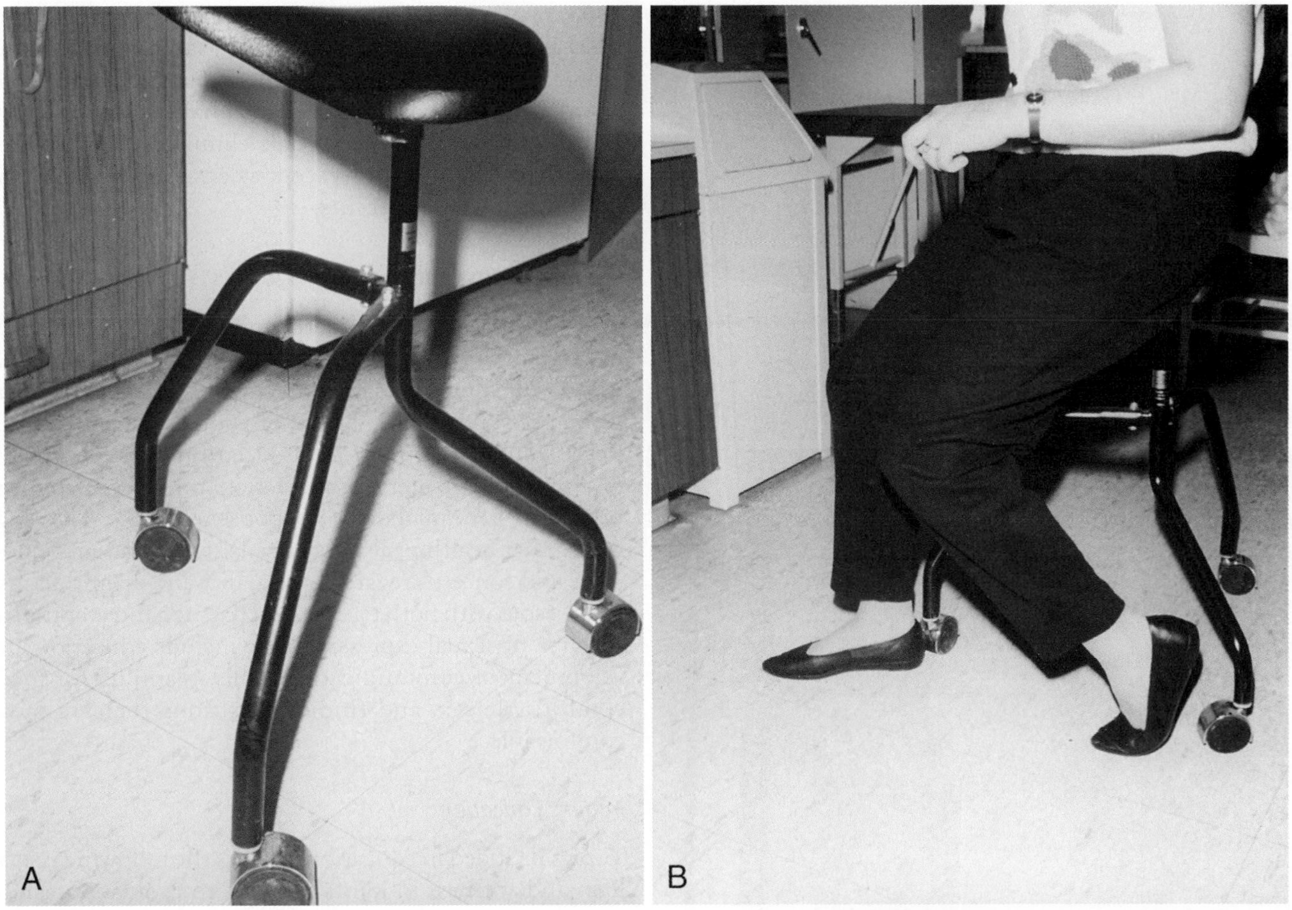

Figure 44-9 EZ Stand Mobile Stool. (Courtesy of the Collection of Rancho Los Amigos National Rehabilitation Center, Downey, CA.)

occupational therapy clinic to have an array of devices for trial use (Mann, 1998). Keeping current equipment catalogs and using the Internet to assist patients in finding appropriate items helps patients perform meaningful occupations. When none of the products available in the general or specialty market solves the problems, the occupational therapist can customize tools in the clinic. Common methods of customizing tools are building up or lengthening handles with materials such as foam tubing, low temperature thermoplastics, plastic tubing, or wooden dowels. Creativity on the part of the therapist is needed to meet the patient's requirements.

People with OA who have significant involvement of only a few joints may not seek out rehabilitation care and may be unaware of and reluctant to use assistive devices that can prevent loss of participation in meaningful occupations. Instead, it is fairly common to hear about continued use of involved joints with pain until there is sudden termination of important occupations, when the use of assistive devices could have prevented aggravation to joints. For example, elevated toilet seats and tub benches can be used to eliminate the stress on knees and hips of arising from low surfaces. Using a reacher and dressing stick to pick up items from the floor prevents stooping.

Assist the Patient to Recognize and Choose Work or Leisure Environments that Accommodate the Disability

To change previously comfortable daily life routines to accommodate disability requires significant effort. The methods used in a study to enable individuals to implement lifestyle redesign can apply to individuals with RA. Lifestyle redesign suggests that people can achieve greater meaning in their lives by examining the occupations that are most meaningful to them and identifying what prevents them from performing these occupations (Clark et al., 1997). In lifestyle redesign, the individual, through a process facilitated by the occupational therapist, determines what is needed to perform these important occupations and develops solutions to overcome these barriers to occupational functioning. Although this was intuitively known by occupational therapists, Clark et al. (1997) showed that, as a result of this lifestyle redesign intervention, people were healthier as demonstrated by scores on tools such as the *Short Form-36*, a quality-of-life measure, in

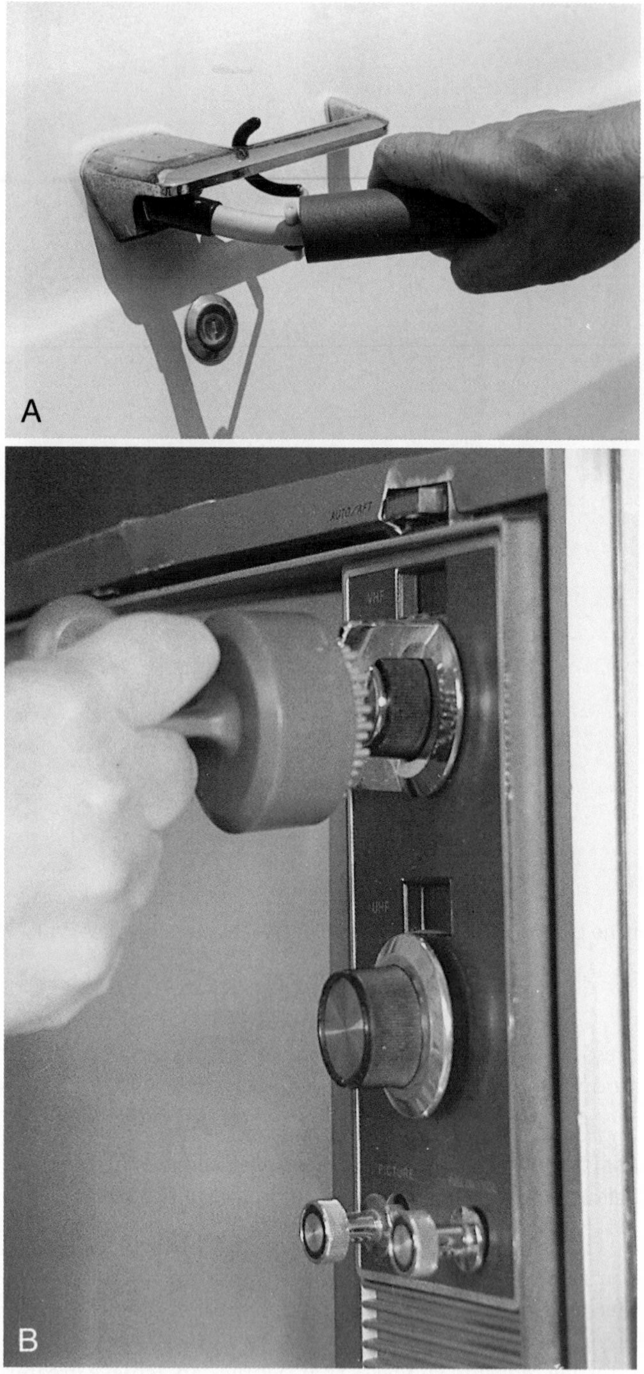

Figure 44-10 Car door opener (**A**) and multipurpose knob turner (**B**). (Courtesy of Rancho Los Amigos National Rehabilitation Center, Downey, CA. Paul Weinreich, photographer.)

contrast to those who did not have this intervention. The intervention included exposure to a number of tasks and activities in small groups. At the same time, each individual approached the task determining what had to be done to meet his or her own needs to perform the task again, independent of the group (Jackson et al., 1998).

In those with RA, these principles of implementing lifestyle changes proposed by Clark et al. (Jackson et al., 1998) may have to be done periodically or on an ongoing basis as the disease progresses or as exacerbations and remissions occur. Teaching people to implement lifestyle changes by emphasizing occupational self-analysis and achievement of individual goals eliminates the need for professional intervention except when a major crisis in the life of the individual occurs.

Sexual Expression

An area of occupational performance that is sometimes overlooked is sexual expression. The focus of assessment is identifying hindrances to sexual expression related to performance skills, client factors, or context. Majerovitz and Revenson (1994) found an association between greater disability and greater dissatisfaction among 113 couples, of whom 79.6% included one spouse with RA, . They suggested that health providers be sensitive to patients' questions and concerns regarding sexuality and openly discuss these issues with both patient and partner. Intervention in the area of sexual expression may include education, development of communication skills, planning for more comfortable sex, and finding positions that are more comfortable.

Patient Education

Topics included in education address the following issues. Pain and stiffness in joints can lead to avoidance or limited sex. Partners may also fear causing pain. Fatigue, which may be part of the disease process, can reduce desire for sex. Some medications cause fatigue or reduce sexual desire.

Development of Communication Skills

Discussion of sex with a partner is difficult for some. Discussion of needs for intimacy and how a partner feels can lead to more extensive discussion of the effects of disease on sexual performance.

Planning for More Comfortable Sex

The following suggestions are from the Arthritis Foundation (1993):

- Plan for sex at a time of day when you generally feel best.
- Time your dose of pain relief medication so that its effect will occur during sexual relations.
- Pace your activities during the day to help avoid extreme fatigue.
- Practice ROM exercises to relax your joints.
- Warm the bed ahead of time with an electric blanket.
- Take a warm bath or shower before sex to relax.
- Find more comfortable positions.

CASE EXAMPLE #1

Ms. B.: Rheumatoid Arthritis

Occupational Therapy Intervention Process	Clinical Reasoning Process: Objectives	Clinical Reasoning Process: Examples of Therapist's Internal Dialogue
Patient Information Ms. B. is 45 years old and has a 3-year history of rheumatoid arthritis (RA). She has been followed by a rheumatologist for the entire period, with ongoing use of anti-inflammatory medication. Her current major complaint is bilateral wrist pain. The finger MCPs show very mild inflammation, and she does not report pain in them. There are no other notable pain complaints in other joints. Grasp strength is 20 pounds bilaterally. She is a full-time fourth grade school teacher and lives alone in a one-bedroom apartment on the first floor.	Understand the patient's diagnosis or condition	"Ms. B. has a mild inflammatory process with localized joint problems interfering with occupational functioning at this time."
	Know the person	"Ms. B. enjoys teaching and looks forward to seeing children learn. Her desire to stay independent throughout the 3-year history of RA is a positive characteristic that makes her a good candidate for rehabilitation."
Reason for Referral to Occupational Therapy Ms. B. was referred to occupational therapy to address her complaint of bilateral wrist pain, which is beginning to interfere with her teaching, although she has not had to take time off work. Ms. B. desires to continue to work full time.	Appreciate the context	"Because Ms. B implemented OT recommendations when seen 2 years ago, it is likely that she will do well again with OT recommendations and most likely will be able to continue full-time work as a school teacher.
Assessment Process and Results Interview with Ms. B. showed that Ms. B. has increased pain after working a full day. Her daily teaching schedule includes an approximate total time of 2 hours writing on the blackboard. She also opens and closes heavy institutional doors at least twice a day. She drives her car to and from work. She carries a full briefcase to and from work. She buys her lunch at the cafeteria daily. The pain subsides over the weekend, when she engages in very few active tasks, such as housecleaning or cooking. She has been having friends cook for her and has let her housecleaning go. Her wrist pain is eliminated over 2-week vacations and the summers, when she is not teaching. Physical examination of Ms. B.'s wrist showed a mild inflammatory process and no deformity. On a *Visual Analog Scale* for pain, Ms. B scored an 8 (out of 10) at her highest level of pain, which occurs following a day of using the blackboard.	Consider evaluation approach and methods	"Reviewing Ms. B.'s typical day schedule revealed problems with occupational functioning. Focusing on her daily schedule enabled me to understand what exacerbated her bilateral wrist pain, which could not easily be understood through physical examination of her wrists, which showed a mild inflammatory process."
	Interpret observations	"It appears that Ms. B.'s wrists have increased pain as a result of aggravation of her inflammatory process through daily overuse. This suspicion is further verified by her discussion that the pain is decreased on weekends and summers when she is not performing continued resistive motions to her wrist in her daily activities."
Occupational Therapy Problem List 1. Bilateral wrist pain exacerbated in the course of her work day, especially when she writes on the blackboard. 2. Inability to perform home maintenance. 3. Inability to prepare meals.	Synthesize results	"If Ms. B. continues to aggravate her wrist pain through activity, it may be increasingly difficult for her to continue working full time and to return to performing home maintenance and meal preparation."

Occupational Therapy Goal List

1. Wear bilateral wrist orthoses for use during performance of occupational tasks.
2. Apply alternative means to writing on the blackboard.
3. Use joint protection techniques to prevent increased wrist pain during work day and during performance of home maintenance and meal preparation tasks and activities.

Develop intervention hypotheses

"I believe that educating Ms. B. about the potential positive effects of wearing wrist orthoses will make her a good candidate to wear the orthoses and to benefit. With her desire to continue teaching, helping her to find a comfortable alternative solution to the use of the blackboard will lead to an outcome that will be carried out. Since it can be difficult to understand the application of joint protection principles easily to all activities, focusing specifically on her goals and helping her to problem-solve application should help her in new situations as they arise."

Select an intervention approach

"Occupational therapy intervention will focus on **compensatory, adaptive, and preventive** approaches."

Consider what will occur in therapy, how often, and for how long

"Ms. B. will be seen in occupational therapy as an outpatient for six sessions over 6 weeks. The sessions will focus on splinting, finding an alternative method to blackboard use, and problem-solving joint protection methods to apply to critical tasks."

Intervention

1. Determine and fit appropriate bilateral wrist orthoses to use during function.
2. Explore alternatives for writing on blackboard, such as use of overhead projector and transparency pens or chalk holders, to diminish prolonged tight pinch with its secondary effect on intercarpal pressures.
3. Explore use of adapted equipment for carrying heavy loads, such as a briefcase. This may include use of a luggage roller, special shoulder straps for carrying the briefcase, or a canvas pack on wheels.
4. Review meal preparation activities and adapted aids to decrease use of prolonged grasp and stress to wrists. This may include use of special jar openers, can openers, and knives that use arms instead of the wrists for power.
5. Review use of tools that can decrease stress to wrists, such as a rolling cart in the kitchen.
6. Identify which activities are the most important to Ms. B. to accomplish each day at work, home, and in the community. Reexamine whether priorities need to be set and whether stress to wrist joints is exacerbated with any of these activities.
7. Provide ongoing education on joint protection techniques that emphasize self-analysis of each activity and examination of alternative methods to accomplish important tasks without undue stress to wrist joints.
8. Explain wearing time of splints and purpose of splints. Train in appropriate donning, doffing and general care of splints.

Assess the patient's comprehension

"Teaching Ms. B. strategies for joint protection during occupational performance allowed the patient to learn self-analysis with each new activity that she could continue after the end of therapy. Because of the visibility of splinting, which may have negative connotations at work, education was important to assure that Ms. B. was comfortable wearing the splints in the classroom and that she recognized that the splints allowed performance in the classroom without increased pain at the end of the work day. It was important to teach Ms. B. to identify activities that aggravated wrist pain and find alternative ways to perform or use special tools or adapt the environment so that she could assume control over her disease."

"Upon Ms. B.'s return following each visit, Ms. B. demonstrated and described how she applied what she had gained from the previous session. At the end of the sixth visit, the *Visual Analog Scale* of pain was readministered, and the score was now 1 (out of 10) following a day at work teaching and using an overhead projector instead of a blackboard."

Next Steps

Ms. B. does not need to return to occupational therapy unless she finds that she has further occupational functioning problems.

Anticipate present and future patient concerns

"Ms. B. understands that she can request an OT referral from her rheumatologist if she has further occupational functioning problems. I believe that Ms. B. will continue to teach full time and enjoy being with her friends on the weekends. She will likely wear her bilateral wrist orthoses during task performance until the inflammatory process subsides. She will likely resume performance of work tasks, home maintenance activities, and meal preparation, applying joint protection principles."

CASE EXAMPLE #2

Mrs. S.: Osteoarthritis

Occupational Therapy Intervention Process	Clinical Reasoning Process: Objectives	Examples of Therapist's Internal Dialogue
Patient Information Mrs. S. is 55 years old and lives with her husband in their own home. They owned and operated a small café for 15 years until they retired 5 years ago. Mrs. S. has bilateral osteoarthritis (OA) of the knees that has progressed to the degree that she can walk only short distances at home without incurring knee pain that requires sitting or lying down. She also has pain in the CMC joint of the right thumb, which is noted especially when she is attempting to cook or garden. On a *Visual Analog Scale* for knee pain, her scores after walking short distances in her home are 8 to 10. Her right palmar and lateral pinch strength ranges between 3 and 5 pounds.	Understand the patient's diagnosis or condition	"X-rays showed that the patient had significant joint narrowing in both knees and the CMC joint of the right thumb. Excessive weight-bearing and resistive use of the right thumb aggravated joint pain secondary to severity of the disease."
	Know the person	"I questioned whether her dependency was secondary to lack of desire or lack of knowledge on how to perform tasks without aggravating pain. Mrs. S. had given up many cherished activities because of bilateral knee pain and right CMC joint pain. She had not personally attempted to use methods to control pain through use of alternative methods to perform important occupations."
Reason for Referral to Occupational Therapy Mrs. S. was referred to outpatient occupational therapy because of her complaints about difficulty managing self-care, home skills, and gardening.	Appreciate the context	"The physicians felt that Mrs. S. would benefit from knee arthroplasties, but she refused. Occupational therapy could perhaps improve her occupational functioning, despite continuing knee pain.
	Develop provisional hypotheses	Because of her expressed interest in returning to participation in important occupations and no previous OT intervention, she should be a good candidate to benefit from use of assistive devices, adapted methods, and right CMC thumb splint."
Assessment Process and Results Self-report ADL assessment and verification by observation reveals that Mrs. S. cannot transfer into and out of the bathtub without her husband's assistance. She prefers to stay in her night clothes all day because of knee discomfort when donning and doffing her pants to dress or to use the toilet. There is loss of interest and need to wear day clothes. She has problems grasping and pinching items in her right hand that require any degree of resistance. This includes opening jars, turning doorknobs, managing can openers, and managing dials that require twisting, such as stove knobs.	Consider evaluation approach and methods	"With limited evaluation time, I focused on observation of simulated occupations of importance, self-reported ADL, IADL measures, information obtained from interview for description of a typical day, and physical assessment of the CMC joint of the right thumb."
	Interpret observations	"Mrs. S. had significant knee pain with prolonged ambulation and movement that required extremes of knee flexion, such as transferring to the bottom of a bathtub. She also demonstrated pain on use of the right thumb in resistive tasks. I do not believe that Mrs. S. is avoiding performance of tasks secondary to dependency or lack of desire. Mrs. S. lacks knowledge of assistive devices, splinting, and joint protection methods that can enable engagement in important occupations."
Occupational Therapy Problem List Reduced occupational functioning in ADL/IADL areas listed in the assessment process.	Synthesize results	"I believe that problems are related to joint pain from overuse or resistive use of unstable, narrowed joints."

Occupational Therapy Goal List

1. Educate in joint protection principles related to Mrs. S.'s problems.
2. Explore use of right CMC thumb splint.
3. Explore use of assistive devices and alternative ways to accomplish important occupations.

Develop intervention hypotheses	"I believe that Mrs. S. will start dressing herself daily in day clothes and participate in occupations of interest once she understands how to avoid aggravating pain in affected joints."
Select an intervention approach	"Occupational therapy intervention will focus on **compensatory, adaptive, and preventative** approaches."
Consider what will occur in therapy, how often, and for how long	"Six sessions of 1 hour, one time per week, in outpatient occupational therapy with home assignments after each session should enable Mrs. S. to meet her occupational goals. Because this is the first time that Mrs. S. has had occupational therapy, time will need to be spent educating her and her husband, who is very supportive, on how goals can be achieved and maintained post intervention. It is also important in the therapy sessions that she actually practice her occupations of choice to understand how pain can be reduced through alternative methods to task performance."

Intervention

1. Educate patient and husband regarding the value of thumb CMC splinting. Provide a thumb CMC splint.
2. Provide joint protection education for patient and husband. Have patient practice use of joint protection methods.
3. Teach use of assistive devices for bathing and use of the EZ Stand Mobile Stool (TM) and educate on their value for joint protection.
4. Practice preparing a light meal using the EZ Stand Mobile Stool (TM) and other joint protection methods in the clinic kitchen.
   Example of Mrs. S.'s Home Program for Joint Protection:
   A. Use EZ Stand Mobile Stool (TM) to prepare a light lunch at least 3 times during the next week (to decrease excess loading to knee joints).
   B. Use thumb CMC splint during task performance (to stabilize thumb joint and to decrease excess loading to CMC joint).
   C. Use adapted equipment (multipurpose knob turner, Zim jar opener, and right-angled knife) to decrease excess loading to thumb CMC joint.
   D. Avoid pain in activities (e.g., holding pot with handle with 2 hands).
5. Practice gardening with walker and long-handled gardening tools in the clinic environment.

Assess the patient's comprehension	"Mrs. S. expressed surprise that her pain was not aggravated throughout the practice sessions in the model kitchen, in which she prepared a light meal, and when she performed gardening tasks in the outdoor garden area at the clinic. I felt this gave Mrs. S. the confidence to perform these occupations at home. Her husband was present throughout the sessions and provided her with additional encouragement."

Next Steps

Discharge from occupational therapy.

Note: Three months after discharge, Mrs. S.'s community rheumatologist reported to the occupational therapist that Mrs. S. has been going to an Arthritis Foundation swim program with her husband weekly and that she is cooking everyday and doing some gardening. She is seriously thinking about having knee arthroplasties soon.

Anticipate present and future patient concerns	"Since Mrs. S. followed through on homework assignments after each session, I felt that Mrs. S. will continue to use her equipment and practice joint protection principles to accomplish her cherished occupations. I did not feel that follow-up sessions were indicated, unless Mrs. S. found a need for further intervention."

CLINICAL REASONING IN OCCUPATIONAL THERAPY PRACTICE

Joint Protection Principles Applied to Leisure Skills

Mrs. S. has returned to cooking for herself and her husband. She also goes out to the garden two or three times a week to water the plants. She has told the therapist that she would like to participate in leisure activities in the community. What kinds of activities would you suggest and for what reasons?

The Arthritis Foundation brochure *Guide to Intimacy and Arthritis* describes positions for sex that reduce stress to commonly involved lower extremity joints (see Resources 44-1). Individuals may use the brochure to identify which postures are the least stressful for them. Communicating with a partner is important for trying new postures, letting the partner know what feels good, and finding alternative ways to enjoy sex.

FIBROMYALGIA

Three symptoms are commonly seen in patients with fibromyalgia (FM): widespread soft tissue pain, fatigue, and non-restorative sleep; these symptoms are accompanied by diffuse tender points. FM is reported to occur in 3.4% of women and 0.5% of men (Silver & Wallace, 2002; Wolfe et al., 1995). The prevalence of the syndrome increases with age but is also seen in children. The typical FM patient is a woman between 30 and 50 years of age (Burckhardt, 2001). Melvin (1998) reports that it is likely that many people go in and out of symptoms of FM and never seek a diagnosis and that OT practitioners are likely to see only the most severe cases. The diffuse, soft tissue pain is characteristically concentrated in axial locations such as the neck and lower back, with the proximal trapezius muscles commonly involved. Individuals often report stiffness in the morning, which dissipates with possibly a remaining sensation of joint swelling. The symptoms are chronic but can vary in intensity from day to day. They are commonly exacerbated by various factors, such as moderate physical exercise, inactivity, poor sleep, emotional stress, and humid weather. Despite a common complaint of paresthesias in the upper extremities and swelling in the hands, results on nerve conduction studies are usually normal, and examination of the hands usually fails to confirm actual swelling (Burckhardt, 2001; Freundlich & Leventhal, 1997). A number of conditions are associated with FM, such as chronic fatigue syndrome (50%), bowel disorders (e.g., irritable bowel syndrome, etc.) (40%), increased cardiac awareness (20%), headache (53%), and temporal-mandibular joint dysfunction (75%); other conditions at lesser percentages include, but are not limited to, heat and cold intolerance, subjective sensation of weakness, and mood disorders (Clauw, 2001; Silver & Wallace, 2002). Approximately 20–40% of people with FM have been reported to have identifiable current mood disorders such as depression or anxiety (Burckhardt, 2001). Cognitive dysfunction, such as forgetfulness and inability to think clearly or work effectively, is among the most distressing symptoms. Onset is usually gradual over a period of months or years, during which time localized or regional pain becomes widespread, although some patients begin with widespread pain after a febrile illness (Burckhardt, 2001). Spontaneous remissions and exacerbations are the rule (Turk, Monarch, & Williams, 2002). A unifying hypothesis is that FM results from sensitization of the CNS leading to expression of symptoms (Dworkin & Fields, 2005; Mease, 2005;). The central sensitization effect includes stimulus-evoked pain including **allodynia**, which is pain in response to a normally non-painful stimulus, an increased response to painful stimuli (**hyperalgesia**), and an increase in the duration of pain after the stimulation.

Rehabilitation Team Management

Nonpharmacologic therapies found to be helpful include an aerobic exercise program, gentle daily stretching and strengthening, cognitive behavioral therapy, alternative medicine approaches, and occupational therapy. Coordinated effort by a multidisciplinary team is important to achieve outcomes.

Assessment

In obtaining an occupational profile with this population, it is important to examine the patient's occupational history throughout a 24-hour period, since sleep disturbance is a common feature of the condition (Kornblau & Kasyan-Itzkowitz, 2002). During this process, a **daily activity log** and interview will provide clues as to whether there is significant fatigue, sleep disturbance, cognitive dysfunction, mood disorders, musculoskeletal symptoms, and other related problems. Additionally, this typical day examination may also describe at what hours of the day the person's highest energy for performance occurs. If some answers to questions relating to understanding of interfering factors contributing to patient's dissatisfaction with occupational functioning are not obtained from team information or the occupational profile, interview questions might include (Turk, Monarch, & Williams, 2002): (1) What do you do when your pain is bothering you? (2) What activities do you avoid that you used to do? (3) What aggravates symptoms? (4) What makes them better? Answers to these questions can assist with treatment planning. Some upper extremity symptoms associated with FM can be confused with a variety of nerve entrapment syndromes and inflammatory disorders, and a skilled therapist can help evaluate for this difference through a musculoskeletal exam (Russell, Melvin, & Siegel, 2000).

Goal Setting

Using the results obtained from an occupational profile, goal setting can be further identified using an instrument such as the *Canadian Occupational Performance Measure*. In goal setting, not only are the physiological and psychological symptoms important to consider, but it is also important to consider how readily the individual is able to incorporate changes into his/her life. Some studies have addressed this issue. For example, Finset, Wigers, and Gotestam (2004) found that depression is a predictive factor for limited treatment response.

Intervention

Self-Management Approaches

Self-management approaches, which include encouraging self-efficacy beliefs, have been found to be useful with clients with FM and would be important to use with all occupational therapy interventions (Burckhardt, 2001). Self-management can be taught by teaching patients to self-monitor occupational functioning that increases or decreases symptoms. Buckelew et al.'s (1995) study of patients with FM found that higher self-efficacy was associated with less pain and less impairment on a physical activities measure.

Simple scales on which patients as well as health professionals measure changes in pain, fatigue, sleep, anxiety, or mood from day to day can help them to recognize when self-management techniques are working (Burckhardt, 2001). Examples of useful scales include: (1) rating on a 10-point scale (10 = great deal, 0 = none) the extent that fatigue limits the ability for self-care (bathing, dressing, and grooming), work (either employment or activities around the home), and community activities; and (2) ongoing rating of morning fatigue, mood, and pain on a 10-point scale (10 = the most severe or worst) for tracking improvements in quality of sleep (Russell, Melvin, & Siegel, 2000).

Several authors (Guymer & Clauw, 2002; Melvin, 1998) suggest that patients should keep an activity log to monitor various aspects of symptom management, such as a sleep log to collect data on how their activities and behavioral interventions are altering their sleep or a fatigue journal to aid symptom assessment, which will help design interventions for lifestyle changes to assist with symptom reduction.

Patient Education

Principles of patient education are similar to those described for RA and OA and need to be specific to the intervention being provided (e.g., fatigue management, energy conservation, etc.) (Russell, Melvin, & Siegel, 2000). A useful teaching technique found by Goldenberg (2002) was the use of homework assignments following occupational therapy education sessions, which led to incorporation of appropriate body mechanics, energy conservation, and pacing of activities into the patients' daily routine.

Lifestyle Changes

An overarching occupational therapy intervention is changes to allow engagement in occupations, stay healthy, and control symptoms. By helping patients modify their lifestyle, practitioners can enable participation in valued occupations. The interventions that follow are some of the methods used to manage the major symptoms of the condition, with lifestyle changes as a desired outcome.

Sleep Hygiene

More than 90% of patients with FM describe disturbed sleep (Moldofsky, 2002). Clinical studies have shown that the soft tissue pain and tender points in specific anatomic regions are related to unrefreshing sleep. Following an occasional night of restful sleep, the patient often finds that pain and fatigue are substantially improved (Moldofsky, 2002). Russell, Melvin, and Siegel (2000) suggest that sleep retraining involves teaching patients about sleep physiology and the skills necessary to implement the recommendations, which may include relaxation training, cognitive behavioral techniques, time management, and how to self-manage depression and anxiety. Sleep hygiene has been included in programs by various health professionals, and occupational therapy practitioners can integrate this into their programs because it is related to helping clients to manage everyday (and evening) tasks for satisfactory performance of daily occupations. A number of basic sleep hygiene measures are advocated by various authors, including the Arthritis Foundation (see Resources 44-1), Guymer and Clauw (2002), Kornblau and Kasyan-Itzkowitz (2002), Russell, Melvin, and Siegel (2000), Moldofsky (2002), the National Sleep Foundation (2006), and Silver and Wallace (2002). A few examples include: (1) develop a regular sleep-wakefulness schedule; (2) develop a relaxing routine before bedtime; (3) reduce the irritation of noises inside or outside the room and/or use ear plugs and white noise machines, if needed; and (4) spend some quiet time by one's self before going to bed.

Fatigue Management

Chronic fatigue and easy fatigability in FM may be more problematic than pain (Burckhardt, 2001). The techniques described for intervention for fatigue management for patients with RA and OA apply to those with FM, namely, interventions that enable appropriate pacing, prioritizing, body mechanics, pre-planning, and work simplification (Burckhardt, 2002).

Cognitive Dysfunction

Cognitive dysfunction, especially decreased attention span and short-term memory, may be the most disabling aspect of FM (Clauw, 2001; Melvin, 1998). The causes of these problems are likely related to fatigue, unrefreshing sleep, chronic pain, and psychological distress (Burckhardt, 2001). Until cognitive disturbances are resolved, occupational therapists can recommend memory aids to compensate for memory difficulties, such as the use of personal data assistants (PDAs) for schedules and alarms to reduce forgetfulness, use of notes posted in prominent places, and keeping a list of tasks to be accomplished (Kornblau & Kasyan-Itzkowitz, 2002). See Chapter 29 for further suggestions.

Pain Management

Progressive increase in response to peripheral stimuli reflects slow temporal summation and has been termed "windup" (Price & Staud, 2005). Windup is likely to be related to mechanisms of central sensitization resulting in some persistent pain frequently reported as dull, aching, or burning. This allodynia of patients with FM, however, is not limited to tender points but, instead, appears to be widespread. Price and Staud (2005) report that almost all studies of patients with FM showed abnormalities of pain sensitivity while using different methods of psychophysical testing, for example, thermal (heat and cold), mechanical, chemical, or electrical stimuli to the skin or muscles. This suggests that teaching avoidance of triggers for pain response through lifestyle changes using any of the occupational therapy interventions described can assist with pain management.

Stress Management

Depending on the role of other team members and the skills of the occupational therapist, the occupational therapist's role may include stress management training to reduce influences that contribute to symptoms. These might include relaxation training, assertiveness training, guided imagery, and biofeedback (Russell, Melvin, & Siegel, 2000).

Modify or Adapt the Environment

Reisine et al. (2003) found that employed women with FM reported significantly less pain, less fatigue, and better functional status than women who were not employed outside the home. Thus, modifications in lifestyle and management at work as well as in the home need to be addressed. Reisine et al. (2003) noted that the absolute number of hours devoted to family work is not the critical element, but rather, it is the perceived demands associated with family work and ability to control the pace of family work. Henriksson and Liedberg's (2000) study of working women with FM showed that it is not only the heavy and physically difficult tasks that cause problems. Short periods of static movements or movements requiring only limited endurance are frequently experienced as difficult to perform and cause increased pain. Many tasks that are considered "light" tend to be highly repetitive and increase the possibility of musculoskeletal pain, suggesting the "windup" phenomenon in action. When necessary, interventions in the work place should be performed and the patient should be advised and supported to carry out necessary changes in daily habits and routines. Examples of employment and home modifications include adjusting the height of a desk and chair, altering the work schedule, avoiding prolonged static sitting by mixing tasks, planning on sharing baby sitting with neighbors to provide time for self, and modifying play with young children by sitting on a sofa with them instead of on the floor.

Clinical Outcomes

The described interventions require that the recipient of services redesign his or her life in a variety of ways, from wearing a hand splint to use of assistive devices or changing the routine patterns of daily living. Change of typical routine is not easy, and it has been estimated that at least 50% of patients with RA are non-compliant with therapy, irrespective of the nature of the intervention (Belcon, Haynes, & Tugwell, 1984; Feinberg & Trombly, 1995). In a study designed to examine the effect of interaction between the patient and the occupational therapist on subsequent splint use, splint use was greater in a group of patients who were treated by a therapist using compliance-enhancing behaviors that included the suggestions in Procedures for Practice 44-4.

PROCEDURES FOR PRACTICE 44-4

Clinical Suggestions for Enhancing Compliance (Feinberg & Trombly, 1995)

Apply Learning Principles to Patient Education

- Patients best remember instructions presented first.
- Emphasized instructions are recalled better.
- The fewer the instructions, the greater the proportion remembered.
- Pace the amount of information to avoid overload.
- Use simple, understandable language without medical jargon.
- Individualize teaching methods to the patient.
- Reinforce essential points by review, discussion, or summary.
- Ask the patient to repeat essential elements of the message.
- Provide written instructions for home reference.
- Devise mechanisms for helping patients to remember advice.

Assess the Patient's Expectations and Experience Concerning the Following

- The clinical encounter
- His or her beliefs and misconceptions about the cause, severity, and symptoms of the illness and susceptibility to complications or exacerbations
- Goals of treatment
- Perceptions about the costs and risks versus the benefits of treatment
- Existing health-related knowledge, skills, and practices
- Degree of adaptation to the disease
- Sense of self-efficacy or lack of control and hopelessness
- Learning limitations
- Extent of family involvement and influence

Encourage the Patient to Assume Responsibility for Disease Management

- Use behavioral contracts if necessary.
- Use other motivational techniques.
- Encourage the patient that he or she can be successful with self-management.
- Use a facilitating affective tone.
- Listen to the patient.
- Be approachable.
- Appear knowledgeable.
- Inspire trust and confidence.
- Be enthusiastic and expect positive results.

RESEARCH NOTE

Abstract: Reisine, S., Fifield, J., Walsh, S. J., & Feinn, R., (2003). Do employment and family work affect the health status of women with fibromyalgia? *The Journal of Rheumatology, 30,* 2045–2053.

To assess health status differences of women with FM who are employed and not employed and to evaluate whether employment and family work influence the health status of women with FM as it does for women in community studies, 287 women with FM (137 employed and 150 not employed) were compared through completed telephone interviews that collected data on demographic characteristics, health status, symptoms, family work, and social support. The majority of employed and not employed participants reported high levels of symptoms and poor health status. Despite having similar disease duration, employed women reported significantly less pain, less fatigue, and better functional status than those who were not employed. Employment remained a significant factor in explaining number of painful areas, functional status, and fatigue, with employed women reporting better health status than those not employed. The psychological demands of family work were consistently related to all dependent measures of health status, as those with greater psychological demands reported worse health status.

Implications for Practice

- During the occupational therapy assessment process, the importance of work to patients is important to assess. For example, has meaningful employment been abandoned secondary to FM symptoms? Or is current employment becoming compromised secondary to FM symptoms?
- If the patient is working and work is highly valued, FM symptoms interfering with occupational functioning at work need to be closely reviewed, and alterations to the work environment should be recommended.
- If the patient preference is to not be employed outside of the home, the home environment needs to be scrutinized for problems that may be aggravating symptoms, such as fatigue, pain, and/or sleep disturbance. Energy conservation, fatigue management, and other interventions need to be considered to enable successful engagement in occupations related to home management.

Evidence Table 44-1
Best Evidence for Occupational Therapy Practice Regarding Rheumatoid Arthritis (RA), Osteoarthritis (OA), and Fibromyalgia (FM)

Intervention	Description of Intervention Tested	Participants	Dosage	Type of Best Evidence and Level of Evidence	Benefit	Statistical Probability and Effect Size of Outcome	Reference
Joint protection (RA)	Standard arthritis education program vs. a joint protection program, using educational, behavioral, motor learning, and self-efficacy–enhancing strategies.	65 people were randomly assigned to a joint protection program, and 62 were assigned to the standard program. Groups were similar in age, disease duration, and use of arthritis medications.	Standard: 2.5 hours of joint protection based on typical United Kingdom OT practice (plus 5.5 hours on RA, exercise, pain management, diet, and foot care). Joint protection: four 2-hour weekly meetings as described.	Randomized controlled trial. IA2a	Yes. At 4 years post treatment, the joint protection group continued to have better joint protection adherence, early morning stiffness, and activities of daily living (ADL) scores.	Joint protection behavioral assessment: $p = 0.001$, $r = 0.27$; stiffness: $p = 0.001$, $r = 0.27$; ADL: $p = 0.04$, $r = 0.15$.	Hammond and Freeman (2004)

Evidence Table 44-1 (*continued*)

Intervention	Description of Intervention Tested	Participants	Dosage	Type of Best Evidence and Level of Evidence	Benefit	Statistical Probability and Effect Size of Outcome	Reference
Splinting the first CMC joint (OA)	Short opponens splint that maintained the web space and immobilized the CMC vs. long opponens splint that immobilized the wrist, CMC, and first MCP joints. All patients wore both in random sequence.	26 patients (5 men and 21 women) who had radiographic evidence of first CMC OA and joint pain (age, 36 to 88 years; mean age = 57 years). 80% were right-hand dominant; 60% had right-hand involvement. Duration of symptoms ranged from <1 year to >5 years. 8 patients had concomitant diagnoses of other impairments.	Patients wore each splint for 1 week at times of feeling symptoms day or night.	Pre–post design; each group and subgroup tested separately before and after splint use. IIIB2b	Yes. Splinting significantly reduced pain in patients with first CMC joint OA. Splinting also significantly reduced subluxation (under stress), especially in the early stages of OA. The splints did not significantly increase pinch strength or lessen the pain associated with pinch, after the splint was removed. Neither splint was more effective than the other. The shorter splint was preferred by most patients.	Pain (*Visual Analog Scale*): $\chi^2 = 14.0$, $p = 0.001$, $r = 0.73$. Percentage of subluxation of first CMC: $F_{(2,26)} = 4.38$, $p = 0.01$, $r = 0.45$. Pinch strength: $F_{(1,24)} = 1.38$, $p = 0.26$, $r = 0.23$. Pain after 1 week of splint wear: $\chi^2 = 3.92$, $p = 0.28$, $r = 0.38$. No significant differences between splints in any tests. ADL (self-rated): 93% of 22 ADLs were easier with the short splint compared with no splint, but 7% were harder; with the long splint compared with no splint, only 16% were reported to be easier. 73% preferred the short splint; 27% preferred the long splint.	Weiss et al., 2000

Interdisciplinary treatment for FM	4-week outpatient program consisting of medical, physical, psychological, and occupational therapies.	67 outpatients with FM (mean age = 48.37 years; SD = 10.99 years).	Pre-treatment 3-hour evaluation (medical, physical, psychological, and self-report inventories). Program was 6.5 day sessions, spaced over a period of 4 weeks. Groups of 4–7 patients attended the program 3 times a week during the first week and once a week for the next 3 weeks. All 4 therapies were administered at each session. OT offered six 1-hour educational sessions regarding body mechanics, energy conservation, and pacing. Patients were given home assignments that were reviewed by the OT at the next session.	One group pre- and post-test design. IIIA3b	Partially. Significant decrease in depression with significant increase in sense of life control (strong effect) and non-significant decrease in sense of perceived disability (small effect).	Results at post treatment significant to OT: *Oswestry Disability Index* at post treatment: $t_{(66)} = 2.14$, not significant, $r = 0.25$; *Multidimensional Pain Inventory–Life Control Subtest*: $t_{(66)} = -5.47$, not significant, $r = 0.56$.	Turk et al., 1998

SUMMARY REVIEW QUESTIONS

1. List the primary differences between RA and OA.
2. Describe joint problems that can lead to diminished occupational functioning for people with RA and OA
3. Besides joint problems, what clinical problems can affect occupational functioning for people with RA?
4. Is a patient with only thumb CMC joint involvement and resultant pain on resistive motion more likely to have OA or RA?
5. Describe joint protection techniques used for people with RA to prevent or restore occupational functioning.
6. Name several resources for patients with RA and OA to find adapted tools to enhance their occupational functioning.
7. How is splinting used for people with RA and OA to enhance occupational functioning?
8. What assessments are used to optimize occupational functioning for people with RA, OA, and FM?
9. What are the major symptoms of FM that lead to diminished occupational functioning?

References

Altman, R., Alarcon, G., Appelrouth, D., Bloch, D., Borenstein, D., Brandt, K., Brown, C., Cooke, T. D., Daniel, W., & Gray, R. (1990). The American College of Rheumatology criteria for the classification and reporting of osteoarthritis of the hand. *Arthritis and Rheumatism, 33,* 1601–1610.

Arthritis Foundation. (1993). *Living and loving.* Atlanta: Arthritis Foundation.

Axtell, L. A., & Yasuda, Y. L. (1993). Assistive devices and home modification in geriatric rehabilitation. *Clinical Geriatric Medicine, 9,* 803–821.

Backman, C. (1998). Functional assessment. In J. Melvin & G. Jensen (Eds.), *Rheumatologic rehabilitation series* (Vol. 1, pp. 157–194). Bethesda, MD: American Occupational Therapy Association.

Backman, C., & Mackie, H. (1995). Arthritis hand function test: Inter-rater reliability among self-trained raters. *Arthritis Care and Research, 8,* 10–15.

Belcon, M. C., Haynes, R. B., & Tugwell, P. (1984). A critical review of compliance studies in rheumatoid arthritis. *Arthritis and Rheumatism, 27,* 1227–1233.

Belza, B. L. (1995). Comparison of self-reported fatigue in rheumatoid arthritis and controls. *Journal of Rheumatology, 22,* 639–643.

Belza, B. L. (2001). Fatigue. In L. Robbins (Ed.), *Clinical care in the rheumatic diseases* (2nd ed., pp. 251–253). Atlanta: Association of Rheumatology of Health Professionals.

Brandt, K. D., & Slemenda, C. W. (1993). Osteoarthritis: Epidemiology, pathology, and pathogenesis. In H. R. Schumacher (Ed.), *Primer on the rheumatic diseases* (10th ed., pp. 184–187). Atlanta: Arthritis Foundation.

Buckelew, S. P., Murray, S. E., Hewett, J. E., Johnson, J., & Huyser, B. (1995). Self-efficacy, pain, and physical activity among fibromyalgia patients. *Arthritis Care and Research, 8,* 43–50.

Burckhardt, C. S. (2001). Fibromyalgia. In L. Robbins (Ed.), *Clinical care in the rheumatic diseases* (2nd ed., pp. 135–153). Atlanta: Association of Rheumatology of Health Professionals.

Burckhardt, C. S. (2002). Nonpharmacologic management strategies in fibromyalgia. *Rheumatic Disease Clinics of North America, 28,* 291–304.

Clark, F., Azen, S. P., Zemke, R., Jackson, J., Carlson, M., Mandel, D., Hay, J., Josephson, K., Cherry, B., Hessel, C., Palmer, J. M., & Lipson, L. (1997). Occupational therapy for independent-living older adults. *Journal of American Medical Association, 278,* 1321–1326.

Clauw, D. J. (2001). Fibromyalgia and diffuse pain syndromes. In J. H. Klippel (Ed.), *Primer in rheumatic diseases* (12th ed., pp. 188–193). Atlanta: the Arthritis Foundation.

Coppard, B. M., Gale, J. R., & Jensen, G. M. (1998). Therapeutic exercise. In J. Melvin & G. Jensen, (Eds.), *Rheumatology rehabilitation series, vol. 1: Assessment and management* (pp. 335–350). Bethesda, MD: American Occupational Therapy Association.

Cordery, J., & Rocchi, M. (1998). Joint protection and fatigue management. In J. Melvin & G. Jensen (Eds.), *Rheumatologic rehabilitation series, vol. 1: Assessment and management* (pp. 279–321). Bethesda, MD: American Occupational Therapy Association.

Dubouloz, C., Laporte, D., Hall, M., Ashe, B., & Smith, C. D. (2004). Transformation of meaning perspectives in clients with rheumatoid arthritis. *The American Journal of Occupational Therapy, 58,* 398–407.

Dworkin, R. H., & Fields, H. L. (2005). Introduction. Fibromyalgia from the perspective of neuropathic pain. *The Journal of Rheumatology, 32,* 1–5.

Falconer, J. (1990). Hand splinting in rheumatoid arthritis. *Arthritis Care and Research, 4,* 81–86.

Feinberg, J. (1992). Effect of the arthritis health professional on compliance with use of resting hand splints by patients with rheumatoid arthritis. *Arthritis Care and Research, 5,* 17–23.

Feinberg, J. R., & Brandt, K. D. (1984). Allied health team management of rheumatoid arthritis patients. *American Journal of Occupational Therapy, 38,* 613–620.

Feinberg, J. R., & Trombly, C. A. (1995). Arthritis. In C. A. Trombly (Ed.), *Occupational therapy for physical dysfunction* (4th ed., pp. 815–830). Baltimore: Williams and Wilkins.

Finset, A., Wigers, S. H., & Gotestam, K. G. (2004). Depressed mood impedes pain treatment response in patients with fibromyalgia. *The Journal of Rheumatology, 31,* 976–980.

Freundlich, B., & Leventhal, L. (1997). Diffuse pain syndromes. In J. H. Klippel (Ed.), *Primer on the rheumatic diseases.* Atlanta: Arthritis Foundation.

Furst, G. P., Gerber, L. H., Smith, C. C., Fisher, S., & Shulman, B. (1987). A program for improving energy conservation behaviors in adults with rheumatoid arthritis. *American Journal of Occupational Therapy, 41,* 102–111.

Gerber, L., Furst, G., Shulman, B., Smith, C., Thornton, B., Liang, M., Stevens, M. B., & Gilbert, N. (1987). Patient education program to teach energy conservation behaviors to patients with rheumatoid arthritis: A pilot study. *Archives of Physical Medicine and Rehabilitation, 68,* 442–445.

Goldenberg, D. L. (2002). Office management of fibromyalgia. *Rheumatic Disease Clinics of North America, 28,* 437–446.

Goldenberg, D. L., Burckhardt, C., & Crofford, L. (2004). Management of fibromyalgia syndrome. *Journal of American Medical Association, 292,* 2388–2395.

Gornisiewicz, M., & Moreland, L. W. (2001). Rheumatoid arthritis. In L. Robbins (Ed.), *Clinical care in the rheumatic diseases* (2nd ed., pp. 89–112). Atlanta: Association of Rheumatology of Health Professionals.

Goronzy, J. J., & Weyand, C. M. (2001). Rheumatoid arthritis. In J. H. Klippel (Ed.), *Primer on the rheumatic diseases* (12th ed., pp. 209–217). Atlanta: Arthritis Foundation.

Guymer, E. M., & Clauw, D. J. (2002). Treatment of fatigue in fibromyalgia. *Rheumatic Disease Clinics of North America, 28,* 367–378.

Hammond, A., & Freeman, K. (2004). The long-term outcomes from a randomized controlled trial of an educational-behavioural joint protection programme for people with rheumatoid arthritis. *Clinical Rehabilitation, 18,* 520–528.

Henriksson, C., & Liedberg, G. (2000). Factors of importance for work disability in women with fibromyalgia. *The Journal of Rheumatology, 27,* 1271–1276.

Hochberg, M. C. (2001). Osteoarthritis. In J. H. Klippel (Ed.), *Primer on the rheumatic diseases* (12th ed., pp. 289–293). Atlanta: Arthritis Foundation.

Huskisson, E. C. (1974). Measurement of pain. *Lancet, 2,* 1127–1131.

Jackson, J., Carlson, M., Mandel, D., Zemke, R., & Clark, F. (1998). Occupation in lifestyle redesign: The well elderly study occupational therapy program. *American Journal of Occupational Therapy, 52,* 326–335.

Kjeken, I., Moller, G., & Kvien, T. K. (1995). Use of commercially produced elastic wrist orthoses in chronic arthritis: A controlled study. *Arthritis Care and Research, 8,* 108–113.

Komatireddy, G. R., Leitch, R. W., Cella, K., Browning, G., & Minor, M. (1997). Efficacy of low load resistive muscle training in patients with rheumatoid arthritis functional class II and III. *Journal of Rheumatology, 24,* 1531–1539.

Kornblau, B. L., & Kasyan-Itzkowitz, P. (2002). Fibromyalgia syndrome: A comprehensive approach. *OT Practice, 7,* 18–23.

Law, M., Baptiste, S., Carswell, A., McColl, M. A., Polatajko, H., & Pollock, N. (1994). *Canadian Occupational Performance Measure* (2nd ed.). Toronto, Ontario, Canada: Canadian Association of Occupational Therapists.

Lozada, C. J., & Altman, R. D. (2001). Osteoarthritis. In L. Robbins (Ed.), *Clinical care in the rheumatic diseases* (2nd ed., pp. 113–133), Atlanta: Association of Rheumatology Health Professionals.

Majerovitz, S. J., & Revenson, T. A. (1994). Sexuality and rheumatic disease. *Arthritis Care and Research, 7,* 29–34.

Mann, W. (1998). Assistive technology for persons with arthritis. In J. Melvin & G. Jensen (Eds.), *Rheumatology rehabilitation series, vol. 1: Assessment and management* (pp. 369–392). Bethesda, MD: American Occupational Therapy Association.

Mathiowetz, V., Kashman, N., Volland, G., Weber K., Dowe, M., & Rogers, S. (1985). Grip and pinch strength, normative data for adults. *Archives of Physical Medicine and Rehabilitation, 66,* 69–74.

McFarlane, D. G., Buckland-Wright, J. C., Emery, P., Fogelman, I., Clark, B., & Lynch, J. (1990). Comparison of clinical, radionuclide, and radiographic features of osteoarthritis of the hands. *Annals of the Rheumatic Diseases, 50,* 623–626.

Mease, P. (2005). Fibromyalgia syndrome: Review of clinical presentation, pathogenesis, outcome measures, and treatment. *The Journal of Rheumatology, 32,* 6–21.

Melvin, J. L. (1998). Self-management for fibromyalgia. *OT Practice, 3,* 39–43, 45.

Minor, M. A. (1996). Rest and exercise. In S. T. Wegener, B. L. Belza, & E. P. Gall (Eds.), *Clinical care in the rheumatic diseases* (pp. 79–82). Atlanta: American College of Rheumatology.

Moldofsky, H. (2002). Management of sleep disorders in fibromyalgia. *Rheumatic Disease Clinics of North America, 28,* 353–365.

Nalebuff, E. A. (1984). The rheumatoid thumb. *Clinics in Rheumatic Diseases, 10,* 589–608.

National Sleep Foundation. (2006). Healthy sleep tips. www.sleepfoundation.org

Nordenskiold, U. M., & Grimby, G. (1993). Grip force in patients with rheumatoid arthritis and fibromyalgia and in healthy subjects. A study with the Grippit instrument. *Scandinavian Journal of Rheumatology, 22,* 14–19.

Nordenskiold, U., Grimby, G., & Dahlin-Ivanoff, S. (1998). Questionnaire to evaluate the effects of assistive devices and altered working methods in women with rheumatoid arthritis. *Clinical Rheumatology, 17,* 7–16.

Palchik, N. S., Mitchell, D. M., Gilbert, N. L., Schulz, A. J., Dedrick, R. F., & Palella T. D. (1990). Nonsurgical management of the boutonniere deformity. *Arthritis Care and Research, 3,* 227–232.

Partridge, R. E. H., & Duthie, J. J. R. (1963). Controlled trial of the effect of complete immobilization of the joints in rheumatoid arthritis. *Annals of Rheumatic Disease, 22,* 91–96.

Price, D. D., & Staud, R. (2005). Neurobiology of fibromyalgia syndrome. *The Journal of Rheumatology, 32,* 22–28.

Reisine, S., Fifield, J., Walsh, S. J., & Feinn, R. (2003). Do employment and family work affect the health status of women with fibromyalgia? *The Journal of Rheumatology, 30,* 2045–2053.

Rizio, L., & Belsky, M. R. (1996). Finger deformities in rheumatoid arthritis. *Hand Clinics, 22,* 531–540.

Russell, I. J., Melvin, J. L., & Siegel, M. (2000). Fibromyalgia syndrome. In J. L. Melvin & K. M. Ferrell (Eds.), *Rheumatologic rehabilitation series, vol. 2. Adult rheumatic diseases.* Bethesda, MD: The American Occupational Therapy Association.

Shapiro, J. S. (1996). The wrist in rheumatoid arthritis. *Hand Clinics, 12,* 477–498.

Silver, D. S., & Wallace, D. J. (2002). The management of fibromyalgia-associated syndromes. *Rheumatic Disease Clinics of North America, 28,* 405–417.

Stein, A. B., & Terrono, A. L. (1996). The rheumatoid thumb. *Hand Clinics, 12,* 541–550.

Stern, E. B., Ytterberg, S. R., Krug, H. E., Mullin, G. T., & Mahowald, M. L. (1996). Immediate and short-term effects of three commercial wrist extensor orthoses on grip strength and function in patients with rheumatoid arthritis. *Arthritis Care and Research, 9,* 42–50.

Stern, E. B., Ytterberg, S. R., Larson, L. M., Portoghese, C. P., Kratz, W. N. R., & Mahowald, M. L. (1997). Commercial wrist extensor orthoses: A descriptive study of the use and preference in patients with rheumatoid arthritis. *Arthritis Care and Research,* 10(1), 27–35.

Taliesnik, J. (1989). Rheumatoid arthritis of the wrist. *Hand Clinics, 5,* 257–277.

Ter Schegget, M., & Knipping, A. (2000). A study comparing the use and effects of custom-made versus prefabricated splints for swan neck deformity in patients with rheumatoid arthritis. *British Journal of Occupational Therapy, 5,* 101–107.

Tijhuis, G. J., Vlieland, T. P. M., Zwinderman, A. H., & Hazes, J. M. W. (1998). A comparison of the Futuro wrist orthosis with a synthetic Thermolyn orthosis: Utility and clinical effectiveness. *Arthritis Care and Research, 11,* 217–222.

Turk, D. C., Monarch, E. S., & Williams, A. D. (2002). Psychological evaluation of patients diagnosed with fibromyalgia syndrome: A comprehensive approach. *Rheumatic Disease Clinics of North America, 28,* 219–233.

Turk, D. C., Okifuji, A., Sinclair, J.D., & Starz, T. V. (1998). Interdisciplinary treatment for fibromyalgia syndrome: Clinical and statistical significance. *Arthritis Care and Research, 11,* 186–195.

van Lankveld, W. G. J. M., Graff, M. J. L., & van't Pad Bosch, P. J. I. (1999). The short version of the Sequential Occupational Dexterity Assessment based on individual tasks' sensitivity to change. *Arthritis Care and Research, 12,* 417–424.

Weiss, S., LaStayo, P., Mills, A., & Bramlet, D. (2000). Prospective analysis of splinting the first carpometacarpal joint: An objective, subjective, and radiographic assessment. *Journal of Hand Therapy, 13,* 218–227.

Wilson, R. L. (1986). Rheumatoid arthritis of the hand. *Orthopedic Clinics of North America, 17,* 313–343.Wolfe, F., Ross, K., Anderson, J., Russell, I. J., & Hebert, L. (1995). The prevalence and characteristics of fibromyalgia in the general population. *Arthritis and Rheumatism, 38,* 19–28.

CHAPTER 45

Burn Injuries

Monica A. Pessina and Amy C. Orroth

LEARNING OBJECTIVES

After studying this chapter, the reader will be able to do the following:

1. Differentiate between superficial, superficial partial-thickness, deep partial-thickness, and full-thickness burn injuries.
2. Explain the rationale for splinting and positioning programs for patients with burn injuries.
3. Outline occupational therapy treatment techniques for each phase of burn recovery.
4. Describe potential complications and treatment strategies for hand burns.
5. Discuss the effects of a burn injury on a patient's psychosocial functioning.

Glossary

Anti-deformity positions—Positions opposite to common patterns of deformity used to prevent contractures.

Blanch—Apply sufficient pressure to interrupt blood flow temporarily: an assessment of capillary flow rate.

Deep partial-thickness burn—Thermal injury that destroys cells from the epidermis to the deep dermal layer.

Debride—Remove eschar and loose or necrotic tissue to prevent infection and promote healing.

Dermis—Layer of skin below the epidermis that contains blood vessels, nerve endings, hair follicles, and sweat and oil glands; supports the regrowth of new epithelial tissue.

Epidermis—Most superficial layer of the skin; acts as a barrier. It is continually sloughed and replaced.

Eschar—Burned tissue.

Full-thickness burn—Thermal injury in which the epidermis and dermis are destroyed.

Superficial burn—Thermal injury that involves only cells in the epidermis.

Superficial partial-thickness burn—Thermal injury in which the epidermis and upper portion of the dermal layer are destroyed.

Wound contracture—Part of normal healing in which myofibroblasts in the wound bed contract to minimize the skin defect

Z-plasty—Surgical procedure in which a Z-shaped incision is made and tissue is transposed to increase tissue length.

Approximately 1.25 million burn injuries occur in the United States each year, resulting in 5,500 fire- and burn-related deaths (Brigham & McLoughlin, 1996). Thermal damage to the skin can be caused by fire, contact with a hot object or hot liquid (scald burn), radiation, chemicals, or electricity. Almost 80% of burn injuries occur in and around the home, and hot food and liquid spills are the most common source of burns to children (Brigham & McLoughlin, 1996) On average, 45,000 acute hospital admissions occur annually for burn injuries. Approximately half of these patients are admitted to regional burn centers designated by the American Burn Association; the remainder are treated at local or regional hospitals (Burn Foundation, 1999). Therefore, every occupational therapist should understand the principles of care and rehabilitation of patients with burn injuries. Treatment of these injuries requires a comprehensive approach by a qualified burn treatment team, including a skilled occupational therapist. This chapter explores the unique role of occupational therapy in treatment of burn patients, from the initial injury to the patient's return to independent function. Topics include various phases of burn rehabilitation, scar management, psychosocial issues, and reconstructive surgery. We hope to convey the unique and rewarding aspects of working with patients with burn injuries.

BURN CLASSIFICATION

In the past, burn depth was classified as first, second, or third degree. Today, the preferred classification system more accurately describes the level of cellular injury. The terms in use are superficial, superficial partial-thickness, deep partial-thickness, and full-thickness. Burns typically have mixed depths, which necessitates that the burn team carefully assess the appearance and progress of each area of the wound site. Disruption of any portion of the skin has the potential to interfere with its normal functions, which include temperature regulation, excretion, sensation, vitamin D synthesis, and acting as a barrier against infection and dehydration (Falkel, 1994). Occupational therapists may treat patients with all levels of thermal injury. It is important to differentiate among the classifications to plan appropriate intervention.

Superficial Burns

Superficial burns damage cells only in the epidermis (Malick & Carr, 1982; Staley, Richard, & Falkel, 1994) (Fig. 45-1). These injuries are painful and red. They heal spontaneously within approximately 7 days and leave no permanent scar (Malick & Carr, 1982).

Superficial Partial-Thickness Burns

Superficial partial-thickness burns damage cells in the epidermis and the upper level of the **dermis** (Malick & Carr, 1982; Staley, Richard, & Falkel, 1994). The most common sign of a superficial partial-thickness burn is intact blisters over the injured area (Staley, Richard, & Falkel, 1994). These injuries are also painful because of the irritation of the nerve endings in the dermal layer. Superficial partial-thickness burns heal spontaneously within 7–21 days and leave minimal or no scarring (Staley, Richard, & Falkel, 1994).

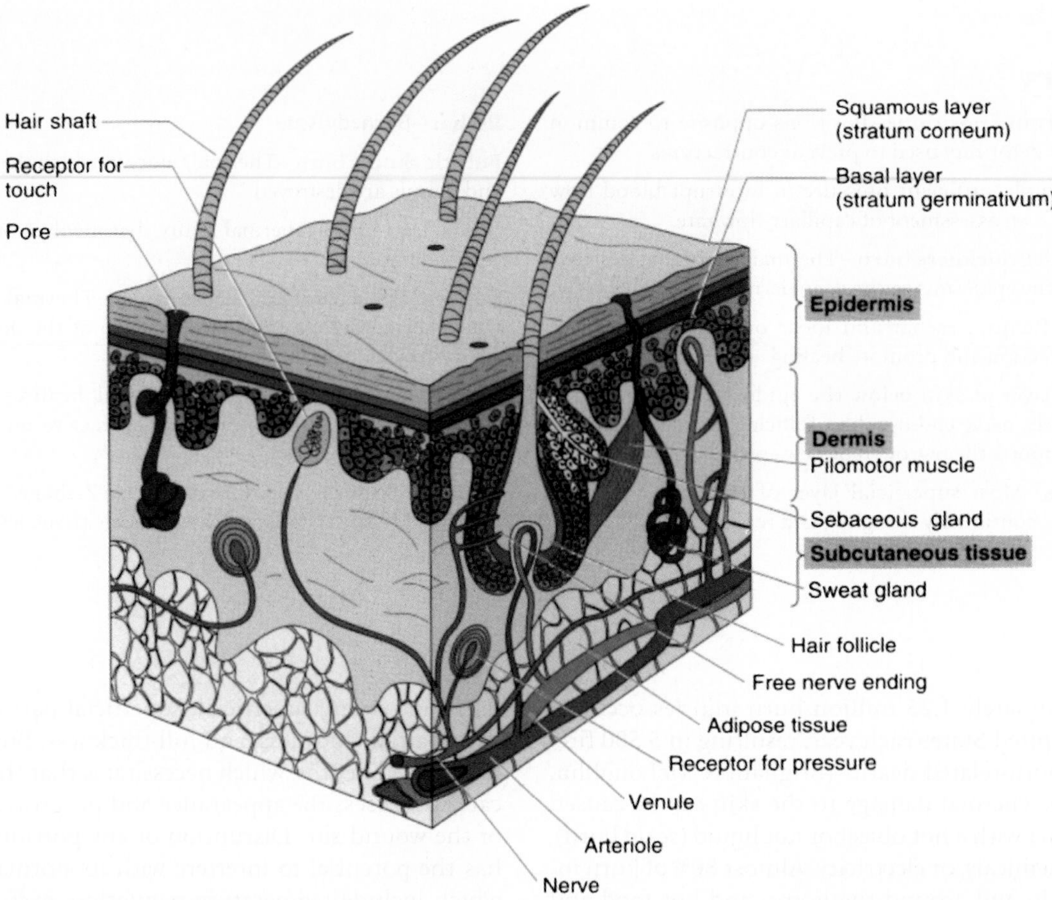

Figure 45-1 Cross-section of the skin. (From Willis, M. C. [1996]. *Medical terminology: The language of health care* [p. 90]. Baltimore: Williams & Wilkins.)

Deep Partial-Thickness Burns

Deep partial-thickness burns cause cell injury in the **epidermis** and severe damage to the dermal layer (Malick & Carr, 1982; Staley, Richard, & Falkel, 1994). These injuries appear blotchy, with areas of whitish color interspersed throughout the wound (Malick & Carr, 1982). The injury site is painful. Pressure sensation is intact, but light touch is diminished (Staley, Richard, & Falkel, 1994). Spontaneous healing of deep partial-thickness burns is sluggish (3–5 weeks) because vascularity in the dermal layer is impaired. Therefore, the risk of significant scarring is increased (Staley, Richard, & Falkel, 1994). For this reason, deep partial-thickness burns are often grafted to expedite healing and minimize scarring.

Full-Thickness Injury

In a full-thickness injury both the epidermis and the dermal layer are destroyed (Malick & Carr, 1982; Staley, Richard, & Falkel, 1994). These wounds appear white or waxy and are inherently insensate because of the complete destruction of the dermal nerve endings (Malick & Carr, 1982). Full-thickness burns require surgical intervention, such as skin grafting (Malick & Carr, 1982; Staley, Richard, & Falkel, 1994), since there are no dermal elements to support the regrowth of epithelial tissue. Some burns, such as electrical burns, may damage structures below the dermis, including subcutaneous fat, muscle, or bone.

RULE OF NINES

A commonly used technique to determine burn size in adults is the rule of nines (Fig. 45-2). To determine burn size in children and infants, a modification of this technique, the Lund-Browder chart, is used. The percentage of total body surface area (TBSA) that has been burned is used for the following:

- Calculating nutritional and fluid requirements
- Determining level of acuity to establish the level of medical treatment needed (i.e., admission to an intensive care unit)
- Classifying patients for use of standardized protocols

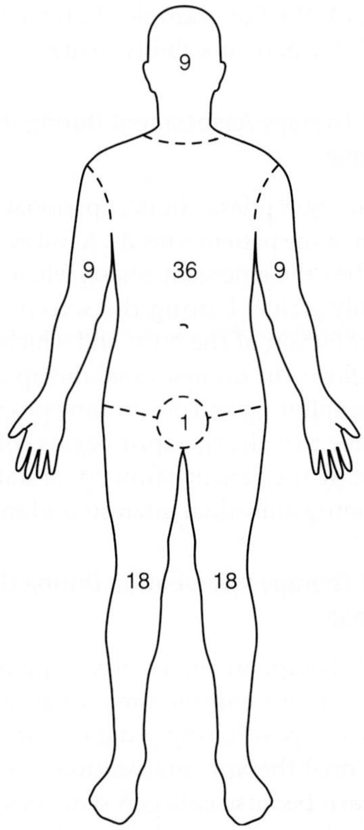

Figure 45-2 Rule of nines. (Reprinted with permission from Malick, M. H., & Carr, J. A. [1982]. *Manual on management of the burn patient* [p. 10]. Pittsburgh: Harmarville Rehabilitation Center.)

PHASES OF BURN MANAGEMENT AND REHABILITATION

Identifying specific phases of burn management helps to describe the role of occupational therapy for patients with burn injuries. These include the emergent, acute, and rehabilitation phases. Each of the phases, along with accompanying occupational therapy considerations, are described.

Emergent Phase

The emergent phase of a burn injury is considered to be from initial injury to approximately 72 hours post burn (Grigsby deLinde & Miles, 1995).

Medical Management

During the emergent phase, the medical team attempts to stabilize the patient. This may include fluid resuscitation, establishment of adequate tissue perfusion, and achievement of cardiopulmonary stability. Associated injuries, such as fractures, are evaluated and treated during this time.

Inhalation Injury

An important consideration in the emergent phase is the possibility of an inhalation injury. Damage to the upper airway as a result of inhaling either hot particles or noxious gases results in an inhalation injury. This damages the respiratory epithelium and can impair gas exchange. Inhalation injuries can significantly increase mortality rate (Cioffi & Rue, 1991). Singed eyebrows, soot around the nares, and facial edema are indications of an inhalation injury (Cioffi & Rue, 1991). Diagnosis is confirmed by analysis of arterial blood gases, chest radiographs, and bronchoscopy. In addition, edema can quickly develop in the airway and constrict breathing. Therefore, patients with significant burn injuries are usually intubated (placed on mechanical ventilation) to maintain an open airway until the risk of airway closure due to edema has diminished.

Escharotomy and Fasciotomy

Circulation can be compromised when burn injuries girdle a body segment. This is due to the inelasticity of the **eschar** (burned tissue) combined with increased internal pressure within fascial compartments. Local increase in pressure in the extremities compresses blood vessels and reduces blood flow (Sheridan et al., 1995). Symptoms of increased compartmental pressure include paresthesias, coldness, and decreased or absent pulses in the extremities. In the trunk, inelastic eschar can act as a corset, limiting lung expansion and preventing adequate respiration. In both cases, surgical intervention (escharotomy and/or fasciotomy) is required to relieve the pressure and prevent tissue death. An escharotomy is a surgical incision through the eschar, whereas a fasciotomy is a deeper incision extending through the fascia. Unless exposed tendon is present, the escharotomy region can be mobilized during therapy (Grigsby deLinde & Miles, 1995).

Dressings

After the initial burn assessment, the nursing staff applies dressings. The functions of dressings include protecting the wound against infection, maintaining contact between the topical agent and the wound, superficially **debriding** the wound, and providing comfort for the patient (Grigsby deLinde & Miles, 1995). Debriding is the removal of devitalized tissue from the wound site. Types of topical agents vary widely, although most are wide-spectrum antimicrobials. Examples include mafenide acetate (Sulfamylon), silver sulfadiazine (Silvadene), and 0.5% silver nitrate solution (Duncan & Driscoll, 1991). As a rule, the nursing staff changes the dressings; however, by periodically participating in dressing removal and application, the occupational therapist makes opportunities to view the healing wounds. This allows the therapist to monitor healing and adjust the therapy program accordingly.

PROCEDURES FOR PRACTICE 45-1

Hand Washing

Hand washing is the easiest and most effective thing you can do to prevent infections for you and your patients.

When to Wash

- Before and after all patient contact
- After removing gloves used to perform a task involving contact with blood, body fluids, or infectious material
- After handling possibly infectious devices or equipment
- Before and after preparing and eating food

General Procedure

- Dispense paper towel
- Push up long sleeves
- Wet hands and wrists
- Apply antiseptic solution or soap
- Use friction to clean between fingers, under nails, and palms and backs of hands; effective scrubbing lasts at least 20–30 seconds
- Rinse hands and towel dry
- Turn off faucet using paper towel
- Dispose of paper towel in appropriate trash barrel
- Waterless hand cleaner can be used until hand washing facilities are available

Infection Control

One of the functions of the skin is to act as a barrier against infection (Falkel, 1994). Therefore, a patient with a burn injury is susceptible to infection. It is essential that all staff, family, and visitors adhere to infection control procedures. This includes frequent hand washing, use of gloves when necessary, and avoiding cross-contamination through instruments and equipment (Procedures for Practice 45-1).

Contracture Formation

Patients with burn injuries are at significant risk for contractures. **Wound contracture**, a normal physiological response to an open wound (Greenhalgh & Staley, 1994; Staley, Richard, & Falkel, 1994), combined with prolonged immobilization, creates an opportunity for permanent soft tissue contracture. Contractures tend to occur in predictable patterns, usually flexed, shortened positions (e.g., elbow flexion, shoulder adduction, knee flexion) and can considerably limit the patient's ability to perform activities of daily living (ADL). For example, decreased elbow extension may limit the patient's ability to dress.

Occupational Therapy Assessment During the Emergent Phase

During the emergent phase, the occupational therapist performs a screen of the patient's needs. A full evaluation is deferred until after the emergent phase, when the patient is more medically stable. During the screen, the therapist notes the distribution of the burn and which joints are involved. This allows the occupational therapist to establish an appropriate splinting and positioning program. It is also during this time that the therapist begins collecting information regarding the patient's functional status before admission, including individual interests and social supports.

Occupational Therapy Intervention During the Emergent Phase

Occupational therapy in the emergent phase focuses on the prevention of early contracture formation through the use of splints and positioning programs. It is ideal to initiate occupational therapy intervention as early as 24–48 hours after burn because collagen synthesis and contracture formation begin during the initial response to thermal injury (Evans & McAuliffe, 1995; Institute for Healthcare Quality [IHQ], 1997).

Splinting

Ideally, splints are fabricated and applied in the initial visit, and a positioning program is established and communicated to the team. Table 45-1 describes common contracture patterns, **anti-deformity positions**, and appropriate splints. Generally, any joint involved in a superficial partial-thickness injury or worse has the potential for contracture and is usually splinted. Splint wearing times are determined by the patient's ability to use the involved extremity. That is, a decrease in active movement indicates the need for increased splint wearing time. For example, a heavily sedated patient cannot perform active movement and, therefore, requires splinting at all times except for therapy and dressing changes. An alert patient who can use his or her affected extremity for functional tasks, such as self-feeding or prescribed exercises, may require the use of splints only at night. Splints are applied over the burn dressing and secured with either gauze wrap or Velcro straps.

Positioning

Anti-deformity positioning, which is used as an adjunct to splinting for prevention of contractures, can be initiated in the first visit. For example, if a patient is unable to be fitted with a custom wrist extension splint, supporting the hand on a rolled pillow can, at least temporarily, maintain appropriate joint position. Elevating the upper extremi-

Table 45-1. Anti-Contracture Positioning by Location of Burn

Location of Burn	Contracture Tendency	Anti-Contracture Positioning and/or Typical Splint
Anterior neck	Neck flexion	Remove pillows; use half-mattress to extend the neck; neck extension splint or collar
Axilla	Adduction	120° abduction with slight external rotation; axilla splint or positioning wedges; watch for signs of brachial plexus strain
Anterior elbow	Flexion	Elbow extension splint in 5–10° flexion
Dorsal wrist	Wrist extension	Wrist support in neutral
Volar wrist	Wrist flexion	Wrist cockup splint in 5–10° flexion
Hand dorsal	Claw hand deformity	Functional hand splint with MP joints 70–90°, IP joints fully extended, first web open, thumb in opposition (safe position; see Chapter 42)
Hand volar	Palmar contracture	Palm extension splint
	Cupping of hand	MPs in slight hyperextension
Hip-anterior	Hip flexion	Prone positioning; weights on thigh in supine; knee immobilizers
Knee	Knee flexion	Knee extension positioning and/or splints; prevent external rotation, which may cause peroneal nerve compression
Foot	Foot drop	Ankle at 90° with foot board or splint; watch for signs of heel ulcer

Reprinted with permission from Pessina, M. A., & Ellis, S. M. (1997). Rehabilitation. *Nursing Clinics of North America, 32,* 367.

ties can also help to minimize upper extremity edema. Elevation can be done with foam wedges, pillows, or specialized arm troughs attached to the bed. A risk of upper extremity elevation is the potential for brachial plexus strain. Symptoms of brachial plexus strain include tingling, numbness, and cold fingers.

Acute Phase

The acute phase begins after the emergent phase and continues until the wound is closed, either by spontaneous healing or skin grafts (Grigsby deLinde & Miles, 1995). The acute phase can last several days to several months, depending on the extent of the burn and the amount of grafting required.

Support and Psychosocial Adjustment in the Acute Phase

All patients with burn injuries, regardless of age, exhibit some of the same psychological responses, including withdrawal, denial, fear of death, regression, anxiety, depression, and grief (Wright, 1984). In addition, various factors can influence a burn patient's psychological status. These include emotional trauma arising from the hospital stay, the length of the hospital stay, adjustment to physical changes, adjustment to others' reactions, and location and depth of the burn injury (Baker et al., 1996; LeDoux et al., 1996). Baker et al. (1996) refer to two stages of psychosocial recovery: the first alert stage and the pre-discharge stage. Performance can vary considerably between the two phases. During the first alert stage, the patient initially orients to the burn injury; a severely burned patient may simply be happy to be alive (Baker et al., 1996). It may not be until later, as the patient enters the rehabilitation phase and approaches the pre-discharge stage, that he or she begins to deal with the limitations in physical function. The patient, however, may also exhibit early signs of depression and withdrawal, and early assessment of the patient's psychosocial status is essential. LeDoux et al. (1996) state that the burn team can foster healthy coping strategies while working with the burn patient by using these techniques:

1. Identify strengths that each patient can emphasize, reminding him or her of the strength already involved in surviving a painful and frightening experience.
2. Validate sadness and fear.
3. Assist patient to achieve goals; this helps to show hope for the future.
4. Instill a belief that the patient can succeed.

Team Communication

Communication with all members of the team, including the patient and the patient's family and/or support system, throughout hospitalization is essential. During this acute phase, collaboration between the occupational therapist and the burn team is essential for several reasons, including (Pessina & Ellis, 1997):

1. Alerting the team to developing contractures and response to therapeutic intervention
2. Planning for perioperative splinting

3. Clarifying range-of-motion orders based on graft integrity
4. Teaching the team about environmental modifications or communication systems
5. Advocating on the patient's behalf regarding eventual outpatient needs

Medical Management

Skin grafting, which occurs primarily in the acute phase, is required when the dermal bed is sufficiently destroyed to prevent or significantly impair spontaneous regrowth of the epithelial tissue (Grigsby deLinde & Miles, 1995). If reepithelialization of the burn site has not occurred within 14 days of the injury or is not expected, grafting would be considered (Kagan & Warden, 1994). Skin grafting is generally performed for all **full-thickness burns** and for large, deep partial-thickness burns. Skin grafting entails both excision of necrotic (dead) tissue and the placement of skin or a skin substitute over the wound bed.

Types of Grafts

A variety of grafting procedures are available to the burn team. According to the size of the burn and the medical stability of the patient, the team may opt to use one or more of the graft types described next.

Autografts

Skin harvested from an unburned area of the patient is an autograft. Split-thickness autografts, the most frequently used, are taken at the level of the mid dermis (IHQ, 1997; Staley, Richard, & Falkel, 1994). Donor sites are ideally selected for the best match of color and texture to the affected area. As donor sites produce mild scarring, their location, when possible, is in an inconspicuous site, such as the upper thigh. The harvested skin can be left as a solid sheet (sheet graft) or perforated to increase surface area (meshed graft) (Staley, Richard, & Falkel, 1994). Meshing allows the surface area of the harvested skin to cover up to four times the original area. Both sheet and meshed grafts have advantages and disadvantages. A sheet graft has the best cosmetic outcome and is thus preferred for the face and hands (Duncan & Driscoll, 1991). Infection and the development of hematoma under a sheet graft, however, can cause complete graft loss and require regrafting. A meshed graft, although less cosmetically appealing (the meshed pattern is retained permanently), covers large areas when the donor site is limited. In addition, meshed grafts allow drainage of blood and exudate, which prevents hematomas and improves graft adherence (Duncan & Driscoll, 1991).

Temporary Grafts

In cases of extensive burn injuries, where there is not sufficient donor skin to cover all of the affected area with autograft, the burn team may opt to use temporary grafts until the donor site has healed sufficiently for reharvesting. These temporary dressings aid in wound management by decreasing infection, stimulating healing and preparing the wound bed for autograft skin, decreasing pain, and protecting exposed tendons, nerves, and blood vessels (Duncan & Driscoll, 1991). Examples include xenografts (medically manipulated bovine skin), allografts (cadaver skin), and biological dressings, such as Biobrane.

Occupational Therapy Assessment During the Acute Phase

During the acute phase, the occupational therapist performs a detailed initial evaluation. This includes a thorough chart review to determine the history of the wound and associated injuries. Previous medical history is also important. Associated diagnoses that may limit occupational performance, such as psychiatric illness, diabetes, or lung disease, are to be noted and accounted for during occupational therapy treatment planning. Areas specifically assessed by the occupational therapist during the initial evaluation include:

- ADL and instrumental activities of daily living (IADL)
- Psychosocial status and support systems
- Behavior and communication
- Cognitive-perceptual status
- Neuromuscular status (range of motion, strength, sensation)
- Activity tolerance

Evaluation can consist of observation during task performance, interviews with patient and family, and the use of standardized tests such as the *Functional Independence Measure* (Uniform Data System for Medical Rehabilitation, 1997). The potential for permanent scarring and disfigurement may cause significant anxiety and limit the patient's ability to participate in rehabilitation. Thus, early identification of the patient's support systems can improve functional outcomes.

Occupational Therapy Intervention During the Acute Phase

Due to the acute medical nature of many burn injuries, treatment in the acute phase focuses on capacities and abilities such as range of motion and strength. These are addressed through continued splinting, positioning, exercise, and activity. Other potential treatment activities include environmental modifications, pain remediation, environmental adaptation, and patient and family education. In the acute phase, the individual's ability to participate in treatment related to self-care and functional retraining is often limited by complex medical issues. These areas are addressed in detail during the rehabilitation phase.

Splinting and Positioning

During the acute phase, the splinting and positioning programs established in the emergent phase are continually monitored and adjusted. Splinting schedules are adjusted according to the individual's ability to participate in an exercise and positioning program. For example, if a patient consistently uses an affected elbow for self-feeding and ADL during the day, decreasing the wearing time for the elbow splint to nights and rest periods is appropriate. Conversely, a patient who cannot follow through with an exercise and positioning program because of impaired alertness or poor motivation should wear a splint continuously except for dressing changes and therapeutic activity. It is imperative to check all splints daily to ensure proper fit and function. In addition, teaching the nursing staff proper fit and application of splints can decrease the potential for complications (Pessina & Ellis, 1997).

Exercise and Activity

In the acute phase, splinting and positioning are used in combination with exercise and activity. Exercise is especially important to control edema and prevent muscle atrophy, tendon adherence, joint stiffness, and capsular shortening (Harden & Luster, 1991). Exercise types include passive range of motion, active range of motion, active assistive range of motion, and functional activity. If the patient cannot participate in active exercise or activity because of poor medical status or impaired level of alertness, passive range of motion is indicated. Active exercise is encouraged whenever possible, however, (Burke Evans et al., 1996; Wright, 1984), and it is the role of the therapist to guide the patient toward function. Within a single treatment session, a patient may participate in all of these forms of exercise. In fact, functional activities may be used to improve active range of motion. Exercise and activity programs are performed up to five times daily (Wright). Contraindications to exercise include exposed tendons, recent autografts (approximately 5–10 days), acute medical complications, and fractures (Duran-Coleman, 1991; Grigsby deLinde & Miles, 1995; Staley, Richard, & Falkel, 1994). In addition, periodic inspection of the wound by the occupational therapist is essential to determine status of wound healing and skin integrity as related to tolerance of the exercise program.

Perioperative Care

The 5–10 days after a skin graft procedure is the perioperative period. A patient with a large burn injury may make many trips to the operating room for skin grafting. Each surgical procedure begins a new perioperative stage. For example, a patient needing grafting on the trunk, arms, and legs may make three trips to the operating room, with each successive area requiring proper perioperative care. The role of the occupational therapist in the perioperative period is to fabricate custom splints to immobilize the newly grafted areas in anti-deformity positions. Ideally, splints are fabricated immediately prior to or during surgery and applied at the conclusion of the surgery. These splints usually stay in place, along with the primary dressing, for 5–10 days (Duran-Coleman, 1991; Grigsby deLinde & Miles, 1995). During this time, range-of-motion exercises are contraindicated to allow for graft adherence. After the primary dressing is removed, the burn team assesses the graft adherence, and a determination is made regarding the appropriateness of resuming exercise.

Pain Management

The occupational therapist must address pain issues that arise during treatment. Many patients in intensive care cannot verbalize subjective response to manipulation, such as during dressing changes or exercise. In these cases, the therapist monitors objective responses to pain, such as blood pressure, heart rate, and respiratory rate, and adjusts the treatment accordingly. If necessary, the time of the treatment may be changed to allow pain medication to be administered. Decreased repetitions and increased rest breaks during exercise sessions may also be appropriate. Other techniques used to manage pain throughout recovery include distraction techniques, meditation, and visualization. Activity context and emotional state can also affect perception of pain (Dubner & Ren, 1999).

Environmental Adaptation

Beginning in the acute phase and throughout recovery, the occupational therapist provides modified call buttons and bed controls, voice-activated telephone systems, and modified utensils (Fig. 45-3) and self-care items. These modifications, combined with patient, staff, and family education, can increase a patient's sense of control and independence. The development of environmental modifi-

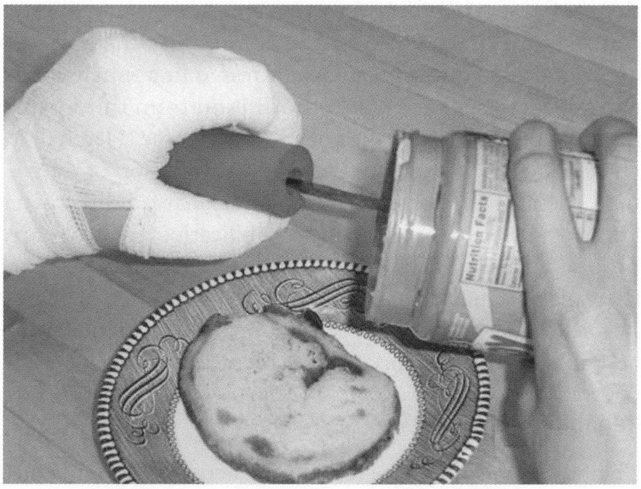

Figure 45-3 Modified utensils can increase independence in the acute phase.

cations is limited only by the patient's motivation and the therapist's creativity.

Patient and Family Teaching

The occupational therapist provides members of the patient's support system with guidance regarding ways to interact with and support the patient during recovery. They may be encouraged to make tape recordings and posters or to bring in favorite music or foods. They may need to learn new ways to touch or comfort their loved one. In addition, the family and friends provide a source of information regarding the patient's vocational and avocational roles and available community resources if the patient cannot communicate this information. An educated family and/or support system can be an important asset for ensuring follow-through of exercise and splinting programs and for encouraging participation in functional activities (Duran-Coleman, 1991).

Discharge Planning

Since hospital stays are generally short, discharge planning begins as soon as possible after admission (Fletchall & Hickerson, 1995; Rivers & Jordan, 1998). Many patients in the acute phase are discharged directly home or leave a burn center for continued care on a rehabilitation unit. Elements to consider during discharge planning are the availability of community resources for outpatient or follow-up care, support systems available to the patient, and physical demands of the home environment. When patients who have sustained major burns cannot return to the hospital where they received acute care, it is important for the inpatient occupational therapist to establish a relationship with a therapist in the patient's community to ensure continuity of care throughout the rehabilitation phase. In accordance with the knowledge and experience of the community therapist, the discharging therapist provides appropriate literature and written, photographic, and/or videotaped descriptions of the rehabilitation program. This establishes a communication channel for the community therapist so questions and concerns can be addressed in a timely manner. Whenever possible, all authorization from third-party payers should be established prior to discharge (Fletchall & Hickerson, 1995) to avoid delays in the initiation of outpatient therapy. If a patient cannot be discharged directly to home, transfer to an inpatient rehabilitation facility is appropriate; again, early communication with the receiving therapist is necessary to ensure continuity of care. Regardless of the discharge setting, well-briefed patients are best able to advocate for appropriate care.

Rehabilitation Phase

The rehabilitation phase follows the acute phase and continues until scar maturation (Rivers & Jordan, 1998). Scar maturation can take 6 months to 2 years (Rivers & Jordan, 1998; Staley, Richard, & Falkel, 1994). It is considered complete when the scar becomes pale and the rate of collagen synthesis levels off (Grigsby deLinde & Miles, 1995). The level of direct involvement of the occupational therapist during this extended time is varied. It may range from daily inpatient treatment to weekly outpatient treatment to annual clinic visits.

Occupational Therapy Assessment During the Rehabilitation Phase

During the rehabilitation phase, the occupational therapist continues to assess capacities and abilities such as range of motion and strength. In addition, functional assessments specific to self-care and homemaking are valuable in guiding treatment planning and preparing for discharge. Standardized tests, such as the *Functional Independence Measure* (Uniform Data System for Medical Rehabilitation, 1997) and the *Valpar Work Samples* (Resources 45-1) are important because they provide objective data.

Occupational Therapy Intervention During Rehabilitation Phase

The overall goal of this phase is to facilitate the patient's return to his or her previous level of occupational performance. Patients are encouraged to take increasing responsibility for their care, including helping to establish meaningful goals. In addition to range of motion and strength, occupational therapy also focuses on activity tolerance, sensation, coordination, scar management, and self-care and home management skills.

Range of Motion

In the rehabilitation stage, the patient continues to benefit from daily stretching routines established in the acute

RESOURCE 45-1

Burns
American Burn Association (ABA)
ABA Central Office – Chicago
625 N. Michigan Avenue, Suite 2550
Chicago, IL 60611
Phone: (312) 642-9260
E-mail: info@ameriburn.org
www.ameriburn.org

Burn Survivors Online
E-mail: info@burnsurvivor-sonline.com
www.burnsurvivors online.com

Journal of Burn Care and Rehabilitation
Published by Lippincott Williams and Wilkins
Glenn D. Warden, MD, Editor in Chief
Shriners Burns Hospital
3229 Burnet Avenue
Cincinnati, OH 45229
Phone: (513) 872-6202
www.burncarerehab.com

Valpar Work Samples
Valpar International Corporation
P.O. Box 5767
Tucson, AZ 85703-5767

phase of care. In the early part of this phase, the rate of collagen synthesis is increased (Staley, Richard, & Falkel, 1994), requiring the patient to stretch frequently throughout the day. As the scar matures and collagen synthesis slows, decreased frequency of stretching is required. At all times, skin integrity must be monitored during stretching to prevent tearing. Massage using a non–water-based cream should precede stretching to help prevent dry skin from rupturing (Rivers & Jordan, 1998). An appropriate stretch consists of bringing the tissue to the point of **blanching**, or becoming pale, and holding it in that position for several seconds. The patient should report tension but not pain. Overzealous stretching can result in tissue tears and edema, which increase joint stiffness. Stretching is initially performed by the occupational therapist. With training, however, the patient and/or caregiver can also complete stretching routines.

Strength

Resistive exercise and graded functional activities can improve strength. For example, a patient may be taught an independent exercise program with resistive rubber ribbon or tubing, such as Theraband, to increase proximal upper body strength. Patients also gain strength as they perform self-care activities, such as progressing from sitting to standing for hygiene activities.

Activity Tolerance

A key feature of rehabilitation is mobilizing the patient as much as possible, thereby increasing the patient's activity tolerance. For an inpatient, this includes increased time spent out of bed and trips to the gym and off the nursing unit. For an outpatient, this may mean resuming leisure activities and going on community outings.

Sensation

Newly healed skin and grafted skin may be hypersensitive. Hypersensitivity can be addressed effectively by systematic desensitization. This can be achieved by asking the patient to manipulate objects with varying textures in the environment. Initially, the patient practices holding soft textures, such as cotton balls or lambswool, and then progresses to manipulating objects with rougher textures, such as Velcro or burlap. Sometimes a formal system such as the Downey desensitization program (Barber, 1990) is used (see Chapter 27).

Coordination

Coordination can be impaired by a variety of factors, including limited range of motion, strength, or sensation. Coordination can be improved through the use of selected progressive tasks designed to challenge the patient's skills. For example, a patient may be asked first to take lids off large jars and then smaller containers (Fig. 45-4). The patient may also trace large letters or patterns before attempting to work a crossword puzzle.

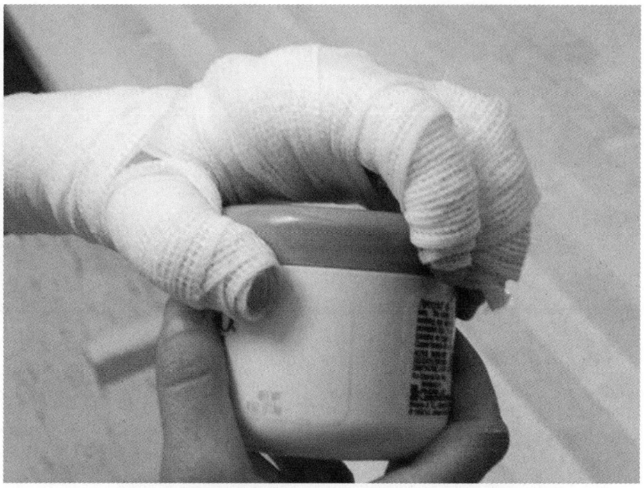

Figure 45-4 Coordination can be addressed with use of simulated or actual functional tasks.

Scar Management

Scar tissue formation is a natural response to wound healing (Grisby deLinde & Miles, 1995). It begins in the emergent phase and may take up to 2 years (Poh-Fitzpatrick, 1992). A hypertrophic scar is an aberration of the normal healing process and presents as a red, raised, and inelastic scar (Abston, 1987) (Fig. 45-5). A hypertrophic scar contains an increased number of fibroblasts as compared to normal skin, and the collagen fibers are arranged in a nodular as opposed to parallel fashion (Abston, 1987). There is thought to be a disruption in the balance between collagen synthesis and lysis (Grigsby deLinde & Miles, 1995). The tendency for hypertrophic scarring is unique to each individual. In general, patients with large amounts of pigment in the skin and young patients are most prone to hypertrophic scarring. Hypertrophic scarring is also inversely related to the depth of the initial burn wound (Staley, Richard, & Falkel, 1994). In addition to being cosmetically unappealing, hypertrophic scars can limit functional skills by restricting joint range of motion.

Occupational Therapy Assessment of Scars

The *Burn Scar Index* (*Vancouver Scar Scale*) is the most widely used standardized scar assessment tool and is used to rate the pliability, vascularity, height, and pigmentation of scars (Sullivan et al., 1990). Used periodically, the *Burn Scar Index* can help guide the occupational therapist in determining effective scar management and evaluating the stage of scar maturation. Other assessments include the *Patient and Observer Scar Assessment Scale* (Draaijers et al., 2004) and the *Matching Assessment of Scars and Photographs* (Masters, McMahon, & Svens, 2005).

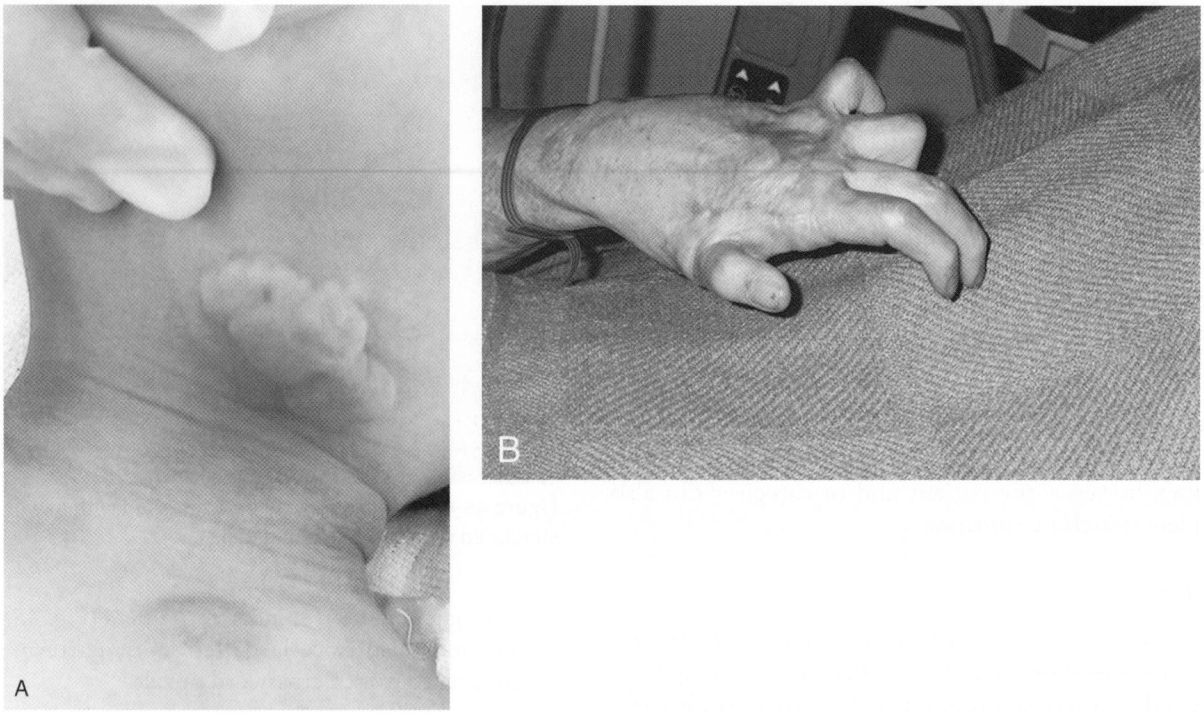

Figure 45-5 Hypertrophic scars on the neck (**A**) and hand (**B**). The hypertrophic scar on the dorsum of the hand causes claw hand deformity.

Occupational Therapy Intervention and Scar Management

The occupational therapist attempts to prevent or limit the development of hypertrophic scars. Treatment methods include a combination of techniques, including massage, pressure therapy, and the use of specialized inserts.

Massage

Massage may be useful in reducing scar contracture (Staley, Richard, & Falkel, 1994). Scar massage is initiated when it is determined that the injured area can withstand slight friction. In addition, scar massage maintains suppleness, as normal sweat and oil gland function is often disrupted. Scar massage also aids in desensitization. Scar massage is performed several times daily with deep pressure (enough to blanch the scar temporarily) in either a circular pattern or perpendicular to the long axis of the scar. Lotion is used during massage to reduce friction. Perfume-free lotions are preferred to decrease potential irritation to newly healed skin. Initially, scar massage is the responsibility of the occupational therapist so that skin integrity and tolerance can be monitored. Once an established routine has been developed, the therapist teaches the patient and/or caregivers to assume responsibility for daily scar massage.

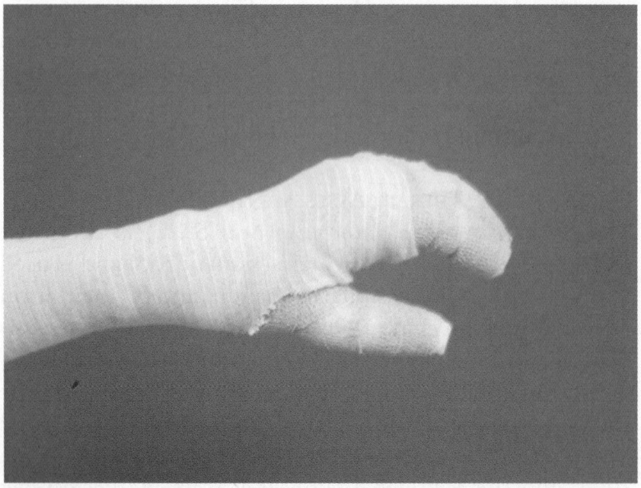

Figure 45-6 Gentle pressure is applied using Coban and Tubigrip.

Pressure Dressings and Garments

Pressure dressings and garments are another form of scar management that has been advocated in the literature (Chang et al., 1995; Ward, 1991). The flattened, smooth, supple appearance of the scar after application of pressure has been reported clinically, but objective support has been inconclusive (Grigsby deLinde & Miles, 1995; Ward, 1991). The occupational therapist initiates the application of gentle pressure via Tubigrip, elastic bandage wraps, Coban, or Isotoner gloves (Fig. 45-6). Initially pressure dressings are applied for 2-hour intervals. Wearing time is gradually increased by 2-hour increments until 24-hour wear is tolerated. Tolerance is determined by lack of blisters or open areas. At this point, increased pressure using customized products such as Jobst or Bioconcepts garments is indicated (Fig. 45-7). Staley, Richard, and Falkel (1994) suggest that the application of 25 mm Hg of pres-

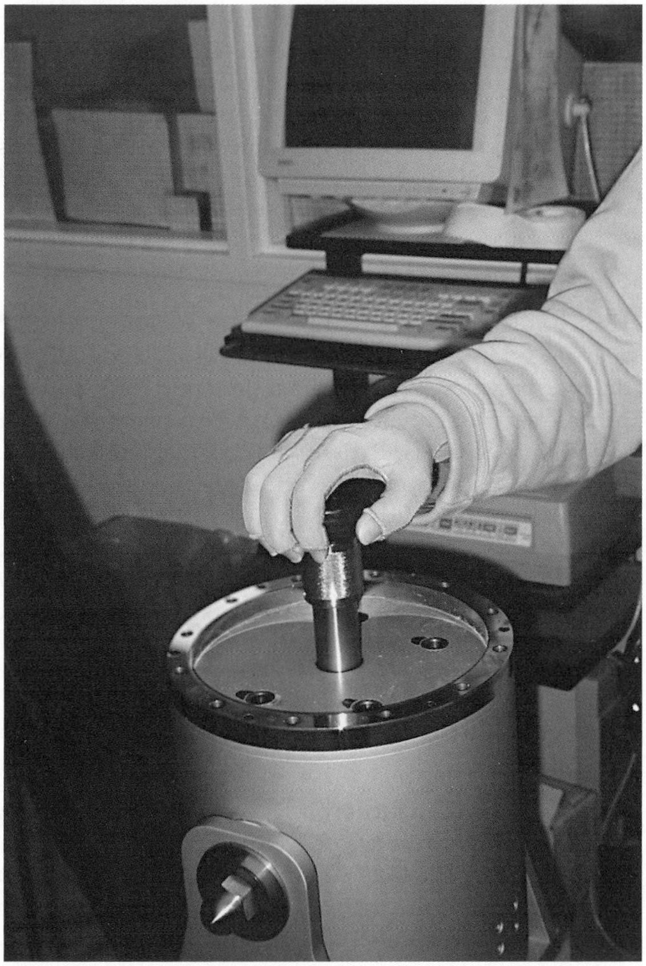

Figure 45-7 Custom pressure garments can be worn while performing simulated functional activity.

sure is ideal to aid in collagen organization, which ultimately helps decrease scar tissue formation. Custom garments cause notable shearing during application and removal and thus should be used only when the skin is healed sufficiently to withstand these forces. Wearing of custom garments continues until the scar is inactive, or mature, as described earlier. The therapist's role is to initiate the ordering of custom garments and oversee their use. Most providers of custom garments send trained personnel to measure the patient for custom fitting. For facial burns, the patient may use a transparent facial orthosis secured by elastic straps to provide even pressure distribution. These orthoses are usually fabricated by a specially trained orthotist at the request of the therapist.

Inserts are often used in conjunction with pressure garments. They may be constructed from products such as Otoform, Elastomere, or closed cell foam. Their purpose is to increase pressure in concave areas, such as the web spaces and the sternoclavicular depression. Silicone inserts have also been demonstrated to be effective in improving some characteristics of hypertrophic scars (Ahn, Monafo, & Mustoe, 1989), although the mechanism of action remains to be determined. The design of a scar management program is determined by the available resources, careful clinical observation, and the patient's ability to comply with the program (Evans & McAuliffe, 1995). Periodic outpatient visits to occupational therapy or an established burn clinic throughout the rehabilitation phase allow for monitoring and adjustments of the scar management program.

Self-Care and Home Management Skills

If neuromuscular limitations impede the patient's performance of functional tasks, the therapist may provide adaptive equipment, such as built-up handles for impaired grasp or long-handled utensils for decreased elbow flexion. Teaching adaptive techniques, such as performing certain activities using two hands for extra support, may also improve function.

Patient and Family Teaching

Patients should understand the rationale for each of the splints and techniques used in their care. They participate in the development of goals, so that they are invested in achieving them. Skin care is an important element in discharge teaching. Patients practice monitoring their skin for breakdown and caring for their skin, including the daily use of a moisturizer. They learn to use a sunscreen with an SPF of at least 15 (reapplied frequently) if they anticipate exposure to the sun (Staley, Richard, & Falkel, 1994). In addition, patients should have a basic understanding of wound healing and tissue response to exercise and scar management techniques.

Support and Psychosocial Adjustment During the Rehabilitation Phase

Although the patient and family typically focus on survival immediately after injury, many other issues arise during rehabilitation. For example, guilt or embarrassment regarding the injury may lead the patient to withdraw. The patient may also begin questioning his or her ability to return to the role of a parent or provider, which creates anxiety. Patients may have fear about their ability to maintain relationships and be concerned regarding sexual functioning. The increase in activity in the rehabilitation phase not only assists physical rehabilitation but also assists patients to discover how their injury affects their daily lives. Emotional reactions to the realization of loss may produce a wide range of behaviors, such as crying and expression of anger. Patients may also have responses related to post-traumatic stress disorder, such as flashbacks.

One of the most difficult challenges for the burn therapist is caring for patients as they grieve for a functional limitation or alteration in body image (Pessina & Ellis, 1997). The occupational therapist supports the patient by encouraging questions and verbalization of feelings about the burn injury (Pessina & Ellis, 1997). The occupational therapist also chooses treatment activities to restore confidence and self-esteem. Group activities provide opportunities for socialization and sharing of concerns in a safe environment (Summers, 1991). Given the extensive contact with the patient throughout all phases of recovery, the occupational therapist is in a unique position to identify and address psychosocial issues, but consultation with other specialists on the burn team (e.g., nursing staff, family members, social workers, and psychologists) is essential.

Potential Complications

In addition to the potential for soft tissue contractures and loss of joint range of motion, other complications may occur in any phase of burn recovery.

Pruritus

Pruritus (persistent itching) is a common complication (IHQ, 1997; Staley, Richard, & Falkel, 1994), presumably due to nerve regeneration. It usually resolves within 2 years of the initial injury (Poh-Fitzpatrick, 1992). The use of compression garments, skin moisturizers, cold packs, and medications such as antihistamines may alleviate itching (IHQ, 1997).

Microstomia

Patients with facial burns in the area of the mouth are at risk for oral commissure contracture (microstomia) (Rivers & Jordan, 1998), which is tightening of the musculature around the lip area that limits mouth opening. In extreme cases, urgent surgical revision is required. This risk is exaggerated if the patient has undergone prolonged periods without eating or speaking because of intubation or respiratory compromise. In addition to daily scar massage, the therapist can teach the patient facial stretching exercises, such as yawning or grinning widely and pursing lips together. The exercises can be combined with the wearing of a microstomia splint to stretch the oral commissure. The splint may be worn as tolerated, usually starting with 10 minutes and gradually increasing to 60 minutes twice a day. These devices can be purchased or constructed by the occupational therapist. The cognitive level of the patient is an extremely important factor in use of a microstomia device because of the risk of an unexpected airway emergency. For example, a heavily sedated or confused patient may attempt to swallow the device.

Heterotopic Ossification

Heterotopic ossification, or myositis ossificans, is the development of new bone in tissues that normally do not ossify. It occurs in up to 13% of patients with major burns (Dutcher & Johnson, 1994). The most common location in the burn-injured population is the elbow, although the shoulder, knee, and hip can also be affected (Dutcher & Johnson, 1994). Heterotopic ossification causes pain, swelling, and rapid loss of range of motion. The therapist must be aware of the symptoms and alert the team so treatment options, including medications and surgery, can be discussed. ***Aggressive range of motion is contraindicated.***

Heat Intolerance

Heat intolerance is caused by loss of sweating, as split-thickness skin grafts do not contain sweat glands (Grigsby deLinde & Miles, 1995; Rivers & Jordan, 1998). To compensate for this, patients may sweat excessively in remaining unburned areas. Patients in extremely hot climates may require additional air conditioners in the home to maintain comfort (Rivers & Jordan, 1998). The lack of sweat glands also makes healed grafts susceptible to extreme dryness (Grigsby deLinde & Miles, 1995; Staley, Richard, & Falkel, 1994), and patients are encouraged to use moisturizing cream often throughout the day.

RECONSTRUCTIVE SURGERY

An important element in burn recovery is the planning and execution of reconstructive procedures. Despite diligent efforts by the burn team and patient, contractures may develop. Reconstructive surgery can be useful in correcting these deformities. Surgery is typically performed once the scar tissue is mature; however, it may be necessary to perform reconstructive surgery before scar maturation if a severe functional deficit is present (Robson et al., 1992). For example, an axillary contracture, which limits abduction to 80°, may significantly interfere with dressing and hygiene. A surgical procedure, a **Z-plasty**, can be performed to elongate soft tissue (Robson et al., 1992; Staley, Richard, & Falkel, 1994). A skin graft to cover the deficit may be necessary once the contracture is released.

Occupational Therapy Assessment Related to Reconstructive Procedures

When results of functional assessment suggest that the patient's progress toward his or her self-management goals has ceased because of a contracture, the occupational therapist communicates to the burn team the possible need for surgical release of the contracture.

Occupational Therapy Intervention Related to Reconstructive Procedures

Post-operatively, the occupational therapist provides a custom splint to immobilize and protect the graft in its new lengthened position. After approximately 10–14 days, the therapist initiates an exercise program beginning with gentle active range of motion and progressing to more aggressive exercise and activity as skin integrity tolerates. Pressure therapy over the newly grafted area minimizes scarring. This includes the use of a pressure garment and an insert fabricated to match the contours of the new graft.

RETURN TO WORK

Returning to work before final scar maturation preserves function and improves the patient's self-concept (Rivers & Jordan, 1998). The physician provides medical clearance for return to work. During the initial evaluation in the acute phase, the occupational therapist gathers information regarding the work history of the patient and specific job demands the patient previously encountered daily. With this information, the occupational therapist can guide treatment activities to prepare for return to the previous level of functioning. For example, if the patient was employed as a mechanic prior to injury, tool use should be incorporated into treatment activities as soon as possible. Patients may need job retraining if the extent of the injury renders the original job demands now unrealistic. In this case, the occupational therapist works with the patient and employer to explore appropriate job modifications.

Return-to-work parameters are ideally based on the percentage of body surface area affected, whether the job requires the use of the affected body part, and the depth of the burn (IHQ, 1997). Fletchall and Hickerson (1995) investigated the effectiveness of a daily 6-hour outpatient program beginning immediately after discharge. Patients in this program, with burns to the upper extremity and hands averaging less than 25% of TBSA, returned to work in an average of 8 weeks; patients in a similar population who participated in traditional outpatient therapy returned in an average of 19 weeks. In addition, the experimental program was shown to reduce the overall costs to the health care payer (Fletchall & Hickerson). Assignment of a case manager early during the inpatient phase also facilitated the progression from rehabilitation to return to work (Fletchall & Hickerson).

SPECIAL CONSIDERATIONS FOR HAND BURNS

Hand burns resulting in significant functional limitations occur quite frequently (Wright-Howell, 1989). The high rate of injury to the hand is because individuals use their hands to protect themselves or to extinguish the fire (Tanigawa, O'Donnell, & Graham, 1974). Dorsal hand burns occur more frequently than palmar injuries (Tanigawa, O'Donnell, & Graham, 1974). As previously noted, significant edema usually occurs in response to thermal injury. This pulls the hand into a position of deformity (Sheridan et al., 1995) characterized by thumb radial abduction, digital metacarpal hyperextension, interphalangeal joint flexion, and flattening of the palmar arches (Wright-Howell, 1989). If this position is maintained, the result is joint contracture and severe functional limitation.

Evaluation of Hand Burns

A comprehensive hand evaluation includes determination of whether range-of-motion limitations are due to joint stiffness, intrinsic muscle tightness, extrinsic muscle tightness, or inelasticity of skin. Other factors that limit hand flexibility and decrease range of motion include pain, bulky dressings, exposed tendons, and the presence of eschar, which is inelastic. Once the clinician determines the cause of range-of-motion limitations, an effective treatment plan can be devised.

Treatment of Hand Burns

The occupational therapist must provide appropriate splinting and exercise programs to prevent contracture and expedite functional use of the burned hand. The appropriate splinting position of the hand is described in Table 45-1. In this position, the collateral ligaments of the metacarpophalangeal (MP), proximal interphalangeal (PIP), and distal interphalangeal joints are positioned at length, preventing ligamentous contracture so that maximum digital range of motion is preserved.

Two distinct options exist for thumb position. Radial abduction maintains the first web space at maximum length. We prefer palmar abduction, however, as this is a position of function. Hand burns are typically dorsal. When present, a deep palmar burn can lead to palmar contracture. In this case, a volar hand extension splint is appropriate. When using this position, however, careful monitoring of MP flexion is critical to prevent shortening of the collateral ligaments. Unfortunately, evidence is lacking regarding specific splint positions and schedules. According to Richard and Ward (2005), "Controversy about splinting in burn care is not based on the rationale for and success of splinting, but exists because of the paucity of validation of its use." A list of splinting options for the conditions previously discussed follows (see Chapter 16 for splint illustrations):

- Dynamic PIP extension splint such as Capaner, LMB, or banana splints for PIP stiffness: start 10 minutes three times a day, increase wearing time as tolerated, not to exceed 60 minutes at a time.

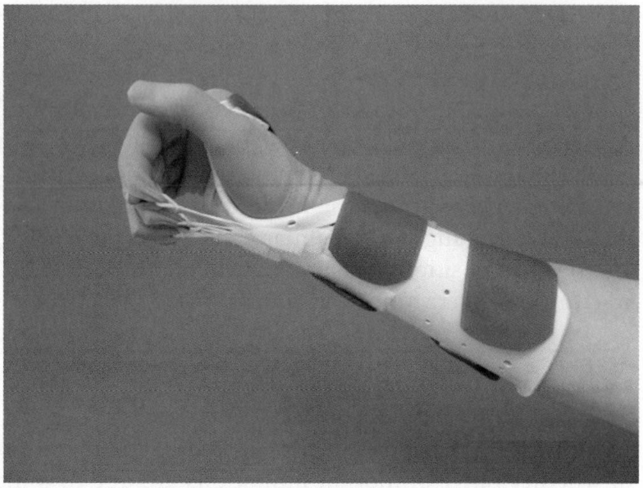

Figure 45-8 Dynamic flexion glove.

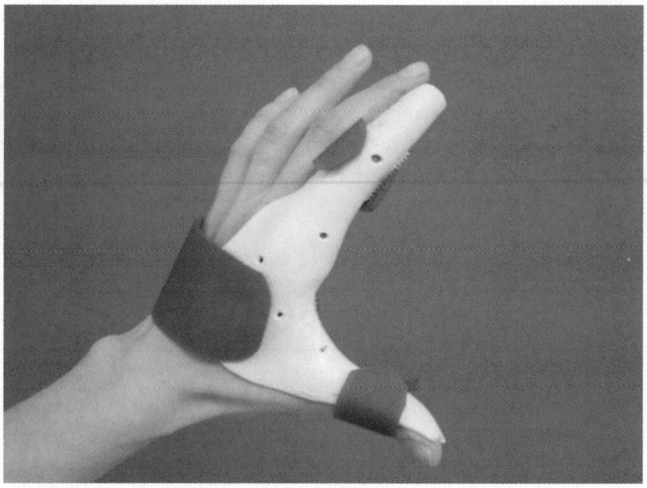

Figure 45-9 C-splint in radial abduction.

- Dynamic flexion splint in which the MPs are blocked in full extension while the IPs are passively flexed (for intrinsic muscle tightness): start 10 minutes three times a day, increase wearing time as tolerated, not to exceed 60 minutes at a time.
- Forearm-based dynamic flexion splint that offers composite MP-IP flexion (Fig. 45-8) (for extrinsic extensor tightness or inelastic skin that limits composite flexion): start 10 minutes three times a day, increasing as tolerated but not to exceed 45 minutes.
- Volar forearm-based static extension splint (for extrinsic flexor tightness): wear at night.
- Forearm-based dynamic extension splint (for extrinsic flexor tightness): wear periodically during the day, starting with 10 minutes three times per day and progressing to 45 minutes as tolerated.

Often, individuals do not present with a single limitation; rather, a combination of factors limits the individual's range of motion. The clinician must determine which factor is the primary source of dysfunction and modify the treatment accordingly. Appropriate splints are always used in conjunction with exercises, functional activities, and scar management techniques. Splints should never be used to the extent that they limit or prevent performance of ADL activities.

Potential Complications of Hand Burns

Normal hand anatomy can be characterized by a balance of levers and pulleys that work harmoniously to achieve motion. Damage to this balanced network results in significant functional limitations.

Extensor Tendon Injury

Extensor tendon injury is often associated with dorsal hand burns because they lie superficially on the dorsal aspect of the hand. Limitations can be due to direct thermal injury or tendon ischemia (Wright-Howell, 1989). Due to the close proximity of structures, the formation of scar tissue can greatly limit tendon excursion and create imbalance. This can result in contracture development. Boutonniere and swan-neck deformities are the result of extensor tendon damage (Evans & McAuliffe, 1995; Rosenthal, 1995; Wright-Howell, 1989).

Web Space Contractures

Web space contractures can be due to overgrafting of the web spaces, muscle shortening (contracture of the adductor pollicis brevis resulting in a first web space contracture), joint stiffness, or skin graft contracture in a normal response to tissue healing. Splints, scar management, and exercise are effective treatment modalities. First web space contractures (between the thumb and index finger) respond well to a web space C-splint (Fig. 45-9) that is lined with Otoform, a silicon gel sheet, or Elastomere. This is usually worn at night for 6–8 hours. During the day, the individual performs stretching, massage, and functional activities that encourage full range of motion of the affected area. For example, an individual with a first web space contracture is asked to pick up containers of various sizes, using palmar abduction to promote full abduction of the thumb. A dynamic splint with an insert that exerts pressure over the second, third, and fourth web spaces can be appropriate for digital web space contractures. Another option is the addition of web space inserts under a Jobst or Isotoner glove.

OUTCOME STUDIES

Long-term outcomes and quality of life after major burn injuries are of significant concern to those working in the field of burn rehabilitation. A research tool that has been established to address this issue is the *Burn Specific Health Scale* (*BSHS*) (Blalock, Bunker, & DeVellis, 1994). This scale is a 31-item instrument that includes items in seven categories: simple functional abilities, work, body image, interpersonal relationships, affect, heat sensitivity, and treatment programs. When the scale was administered to 244 patients from eight burn centers, it was found both reliable and valid (Blalock, Bunker, & DeVellis, 1994). Subjects were asked to report their functioning using a 5-point scale, with 1 indicating extremely good function and 5 indicating none at all. The mean values for employed patients in the categories of simple functional abilities, body image, and interpersonal relationships were 4.77, 3.74, and 4.60, respectively (Blalock, Bunker, & DeVellis, 1994).

Baker et al. (1996) performed an outcome study using the *Burn Specific Health Scale* to identify factors affecting physical functioning and psychological status of 31 adult patients who had sustained burn injuries. The study concluded that minor first-degree burns can significantly affect an individual's physical and psychological functioning (Baker et al., 1996). These results highlight the fact that patients whose burns are not severe may undergo physical and psychological ramifications similar to those of patients with major burn injuries (Baker et al., 1996). Baker et al. also state that the psychosocial influence of a burn injury may, in some cases, provide a growth experience and actually enhance self-esteem as the patient takes pride in the tremendous accomplishment of recuperation.

LeDoux et al. (1996) administered to 32 burn survivors two standardized instruments that measured self-perception of competence and adequacy. Many of the patients used denial as a coping mechanism, and this was found to be beneficial to their perception of competence. The study demonstrated that the patients did not accept feelings of being helpless or hopeless but rather seemed to change their value systems to reflect areas they could control. They placed less value on social acceptance, athletic competence, and physical appearance and more value on job competence, romantic appeal, and scholastic appeal—areas they believed they could control and develop (LeDoux et al., 1996).

Another study investigated hand function after acute hand burns (Sheridan et al., 1995). The study examined 659 patients with a total of 1047 hand burns. It was reported that normal function was resumed in 97% of patients with superficial injuries and 81% of patients with deep dermal or full-thickness injuries. Of the patients with severe injuries, which included tendon damage or joint capsule or bone involvement, only 9% had normal function, while 90% were able to compensate for this and independently perform ADL (Sheridan et al., 1995).

A more recent study published by Sheridan et al. in 2000 investigated the long-term outcome of children surviving major burn injuries (>70% TBSA) using a validated quality-of-life scale administered an average of 14 years post injury. The authors reported that most children had a satisfying quality of life. The majority of the subjects (72%) were either full-time students or gainfully employed. Statistical analysis revealed that key factors such as early return to pre-burn activities and comprehensive burn care that included experienced multidisciplinary aftercare played an important role in recovery (Sheridan et al., 2000). The authors are careful to note that, "Children who survive massive burns will have major cosmetic and functional impairments that can never be completely corrected" (Sheridan et al., 2000).

When outcomes were assessed in adult survivors of severe burn injuries, the results were similar (Druery et al., 2005). Using an abbreviated form of the *BSHS* to assess function and quality of life in adults surviving burns >40% TBSA, it was determined that the majority of these burn survivors developed functional independence and a good quality of life (Druery et al., 2005).

Although evidence is growing that patients who sustain burn injuries can expect generally positive outcomes, little evidence is available to guide the occupational therapy clinician in choosing specific treatment approaches and modalities. The lack of evidence in this field prevents a formal assessment of evidence related to occupational therapy practice. It highlights the need of occupational therapists to participate in outcome-based research related to the treatment of patients with burn injuries. As specialists in the evaluation and treatment of function, occupational therapists have a responsibility to continue to enhance the knowledge base in this area (see Resources 45-1).

CASE EXAMPLE

Mrs. J.: Burn Rehabilitation

Occupational Therapy Process	Objectives	Clinical Reasoning Process Examples of Therapist's Internal Dialogue
Patient Information Mrs. J. is a 42-year-old woman who sustained a 45% TBSA burn as a result of a house fire. She presented to the emergency department with superficial and superficial partial-thickness burns to her face and neck and deep partial- and full-thickness burns to both upper extremities and hands (dorsal aspect only), chest, and proximal aspect of her bilateral lower extremities. She also sustained an inhalation injury and was intubated and sedated. She was admitted to the intensive care unit. No significant medical history was reported. Split-thickness skin grafts (STSGs) were performed to her chest and upper thighs 3 days after admission. STSGs were performed to her arms and hands 10 days after admission. After skin grafting was complete, Mrs. J. was extubated and moved to a private room. She was on a regular diet and could walk independently. She was noted to be withdrawn and was concerned regarding her ability to care for her 3-year-old daughter. Her husband and sister were present and supportive throughout her hospitalization.	Understand the patient's diagnosis or condition Know the person	"Split-thickness skin grafts have the potential for contracture, which means we will have to work hard to ensure full return of her upper extremity function. In addition, STSGs may result in some scarring, which means a scar management program will need to begin as soon as possible." "From the pictures her family has brought in, it seems she took great pride in caring for her daughter—doing her hair, getting her dressed, etc. I can work with her to create goals related to care for her daughter that will be motivating for her and will reassure her that she will, in fact, be able to resume care for her child. Also, it appears that Mrs. J. has good family support. I wonder how available her husband and sister will be now that Ms. J. is beginning rehabilitation. It seems that often, after the acute crisis is over, many family members need to return to their jobs, at least to some extent."
Reason for Referral to Occupational Therapy Mrs. J. was referred to occupational therapy during the acute phase to prevent contractures that might result in deficits in occupational functioning, to provide patient and family education, and to address psychosocial sequelae related to the burn injury.	Appreciate the context Develop provisional hypotheses	"I am going to suggest regular team meetings to discuss goals and monitor Mrs. J.'s progress. It will be important for the team to recognize if she is becoming more withdrawn or depressed. I will also need to know what services will be available as she prepares for discharge. I anticipate that OT intervention can help in many aspects of recovery, from restoring performance skills, such as range of motion, to returning to important life roles such as caring for her family."
Assessment Process and Results (performed on transition to rehabilitation phase) Assessment of wound healing: Immature scar noted on bilateral forearms and dorsum of both hands Assessment of cognitive/social status: Awake and alert for several short periods throughout the day; also noted to appear withdrawn, not seeking social interaction Biomechanical assessment—range of motion (ROM) and strength: Decreased elbow flexion, decreased grasp (MP flexion limited) and decreased upper extremity strength bilaterally Role and interest assessment: Ability to care for daughter is of primary importance Functional assessment: Observed having difficulty using utensils and difficulty using nurse call button and observed to fatigue easily	Consider evaluation approach and methods Interpret observations	"Mrs. J. has many services throughout the day and has limited activity tolerance. In my experience, observational methods are the most efficient way to gather this information during this phase of burn recovery." "Mrs. J.'s limited ROM is not unexpected at this stage of recovery. Fortunately, these patients usually respond well to OT treatment. In addition to working to remediate her biomechanical limitations, I would like to try to quickly improve her independence in activities by issuing some adaptive equipment as well. This may help her feel more in control and less dependent."

Occupational Therapy Problem List • Unable to feed or dress independently because of impaired strength and range of motion in both upper extremities • Impaired ability to care for her daughter • Withdrawn behavior • Activity tolerance limited to 5 minutes	Synthesize results	"Biomechanical limitations are affecting her ability to perform tasks independently. Before the fire, Mrs. J. was so competent and in control of her activities. I'm sure that her current functional status is also contributing to feelings of dependence and poor self-esteem."
Occupational Therapy Goal List • Mrs. J. will use splinting, positioning, exercise, and activity to prevent loss of ROM in her upper extremities. • Mrs. J. will be able to perform 10 repetitions of active assistive ROM of bilateral upper extremities. • Mrs. J. will improve ability to grasp utensils by increasing flexion in her right MP joints from 40 to 75°. • Mrs. J. will eat 90% of her meal independently, using adaptive equipment as needed. • Ms. J. will be able to comb her daughter's hair for 5 minutes while sitting independently. • Mrs. J. will cope with anxiety and withdrawal by attainment of goals and through increased knowledge of the burn recovery process.	Develop intervention hypotheses Select an intervention approach Consider what will occur in therapy, how often, and for how long	"I believe that through the use of carefully selected activities, Mrs. J. will regain basic skills, as well as quickly gain confidence in her ability to perform tasks that are important to her." "The most limiting factors in her task performance are her biomechanical limitations. Therefore, I need to address these as a priority. However, I will accomplish biomechanical goals by using activities that also address psychosocial needs." "In my experience, OT treatment six times a week is appropriate for the remainder of Mrs. J.'s acute hospitalization (2–3 weeks). Initially, she may be frustrated and discouraged. However, I expect that, with the proper motivation, she will quickly regain function. This means that her goals will need to be continually reviewed and adjusted appropriately. I really want her to feel like she is part of setting the goals for treatment, so she can take pride in her achievements in therapy."
Intervention Occupational therapy occurred six times a week. Bilateral elbow and hand splints were fabricated. Adaptive equipment, such as modified call button and built-up utensils, were provided. The therapist encouraged the family to bring in tapes of get-well messages that Mrs. J. could listen to with headphones. Mrs. J. was taken to the occupational therapy gym as much as possible, and private time with her daughter was added to her daily schedule.	Assess the patient's comprehension Understand what she is doing Compare actual to expected performance Know the person Appreciate the context	"Mrs. J. is slowly beginning to ask me and the other team members appropriate questions regarding her treatment. She is demonstrating beginning awareness of the course of recovery and expected outcomes from this type of injury. She is smiling more and appears more open as she realizes that she will be able to resume activities that are meaningful to her. Her family is responding well to her new brightness. This is a nice cycle that is further motivation for Mrs. J."
Next Steps As the scars matured, Mrs. J. was provided with both verbal and written instructions regarding scar management and skin care. As discharge neared, a local therapist was contacted to follow Mrs. J. three times a week.	Anticipate present and future patient concerns Analyze patient's comprehension Decide if the patient should continue or discontinue therapy and/or return in the future	"As Mrs. J. transitions to home, she may be initially fearful of being home again, but we will plan close follow-up to quickly address any new issues that arise. Also, as she becomes more competent in her daily activities, her focus may shift to concerns about her appearance. She will likely have many questions in the next few months. I believe that the more she knows about the scar maturation process and scar management treatments, the more empowered she will feel. A burn garment will be needed, and I will order it prior to discharge, so trials can begin under the supervision of an experienced therapist." "I will need to be sure that I have opened the lines of communication with her local therapist who may also have questions about types of treatment, appropriate goals, and so on." "In addition to local follow-up, I would like to see Mrs. J. in the Burn Clinic in 1 month to assess outpatient care and provide additional recommendations as needed."

CLINICAL REASONING IN OCCUPATIONAL THERAPY PRACTICE

Outpatient Occupational Therapy after Burn Injury

As Mrs. J. is discharged home, she continues to have limitations that affect her ability to resume tasks and roles of importance. How would you characterize her phase of recovery once she is discharged home? Based on the description of her background, scope of injury, and progress to date, write three possible short-term goals as she begins outpatient treatment.

SUMMARY REVIEW QUESTIONS

1. In your own words, what is the primary goal of burn care?
2. How is the role of the occupational therapist unique to the burn team?
3. Describe key differences between superficial, superficial partial-thickness, deep partial-thickness, and full-thickness burns.
4. What splinting and positioning program would you establish for a patient who is intubated in the intensive care unit with deep partial-thickness burns to the axilla, elbow, and wrist?
5. How would your approach differ with the same patient awake and alert?
6. Describe the correct positioning for a deep dorsal hand burn and explain the anatomical justification behind your answer.
7. What factors would you consider when designing a scar management program for your patient?
8. As the occupational therapist on the burn unit, how would you help to address the psychosocial issues of your patients?
9. List five complications you might encounter as your patient recovers from a significant burn injury.
10. What might you, as an occupational therapist, find difficult about treating a patient with a burn injury? How would you address these issues?

ACKNOWLEDGMENT

We thank the patients, physicians, and staff of the Sumner Redstone Burn Unit at Massachusetts General Hospital and the staff of the occupational therapy and hand therapy departments.

References

Abston, S. (1987). Scar reaction after thermal injury and prevention of scars and contractures. In J. A. Boswick Jr. (Ed.), *The art and science of burn care* (pp. 359–371). Rockville, MD: Aspen.

Ahn, S. T., Monafo, W. W., & Mustoe, T. A. (1989). Topical silicone gel: A new treatment for hypertrophic scars. *Surgery, 106,* 781–787.

Baker, R. A., Jones, S., Sanders, C., Sadinski, C., Martin-Duffy, K., Berchin, H., & Valentine, S. (1996). Degree of burn, location of burn, and length of hospital stay as predictors of psychosocial status and physical functioning. *Journal of Burn Care and Rehabilitation, 17,* 327–333.

Barber, L. M. (1990). Desensitization of the traumatized hand. In J. M. Hunter, E. J. Mackin, & A. D. Callahan (Eds.), *Rehabilitation of the hand* (p. 721). St. Louis: Mosby.

Blalock, S. J., Bunker, B. J., & DeVellis, R. F. (1994). Measuring health status among survivors of burn injury: Revisions of the Burn Specific Health Scale. *Journal of Trauma, 36,* 508–515.

Brigham, P. A., & McLoughlin, E. (1996). Burn incidence and medical care use in the United States: Estimates, trends, and data sources. *Journal of Burn Care and Rehabilitation, 17,* 95–107.

Burke Evans, E., Alvarado, M. I., Ott, S., McElroy, K., & Irwin, C. (1996). Prevention and treatment of deformity in burned patients. In D. N. Herndon (Ed.), *Total burn care* (pp. 443–454). Philadelphia: Saunders.

Burn Foundation. (1999). Burn Incidence Fact Sheet, 1999. Retrieved December 12, 2005 from http://www.burnfoundation.org/content/view/94/102/

Chang, P., Laubenthal, K. N., Lewis, R. W, Rosenquist, M. D., Lindley-Smith, P., & Kealy, G. P. (1995). Prospective, randomized study of the efficacy of pressure garment therapy in patients with burns. *Journal of Burn Care and Rehabilitation, 16,* 473–475.

Cioffi, W. G., & Rue, L. W. (1991). Diagnosis and treatment of inhalation injuries. *Critical Care Nursing Clinics of North America, 3,* 191–198.

Draaijers, L. J., Tempelman, F. R., Botman, Y. A., Tuinebreijer, W. E., Middelkoop, E., Kreis, R. W., & van Zuijlen, P. P.(2004). The patient and observer scar assessment scale: A reliable and feasible tool for scar evaluation. *Plastic and Reconstructive Surgery, 113,* 1960–1965.

Druery, M., La, H., Brown, T., & Muller, M. (2005). Long term functional outcomes and quality of life following severe burn injury. *Burns, 31,* 692–695.

Dubner, R., & Ren, K. (1999). Endogenous mechanisms of sensory modulation. *Pain, Suppl 6,* S45–S53.

Duncan, D. J., & Driscoll, D. M. (1991). Burn wound management. *Critical Care Nursing Clinics of North America, 3,* 199–220.

Duran-Coleman, L. A. (1991). Rehabilitation of the burn survivor. *Progress Report: A Rehabilitation Journal, 3,* 1–8.

Dutcher, K., & Johnson, C. (1994). Neuromuscular and musculoskeletal complication. In R. L. Richard & M. J. Staley (Eds.), *Burn care and rehabilitation: Principles and practice* (pp. 576–602). Philadelphia: Davis.

Evans, R. B., & McAuliffe, J. A. (1995). Wound classification and management. In J. M. Hunter, E. J. Mackin, & A. D. Callahan (Eds.), *Rehabilitation of the hand: Surgery and therapy* (pp. 217–235). St. Louis: Mosby Year Book.

Falkel, J. E. (1994). Anatomy and physiology of the skin. In R. L. Richard & M. J. Staley (Eds.), *Burn care and rehabilitation: Principles and practice* (pp. 10–18). Philadelphia: Davis.

Fletchall, S., & Hickerson, W. L. (1995). Quality burn rehabilitation: Cost-effective approach. *Journal of Burn Care and Rehabilitation, 16,* 539–542.

Greenhalgh, D. G., & Staley, M. J. (1994). Burn wound healing. In R. L. Richard & M. J. Staley (Eds.), *Burn care and rehabilitation: Principles and practice* (pp. 70–102). Philadelphia: Davis.

Grigsby deLinde, L., & Miles, W. K. (1995). Remodeling of scar tissue in the burned hand. In J. M. Hunter, E. J. Mackin, & A. D. Callahan (Eds.), *Rehabilitation of the hand: Surgery and therapy* (pp. 1265–1303). St. Louis: Mosby Year Book.

Harden, N. G., & Luster, S. H. (1991). Rehabilitation considerations in the care of the acute burn patient. *Critical Care Nursing Clinics of North America, 3,* 245–253.

Institute for Healthcare Quality [IHQ]. (1997). *Quality first position paper: Burns*. Minneapolis: Institute for Healthcare Quality.

Kagan, R. J., & Warden, G. D. (1994). Management of the burn wound. *Clinical Dermatology, 12,* 47–56.

LeDoux, J. M., Meyer, W. J., Blakeney, P., & Herndon, D. (1996). Positive self-regard as a coping mechanism for pediatric burn survivors. *Journal of Burn Care and Rehabilitation, 17,* 472–476.

Masters, M., McMahon, M., & Svens, B. (2005) Reliability testing of a new scar assessment tool, Matching Assessment of Scars and Photographs (MAPS). *Journal of Burn Care and Rehabilitation, 26,* 273–284.

Malick, M. H., & Carr, J. A. (1982). *Manual on management of the burn patient*. Pittsburgh: Harmarville Rehabilitation Center.

Pessina, M. A., & Ellis, S. M. (1997). Rehabilitation. *Nursing Clinics of North America, 32,* 365–374.

Poh-Fitzpatrick, M. B. (1992). Skin care of the healed burn patient. *Clinical Plastic Surgery, 19,* 745–751.

Richard, R., & Ward R. S. (2005). Splinting strategies and controversies. *Journal of Burn Care and Rehabilitation, 26,* 392–396.

Rivers, E. A., & Jordan, C. L. (1998). Skin system dysfunction: Burns. In M. J. Neistadt & E. B. Crepeau (Eds.), *Willard and Spackman's occupational therapy* (9th ed., pp. 741–755). Philadelphia: Lippincott.

Robson, M. C., Barnett, R. A., Leitch, I. O., & Hayward, P. G. (1992). Prevention and treatment of postburn scars and contracture. *World Journal of Surgery, 16,* 87–96.

Rosenthal, E. A. (1995). The extensor tendons: Anatomy and management. In J. M. Hunter, E. J. Mackin, & A. D. Callahan (Eds.), *Rehabilitation of the hand: Surgery and therapy* (pp. 519–564). St. Louis: Mosby.

Sheridan R. L, Hinson, M. I., Liang, M. H., Nackel, A. F., Schoenfeld, D. A., Ryan, C. M, Mulligan, J. L., & Tompkins, R. G. (2000). Long-term outcome of children surviving massive burns. *Journal of the American Medical Association, 283,* 69–73.

Sheridan, R. L., Hurley, J., Smith, M. A., Ryan, C. M., Bondoc, C. C., Quinby, W. C., Tompkins, R. G., & Burke, J. F. (1995). The acutely burned hand: Management and outcome based a ten-year experience with 1047 acute hand burns. *Journal of Trauma, 38,* 406–411.

Staley, M. J., Richard, R. L., & Falkel, J. E. (1994). Burns. In S. B. O'Sullivan, & T. J. Schmitz (Eds.), *Physical rehabilitation: Assessment and treatment* (pp. 509–532). Philadelphia: Davis.

Sullivan, T., Smith, J., Kermode, J., McIver, E., & Courtemanche, D. J. (1990). Rating the burn scar. *Journal of Burn Care and Rehabilitation, 3,* 256–260.

Summers, T. M. (1991). Psychosocial support of the burned patient. *Critical Care Nursing Clinics of North America, 3,* 237–244.

Tanigawa, M. C., O'Donnell, O. K., & Graham, P. L. (1974). The burned hand: A physical therapy protocol. *Physical Therapy, 54,* 953–958.

Uniform Data System for Medical Rehabilitation. (1997). *Guide for the Uniform Data Set for Medical Rehabilitation*. Buffalo: University of New York.

Ward, R. S. (1991). Pressure therapy for the control of hypertrophic scar formation after burn injury: A history and review. *Journal of Burn Care and Rehabilitation, 12,* 257–262.

Wright, P. C. (1984). Fundamentals of acute burn care and physical therapy management. *Physical Therapy, 64,* 1217–1231.

Wright-Howell, J. (1989). Management of the acutely burned hand for the non-specialized clinician. *Physical Therapy, 69,* 1077–1089.

Supplemental Reference

Choctaw, W. F., Eisner, M. E., & Wachtel, T. L. (1987). Causes, prevention, pre-hospital care, evaluation, emergency treatment, and prognosis. In B. M. Achauer (Ed.), *Management of the burned patient* (pp. 3–19). Los Altos, CA: Appleton & Lange.

CHAPTER 46

Amputations and Prosthetics

Kathy Stubblefield and Anne Armstrong

LEARNING OBJECTIVES

After studying this chapter, the reader will be able to do the following:

1. Discuss prosthetic components available and appropriate for upper limb amputation levels.
2. State options for creating prosthetic prescriptions.
3. Plan treatment programs for persons with transradial and transhumeral amputations.
4. Design treatment for pre-prosthetic and prosthetic management of upper and lower limb amputation.
5. Describe the psychological implications of amputation for the patient in social and other contexts and their impact on therapeutic management.

Glossary

Acquired amputation—Surgical amputation after birth as a result of trauma or disease.

Body power (BP)—Person's own effort, without an external power source.

External power—Electric or other motor that provides impetus to move the prosthesis or terminal device.

Pre-prosthetic therapy program—Period from the post-surgical procedure until the permanent prosthesis is received.

Terminal device (TD)—Prosthetic hook, hand, or other prehensile device that is inserted into the wrist unit of the prosthesis.

Transfemoral amputation—Amputation across the axis of the femur; previously called above knee (AK).

Transhumeral amputation—Amputation across the axis of the humerus; previously called above elbow (AE).

Transradial amputation—Amputation across the axis of the radius and ulna; labeled by the larger of two adjacent bones; previously called below elbow (BE).

Transtibial amputation—Amputation across the axis of the fibula and tibia; labeled according to the larger of two adjacent bones; previously called below knee (BK).

Voluntary closing (VC) mechanism—TD that remains open until tension is applied to the control cable for grasp.

Voluntary opening (VO) mechanism—TD that remains closed until tension is applied to the control cable to open it.

Amputation can result from several causes:

- Traumatic injury that occurs as a result of accidents as in the use of machinery or motor vehicle accidents
- Disease such as vascular disease, tumors, or infection
- Congenital limb deficiencies that present as missing or partially developed limbs

This chapter addresses only adults with **acquired amputation**, that is, amputations that occurred after birth. Discussion of the role of the occupational therapist in providing therapy for adults with lower limb amputation is also included.

INCIDENCE, LEVELS, AND CLASSIFICATION OF AMPUTATION

More than 150,000 persons in the United States have amputations, with the ratio of arm to leg amputations estimated to be 1:3. Some 57% of arm amputations are transradial, that is, below the elbow through the radius and ulna (Esquenazi, 1996; Leonard & Meier, 1998). Trauma rather than disease is the primary cause (close to 75%) of upper limb amputations in adults, with injury occurring primarily to males aged 15–45 years in work-related accidents (Leonard & Meier, 1998). Amputations of upper limbs can also result from other events, such as gunshot wounds and electrical burns. Disease is the primary reason for lower limb amputations, with peripheral vascular disease and diabetes being the most common causes in people over 60 years of age. Trauma causes 20% of acquired lower extremity amputations, with 5% due to tumors (Leonard & Meier, 1998). Currently available official statistics do not reflect war-related injuries since Vietnam. It is known, however, that the incidence of amputation has steadily declined since the Civil War due to improved management of extremity trauma resulting in limb salvage. In more recent conflicts, the survival of combatants has increased with the use of body armour, so the number of individuals surviving the loss of limbs has increased the number of amputated individuals in the general population (Ramalingan, Pathak, & Barker, 2005).

When amputation is necessary, the surgeon's aim is to preserve as much limb length as possible and still retain healthy skin, soft tissue, blood supply, sensation, muscles, bones, and joints (Leonard & Meier, 1998). A residual limb that is pain free and functional is the final surgical goal.

Acquired amputations were previously described by such terms as short above elbow (AE), standard AE, very short below elbow (BE), and long BE. Other terminology has been adopted by the International Standards Organization and endorsed by the American Academy of Orthotists and Prosthetists, the American Academy of Orthopedic Surgeons, and the International Society for Prosthetics and Orthotics (Schuch & Pritham, 1994). The term *trans* is now used to describe an amputation across the axis of a long bone, as with **transhumeral** to replace AE, or **transradial** for radius-ulna, or BE. The levels of amputation for the upper extremity are illustrated in Figure 46-1. Often the level of amputation directly affects the use of a prosthesis. The higher the amputation, the more difficult it is to use a prosthesis because fewer joints and muscles are available for control. Furthermore, the weight of the prosthesis is greater, and more complex systems are needed for active control. A patient may choose not to wear a prosthesis for many reasons, including the individual's psychological reaction to the amputation.

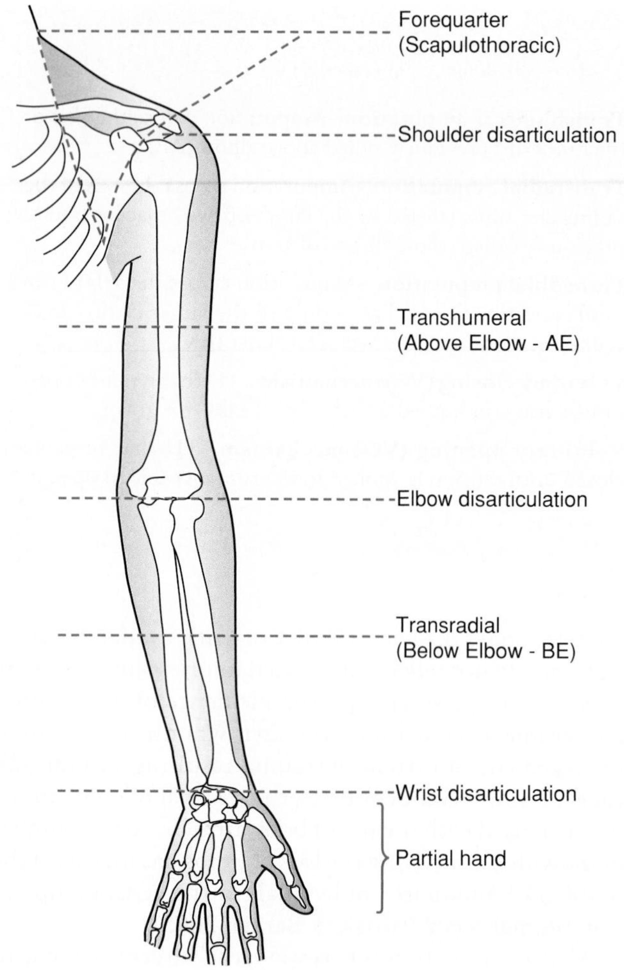

Figure 46-1 Levels of amputations.

PSYCHOLOGICAL ASPECTS OF LIMB LOSS

Amputation of an upper limb results in a change in the ability to grip, feel, and manipulate objects; physically engage in social interaction; and communicate through gestures. This loss can profoundly influence the person's body scheme, self-esteem, and sense of efficacy. Reactions to amputation are as complex as the unique nature of each human, and an individual's personality and belief system influence how he or she responds to amputation. Often, an early response to limb amputation is shock and disbelief; when both upper extremities are amputated, a feeling of helplessness is common. It is also natural for the person to grieve (Dise-Lewis, 1989; Winchell, 1995) and feel a multitude of painful emotions. For example, some may respond with anger, feelings of guilt, denial, hopelessness, bitterness, revulsion, or depression. Sometimes the patient may project negative feelings onto the therapist. The therapist must encourage open discussion, instill a climate of trust and respect, and work with the team members to facilitate the patient's psychological adjustment and reintegration into previous roles. Amputation affects not only physical function but also the patient's competence and satisfaction in life roles: maintenance of self, family, and home; self-enhancement, such as engaging in leisure and community activities; and self-advancement as a worker or student (see Chapter 1). What can the occupational therapist do?

- Give the patient information. Explanation of therapy and realistic outcomes can clarify the patient's expectations and reduce the patient's fear and anxiety. The therapist can prepare the patient during the preprosthetic phase by showing prostheses that are appropriate to the amputation level and by discussing their features while listening to the patient and understanding the patient's life roles. A collaborative relationship between therapist and patient instills a sense of control in the patient.
- Introduce the patient to another person with a similar amputation to facilitate sharing of life and recovery experience, as well as problem-solving strategies. This is an important action the therapist can take to help the patient adjust. Referring the patient to self-help amputee support groups in the area and recommending internet resources can acquaint the patient with several perspectives.
- Provide the patient with reference material; topics can include information on coping and adjusting to the amputation, information on prosthetic options, tips on how to manage one's occupations (daily life skills) independently, and a list of organizations for persons with upper and lower limb amputation (Resource 46-1).
- Communicate with (and, when necessary, refer the patient to) the psychologist, spiritual counselor, and other team members throughout the psychosocial intervals, described by Van Dorsten (2004), of survival, recovery, and reintegration after amputation.

REHABILITATION: A TEAM APPROACH

The core members of the professional team are the physician, prosthetist, occupational therapist, and physical therapist. The social worker, psychologist, and vocational counselor should be called in as needed. Patients are always active, equal members of the team and must be given the opportunity to explain their needs, preferences, and goals. The occupational therapist is critical to the rehabilitation process, since this professional works so closely with the patient and can influence the patient's adjustment. Some aspects of the rehabilitation program may be addressed by other team members, as in the acute post-operative period, when management of the

RESOURCE 46-1

Publications for Consumers and Professionals

Challenge Magazine: a publication of Disabled Sports USA
451 Hungerford Drive,
Suite 100
Rockville, MD 20850
Phone: (301) 217-9841
E-mail: disuse@dsusa.org
www.dsusa.org

First Step: a biennial publication of the Amputee Coalition of America
900 E. Hill Avenue, Suite 285
Knoxville TN, 37915-2568
Phone: (865) 524-8772
E-mail: editor@amputee-coalition.org

In Motion: a publication of the Amputee Coalition of America
900 E. Hill Ave, Suite 285
Knoxville, TN 37915-2568

One-Handed in a Two-Handed World, 2nd ed revised August, 2001, Prince-Gallison Press
P.O. Box 23, Hanover Station
Boston, MA 02113
Phone: (607) 367-5815

Organizations

American Amputee Foundation
P.O. Box 250218
Little Rock, AK 72225
Phone: (501) 666-2523
E-mail: Americanamputee foundation@hotmail.com.
www.americanamputee.org

Amputee Coalition of America
900 E. Hill Avenue, Suite 285
Knoxville, TN 37915-2568
Phone: (888) 267-5669
www.amputee-coalition.org;
Spanish/English

National Amputation Foundation
40 Church Street
Malvern, NY 11565
Phone: (516) 887-3600
www.nationalamputation.org

Web Sites on Topics Related to Limb Loss

Amputee Information Network: www.amp-info.net
Amps76@aol.com
acainfo@amputee-coalition.org
www.amputeeonline.com
www.activeamp.org

Manufacturers and Distributors

Hosmer-Dorrance Corp.
561 Division Street
Campbell, CA 95008
Phone: (800) 827-0070
www.hosmer.com
Manufactures primarily BP components.

Liberty Mutual Research Center
71 Frankland Road
Hopkinton, MA 01748
Phone: (800) 437-0024
www.Libertytechnology.com
Manufactures electronic elbows, control systems, hands, and gloves.

Motion Control, Inc.
2401 South 1070 West,
Suite B
Salt Lake City, UT 84119
Phone: (888) 696-2767
www.utaharm.com/
Manufactures the Utah electronic elbow and other electronic systems.

Otto Bock Orthopedic Industry
300 Xenium Lane N.
Minneapolis, MN 55441
Phone: (800) 328-4058
www.ottobock.com
Manufactures electronic hands and hooks; wrist, elbow, and other electronic systems; and BP components.

Ross Prosthetics
17 Lynwood Road
Scarsdale, NY 10583
Phone: (914) 725-7785.
Manufactures anatomical hand covers.

TRS, Inc. (Therapeutic Recreation Systems)
2450 Central Avenue, Unit D
Boulder, CO 80301-2844
Phone: (800) 279-1865.
www.oandp.com/products/trs/
Manufactures VC terminal devices and adaptations for sports activities and musical instruments.

residual limb may be rendered by a physical therapist or a nurse.

PRE-PROSTHETIC THERAPY

The **pre-prosthetic** therapy program occurs from the post-surgical period until the patient receives the permanent prosthesis. This is a preparatory time for emotional and physical healing.

Post-Operative Care

Post-operative care, required immediately after surgery, addresses wound care, maintenance of skin integrity, joint mobility, reduction of edema, prevention of scarring, and control of pain (Atkins & Meier, 2004a; Malone, Fleming, & Robinson, 1984). This usually occurs in an acute-care setting, with surgeon, nurse, and physical therapist most involved, and continues in an outpatient setting. Outpatient therapy can be provided in a rehabilitation unit, rehabilitation center, or hand clinic. Inpatient admission may be necessary for multiple amputations or other complications, such as extensive burns.

Phantom Limb Sensation

The perception of the presence of the amputated limb is a universal phenomenon that is remarkably real to the patient. The cause of phantom limb sensation is still not clearly understood and research into it is continuing (Hunter, Katz, & Davis, 2003). Phantom limb sensation is most common in traumatic amputations. According to Melzack (1989), the neural system exists within the brain even when the body input is cut off by amputation. These perceptions are strongest with amputations of upper extremities, and the hand and fingers are felt more vividly than the arm.

With time, the patient may feel that the distal portions of the phantom limb have moved closer to the site of the amputation. Phantom limb sensation often remains, and ordinarily, the patient accepts it. The patient may view it as an annoyance if the sensation is mild burning or tingling or may find it useful, as when learning myoelectric control for externally powered prostheses.

Open discussion with the patient regarding this common phenomenon is imperative.

Phantom Limb Pain

Phantom limb pain is even less clearly understood, and its causation and management remain controversial; again, research continues (Hompland, 2004). This pain can be felt as extremely intense burning or cramping sensations or shooting pain and is most common in traumatic amputations. Peripheral nerve irritation, abnormal sympathetic function, and psychological factors are thought to be contributory factors.

Often, pain increases with stress. The therapist is advised to avoid emphasizing pain when possible. Treatments for those with severe pain include analgesics and surgery, such as nerve blocks and neurectomies. In the rehabilitation setting, limb percussion, ultrasound, and transcutaneous electrical nerve stimulation (TENS) have been used (Jones & Davidson, 1996). Acupuncture, psychotherapy, hypnotherapy, and relaxation techniques have also been instituted. No one approach, however, has proven to be clearly successful.

Pre-Prosthetic Program Guidelines

Occupational therapy during the pre-prosthetic period for the upper extremity includes providing emotional support, ensuring maximal limb shrinkage and shaping, desensitizing the residual limb, maintaining range of motion and strength, and facilitating independence in activities of daily living.

Provide Emotional Support

Establish an ongoing supportive, trusting relationship with the patient and family to facilitate open discussion (see Chapter 15). Collaborate with the team regarding the patient's needs, and refer the patient for counseling if needed. Introduce the patient to others with similar amputations and comparable circumstances, such as similar levels of amputation or vocation.

Instruct in Limb Hygiene and Expedite Wound Healing

- Instruct the patient to wash the limb daily with mild soap and dry it thoroughly.
- Provide wound cleansing, such as debridement or use of a whirlpool; this may be the responsibility of the physical therapist or nurse.
- Use creams to massage at the suture line to loosen crustlike formations.

Maximize Limb Shrinkage with Limb Shaping

The goal is to shrink and shape the residual limb so that it is tapered at the distal end; this allows for optimal prosthetic fit. The following interventions can be used to achieve this goal.

- *Elastic bandage.* The patient is taught to wrap the limb and is expected to do so independently unless physical or mental limitations prevent it. In this case, a family member, friend, or caregiver is instructed in the process. The residual limb must be wrapped in a figure-of-eight diagonal configuration, with most pressure applied at the end of the limb. ***The limb must never be wrapped in a circular manner, as this causes a tourniquet effect and restricts circulation.*** The bandage must conform firmly to the limb and be wrapped in a distal to proximal direction (Fig. 46-2). The wrap should be worn continuously and reapplied immediately if it loosens. ***The patient is advised to remove the bandage two to three times daily to examine the skin for any redness or excessive pressure. A clean bandage should be applied at least every 2 days.*** Bandages can be washed with mild soap and laid flat to dry but not squeezed or machine dried.
- *Elastic shrinker.* An elasticized sock can be worn in lieu of the bandage if the patient or family members have difficulty following proper wrapping procedures using the elastic bandage. The shrinker tends to loosen, however, as the limb shrinks. Although the shrinker can be less effective than the bandage, it is preferable to improper application of the elastic bandage.
- *Removable rigid dressing.* A socket can be fabricated using plaster bandages or fiberglass casting tape. This may be the method of choice for those unable to wrap the limb (Olivett, 1995); however, this cast must be replaced or altered frequently as the limb shrinks.
- *Immediate post-operative prosthesis.* The immediate post-operative prosthesis is, as the name suggests, applied directly after surgery (Maiorano & Byron, 1995; Malone, Fleming, & Robinson, 1984). This is probably the ideal approach if the rehabilitation team members are available to ensure success.
- *Early post-operative prosthesis.* The early post-operative prosthesis is strongly recommended for bilateral amputations (Uellendahl, 2004) to reduce dependency for self-care activities. This temporary prosthesis may ensure acceptance and use of the permanent prosthesis. Studies support the premise that early fitting tends to ensure acceptance of the prosthesis and its use (Kejlaa, 1993; Pinzur & Angelats, 1994).

Desensitize the Residual Limb

The aim is to desensitize the residual limb so that it will accommodate touch and pressure in preparation for encasement in the socket. This goal can be met through the following interventions (see also Chapter 27).

- The patient bears weight on the end of the limb against various surfaces. These surfaces are graded from very

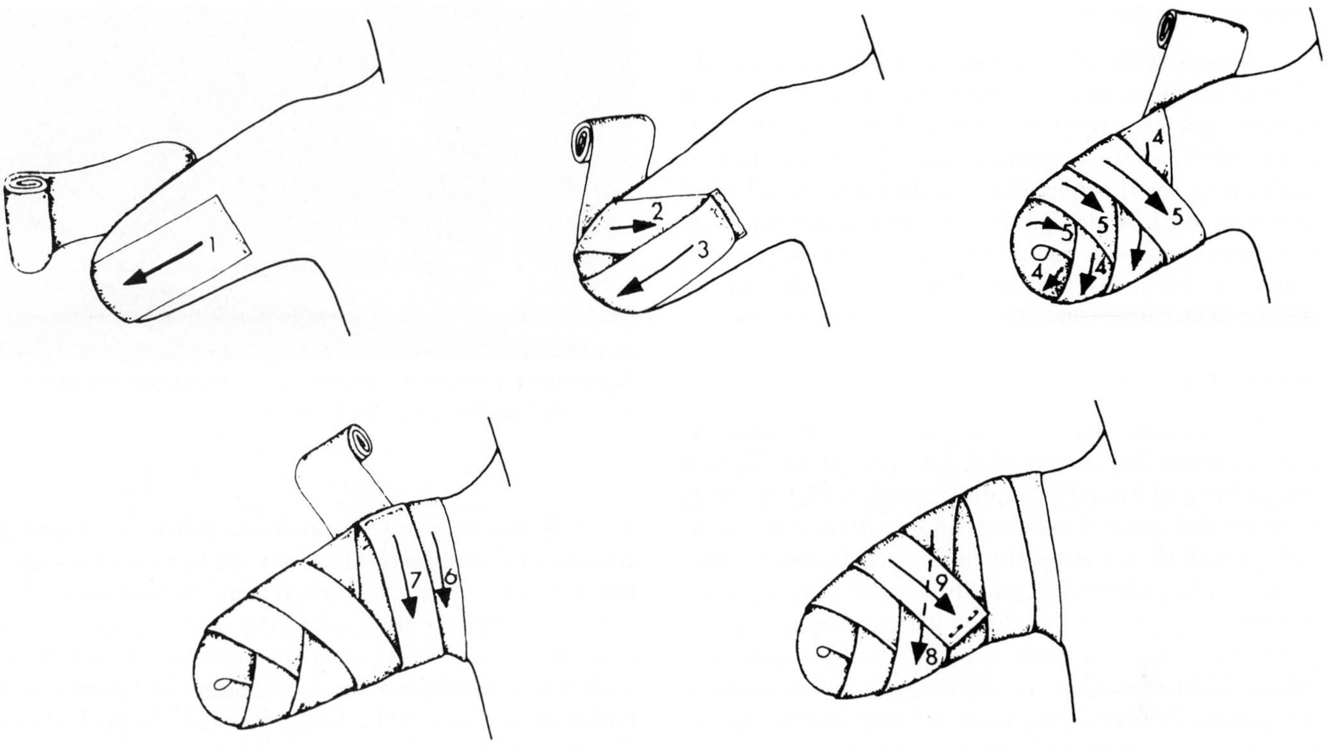

Figure 46-2 Wrapping technique for transhumeral amputation. Repeat diagonal turns as necessary to cover the limb with no constriction.

resilient, such as soft foam, to variously resistant and textured, such as layers of felt, rice, and clay (Fig. 46-3). The patient is to push the limb down into the surface for 5-second intervals and increase the contact time and pressure as tolerated.

- Massage is useful for desensitizing but is primarily used to prevent or release adhesions and soften scar tissue.

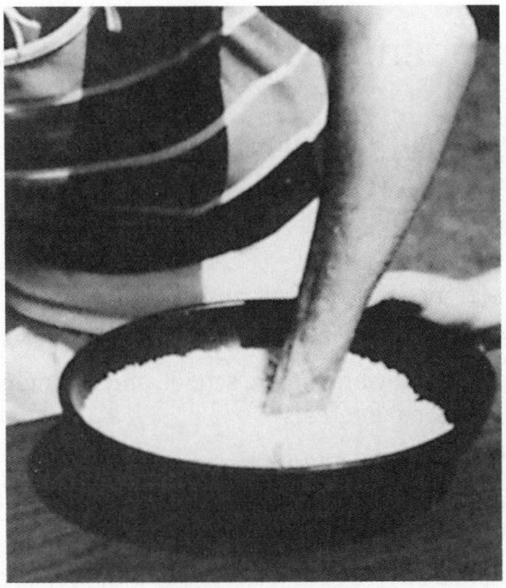

Figure 46-3 Weight bearing into materials of various textures (here, rice) to desensitize limb.

- Tapping and rubbing the residual limb and applying a vibrator are also useful.
- Residual limb wrapping contributes to desensitizing the limb.

Maintain or Increase Range of Motion and Strength of the Limb

A physical conditioning regimen can be instituted to increase or maintain the range of motion of all joints proximal to the amputation. Increasing muscle strength of the residual limb and shoulder area are also goals. Include the contralateral side if limitations are noted. For patients with high-level amputations, a shift of weight and center of gravity can occur. Core strengthening will promote postural control, balance, and endurance and prevent asymmetry. Mobilization of the limb also increases circulation and reduces edema. This conditioning regimen should be practiced at home. Encourage the patient with unilateral limb loss to incorporate the residual limb into bilateral tasks during daily activities.

Facilitate Independence in Daily Living Activities

It is important that the patient develop skills to be proficient without the prosthesis. Ordinarily, the patient with a unilateral amputation receives only one prosthesis; therefore, there may be times when the prosthesis is being repaired and the patient will have to manage without it.

Unilateral Amputation

For persons with amputation of the dominant limb, change of dominance activities, such as writing, must receive special attention. Although the patient will instinctively use the remaining extremity for activities of daily living, the therapist can introduce a wide variety of activities and provide tips for one-handed techniques or recommend adaptive equipment for home management, communication, desk activities, and community participation (see Chapters 30–32).

Bilateral Amputation

Establishing some degree of independence is essential for the patient who has undergone bilateral amputations, and this must be addressed promptly (Lehneis & Dickey, 1992) to lessen feelings of dependency and frustration. Immediately provide the patient with a universal cuff, which is useful for holding a utensil or toothbrush; this is a temporary substitute for grasp. Early fitting with a temporary prosthesis on at least one limb is by far the best approach. Adapted devices may be needed (Friedmann, 1989) to assist the patient in performing basic self-maintenance tasks, such as eating, toileting, grooming, and some dressing. Use of the feet should be encouraged if at all possible, and other modifications of performance can be suggested, such as use of the chin, knees, and teeth (Edelstein, 2004). The therapist and patient can analyze tasks and solve problems together. Ordinarily, the longer limb will be chosen as the dominant extremity.

Explore Prosthetic Options

The occupational therapist and prosthetist educate the patient about prostheses appropriate to the level of amputation to guide the patient to establish realistic expectations. If appropriate, a meeting can be arranged between this patient and a former one, preferably someone with a similar level of amputation, so that they can talk candidly about any issues of concern, including negative and positive features of prostheses.

Myoelectric Site Testing and Training

Muscle site testing must be instituted for patients choosing a myoelectric prosthesis. The prosthetist and therapist can collaborate to determine whether the patient is a candidate by evaluating electromyographic (EMG) signals. At that time, the optimal location for the control site or sites is chosen. The goal is to find a site where the patient can hold a steady contraction for at least 1–2 seconds and relax for that time. A myotester or computer program can be used as well as the electronic hand. Ordinarily, the agonist and antagonist are chosen, such as biceps and triceps for transhumeral amputation and typically wrist extensors and flexors for transradial amputation. It is possible to use only one muscle to control two functions: a strong contraction controls one function, and a weaker contraction controls another; relaxation turns the system off. The skin electrodes are strapped to the limb or encased in a test socket (Fig. 46-4), with the electronic controls attached to a motorized hand, computer, or myotester. A biofeedback unit can also be used to train the patient (see Chapter 20).

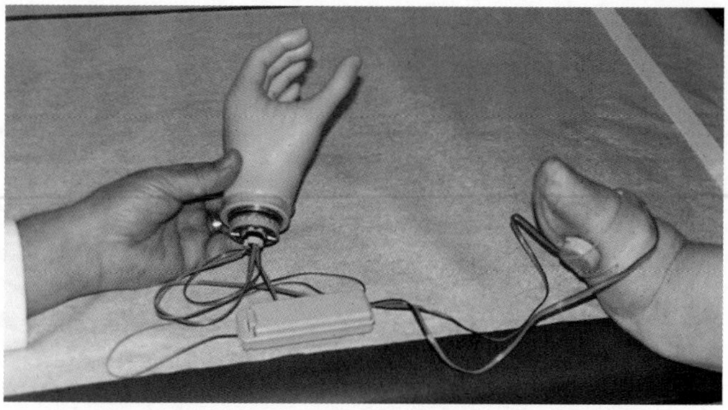

Figure 46-4 Finding the best site for electrode placement for consistent control of electric hand.

PRESCRIBING THE PROSTHESIS

As a member of the prosthetic team, the occupational therapist contributes to the prescription of the prosthesis. The therapist has come to know the patient in some depth during the pre-prosthetic program and can contribute information regarding the patient's social and cultural contexts (Procedures for Practice 46-1).

PROCEDURES FOR PRACTICE 46-1

Prescribing the Prosthesis

Consider these factors:

- Residual limb: length, range of motion, skin integrity, strength
- Preference for cosmesis and function
- Hand dominance
- Activities at work, home, school, and community and recreational interests
- Motivation and attitude
- Financial coverage: health care insurance, ability to pay privately, and alternative funding sources
- Cognitive abilities to learn to use prosthetic controls

Prosthetic Components

The components of a prosthesis are frequently categorized in the following sequence, from distal to proximal:

1. **Terminal devices (TD)**
   - Active prehensors
   - Passive terminal devices
2. Wrist units
3. Forearm component or sockets
4. Elbow units or hinges
5. Upper arm component or sockets
6. Shoulder units or hinges
7. Suspension or harness

Prosthetic Control Choices: Body Powered (Definition 46-1)

Terminal Devices

Terminal devices (TD) are considered the most important components of the prosthesis. The components for the wrist, elbow, and upper arm are needed to position the arm in space to enable efficient TD use.

TD Prehensors

TD prehensors can be classified as operating by a **voluntary opening (VO) mechanism** or **voluntary closing (VC) mechanism** (Table 46-1). The fingers of a VO device remain closed by springs for a mechanical hand or by rubber bands for a hook. The force of pinch on the hook can be increased by adding rubber bands, approximately 1 pound for each band, and by adjusting the spring mechanism for the hands. The Therapeutic Recreational Systems (TRS) VC mechanism adjusts the amount of pinch force by decreasing or increasing the amount of tension the patient applies on the cable to close the TD.

Voluntary Opening Hooks

The voluntary opening hook is most widely used, and Hosmer-Dorrance is the primary manufacturer (Fig. 46-5). Hooks of aluminum, titanium, or stainless steel come in several sizes; some have neoprene rubber-lined fingers. The neoprene lining provides a firm grip and prevents slippage. Aluminum hooks are lighter (4 ounces) than stainless steel (8 ounces) and are used for routine activities.

The stainless steel work hook has special features that facilitate holding tools and can withstand the rigors of heavy mechanical activity; however, it weighs 10 ounces. The Hosmer hooks come in right or left and can be differentiated by holding the hook with fingers in pronation; the thumb post closest to the midline indicates its orientation to side. For example, a right hook, when pronated, has the thumb post closest to the body or midline.

Voluntary Closing Terminal Devices

The TRS GRIP voluntary closing terminal device is fast becoming the TD of choice in this category (Fig. 46-6). Strong variable prehension is controlled by the amount of force the individual can exert. It is conceivable that a grasp of more than 30 pounds can be attained. A locking mechanism is employed to sustain grip. These devices are available in aluminum and steel and can be plastic coated. This TD is particularly appealing for people who are active in sports, heavy physical work, or recreational activities.

Voluntary Opening Mechanical Hands

The Hosmer-Dorrance or Otto Bock mechanical hand is most frequently selected. The VO hands operate similarly to the VO hooks except that, in the hand, the thumb and first two fingers open when the cable is pulled. These fingers oppose in a three-point prehension pattern. This is different from the Hosmer hook, in which the cable is attached only to the thumb post so that one finger moves while the other finger remains stationary.

Voluntary Closing Mechanical Hands

The APRL VC hand is available only in men's sizes. The thumb can be manually adjusted and locked in two positions to achieve a 1.5- or 3-inch opening. Otto Bock offers VC hands in several sizes, all of which weigh less than the APRL hand. The VC hands are less popular than the VO hands. TRS also provides VC hands.

Cosmetic Gloves

All prosthetic hands have rubberized coverings (Fryer, Michael, & Stark, 2004). These gloves are available in a

DEFINITION 46-1

Types of Prostheses

Body-Powered (BP) Prosthesis

Body motion is used to apply tension on the control cable to activate the TD and elbow unit.

Externally Powered Prosthesis

Motors for the TD, wrist unit, and elbow components are electrically controlled either by a microswitch or by electromyographic (EMG) signals.

Myoelectric Prosthesis

This externally powered prosthesis uses EMG signals to activate electric components. Electrodes embedded inside the prosthetic socket are in contact with the patient's skin and pick up EMG signals as the muscle contracts. The signals are amplified and relayed to the electronic TD, wrist unit, or/and elbow unit.

Hybrid Prosthesis

Hybrid prostheses combine BP and electrical power control systems.

Table 46-1. Hooks and Hands Compared

Features	Hooks VO (Body Power)	VC TRS Grip (Body Power)	Hands (External Power)	Hands VO (Body Power)	Greifer (External Power)
Cosmesis	Unfavorable	Unfavorable	Favorable	Favorable	Unfavorable
Pinch force	1 lb/rubber band; more rubber bands yield stronger grip but require more effort to open	Controlled strong grip >40 lb dependent on force exerted on cable	Strong grip, 22 lb; may have proportional control	Pinch stronger than VO hook but weaker than externally powered TD; relies on internal springs, adjustable	Strong pinch, 32 lb
Prehension pattern	Precise, exact pinch	Pinch more precise than hand, less than hook	Cylindrical grasp 3-point pinch; configuration same as BP hand	Cylindrical grasp, 3-point pinch; configuration same as external powered hand	Precise pinch and cylindrical grasp
Weight	Lighter than hands; aluminum to stainless steel; 3–8.7 oz	Aluminum, polymer, stainless steel; 4–16 oz	Heavy; 16.2 oz	Heavy; 10.5–14 oz	Heavy; 19 oz
Durability	Durable; stainless steel is strongest	Durable and rugged; especially stainless	Not durable; delicate internal electronics and glove	Not durable; delicate inner spring mechanism and glove	Durable and rugged
Reliability	Very good; requires minimal service	Very good; requires minimal service	Good if not used for rugged activities	Good if not used for rugged activities	Very good
Feedback	Some proprioceptive feedback from tension on harness and limb in socket when operating TD/elbow	Better proprioceptive feedback, as tension on cable must be maintained for sustained grasp	Some feedback through intensity of muscle contraction, particularly for proportional control	Feedback similar to VO hook	Same as externally powered hand
Ease of use	Effort increases with more rubber bands	More effort to sustain grasp; lock available	Low effort to activate	More effort to open; can relax for grasp	Same as externally powered hand
Use in various planes	Difficult for high planes	Similar to VO hook	Very good for transradial amputation	Similar to VO hook/hand because of harness	Same as externally powered hand
Visibility of items grasped	Very good	Good; less than VO	Poor for small items	Poor for small items	Poor for small items
Cost	Lowest	Higher than hook, less than hand	Highest cost	Higher than hooks; lower than externally powered hand	About the same as externally powered hand

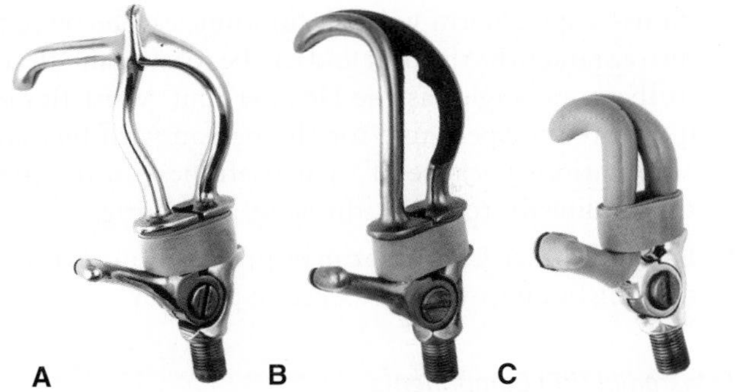

Figure 46-5 Hooks. A. Stainless steel work hook. B. Titanium hook; as strong as steel but less weight. C. Aluminum plastisol coated with canted fingers. (Photo courtesy of Hosmer-Dorrance Corp., Campbell, CA.)

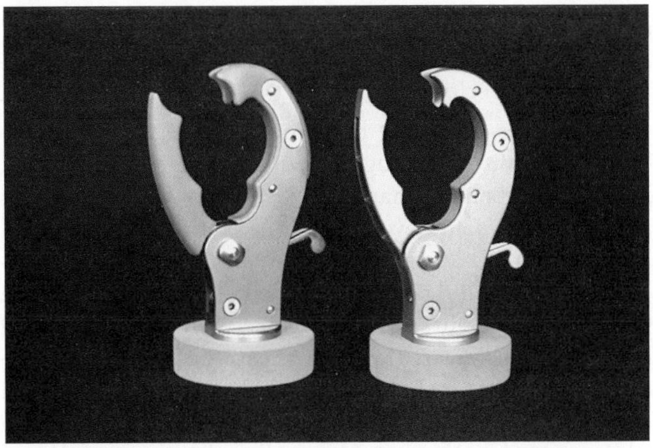

Figure 46-6 Voluntary closing prehensors. A. Grip 3 with polyethylene gripping surface. B. Grip 2S made with titanium, stainless steel, and aluminum materials. (Photo courtesy of TRS, Inc., Boulder, CO.)

variety of colors and sizes to cover mechanical, passive, and electric hands. A reverse mold of the remaining hand is sent to the manufacturer. The glove is replaced by the prosthetist when damaged. Some of the available choices are described here.

A stock (production) glove is ordered by the prosthetist. The skin color choices are made from a selection of sample swatches. These polyvinyl chloride (PVC) gloves are the least expensive but are susceptible to staining from contact with such items as newsprint, clothing dyes, and ballpoint ink. The glove can deteriorate with temperature extremes and in sunlight.

A silicone covering is more expensive than PVC. A wider range of color choices is available, and details, such as veins, are painted on the glove to render a more realistic covering. These silicone gloves can withstand extremes of temperature and do not stain as easily as those of PVC.

A custom-sculpted silicone glove, also called an anatomical cover, truly attempts to replicate the individual's remaining hand (Figs. 46-7 and 46-8). The remaining hand is cast in silicone, which duplicates its contours in great detail. It is then reversed. A cosmetic restorationist adds to the realistic appearance of the hand by painting the glove and adding veins and other features. This glove is the most costly.

Passive cosmetic hands and prostheses are chosen when appearance is valued more than function. These prostheses are available to replace any part of a limb, from a single digit to a whole arm.

The Final Choice: Hooks or Hands?

Fortunately, the patient can choose from several TDs. It is possible to have several interchangeable hooks and hands. The hook is viewed as most functional for the following reasons:

- Small items can be grasped with precision.
- Visibility is good, an extremely important feature, since tactile sensation is absent.
- It weighs less than the hand.
- It costs less than the hand.

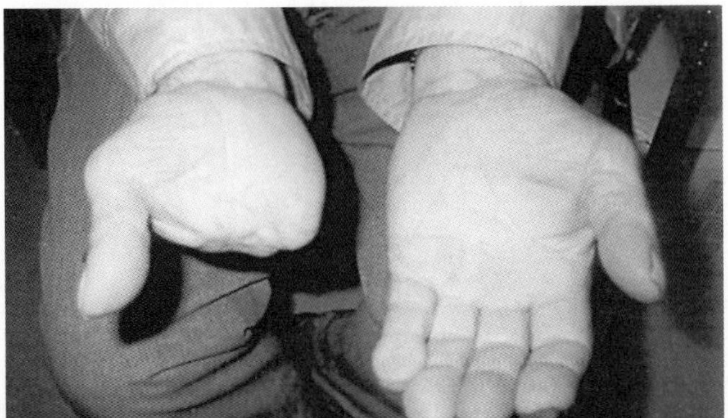

Figure 46-7 Partial hand amputation.

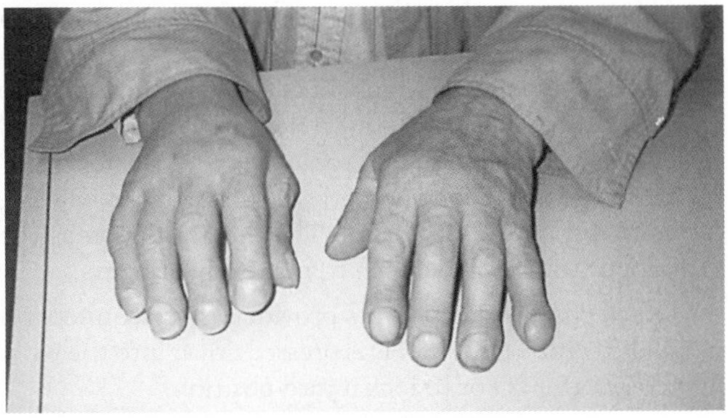

Figure 46-8 Cosmetic anatomical covering for this partial hand. (Courtesy of Michael Curtain, Alternative Prosthetic Services, Southport, CT.)

- It is more reliable and requires less maintenance than the hand.
- It can fit in close quarters.

Many people prefer the hand, however, because it is cosmetically more appealing, although heavier, more delicate, and more expensive than hooks.

The continued development and refinement of externally powered hands has led to electric hands being chosen over mechanical hands, particularly by those with transradial amputations, since they offer greater pinch force, can be activated with more ease, and do not require a harness. A mistaken notion is that the electric hand provides more dexterity than the mechanical hand. To the contrary, both move identically, with the thumb and first two fingers moving as a unit, in a three-point prehension pattern. They differ in the control system only; the mechanical hand is controlled through cable or **body power (BP)**, and the electric hand is controlled through myoelectric signals or switches, that is, **external power**. Individuals with bilateral amputations continue to prefer BP hooks because function is of paramount importance. Some individuals choose a different TD for each limb, for example, a BP hook for the dominant side and a myoelectric hand for the other. How can the ideal TDs be chosen? Listen to the patient and consult with the other team members to get varied perspectives. These options are presented to the patient, who makes the ultimate choice.

Wrist Units

The wrist unit provides a means to attach the TD to the forearm. It also provides an important function: the terminal device can be rotated to positions of supination, pronation, or midposition before engaging in an activity. This pre-positioning is an important substitution movement for reduced or absent active forearm rotation. Several types of wrist units are available; the ones described here are the most popular:

- Constant friction. This wrist unit contains a nylon threaded insert that surrounds the stud of the TD to hold it in place. An Allen wrench is used to turn a small set screw that applies pressure against the nylon insert, which causes constant pressure against the stud of the TD. Just enough friction must be applied to allow the individual to rotate the TD but not so little that the TD inadvertently rotates while it is being activated by the cable pull. The therapist teaches the patient to use the wrench to make adjustments.
- Quick change. These units provide easy disconnection of different TDs. The TD is pressed down into the wrist to eject the TD or to lock it into position.
- Wrist flexion. There are two versions of this unit: (1) The Hosmer wrist flexion unit can be manually placed in neutral, 30° of flexion, or 50° of flexion. (2) The dome-shaped Sierra wrist flexion unit can be screwed into a standard wrist unit and can be rotated and flexed to the same angles as the Hosmer unit. Wrist flexion units are indispensable for the person with bilateral amputations because of their usefulness in reaching the midline for toileting, dressing, and eating.
- Ball and socket. This unit can be pre-positioned around the ball, but it cannot be locked in position.

Transradial (BE) Components

Forearm Socket Designs

The residual limb is encased in the socket of the prosthesis with total contact. A standard forearm socket (Fig. 46-9) encases two-thirds of the arm length but can be cut down to allow for more active pronation and supination for a long limb. The supracondylar socket (modified Muenster) is a frequent choice for the short transradial limb; the proximal brim grips the humeral lateral and medial epicondyles and the posterior olecranon (Fig. 46-10). This design is widely used for the myoelectric prostheses. It is self-suspending, with no harnessing necessary.

Elbow Hinges

Elbow hinges connect the socket to the triceps cuff or pad on the upper arm. These can be flexible straps of Dacron or leather or rigid metal hinges. The flexible hinge allows for flexibility around the joint, whereas the rigid hinge offers stability at the elbow joint.

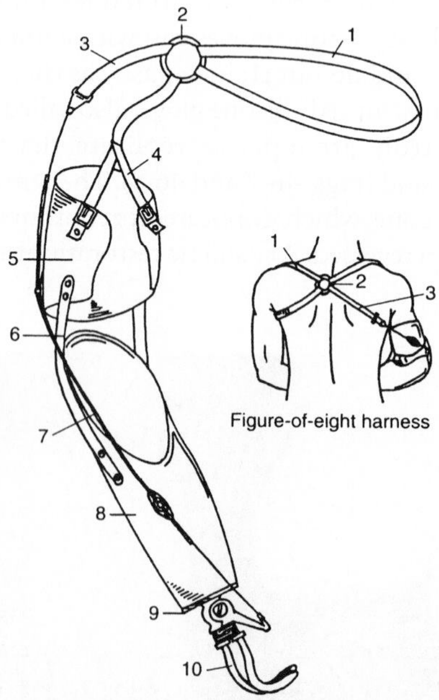

Figure 46-9 Standard transradial prosthesis. 1, Axilla loop; 2, Northwestern University (NU) ring; 3, Control-attachment strap; 4, Inverted Y strap; 5, Triceps cuff; 6, Flexible elbow hinge; 7, Cable; 8, Socket; 9, Wrist unit; and 10, TD. (Illustration by Gregory Celikyol.)

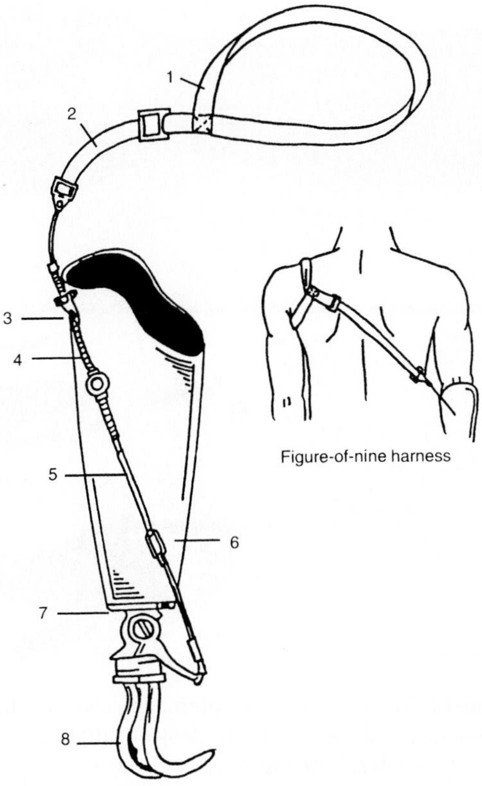

Figure 46-10 Supracondylar prosthesis. 1, Figure-of-nine harness; 2, Control attachment strap; 3, Lift loop; 4, Housing; 5, Cable; 6, Supracondylar socket; 7, Wrist unit; and 8, TD. (Illustration by Gregory Celikyol.)

Triceps Cuff

The triceps cuff on the upper arm is connected to the socket by the elbow hinge. It serves as a point of attachment for the cable housing of the control attachment strap.

Harness and Control System

The harness serves two purposes: (1) to suspend, or hold, the prosthesis firmly on the residual limb and (2) to allow for force (through body motion) to be transmitted to the control cable that operates the terminal device. Three types of harnesses are most popular for the transradial prosthesis: figure-of-eight, figure-of-nine, and chest strap with a shoulder saddle. The figure-of-eight harness is most often used. Its axilla loop serves as the anchor point (reaction point) from which the other straps are attached; the inverted **Y** support strap attaches to the anterior support strap of the harness. These two attachments are important because they stabilize the socket to the harness and prevent displacement when heavy loads are carried or lifted. The chest strap with shoulder saddle may be suitable for the patient who cannot tolerate the axilla loop pressure or when stability is needed for heavy work. The shoulder saddle distributes the pressure over a larger area. The figure-of-nine harness is used with the supracondylar socket. Since the socket configuration provides self-suspension, only a control attachment strap is needed to attach the axilla loop to the cable control system.

Transhumeral (AE) Components

Socket Designs

The conventional socket edge is generally just near or above the acromion, depending on limb length. Another design is often selected because it provides more rotational stability, as with the Utah arm. A transhumeral prosthesis with an internal locking elbow is shown in Figure 46-11.

Elbow Units

Two elbow units are available for the AE prosthesis: (1) an internal elbow locking unit for a standard or short transhumeral amputation and (2) an external elbow locking unit for a long transhumeral or elbow disarticulation amputation.

Friction Units

The friction unit must be manually flexed into place. It is lightweight and is used with passive prosthetic arms. Manual elbow components are also available with a locking mechanism.

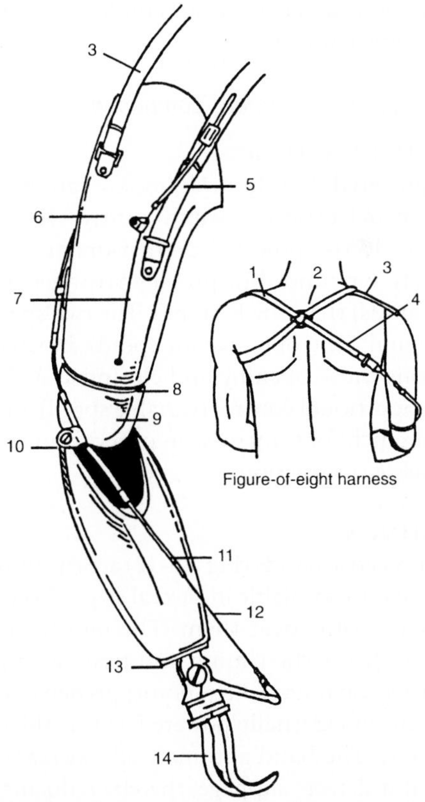

Figure 46-11 Standard transhumeral prosthesis. 1, Axilla loop; 2, Northwestern University (NU) ring; 3, Lateral support strap; 4, Control attachment strap; 5, Elastic anterior support strap; 6, Socket; 7, Elbow lock cable; 8, Turntable; 9, Internal elbow lock unit; 10, Lift loop; 11, Housing; 12, Cable; 13, Wrist unit; and 14, TD. (Illustration by Gregory Celikyol.)

EXTERNAL SPRING LIFT ASSIST
The external spring lift assist is a clock spring mechanism that is added to the medial side of the elbow. Tightening the mechanism causes increased tension for elbow flexion and assists in initiating this motion. The patient can adjust it.

SHOULDER HINGES
The shoulder hinges can be manually positioned into flexion or extension or abduction or adduction for placement of the arm in space.

Shoulder Disarticulation and Scapulothoracic Components

Most socket designs for shoulder disarticulation and scapulothoracic protheses consist of a plastic laminated shoulder cap or frame socket with carbon fiber reinforcements. Another choice is an endoskeletal passive arm that is lightweight and contains an internal pylon shaft. It is covered with resilient foam contoured to the shape of the arm. A chest strap harness suspends the prosthesis.

HARNESS AND CONTROL SYSTEMS
The harness and control systems for a transhumeral amputation are usually of the figure-of-eight or chest strap design. For a shoulder disarticulation prosthesis, the elbow lock can be activated using a chin nudge lever or a manual elbow lock mechanism.

Externally Powered Prosthetic Components

ELECTRIC TERMINAL DEVICES
Electric-powered hands and hooks can be activated through myoelectric or switch control (Heckathorne, 2004). The electric-powered prehensors are heavier (approximately 1 pound) but provide stronger pinch force (20–32 pounds) than the BP types. The two speed systems are: (1) digital control (constant speed), in which muscle contractions cause opening and closing at a given speed; and (2) proportional control (variable speed), in which the speed and pinch force increase in proportion to the intensity of muscle contraction.

ELECTRIC HANDS
Otto Bock electric hands (Fig. 46-12) are the most popular models. They are available in several sizes. Either a PVC or silicone glove can cover them. The motor in the hand mechanism drives the thumb and first two fingers as a unit to provide palmar (three-point) prehension. A recent development in externally powered TDs is the Otto Bock Sensor Hand. The hand automatically increases force on an object if it detects slippage, thereby reducing the mental load of the user. Constant visual contact with the object in the hand is unnecessary.

ELECTRIC HOOKS
The Otto Bock electric Greifer TD is interchangeable with the Otto Bock hand and may be preferred for work that requires prehension force up to 32 pounds. It is bulky, encased in a hard plastic shell with no glove covering, and is less delicate than the hand. It is available in one size. The two "fingers" move symmetrically in opposition to one another for precision pinch while a more proximal, expanded contact area provides for a cylindrical grasp (Fig. 46-13).

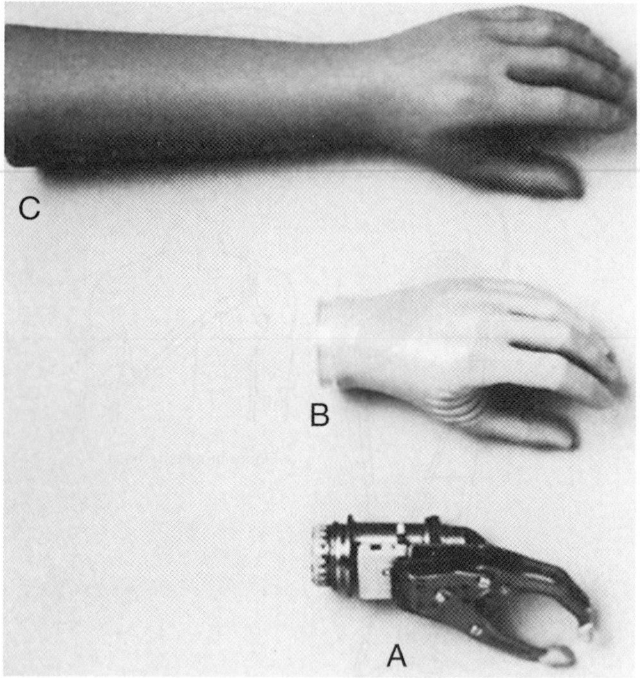

Figure 46-12 Electronic hand. **A.** Internal mechanism. **B.** Hand shell covering. **C.** Glove. (Photo courtesy of Otto Bock Orthopedic Industry, Minneapolis, MN.)

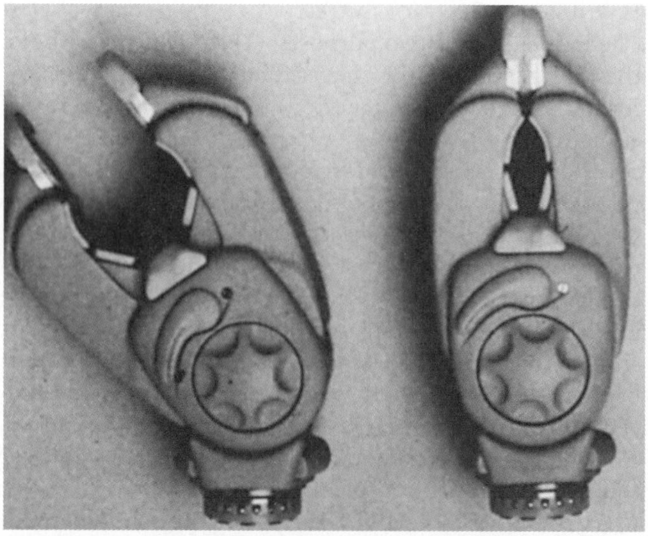

Figure 46-13 Electric Greifer TD in open and closed position. (Photo courtesy of Otto Bock Orthopedic Industry, Minneapolis, MN.)

The Hosmer NU-VA Synergetic Prehensor contains two motors geared to drive each of the two hook fingers differently. One finger can be made to move quickly for fast opening and closing, while the other finger applies the force for secure grip. Therefore, in grasping, one finger closes quickly on an object while the other finger applies the force for secure grip.

Electric Wrist Rotation Units

Wrist rotation units, used for pronation and supination, are being prescribed more often. Sears and Shaperman (1998) present a strong case for their use by persons with unilateral and bilateral amputations.

Electric Elbows

The following three electric elbow mechanisms are the most popular: the Boston elbow, the NY electric elbow (Hosmer), and the Utah (Motion Control) elbow (Fig. 46-14). These elbows can be controlled by electromechanical switches or by myoelectric control. The Boston and Motion Control elbows can accommodate wrist and hand components as well.

The Final Prescription: A Discussion

> "In the upper extremity, the prosthesis meets its greatest challenge. Here the lost function can only be imitated. . . . We must fit the prosthesis not only to the patient's limb but to his whole personality." (Kessler, 1947, p. 5)

Motivation is the most important factor in the acceptance and use of the prosthesis. In addition, clinician expertise, appropriateness of the prosthetic prescription to meet patient goals, and the final fit and function of the artificial limb contribute to the ultimate outcome. The prosthesis is chosen just when the patient is most confused and vulnerable. The patient's desire for a prosthesis is strongest after surgery and may wane as time passes, particularly for those with unilateral amputations, since compensatory one-handed techniques are soon perfected. The patient with a bilateral amputation needs function and is likely to accept and use the prostheses.

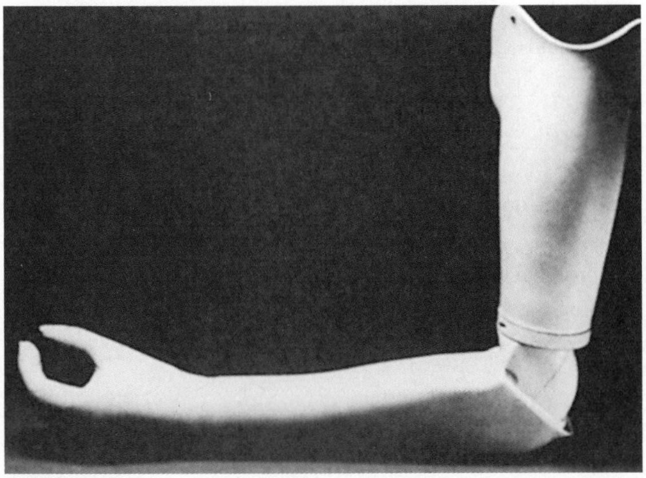

Figure 46-14 Utah arm with externally powered hand and elbow. (Photo courtesy of Motion Control, Salt Lake City, UT.)

What defines a successful wearer? When the prosthesis is viewed as necessary or meaningful for any activity, such as leisure activities, or for cosmesis, it has added to the quality of life and is therefore successful (Fraser, 1998; Wright & Hagen, 1995). A patient with a unilateral amputation may use the prosthesis for particular activities, such as for sports, and these interests can change with time. Two sets of prostheses are strongly recommended for the person with high-level bilateral amputations; this ensures that the patient will always have use of the prostheses should one set need repairs.

The end goal of a therapeutic program is to ensure the highest level of independence and competency in life roles that the patient views as meaningful. This does not always assume prosthetic use. It is, however, the team's responsibility to present the options to the patient.

PROSTHETIC TRAINING PROGRAM

The minimal training time is 6 hours for persons with transradial amputation; 15 hours for transhumeral, shoulder disarticulation, and bilateral transradial amputations; and 20 hours for bilateral transhumeral amputations.

Initial Stage of Treatment

The initial stage of treatment can generally be covered in one or two therapy sessions. Procedures for Practice 46-2 has treatment guidelines for this stage.

PROCEDURES FOR PRACTICE 46-2

Treatment Guidelines for Initial Stage of Treatment (ideally within 4–12 weeks of surgery)

- Evaluate the prosthesis.
- Explain program goals to the patient.
- Describe the functions of each component; give the patient an illustration of the prosthesis with components labeled.
- Teach the patient to don and doff the prosthesis.
- Discuss the wearing schedule with the patient.
- Teach limb hygiene care.
- Teach care of the prosthesis.
- Begin controls training using the terminal device.

Evaluation of the Prosthesis

On the first visit, the therapist checks out and evaluates the prosthesis before instituting training. The evaluation's purpose is to determine (1) compliance with the prescription, (2) comfort of fit of the socket and harness, (3) satisfactory operation of all components, and (4) appearance (features) of the prosthesis and its parts. Table 46-2 lists methods and standards for evaluation.

First Therapy Session

Generally, patients with unilateral amputations attend therapy on an outpatient schedule of 2 or 3 days a week; therefore, the first visit is a critical one. The aim from the outset is to minimize negative experiences to ensure acceptance and use of the prosthesis. In addition to evaluation of the prosthesis, the following must also be covered during the first visit: (1) donning and removing the prosthesis, (2) wearing schedule, and (3) hygienic care of the residual limb if the patient did not receive pre-prosthetic care in the clinic.

Donning and Removing the Prosthesis

Donning and removing the prosthesis can be achieved by one of two methods that simulate putting on a coat or pullover shirt. To use the coat method, the residual limb is inserted into the socket (Fig. 46-15), which is held in place with the intact hand, with the harness and axilla loop

Table 46-2. Chart for Evaluating a Prosthesis

Activity	Y	N	Comments
1. Does the prosthesis comply with the written prescription?			
2. Is the length of the prosthesis equal to the length of the sound arm? (Measure tip of TD to ground and compare to tip of thumb of sound hand to ground when the patient is standing. Compare elbow length for each side.)			
3. Are appearance and workmanship satisfactory? (Examine for smooth edges, smooth interior of socket, no loose rivets or screws, finished harness edges, and satisfactory arm color.)			
4. Can the socket tolerate a downward pull of 50 lb without displacing more than 1 in?			
5. a. Is there pain or discomfort while the limb is in the socket? b. Does the limb show abrasions or discoloration when the prosthesis is removed?			
6. a. Does the housing cover the cable without restricting elbow flexion? b. Is the cable free of sharp bends?			
7. a. Is the axilla loop small enough to keep the figure-eight harness below the seventh cervical vertebra and slightly to the unamputated side? b. Is the axilla loop covered and comfortable? c. Are all straps of adequate length and in proper alignment?			
8. a. Does the triceps cuff fit firmly without gapping? b. Can the turntable be rotated manually with relative ease and remain in position?			
9. a. Do the TDs and wrist unit function smoothly? b. Is the glove covering for the hand satisfactory in color and fit? c. Does the TD have full opening, closing? d. Can the TD be fully opened and closed at the hip, at 90° of elbow flexion, and at the mouth?			
10. Can forearm rotation that is at least 50% of rotation without the prosthesis be achieved?			
11. Can elbow flexion that is only 10° less than flexion with prosthesis off be achieved?			
12. For transhumeral amputation: a. Can 90° of shoulder abduction and flexion and 30° of arm extension be achieved? b. Can the prosthetic elbow be flexed by flexing the humerus 45° or less?			

Adapted from Department of Prosthetics and Orthotics. (1986). *Upper limb prosthetics.* New York: New York University Medical Center, Postgraduate Medical School.

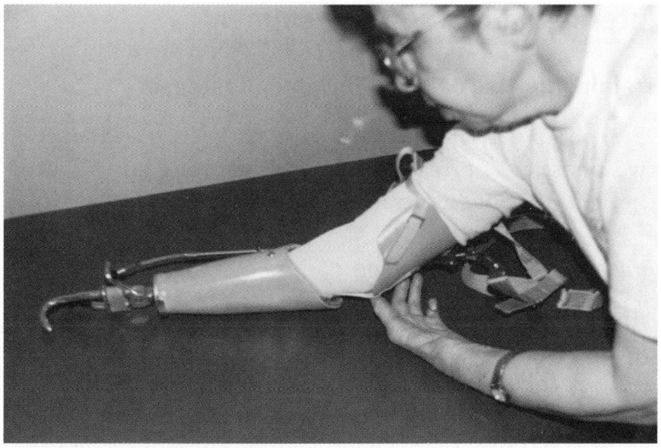

Figure 46-15 One method of donning a unilateral prosthesis.

dangling behind the back. The intact arm reaches behind and slips into the axilla loop; a forward shrug of the shoulders positions the prosthesis in place. For the pullover method, the patient places the prosthesis in front of him or her, and the intact arm is placed through the axilla loop while the residual limb is placed into the socket. Both limbs are raised to lift the prosthesis and harness over the head as the harness falls into place (Fig. 46-16). Initially, the prosthesis can be placed on a bed or dresser to support it as the patient slips into the prosthesis.

Wearing Time

The patient must increase wearing time gradually to develop tolerance to the socket and harness. The initial wearing time may be 15–30 minutes. Each time the prosthesis is removed, the residual limb must be examined for excessive redness or irritation, and it must not be reapplied until any redness subsides. ***Redness that does not disappear after approximately 20 minutes should be reported to the prosthetist for adjustment to the prosthesis.*** Otherwise, prosthetic wearing time can be increased in 30-minute increments until the prosthesis can be worn all day. The importance of gradually increasing the wearing time cannot be overemphasized, particularly for patients with decreased sensation and scar tissue.

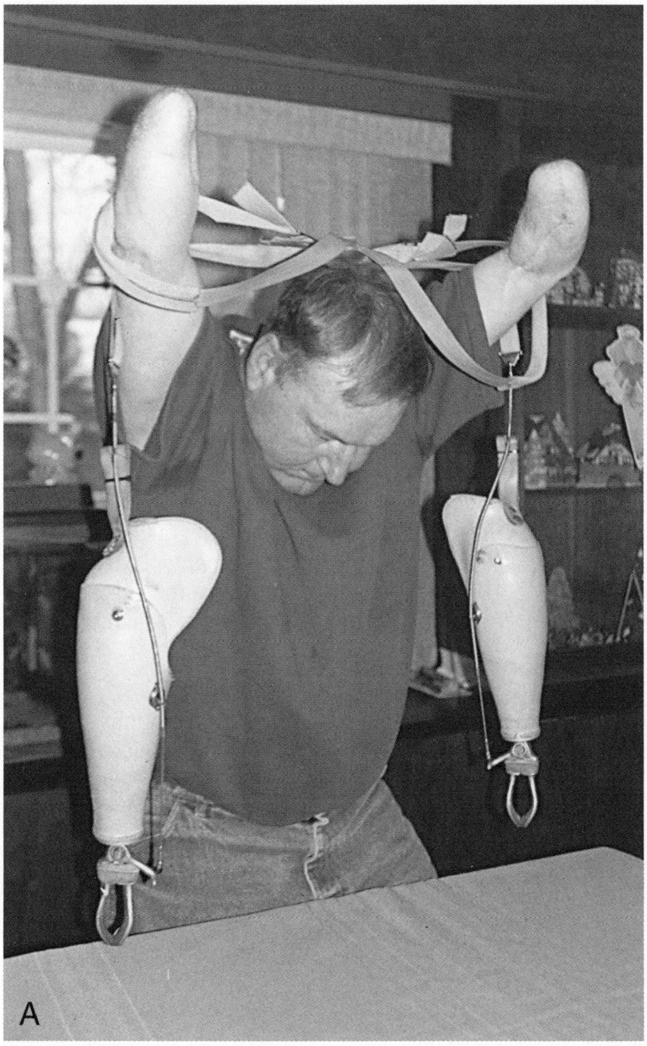

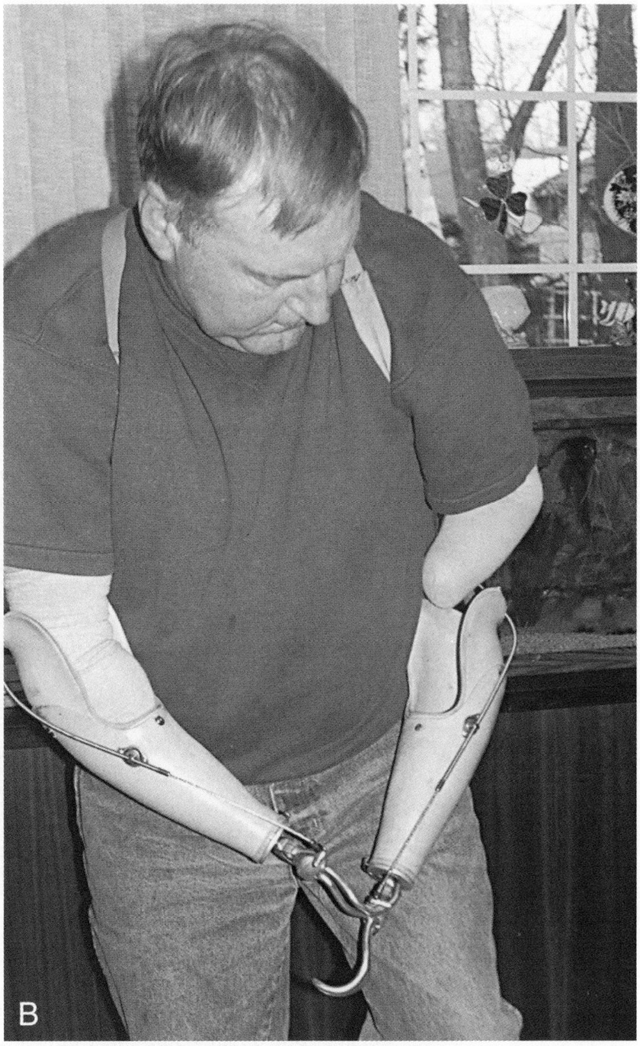

Figure 46-16 **A.** Donning bilateral harness overhead. **B.** Completing the process by inserting limbs into the sockets.

Limb Hygiene

Since the residual limb is enclosed in a rigid socket where excessive perspiration can macerate the skin, it is important to instruct the patient to wash the limb daily with mild soap and lukewarm water and pat dry. The therapist can recommend that the patient wear a tee shirt or equivalent covering so that the harness system of a BP prosthesis is not in direct contact with the skin. This provides padding and absorbs perspiration. For the same reason, the patient is instructed to wear a sock over the residual limb. A roll-on silicone liner may be issued to those who perform heavy work; it provides secure suspension and minimizes piston action, but can cause excessive perspiration.

Care of Prosthesis

Mild soap and warm water are recommended to clean the interior of the socket. It can also be wiped with rubbing alcohol every several weeks. The patient must be cautioned about agents that may stain or damage gloves. The hook is more rugged, but care must be taken during work in areas where there is excessive dirt, grease, or water. The patient must be especially careful with externally powered components.

Intermediate Stage of Treatment

Training for Use of Body-Powered Prosthesis

The therapy program for the BP prosthesis is addressed in two phases: (1) prosthetic controls training and (2) prosthetic functional use training.

Prosthetic Controls Training

Therapy for controls training begins with teaching the operation of each control, beginning with the TD (Procedures for Practice 46-3). The therapist guides the patient to practice repetitive activation of each component. Transradial prostheses have a single control system that activates the TD by cable pull. Patients are instructed to activate the TD (Figs. 46-17 and 46-18) by using humeral flexion and scapular abduction (protraction). Transhumeral prostheses have a dual control system for the TD and elbow. The motions required to lock and unlock the elbow are a combination of humeral extension, abduction, and depression (Fig. 46-19). TD activation is achieved in the same manner as with the transradial controls except that the elbow must be locked. The patient with a transhumeral prosthesis may also have to learn to

PROCEDURES FOR PRACTICE 46-3

Controls Training for Body Powered Prostheses

Component	Movement	Intervention
Terminal device	Humeral flexion with scapular abduction (protraction) on side of amputation; bilateral scapular abduction for midline use of TD or when strength is limited.	Manually guide patient through motions. For transhumeral prostheses, keep elbow unit locked in 90° flexion; teach TD control first.
Wrist unit	Rotate TD to supination (fingers of hook up), midposition (fingers toward midline), or pronation (fingers down). For unilateral amputation, patient uses sound hand to rotate TD. For bilateral amputation, rotate TD against stationary object, between knees, or with contralateral TD.	Have patient analyze the task and determine the most efficient approach for grasp, avoiding excessive or awkward movements. Examples: TD in midposition for carrying a tray, in pronation for grasping small box from table.
Elbow unit	Depress arm while extending and abducting humerus to lock or unlock elbow mechanism.	Manually guide patient through motions. Begin with elbow unlocked. Patient listens for click as lock activates. Have patient exaggerate movements initially. Use a mirror.
	Practice flexing and locking elbow in several planes.	Use humeral flexion to flex the elbow; go beyond desired height, since the arm will drop with gravity pull as patient is in process of locking the elbow unit.
Turntable	Rotate elbow turntable toward or away from body using sound hand. With bilateral amputations, push or pull against stationary object to rotate.	Teach patient to analyze task to determine need to use this component for more efficiency.

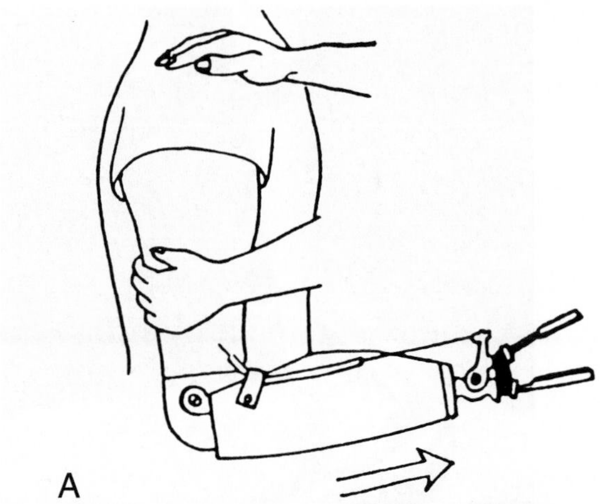

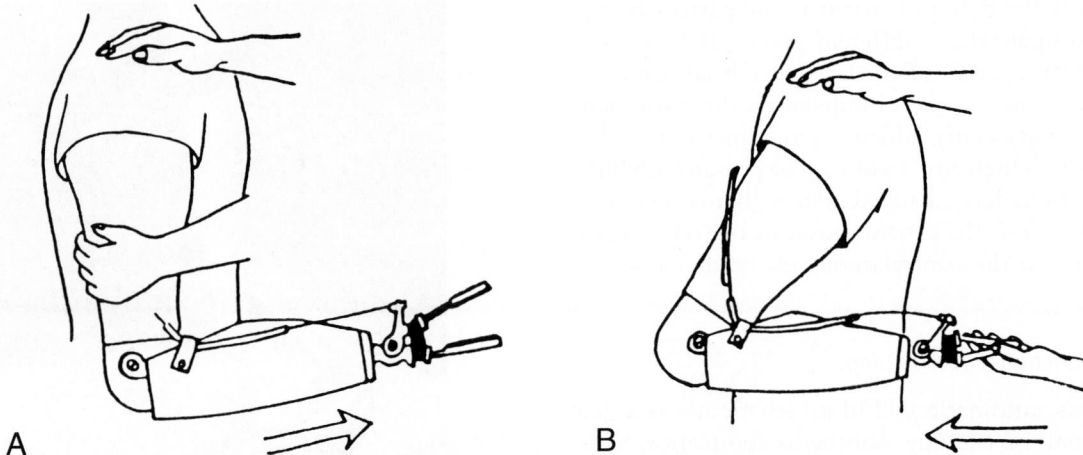

Figure 46-17 **A.** Teaching activation of VO TD. With elbow locked, therapist pulls the patient's upper arm forward to open TD. **B.** Teaching elbow lock and unlock. The therapist pushes the patient's arm back (*arrow*) into extension, abduction, and depression. It is brought back to the vertical plane between cycles. (Illustration by Gregory Celikyol.)

use the turntable to rotate the arm and possibly a shoulder joint to position the shoulder.

Practice in control drills requires coaching the patient in patterns of reach, grasp, and release for objects that vary in weight, size, texture, and configuration. Ordinarily, the sequence is from large, hard objects to small, fragile ones. These assortments are subject to the therapist's ingenuity and patient's interests. Initially, objects are placed on a tabletop for prehension practice; they are then transported to various locations in the room. The therapist instructs the patient to determine the most natural and efficient position for the TD before grasping an item and to rotate it in the wrist unit. This is called pre-positioning the TD.

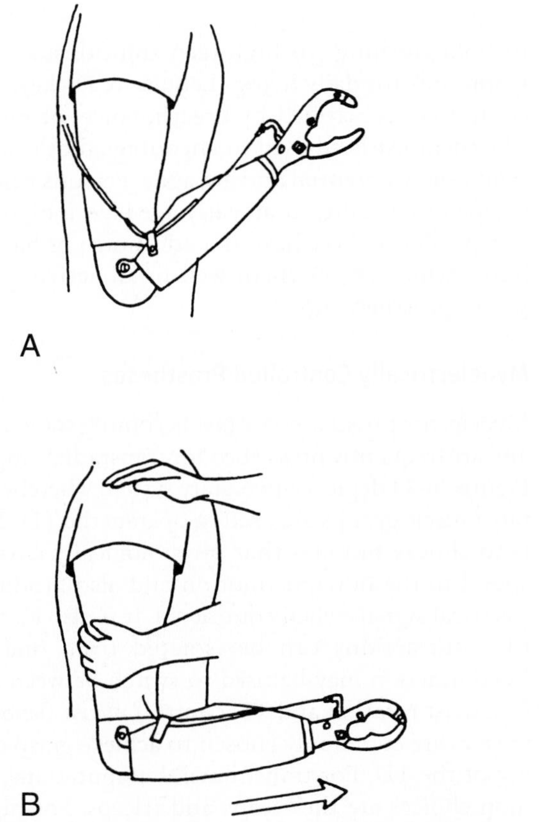

Figure 46-18 Activation of voluntary closing TD. **A.** The TD remains open at rest **B.** The TD closes with forward flexion. (Illustration by Gregory Celikyol.)

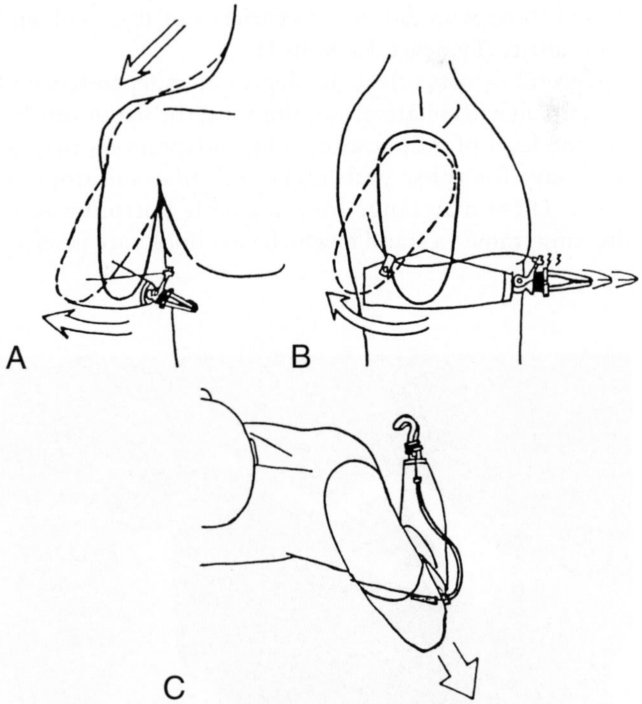

Figure 46-19 Motions (*arrows*) necessary for elbow lock or unlock for a transhumeral prosthesis. **A.** Abduction with depression. **B.** Extension. **C.** Combined movement pattern of extension, depression, and abduction. (Illustration by Gregory Celikyol.)

Eventually the therapist instructs the patient to perform motion patterns in different planes, such as overhead, at tabletop, and at floor level. Overhead use is the most difficult because it is hindered by the harnessing system; it is particularly difficult, sometimes impossible, for persons with high amputations. The person with bilateral amputations has a harness system that is bilaterally attached; therefore, the patient must practice relaxing the musculature on the contralateral side while using one prosthesis.

Prosthetic Functional Use Training

Spontaneous, automatic skillful prosthetic use is a goal for functional use training. Another is completion of activities within a reasonable length of time while using minimal extraneous movement and energy expenditure. Figures 46-20 to 46-23 show functional tasks. The therapist encourages patients to analyze and see similarities among situations and reminds them of relevant principles. This prepares the patient to respond with a sense of control in unpredictable situations.

A person with a unilateral amputation can be expected to use the prosthesis primarily for sustained holding or for stabilization and to use it more slowly compared to the unaffected extremity. Table 46-3 suggests how some activities can be accomplished; Atkins and Meier (2004b) offer more comprehensive lists. An interesting study (Lake, 1997) revealed that individuals who received training surpassed those who did not in efficiency of use, skill, and spontaneity (Evidence Table 46-1).

Several factors affect the degree of independence of the person with bilateral amputations, the major one being the level of amputation. Some adaptations may be necessary for those with high-level bilateral amputations. These may range from a simple buttonhook or dressing frame—a stand in which coat hooks are inserted to hold clothing—to high-tech solutions, such as electronic aids for daily living (Lehneis & Dickey, 1992) and computers controlled by breath, voice, or mouthstick. The therapist is advised to encourage foot use when patients show potential and are agile. Persons who have developed this ability at an early age have a high degree of independence. Feet have the advantage of having sensibility, which serves them well in all activities and surpasses prosthetic use.

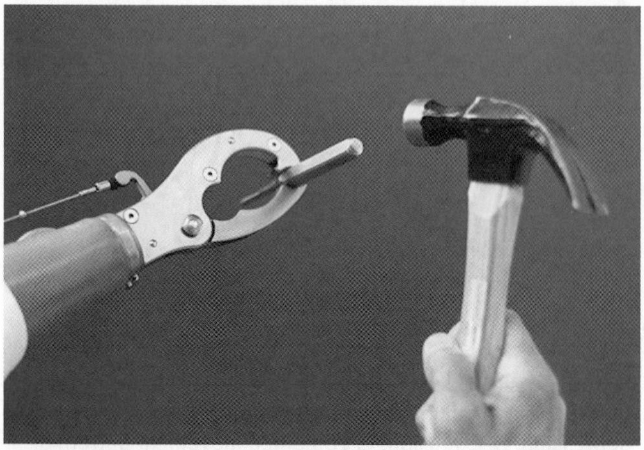

Figure 46-20 Use of the voluntary closing TRS Grip for bimanual task. (Photo courtesy of TRS, Inc., Brooklyn, NY.)

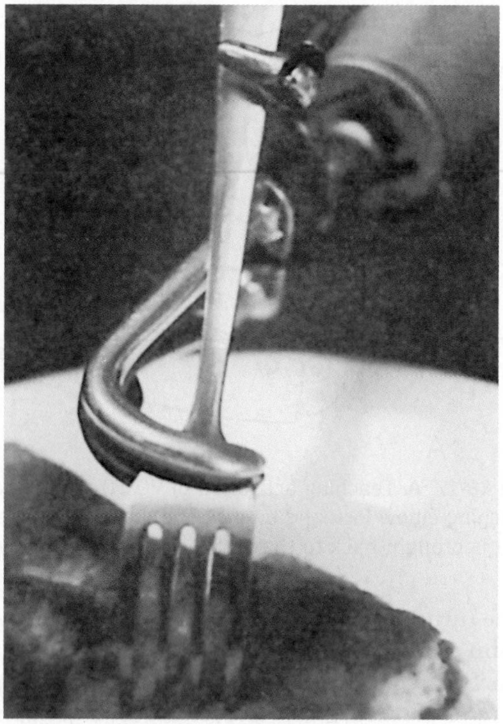

Figure 46-21 Grasping a fork using this method provides stability while the sound hand cuts the food.

Myoelectrically Controlled Prostheses

Myoelectric prostheses are fast becoming standard choices and are frequently prescribed for transradial amputations. Figure 46-24 depicts a two-state system whereby two separate muscle groups are used to operate the TD. The intent is to choose muscles that physiologically closely correspond to the outcome motion and also produce strong electrical signals when contracted. It is also essential that the contractions can be isolated from one another. Cocontraction may be used to switch between functions (i.e., wrist rotation and TD control). Wrist flexors and extensors are commonly chosen to achieve grasp and opening of the TD. For transhumeral amputations, the common choices are the biceps and triceps. For higher level amputations, as in shoulder disarticulation or forequarter amputations, the choices for control may be trapezius, latissimus, infraspinatus, or pectoralis muscles.

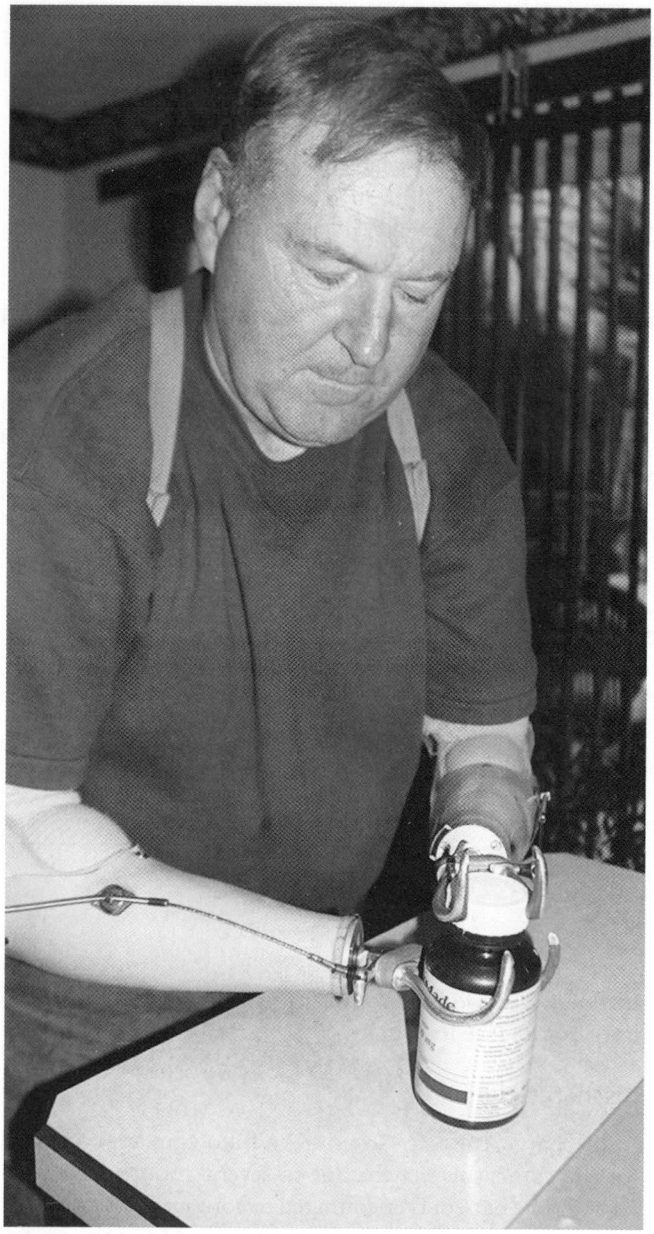

Figure 46-22 One way to open a jar using bilateral prostheses.

Most of the principles and treatment goals previously mentioned for BP prosthesis training apply to myoelectrically controlled prostheses. The therapy program begins with evaluation of the prosthesis, with special emphasis on the control system (Spiegel, 1989). Factors to be addressed include:

- Are the electrodes aligned along the direction of the muscle fiber and placed over the site offering the best muscle control potential?
- Is there good contact between the electrodes and the skin? (An imprint should be visible on the skin when the prosthesis is removed but should not be deep enough to cause irritation.)
- Can the patient open and close the hand in various planes?
- Can the patient remove and replace the battery with ease?

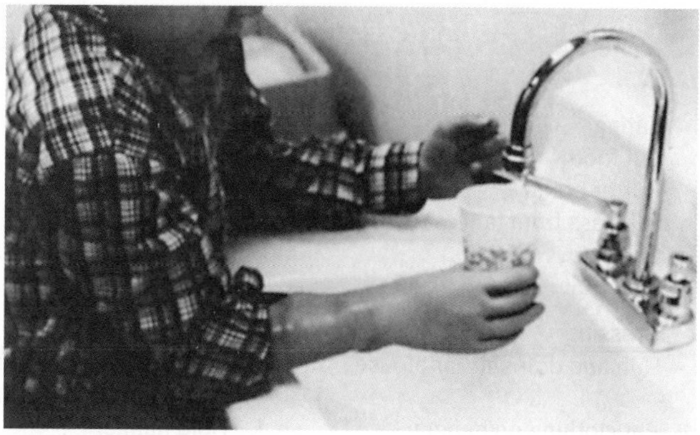

Figure 46-23 The myoelectric hand can hold delicate objects in bimanual activities.

The therapist should consult with the prosthetist for guidance with any concerns. Donning and removing the prosthesis may require collaboration with the prosthetist to determine the simplest method for the patient. Often, a slight twisting of the forearm when inserting the limb is helpful. Sometimes baby powder or a lubricant can be used to ease donning, but these may inhibit electrode functioning.

Care of the socket requires daily cleansing with a damp cloth and mild soap to remove any residues of powder, lubricants, and perspiration. Other special concerns are care of the batteries, methods of charging the batteries, and operation of the on-off switch. Care of the glove was discussed earlier.

Controls and functional use training goals are similar to those for the BP prosthesis. This assumes that the patient has already received muscle site controls training during the pre-prosthetic period. When a myoelectric tester is used (a biofeedback unit can also be used), the goals are to isolate muscle contractions and increase muscle strength (see Chapter 20). If sustained grasp is required for an extended period, when one might inadvertently contract muscles that open the hand, a manual lock mechanism can be installed in the hand. This can be controlled by pushing it in with the remaining hand.

Final Stage of Treatment: IADLs

In the final stage, prosthetic functional use skills are further refined, and daily living activities that are more demanding are introduced. Discharge planning should

Table 46-3. Suggested Approaches for Functional Activities: Unilateral Upper Limb Amputation

Task	Prosthesis	Sound Limb
Eating		
Cut food	Hold fork	Cut with knife
Butter bread	Stabilize bread	Spread toward body
Fill glass from faucet	Hold glass	Turn knob or lever
Carry tray	TD in midposition to hold	Hold in midposition
Peel fruit	Stabilize with TD	Peel
Dressing		
Don and doff shirt or blouse	Don: prosthesis in sleeve first; doff: remove sound arm first	Don: sound arm last; doff: remove prosthesis last
Put clothing on hanger	Hold hanger	Place clothing on hanger
Buckle belt	Stabilize belt	Push belt through buckle
Tie bow	Stabilize lace	Manipulate and make loops
Button cuff on sound side	Use buttonhook (or sew on button with elastic thread)	Hold cuff in place with fingertips while using buttonhook
Use zipper	Hold fabric with TD	Pull zipper
Desk skills		
Write	Stabilize paper	Write
Insert letter in envelope	Hold, stabilize envelope at end	Insert letter and seal
Use phone, dial, take notes	Hold receiver: TD or with chin and shoulder	Dial and write
Draw line with ruler; use paper clip	Stabilize ruler; hold paper	Draw line; apply clip
General skills		
Take bill from wallet	Hold wallet or stabilize on table	Manipulate wallet and remove bill
Wrap and unwrap package	Stabilize box and paper	Manipulate box, paper; tie
Thread needle	Hold needle	Thread needle

include exploration of vocational and recreational interests and driving and/or the use of public transportation. An adaptation for driving may be a simple knob or driving ring attached to the steering wheel. Foot controls can be installed for those with very high level bilateral amputations. The therapist can consult companies that do van conversions (see Chapter 31).

Visits to the community, home, school, and work are strongly advised. This brings the patient and therapist into the actual environment, away from simulated, static settings. Patients may be referred to a self-help group. These organizations vary in their goals, but most provide a forum wherein people can interact and share experiences. Many groups provide ongoing educational programs on new prosthetic developments or on sports and recreational activities.

Sports and Recreation

Increasing numbers of individuals with amputations are pursuing recreational activities, and as a result, several customized prosthetic components are available for sports and recreational activities (Radocy, 2004; Radocy & Furlong, 2004). Figures 46-25 to 46-27 show modifications used to enable participation in sports activities. The Internet is a good source of information for this and related topics (see Resources 46-1).

Discharge Planning

At discharge, the team schedules a follow-up appointment for the clinic; this may be one to several months after discharge. The patient is encouraged to contact the prosthetist for repairs or maintenance as needed and to make an appointment for a clinic visit at any time. Patients' needs do not remain constant; as they resume their lives, they may want special modifications or different prostheses.

PARTIAL HAND AMPUTATIONS

As with any amputation, the surgeon performing a partial hand amputation attempts to preserve length with intact sensibility. At this level, retaining residual digits with adequate skin coverage and some degree of mobility and sensation is far superior to any prosthesis (Bunnell, 1990) and is the goal. The principles of pre-prosthetic therapy (discussed earlier) apply to this level of amputation as well. Devices available for persons with partial

CASE EXAMPLE

Mr. C.: Training with a Myoelectric Prosthesis for Transradial Amputation

Occupational Therapy Process	Clinical Reasoning Process: Objectives	Clinical Reasoning Process: Examples of Therapist's Internal Dialogue
Patient Information Mr. C., aged 53 years, sustained a crush injury of his dominant right arm in machinery at work that required a transradial (BE) amputation. His role as plant manager in a recycling plant is comprised of tasks including worker supervision, activities including machinery adjustment, and habits including lifting. Other self-maintenance roles are husband, parent of two teenaged children, and sole wage earner for the family.	Understand the patient's diagnosis or condition	"Mr. C. has experienced a type of amputation that is not uncommon for workplace injuries and has achieved appropriate goals, which include dominance retraining for fine motor demands, tolerance and control of a body-powered prosthesis, and independence in self-care activities. Harnessing configuration that is used for a transradial body-powered prosthesis interfered with overhead reach and made it difficult to maintain grasp on items at floor level."
Mr. C. received occupational therapy to use a body-powered prosthesis with interchangeable hook and hand. He chose to use the hand rather than the hook, as appearance was important to him. He developed exceptional dexterity in his remaining hand and has continued to improve writing skills. Full day–wearing tolerance and independence in self-care skills were achieved with the body-powered prosthesis. However, Mr. C. continued to have difficulty grasping objects above shoulder level and occasionally grasping items at floor level because of harnessing strap restrictions. Mr. C. has returned to work part time and resumed his position as plant manager.	Know the person	"Mr. C. had demonstrated his motivation to integrate prosthesis use into job tasks but desired improved performance with some job tasks. As sole wage earner of his family, successful job performance is critical. Cosmesis is also important as indicated by Mr. C.'s choice of a hand rather than a hook terminal device."
Reason for Referral to Occupational Therapy Mr. C. has requested a myoelectrically controlled prosthesis with a hand terminal device. Approval was received from the insurance company for the prosthesis and indicated therapy services. Mr. C. was scheduled for occupational therapy to determine whether he is a candidate and to provide training if eligible.	Appreciate the context Develop provisional hypotheses	"During the 2 months that Mr. C. received occupational therapy, I consulted and treated with the prosthetist as needed to ensure best results with prosthesis fit and use. It was helpful to further discuss Mr. C.'s vocational requirements and performance with his employer, ensure that Mr. C.'s expectations were realistic, and arrange for a job site visit. Because Mr. C. had expressed some anxiety about returning to work full time, a psychologist's consultation was arranged. Based on his desire and ability to complete most job responsibilities with a body-powered prosthesis, I anticipated that Mr. C. would successfully incorporate his requested myoelectric prosthesis into self-advancement activities."
Assessment Process and Results Mr. C. was tested with the myotester and was able to achieve a sufficient, although inconsistent, level of muscle contraction in wrist flexors and extensors.	Consider evaluation approach and methods	"The myotester provided more accurate measurement of isolated and sustained muscle contraction than palpation or manual muscle testing so that the prosthetist and I could determine the best positions for the electrode placement."

Interpret observations	"Because he demonstrated sufficient muscle contraction in the desired muscle groups, I focused Mr. C.'s pre-prosthetic training on improving consistency, endurance, and control of these contractions."

Occupational Therapy Problem List

- Inconsistent demonstration of developed capacity to maintain strong muscle contractions
- Inconsistent demonstration of developed capacity to isolate muscle contractions
- Inability to demonstrate developed capacity of grading (increasing or decreasing) volitional muscle contractions, which relates to use of proportional control in the prosthesis
- Decreased ability to reach overhead or to floor with body-powered prosthesis, especially during vocational activities

Synthesize results	"The inconsistency of maintained and isolated muscle contractions was a result of fatigue and disuse of the wrist flexors and extensors while the body-powered prosthesis was worn. Mr. C. benefited from the visual feedback available during pre-prosthetic training as well as use of simulated and actual self-advancement activities."

Occupational Therapy Goal List

Pre-Prosthetic Goals (anticipated length of treatment: six 1-hour sessions)

1. Mr. C. will achieve maximal muscle contraction (as measured by myotester or myosoftware) of wrist flexors and extensors.
2. Mr. C. will maintain the level of contraction of the agonist while relaxing the antagonist muscle.
3. Mr. C. will control (or grade) the magnitude of contractions.
4. Mr. C. will demonstrate improved performance of identified tasks with dominant left hand.

Myoelectric Prosthetic Training Goals (anticipated length of treatment: eight 2-hour sessions)

1. Mr. C. will demonstrate control of the myoelectric hand during clinic drills.
2. Mr. C. will use the prosthesis during self-maintenance and self-enhancement task-specific training.
3. Mr. C. will consistently use the prosthesis as a functional assist at work.

Develop intervention hypotheses	"Mr. C.'s ability to achieve isolation, consistency, and control of wrist contractions during the pre-prosthetic training allowed for optimal prosthetic outcomes. Prosthetic training progressed from demonstration of basic skills to consistent incorporation of the myoelectric hand as a functional assist during work tasks."
Select an intervention approach	"Visual feedback from the myotester and myosoftware not only promoted Mr. C.'s learning, but also provided positive feedback, which encouraged him to participate and improve during the sessions. Because I had experience and training with myotesters and myosoftware programs, I was able to provide the treatment recommended. Contact was made with the prosthetist as questions or problems arose." "I chose clinical drills and task-specific training that allowed Mr. C. to master control of the myoelectric hand when grasping, holding, releasing, and reaching for different objects. When indicated, I increased the level of difficulty, requiring him to handle crushable objects and perform manipulative bilateral tasks before performing occupational tasks. In the clinic environment, I instructed and observed Mr. C., analyzing and grading his tasks and activities."
Consider what will occur in therapy, how often, and for how long	"The intervention approaches I chose could be completed in the 2-month time frame anticipated."

Intervention

Pre-Prosthetic Intervention

Mr. C. was instructed to flex and extend the sound wrist/hand and imitate the contractions with the residual limb. The visual feedback of the myotester and training software allowed Mr. C. to improve proportional control, isolation, and endurance of muscle contractions. Mr. C. was able to open and close an electronic hand (held by therapist or placed on a stand) using refined muscle contractions. Mr. C. received the permanent myoelectric prosthesis, which contains a supracondylar socket without harness straps and a proportionally controlled electronic hand.

Assess the patient's comprehension Understand what he is doing Compare actual to expected performance Know the person Appreciate the context	"Mr. C. was able to demonstrate understanding of specific muscle contractions of the wrist flexors and extensors by producing these movements consistently during pre-prosthetic training. The visual feedback provided by the myotester and myosoftware engaged him in the training process as he improved his muscle strength and control. By using the practice electronic hand, Mr. C. further refined the natural movement speed and appearance required for grasp and release of objects. The myoelectric prosthesis socket fit Mr. C. comfortably. He was able to open and close his hand consistently, indicating accurate placement and contact of the electrodes on the muscles."

Prosthetic Intervention

Mr. C. learned to don and remove the prosthesis, clean the socket and electrodes, and change the battery. Instruction was given for precautions with prosthesis use and care of the prosthesis glove. He practiced maintaining grasp and grading control of pressure on objects.

The therapist obtained job requirements from Mr. C.'s employer, and Mr. C. simulated tool use and lifting/placement of items from floor to shelves at shoulder height.

During a job site visit, Mr. C. was observed performing his job tasks, and recommendations for modification of activity or environment were discussed with Mr. C. and his employer. A plan for gradually increasing Mr. C.'s hours and responsibilities were also discussed, decreasing the anxiety he initially expressed.

"Following instruction from the prosthetist and therapist, Mr. C. independently cared for and wore his prosthesis. He understood the progression of occupational therapy treatment, demonstrating controlled grasp and release of various items in all arm movement ranges before practicing simulated work tasks. In the clinic, adaptive equipment or techniques were used when needed so that Mr. C. could incorporate his myoelectric hand as an assist when using tools, performing desk activities, and lifting items unilaterally or bilaterally.

The job site visit allowed Mr. C. to demonstrate his competence with the performance of self-advancement activities to his employer. Mr. C. was encouraged by the support of his employer and actively participated in applying the activity and environmental modification recommendations.

Mr. C. was no longer apprehensive about returning to work because he was confident about the cosmesis and function of his myoelectric hand."

Next Steps

- Mr. C. was discharged from occupational therapy but was encouraged to contact the therapist for problems or questions if needed.
- Mr. C. saw his psychologist to address any remaining concerns about occupational adjustment and participated in a monthly support group for amputees.
- Mr. C. continued with periodic doctor and prosthetist appointments as indicated. The myoelectric prosthesis needed to be replaced within 2 years, and the gloves were replaced more frequently.
- Mr. C. was given a list of written and Internet resources so that he could increase his knowledge about myoelectric prostheses and, if desired, contact others with similar life circumstances.

Anticipate present and future patient concerns

Analyze patient's comprehension

Decide if the patient should continue or discontinue therapy and/or return in the future

"After observing Mr. C. at work, I was confident that he would successfully use his myoelectric prosthesis effectively. He had expressed satisfaction with the appearance and performance of the myoelectric hand. He had demonstrated good generation and application of adaptive problem-solving during his therapy course. Mr. C. had established a strong support network and was motivated to use the appropriate resources so that he could achieve the best possible outcome in his occupational roles."

? CLINICAL REASONING IN OCCUPATIONAL THERAPY PRACTICE

Myoelectric Prosthesis Training

Mr. C. has demonstrated effective use of a body-powered hand prosthesis but is challenged by lifting items that require bimanual grasp in various planes and in maintaining a firm grasp when adjusting machinery.

How can the therapist design a program that will address these issues? What information is necessary to quantify the job requirements?

Evidence Table 46-1
Best Evidence for Occupational Therapy Practice Regarding Upper Extremity Amputations

Intervention	Description of Intervention Tested	Participants	Dosage	Type of Best Evidence and Level of Evidence	Benefit	Statistical Probability and Effect Size of Outcome	Reference
Training with bilateral training prostheses	One group received training at home, while the control group was given the same tools and activities but not specific training.	10 individuals without amputations, using training prostheses, randomized to experimental and control groups. Mean age = 48.5 years.	Four sessions of 2 hours each.	Randomized trial. IC2b	Greater improvement in efficiency and skill in the group who received training as reflected on the *University of New Brunswick (UNB) Test of Prosthetic Function* (Sanderson & Scott, 1985; Burger, Brezovar, & Marinček, 2004).	The trained group performed significantly more skillfully than the untrained group on one of the subtests ($p = 0.03$, $r = 0.59$) and significantly more efficiently on two of the subtests ($p = 0.006$, $r = 0.79$; $p = 0.04$, $r = 0.55$). Statistical significance was not attained on all subtests, however, probably due to small sample size.	Lake, 1997
Fitting of bilateral transhumeral, low-temperature plastic prostheses with utensils to address specific patient goals: feeding, dressing, and writing	Patient was fit with 2 sockets, figure-eight harness, 2 utensil holders and several utensil devices, a dressing hook, and a typing bar. Patient was trained to change and adjust utensils.	One right-handed subject with bilateral transhumeral amputations resulting from electrical burn injury. Initially fitted with bilateral transhumeral body-powered prostheses.	10 hours of training with initial prosthetic prescription, spread over 1 month; 1 hour of training with "utensil" prostheses.	Single-subject case report. Unrated.	After 10 years, subject reports successfully using the "utensil" prostheses to accomplish his stated goals more than 8 hours per day. He scored 100 (highest score) on the *Barthel Index*.	Not applicable.	Hung & Wu, 2005

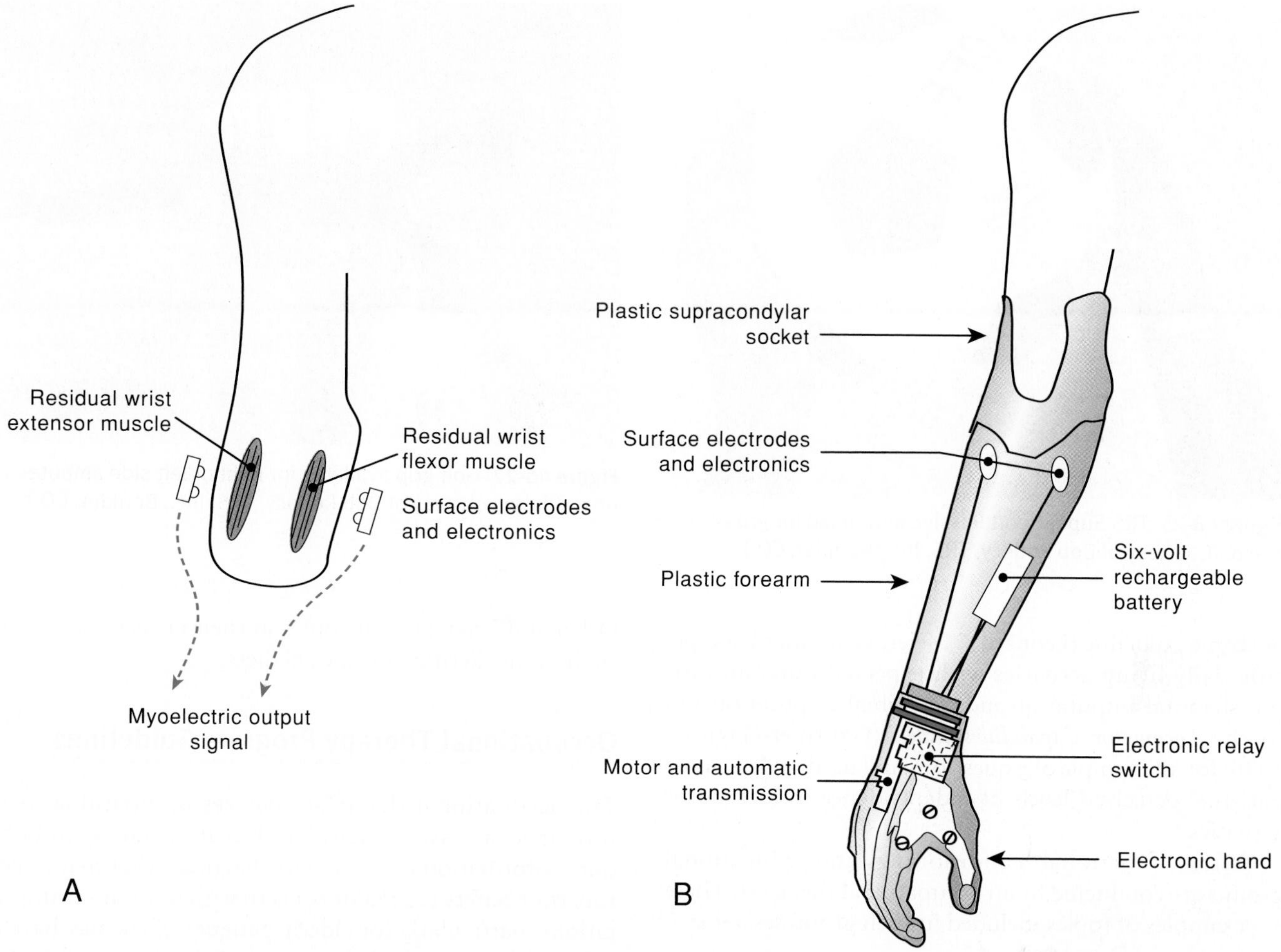

Figure 46-24 Myoelectric prosthesis, a two-state system in which two separate muscle groups operate the terminal device. **A.** 1. The muscle contracts and creates an electrical signal that can be measured in microvolts (1 millionth of a volt). 2. The EMG signal is detected by the surface electrode. 3. The EMG signal is processed by the electronics and transmitted to the electronic relay in the hand. **B.** 1. When the electronic relay receives an EMG signal from the wrist flexors, the circuit is complete, and the electricity from the battery runs the motor to close the hand. 2. When the relay receives an EMG signal from the wrist extensors, the motor runs in the opposite direction to open the hand. (Illustration courtesy of Jack Hodgins, CPO, Kessler Institute for Rehabilitation, West Orange, NJ.)

hand amputations can be described as cosmetic, passive functional, or active functional prostheses.

Some patients with a partial hand amputation want a prosthesis that closely replicates the look of the hand and provides dexterity as well. Although cosmetic hand coverings are truly artistic endeavors, once they fit over the residual hand, tactile sensation is lost, which limits function. The passive functional prosthesis may be a highly specialized device that is task specific, or it may be a simple post to provide opposition.

An active functional prosthesis may be cable driven by scapular or humeral movements, requiring restrictive harnessing. This, however, may be the best option for the person with bilateral amputations (Weir, Grahn, & Duff, 2001).

MANAGEMENT OF LOWER LIMB AMPUTATIONS

The therapeutic program for persons with lower limb amputations requires collaboration between the physical therapist and occupational therapist. The physical therapist is responsible for skin care, limb wrapping, lower limb strengthening exercises, range of motion, and ambulation training. Training in some daily living activities may be shared, for example limb bandaging, bed mobility, and transfers. Critical care pathways can identify specific goals within a time frame for all professionals involved with patient care, ensuring maximum functional outcome (Esquenazi, 1996). The therapist can refer to a functional

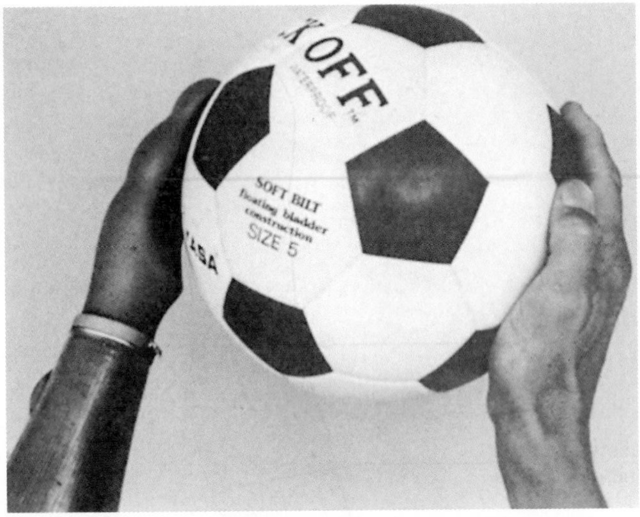

Figure 46-25 TRS Super Sport Passive Mitt, used for gross grasp. (Courtesy of Bob Rodocy, TRS, Inc., Boulder, CO.)

outcome guideline (Leonard & Meier, 1998) that lists specific daily living activities with expected outcomes for transfemoral amputation and transtibial amputation and to the *Locomotor Capabilities Index* (Gauthier-Gagnon, 1998) for an example of a questionnaire used to determine patients' perceived levels of independence in locomotor activities.

Often, functional conditioning and educational groups are conducted by an occupational therapist. These are examples of topics included in such group sessions:

- Upper extremity strengthening exercises
- Safety precautions related to specific activities
- Principles of energy conservation and body mechanics
- Use of adaptive devices
- Review of dietary restriction when appropriate

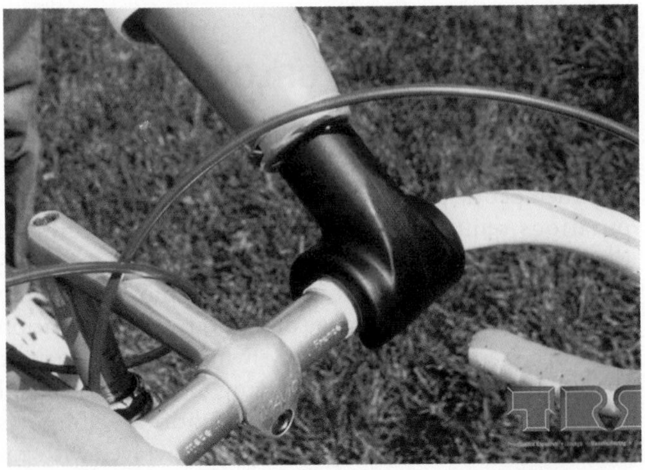

Figure 46-26 Handlebar adapter. (Photo courtesy of Bob Rodocy, TRS, Inc., Boulder, CO.)

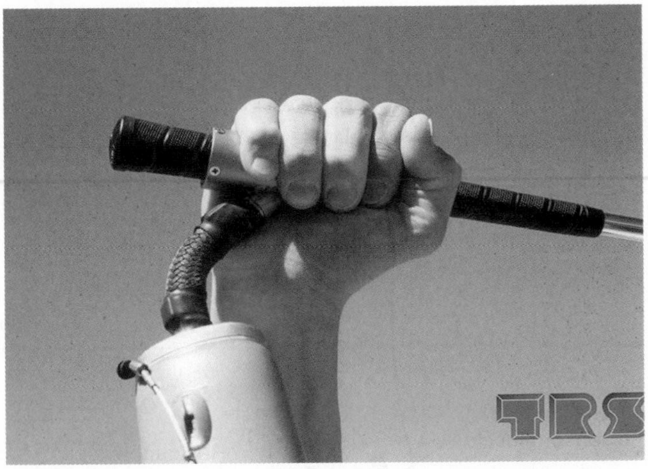

Figure 46-27 Golf grip available for right or left side amputation. (Photo courtesy of Bob Rodocy, TRS, Inc., Boulder, CO.)

Other staff may present topics in their areas of expertise, such as the dietitian on special diets.

Occupational Therapy Program Guidelines

The occupational therapist analyzes occupational performance, assesses physical and mental status, and obtains information on secondary diagnoses that may affect function. Safety is a major concern with lower limb amputations, particularly for elderly patients. They may have a primary diagnosis of diabetes or vascular disease with secondary complicating factors that affect therapy, such as kidney disease, cardiovascular disease, chronic infection, respiratory disease, and arthritis. In the elderly, impaired vision and memory deficits may influence safe performance in activities of daily living. Energy expenditure 25–40% above normal can be expected for unilateral transtibial amputation, 68–100% above normal for unilateral transfemoral, more than 40% above normal for bilateral transtibial, and 100% above normal for bilateral transtibial-transfemoral amputation (Esquenazi, 1996).

From the outset, coordination with the physical therapist will determine the wearing schedule and the amount of assistance or assistive device needed, as well as readiness for any standing or ambulation activities. The occupational therapist and physical therapist can address activities of daily living in the following sequence: bed mobility; hygiene and grooming; dressing, including donning and removing the leg prosthesis; and wheelchair propulsion and management. Transfer skills are practiced with and without the prosthesis. Practice sessions include transfers to the bed, toilet, furniture, and car. The therapists teach the family the transfer techniques when safety is a concern. The occupational therapist addresses energy, effort, and mobility skills in the kitchen while the patient is using a wheelchair and/or ambulating with the prosthesis. The therapist includes other self-maintenance skills as appropriate, such as housecleaning and bed making. Home and community visits with the patient and a staff member may be indicated. During standing and ambulation, special attention is paid to balance, posture, and equal weight bearing through both legs.

Appropriate application of the prosthesis is crucial and always begins with skin inspection. Stump socks, liners, or sheaths and inserts are applied, and then the hard socket (Fig. 46-28). The socks should have no wrinkles, and seams should not be over bony areas or the scar. The transfemoral prosthesis should be applied in standing because weight bearing will ensure total contact. This may be challenging for the elderly individual. Consultation with the physical therapist should be ongoing to determine the amount of support and assistance the patient requires in this process.

The therapist may recommend home modifications and equipment to the patient and family. Equipment often includes transfer tub bench or seat and toilet safety arm rails. These rails fit around the toilet and provide a means of arm support that assists with lowering and coming to standing. The therapist makes the referral for driving assessment and training when appropriate. Installation of a left-foot accelerator bar and pedal is necessary for a person with a right-leg amputation. Hand controls can be installed for persons with bilateral leg amputations (see Chapter 31).

EMERGING TRENDS IN PROSTHETICS

Recent improvements in lower extremity prosthetic devices related to materials include suspension sleeves and gel interfaces in direct contact with the skin and the use of carbon fiber and graphite combined with improved mechanical and electro-mechanical components. Innovations have enabled more successful participation in ADLs, including recreational sports activities.

As mentioned in the introduction to this chapter, the ratio of upper to lower limb amputations is about 1:3; this ratio is reflected in the motivation for research in lower limb prosthetics. Research and development activities increase

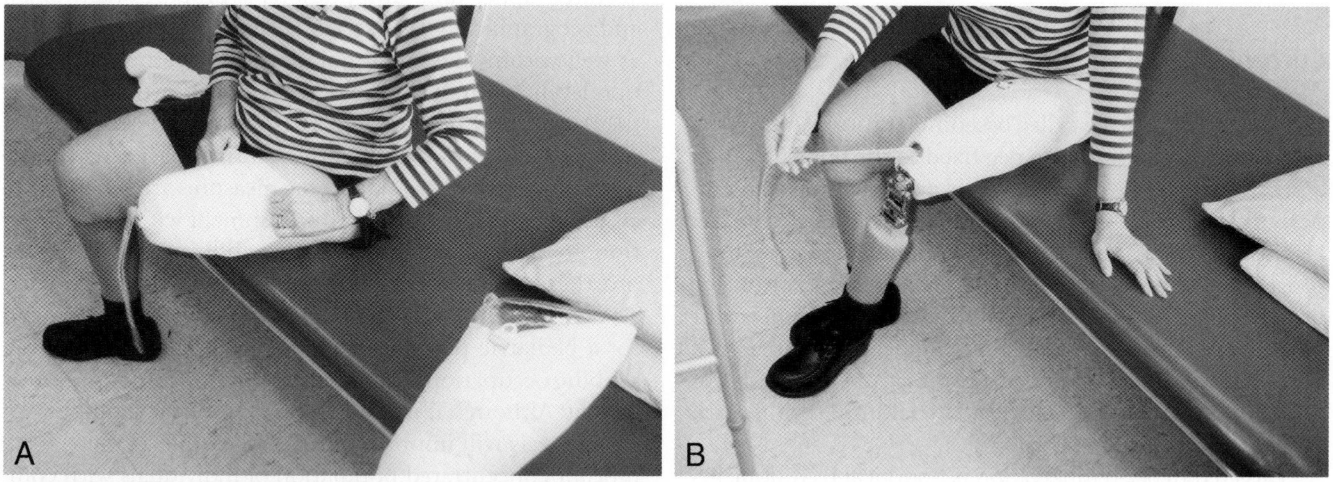

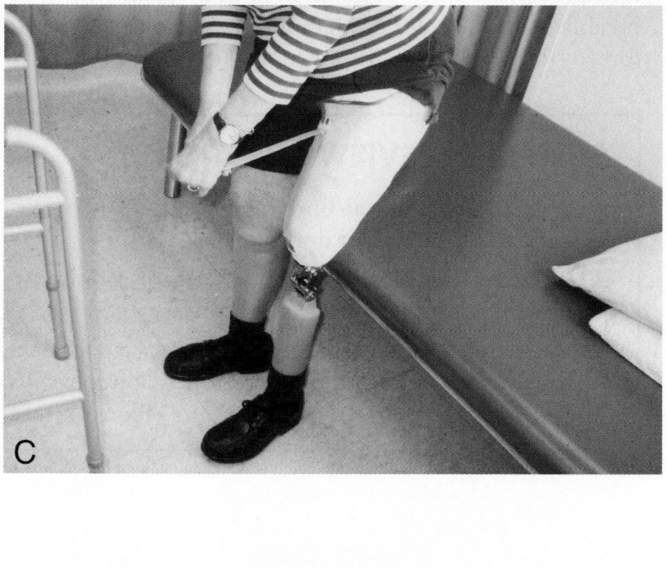

Figure 46-28 **A.** Donning the transfemoral prosthesis beginning with the silicone liner with attached lanyard, and socks (to compensate for volume changes in the residual limb). **B.** Donning the transfemoral socket. **C.** Securing the suspension of the transfemoral prosthesis is done in standing to ensure total contact in the socket. The lanyard attaches with Velcro.

during times of armed conflict, as is currently the case in the Iraq war. As a result, attention is focused on the increase in numbers of amputations in a young, previously healthy population, whose members will hopefully live long, productive lives using prosthetic devices. The infusion of funds may further develop the technology supporting upper limb prosthetics (signal processing, electronics, and microprocessors) while fostering development of improved hardware. In articles by Atkins and Heard (1996) and by Kyberd and Beard (1998), users identified the following features needing improvement: better suspension and cable systems, additional wrist movement, more precision of pinch with more dexterity, coordinated motions of two joints, and improved reliability for electronic hands.

Recent developments include the Otto Bock Sensor Hand, which incorporates "reflex" action, that is, sensors in the hand can detect slip and automatically adjust grip, thereby reducing the mental load required of the user to visually monitor grasp. Although no commercial electric shoulder is currently available, LTI-Collier has developed an electric lock actuator to lock the manually positioned shoulder. Wrist flexion and rotation units are available on both body-powered as well as electric TDs. Motion Control has a mechanical flexion/rotation component to incorporate with the electric TD.

Current Research Topics

The surgical approach called osseointegration requires the implantation of a titanium peg fixed to the bone to which a prosthesis can be attached. This approach has been reportedly successful for lower limb amputations (Jones & Davidson, 1996) and has further potential for upper limb prosthetics. This approach provides a stable fixation for prosthetic attachment and would eliminate the need for harness suspension if successful in higher level upper limb amputations. It has the added advantage of enhanced proprioceptive feedback from the artificial limb (Brånemark et al., 2001).

Targeted hyper-reinnervation is a surgical technique being pursued to increase the number of myoelectric control sites available in a higher level amputation. After limb loss, the brachial plexus and peripheral nerves may remain intact in the residual limb. This procedure takes advantage of expendable regions of remaining muscle by denervating and hyper-reinnervating sections of tissue. When successful, this can result in myoelectric sites that correlate physiologically with prosthetic functions: the radial nerve innervates musculature that contracts when the subject attempts to extend the elbow; the distal radial nerve reinnervated area contracts to open the hand; the median nerve area contracts to close the hand. Early indications are that sensory reinnervation may be tapped to enhance control of multiple functions in the artificial arm (Kuiken et al., 2004).

Currently, surface EMG will only allow up to four channels of control in the forearm, but 18 extrinsic muscles supply the hand and wrist. Development is proceeding on implantable myoelectric sensors (IMES) small enough to be injected. The potential is for myoelectric control of multiple degrees of freedom in the hand, simultaneously (Weir et al., 2003).

Future advances in engineering, medicine, and prosthetics promise technical improvements in the fit and function of artificial limbs. As with research and development, the therapeutic program must be driven by the patient's needs. As the patient masters the basics of prosthetic control systems and practices their use in activities, with the therapist's guidance as facilitator or teacher, the patient chooses tasks that he or she values. The approach of analyzing tasks and problem solving on how best to use this tool, the prosthesis, regardless of its complexity, serves the patient well throughout life.

EVIDENCE

Research addressing upper limb prosthetics in occupational therapy literature is limited because the incidence of acquired upper limb amputations is proportionally small and geographically diverse. Considerable variation is found as well within that small population concerning amputation level, dominance, etiology, post-operative or pre-prosthetic care, and prosthetic prescription, with occupational therapy intervention frequently occurring only after the delivery of the prosthesis. Outcome measures are generally focused on functional task accomplishment with some attention to quality of performance, ability to incorporate prosthesis, and wearer satisfaction with task performance. To date, most formal assessment tools have been developed for a pediatric population. Frequently, the literature describing occupational therapy intervention is in a case study format. Although it is generally accepted that training with a prosthesis will improve outcomes, seldom is there a significant concentrated population of individuals with comparable levels of recent arm amputation who are willing to forego training to constitute a control group.

SUMMARY REVIEW QUESTIONS

1. Why is the residual limb wrapped with elastic bandaging? How is it done?
2. What are the most common causes of acquired upper and lower limb amputations?
3. Which body movements are required for a patient with a transhumeral amputation to operate a conventional BP terminal device and elbow unit?

4. What are the positive and negative features of a hook? A hand?
5. Describe the differences between a VO and a VC terminal device.
6. What is myoelectric control?
7. What is the purpose of controls training and use training?
8. Why might a prosthesis be rejected?
9. What are the functional expectations for a person with a unilateral transhumeral amputation or a bilateral transhumeral amputation?
10. What is the role of the occupational therapist in the rehabilitation of the patient with lower extremity amputations?

ACKNOWLEDGMENT

The authors wish to acknowledge the work of Felice Gadaleta Celikyol, the author of this chapter for the fourth and fifth editions.

References

Atkins, D. J., & Heard, D. C. Y. (1996). Epidemiologic overview of individuals with upper-limb loss and their reported research priorities. *Journal of Prosthetics and Orthotics, 8,* 2–11.

Atkins, D. J., & Meier, R. H. (2004a). Postoperative and preprosthetic preparations. In D. J. Atkins & R. H. Meier III (Eds.), *Functional restoration of adults and children with upper extremity amputation* (pp. 135–138). New York: Demos Medical Publishing.

Atkins, D. J., & Meier, R. H. (2004b). Functional skills training with body-powered and externally powered prostheses. In D. J. Atkins & R. H. Meier III (Eds.), *Functional restoration of adults and children with upper extremity amputation* (pp. 139–157). New York: Demos Medical Publishing.

Brånemark, R., Brånemark, P.-I., Rydevik, B., & Myers, R. R. (2001). Osseointegration in skeletal reconstruction and rehabilitation. *Journal of Rehabilitation Research and Development, 38,* 175–181.

Bunnell, S. (1990). The management of the non-functional hand: Reconstruction versus prosthesis. In J. M. Hunter, L. H. Schneider, E. J. Mackin, & A. D. Callahan (Eds.), *Rehabilitation of the hand* (pp. 997–1017). St. Louis: Mosby.

Burger, H., Brezovar, D., & Marin⁻ek, C. (2004). Comparison of clinical test and questionnaires for the evaluation of upper limb prosthetic use in children. *Disability and Rehabilitation, 26,* 911–916.

Dise-Lewis, J. E. (1989). Psychological adaptation to limb loss. In D. J. Atkins & R. H. Meier III (Eds.), *Comprehensive management of the upper-limb amputee* (pp. 165–172). New York: Springer-Verlag.

Edelstein, J. E. (2004). Rehabilitation without prostheses. In D. G. Smith, J. W. Michael, & J. H. Bowker (Eds.), *Atlas of amputations and limb deficiencies: Surgical, prosthetic and rehabilitation principles* (pp. 745–755). Rosemont, IL: American Academy of Orthopaedic Surgeons.

Esquenazi, A. (1996). Rehabilitation in limb deficiency: 4. Limb amputation. *Archives of Physical Medicine and Rehabilitation, 77,* S-18–S-28.

Fraser, C. M. (1998). An evaluation of the use made of cosmetic and functional prostheses by unilateral upper limb amputees. *Prosthetics and Orthotics International, 22,* 216–223.

Friedmann, L. (1989). Functional skills in multiple limb anomalies. In D. J. Atkins & R. H. Meier III (Eds.), *Comprehensive management of the upper limb amputee* (pp. 150–164). New York: Springer-Verlag.

Fryer, C. M., Michael, J. W., & Stark, G.E. (2004). Body-powered components. In D. G. Smith, J. W. Michael, & J. H. Bowker (Eds.), *Atlas of amputations and limb deficiencies: Surgical, prosthetic and rehabilitation principles* (pp. 117–143). Rosemont, IL: American Academy of Orthopaedic Surgeons.

Gauthier-Gagnon, C. (1998). The Locomotor Capabilities Index: Content validity. *Journal of Rehabilitation Outcomes Measures, 2,* 40–46.

Heckathorne, C. W. (2004). Components for electric powered systems. In Smith, D.G., Michael, J.W., & Bowker, J.H. (Eds.), *Atlas of amputations and limb deficiencies: Surgical, prosthetic and rehabilitation principles* (pp.145–171). Rosemont, IL: American Academy of Orthopaedic Surgeons.

Hompland, S. (2004). Pain management for upper extremity amputation. In D. J. Atkins & R. H. Meier III (Eds.), *Functional restoration of adults and children with upper extremity amputation* (pp. 89–105). New York: Demos Medical Publishing.

Hung, J. W. & Wu, Y. H. (2005). Fitting a bilateral transhumeral amputee with utensil prostheses and their functional assessment 10 years later: A case report. *Archives of Physical Medicine and Rehabilitation, 86,* 2211–2213.

Hunter, J. P., Katz, J., & Davis, K. D. (2003). The effect of tactile and visual sensory inputs on phantom limb awareness. *Brain, 126,* 579–589.

Jones, L. E., & Davidson, J. (1996). A review of the management of upper-limb amputees. *Critical Review in Physical and Rehabilitation Medicine, 8,* 297–322.

Kejlaa, G. H. (1993). Consumer concerns and the functional value of prostheses to upper limb amputees. *Prosthetics and Orthotics International, 17,* 157–163.

Kessler, H. H. (1947). *Cineplasty*. Springfield, IL: Charles C. Thomas.

Kuiken, T. A., Dumanian, G. A., Lipschutz, R. D., Miller, L. A., & Stubblefield, K. A. (2004). The use of targeted muscle reinnervation for improved myoelectric prosthesis control in a bilateral shoulder disarticulation amputee. *Prosthetics and Orthotics International, 28,* 245–253.

Kyberd, P. J., & Beard, D. J. (1998). A survey of upper-limb prosthetic users in Oxfordshire. *Journal of Prosthetics and Orthotics, 10,* 85–91.

Lake, C. (1997). Effects of prosthetic training on upper-extremity prosthetic use. *Journal of Prosthetics and Orthotics, 9,* 3–9.

Lehneis, H. R., & Dickey, R. (1992). Fitting and training the bilateral upper limb amputee. In *Atlas of limb prosthetics: Surgical, prosthetic and rehabilitation principles* (pp. 311–323). St. Louis: Mosby-Year Book.

Leonard, J. A., & Meier, R. H. (1998). Upper and lower extremity prosthetics. In J. DeLisa & B. M. Gans (Eds.), *Rehabilitation medicine: Principles and practice* (pp. 669–696). Philadelphia: Lippincott-Raven.

Maiorano, L. M., & Byron, P. M. (1995). Fabrication of an early-fit prosthesis. In J. M. Hunter, E. J. Mackin, & A. D. Callahan (Eds.), *Rehabilitation of the hand: Surgery and therapy* (pp. 1211–1221). St. Louis: Mosby.

Malone, J. M., Fleming, L. L., & Robinson, J. (1984). Immediate, early, and late post-surgical management of upper-limb amputations. *Journal of Rehabilitation, 21,* 33–41.

Melzack, R. (1989). Phantom limbs, the self and the brain. *Journal of Canadian Psychology, 30,* 1–16.

Olivett, B. L. (1995). Conventional fitting of the adult amputee. In J. M. Hunter, E. J. Mackin, & A. D. Callahan (Eds.), *Rehabilitation of the hand: Surgery and therapy* (pp. 1223–1240). St. Louis: Mosby.

Pinzur, M. S., & Angelats, J. (1994). Functional outcome following traumatic upper limb amputation and prosthetic limb fitting. *Journal of Hand Surgery, 19A,* 836–839.

Radocy, R. (2004). Prosthetic adaptations in competitive sports and recreation. In Smith, D. G., Michael, J. W., & Bowker, J. H. (Eds.), *Atlas of amputations and limb deficiencies: Surgical, prosthetic and rehabilitation principles* (pp. 327–338). Rosemont, IL: American Academy of Orthopaedic Surgeons.

Radocy, R., & Furlong, A. (2004). Recreation and sports adaptations. In D. J. Atkins & R. H. Meier III (Eds.), *Functional restoration of adults and children with upper extremity amputation* (pp. 251–272). New York: Demos Medical Publishing.

Ramalingam, T., Pathak, G., & Barker, P. (2005). A method for determining the rate of major limb amputations in battle casualties: Experiences of a British field hospital in Iraq, 2003. *Annals of the Royal College of Surgeons of England, 87,* 113–116.

Sanderson, E. R., & Scott, R. N., (1985). *UNB test of prosthetic function: A test for unilateral amputees, test manual.* Fredricton, New Brunswick, Canada: Bio-Engineering Institute, University of New Brunswick.

Schuch, C. M., & Pritham, C. H. (1994). International organization terminology: Application to prosthetics and orthotics. *Journal of Prosthetics and Orthotics, 6,* 29–33.

Sears, H. H., & Shaperman, J. (1998). Electric wrist rotation in proportional-controlled systems. *Journal of Prosthetics and Orthotics, 10,* 92–98.

Spiegel, S. R. (1989). Adult myoelectric upper-limb prosthetic training, In D. J. Atkins & R. H. Meier III (Eds.), *Comprehensive management of the upper limb amputee* (pp. 60–71). New York: Springer-Verlag.

Uellendahl, J. E. (2004). Bilateral upper limb prostheses. In D. G. Smith, J. W. Michael, & J. H. Bowker (Eds.), *Atlas of amputations and limb deficiencies: Surgical, prosthetic and rehabilitation principles* (pp. 311–325). Rosemont, IL: American Academy of Orthopaedic Surgeons.

Van Dorsten, B. (2004). Common emotional concerns following limb loss. In D. J. Atkins & R. J. Meier III (Eds.), *Functional restoration of adults and children with upper extremity amputation* (pp. 73–78). New York: Demos Medical Publishing.

Weir, R. F., Grahn, E. C., & Duff, J. (2001). A new externally powered myoelectrically controlled prosthesis for persons with partial-hand amputations at the metacarpals. *Journal of Prosthetics and Orthotics, 13,* 26–31.

Weir, R. F., Troyk, P. R., DeMichele, G., & Kuiken, T. (2003). Implantable myoelectric sensors (IMES) for upper-extremity prosthesis control-preliminary work. From *Proceedings of the 25th Annual International Conference of the IEEE EMBS*, Cancun, Mexico, September 17–21, 2003; pp. 1562–1565.

Winchell, E. (1995). *Coping with limb loss.* Garden City Park, NY: Avery.

Wright, T. W., & Hagen, A. D. (1995). Prosthetic usage in major upper extremity amputations. *Journal of Hand Surgery, 20A,* 619–622.

Supplemental References

Ehde, D. M., & Smith, D. G. (2004). Chronic pain management. In D. G. Smith, J. W. Michael, & J. H. Bowker (Eds.), *Atlas of amputations and limb deficiencies: Surgical, prosthetic and rehabilitation principles* (pp. 711–726). Rosemont, IL: American Academy of Orthopaedic Surgeons.

Kuiken, T., Edwards, M., & Miceli, N. (2002). *Below-knee amputation: A guide for rehabilitation.* Chicago: Rehabilitation Institute of Chicago.

Kuiken, T., Edwards, M., & Soltys, N. (2002). *Above-knee amputation: A guide for rehabilitation.* Chicago: Rehabilitation Institute of Chicago.

Liaw, M. Y. (1998). Central representation of phantom limb phenomenon in amputees studied with single photon emission computerized tomography. *American Journal of Physical Medicine and Rehabilitation, 77,* 368–375.

Trombly, C. A., & Ma, H.-I. (2002). A synthesis of effects of occupational therapy for persons with stroke. Part I: Restoration of roles, tasks, and activities. *American Journal of Occupational Therapy, 56,* 250–259.

LEARNING OBJECTIVES

After studying this chapter, the reader will be able to do the following:

1. Recognize the signs and symptoms of exercise/activity intolerance.
2. Identify the common cardiac diagnoses and their treatment in occupational therapy.
3. Understand various cardiac and pulmonary diagnostic studies and how these tests assist with treatment planning in occupational therapy.
4. Know the controllable risk factors for heart disease and ways to ameliorate their effect.
5. Be able to instruct patients with pulmonary disease in breathing techniques.
6. Know resources for further guidelines in cardiac and pulmonary rehabilitation.

CHAPTER 47

Cardiac and Pulmonary Diseases

Nancy Huntley

Glossary

Acute coronary syndrome (ACS)—A term including unstable angina and myocardial infarction (MI), both non-ST elevation MI (non-STEMIs) and ST elevation MIs (STEMIs). This designation is used to triage and manage patients with symptoms of myocardial ischemia (Kim, Kine, & Fuster, 2004).

Angina—A temporary lack of blood flow to the myocardium, which causes the sensation of chest pain, fullness, tightness, or pressure. The pain or discomfort from angina can be referred to the teeth, jaw, back, ear, or arm. Angina is relieved with nitroglycerin or rest.

Atherogenic—Causing the development of plaque in an artery.

Atrial fibrillation—A rapid firing of cells in the atria of the heart with irregular response of the ventricles causing a fast irregular heart rhythm. With uncontrolled atrial fibrillation, the patient often feels short of breath and fatigued.

Cardioversion—Electrical shock delivered to the heart to stop a serious dysrhythmia, with the hope that the heart will restart in a normal sinus rhythm.

Congestive heart failure (CHF)—A condition where the heart's pumping function is impaired from a variety of etiologies. This impairment results in the heart's inability to rid the body of excess fluid, which then collects in the lungs and extremities.

Diaphoresis—A cold clammy sweat that comes on suddenly.

Oxygen saturation (O_2 Sat)—Measurement of the amount of oxygen carried by the hemoglobin in the blood. A normal O_2 Sat is greater than 95%.

Sternotomy—A procedure used in open heart surgery where the sternum is split in half to allow the surgeon access to the chest cavity. After surgery, it is wired together.

Tachypnea—Rapid shallow breathing.

INCIDENCE OF CARDIAC AND PULMONARY DISEASE

Heart disease is the leading cause of death in the United States. Annually, 41% of all deaths in the United States are caused by coronary artery disease. Fifty-seven million, or 45%, of all Americans are living with some form of the disease (American Heart Association [AHA], 2005). According to 1998 Heart and Stroke Statistical Update, "about two thirds of the people who survive a heart attack do not make a complete recovery, but 88% of those people under the age of 65 years will be able to return to their usual work" (AHA, 1998, p. 11).

Pulmonary disease is also a significant cause of death in the United States. Chronic Obstructive Pulmonary Disease (COPD) is the fourth leading killer of Americans (American Lung Association, 2004). Lung disease is not only a killer; it is also chronic and significantly alters the lives of those who have it. Seventy percent of persons with COPD say it limits their ability to do normal exertion (American Lung Association, 2004).

Even though a clinician is not working in either cardiac or pulmonary rehabilitation, the diagnosis of cardiac or pulmonary disease in a patient's medical history has implications for the occupational therapist's treatment plan. For instance, a patient may carry the primary diagnosis of a recent stroke. If that stroke occurred shortly after coronary artery bypass surgery, certain precautions should be taken to protect the patient's sternum. When the patient has a history of heart disease, the therapist should also routinely measure their heart rate and blood pressure both at rest and with activity to determine the patient's cardiovascular response to rehabilitation. The occupational therapist must, therefore, be aware of these disease processes and know how they will influence treatment.

HEART DISEASE

Heart disease may be due to a blockage of the coronary arteries, diseases of the heart muscle, or structural anomalies of the heart. Heart attacks are the single leading cause of death in men and women in the United States (AHA, 2005). A **myocardial infarction (MI)**, or heart attack, is death of the heart muscle caused by lack of blood flow due to an obstruction of a coronary artery by plaque or spasm. The patient's clinical history, along with several diagnostic tests, is considered when diagnosing a heart attack. The patient may first have an onset of symptoms known as **acute coronary syndrome (ACS)**, which indicates acute myocardial ischemia (Kim, Kine, & Fuster, 2004). The patient may first have symptoms such as chest pain or pressure, which may radiate to the teeth, jaw, ear, arm, or midback. These symptoms may be accompanied by **diaphoresis**, shortness of breath (SOB), nausea, vomiting, and/or fatigue. The patient may present with one or more of these symptoms, and the severity and intensity varies from person to person. (Not everyone who has these symptoms will have a heart attack, but it helps to triage them to the appropriate treatment.) An electrocardiogram (EKG) will show where the damage to the heart muscle occurred. Meanwhile, blood tests for certain structural proteins and cardiac enzymes will confirm a heart attack and give an idea of the amount of damage done to the heart muscle.

If a person realizes he or she is having a heart attack and comes to the hospital immediately, a drug called a thrombolytic agent may be given to stop the damage to the heart muscle. Thrombolytics break up the clot in the coronary artery, thus restoring blood flow. They must be given quickly after the onset of symptoms and are most effective within the first hour. The benefit decreases incrementally from 1–12 hours post symptom onset. From 12–24 hours, thrombolytics have only a minimal effect (Antman, 2005), so the sooner the patient receives the thrombolytic, the more heart muscle can be saved.

The left ventricle is the main pump of the heart. It pumps the blood from the heart to the rest of the body. Since the left ventricle does more work, it has a higher oxygen requirement than the rest of the heart. It is usually the first area of the heart to suffer from any coronary artery perfusion deficiency.

Types of MI

In evaluating an MI, an EKG is an important adjunct in determining the location of the MI and the severity of the infarction. An MI that involves all three layers of the heart muscle is called transmural, and it usually produces ST elevation on the EKG. It is referred to as an ST elevation MI, or STEMI. Three fourths of these MIs will later produce a Q wave over EKG leads affected by the MI (Antman & Braunwald, 2005). A Q wave is an identifying characteristic showing where damage occurred. In STEMI MIs, the size of the infarct is important. If the STEMI is large or if the STEMI is small to moderate in a person with previous STEMIs, the prognosis is poor (Antman, 2005). An anterior STEMI is considered the most serious because of the large amount of muscle mass lost and decrease in the effectiveness of ventricles pumping action (Meyers, 2005). (See Definition 47-1 for a review of common diagnostic procedures.)

When the thrombus in the coronary artery is incomplete, less damage is done, and it is called a non-ST elevation MI or a non-STEMI. The majority of these MIs do not develop a Q wave. These MIs are called non-STEMIs or non–Q wave MIs (Antman & Braunwald, 2005). Although the immediate prognosis is better in patients with a non-STEMI, their future risk is often higher for death or further cardiac events because of a history of previous heart events or due to the extent of their underlying heart disease (Cannon & Braunwald, 2005).

Blockage in the left main or left anterior descending artery of the heart will cause damage to the front of the left ventricle and is called an anterior MI. When the right coronary artery is involved, the back and bottom of the left ventricle are damaged; this is called an inferior MI. The circumflex artery feeds the lateral wall of the heart, and blockage in this artery results in a lateral MI (Fig. 47-1).

Open Heart Surgery

Open heart surgery is a procedure that usually involves a **sternotomy** and allows the surgeon to work on the heart. There are several types of open heart surgery.

Coronary artery bypass graft (CABG) is the replacement of occluded coronary arteries with artery or vein grafts. These grafts are attached to the aorta and reconnected below the occlusion in the coronary artery. Sometimes the mammary artery, which comes directly off the aorta, is dissected from its original destination and used as a graft. Another arterial graft is the radial artery. Arteries are preferred as grafts because they stay patent longer than vein grafts. Vein grafts are usually harvested from the legs.

Valve replacement and/or repair may be necessitated by destruction of a heart valve due to disease or congenital malformation. If the surgeon is unable to repair the valve, it is replaced with a prosthetic or tissue valve. If a prosthetic valve is used, patients will have to take thrombolytics for the rest of their lives. The thrombolytics will prevent blood from clotting as it goes through the valve. A tissue or biothesis valve is from humans or pigs. These valves do not require the patient to be on thrombolytic therapy, and they usually last about 10–15 years before they need to be replaced (Gersh, 2000).

Twenty-five percent of the congenital heart defects in adolescents and adults are atrial septal defects (Gersh, 2000). About 30% of people with atrial septal defect will develop symptoms in the third decade of life, but 75% will have symptoms by their fifties (Webb et al., 2005). When the heart has been attempting to compensate for a defect for a long time, it may become enlarged, and the patient may complain of fatigue and shortness of breath. The current standard of practice is to repair these heart defects before the patient has significant symptoms or sustains myocardial damage.

Other Heart Diagnoses and Procedures

Congestive heart failure (CHF) describes the inability of the heart to function as an effective pump. The heart muscle becomes stretched beyond its ability to contract efficiently, resulting in the collection of fluid in the lungs or the extremities. Seventy-five percent of patients with CHF have a previous history of hypertension (AHA, 2005). CHF may also result from a number of other disease processes such as multiple MIs, incompetent valves, cardiomyopathy, and so on. Patients with CHF experience SOB and fatigue and may have an increase in weight and a dry hacking cough. Often they complain of coughing or being SOB in a recumbent position (see Safety

DEFINITION 47-1

de·fin·i·tion

Common Diagnostic Studies for Heart Disease

Blood Tests

Blood tests are usually drawn on patients with symptoms of a probable heart attack. The cells of the heart contain isoenzymes and structural proteins, which are specific to that organ. Death of the heart's cells causes those isoenzymes and structural proteins to be released into the blood stream where an increase in their levels can be measured. CPK MB is an isoenzyme that shows up in the blood within 4–6 hours after a heart attack (Maltas, 2003). Troponin I and troponin T are two structural proteins whose levels rise with heart damage. Troponin is specific to heart muscle. Troponin levels start rising after 3–6 hours and stay elevated for up to 14 days, allowing detection of an MI in patients who wait to seek treatment (Maltas, 2003).

Stress Echocardiogram

A stress echocardiogram is an exercise test usually conducted on a treadmill. Before starting the test, an ultrasound recording is taken of the function of the heart at rest. The patient is then exercised to his or her maximum capacity. After exercising, another ultrasound recording of the heart is done to show how the heart responds to work. It will show whether the heart muscle and valves work normally under pressure or if some parts respond suboptimally. It is also possible to measure how much blood the heart ejects with each beat. This number is the ejection fraction (EF).

A normal EF is >60%. A person is mildly impaired with an EF of 50–59%. A person with an EF of 40–50% has moderate impairment. An EF below 40% is considered significant impairment. The lower the EF, the higher the risk the patient has for further events and complications. If individuals who have a low EF can tolerate mild-to-moderate exercise, they have a better long-term outcome than those who cannot tolerate exercise well (Antman, 2005). The EF does not always accurately reflect an individual patient's ability to work, but the EF is helpful as a starting point for making appropriate exercise and activity recommendations and precautions.

A stress echocardiogram will also reveal the maximum exercise capacity of an individual. Using 60–85% of the maximum heart rate attained during the stress test, the therapist can determine an appropriate level to start exercise and activity.

Stress echocardiography is approximately 88% accurate in predicting coronary ischemia depending on the cohort of the study (Barasch, 2000). When a stress test is given without the echo, the accuracy is reduced to 75% in predicting heart disease, but patient's maximum exercise capacity and their maximum heart rate with exercise is known.

Nuclear Stress Test

A nuclear stress test is conducted with a 12-lead EKG as patients exercise to their maximum capacity on a treadmill. During this test, the patient is injected with a radioactive isotope when the patient feels only able to exercise for one more minute. The patient is then placed under a special instrument called a scintillation camera, which can detect the presence of the radioactive isotope in the heart muscle. This isotope has special properties, which allows it to be readily picked up by healthy myocardium cells, more slowly by cells with poor perfusion, and not at all by infarcted myocardium. The radioactive isotope stays in the blood stream for approximately 72 hours. Those areas with restricted blood flow may eventually "fill in" with the radioactive isotope, and these areas are said to have a reversible defect. Areas that do not "fill in" are infarcted, and the deficit is permanent. Since this process may take several hours, the nuclear test usually has an initial scan, and then another scan is administered 2–3 hours later (Maltas, 2003).

Coronary Angiography

Coronary angiography is currently the most definitive test in the diagnosis of coronary artery disease. A catheter is inserted into a blood vessel in the groin and threaded back into the heart, and a radiopaque dye is injected through it into the coronary blood vessels. The extent of the obstruction in any coronary blood vessel can be visualized. A blockage must be greater than 70–75% of the lumen to be considered significant. A lesion greater than 50% in the left main artery is considered equivalent to two-vessel disease. The length of coronary artery lesion(s) is also taken into consideration. In addition, heart valve function, ventricular wall motion abnormalities, and some heart defects can be detected (Paganda & Paganda, 2001).

Note 47-1 for signs and symptoms). Recent medication treatment options for patients with CHF have increased significantly. Yet even with treatment, 40% of patients will die within 4 years (Yakubov & Bope, 2002).

Cardiomyopathies (CMs) are diseases of cardiac muscle. The three main types of cardiomyopathy are dilated, hypertrophic, and restrictive. Dilated cardiomyopathy is the most common type, comprising over 75% of the cases. Seventy-five specific diseases can cause dilated cardiomyopathy, but symptoms are an enlarged heart with decreased pumping capacity that usually results in congestive heart failure. Depending on the cohort of the study, 10–50% of people with cardiomyopathy who are hospitalized due to CHF will die within 1 year (Wynne & Braunwauld, 2005); other patients with cardiomyopathy, for unknown reasons, improve over time. An enlarged left

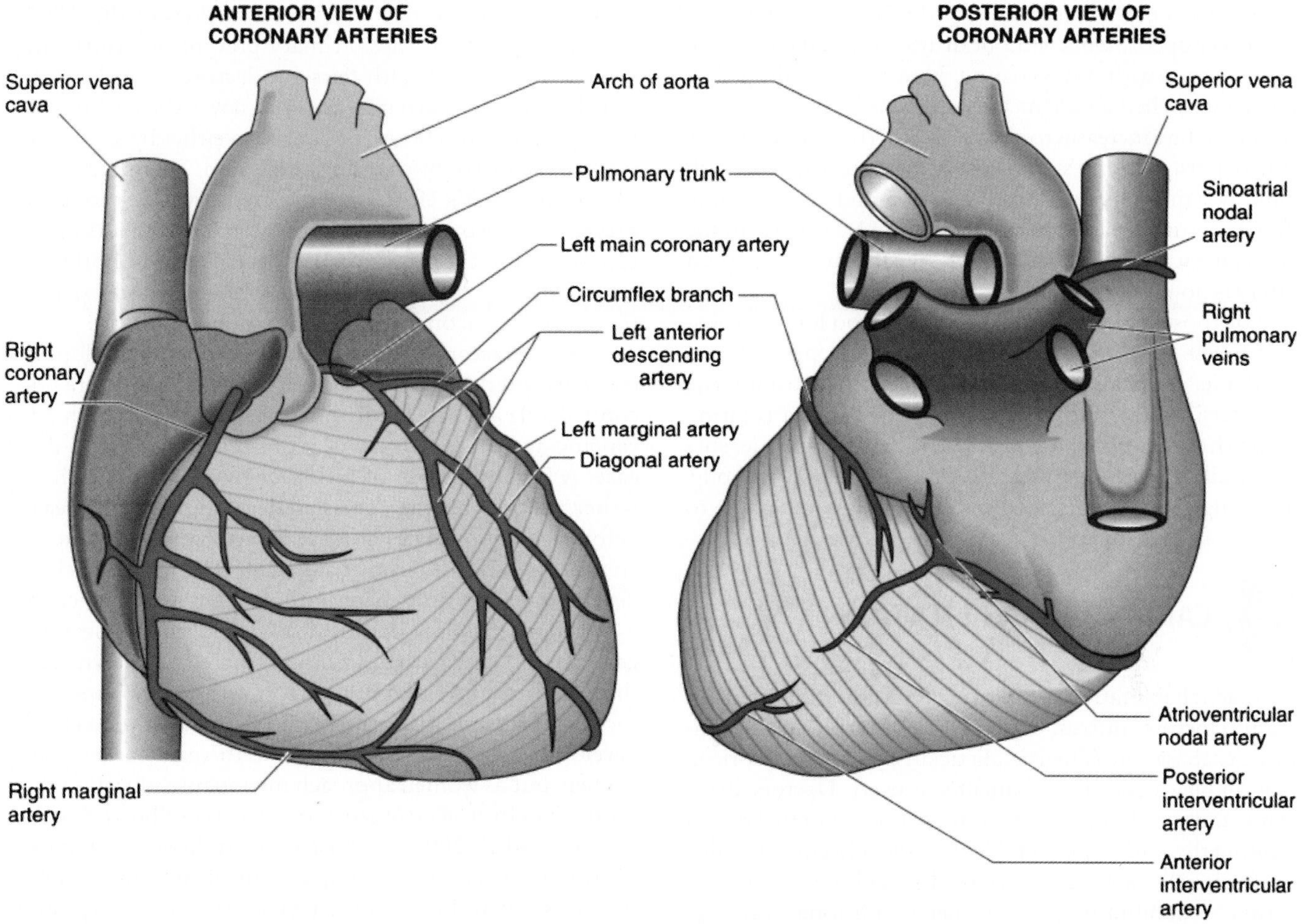

Figure 47-1 Coronary arteries. Location of damage to the heart depends on which coronary arteries are blocked. (From Willis, M. C. [1996]. *Medical terminology: The language of health care* [p. 160]. Baltimore: Williams & Wilkins.)

ventricle and decreased heart function are indicators of a poorer prognosis (Wynne & Braunwald, 2005).

Angina pectoris is heart pain caused by a temporary inadequate supply of blood to the heart muscle. Angina might be described as pain, aching tightness, or pressure. It is usually diffuse and located in the mid chest, but it may radiate to the mid back, teeth, ear, jaw, or arm. Typically, angina comes on with increased activity and is relieved with rest. Some people, however, may develop angina after a heavy meal or while resting. Nitroglycerin, taken by pill or spray under the tongue, usually relieves angina quickly. Angina is an indication of coronary artery disease; it is not uncommon to have angina after a heart attack. If the frequency or intensity of angina changes, the physician should be notified.

Percutaneous transluminal coronary revascularization (PTCR) or angioplasty is a procedure used to improve the blood flow through an occluded artery and reduce the symptoms of angina. Angioplasty requires the insertion of a catheter into the coronary artery at the site of the occlusion. On the end of the catheter is a balloon that is inflated until the arterial walls at the point of the occlusion are pushed out to allow more blood flow through the area. The initial success rate with angioplasty is 90%, but approximately 30–40% of all angioplasties close within 6 months (Baim, 2005). Sometimes a stent, which resembles a spring in a ballpoint pen, may be used. The stent lies over the balloon, and when the balloon is inflated, the stent opens and

SAFETY NOTE 47-1

Signs and Symptoms of Congestive Heart Failure

- Increase in weight of 2–5 pounds or more over several days
- Inability to sleep
- Persistent dry hacking cough
- Shortness of breath with normal activity
- Swelling in ankles or feet
- Fatigue

Reprinted with permission from Huntley, 1998.

imbeds itself in the artery wall, forming a structure to keep the artery open. Stents without drugs are called bare metal stents. Stents with drugs coating them are called drug-eluting stents. When a bare metal stent is used, the success of the procedure increases to about 70–80% (Lowe et al., 2005). When a drug-eluting stent is used, the restenosis rate with clinical symptoms drops to between 5 and <10% (Baim, 2005). Getting a patient who is having an MI quickly to the catheterization lab for an angioplasty/stent to the involved artery is now considered the standard of care.

For those patients whose lesions are too long or calcified to use the angioplasty balloon, another procedure is available. It is called atherectomy. In atherectomy, the catheter inserted into the coronary artery has a rotating blade that cuts out the plaque. As it cuts the plaque, suction pulls the plaque through a tube and out of the body. The long-term success of this procedure is comparable to angioplasty (Baim, 2005).

CARDIAC REHABILITATION

Cardiac rehabilitation usually involves a multidisciplinary team. Doctors, nurses, occupational and physical therapists, exercise physiologists, dieticians, and social workers may all play a part in the patient's recovery. Doctors, dieticians, and social workers perform their conventional role in treating the cardiac patient. None of the other allied health professionals, however, are trained specifically to work in cardiac rehabilitation, and all need additional training. Geographical tradition and availability of staff seem to determine what role each allied health professional plays. Each discipline uses their own special skills in dealing with patients with heart disease, but their job expectations and responsibilities may essentially be the same. (See Resource 47-1 for information on organizations that dominate policies and certifications in cardiac rehabilitation.)

Occupational therapists are invaluable when treating the patient with heart disease. Therapists are able to evaluate and analyze the patient's activities of daily living. The therapist can then assist patients in modifying activities, if necessary, so they can resume those activities they previously enjoyed. The occupational therapist's expertise in the rehabilitative process and knowledge of comorbid diseases is extremely important when evaluating and adapting treatment for the individual needs of the patient. Patients who have undergone lifestyle changes and experienced life-threatening diseases also benefit from occupational therapy intervention to help with psychosocial adjustment to their new situation.

Risk Factors for Heart Disease

One of the main goals of all phases of cardiac rehabilitation is primary and secondary prevention of heart disease. Primary prevention refers to efforts to prevent the development of heart disease. Primary prevention efforts are usually limited to health fairs and lecture series because health insurance currently does not cover the cost of primary prevention. Those costs are born either by a sponsor (i.e., a hospital) or by charging admission. Therefore, most of the therapist's efforts are directed toward secondary prevention. Secondary prevention pertains to efforts made to stop or slow the progression of heart disease. Improving an individual's risk factor profile is the method used by therapists for secondary prevention of heart disease.

Ten risk factors increase one's likelihood of developing coronary artery disease. The three risk factors that are not controllable are age, family history, and gender. With advancing age, an individual is at greater risk for heart disease. A family history of a first-degree relative, such as father, mother, brother, or sister, developing heart disease before age 55 for males and before age 65 for females increases one's risk (Maron et al., 2004). The highest risk of developing heart disease for both men and women occurs when another sibling has the disease. Indeed, studies suggest that a sibling with heart disease increases one's risk by three to four times that of a person without a sibling history of the disease (Jairath, 1999). Men are more likely to develop heart disease an average of 10 years earlier than women, but as women approach menopause, they lose the protective effect of estrogen, and their risk of heart disease increases (AHA, 2005). The risk of heart disease in women continues to rise after menopause until they are in their seventies. Then their incidence of heart disease surpasses that in men (AHA, 2005). Although heart disease is commonly considered a male problem, it is an equal opportunity killer. It remains the number one cause of death for both men and women (AHA, 2005).

Controllable Risk Factors

The risk factors one can control are smoking, hyperlipidemia, hypertension, sedentary lifestyle, obesity, diabetes, and psychological stress.

Smoking is a major modifiable risk factor in heart disease that contributes to heart disease in multiple ways. People who smoke have a two to three times greater risk of dying of heart disease (AHA, 2005). Smoking damages the endothelial lining of the coronary arteries, making them more susceptible to plaque formation. Nicotine causes vasoconstriction of the arteries and increases heart rate. Smoking makes the heart more susceptible to lethal ventricular arrhythmias and predisposes it to coronary artery spasm (Ricker & Libby, 2005). Carbon monoxide in cigarette smoke binds with the hemoglobin faster than oxygen, resulting in less oxygen being distributed to the tissues. Nicotine also alters the metabolism of fats, increasing the levels of **atherogenic** LDL cholesterol and decreasing the levels of the heart-protective HDL cholesterol. Smoking causes the blood to coagulate more quickly and promotes thrombus formation (Ricker & Libby, 2005).

Hyperlipidemia or a high lipid level is a major risk factor among Americans. It has been demonstrated that a total cholesterol level above 200 mg/dL, an LDL cholesterol above 130 mg/dL, and an HDL cholesterol of less than 37 mg/dL for men and 47 mg/dL for women significantly increases the risk of heart disease (AHA, 2005). Fifty-one percent of American adults have cholesterol levels above 200 mg/dL (AHA, 2005). Patients with known coronary artery disease should have an LDL cholesterol below 100 mg/dL. Cholesterol levels may be lowered through a low-fat diet, regular aerobic exercise, and weight loss. If these options are unsuccessful, the physician will put a patient on a lipid-lowering drug. Some individuals inherit an inability to metabolize lipids normally. They have very high lipid levels in their blood because they manufacture their own cholesterol. These patients will never be able to lower their blood lipids sufficiently without medication. When their lipid level is lowered using medication, they have fewer coronary events (Libby, 2005).

Patients with hypertension have two to three times the risk of developing cardiovascular disease (AHA, 2005). The American Heart Association classifies blood pressures greater than 140/90 at rest as being hypertensive. Hypertension causes damage to the arterial walls and causes increased myocardial oxygen consumption due to the need for the heart to do more work against high pressures. High blood pressure may be diagnosed after several elevated blood pressure readings. Other than taking medication, individuals can improve their blood pressure by weight loss, dietary management, regular aerobic exercise, relief of stress, and controlling other risk factors for coronary artery disease (Fisher & Williams, 2005).

Sedentary lifestyle is a risk factor for heart disease. The relative risk of a sedentary lifestyle for heart disease is comparable to the risk associated with smoking, hypercholesterolemia, and high blood pressure (AHA, 2005). People who are physically inactive have twice the rate of heart disease as those who exercise regularly (McArdle, Katch, & Katch, 2001). Regular physical exercise assists with weight control, lowering blood pressure, and improves the lipid profile and glucose tolerance (McArdle, Katch, & Katch, 2001). The Center for Disease Control (CDC) and the American College of Sports Medicine (ACSM) recommend that American adults get 30 minutes or more of moderate physical activity on most and preferably all days of the week (American College of Sports Medicine, 2000). After an MI, those patients who undergo cardiac rehabilitation exercise training have 20–25% fewer MIs than those who do not exercise (Franklin, 2003). Due to the effect of exercise on the heart, circulatory system, and other risk factors, aerobic exercise is an effective weapon against heart disease.

In the United States, seven of every 10 adults are overweight, and three of those are obese. Obesity is now the second leading preventable cause of death (AHA, 2005). Obesity is closely related to and influences negatively a number of risk factors for heart disease such as hypertension, diabetes, hyperlipidemia, and physical activity. The distribution of body fat is important in disease promotion. Central or abdominal obesity is linked to increased risk of coronary artery disease (CAD) (Wallace, 2003). The loss of even 5–10% of one's weight, however, can have a positive influence on risk factors such as hypertension, lipid levels, and sleep apnea (Gaziano, Monson, & Redker, 2005).

Diabetes has long been recognized as a risk factor for heart disease. The incidence of diabetes increased 8.2% from the year 2000 to 2001. Since 1991, the diagnosis of diabetes has increased 61% primarily due to the increase in obesity in the United States (Mokdad et al., 2001). Women who have diabetes lose the protective effect of their hormones against heart disease, and their risk of CAD increases to five times that of non-diabetic women (Foody & Pordon, 2001). Some form of heart or blood vessel disease will kill two thirds to three fourths of persons with diabetes (AHA, 2005). Keeping blood sugar levels in tight control through medication, diet, and exercise reduces macro- and microvascular disease in patients with type I and type II diabetes and thus reduces risk of heart disease (Powers, 2005).

Stress is also considered to be a risk factor for heart disease, but its effect is difficult to quantify. What is stressful for one individual is not for another. Chronic stress, however, negatively affects the cardiovascular system. Stress increases the heart rate, blood pressure, blood lipid levels, and blood clotting. Managing chronic stressors with relaxation techniques or through behavioral change is helpful in eliminating or minimizing the effect of stress on the body.

As part of secondary prevention, the therapist must direct considerable energy toward educating the patient regarding the significance of these risk factors and methods of ameliorating them. Education may take place in one-on-one sessions, such as with the patient while doing a home program, or with groups of patients before, during, or after exercise.

Inpatient Cardiac Rehabilitation or Phase I

The goals of inpatient cardiac rehabilitation are to prevent muscle loss from bedrest, monitor and assess the patient's ability to function, instruct the patient in appropriate home activities, educate the patient about individual risk factors, and teach methods to lessen these risks.

Therapists treat each patient at least once a day and usually twice daily as soon as the patient's medical status has stabilized, often within the first 24–48 hours after admission. Hospital stays for coronary events have declined significantly in the past 10 years. The average stay for the uncomplicated non-STEMI is 1–2 days; for STEMIs and open heart surgery, it is 3–7 days.

The occupational therapist working in cardiac rehabilitation initiates therapy on a one-on-one basis so that the therapist can interview the patient regarding lifestyle and assess the patient's cardiovascular response to exercise. During exercise, physical measurements of heart rate, blood pressure, EKG response, and symptoms are noted. (Occupational therapists working in cardiac rehabilitation need to take an EKG reading course.) (See Procedures for Practice 47-1 for instructions regarding blood pressure measurement and pulse taking.)

Those patients who are stable are subsequently seen for group treatment. Although programs vary in the type of exercise done, many begin with mild calisthenics for 2-minute bouts with a 1-minute rest. Initially the total time of the calisthenics added together is 4–8 minutes, depending on the patient's tolerance. As the patient progresses, the amount of time the patient may spend doing calisthenics typically increases to 8–10 minutes. Programs may include other modalities such as stair climbing, treadmill, bicycle ergometer, and/or hall walking (Fig. 47-2). Regardless of the modality used, each is started gradually (i.e., treadmill walking at 1–1.5 mph or less for about 3–5 minutes, with progression based on the patient's tolerance). It is important for the therapist to assess the patient's heart rate, blood pressure, EKG, and symptoms to establish the patient's tolerance for exercise (see Safety Note 47-2).

Clinical Pathways

A clinical pathway is a tool that describes a comprehensive program for a patient with a particular diagnosis such as a myocardial infarction pathway, a coronary artery bypass graft pathway, or a congestive heart failure pathway. The

PROCEDURES FOR PRACTICE 47-1

Measuring Blood Pressure and Pulse

Measuring Blood Pressure

1. Wrap blood pressure cuff 1 to 1 1/2 inches above the antecubital space.
2. The cuff should be wrapped smoothly and firmly around the arm.
3. The bladder of the cuff should cover 80% of the arm circumference.
4. Palpate the brachial pulse on the medial aspect of the arm.
5. Place the stethoscope over the pulse.
6. Close the valve on the inflation ball.
7. Inflate the cuff 20 mm Hg greater than the point where you heard the pulse obliterated.
8. Slowly open the valve on the inflation ball so the mercury or arrow drops at the rate of 2–3 mm per second.
9. The first sound heard is the systolic pressure; make a note of that number.
10. Continue to listen until the pulse starts to muffle and finally disappears.
11. The point at which the pulse disappears is the diastolic pressure; make a note of that number.
12. Be sure to listen for 20 mm Hg longer to make sure you heard the exact last pulsation.
13. Completely deflate the cuff and remove from the patient (Rayman, 2004).

To be considered normal, blood pressure must be under 140/90 at rest. Systolic blood pressure should rise with exercise. Diastolic blood pressure should stay the same or drop slightly. With exercise, diastolic blood pressure should not increase more than 10 mm of mercury compared with resting. The blood pressure response of patients with a history of high blood pressure is likely to be exaggerated with exercise.

Pulse Taking

1. Locate indentation on lateral side of wrist about 1/2 inch proximal to the wrist crease.
2. Palpate the radial artery with the index and middle finger.
3. Count the number of pulsations for 10 seconds.
4. Multiply that number by 6 to determine the number of beats per minute.
5. Notice if the pulse is regular or irregular.
6. Also note any "skipped" or early beats.

A normal heart rate (HR) range at rest is between 60–100 beats per minute (bpm). Someone who is very fit, such as a runner, may have a heart rate in the 40s or 50s. After open heart surgery, a patient often has a heart rate in the low 100s. During exercise in the first 2 weeks of convalescence, the heart rate should not increase more than 20 bpm above resting for a patient with an MI and about 30 bpm for a patient after surgery (ACSM, 2000). (Note that these are relative guidelines and not absolute.) It is not uncommon for patients who have valve repair or replacement to develop a rapid heart rhythm called atrial fibrillation. This rhythm is usually controlled with medication or by **cardioversion**. If the patient's HR is uncontrolled and is 120 bpm or higher at rest, exercise is contraindicated.

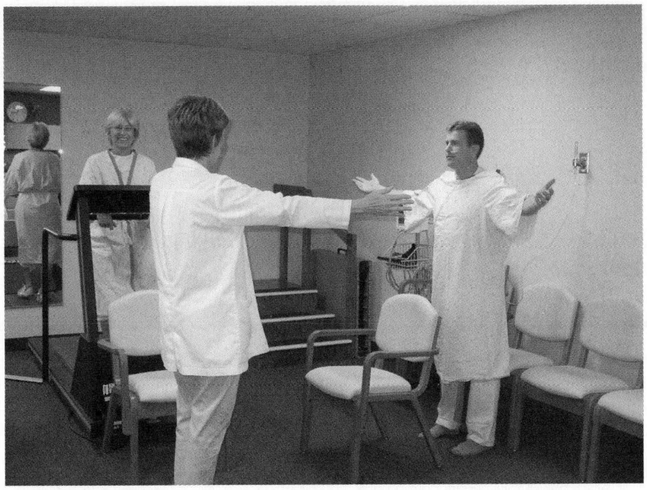

Figure 47-2 Patients exercising in inpatient cardiac rehabilitation to maintain muscle tone and endurance. The exercises also allow the therapist to evaluate the patients' cardiovascular response to light-to-moderate activity while they recuperate from a myocardial infarction, congestive heart failure, or open heart surgery.

treatment plan for a patient with a particular diagnosis is delineated in a grid format. During each day of the hospitalization, the grid lists the treatment that the patient should receive. Areas included in a pathway are IADLs, rehabilitation, nutrition, interventions, patient education, treatments, psychosocial/spiritual counseling, and discharge planning. Daily the various disciplines record, in checklist fashion, the care given. Deviations from the expected routine are recorded as variances in the progress record of the chart. Clinical pathways thus assist in evaluating outcomes and ensure a standard level of care (American Association of Cardiovascular and Pulmonary Rehabilitation [AACVPR], 2004a).

SAFETY NOTE 47-2

Signs and Symptoms of Exercise Intolerance

- Chest pain or pain referred to the teeth, jaw, ear, or arm
- Excessive fatigue
- Shortness of breath
- Lightheadedness or dizziness
- Nausea or vomiting
- Unusual weight gain of 3–5 lbs in a 1- to 3-day period

If a Patient Needs to Take Nitroglycerin

A patient with chest pain or angina who has a prescription for nitroglycerin should try a nitroglycerin pill under the tongue. If the chest pain has not disappeared within 3–5 minutes, another nitroglycerin pill should be tried. Continue until a total of three nitroglycerin pills have been taken over a 15-minute period. If the chest pain persists, call 911. The doctor should be notified when the patient first has angina or if there are changes in the frequency or intensity of episodes of angina. Notify the physician if other symptoms of exercise intolerance persist after resting.

Home Programs

Each patient is given a home program before discharge from the hospital. The type of program given is individualized to the patient and his or her particular diagnosis. The general components of a home program are activity and exercise guidelines, work simplification, pacing, temperature precautions, social activity, sexuality, signs and symptoms of exercise intolerance, and/or a discussion of risk factors. Depending on the diagnosis, certain aspects of the home program are emphasized or minimized. The information should be pertinent to the patient's lifestyle, including favorite activities, work, and/or hobbies with suggestions for resuming these activities.

MI Home Program

The home program of a patient who has had an STEMI will tend to highlight how to evaluate activity/exercise and determine the correct energy expenditure during the patient's recovery. Healing of the heart muscle takes about 4–8 weeks depending on the amount of damage sustained. Patients are usually asked to restrict their activities to the 2–4 MET range during this time (Definition 47-2 and Table 47-1). Pacing and work simplification may also be explained. This is especially important when the patient has had a significant amount of heart damage. (It should be remembered, however, that 88% of those under age 65 eventually will return to work, according to the AHA [1998].) A walking or biking exercise schedule is given. Depression and sexuality are discussed because certain cardiac medications can play a significant role in mood as well as sexual function and desire. Patients should be told that, if

DEFINITION 47-2

METs

METS are a unit of measure used to describe the amount of oxygen the body needs for a given activity (DeBusk, 2003). One MET is equal to oxygen consumption at rest or 3.5 ml of oxygen/kg of body weight/min. Extensive oxygen consumption tests have been done on a number of activities, and a small sampling of activities is included in Table 47-1. These values are still approximate because they do not take into account environmental factors or skill. The more the body moves and has to work against resistance, the higher the MET level.

Table 47-1. MET Values for Various Activities

Home	Leisure and Vocational	Exercise and Sports
1.0–2.5 METS		
Sweeping floors Dusting Straightening up Serving food Table setting Knitting and crocheting Putting away groceries Making bed Standing quietly in line Mowing lawn with a riding mower Casino gambling–standing Sexual activity Dressing and undressing Sleeping Watching TV Dish washing	Power boating Fishing from boat Pumping gas Changing light bulbs Typing, computer Sitting for light office work Card playing, sitting Board games Playing piano or organ Driving tractor Sewing with a machine Driving an auto or truck Sitting to study, read, or write	Walking at slow pace Playing catch with a baseball or football Horseback riding, walking
2.6–4.0 METS		
Child care, bathing, and grooming Walk, run, and play with children (moderate) General house cleaning Walking downstairs Sweeping garage or sidewalk Raking lawn Walking and carrying load of 15 lbs	Pitching horseshoes Home auto repair Planting seedlings and shrubs Playing the drums Home wiring or plumbing Feeding small farm animals Standing to pack light to moderate boxes Bartending–standing Walking and picking up yard	Very light stationary biking Weight lifting of light to moderate effort Stretching, yoga Golf using a cart Snowmobiling Walking at moderate speed Water aerobics
>4.0–6.0 METS		
Major house cleaning, such as washing windows, vigorous effort Moving furniture Scrubbing floors on hands and knees Cleaning gutters Painting the outside of house Painting and wallpapering inside of house Weeding or cultivating	Laying carpet or tile Slow wood chopping Farming, feeding cattle Carpentry on outside of house Carpentry, refinishing surfaces Hunting–general Road building, carrying heavy loads Roofing	General calisthenics, moderate effort Shooting hoops Golf, carrying clubs Softball, fast or slow pitch Low-impact or dance aerobics Dodgeball or hopscotch Bicycling at 10–11.9 mph
<6.0–10 METS		
Carrying groceries upstairs Moving household items in boxes Shoveling more than 16 lbs per minute (heavy) Walking or standing with objects weighing 50–74 lbs	Farming, bailing hay Concrete masonry Moving heavy objects such as furniture Firefighter carrying hoses	High-impact aerobics Running 10–12 min/mile Basketball game Jump roping Race walking Swimming laps at a moderate pace Bicycling at moderate pace >12 mph

From Ainsworth et al., 1998.

there is a change in sexual ability or desire after their cardiac event, they should talk to their doctor to explore the role of any new medications in those changes. When a patient can climb two flights of stairs without symptoms of intolerance, they can usually resume sexual relations without cardiovascular symptoms (DeBusk, 2003).

Open Heart Surgery Home Program

Patients who have had open heart surgery are given directions that are more specific. They are in pain and under the influence of analgesics, which may affect retention of information. They are told specifically what to do and what to avoid. They are also given information on stretches and mild exercises to assist in incisional pain management. In these patients, the sternum has been broken and it must be treated like any other broken bone. Surgical patients are to avoid lifting, pushing, or pulling, especially one-sided lifting or pulling, of greater than 10 lbs for 6–12 weeks. Therapists should make recommendations for alternative ways of doing activities to avoid one-sided pulling. For example, when pulling open a heavy door, it is desirable to use two hands, or when picking up a heavy coffeepot, put one hand covered with an oven mitt on the bottom of a coffee pot and the other hand on the handle. Patients who complain of feeling sternal shifting or clicking are told to try to avoid the activity that causes it and to stop any upper extremity exercises. Usually the clicking goes away with just a little care. Be aware that individual surgeons have their own views regarding the exact length of time to avoid lifting and the amount of arm activity they will allow. Walking schedules per patient tolerance are given. Patients are also given information regarding the possible emotional and physical responses they may expect during the healing process, such as easy fatigability or depression. Patients are encouraged to express their affection. If they have sexual intercourse, they may wish to try positions that avoid strain on the sternum, such as side-lying or sitting in a chair facing each other.

CHF Home Program

Patients with CHF and/or cardiomyopathy often have limited endurance. Their home program puts heavy emphasis on pacing and work simplification. It also includes a mild exercise program. Information regarding their diagnosis is given to help these patients understand that overexertion could put them back into heart failure. Signs and symptoms of CHF are included to alert the patient to signs of worsening medical status (see Safety Note 47-1).

Angioplasty Home Program

Patients admitted solely for an angioplasty/stent or atherectomy are usually seen for home instruction. The goal of this home program is to teach risk factor recognition and patient awareness of ways to modify these risks. An aerobic exercise program positively affects most risk factors for heart disease. Therefore, a variety of ways to exercise are discussed, with the goal of finding one or several modes of aerobic exercise that might interest the patient. For example, if the patient chooses walking, options such as mall walking, treadmill and video walking programs, and outdoor walking are explored. Patients are given instruction in how to start an exercise program and taught how to assess their physical response to exercise using the *Borg Rating of Perceived Exertion Scale* (*RPE*) (ACSM, 2000) and heart rate monitoring, if appropriate. Again, the therapist reviews signs and symptoms of exercise intolerance. Stress reduction techniques may be covered, and other resources for stress reduction are given. If the patient is a smoker, his or her willingness to quit is assessed. If the patient is in the planning or action phase of quitting, information regarding the effects of nicotine on the body is given, as well as assistance in planning how to beat the urge to smoke and resources for support groups. All information is written so that the patient may refer to it later.

Discharge Planning

Discharge planning begins early due to the shortened hospital stays. The cardiac occupational therapist provides information regarding the level of physical function the patient tolerates at discharge. The therapist also makes recommendations for further therapies and gives input regarding the possible need for home health or extended care facility.

Outpatient Cardiac Rehabilitation or Phase II

Outpatient cardiac rehabilitation is a multifaceted program of EKG-monitored exercise and education for secondary prevention of heart disease. The goals for outpatient cardiac rehabilitation are:

1. Continue medical surveillance and assessment of an individual's cardiovascular response to exercise
2. Limit the physiological and psychological effects of heart disease
3. Instruct on risk factors for heart disease and how to reduce their impact
4. Maximize psychosocial and vocational status

Patients are usually started in outpatient cardiac rehabilitation 1–2 weeks after discharge from the hospital. The program runs 3 days a week for 4–8 weeks. It would be ideal if each patient had a stress test prior to starting rehabilitation so that the results could be used in developing an exercise prescription. Many patients, however, will not have a stress test until 3–6 months after a STEMI or percutaneous transluminal coronary revascularization (PTCT)/stent and a year after a bypass. Often the therapist must take a careful history to determine risk stratification based on the

PROCEDURES FOR PRACTICE 47-2

Determining the Maximum Age-Adjusted Heart Rate (MAHR)

1. Take the number 220.
2. Subtract the patient's age.
3. The difference is that patient's MAHR.
4. To establish his or her exercise heart range, multiply the MAHR by 50–85% to obtain the heart rate for exercise.

For example, a 50-year-old patient's MAHR would be 170 (220–50). To determine the exercise heart rate, multiply 170 by 0.50 and 0.85. The 50-year-old patient's exercise heart rate range is 85–149 bpm.

patient's ejection fraction, hospital course, heart rate and blood pressure response, symptoms, and/or possible EKG changes with exercise. (Risk stratification refers to determination of the patient's risk for further cardiac events based on the past medical history.)

After assessing the patient's risk stratification, the therapist will need to determine the appropriate exercise intensity using one of the following means. The therapist could determine 50–85% of the patient's maximum age-adjusted heart rate (MAHR) (ACSM, 2000) (see Procedures for Practice 47-2 regarding how to calculate MAHR). If, however, the patient is on a beta blocker medication, such as atenolol or metoprolol, his or her heart rate response will be blunted, making the heart rate calculation inaccurate. Using the *Borg RPE Scale* is an additional way to measure the patient's tolerance of exercise. The patient is usually asked to rate the intensity of the exercise on the *Borg RPE Scale*. Initially the patient should try to keep the score between 11 and 13; later in the rehabilitation program, a score between 12 and 15 may be appropriate (ACSM, 2001). The patient's cardiovascular response and/or symptoms all assist in formulating the exercise prescription.

The exercise goal varies per individual depending on the function of his or her heart and physical condition. Usually those with good heart function and physical condition achieve between 5–6 METS. The patient's previous vocational and leisure interests, however, must also be considered in determining the patient's exercise goal.

The elderly, those who are sedentary, or those who have low functional capacity can still benefit by increasing their maximum MET level. For example, a patient with CHF may have a functional capacity of 2.5 METs after a hospitalization. If they can increase their MET level to 3.5–4 METs, they have significantly increased the number of activities or tasks they can do.

The two primary methods of achieving exercise goals are continuous and discontinuous exercise. For some, continuous exercise works well. For others, short bouts of exercise on various pieces of equipment followed by a short rest of 1–2 minutes are preferable. With continuous exercise, increasing the total duration of the exercise to at least 20–40 minutes is the first goal. Later, intensity is gradually increased. The advantages of continuous exercise are that less equipment and space are needed and the exercise more closely mimics what the patient will be doing at home. The disadvantages are that only certain muscle groups are targeted on one piece of equipment and the patient is exposed to just one form of aerobic exercise.

In discontinuous exercise, the amount of time a patient stays on a piece of equipment remains the same, but the intensity gradually increases. After finishing the allotted time on one piece of equipment, the patient then switches to another; this process is repeated several times. The advantages of discontinuous exercise are that the patient is exposed to a variety of equipment, boredom is minimized, and multiple muscle groups are used. The disadvantages are that discontinuous exercise takes a lot of space and equipment, it is sometimes hard to coordinate patients shifting equipment at the same time, and it does not reflect what the patient will be doing for aerobic exercise at home. With both methods of conditioning, however, the patients achieve the same MET levels.

In outpatient cardiac rehabilitation, a variety of exercise equipment may be used. Treadmills, bicycle ergometers, recumbent bikes, rowing machines, arm ergometers, and so on are used, depending on the patient's preference and to accommodate any existing orthopedic problem the patient may have. Weight training is usually started 2–4 weeks post event. Prior to weight training, patients must meet certain criteria regarding their exercise capacity, blood pressure (BP) control, and ejection fraction (ACSM, 2000).

Risk factor modification is a key focus of outpatient cardiac rehabilitation. Therapists help patients identify their own risk factors and choose which risk factors they would like to try to modify or eliminate. Risk factor education occurs in a variety of ways. Some centers have specific times on various days where health professionals will lecture on a particular topic. Other hospitals have short education sessions before, during, or after exercise sessions. The goal of these educational sessions is to give patients the information they need to modify their risk factors.

Psychosocial issues must be evaluated with the patient who has heart disease because depression, post MI, has been linked to increased mortality (Musselman, 2004). Many centers use standardized questionnaires to determine depression or anxiety such as the *Symptom Checklist-90-Revised*, *Beck Depression Inventory*, or the *Profile of Mood States* (AACVPR, 2004b). The results of testing will indicate if the patient needs referral to a chaplain, social worker, or psychologist based on their circumstance or preference.

Some patients have very physical jobs, which require heavy lifting. Feedback is given to the physician regarding the patients' exercise capacity and cardiovascular response to aerobic exercise in cardiac rehabilitation. Following the outpatient cardiac rehabilitation program, these individuals may also need to be referred to a work-hardening program to further ready them to return to work.

Community-Based Phase III Cardiac Rehabilitation

Phase III is a community-based cardiac rehabilitation with larger groups of patients and fewer staff members per participant. Phase III programs are often located in community centers, school gyms, or YMCAs. Such programs may follow outpatient or phase II cardiac rehabilitation. Patients may skip phase II, however, and go directly to phase III if they are low risk and have been active in the past. Only a small percentage of patients go to phase III after phase II because it is generally not covered by insurance. Since reimbursement is difficult, it also means that these programs run on a very low budget and usually are lucky to break even.

A physician must refer a participant to a phase III program. Usually a stress test is required, or the physician establishes heart rate guidelines. Trained personnel monitor BP response and assist patients with monitoring their heart rate. EKG monitoring is typically limited to once per month. Goal setting for risk management continues, as does the education component, although the education may be more informal. Participants also enjoy the support and encouragement of others who have a common goal of reducing their incidence of heart disease.

CHRONIC OBSTRUCTIVE PULMONARY DISEASE

Chronic obstructive pulmonary disease (COPD) is a combination of emphysema and bronchitis (MedicineNet, 2005). Emphysema is the progressive and irreversible destruction of the alveoli walls (Etkin, Lenker, & Mills, 2005). The walls of the alveoli have elastic fibers, and when these are destroyed, the lung loses some of its elasticity, resulting in air trapping. This air trapping reduces the ability of the lung to shrink during exhalation; the lung then inhales less air with the next breath (MedicineNet, 2005). Chronic bronchitis is defined as excessive sputum production and cough of at least 3 months in duration occurring 2 years in a row (MedicineNet, 2005). This inflammation also causes the bronchial tubes to increase their production of mucus. The result of these processes is that the patient experiences sudden shortness of breath and may wheeze or cough (MedicineNet, 2005). Patients with COPD have characteristics of all these diseases (see Definition 47-3 for a description of pulmonary function tests). COPD is a chronic and progressive condition (MedicineNet, 2005). Medications and good health habits can lessen the symptoms and maximize function.

> **DEFINITION 47-3**
>
> **Pulmonary Function Tests**
>
> - Patients are asked to exhale forcefully as much air as possible into a spirometer. The amount of air exhaled in l second is called the forced expiratory volume (FEV1). Age-related norms for the FEV1 are available (Couch & Ryan, 2000).
> - Arterial blood gases are drawn to determine the lungs' ability to oxygenate blood, remove CO_2, and maintain the body's acid-base status (Couch & Ryan, 2000). It is helpful to draw blood gases before and after exercise to see how well oxygenation is maintained during activity.
> - A pulse oximeter is a non-invasive test to determine the amount of oxygen in the blood. A probe is wrapped around a fingertip. A light shines through the finger, and the amount of light reaching the other side indicates the amount of oxygen in the blood. Hemoglobin is red, and the more hemoglobin in the blood, the less light is able to penetrate the fingertip (MedicineNet, 2005). The oximeter can occasionally give false readings. If the patient is anemic, wears nail polish, or has poor circulation, the pulse oximetry may be inaccurate. Often the oximetry machine will also determine the patient's pulse. If the palpated pulse and the oximetry machine pulse match, it is likely that the **oxygen saturation (O_2 Sat)** will be accurate.

The feeling of breathlessness, called dyspnea, is a key feature of COPD. Damage to the lung results in a flattening of the diaphragm due to hyperinflation. This flattening takes away the ability of the diaphragm to act effectively in assisting with expansion of the lungs during inspiration. To compensate for the lack of inspiratory pressure, patients with COPD tend to use their shoulder girdle muscles to expand their lungs, making it difficult to use those muscles in unsupported upper extremity activities (Coppola & Wood, 2000).

Dyspnea, fatigue, cough, and sputum production are part of the disease process. The effort of breathing takes so much energy that often COPD patients find themselves without enough energy to do their daily tasks, including ADLs and vocational and leisure endeavors. They are unable to increase their ventilation enough to meet physiological demands. Due to the unpleasant sensation of shortness of breath (SOB), patients reduce their physical activities, resulting in muscle weakness and the inability to use oxygen efficiently (Jackson & Horn, 1998). Eating is an activity made difficult by lack of air. Maintaining adequate nutrition is a problem for 40–60% of patients with COPD, and nutrition problems are independent predictors of mortality (AACVPR, 2004b). Some patients lose weight because of the excessive energy costs of their breathing efforts (AACVPR, 2004b). Others use steroids to reduce lung inflammation, resulting in weight gain that contributes to additional problems. Weight gain exacerbates the problem of not having enough oxygen to metabolize food, and extra weight requires more oxygen to do any activity including eating.

Depression is common with COPD. Between 7 and 42% of patients with moderate to severe COPD experience depression (AACVPR, 2004b). As with any chronic disease process, the changes in lifestyle, the struggle to accomplish normal daily activities, the fear of extreme SOB, and feelings of hopelessness all contribute to the depression that many patients with COPD feel.

PULMONARY REHABILITATION

The American Association of Cardiovascular and Pulmonary Rehabilitation (AACVPR) sets standards of practice for pulmonary rehabilitation, which are used by insurers and the Joint Commission of Hospital Organizations. The AACVPR has published a book called *Guidelines for Pulmonary Rehabilitation Programs* to guide practice (2004b). It has also instituted a certification for pulmonary rehabilitation programs (see Resources 47-1). A team of health professionals, including doctors, respiratory therapists, dieticians, pharmacists, and occupational and physical therapists, is ideally involved in the pulmonary rehabilitation program. As with other diagnostic categories, the roles may overlap in reinforcing behaviors to enhance function.

The goals of the occupational therapist in pulmonary rehabilitation are (AACVPR, 2004b; O'Dell-Rossi et al., 1999):

1. ADL evaluation and training to increase functional endurance
2. Instruction and training in appropriate breathing techniques with ADLs
3. Evaluation and strengthening of the upper extremity
4. Work simplification and energy conservation
5. Evaluation of the need for adaptive equipment
6. Assistance in adapting leisure activities
7. Education in stress management and relaxation techniques.

ADL Evaluation and Training

Patients with COPD are often limited in their ability to perform their ADLs due to dyspnea. It is common to have significant muscle wasting from disuse. The therapist should note during the ADL evaluation the patient's breathing pattern. Often patients with COPD hold their breath, breathe shallowly and fast, or elevate their shoulders as they breathe. The amount of oxygen in the blood or oxygen saturation (O_2 Sat) with activity should also be measured by pulse oximetry (Procedures for Practice 47-3). If the O_2 Sat falls below 90% with a patient's ADLs, the use of oxygen with activity should be considered. If the patient does not have home oxygen, the physician should be informed of the patient's low oxygen saturation. Currently the O_2 Sat must be below 88% to qualify for reimbursement for home oxygen from Medicare or other supplemental insurances (Couch & Ryan, 2000). As part of the functional assessment, measurements of heart rate and blood pressure should also be taken.

RESOURCE 47-1

Two organizations dominate the administration and policies of cardiac rehabilitation. One is the American Association of Cardiovascular and Pulmonary Rehabilitation (AACVPR), which published the book *Guidelines for Cardiac Rehabilitation and Secondary Prevention Programs*. Government agencies and third-party payers use this publication to determine appropriate cardiac rehabilitation policies and procedures. The second is the American College of Sports Medicine (ACSM), which has several nationally recognized certifications for health professionals who wish to work in cardiac rehabilitation. Both organizations offer continuing education courses in cardiac rehabilitation. Together these two organizations shape the practice of cardiac rehabilitation.

AACVPR
401 North Michigan Avenue, Suite 2200
Chicago, IL 60611
Phone: (312) 321-5146
E-mail: aacvpr@smithbucklin.com
www.aacvpr.org

ACSM National Center
401 West Michigan Street
Indianapolis, IN 46202-3233
Phone: (317) 637-9200
E-mail: crt2acsm@acsm.org
www.acsm.org/sportsmed

Breathing Techniques

It is important that the patient practice use of breathing techniques with ADLs. After becoming familiar with diaphragmatic and pursed lip breathing, the patient should attempt tasks using these breathing techniques that previously caused them to be breathless. The pulse oximeter helps to reinforce the improvement in the O_2 Sat with use of a breathing technique. Timing the breath with work is also helpful. For example, the patient should breathe out with pushing the vacuum cleaner, and breathe in while pulling the vacuum cleaner. Exhaling with the exertion of lifting is less taxing not only on the lungs but also on the cardiovascular system because it prevents the Valsalva

PROCEDURES FOR PRACTICE 47-3

Breathing Techniques

Patients are instructed to practice these techniques while sitting in a relaxed position preferably with feet elevated. After they become proficient using these breathing methods at rest, patients should try using them while doing pleasant activities such as reading or watching television. Finally, patients should try using one of these techniques while doing a task that is difficult, such as stair climbing (Coppola & Wood, 2000).

Pursed Lip Breathing

- Breathe in through your nose.
- With lips pursed, exhale air slowly.
- Try to take twice as much time to exhale as it did to inhale.

Diaphragmatic Breathing

- Sit in a relaxed position preferably with feet elevated.
- Place your hand on your abdomen.
- As you inhale through your nose, try to feel your stomach push out as your lungs fill with oxygen.
- Next, feel your stomach go down as you slowly breathe out through pursed lips.
- Continue to repeat this process until you become comfortable doing it.
- Stop the diaphragmatic breathing if you become lightheaded or fatigued.

maneuver (see Procedures for Practice 47-3 for breathing techniques).

Upper Extremity Function

Muscle strength of the upper extremity must be evaluated. Since pulmonary patients are often on steroids, their shoulder girdle, trunk, and hip muscles are usually weak (Coppola & Wood, 2000). Patients with COPD commonly use the accessory muscles of the shoulder girdle to help them breathe, which makes it difficult for them to use these muscles in unsupported upper extremity activity. Upper extremity (UE) strengthening has been found to improve the quality of life by increasing the capacity to work and reducing the oxygen requirement of upper extremity activity (Couch & Ryan, 2000). Use of free weights, Theraband, an arm ergometer, and other upper body strengthening techniques are all helpful in increasing upper body strength. Additional improvement in functional status is seen when leg training is added (Couch & Ryan, 2000).

Work Simplification and Energy Conservation

Since their work capacity is significantly reduced, patients with COPD will benefit from instruction in work simplification and energy conservation. Bathing is a particularly strenuous activity because the hot humid air makes breathing difficult. Therapists encourage patients to use the ventilation fan or leave the door open while bathing to keep the humidity level down. Recommending the use of a chair in the shower and using a thick terry robe after showering instead of toweling off are two suggestions that are helpful in reducing energy expenditure. Unsupported upper extremity activity is very fatiguing for patients with COPD. It is important to teach these patients to support their arms during upper extremity activities such as hair combing or shaving. Sometimes a machine like an electric toothbrush can be of assistance. Scheduling of activities that require more energy expenditure for the time following the use of an inhaler will also allow patients to accomplish more (Couch & Ryan, 2000).

Not all patients with COPD will need adaptive equipment. As the disease progresses in severity, however, some adaptive equipment is useful (Fig. 47-3). Since bending over to tie shoes or put on pants may cause significant SOB, elastic shoe laces, a long-handled shoe horn, or a reacher to assist with putting on slacks may be helpful.

Promoting Self-Enhancement Roles

Having COPD tends to isolate those who have it. Just completing daily necessities takes so much energy that little, if any, is left for leisure activities. Many patients fear becoming very SOB in front of others or are embarrassed using

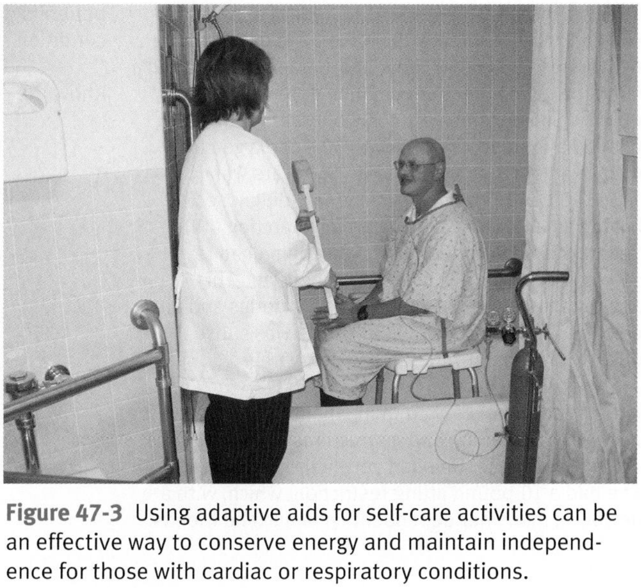

Figure 47-3 Using adaptive aids for self-care activities can be an effective way to conserve energy and maintain independence for those with cardiac or respiratory conditions.

oxygen. The occupational therapist can help the patient evaluate previously enjoyed activities and see if those activities can be adapted to fit the current health status. Providing patients with information regarding programs or activities available in their community is also helpful. Sometimes involving a helper or companion may make an activity more feasible.

Stress Management

The feeling of being unable to get enough air is truly frightening. Patients with COPD often experience a sense of panic with breathlessness. Teaching patients methods to cope with extreme SOB can lessen their fear. Leaning forward and resting their arms on the table releases the diaphragm and makes breathing easier. Using pursed lip and/or diaphragmatic breathing helps to slow the pace of breathing so that the patient is not breathing so shallowly and rapidly. A stress management technique such as visualization may help patients calm themselves by mentally transporting them out of the stressful situation. It is important that the patient practice these options prior to actually needing them. Having a well-practiced plan of action for the panic associated with breathlessness will give patients confidence in their ability to control the situation.

Heart disease and pulmonary disease, as the first and fourth leading causes of death, respectively, pose a major health problem. As either a primary or a secondary diagnosis, both heart disease and COPD require specialized attention in planning occupational therapy intervention. If a patient has a history of heart disease or COPD, the occupational therapy practitioner must assess the patient's cardiovascular response to activity or exercise. Precautions for the patient's cardiac or pulmonary problem must be incorporated into the treatment program.

CASE EXAMPLE #1

K. M.: Cardiac Rehabilitation

Occupational Therapy Process	Clinical Reasoning Process: Objectives	Clinical Reasoning Process: Examples of Therapist's Internal Dialogue
Patient Information K.M. is a married, 32-year-old mother of a 3-year-old child and a full-time health worker. The day after the delivery of her second child, she suddenly developed a migraine headache. Her condition deteriorated quickly. She became very short of breath (SOB) and needed a rebreather mask with 10 L of oxygen to maintain her O_2 saturation. Her heart rate was 135–140 bpm. The next day, she was diagnosed as having an anterior wall myocardial infarction (MI). Several days later, her pulmonary edema had resolved, and she had a coronary angiogram. The angiogram showed normal coronary arteries and an ejection fraction (EF) of 25–30%. She was subsequently diagnosed with a cardiomyopathy.	Understand the patient's diagnosis or condition	"Cardiomyopathy after pregnancy is rare. If she improves within the 6 months after diagnosis, she will probably be able to lead a normal life."
	Know the person	"K.M. will be a busy lady, working and taking care of two children under 3 years old. She works in the health care system and has some knowledge of health issues. K.M. is used to a full-time income and taking care of herself, her home, and family. It must be stressful to have to rely on others to take care of something she normally did herself."
Initially, she was referred to inpatient cardiac rehab for general conditioning and instructions for appropriate activities at home. She had very limited endurance. She had a 10-pound lifting restriction, which, with a newborn, made her dependent on family and friends.		

She was seen by home health occupational therapy for several weeks. She was given exercises to increase her endurance and instructed in energy conservation techniques. Although she became somewhat stronger, she was still dependent on volunteers around the clock to do the majority of household tasks and take care of the children. This caused her a great deal of stress. Her therapist instructed her in stress management techniques and practiced them with K.M.

Reason for Referral to Cardiac Occupational Therapy Phase II K.M. was referred to outpatient cardiac rehabilitation for physical conditioning and education.	Appreciate the context Develop provisional hypotheses	"I will talk with the husband to get his view of how things are going at home and get a feel of how supportive he is to K.M. I will also need to consider if K.M. is getting secondary gain from all the attention."
Assessment Process and Results K.M. arrived in outpatient cardiac rehabilitation via wheelchair because she felt she was too weak to walk from the car and exercise. She was now doing her own self-care but still relied on volunteers for most of her household chores and caring for her children. She admitted she was stressed by her diagnosis, the number of volunteers in her home, and financial worries. She reported that she slept excessively and was exhausted with exercise. She also reported that she had a history of depression and complained of being somewhat depressed. She was able to walk slowly on the treadmill at 2.0 mph for 20 minutes with normal cardiovascular response. A recent echocardiogram revealed her EF to now be up to 50%.	Consider evaluation approach and methods Interpret observations	"Initially, K.M. is allowed to demonstrate what she can comfortably do physically. After 20 minutes of walking, she still is tolerating the exercise well." "K.M. doesn't seem to correlate her ability to easily walk 20 minutes at a strolling pace as indicative of her ability to do many household chores, such as dishwashing, folding clothes, making beds, etc. I will continue to assess K.M. to see if she may need referral for psychiatric help."
Occupational Therapy Problem List • Low physical capacity for work less than 3 METS. • Inability to engage in previous work and leisure pursuits due to decreased endurance. • Depression over feelings of dependency and concern over cardiac diagnosis. • Dependence on volunteers for most IADLs.	Synthesize results	"K.M. seems to be overwhelmed with her diagnosis and has not assimilated that her heart function has now improved to near normal. With an exercise program to increase her physical capacity, she should be able to return to her job and all her IADLs. Stress management technique training will assist her to cope with difficulties caused by illness."
Occupational Therapy Goal List • Learn to monitor physical response to exercise and activity through use of *Borg RPE Scale* and pulse monitoring. • Gradually increasing capacity for work through aerobic exercise and strengthening exercises (2–5 METS). • Gradually resume household and leisure pursuits (1.5–5 METS). • Learn to pace household activities. • Learn stress management techniques to cope with difficulties caused by illness. • Instruct patient in risk factors for heart disease. • Identify patient's personal risk factors and ways to ameliorate their effects. • Start a regular home aerobic exercise program.	Develop intervention hypotheses Select an intervention approach Consider what will occur in therapy, how often, and for how long	"As K.M. increases her endurance, we can gradually shift her back to some of her household responsibilities of the same energy or MET level. In the meantime, learning stress techniques will help her handle her current situation. Education about her current health problem will help her understand that she is truly getting better." "Cardiac rehabilitation will concentrate on an aerobic exercise and strengthening program. Brief educational sessions will be conducted as she exercises or after the exercise session." "K.M. is highly motivated to improve, but conditioning takes time. I will see her three times a week for 6 weeks. During that time, I will help her understand the connection between workload on treadmill or exercise cycle and home activities. Together we can develop a plan on how she will start resuming household tasks. I will also instruct her in a home exercise program to assist in improving her conditioning. After exercising, we will practice some stress management techniques."

Intervention As she regained physical strength through exercise, K.M. could start resuming more of her usual activities and reduce her dependence on volunteers. Instructing K.M. in how to assess her own physical response to exercise and activity gave her confidence that she was in control. Since K.M. had difficulty with pacing, the therapist had her keep a diary of her daily routine. Later, they reviewed it, and the occupational therapist reviewed work simplification techniques and methods of pacing. The therapist also assigned her tasks within her current aerobic capacity to assist her in resuming her home responsibilities. K.M. was also instructed in stress management techniques to help her deal with the stresses of her illness. Due to her previous history of depression, the therapist reviewed information about the relationship of depression and fatigue. The occupational therapist explored with K.M. the possibility of seeking professional help and/or medication to deal with her depression. Additionally, K.M. was instructed in the risk factors for heart disease. Her individual risk factors were identified, and information was provided on how to ameliorate their effects. As part of her risk factor reduction, K.M. initiated a walking program.	Assess the patient's comprehension Understand what she is doing Compare actual to expected performance Know the person Appreciate the context	"K.M. was a quick learner. As she fully understood that her heart function was near normal, she really started to gain confidence that her life could return to normal. However, she needed some concrete direction to translate what she was learning into action. Adding the additional home exercise program helped to increase her capacity more quickly, but depression was holding her back from making a complete recovery. Even with her health care background, she did not realize the effect of depression on her physically. With more information about depression, she was more willing to seek professional help."
Next Steps Discharge from outpatient cardiac rehabilitation.	Anticipate present and future patient concerns Analyze patient's comprehension Decide if the patient should continue or discontinue therapy and/or return in the future	"K.M. was making significant strides in returning to her previous activity level. She seemed to benefit significantly from activity modification, education, and information on heart disease. She had initiated a home walking program, and she planned to return to work within a month."

CLINICAL REASONING IN OCCUPATIONAL THERAPY PRACTICE

Implications of a Diagnosis

K.M. was initially diagnosed as having an anterior MI and, later, was also given a diagnosis of cardiomyopathy.

If a patient has had an MI, what symptoms or signs would you look for to determine if he or she is tolerating an activity or exercise? Would those signs and symptoms be different if the patient has a diagnosis of cardiomyopathy without an STEMI?

CASE EXAMPLE #2

Pulmonary Rehabilitation

Occupational Therapy Process	Clinical Reasoning Process: Objectives	Clinical Reasoning Process: Examples of Therapist's Internal Dialogue
Patient Information Mr. M. is an 85-year-old male with a medical history of congestive heart failure, chronic obstructive pulmonary disease (COPD), and diabetes. He also has a history of coronary artery disease and has had a myocardial infarction in the past. He has been on home oxygen but reports he was not always using it despite it being prescribed. He lives alone in an apartment building with an elevator. Prior to this hospitalization, he had recently begun receiving home visits from an RN and was getting meals-on-wheels. Up until this point, he has been independent with dressing, toileting, bathing, laundry, and finances. He is ambulating without an assistive device but owns a front-wheeled walker and a wheelchair. He also stated that he owns a shower chair and has a hand-held shower but has not needed to use the shower chair for bathing. He does not drive and is provided with transportation by various family members. He is currently on 6 L of oxygen and is receiving steroids and inhalers to improve breathing. He states that he has had "a little" education for COPD/congestive heart failure (CHF) management in the past. His goal was to return to his apartment at discharge from the hospital, to which he was admitted for increased shortness of breath. He was open to receiving more assistance from family or outside agencies if necessary.	Understand the patient's diagnosis or condition Know the person	"Mr. M. has been on 6 L of oxygen chronically at home and has other medical conditions that indicate to me that he likely has poor endurance and may have had some difficulty managing ADLs at home." "The lack of Mr. M.'s use of energy conservation techniques and his prescription for oxygen during daily activities suggests that he would benefit from education in these areas. His daughter reports some forgetfulness in the patient, and therefore, I need to keep in mind that he may need to have education repeated and in written form, as well as hands-on practice and demonstration, for the most success in learning new information."
Reason for Referral to Occupational Therapy Mr. M. was admitted to the hospital due to increased shortness of breath. He was referred to occupational therapy for an evaluation and further treatment to improve efficiency with functional activities. Because Mr. M. lives alone, it is especially important that he be as independent as possible to allow him to reach his goal of returning to his apartment.	Appreciate the context Develop provisional hypotheses	"I feel that Mr. M. will benefit from the combination of education and adaptive equipment use, as well as exercise to improve his activity tolerance at home. I am hoping that, as Mr. M. gets more fluent with using breathing techniques, he will be more inspired to combine them with the adaptive equipment use to improve his efficiency. I am glad that he has a supportive family that is working to keep Mr. M. as independent as possible."

Assessment Process and Results Mr. M.'s assessment took place in his hospital room. He was on 6 L of oxygen via nasal cannula. He appeared to be comfortable at rest, but following activity, his oxygen saturations decreased to 85%. He was able to complete pursed lip breathing with cues, and his saturations increased to 93% after 90 seconds of rest and pursed lip breathing. His upper body strength and range of motion were within functional limits. He was able to demonstrate ability to physically complete grooming, dressing, and toileting independently but was limited by decreased endurance and rapid shortness of breath. He frequently had to stop what he was doing to rest and, for that reason, took extra time or chose not to complete some tasks. He was able to complete basic transfers and ambulate in his room with stand-by assistance and no assistive device. Basic cognitive screen indicated that Mr. M.'s cognition was intact. His daughter did report that he has been more forgetful lately.	Consider evaluation approach and methods Interpret observations	"My focus was primarily on Mr. M.'s functional status and assessing his level of fatigue during functional tasks. I did spend some time observing him completing ADLs as well as interviewing him about his perceived level of fatigue and level of difficulty completing tasks. I monitored his oxygen saturations throughout our treatment sessions and observed his levels of dyspnea." "We discussed what ADLs were a priority to him versus less important tasks, and we were able to narrow our focus and set specific goals."
Occupational Therapy Problem List • Limited endurance affecting ADL performance • Limited education of energy conservation and work simplification techniques and pursed lip and diaphragmatic breathing • Decreased awareness of adaptive equipment resources and oxygen utilization • Mild memory impairments	Synthesize results	"It was apparent to me that Mr. M. was not conserving the maximum amount of his energy during certain functional tasks. Occasionally when he was fatigued, he would not complete grooming or hygiene tasks at all. I feel that, because he lives alone, we needed to focus on being able to complete his basic self-care activities efficiently and independently. At this point, he was not able to complete all self-care activities due to fatigue and shortness of breath."
Occupational Therapy Goal List (anticipated length of treatment: 4–5 sessions) • Patient will be able to verbalize and demonstrate understanding of pursed lip breathing and diaphragmatic breathing during functional activities by discharge. • Patient will verbalize or demonstrate understanding of 2–3 work simplification and energy conservation techniques during self-care activities, community activities, and laundry and other homemaking tasks by discharge. • Patient will complete tub transfer independently using adaptive equipment to increase activity tolerance by discharge. • Patient will have all recommended adaptive equipment or resources for pursuing purchase of equipment by discharge. • Patient will be independent with a 10- to 15-minute upper extremity exercise program while using pursed lip breathing to improve overall endurance and ability to tolerate ADLs.	Develop intervention hypotheses Select an intervention approach Consider what will occur in therapy, how often, and for how long	"I plan on providing Mr. M. with instruction on breathing techniques, energy conservation, adaptive equipment recommendations, and resources. This education will provide him with improved activity tolerance and give him a greater sense of independence. I believe that it is important to provide him with the opportunity to prioritize the importance of completing certain tasks and allowing him to participate in the goal-setting process. "My intervention will primarily focus on an adaptive approach with a focus on patient education." "Mr. M. will likely only be hospitalized for 5 to 6 days, and therefore, we will need to strive to meet our goals in that timeframe. I will focus mostly on completing functional tasks while providing education throughout the sessions. Written materials will also be provided, as well as family education when possible."

Intervention Mr. M.'s treatment plan consisted of education for specific breathing techniques (pursed lip and diaphragmatic). He was instructed on how to incorporate these breathing techniques into his daily routine. He was then provided with more education in energy conservation and work simplification to allow him to be more efficient. Discussion about adaptive equipment needs took place, and recommendations were made. He was instructed in an upper extremity exercise program to increase endurance, and he was provided with a handout to encourage him to continue with the exercises after he was discharged. Mr. M. was provided with written instruction for all education due to memory impairments. Repetition and hands-on training were also provided whenever possible. Providing education was key to allow Mr. M. to understand how to manage his COPD symptoms better. He was better able to manage his shortness of breath and fatigue during activities by using pursed lip breathing combined with work simplification and energy conservation techniques. Discussion about the benefits of adaptive equipment use and incorporation into Mr. M.'s daily routine has allowed him to complete more tasks independently and with less fatigue. He was in agreement with using a shower chair, hand-held showerhead, and long-handled bath sponge to ease the burden that bathing once had been. Mr. M. elected to purchase a long-handled bath sponge from the hospital before discharge, and he already had a shower chair and hand-held showerhead at his apartment. He was encouraged to use his oxygen for all activities, including showering, to maintain a desirable oxygen saturation level for his safety. By participating in a daily exercise program, Mr. M.'s endurance improved, which allowed him to complete his ADLs with much less shortness of breath and fewer rest breaks. Mr. M. was seen for six sessions by occupational therapy. He met all of his established goals and was discharged back to his apartment	Assess the patient's comprehension Understand what he is doing Compare actual to expected performance Know the person Appreciate the context	"I could see the initial frustration that Mr. M. had when he was not fully able to complete tasks due to dyspnea. He was hesitant to try pursed lip breathing initially due to thinking it was 'too confusing' and that he would 'forget how to do it.' But with repetition and encouragement, he was able to quickly learn the technique and feel the benefits. Once we started to incorporate the use of adaptive equipment (such as a shower chair, hand-held showerhead, and long-handled bath sponge), Mr. M. was appearing more positive and confident in his abilities. He really was a rewarding patient to work with because he dramatically improved with simple modifications to his routine."
Next Steps Discharge to his apartment with recommendation of home occupational therapy evaluation and to resume meals-on-wheels as was established previously.	Anticipate present and future patient concerns Analyze patient's comprehension Decide if the patient should continue or discontinue therapy and/or return in the future	"I am recommending a home occupational therapy evaluation to reinforce the use of adaptive equipment and oxygen in Mr. M.'s home setting. I feel that Mr. M. was able to fully appreciate the benefits of using pursed lip breathing and oxygen to extend his endurance. He was comfortable with the idea of using adaptive equipment and work simplification techniques incorporated into his everyday routine. He is confident in his abilities to complete his daily activities and to return to his apartment independently. His family is comfortable with his abilities to care for himself, and they feel he has the resources he needs to be successful."

? CLINICAL REASONING IN OCCUPATIONAL THERAPY PRACTICE

Implications of a Diagnosis

Mr. M. has COPD, but he also has several other comorbid diseases. How would these other conditions potentially affect your treatment?

Evidence Table 47-1
Best Evidence for Occupational Therapy Practice Regarding Cardiac Rehabilitation

Intervention	Description of Intervention Tested	Participants	Dosage	Type of Best Evidence and Level of Evidence	Benefit	Statistical Probability and Effect Size of Outcome	Reference
Any form of supervised or unsupervised structured exercise program (compared with usual care)	Inpatient, outpatient, or community- or home-based setting exercise program either with or without psychosocial and educational interventions.	8,940 patients.	Varied from study to study. Median intervention time was 3 months.	Meta-analysis of 48 trials.	Yes, significant reduction in all-cause mortality and total cardiac mortality, a significant reduction in total cholesterol and triglycerides and systolic blood pressure, and lower self-reports of smoking.	Reduction in all-cause mortality (odds ratio [OR] = 0.80; 95% confidence interval [CI]: 0.68 to 0.93). Reduction in cardiac mortality (OR = 0.74; 95% CI: 0.61 to 0.96). Reduction in total cholesterol level (weighted mean difference, −0.37 mmol/L; 95% CI: −0.63 to −0.11 mmol/L). Reduction in total triglyceride level (weighted mean difference, −0.23 mmol/L; 95% CI: −0.39 to −0.07 mmol/L).	Taylor et al., 2004

						Reduction in systolic blood pressure (weighted mean difference, −3.2 mm Hg; 95% CI: −5.4 to −0.9 mm Hg). Reduction in smoking (OR = 0.64; 95% CI: 0.50 to 0.83).	
Inpatient and extended cardiac counseling and rehabilitation	Inpatient rehabilitation and extended cardiac rehabilitation consisting of exercise and education on resumption of activities, emotional effects of heart disease, risk factors, and coronary anatomy and physiology.	100 patients post myocardial infarction (MI) and <70 years old.	Inpatient group received 5.5 sessions and extended group received 9.55 sessions over 6 weeks.	Randomized, controlled study. IA2a. Therapists and subjects unblinded.	Yes. The cardiac rehabilitation groups (inpatient and extended) did better than the control group in knowledge, less depression, less physical disability, and less anxiety (persons in the control did not receive any formal programming).	Inpatient rehabilitation: knowledge, $p < 0.005$; depression, $p = 0.009$; anxiety, $p = 0.001$; and disability, $p < 0.009$. Extended treatment: knowledge, $p = 0.002$; depression, $p = 0.001$; anxiety, $p = 0.013$; and disability, $p < 0.005$.	Johnston et al., 1999

Evidence Table 47-2
Best Evidence for Occupational Therapy Practice Regarding Pulmonary Rehabilitation

Intervention	Description of Intervention Tested	Participants	Dosage	Type of Best Evidence and Level of Evidence	Benefit	Statistical Probability and Effect Size of Outcome	Reference
Patients seen in hospital-based program	Rehabilitation group was seen repeatedly for exercise and education. Brief advice group was given written educational materials and advice.	103 patients with severe chronic obstructive pulmonary disease (COPD) having a forced expiratory volume in 1 second (FEV1) <40% predicted value; 54 in exercise group; 49 in advice group.	Rehabilitation group was seen 2 times a week for 6 weeks. Brief advice group was seen once for 1 hour.	Randomized controlled study. IA2a (lacked blinded subjects and instructors)	Yes, the rehabilitation group did significantly better on the shuttle walk test. Improvements in quality of life were not significant.	$p < 0.001$	White et al., 2002
Exercise for pulmonary rehabilitation	Studies included in meta-analysis involved exercise (upper extremity, lower extremity, or respiratory muscle).	979 patients having COPD with an FEV1 <70% predicted in exercise trials. 723 patients meeting the above criteria participated in trials in which shortness of breath (SOB) was an outcome measure.	Experimental groups participated in exercise 3 times per week for at least 4 weeks.	Meta-analysis of 20 trials.	Yes, the rehabilitation group did significantly better in exercise capacity (walking test) and improvement in SOB than the control group.	Effect size for walking test = 0.71; 95% confidence interval (CI): 0.43 to 0.99. Effect size for SOB (12 trials) = 0.62; 95% CI: 0.35 to 0.89.	Salman et al., 2003

SUMMARY REVIEW QUESTIONS

1. A person is admitted to the hospital with an acute STEMI. He is given thrombolytics to reverse clot formation in his coronary arteries, but the thrombolytics cause a cerebral bleed. In evaluating and treating for stroke-related deficits, what physiological parameters should the therapist take to measure the workload on the patient's heart? What factors might increase these parameters?
2. What cardiac symptoms might a patient who has a previous heart history exhibit if he or she were not tolerating the treatment you prescribed for the patient's current shoulder injury?
3. What symptoms would a person going into CHF exacerbation exhibit?
4. In reviewing a patient's medical record after hip replacement surgery, what cardiac diagnoses might impinge on your treatment? What cardiac diagnostic tests might provide information to help you make decisions about the severity of his or her heart disease?
5. Describe in detail the differences between a home program for a patient with an STEMI, a coronary artery bypass graft, and an angioplasty. How would you customize the program for the individual?
6. Describe the different ways of conditioning an outpatient in cardiac rehabilitation. What are the advantages and disadvantages of each method?
7. List the risk factors for heart disease. What methods might an occupational therapist use to decrease a patient's risk for coronary artery disease?
8. Develop a treatment plan for a patient with COPD who is having problems with SOB while doing her ADLs.
9. Describe pursed lip and diaphragmatic breathing. How would you teach it to a patient with COPD?
10. If you were the only occupational therapist in a small rural hospital, where could you find information pertaining to the treatment of the patient with cardiac or pulmonary disease?

ACKNOWLEDGMENT

Thanks to Stacey Larson, MA, OTR/L, staff therapist from Fairview Southdale Hospital in Edina, Minnesota, for submitting the case study on COPD.

References

Ainsworth, B., Haskell, W., Leon, A., Jacobs D. Jr., Montoye, H., Sallis, J., & Paffenbarger R. Jr. (1998). Compendium of physical activities: Classification of energy costs of human physical activities. In J. Roitman (Ed.), *ACSM's resource manual for exercise testing and prescription* (pp. 657–665). Baltimore: Williams & Wilkins.

American Association of Cardiovascular and Pulmonary Rehabilitation [AACVPR]. (2004a). *Guidelines for cardiac rehabilitation programs and secondary prevention programs*. Champaign, IL: Human Kinetics.

American Association of Cardiovascular and Pulmonary Rehabilitation [AACVPR]. (2004b). *Guidelines for pulmonary rehabilitation programs*. Champaign, IL: Human Kinetics.

American College of Sports Medicine. (2000). *ACSM's guidelines for exercise testing and prescription*. Philadelphia: Lippincott, Williams & Wilkins.

American Heart Association. (1998). *Heart and stroke statistical update*. Dallas: American Heart Association.

American Heart Association. (2005). *Heart and stroke statistics–2005 update*. Dallas: American Heart Association.

American Lung Association. (2004). Chronic pulmonary disease (COPD) fact sheet. Retrieved September 1, 2005 from http://www.lungusa.org

Antman, E. (2005). ST elevation myocardial infarction management. In D. Zipes, P. Libby, R. Bonow, & E. Braunwald (Eds.), *Braunwald's heart disease* (pp. 1167–1226). Philadelphia: Elsevier Saunders.

Antman, E., & Braunwald, E. (2005). ST elevation, myocardial infarction, pathology, pathophysiology and clinical features. In D. Zipes, P. Libby, R. Bonow, & E. Braunwald, (Eds.), *Braunwald's heart disease* (pp. 1141–1165). Philadelphia: Elsevier Saunders.

Baim, D. (2005). Percutaneous coronary revascularization. In D. Kasper, A. Fauci, D. Longo, E. Braunwald, S. Huser, & J. L. Stephen (Eds.), *Harrison's principles of internal medicine* (pp. 1454–1462). New York: McGraw Hill.

Barasch, E. (2000). Echocardiography. In J. Willerson & J. Cohn (Eds.), *Cardiovascular medicine* (pp. 76–98). Philadelphia: Churchill Livingston.

Cannon, C., & Braunwald, E. (2005). Unstable angina and non ST elevation MI. In D. Zipes, P. Libby, R. Bonow, & E. Braunwald (Eds.), *Braunwald's heart disease* (pp. 1243–1279). Philadelphia: Elsevier Saunders.

Coppola, S., & Wood, W. (2000). Occupational therapy to promote function and health related quality of life. In J. Hodgkin, R. C. Bartholome, & G. Connors (Eds.), *Pulmonary rehabilitation: Guidelines to success* (pp. 213–245). Philadelphia: Lippincott.

Couch, R., & Ryan, K. (2000). Physical therapy and respiratory care: Integration as a team in pulmonary rehabilitation. In J. Hodgkin, R. C. Bartholome, & G. Connors (Eds.), *Pulmonary rehabilitation: Guidelines to success* (pp. 173–211). Philadelphia: Lippincott.

DeBusk, R. (2003). Sexual activity in patients with angina. *Journal of the American Medical Association, 290,* 3129–3132.

Etkin, S., Lenker, D., & Mills, J. (2005). *Professional guide to diseases*. Philadelphia: Lippincott.

Fisher, N., & Williams, G. (2005). Hypertensive vascular disease. In D. Kasper, A. Fauci, D. Longo, E. Braunwald, S. Hauser, & J. L. Jameson (Eds.), *Harrison's principles of internal medicine* (pp. 1463–1481). New York: McGraw Hill.

Foody, J., & Pordon, C. (2001) Women and cardiovascular disease. In J. Foody (Ed.), *Preventive cardiology strategies for prevention and treatment of cardiovascular disease* (pp. 193–219). Totowa, NJ: Humana Press.

Franklin, B. (2003). Myocardial infarction. In L. Durstine & G. Moore (Eds.), *ACSM's exercise management for persons with chronic diseases and disability* (pp. 24–31). Champaign, IL: Human Kinetics.

Gaziano, J. M., Monson, J., & Redker, P. (2005). Primary and secondary prevention of coronary heart disease. In D. Zipes, P. Libby, R. Bonow, & E. Braunwald (Eds.), *Braunwald's heart disease* (pp. 1057–1084). Philadelphia: Elsevier Saunders.

Gersh, B. (Ed.) (2000). *Mayo Clinic heart book*. New York: William Morrow and Company.

Huntley, N. (1998). Reading the signs of heart disease. *OT Practice, 3,* 38–41.

Jackson, C. T., & Horn, S. (1998). *Practical manual of physical medicine and rehabilitation.* St. Louis: Mosby.

Jairath, N. (1999). *Coronary heart disease and risk factor management.* Philadelphia: Saunders.

Johnston, M., Foulkes, J., Johnston, D., Pollard, B., & Gudmundsdottir, H. (1999). Impact on patients and partners of inpatient and extended cardiac counseling and rehabilitation: A controlled trial. *Psychosomatic Medicine, 61,* 225–233.

Kim, M., Kine, A., & Fuster, V. (2004). Definitions of coronary syndromes. In V. Fuster, R. W. Alexander, R. O'Rourke, R. Robert, S. King, I. Nash, & E. Prystowsky, E. (Eds.), *Hurst's the heart* (pp. 1215–1222). New York: McGraw Hill.

Libby, P. (2005). Prevention and treatment of atherosclerosis. In D. Kasper, A. Fauci, D. Longo, E. Braunwald, S. Hauser, & J. L. Jameson (Eds.), *Harrison's principles of internal medicine* (pp. 1430–1433). New York: McGraw Hill.

Lowe, R., Menown, I., Nogareda, G., & Penn, I. (2005). Coronary stents: In these days of climate change, should all stents wear coats? *British Heart Journal, 91, (Suppl. III),* iii20.

Maltas, J. (2003). Cardiac disorders. In A. Linton & N. Maebus (Eds.), *Introduction to Medical surgical nursing* (pp. 555–607). Philadelphia: Saunders.

Maron, D., Grundy, S., Ridker, P., & Pearson, T. (2004). Dyslipidemia, other risk factors, and the prevention of coronary heart disease. In V. Fuster, R. W. Alexander, R. O'Rourke, R. Robert, S. King, I. Nash, & E. Prystowsky, E. (Eds.), *Hurst's the heart* (pp. 1093–1122). New York: McGraw Hill.

McArdle, W., Katch, F., & Katch, V. (2001). *Exercise physiology: Energy, nutrition and human performance.* Philadelphia: Lippincott, Williams & Wilkins.

MedicineNet. (2005). Chronic obstructive pulmonary disease (COPD). Retrieved on October 4, 2005 from http://www.medicinenet.com/chronic_obstructive_pulmonary_disease_copd/page3.htm.

Meyers, J. (2005) Exercise and activity. In S. Woods, E. Froelicher, S. Mozer, & E. Bridges (Eds.), *Cardiac nursing* (pp. 916–936). Philadelphia: Lippincott, Williams & Wilkins.

Mokdad, A., Ford, E., Bowman, B., Dietz, W., Vinicor, F., Bales, V., & Marks, J. (2001). Prevalence of obesity, diabetes, and obesity-related health risk factors, 2001. *Journal of the American Medical Association, 289,* 76–79.

Musselman, D. (2004). Effects of mood and anxiety disorders on the cardiovascular system. In V. Fuster, R. W. Alexander, R. O'Rourke, R. Robert, S. King, I. Nash, & E. Prystowsky, E. (Eds.), *Hurst's the heart* (p. 2189). New York: McGraw Hill.

O'Dell-Rossi, P., Browning, G., Barry, J., & Sahgal, V. (1999). Occupational therapy in pulmonary rehabilitation. In N. Cherniack, M. Altose, & I. Homma (Eds.), *Rehabilitation of the patient with respiratory disease* (pp. 679–681). New York: McGraw-Hill.

Paganda, K., & Paganda, T. (2001). *Mosby's diagnostic laboratory and test reference.* St. Louis: Mosby.

Powers, A. (2005). Diabetes mellitus. In D. Kasper, A. Fauci, D. Longo, E. Braunwald, S. Hauser, & J. L. Jameson (Eds.), *Harrison's principles of internal medicine* (pp. 2152–2180). New York: McGraw Hill.

Rayman, S. (2004). Health assessment. In R. Daniels (Ed.), *Nursing fundamentals: Caring and clinical decision making* (pp. 546–650). Victoria, Australia: Delmar Learning.

Ricker, P., & Libby, P. (2005). Risk factors for atherothrombotic disease. In D. Zipes, P. Libby, R. Bonow, & E. Braunwald (Eds.), *Braunwald's heart disease* (pp. 939–958). Philadelphia: Elsevier Saunders.

Salman, G., Mosier, M., Beasley, B., & Calkins, D. (2003). Rehabilitation for patients with chronic obstructive pulmonary disease: Meta-analysis of randomized controlled trials. *Journal of General Internal Medicine, 18,* 213–221.

Taylor, R., Brown, A., Ebrahim, S., Jolliffe, J., Moorani, H., Rees, K., Skidmore, B., Stone, J., Thompson, D., & Oldridge, N. (2004). Exercised-based rehabilitation for patients with coronary heart disease: Systemic review and meta-analysis of randomized controlled trials. *American Journal of Medicine, 116,* 682–692.

Wallace, J. (2003). Obesity. In G. Moore & J. L. Durstine (Eds.), *ACSM's exercise management for persons with chronic disabilities* (pp. 149–156). Champaign, IL: Human Kinetics.

Webb, G., Smallhorn, J., Tirrien, J., & Reddington, A. (2005). Congenital heart disease. In D. Zipes, P. Libby, R. Bonow, & E. Braunwald (Eds.), *Braunwald's heart disease* (pp. 1489–1552). Philadelphia: Elsevier Saunders.

White, R., Rudkin, S., Harrison, S., Day, K., & Harvey, I. (2002). Pulmonary rehabilitation compared with brief advice given for severe chronic obstructive pulmonary disease. *Journal of Cardiopulmonary Rehabilitation, 22,* 338–344.

Wynne, J., & Braunwald, E. (2005). The cardiomyopathies. In D. Zipes, P. Libby, R. Bonow, & E. Braunwald (Eds.), *Braunwald's heart disease* (pp. 1659–1696). Philadelphia: Elsevier Saunders.

Yakubov, S., & Bope, E. (2002). Cardiovascular disease. In R. Rakel (Ed.), *Textbook of family practice* (pp. 752–787). Philadelphia: W.B. Saunders.

Supplemental Reference

Gordon, N. F. (2003). Hypertension. In L. Durstine & G. Moore (Eds.), *ACSM's exercise management for persons with chronic diseases and disabilities* (pp. 76–80). Champaign, IL: Human Kinetics.

LEARNING OBJECTIVES

After studying this chapter, the reader will be able to do the following:

1. Discuss normal swallowing.
2. Identify types of dysphagia and their presentation.
3. Describe how to perform a clinical dysphagia assessment.
4. Employ basic compensatory and rehabilitative strategies to treat dysphagia.
5. Describe instrumental evaluation procedures for dysphagia.

CHAPTER 48

Dysphagia

Wendy Avery

Glossary

Aspiration—Entrance of food or secretions into the larynx below the level of the vocal cords.

Bolus—Food or liquid in the mouth.

Deglutition—The act of swallowing.

Direct therapy—Therapeutic techniques involving ingestion of food or liquids.

Dysphagia—Difficulty with any stage of swallowing.

Eating—Ingestion of food and liquid, including the pre-oral, oral preparatory, oral, pharyngeal, and esophageal stages.

Feeding—Taking or giving nourishment.

Fiberoptic endoscopic evaluation of swallowing (FEES)—Direct visualization of the swallow using a small illuminated camera at the end of a flexible tube (endoscope), which is introduced into the pharynx through the nose

Indirect therapy—Therapy addressing the prerequisite capacities associated with swallowing without ingestion of food or liquid.

Instrumental evaluation—Use of technology to assess aspects of swallowing.

Laryngeal penetration—Entrance of food or secretions into the larynx above the level of the vocal cords.

NPO (nil per os)—Latin for "nothing by mouth": no food or medication to be administered orally.

Swallowing—Ingestion of nourishment, beginning with introduction of food into the mouth and ending with reception of food into the stomach; includes the pre-oral, oral preparatory, oral, pharyngeal, and esophageal stages.

Videofluoroscopy—Moving radiographic images of swallowing structure and physiology, also known as "modified barium swallow study," recorded on videotape or DVD.

Dysphagia, or difficulty with any stage of **swallowing**, interferes with functional independence for many recipients of occupational therapy services; 33% of acute-care hospital inpatients (Groher & Bukatman, 1986), 32% of rehabilitation hospital inpatients (Cherney, 1994), and 59% of nursing home residents (Siebens, Trupe, & Siebens, 1986) may be dysphagic. Dysphagia care is a rapidly evolving science. Safe swallowing is a critical and life-supporting activity of daily living that is addressed by occupational therapists in many environments, including acute-care and psychiatric hospitals, rehabilitation centers, outpatient clinics, nursing homes, and schools.

Occupational therapists assist patients with dysphagia in rehabilitation of abilities that affect swallowing, including self-feeding, cognition, perception, sensory and motor skills, and postural control. Patients with acute, chronic, congenital, and acquired dysphagias may all benefit from intervention. In some settings, occupational therapists serve as the primary swallowing therapist (Avery-Smith, 1998); in other settings, speech and language pathologists serve as the primary swallowing therapist. Dysphagia care may be provided by a multidisciplinary dysphagia team.

This chapter introduces the entry-level skills required for the evaluation and treatment of dysphagia in adults. Independent intervention with the dysphagic patient requires advanced knowledge and skills on the part of the occupational therapy clinician. The American Occupational Therapy Association (2000) delineates entry-level and advanced-level skills in dysphagia care for occupational therapists and assistants. Further information about dysphagia can be acquired by seeking basic and advanced learning opportunities, researching new developments, attending workshops and conferences, and receiving mentoring.

NORMAL SWALLOWING

Deglutition is a complex process involving both volitional and non-volitional behaviors. The cranial nerves execute the sensory and motor processes that constitute swallowing. Cortically mediated factors, including appetite, attitude, attention span, appreciation of food, and body position, influence swallowing and must be considered in evaluation and treatment. Oral, pharyngeal, and esophageal structures involved in swallowing are shown in Figure 48-1.

The stages of swallowing include the pre-oral, oral preparatory, oral, pharyngeal, and esophageal stages (Definition 48-1). The pre-oral, oral preparatory, and oral stages are voluntary. The length of the oral preparatory stage varies considerably with the type of **bolus** (Hiiemae et al., 1996) and age (Logemann, 1998). Oral transit time, the length of time to accomplish the oral stage, is normally 1–1.5 seconds (Tracy et al., 1989). The pharyngeal stage is involuntary, although volitional movements can alter it. Normal pharyngeal transit time is 1 second (Tracy et al., 1989). Although the patient's position may affect the esophageal stage because of the effects of gravity, this stage is involuntary.

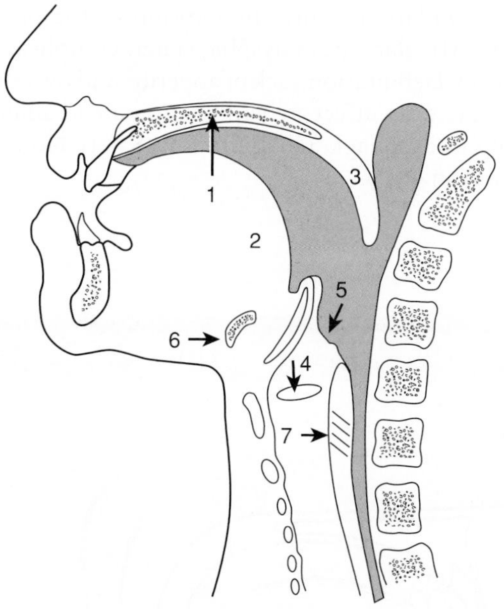

Figure 48-1 The oral, pharyngeal, and esophageal structures involved in swallowing. 1. The hard palate. 2. The base of the tongue. 3. The soft palate and uvula. 4. The vocal cords. 5. The laryngeal vestibule. 6. The hyoid bone. 7. The upper esophageal sphincter. (Adapted with permission from Groher, M. E. [1997]. *Dysphagia: Diagnosis and management* [3rd ed.]. Boston: Butterworth-Heinemann.)

IMPAIRED SWALLOWING

Many disease processes cause dysphagia, including those that affect the central nervous system, peripheral nervous system, motor end plate, muscles, and other anatomical structures. Trauma may affect anatomy and physiology, resulting in dysphagia. Dysphagia can lead to dehydration (Musson et al., 1990), malnutrition (Finestone et al., 1995), and pulmonary complications due to aspiration, including aspiration pneumonia (Schmidt et al., 1994), airway obstruction (Eckberg & Feinberg, 1992), adult respiratory distress syndrome (Garber et al., 1996), and death (Schmidt et al., 1994). The limited ability to participate in social and cultural activities because of chronic dysphagia can profoundly affect an individual.

Types of Dysphagia

Dysphagia occurs in three types: paralytic, pseudobulbar, and mechanical. Paralytic dysphagia results from lower motor neuron involvement that causes weakness and sensory impairment of oral and pharyngeal structures, including weakness or absence of the swallowing reflex. Pseudobulbar dysphagia results from upper motor neuron

DEFINITION 48-1

The Stages of Swallowing

Pre-Oral Stage

The food is visually and olfactorily appreciated. This stimulates salivation, and there are preparatory movements of the mouth to ready the oral cavity to receive and mobilize the food or liquid. Spontaneous upper extremity movements occur as the person reaches for and grasps the utensil, cup, or finger food and brings it to the mouth.

Oral Preparatory Stage

The food is received and contained by the mouth. It is then formed into a bolus of food and mixed with saliva. Pureed or liquid boluses require little mastication and may briefly be held centrally in the mouth by the tongue and cheek musculature. If solid, the food may need to be bitten off to be contained in the mouth. The bolus is chewed in a rotary motion by the molars and is moved between the left and right molars. The buccal muscles contract to prevent food from pocketing between the cheeks and the teeth. Once masticated or formed, the bolus is brought to the center of the tongue.

Oral Stage

As the cheek and tongue muscles retain the bolus centrally in the mouth, the tongue squeezes it against the hard palate, moving it posteriorly to the level of the faucial arches.

Pharyngeal Stage

The soft palate elevates to close off the nasopharynx. The larynx and hyoid elevate and protract, minimizing the size of the laryngeal vestibule (its opening) as the epiglottis tips to cover the vestibule. Breathing stops (termed "swallowing apnea"), which reduces the possibility of **aspiration** or laryngeal penetration of food or liquid. The vocal cords close. Simultaneously, the pharyngeal constrictor muscles sequentially contract to propel the bolus through the pharynx. The elevation of the larynx causes the upper esophageal sphincter (UES) to relax, allowing the bolus to pass through it.

Esophageal Stage

The UES returns to its normal tonic state, and the bolus is transported through the esophagus via esophageal peristalsis and gravity. The lower esophageal sphincter relaxes, allowing the bolus to pass through into the stomach.

involvement, causing hypotonicity or hypertonicity of oral and pharyngeal structures and a slow or poorly coordinated swallowing reflex. Paralytic and pseudobulbar dysphagia are neurological dysphagias. Mechanical dysphagia is caused by loss of oral, pharyngeal, or esophageal structures; weakness; and/or sensory deficits due to trauma or surgery. Secondary disorders in addition to the primary cause of a particular type of dysphagia may complicate the presentation. Debilitation, lack of appetite, and overall nutritional status can affect a client's stamina and ability to participate in dysphagia rehabilitation (Safety Note 48-1 and Definition 48-2).

SAFETY NOTE 48-1

Pulmonary Concerns

Respiratory problems may contribute to dysphagia and vice versa because the respiratory and swallowing mechanisms share anatomy and physiology,

Secretion Management

The patient's airway must be clear of excessive secretions. Intermittent suctioning through the nose or tracheostomy may be needed to clear the airway. The swallowing therapist should work closely with nursing and respiratory staff to assess whether airway protection and the ability to maintain oxygenation are adequate. Personnel should be available to suction the airway as necessary.

Tracheostomy

A tracheostomy tube reroutes breathing through a stoma in the neck. Tracheostomy tubes may be temporary or permanent and are used to keep the airway open (Fig. 48-2). Tracheostomies provide easy access for suctioning or ventilator use but can cause or exacerbate dysphagia. They cause reduced smell and taste sensation because the patient is not breathing through the nose. Tracheostomy reduces the ability to clear the upper airway if laryngeal penetration occurs. It increases the risk of aspiration due to pooling in the pharynx, delays trigger of the swallow reflex (Devita & Spierer-Rundback, 1990), decreases duration of vocal cord closure (Shaker et al., 1995), and reduces laryngeal movement. An "open" tracheostomy in which the tube is not covered or "capped" eliminates the subglottic pressure, reducing the force of the swallow response (Gross, Mahlmann, & Grayhack, 2003).

Mechanical Ventilators

Ventilators are machines that assist patients to breathe if they cannot do so on their own. Positive pressure ventilators may be used temporarily, to assist a patient through an acute illness, or chronically, for a patient with a long-term respiratory deficit. Positive pressure ventilators deliver breaths to patients through a tube in the nose or mouth or through a tracheostomy. Patients who use a ventilator to breathe via a tracheostomy may be able to eat by mouth. Breathing and swallowing alternate (Logemann, 1998). A well-coordinated swallow is needed to interpose the swallow between inhalation and exhalation. Patients who have had mechanical ventilation for more than a week have been shown to have multiple swallowing deficits once the ventilator is removed (Tolep, Getch, & Criner, 1996). Patients who are ventilator dependent via tracheostomy are prone to aspiration during eating (Elpern et al., 1994).

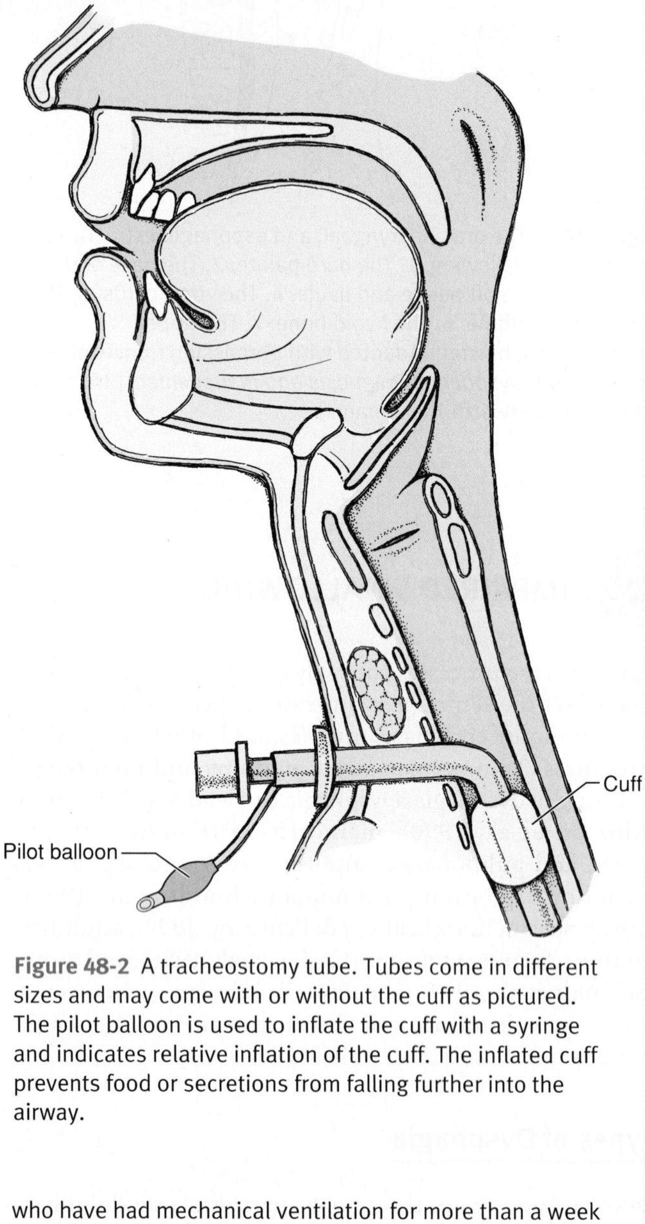

Figure 48-2 A tracheostomy tube. Tubes come in different sizes and may come with or without the cuff as pictured. The pilot balloon is used to inflate the cuff with a syringe and indicates relative inflation of the cuff. The inflated cuff prevents food or secretions from falling further into the airway.

DEFINITION 48-2

de·fin·i·tion

Clinical Dysphagia Presentation for Various Diagnostic Groups

Alzheimer's Disease: Pseudobulbar Dysphagia

- Decreased attention span and apraxia for swallowing and self-feeding may be seen.
- Oral and pharyngeal responses slow and a need for physical and verbal cues to self-feed are needed (Priefer & Robbins, 1997).
- Difficulty with self-feeding is common.
- Clients prefer sweet flavored and pureed foods.
- Clients are prone to aspiration in later stages of the disease (Horner et al., 1994).

Brain Injury: Pseudobulbar, Paralytic Dysphagia

- Type and severity of dysphagia in brain injury depends on the cause of the injury and location and size of brain lesions.
- Behavioral and cognitive problems affect self-feeding and swallowing.
- Abnormal pathological reflexes can affect oral and pharyngeal control (Logemann, Pepe, & Mackay, 1994).
- Increased or reduced muscle tone may cause decreased mouth opening, decreased lip closure, drooling, decreased tongue control, and pocketing of the bolus in the cheek (Logemann, Pepe, & Mackay, 1994; Mackay, Morgan, & Bernstein, 1999).
- Delayed pharyngeal swallow trigger, nasal regurgitation, decreased base of tongue movement, and decreased laryngeal elevation with resulting pharyngeal residue may be seen (Logemann, Pepe, & Mackay, 1994).
- Overall mealtime may be slow (Mackay, Morgan, & Bernstein, 1999).

Cerebrovascular Accident: Pseudobulbar and Paralytic

- Pharyngeal and laryngeal sensory deficits may occur in right and left hemispheric as well as subcortical strokes (Aviv et al., 1996).
- Symptoms vary with lesion location and size.
- Patients with right hemispheric stroke (pseudobulbar dysphagia) display mild oral transit delays and some delay in pharyngeal trigger and laryngeal elevation (Lazarus, 1995). The pharyngeal stage lasts longer, and there may be penetration of the larynx and aspiration (Robbins et al., 1993). There may be neglect or denial of swallowing problems.
- Patients with left hemispheric stroke (pseudobulbar dysphagia) display delays in initiating the oral stage and in triggering the pharyngeal stage (Lazarus, 1995). The pharyngeal stage takes longer (Robbins et al., 1993). There may be apraxia for eating and swallowing.
- Patients with subcortical stroke (paralytic dysphagia) demonstrate mild oral transit delays and a delay in triggering the swallow. There is general weakness of pharyngeal swallow, as seen in reduced laryngeal elevation, reduced tongue base retraction, and unilateral pharyngeal weakness (Horner et al., 1991; Robbins et al., 1993). There may also be reduced upper esophageal sphincter (UES) opening (Horner et al., 1991).

Developmental Disabilities: Pseudobulbar, Paralytic Dysphagia

- Cerebral palsy (CP) and mental retardation, together or in isolation, may present deficits of bolus formation and transit, delayed swallow reflex, pharyngeal dysmotility, esophageal disease, and aspiration (Rogers et al., 1994).
- Abnormal oral reflexes, oral hyposensitivity or hypersensitivity, pharyngeal stage delay, decreased laryngeal elevation, and aspiration may be observed (Logemann, 1998).
- Poor postural, head, neck, and limb control can affect swallowing.

Head and Neck Cancer: Mechanical Dysphagia

- Swallowing problems with head and neck cancer vary with tumor type, size, and location.
- Bolus control and containment problems result from surgery to the lip (McConnel & O'Connor, 1994).
- Resection of tumor from the floor of the mouth causes difficulty with bolus control, reduced laryngeal elevation, and its accompanying reduction in UES opening (McConnel & O'Connor, 1994).
- Glossectomy, or removal of some or all of the tongue, causes difficult or absent bolus mobilization; a resection of the tongue base limits the elevation needed to initiate the pharyngeal swallow (McConnel & O'Connor, 1994).
- Unilateral laryngeal cancer may require a vertical laryngectomy or hemilaryngectomy; this may cause reduced vocal cord closure, reduced posterior tongue movement, and reduced UES opening (McConnel & O'Connor, 1994).
- Supraglottic laryngectomy reduces glottic closure, laryngeal elevation, and opening of the UES (McConnel & O'Connor, 1994).
- Extensive cancer of the larynx necessitates a total laryngectomy, which separates the foodway and airway tracts and creates a permanent anatomical tracheostomy. Although aspiration is no longer a threat, there is no laryngeal elevation, hence there is a reduced movement and force of the UES (McConnel & O'Connor, 1994).

(continued)

DEFINITION 48-2 *(continued)*

- Adjunctive radiation therapy causes edema in areas adjacent to the radiation field, fibrosis, and reduced salivary flow, causing dry mouth or xerostomia.
- Radiation therapy combined with chemotherapy without surgery can reduce tongue base movement, laryngeal elevation, and pharyngeal range of motion and speed (Lazarus et al., 1996).
- Radiation therapy combined with surgery can cause longer oral transit time, increased pharyngeal residue, and reduced UES opening (Pauloski et al., 1998).

Multiple Sclerosis: Pseudobulbar, Paralytic Dysphagia

- Dysphagia symptoms vary with location of plaques in the central and peripheral nervous systems.
- Weakness of the oral structures and the neck muscles may be seen (Thomas & Wiles, 1999).
- Delayed pharyngeal swallow and weakness of pharyngeal contractions may be seen (Logemann, 1998).

Neoplasms of the Brain: Pseudobulbar, Paralytic Dysphagia

- Dysphagia may be due either to a tumor or to metastasis in the brain or to medical or surgical interventions (Newton et al., 1994).
- Symptoms vary with the location and extent of the client's neoplasm and interventions, and symptoms may be similar to those found in clients with stroke (Wesling et al., 2003).

Parkinson's Disease: Pseudobulbar Dysphagia

- Impulsiveness and poor judgment can affect swallowing (Leopold & Kagel, 1996).
- Jaw rigidity, abnormal head and neck posture, impaired coordination of tongue movements and mastication, and difficulty with coordination of upper extremity movements for self-feeding are seen (Leopold & Kagel, 1996).
- **Feeding** and swallowing may be too slow and laborious to allow sufficient nutritional intake.
- There may be oral residue, poor oral bolus manipulation, residue in the pharynx, delayed laryngeal elevation, and delayed oral and pharyngeal transit times (Nagaya et al., 1998).
- Impaired pharyngeal motility and aspiration may be seen (Leopold & Kagel, 1997).

Psychiatric Disorders: Pseudobulbar Dysphagia

- Tardive dyskinesia caused by long-term use of neuroleptic agents causes dystonia of the tongue and larynx and hyperkinesis of the face, jaw, tongue, and UES (Groher, 1997; Sokoloff & Pavlakovic, 1997).
- There can be choking due to eating too quickly (Fioretti, Giacotto, & Melega, 1997).

DYSPHAGIA ASSESSMENT

A dysphagia assessment involves two components, a clinical assessment and an **instrumental evaluation**.

Clinical Assessment

Clinical assessment of dysphagia must be thorough, with examination of all areas relevant to swallowing. It is best done using a reliable and valid tool (Avery-Smith, Rosen, & Dellarosa, 1997). A reliable and valid tool allows for accurate assessment and reassessment by different test administrators and ensures that each test item provides accurate assessment of performance components. Figure 48-3 illustrates the use of a chartable form to document evaluation results.

History, Nutrition, and Respiratory Considerations

The clinician reviews the patient's medical and surgical history, with special attention to any diagnoses and procedures that are relevant to dysphagia. The patient and caregiver also provide information about any history of swallowing disorders. Specific signs and symptoms and modifications in behaviors relevant to mealtime are noted, as are changes in food intake and weight loss. The current nutritional sources are recorded, including the length of time the patient has been **NPO**, or not eating by mouth, if applicable. The therapist also documents any cultural and religious dietary preferences and practices. Information regarding respiratory status is gathered from the hospital chart and staff, especially any tracheostomy and/or mechanical ventilation and the level of independence with secretion management.

Assessment of Cognitive, Perceptual, and Physical Abilities

Important cognitive and perceptual considerations include the level of alertness and arousal, orientation, ability to attend to a feeding session or meal, ability to follow multistep commands, and any visual deficits or neglect. The clinician notes the patient's insight into his or her dysphagia and observes head, neck, trunk, and limb control and endurance for being out of bed at mealtimes. The ability to self-position and self-feed and need for or use of adaptive eating equipment are assessed.

DYSPHAGIA
Evaluation Protocol
RECORD FORM

Client name: Doe, John DOB: 1/1/20 Age: 80 Date: 1/1/00
Physician: Dr. Physician Location: bedside Type of service: Neuro
Type of eval ☑ Initial ☐ Re-eval Assistive or postural devices used: Wheelchair
Diagnosis: Ⓛ CVA, Ⓡ heme Date of onset: 12/25/99 Reason for referral: S/S dysphagia
Last oral feeding: breakfast Clinician/Title: Wendy Avery-Smith, OTR

HISTORY AND OBSERVATIONS

Feeding History

Normal preexisting function? ☑ No ☐ Yes
When did change occur? Describe change. Coughing with all textures, p̄ CVA
Has consistency of food changed? ☐ No ☑ Yes
When, and how did client compensate? MD ordered Level I Aspiration Prevention Diet
Has food intake changed? ☐ No ☑ Yes
When, and how? Reduced, p̄ CVA
Weight loss? ☑ No ☐ Yes
Number of lbs: ______ When? ______
Other changes: ______

Nutritional Status

Nutritional Route:
☐ NPO ☑ PO
Alternative feeding method used:
☐ NGT ☐ PEG ☐ TPN ☑ Other: IV for fluids
Current diet:
☐ Regular ☑ Other: Level I, Aspiration Prevention
Special dietary requirements:
☐ No concentrated sweets ☐ Low salt ☐ Kosher
☐ Other: none

Respiratory Status

Auscultation of pooling? ☑ No ☐ Yes
Suctioning required? ☑ No ☐ Yes
Frequency: ______ Route: ______
Tracheostomy? ☑ No ☐ Yes
Type: ☐ Cuffed ☐ Cuffless
☐ Fenestrated Size: ______
Position of cuff:
☐ Fully inflated ☐ Partially inflated ☐ Deflated
Comments: ______

Ventilator? ☑ No ☐ Yes ☐ Cannot be removed
Weaning parameters: ______

Receiving chest physical therapy? ☑ No ☐ Yes
Type of treatment: ______
Comments: ______

General Status

Alertness:
☑ No deficit ☐ Partial deficit ☐ Moderate/Severe deficit
Follows directions:
☑ verbal ☐ gesture
☑ 3-step ☐ 2-step ☐ 1-step ☐ Unable
If client responds to fewer than 3-step directions, note reason for difficulty: ______

If the client has difficulty with two- or three-step directions, see Alternative Administration Protocol section of the manual for information about continuing the evaluation.

Recognizes swallowing problems:
☑ Good insight ☐ Partial insight ☐ No insight

Record the appropriate rating of this item after observing client's performance during the Feeding Trial portion of the evaluation.

Perceptual/Cognitive observations:
☑ No deficit ☐ Partial deficit ☐ Severe deficit
Comments: ______

Physical Status

Assistance needed to attain and maintain position:
☑ Independent ☐ Minimal/Moderate assistance
☐ Maximal assistance
Comments: ______

Head and neck control
Range of motion: ☐ Normal ☑ Impaired
Manual muscle testing ☐ Normal ☑ Impaired
☐ Nonfunctional for eating

If head and neck control is nonfunctional for eating, stop the evaluation and refer to the Manual for additional information.

Upper-extremity control for self-feeding: ☐ Normal ☑ Impaired
☐ Nonfunctional

Record rating for upper-extremity control during the feeding trial.

Comments: ↓ tone R side of neck; needs cues to keep head erect; decreased RUE tone for utencil manipulation.

1

Figure 48-3 A completed evaluation for the case example from the *Dysphagia Evaluation Protocol.* (Copyright 1997 by Harcourt Assessment, Inc. Reproduced with permission. All rights reserved.)

CLINICAL EVALUATION OF SWALLOWING

Observations

☐ Drooling	☐ Tongue or lip biting
☑ Excessive oral secretions	☐ Tongue thrust
☐ Dry mouth	☐ Oral-motor apraxia
☑ Poor oral hygiene	☐ Excessive coughing (more than twice)
☐ Residual food in the oral cavity	☐ Hoarse or wet voice
☐ Food remnants on the lips	☐ Frequent clearing of throat
☐ Dentures	☑ Other observations: *Dentition intact*

Oral Control

	Tone		ROM		Strength		Sensation		Comments
	Intact	Impaired	Intact	Impaired	Intact	Impaired	Intact	Impaired	
Lips		✓R		✓		✓	✓		
Cheeks		✓R		✓		✓	✓		
Jaw	✓		✓		✓		✓		
Tongue		✓R		✓		✓	✓		

Primitive and Abnormal Reflexes

Jaw jerk	☑ Absent	☐ Present
Rooting	☑ Absent	☐ Present
Sucking	☑ Absent	☐ Present
Bite	☑ Absent	☐ Present

Pharyngeal Control

	Normal	Impaired	Absent	Comments
Soft palate function		✓		
Gag reflex		✓		
Vocal quality			✓	*Unable to phonate 2° vocal cord weakness*
Volitional cough		✓		

2

Figure 48-3 *(continued)*

FEEDING TRIAL

Appetite/Willingness to Participate

- ☑ Positive
- ☐ Neutral
- ☐ Negative

Consistencies Used: (Description)

- ☑ Moist, cohesive Applesauce, pudding
- ☐ Soft, chewable
- ☐ Thick liquid
- ☐ Thin liquid
- ☐ Crunchy, chewable

Special Tools and Techniques: Hand over hand guiding to self-feed c̄ (R) hand, use (L) hand to maintain lip closure and massage (R) cheek to prevent pocketing of food in cheek

Ability to Swallow Without Food Bolus: ☐ Normal ☑ Impaired ☐ Absent

Oral Stage

	Normal	Impaired	Absent	Comments
Bolus containment in oral cavity		✓		
Bolus formation		✓		
Bolus propulsion		✓		
Mastication				Not tested

Pharyngeal Stage

Laryngeal elevation ☑ Normal ☐ Impaired ☐ Absent

Voice quality after swallow ☐ Normal ☐ Impaired ☑ Absent (was not present pre-swallow)

Auscultation:

Audibility of upper esophageal sphincter: ☐ No ☑ Yes

Pooling ☑ No ☐ Yes

Comments: Delay in trigger of pharyngeal swallow response.

Repetitive swallows ☐ No ☑ Yes Number of swallows: 1

Cough reflex ☑ No ☐ Yes

☐ Before swallow ☐ During swallow ☐ After swallow

Other Observations:

O_2 saturation level remained at 96 % before, during and immediately after feeding trial

During the feeding trial, record the patient's recognition of swallowing problems and upper extremity control for self-feeding.

Comments:

Pt is aware of inability to swallow fluids and chewable solids. He required hand over hand assistance to load spoon and bring to mouth. Able to hold a plastic cup with two hands, and bring to mouth.

Figure 48-3 *(continued)*

IMPRESSIONS

Summary

This 80 yo gentleman is s/p CVA c̄ Ⓡ hemiplegia and aphasia. He shows reduced oral tone and control in the Ⓡ tongue and cheek. He is managing soft, formed boluses with extra time for oral manipulation and a slowed swallow response. No pooling or coughing was noted after swallowing. There were no clinical signs of laryngeal penetration or aspiration.

Functional Level (Physical and verbal assistance needed for positioning, hand-to-mouth movements, and swallowing):

Pt was able to self-feed c̄ hand over hand guidance to use utensil, but was able to use cup Ⓘ c̄ 2 hands. He needed supervision to transfer to the wheelchair to eat and verbal cues to prepare his tray to eat.

Intermittent supervision at meals and snacks, as well as assistance to self-feed c̄ Ⓡ hand is recommended

Recommendations/Plan:

- ☐ NPO (No food by mouth)
- ☐ Nutrition consultation:
- ☑ Videofluoroscopy To assess laryngeal protection c̄ fluids.
- ☐ Prefeeding program
- ☑ Special positioning, Adaptive equipment: Seated to eat
- ☑ Mealtime supervision ☐ Constant ☑ Intermittent ☐ Set-up
- ☑ Diet recommendation: Continue c̄ Level I, Aspiration Prevention
- ☑ Other: Short term goals:
  1. Advance diet to Level II, including cooked fruit and pasta.
  2. Tolerate soft chewables without s/s aspiration
  3. Ⓘ use of techniques to maintain lip closure and prevent food pocketing
  4. Ⓘ vocal cord adduction exercises
  5. Modified Ⓘ self-feeding c̄ equipment and adapted tech.

Copyright © 1997 by

Therapy Skill Builders™
a division of
The Psychological Corporation
555 Academic Court
San Antonio, Texas 78204-2498
1-800-228-0752

0761644121
Printed in the U.S.A.
1 2 3 4 5 6 7 8 9 10 11 12 A B C D E

4

Figure 48-3 *(continued)*

Assessment of Oral and Pharyngeal Abilities

Once direct physical assessment begins, the clinician must observe universal precautions to prevent exposure to pathogens for both the clinician and the patient (Safety Note 48-2). The occupational therapist begins by assessing oral and pharyngeal control, including tone, range of motion, strength, and sensation of the lips, tongue, jaw, and cheeks and any abnormal oral reflexes. To assess pharyngeal control, the therapist observes soft palate movement, gag reflex, vocal quality, and volitional cough. A stethoscope may be used to listen for pooling of fluid above the level of the vocal cords, as pooled liquids resonate during breathing. The therapist rates the patient's hunger and level of enthusiasm for a snack or meal.

The Feeding Trial

Interventions that maximize performance can be initiated before the feeding trial begins (Procedures for Practice 48-1). The safest food textures are chosen for the trial. Easy-to-manage foods and thick fluids are attempted first, especially if the patient has been NPO and/or has a diagnosis or clinical picture that suggests a high risk of aspiration. During the oral stage, the clinician observes bolus containment, formation, propulsion, and mastication. During the pharyngeal stage, the clinician assesses laryngeal elevation, voice quality after swallow, repetitive swallows, and cough reflex. The therapist should observe for signs and symptoms of **laryngeal penetration** or aspiration, especially during the first feeding trial (Safety Note 48-2). The evaluation concludes with a summary, recommendations, and a plan (Avery-Smith, Rosen, & Dellarosa, 1992).

Specific techniques are helpful during the feeding trial. Auscultation of the swallow with a stethoscope (Fig. 48-5) can reveal the efficiency and safety of the oral and pharyngeal stages (Zenner, Losinski, & Mills, 1995). Gentle palpation of the neck (Fig. 48-6) during the swallow reveals symmetry, strength, and speed of oral pharyngeal movement and may be done simultaneous to auscultation. Use of a pulse oximeter, a non-invasive monitoring device that measures the patient's oxygen saturation in the bloodstream, may be effective in assessing whether aspiration or respiratory difficulties are occurring (Sherman et al., 1999). Normal oxygen saturation in the bloodstream falls in between 93 and 98%; a level below 92% after swallowing suggests aspiration. If the patient can self-feed, palpation and auscultation may be done simultaneously. If the patient needs help to self-feed, auscultation and guiding with hand-to-mouth efforts may be done simultaneously.

Recommendations and Plan

Once the clinical evaluation is complete, recommendations and a plan are formulated. As seen in Figure 48-4, recommendations may include: whether eating by mouth is

SAFETY NOTE 48-2

Precautions for the Therapist and Patient

The swallowing therapist stays close to the patient during eating and is exposed to oral secretions and respirations. Likewise, the patient is exposed to pathogens on the therapist's clothing and hands and in the therapist's respiratory tract. Universal (also called standard) precautions should be used. The use of gloves is mandatory anytime the therapist touches the face or inside the oral cavity.

Dysphagia patients are prone to difficulty with airway obstruction and aspiration during eating. For the safety of the patient, the swallowing therapist should be trained in suctioning of the airway, the Heimlich maneuver, and cardiopulmonary resuscitation.

Signs and Symptoms of Potential or Actual Aspiration

Although laryngeal penetration or aspiration may be silent, occurring without overt warning signs and symptoms, the following indicate that it may occur or be occurring. If observed during a dysphagia evaluation, these signs or symptoms can indicate that a feeding trial should not be initiated or should be discontinued. Specific items of concern are as follows (Avery-Smith, Rosen, & Dellarosa, 1997):

1. The patient cannot remain awake for the clinical evaluation.
2. The oral and/or pharyngeal sensation and motion assessment reveal poor ability to manipulate and contain the bolus.
3. The bolus remains in the mouth, and the patient cannot initiate or complete the oral preparatory stage within a reasonable time.
4. There is excessive coughing or choking before, during, or after swallowing.
5. There is no swallow response once the oral stage is completed.
6. There is a change in voice quality, often wet, or no voice after swallowing.
7. Severe pooling or wetness is heard on auscultation or by the naked ear; secretions are poorly managed.
8. Silent aspiration is suggested by a change in the patient's color and/or respiratory rate, increased congestion on auscultation of the chest, and/or a reduction in oxygen level in the blood as recorded by pulse oximetry.

PROCEDURES FOR PRACTICE 48-1

Preparation for Eating

Prior to the feeding trial portion of an evaluation and snacks or meals, measures must be taken to optimize the patient's swallowing performance. As these strategies do not involve ingestion of food, they are **indirect therapy** techniques.

- Provide a quiet environment to encourage concentration.
- Position the patient upright in a chair to minimize the risk of aspiration. The feet should be supported, and the arms should be free for self-feeding. Patients with pseudobulbar dysphagia may need special attention to positioning before eating and special positioning devices; they may need assistance to maintain head and neck alignment and facilitation to stimulate oral and pharyngeal motions prior to and during eating (Fig. 48-4).
- Complete oral hygiene activities before the trial because this stimulates sensation and range of motion in oral structures.
- Present a simplified visual array of food and utensils for the patient with visual neglect and/or other visual deficits. Anchors, colorful cues to call attention to the side of the plate, are helpful for patients with neglect.
- Present appetizing, culture-specific foods, utensils, and tableware.
- Provide adaptive equipment and/or use hand-over-hand guiding to facilitate self-feeding.
- Provide simple explanations and one-step verbal directions if necessary.
- If the patient eats too quickly or is confused by multiple food choices, present one food at a time.
- Use small-bowled utensils and verbal or manual assistance to load just a teaspoon-sized bolus. Pinch the straw to limit the amount of liquid consumed or use a covered cup with a small opening.

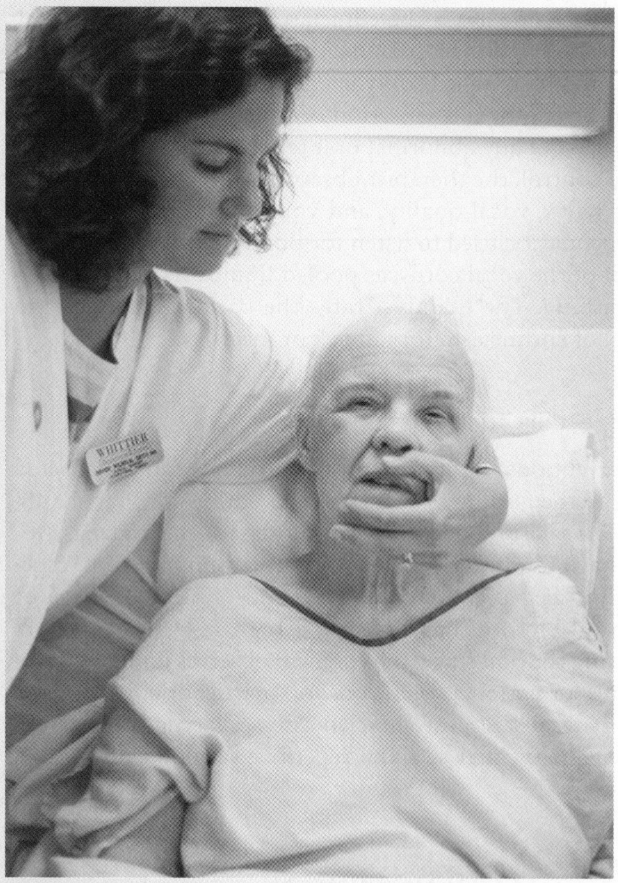

Figure 48-4 Using the half-nelson position to assist with head and neck control. The therapist can also assist with jaw, cheek, and lip control at the same time.

advisable; whether an instrumental evaluation is advised; whether a nutritional consultation with a dietitian is needed; recommended diet type; mealtime positioning and supervision; adaptive equipment; and type and amount of assistance. Evaluation of the patient is ongoing, and with additional information from clinical observations, instrumental evaluations, and input from other dysphagia team members, the treatment plan and goals change.

Instrumental Evaluation

Clinical assessment goes hand in hand with instrumental evaluation, which uses imaging and diagnostic studies to provide critical information about the unseen parts of the oral, pharyngeal, and esophageal stages of swallowing. Various types of instrumental evaluations for dysphagia are discussed in Definition 48-3. These evaluations are usually performed by physicians, often together with a swallowing therapist. Aspiration of food or fluid may be silent (Linden, Kuhlemeier, & Patterson, 1993). Imaging studies, such as **videofluoroscopy**, are needed to identify aspiration (Splaingard et al., 1988), but they may not identify aspiration in all instances, as client skills can vary, and the testing situation in the radiology suite may not approximate an actual eating situation very closely. However, these studies do provide important information about the quality of the swallow and the efficacy of compensatory therapy techniques used during swallowing.

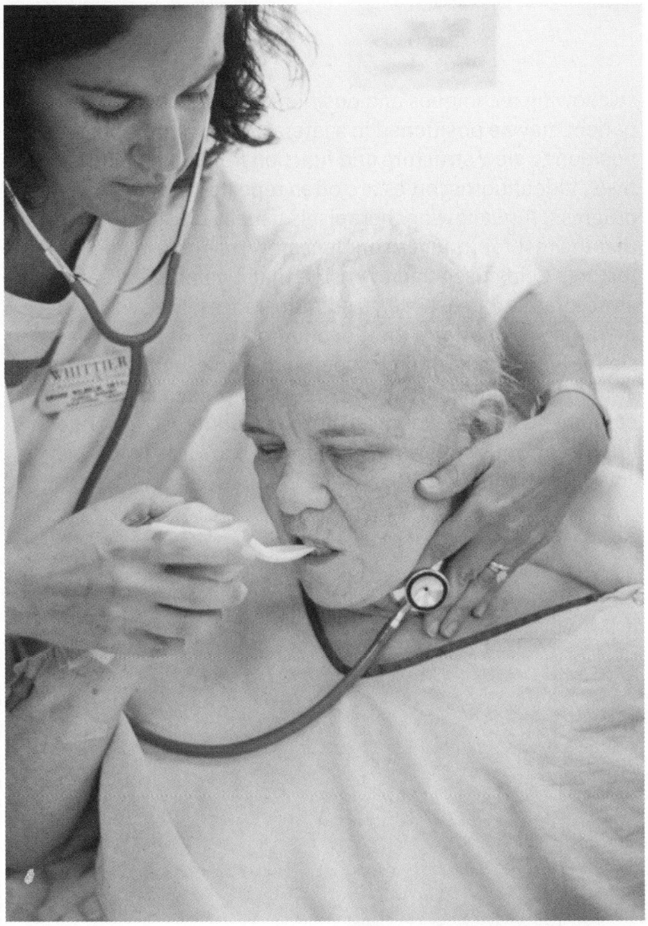

Figure 48-5 Auscultation of the swallow using a stethoscope. The therapist may be able to facilitate head position and guide self-feeding while listening to the sounds of the swallow.

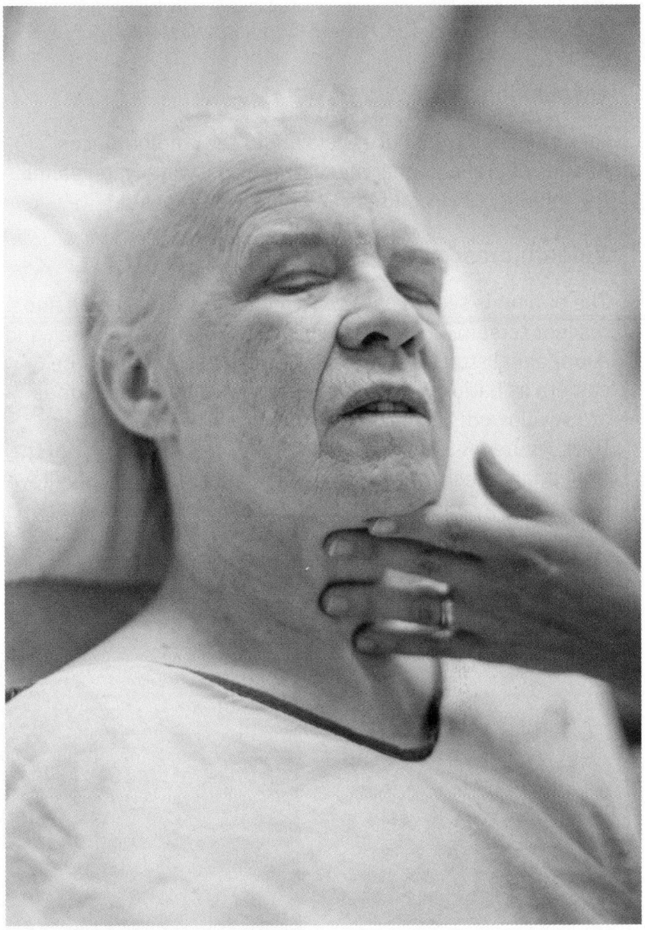

Figure 48-6 Palpation of the neck during swallowing. The first finger is under the chin; the second finger is at the base of the tongue; the third finger is over the thyroid cartilage; and the fourth finger is at the base of the throat. A very light touch should be used so as not to inhibit motion.

DEFINITION 48-3

de·fin·i·tion

Instrumental Evaluation of Swallowing

Instrumental evaluation uses technology, including the following.

Electromyography

Electrodes are placed either into the muscle via a small needle or on the skin over a muscle to record contractions of the muscle. Surface electrodes have been used to assess aspects of oral bolus management in neurological dysphagia patients and pharyngeal, laryngeal, and esophageal activity (Ertekin et al., 1998).

Fiberoptic Endoscopic Swallowing Study

A fiberoptic laryngoscope, a narrow flexible tube with a small camera on its tip, is introduced through the nose into the nasopharynx, where structures including the palate, pharynx, and larynx are viewed for assessment of anatomy and movement. Food is administered in different consistencies to observe posterior oral and pharyngeal function and airway protection during eating.

Manometry

A catheter with transducers to measure pressure is introduced into the esophagus. The force, timing, and sequence of the esophageal contractions are measured.

Scintigraphy

A radioactive isotope is mixed with food. As the bolus is swallowed, a gamma camera tracks the radioactive particles. This test measures the speed of bolus transit and can accurately measure the amount of bolus that is aspirated.

(continued)

DEFINITION 48-3 *(continued)*

Ultrasonography

An ultrasound transducer held under the chin produces images of oral and pharyngeal stages of swallow, revealing the mobility of structures and boluses swallowed.

Videofluoroscopy

The patient is seated between a movable camera and a fluorescent screen. Radiographic images of oral, pharyngeal, and esophageal structures are delivered to a screen from the camera as barium or barium-impregnated fluids and foods are swallowed. The images are recorded on videotape or DVD. Figure 48-7 illustrates a videofluoroscopic image of the oral, pharyngeal, and upper esophageal structures. Swallowing pathology and the effectiveness of compensatory swallowing techniques and positions can be observed. The patient may be positioned in a lateral and/or anteroposterior position to view structure and function from both perspectives. Videofluoroscopies are often repeated to assess progress. A swallowing therapist is usually present to ensure that the test reproduces compensatory maneuvers and food textures being used and to ensure that it mimics real eating as accurately as possible. In some instances, the swallowing therapist may perform the videofluoroscopy. Therapists assisting with or performing videofluoroscopies must be expert swallowing clinicians; they must be fully trained in use of the equipment and procedures used in videofluoroscopy. Videofluoroscopy of swallowing may also be known as "MBS" or "modified barium swallow."

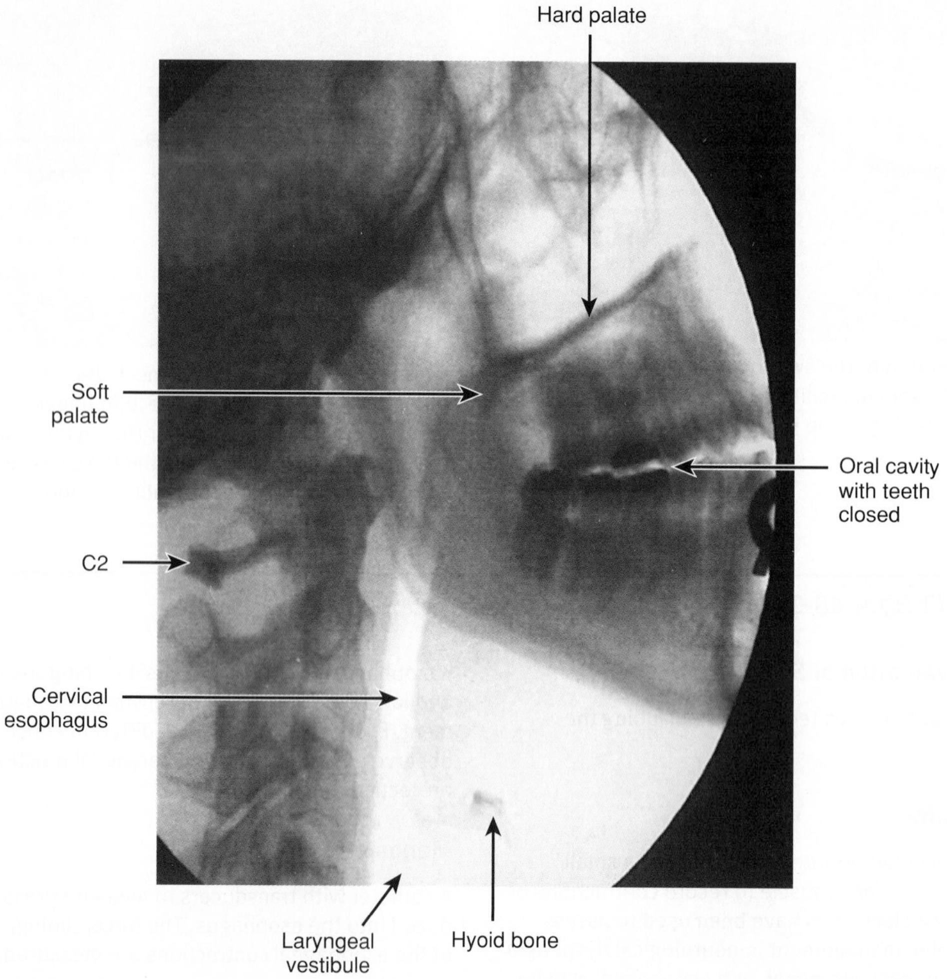

Figure 48-7 A videofluoroscopic image of the oral, pharyngeal, and esophageal structures. (Videoprint image courtesy of Bette Pomerleau, MS, SLP, and Ray Autiello, LPN, RT, of Universal Mobile Services, Haverhill, MA.)

DYSPHAGIA INTERVENTION

One consideration in treatment is remedial versus compensatory goals. Remedial treatment focuses on restoring a normal level of swallowing function. Potential for partial or full recovery is anticipated when goals are remedial. Compensatory treatment circumvents a problem with the use of alternative strategies and techniques. Use of these techniques implies either that full recovery is not anticipated or that these techniques are necessary for a safe, functional swallow prior to recovery of normal swallowing. Table 48-1 discusses compensatory and remedial interventions for specific swallowing deficits. Compensatory swallowing maneuvers and their indications are discussed in Definition 48-3. Goals may be remedial and then change to compensatory once a plateau in function is reached.

Another consideration is the type of therapeutic techniques used. **Indirect** therapy addresses the prerequisite abilities or the capacity to swallow without ingestion of food or liquid. Patients who are at high risk for aspiration often begin with indirect therapy only. Indirect therapy can include range of motion, strengthening, and coordination exercises for weak or hypotonic oral and pharyngeal musculature; strengthening of pharyngeal and laryngeal structures; techniques to reduce or stimulate sensitivity of oral musculature; and techniques to improve the pharyngeal swallowing response. Indirect therapy also involves manipulating the environment to optimize behaviors that affect swallowing (see Procedures for Practice 48-1).

Direct therapy rehabilitates prerequisite abilities or the capacity to swallow during therapeutic snacks or meals. This entails exercises and/or the use of compensatory swallowing maneuvers that include ingestion of food. Indirect therapy may continue once direct therapy has begun. An individualized treatment plan usually includes a selection of direct and indirect techniques. The complexity of a treatment plan depends on the ability of the patient and/or caregiver to process complex information. Treatment techniques, especially in the pharyngeal stage, where the effect of techniques are unseen, should be evaluated by videofluoroscopy or fiberoptic endoscopy to assess their efficacy. Although not discussed in depth here, for many patients, optimizing self-feeding skills is an important goal to address hand-in-hand with swallowing goals. Although not yet proven in the literature, the sensory inputs and motor patterns used for self-feeding are probably related to those used in the partly voluntary swallow, and facilitating both skills enhances each.

Progression of Diet with Swallowing Therapy

As indirect therapy begins, some patients may receive all nutrition, hydration, and medication via a non-oral source, such as intravenous or gastrostomy tube feedings. As the patient recovers the ability to swallow without laryngeal penetration or aspiration, direct therapy with the therapist present begins during snacks and progresses to meals. As improvement continues and the patient learns compensatory techniques, he or she may progress to eating under the supervision of nursing personnel and trained significant others and then progress to eating independently. Calorie counts are initiated by the dietitian to assess the adequacy of oral intake. Once food intake improves and calories are consistently sufficient, non-oral feeding sources may be used only for hydration and/or medication. Finally, as the patient improves and fluids and medications are safely ingested by mouth, the use of non-oral feeding sources can be discontinued. Diet textures are upgraded as skills develop. Depending on the diagnosis and potential for recovery, patients may level off at any point in the described progression (Procedures for Practice 48-2).

Dysphagia Diets

Dysphagia diets are designed to provide stepwise gradation of food and fluid textures that are matched to the patient's improving oral and pharyngeal skills. Groher (1987) found that a diet of mechanical soft foods that form a cohesive bolus and thickened fluids significantly reduced the incidence of aspiration in a group of patients with pseudobulbar dysphagia compared with pureed food and thin fluids. Specific textures and flavors can stimulate optimal oral and pharyngeal motion; for example, sour flavors may stimulate movement responses (Pelletier & Lawless, 2003). Patients may have strong preferences; those with dementias may prefer sweet flavors and reject foods that require chewing. Dysphagia diets for most patients follow this general progression:

1. Thick purees, such as pudding and applesauce
2. Very soft moist chewables, such as soft cooked vegetables, fruits, and soft pastas
3. Drier chewables, such as cookies and breads
4. Foods requiring biting, firmer chewables such as meats, and mixed textures like cereals and milk or pills and water.

The progression of fluids advances thus:

1. No fluids at all
2. Honey-thick fluids
3. Nectar-thick fluids
4. Thin, flavored fluids
5. Water

Fluids are easily thickened with commercial thickeners, which can be mixed with hot or cold beverages. Unthickened or "free" water is sometimes provided to dysphagia clients on the assumption that consuming small amounts of water creates little risk of pneumonia and can improve

Table 48-1. Compensatory and Remedial Interventions for Specific Problems

Patient Problem	Compensatory Intervention	Remedial Intervention
Swallowing apraxia		Provide a natural mealtime setting; enhance self-feeding skills to facilitate oral skills. Provide a variety of boluses to stimulate oral movements (Logemann, 1998).
Weakness of cheeks, lips	Provide soft solids and thick fluids for easy oral manipulation; place food at back and stronger side of mouth; tilt head toward stronger side; massage cheek to prevent pocketing; hold lips closed; inspect mouth after meals to check for residue.	Use tapping, vibration, and quick stretch to stimulate movement; provide range-of-motion and stretching exercises progressing to resistive sucking and blowing exercises.
Abnormal oral reflexes	Avoid stimuli that provoke rooting, bite, tongue thrust, sucking, and hyperactive gag. Elicit movements antagonistic to undesirable reflex; for example, encourage mouth opening to weaken bite reflex. Seat patient with body well supported to minimize proximal extensor tone, which can provoke abnormal distal movements and reflexes.	
Facial, intra-oral hypersensitivity		Provide systematic desensitization to face and intra-oral area. If sensory defensiveness affects whole body, a program of sensory diet and graded sensory stimulation to body should precede stimulation to oral area, followed by careful introduction of food. Use systematic desensitization with guided imagery to reduce muscle tone and anxiety regarding eating and mouth.
Oral hyposensitivity	Place bolus on more sensitive areas of mouth; use warmer or colder bolus and flavorful food to stimulate sensation (Logemann, 1998). Use heavy or viscous boluses.	Sensory diet providing heightened tactile and proprioceptive input to intra-oral structures may stimulate sensation and movement before and during a meal or snack.
Reduced lingual control	Introduce diet requiring little oral manipulation, including soft solids and thick fluids; use posterior and/or lateral placement of food on stronger side; inspect mouth for residue after meals.	Introduce active and passive tongue range-of-motion exercises, activities; provide quick stretch to tongue with tongue depressor or gloved fingers; provide articulation and tongue-strengthening exercises (Robbins et al., 2005)
Slow oral transit time	Use cold boluses to hasten oral transit time; take care in case they melt into a difficult-to-manage liquid. Sour boluses, such as those infused with lemon juice, can speed oral manipulation.	
Delayed swallow	Use a sour bolus to reduce swallow delay (Logemann et al., 1995). Try chin tuck to enhance airway protection; increase bolus volume and viscosity to reduce pharyngeal delay time (Bisch et al., 1994).	Try thermal-tactile stimulation: stroke anterior faucial arches with iced laryngeal mirror (Fig. 48-8); hastens initiation and overall speed of swallow immediately after application (Rosenbek et al., 1996).
Reduced laryngeal elevation	Use Mendelsohn maneuver to prolong laryngeal elevation or chin tuck to elevate larynx; use supraglottic or supersupraglottic swallow to clear or minimize any material in airway (Logemann, 1998).	Use "Shaker" exercises (a program of head raising exercises) to strengthen suprahyoid musculature and prolong opening of the UES (Shaker et al., 2002).
Reduced laryngeal closure	Use supraglottic or super supraglottic swallow to enhance airway protection (Logemann, 1998) or chin tuck to elevate and close off larynx.	Introduce vocal cord adduction exercises (Logemann, 1998).
Tracheostomy	Occlusion of tracheostomy tube minimizes aspiration and improves swallow biomechanics (Logemann, Pauloski, & Colangelo, 1998); use of one-way speaking valve can decrease frequency of aspiration (Dettelbach et al., 1995). Chin tuck may be useful.	

The swallowing therapist typically has to try several interventions, preferably with the assistance of videofluoroscopy, to assess which techniques work most effectively. Clinicians should work under the guidance of an experienced therapist when using a technique that is new to them.

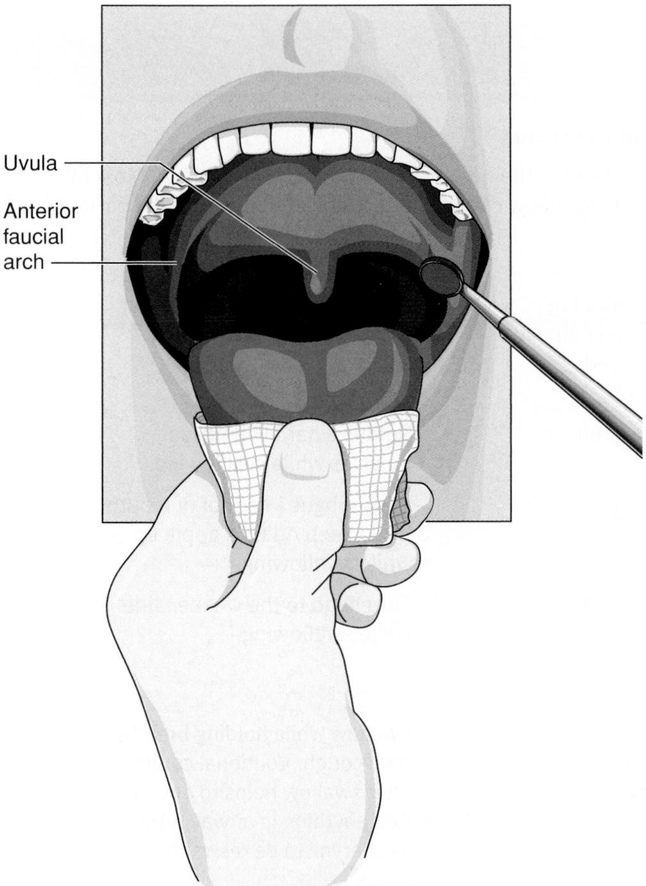

Figure 48-8 Thermal-tactile stimulation of the swallow. An iced laryngeal mirror is used to stroke the faucial arches to elicit or improve strength of the swallowing reflex.

hydration (Garon, Engle, & Ormiston, 1997). As bacterial pathogens in the mouth may be aspirated into the lungs, meticulous oral hygiene is needed with any diet and free water to reduce the risk of pneumonia (Yamaya et al., 2001).

Patient and Caregiver Training

Although the occupational therapist alone may carry out treatment, the plan for intervention also includes education of the patient, nursing staff, and caregivers (Definition 48-4). The patient and family should understand the cause of and prognosis for the patient's dysphagia and the importance of strategies to be carried out at home. It may be helpful to have the patient view the videofluoroscopy or fiberoptic endoscopy to clarify his or her condition and the benefits of compensatory techniques. Mealtime positioning, adaptive equipment, and the type and amount of assistance must be taught to caregivers. Meal preparation practice and community outings can reinforce diet modifications, enhance patient and family education in various settings, and motivate the patient.

Efficacy of Dysphagia Intervention

Numerous studies cite the efficacy of dysphagia intervention in both acute and chronic populations with a variety of diagnostic cohorts. Odderson, Keaton, and McKenna (1995) found that early management of dysphagia in the acute-care setting prevents incidents of aspiration and is cost effective. Dysphagia intervention has been shown to be effective for patients with traumatic brain injury (Shurr et al., 1999), acute neurogenic dysphagia (Bartolome, Prosiegal, & Yassouridis, 1997), stroke (Elmstahl et al., 1999), chronic dysphagia following brainstem lesions (Huckabee & Cannito, 1999), and head and neck cancer (Dejonckere & Hordijk, 1998) and for the profoundly mentally retarded cerebral palsy population (Helfrich-Miller, Rector, & Straka, 1986). Examples of proven therapeutic techniques to manage dysphagia are presented earlier in the chapter.

As the emphasis on evidence-based medicine and rehabilitation advances, clinicians must keep abreast of new knowledge. Useful resources on dysphagia care for both beginning and advanced-level swallowing therapists are noted under Resource 48-1. The author encourages the reader to explore further learning and expertise in dysphagia care. In many facilities, problem-oriented rehabilitation team goals are supplanting discipline-specific goals to target improvement of specific abilities that pose barriers to discharge, creating a need for occupational therapists versed in dysphagia management. Early discharge from acute care and rehabilitation hospitals and minimized staffing in health care facilities create situations in which competence in dysphagia intervention has become a mandatory skill for occupational therapy practitioners. Occupational therapists, with their background in the many abilities and capacities that influence eating and swallowing, make logical primary swallowing therapists.

PROCEDURES FOR PRACTICE 48-2

Compensatory Swallowing Maneuvers: Their Purpose and Execution

The following techniques are ways to use volitional movement to improve the quality of the pharyngeal swallow. Most of them are complex and require a good attention span and the ability to follow complex directions on the part of the patient.

Maneuver	Purpose	Execution
Chin tuck	Moves base of tongue back; narrows opening to larynx, protecting airway; helps protect airway when larynx is low and swallow is delayed (Ohmae et al., 1996; Welch et al., 1993).	Tuck chin down toward chest while swallowing.
Effortful swallow	Helps to elevate base of tongue (Pouderoux & Kahrilas, 1995).	Squeeze hard with throat muscles while swallowing.
Mendelsohn maneuver	Prolongs opening of UES when larynx is low (Logemann, 1998).	Push tongue into roof of mouth; try to keep Adam's apple up while swallowing.
Neck rotation	Closes weaker side of pharynx; uses stronger intact musculature in cases of unilateral weakness of pharynx and/or vocal folds (Logemann et al., 1989).	Turn head to the weaker side while swallowing.
Supraglottic swallow	Compensates for weak vocal cord closure, reduces penetration of food into larynx during swallow by closing vocal cords (Ohmae et al., 1996).	Swallow while holding breath; then cough. Volitional cough after swallow helps to ensure that anything in airway returns to pharynx to be reswallowed.
Super supraglottic swallow	Reduces penetration of food into larynx during swallow by narrowing opening to airway (Ohmae et al., 1996).	Hold breath and bear down; maintain breath-hold, keep bearing down while swallowing; cough after swallowing.

RESOURCE 48-1

American Dietetic Association
Offers *National Dysphagia Diet: Standardization for Optimal Care*
Phone: (800) 877-1600
http://www.eatright.org

Dysphagia Resource Center
www.dysphagia.com
Web site provides information and links on anatomy and physiology pertinent to dysphagia, organizations, print materials, case studies, research information, and funding. Information for clinicians and lay persons.

Dysphagia Evaluation Protocol
Assessment of dysphagia in adults developed by occupational therapists and tested for reliability and validity. Chartable record form and easy-to-use flip book format.

Harcourt Assessment
Phone: (800) 211-8378
http://www.harcourtassessment.com

Dysphagia Research Society
Houston, TX.
http://www.uiuc.edu/drs/

Dysphagia
Official journal of the Dysphagia Research Society
Springer-Verlag
Phone: (713) 965-0566
http://www.springer.de/
Peer-reviewed journal devoted to publication of scholarly articles about dysphagia. Abstracts and subscription information available online. Subscription information available by telephone.

DEFINITION 48-4

de·fin·i·tion

Instrumental Intervention

Surface electromyography provides patients with improved awareness of swallowing function, providing for better swallowing. This intervention has been shown to be useful in populations with stroke (Crary et al., 2004; Freed et al., 2001). One example of this is VitalStim Therapy, which uses a specially designed electrical stimulation unit with surface electrodes placed on the neck (Fig. 48-9).

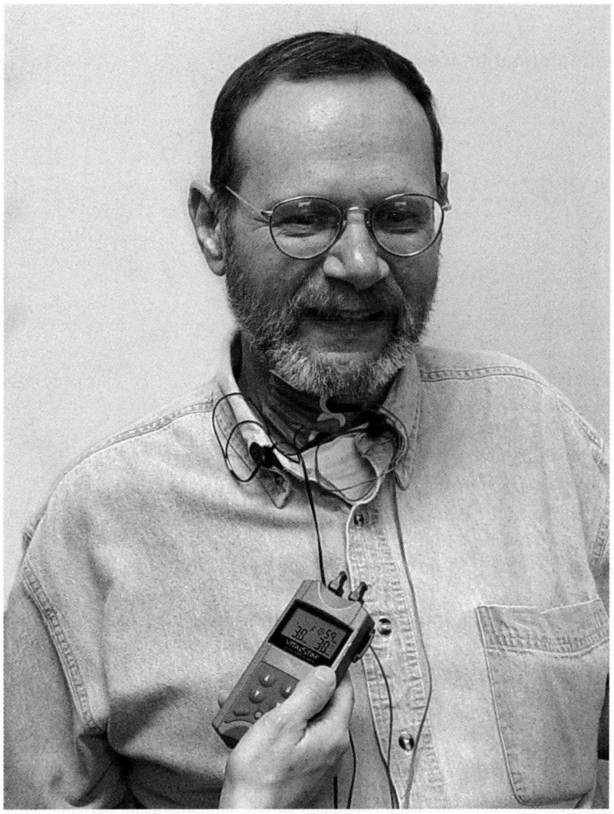

Figure 48-9 VitalStim, a specially developed neuromuscular stimulation unit that facilitates contraction of the muscles used in swallowing, in place on a dysphagic patient's neck. (©2005 Encore Medical, L.P. VitalStim is a registered trademark of VitalStim, LLC.)

CASE EXAMPLE

Mr. D.: Dysphagia Evaluation and Treatment for a Patient with Left Cerebrovascular Accident (CVA)

Occupational Therapy Process	Clinical Reasoning Process: Objective	Clinical Reasoning Process: Examples of Therapist's Internal Dialogue
Patient Information Mr. D. is an 86-year-old man with a left hemispheric CVA. He was admitted to an acute-care hospital with aphasia and right upper extremity weakness, with a prior history of hypertension and transient ischemic attacks (TIAs) with aphasia.	Understand the patient's diagnosis or condition	"According to my experience and the literature, patients with dysphagia due to an acute single stroke eventually swallow safely without compensatory techniques. However, Mr. D. has had prior TIAs (possible permanent damage), which may limit his swallowing recovery. I expect that his symptoms will resolve, at least in part. He does have some control of his lips, cheek, and tongue, and reduced competence of his airway protection skills indicate that oral feeding should proceed cautiously."

Patient Information (cont'd)	Know the person	"Although he is frail, Mr. D. is enthusiastic about advancing his diet and participates fully in his dysphagia intervention, and I believe that he will take responsibility for following through with his rehabilitation program. He enjoys meals at home and assists with meal preparation. He has a supportive spouse who will help to carryover mealtime recommendations and exercise programs. Because he is ambulatory, I believe that follow-up dysphagia therapy will occur on an outpatient basis."
Reason for Referral to Occupational Therapy Mr. D. was referred to occupational therapy for dysphagia intervention, as well as to improve his upper extremity skills including self-feeding. The medical staff wants to be sure that he does not need alternative nutritional routes (nasogastric feedings or IVs) to nourish and hydrate himself while in the hospital and wants assurance that he is not at risk for aspiration. The doctors also want to assure that he can maintain his nutritional requirements so that he can safely be discharged home.	Appreciate the context Develop the provisional hypotheses	"Mr. D. is being seen as a hospital inpatient. Although eating and mealtime in this setting is very different from being home, due to natural recovery, his level of function may improve quickly, and I should be alert to update goals on a daily basis. I'll be working together with the dietician to care for Mr. D.; she will monitor that he is eating and drinking enough and initiate any changes in diet that I recommend." "Because Mr. D.'s muscle tone is low, I may be working with him to reinforce muscle activity for both muscles involved in swallowing and his upper extremity muscles involved in self-feeding."
Assessment Process and Results A dysphagia evaluation was done using the *Dysphagia Evaluation Protocol* (see Resources 48-1). The evaluation (Fig. 48-3) revealed that Mr. D. had hypotonicity and reduced control of his lips, cheek, and tongue on the right side. Decreased airway protection skills were evidenced by his inability to phonate because of vocal cord weakness, inability to cough volitionally, and reduced laryngeal elevation during swallowing. He was not aphasic. Mr. D. was able to swallow foods from the beginning level dysphagia diet, including foods with soft, moist textures, such as pudding and applesauce, with mild food spillage out of the mouth due to poor lip control, delayed formation and propulsion of the bolus, and delayed initiation of the swallow. He had difficulty grasping utensils and cups because of hypotonicity of his dominant right hand.	Consider evaluation approach and methods Interpret observations	"I have chosen a standardized evaluation of dysphagia skills that also examines self-feeding and includes all components of swallowing that I need to assess." "Given the evaluation results and observation over the course of several meals, Mr. D. should be able to nourish and hydrate himself with supplementary (not by mouth) nutrition or hydration."
Occupational Therapy Problem List 1. Hypotonicity of oral, pharyngeal, and laryngeal structures, resulting in: • Delay in and reduced coordination of bolus control both in the mouth and in propelling the bolus posteriorly to initiate the swallow • Delayed initiation of the swallow 2. Reduced upper extremity control, making use of his dominant arm to self-feed awkward	Synthesize results	"Reduced muscle tone is evidenced with both his swallowing and self-feeding."
Occupational Therapy Goal List (five daily treatments prior to discharge) 1. Mr. D. will tolerate a more advanced dysphagia diet, adding soft chewables such as cooked fruit and soft pasta.	Develop intervention hypotheses	"I believe that focusing occupational therapy within a functional mealtime context can efficiently address both swallowing and self-feeding."

Occupational Therapy Goal List (cont'd)

2. Mr. D. will tolerate these textures without clinical signs of aspiration (see Safety Note 48-2).
3. Mr. D. will be independent in vocal cord adduction exercises.
4. Mr. D. will support the right side of his lower lip and massage the right cheek during the oral preparatory stage to prevent food spillage and pocketing in his right cheek.
5. Mr. D. will feed himself with his right hand with built-up utensils and an adapted cup while weight bearing on his right elbow.

Select an intervention approach

"Because Mr. D.'s stroke is acute and has great potential for improvement, the initial approach will be remedial, although a compensatory dysphagia modification will be used to reduce any possible risk of aspiration or laryngeal penetration at meal or snack time."

Consider what will occur in therapy, how often, and for how long

"Because Mr. D. has an acute stroke, the intervention plan should be intensive; exercises should be done once or twice daily, and mealtime techniques be employed each time he eats, for both safety and to facilitate improvement."

Intervention

Mr. D. was seen daily for occupational therapy during a week as a hospital inpatient. Constant supervision at mealtime was accomplished, and all meals and snacks took place with him seated upright in the chair. Occupational therapy intervention addressed exercises and positioning to enhance tone and control of oral motor skills, laryngeal exercises to strengthen his vocal cords and improve laryngeal elevation, and facilitation of tone and movement in his hypotonic right upper extremity to improve self-feeding skills. Mr. D. and his caregiver were educated and given handouts on the nature of his dysphagia, exercises, and mealtime procedures and precautions.

Assess the patient's comprehension

Understand what he is doing

Compare actual to expected performance

Know the person
Appreciate the context

"Mr. D., with the help of his wife, was able to understand all instructions and followed through with the treatment plan. He was anxious to progress to his normal diet and eating habits. He understood that the supervision at mealtime and exercises would help him to improve and prevent complications such as aspiration. He demonstrated improvements daily, and although his appetite initially was limited, he showed definite improvement through the week in terms of his intake. His progress was on target with what I expected, given that he developed no further medical complications. Happily, he achieved his short-term goals within a week."

Next Steps

Mr. D. was discharged from the hospital to home in the company of his wife. He and his wife were taught to thicken fluids with commercial thickeners at home. As his vocal cord strength returned, his volitional cough became stronger, and he gradually became able to speak in a loud whisper; laryngeal strengthening exercises continued. Mr. D. was able to discontinue use of external lip control strategies as oral motor control returned. He continued use of built-up utensils and weight bearing at the elbow while self-feeding. He continued with outpatient occupational therapy for 4 more weeks. During that time, the following long-term goals were accomplished:

1. Mr. D. will tolerate a regular diet consisting of a variety of solid and liquid textures, dry cut-up chewable solids, and thin liquids without signs or symptoms of aspiration.
2. Mr. D. will eat independently with his right upper extremity without use of adaptive equipment and without compensatory movements.

Anticipate present and future patient concerns

Analyze the patient's comprehension

Decide if the patient should continue or discontinue therapy and/or return in the future

"I know that Mr. D. will be anxious to resume a normal diet and enjoy a normal range of food textures. He will also be concerned about being able to eat in a restaurant or with friends without his 'elbow on the table' weight-bearing strategy to improve his upper extremity control. For this reason and because of continued expected improvement, I'll continue to see him as an outpatient until the remedial long-terms goals are accomplished. Once he has regained 'normal' function, I'll discharge him."

CLINICAL REASONING IN OCCUPATIONAL THERAPY PRACTICE

Dysphagia Evaluation and Intervention for Stroke Patients

Patients with cerebrovascular accidents (CVA) due to a left-hemisphere lesion (right hemiplegia) can demonstrate slow initiation of the oral stage of the swallow and slowed trigger of the swallow response. There may be reduced muscle tone in the right-side oral structures. The pharyngeal stage may be slowed. There may be apraxia for feeding and swallowing. Intervention focuses on activities to stimulate motion in the oral structures, providing a modified diet for safe swallowing, and creating a naturalistic setting at meals to stimulate motor planning. How are symptoms different in a patient with right-hemisphere stroke? How are they similar? How is intervention different?

Evidence Table 48-1
Best Evidence for Dysphagia Interventions Used in Occupational Therapy

Intervention	Description of Intervention Tested	Participants	Dosage	Type of Best Evidence and Level of Evidence	Benefit	Statistical Probability and Effect Size of Outcome	Reference
Remedial Approach	Oral motor exercises, compensatory swallowing techniques, positioning, dysphagia diet.	38 stroke patients.	Not provided.	Level IIIB3a	Yes; 61% of patients showed overall improvement on modified barium swallow testing and improved levels of nutrition.	Standardized assessment of videofluoroscopic swallow performance improved significantly, $p < 0.001$; a calculated overall dysphagia score showed significant improvement, $p < 0.05$; body weight showed significant improvement, $p < 0.05$.	Elmstahl et al., 1999
Remedial Approach	Individualized program that may include: remedial techniques such as oral motor exercises, laryngeal adduction and elevation exercises, and other remedial techniques including: Mendelsohn maneuver, supraglottic swallow, repeated swallows, postural techniques, thermal stimulation, and diet modification.	63 patients with neurogenic dysphagia.	Not provided.	Level IIIA3b	Yes; 70% of patients showed immediate improvement, 43% showed improvement on follow-up; no deterioration was reported for any patient.	Improved feeding ability over time, $p < 0.05$; the relationship between post-intervention outcome and type of feeding at discharge and during follow-up, $p < 0.05$.	Bartolome, Prosiegel, & Yassouridis, 1997

SUMMARY REVIEW QUESTIONS

1. What are the stages of swallowing, and what events occur during each stage? Which stage or stages are most amenable to therapeutic intervention, and why?
2. What is aspiration, and what are its warning signs and symptoms?
3. Outline the three types of dysphagia; compare the specific dysphagia symptoms of selected diagnoses with the typical manifestations of the appropriate category: paralytic, pseudobulbar, and mechanical dysphagia.
4. Which components of a thorough dysphagia evaluation are most accurately completed with a patient who can follow multistep commands? How would you alter bedside evaluation for patients with various cognitive and perceptual deficits?
5. What are the instrumental evaluations for dysphagia, and how does the information that each provides assist in dysphagia rehabilitation?
6. What recommendations should a dysphagia evaluation provide?
7. Define compensatory and remedial and direct and indirect dysphagia treatments and provide examples of each for specific diagnoses.

ACKNOWLEDGMENT

I thank Denise Jules Wilhelm, OTR, for her assistance with photographs used in this chapter. Thanks also to Bette Pomerleau, MS, SLP, and Ray Autiello, LPN, RT, formerly of Universal Mobile Services in Haverhill, Massachusetts, for their assistance with the videofluoroscopic image reproduced in this chapter.

References

American Occupational Therapy Association. (2000). Specialized knowledge and skills for eating and feeding in occupational therapy practice. *American Journal of Occupational Therapy, 54,* 629–640.

Avery-Smith, W. (1998). An occupational therapist-coordinated dysphagia program. *OT Practice, 3,* 20–23.

Avery-Smith, W., Rosen, A. B., & Dellarosa, D. (1992). Clinical assessment of dysphagia in adults. *Occupational Therapy Practice, 3,* 51–58.

Avery-Smith, W., Rosen, A. B., & Dellarosa, D. (1997). *Dysphagia evaluation protocol.* San Antonio, TX: Harcourt Assessment.

Aviv, J. E., Martin, J. H., Sacco, R. L., Zagar, D., Diamond, B., Keen, M. S., & Blitzer, A. B. (1996). Supraglottic and pharyngeal sensory abnormalities in stroke patients with dysphagia. *Annals of Otology, Rhinology and Laryngology, 105,* 92–97.

Bartolome, M., Prosiegal, M., & Yassouridis, A. (1997). Long-term functional outcome in patients with neurogenic dysphagia. *Neurorehabilitation, 9,* 195–204.

Bisch, E. M., Logemann, J. A., Rademaker, A. A. W., Kahrials, P. J., & Lazarus, C. L. (1994). Pharyngeal effects of bolus volume, viscosity, and temperature in patients with dysphagia resulting from neurologic impairment and in normal subjects. *Journal of Speech and Hearing Research, 37,* 10541–1059.

Cherney, L. R., (1994). Dysphagia in adults with neurologic disorders: An overview. In L. R. Cherney (Ed.), *Clinical management of dysphagia in adults and children.* Gaithersburg, MD: Aspen.

Crary, M. A., Carnaby Mann, G. D., Groher, M. E., & Helseth, E. (2004). Functional benefits of dysphagia therapy using adjunctive sEMG biofeedback. *Dysphagia, 19,* 160–164.

Dejonckere, P. H., & Hordijk, G. K. (1998) Prognostic factors for swallowing after treatment of head and neck cancer. *Clinical Otolaryngology, 23,* 218–223.

Dettelbach, M. A., Gross, R.D., Mahlman, J., & Eibling, D. E. (1995). Effect of the Passy-Muir valve on aspiration in patients with tracheostomy. *Head and Neck, 17,* 297–302.

Devita, M. A., & Spierer-Rundback, L. (1990). Swallowing disorders in patients with prolonged orotracheal intubation or tracheostomy tubes. *Critical Care Medicine, 18,* 1328–1330.

Eckberg, O., & Feinberg, M. (1992). Clinical and demographic data in 75 patients with near-fatal choking episodes. *Dysphagia, 7,* 205–208.

Elmstahl, S., Bulow, M., Ekberg, O., Petersson, M., & Tegner, H. (1999). Treatment of dysphagia improves nutritional conditions in stroke patients. *Dysphagia, 14,* 61–66.

Elpern, E. H., Scott, M. G., Petro, L., & Ries, M. H. (1994). Pulmonary aspiration in mechanically ventilated patients with tracheostomies. *Chest, 105,* 563–566.

Ertekin, C., Aydogdu, I., Yuceyar, N., Tarlaci, S., Kiylioglu, N., Pehlivan, M., & Celebi, G. (1998). Electrodiagnostic methods for neurogenic dysphagia. *Electroencephalography and Clinical Neurophysiology, 109,* 331–340.

Finestone, H. M., Greene-Finestone, L. S., Wilson, E. S., & Teasell, R. W. (1995). Malnutrition in stroke patients on the rehabilitation service and at follow-up: Prevalence and predictors. *Archives of Physical Medicine and Rehabilitation, 76,* 310–316.

Fioretti, A., Giacotto, L., & Melega, V. (1997). Choking incidents among psychiatric patients: Retrospective analysis of thirty-one cases from the west Bologna psychiatric wards. *Canadian Journal of Psychiatry, 42,* 515–520.

Freed, M. L., Freed, L., Chatburn, R. L., & Christian, M. (2001). Electrical stimulation for swallowing disorders caused by stroke. *Respiratory Care, 46,* 466–474.

Garber, B. G., Hebert, P. C., Yelle, J. D., Hodder, R. V., & McGowan, J. (1996). Adult respiratory distress syndrome: A systemic overview of incidence and risk factors. *Critical Care Medicine, 24,* 555–556.

Garon, B. R., Engle, M., & Ormiston, C. (1997). A randomized control study to determine the effects of unlimited oral intake of water in patients with identified aspiration. *Journal of Neurologic Rehabilitation, 11,* 139–148.

Groher, M. E. (1987). Bolus management and aspiration pneumonia in patients with pseudobulbar dysphagia. *Dysphagia, 1,* 215–216.

Groher, M. E. (1997). *Dysphagia: Diagnosis and management* (3rd ed.). Boston: Butterworth-Heinemann.

Groher, M. E., & Bukatman, R. (1986). Prevalence of dysphagia in two teaching hospitals. *Dysphagia, 1,* 30–35.

Gross, R. D., Mahlmann, J., & Grayhack, J. P. (2003). Physiologic effects of open and closed tracheostomy tubes on the pharyngeal swallow. *Annals of Otology, Rhinology, and Laryngology, 112,* 143–152.

Helfrich-Miller, K. R., Rector, K. L., & Straka, J. A. (1986). Dysphagia: Its treatment in the profoundly retarded patient with cerebral palsy. *Archives of Physical Medicine and Rehabilitation, 67,* 520–525.

Hiiemae, K., Heath, M. R., Heath, G., Kazazoglu, E., Murrary, J., Snapper, D., & Hamblett, K. (1996). Natural bites, food consistency and feeding behaviour in man. *Archives of Oral Biology, 41,* 175–189.

Horner, J., Alberts, M. J., Dawson, D. V., & Cook, G. M. (1994). Swallowing in Alzheimer's disease. *Alzheimer Disease and Associated Disorders, 8,* 177–189.

Horner, J., Buoyer, F. G., Alberts, M. J., & Helms, M. J. (1991). Dysphagia following brainstem stroke. *Archives of Neurology, 48,* 1170–1173.

Huckabee, M. L., & Cannito, M. P. (1999). Outcomes of swallowing rehabilitation in chronic brainstem dysphagia: A retrospective evaluation. *Dysphagia, 14,* 93–109.

Lazarus, C. L. (1995). Conference notes from Dysphagia Symposium: Management of Swallowing Disorders in the Medical Setting. Salem, MA: North Shore Medical Center.

Lazarus, C. L., Logemann, J. A., Pauloski, B. R., Colangelo, L. A., Kahrilas, P. J., Mittal, B. B., & Pierce, M. (1996). Swallowing disorders in head and neck cancer patients treated with radiotherapy and adjuvant chemotherapy. *Laryngoscope, 106,* 1157–1166.

Leopold, N. A., & Kagel, M. C. (1996). Prepharyngeal dysphagia in Parkinson's disease. *Dysphagia, 11,* 14–22.

Leopold, N. A., & Kagel, M. C. (1997). Pharyngo-esophageal dysphagia in Parkinson's disease. *Dysphagia, 12,* 11–20.

Linden, P., Kuhlemeier, K. V., & Patterson, C. (1993). The probability of correctly predicting subglottic penetration from clinical observations. *Dysphagia, 8,* 170–179.

Logemann, J. A. (1998). *Evaluation and treatment of swallowing disorders.* Austin: Pro-Ed.

Logemann, J. A., Kahrilas, P. J., Kobara, M., & Vakil, N. B. (1989). The benefit of head rotation on pharyngoesophageal dysphagia. *Archives of Physical Medicine and Rehabilitation, 70,* 767–771.

Logemann, J. A., Pauloski, B. R., & Colangelo, L. (1998). Light digital occlusion of the tracheostomy tube: A pilot study of effects on aspiration and biomechanics of the swallow. *Head and Neck, 20,* 52–57.

Logemann, J. A., Pepe, J., & Mackay, L. E. (1994). Disorders of nutrition and swallowing: Intervention strategies in the trauma center. *Journal of Head Trauma Rehabilitation, 9,* 43–56.

Mackay, L. E., Morgan, A. S., & Bernstein, B. A. (1999). Swallowing disorders in severe brain injury: Risk factors affecting return to oral intake. *Archives of Physical Medicine and Rehabilitation, 80,* 365–371.

McConnel, F. M. S., & O'Connor, A. (1994). Dysphagia secondary to head and neck cancer surgery. *Acta Oto-Rhino-Laryngologica Belgica, 48,* 165–170.

Musson, N. D., Kincaid, J., Ryan, P., Glussman, B., Varone, L., Gamarra, N., Wilson, R., Reefe, W., & Silverman, M. (1990). Nature, nurture, nutrition: Interdisciplinary programs to address the prevention of malnutrition and dehydration. *Dysphagia, 5,* 96–101.

Nagaya, M., Kachi, T., Yamada, T., & Igata, A. (1998). Videofluorographic study of swallowing in Parkinson's disease. *Dysphagia, 13,* 95–100.

Newton, H. B., Newton, C., Pearl, D., & Davidson, T. (1994). Swallowing assessment in primary brain tumor patients with dysphagia. *Neurology, 44,* 1927–1932.

Odderson, I. R., Keaton, J. C., & McKenna, B. S. (1995). Swallow management in patients on an acute stroke pathway: Quality is cost effective. *Archives of Physical Medicine and Rehabilitation, 76,* 1130–1133.

Ohmae, Y., Logemann, J. A., Kaiser, P., Hanson, D. G., & Kahrilas, P. J. (1996). Effects of two breath-holding maneuvers on oropharyngeal swallow. *Annals of Otology, Rhinology, & Laryngology, 105,* 123–131.

Pauloski, B. R., Rademaker, A. W., Logemann, J. A., & Colangelo, L. A. (1998). Speech and swallowing in irradiated and nonirradiated postsurgical oral cancer patients. *Otolaryngology—Head and Neck Surgery, 118,* 616–614.

Pelletier, C. A., & Lawless, H. T. (2003). Effect of citric acid and citric acid-sucrose mixtures on swallowing in neurogenic oropharyngeal dysphagia. *Dysphagia, 18,* 231–241.

Pouderoux, P., & Kahrilas, P. J. (1995). Deglutitive tongue force modulation by volition, volume, and viscosity in humans. *Gastroenterology, 108,* 1418–1426.

Priefer, B. A., & Robbins, J. (1997). Eating changes in mild-stage Alzheimer's disease: A pilot study. *Dysphagia, 12,* 212–221.

Robbins, J., Gangnon, R. E., Theis, S. M., Kays, S. A., Hewitt, A. L., & Hind, J. A. (2005). The effects of lingual exercise on swallowing in older adults. *Journal of the American Geriatrics Society, 53,* 1483–1489.

Robbins, J., Levine, R. L., Maser, A., Rosenbek, J. C., & Kempster, G. B. (1993). Swallowing after unilateral stroke of the cerebral cortex. *Archives of Physical Medicine and Rehabilitation, 74,* 1295–1300.

Rogers, B., Stratton, P., Msall, M., Andres, M., Champlain, M. K., Koerner, P., & Piazza, J. (1994). Long-term morbidity and management strategies of tracheal aspiration in adults with severe developmental disabilities. *American Journal of Mental Retardation, 98,* 490–498.

Rosenbek, J. C., Roecher, E. B., Wood, J. L., & Robbins, J. (1996). Thermal application reduces the duration of stage transition in dysphagia after stroke. *Dysphagia, 11,* 225–233.

Schmidt, J., Holas, M., Halvorson, K., & Reding, M. (1994). Videofluoroscopic evidence of aspiration predicts pneumonia and death but not dehydration following stroke. *Dysphagia, 9,* 7–11.

Shaker, R., Easterling, C., Kern, M., Nitschke, T., Massey, B., Daniels, S., Grande, B., Kazandjian, M., & Dikeman, K. (2002). Rehabilitation of swallowing by exercise in tube-fed patients with pharyngeal dysphagia secondary to abnormal UES opening. *Gastroenterology, 122,* 1314–1321.

Shaker, R., Milbrath, M., Ren, J., Campbell, B., Toohill, R., & Hogan, W. (1995). Deglutitive aspiration in patients with tracheostomy: Effect of tracheostomy on the duration of vocal cord closure. *Gastroenterology, 108,* 1357–1360.

Sherman, B., Nisenboum, J. M., Jesberger, B. L., Morrow, C. A., & Jesberger, J. A. (1999). Assessment of dysphagia with the use of pulse oximetry. *Dysphagia, 14,* 152–156.

Shurr, M. J., Ebner, K. A., Maser, A. L., Sperling, K. B., Helgerson, R. B., & Harms, B. (1999). Formal swallowing evaluation and therapy after traumatic brain injury improves dysphagia outcomes. *Journal of Trauma, 46,* 817–821.

Siebens, H., Trupe, E., & Siebens A. A. (1986). Correlates and consequences of eating dependency in institutionalized elderly. *Journal of the American Geriatrics Society, 34,* 192–198.

Sokoloff, L. G., & Pavlakovic, R. (1997). Neuroleptic-induced dysphagia. *Dysphagia, 12,* 177–179.

Splaingard, M. L., Hutchins, B., Sulton, L. D., & Chaudhuri, G. (1988). Aspiration in rehabilitation patients: Videofluoroscopy vs. bedside clinical assessment. *Archives of Physical Medicine and Rehabilitation, 69,* 637–640.

Thomas, F. J., & Wiles, C. M. (1999). Dysphagia and nutritional status in multiple sclerosis. *Neurology, 246,* 677–682.

Tolep, K., Getch, C. L., & Criner, G. J. (1996). Swallowing dysfunction in patients receiving prolonged mechanical ventilation. *Chest, 109,* 167–172.

Tracy, J., Logemann, J., Kahrilas, P., Jacob, P., Kobara, M., & Krugler, C. (1989). Preliminary observations on the effects of age on oropharyngeal deglutition. *Dysphagia, 4,* 90–94.

Welch, M. V., Logemann, J. A., Rademaker, A. W., & Kahrilas, P. J. (1993). Changes in pharyngeal dimensions effected by chin tuck. *Archives of Physical Medicine and Rehabilitation, 74,* 178–181.

Wesling, M., Brady, S., Jensen, M., Nickell, M., Starkus, D., & Escobar, N. (2003). Dysphagia outcomes in patients with brain tumors undergoing inpatient rehabilitation. *Dysphagia, 18,* 203–210.

Yamaya, M., Yanai, M., Ohrui, T., Arai, H., & Sasaki, H. (2001). Interventions to prevent pneumonia among older adults. *Journal of the American Geriatrics Society, 49,* 85–90.

Zenner, P. M., Losinski, D. S., & Mills, R. H. (1995). Using cervical auscultation in the clinical dysphagia examination in long term care. *Dysphagia, 10,* 27–31.

LEARNING OBJECTIVES

After studying this chapter, the reader will be able to do the following:

1. Convey the social and epidemiological history of HIV/AIDS in the United States, focusing on the populations most prevalently infected.
2. Summarize the natural history of HIV and its concomitant social trajectory.
3. Extrapolate the impact of HIV/AIDS at points along the disease trajectory on the occupations of people within different populations.
4. Select tools and assessment strategies to ascertain the specific occupational needs of individuals living with HIV/AIDS.

CHAPTER 49

Human Immunodeficiency Virus

Karin J. Opacich

Glossary

Global pandemic—An epidemic that affects many countries similarly.

HAART—An acronym for *highly active antiretroviral therapy*; combinations of pharmaceutical interventions configured to act on HIV at different points of reproduction.

Health disparities—Unintended differences in health status or health outcomes; seemingly associated with race/ethnicity, socioeconomic status, education, and access to health care.

Naturalistic paradigm—Research methodology that focuses on the lived experience, people in their natural environments; generally yields qualitative data rather than quantitative data from which themes or meanings are extracted.

Occupational competencies—Skills and abilities associated with effective execution of occupations and occupational roles.

Occupational coherence—Fluidity and complementarity of occupations that make outcomes predictable.

Occupational role integrity—Clusters of skills and abilities that support the tasks and activities associated with a given role; intactness of an occupational role.

Opportunistic illness—Infections and diseases that manifest because the normal protective responses of the immune system have been disabled.

Retrovirus—A virus that replicates itself using the mechanisms of host cells to convert RNA to DNA.

Since the symptoms associated with human immunodeficiency virus (HIV) were first described in 1981 (Masur et al., 1981; Siegal et al., 1981; Gottlieb et al., 1981), nearly a million cases have been recorded in the United States alone. Acquired immunodeficiency syndrome (AIDS) was officially defined in 1993 and periodically updated (Centers for Disease Control and Prevention [CDC], 1993), and surveillance systems for both HIV and acquired immunodeficiency syndrome (AIDS) have been established and revised by the Centers for Disease Control and Prevention (CDC, 1999; Nakashima & Fleming, 2003). HIV/AIDS is regarded as a **global pandemic** because it has dramatically affected nations and populations throughout the world. Initially thought to be a fatal diagnosis, life expectancies have increased due to advances in medical management. HIV/AIDS is now considered a chronic disease. Although the science associated with HIV/AIDS has rapidly compounded, arresting the disease still depends largely upon individual compliance with prevention strategies. Biological and physical aspects of HIV/AIDS have been systematically studied and documented, but the more variable social trajectory is shaped by the sociopolitical context in which individuals experience the disease. Consequently, quality of life after diagnosis is highly contingent upon resources, support, and access to relevant treatment. Among the services that can impact the lives of people with HIV/AIDS, occupational therapy can be valuable.

EPIDEMIOLOGICAL HISTORY

Epidemiologists have now established that HIV and AIDS are the result of human exposure to a chimpanzee virus in Africa that mutated perhaps as early as the 1920s. It is conjectured that this mutant viral strain has spread in modern times due to increased slaughter and consumption of primate meat, widespread prostitution, and use of contaminated needles. After reexamination of stored specimens, it appears that HIV entered the United States sometime in the 1970s (Armstrong, Calabrese, & Taege, 2005). In the ensuing years, an increasing incidence of rare cancers and opportunistic infections precipitated curiosity among health scientists (Fan, Connor, & Villareal, 2004).

THE GLOBAL PICTURE

According to cumulative surveillance data, 42 million people in the world are living with HIV/AIDS. Of those, 29.4 million are from sub-Saharan Africa; 1.4 million are from Eastern Europe and Central Asia; and over 950,000 live in the United States (CDC, 2004; Joint United Nations Program on HIV/AIDS [UNAIDS], 2004). New infections are estimated to occur at a rate of 5 million per year. The most common route of transmission, based on global data, is heterosexual sex. In 2002, 3.1 million people died from AIDS (Curran, 2003; Ogunbodede, 2004).

HIV/AIDS in the United States

Unlike the epidemiological history in Africa, HIV/AIDS in the United States first manifested among gay men. In the early years of the epidemic in the United States, those considered most at risk for infection were gay men, people requiring blood products, and users of injected drugs (Fan, Connor, & Villareal, 2004). Women and children initially represented a very small proportion of those infected. Although predicted transmission has been contained, men who have sex with men still comprise the largest cohort of people with HIV/AIDS in the United States (CDC, 2004).

Data accumulated through 2002 show that women now represent nearly 25% of all people with HIV/AIDS and 30% of the new cases in the United States (National Institute of Allergy and Infectious Diseases [NIAID], 2005). Incidence among children rose until studies in the late 1990s demonstrated that drug therapies administered during the perinatal period could reduce transmission from mother to child. HIV infection among infants has nearly been eliminated, with only 59 new cases reported in children under age 13 in 2003 (CDC, 2004).

THE DISEASE MECHANISM

HIV is a **retrovirus** that results in a gradual deterioration of the immune system. Once the virus enters the human body, it overwhelms the $CD4^+$ T cells that usually defend the body against viruses. HIV uses the cell machinery to convert its own RNA into a form that can be recognized and replicated using the DNA of the host, a process called transcription. Once emitted into the cytoplasm of the cell, this reconfigured virus translates itself prolifically, producing new copies and long chains of viral proteins that mature into new infectious particles that are emitted into other cells (NIAID, 2005). The most efficient vehicle for transmission is blood and contact with delicate mucosal tissue susceptible to cuts and tears. Studies have shown that HIV is not spread through casual contact with saliva, sweat, tears, urine, or feces. HIV status is confirmed by blood tests such as the enzyme-linked immunosorbent assay (ELISA), which detects exposure to the HIV virus via the presence of antibodies, or the Western blot, which targets the presence of the virus itself. Home screening kits are now available as well. Despite the availability of laboratory tests, initial diagnosis is sometimes not made until a person is hospitalized for pneumonia, persistent diarrhea, or other AIDS-related illness.

Although it is rare for health care providers to contract HIV through patient contact or even accidental needle sticks (NIAID, 2004), universal precautions (Safety Note 49-1) are advised, particularly if the provider is handling blood and blood products. Surgeons performing extraordinarily bloody procedures (e.g., orthopedists) are at greatest risk. Special care should be taken to avoid exposing HIV-positive persons to infectious agents because their compromised immunity makes them more vulnerable to serious infections.

SYMPTOMS

Within 2–4 weeks of initial exposure, most, although not all, people infected with HIV experience flu-like symptoms, such as fever, headache, fatigue, and enlarged lymph

SAFETY NOTE 49-1

Standard Precautions

You must routinely use standard precautions to protect yourself from exposure to blood or body fluids from all patients, regardless of their diagnosis. Standard precautions consist of the use of protective barriers to prevent contamination of the skin, clothing, and mucous membranes (eyes, ears, and nose). Hepatitis B virus, hepatitis C virus, and HIV are communicated through blood-borne pathogens. Modes of transmission include sexual contact involving the sharing of body fluid, needlestick, contact with blood through mucous membranes or broken skin, childbirth, receiving blood or blood products, and organ transplantation. Proper use of protective barriers prevents exposure. Protect yourself by always following these recommendations.

- Wear and change gloves.
- Do not wash or decontaminate disposable (single-use) gloves.
- Wear fluid- or moisture-resistant gown, apron, or lab coat when you anticipate contact with bodily fluids.
- Wear surgical cap and/or hood and shoe covers and/or boots when gross contamination is likely.
- Wear mask and eye protection with side shields and face shield when there is potential for splash, spray, or splattering of body fluids to the eyes, nose, or mouth.
- Wash your hands before and after contacting patients.
- Use a pocket mask or other ventilation guard device when doing CPR.

Needlestick or puncture is the most common mechanism for transmission for occupational therapists. To minimize risk use these precautions used by medical personnel:

- Use caution when handling all sharp objects.
- Do not bend, break, or manipulate items by hand.
- Place disposable sharp objects in puncture-resistant container immediately after use.
- Do not recap or remove needles from syringe by hand unless no alternative exists.
- Use a device instead of your hand to pick up or remove contaminated needles or other sharp objects.
- Place reusable sharp objects in containers that are puncture resistant, leak-proof on sides and bottom, and labeled.
- Use a mechanical device to clean up broken glassware.
- *Promptly* report all exposures to your supervisor and health care authorities.

nodes. Until the body's immune system is depleted of resources to combat the virus, the infected person may not experience further symptoms. Symptoms reported before progression to full-blown AIDS include lack of energy, weight loss, fevers and sweats, yeast infections, skin rashes, pelvic inflammatory disease unresponsive to treatment, and short-term memory loss. In many people, progression to AIDS takes 10–12 years, although approximately 10% of those who are HIV positive will progress to AIDS within 2–3 years of infection (NIAID, 2005). According to the prevailing CDC definition (CDC, 1993), HIV-infected people with fewer than 200 $CD4^{+}$ T cells per cubic millimeter of blood and manifesting at least one Category C **opportunistic illness** are considered to have AIDS. As the disease progresses and opportunistic illnesses accrue, people with HIV often experience cognitive, motor, and behavioral manifestations including memory impairment, poor concentration, incoordination, weakness, irritability, and depression. More severe neurological deterioration may occur, especially with high viral loads (NIAID, 2005).

MEDICAL INTERVENTIONS AND ADVANCES

Clearly the best treatment for HIV is prevention. Prevention strategies entail raising public awareness, providing education, and promoting individual behaviors that avoid risk or minimize harm. Prevention strategies can have a dramatic impact as illustrated by the reduction in the rates of new infection among gay men and in Thailand, where safe sex campaigns have been successful (Curran, 2003). Scientists continue to focus on developing effective barriers to the virus and vaccinations that would protect people from sexual transmission (Armstrong, Calabrese, & Taege, 2005).

For those infected with HIV, advances in pharmaceutical interventions have made notable impact upon survival and extended years of quality life. It is no longer unusual for people to experience 15 or more years of quality life from the time of diagnosis. The use of zidovudine during pregnancy (CDC, 1994) is among the most successful advances; it dramatically reduces transmission of the virus to infants born to HIV-positive mothers to a rate of about 1% (NIAID, 2005). Even though they may test positively for antibodies to HIV at birth, only a very small number of newborns now go on to develop the disease. As women tend to underestimate their risk and because prenatal transmission to infants can be prevented, in 2001 the CDC recommended that all pregnant women be routinely tested for HIV (CDC, 2001).

For infected adults, three categories of drugs have evolved and are currently used to treat HIV. Reverse transcriptase inhibitors interrupt the viral cycle early in its proliferation, and protease inhibitors interrupt it later. The third class of drugs, fusion inhibitors, interferes with viral reproduction by blocking the cell membrane, preventing permeation of HIV. Combination therapies, called highly active antiretroviral therapy or **HAART**, are aimed at curtailing HIV at multiple points along its reproductive cycle. For those who tolerate and respond to HAART, the drugs can retard the progression of HIV and even restore some immune functions for those with AIDS (NIAID, 2005). Long-term use of HAART does seem to be associated with detrimental side effects including fat redistribution, insulin resistance, poor lipid profiles, and increased risk of myocardial infarction (Armstrong, Calabrese, & Taege, 2005; NIAID, 2005).

PROGNOSIS AND MITIGATING FACTORS

Numerous strains of HIV have been identified, and the virus tends to customize itself within the individual. Some people seem to be more resistant to rapid translation than others. Viral load and strength of the particular HIV strain also seem to be associated with the rate of progression of the disease. Concurrent diseases or poor health status before infection can increase vulnerability and complicate medical interventions. Early detection of infections and adherence to medication regimens can prevent or slow the virus from usurping the entire immune system. Unfortunately, not everyone has access to testing, and not everyone responds positively to the drugs. For many people infected with HIV, sociopolitical circumstances erect barriers to health.

THE SOCIOPOLITICAL CONTEXT OF HIV/AIDS

HIV infection is most frequently attributed to unprotected sexual intercourse and behaviors that are generally not socially acceptable, such as illegal intravenous drug use and commercial sex. History demonstrates that people tend to underestimate their risk of exposure, and HIV infections are now permeating the mainstream heterosexual population in the United States. People with HIV often report being stigmatized or marginalized, and the potential for discrimination is very real. In the United States, HIV is most prevalent among men who have sex with men. Minorities, especially poor women of color, are disproportionately infected and vulnerable to exclusion, stigmatization, and discrimination (Dean et al., 2005; Duffy, 2005). The distribution of HIV represents one among many disconcerting **health disparities** in the United States.

Gay Men

Although discrimination against gay men has long been an issue, the gay community has some attributes that yielded some positive preventive responses. Higher levels of education, access to resources, and community mobilization allowed the gay community to promote education and prevention strategies (Curran, 2003; Fan, Connor, & Villareal, 2004). Concerns about confidentiality and employer discrimination may deter access to appropriate health care. To be effective, occupational therapists providing treatment to gay and bisexual men must be culturally sensitive. Unconventional life partners and families are likely to be involved in care, and the occupational therapist should be aware that the gay community has established many agencies, programs, and support networks that can enhance quality of life for people living with HIV/AIDS.

Women with HIV/AIDS

Poor women of color are disproportionately represented among those with HIV infection. According to the 2000 census data, African American and Hispanic women constitute approximately 25% of the total population but represent over 83% of HIV cases among women (CDC, 2006; United States Census Bureau, 2000). These women are generally socioeconomically disadvantaged and often disempowered. Their stories often reveal family violence, disrupted education, dependency upon exploitive men, and engagement in high-risk behaviors such as drug and alcohol use and commercial sex. General health literacy is poor, and health status even before infection may have been compromised. Therapists need to be particularly sensitive to the context in which these women live to avoid unreasonable expectations of them and exposure to increased harm from unempathic people. To attend to their own health, these women may need housing and transportation assistance, childcare, and partner or family counseling.

People Who Abuse Drugs and Alcohol

For people who have been actively using drugs and/or alcohol, sobriety is critical to improving health. HIV infection often leads to an epiphany that provides a powerful incentive for getting clean and sober (Opacich, 2004). Since chemical dependency is a complex biopsychosocial phenomenon, it is important to collaborate closely with expert colleagues and to encourage participation in programs designed to support sobriety.

Impact on Scientific and Health Resources

Despite the tremendous social and economic impact of HIV/AIDS on nations worldwide, resources are still inadequate to meet needs. Over the years, programs have emerged that attend to the social complexities as well as the medical needs of people with HIV/AIDS. Many of these programs rely on grants and resources from state, federal, and private agencies. Treating HIV/AIDS successfully requires an array of health and human services and a culturally competent workforce to deliver those services. Labor statistics reveal shortages in many of those disciplines.

In 2004, $415 billion were allocated to state and local health departments for AIDS prevention (Rand Health, 2005). Along with other sexually transmitted diseases, AIDS prevention efforts in the United States have largely been funded by the CDC. It appears that these efforts have been somewhat successful in containing gonorrhea, but their cost effectiveness in curtailing AIDS is yet unknown (Chesson et al., 2005). Cost of treatment for each person with HIV/AIDS has been estimated to be $20,000 to $100,000 each year (Schackman, Feedberg, & Goldie, 2005). Given the demographics of those infected in the United States, a large proportion of those who are HIV positive are uninsured. The Ryan White Comprehensive AIDS Resources Emergency Act (CARE Act) provided over $2 billion in assistance to individuals and families through state-administered programs in 2004 (Government Accounting Office, 2005); however, poor health literacy, disempowerment, and stigmatization may still limit access to health resources.

CONTRIBUTION OF OCCUPATIONAL THERAPY IN THE TREATMENT OF HIV/AIDS

A growing body of professional literature attests to successful and potential occupational therapy contributions in addressing the needs of people with HIV/AIDS. Disease trends have stimulated research about the particular needs of women and the challenges people with HIV face in returning to work. To date, most of the literature has yielded program recommendations and educational strategies rather than evidence of effectiveness. Occupational therapy interventions for HIV/AIDS can be enhanced by the use of instruments that address underlying abilities and capacities that lead to competency in occupational performance and that measure outcomes of therapy.

Framing Occupational Problems and Developing Interventions

HIV insinuates itself into the human body and into every aspect of daily life. Although the diagnosis of HIV is devastating to some people, it becomes the vehicle to a more meaningful and productive life to others. An individual's response to untoward events, including HIV infection, seems to depend on both internal and external resources and individual capacities. When establishing goals for occupational therapy treatment, it will help the therapist to think in terms of **occupational role integrity**, **occupational competencies**, and overall **occupational coherence**.

Since occupational functioning is the culmination of abilities and capacities that shape activities, tasks, and roles, multiple strategies may be needed to sort out occupational dysfunction. Although some problems in occupation may be directly attributable to AIDS-related illness, others may reflect contextual challenges or histories that prevented the development of occupational competency.

Neurobiological Changes That Affect Occupation

At times, it can be difficult to distinguish symptoms associated with HIV/AIDS and those related to the treatment of the virus. Nevertheless, these symptoms can impact quality of life. For many years, the *Whalen Symptom Index* (Whalen et al., 1994) has been used to indicate how frequent and troublesome the symptoms are. The index focuses on 12 of the most commonly experienced symptoms: fatigue, fevers, imbalance, paresthesias, memory loss, nausea, diarrhea, sadness, sleep disturbance, skin problems, cough, and headache. The client is asked about the frequency of these symptoms over a 2-week period, and each symptom is scored on a 3-point scale. Cumulative scores are thought to vary proportionally with the impact of symptoms on the person's life. Combined with other data, the index informs the occupational therapist and other health providers so they may help the person with HIV to manage symptoms. Occupational therapists can recommend lifestyle modifications and compensatory strategies to cope with a number of symptoms.

Psychosocial Manifestations

Awareness of the social trajectory is equally important in the treatment of people with HIV/AIDS. As with any serious illness, initial diagnosis is usually followed by a grief response. Depression is common both initially and intermittently throughout the disease process. Education is vitally important at this time because many misperceive HIV as a certain and imminent death sentence. Some programs link newly diagnosed people with a peer outreach worker who can comfort and inform them about HIV and helpful resources. If connected to relevant services, the person with HIV is less likely to become socially isolated or marginalized. As the disease progresses, neurological changes may predispose the person with HIV to mood swings, prolonged depression, and cognitive impairment. Occupational therapists should be prepared to employ psychosocial strategies to combat psychomotor retardation that often accompanies depression and to facilitate participation in family and community life (see Chapters 35 and 36).

Qualitative Assessment Strategies

Each theoretical model of occupation is associated with instruments and strategies for framing occupation. An array of qualitative tools reflecting the **naturalistic paradigm** can be useful to reveal the nature of experience, in this case how an individual experiences HIV. Among these strategies, semi-structured interviews can elicit narrative reflecting occupations; one of the published narrative tools, the *Occupational Performance History Interview II*, is reflective of the Model of Human Occupation (Kielhofner et al., 1998). This particular template is used to probe how a given illness, condition, or untoward event shaped or altered the person's occupations. This narrative data can be analyzed a number of ways and used to generate plans and strategies for reconstructing occupation.

Quantitative Assessment Strategies

Quantitative strategies are useful when the phenomenon in question is well defined and the query is focused. An example of a quantitative criterion-referenced tool useful for people with AIDS is the *Assessment of Motor and Process Skills* (Fisher, 1997). This tool enables the therapist to observe the person with HIV engaging in familiar tasks, to quantify, and compare the person's occupational performance, and to recommend strategies and levels of support necessary for safe living. The therapist might consider incorporating quality-of-life measures that reflect occupations and inform decision making (Robinson, 2004).

Preserving, Restoring, and Adapting Meaningful Doing

The Occupational Functioning Model organizes roles and the definition of self into self-maintenance, self-advancement, and self-enhancement (see Chapter 1). Occupational therapy may address any or all of these aspects with the person with HIV/AIDS, depending on the occupational status of that person both before and after HIV infection. As previously noted, some cohorts of people with HIV have led marginal lives that are likely to have stymied their occupational potential.

Preservation

In the early stages of HIV infection, it is important that the individual resume or establish routines, habits, and behaviors that preserve healthfulness. Along with established roles, the newly diagnosed person must now incorporate medication regimens and attend appointments for regular lab tests and check-ups. For those whose lifestyles involved drug use or commercial sex, HIV treatment also entails intensive redirection, psychotherapy, and peer support. If pharmaceutical interventions or the virus itself results in symptoms, the person with HIV can face additional challenges in work, parenting, self-care, or other occupational pursuits. Whether the patient is a child or an adult, preserving and adapting occupational roles is critically important for both physical and mental health. For people whose lifestyles entailed maladaptive behaviors, occupational therapy may well require role exploration that may have been derailed in childhood or adolescence or abandoned in adulthood. Strategies may include parenting classes, practicing independent living skills (e.g., laundry), and job training/retraining.

Restoration

As the disease progresses, it is common for people to experience periods of ill health and disruption of normal routines. Those with HIV/AIDS are immunocompromised and are therefore susceptible to illness and opportunistic infections. Improvement in health can occur when symptoms are addressed and HIV medication regimens bolster the immune system. Similar to cardiac rehabilitation, occupational therapy can be useful while the person is reconditioning and illness abates. During these times, therapy may entail work simplification or rebuilding endurance. Roles, routines, and habits related to work, self-care, and leisure may need to be negotiated and adjusted. When symptoms persist or abilities are permanently altered, the occupational therapist and the HIV-positive client should focus on adaptation.

Adaptation

As the immune system is overwhelmed, the person with HIV/AIDS is likely to lose abilities. Sensory deficits, weakness, incoordination, compromised memory, and other sequelae can compromise occupational roles and independent living. During this stage of illness, occupational therapy can facilitate adaptations that enable the person with HIV/AIDS to participate in daily life as fully as possible. This may entail environmental adjustments, adaptive strategies or assistive devices, personal assistance, or changes in living situation (see Chapters 19, 30, 32, and 33).

Integrity of Occupational Roles

In the initial interview, the occupational therapist working with a person with HIV/AIDS needs to develop a clear picture of the roles that characterize the person's life. Depending on the point along the disease trajectory at which the therapist encounters the recipient of services, evidence of role strain, role disruption, or role abandonment may be present. The therapist may find it useful to plot the person's role status on the Matrix of Occupational Status (Table 49-1) to establish a baseline for decision making and intervention.

Table 49-1. Matrix of Occupational Status for People with HIV/AIDS

Occupational Domain	Occupational Role	Discontinued	Disrupted	Adapted	No Change	Expanded
WORK	Parent/Caregiver Homemaker (IADL) Employee Entrepreneur Vocational Trainee Student					
PLAY/LEISURE	Participant/Observer Spectator Hobbyist Athlete					
SELF-CARE	Personal Care (ADL) Instrumental Activities of Daily Living (IADL) Health-Related Care Self-Advocacy Intimacy/Sexual Expression Spiritual/Devotional Expression					
Description of Occupational Context	Neighborhood/Community Home Environment Health Care Setting Social Network Employment Setting					

Role Strain

The occupational therapist should ascertain whether the HIV-positive person is responsible for the care of others. If there are children, life partners, elderly adults, or even pets in the household, the person with HIV may be experiencing the strain of taking care of others given the added burden of managing HIV. In addition, others in the family, however that family is constituted, may also have HIV.

Most people sustain multiple roles, and life is an exercise of juggling priorities and meeting obligations. Some individuals are very tenacious about their roles, even when their health is compromised. Since those with HIV frequently experience fatigue, it is important to designate time for rest and restoration throughout the day. The occupational therapist can help the person with HIV to establish role priorities, reserving time and energy to attend to personal health needs. This may entail negotiating and relinquishing some responsibilities and tasks to others or arranging for support (e.g., homemaker services).

Role Disruption

When immune system failure results in illness, the person with HIV might be confined to bed or hospitalized for brief or extended periods of time. This is not an unusual pattern and should be anticipated. The occupational therapist can help to plan strategies for dealing with health emergencies. Such strategies may include identifying babysitters, notifying family members, enlisting help from neighbors, calling health care providers, and arranging sick leave. When the individual with HIV is ready to resume a former role after a period of illness, the occupational therapist can assess, modify, and design rehabilitative strategies consistent with the person's state of health and abilities.

Role Abandonment

Many stories elicited from people with HIV reveal role abandonment. For those whose lives were dominated by chemical dependency, development may have been arrested and efforts diverted to the procurement of drugs or alcohol. For others who are HIV positive, depression or shame may have interrupted life plans. For still others, the symptoms and sequelae of HIV itself may have prevented full participation. Whatever the case, if reasonable health can be restored, then the occupational therapist may be the primary facilitator of role resumption or role exploration.

Occupational Competencies

At the start of therapy, the occupational therapist should generate a list of **occupational competencies** or skills relative to the roles the client fulfills. For example, if remunerative employment is relevant, the occupational therapist can help to delineate the skills the client has or needs to acquire to resume or pursue work. Some people with HIV/AIDS who had been unable to work have been restored to a level of health through HAART that makes employment feasible again (Kielhofner et al., 2004). The therapist might advocate on behalf of the client to accommodate special needs (e.g., flexible work schedules, longer rest periods, or accommodations for adaptive equipment). The occupational therapist may need to assist clients to develop strategies to compensate for low vision or for poor coordination

If the HIV-positive person is a homemaker, establishing routines to accomplish cleaning, shopping, laundry, and so on will be important. Safety in the kitchen, especially when handling sharp utensils, will prevent exposure of others to HIV-positive blood. If the person is living with family members or friends, the occupational therapist can help the individual to negotiate household responsibilities, rest and privacy needs, and accurate understanding of HIV/AIDS and healthy behaviors. Work simplification and energy conservation principles may be useful for coping with changes in strength, endurance, and sequencing tasks and activities. It is important to acknowledge that many people living with HIV/AIDS are impoverished and may be living in poor housing and unsafe environments, which pose additional challenges. For some, the social assistance surrounding HIV care may present new housing opportunities; the occupational therapist can guide the person through the establishment of a household, from obtaining utilities to paying bills to preparing meals.

Occupational Coherence

Occupational coherence speaks to the complementarity of roles, routines, habits, and behaviors that contribute to a progenerative life that, in totality, makes sense (Opacich, 2004). Coherence is a notion introduced by Antonovsky (1987), a sociologist, and later expanded by Nyamathi (1993). Coherence was first applied to occupations by Christiansen and colleagues (Christiansen, 1999; Christiansen, Little, & Backman, 1998) as an indicator for outcomes in the face of threats to health. Research on women with HIV/AIDS illustrates the construct by contrasting the lives of women living amidst chaos and uncertainty with those whose lives were more coherent (Opacich, 2004). If a person is ill with HIV, actively chemically dependent, and homeless, one would not describe that person as leading an occupationally coherent life. If that same person became sober, adhered to medical recommendations for arresting HIV, procured safe housing, and resumed remunerative employment, life would appear to be occupationally coherent and built upon meaningful doing. The ultimate goal of occupational therapy with people with HIV might well be the achievement of occupational coherence.

EVIDENCE OF EFFECTIVENESS OF OCCUPATIONAL THERAPY FOR PERSONS WITH HIV/AIDS

The literature pertaining to HIV/AIDS in occupational therapy is largely conceptual or phenomenological. It reflects the experience of people with HIV/AIDS and informs the development of programs and services. A number of those studies have been mentioned in this chapter. Very few studies have been designed to examine particular interventions or to quantitatively measure effectiveness of occupational therapy interventions.

CASE EXAMPLE

N.J.: Acquired Immunodeficiency Syndrome (AIDS)

Occupational Therapy Intervention Process	Clinical Reasoning Process: Objectives	Clinical Reasoning Process: Examples of Therapist's Internal Dialogue
Patient Information N.J. (a 49-year-old African American female with AIDS) participated in an outpatient occupational therapy assessment. The following problems were identified: (1) insufficient endurance for some ADL and IADL; (2) mild memory impairment and confusion that interferes with self-care; (3) ambiguity of roles and routines; (4) intermittent loss of balance impacting environmental mobility; and (5) paresthesias that affect the execution of fine motor tasks.	Appreciate the context	(The assessment process in general, including ascertaining personal background information, is described in Chapters 4–11).
	Develop intervention hypotheses	"N.J.'s poor endurance is a direct result of her extended hospitalization and convalescence, during which she was bedridden and tube fed. Since her recovery, she has abandoned former dysfunctional pursuits, leaving her to redefine her roles, habits, and routines. Her remaining symptoms are natural sequelae of HIV/AIDS and/or drug interventions."
	Select an intervention approach	"The first order of therapy will be to identify critical ADL and IADL that support recovery, such as adherence to medication regimens, establishing intermittent rest periods, and planning for proper nutrition. Given the reported sensory and cognitive issues, precautions and compensatory strategies need to be implemented to assure the patient's safety. Finally and probably most importantly, the patient needs to be supported in her role exploration and resumption for maximal participation in family and community life."
	Reflect on competence	"Do I have adequate understanding of the relevant epidemiology, neurobiology, pharmacology, and psychodynamics? Am I sufficiently culturally competent, and can I be effective with this patient? I will need to collect tools and strategies for role exploration and practice any specific administration protocols."

Recommendations

The occupational therapist recommended home-based care two times a week initially for 4 weeks and one time a week for the next 2 months. In collaboration with N.J., long-term goals for treatment were established as follows: (1) N.J. will identify which ADL and IADL tasks are indispensable to her management of HIV and will establish a daily schedule and record system for these; (2) N.J. will learn and implement home safety strategies relying on cue cards posted where most needed; and (3) N.J. will explore two roles or interests that will lead to safe and productive use of time.

Consider the patient's appraisal of performance

Consider what will occur in therapy, how often, and for how long

Ascertain the patient's endorsement of plan

"Since the initiation of the HAART protocol, N.J. has been slowly regaining her health and is more hopeful than she has been in years. She describes herself as having died and been reborn to a different life, and she says that she is actually grateful for HIV. She sees herself as having some special purpose. Since she once had many occupational competencies, she seems eager and able to reach her goals. N.J. is currently residing with her daughter and young grandchildren; they have agreed to support her in these goals and to be present for at least one in-home occupational therapy session each week."

Summary of Short-Term Goals and Progress

1. N.J. will identify which ADL and IADL tasks are indispensable to her management of HIV and will establish a daily schedule and a record system for these.

N.J. and her therapist identified the following ADL and IADL tasks as indispensable: 15 minutes of morning meditation, showering once a day, preparing her own breakfast and lunch, eating her evening meal with the family, taking her medications at 6-hour intervals, and taking a nap for 1 hour in the afternoon. N.J. developed a schedule for herself that she kept next to her bed and checked off after completing each task. At each occupational therapy session, the therapist reviewed these with N.J. and addressed any problems.

2. N.J. will learn and implement home safety strategies relying on cue cards posted where most needed.

N.J. and her therapist practiced safe methods of handling sharp objects in the kitchen and posted pictures of her using these procedures under the cabinets. With the assistance of the therapist, the family installed grab bars in the bathroom. The therapist also instructed N.J. in the use of a walker for those days when her balance felt precarious. N.J. also generated a list of emergency numbers that she programmed into her cell phone. The family also established a call system to check on her well-being.

3. N.J. will explore two roles or interests that will lead to safe and productive use of time.

Through interviews with the therapist, N.J. will tell stories of things that she did in the past that she found enjoyable and fulfilling. Responding to the Occupational Performance History Interview, N.J. related that she loved to sing, and she began attending choir practice one evening a week and singing in the church choir on Sundays. She also decided that she would like to try working in her daughter's grocery store, and she began doing this for 2 hours two times a week in the early afternoon.

Assess the patient's comprehension

Understand what she is doing

Compare actual to expected performance

Know the person

Appreciate the context

"As N.J. began to feel better, she seemed genuinely happy to have a structure to her life. She would relate stories of how dysfunctional she had become before she got so sick. Even on the days when she was very tired or experienced a setback, she expressed gratitude for being here to help raise her grandchildren."

"N.J. felt that she didn't need the safety procedures most of the time, but she began to accept that it was better to be cautious than to have an unnecessary accident. Even her family members would remind her to do things 'like in the pictures.' N.J. took the walker with her when she left the house because it just made her feel a little safer if she got dizzy."

"N.J. really enjoyed singing in church, and joining the choir gave her the opportunity to make some new friends who were very supportive. Working in her daughter's grocery store was tiring at first, but N.J. felt like she was able to help out and even began to repair the strained relationship with her eldest child. Even though she shares a room with her grandchildren in her youngest daughter's apartment, she seems very happy to be there."

Next Steps Revised short-term goals (1 month): • N.J. will identify one household task for which she will take responsibility on a daily basis. • N.J. will continue to adhere to established safety strategies and will report to the therapist any problems or other situations that seem to pose a threat to safety. • N.J. will increase her hours at the grocery store to a maximum of 3 hours daily depending on the state of her health.	Anticipate present and future patient concerns Analyze patient's comprehension Decide if the patient should continue or discontinue therapy and/or return in the future	"N.J. seems much healthier in a short period of time. She is enthusiastic about the church choir, and a few of the ladies have even begun to visit her at home. She is acutely aware of how important it is for her to eat well, rest, and take her medication. She has a frank and wonderful rapport with her physician, and she trusts her advice. N.J. has a tendency to do a little too much, and she needs to be reminded to add things into her schedule gradually. Despite everything that has happened to her, she is not at all bitter and seems to have accepted her diagnosis and its implications in her life."

CLINICAL REASONING IN OCCUPATIONAL THERAPY PRACTICE

HIV and Health Disparities

N.J. is representative of a group of people (poor women of color) known to manifest health disparities. What social, economic, and political conditions may contribute to disparities in health? How might these have affected the course of N.J.'s illness to date? How might occupational therapy address some of the consequences of health disparities in this case?

Evidence Table 49-1
Best Evidence for Occupational Therapy Practice Regarding HIV/AIDS

Intervention	Description of Intervention Tested	Participants	Dosage	Type of Best Evidence and Level of Evidence	Benefit	Statistical Probability and Effect Size of Outcome	Reference
Four-phase vocational program: (1) 8 weeks of self-assessment and preparation for work; (2) effort to reacquire productive roles through experiences; (3) support successful employment; (4) support sustained employment	Model of Human Occupation (MOHO)-based program customized to individual needs to explore, develop skills, and seek employment.	Convenience sample of 129 men and women with HIV/AIDS (106 males, 21 females, and 2 transgendered persons; mean age = 41 years); 30% attrition rate (39 of 129 participants).	Phase 1: 8 weeks, group session 1 time a week plus individual sessions. Length of subsequent phases varied by individual.	Qualitative research. Participatory action research to examine and improve the program as it unfolded. Level of evidence not rated.	Yes; 50 participants achieved employment, 2 returned to school, and 8 participated in volunteer or internship programs from 6–24 months after the program. Persons with a history of mental illness were *more likely* to benefit.	90 participants completed program; 67% of those achieved successful outcome. Effect size not reported.	Kielhofner et al., 2004

SUMMARY REVIEW QUESTIONS

1. How does the epidemiology of HIV differ in the United States compared with other countries?
2. By what mechanisms does HIV overwhelm the immune system?
3. What are the routes of transmission for HIV?
4. Which populations are most vulnerable to HIV/AIDS and why?
5. What information is yielded from particular qualitative strategies and quantitative measures that is useful for developing interventions for people with HIV/AIDS?
6. How are occupational roles affected by HIV/AIDS?
7. How does the illness trajectory impact occupational therapy interventions?

References

Antonovsky, A. (1987). *Unraveling the mystery of health: How people manage stress and stay well.* San Francisco: Jossey-Bass.

Armstrong, W., Calabrese, L., & Taege, A. J. (2005). HIV update 2005: Origins, issues, prospects, and complications. *Cleveland Clinic Journal of Medicine, 72,* 73–78.

Centers for Disease Control and Prevention [CDC]. (1993). *Revised classification system for HIV infection and expanded surveillance case definition for AIDS among adolescents and adults.* Washington, DC: United States Government Printing Office.

Centers for Disease Control and Prevention [CDC]. (1994) Recommendations of the U.S. Public Health Service Task Force on the use of zidovudine to reduce perinatal transmission of human immunodeficiency virus. *Morbidity and Mortality Weekly Report, 43,* RR-11.

Centers for Disease Control and Prevention [CDC]. (1999). *CDC guidelines for national human immunodeficiency virus case surveillance, including monitoring for human immunodeficiency virus infection and acquired immunodeficiency syndrome.* Washington, DC: United States Government Printing Office.

Centers for Disease Control and Prevention [CDC]. (2001). *Revised recommendations for HIV screening of pregnant women.* Washington, DC: United States Government Printing Office.

Centers for Disease Control and Prevention [CDC]. (2004). Division of HIV/AIDS Prevention: Basic statistics. Retrieved November 11, 2005 from http://www.cdc.gov/hiv/stats.htm.

Centers for Disease Control and Prevention [CDC]. (2006). Division of HIV/AIDS Prevention: Fact sheet-HIV/AIDS among women. Retrieved November 16, 2005 from
http://www.cdc.gov/hiv/pubs/facts/women.htm.

Chesson, H. W., Harrison, P., Scotton, C. R., & Varghese, B. (2005). Does funding for HIV and sexually transmitted disease prevention matter? Evidence from panel data. *Evaluation Review, 29,* 3–23.

Christiansen, C. H. (1999). Defining lives: Occupation as identity: An essay on competence, coherence, and the creation of meaning. *American Journal of Occupational Therapy, 53,* 547–558.

Christiansen, C. H., Little, B. R., & Backman, C. (1998). Personal projects: A useful approach to the study of occupation. *American Journal of Occupational Therapy, 52,* 439–446.

Curran, J. W. (2003). Reflections on AIDS, 1981-2031. *American Journal of Preventive Medicine, 24,* 281–284.

Dean, H., Steele, C., Satcher, A., & Nakashima, A. (2005). HIV/AIDS among minority races and ethnicities in the United States, 1999–2003. *Journal of the National Medical Association, 97 (Suppl.),* 5S–12S.

Duffy, L. (2005). Suffering, shame, and silence: The stigma of HIV/AIDS. *Journal of the Association of Nurses in AIDS Care, 16,* 13–20.

Fan, H. Y., Connor, R. F., & Villareal, L. P. (2004). *AIDS science and society* (4th ed.). Sudbury, MA: Jones and Bartlett Publishers, Inc.

Fisher, A. G. (1997). *Assessment of motor and process skills* (2nd ed.). Fort Collins, CO: Three Star Press.

Government Accounting Office. (2005). Ryan White CARE Act: Factors that impact HIV and AIDS funding and client coverage. (GAO-05-841T). Washington, DC: United States Government Accounting Office.

Gottlieb, M. S., Schroff, R., Schanker, H. M., Weisman, J. D., Fan, P. T., Wolf, R. A., & Saxon, A. (1981). *Pneumocystis carinii* pneumonia and mucosal candidiasis in previously healthy homosexual men: Evidence of a new acquired cellular immunodeficiency. *New England Journal of Medicine, 305,* 1425–1431.

Joint United Nations Program on HIV/AIDS [UNAIDS]. (2004). *Eastern European and Central Asia fact sheet.* Retrieved November 11, 2005 from http://www.unaids.org/bangkok2004/report.html.

Kielhofner, G., Braveman, B., Finlayson, M., Paul-Ware, A., Goldbaum, L., & Goldstein, K. (2004). Outcomes of a vocational program for persons with AIDS. *American Journal of Occupational Therapy, 58,* 64–72.

Kielhofner, G., Mallinson, T., Crawford, C., Nowak, M., Rigby, M., Henry, A., & Walens, D. (1998). *The user's manual for the Occupational Performance History Interview (Version 2) OPHI-II.* Chicago: University of Illinois at Chicago.

Masur, H.., Michelis, M. A., Greene, J. B., Onorato, I., Stoue, R.A., Holzman, R. S., Wormser, G., Brettman, L., Lange, M., Murray, H. W., & Cunningham-Rundles, S. (1981). An outbreak of community-acquired *Pneumocystis carinii* pneumonia: Initial manifestation of cellular immune dysfunction. *New England Journal of Medicine, 305,* 1431–1438.

Nakashima, A. K., & Fleming, P. L. (2003). HIV/AIDS surveillance in the United States, 1981–2001. *Journal of Acquired Immune Deficiency Syndrome, 32 (Suppl. 1),* S68–S85.

National Institute of Allergy and Infectious Diseases [NIAID]. (2004). How HIV causes AIDS. Retrieved November 11, 2005 from http://www.niaid.nih.gov/factsheets/howhiv.htm.

National Institute of Allergy and Infectious Diseases [NIAID]. (2005). HIV infection and AIDS: An overview. Retrieved November 11, 2005 from http://www.niaid.nih.gov/factsheets/hivinf.htm.

Nyamathi, A. M. (1993). Sense of coherence in minority women at risk for HIV infection. *Public Health Nursing, 10,* 151–158.

Ogunbodede, E. O. (2004). HIV/AIDS situation in Africa. *International Dental Journal, 54 (Suppl. 1),* 352–360.

Opacich, K. J. (2004). Reconstructing occupation after HIV infection: Lessons from women's experiences. *International Journal of Therapy and Rehabilitation, 11,* 516–524.

Rand Health. (2005). Fact sheet: Cost-effective allocation of Government funds for preventing HIV. Retrieved November 16, 2005 from http://www.rand.org/pubs/research_briefs/RB9132/RAND_RB9132.pdf.

Robinson, F. (2004). Measurement of quality of life in HIV disease. *Journal of the Association of Nurses in AIDS Care, 15 (Suppl.),* 14S–19S.

Schackman, B. R., Feedberg, K. A., & Goldie, S. J. (2005). Budget impact of Medicaid section 1115 demonstrations for early HIV treatment (maybe). *Health Care Financing Review, 26,* 67–80.

Siegal, F. P., Lopez, C., Hammer, G. S., Brown, A. E., Kornfeld, S. J., Gold, J., Hassett, J., Hirschman, S. Z., Cunningham-Rundles, C., Adelsberg, B. R., et al. (1981). Severe acquired immunodeficiency in male homosexuals, manifested by chronic perianal ulcerative herpes simplex lesions. *New England Journal of Medicine, 305,* 1439–1444.

United States Census Bureau. (2000). Census brief: Women in the United States: A profile. Retrieved November 16, 2005 from www.census.gov/prod/2000pubs/cenbr001.pdf.

Whalen, C., Antani, M., Carey, J., & Landefeld, C. (1994). An index of symptoms for infection with human immunodeficiency virus: Reliability and validity. *Journal of Clinical Epidemiology, 47,* 537–546.

CHAPTER 50

Oncology

Margarette L. Shelton, Joanna B. Lipoma, and E. Stuart Oertli

LEARNING OBJECTIVES

After studying this chapter, the reader will be able to do the following:

1. Understand the role of occupational therapy in cancer rehabilitation.
2. Identify role, tasks, and activity deficits that may affect occupational functioning, regardless of type of cancer diagnosis.
3. Identify types of interventions that may improve occupational functioning.
4. Become aware of some safety concerns when treating a person who has cancer.
5. Know how to access resources to improve the quality of care that one offers to a person who has cancer.

Glossary

Carcinoma—Cancers originating in the tissues of the body's organs.

Hematopoiesis—The process of blood formation.

Leukemia—Cancers involving the blood cells and blood-forming organs.

Lymphoma—Cancers arising in the lymphatic system; affect the B and/or T lymphocytes.

Lytic—Breakdown of bone marrow due to tumor invasion, putting person at risk of pathological fracture.

Palliative (care)—Supportive care aimed at symptom relief; relevant along the entire continuum of care; typically used at end of life when all other treatment has failed.

Sarcomas—Cancers of the bones and/or connective tissues.

Cancer: The word alone evokes fear and stigma. People equate the diagnosis of cancer with death. Yet heart diseases, not cancer, are the leading causes of death in the United States (American Cancer Society, 2006). One of two men and one of three women in the United States may be diagnosed with cancer in their lifetime. All ethnic groups are affected by the diagnosis, although some groups access screening and intervention earlier than others. Access to screening and intervention are among the determinants of prognosis and survival.

A diagnosis of cancer, then, challenges meanings and priorities in life. The person who lives with the diagnosis, as well as members of his or her support system, must adjust to changes and losses. The person with cancer (and this support system) is considered to be a survivor from the moment of diagnosis throughout the remainder of his or her life. Both the disease and its treatment can disrupt occupational functioning of the individual and his or her support system. Routines can be disrupted, valued roles and the activities associated with these roles can be lost, and impairments can lead to long-term disability in some cases.

Although this chapter focuses on the individual who has cancer, occupational therapists who work with this diagnostic population should also be aware of the impact the diagnosis has on the individual's social support system. Moreover, treatment of the person with cancer must take into account physical, emotional, cognitive, and spiritual needs to facilitate adjustment and maximize occupational performance.

CANCER STATISTICS: INCIDENCE AND ETIOLOGY

The American Cancer Society (ACS) (2006) predicted that 1.4 million new cases of cancer would be reported in 2006. Most new cases are **carcinomas**, cancers originating in the body's organs (The University of Texas M. D. Anderson Cancer Center [MDACC], 2006). In terms of reported incidences, men are most often affected by prostate (33% of predicted cases), lung (13%), and colorectal cancers (10%), while women are at greatest risk for breast (31%), lung (12%), and colorectal (10%) cancers. Other types of cancer, such as **leukemias** (cancers involving the blood cells, bone marrow, and other blood-forming organs), **lymphomas** (cancers arising in the lymphatic system), and **sarcomas** (cancers of the bones and/or connective tissues), have lower rates of incidence (ACS, 2006).

Cancers ultimately involve diseases of the body's cells. Anything that affects cells' reproductive function, altering genetic structures, can be considered a risk factor or cause for cancer. Environmental and cellular factors constitute the two primary sources of risk for developing cancer and contribute to cancers' underlying causes (ACS, 2006; Heath & Fontham, 2001; MDACC, 2006; Rohan & Budds, 2004).

Environmental factors may be considered in terms of lifestyle and environmental exposure. Lifestyle-related risk factors include diet (i.e., dietary exposure to carcinogens), obesity, and level of physical or leisure activity (ACS, 2006; Heath & Fontham, 2001). Smoking is part of the lifestyle of 90% of persons diagnosed with lung cancer (Van Cleave & Cooley, 2004). Other environmental factors include exposure to chemicals, such as asbestos or benzene; to radiation sources, as in ultraviolet rays present in sunlight; or to infectious processes, such as Epstein-Barr virus or hepatitis C virus. Cellular (or molecular) factors include genetic predisposition to cancer due to heredity or impaired immune system function (Heath & Fontham, 2001).

MECHANISMS OF CANCER: PATHOLOGICAL BASIS OF DIMINISHED CAPACITIES AND ABILITIES

Once a cell's DNA or genetic components change, those changes are copied in new cells as the altered cell divides. If the body does not have sufficient immune function or capability to repair its DNA and stop the cell division of the mutated cells, then cancer forms. The mutated cells subsequently lose functions and characteristics that define them histologically as a certain type of cell. They then proliferate to impinge on other cells or organs (Workman, 2004).

Cancers can be graded and staged. Tumors are graded in terms of degree of differentiation, that is, the degree to which the cell resembles the source tissue (Hutson, 2004). Staging is the process of determining the degree to which a cancer has progressed (Lenhard & Osteen, 2001). The TNM staging system, adopted by the International Union Against Cancer and the American Joint Committee on Cancer, is the most common method. It involves identification of (1) tumor size, (2) the number of lymph nodes to which the cancer has locally spread, and (3) the presence of metastasis (spread to more remote areas of the body). Staging helps physicians select the type of treatment that will be most appropriate for the patient, and it contributes to the estimate of prognosis. A stage I, grade 1 cancer is one where a tumor is present but has not infiltrated surrounding tissues, and its cells are well differentiated. In a stage III, grade 3 cancer, a tumor is large, has invaded other tissues and lymph nodes, and has poorly differentiated cells. Although they are beyond the scope of this chapter, the occupational therapist who works in oncology should know about the specific processes that occur in tumor formation and growth (angiogenesis) and during metastasis (Resources 50-1).

RESOURCE 50-1

Essential Resources for the Entry Level Occupational Therapist

Recommended Texts

These books will help you get started working with people who have cancer.

Cooper, J. (Ed.). (1997). *Occupational therapy in oncology and palliative care*. London: Whurr Publishers Ltd.
Treatment suggestions across the continuum of cancer care.

Kumiega, K. (1997). *Windows to cancer care: An occupational therapy treatment guide*. Bisbee, AZ: Imaginart.
Overview of oncology, assessment, treatment planning, and intervention.

Lenhard, R. E., Osteen, R. T., & Gansler, T. (2001). *The American Cancer Society's clinical oncology*. Atlanta: American Cancer Society.
Medical overview of various cancers, medical treatment, and symptom management; includes a chapter on cancer-related emergencies; good for more in-depth perspective.

Varricchio, C., Ades, T. B., Hinds, P. S., & Pierce, M. (Eds.). (2004). *A cancer source book for nurses* (8th ed.). Atlanta: American Cancer Society.
Comprehensive overview of cancers and treatment, treatment-related problems, and ancillary treatment.

Web Sites

The following are sites to help you access cancer information easily. These will also lead you to different topics, such as research, prevention, monitoring, and survivorship.

National Cancer Institute:
http://www.cancer.gov

Centers for Disease Control and Prevention:
http://www.cdc.gov/cancer/

American Cancer Society:
http://www.cancer.org

Lance Armstrong Foundation:
http://www.livestrong.org

Hospital Web Sites

The following web sites provide patient information and information about clinical trials.

Mayo Clinic:
http://www.mayoclinic.com/health/cancer/CA99999

Memorial Sloan-Kettering Cancer Center:
http://www.mskcc.org

The University of Texas M.D. Anderson Cancer Center:
http://www.mdanderson.org

Lung Cancers

Thomas et al. (2001) and Van Cleave and Cooley (2004) describe two classes of lung cancer. Small-cell lung cancers (SCLC) are derived from neuroendocrine cells, while non–small-cell lung cancers (NSCLC) arise from the epithelial types of tissues that line the lungs. Lung cancers tend to be diagnosed at later stages, when the cancer has metastasized to other sites and when other symptoms, such as weight loss, fatigue, pain, or osteoarthropathy (arthritis-like bone and joint pain), have become more prevalent and affect the individual's daily routines. These and other symptoms, such as weakness, shortness of breath, dyspnea, or neurologic changes indicative of brain metastasis, contribute to individuals' diminished capacities and abilities. Occupational therapists can intervene to help persons with lung cancers modify their lifestyles to accommodate these changes in bodily function, as seen in Case Example 50-1 about Joan.

Hematological Cancers

Hematological cancers consist of three major classes of stem cell diseases: leukemias, lymphomas, and multiple myeloma. As a group, these cancers comprise the fifth most commonly occurring cancers and the second leading cause of cancer deaths in the United States (Hematological Cancer Research Investment and Education Act of 2001: S1094, 2002). More than 100,000 U.S. residents are diagnosed each year with blood cancers, and 60,000 people die annually. At any one time, about 700,000 individuals are living with blood cancers in the United States, and management of their cancers is a monumental task. Typically, patients diagnosed with blood cancers are managed by

CASE EXAMPLE # 1

Joan: A Patient with Lung Cancer

Occupational Therapy Process	Clinical Reasoning Process: Objectives	Clinical Reasoning Process: Examples of Therapist's Internal Dialogue
Patient Information Joan is a 60-year-old woman who has a history of metastatic lung cancer that was diagnosed 3 years ago. Prior to the diagnosis, she worked as a high-level manager with a premier telecommunications company; she retired after she was diagnosed with cancer.	Understand the patient's diagnosis or condition	"Given the presence of brain and liver metastases, along with ascites and lymphedema, this cancer appears to be in advanced stages. Her doctor will not indicate her prognosis."
The cancer was treated with chemotherapy and radiation. Most recently, she received whole-brain radiation to treat metastases in the brain. She has a history of liver metastases (mets), bilateral pleural effusions, and ascites (accumulation of fluid in the abdomen). She currently has mets to her lumbar spine, left ribs, left iliac crest, both femora, and her sacrum. She presents with fatigue, lymphedema, and decreased appetite. Joan lives alone. She arrived for her appointment in the company of her brother, who lives about an hour from her in another community.	Know the person	"Joan's background indicates that she is someone who is used to being in control. She is also used to living alone, which might be compromised if she has any problems with self-care or mobility."
Reason for Referral to Occupational Therapy Joan was referred to outpatient occupational therapy to assess her equipment needs.	Appreciate the context Develop provisional hypotheses	"I wonder what equipment she might need and what she would be willing to accept. I will plan for possible wheelchair, bathroom equipment, and assistive devices for ADL; possibly other interventions are needed as well."
Assessment Process and Results This setting uses a non-standardized, structured evaluation that includes measures of self-care, mobility, and sensorimotor and cognitive components and allows for interview. Findings are noted as follows:	Consider evaluation approach and methods	"Using the center's evaluation lets me explore not just the problem that brought Joan to the clinic but also to make sure there are no other functional problems that might otherwise not be addressed. Time constraints may prevent selection of other standardized assessments."
• Joan's chief complaints are lymphedema and difficulty with mobility and transfers. For example, she has difficulty getting in and out of her bed, the top of which is 28″ from the floor; she has difficulty rising from the built-in shower bench she sits upon when she bathes; and she is unable to walk the length of her home without experiencing severe shortness of breath and fatigue. • Her home and support system: Joan lives alone in a two-story home; her bedroom and bathroom are on the first floor. Doorways are wide for wheelchair accessibility, but the thresholds range in height from 3.5″ to 6.0″. Her shower has a 6″ threshold, and there is a low built-in bench for her to sit on when she bathes. The shower walls are lined with marble, which she refuses to mar/modify. Her brother and her friends check on her regularly.	Interpret observations	"Joan has a strong desire to remain in her home and to be safe there. We will have to work together within the boundaries of what she is willing to accept. She may accept ramps for thresholds to the outdoors, for example, but not grab bars in the shower. Will she accept a wheelchair?"

- Sensorimotor and cognitive capacities: Joan has a history of falls and has a call alert system. She rates her shortness of breath as 10/10 after activity. Her fatigue is 8/10 at rest and 10/10 after activity. Endurance is poor. She has no complaints of pain. Standing (static and dynamic) balance is impaired. She lacks approximately 50% of full ROM in both shoulders, her gross upper extremity strength ranges from 4 to 4–/5 (left weaker than right), and her grip strength is in the 25th percentile (35 lb on left; 40 lb on right). She has lymphedema in all extremities, and she has ascites. She complains of chemotherapy-induced neuropathy in both feet and is most comfortable walking barefooted. Joan is cognitively intact.
- Self-care and home management: Joan is modified independent in most ADL and prefers to bathe with supervision. She has altered her clothing preference to accommodate limitations in upper/lower extremity dressing as well as the lymphedema and ascites, and she takes longer to perform self-care activities. She prepares meals in a microwave oven, "not doing normal cooking." She requires assistance with housekeeping and grocery shopping. She has a dog that is staying with her brother, and she would like for her pet to return home if she could care for it and walk it. She enjoys doing needlepoint, reading, and gardening.
- Other: Joan lives in a community that is about an hour away from the medical center, and she is unwilling to come for outpatient treatment on a regular basis. She would be willing to come for 1–2 visits to plan for equipment.

Occupational Therapy Problem List

- Severe fatigue and poor endurance
- Limited mobility: getting in and out of bed, getting in and out of shower, moving about her home
- Needs wheelchair
- Consider home modifications

Synthesize results

"Besides problems with falling, her function is affected by severe fatigue and poor endurance. The lymphedema is not a problem that can be addressed; it is widespread, and there is no place for the fluid to go. The lymphedema limits her ROM. Distance and desire prevent her from attending many sessions, so treatment must be focused on issues and brief."

Occupational Therapy Goal List

1. Joan will use adaptive equipment and assistive devices of her own choosing to move about her home with modified independence.
2. Joan will make changes in her daily routines to assure that she has adequate energy to complete desired activities.
3. Joan will identify acceptable home modifications to ensure her safety.

Develop intervention hypotheses

"Joan is cognitively able to grasp instruction in energy conservation and suggestions for home modification. She has her brother's support to remain in her home safely."

Select an intervention approach

"My intervention approach is based on the theory of Occupational Adaptation (Schkade & Schultz, 1992). The individual selects the activities and goals that are important to her, and my role is to facilitate her internal process. In this way, I can honor Joan's autonomy and her ability to decide what is best for her by providing her sets of realistic choices."

Consider what will occur in therapy, how often, and for how long

"In accordance with her wishes and goals, Joan will be seen for one to two visits, each lasting 1 hour, for the next 2 weeks."

Intervention • As part of the evaluation, Joan demonstrated the difficulty she had getting into and out of bed, which was fairly high. She and the occupational therapist used a hydraulic mat to simulate the bed height and were able to determine that a wide 6″ high step would facilitate her mobility. Her brother constructed the step for her after the session. The occupational therapist also consulted with one of the staff physical therapists about using a standard walker with no wheels to step into and out of the shower and to help her rise from sitting on the built-in bench. After practicing, she purchased the walker as an out-of-pocket expense. Joan and her therapist reviewed principles of energy conservation, and the therapist provided her with written instructions about energy conservation. • The occupational therapist arranged for an outside consulting occupational therapist to provide a "pro bono" home assessment. This occupational therapist visited her home between her outpatient sessions and also built a ramp for outdoor access. • Joan would not accept a manual wheelchair, but she did accept powered mobility. At the last session, an assistive technology specialist worked with the occupational therapist to fit her in a power wheelchair. The occupational therapist drafted a letter of medical necessity, which was signed by the referring physician. Joan did accept a manual wheelchair as a "loaner" while she waited for the power wheelchair to be delivered.	Assess the patient's comprehension Understand what she is doing Compare actual to expected performance Know the person Appreciate the context	"Joan clearly comprehended solutions and instructions. She provided directions regarding her needs to climb into and out of bed, which her brother could address. She offered her own strategies regarding energy conservation." "I was fortunate to be able to enlist the assistance of the outside consultant. We worked together to gain an appreciation of her home environment, and Joan appreciated his level of professionalism and service." "Joan viewed the powered wheelchair as a means of remaining independent in her home and in her community. Furthermore, it would not deplete her energy as a manual wheelchair would."
Next Steps Discontinue services.	Anticipate present and future patient concerns Analyze patient's comprehension Decide if the patient should continue or discontinue therapy and/or return in the future	"Joan felt that she had satisfactorily achieved her goals and expressed no other concerns. Her brother informed me that she died about 1 month after our visits. I canceled the power chair order, and the "loaner" chair was returned. Should I have ordered the power chair? I think so. First, her prognosis was not clear, and her doctor could not offer clarification. Second, she was able to accept an alternative arrangement that helped her to move around safely in her home. Finally, the diagnosis should not prevent me from facilitating the amelioration of an individual's quality of life."

CLINICAL REASONING IN OCCUPATIONAL THERAPY PRACTICE

Building Rapport

Joan's case depicts a situation where the evaluation (and treatment) needs to be comprehensive yet focused. How does a clinician build rapport in such a short period of time? How can the clinician stay focused in his or her treatment?

multidisciplinary teams of health care professionals; occupational therapists are often key members of these treatment teams.

Hematopoiesis (blood formation) is an orderly biological process by which pluripotent stem cells form normal and mature blood cells including lymphocytes, granulocytes, erythrocytes, and platelets (Weisman, 2000). With hematological cancers, abnormalities in cell signaling result in uncontrolled cell growth or division, followed by "arrested development" or poor differentiation of cells during the conversion of the stem cells into mature blood cells. These changes often result in an accumulation of immature blood cells that cannot perform normal physiological functions of blood cells. In addition, the proliferation of one type of cell overwhelms the normal physiological functions of other cells, resulting in disease. The remainder of this discussion will focus on leukemia.

Leukemias are blood diseases originating in the blood-forming organs (Mandrell, 2004; Miller & Grodman, 2001). They can affect lymphocytes, white blood cells, red blood cells, or platelets. They are acute or chronic in nature. In acute leukemias, the cells fail to mature as they proliferate and infiltrate the bone marrow and other organs, particularly the lymph nodes, spleen, and liver, as well as the central nervous system (CNS) in some types of disease. In chronic leukemias, the cells proliferate, but they reach maturity and differentiate into distinct functional components (Mandrell, 2004; Miller & Grodman, 2001). The proliferation of cells still affects organs. Cell maturation and differentiation can continue for several years before a blast crisis (proliferation of cells that fail to mature) occurs.

In the case of acute leukemias, numerous symptoms can limit an individual's capacities and abilities. Anemia augments one's sense of fatigue and lack of activity tolerance due to poor endurance. Edema can occur that limits mobility. When cells infiltrate the bone marrow, the person may experience bone and joint pain or be at risk for pathologic fractures (Safety Note 50-1). When cells infiltrate the CNS, one's cognitive function may be affected. Susceptibility to infection and to bruising also affects functional capacities. With chronic leukemias, fatigue primarily affects individuals' functional capacities and abilities.

SAFETY NOTE 50-1

General Precautions in Treatment

- Before you enter a patient's room, read the chart and check with the patient's nurse to find out if any events or changes have occurred since your last visit.
- Practice universal precautions. You will protect the patient and prevent spread of infection to others.
- Be familiar with handling oncological emergencies (See Resource 50-1), and observe precautions as necessary. Categories of oncological emergencies include: obstructive/compressive, hematological/immune, metabolic, those related to increased pressure or fluid accumulation, and pathological fractures (Garrett & Kirchner, 1995; Hockett, 2004; Tatu, 2005). Although some of these conditions/emergencies may not prevent you from working with individuals who have cancer, you should know how to respond should one occur.
- Regarding the use of physical agent modalities:
  - Follow all standard precautions regarding their use.
  - Do NOT apply thermal or electrical modalities over areas of active or potential malignancies.
  - Avoid areas with altered skin integrity (i.e., radiation sites, graft vs. host disease, chemotherapy burns, etc.).
  - Inappropriate use of modalities may exacerbate conditions, such as lymphedema.
- Regarding the use of exercise:
  - Consider the impairment or condition. Aggressive exercise may be contraindicated, as in the presence of spinal cord compression, lymphedema, or pathologic fracture.
  - With myelosuppression, platelet counts are of concern. It IS safe to engage the patient in light ADL or to provide up to 5 lb of resistance when platelet counts are lower than 20 k/μL.
- When in doubt, consult with your clinical instructor or supervisor.

Sarcoma

As a collection of diseases, sarcomas include both soft tissue sarcomas and primary bone tumors. Of the two, soft tissue sarcomas are nearly four times more common (American Cancer Society, 2005), but they are rare in adults (Yasko et al., 2001). Soft tissue sarcomas include tumors that develop from fat, muscle, nerve, fibrous tissues surrounding joints, blood vessels, and deep skin tissues. Primary bone tumors arise from both bone and cartilage. Most sarcomas are found in the legs, but they can arise in any part of the body. According to Yasko et al. (2001), soft tumor sarcomas have no identified etiological factor, although some genetic conditions and previous treatment for cancer have been identified as predisposing factors. People who have either primary bone tumors or soft tissue sarcomas typically require the services of rehabilitation professionals during the course of treatment, particularly in the post-operative period.

The primary pathological basis of diminished capacities related to engagement in occupation for persons with sarcoma can be directly attributed to tumor growth at the primary site of disease and metastatic disease spread to secondary sites. Treatment of the disease itself can result in a secondary pathological basis for diminished capacities in that it frequently alters body structures and/or functions to the point of disability.

Tumor growth, whether at the primary site or in the form of a metastatic lesion, will frequently result in weakened body structures. Primary and metastatic bone tumors, particularly **lytic** lesions, may weaken the bone to the point of pathological fracture. Tumor growth may also impair circulatory function, resulting in edema, and can compress nerves and invade muscle or joint structures, causing pain or altered sensory perception and limiting range of motion.

Effects of Treatment on Functional Capacities and Abilities

As noted earlier, not only do the various cancers affect individuals' functional capacities, but treatment for those cancers can also affect individuals' function and ability to engage in valued roles and activities. The course of treatment for different cancers can involve multiple modalities, such as surgery, chemotherapy, and/or radiation, as well as experimental therapies. These treatments occur at different intervals and present individuals with physical, cognitive, and emotional challenges. Treatment can lead to frequent disruptions of lifestyle and activities. Furthermore, cancer and its treatment generate feelings of uncertainty with regard to the future, which makes it difficult for some individuals to engage in planning daily activities and routines. Finally, in cases where the cancer is progressing or the treatment produces side effects, individuals experience progressive functional loss (Bertero, Eriksson, & Ek, 1997; Schumacher et al., 1998).

In general, people with cancers may present to the occupational therapy clinic with a myriad of somatic, cognitive, and psychosocial problems. Impairments that impact the body's structures and functions can limit performance patterns and hinder performance in areas of occupation (American Occupational Therapy Association [AOTA], 2002). Chemotherapy-induced peripheral neuropathy can be extremely painful and limit mobility as well as hand dexterity. People may also display tremors following chemotherapy, which interfere with fine motor function. Radiation causes fibrosis (scarring of internal structures), which can limit movement and can sometimes impinge upon nerves to cause peripheral nerve injury (Cooper, 1998). Edema can occur independently of cancer treatment, while lymphedema is typically a sequela to surgery and/or radiation that involves one or more lymph nodes. Incidentally, lymphedema is a lifetime risk, and occupational therapists should seek training to provide specialized treatment (see Case Example 50-2). It is not uncommon to observe musculoskeletal changes, such as arthritis or arthropathy, fascial tightening, or frozen shoulder, in persons who undergo cancer treatment. Fatigue, pain, and nausea are frequent side effects of treatment.

CASE EXAMPLE #2

Mrs. K.: Assessing One's Clinical Competence

Occupational Therapy Intervention Process	Objectives	Clinical Reasoning Process: Examples of Therapist's Internal Dialogue
Patient Information Mrs. K. is a 50-year-old woman with a diagnosis of left postmastectomy lymphedema with multiple infections and fibrosis. Mrs. K. underwent mastectomy for left breast cancer 15 months ago and had 20 of her lymph nodes removed on the left side. She had chemotherapy and irradiation and now shows no evidence of disease. She recently saw her oncologist with complaints of left upper extremity swelling and aching heaviness in the arm and across her chest and back. She reported difficulty with fit of clothing on the left, which causes her increasing embarrassment at work. Her sleep is also disturbed because of left arm discomfort. She is referred to outpatient occupational therapy for evaluation and treatment of lymphedema, including manual lymph drainage, compressive bandaging, fitting of custom compressive garments, and instruction in home exercises and skin care.	Appreciate the context	"I wonder how much Mrs. K. knows about lymphedema and how to manage it. I wonder what kind of work she does along with other kinds of activities. Do any of these need to be modified in order to prevent recurrence of lymphedema once it is under control? Does Mrs. K. have a support system in place to which she can delegate tasks to prevent further exacerbation of the lymphedema?"

While the occupational therapist had previous experience treating cancer patients and instructing in self-care, home management, and work simplification strategies, she had no specific or specialized training in the area of lymphedema management. Because this new area of practice interested her, she searched the internet for information. She readily found information on lymphedema and its treatment (www.cancer.org) and guidelines for contacting a lymphedema treatment center, information about training programs, and names of clinicians with specialized training (www.lymphnet.org). She searched the National Library of Medicine (www.nlm.nih.gov) for abstracts of research regarding treatment of lymphedema.	Develop intervention hypotheses	"It appears that Mrs. K. needs a specialized form of intervention."
	Reflect on competence	"I am an occupational therapist working in a small physical disabilities setting at a suburban hospital in the Midwest. I have 5 years of experience, working in long-term care for 1 year and for 4 years in my present position. I typically work with both inpatients and outpatients, primarily with orthopedic or neurological problems. I am concerned that I don't have the expertise that is required to perform the manual lymph drainage or the fitting for a compression garment in this case."

Recommendations

Having some preliminary information, the occupational therapist used American Occupational Therapy Association Standards of Continuing Competence to assess her competence to treat Mrs. K. She concluded that she did not have the knowledge, critical reasoning, or performance skills necessary to assess and treat Mrs. K. She used information from her internet search to provide Mrs. K. with suggestions to help minimize the impact of lymphedema in her daily life and to refer Mrs. K. to another facility with specially trained therapists. She also decided to pursue training herself to make these services available to patients at her hospital.

Cognitive dysfunction is also a byproduct of cancer treatment. Patients who are in isolation sometimes experience the effects of sensory deprivation. In some, dysfunction manifests itself as impaired executive functions, slowed information processing, short attention spans, and impaired short-term memory. The symptoms may lead to social withdrawal. An occupational therapist might also observe altered safety awareness, judgment, and problem solving in some individuals. At times, cancer treatment can unmask underlying cognitive disorders, such as dementia, or neurological disorders, such as parkinsonism. Effects of treatment on psychosocial adjustment will be discussed later.

As one becomes more familiar with different types of cancer, one can begin to anticipate diagnosis- and treatment-related problems, just as one would with other conditions. For example, in the case of sarcoma, treatment-related changes to body structures may also limit engagement in occupation. Surgery may require amputation of all or part of an extremity. A limb salvage procedure, on the other hand, often results in significant, often lifelong, post-operative restrictions. Less invasive treatments for sarcoma, such as chemotherapy, are frequently associated with such symptoms as fatigue, nausea and vomiting, alopecia, and neutropenic fever related to anemia, leukopenia, and thrombocytopenia. Chemotherapy may also result in neurological changes such as hearing loss and peripheral neuropathy. External-beam radiation, a frequently used pre-operative treatment (Yasko et al., 1997), may result in decreased elasticity of the skin or other soft tissues and in diminished or absent protective responses at the irradiated site.

EXPECTED COURSE OF RECOVERY (OR DECLINE)

The expected course of recovery depends on when cancer is detected and staged and on the individual's response to treatment. Generally, the earlier the cancer is detected and treated, the better the prognosis is for the individual. Trends suggest that long-term survival is improving for many types of cancer (ACS, 2006).

Morbidity associated with cancer treatment can be debilitating if not addressed appropriately. One's future ability to engage in occupation may be directly related to the intervention provided, and occupational therapists are instrumental in their understanding of the client factors that will influence performance. Unfortunately, stigma persists regarding the rehabilitation potential of cancer patients, which can subsequently limit their access to care. Pandey and Thomas (2001) identified the need to promote both physical and psychosocial rehabilitation for cancer patients while providing a comprehensive, multidisciplinary approach to prevent and treat disability. Occupational therapists need to be cognizant of their role in the rehabilitation of patients who have chronic conditions.

Lung Cancers

Lung cancers may be curable in early stages, but there is no effective screening method to detect them. They tend to be detected at advanced stages and have an overall 15% 5-year relative survival rate (ACS, 2006). Treatment of these cancers may entail surgery, chemotherapy, and/or radiation, which is determined by the type and stage of cancer and the goals of treatment (i.e., curative or **palliative**). People with lung cancer tend to be referred to occupational therapy to address quality-of-life issues related to maximizing performance in light of steady decline.

Hematological Cancers

People who have hematological cancers have periods of functional stability interspersed with varying rates of decline. Initially, they may attempt to remain engaged in areas of occupational performance, but immunosuppression, fatigue, and emotional distress may prevent them from doing so (Mandrell, 2004). This group of cancers has a 5-year relative survival rate of 49% (ACS, 2006). The trajectory of these cancers varies from person to person, depending upon exacerbations, type of treatment, and response to treatment. Leukemias are typically treated with multiple chemotherapies to induce and maintain remission or to reinduce remission should relapse occur. Following this course, the person may consider options for allogeneic (related or matched unrelated donor) bone marrow or peripheral-blood stem cell transplantation. Treatment can lead to debility, and people with hematological cancers benefit from rehabilitation and from interventions designed to facilitate psychosocial adjustment and activity planning.

Sarcoma

Sarcomas, too, can be cured if caught early. The 5-year survival rate for soft tissue sarcomas exceeds 90%. As previously discussed, the expected course of recovery is directly related to the severity and extent of treatment required to achieve complete tumor removal (if possible). In the past, amputation was thought to be the only surgical treatment option. Recent studies, however, have shown no significant differences between 5-year survival rates of amputation versus limb salvage (Bacci et al., 2002; Veth et al., 2003).

Limb salvage is surgery that preserves, repairs, or reconstructs critical structures needed for limb function (Yasko et al., 1997). The typical rehabilitation period for limb salvage is longer than that for an amputated limb. In the long run, whether amputation or limb salvage is chosen, individuals typically resume engagement in occupation. For example, people with limb salvage and those with amputation reported high levels of return to driving, relatively high levels of employment and participation in sexual relations, and moderate levels of participation in sports (Table 50-1) (Refaat et al., 2002).

PSYCHOSOCIAL ADJUSTMENT ISSUES

Many people view their experience of cancer as life altering. Some use the diagnosis as a springboard for growth and development, regardless of outcome. Almost all the people that we have encountered in our practices have experienced psychosocial adjustment issues, and many of them note that intervention and support to help with the resolution of these issues is lacking among health care professionals. Occupational therapists are well-equipped to address these issues.

One of the most challenging issues that patients face is the loss of control (Bertero, Eriksson, & Ek, 1997; Schumacher et al., 1998). Cancer and its treatment disrupt performance patterns, leading to occupational deprivation and loss of valued routines and roles. Moreover, people report distress when they lose control of their bodily functions due to side effects of treatment, such as nausea, vomiting, and diarrhea. Changes in one's body—weight loss due to disease, weight gain due to the use of

Table 50-1. Percentages of People Returning to Occupational Function after Limb Amputation Versus Limb Salvage Associated with Sarcoma

Activity	Limb Amputation (%)	Limb Salvage (%)
Require device for ambulation	83	50
Employed	74	77
Able to drive	90	92
Engaging in sports	68	58
Participating in sexual relations	88	75

From Refaat et al., 2002.

steroids, hair loss—also affect one's sense of well-being. Loss of control may induce a sense of helplessness and dependence, especially when one is unable to perform activities previously taken for granted or to meet role expectations. Some people express uncertainty about the future in light of disease progression and the frequency and effects of treatment.

Persons with cancer also experience disruption of their social and cultural contexts. They may be physically removed from their support systems should they have to seek treatment in a distant community, state, or country. The stigma of cancer or the perceived burden of care may result in the loss of key social supports or, conversely, in the person's own social withdrawal. Finally, prolonged hospitalization, particularly when isolation is involved, may result in institutionalization, where the person becomes habituated to and dependent upon the hospital environment and fearful about leaving that environment.

Robinson et al. (1991) studied a group of 54 patients status post limb salvage to determine perceived quality of life and limb function 2 years after their procedure. The authors found that the most frequently reported deficit was decreased participation in leisure activities, an area of occupation frequently overlooked by clinicians working with cancer patients. Yet, the occupational therapist can facilitate psychosocial adjustment to changes in performance patterns by helping the client to identify alternative leisure opportunities and to develop the coping skills needed to deal with the reality of the expected outcomes of treatment.

Psychosocial adjustment certainly appears to be an area that needs attention. Nearly 25% of individuals studied after undergoing surgical treatment for sarcoma reported adjustment-related issues, such as depression, anxiety, sleep disturbance, need for pain medication, and diminished life satisfaction (Lane et al., 2001; Refaat et al., 2002). Procedures for Practice 50-1 provides further discussion about adjustment to loss.

PROCEDURES FOR PRACTICE 50-1

Adjustment to Loss

Cancer, regardless of its type, treatment, or course, can result in loss. Many of those losses are obvious and often temporary, such as the physical changes due to chemotherapy treatment (i.e., hair loss or peripheral neuropathy). Other losses are permanent. They are not only physical, but they also affect one's sense of identity. One's sense of self or body image may be altered as a result of mastectomy, orchiectomy, or limb amputation/salvage. Additional losses may include a loss of locus of control, social isolation or withdrawal, role changes, and impaired or absent body functions.

Interventions aimed at facilitating the adjustment to loss are well documented and include strategies ranging from patient journaling (Smith et al., 2005) to teaching caregivers stress management techniques (Kurtz et al., 2005). Some research suggests that a younger age at diagnosis is predictive of better long-term adjustment (Schroevers, Ranchor, & Sanderman, 2004).

Adjustment to loss is an important consideration for any occupational therapist working with the person who has cancer. Carver (2005) describes individuals as "goal-seeking beings whose efforts toward desired outcomes are threatened by diagnosis and treatment of cancer" (p. 2602). Carver believes that adaptation allows a person to remain engaged in the pursuits that form his or her life. Loss, however, is not only perceived by the individual diagnosed with cancer, but also by family, friends, and caregivers, and the occupational therapist must consider this when planning treatment.

MEMBERS OF THE TREATMENT TEAM AND THEIR ROLES

As with many diagnoses, the team involved in a person with cancer's care can be extensive. The staff involved in a person's care may vary according to the person's specialized needs (Figs. 50-1 and 50-2). The individual with cancer and his or her support system constitute the core of the team. Family members or other caregivers are often the primary providers of routine care at home and, to some extent, while the person is hospitalized.

Nursing staff—registered nurses and licensed vocational nurses—are essential care providers when people are hospitalized. They are frequently the primary contact at all points of patient care in both the inpatient and outpatient settings. A wound, ostomy, and continence nurse (WOCN) may be consulted to address wound care concerns and educate care providers in the management of poorly healing sores, incision sites, and ostomy sites. The certified nursing assistant attends to the day-to-day care of patients and as-

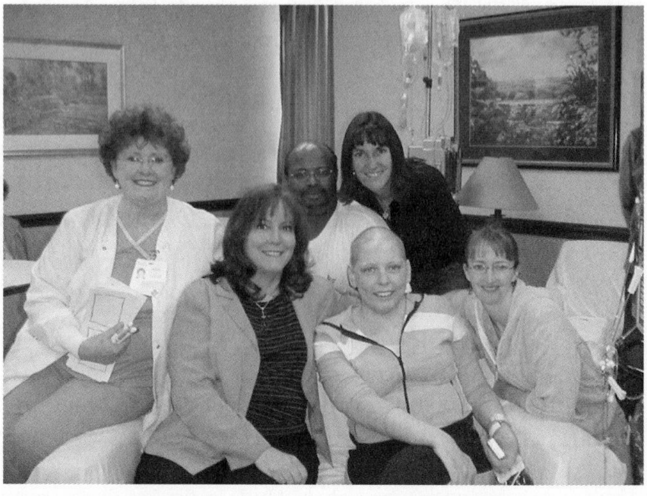

Figure 50-1 A patient with leukemia and her rehabilitation team.

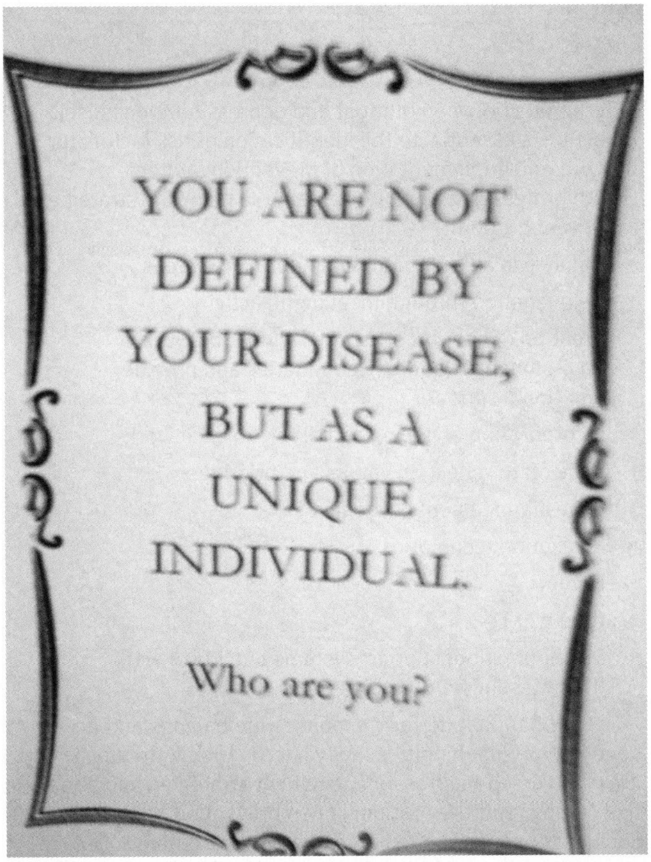

Figure 50-2 Patient-generated occupational therapy project to engage other patients.

sists them with many self-care tasks, including bathing and dressing.

Physicians tend to specialize in specific treatment domains, such as neurology, orthopedics, cardiopulmonary, physiology, and psychiatry. Other specialists include the following. Pathologists determine the type, stage, and grade of cancer. Medical oncologists direct the treatment of primary disease. Surgical oncologists treat cancer by resecting tumors and reconstructing damaged sites. Radiation oncologists design and implement high-energy radiation to treat cancer. Pain and palliative care specialists manage symptoms related to cancer and its treatment, and often help the individual and his or her support system to deal with end-of-life issues and transitions.

In addition to occupational therapists, physical therapists, and speech and language pathologists, professionals in other services may be consulted during the course of an individual's treatment. These may include orthotists or prosthetists, audiologists, case managers, chaplains, child life and young adult specialists, dieticians, massage therapists, music therapists, patient advocates, nurse practitioners, physician assistants, neuropsychologists, respiratory therapists, and social workers.

Finally, volunteers, particularly those who are cancer survivors, are vital partners of the medical team. They serve as friendly visitors in some instances, and as peer counselors and support group leaders in others. They help meet the needs of current patients through numerous hospital- or community-sponsored programs.

All team members are advised to recognize and try to prevent burnout so that they may best serve their patients (Procedures for Practice 50-2).

OVERVIEW OF OCCUPATIONAL THERAPY EVALUATION AND INTERVENTION PROCESS

Ideally, occupational therapy evaluation and treatment are guided by models of practice and evidence-based guidelines. A top-down approach allows the therapist and client to identify meaningful roles, levels of competency, and levels of satisfaction in carrying out the tasks and activities that support these roles. The therapist and client also identify the contexts in which valued roles are enacted. The client defines his or her values, goals, and quality of life.

Individuals with cancer have complex needs and priorities that can change, sometimes rapidly, depending on severity of illness, response to treatment, stage of cancer, stage of treatment, and so forth. The diversity of cancers and treatment regimens makes it challenging to establish definitive guidelines for practice. It is essential to continually reevaluate the client's performance, adaptation, goals, and plan of care.

Occupational Therapy Evaluation

Occupational therapists can establish rapport with a client by addressing immediate needs and by understanding who this person is, was, and wants to be through his or her narrative. The type of assessment chosen and the length of the evaluation process depend upon the individual's medical and cognitive status. Information can be collected from significant others, team members, and chart review. The clinician needs to understand the client's medical history, previous responses to and side effects of treatments, prognosis, and the current and potential impact of the disease and treatment on performance areas. In addition, precautions, such as immunosuppression, thrombopcytopenia, isolation (to prevent exposure to vancomycin-resistant *Enterococcus*, *Clostridium difficile*, fungoides, etc.), and anemia should be noted because these factors impact functioning and occupational therapy treatment.

The *Canadian Occupational Performance Measure* (Law et al., 1998) and the *Occupational Performance History Interview II* (Kielhofner et al., 1998) are occupation-based assessments that facilitate identification of a client's sense of

PROCEDURES FOR PRACTICE 50-2

Recognizing and Preventing Burnout

Health care providers who specialize in oncology are susceptible to chronic work-related stress and resulting burnout. Burnout is a syndrome identified by three components: emotional exhaustion, depersonalization, and diminished feelings of personal accomplishment. The 22-item *Maslach Burnout Inventory–Human Services Survey* (*MBI-HSS*) is commonly used to assess burnout (Chopra, Sotile, & Sotile, 2004; Maslach, Schaufeli, & Leiter, 2001).

Burnout is a function of both individual and contextual factors. Individual factors include one's personality traits, attitudes, and perceptions, such as locus of control and sense of mastery. Maslach and Leiter (1997) identified workload, control, reward or recognition, community, fairness, and values as six contextual factors that, when mismatched with the individual, contribute to burnout. Other contextual factors contributing to burnout in oncology include exposure to issues of death and dying; patients' emotional distress; conflict between curative goals of medicine, patients' prognosis, and the functional desires and goals of the patient and therapist; and exposure to the sometimes painful, debilitating, and disfiguring consequences of medical treatment. In short, occupational therapists can themselves be traumatized when working with medically traumatized patients.

Symptoms of burnout may include somatic complaints (e.g., headaches, joint pain, etc.), withdrawal behaviors, lack of creativity, and decreased quality of care. Burnout can also be related to major depression. It is important to differentiate between burnout and depression. Honest self-reflection is essential to the identification of risk factors for burnout and implementation of prevention strategies. Health professionals can implement the following strategies to prevent burnout:

- Balance in all occupational performance areas
- Rejuvenation through meaningful activity
- Creation of support structures within the work environment to address boundaries and provide emotional support
- Incorporation of pacing and break times at work
- Time off to reflect on values and priorities
- Time management strategies
- Relaxation techniques
- Humor
- Grief work
- Development of support systems outside of work (Brachtesende, 2004; Lyckholm, 2001)

Occupational therapy espouses life balance and engagement in meaningful activity. Occupational therapists are well versed in stress management strategies and adaptive coping, and they routinely use prevention strategies, such as those mentioned above, with their patients (Painter et al., 2003). The challenge then is for occupational therapists to routinely use these strategies with themselves.

self-efficacy and self-esteem, as well as satisfaction with life roles in self-maintenance, self-advancement, and self-enhancement. Observing clients as they perform tasks and activities provides information about performance levels, abilities, and habits. Other assessments may be indicated to determine limiting factors and underlying reasons for diminished ability to meet activity demands.

Individuals' motor, process, and/or communication performance skills may be affected by the side effects of treatment or by the effects of primary tumor or metastases. Assessment of these skills and of specific client factors (AOTA, 2002), such as mental functions, sensory functions and pain, neuromusculoskeletal and movement-related functions, skin and related structures, and cardiovascular, hematological, immunological, and respiratory system functions may be warranted. Specific assessments of performance skills and client factors have been described in detail in other chapters of this text. Some instruments that have been developed to monitor cancer-related symptoms and the effects of cancer on quality of life are described here.

Fatigue is the most common problem reported by individuals with cancer. The *Brief Fatigue Inventory* (Mendoza et al., 1999) provides a quick assessment of the severity of fatigue and its impact on daily function. Cleeland et al. (2000) also developed a global symptoms assessment, the *M. D. Anderson Symptom Inventory*, which measures the severity of many cancer-related symptoms and the degree to which they interfere with daily function. Either of these tools can be used routinely to monitor changes in the individual's status, side effects of treatment, and effectiveness of rehabilitation.

The *Functional Assessment of Cancer Therapy* (*FACT*) measures quality of life in persons undergoing cancer treatment (Cella et al., 1993). Several versions have been developed that are specific to different types of cancer. As clinicians develop their practice in oncology or with people who have other challenging conditions, they might consider incorporating instruments that measure psychosocial factors, such as locus of control, meaning-making, self-efficacy, or hope, into their repertoires. Finally, assessment should include exploration of the social support that is available as well as environmental barriers and supports.

Goals and Moderating Variables that Affect Realistic Goal Setting across the Continuum of Care

The goal of therapy is to enable clients to optimize their quality of life by engaging in meaningful occupations and to facilitate living regardless of life expectancy. Many of the goals that are meaningful to the client who has cancer are the same as those encountered with persons who have other diagnoses. With cancer, however, distinct moderating variables may affect realistic goal setting. People with cancer experience rapid changes in medical and functional status across the continuum of care. It is sometimes difficult for the person and the therapist to determine how permanent these changes might be. The severity of the disease and the individual's expectations regarding function and recovery may be incongruous. The occupational therapist should continually monitor these changes and help the individual to modify valued goals and roles accordingly. At the same time, the therapist must walk a fine line to avoid dispelling hope.

The role of the occupational therapist varies according to the point at which he or she enters the patient's course of treatment. Duration of treatment depends on acuity of the condition and severity of the disease, along with the patient's wishes. Regardless, the treatment plan should be individualized and address the performance skills required to function at that point in the continuum of care.

In cases where surgery is involved, pre-operative goals typically focus on facilitating continued engagement in activities by managing or compensating for the side effects of treatment. Energy conservation, fatigue management, and exercise are common strategies aimed at improving the ability to manage daily life despite the side effects of chemotherapy and/or radiation. Another important aim of early treatment is to identify the performance patterns that may be altered by future medical treatment. Post-operatively, the therapist and patient generally focus on increasing independence in activities of daily living (ADLs) and instrumental activities of daily living (IADLs). Decreased performance skills related to changes in body structures can make engagement in these activities quite difficult. As the person becomes able or in the outpatient setting, treatment shifts to focus on social participation.

In the post-operative period, the therapist should also address the psychosocial factors related to altered body structures and/or body functions. It may be necessary to assist the patient in understanding the realistic expectations for functional recovery as a result of the procedure and to help him or her identify methods of coping with these changes.

The patient's long-term goals should guide him or her toward resuming activities such as work, driving, leisure, social interaction, play, and education. Although some procedures may permanently restrict the activities of some patients, most patients are able to resume normal activities with few, if any, long-term restrictions. Similar goals may be considered for patients who do not undergo surgery. The various cancers and their treatment have similar impacts on function and body image.

Occupational Therapy Intervention

The types of intervention that occupational therapists employ with individuals who have cancer do not differ much from those used with persons who have other conditions. Interventions focus on promoting health in the face of disease; restoring performance skills and patterns; preventing disability; modifying contexts, activity demands, or performance patterns; and providing supports that help patients maintain function (AOTA, 2002). Thus, interventions include fatigue management and energy conservation; sensory reeducation or desensitization; wheelchair seating and positioning; scar management, including fibrosis; conditioning (endurance, range of motion, and strengthening); and fall prevention and other activities to promote home safety. Some interventions, such as physical agent modalities (see Safety Note 50-1) or lymphedema management, require specialized training (see Case Example 50-2 on clinical competence).

Occupational therapists also provide cognitive intervention, as warranted by specific problems. Intervention can address psychosocial issues, such as caregiver concerns regarding the activities of caregiving, stress and anxiety management, relaxation techniques, and pain management. Occupational therapists may be called upon to provide interventions at the end of a person's life, as exemplified by referrals from palliative care physicians during a person's advanced stages of cancer. Even at the end of life, some people struggle to remain productive, and occupational therapists can help these people plan and engage in realistic levels of activity. Furthermore, the use of purposeful activity can facilitate closure to the relationship between the person who is dying and members of his or her support system.

In all phases of intervention, one needs to be able to clearly articulate the rationale for the intervention. To do this, it may be helpful to adopt a stance that rehabilitation is helpful even with declining patients (Procedures for Practice 50-3).

PROCEDURES FOR PRACTICE 50-3

Reframing a Mindset for Rehabilitation with Declining Patients

There has been discussion about the rationale for treating people who have progressive and degenerative disease processes. With some diagnoses, such as neurodegenerative diseases, health care professionals have adopted the stance that these are chronic conditions with periods of remission, relapse, and progression. Cancers, too, can be viewed in a similar manner. Thus people with cancer have different occupational needs throughout the trajectory of the disease and treatment process.

Some of the factors that compel one to consider treating cancers as chronic conditions are:

- Public awareness campaigns promote screening and prevention of certain cancers.
- For some cancers, medical treatment has advanced, introducing hormonal therapies, biotherapies, tumor vaccines, and innovative surgical techniques.
- More people are achieving 5-year survival, from 50% relative survival in 1974–1976 to 65% in 1995–2001 (ACS, 2006).
- There is greater interest in studying and promoting health-related quality of life in persons with cancer.

Furthermore, disease and the treatment of disease can adversely affect people's function and participation in valued roles and activities:

- Treatment frequency and side effects can cause frequent disruptions of lifestyle and activities.
- Disease progression and/or side effects of treatment can cause progressive functional loss at varying rates.
- Psychologically, people experience uncertainty about the future, potential relapse, and/or death.

To cultivate a mindset for rehabilitation with declining patients, it is important for occupational therapists to:

- Recognize that, although medical treatment can deplete a person's energy during hospitalization, the person will recover some (not necessarily all) energy as blood counts recover
- Be aware that individuals with cancer may have phases of decline and then stabilization, where realistic activity planning, focused on short-term aspects of function and quality of life, can be facilitated by an occupational therapist
- Recognize that, even at the end of life, many people with cancer wish to engage in occupations, however limited
- Become aware of their feelings about their clients' adjustment to loss and about death and dying
- Keep in mind a goal of rehabilitation for persons with cancer, stated by Cheville (2001): "While rehabilitation cannot eliminate cancer's assaults on functional autonomy, it can certainly attenuate and decelerate them. It can also engage patients and families in constructive purpose such that functional decline is not experienced as helplessness" (p. 1040)

EVIDENCE FOR OUTCOMES OF REHABILITATION

Although the evidence supporting rehabilitation of the cancer patient is limited when compared to other diagnoses, what evidence exists supports its efficacy when used with this population. Most of the identified research focuses on quality of life and does not identify the specific aspects of rehabilitation that led to its improvement. Some authors, however, have described the impact of specific interventions on functional outcome. The evidence is, in some cases, qualitative in nature. Evidence Table 50-1 includes an example of literature that comes from outside of occupational therapy and two studies by occupational therapists. Until more evidence is generated by occupational therapists, studies generated outside the profession should be examined, including studies by psychosocial and behavioral scientists, physicians, nurses, exercise physiologists, and physical therapists. The problem with such studies is that the unique perspective of occupational therapy is missing, and the clinician must add his or her own interpretation to the findings.

Evidence Table 50-1
Best Evidence for Occupational Therapy Practice Regarding Cancer

Intervention	Description of Intervention Tested	Participants	Dosage	Type of Best Evidence and Level of Evidence	Benefit	Statistical Probability	Reference
Fatigue	Aerobic exercise (stationary bike) vs. progressive relaxation.	72 post-operative lung cancer (n = 27) and gastrointestinal cancer (n = 42) patients.	Aerobic exercise group: 30 minutes, 5 times a week; relaxation group: 45 minutes, 3 times a week; both for 3 weeks.	Randomized comparison group study. IA2a	Both groups reported similar improvements in fatigue: no difference between interventions; exercise group improved physical performance.	Fatigue rating (*European Organization for Research and Treatment of Cancer Quality of Life Questionnaire Core Module*): Exercise group improved 21%, $p = 0.01$; relaxation group improved 19%, $p = 0.01$. No difference between groups: $p = 0.67$.	Dimeo et al., 2004
Treatments used with patients with breast cancer	Survey of assessments, intervention, and time allocation.	5 occupational therapists at 2 sites, treating patients with breast cancer; interventions with 35 women recorded.	Log sheet completed daily for 1 month.	Survey (design not rated). A3c	Treatment is individualized. Most common interventions: educational program, support groups; relaxation training; wheelchair assessment and provision; transfer training; and equipment provision.	Descriptive study; unable to calculate.	Vockins, 2004
Treatment of brachial plexopathy	Activity modification using assistive devices; environmental modification (offered but declined).	One 67-year-old woman, treated for breast cancer with mastectomy and radiation 12 years prior to intervention under study.	Documentation of assessment and treatment.	Narrative case study. VC3c	Treatment is based on client's values; individualized due to nature of condition.	Narrative study; unable to calculate.	Cooper, 1998

SUMMARY REVIEW QUESTIONS

1. At what points in the care continuum might patients be referred to occupational therapy?
2. What issues might arise for patients regarding loss or loss of control during the course of their cancer experience?
3. How does loss of control affect a person's role and occupational performance?
4. The clinician is working with a person who has been treated with limb salvage for sarcoma. What general safety precautions should he or she be aware of? Would the application of physical agent modalities be appropriate? Justify.
5. What presenting symptoms would a clinician expect in a person who has acute leukemia? How might these symptoms affect occupational performance?
6. In what ways, if any, do symptoms and occupational performance in a person with lung cancer differ from those in a person with sarcoma? From those in a person with leukemia?
7. Discuss three interventions used by occupational therapists in cancer settings, and describe how they are used to improve occupational functioning.
8. How might a clinician best address patients' fatigue?
9. Based on the boxes and references in this chapter, what three resources might you use to improve the quality of the care you would offer to a person who has cancer?
10. In your opinion, what is the unique perspective that occupational therapy can add to the evidence regarding treatment effectiveness?

ACKNOWLEDGMENT

We wish to acknowledge and thank our patients, who have courageously shared their life experiences with us, and our students, who strive to master the complexities of practice. Both of these groups helped us to realize the importance of sharing more information about the role of occupational therapy in cancer care.

References

American Cancer Society [ACS]. (2005). Key statistics for Ewing's family of tumors. Retrieved October 15, 2005 from http://www.cancer.org.

American Cancer Society [ACS]. (2006). Cancer statistics 2006: A presentation from the American Cancer Society. Retrieved March 19, 2006 from http://www.cancer.org.

American Occupational Therapy Association [AOTA]. (2002). Occupational therapy practice framework: Domain and process. *American Journal of Occupational Therapy, 56,* 609–639.

Bacci, G., Ferrari, S., Lari, S., Mercuri, M., Donati, D., Longhi, A., Forni, C., Bertoni, F., Versari, M., & Pignotti, E. (2002). Osteosarcoma of the limb: Amputation or limb salvage in patients treated by neoadjuvant chemotherapy. *Journal of Bone and Joint Surgery, 84-B,* 88–92.

Bertero, C. R. N., Eriksson, B.-E., & Ek, A.-C. (1997). Explaining different profiles in quality of life experiences in acute and chronic leukemia. *Cancer Nursing, 20,* 100–104.

Brachtesende, A. (2004). Coping with burnout. *OT Practice, 9,* 14–18.

Carver, C.S. (2005). Enhancing adaptation during treatment and the role of individual differences. *Cancer, 104 (Suppl. 11),* 2602–2607.

Cella, D. F., Tulsky, D. S., Gray, G., Sarafian, B., Linn, E., Bonomi, A., et al. (1993). The functional assessment of cancer therapy scale: Development and validation of the general measure. *Journal of Clinical Oncology, 11,* 570–579.

Cheville, A. (2001). Rehabilitation of patients with advanced cancer. *Cancer, 92 (Suppl. 4),* 1039–1048.

Chopra, S. S., Sotile, W. M., & Sotile, M. O. (2004). Physician burnout. *Journal of the American Medical Association, 291,* 633.

Cleeland, C. S., Mendoza, T. R., Wang, X. S., Chou, C., Harle, M., Morrissey, M., & Engstrom, M. C. (2000). Assessing symptom distress in cancer: The M. D. Anderson symptom inventory. *Cancer, 89,*1634–1646.

Cooper, J. (Ed.). (1997). *Occupational therapy in oncology and palliative care.* London: Whurr Publishers Ltd.

Cooper, J. (1998). Occupational therapy intervention with radiation-induced brachial plexopathy. *European Journal of Cancer Care, 7,* 88–92.

Dimeo, F. C., Thomas, F., Raabe-Menssen, C., Propper, E., & Mathias, M. (2004). Effect of aerobic exercise and relaxation training on fatigue and physical performance of cancer patients after surgery: A randomized control trial. *Supportive Care in Cancer, 12,* 774–779.

Garrett, K., & Kirchner, S. (1995). Oncologic emergencies: The role of physical therapy and occupational therapy. *Rehabilitation in Oncology, 13,* 10–24.

Heath, C. W., & Fontham, T. H. (2001) Cancer etiology. In R. E. Lenhard, R. T. Osteen, & T. Gansler (Eds.), *The American Cancer Society's clinical oncology* (pp. 37–54). Atlanta: The American Cancer Society.

Hematological Cancer Research Investment and Education Act of 2001: S1094. (2002). Retrieved November 22, 2006, from http://www.congress.gov/cgi-bin/query/R?107:FL001:H51723.

Hockett, K. (2004). Oncologic emergencies. In C. Varricchio, T. B. Ades, P. S. Hinds, & M. Pierce (Eds.), *A cancer source book for nurses* (8th ed., pp. 447–465). Atlanta: American Cancer Society.

Hutson, L. M. (2004). Breast cancer. In C. Varricchio, T. B. Ades, P. S. Hinds, & M. Pierce (Eds.), *A cancer source book for nurses* (8th ed., pp. 173–185). Atlanta: American Cancer Society.

Kielhofner, G., Mallinson, T., Crawford, C., Nowak, M., Rigby, M., Henry, A., & Walens, D. (1998). *A user's manual for the Occupational Performance History Interview (Version 2.0).* Chicago: University of Illinois at Chicago.

Kumiega, K. (1997). *Windows to cancer care: An occupational therapy treatment guide.* Bisbee, AZ: Imaginart.

Kurtz, M. E., Kurtz, J. C., Given, C. W., & Given, B. (2005). A randomized, controlled study of a patient/caregiver symptom control intervention: Effects of depressive symptomatology of caregivers of cancer patients. *Journal of Pain and Symptom Management, 30,* 112–122.

Lane, J. M., Christ, G. H., Khan, S. N., & Backus, S. I. (2001). Rehabilitation for limb salvage patients: Kinesiologic parameters and psychologic assessment. *Cancer, 92 (Suppl. 4),* 1013–1019.

Law, M., Baptiste, S., Carswell, A., McColl, M. A., Polatajko, H., & Pollock, N. (1998). *Canadian occupational performance measure* (3rd ed.). Toronto, Ontario, Canada: Canadian Association of Occupational Therapists.

Lenhard, R. E., & Osteen, R. T. (2001). General approach to cancer patients. In R. E. Lenhard, R. T. Osteen, & T. Gansler (Eds.), *The American Cancer Society's clinical oncology* (pp. 149–158). Atlanta: American Cancer Society.

Lenhard, R. E., Osteen, R. T., & Gansler, T. (2001). *The American Cancer Society's clinical oncology*. Atlanta: American Cancer Society.

Lyckholm, L. (2001). Dealing with stress, burnout and grief in the practice of oncology. *Lancet Oncology, 2,* 750–755.

Mandrell, B. (2004). Leukemia. In C. Varricchio, T. B. Ades, P. S. Hinds, & M. Pierce (Eds.), *A cancer source book for nurses* (8th ed., pp. 251–263). Atlanta: American Cancer Society.

Maslach, C., & Leiter, M. P. (1997). The truth about burnout: How organizations cause personal stress and what to do about it. San Francisco: Jossey-Bass Publishers.

Maslach, C., Schaufeli, W. B., & Leiter, M. P. (2001). Job burnout. *Annual Review of Psychology, 52,* 397–422.

Mendoza, T., Wang, X. S., Cleeland, C. S., Morrissey, M., Johnson, B. A., Wendt, J. K., & Huber, S. L. (1999). The rapid assessment of fatigue severity in cancer patients: Use of the Brief Fatigue Inventory. *Cancer, 85,* 1186–1196.

Miller, K. B., & Grodman, H. M. (2001). Leukemia. In R. E. Lenhard, R. T. Osteen, & T. Gansler (Eds.), *The American Cancer Society's clinical oncology* (pp. 527–551). Atlanta: American Cancer Society.

Painter, J., Akroyd, D., Eliot, S., & Adams, R. D. (2003). Burnout among occupational therapists. *Occupational Therapy in Health Care, 17,* 63–78.

Pandey, M., & Thomas, B. C. (2001). Rehabilitation of cancer patients. *Journal of Postgraduate Medicine, 47,* 62–65.

Refaat, Y., Gunnoe, J., Hornicek, F. J., & Mankin, H. J. (2002). Comparison of quality of life after amputation or limb salvage. *Clinical Orthopedics and Related Research, 397,* 298–305.

Robinson, M. H., Spruce, L., Eeles, R., Fryatt, I., Harmer, C. L., Thomas, J. M., & Westbury, G. (1991). Limb function following conservation treatment of adult soft tissue sarcoma. *European Journal of Cancer, 27,* 1567–1574.

Rohan, K., & Budds, S. (2004). Epidemiology of cancer. In C. Varricchio, T. B. Ades, P. S. Hinds, & M. Pierce (Eds.), *A cancer source book for nurses* (8th ed., pp. 29–39). Atlanta: American Cancer Society.

Schkade, J., & Schultz, S. (1992). Occupational adaptation: Toward a holistic approach for contemporary practice, part 1. *American Journal of Occupational Therapy, 46,* 829–837.

Schroevers, M., Ranchor, A. V., & Sanderman, R. (2004). The role of age at the onset of cancer in relation to survivors' long-term adjustment: A controlled comparison over an eight-year period. *Psychooncology, 13,* 740–752.

Schumacher, A., Kessler, T., Buchner, T., Wewers, D., & van de Loo, J. (1998). Quality of life in adult patients with acute myeloid leukemia receiving intensive and prolonged chemotherapy: A longitudinal study. *Leukemia, 12,* 586–592.

Smith, S., Anderson-Hanley, C., Langrock, A., & Compas, B. (2005). The effects of journaling for women with newly diagnosed breast cancer. *Psychooncology, 14,* 1075–1082.

Tatu, B. (2005). Physical therapy intervention with oncological emergencies. *Rehabilitation Oncology, 23,* 4–17.

Thomas, C. R., Williams, T. E., Cobos, E., & Turrisi, A. T. (2001). Lung cancer. In R. E. Lenhard, R. T. Osteen, & T. Gansler (Eds.), *The American Cancer Society's clinical oncology* (pp. 269–295). Atlanta: American Cancer Society.

The University of Texas M. D. Anderson Cancer Center. (2006). About cancer. Retrieved March 19, 2006 from http://www.mdanderson.org/patients_public/about_cancer/.

Van Cleave, J. H., & Cooley, M. E. (2004). Lung cancer. In C. Varricchio, T. B. Ades, P. S. Hinds, & M. Pierce (Eds.), *A cancer source book for nurses* (8th ed., pp. 215–227). Atlanta: American Cancer Society.

Varricchio, C., Ades, T. B., Hinds, P. S., & Pierce, M. (Eds.). (2004). *A cancer source book for nurses* (8th ed.). Atlanta: American Cancer Society.

Veth, R., van Hoesel, R., Pruszczynski, M., Hoogenhout, J., Schreuder, B., & Wobbes, T. (2003). Limb salvage in musculoskeletal oncology. *Lancet Oncology, 4,* 343–350.

Vockins, H. (2004). Occupational therapy intervention with patients with breast cancer: A survey. *European Journal of Cancer Care, 13,* 45–52.

Weisman, I. L. (2000). Stem cells: Units of development, units of regeneration, and units in evolution. *Cell, 100,* 157–168.

Workman, M. L. (2004). The biology of cancer. In C. Varricchio, T. B. Ades, P. S. Hinds, & M. Pierce (Eds.), *A cancer source book for nurses* (8th ed., pp. 13–28). Atlanta: American Cancer Society.

Yasko, A. W., Reece, G. P., Gillis, T. A., & Pollock, R. E. (1997). Limb-salvage strategies to optimize quality of life: The M. D. Anderson Cancer Center experience. *CA: A Cancer Journal for Clinicians, 47,* 226–238.

Yasko, A. W., Shreyaskumar, R. P., Pollack, A., & Pollock, R. E. (2001). Sarcomas of soft tissue and bone. In R. E. Lenhard, R. T. Osteen, & T. Gansler (Eds.), *The American Cancer Society's clinical oncology* (pp. 611–631). Atlanta: American Cancer Society.

Index

C

M

RRS1001

[redacted]

[redacted]

615.8515 O15tp6
Radomski, Mary V
Occupational therapy for physical ...